Diagnostic Ultrasound
Abdomen & Pelvis

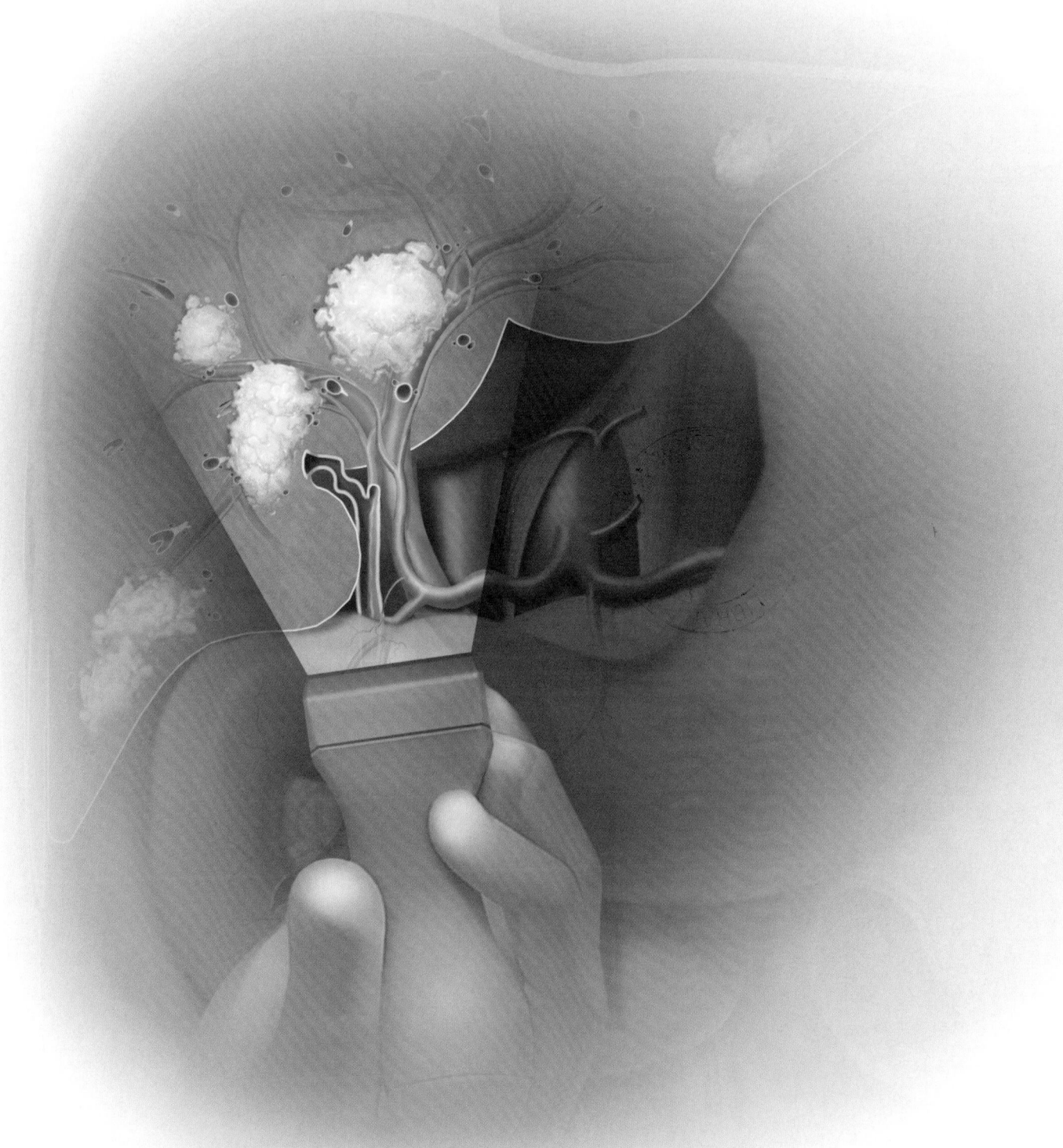

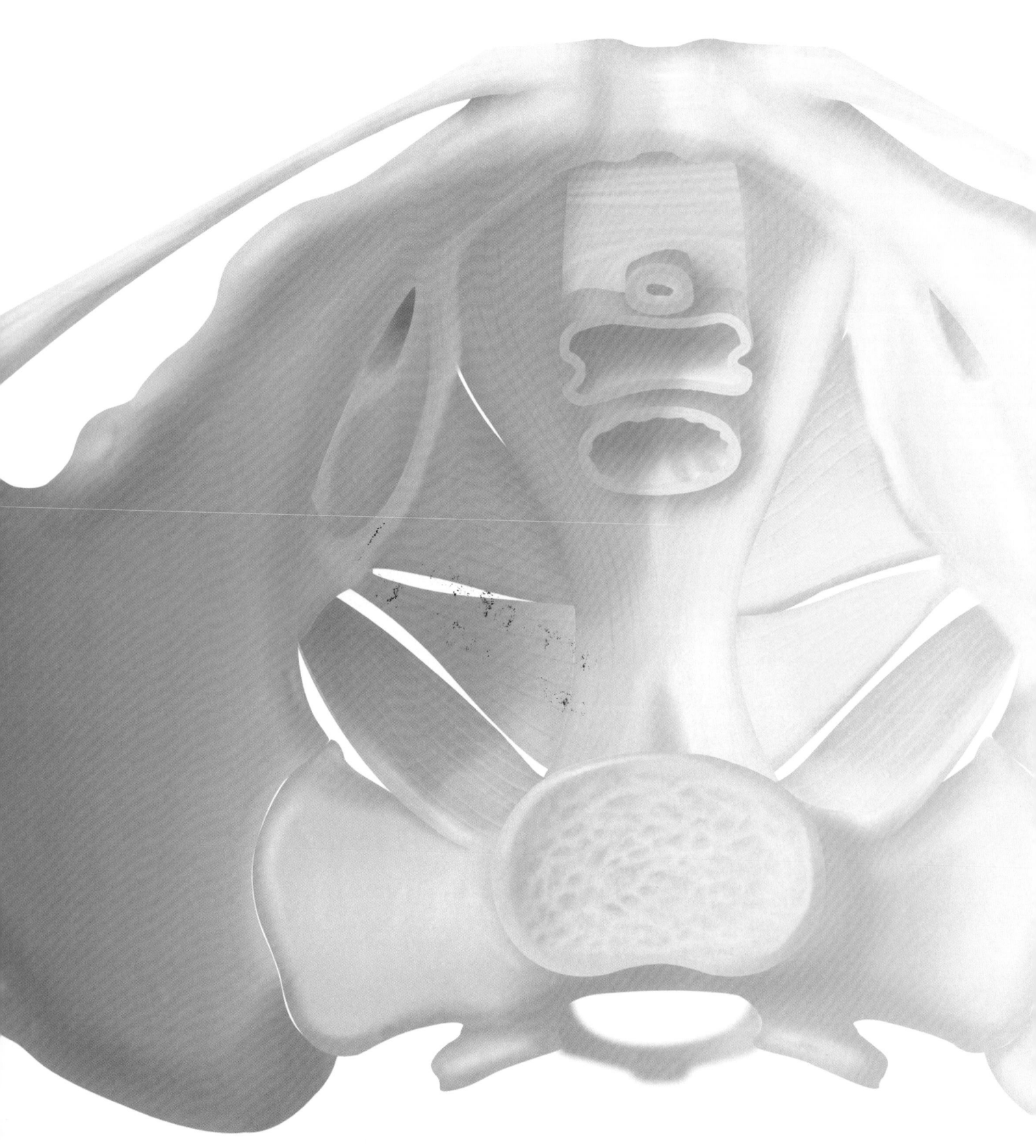

Diagnostic Ultrasound
Abdomen & Pelvis

Aya Kamaya, MD, FSRU, FSAR
Associate Professor of Radiology
Associate Director, Stanford Body Imaging Fellowship
Stanford University School of Medicine
Stanford, California

Jade Wong-You-Cheong, MBChB, MRCP, FRCR
Professor
Department of Diagnostic Radiology and Nuclear Medicine
University of Maryland School of Medicine
Director of Ultrasound
University of Maryland Medical Center
Baltimore, Maryland

Hee Sun Park, MD, PhD
Visiting Associate Professor
Department of Radiology
Stanford University School of Medicine
Stanford, California

Barton F. Lane, MD
Assistant Professor
Clinical Director of CT
Department of Diagnostic Radiology and Nuclear Medicine
University of Maryland School of Medicine
Baltimore, Maryland

Fauzia Vandermeer, MD
Assistant Professor of Diagnostic Radiology
Associate Program Director, Radiology Residency
Department of Diagnostic Radiology and Nuclear Medicine
University of Maryland School of Medicine
Baltimore, Maryland

Katherine E. Maturen, MD, MS
Associate Professor
Abdominal Radiology Fellowship Director
University of Michigan Hospitals
Ann Arbor, Michigan

Shweta Bhatt, MD
Associate Professor
Department of Imaging Sciences
University of Rochester Medical Center
Rochester, New York

Bryan R. Foster, MD
Assistant Professor
Department of Radiology
Oregon Health & Science University
Portland, Oregon

Sathi A. Sukumar, MBBS, FRCP (UK), FRCR
Consultant Radiologist
University Hospital of South Manchester
Manchester, United Kingdom

Ashish P. Wasnik, MD
Assistant Professor
Department of Radiology
Division of Abdominal Imaging
University of Michigan Health System
Ann Arbor, Michigan

ELSEVIER

1600 John F. Kennedy Blvd.
Ste 1800
Philadelphia, PA 19103-2899

DIAGNOSTIC ULTRASOUND: ABDOMEN AND PELVIS

ISBN: 978-0-323-37643-3

Publisher Cataloging-in-Publication Data

Diagnostic ultrasound. Abdomen and pelvis / [edited by] Aya Kamaya and Jade Wong-You-Cheong.
   pages ; cm
   Abdomen and pelvis
   Includes bibliographical references and index.
 ISBN 978-0-323-37643-3 (hardback)
  1. Abdomen--Ultrasonic imaging--Handbooks, manuals, etc. 2. Pelvis--Ultrasonic imaging--Handbooks, manuals, etc. 3. Diagnostic ultrasonic imaging--Handbooks, manuals, etc.
 I. Kamaya, Aya. II. Wong-You-Cheong, Jade. III. Title: Abdomen and pelvis.
 [DNLM: 1. Abdomen--ultrasonography--Atlases. 2. Pelvis--ultrasonography--Atlases.
 3. Ultrasonography--Atlases. WN 208]
  RC78.7.U4 D515 2015
  616.07/543--dc23

International Standard Book Number: 978-0-323-37643-3

Cover Designer: Tom M. Olson, BA
Cover Art: Lane R. Bennion, MS

Printed in Canada by Friesens, Altona, Manitoba, Canada

Last digit is the print number: 9 8 7 6 5 4 3 2 1

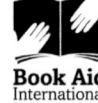

Dedications

To my sweet and supportive husband, Yuji, who makes me feel like the luckiest person in the world; our kids, Mika (2) and Kenzo (5); my wonderful parents, Yoko and Hiroshi; and my mentors, Brooke Jeffrey and Jon Rubin, who inspired my passion for ultrasound.
AK

To my family: my parents and siblings, who have helped shape who I am, and my boys (now men), who make my life complete. I also want to thank all the radiologists, sonographers, and technologists I have had the privilege of working with and learning from.
JWYC

Dedicated to my two adorable children, Raymond and Justin, for their unconditional love, and to my husband, Joonsung, for his enduring support from across the ocean.
HSP

Dedicated to my family: my parents who have always supported me despite tangential endeavors, my wife, Akiko, who manages to keep me together, and my daughters, Charlotte and Delaney, who are my daily inspiration.
BFL

To my parents, my first and best teachers.
To Elianna, Noah, Hanna, & Nyla, who continue my education of life's most important lessons everyday.
And to Peter, my love and wise counsel.
FV

Thank you to all of the mentors, friends, and trainees who teach me so much and make my job fun. Much love and appreciation to my very supportive husband, Geoff, and my two fantastic kids, Iris and Julian.
KEM

Dedicated to my parents for their constant support and encouragement, and to my teacher and mentor, Vikram Dogra, for teaching me the skills of being an academic radiologist.
SB

To my many mentors from east coast to west. To my parents, who sparked the teaching interest. Most of all to my 2 future radiologists, Nolan and Bennett, and incredible wife, Sarah.
BRF

This is for my wife, Jino, and sons, Nim and Siv. Thanks for being supportive and understanding.
SAS

To my mom, Sushila, and my wife, Usha, for their unconditional love, support, and inspiration!
APW

Contributing Authors

Katherine To'o, MD
Staff Radiologist
Veterans Affairs Palo Alto Health Care System
Palo Alto, California

Ali M. Tahvildari, MD
Staff Radiologist
VA Palo Alto Healthcare System
Palo Alto, California
Clinical Instructor (Affiliated)
Department of Radiology
Stanford University School of Medicine
Stanford, California

Maria A. Manning, MD
Section Chief, Gastrointestinal Radiology
American Institute of Radiologic Pathology
Associate Professor
Georgetown University School of Medicine
Washington, DC

Karen Y. Oh, MD
Associate Professor
Chief of Women's Imaging
Department of Radiology
Department of Obstetrics and Gynecology
Oregon Health & Science University
Portland, Oregon

Mariam Moshiri, MD, FSAR
Associate Professor
University of Washington Medical Center
Seattle, Washington

L. Nayeli Morimoto, MD
Clinical Instructor
Department of Radiology
Stanford University School of Medicine
Stanford, California

Hammed Ninalowo, MD
Fellow, Interventional Radiology
University of Pennsylvania
Philadelphia, Pennsylvania

Nicole Roy, MD
Assistant Professor
Diagnostic Radiology
Oregon Health & Science University
Portland, Oregon

Adnaan Moin, MD
Fellow
Department of Interventional Radiology
McGaw Medical Center of Northwestern University
Chicago, Illinois

Sonya Y. Khan, MD
Diagnostic Radiology Resident
Department of Diagnostic Radiology and
Nuclear Medicine
University of Maryland Medical Center
Baltimore, Maryland

Jane S. Kim, MD
Assistant Professor
Department of Diagnostic Radiology and
Nuclear Medicine
University of Maryland Medical Center
Baltimore, Maryland

Narendra Shet, MD
Assistant Professor
Department of Diagnostic Radiology and
Nuclear Medicine
University of Maryland School of Medicine
Baltimore, Maryland

Amit B. Desai, MD
Radiology Resident
Department of Imaging Sciences
University of Rochester Medical Center
Rochester, New York

Richard E. Fan, PhD
Engineering Research Associate
Department of Urology
Stanford University School of Medicine
Stanford, California

Asef Khwaja, MD
Assistant Professor of Clinical Radiology
Perelman School of Medicine
University of Pennsylvania
Department of Radiology at The Children's Hospital of
Philadelphia
Philadelphia, Pennsylvania

Priya Menon Krishnarao, MD
Diagnostic Radiology Resident
Department of Radiology
Santa Clara Valley Medical Center
San Jose, California

Velauthan Rudralingam, MBBCh, FRCR (UK)
Consultant Radiologist
Department of Radiology
University Hospital of South Manchester
Manchester, United Kingdom

Tanzilah Afzal Barrow, MBChB, BA, MA (Oxon), FRCR
Radiology Resident
University Hospital of South Manchester
Manchester, United Kingdom

Geoffrey Sonn, MD
Assistant Professor
Department of Urology and Radiology (by Courtesy)
Stanford University School of Medicine
Stanford, California

Tapas K. Tejura, MD
Assistant Professor of Clinical Radiology
Department of Radiology
Keck Medical Center of USC
University of Southern California
Los Angeles, California

Thomas Westwood, MBBS, FRCR
Consultant Radiologist
The Christie NHS Foundation Trust
Manchester, United Kingdom

Keegan Hovis, MD
PGY-1 Preliminary Intern
Department of Internal Medicine
Kaiser San Francisco
San Francisco, California

Rachel F. Magennis, MBChB, DMRD, FRCR
Consultant Radiologist
Department of Radiology
University Hospital of South Manchester
Manchester, United Kingdom

Sue Liong, MBChB (Hons), FRCR
Consultant Radiologist
Department of Clinical Radiology
University Hospital of South Manchester
Manchester, United Kingdom

Terry S. Desser, MD
Professor
Department of Radiology
Stanford University School of Medicine
Stanford, California

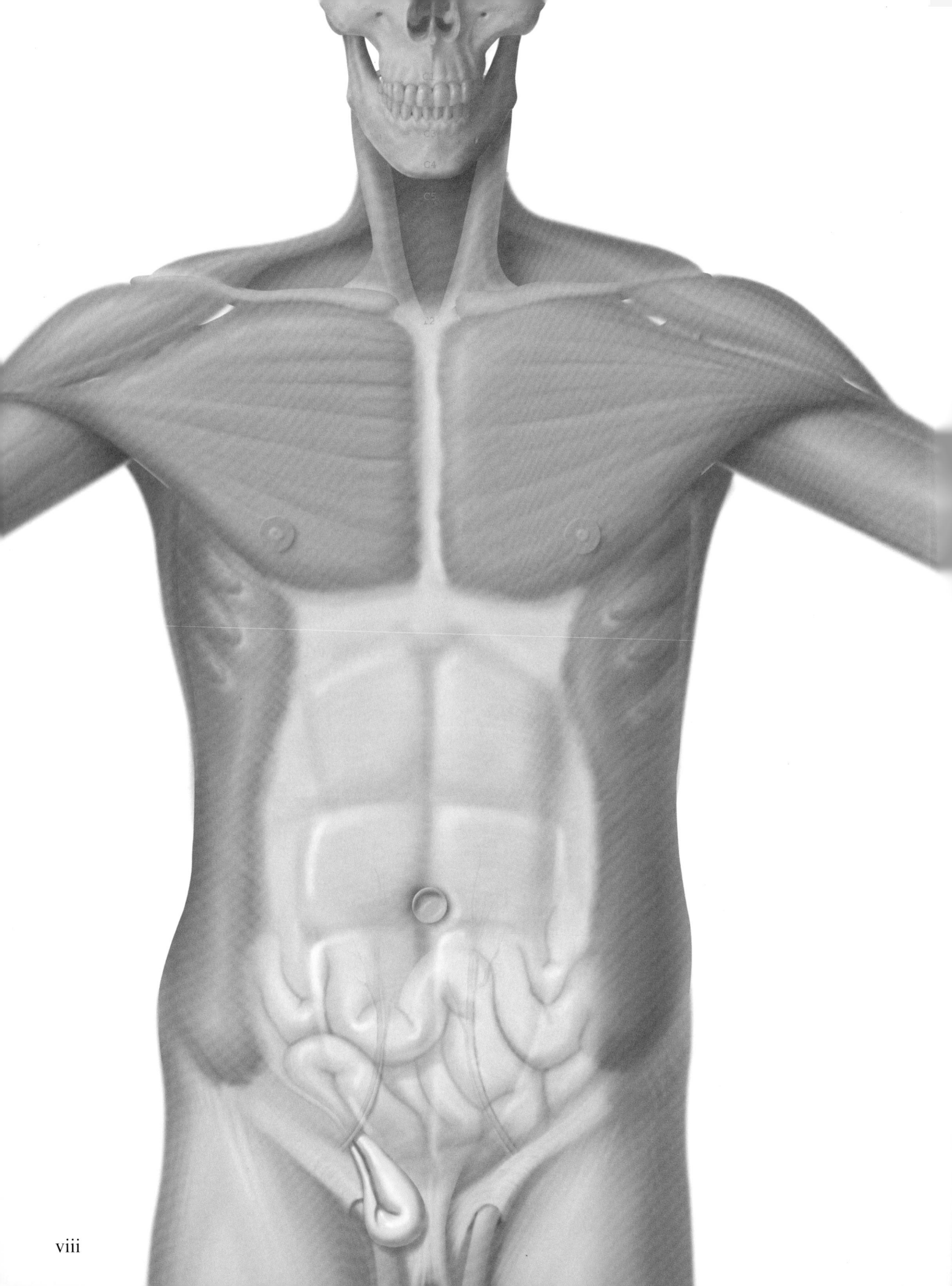

Preface

Ultrasound is often the first imaging study for evaluation of patients presenting with abdominal or pelvic pain, abnormal biochemical tests, suspected mass, or gynecologic symptoms. Depending on the ultrasound findings, patients may go on to further imaging or, in many cases, the clinical decision is based on ultrasound findings alone. It is therefore imperative for the radiologist to confidently recognize the sonographic appearance of specific diagnoses. The more the radiologist knows about the sonographic appearance of specific entities, the less likely a patient will be referred for potentially unnecessary imaging.

We hope this book highlights this information in an easily digestible and image-focused format. We have tailored this book for the well-rounded abdominal radiologist who uses all imaging modalities in evaluation of the abdomen and pelvis but with a focus on ultrasound. You will find numerous examples of grayscale, color, power, and spectral (pulsed) Doppler imaging in each chapter and, when applicable, contrast-enhanced ultrasound. Correlation with CT and MR is provided in many chapters. Detailed artistic renderings of each disease entity further complement the visual splendor of the book.

In this era, when conservative use of radiation exposure from CT as well as minimization of iodinated- or gadolinium-based contrast are increasingly important, ultrasound is reemerging as an extremely attractive and optimal imaging modality. Moreover, ultrasound technology continues to improve, resulting in dramatic changes in image quality in the last decade. New transducer materials, improved image quality with higher resolution, noise-reduction techniques, increased Doppler sensitivity, together with widespread use of 3D transducers have significantly impacted our daily ultrasound practice. It is thus time for a book dedicated to the abdomen and pelvis in the highly acclaimed Amirsys series. *Diagnostic Ultrasound: Abdomen & Pelvis* presents dedicated sections on ultrasound anatomy, diagnoses, and differential diagnoses, organized by organ. Ultrasound images, text, and references have been extensively updated, and new chapters have been added to reflect current ultrasound practice.

We hope that you enjoy this book as much as we have enjoyed presenting it to you.

Aya Kamaya, MD, FSRU, FSAR
Associate Professor of Radiology
Associate Director, Stanford Body Imaging Fellowship
Stanford University School of Medicine
Stanford, California

Jade Wong-You-Cheong, MBChB, MRCP, FRCR
Professor
Department of Diagnostic Radiology and Nuclear Medicine
University of Maryland School of Medicine
Director of Ultrasound
University of Maryland Medical Center
Baltimore, Maryland

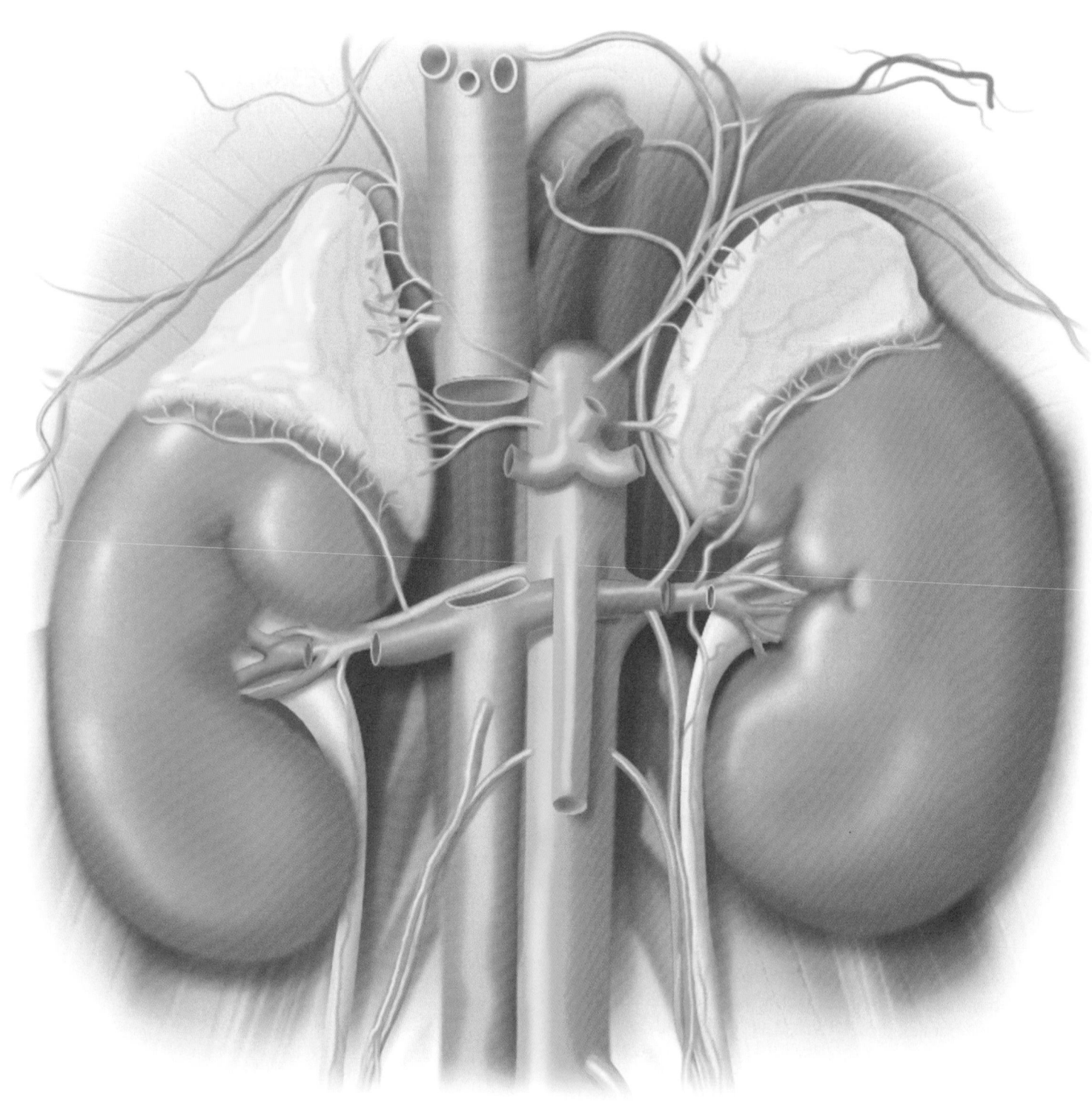

X

Acknowledgements

Text Editors
Nina I. Bennett, BA
Sarah J. Connor, BA
Tricia L. Cannon, BA
Terry W. Ferrell, MS
Lisa A. Gervais, BS
Karen E. Concannon, MA, PhD

Image Editors
Jeffrey J. Marmorstone, BS
Lisa A. M. Steadman, BS

Medical Editor
Ann E. Podrasky, MD, FSRU

Illustrations
Lane R. Bennion, MS
Laura C. Sesto, MA
Richard Coombs, MS

Art Direction and Design
Laura C. Sesto, MA
Tom M. Olson, BA

Lead Editor
Arthur G. Gelsinger, MA

Production Coordinators
Rebecca L. Hutchinson, BA
Angela M. G. Terry, BA

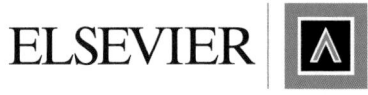

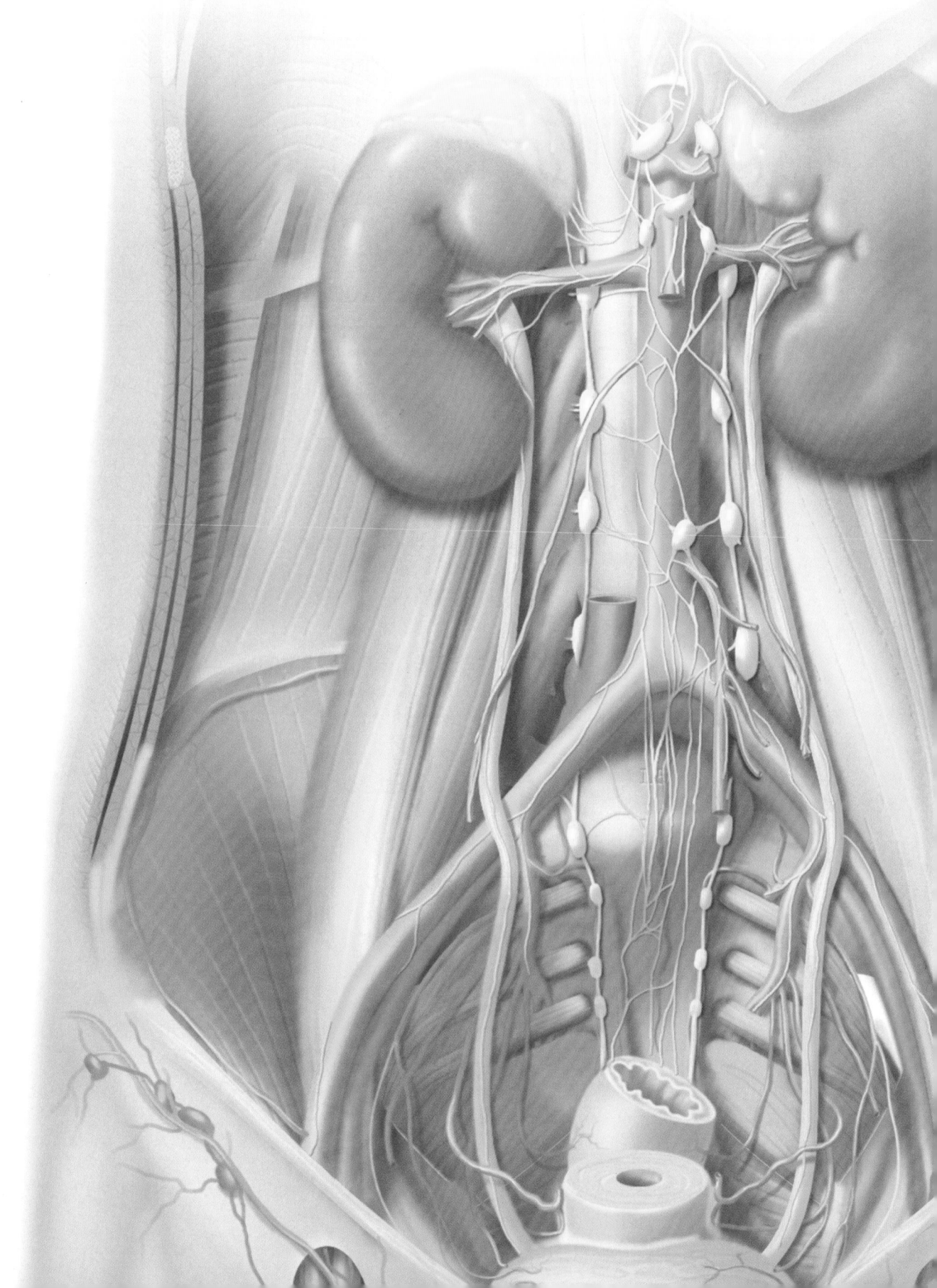

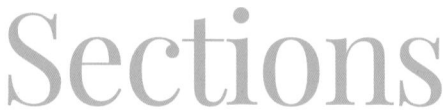

Sections

TABLE OF CONTENTS

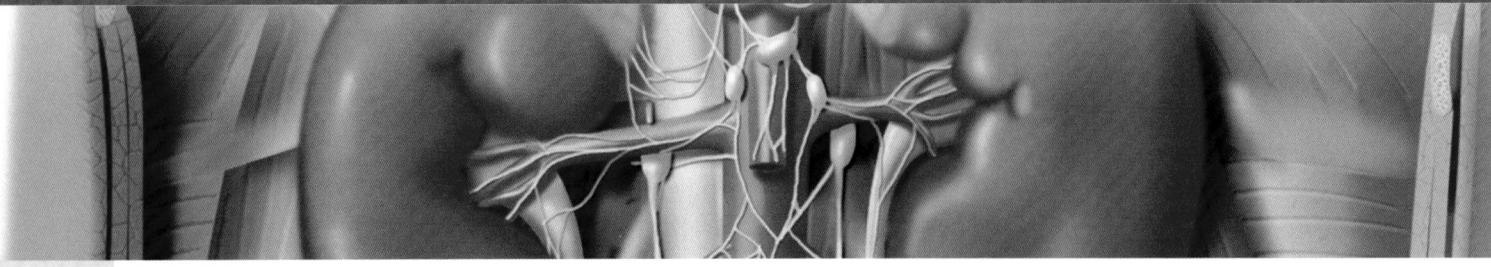

Part I: Anatomy

Part II: Diagnoses

TABLE OF CONTENTS

TABLE OF CONTENTS

TABLE OF CONTENTS

TABLE OF CONTENTS

Part III: Differential Diagnoses

TABLE OF CONTENTS

Diagnostic Ultrasound
Abdomen & Pelvis

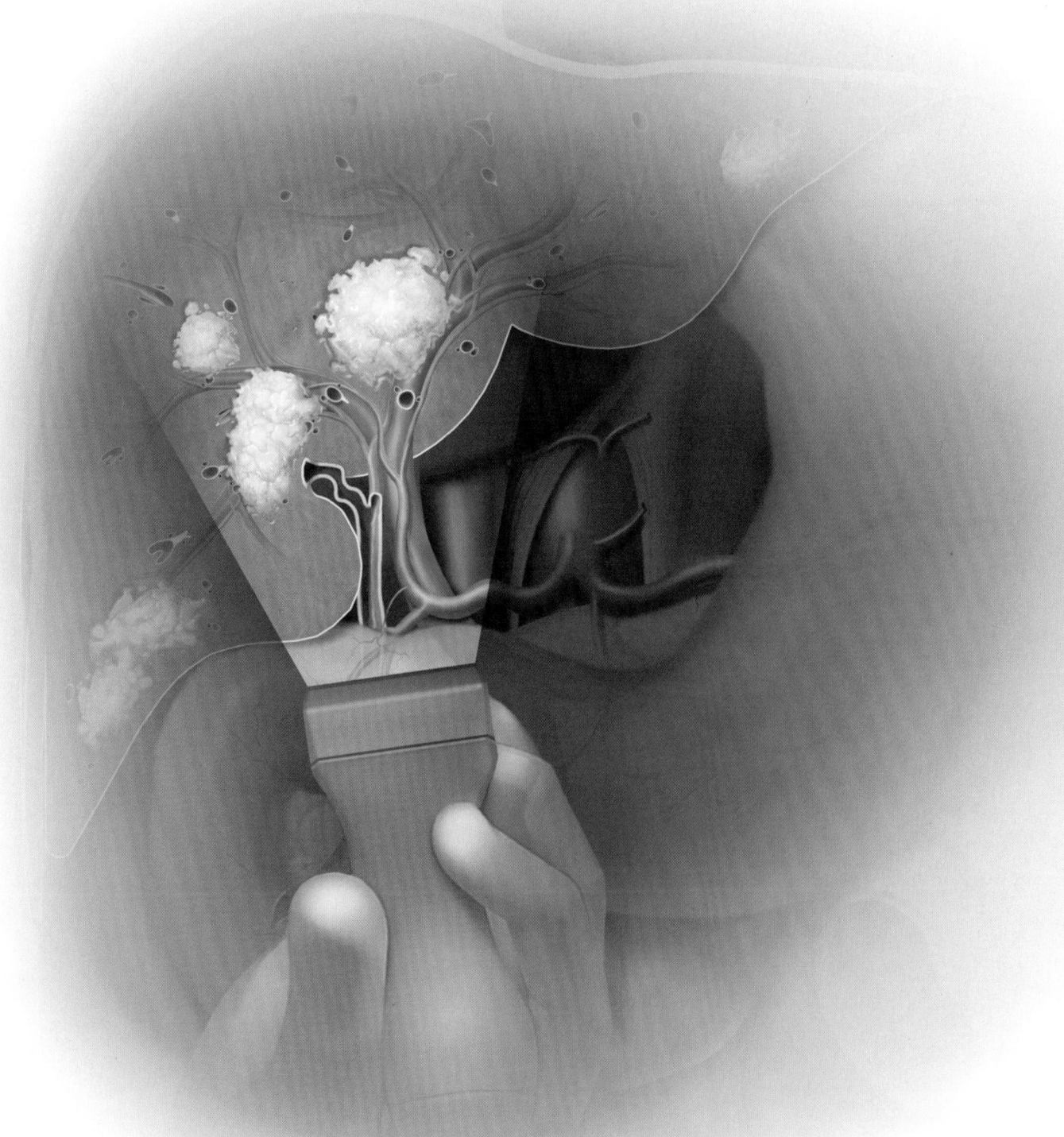

PART I
SECTION 1

Abdomen

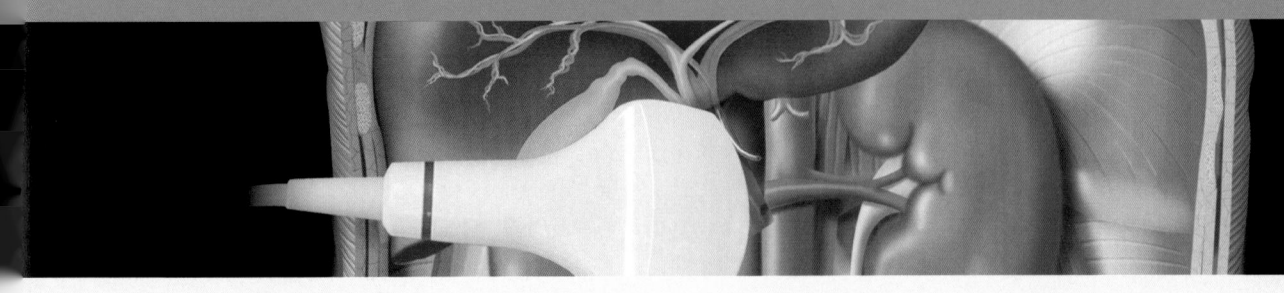

GROSS ANATOMY

Overview

- Liver is largest gland and largest internal organ (average weight: 1,500 grams)
  - Functions
    - Processes all nutrients (except fats) absorbed from GI tract; conveyed via portal vein
    - Stores glycogen, secretes bile
  - Relations
    - Anterior and superior surfaces are smooth and convex
    - Posterior and inferior surfaces are indented by colon, stomach, right kidney, duodenum, inferior vena cava (IVC), gallbladder
  - Covered by peritoneum except along gallbladder fossa, porta hepatis, and bare area
    - Bare area: Nonperitoneal posterior superior surface where liver abuts diaphragm
    - Porta hepatis: Portal vein, hepatic artery, and bile duct are located within hepatoduodenal ligament
  - Falciform ligament: Extends from liver to anterior abdominal wall
    - Separates right and left subphrenic peritoneal recesses (between liver and diaphragm)
    - Marks plane separating medial and lateral segments of left hepatic lobe
    - Carries round ligament (ligamentum teres), fibrous remnant of umbilical vein
  - Ligamentum venosum: Remnant of ductus venosus
    - Separates caudate from left hepatic lobe
- Vascular anatomy (unique dual afferent blood supply)
  - Portal vein
    - Carries nutrients from gut and hepatotrophic hormones from pancreas to liver along with oxygen (contains 40% more oxygen than systemic venous blood)
    - 75-80% of blood supply to liver
  - Hepatic artery
    - Supplies 20-25% of blood
    - Liver is less dependent than biliary tree on hepatic arterial blood supply
    - Usually arises from celiac artery
    - Variations are common, including arteries arising from superior mesenteric artery
  - Hepatic veins
    - Usually 3 (right, middle, and left)
    - Many variations and accessory veins
    - Collect blood from liver and return it to IVC at confluence of hepatic veins just below diaphragm and entrance of IVC into right atrium
  - Portal triad
    - At all levels of size and subdivision, branches of hepatic artery, portal vein, and bile ducts travel together
    - Blood flows into hepatic sinusoids from interlobular branches of hepatic artery and portal vein → hepatocytes (detoxify blood and produce bile) → bile collects into ducts, blood collects into central veins → hepatic veins
- Segmental anatomy of liver
  - 8 hepatic segments
    - Each receives secondary or tertiary branch of hepatic artery and portal vein
    - Each is drained by its own bile duct (intrahepatic) and hepatic vein branch
  - Caudate lobe = segment 1
    - Has independent portal triads and hepatic venous drainage to IVC
  - Left lobe
    - Lateral superior = segment 2
    - Lateral inferior = segment 3
    - Medial superior = segment 4A
    - Medial inferior = segment 4B
  - Right lobe
    - Anterior inferior = segment 5
    - Posterior inferior = segment 6
    - Posterior superior = segment 7
    - Anterior superior = segment 8

IMAGING ANATOMY

Internal Contents

- Capsule
  - Reflective Glisson capsule making borders of liver well defined
- Left lobe
  - Contains segments 2, 3, 4A, and 4B
  - Longitudinal scan
    - Triangular in shape
    - Rounded upper surface
    - Sharp inferior border
  - Transverse scan
    - Wedge-shaped tapering to left
  - Liver parenchyma echoes are mid gray with uniform sponge-like pattern interrupted by vessels
- Right lobe
  - Contains segments 5, 6, 7, and 8
  - Liver parenchymal echoes similar to left lobe
  - Sections of right lobe show same basic shape, though right lobe is usually larger than left
- Caudate lobe
  - Longitudinal scan
    - Almond-shaped structure posterior to left lobe
  - Transverse scan
    - Seen as extension of right lobe
- Portal veins
  - Have thicker reflective walls than hepatic veins; portal veins have fibromuscular walls
  - Wall reflectivity also depends on angle of interrogation; portal veins cut at more oblique angle may have less apparent wall
  - Can be traced back towards porta hepatis
  - Normal portal flow is hepatopetal on color Doppler; absent or reversal of flow may be seen in portal hypertension
  - Normal velocity 13-55 cm/s
  - Portal waveform has undulating appearance due to variations with cardiac activity and respiration
  - Branches run in transverse plane
  - Hepatic portal vein anatomy is variable
- Hepatic veins

- o Appear as echolucent defects within liver parenchyma with no reflective wall: Large sinusoids with thin or absent wall
- o Branches enlarge and can be traced towards IVC
- o Flow pattern has a triphasic waveform
  - – Resulting from transmission of right atrial pulsations into veins
    - □ A wave: Atrial contraction
    - □ S wave: Systole (tricuspid valve moves toward apex)
    - □ D wave: Diastole
- o Right hepatic vein
  - – Runs in coronal plane between anterior and posterior segments of right hepatic lobe
- o Middle hepatic vein
  - – Lies in sagittal or parasagittal plane between right and left hepatic lobe
- o Left hepatic vein
  - – Runs between medial and lateral segments of left hepatic lobe
  - – Frequently duplicated
- o 1 of 3 major branches of hepatic veins may be absent
  - – Absent right hepatic vein ~ 6%
  - – Less commonly middle and left hepatic vein
- Hepatic artery
  - o Flow pattern has low-resistance characteristics with large amount of continuous forward flow throughout diastole
    - – Normal velocity 30-70 cm/s
    - – Resistive index ranges 0.5-0.8, increases after meal
  - o Common hepatic artery usually arises from celiac axis
  - o Classic configuration: 72%
    - – Celiac axis → common hepatic artery → gastroduodenal artery and proper hepatic artery → latter gives rise to right and left hepatic artery
  - o Variations from classic configuration
    - – Common hepatic artery arising from SMA (replaced hepatic artery): 4%
    - – Right hepatic artery arising from SMA (replaced right hepatic artery): 11%
    - – Left hepatic artery arising from left gastric artery (replaced left hepatic artery): 10%
- Bile ducts
  - o Normal peripheral intrahepatic bile ducts are too small to be demonstrated
  - o Normal right and left hepatic ducts measuring a few millimeters are usually visible
  - o Normal common duct
    - – Most visible in its proximal portion just caudal to porta hepatis: Less than 5 mm
    - – Distal common duct should typically measure < 6-7 mm
    - – In elderly, generalized loss of tissue elasticity with advancing age leads to increase in bile duct diameter: < 8 mm (somewhat controversial)

ANATOMY IMAGING ISSUES

Imaging Recommendations

- Transducer
  - o 2.5-5 MHz curvilinear or vector transducer is generally most suitable

- o Higher frequency linear transducer (i.e., 7-9 MHz) useful for evaluation of liver capsule and superficial portions of liver
- Left lobe
  - o Subcostal window with full inspiration generally most suitable
- Right lobe
  - o Subcostal window
    - – Cranial and rightwards angulation useful for visualization of right lobe below dome of hemidiaphragm
    - – Can sometimes be obscured by bowel gas
  - o Intercostal window
    - – Usually gives better resolution for parenchyma without influence from bowel gas
    - – Right lobe just below hemidiaphragm may not be visible due to obscuration from lung bases
    - – Important to tilt transducer parallel to intercostal space to minimize shadowing from ribs

Imaging Pitfalls

- Because of variations of vascular and biliary branching within liver (common), it is frequently impossible to designate precisely boundaries between hepatic segments on imaging studies

CLINICAL IMPLICATIONS

Clinical Importance

- Liver ultrasound often first-line imaging modality in evaluation for elevated liver enzymes
  - o Diffuse liver disease, such as hepatic steatosis, cirrhosis, hepatomegaly, hepatitis, and biliary ductal dilatation, are well visualized with ultrasound
  - o Documentation of patency of portal vein, hepatic vein waveforms, and hepatic arterial velocities are helpful in evaluation for etiologies of elevated liver function tests
- Liver metastases are common
  - o Primary carcinomas of colon, pancreas, and stomach are common
    - – Portal venous drainage usually results in liver being initial site of metastatic spread from these tumors
  - o Metastases from other non-GI primaries (breast, lung, etc.) commonly spread to liver hematogenously
- Primary hepatocellular carcinoma
  - o Common worldwide
    - – Risk factors include chronic viral hepatitis B or C, alcoholic cirrhosis, or nonalcoholic steatohepatitis
    - – Ultrasound commonly used for screening and surveillance in patients at risk for development of hepatocellular carcinoma (HCC) typically at 6 month intervals

SELECTED REFERENCES

1. Heller MT et al: The role of ultrasonography in the evaluation of diffuse liver disease. Radiol Clin North Am. 52(6):1163-75, 2014
2. McNaughton DA et al: Doppler US of the liver made simple. Radiographics. 31(1):161-88, 2011
3. Kruskal JB et al: Optimizing Doppler and color flow US: application to hepatic sonography. Radiographics. 24(3):657-75, 2004

HEPATIC VISCERAL SURFACE

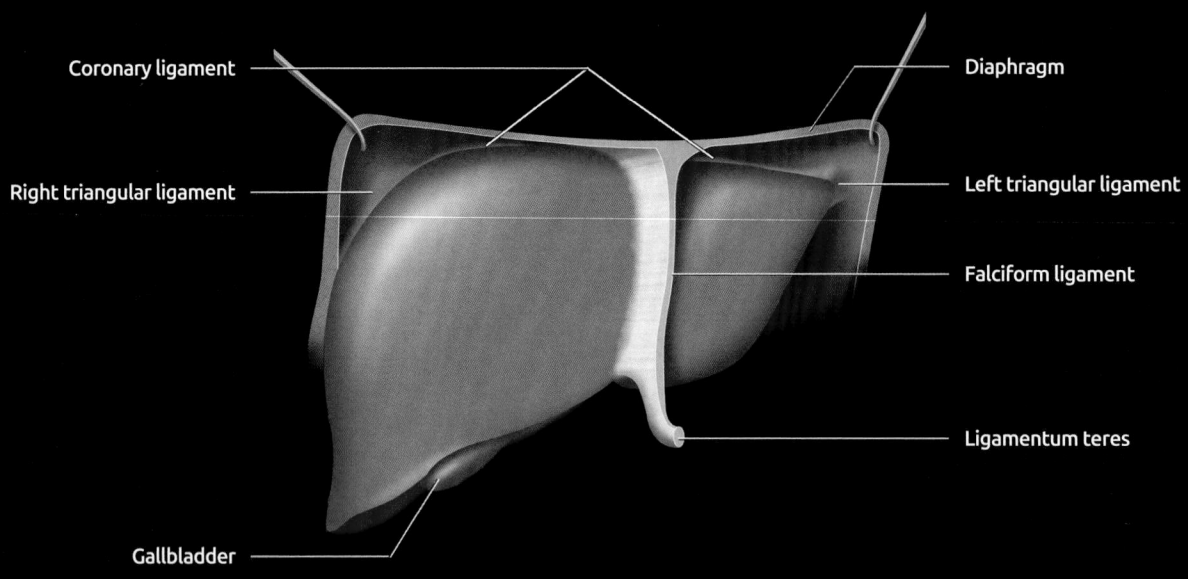

Coronary ligament

Right triangular ligament

Gallbladder

Diaphragm

Left triangular ligament

Falciform ligament

Ligamentum teres

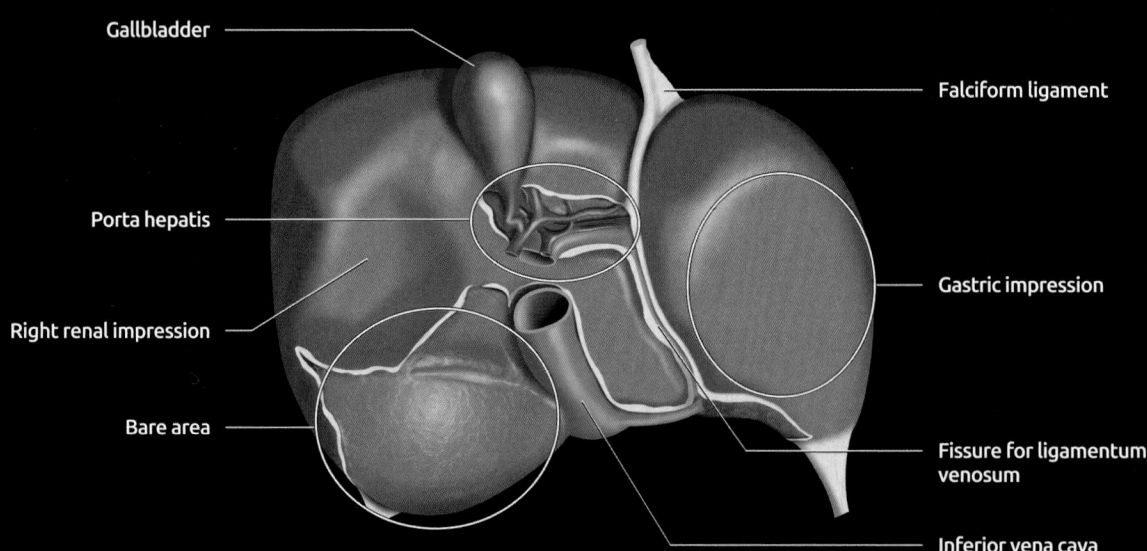

Gallbladder

Porta hepatis

Right renal impression

Bare area

Falciform ligament

Gastric impression

Fissure for ligamentum venosum

Inferior vena cava

(Top) *The anterior surface of the liver is smooth and molds to the diaphragm and anterior abdominal wall. Generally, only the anterior/inferior edge of the liver is palpable on a physical exam. The liver is covered with peritoneum, except for the gallbladder bed, porta hepatis, and the bare area. Peritoneal reflections form various ligaments that connect the liver to the diaphragm and abdominal wall, including the falciform ligament, the inferior edge that contains the ligamentum teres, and the obliterated remnant of the umbilical vein.* (Bottom) *This graphic shows the liver inverted, which is somewhat similar to the surgeon's view of the upwardly retracted liver. The structures in the porta hepatis include the portal vein (blue), hepatic artery (red), and the bile ducts (green). The visceral surface of the liver is indented by adjacent viscera. The bare area is not easily accessible.*

HEPATIC ATTACHMENTS AND RELATIONS

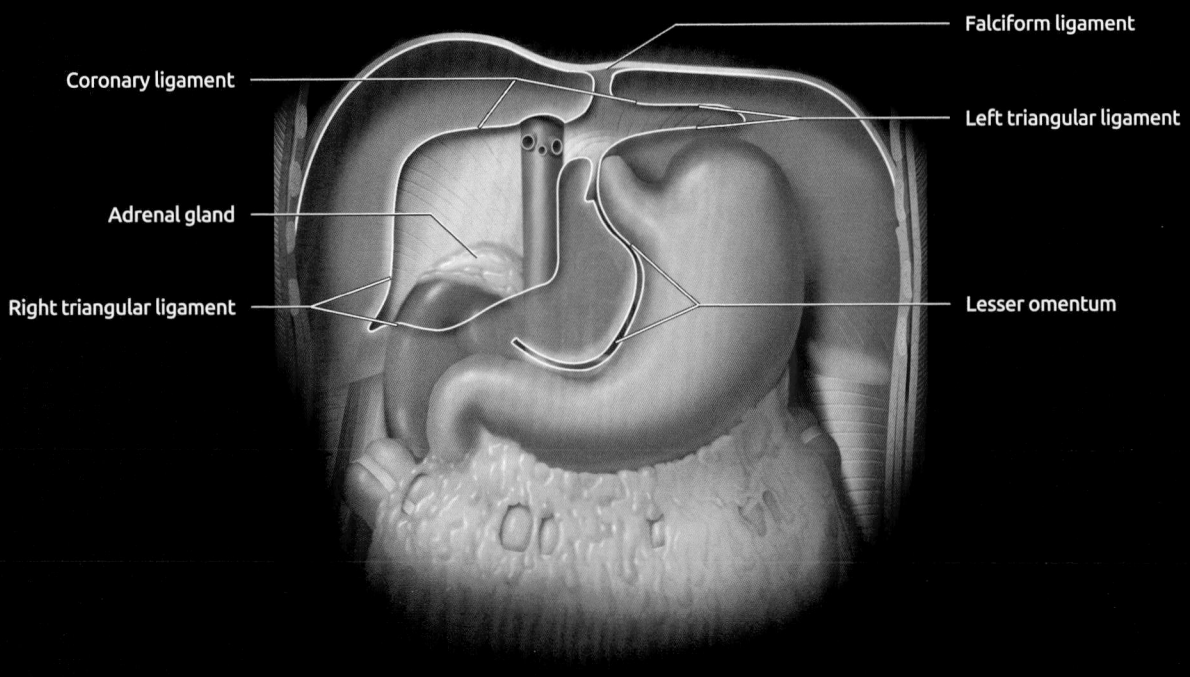

Coronary ligament

Adrenal gland

Right triangular ligament

Falciform ligament

Left triangular ligament

Lesser omentum

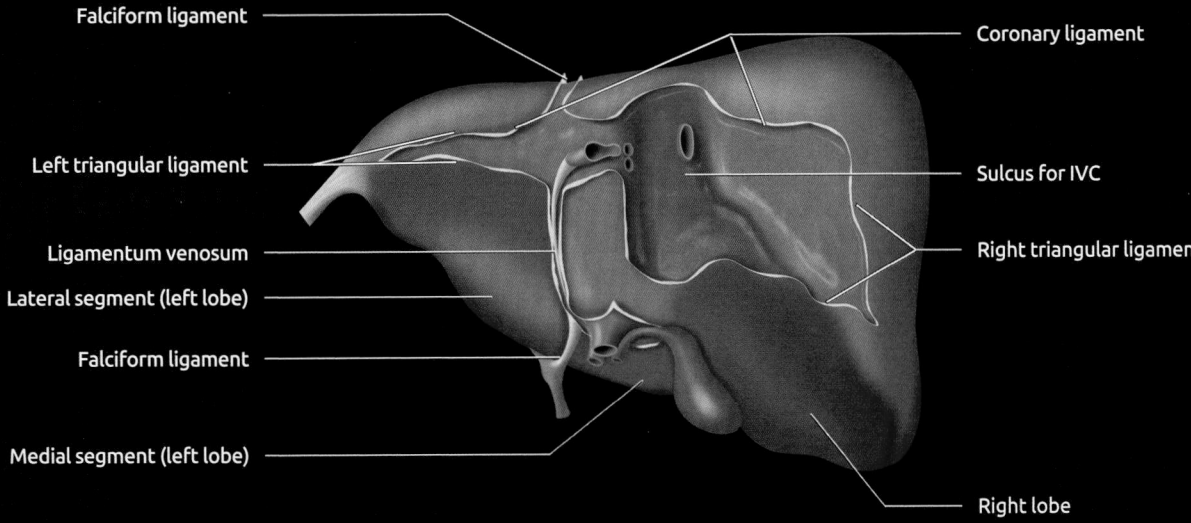

Falciform ligament

Left triangular ligament

Ligamentum venosum

Lateral segment (left lobe)

Falciform ligament

Medial segment (left lobe)

Coronary ligament

Sulcus for IVC

Right triangular ligament

Right lobe

(Top) *The liver is attached to the posterior abdominal wall and diaphragm by the left and right triangular and coronary ligaments. The falciform ligament attaches the liver to the anterior abdominal wall. The bare area is in direct contact with the right adrenal gland, kidney, and inferior vena cava (IVC).* (Bottom) *Posterior view of the liver shows the ligamentous attachments. While these may help to fix the liver in position, abdominal pressure alone is sufficient, as evidenced by orthotopic liver transplantation, after which the ligamentous attachments are lost without the liver shifting position. The diaphragmatic peritoneal reflection is the coronary ligament whose lateral extensions are the right and left triangular ligaments. The falciform ligament separates the medial and lateral segments of the left lobe.*

HEPATIC VESSELS AND BILE DUCTS

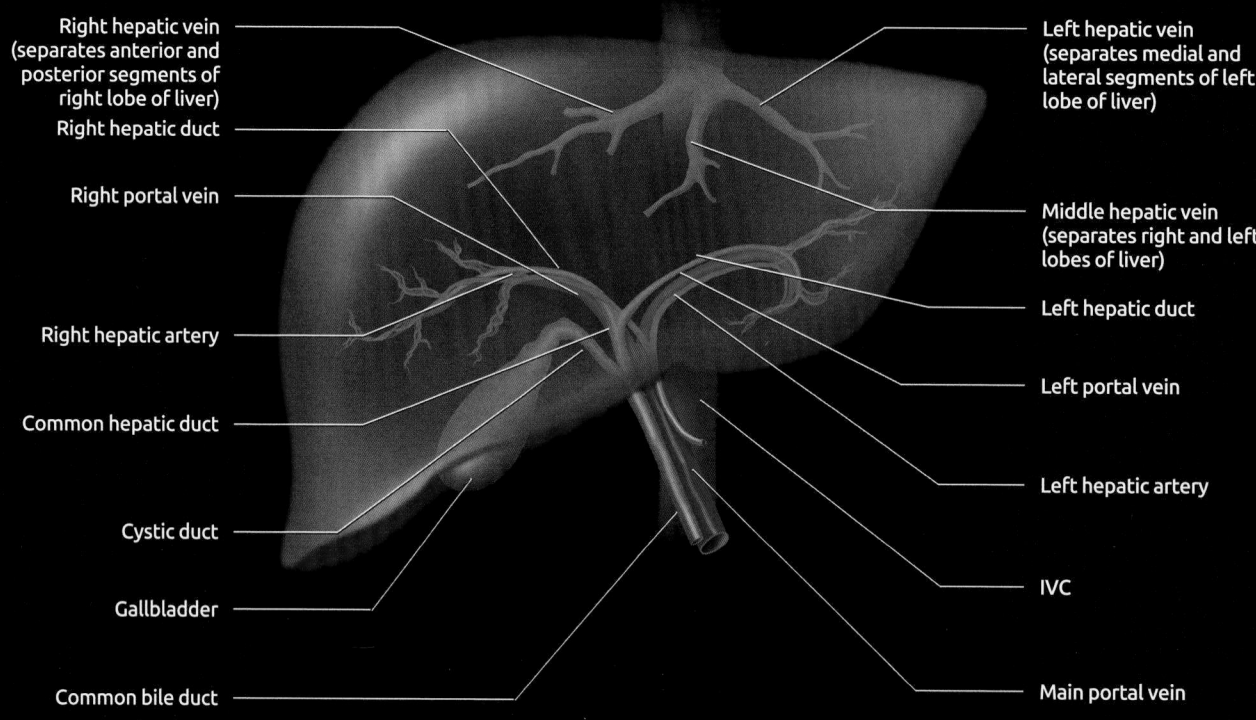

Right hepatic vein
(separates anterior and
posterior segments of
right lobe of liver)

Right hepatic duct

Right portal vein

Right hepatic artery

Common hepatic duct

Cystic duct

Gallbladder

Common bile duct

Left hepatic vein
(separates medial and
lateral segments of left
lobe of liver)

Middle hepatic vein
(separates right and left
lobes of liver)

Left hepatic duct

Left portal vein

Left hepatic artery

IVC

Main portal vein

This graphic emphasizes that at every level of branching and subdivision, the portal veins, hepatic arteries, and bile ducts course together, constituting the "portal triad." Each segment of the liver is supplied by branches of these vessels. Conversely, hepatic venous branches lie between hepatic segments and interdigitate with the portal triads, but never run parallel to them.

HEPATIC SEGMENTS

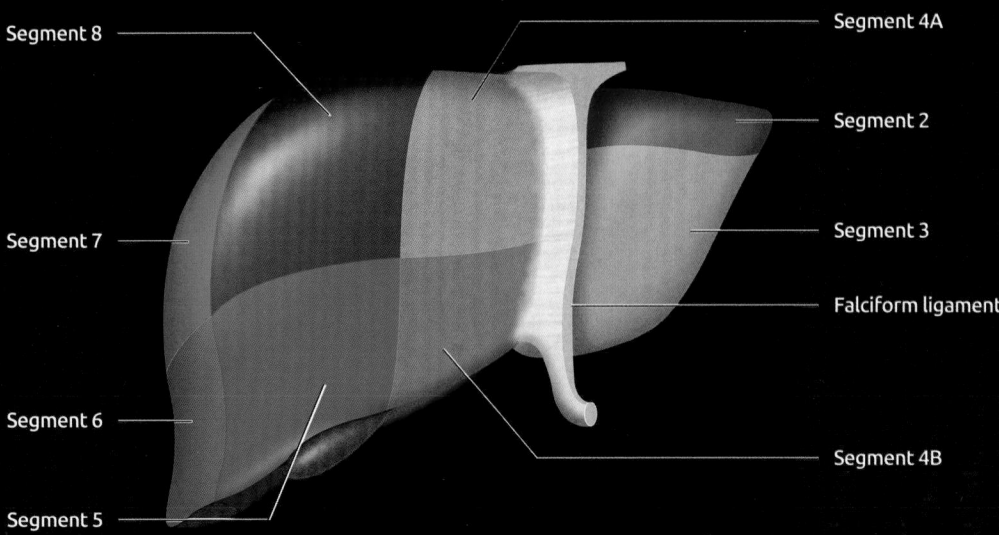

Segment 8 — Segment 4A — Segment 2 — Segment 7 — Segment 3 — Falciform ligament — Segment 6 — Segment 4B — Segment 5

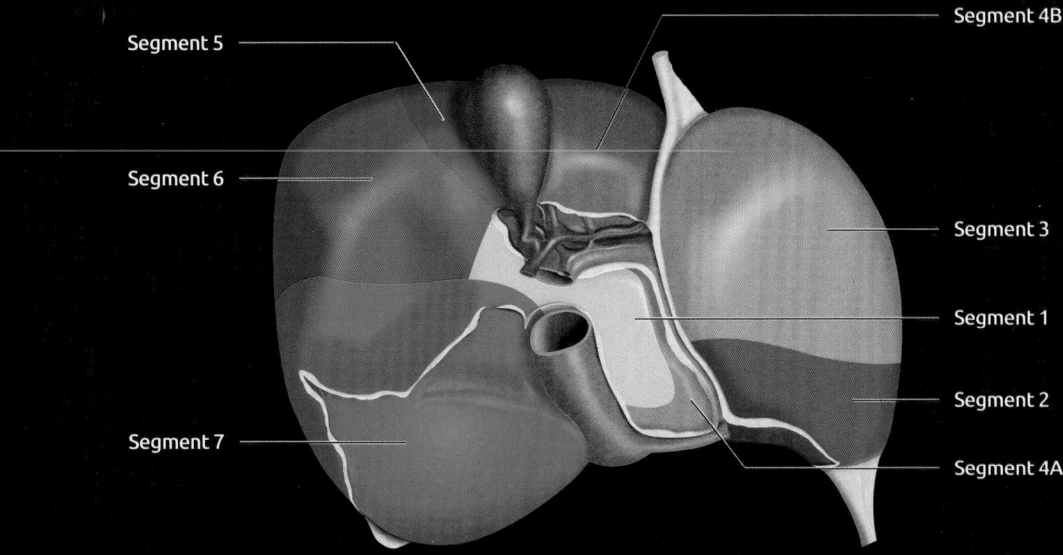

Segment 5 — Segment 4B — Segment 6 — Segment 3 — Segment 1 — Segment 2 — Segment 7 — Segment 4A

(Top) *The 1st of 2 graphics demonstrating the segmental anatomy of the liver in a somewhat idealized fashion is shown. Segments are numbered in a clockwise direction, starting with the caudate lobe (segment 1), which cannot be seen on this frontal view. The falciform ligament divides the lateral (segments 2 and 3) from the medial (segments 4A and 4B) left lobe. The horizontal planes separating the superior from the inferior segments follow the course of the right and left portal veins. An oblique vertical plane through the middle hepatic vein, gallbladder fossa ,and IVC divides the right and left lobes.* **(Bottom)** *Inferior view of the liver shows that the caudate is entirely posterior, abutting the IVC, ligamentum venosum, and porta hepatis. In this view, a plane through the IVC and gallbladder approximately divides the left and right lobes.*

TRANSVERSE VIEW OF LEFT LOBE OF LIVER

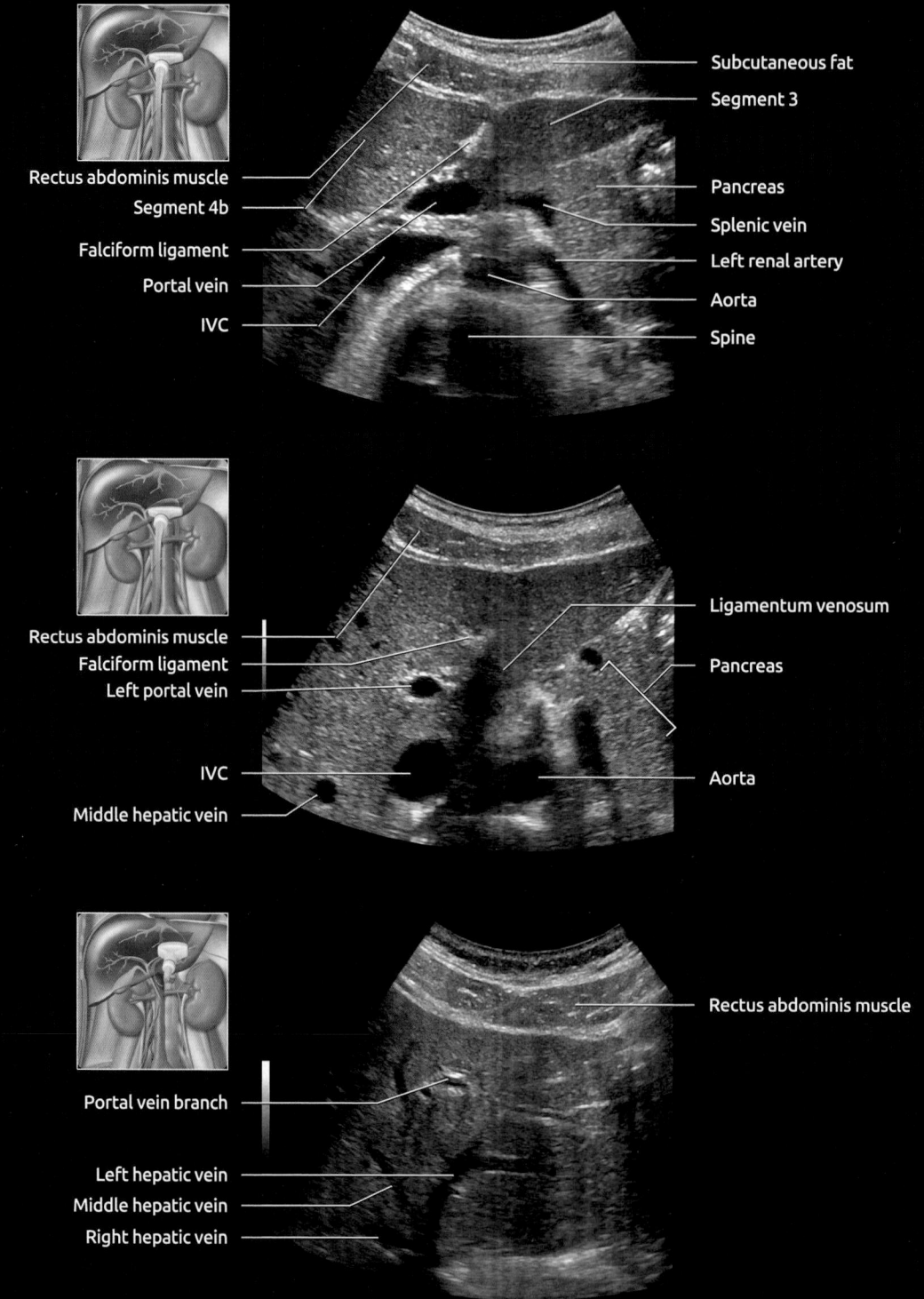

(Top) *Transverse grayscale ultrasound of the left lobe of the liver is shown, centered at the level of the falciform ligament and pancreas.* **(Middle)** *Transverse grayscale ultrasound of the left lobe of the liver is shown.* **(Bottom)** *Transverse grayscale ultrasound of the left lobe of the liver is shown, centered at the level of the left hepatic vein.*

LEFT LOBE OF LIVER: LEFT PORTAL VEIN

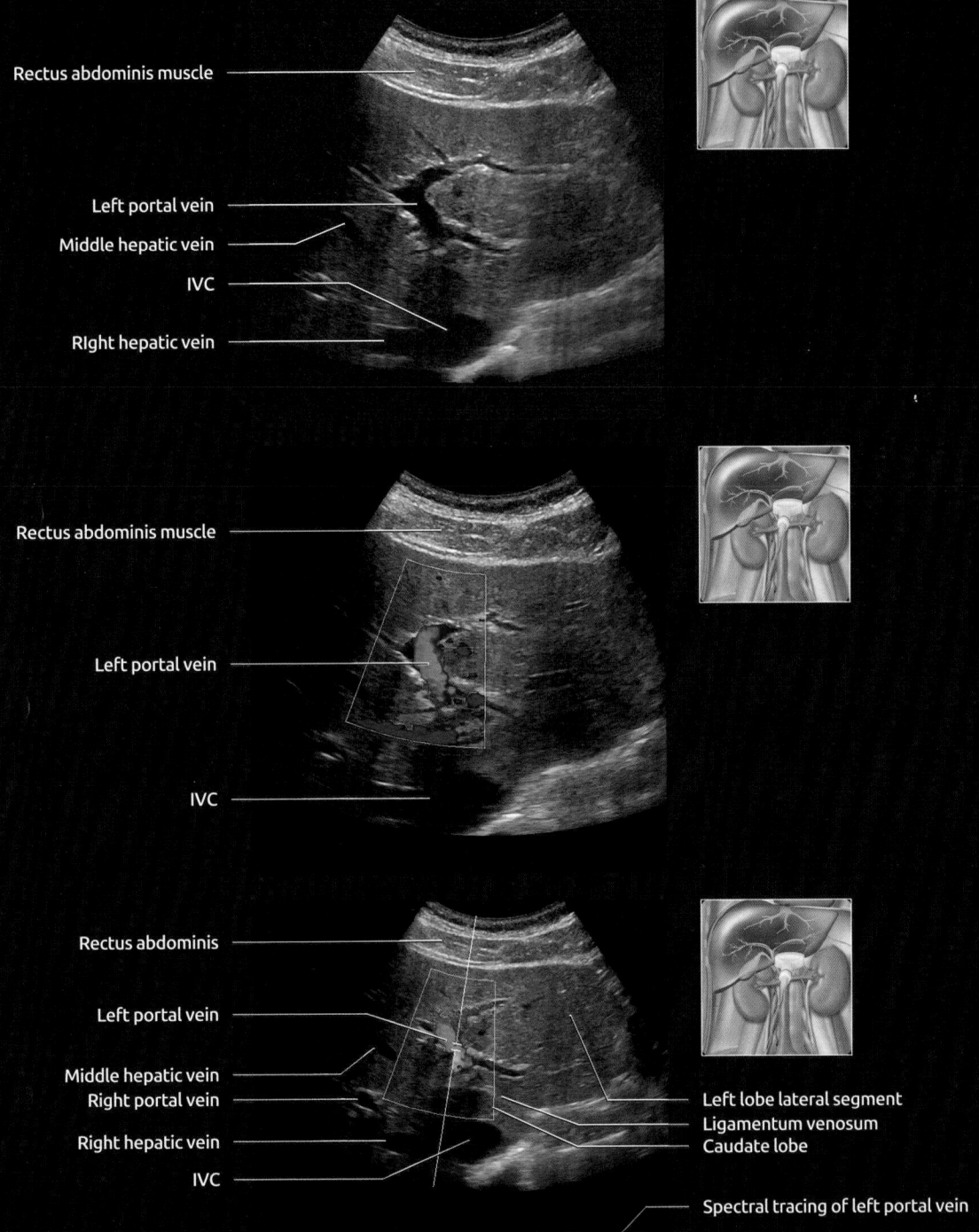

Rectus abdominis muscle

Left portal vein
Middle hepatic vein
IVC
RIght hepatic vein

Rectus abdominis muscle

Left portal vein

IVC

Rectus abdominis

Left portal vein

Middle hepatic vein
Right portal vein

Right hepatic vein

IVC

Left lobe lateral segment
Ligamentum venosum
Caudate lobe

Spectral tracing of left portal vein

(Top) *Transverse grayscale ultrasound of the left lobe of the liver is shown, centered at the left portal vein.* (Middle) *Transverse color Doppler ultrasound of the left lobe of the liver is shown, centered at the level of the left portal vein. Flow in the left portal vein is directed towards the transducer, indicating that the flow is hepatopetal and therefore normal.* (Bottom) *Spectral tracing of the left portal vein on this transverse pulsed Doppler ultrasound shows that the flow is monophasic, directed towards the transducer, with a mildly undulating waveform related to slight transmission of the cardiac cycle, which is a normal appearance for the portal vein.*

LEFT LOBE OF LIVER: LEFT HEPATIC VEIN

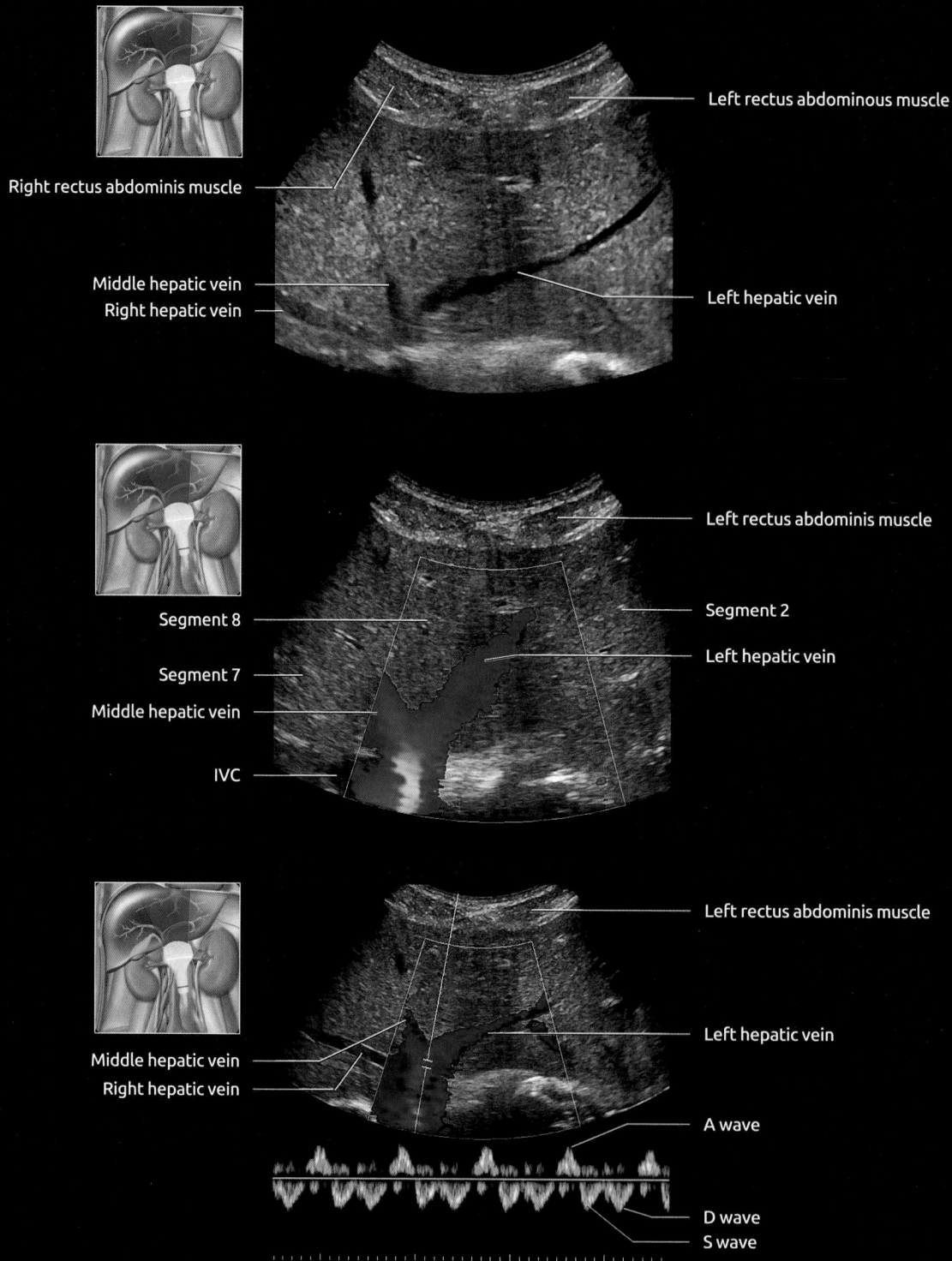

Left rectus abdominous muscle

Right rectus abdominis muscle

Middle hepatic vein
Right hepatic vein

Left hepatic vein

Left rectus abdominis muscle

Segment 8

Segment 2

Segment 7

Left hepatic vein

Middle hepatic vein

IVC

Left rectus abdominis muscle

Middle hepatic vein
Right hepatic vein

Left hepatic vein

A wave

D wave
S wave

(Top) *Transverse grayscale ultrasound of the liver centered at the left hepatic lobe shows the right, middle, and left hepatic veins as they join into the intrahepatic IVC.* (Middle) *Transverse color Doppler ultrasound of the liver, centered at the confluence of the hepatic veins, shows that the flow direction is away from the transducer, directed towards the IVC.* (Bottom) *Spectral tracing the left hepatic vein near the confluence with the IVC shows a characteristic triphasic waveform pattern, which represents reflection of cardiac motion.*

LEFT LOBE OF LIVER: LONGITUDINAL VIEW

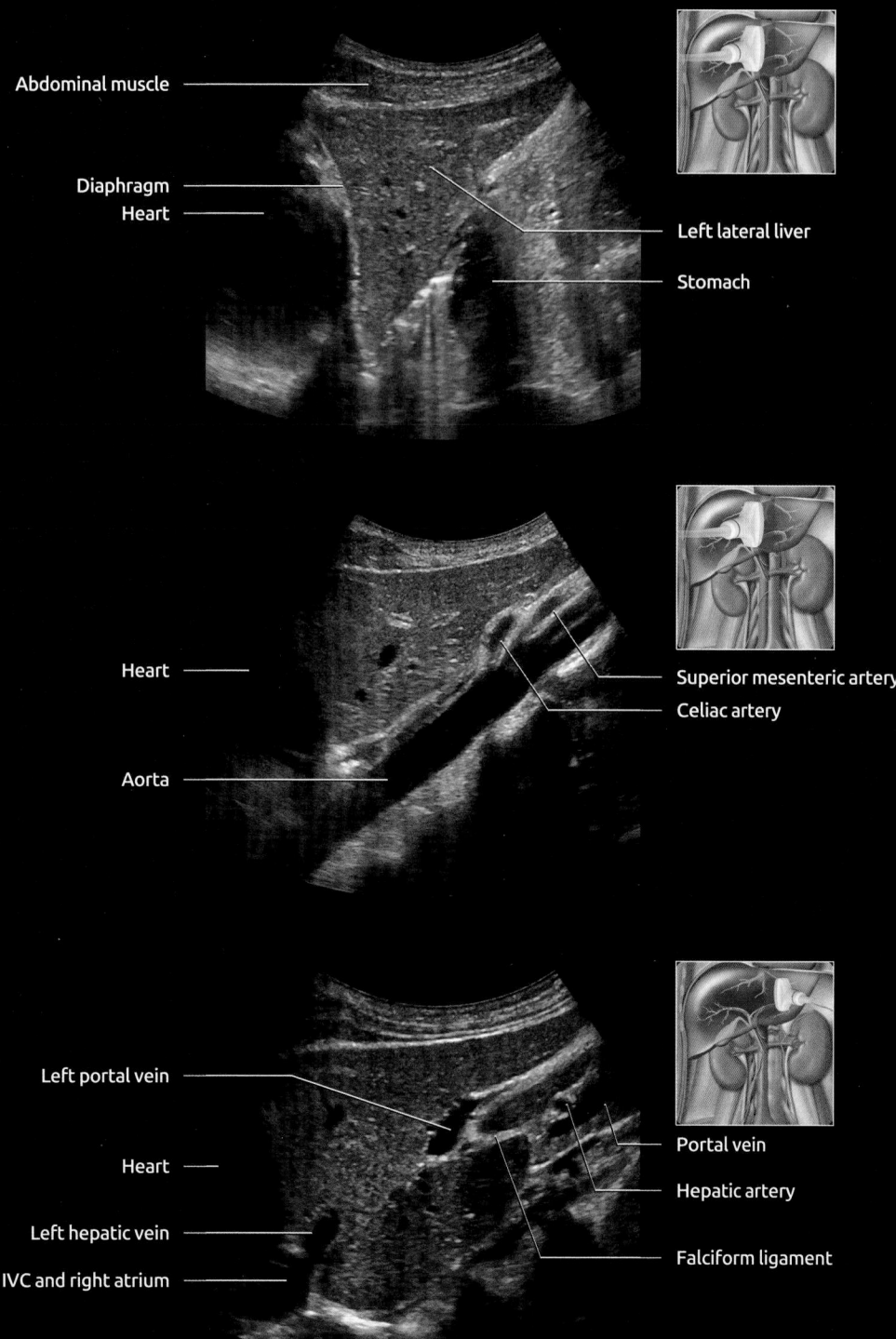

Abdominal muscle

Diaphragm
Heart

Left lateral liver

Stomach

Heart

Aorta

Superior mesenteric artery
Celiac artery

Left portal vein

Heart

Left hepatic vein

Junction of IVC and right atrium

Portal vein

Hepatic artery

Falciform ligament

(Top) *Longitudinal grayscale ultrasound of the left lobe of the liver shows a triangular-shaped cross section. The heart is partially visualized above the diaphragm.* (Middle) *Longitudinal grayscale ultrasound view of the left lobe of the liver at the level of the aorta shows the aorta posterior to the liver, the celiac artery, and superior mesenteric artery arising from the aorta.* (Bottom) *Longitudinal grayscale ultrasound of the left lobe of the liver shows the left hepatic vein and left portal vein in cross section.*

TRANSVERSE RIGHT LOBE OF LIVER

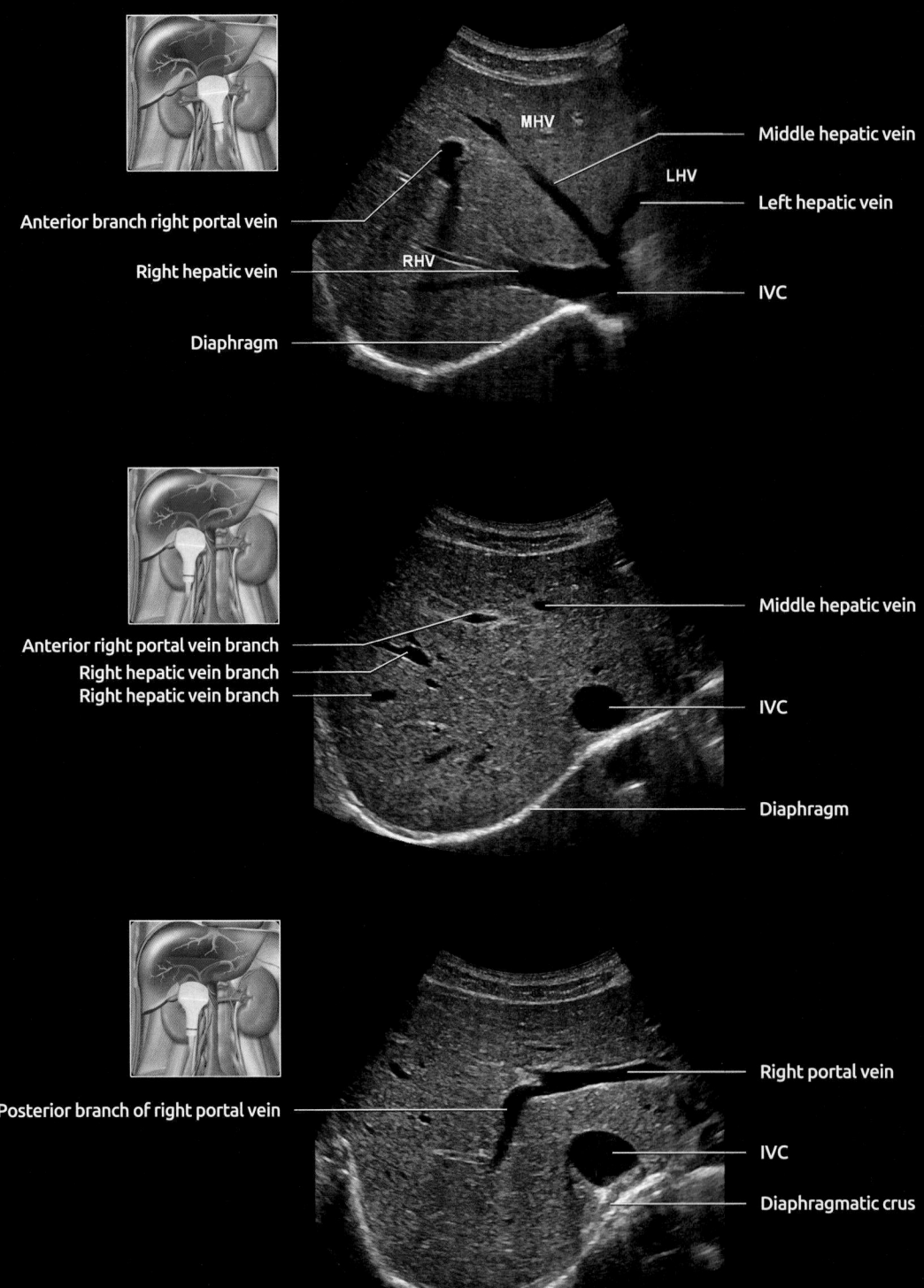

Top image labels:
- Anterior branch right portal vein
- Right hepatic vein
- Diaphragm
- MHV
- LHV
- RHV
- Middle hepatic vein
- Left hepatic vein
- IVC

Middle image labels:
- Anterior right portal vein branch
- Right hepatic vein branch
- Right hepatic vein branch
- Middle hepatic vein
- IVC
- Diaphragm

Bottom image labels:
- Posterior branch of right portal vein
- Right portal vein
- IVC
- Diaphragmatic crus

(Top) *Transverse grayscale ultrasound at the level of the hepatic vein confluence shows the right, middle, and left hepatic veins as they join with the IVC posteriorly.* (Middle) *Transverse grayscale ultrasound of the liver just below the confluence of the hepatic veins shows the IVC and more peripheral portions of the right and left hepatic veins.* (Bottom) *Transverse grayscale ultrasound of the right lobe of the liver, centered at the right portal vein, shows the posterior branch of the right portal vein, which is typically directed away from the transducer.*

RIGHT LOBE OF LIVER: RIGHT HEPATIC VEIN

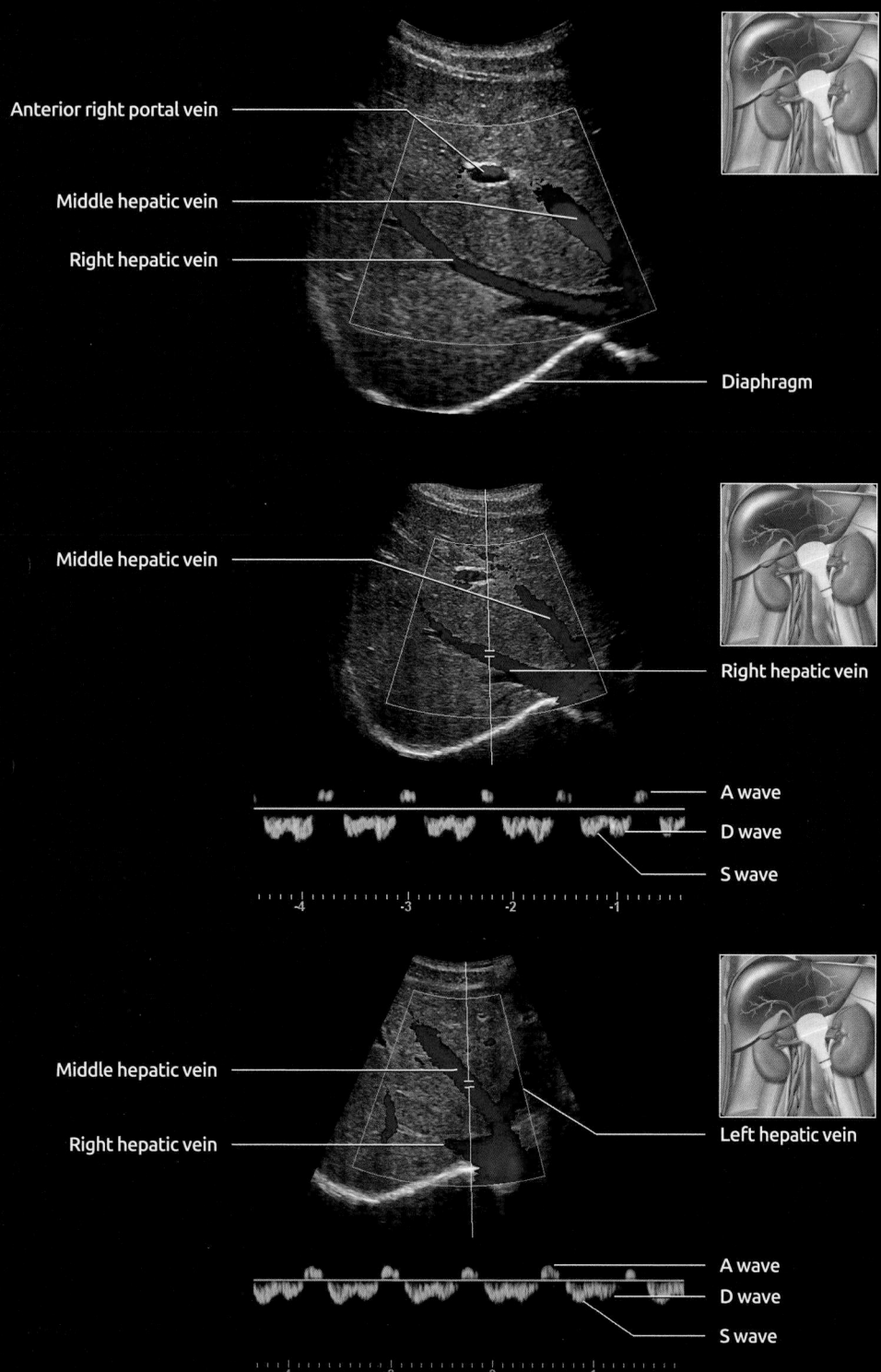

Anterior right portal vein

Middle hepatic vein

Right hepatic vein

Diaphragm

Middle hepatic vein

Right hepatic vein

A wave

D wave

S wave

Middle hepatic vein

Left hepatic vein

Right hepatic vein

A wave

D wave

S wave

(Top) *Transverse color Doppler ultrasound of the right lobe of the liver shows that the right and middle hepatic vein are directed away from the transducer and flowing toward the IVC.* **(Middle)** *Spectral tracing of the right hepatic vein shows a typical triphasic waveform with A, S, and D waves representing reflection of cardiac motion in the hepatic veins.* **(Bottom)** *Spectral tracing of the middle hepatic vein shows a typical triphasic waveform with A, S, and D waves representing reflection of cardiac motion in the hepatic veins.*

MAIN PORTAL VEIN

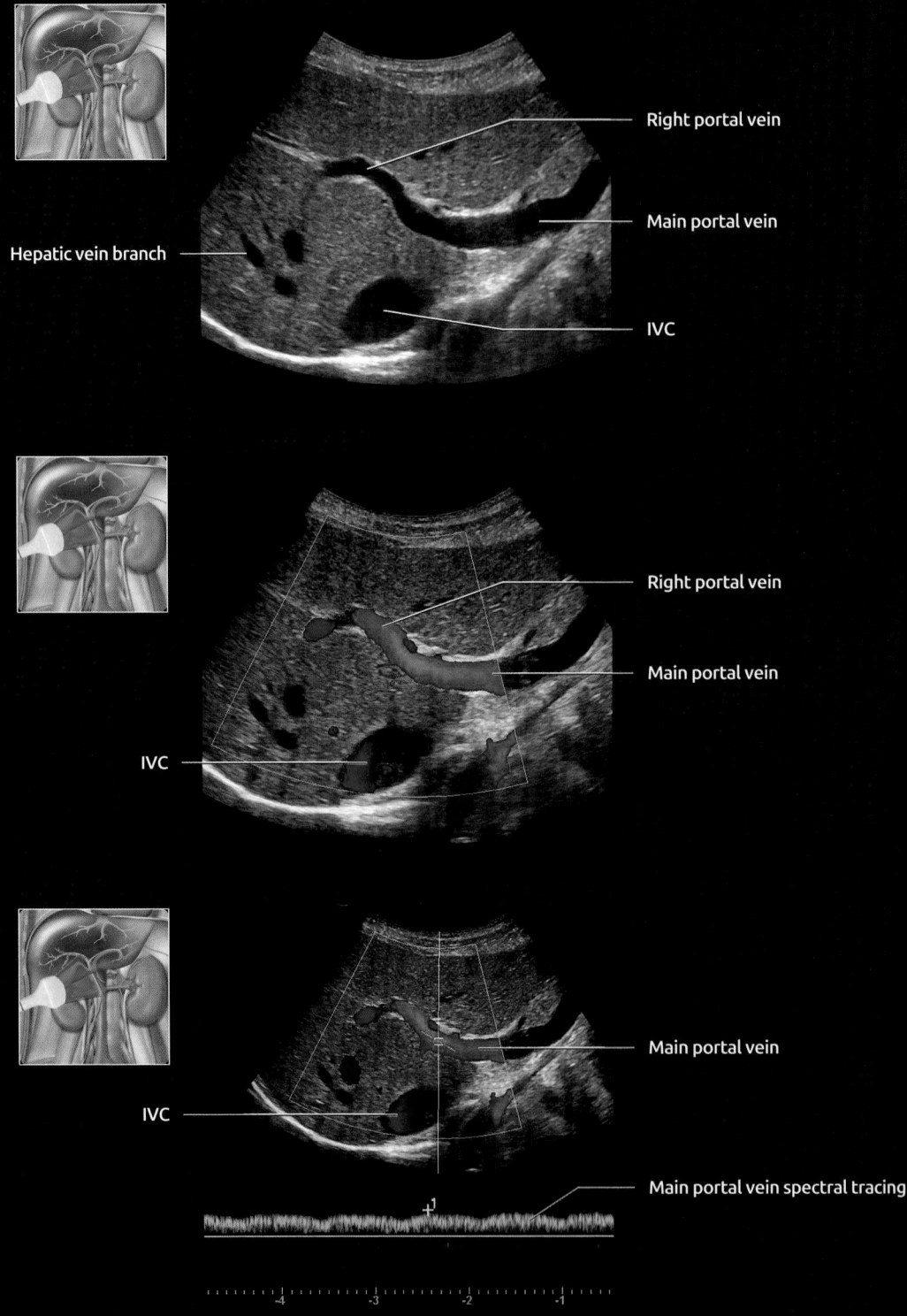

Right portal vein

Main portal vein

Hepatic vein branch

IVC

Right portal vein

Main portal vein

IVC

Main portal vein

IVC

Main portal vein spectral tracing

(Top) *Longitudinal oblique grayscale ultrasound is shown, centered at the level of the main portal and right portal vein.* (Middle) *Longitudinal oblique color Doppler ultrasound, centered at the level of the main portal and right portal vein, shows that flow in the portal vein is directed toward the liver (hepatopetal).* (Bottom) *Longitudinal oblique spectral Doppler ultrasound of the main portal vein shows that the flow is hepatopetal, with gentle undulation reflecting the cardiac and respiratory cycle.*

PORTA HEPATIS

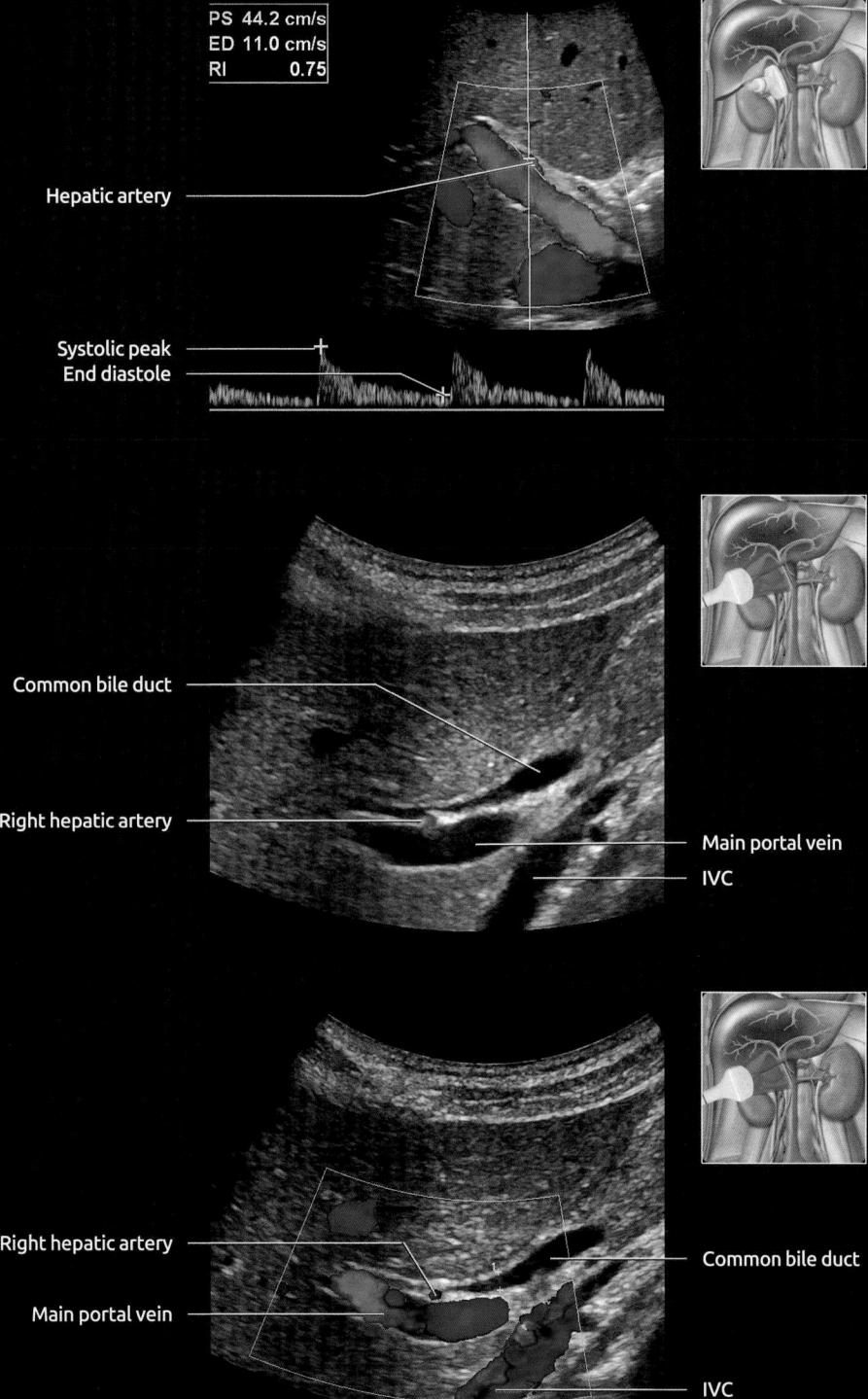

PS 44.2 cm/s
ED 11.0 cm/s
RI   0.75

Hepatic artery

Systolic peak
End diastole

Common bile duct

Right hepatic artery

Main portal vein
IVC

Right hepatic artery

Main portal vein

Common bile duct

IVC

(Top) *Longitudinal oblique spectral tracing of the main hepatic artery shows a typical low-resistance waveform, with brisk upstroke and forward diastolic flow. In this case, the hepatic artery velocity is 44 cm/s, which is normal. When measuring velocity, proper angle correction is the key to obtaining accurate velocities.* **(Middle)** *Oblique grayscale ultrasound of the liver, centered at the porta hepatis, shows the common bile duct anterior to the right hepatic artery and portal vein. The IVC is seen posterior to the portal vein.* **(Bottom)** *Oblique color Doppler ultrasound of the liver, centered at the porta hepatis, shows the common bile duct is anterior to the portal vein and the right hepatic artery is between these 2 structures. This is the typical anatomy in this location, although anatomic variants of the right hepatic artery may occur in which the hepatic artery may be located anterior to the common bile duct.*

LONGITUDINAL LIVER

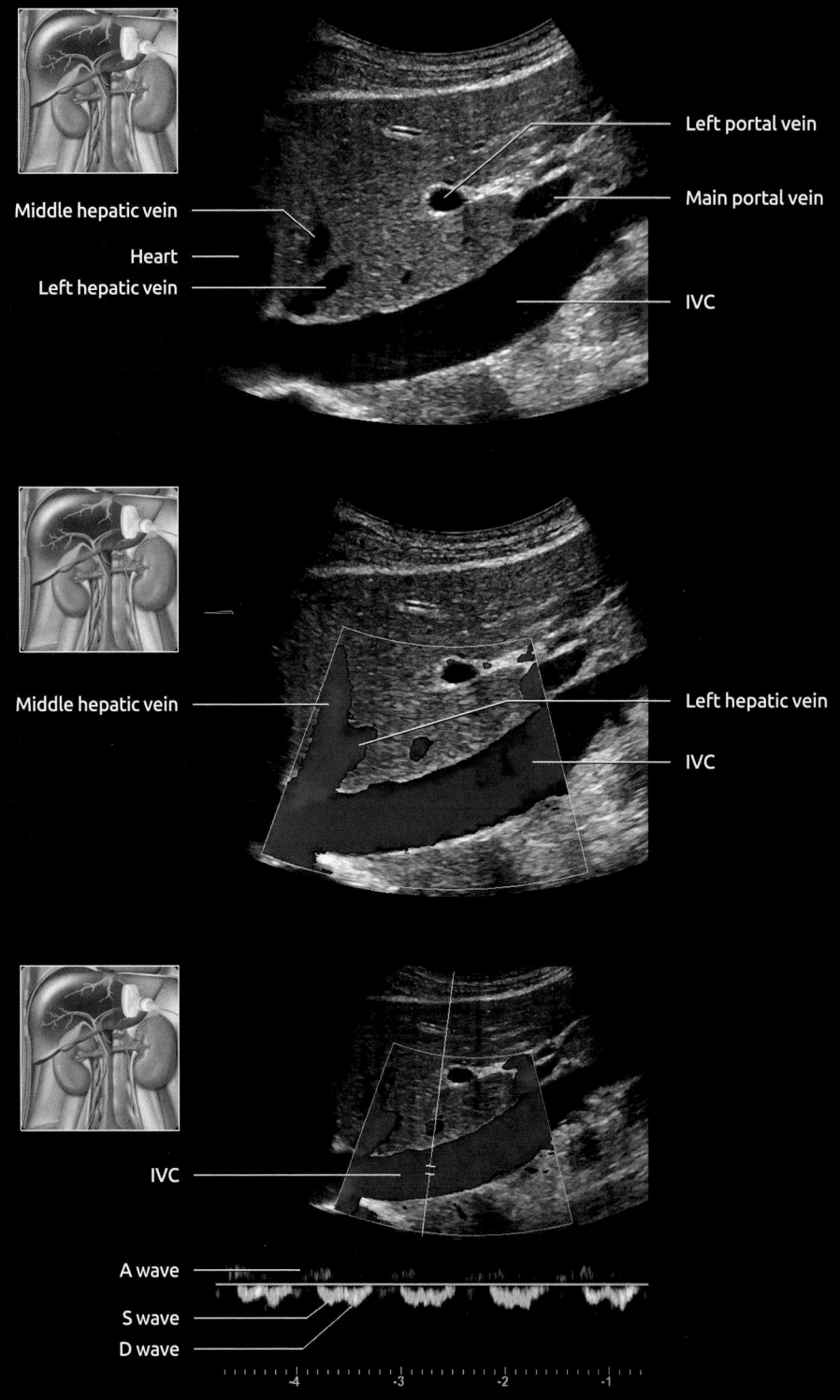

Left portal vein

Main portal vein

Middle hepatic vein

Heart

Left hepatic vein

IVC

Middle hepatic vein

Left hepatic vein

IVC

IVC

A wave

S wave

D wave

(Top) *Longitudinal grayscale ultrasound of the right lobe of the liver is shown, centered at the level of the IVC.* (Middle) *Longitudinal color Doppler ultrasound of the liver is shown at the level of the IVC.* (Bottom) *Spectral tracing of the IVC shows a typical triphasic waveform with A, S, and D waves representing reflection of cardiac motion in the IVC.*

OTHER VIEWS OF LIVER

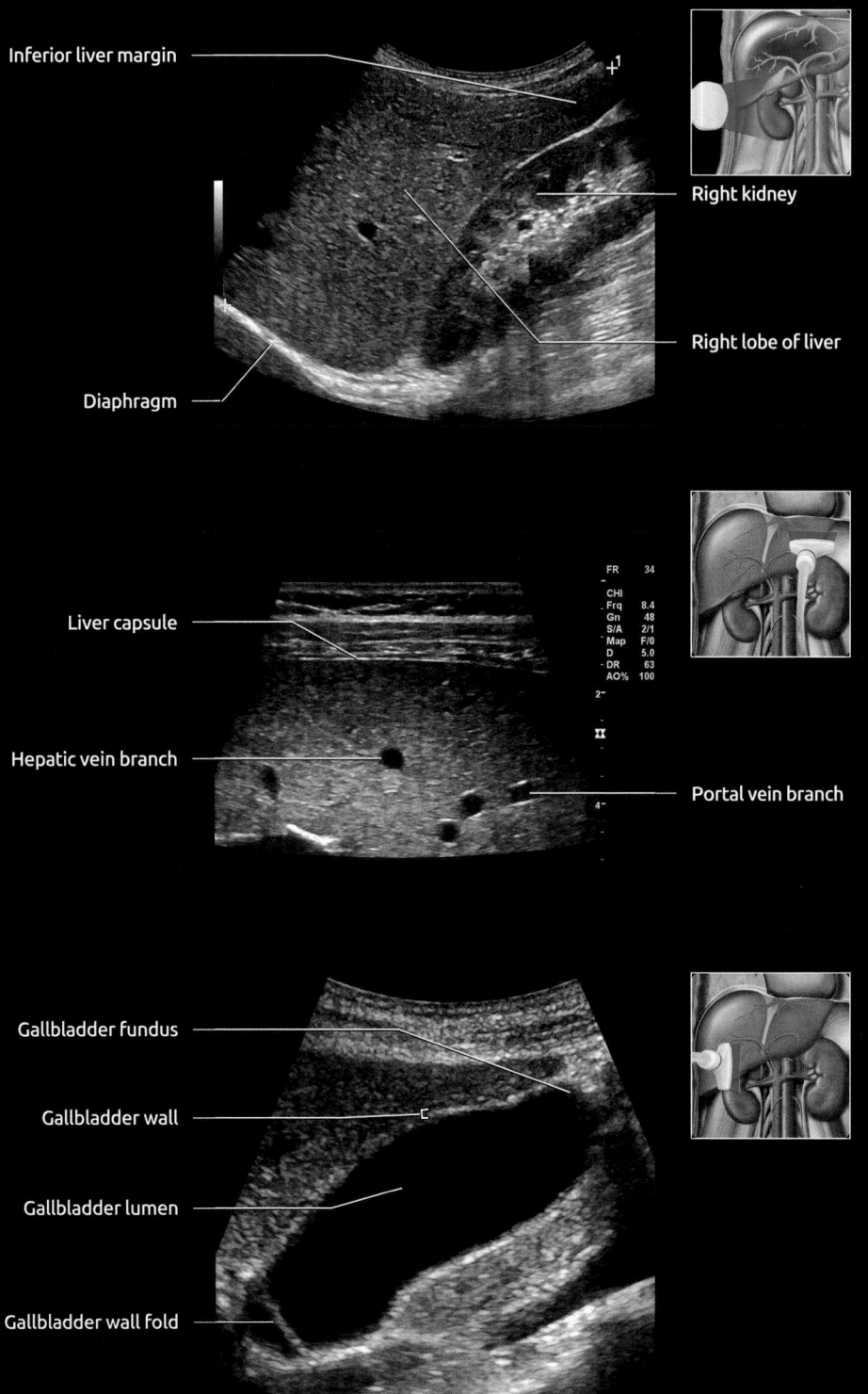

Inferior liver margin

Right kidney

Right lobe of liver

Diaphragm

Liver capsule

Hepatic vein branch

Portal vein branch

FR 34
CHI
Frq 8.4
Gn 48
S/A 2/1
Map F/0
D 5.0
DR 63
AO% 100

Gallbladder fundus

Gallbladder wall

Gallbladder lumen

Gallbladder wall fold

(Top) *Longitudinal grayscale ultrasound of the right lobe of the liver shows the liver ends just above the inferior margin of the right kidney. Normal hepatic length should be < 15-15.5 cm. Notice that the normal hepatic parenchyma is slightly hyperechoic compared to the normal kidney.* (Middle) *Transverse high-resolution ultrasound of the liver capsule, as seen here, is typically obtained with higher frequencies (7-9 MHz). Subtle nodularity of the capsule and small subcapsular liver lesions that may not be as well visualized with standard (3-5 MHz) frequencies are best visualized with this view. Note the hepatic veins have no discernible wall, whereas the portal veins have slightly echogenic walls.* (Bottom) *Longitudinal oblique ultrasound shows a normal gallbladder with anechoic fluid within the lumen and normal appearance of the gallbladder wall. Normal gallbladder wall thickness should be measured at the interface with the liver and should be less than 3 mm in thickness. A fold in the gallbladder neck is incidentally seen in this patient.*

TERMINOLOGY

Abbreviations

- Extrahepatic biliary structures
  - Gallbladder (GB)
  - Cystic duct (CD)
  - Right hepatic (RH) and left hepatic (LH) ducts
  - Common hepatic duct (CHD)
  - Common bile duct (CBD)

Definitions

- Proximal/distal biliary tree
  - Proximal refers to portion of biliary tree that is in closer in proximity to liver and hepatocytes
  - Distal refers to caudal end closer to ampulla and bowel
- Central/peripheral
  - Central refers to biliary ducts close to porta hepatis
  - Peripheral refers to higher-order branches of intrahepatic biliary tree extending into hepatic parenchyma

IMAGING ANATOMY

Overview

- Biliary ducts carry bile from liver to duodenum
  - Bile is produced continuously by liver, stored and concentrated by GB, and released intermittently by GB contraction in response to presence of fat in duodenum
  - Hepatocytes form bile → bile canaliculi → interlobular biliary ducts → collecting bile ducts → right and left hepatic ducts → common hepatic duct → common bile duct → intestines
- Common bile duct forms in free edge of lesser omentum by union of cystic duct and common hepatic duct
  - Length of duct: 5-15 cm, depending on point of junction of cystic and common hepatic ducts
  - Descends posterior and medial to duodenum, lying on dorsal surface of pancreatic head
  - Joins with pancreatic duct to form hepaticopancreatic ampulla of Vater
  - Ampulla opens into duodenum through major duodenal (hepaticopancreatic) papilla
  - Distal common bile duct is thickened into sphincter of Boyden and hepaticopancreatic segment is thickened into a sphincter of Oddi
    - Contraction of these sphincters prevents bile from entering duodenum; forces it to collect in GB
    - Relaxation of sphincters in response to parasympathetic stimulation and cholecystokinin (released by duodenum in response to fatty meal)
- Vessels, nerves, and lymphatics
  - Arteries
    - Hepatic arteries supply intrahepatic ducts
    - Cystic artery supplies proximal common duct
    - RH artery supplies middle part of common duct
    - Gastroduodenal and pancreaticoduodenal arcade supply distal common duct
    - Cystic artery supplies GB (usually from right hepatic artery; variable)
  - Veins
    - From intrahepatic ducts → hepatic veins
    - From common duct → portal vein (in tributaries)
    - From GB directly into liver sinusoids, bypassing portal vein
  - Nerves
    - Sensory: Right phrenic nerve
    - Parasympathetic and sympathetic: Celiac ganglion and plexus; contraction of GB and relaxation of biliary sphincters is caused by parasympathetic stimulation, but more important stimulus is from hormone cholecystokinin
  - Lymphatics
    - Same course and name as arterial branches
    - Collect at celiac lymph nodes and node of omental foramen
    - Nodes draining GB are prominent in porta hepatis and around pancreatic head
- Gallbladder
  - ~ 7-10 cm long, holds up to 50 mL of bile
  - Lies in shallow fossa on visceral surface of liver
  - Vertical plane through GB fossa and middle hepatic vein divides left and right hepatic lobes
  - May touch and indent duodenum
  - Fundus is covered with peritoneum and relatively mobile; body and neck attached to liver and covered by hepatic capsule
  - Fundus: Wide tip of GB, projects below liver edge (usually)
  - Body: Contacts liver, duodenum, and transverse colon
  - Neck: Narrowed, tapered, and tortuous; joins cystic duct
  - Cystic duct: 3-4 cm long, connects GB to common hepatic duct; marked by spiral folds of Heister; helps to regulate bile flow to and from GB
- Normal measurement limits of bile ducts
  - CBD/CHD
    - < 6-7 mm in patients without history of biliary disease in most studies
    - Controversy about dilatation related to previous cholecystectomy and old age
  - Intrahepatic ducts
    - Normal diameter of 1st and higher-order branches < 2 mm or < 40% of diameter of adjacent portal vein
    - 1st (i.e., LH duct and RH duct) and 2nd-order branches are normally visualized
    - Visualization of 3rd and higher-order branches is often abnormal and indicates dilatation

ANATOMY IMAGING ISSUES

Imaging Recommendations

- Patient should fast for at least 4 hours prior to US examination to ensure GB is not contracted after a meal, ideally fasting for 8-12 hours (overnight)
- Complete assessment includes scanning liver, porta hepatis region, and pancreas in sagittal, transverse, and oblique views
- Subcostal and right intercostal transverse views help align bile ducts and GB along imaging plane for optimal visualization
- Usually structures are better assessed and imaged with patient in full suspended inspiration and in left lateral oblique position

- Harmonic imaging provides improved contrast between bile ducts and adjacent tissues, leading to improved visualization of bile ducts, luminal content, and wall
- For imaging of gallstone disease, special maneuvers are recommended
  o Move patient from supine to left lateral decubitus position
    – Demonstrates mobility of gallstones
    – Gravitates small gallstones together to appreciate posterior acoustic shadowing
  o Set focal zone at level of posterior acoustic shadowing
    – Maximizes effect of posterior acoustic shadowing

Imaging Approaches

- Transabdominal ultrasound is ideal initial investigation for suspected biliary tree or GB pathology
  o Cystic nature of bile ducts and GB (especially if these are dilated) provides inherently high-contrast resolution
  o Acoustic window provided by liver and modern state of the art ultrasound technology provides good spatial resolution
  o Common indications of US for biliary and GB disease include
    – Right upper quadrant/epigastric pain
    – Abnormal liver function test or jaundice
    – Suspected gallstone disease
    – Pancreatitis
  o US plays key role in multimodality evaluation of complex biliary problems
- Supplemented by various imaging modalities including MR/MRCP and CT

Imaging Pitfalls

- Common pitfalls in evaluation of GB
  o Posterior shadowing may arise from GB neck, Heister valves of CD, or adjacent gas-filled bowel loops
    – Mimics cholelithiasis
    – Scan after repositioning patient in prone or left lateral decubitus positions
  o Food material within gastric antrum/duodenum
    – Mimics GB filled with gallstones or GB containing milk of calcium
    – During real-time scanning, carefully evaluate peristaltic activity of involved bowel with oral administration of water
- Common pitfalls in US evaluation of biliary tree
  o Redundancy, elongation, or folding of GB neck on itself
    – Mimics dilatation of CHD or proximal CBD
    – Avoided by scanning patient in full suspended inspiration
    – Careful real-time scanning allows separate visualization of CHD/CBD medial to GB neck
  o Presence of gas-filled bowel loops adjacent to distal extrahepatic bile ducts
    – Obscure distal biliary tree and render detection of choledocholithiasis difficult
    – Scan with patient in decubitus positions or after oral intake of water
  o Gas/particulate material in adjacent duodenum and pancreatic calcification
    – Mimic choledocholithiasis within CBD

  o Presence of gas within biliary tree
    – May mimic choledocholithiasis, differentiated by presence of reverberation artifacts
    – Limits US detection of biliary calculus

Key Concepts

- Direct venous drainage of GB into liver bypasses portal venous system, often results in sparing of adjacent liver from generalized steatosis (fatty liver)
- Nodal metastasis from GB carcinoma to peripancreatic nodes may simulate a primary pancreatic tumor
- Sonography: Optimal means of evaluating GB for stones and inflammation (acute cholecystitis); best done in fasting state (distends GB)
- Intrahepatic bile ducts follow branching pattern of portal veins
  o Usually lie immediately anterior to portal vein branch; confluence of hepatic ducts just anterior to bifurcation of right and main portal veins

CLINICAL IMPLICATIONS

Clinical Importance

- In patients with obstructive jaundice, US plays key role
  o Differentiates biliary obstruction from liver parenchymal disease
  o Determines presence, level, and cause of biliary obstruction
- Common variations of biliary arterial and ductal anatomy result in challenges to avoid injury at surgery
  o CD may run in common sheath with bile duct
  o Anomalous right hepatic ducts may be severed at cholecystectomy
- Close apposition of GB to duodenum can result in fistulous connection with chronic cholecystitis and erosion of gallstone into duodenum

Function & Dysfunction

- Obstruction of common bile duct is common
  o Gallstones in distal bile duct
  o Carcinoma arising in pancreatic head or bile duct
  o Result is jaundice due to back up of bile salts into bloodstream

Embryologic Events

- Abnormal embryological development of fetal ductal plate can lead to spectrum of liver and biliary abnormalities including
  o Polycystic liver disease
  o Congenital hepatic fibrosis
  o Biliary hamartomas
  o Caroli disease
  o Choledochal cysts

SELECTED REFERENCES

1. Shackelford RT: Shackelford's Surgery of the alimentary tract. 7th edition. Elsevier/Saunders, 2013
2. Standring S et al: Gray's anatomy: the anatomical basis of clinical practice. Edinburgh: Churchill Livingstone/Elsevier, 2008

GALLBLADDER IN SITU

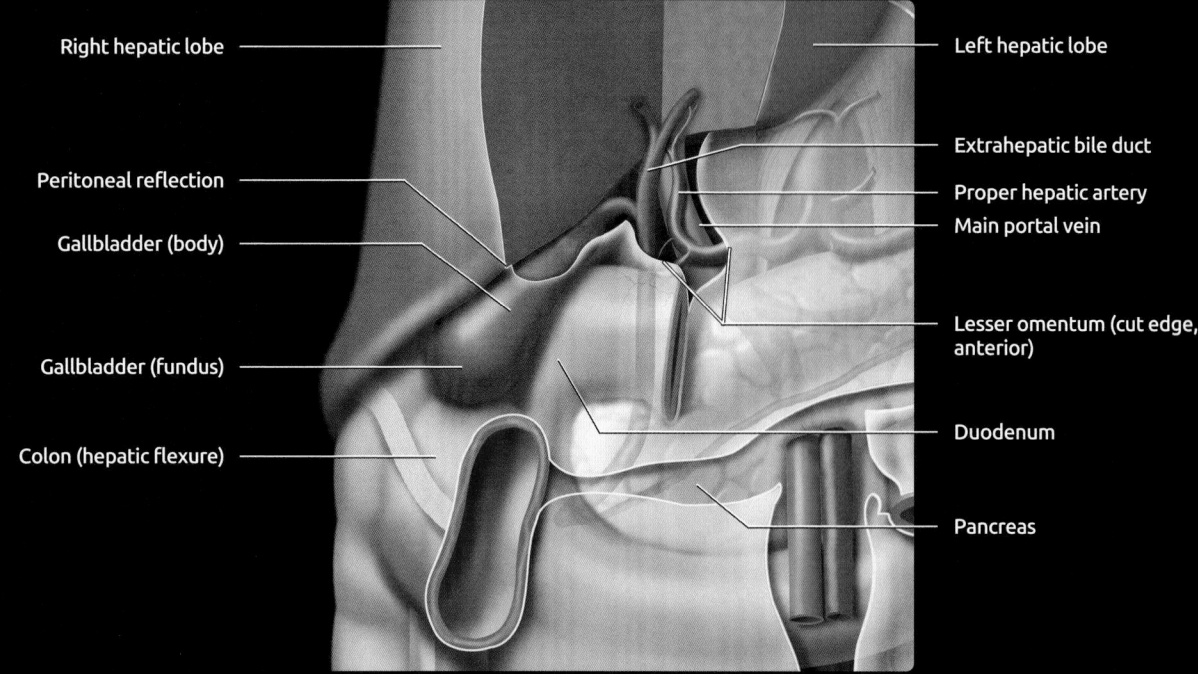

Right hepatic lobe

Left hepatic lobe

Extrahepatic bile duct

Peritoneal reflection

Proper hepatic artery

Gallbladder (body)

Main portal vein

Lesser omentum (cut edge, anterior)

Gallbladder (fundus)

Duodenum

Colon (hepatic flexure)

Pancreas

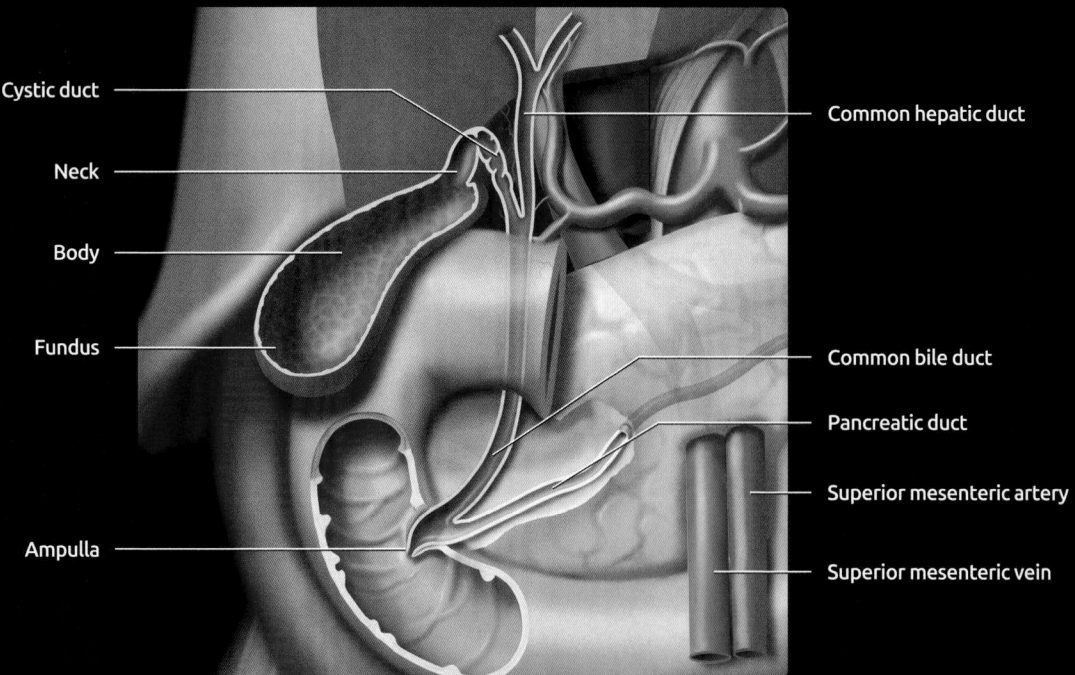

Cystic duct

Common hepatic duct

Neck

Body

Fundus

Common bile duct

Pancreatic duct

Superior mesenteric artery

Ampulla

Superior mesenteric vein

(Top) *Graphic shows that the gallbladder is covered with peritoneum, except where it is attached to the liver. The extrahepatic bile duct, hepatic artery, and portal vein run in the lesser omentum. The fundus of the gallbladder extends beyond the anterior-inferior edge of the liver and can be in contact with the hepatic flexure of the colon. The body (main portion of the gallbladder) is in contact with the duodenum.* (Bottom) *The neck of the gallbladder narrows before entering the cystic duct, which is distinguished by its tortuous course and irregular lumen. The duct lumen is irregular due to redundant folds of mucosa, called the spiral folds of Heister, that are believed to regulate the rate of filling and emptying of the gallbladder. The cystic duct joins the hepatic duct to form the common bile duct, which passes behind the duodenum and through the pancreas to enter the duodenum.*

ANATOMIC VARIATIONS OF BILIARY TREE

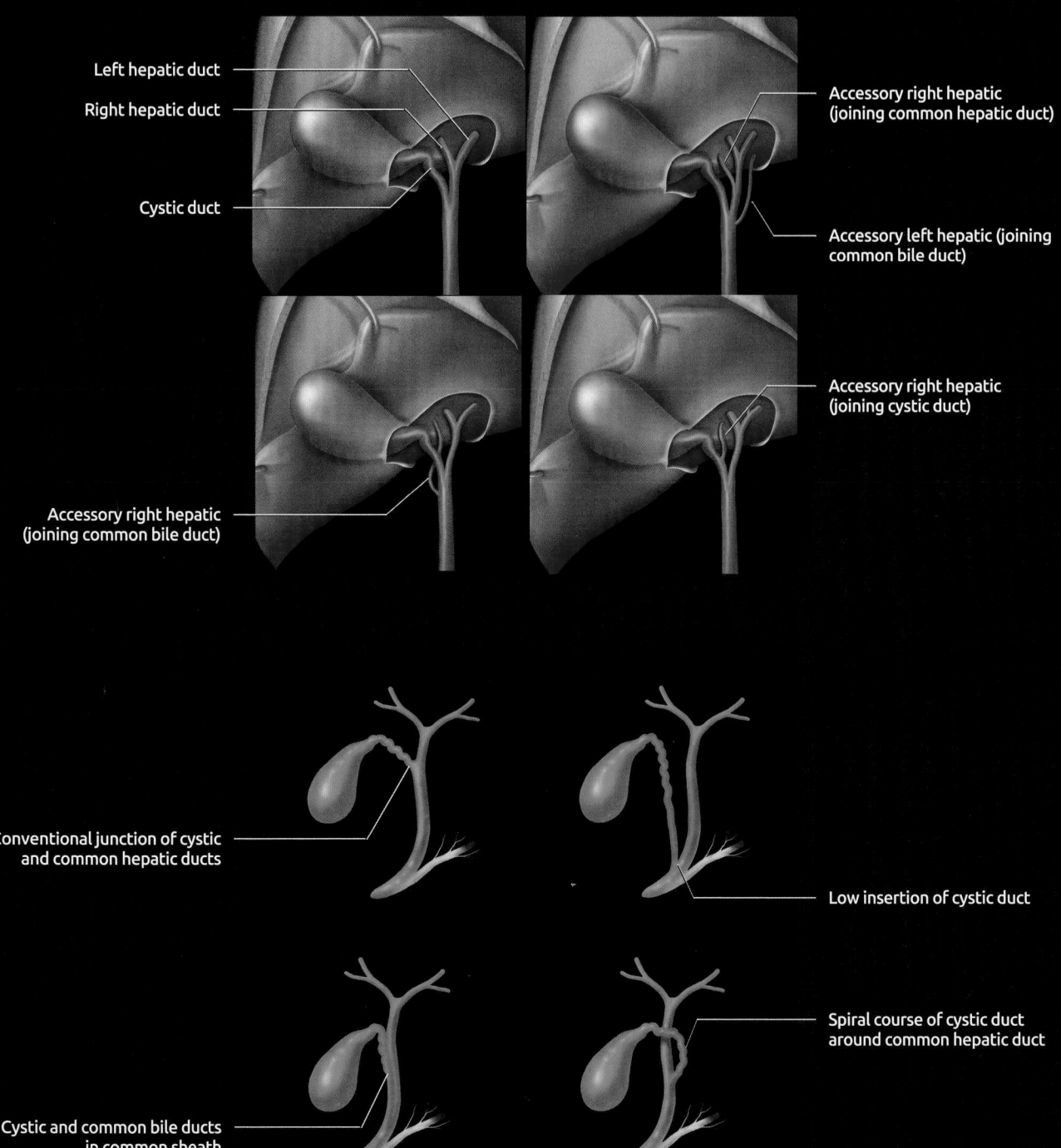

Left hepatic duct

Right hepatic duct

Cystic duct

Accessory right hepatic (joining common hepatic duct)

Accessory left hepatic (joining common bile duct)

Accessory right hepatic (joining cystic duct)

Accessory right hepatic (joining common bile duct)

Conventional junction of cystic and common hepatic ducts

Low insertion of cystic duct

Cystic and common bile ducts in common sheath

Spiral course of cystic duct around common hepatic duct

(Top) *Graphic shows the conventional arrangement of the extrahepatic bile ducts, but variations are common (20% of population) and may lead to inadvertent ligation or injury at surgery (such as during cholecystectomy), where the cystic duct is clamped and transected. Most accessory ducts are on the right side and usually enter the common hepatic duct, but they may enter the cystic or common bile duct. Accessory left ducts enter the common bile duct. While referred to as "accessory," these ducts are the sole drainage of bile from at least 1 hepatic segment. Ligation or laceration can lead to significant hepatic injury or bile peritonitis.* **(Bottom)** *The course and insertion of the cystic duct are highly variable, leading to difficulty in isolation and ligation at cholecystectomy. The cystic duct may be mistaken for the common hepatic or common bile duct.*

RIGHT HEPATIC LOBE

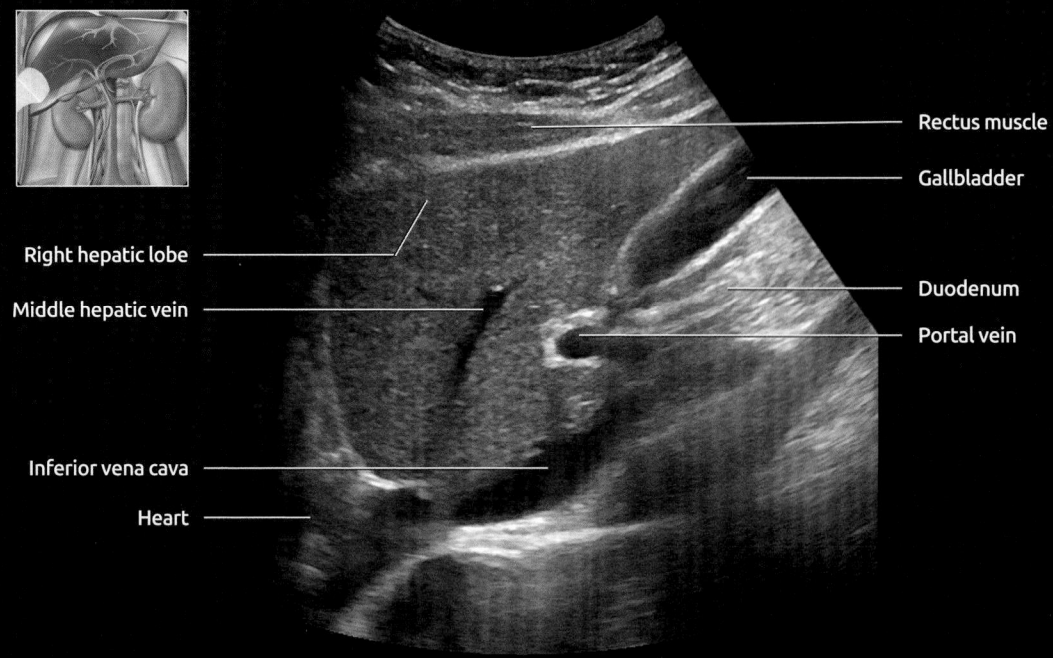

Rectus muscle

Gallbladder

Right hepatic lobe

Middle hepatic vein

Duodenum

Portal vein

Inferior vena cava

Heart

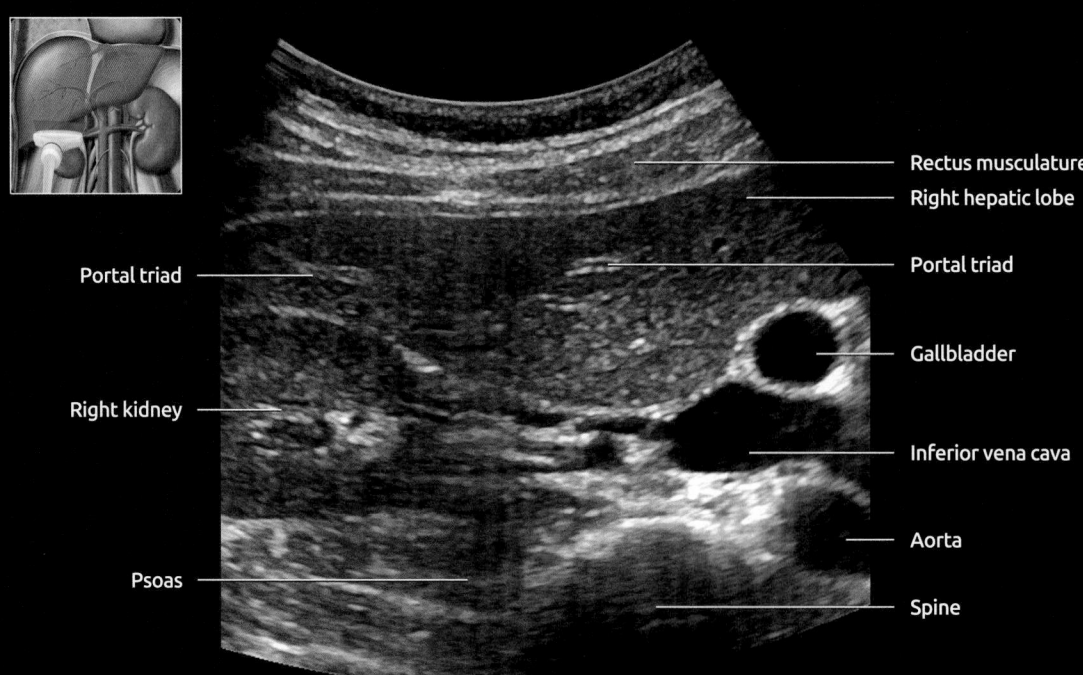

Rectus musculature

Right hepatic lobe

Portal triad

Portal triad

Gallbladder

Right kidney

Inferior vena cava

Aorta

Psoas

Spine

(Top) *Subcostal, longitudinal ultrasound shows the right hepatic lobe and gallbladder with patient in the left lateral decubitus position. Ideally, a patient must fast for at least 4 hours to allow for adequate gallbladder distension.* **(Bottom)** *Subcostal, transverse ultrasound of the right hepatic lobe demonstrates its anatomical relationships with major vessels and the right kidney. The intrahepatic bile ducts are localized within the portal triads, which are visible by the prominent echogenic walls of the portal veins in these triads. The portal triad contains the portal vein, bile duct, and hepatic artery. Normally, the intrahepatic bile ducts and hepatic arteries are not readily visible unless they are dilated.*

LEFT HEPATIC LOBE

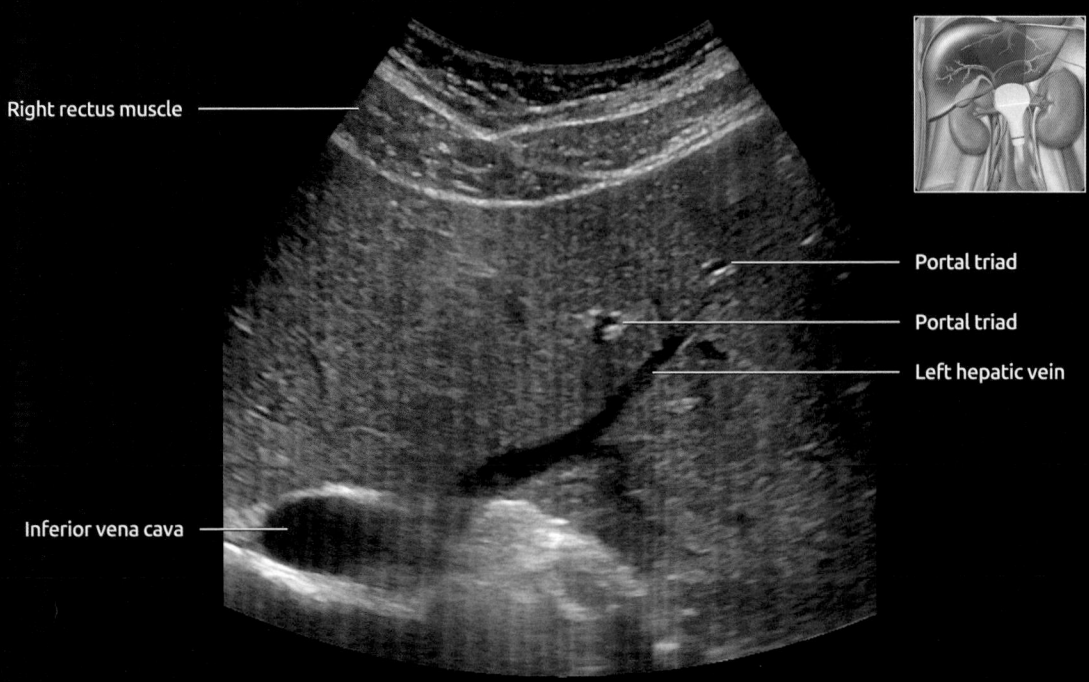

Right rectus muscle

Portal triad

Portal triad

Left hepatic vein

Inferior vena cava

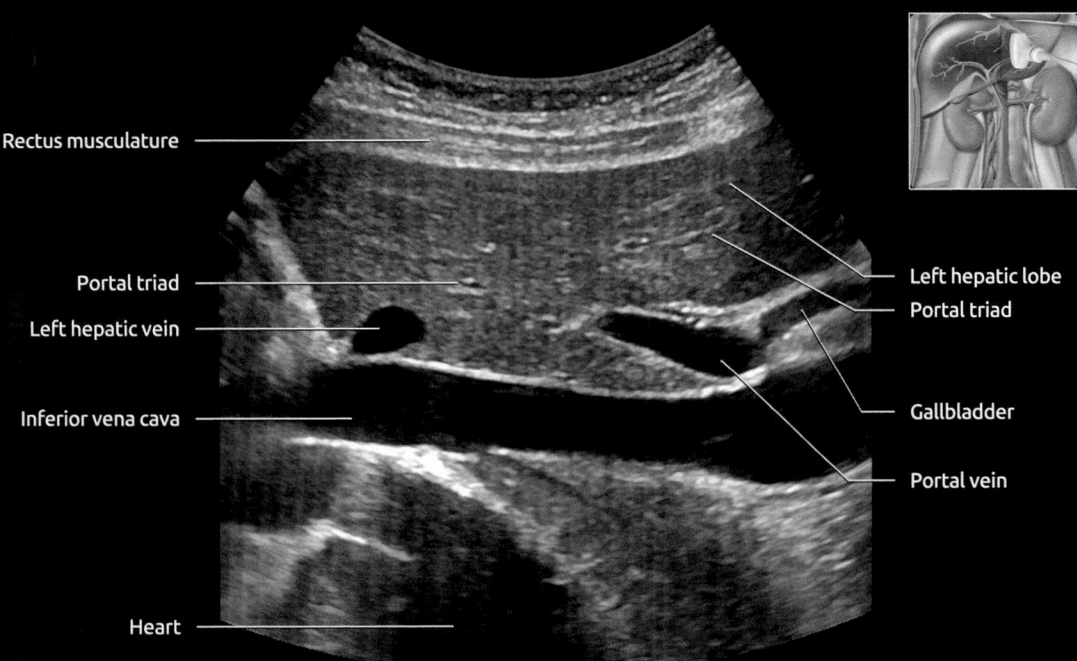

Rectus musculature

Left hepatic lobe

Portal triad

Portal triad

Left hepatic vein

Inferior vena cava

Gallbladder

Portal vein

Heart

(Top) *Subxiphoid, transverse grayscale ultrasound of the left hepatic lobe shows the left hepatic vein and several portal triads. The portal triads are identified by the prominent echogenic walls of the portal veins. The portal triad contains a portal vein, a bile duct, and a hepatic artery. The hepatic artery and bile duct are not readily visible unless they are dilated.* **(Bottom)** *Longitudinal ultrasound of the left hepatic lobe near the confluence of the left hepatic vein with the inferior vena cava is shown. Portal triads are recognizable by the prominent walls of the portal veins.*

GALLBLADDER

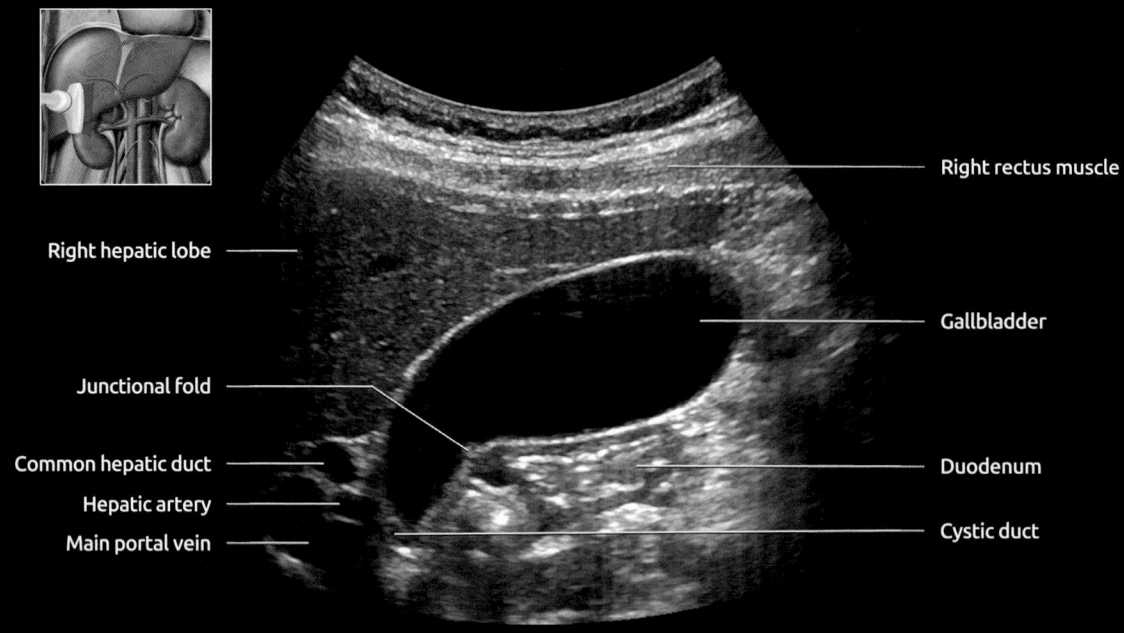

Right rectus muscle

Right hepatic lobe

Gallbladder

Junctional fold

Common hepatic duct

Duodenum

Hepatic artery

Main portal vein

Cystic duct

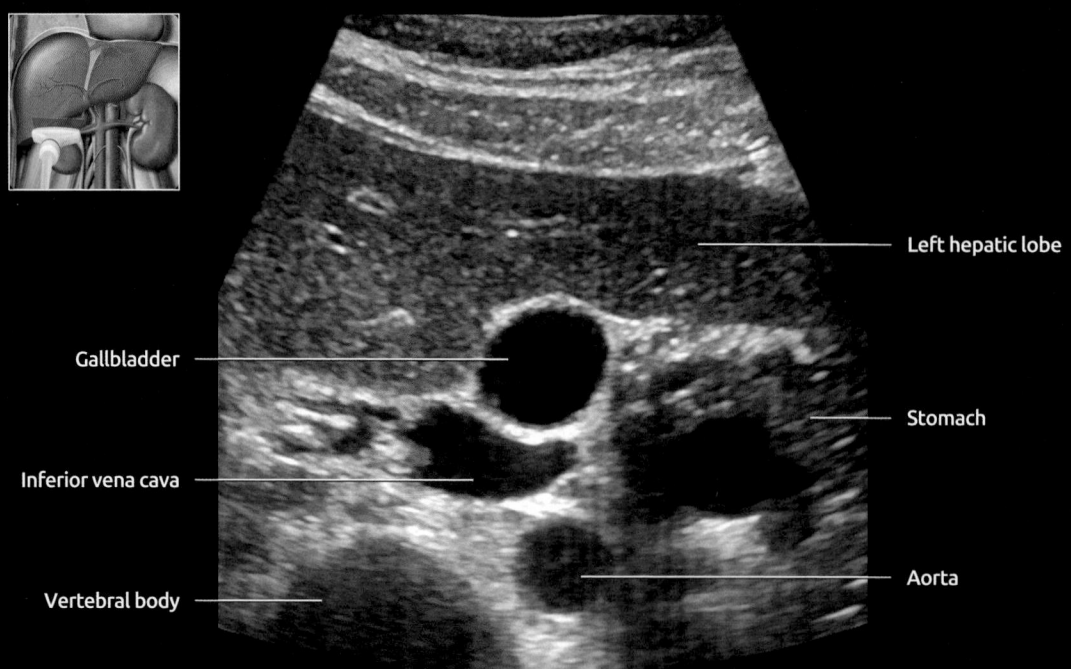

Left hepatic lobe

Gallbladder

Stomach

Inferior vena cava

Vertebral body

Aorta

(Top) *Subcostal, longitudinal grayscale ultrasound shows the gallbladder with patient in the left lateral decubitus position. The gallbladder is distended with bile, causing increased transmission of echoes. A patient must fast for at least 4 hours to allow for adequate gallbladder distension.* (Bottom) *Transverse ultrasound of a distended gallbladder in left lateral decubitus position is shown. The gallbladder is best evaluated if the patient has fasted at least 4 hours, ideally 8-12 hours.*

COMMON BILE DUCT

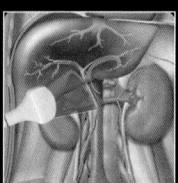

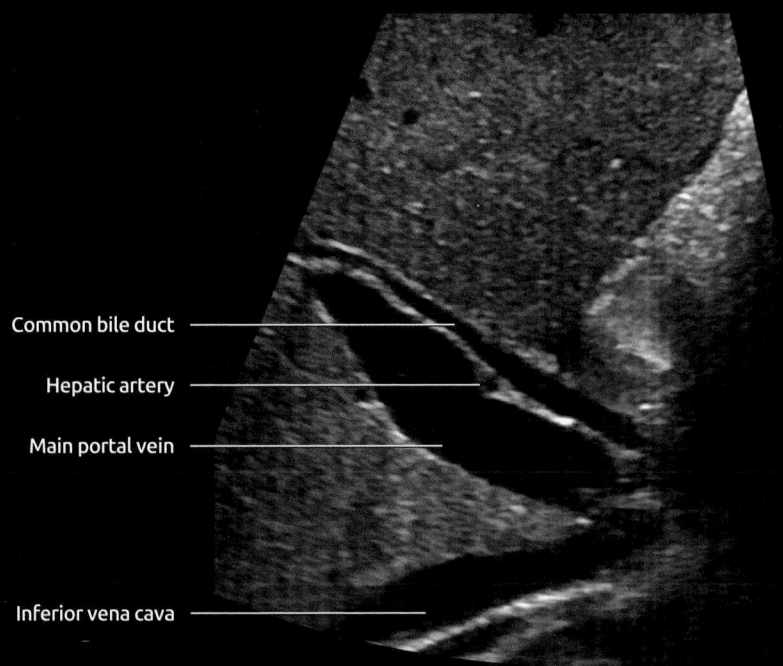

Common bile duct

Hepatic artery

Main portal vein

Inferior vena cava

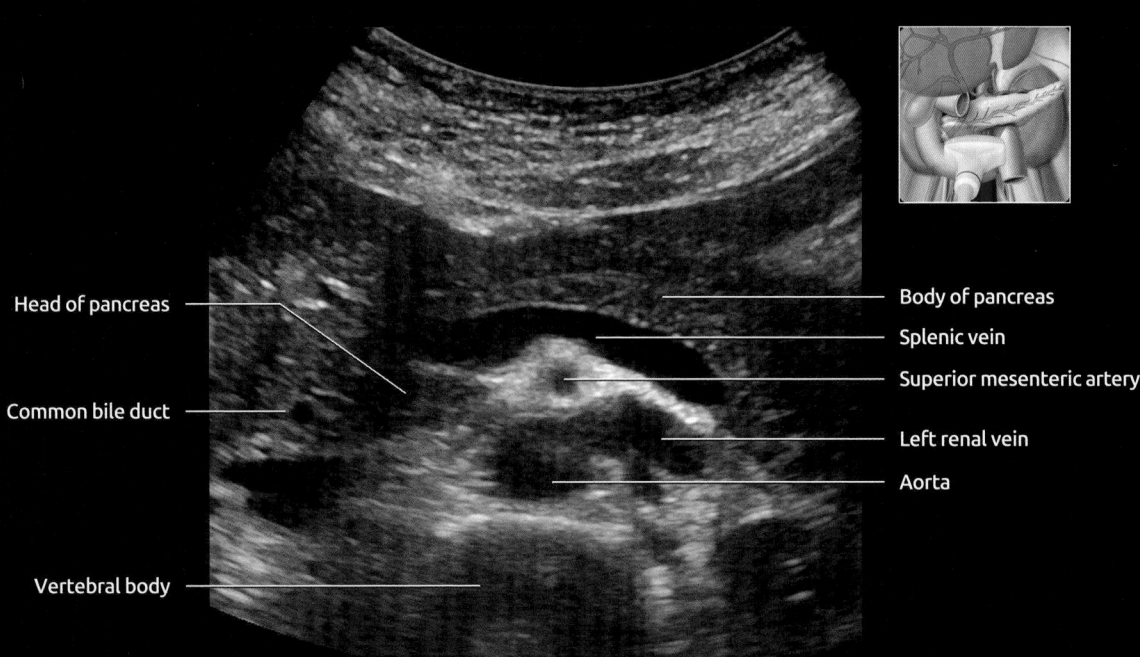

Head of pancreas

Common bile duct

Vertebral body

Body of pancreas

Splenic vein

Superior mesenteric artery

Left renal vein

Aorta

(Top) *Subcostal, longitudinal oblique ultrasound shows the common bile duct and the portal vein in the hepatoduodenal ligament. The common bile duct is normally identified anterior to the portal vein. The distal common bile duct pierces the pancreatic head. Also demonstrated is the hepatic artery, which normally traverses between the portal vein and common bile duct.* (Bottom) *Transverse ultrasound at the level of the pancreas demonstrates the distal common bile duct as it pierces the pancreatic head. Overlying bowel gas may obscure this area; positioning the patient upright or in a left lateral decubitus position may help visualization.*

RIGHT INTRAHEPATIC DUCTS

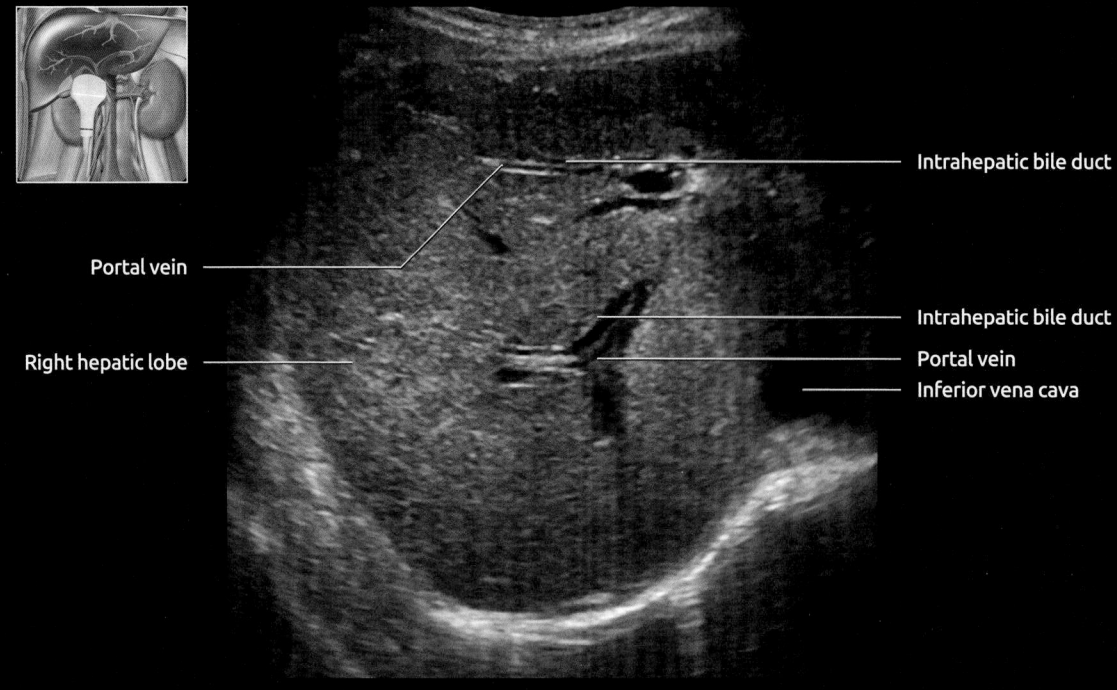

Intrahepatic bile duct

Portal vein

Intrahepatic bile duct

Right hepatic lobe

Portal vein

Inferior vena cava

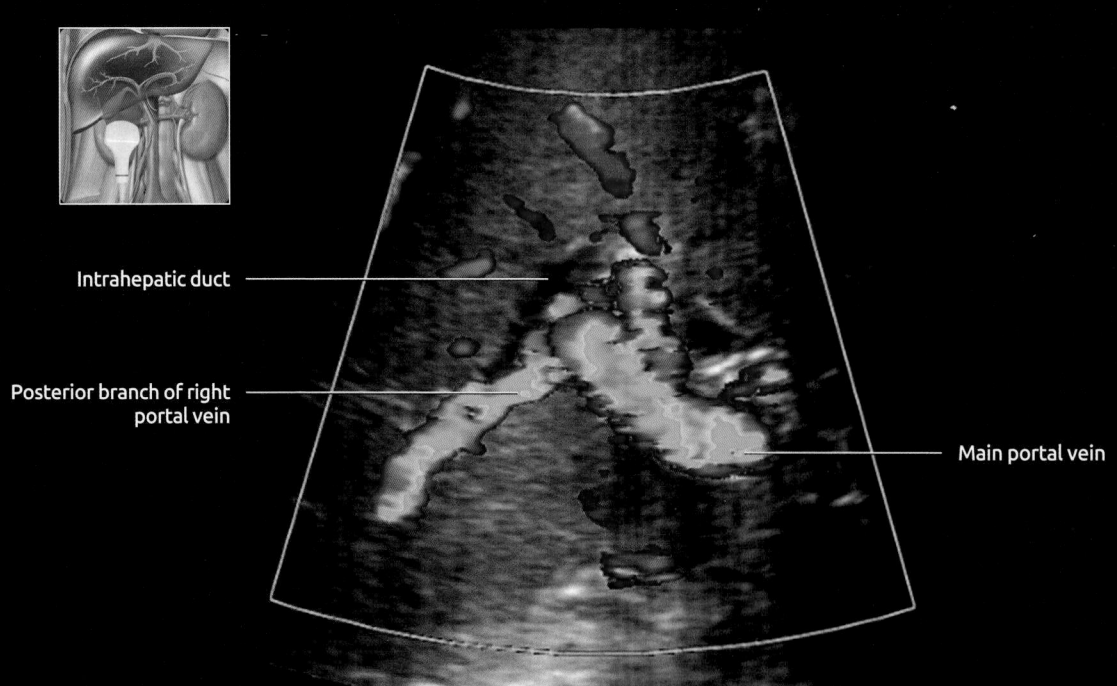

Intrahepatic duct

Posterior branch of right portal vein

Main portal vein

(Top) Transverse ultrasound through the right hepatic lobe in a patient with biliary obstruction demonstrates dilated right intrahepatic bile ducts. Normally, intrahepatic ducts are not readily visualized unless they are dilated. Parallel linear hypoechoic structures are not normally seen in the liver, and this may represent a dilated bile duct or dilated hepatic artery adjacent to the normally visualized portal venous structure in the portal triad. (Bottom) Transverse color Doppler ultrasound through the right hepatic lobe in a patient with biliary obstruction demonstrates dilated right intrahepatic bile ducts. Normally, intrahepatic ducts are not readily visualized unless they are dilated. Color Doppler ultrasound helps to determine whether the dilated structure is a dilated hepatic artery or dilated bile duct.

LEFT INTRAHEPATIC DUCTS

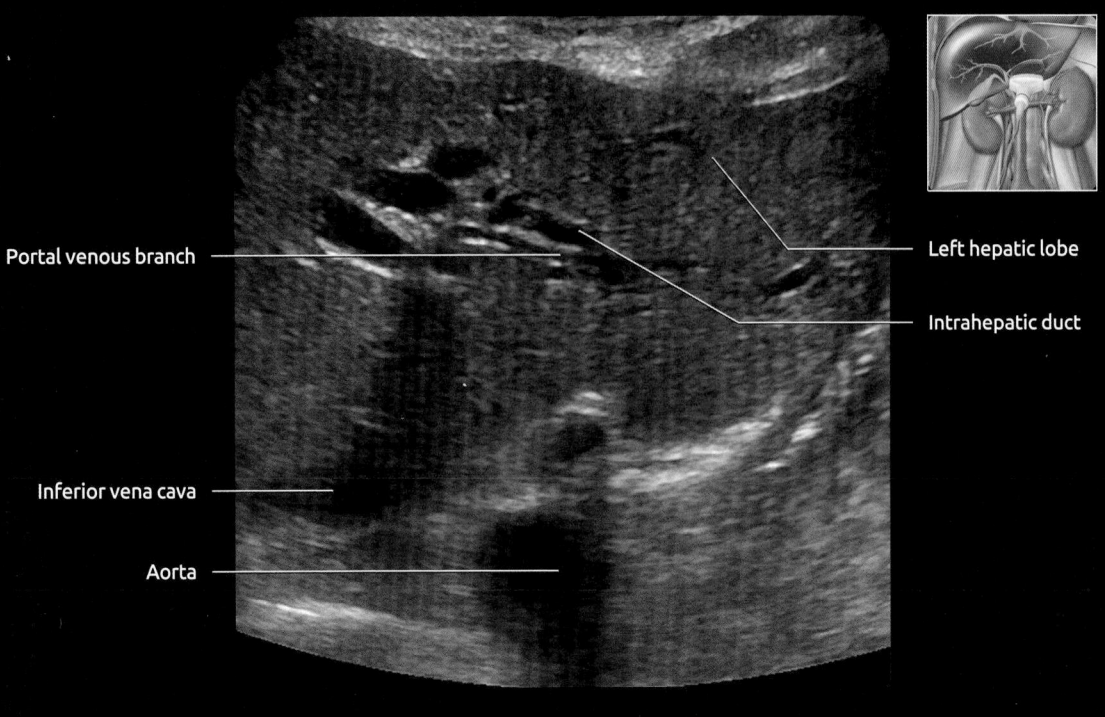

Portal venous branch — — Left hepatic lobe

— Intrahepatic duct

Inferior vena cava

Aorta

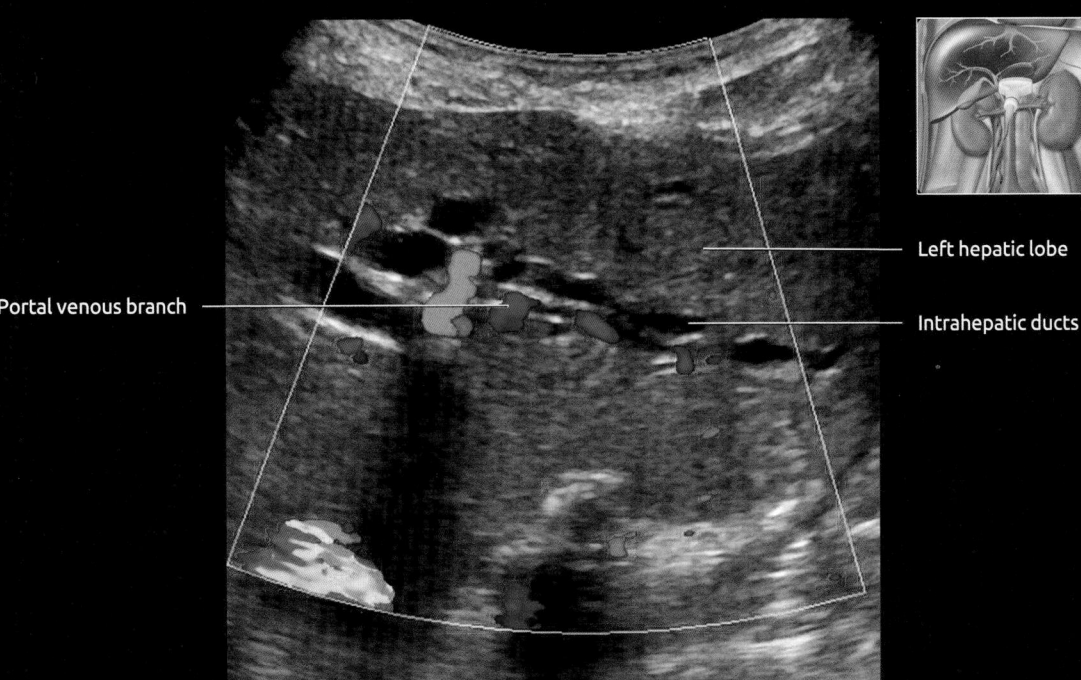

Portal venous branch — — Left hepatic lobe

— Intrahepatic ducts

(Top) *Transverse ultrasound through the left hepatic lobe in a patient with biliary obstruction demonstrates dilated left intrahepatic bile ducts. Normally, intrahepatic ducts are not readily visualized unless they are dilated.* **(Bottom)** *Transverse color Doppler ultrasound through the left hepatic lobe in a patient with biliary obstruction demonstrates dilated left intrahepatic bile ducts. Normally, intrahepatic ducts are not readily visualized unless they are dilated. Color Doppler ultrasound is helpful to determine whether the dilated structure is vascular or biliary, as dilated hepatic arteries can be mistaken for dilated bile ducts. The absence of flow allows one to determine that these are biliary in origin.*

GROSS ANATOMY

Overview

- Spleen is largest lymphatic organ
  - Normal size is variable; no universal consensus
    - Generally, normal adult spleen considered 12 cm length x 4 cm thickness x 7 cm width
    - **Length** = longest diameter in longitudinal plane; **thickness** = transverse measurement from hilum; **width** = longest transverse diameter
    - Splenic index (product of length, thickness, and width): Normally 120-480 cm³
    - Size correlates with height and can exceed these limits in tall, healthy people
  - Functions
    - Manufactures lymphocytes, filters blood (removes damaged red blood cells and platelets)
    - Acts as blood reservoir: Can expand or contract in response to changes in blood volume
- Histology
  - Soft organ with fibroelastic capsule entirely surrounded by peritoneum, except at splenic hilum
  - Trabeculae: Extensions of capsule into parenchyma; carry arterial and venous branches
  - Pulp: Substance of spleen; white pulp = lymphoid nodules; red pulp = sinusoidal spaces containing blood
  - Splenic cords (plates of cells) lie between sinusoids; red pulp veins drain sinusoids
- Relations and vessels
  - Spleen contacts posterior surface of stomach and is connected via gastrosplenic ligament (GSL)
    - GSL is left anterior margin of lesser sac; carries short gastric and left gastroepiploic arteries and venous branches to spleen
  - Contacts pancreatic tail and surface of left kidney and is connected by the splenorenal ligament (SRL)
    - SRL is left posterior margin of lesser sac (omental bursa); carries splenic arterial and venous branches to spleen
  - Splenic vein runs in groove along dorsal surface of pancreatic body and tail
    - Receives inferior mesenteric vein (IMV)
    - Combined splenic vein and IMV join superior mesenteric vein to form portal vein
  - Splenic artery arises from celiac axis in 90%; 8% directly from aorta; often very tortuous

IMAGING ANATOMY

Internal Contents

- Echo pattern
  - Homogenous, similar to liver
  - Echogenicity: Pancreas > spleen > liver > kidney
- Architecture
  - Radiating pattern of segmental arteries and veins
  - Splenic vein
    - Normal diameter 5-10 mm; peak systolic velocity (PSV): 9-18 cm/s
    - Splenic vein at midline is useful landmark for locating pancreas; pancreas lies anterior to splenic vein

- Diameter increases between 50-100% from quiet respiration to deep inspiration; increase of < 20% suggests portal hypertension
    - Spectral Doppler waveform typically shows band-like flow profile with minimal respiratory fluctuations
  - Splenic artery
    - Low-resistance waveform; tortuosity of vessel results in turbulence and spectral broadening
    - Normal diameter: 4-8 mm; PSV: 25-45 cm/sec

ANATOMY IMAGING ISSUES

Imaging Recommendations

- Patient positioned supine or right decubitus position (left side up) with left arm raised
- Place transducer parallel to ribs in 10th or 11th intercostal space at left midaxillary line, searching for best window
  - Due to rib angle this results in oblique view, which by convention is called longitudinal or transverse (depending on transducer orientation)
  - Transverse US view of spleen does not correlate directly to axial CT view
- End expiration may be helpful; lung base may obscure spleen in full inspiration
- Spleen poorly accessed from posterior (obscured by left lung base), anterior, or subcostal approach (obscured by stomach and colon)
- Assess splenic vein at hilum and midline for patency and flow direction

Key Concepts

- Spleen has highly variable size and shape
  - Easily indented and displaced by masses and even loculated fluid collections

EMBRYOLOGY

Practical Implications

- **Accessory spleen** (splenunculus, splenule): Found in 10-30% of population
  - Usually small, near splenic hilum
  - Can enlarge and simulate mass, especially after splenectomy
  - Ectopic intrapancreatic splenule can mimic pancreatic tail mass; should not be more than 3 cm from tail tip
- **Wandering spleen:** Spleen may be on long mesentery; found in any abdominopelvic location; risk of torsion
- **Asplenia and polysplenia** (heterotaxy syndromes)
  - Situs ambiguus; rare congenital conditions of altered left/right orientation of organs; associated with cardiovascular anomalies, intestinal malrotation, etc.
- **Splenosis:** Peritoneal implantation of splenic tissue after traumatic splenic injury, can mimic polysplenia

SELECTED REFERENCES

1. Benter T et al: Sonography of the spleen. J Ultrasound Med. 30(9):1281-93, 2011
2. Kim SH et al: Intrapancreatic accessory spleen: findings on MR Imaging, CT, US and scintigraphy, pathologic analysis. Korean J Radiol. 9(2):162-74, 2008
3. Gillen MA : The spleen. In McGahan JP, Goldberg BB (eds) Diagnostic Ultrasound, 2nd ed, New York, NY: Informa Healthcare:2008: 801-822
4. Applegate KE et al: Situs revisited: Imaging of the heterotaxy syndrome. RadioGraphics 19:837-852, 1999

SPLEEN ANATOMY AND HISTOLOGY

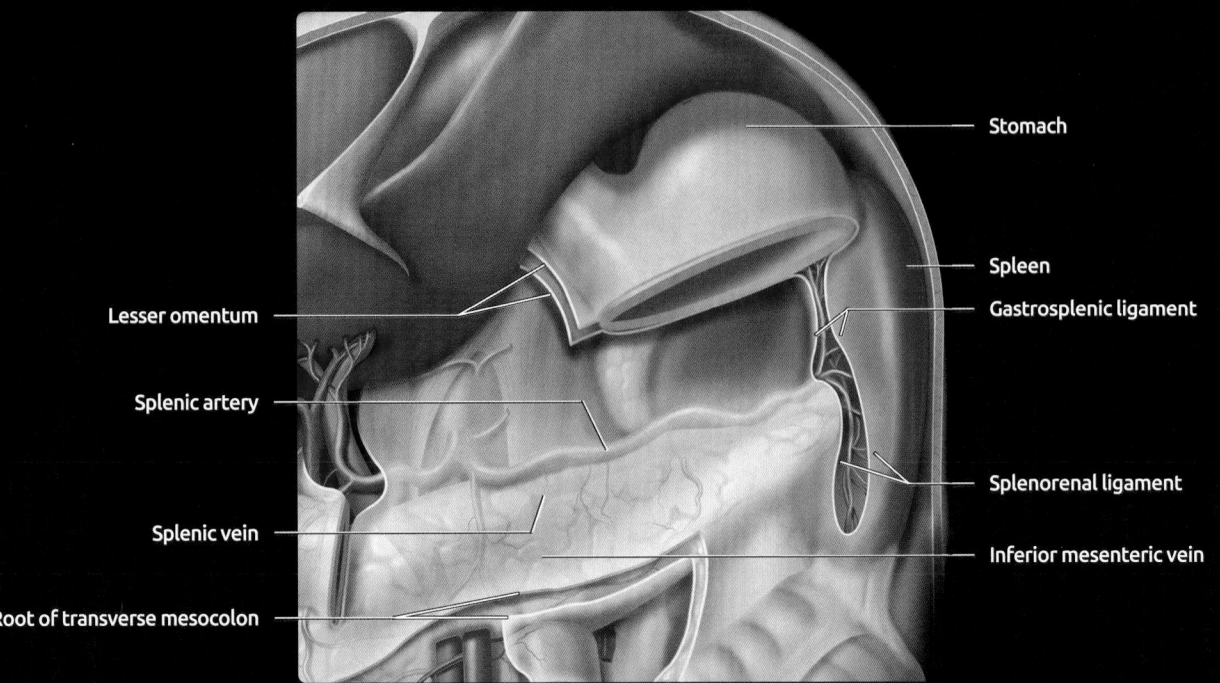

Stomach

Spleen

Gastrosplenic ligament

Lesser omentum

Splenic artery

Splenorenal ligament

Splenic vein

Inferior mesenteric vein

Root of transverse mesocolon

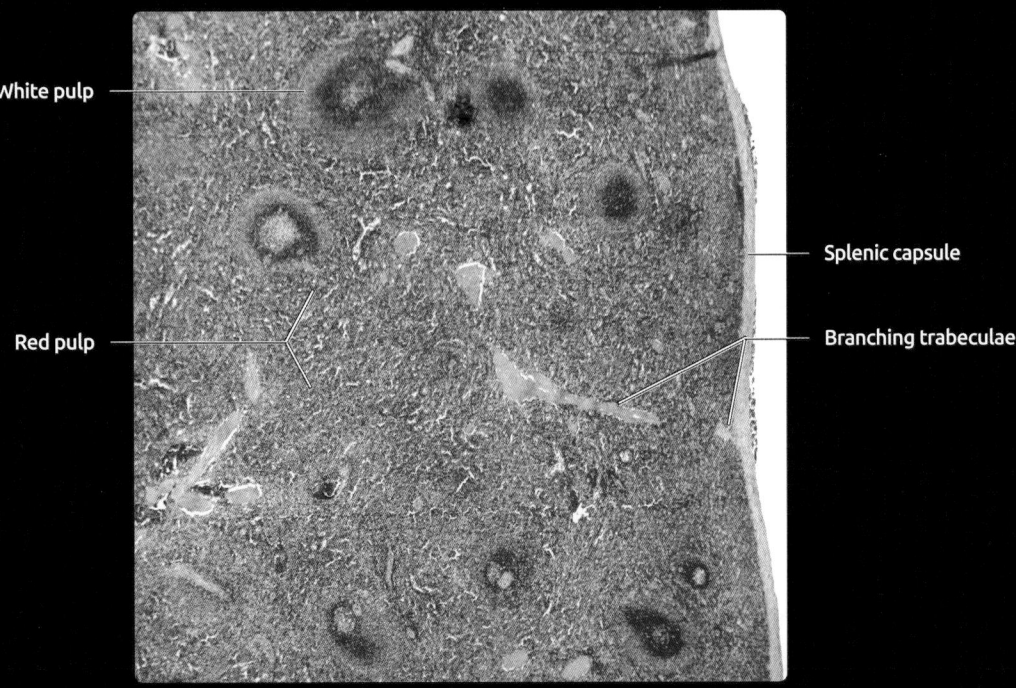

White pulp

Splenic capsule

Red pulp

Branching trabeculae

(Top) *Graphic shows the liver is retracted upward and the stomach transected to reveal the pancreas and spleen. The splenic artery and vein course along the body of the pancreas, and the tail of the pancreas lies within the splenorenal ligament. The gastrosplenic ligament carries the short gastric and left gastroepiploic vessels to the stomach and spleen. The splenic vein receives the inferior mesenteric vein and joins the superior mesenteric vein behind the neck of the pancreas to form the portal vein. (Bottom) Histologic section of a normal spleen viewed at low power shows white pulp and red pulp. A thin splenic capsule with slivers of branching trabeculae is also noted.*

SPLEEN ANATOMY

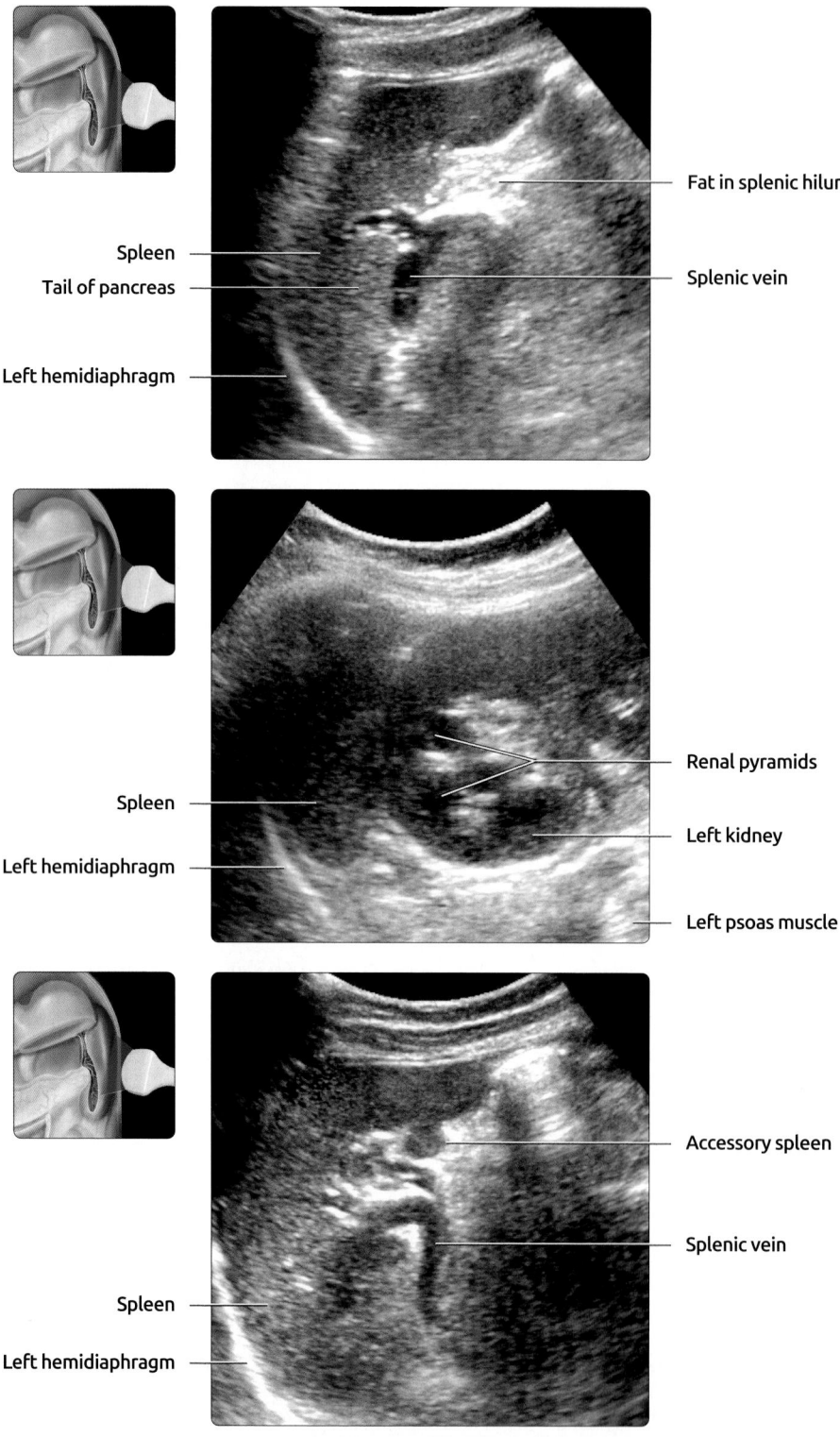

Spleen	Fat in splenic hilum
Tail of pancreas	Splenic vein
Left hemidiaphragm	
Spleen	Renal pyramids
Left hemidiaphragm	Left kidney
	Left psoas muscle
	Accessory spleen
	Splenic vein
Spleen	
Left hemidiaphragm	

(Top) *Longitudinal oblique grayscale ultrasound shows the spleen from a posterolateral intercostal approach. The patient is positioned in the right lateral decubitus position with examination during full expiration. Note that the tail of the pancreas can be imaged using the spleen as an acoustic window.* **(Middle)** *Longitudinal oblique ultrasound shows the spleen and its relationship to the upper pole of the left kidney with the transducer placed parallel to the intercostal space.* **(Bottom)** *Longitudinal oblique grayscale ultrasound of a splenule (accessory spleen) is shown. Splenules are rounded, well-defined masses commonly found (10-30% of population) in or near the splenic hilum. They are homogeneous and isoechoic to the splenic parenchyma.*

CT CORRELATION

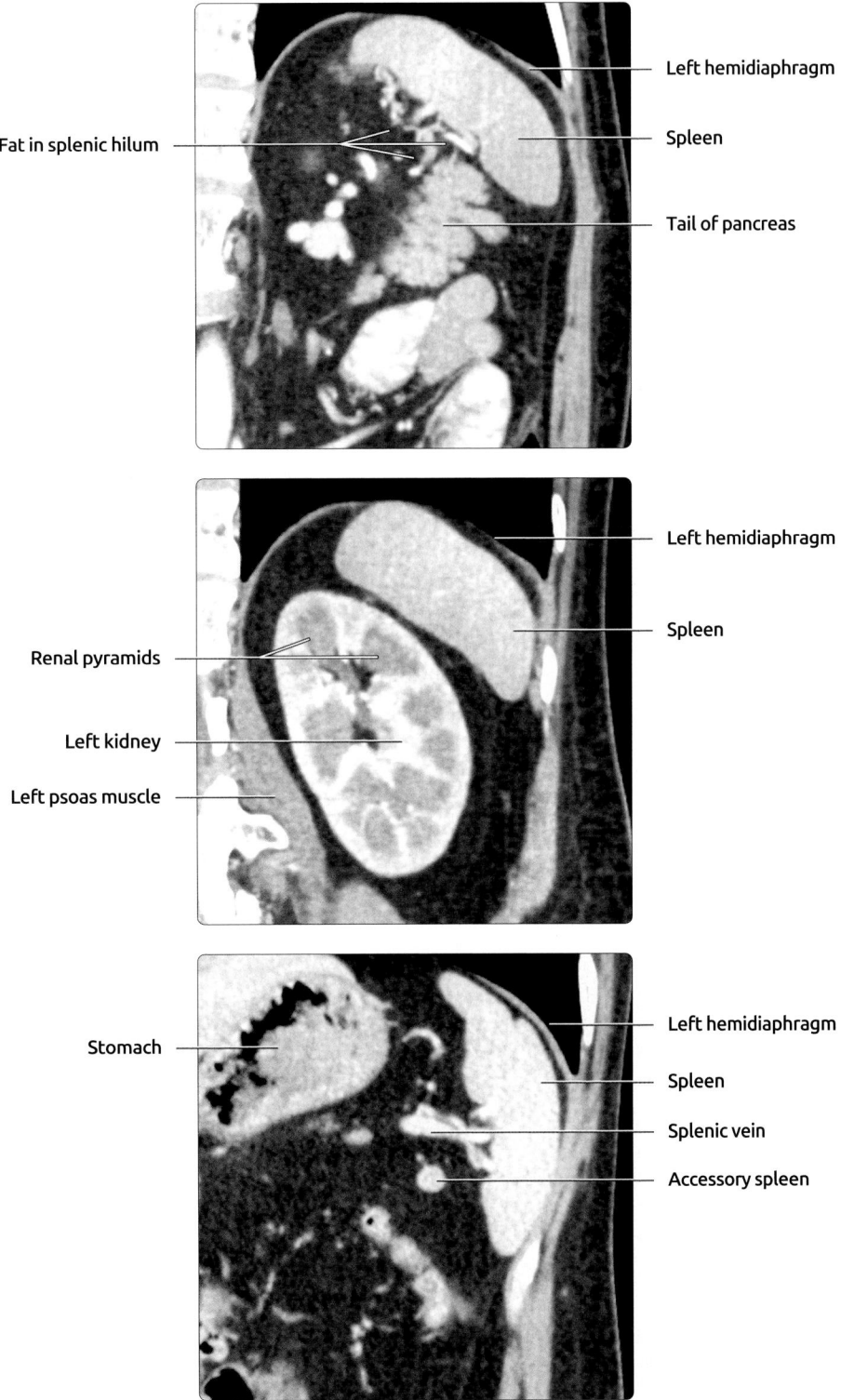

Left hemidiaphragm

Fat in splenic hilum

Spleen

Tail of pancreas

Left hemidiaphragm

Renal pyramids

Spleen

Left kidney

Left psoas muscle

Stomach

Left hemidiaphragm

Spleen

Splenic vein

Accessory spleen

(Top) *Oblique correlative multiplanar reconstruction CT of the spleen is shown. Note the fat around the splenic hilum and the extension of the pancreatic tail towards the splenic hilum. This allows the pancreatic tail to be visualized by ultrasound using the spleen as an acoustic window.* **(Middle)** *Oblique correlative multiplanar reconstruction CT shows the relationship between the spleen and the kidney.* **(Bottom)** *Oblique correlative multiplanar reconstruction CT of the accessory spleen in the splenic hilum is shown. The accessory spleen simulates the appearance of a normal spleen on imaging; this identical appearance prevents it from being mistaken for pathology.*

SPLENIC VESSELS

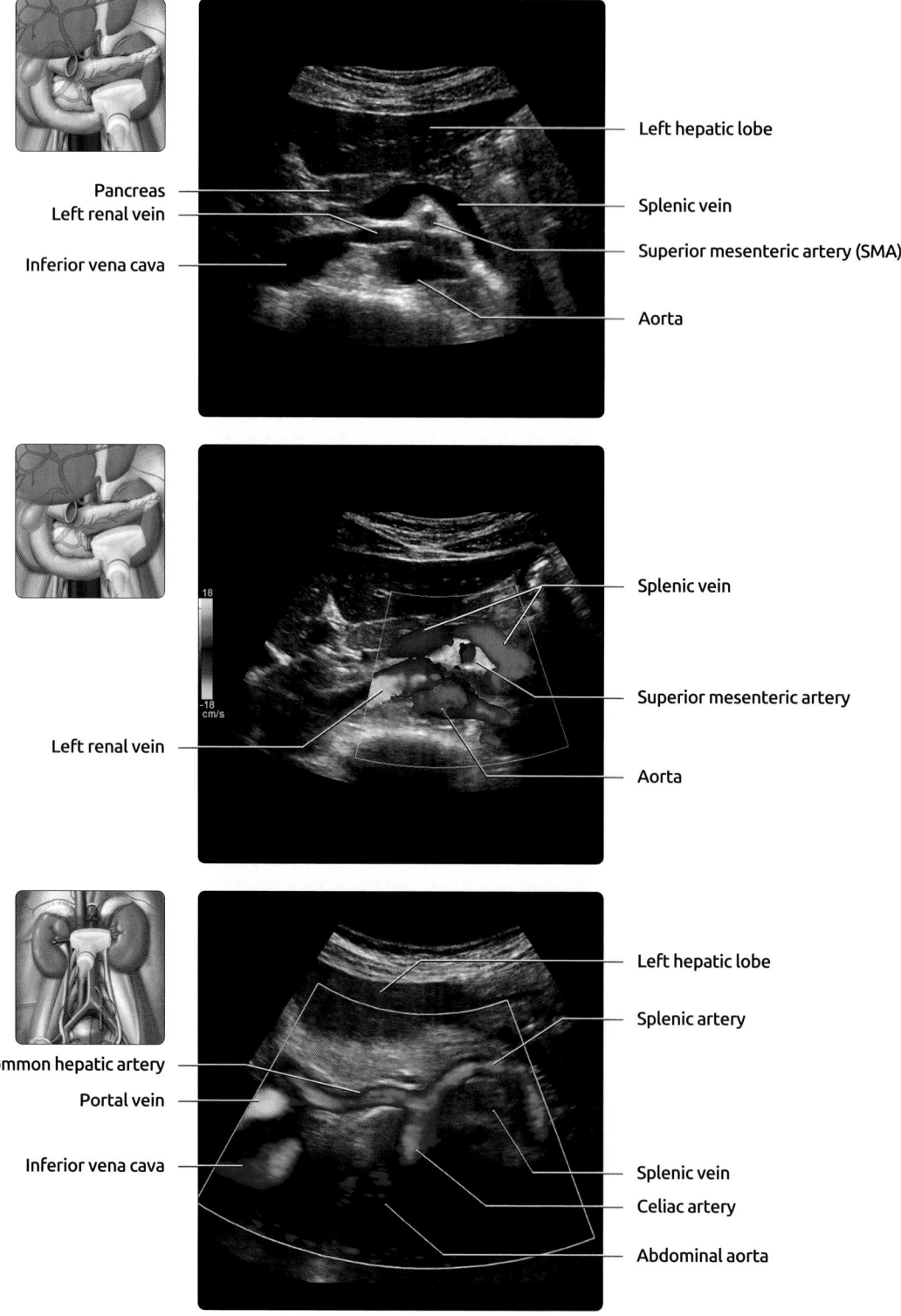

Pancreas
Left renal vein
Inferior vena cava

Left hepatic lobe
Splenic vein
Superior mesenteric artery (SMA)
Aorta

Left renal vein
18
-18 cm/s

Splenic vein
Superior mesenteric artery
Aorta

Common hepatic artery
Portal vein
Inferior vena cava

Left hepatic lobe
Splenic artery
Splenic vein
Celiac artery
Abdominal aorta

(Top) *Midline transverse anterior grayscale ultrasound of the splenic vein is shown. The splenic vein is located deep to the pancreatic body. Note the left renal vein course between the SMA and aorta.* **(Middle)** *Color Doppler of the same area shows the normal direction of flow in the splenic vein, towards the liver (hepatopetal). Note the change in color from red to blue, which is due to the position of the transducer, aligned at the midpoint of the vein. Using the information provided by the color bar, the red portion of the splenic vein is blood flowing towards the transducer (away from the spleen), and the blue is blood flowing away from the transducer (towards the liver).* **(Bottom)** *Power Doppler of the upper abdomen at midline shows the origin of the splenic artery from the celiac axis. The celiac artery branches into the splenic artery, common hepatic artery, and left gastric artery (not shown). After its takeoff, the splenic artery typically has a tortuous course. The branching of the celiac axis, as shown in this image, has been referred to as the "seagull" sign.*

SPLENIC VESSELS

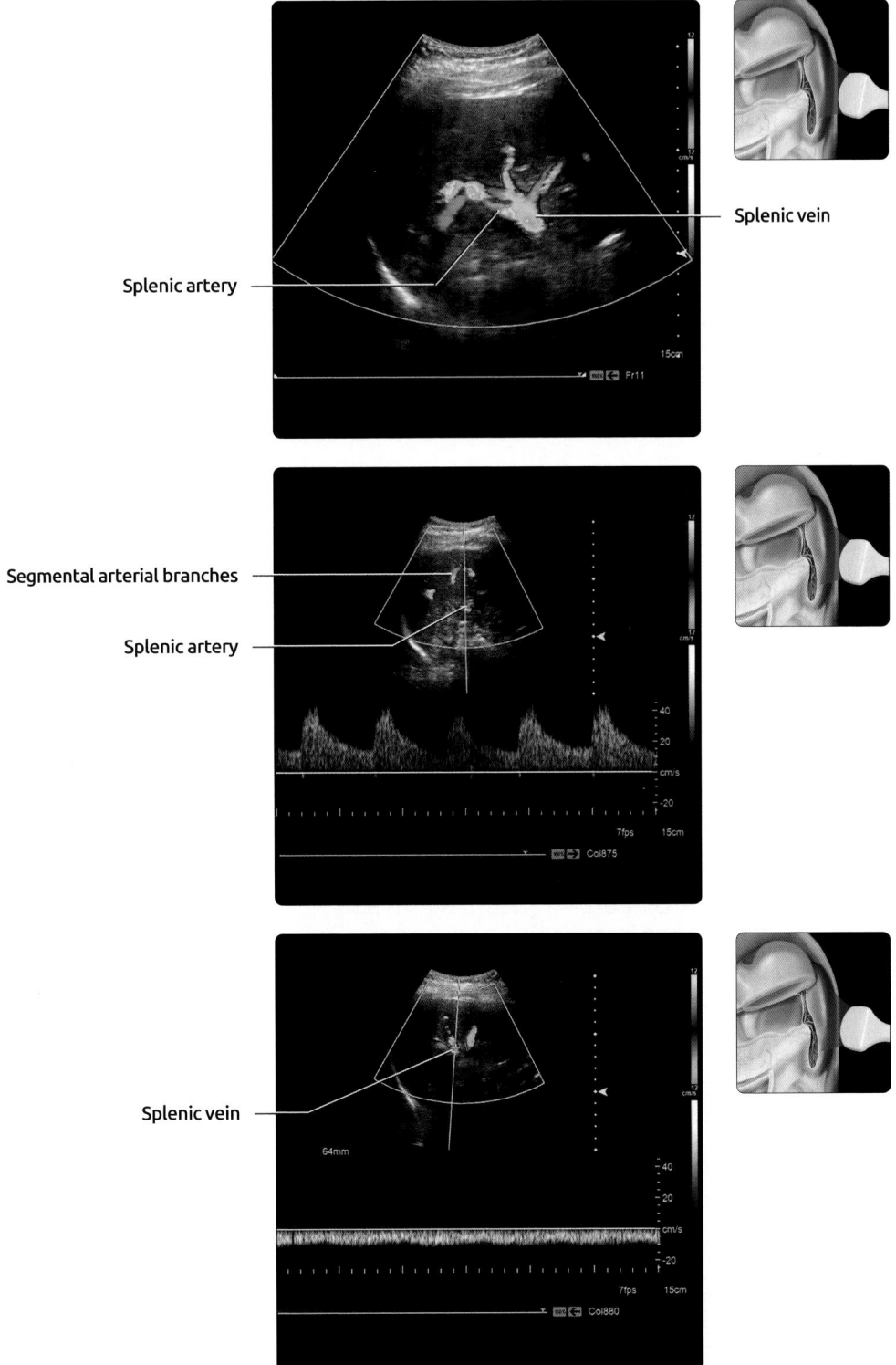

Splenic artery

Splenic vein

Segmental arterial branches

Splenic artery

Splenic vein

(Top) *Longitudinal oblique color Doppler ultrasound demonstrates the branching of the splenic arteries and veins in the splenic hilum.* **(Middle)** *Spectral Doppler waveform of the distal splenic artery at the splenic hilum is shown. Because of a tortuous course, flow in this vessel is typically turbulent. The splenic artery has a low-resistance waveform (ample flow throughout diastole). Normal peak systolic velocity for the splenic artery is 25-45 cm/sec.* **(Bottom)** *Spectral Doppler waveform ultrasound of the splenic vein at the hilum shows a typical band-like flow profile with minimal respiratory fluctuations; flow is directed away from the transducer (away from the spleen). Normal peak systolic velocity of the splenic vein is 9-18 cm/sec.*

ANATOMICAL VARIANTS

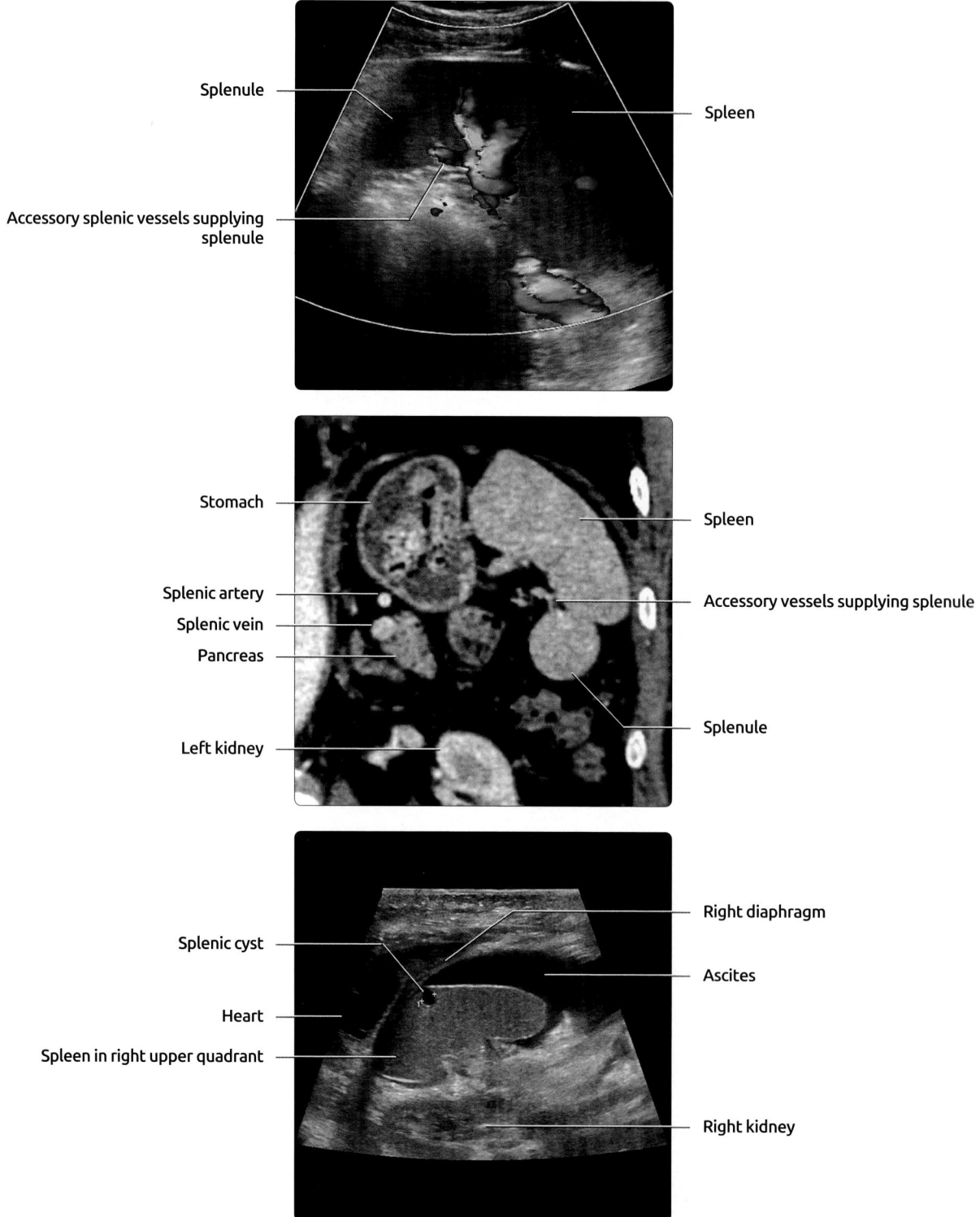

Splenule

Spleen

Accessory splenic vessels supplying splenule

Stomach

Spleen

Splenic artery

Accessory vessels supplying splenule

Splenic vein

Pancreas

Left kidney

Splenule

Splenic cyst

Right diaphragm

Ascites

Heart

Spleen in right upper quadrant

Right kidney

(Top) *Longitudinal oblique intercostal color Doppler ultrasound shows a splenule adjacent to the spleen tip. Splenules should have the same echogenicity and echotexture as the spleen, though this may depend on the sonographic window. The identification of vascular supply from the splenic vessels may also aid in identification of a splenule.* **(Middle)** *Correlative coronal CECT of the left upper quadrant demonstrates a splenule along the inferior tip of the spleen. Branch vessels from the splenic artery and vein supplying the splenule are visualized.* **(Bottom)** *Longitudinal oblique ultrasound of the right upper quadrant in a patient with heterotaxy syndrome (situs ambiguus) demonstrates a right-sided spleen. The classification of heterotaxy syndromes is complex; there is a spectrum ranging from classic asplenia to classic polysplenia. Heterotaxy with polysplenia (i.e., left double-sidedness or left isomerism) may present with multiple spleens (resembling splenules) or a single spleen, as in this case.*

ANATOMICAL VARIANTS

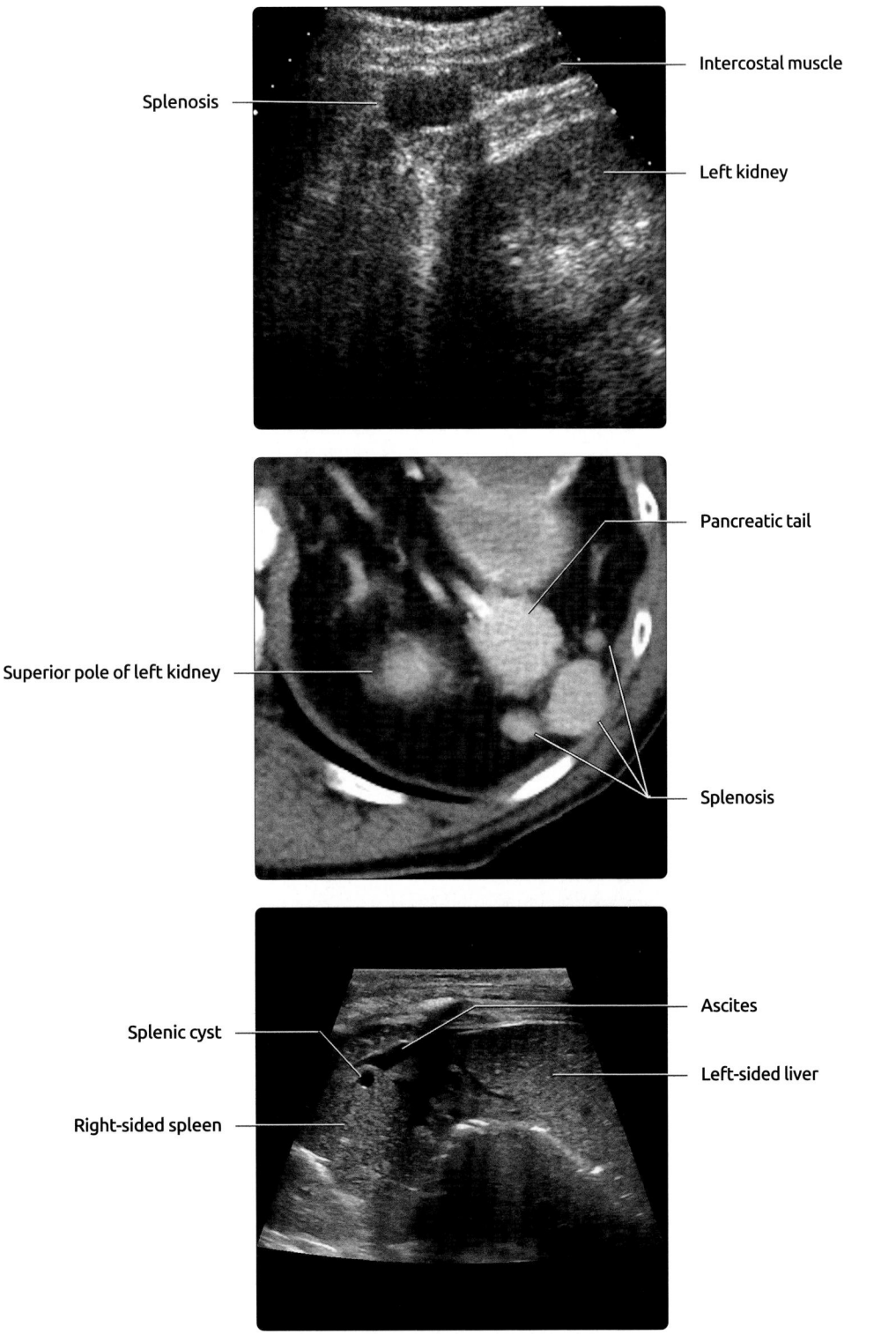

Splenosis — Intercostal muscle — Left kidney

Superior pole of left kidney — Pancreatic tail — Splenosis

Splenic cyst — Ascites — Left-sided liver — Right-sided spleen

(Top) *Longitudinal oblique intercostal grayscale ultrasound through the left upper quadrant shows a round hypoechoic structure adjacent to the upper pole of the left kidney; this represents splenosis.* (Middle) *Correlative axial CECT through the left upper quadrant in a patient with prior splenic trauma and splenectomy shows residual splenosis.* (Bottom) *Transverse anterior ultrasound in the setting of heterotaxy with polysplenia demonstrates the relationship between the right-sided spleen and the left-sided liver.*

GROSS ANATOMY

Overview

- Pancreas: Accessory digestive gland lying in retroperitoneum behind stomach
  - Exocrine function: Pancreatic acinar cells secrete pancreatic juice → pancreatic duct → duodenum
  - Endocrine: Pancreatic islet cells (of Langerhans) secrete insulin, glucagon, and other polypeptides → portal venous system

Divisions

- Head: Thickest part; lies to right of superior mesenteric artery and vein (SMA, SMV)
  - Attached to "C" loop of duodenum (2nd & 3rd parts)
  - Uncinate process: Head extension, posterior to SMV
  - Bile duct lies along posterior surface of head, joins with pancreatic duct (of Wirsung) to form hepatopancreatic ampulla (of Vater)
  - Main pancreatic and bile ducts empty into major papilla in 2nd portion of duodenum
- Neck: Thinnest part; lies anterior to SMA, SMV
  - SMV joins splenic vein behind pancreatic neck to form portal vein
- Body: Main part; lies to left of SMA, SMV
  - Splenic vein lies in groove on posterior surface of body
  - Anterior surface is covered with peritoneum forming back surface of omental bursa (lesser sac)
- Tail: Lies between layers of splenorenal ligament in splenic hilum

Internal Structures

- Pancreatic duct (of Wirsung) runs length of pancreas, turning inferiorly through head to join bile duct
- Accessory pancreatic duct (of Santorini) opens into duodenum at minor duodenal papilla
  - Usually communicates with main pancreatic duct
  - Variations are common, including a dominant accessory duct draining most pancreatic juice
- Vessels, nerves, and lymphatics
  - Arteries to head mainly from gastroduodenal artery
    - Pancreaticoduodenal arcade of vessels around head also supplied by SMA branches
  - Arteries to body & tail from splenic artery
  - Veins are tributaries of SMV and splenic vein → portal vein
  - Autonomic nerves from celiac and superior mesenteric plexus
    - Parasympathetic stimulation of pancreatic secretion, but pancreatic juice secretion is mostly under hormonal control (secretin, from duodenum)
  - Lymphatics follow blood vessels
    - Collect in splenic, celiac, superior mesenteric and hepatic nodes

IMAGING ANATOMY

Overview

- Pancreas can be localized on ultrasound by
  - Typical parenchymal architecture: Homogeneously isoechoic/hyperechoic echo pattern when compared with overlying liver
  - Surrounding anatomical landmarks: Body anterior to splenic vein; neck anterior to SMA/SMV
- Variations in reflectivity related to degree of fatty infiltration; uncinate process and posterior pancreatic head are relatively echo-poor in 25% of subjects (lack of intraparenchymal fat)

ANATOMY IMAGING ISSUES

Imaging Recommendations

- Use 2-5 MHz transducers, or up to 9 MHz for smaller patients
- Techniques to combat overlying stomach and bowel gas include
  - Displacement of intervening bowel gas by gentle firm graded compression with transducer
  - Overnight fasting or fasting > 6-8 hours
  - Non-effervescent fluid can be given orally to fill gastric fundus
    - Scanning delayed for a few minutes to allow fluid to settle
    - Patient can lie on left side to allow imaging of body and tail of pancreas
    - Patient can then be turned right to allow gastric fluid to flow to stomach antrum and duodenum, allowing imaging of head and uncinate process
- CT is preferred imaging modality for imaging of pancreas
- MRCP or ERCP useful for defining pancreatic duct

Imaging Pitfalls

- Ultrasound examination of pancreas is often limited by overlying bowel gas

Key Concepts

- Shape, size, and texture of pancreas are quite variable
  - Largest in young adults
  - Atrophy and fatty infiltration with age (> 70), obesity, diabetes, corticosteroids, Cushing disease
  - Pancreatic duct also becomes more prominent with age (normal < 3 mm diameter)
  - Focal bulge or mass effect is abnormal
- Location behind lesser sac
  - Acute pancreatitis often results in lesser sac fluid (may mimic pseudocyst)
- Pancreas lies in anterior pararenal space (APS)
  - Inflammation (from pancreatitis) easily spreads to duodenum and descending colon; also lie in APS
  - Inflammation easily spreads into mesentery and mesocolon; roots of these lie just ventral to pancreas
- Obstruction of pancreatic duct
  - Relatively common result of chronic pancreatitis (fibrosis &/or stone occluding pancreatic duct), or pancreatic ductal carcinoma
- Acute pancreatitis
  - Relatively common result of gallstone (lodged in hepatopancreatic ampulla causing bile to reflux into pancreas) or damage from alcohol abuse

PANCREAS IN SITU

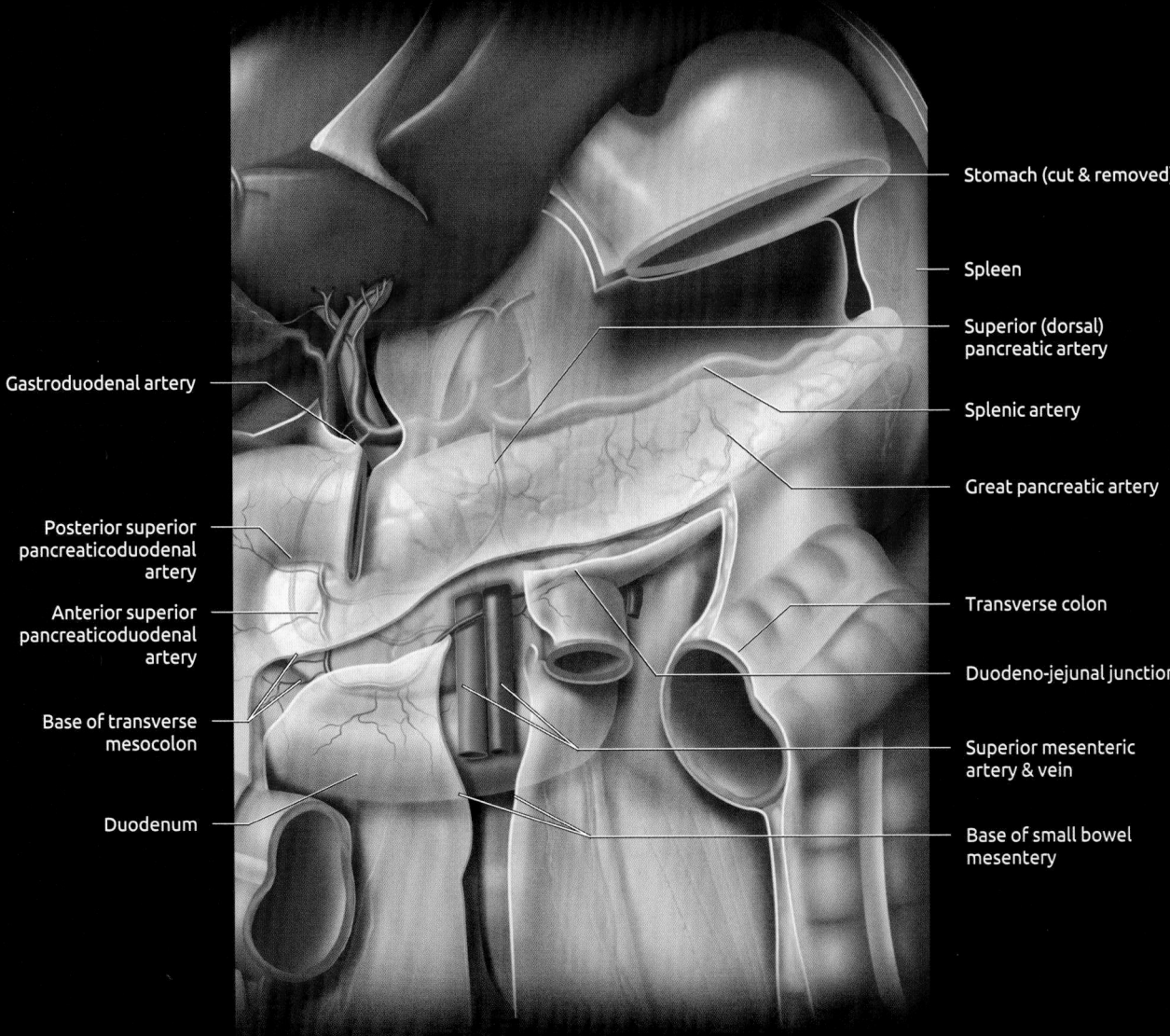

Gastroduodenal artery

Posterior superior pancreaticoduodenal artery

Anterior superior pancreaticoduodenal artery

Base of transverse mesocolon

Duodenum

Stomach (cut & removed)

Spleen

Superior (dorsal) pancreatic artery

Splenic artery

Great pancreatic artery

Transverse colon

Duodeno-jejunal junction

Superior mesenteric artery & vein

Base of small bowel mesentery

Graphic shows the arterial supply to the body & tail of the pancreas through terminal branches of the splenic artery, which are variable in number & size. The two largest are usually the dorsal (superior) and great pancreatic arteries, which arise from the proximal & distal splenic artery, respectively. The arteries to the pancreatic head and duodenum come from the pancreaticoduodenal arcades that receive flow from the celiac and superior mesenteric arteries. The superior mesenteric vessels pass behind the neck of the pancreas and in front of the third portion of the duodenum. The root of the transverse mesocolon and small bowel mesentery arise from the surface of the pancreas and transmit the blood vessels to the small bowel & transverse colon. The splenic vein runs along the dorsal surface of the pancreas. The splenic vessels and pancreatic tail insert into the splenic hilum.

PANCREAS, TRANSVERSE VIEW

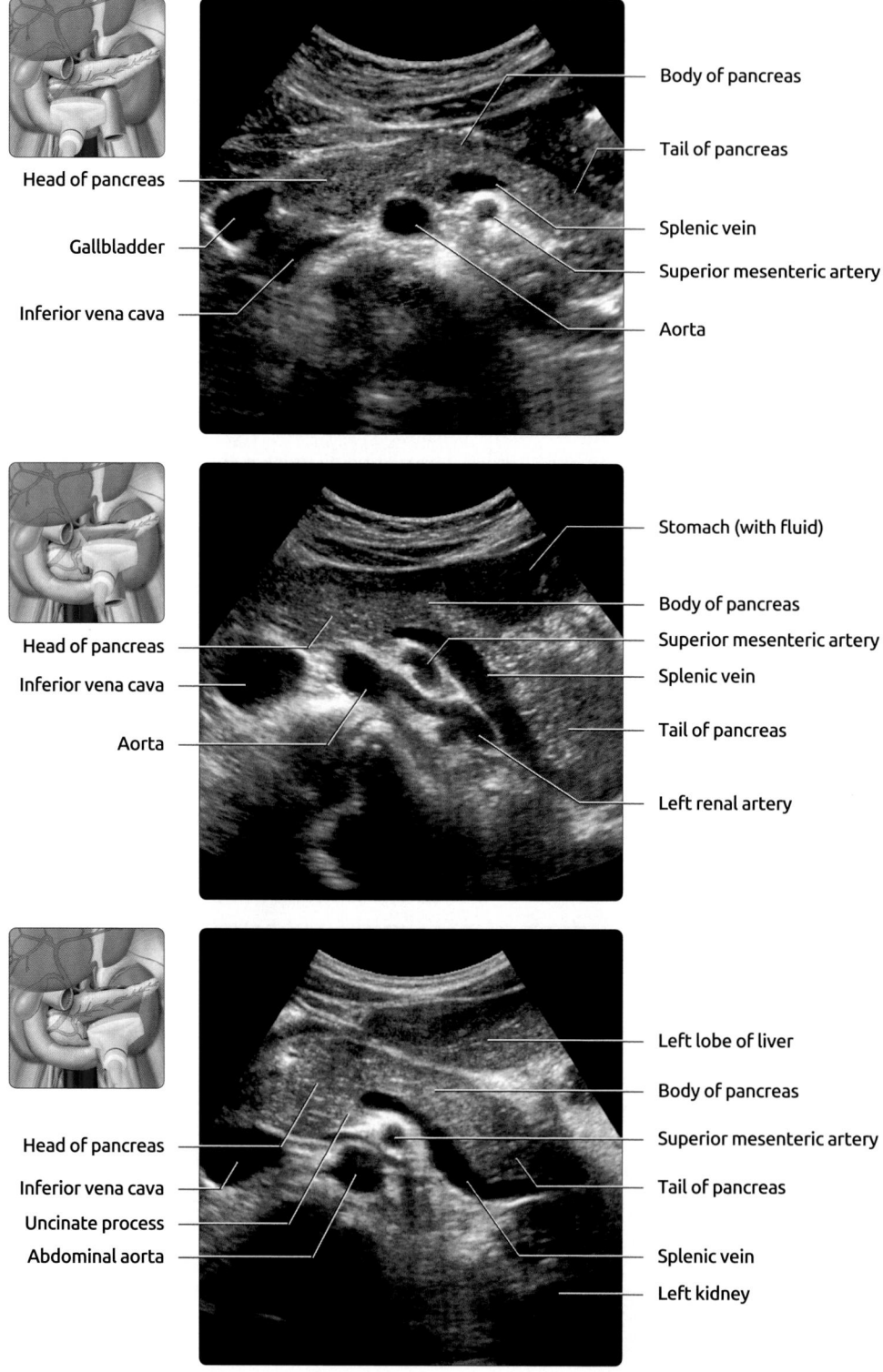

Head of pancreas

Gallbladder

Inferior vena cava

Body of pancreas

Tail of pancreas

Splenic vein

Superior mesenteric artery

Aorta

Head of pancreas

Inferior vena cava

Aorta

Stomach (with fluid)

Body of pancreas

Superior mesenteric artery

Splenic vein

Tail of pancreas

Left renal artery

Head of pancreas

Inferior vena cava

Uncinate process

Abdominal aorta

Left lobe of liver

Body of pancreas

Superior mesenteric artery

Tail of pancreas

Splenic vein

Left kidney

(Top) *Transverse transabdominal grayscale ultrasound at the epigastrium is shown. Anatomically, the pancreatic axis from head to tail is directed superiorly and to the left. This lower transverse section demonstrates the bulk of the pancreatic head.* **(Middle)** *Transverse transabdominal grayscale ultrasound at the epigastrium is shown, slightly higher than the previous image. Note that the pancreatic body and tail have now come into view.* **(Bottom)** *Oblique transabdominal grayscale ultrasound at the epigastrium is shown. The transducer is tilted slightly cranially and laterally to the left to follow the pancreatic axis, thus imaging the pancreas in its entirety. The splenic vein courses along the posterior pancreas and provides an excellent landmark in locating the pancreas. The superior mesenteric artery is more posteriorly located and has a characteristic dot shape as it is imaged end-on.*

PANCREAS, TRANSVERSE VIEW

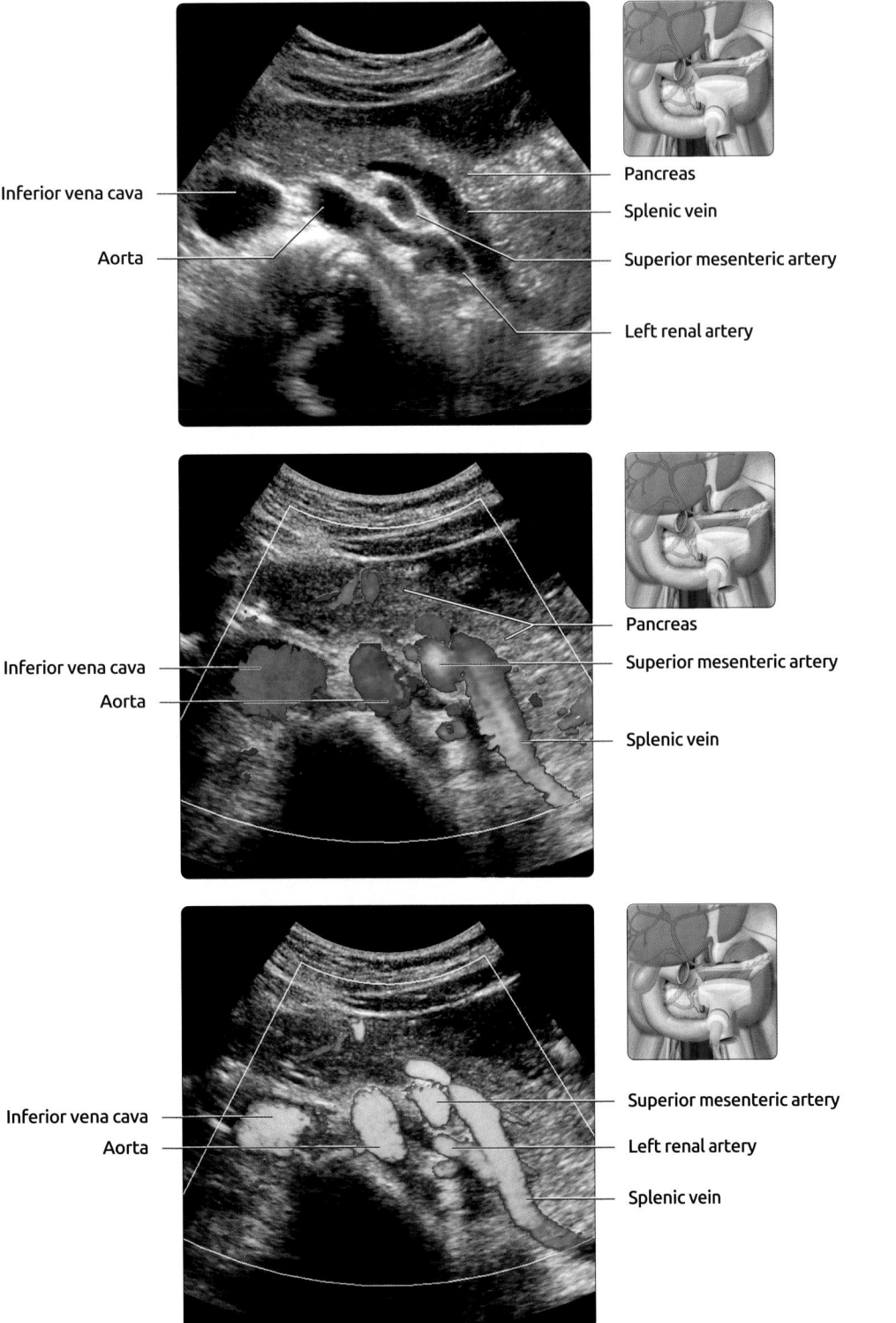

Inferior vena cava — Aorta — Pancreas — Splenic vein — Superior mesenteric artery — Left renal artery

Inferior vena cava — Aorta — Pancreas — Superior mesenteric artery — Splenic vein

Inferior vena cava — Aorta — Superior mesenteric artery — Left renal artery — Splenic vein

(Top) *Transverse subxiphoid grayscale ultrasound shows the left renal artery coursing posterior to the superior mesenteric artery and splenic vein as it descends to enter the left renal hilum.* (Middle) *Transverse subxiphoid color Doppler ultrasound is shown. This image was taken with a small amount of cranial tilt so that blue indicates flow toward the transducer and red away from the transducer. Note therefore that aortic flow is blue and IVC flow is red. The splenic vein is red in its proximal portion but exhibits blue color distally, owing to its course. The left renal artery is almost at right angles to the transducer and therefore flow is not well seen.* (Bottom) *Transverse subxiphoid power Doppler ultrasound demonstrates the vessels posterior to the pancreas. Power Doppler is more sensitive for detecting vascular flow but fails to provide information on flow direction.*

PANCREAS, SAGITTAL VIEW

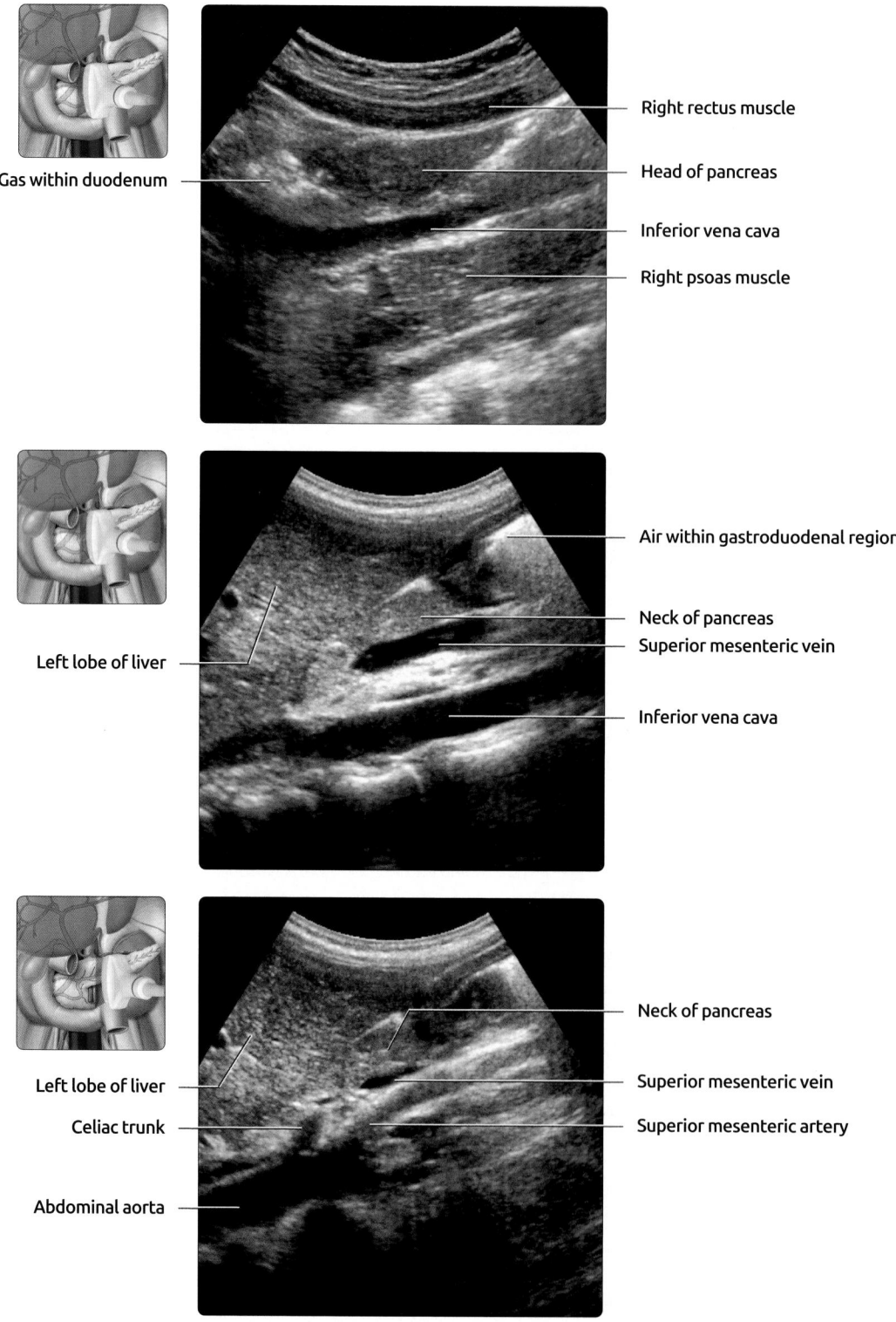

Gas within duodenum

Right rectus muscle

Head of pancreas

Inferior vena cava

Right psoas muscle

Left lobe of liver

Air within gastroduodenal region

Neck of pancreas

Superior mesenteric vein

Inferior vena cava

Left lobe of liver

Celiac trunk

Abdominal aorta

Neck of pancreas

Superior mesenteric vein

Superior mesenteric artery

(Top) *Longitudinal transabdominal grayscale ultrasound at the epigastrium, right paramedian region, is shown. Note the relationship of the pancreatic head with the posteriorly located inferior vena cava.* **(Middle)** *Longitudinal transabdominal grayscale ultrasound at the epigastrium, right paramedian region, is shown continuing medially from the previous image. Note the superior mesenteric vein coming into view; this is a good landmark for locating the neck of the pancreas on the sagittal ultrasound.* **(Bottom)** *Longitudinal transabdominal grayscale ultrasound at the epigastrium, right paramedian region, is shown slightly more medial to the previous image. The origin of the superior mesenteric artery arising from the abdominal aorta is brought into view. The SMA is also a useful marker for identifying the neck of the pancreas on sagittal ultrasound.*

PANCREAS, SAGITTAL VIEW

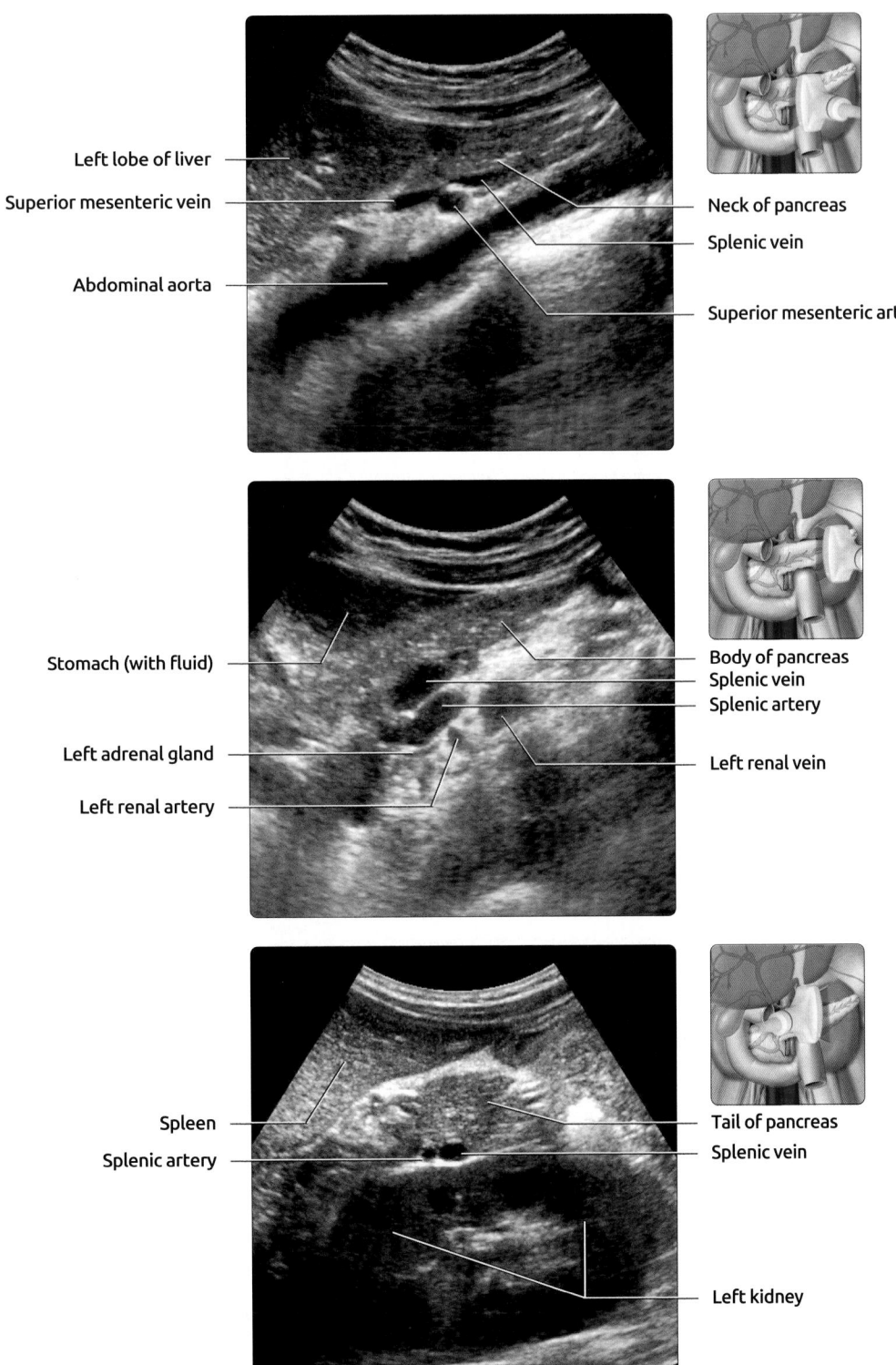

Left lobe of liver

Superior mesenteric vein

Abdominal aorta

Neck of pancreas

Splenic vein

Superior mesenteric artery

Stomach (with fluid)

Left adrenal gland

Left renal artery

Body of pancreas

Splenic vein

Splenic artery

Left renal vein

Spleen

Splenic artery

Tail of pancreas

Splenic vein

Left kidney

(Top) *Longitudinal transabdominal grayscale ultrasound at the midline epigastrium is shown, revealing the SMA that has taken off from the abdominal aorta, its relationship with the splenic vein, and the anteriorly located pancreatic neck. The inferior mesenteric vein joins the splenic vein here.* (Middle) *Longitudinal transabdominal grayscale ultrasound at the epigastrium, left paramedian region, is shown by sweeping the transducer laterally from the top image. The body of the pancreas lies to the left of the SMA (not shown). The stomach lies superiorly and may be filled with fluid for use as an acoustic window. The splenic vein maintains its course behind the pancreas.* (Bottom) *Longitudinal transabdominal grayscale ultrasound at the epigastrium is shown, continuing the scan laterally from the middle image. The pancreatic tail is identified between the spleen and the left kidney.*

GROSS ANATOMY

Overview

- Kidneys are paired, bean-shaped, retroperitoneal organs
  - Function: Remove excess water, salts, and wastes of protein metabolism from blood

Anatomic Relationships

- Lie in retroperitoneum, within perirenal space, surrounded by renal fascia (of Gerota)
- Each adult kidney is ~ 9-14 cm in length, 5 cm in width
- Both kidneys lie on quadratus lumborum muscles, lateral to psoas muscles

Internal Structures

- Kidneys can be considered hollow with renal sinus occupied by fat, renal pelvis, calyces, vessels, and nerves
- Renal hilum: Where artery enters, vein and ureter leave renal sinus
- Renal pelvis: Funnel-shaped expansion of upper end of ureter
  - Receives major calyces (infundibula) (2 or 3), each of which receives minor calyces (2-4)
- Renal papilla: Pointed apex of renal pyramid of collecting tubules that excrete urine
  - Each papilla indents a minor calyx
- Renal cortex: Outer part, contains renal corpuscles (glomeruli, vessels), proximal portions of collecting tubules and loop of Henle
- Renal medulla: Inner part, contains renal pyramids, distal parts of collecting tubules, and loops of Henle
- Vessels, nerves, and lymphatics
  - Artery
    - Usually 1 for each kidney
    - Arise from aorta at about L1-L2 vertebral level
  - Vein
    - Usually 1 for each kidney
    - Lies in front of renal artery and renal pelvis
  - Nerves
    - Autonomic from renal and aorticorenal ganglia and plexus
  - Lymphatics
    - To lumbar (aortic and caval) nodes

IMAGING ANATOMY

Overview

- Well-defined retroperitoneal bean-shaped structures, which move with respiration

Internal Contents

- Renal capsule
  - Normal kidneys are well-defined due to presence of renal capsule and are less reflective than surrounding fat
- Renal cortex
  - Renal cortex has reflectivity that is less than adjacent liver or spleen
  - If renal cortex brighter than normal liver (echogenic), then high suspicion of renal parenchymal disease
- Medullary pyramids
  - Medullary pyramids are less reflective than renal cortex
- Corticomedullary differentiation
  - Margin between cortex and pyramids is usually well-defined in normal kidneys
  - Margin between cortex and pyramids may be lost in presence of generalized parenchymal inflammation or edema
- Renal sinus
  - Echogenic due to fat that surrounds blood vessels and collecting systems
  - Outline of renal sinus is variable, from smooth to irregular
  - Renal sinus fat may increase in obesity, steroid use, and sinus lipomatosis
  - Renal sinus fat may decrease in cachectic patients and neonates
  - If sinus echoes are indistinct in noncachectic patient, tumor infiltration or edema should be considered
- Collecting system (renal pelvis and calyces)
  - Not usually visible in dehydrated patient
  - May be seen as physiological "splitting" of renal sinus echoes in patients with a full bladder undergoing diuresis
  - Physiological "splitting" of renal sinus echoes is common in pregnancy
    - Cause of dilatation of pelvicalyceal system may be due to mechanical obstruction by enlarging uterus, hormonal factors, increased blood flow, and parenchymal hypertrophy
    - May occur as early as 12 weeks into pregnancy
    - Seen in up to 75% of right kidneys at 20 weeks into pregnancy, less common on left side, thought to be due to cushioning of ureter from gravid uterus by sigmoid colon
    - Obvious dilatation of pelvicalyceal system can be seen in 2/3 of patients at 36 weeks
    - Changes usually resolve within 48 hours after delivery
  - Possible obstruction can be excluded by performing post micturition images of collecting system
    - AP diameter of renal pelvis in adults should be < 10 mm
- Renal arteries
  - Normal caliber 5-8 mm
  - 2/3 of kidneys are supplied by single renal artery arising from aorta
  - 1/3 of kidneys are supplied by 2 or more renal arteries arising from aorta
    - Main renal artery may be duplicated
    - Accessory renal arteries may arise from aorta superior or inferior to main renal artery
    - Accessory renal arteries may enter kidney either in hilum or at poles
    - Extrahilar accessory renal arteries may arise from ipsilateral renal artery, ipsilateral iliac artery, aorta, or retroperitoneal arteries
  - Spectral Doppler
    - Open systolic window, rapid systolic upstroke occasionally followed by secondary slower rise to peak systole with subsequent diastolic delay but persistent forward flow in diastole
    - Continuous diastolic flow is present due to low resistance in renal vascular bed
    - Low resistance flow pattern is also present in intrarenal branches

- – Normal peak systolic velocity (PSV) 75-125 cm/s, not more than 180 cm/s
  - □ > 200 cm/s is abnormal
  - – Resistive index (RI) is (peak systolic velocity - end diastolic velocity)/peak systolic velocity; normal < 0.7
  - – Pulsatility index (PI) is (peak systolic velocity - end diastole velocity)/mean velocity, normal < 1.8
- Renal veins
  - ○ Normal caliber 4-9 mm
  - ○ Formed from tributaries that coalesce at renal hilum
  - ○ Right renal vein is relatively short and drains directly into IVC
  - ○ Left renal vein receives left adrenal vein from above and left gonadal vein from below
  - ○ Left renal vein crosses midline between aorta and superior mesenteric artery
  - ○ Spectral Doppler
    - – Normal PSV 18-33 cm/s
    - – Spectral Doppler in right renal vein mirrors pulsatility in IVC
    - – Spectral Doppler in left renal vein may show only slight variability of velocities consequent upon cardiac and respiratory activity

Size

- Bipolar length is found by rotating transducer around its vertical axis such that the longest craniocaudal length can be identified
- Normal size between 10-15 cm
- Volume measurements
  - ○ May be more accurate, but is time consuming
  - ○ 3D ellipsoidal formula can be used for volume estimation
    - – Length x AP diameter x transverse diameter x 0.5
  - ○ Consistency and changes in volume over time more important

ANATOMY IMAGING ISSUES

Imaging Recommendations

- Right kidney
  - ○ Liver used as acoustic window
  - ○ Transducer placed in subcostal or intercostal position
  - ○ Varying degree of respiration is useful
  - ○ Raising patient's right side and scanning laterally/posterolaterally may be useful
- Left kidney
  - ○ More difficult to visualize due to bowel gas from small bowel and splenic flexure
  - ○ Usually easier to search for left kidney using posterolateral approach with left side raised
  - ○ Full right lateral decubitus with pillow under right flank and left arm extended above head may be useful in difficult cases
    - – Spleen can be used as acoustic window for imaging upper pole of left kidney
  - ○ Posterior approach
    - – Useful for intervention procedures (renal biopsy, nephrostomy)
    - – Image quality may be impaired by thick paraspinal muscles and ribs shadowing
- Renal arteries

  - ○ Origins best seen from midline anterior approach
  - ○ Right renal artery can usually be followed from origin to kidney
  - ○ Left renal artery often requires posterolateral coronal transducer scanning position for visualization
- Renal veins
  - ○ Best seen on transverse scan from anterior approach
  - ○ May also be seen on coronal scan from posterolateral coronal

Key Concepts

- Accessory renal vessels
  - ○ Must be accounted for in planning surgery (e.g., resection, transplantation)
  - ○ Often are best seen using multidetector row CT, magnetic resonance angiogram, or digital subtraction angiography rather than ultrasound

EMBRYOLOGY

Embryologic Events

- Congenital anomalies of renal number, position, structure, and form are very common
  - ○ Often accompanied by anomalies of other systems
  - ○ VATER acronym: Vertebral, anorectal, tracheoesophageal, radial ray, renal
  - ○ Congenital absence of kidney
  - ○ Anomalies of position (ectopia) are common
  - ○ Anomalies of structure
    - – Congenitally large septum of Bertin (lobar dysmorphism); asymptomatic
    - – Fetal lobulations (lobation), single or multiple indentations of lateral renal contours
    - – Partial duplication: Commonly results in enlarged kidney with 2 separate hila, 2 ureters (may join downstream or join bladder separately); duplex kidney = bifid renal pelvis, single ureter

KIDNEYS IN SITU

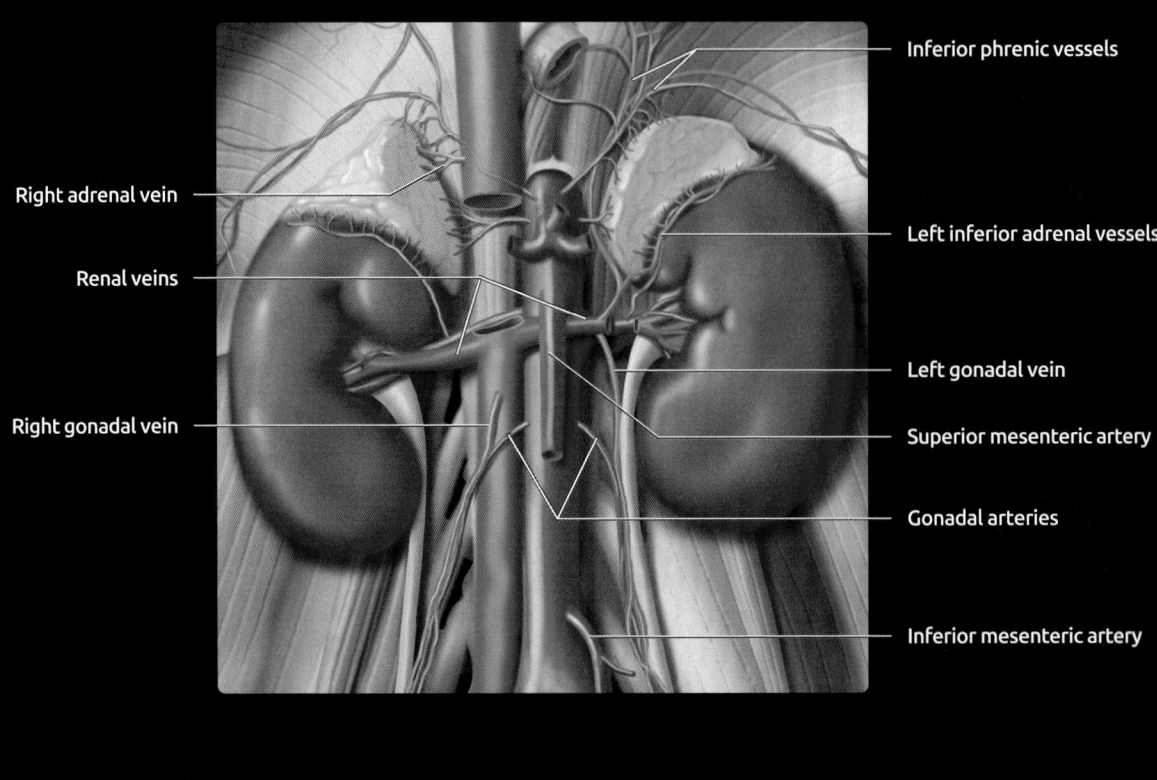

Inferior phrenic vessels

Right adrenal vein

Left inferior adrenal vessels

Renal veins

Left gonadal vein

Right gonadal vein

Superior mesenteric artery

Gonadal arteries

Inferior mesenteric artery

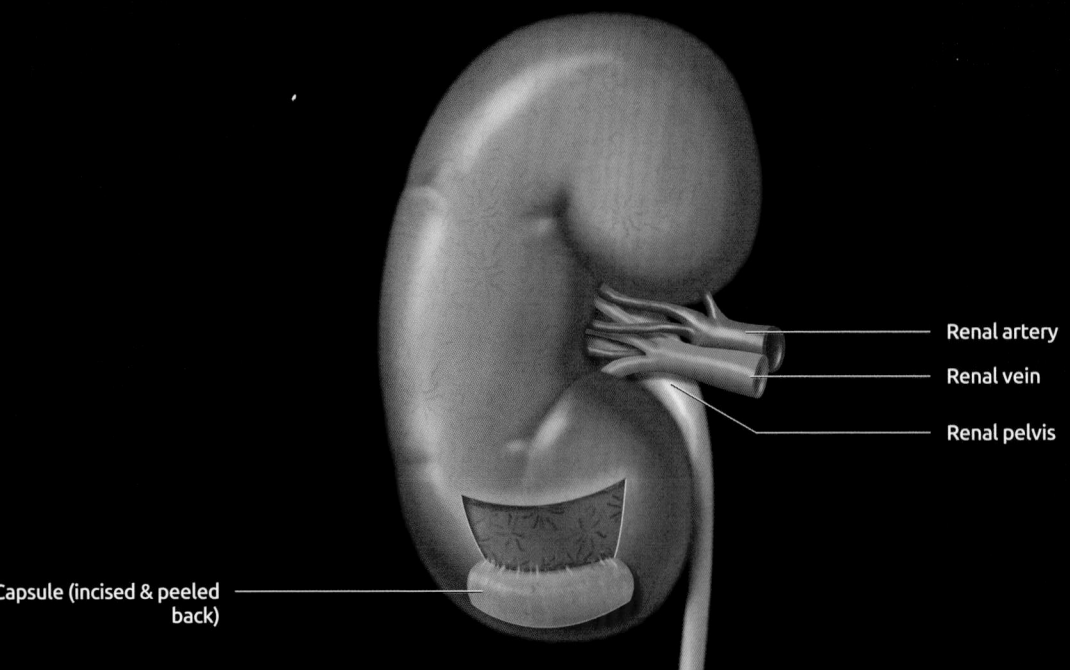

Renal artery

Renal vein

Renal pelvis

Capsule (incised & peeled back)

(Top) *The kidneys are retroperitoneal organs that lie lateral to the psoas and "on" the quadratus lumborum muscles. The oblique course of the psoas muscles results in the lower pole of the kidney lying lateral to the upper pole. The right kidney usually lies 1-2 cm lower than the left, due to inferior displacement by the liver. The adrenal glands lie above and medial to the kidneys, separated by a layer of fat and connective tissue. The peritoneum covers much of the anterior surface of the kidneys. The right kidney abuts the liver and the hepatic flexure of the colon and duodenum, while the left kidney is in close contact with the pancreas (tail), spleen, and splenic flexure.* (Bottom) *The fibrous capsule is stripped off with difficulty. Subcapsular hematomas do not spread far along the surface of the kidney, but compress the renal parenchyma, unlike most perirenal collections.*

KIDNEY ARTERIES AND INTERIOR ANATOMY

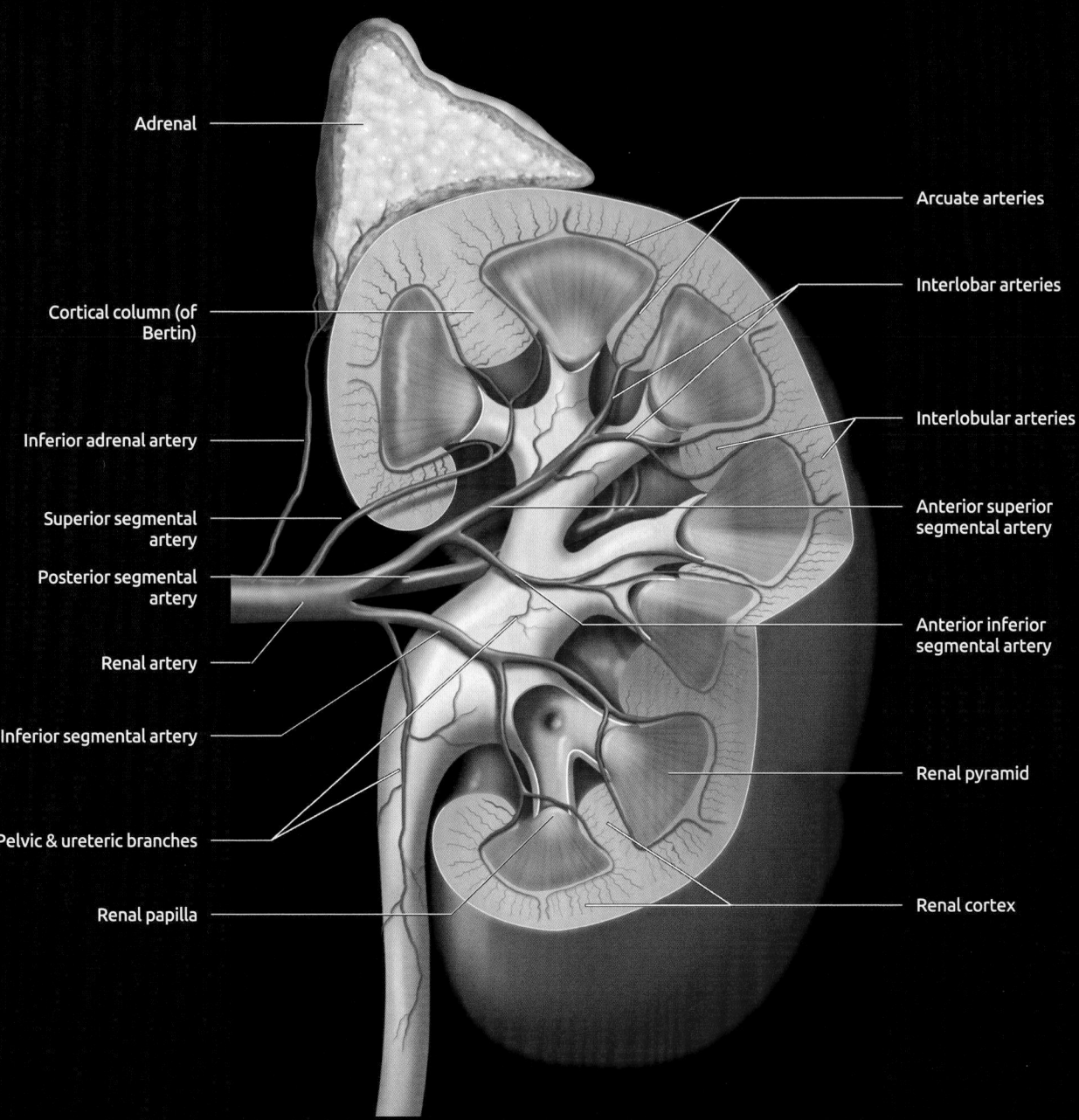

Adrenal

Cortical column (of Bertin)

Inferior adrenal artery

Superior segmental artery

Posterior segmental artery

Renal artery

Inferior segmental artery

Pelvic & ureteric branches

Renal papilla

Arcuate arteries

Interlobar arteries

Interlobular arteries

Anterior superior segmental artery

Anterior inferior segmental artery

Renal pyramid

Renal cortex

The kidney is usually supplied by a single renal artery, the 1st branch of which is the inferior adrenal artery. It then divides into 5 segmental arteries, only 1 of which (the posterior segmental artery) passes dorsal to the renal pelvis. The segmental arteries divide into the interlobar arteries that lie in the renal sinus fat. Each interlobar artery branches into 4 to 6 arcuate arteries that follow the convex outer margin of each renal pyramid. The arcuate arteries give rise to the interlobular arteries that lie within the renal cortex, including the cortical columns (of Bertin) that invaginate between the renal pyramids. The interlobular arteries supply the afferent arterioles to the glomeruli. The arterial supply to the kidney is vulnerable, as there are no effective anastomoses between the segmental branches, each of which supplies a wedge-shaped segment of parenchyma.

CT UROGRAM

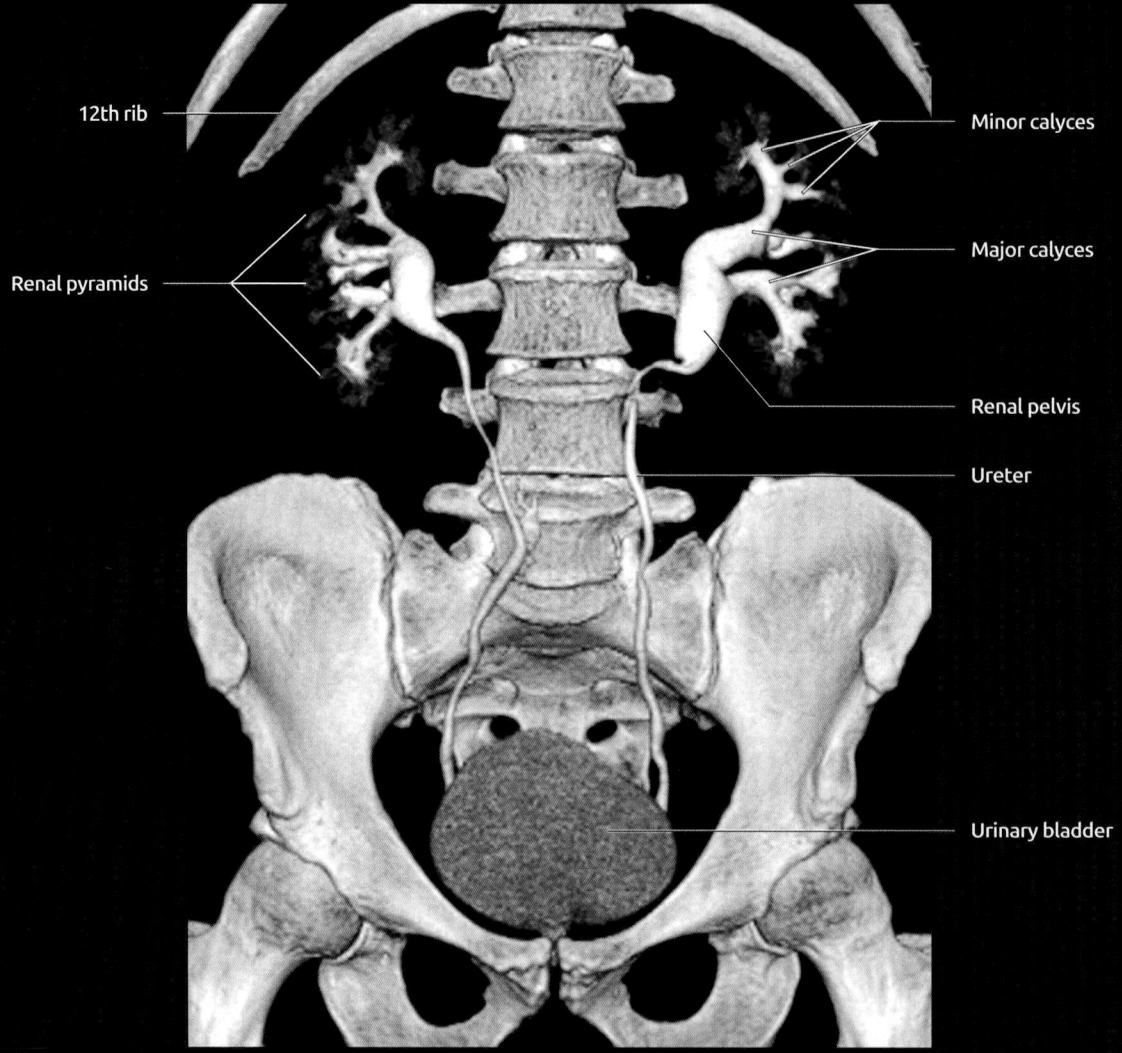

12th rib

Minor calyces

Major calyces

Renal pyramids

Renal pelvis

Ureter

Urinary bladder

A coronal reconstruction of a series of axial CT sections can be viewed as a surface-rendered 3D image to simulate an excretory urogram. The window levels and work station controls have been set to optimally display the renal collecting system. The color scale is arbitrary; in this case, opacified urine is displayed as white. Less dense urine within the renal tubules in the pyramids and the diluted urine within the bladder are displayed as red. The CT scan was obtained in suspended inspiration, resulting in caudal displacement of the kidneys. In the supine position at quiet breathing, the upper poles of the kidneys usually lie in front of the 12th ribs.

RENAL FASCIA AND PERIRENAL SPACE

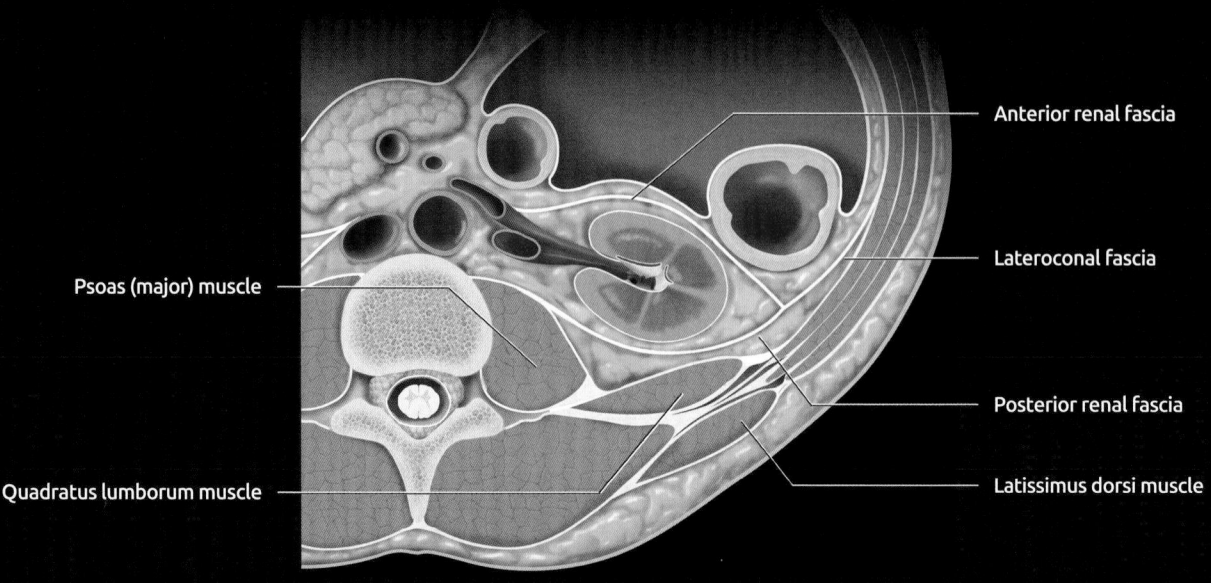

Anterior renal fascia

Lateroconal fascia

Psoas (major) muscle

Posterior renal fascia

Quadratus lumborum muscle

Latissimus dorsi muscle

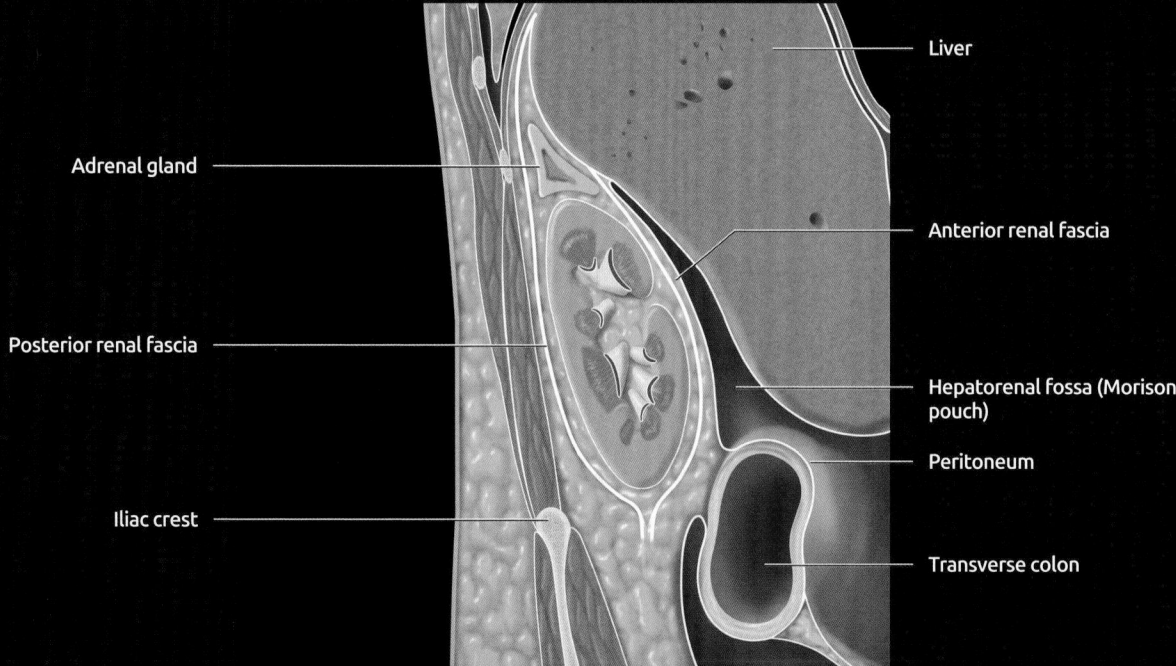

Liver

Adrenal gland

Anterior renal fascia

Posterior renal fascia

Hepatorenal fossa (Morison pouch)

Peritoneum

Iliac crest

Transverse colon

(Top) *The anterior and posterior layers of the renal fascia envelope the kidneys and adrenals along with the perirenal fat. Medial to the kidneys, the course of the renal fascia is variable (and controversial). The posterior layer usually fuses with the psoas or quadratus lumborum fascia. The perirenal spaces do not communicate across the abdominal midline. However, the renal and lateroconal fasciae are laminated structures that may be distended with fluid collections to form interfascial planes that do communicate across the midline and also inferiorly to the extraperitoneal pelvis. **(Bottom)** A sagittal section through the right kidney shows the renal fascia enveloping the kidney and adrenal gland. Inferiorly, the anterior and posterior renal fasciae come close together at about the level of the iliac crest. Note the adjacent peritoneal recesses.*

RIGHT KIDNEY, ANTERIOR ABDOMEN SCAN

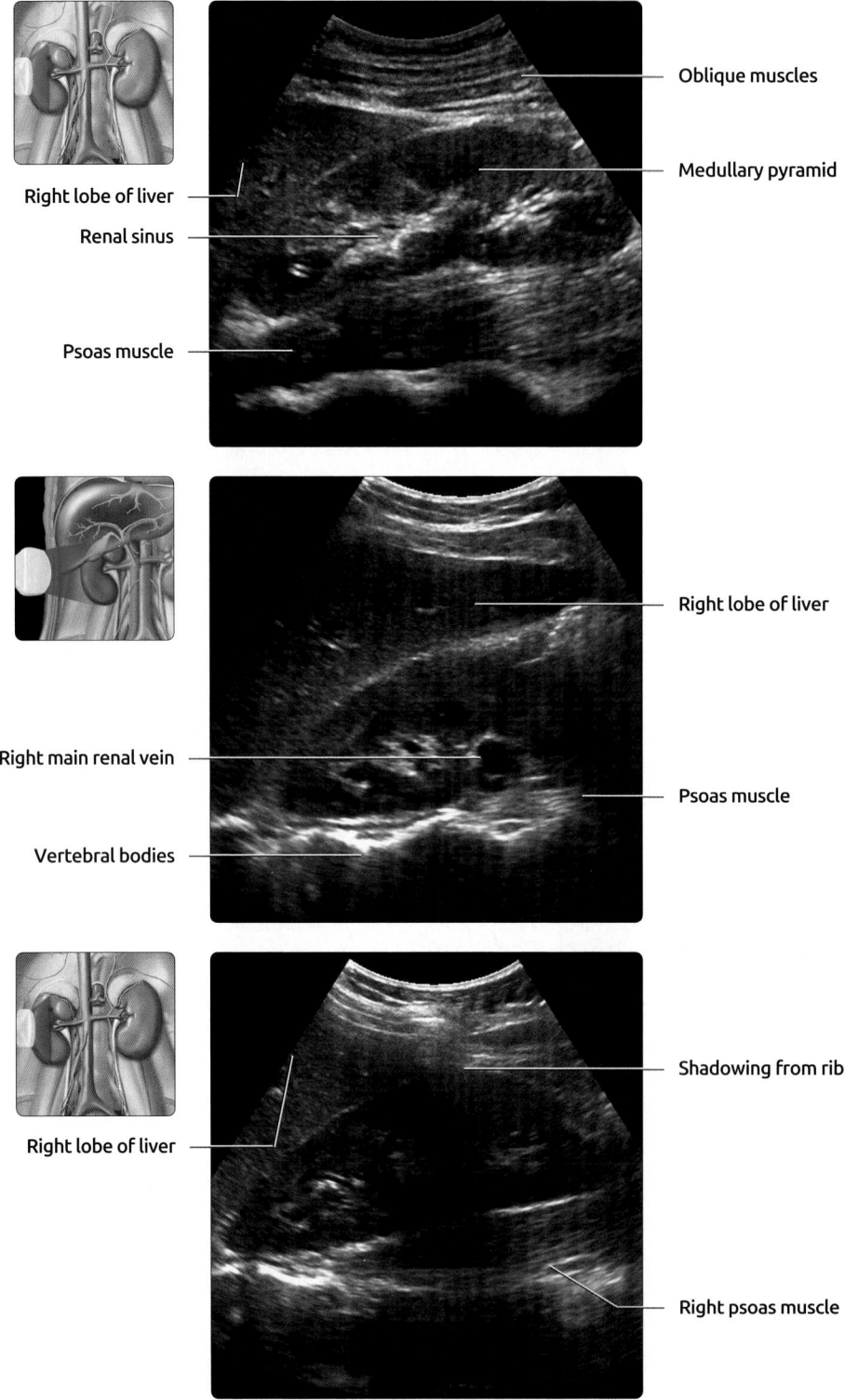

Oblique muscles

Medullary pyramid

Right lobe of liver

Renal sinus

Psoas muscle

Right lobe of liver

Right main renal vein

Psoas muscle

Vertebral bodies

Shadowing from rib

Right lobe of liver

Right psoas muscle

(Top) Longitudinal grayscale ultrasound of the right kidney using the liver as an acoustic window is shown. This approach usually provides excellent visualization of the right kidney and is useful for measuring bipolar renal length. (Middle) Longitudinal oblique grayscale ultrasound of the right kidney using the liver as an acoustic window with the view obtained with a bit more medial angulation (when compared with the previous image). (Bottom) Longitudinal oblique grayscale ultrasound of the right kidney using the liver as an acoustic window with the view obtained with more lateral angulation (when compared with the previous 2 images) cuts through the renal parenchyma on the lateral aspect of the right kidney. Note that the echogenic sinus is not demonstrated and that there is shadowing from ribs.

RIGHT KIDNEY, CT CORRELATION

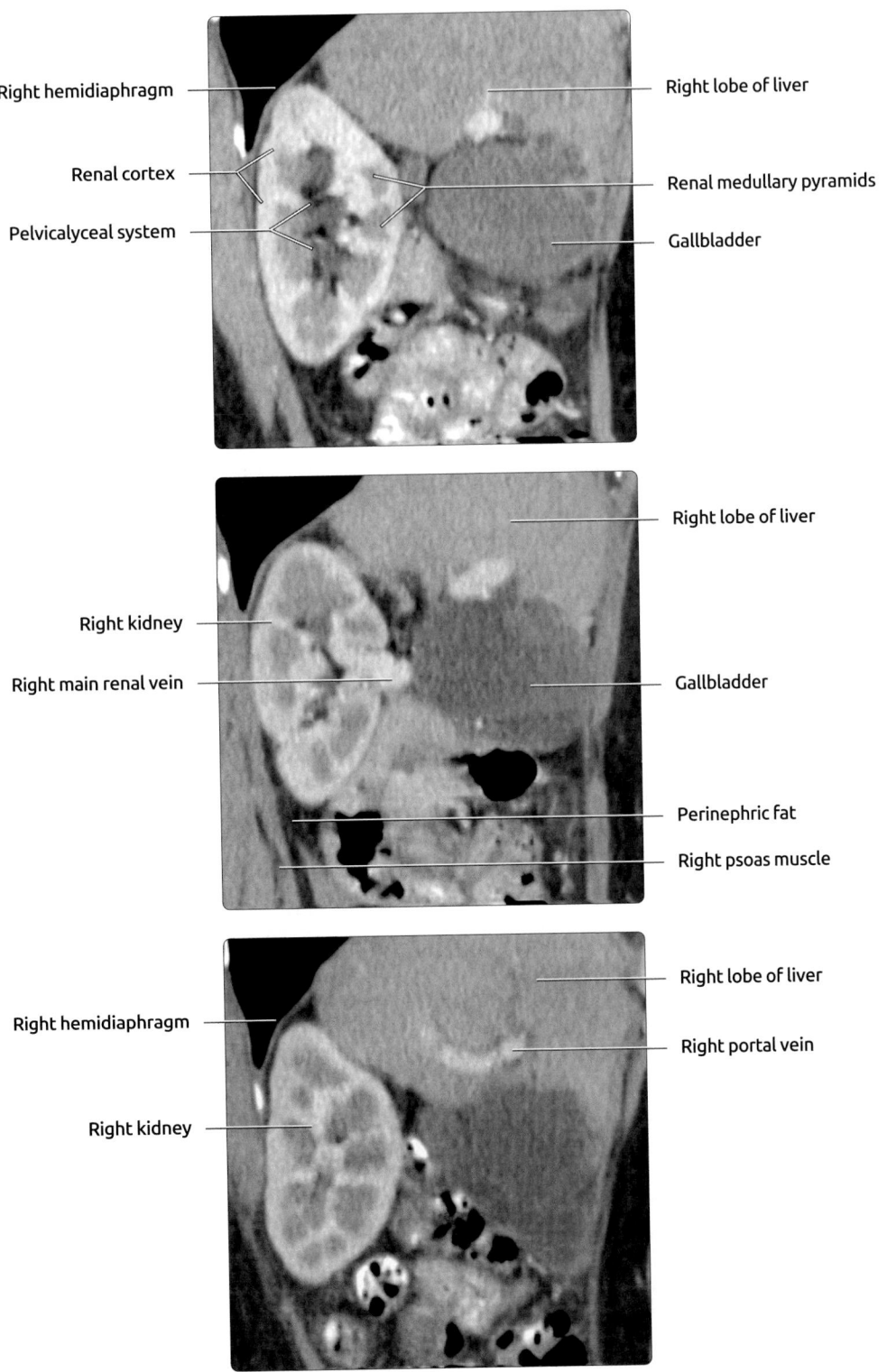

Right hemidiaphragm

Renal cortex

Pelvicalyceal system

Right lobe of liver

Renal medullary pyramids

Gallbladder

Right lobe of liver

Right kidney

Right main renal vein

Gallbladder

Perinephric fat

Right psoas muscle

Right lobe of liver

Right hemidiaphragm

Right portal vein

Right kidney

(Top) *Correlative longitudinal CT multiplanar reconstruction image of the right kidney through planes that are commonly used when examining the patient with ultrasound. Like ultrasound, multidetector row CT now allows evaluation of kidneys in many planes; however, ionizing radiation and the use of intravenous contrast are its limiting factors, particularly in children.* **(Middle)** *Correlative longitudinal oblique CT multiplanar reconstruction image of the right kidney cutting through the right renal vein is shown. The plane of this image is angulated more medially when compared with the previous image.* **(Bottom)** *Correlative longitudinal oblique CT multiplanar reconstruction image of the right kidney cutting through the right portal vein with the plane of this image is angulated more laterally when compared with the previous 2 images.*

RIGHT KIDNEY, ANTERIOR ABDOMEN SCAN

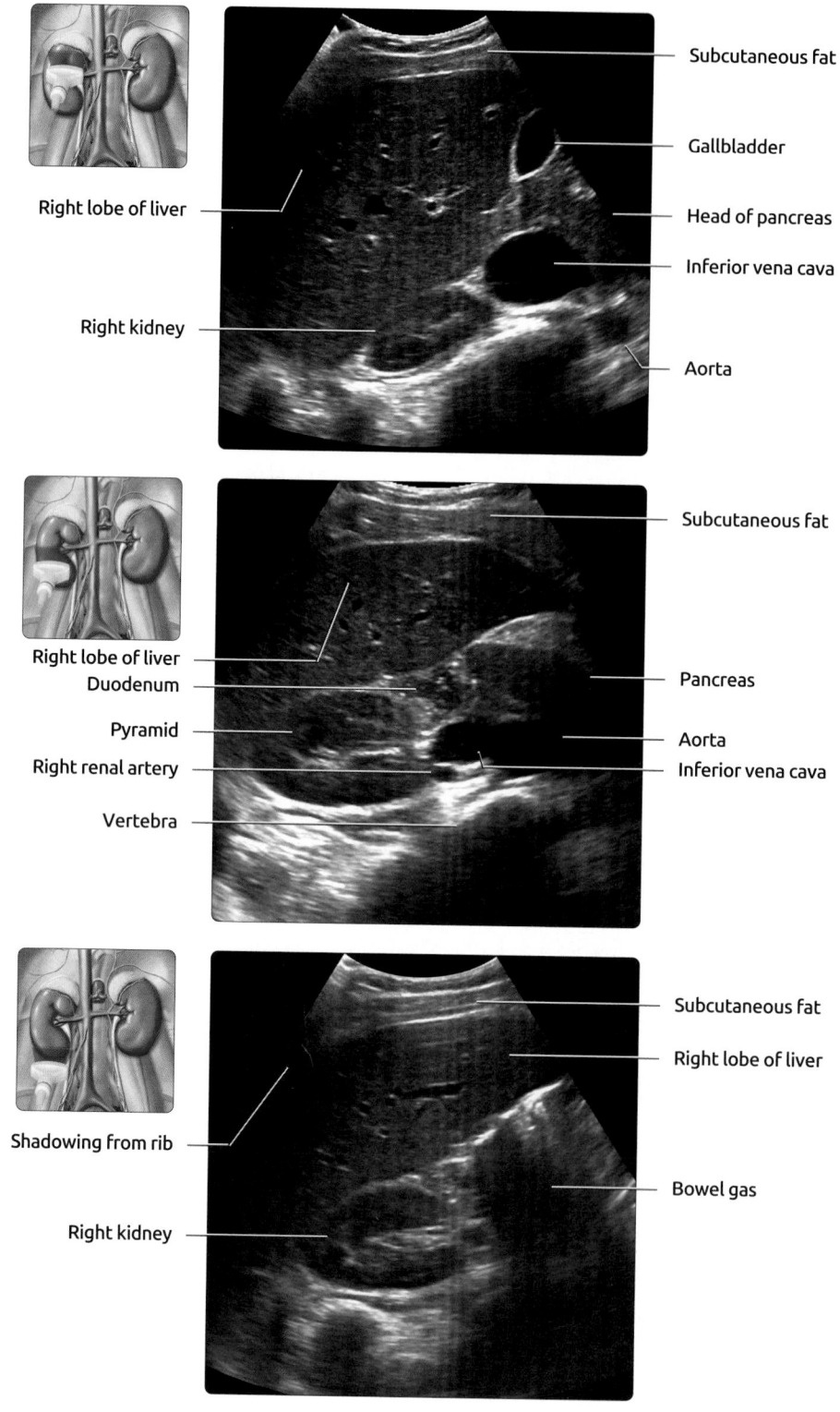

Top panel labels:
- Right lobe of liver
- Right kidney
- Subcutaneous fat
- Gallbladder
- Head of pancreas
- Inferior vena cava
- Aorta

Middle panel labels:
- Right lobe of liver
- Duodenum
- Pyramid
- Right renal artery
- Vertebra
- Subcutaneous fat
- Pancreas
- Aorta
- Inferior vena cava

Bottom panel labels:
- Shadowing from rib
- Right kidney
- Subcutaneous fat
- Right lobe of liver
- Bowel gas

(Top) *Transverse grayscale ultrasound of the upper pole of the right kidney is shown.* **(Middle)** *Transverse grayscale ultrasound of the mid pole of the right kidney shows the renal hilum with the renal vein. Note that the pelvicalyceal system within the renal sinus echoes is not usually visible in the normal individual.* **(Bottom)** *Transverse grayscale ultrasound of the lower pole of the right kidney. The renal parenchymal echogenicity is less than the adjacent liver or spleen. If the renal parenchyma is brighter than normal liver, renal parenchymal disease should be suspected.*

RIGHT KIDNEY, CT CORRELATION

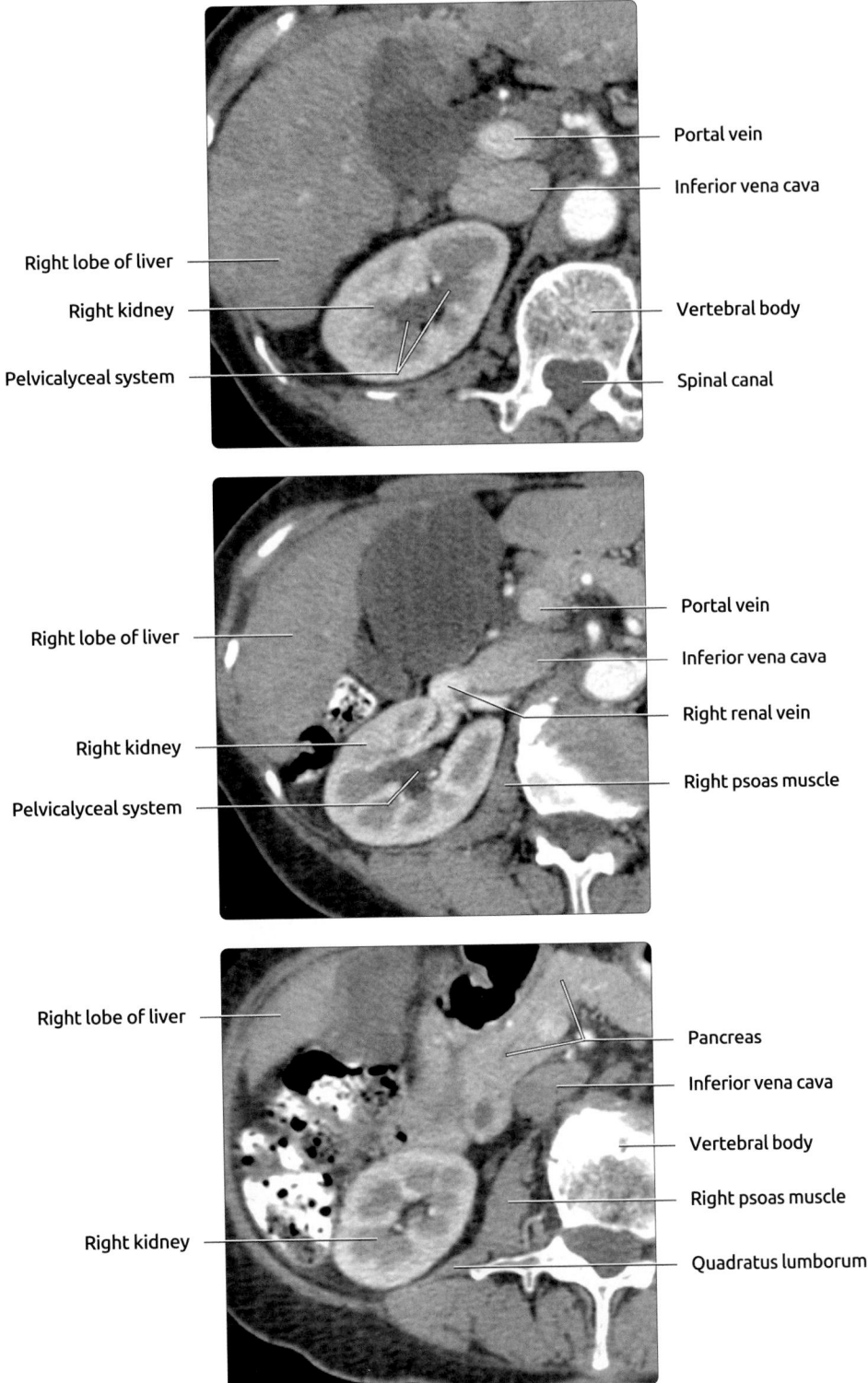

(Top) The 1st in a series of 3 correlative transverse CT images of the right kidney, from the upper pole through the kidney to the lower pole, is shown through planes commonly used when examining the patient with ultrasound. This image shows the upper pole of the right kidney. Multidetector row CT with examination in different phases, following intravenous contrast injection, allows superb differentiation between the renal cortex and medulla. (Middle) Correlative transverse CT of the mid pole of the right kidney shows the renal hilum with the renal vein. (Bottom) Correlative transverse CT image of the lower pole of the right kidney.

RIGHT KIDNEY, POSTERIOR ABDOMEN SCAN

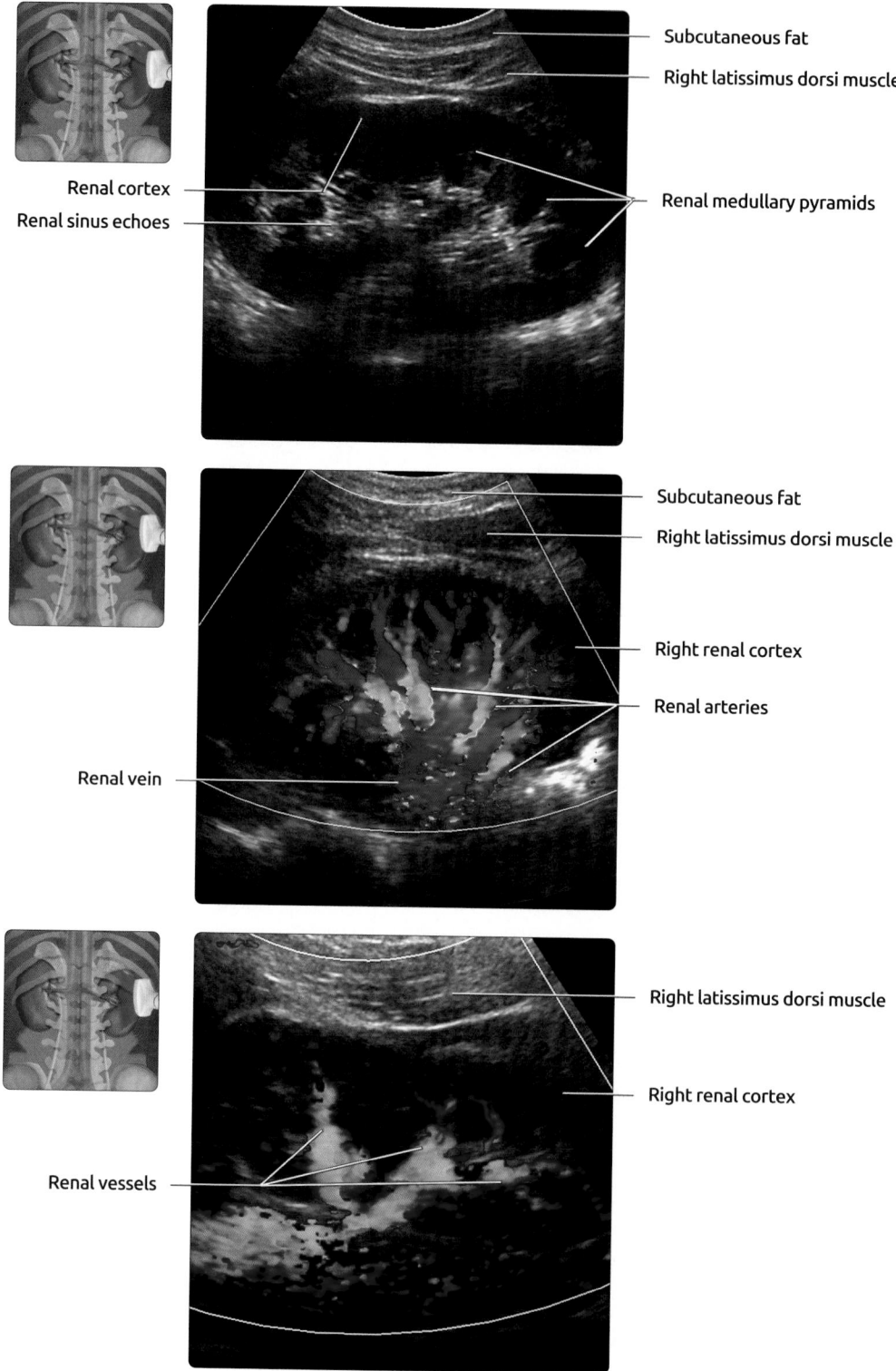

Subcutaneous fat

Right latissimus dorsi muscle

Renal cortex

Renal sinus echoes

Renal medullary pyramids

Subcutaneous fat

Right latissimus dorsi muscle

Right renal cortex

Renal arteries

Renal vein

Right latissimus dorsi muscle

Right renal cortex

Renal vessels

(Top) Longitudinal grayscale ultrasound of the right kidney scanning from the posterior approach shows normal medullary pyramids. It is a good way for standardizing renal length measurements in children. (Middle) Posterior longitudinal color Doppler ultrasound of the right kidney is shown. This evaluation of the position of major vessels is useful to avoid major vessels during renal interventional procedures, such as renal biopsy or nephrostomy. (Bottom) Posterior longitudinal power Doppler ultrasound of the right kidney is shown. Note that power Doppler ultrasound does not provide information about the direction of flow within vessels.

RIGHT KIDNEY, POSTERIOR ABDOMEN SCAN

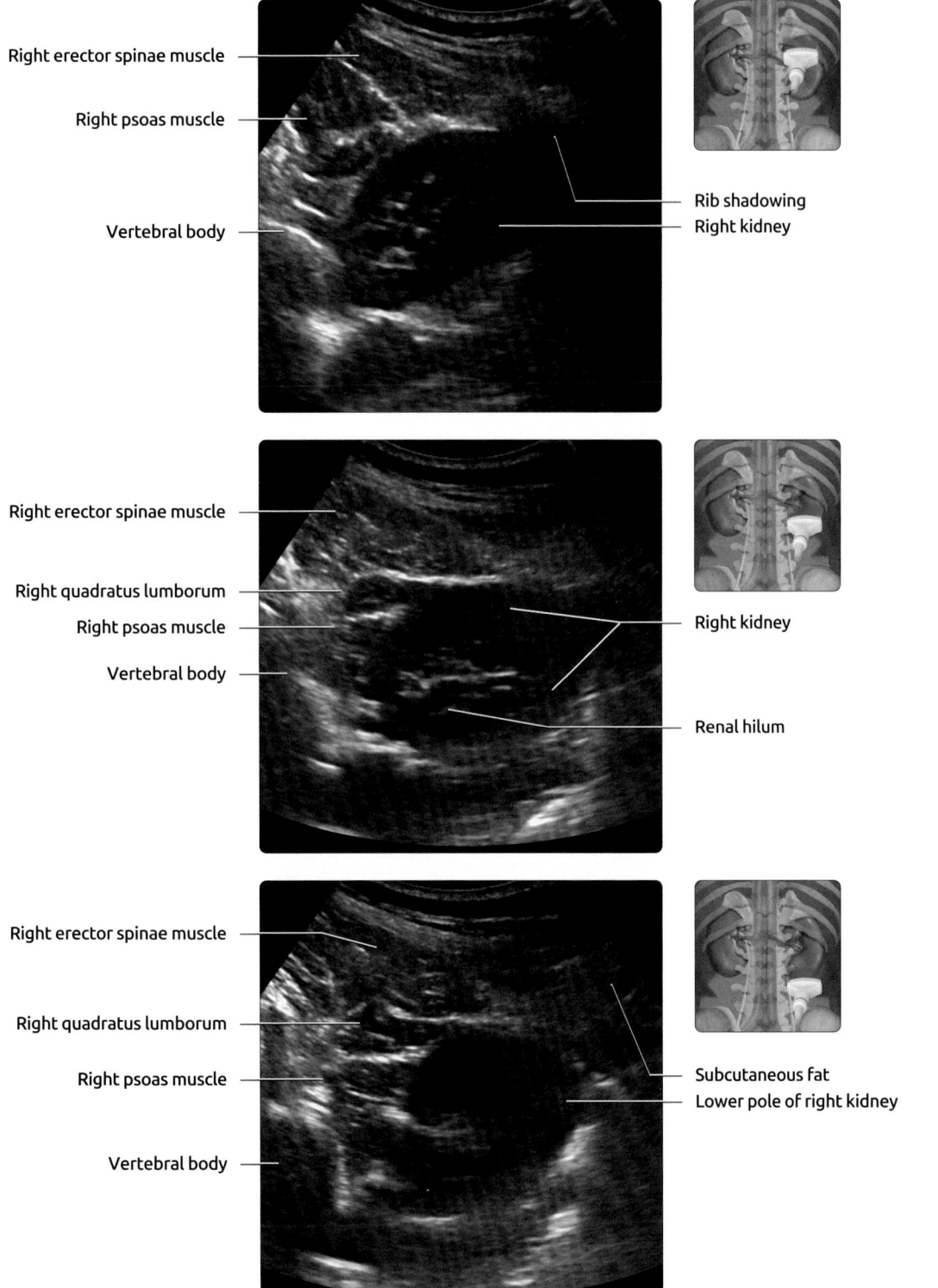

Right erector spinae muscle

Right psoas muscle

Vertebral body

Rib shadowing
Right kidney

Right erector spinae muscle

Right quadratus lumborum

Right psoas muscle

Vertebral body

Right kidney

Renal hilum

Right erector spinae muscle

Right quadratus lumborum

Right psoas muscle

Vertebral body

Subcutaneous fat
Lower pole of right kidney

(Top) *Transverse grayscale ultrasound of the right kidney scanning from the posterior approach is shown. Scanning through the posterior approach is useful while performing interventional procedures, such as nephrostomy or renal biopsy. However, visualization/image quality may be impaired by thick paraspinal muscles and rib shadowing. This image shows the upper pole of the right kidney.* (Middle) *Transverse grayscale ultrasound from the posterior approach shows the mid pole of the right kidney.* (Bottom) *Transverse grayscale ultrasound from the posterior approach shows the lower pole of the right kidney.*

RIGHT MAIN RENAL ARTERY AND VEIN

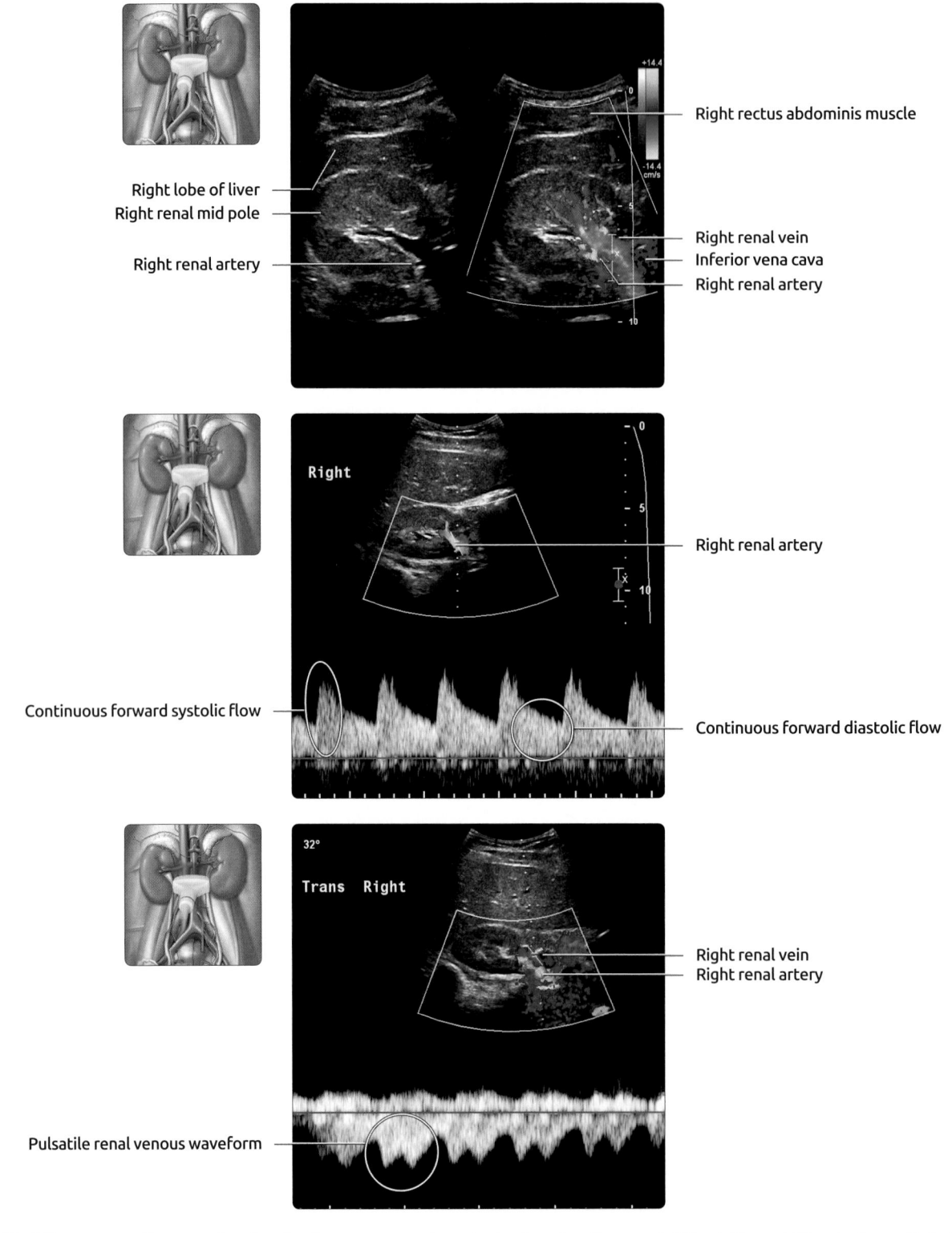

Right rectus abdominis muscle

Right lobe of liver

Right renal mid pole

Right renal artery

Right renal vein
Inferior vena cava
Right renal artery

Right renal artery

Continuous forward systolic flow

Continuous forward diastolic flow

Right renal vein
Right renal artery

Pulsatile renal venous waveform

(Top) *Transverse split screen showing simultaneous grayscale and color Doppler ultrasound of the right renal hilum is shown. Note that the right renal artery lies posterior to the renal vein and inferior vena cava. The renal artery normally measures 5-8 mm in caliber.* (Middle) *In this spectral Doppler waveform of the right renal artery, note the low-resistance renal waveform with continuous forward systolic and diastolic flow. Normal PSV ranges from 60-140 cm/s; not more than 180 cm/s. Normal resistivity index is < 0.7 and normal pulsatility index is < 1.8.* (Bottom) *Spectral Doppler waveform of the right renal vein is shown, which mirrors the pulsatility in the inferior vena cava. The renal vein normally measures 4-9 mm in caliber. Normal PSV ranges from 18-33 cm/s.*

RIGHT INTRARENAL ARTERY AND VEIN

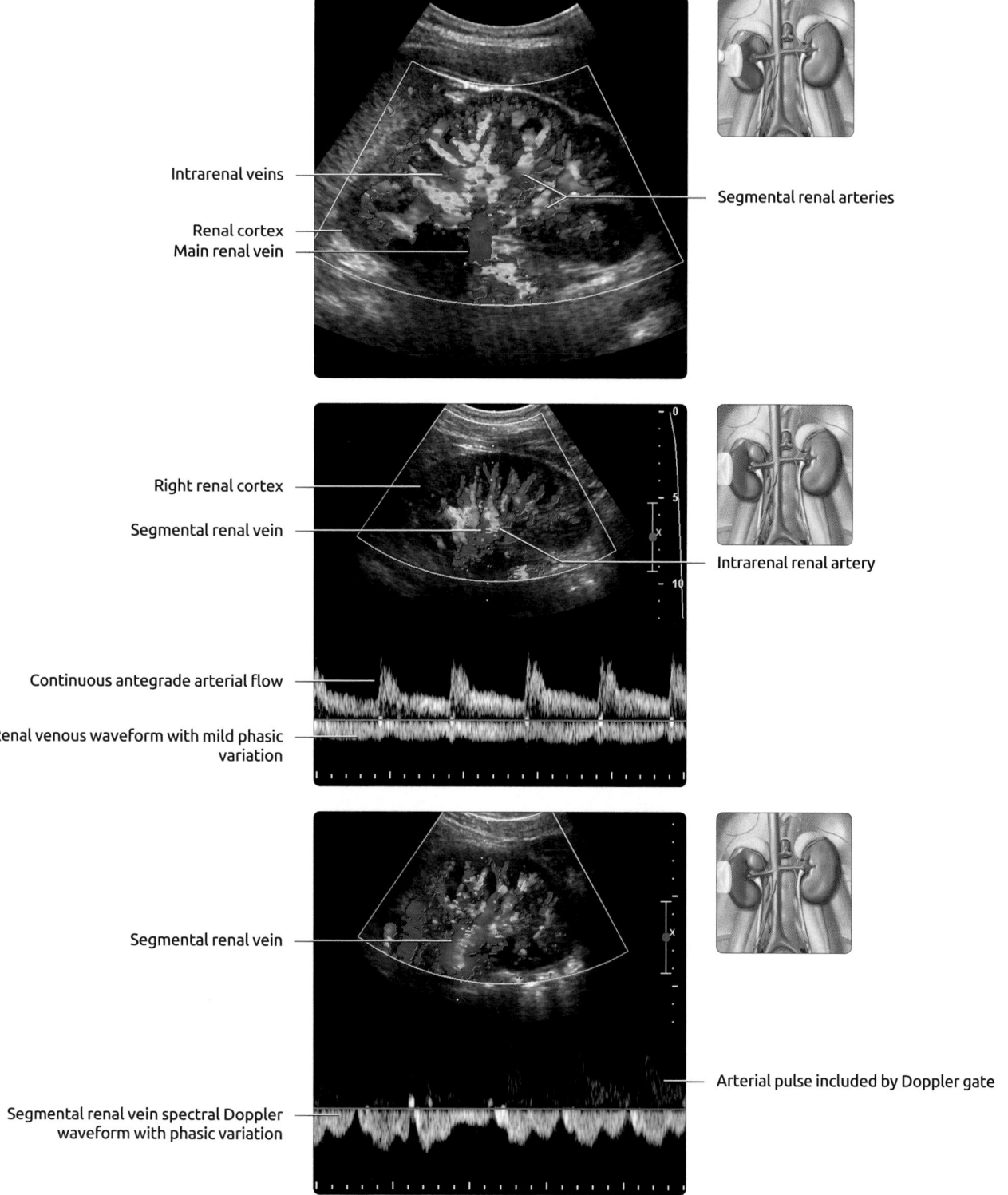

Intrarenal veins

Segmental renal arteries

Renal cortex
Main renal vein

Right renal cortex

Segmental renal vein

Intrarenal renal artery

Continuous antegrade arterial flow

Renal venous waveform with mild phasic variation

Segmental renal vein

Arterial pulse included by Doppler gate

Segmental renal vein spectral Doppler waveform with phasic variation

(Top) *Longitudinal color Doppler ultrasound of the right kidney shows renal artery branches as red and renal vein branches as blue.* **(Middle)** *In this spectral Doppler waveform of a right segmental renal artery branch, note the low-resistance arterial Doppler waveform with continuous diastolic flow, similar to that seen in the more proximal renal artery. The venous waveform shows minimal phasicity.* **(Bottom)** *In this spectral Doppler waveform of a right segmental renal vein branch, note the phasic variation in the renal vein, which can vary depending on systemic venous pressure and cardiac and fluid status.*

LEFT KIDNEY, POSTEROLATERAL SCAN

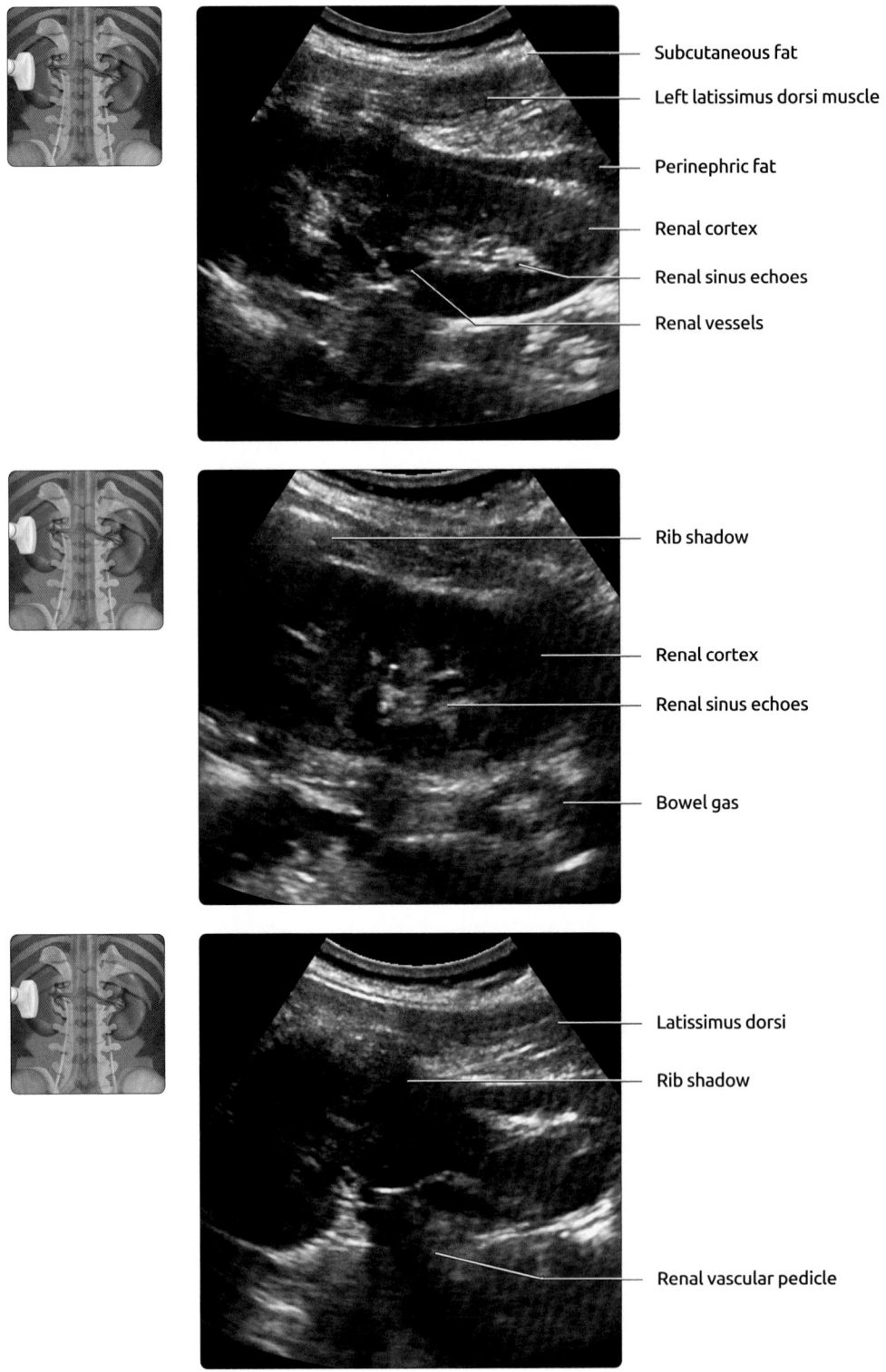

Subcutaneous fat

Left latissimus dorsi muscle

Perinephric fat

Renal cortex

Renal sinus echoes

Renal vessels

Rib shadow

Renal cortex

Renal sinus echoes

Bowel gas

Latissimus dorsi

Rib shadow

Renal vascular pedicle

(Top) *Longitudinal grayscale ultrasound of the left kidney scanning from the posterolateral approach is shown. This approach avoids interference from bowel gas shadowing.* **(Middle)** *Longitudinal grayscale ultrasound of the left kidney scanning from the posterolateral approach with the transducer angling more posteriorly when compared with the previous image. Note shadowing from rib degrading imaging of the upper pole.* **(Bottom)** *Longitudinal grayscale ultrasound of the left kidney scanning from the posterolateral approach with the transducer angling more anteriorly when compared with the previous 2 images.*

LEFT KIDNEY, CT CORRELATION

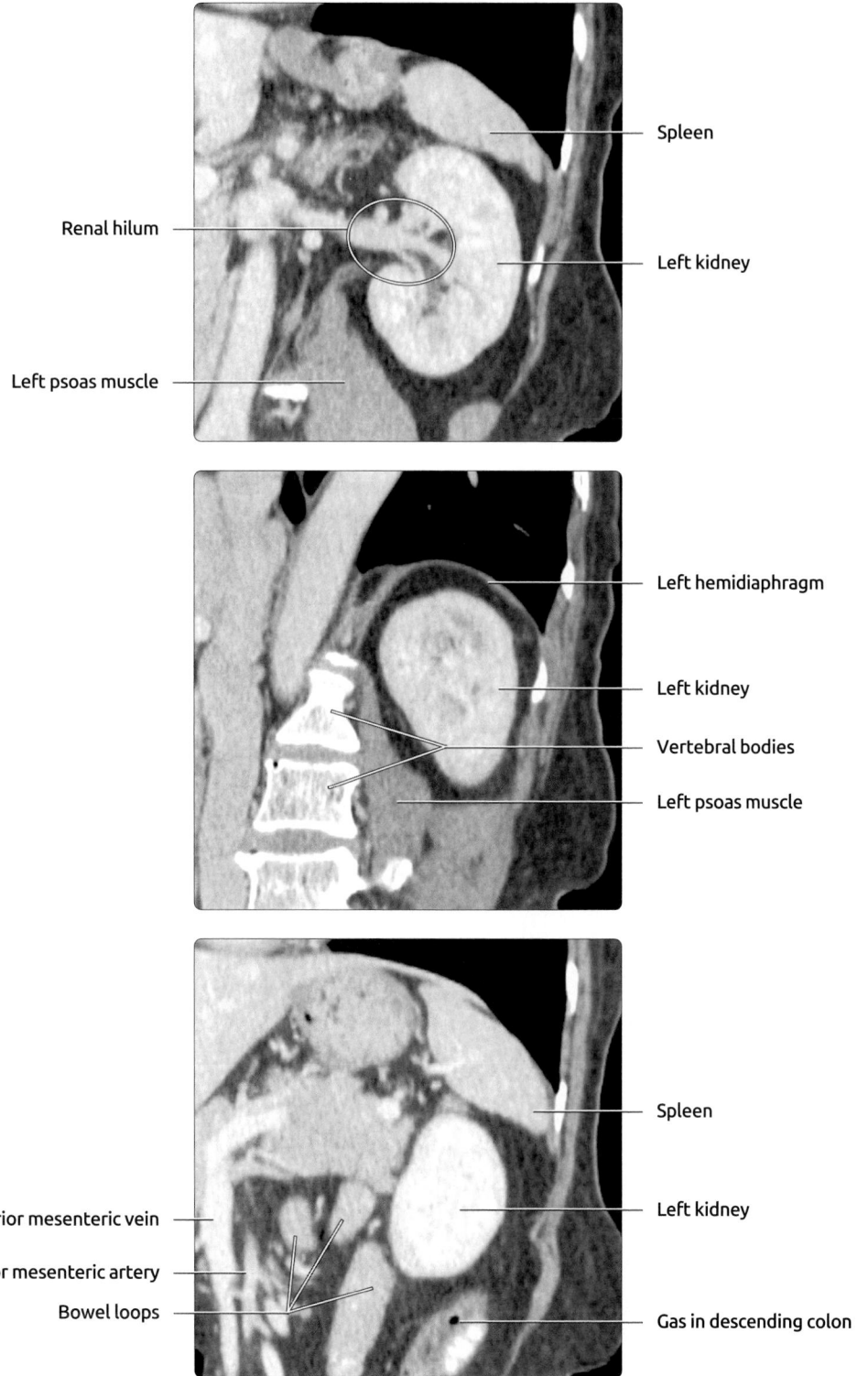

Spleen

Renal hilum

Left kidney

Left psoas muscle

Left hemidiaphragm

Left kidney

Vertebral bodies

Left psoas muscle

Spleen

Superior mesenteric vein

Left kidney

Superior mesenteric artery

Bowel loops

Gas in descending colon

(Top) *The 1st in a series of 3 correlative longitudinal oblique multiplanar reconstruction CT images of the left kidney, through planes commonly used when examining the patient with ultrasound, shows clear visualization of the kidney, renal pedicle, and surrounding structures. This makes multidetector row CT the imaging modality of choice (over ultrasound) in patients suspected to have renal injury.* **(Middle)** *Correlative longitudinal oblique multiplanar reconstruction CT of the left kidney in a plane more posterior to the previous image.* **(Bottom)** *Correlative longitudinal oblique multiplanar reconstruction CT of the left kidney in a plane more anterior than the previous 2 images.*

LEFT KIDNEY, ANTERO LATERAL TRANSVERSE SCAN

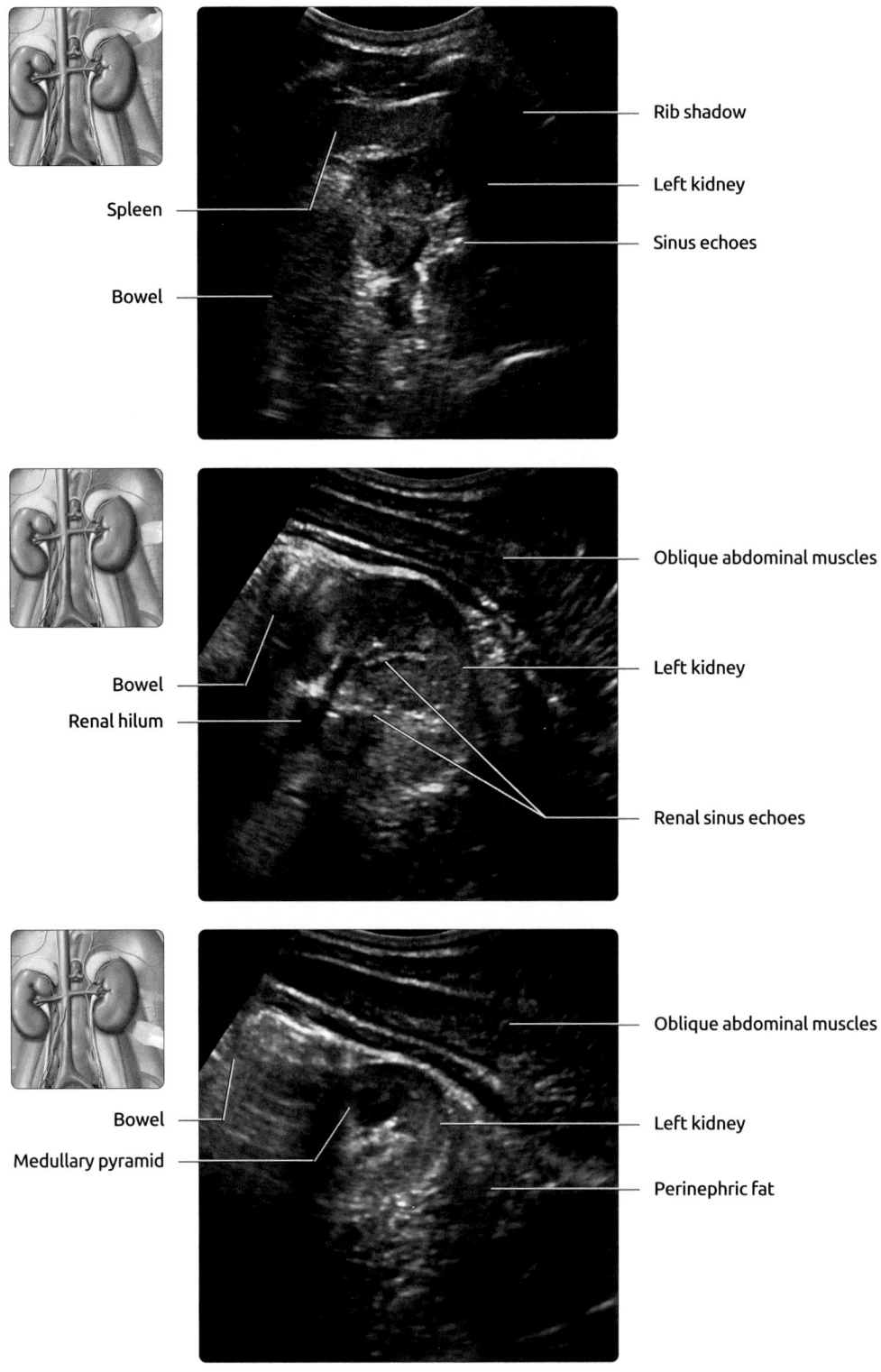

Spleen

Bowel

Rib shadow

Left kidney

Sinus echoes

Bowel

Renal hilum

Oblique abdominal muscles

Left kidney

Renal sinus echoes

Bowel

Medullary pyramid

Oblique abdominal muscles

Left kidney

Perinephric fat

(Top) Transverse grayscale ultrasound of the upper pole of the left kidney using the anterolateral approach. Note that the image quality is limited by interference from gas in the stomach and bowel. The presence of bowel loops anteriorly also limits the use of this approach for interventional procedures on the left kidney. (Middle) Transverse grayscale ultrasound of the mid pole of the left kidney using the anterolateral approach. (Bottom) Transverse grayscale ultrasound of the lower pole of the left kidney using the anterolateral approach.

LEFT KIDNEY, CT CORRELATION

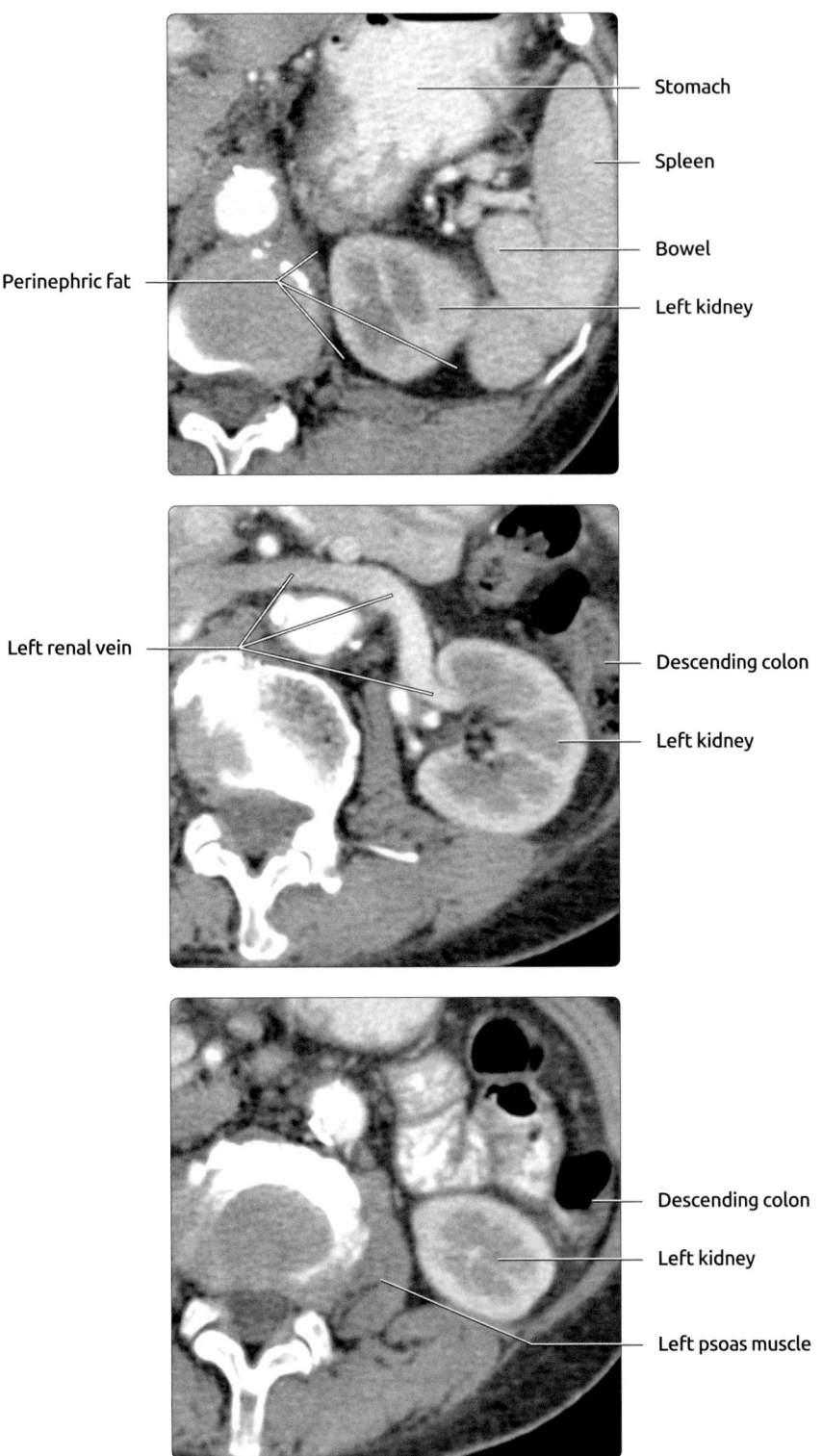

Stomach

Spleen

Bowel

Left kidney

Perinephric fat

Left renal vein

Descending colon

Left kidney

Descending colon

Left kidney

Left psoas muscle

(Top) *The 1st in a series of 3 correlative transverse CT images of the left kidney, through planes commonly used when examining the kidney, is shown using the anterior approach. Note the relationship of the spleen to the upper pole of the left kidney, allowing it to be used as an acoustic window, particularly in patients with splenomegaly. This transverse CT image shows the upper pole of the left kidney.* **(Middle)** *Correlative transverse CT image of the mid pole of the left kidney at the level of the left renal vein.* **(Bottom)** *Correlative transverse CT image of the lower pole of the left kidney.*

LEFT KIDNEY, ANTERIOR TO ANTEROLATERAL TRANSVERSE SCAN

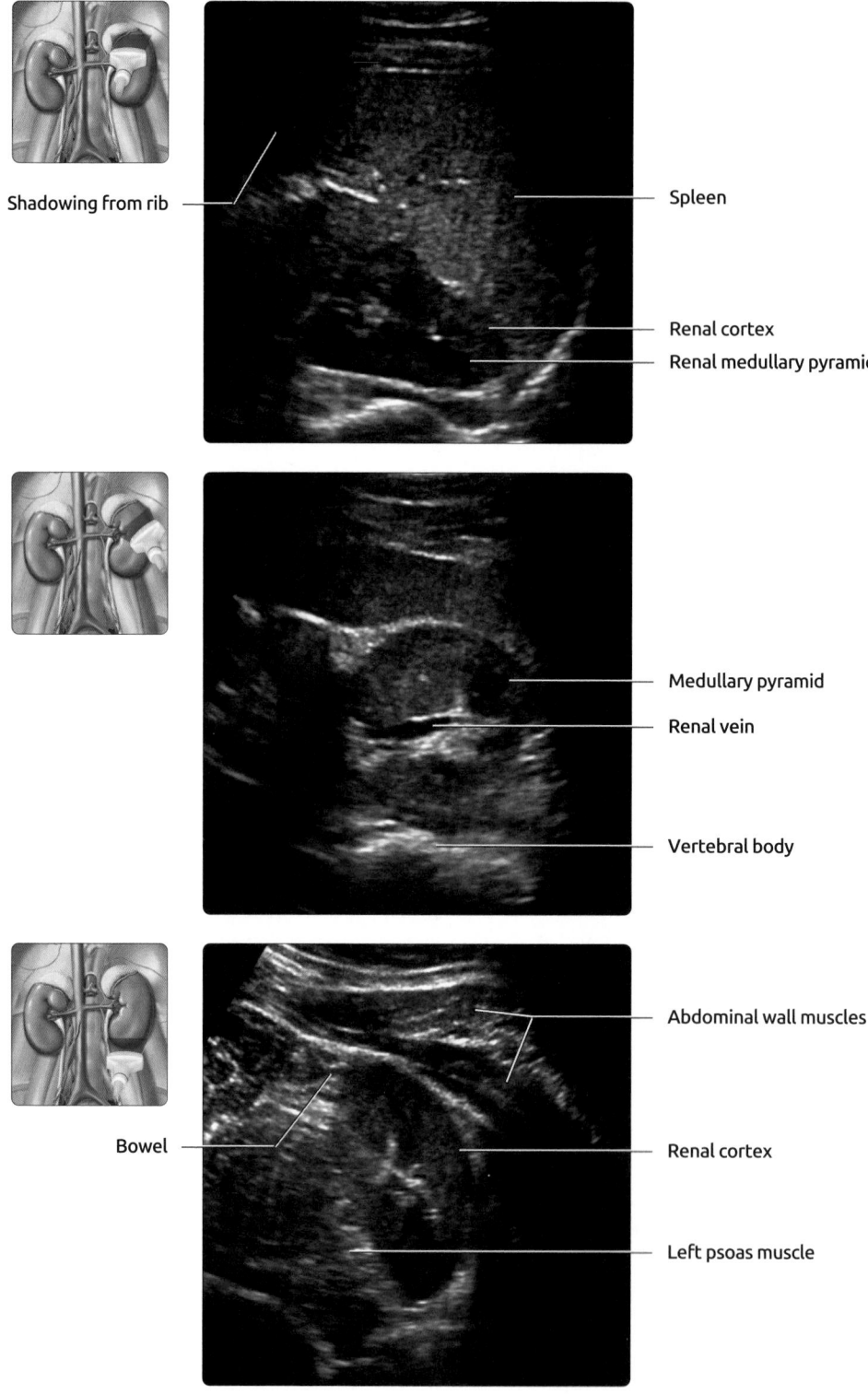

Shadowing from rib

Spleen

Renal cortex

Renal medullary pyramid

Medullary pyramid

Renal vein

Vertebral body

Bowel

Abdominal wall muscles

Renal cortex

Left psoas muscle

(Top) *Transverse grayscale ultrasound of the upper pole of the left kidney using the anterolateral approach. Note the proximity of the kidney to the skin surface and the absence of intervening bowel loops. Adjacent spleen provides an imaging window; however, ribs cast a shadow.* **(Middle)** *Transverse grayscale ultrasound of the mid pole of the left kidney using the posterolateral approach.* **(Bottom)** *Transverse grayscale ultrasound of the lower pole of the left kidney using the posterolateral approach.*

LEFT KIDNEY, POSTERIOR ABDOMEN SCAN

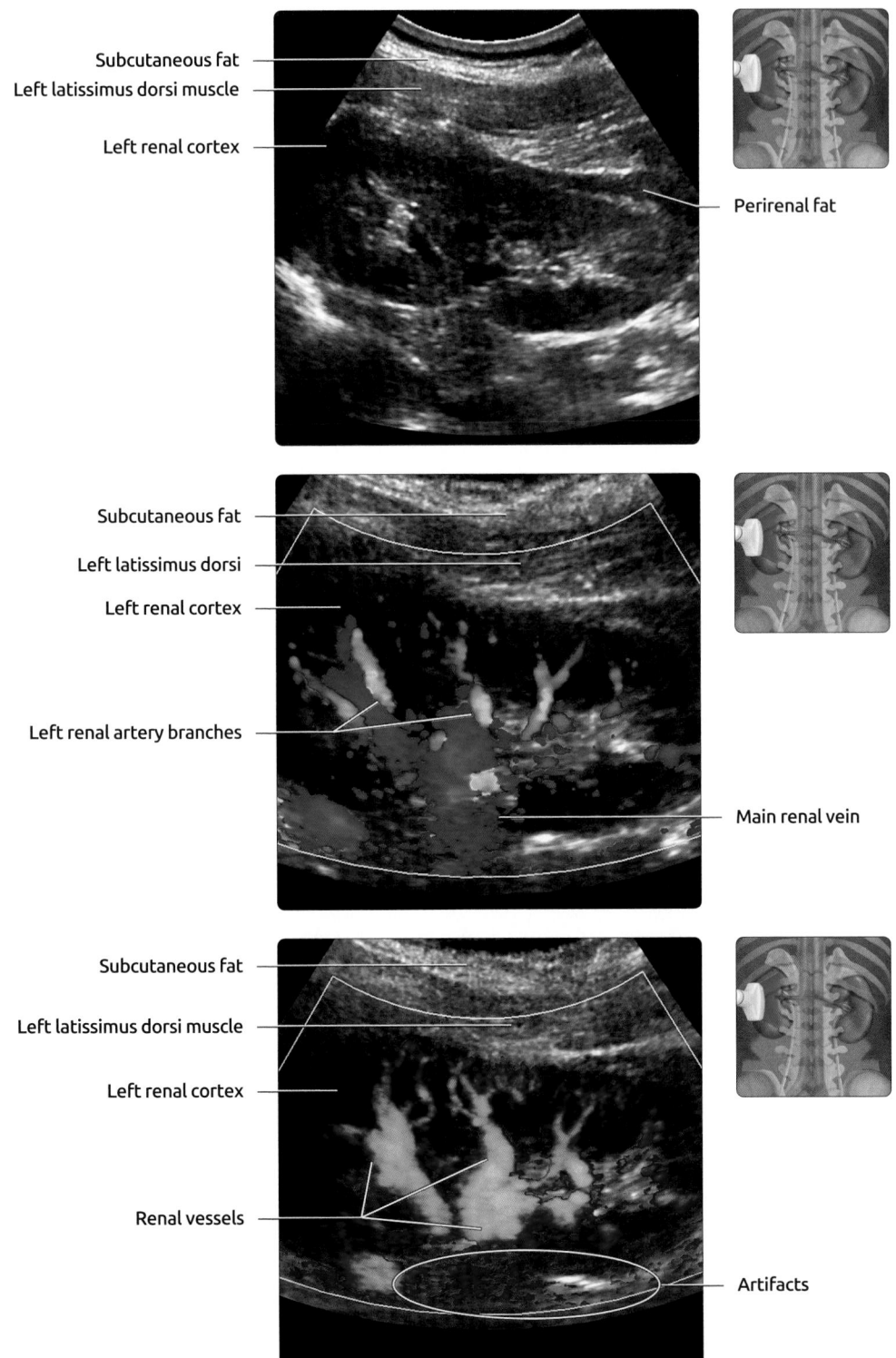

Subcutaneous fat
Left latissimus dorsi muscle
Left renal cortex
Perirenal fat

Subcutaneous fat
Left latissimus dorsi
Left renal cortex
Left renal artery branches
Main renal vein

Subcutaneous fat
Left latissimus dorsi muscle
Left renal cortex
Renal vessels
Artifacts

(Top) *Longitudinal grayscale ultrasound of the left kidney scanning from the posterior approach shows renal veins that may mimic hydronephrosis. Color Doppler ultrasound should be used to differentiate fluid from vessels. This view is useful for performing renal interventional procedures, such as renal biopsy or nephrostomy. It is also a good way for standardizing renal length measurements in children.* (Middle) *Posterior longitudinal color Doppler ultrasound of the left kidney is shown. This assessment of the position of major vessels is useful for avoiding major vessels when performing renal interventional procedures, such as renal biopsy or nephrostomy.* (Bottom) *In this posterior longitudinal power Doppler ultrasound of the left kidney, note the absence of information about flow direction on power Doppler. Motion artifact is more evident on power Doppler.*

LEFT KIDNEY, POSTERIOR ABDOMEN SCAN

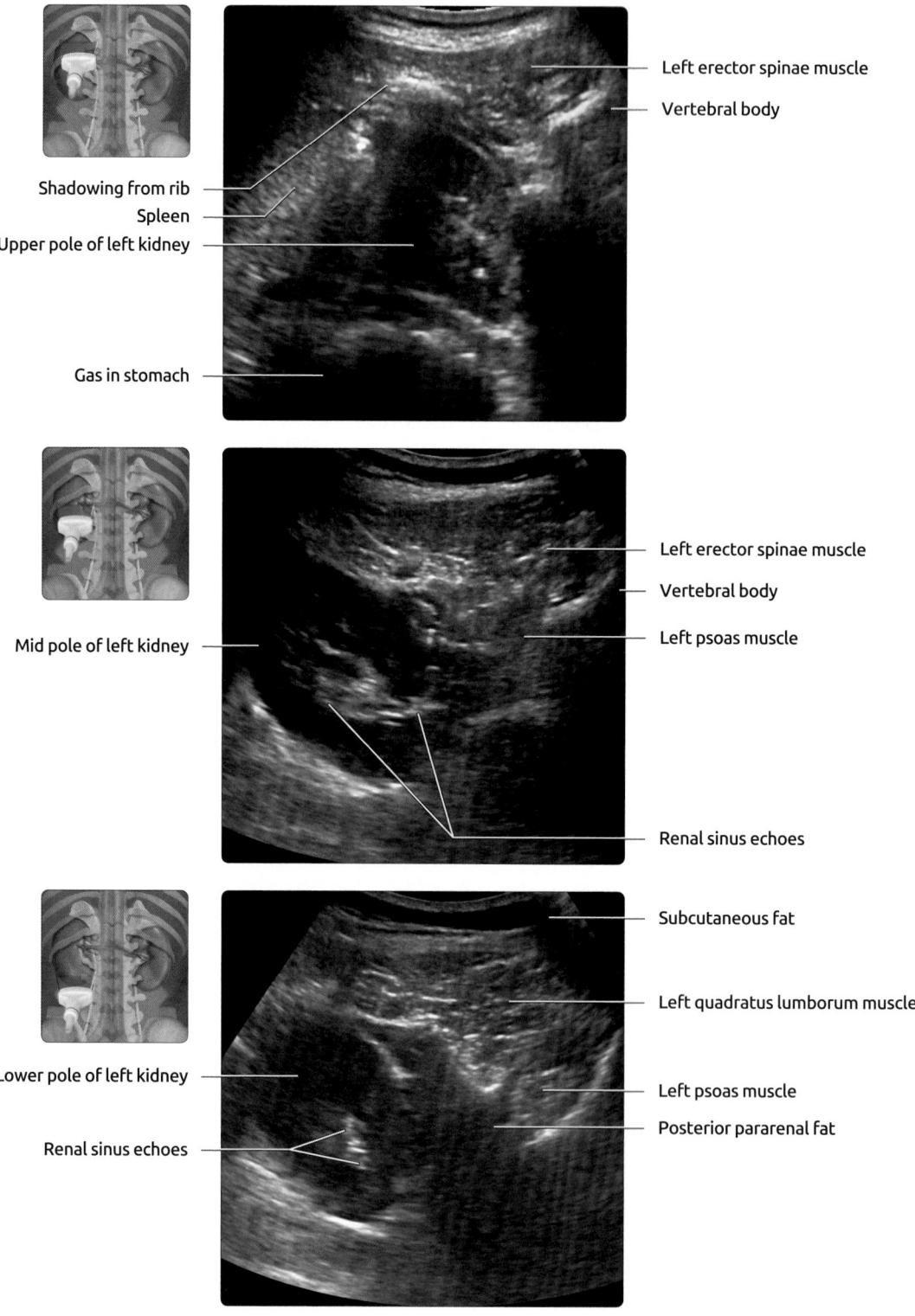

Shadowing from rib

Spleen

Upper pole of left kidney

Gas in stomach

Left erector spinae muscle

Vertebral body

Mid pole of left kidney

Left erector spinae muscle

Vertebral body

Left psoas muscle

Renal sinus echoes

Lower pole of left kidney

Renal sinus echoes

Subcutaneous fat

Left quadratus lumborum muscle

Left psoas muscle

Posterior pararenal fat

(Top) *Transverse grayscale ultrasound of the upper pole of the left kidney using the posterior approach is shown. Note the proximity of the kidney to the skin surface and absence of intervening bowel/other major structures, making this a suitable approach for renal interventional procedures.* **(Middle)** *Transverse grayscale ultrasound of the upper pole of the left kidney using the posterior approach shows the proximity of the kidney to the skin surface and absence of intervening bowel/other major structures, making this a suitable approach for renal interventional procedures.* **(Bottom)** *Transverse grayscale ultrasound of the lower pole of the left kidney using the posterior approach is shown.*

LEFT MAIN RENAL ARTERY AND VEIN

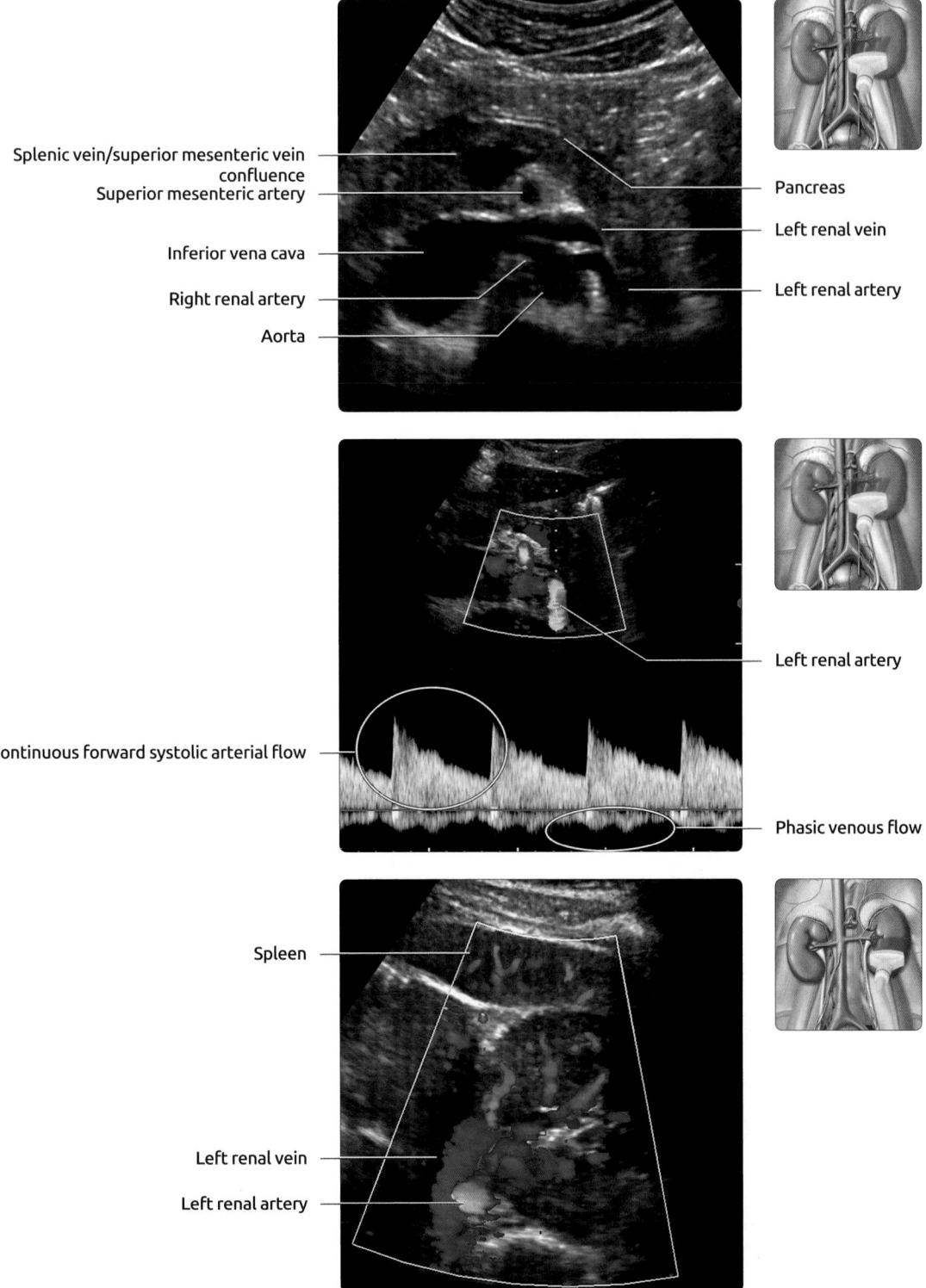

Splenic vein/superior mesenteric vein confluence

Superior mesenteric artery

Inferior vena cava

Right renal artery

Aorta

Pancreas

Left renal vein

Left renal artery

Left renal artery

Continuous forward systolic arterial flow

Phasic venous flow

Spleen

Left renal vein

Left renal artery

(Top) *Transverse ultrasound in the anterior midline shows that the left renal artery arises from the anterolateral aorta just around or below the level of the superior mesenteric artery. The normal caliber of the renal artery ranges from 5-8 mm. The left renal vein courses between the aorta and superior mesenteric artery.* (Middle) *Spectral Doppler waveform of the left renal artery and vein is shown. The normal PSV in the artery ranges from 60-140 cm/s with a normal resistive index < 0.7 and pulsatility index < 1.8. There is variability in venous velocity consequent upon cardiac and respiratory activity. The renal vein normally measures 4-9 mm in caliber with a PSV of 18-33 cm/s.* (Bottom) *Transverse color Doppler waveform of the left renal hilum obtained from an anterolateral approach is shown. An anterior approach may not be feasible secondary to bowel gas. The left renal artery is posterior to the left renal vein.*

LEFT INTRARENAL ARTERY AND VEIN

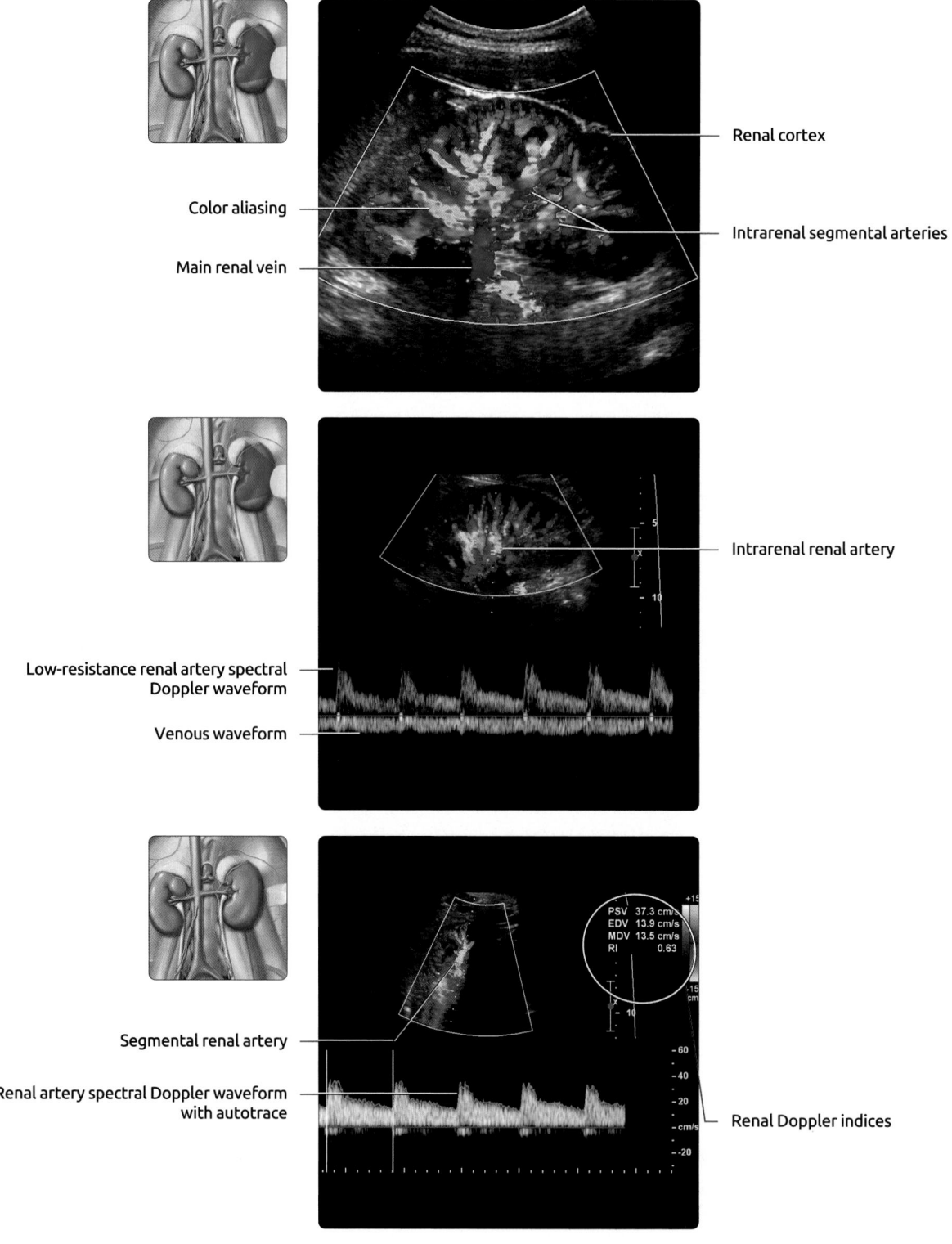

Renal cortex

Color aliasing

Intrarenal segmental arteries

Main renal vein

Intrarenal renal artery

Low-resistance renal artery spectral Doppler waveform

Venous waveform

PSV 37.3 cm/s
EDV 13.9 cm/s
MDV 13.5 cm/s
RI 0.63

Segmental renal artery

Renal artery spectral Doppler waveform with autotrace

Renal Doppler indices

(Top) Longitudinal color Doppler ultrasound of the left kidney shows renal artery branches as red and renal vein branches as blue. There is some color aliasing in the veins, shown as yellow. (Middle) In this spectral Doppler waveform of a left segmental renal artery, there is continuous flow throughout the cardiac cycle with a low-resistance pattern. The segmental renal vein shows mild phasicity. (Bottom) Spectral Doppler waveform of a left segmental renal artery in the transverse plane is shown. Doppler indices are normal: PSV of 37.3 cm/s, EDV of 13.9 cm/s, and resistive index (RI) of 0.63.

MULTIPLANAR ULTRASOUND OF RIGHT KIDNEY

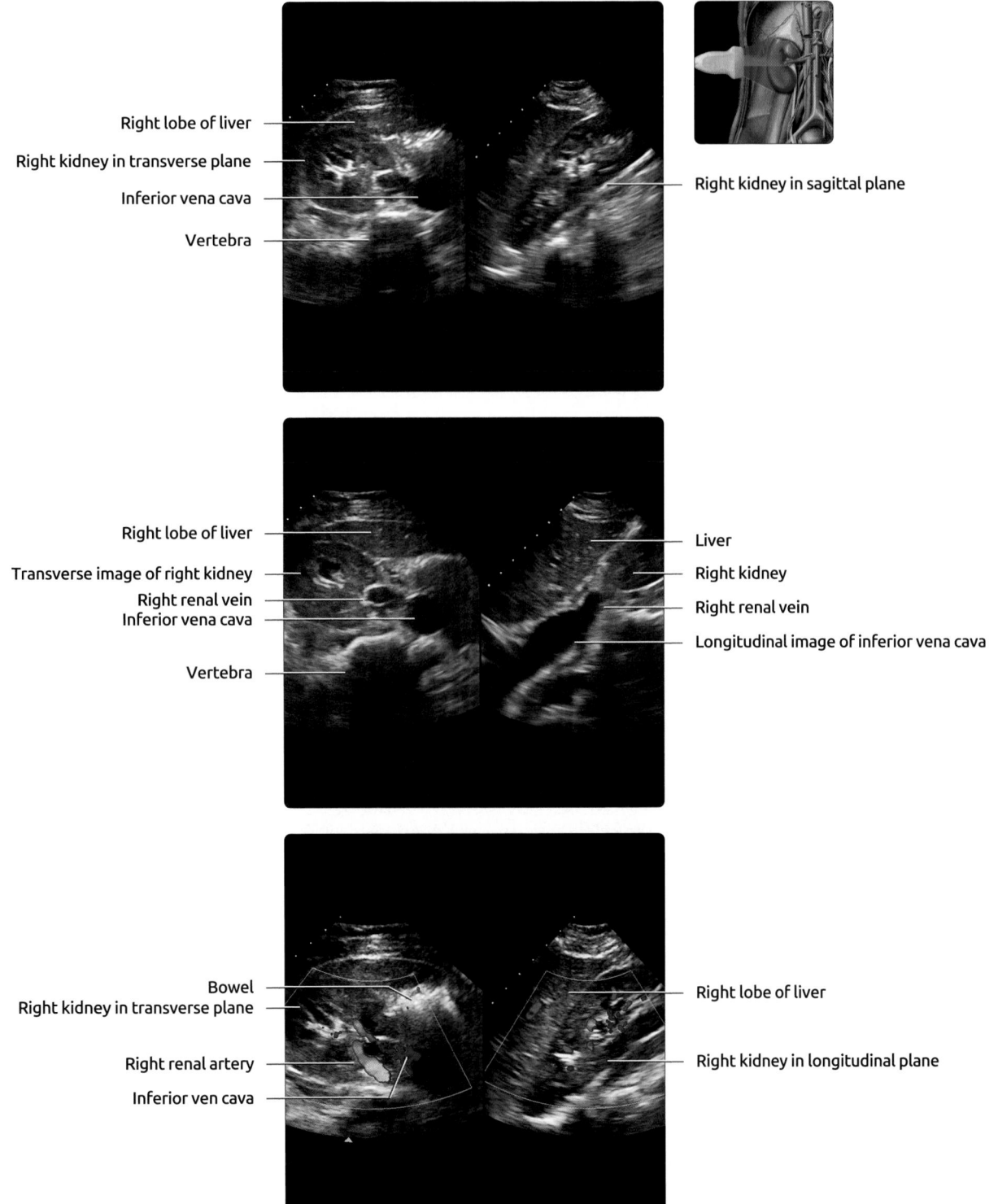

Right lobe of liver

Right kidney in transverse plane

Inferior vena cava

Vertebra

Right kidney in sagittal plane

Right lobe of liver

Transverse image of right kidney

Right renal vein

Inferior vena cava

Vertebra

Liver

Right kidney

Right renal vein

Longitudinal image of inferior vena cava

Bowel

Right kidney in transverse plane

Right renal artery

Inferior ven cava

Right lobe of liver

Right kidney in longitudinal plane

(Top) *3D real-time ultrasound with a matrix probe in shown in which simultaneous axial and sagittal images are obtained. The sagittal plane can be steered electronically to obtain the long axis of the kidney.* (Middle) *In this 3D real-time ultrasound with a matrix probe, the sagittal plane has been steered electronically to obtain a longitudinal view of the inferior vena cava and right renal vein.* (Bottom) *3D real-time ultrasound with a matrix probe in shown in which simultaneous axial and sagittal images are obtained. This technology can enable imaging in planes not otherwise feasible.*

GROSS ANATOMY

Divisions

- Esophagus: Cervical and thoracic segments
- Stomach
  - Hollow muscular organ between esophagus and small intestine
  - Location: Intraperitoneal, in left upper quadrant, bordered superiorly by left hemidiaphragm, posterolaterally by spleen, posteroinferiorly by pancreas
    - Greater omentum attached from greater curvature and drapes over small and large intestines
    - Lesser omentum attached from lesser curvature to porta hepatis, covers lesser sac
  - Function
    - Gastric acid production for breakdown of large molecules of food into smaller molecules in preparation for small intestinal absorption
    - Storage of food
  - Sections
    - Gastroesophageal junction/cardia, lower esophageal sphincter
    - Fundus and body: Delineated by horizontal plane passing through cardia
    - Antrum/pylorus: Lower section facilitating entry of gastric contents into duodenum
  - Curvatures
    - Greater curvature: Lateral wall of stomach
    - Lesser curvature: Medial wall of stomach
  - Rugae/internal ridges increase surface area for digestion
  - Arterial supply
    - Right and left gastric arteries supply lesser curvature
    - Right and left gastroepiploic arteries supply greater curvature
    - Short gastric artery supplies fundus
  - Venous drainage
    - Follow arteries and drain into portal vein and its tributaries
- Small bowel
  - Between stomach and large intestine
  - ~ 4-7 meters in length
  - Centrally located in abdomen
  - Intraperitoneal, except for 2nd-4th portions of duodenum
  - Function: Further breakdown of food molecules from stomach with eventual absorption
  - Intraluminal extensions/folds valvulae conniventes increase surface area for absorption
    - Abundant in proximal small bowel, decrease in number in distal small bowel loops
  - Duodenum
    - C-shaped hollow tube connecting stomach with jejunum
    - Begins with duodenal bulb, ends in ligament of Treitz (duodenojejunal junction)
    - Arterial supply and venous drainage: Superior and inferior pancreaticoduodenal artery, pancreaticoduodenal veins
  - Jejunum
    - Connects duodenum with ileum

- ~ 2.5 meters in length
    - Begins at ligament of Treitz
    - Along with ileum, suspended by mesentery
    - Arterial supply and venous drainage: Superior mesenteric artery and vein
  - Ileum
    - Connects jejunum with ascending colon
    - ~ 3.5 meters in length
    - Along with jejunum, suspended by mesentery
    - Arterial supply and venous drainage: Superior mesenteric artery and vein
- Large bowel
  - Between small bowel and anus
  - ~ 1.5 meters in length
  - Peripherally located in abdomen
    - Cecum and appendix, transverse colon, and rectosigmoid are intraperitoneal
    - Ascending colon, descending colon, and middle rectum are retroperitoneal
    - Distal rectum is extraperitoneal
  - Function: Absorption of remaining water, storage, and elimination of waste
  - Sections
    - Ascending colon: Located in right side of abdomen, includes cecum where appendix arises
    - Hepatic flexure: Turn of colon at liver
    - Transverse colon: Traverses upper abdomen
    - Splenic flexure: Turn of colon at spleen
    - Descending colon: Left side of abdomen
    - Sigmoid/rectum: At posterior pelvis
  - With taenia coli: 3 bands of smooth muscle just under serosa
    - Haustration: Sacculations in colon resulting from contraction of taenia coli
    - Epiploic appendages: Small fat accumulations on viscera
  - Arterial supply
    - Superior mesenteric artery supplies colon from appendix through splenic flexure
    - Ileocolic branch supplies cecum
    - Right colic branch supplies ascending colon
    - Middle colic branch supplies transverse colon
    - Inferior mesenteric artery supplies descending colon through rectum
    - Left colic branch supplies descending colon
    - Sigmoid branches supply sigmoid
    - Superior rectal artery supplies superior rectum
    - Middle and inferior rectum are supplied by arteries of same name originating from internal iliac artery
  - Venous drainage
    - Superior and inferior mesenteric veins
- Anus
  - External opening of rectum
    - Termination of gastrointestinal tract
  - With sphincters for controlling defecation
  - Internal anal sphincter
    - Thin ring of smooth muscle surrounding anal canal, deep to submucosa
    - Under involuntary control
    - Continuous with muscularis propria of rectum

– Forms an incomplete ring in females
- External anal sphincter
  – Thick ring of skeletal muscle around internal anal sphincter
  – Under voluntary control
  – 3 parts from superior to inferior: Deep, superficial, and subcutaneous
- Longitudinal muscle
  – Thin muscle between internal and external anal sphincters
  – Conjoined muscle from muscularis propria of rectum and levator ani

Histology

- Bowel wall throughout GI tract has uniform general histology, comprised of 4 layers
  - Mucosa
    – Functions for absorption and secretion
    – Composed of epithelium and loose connective tissue
    – Lamina propria
    – Muscularis mucosa (deep layer of mucosa)
  - Submucosa
    – Consists of fibrous connective tissue
    – Contains Meissner plexus
  - Muscularis externa
    – Muscular layer responsible for peristalsis or propulsion of food through gut
    – Contains Auerbach plexus
  - Serosa
    – Epithelial lining continuous with peritoneum

IMAGING ANATOMY

Overview

- GI tract extends from mouth to anus
- Esophagus, which is intrathoracic, is difficult to visualize with external ultrasound due to rib cage and air-containing lungs
  - Endoluminal ultrasound performed to assess mural pathology
- Stomach to rectum lie within abdomen and pelvis
- Stomach, 1st part of duodenum, jejunum, ileum, transverse colon, and sigmoid colon suspended within peritoneal cavity by peritoneal folds and are mobile
- 2nd to 4th part of duodenum, ascending colon, descending colon, and rectum are typically extraperitoneal/retroperitoneal
  - Retroperitoneal structures have more fixed position and are easy to locate
- Stomach located in left upper quadrant
  - Identified by presence of rugae/mural folds
  - Prominent muscular layer facilitates identification of pylorus
- Small bowel loops are located centrally within abdomen
  - Abundant valvulae conniventes helps identify jejunal loops
  - Jejunalization of ileum seen in celiac disease to compensate for atrophy of folds in proximal small bowel
  - Contents of jejunal loops are usually liquid and appear hypoechoic/anechoic
- Cecum and colon identified by haustral pattern

- Located peripherally in abdomen
- Contain feces and gas
- Haustra seen as prominent curvilinear echogenic arcs with posterior reverberation
- Cecum identified by curvilinear arc of hyperechogenicity (representing feces and gas) in right lower quadrant blind-ending caudally
- Not uncommonly, cecum high-lying and may be horizontally placed
- Sigmoid colon variable length and mobile
- Junction of left colon with sigmoid colon identified in left iliac fossa by tracing descending colon
- Rectosigmoid junction has fixed position and is identified with full bladder, which acts as acoustic window
- Appendicular base normally located in right lower quadrant
  - Length and direction of tip vary
  - Retrocecal appendix and pelvic appendix can be difficult to locate transabdominally
    – Transvaginal ultrasound examination useful to identify pelvic appendix
- Normal measurements of bowel caliber
  - Small bowel < 3 cm
  - Large bowel
    – Cecum < 9 cm
    – Transverse colon < 6 cm
- Stratified appearance of bowel wall on histology is depicted by 5 distinct layers on ultrasound as alternating echogenic/sonolucent (hypoechoic) appearance (gut signature)
  - Interface of lumen and mucosa: Echogenic
  - Muscularis mucosa: Hypoechoic
  - Submucosa: Echogenic
  - Muscularis propria/externa: Hypoechoic
  - Serosa: Echogenic
- Normal bowel wall thickness < 3 mm

Bowel Motility

- Bowel is hollow viscus and is constantly mobile due to peristalsis
  - Assessing direction of flow of contents often challenging
  - When visibility permits, direction of flow can be determined by following long segments of bowel in continuous fashion
- Fixed points of bowel are easy to assess with transabdominal ultrasound
  - Pylorus, "C loop" of duodenum, and ileocecal junction useful landmarks to assess direction of content flow
- Different bowel pathologies have potential to alter normal gut motility
- Real-time dynamic ultrasound provides useful information regarding bowel mobility, which can aid in diagnosis of underlying condition
  - Cine function useful to store dynamic images for review
- Abnormal bowel identified as thickened or dilated segments
  - Thickened bowel demonstrates reduced peristalsis
    – Stands out among normally peristalsing loops of normal bowel

GASTROINTESTINAL TRACT IN SITU

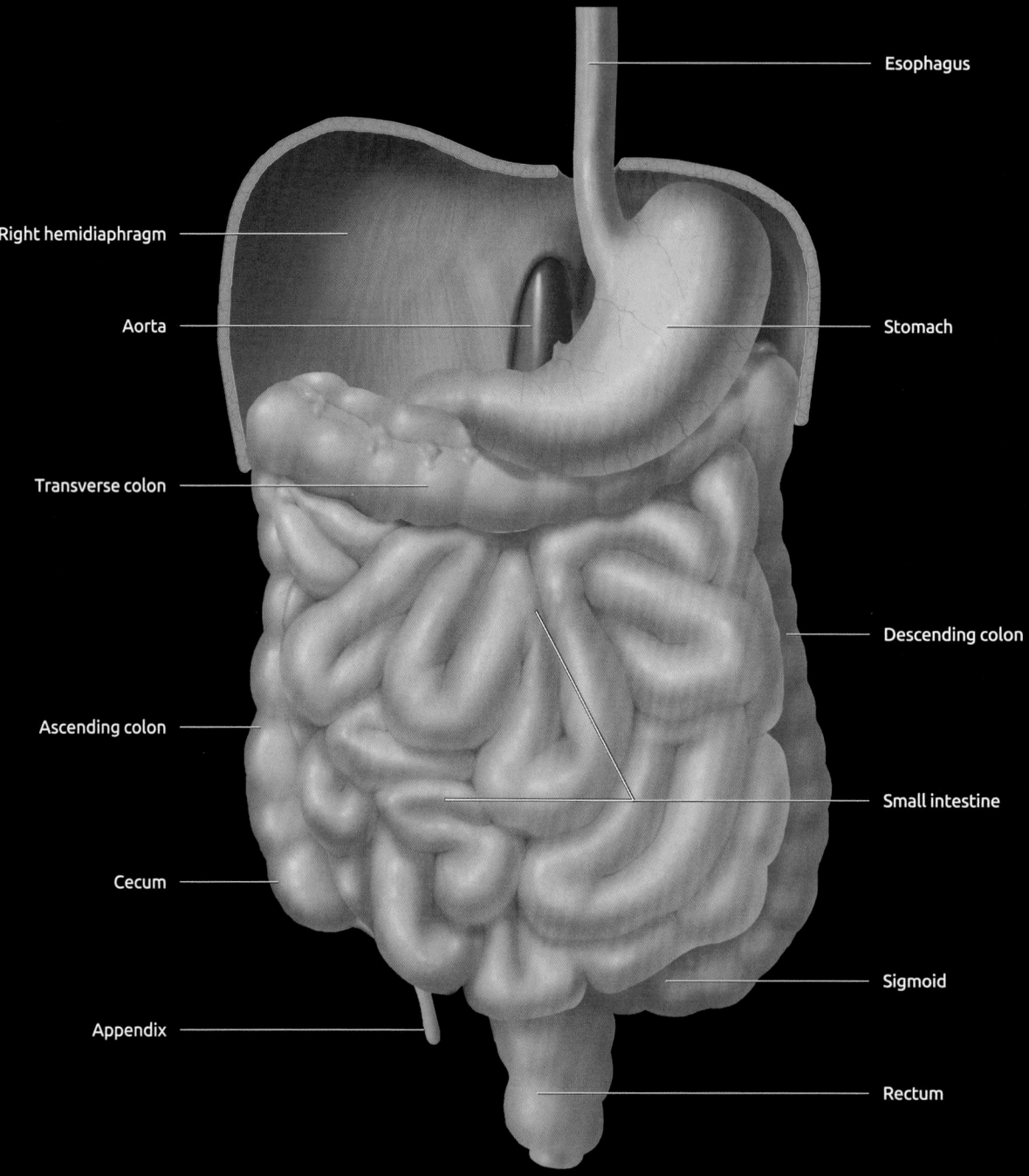

Esophagus

Right hemidiaphragm

Aorta

Stomach

Transverse colon

Descending colon

Ascending colon

Small intestine

Cecum

Sigmoid

Appendix

Rectum

Graphic shows the gastrointestinal tract in situ. The liver and the greater omentum have been removed. Note the relatively central location of the small intestine compared with the peripherally located large intestine. Most of the bowel segments are intraperitoneal, apart from the 2nd to 4th parts of the duodenum, the ascending and descending colon, and middle 1/3 of the rectum, which are retroperitoneal. The distal 1/3 of the rectum is extraperitoneal.

STOMACH AND DUODENUM IN SITU

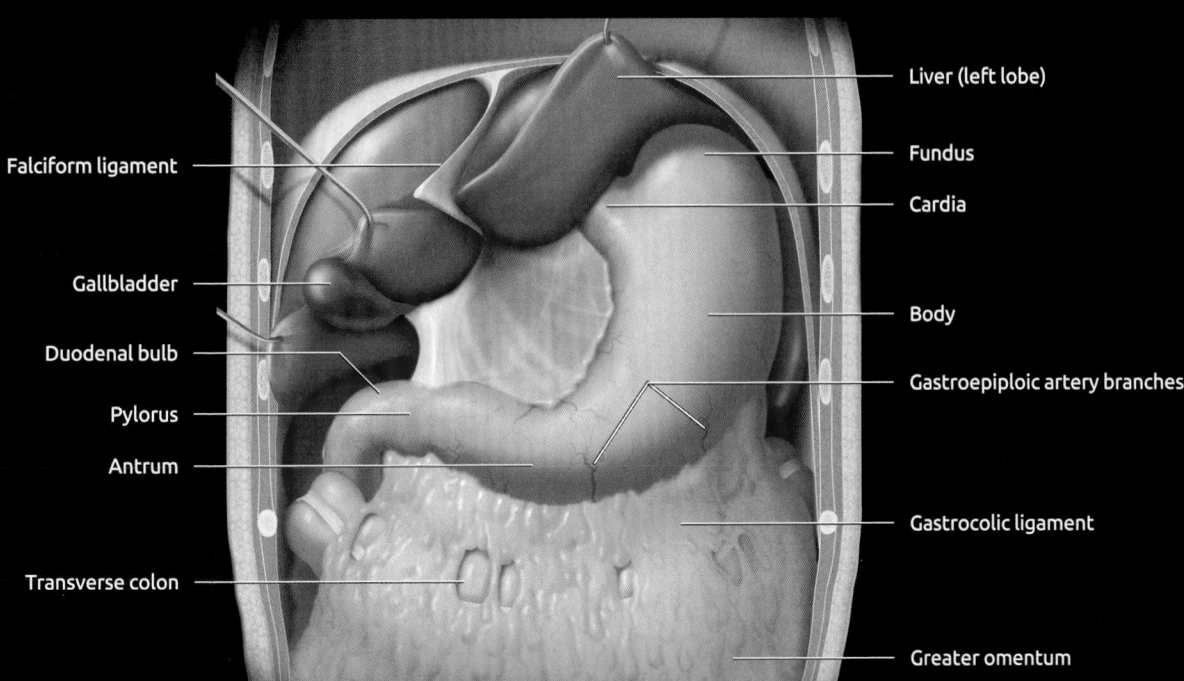

Liver (left lobe)

Fundus

Cardia

Falciform ligament

Body

Gallbladder

Gastroepiploic artery branches

Duodenal bulb

Pylorus

Antrum

Gastrocolic ligament

Transverse colon

Greater omentum

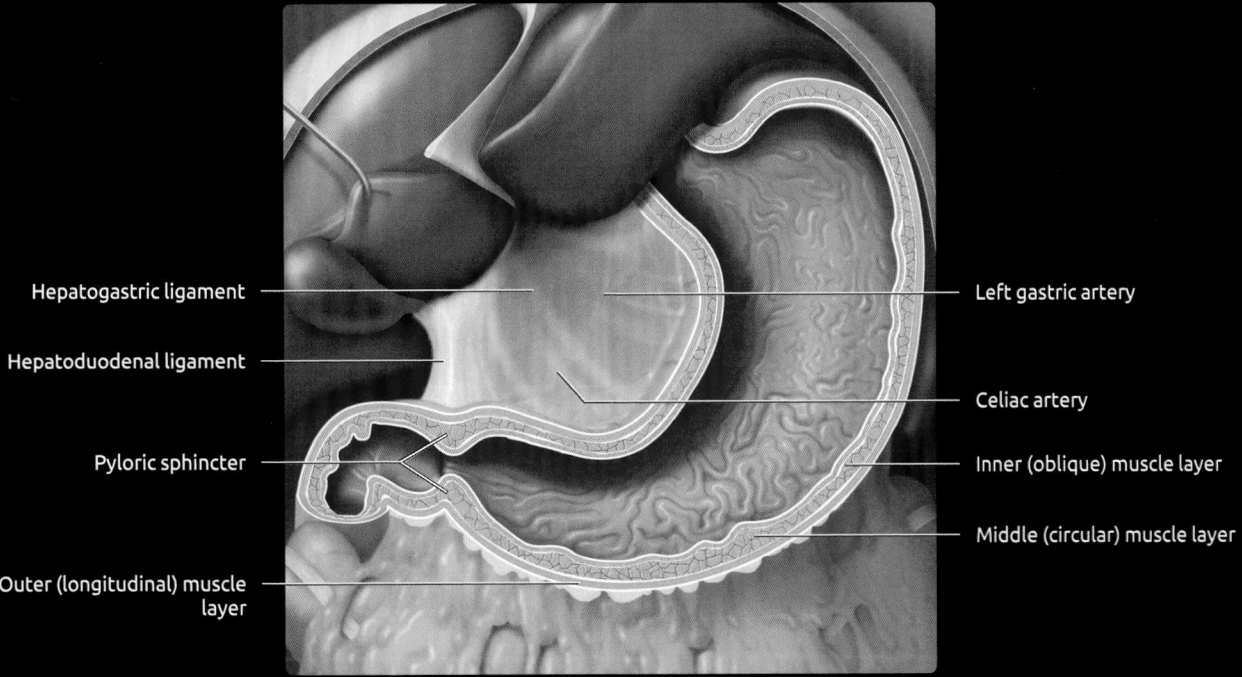

Hepatogastric ligament

Left gastric artery

Hepatoduodenal ligament

Celiac artery

Pyloric sphincter

Inner (oblique) muscle layer

Middle (circular) muscle layer

Outer (longitudinal) muscle layer

(Top) Graphic shows the stomach and proximal duodenum in situ. The liver and gallbladder have been retracted upward. Note that the lesser curvature and anterior wall of the stomach touch the underside of the liver and the gallbladder abuts the duodenal bulb. The greater curvature is attached to the transverse colon by the gastrocolic ligament, which continues inferiorly as the greater omentum, covering most of the colon and small bowel. (Bottom) Graphic shows the lesser omentum extending from the stomach to the porta hepatis, divided into the broader and thinner hepatogastric ligament and the thicker hepatoduodenal ligament. The lesser omentum carries the portal vein, hepatic artery, common bile duct, and lymph nodes. The free edge of the lesser omentum forms the ventral margin of the epiploic foramen. Note the layers of gastric muscle; the middle circular layer is thickest.

DUODENUM

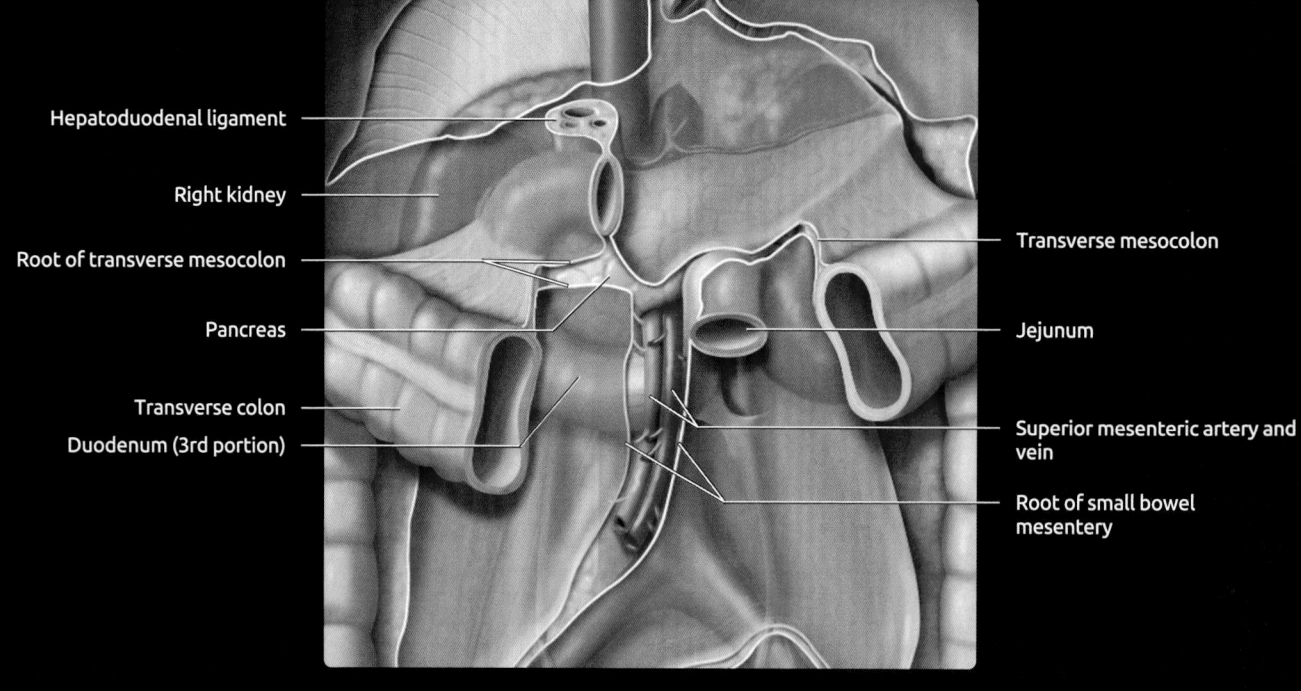

Hepatoduodenal ligament

Right kidney

Root of transverse mesocolon

Pancreas

Transverse colon

Duodenum (3rd portion)

Transverse mesocolon

Jejunum

Superior mesenteric artery and vein

Root of small bowel mesentery

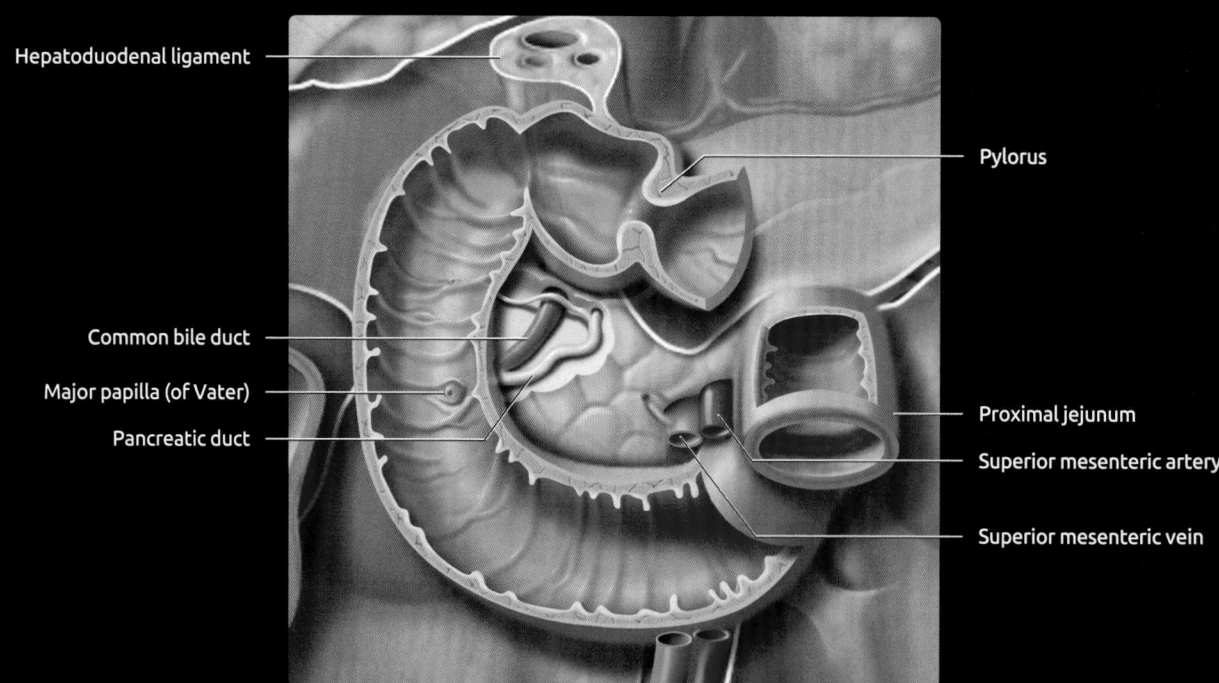

Hepatoduodenal ligament

Common bile duct

Major papilla (of Vater)

Pancreatic duct

Pylorus

Proximal jejunum

Superior mesenteric artery

Superior mesenteric vein

(Top) *The duodenum is retroperitoneal, except for the bulb (1st part). The proximal jejunum is intraperitoneal. The hepatoduodenal ligament attaches the duodenum to the porta hepatis and contains the portal triad (bile duct, hepatic artery, portal vein). The root of the transverse mesocolon and mesentery both cross the duodenum. The 3rd portion of the duodenum crosses in front of the aorta and inferior vena cava (IVC) and behind the superior mesenteric vessels. The 2nd portion of the duodenum is attached to the pancreatic head and lies close to the hilum of the right kidney.* **(Bottom)** *Graphic shows the duodenal bulb suspended by the hepatoduodenal ligament. The duodenal-jejunal flexure is suspended by the ligament of Treitz, an extension of the right crus. The major pancreaticobiliary papilla enters the medial wall of the 2nd portion of the duodenum.*

SMALL INTESTINE

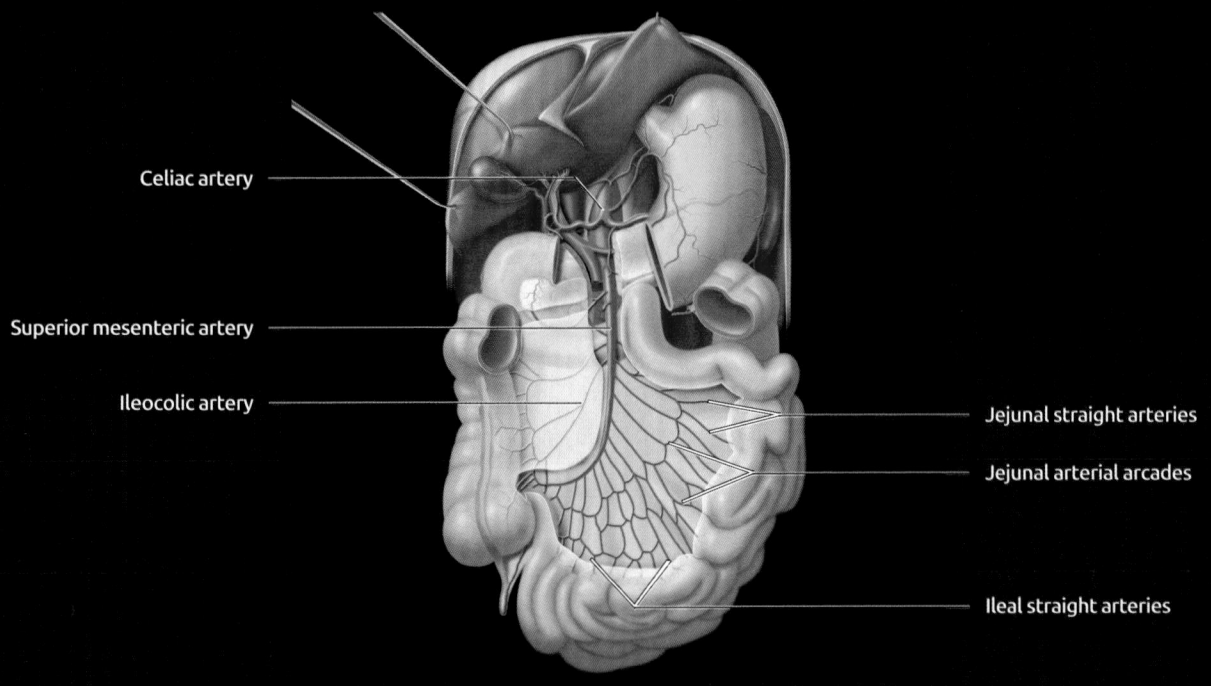

Celiac artery

Superior mesenteric artery

Ileocolic artery

Jejunal straight arteries

Jejunal arterial arcades

Ileal straight arteries

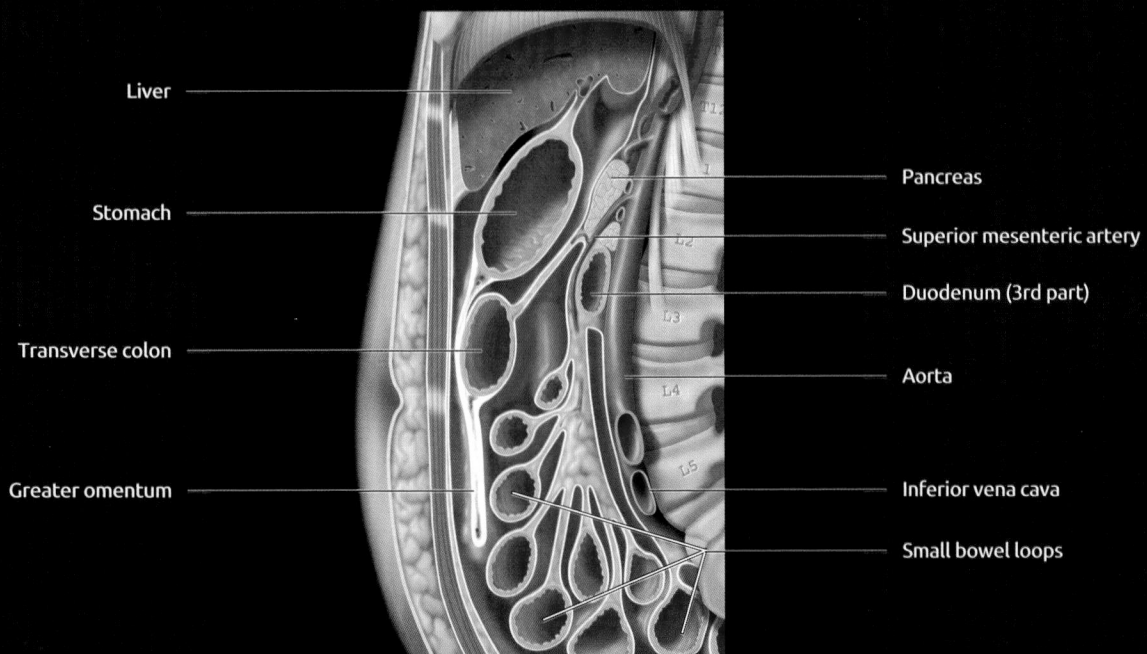

Liver

Stomach

Transverse colon

Greater omentum

Pancreas

Superior mesenteric artery

Duodenum (3rd part)

Aorta

Inferior vena cava

Small bowel loops

(Top) *Graphic shows the vascular supply of the entire small intestine from the superior mesenteric artery (SMA). The small bowel segments are displaced inferiorly. The SMA arises from the anterior abdominal aorta and gives off the inferior pancreaticoduodenal branch that supplies the duodenum and pancreas. Arising from the left side of the SMA are numerous branches to the jejunum and ileum. Jejunal arteries are generally larger and longer than those of the ileum. After a straight course, the arteries form multiple intercommunicating curvilinear arcades.* **(Bottom)** *Graphic shows the sagittal section of the central abdomen, revealing the jejunum and ileum suspended in a radial pattern by the mesentery. Note the overlying greater omentum attached from the inferior portion of the stomach to drape the small bowel segments and transverse colon.*

COLON AND ANUS

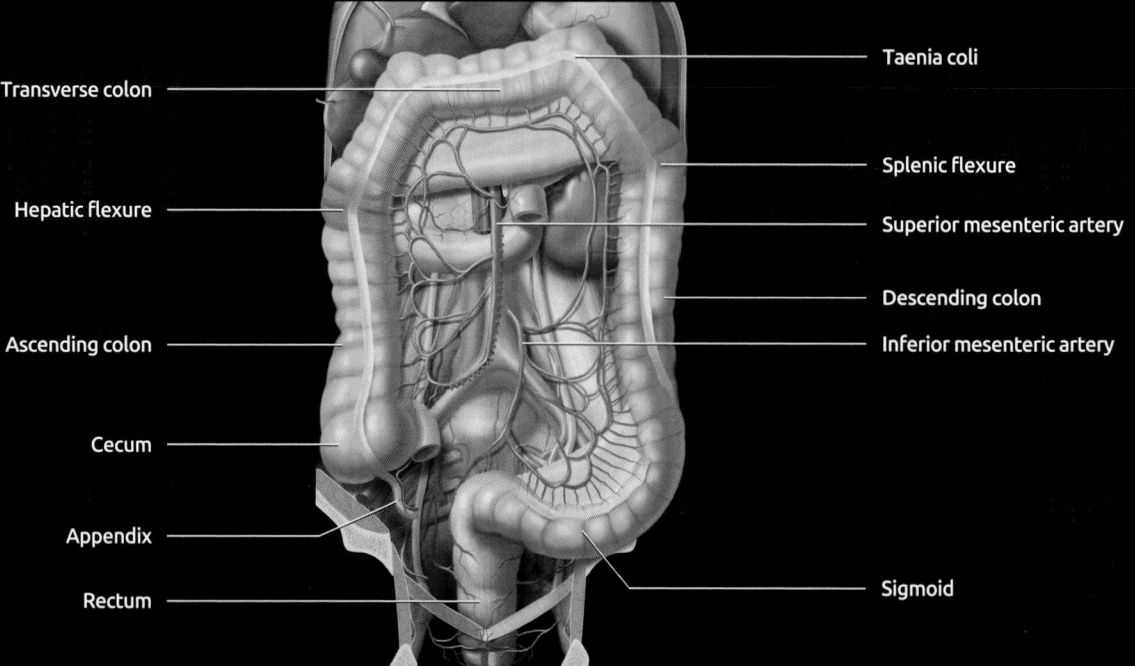

Transverse colon

Hepatic flexure

Ascending colon

Cecum

Appendix

Rectum

Taenia coli

Splenic flexure

Superior mesenteric artery

Descending colon

Inferior mesenteric artery

Sigmoid

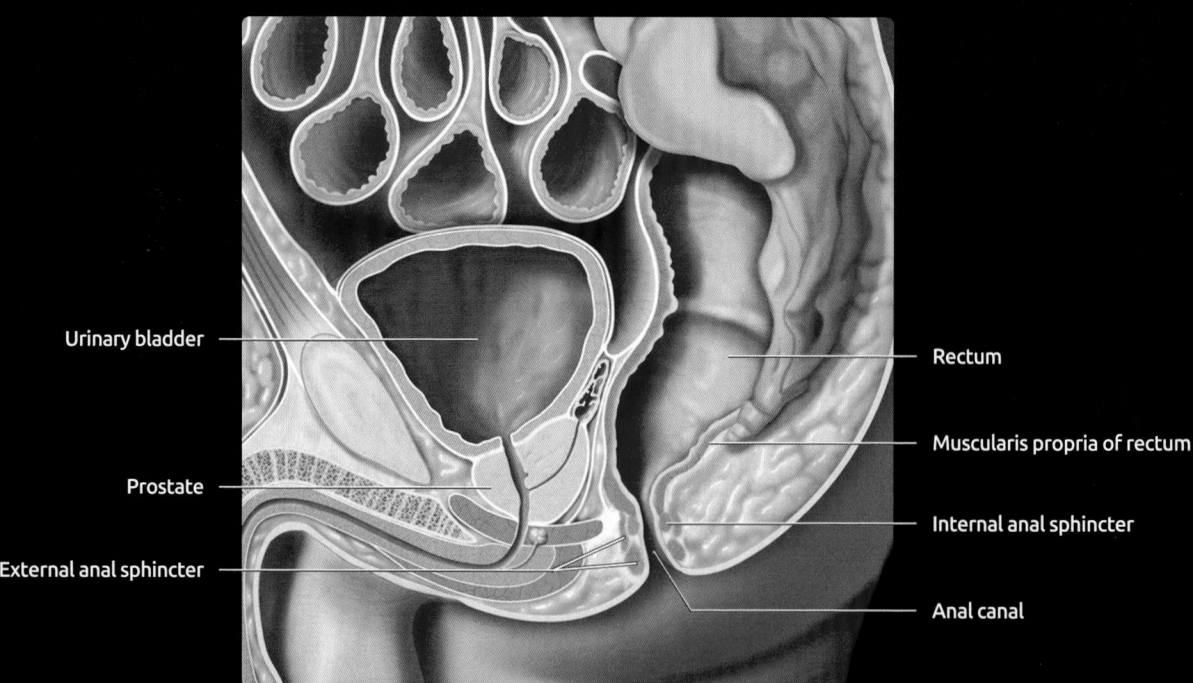

Urinary bladder

Prostate

External anal sphincter

Rectum

Muscularis propria of rectum

Internal anal sphincter

Anal canal

(Top) *Graphic shows the colon in situ. The transverse colon has been retracted upward to demonstrate the arterial supply of the colon from the superior and inferior mesenteric arteries. The SMA supplies the colon from the appendix through the splenic flexure, and the inferior mesenteric artery (IMA) supplies the descending colon through the rectum. Note the band of smooth muscle (taenia coli) running along the length of the intestine, which terminates in the vermiform appendix; these result in sacculations/haustrations along the colon, giving it a segmented appearance.* **(Bottom)** *Graphic shows the longitudinal section of a male pelvis. The anus is the external opening of the rectum and terminal end of the GI tract. The internal anal sphincter (IAS) is a thin involuntary muscle deep to the submucosa. The external anal sphincter is thicker, encircles the IAS, and is under voluntary control.*

STOMACH

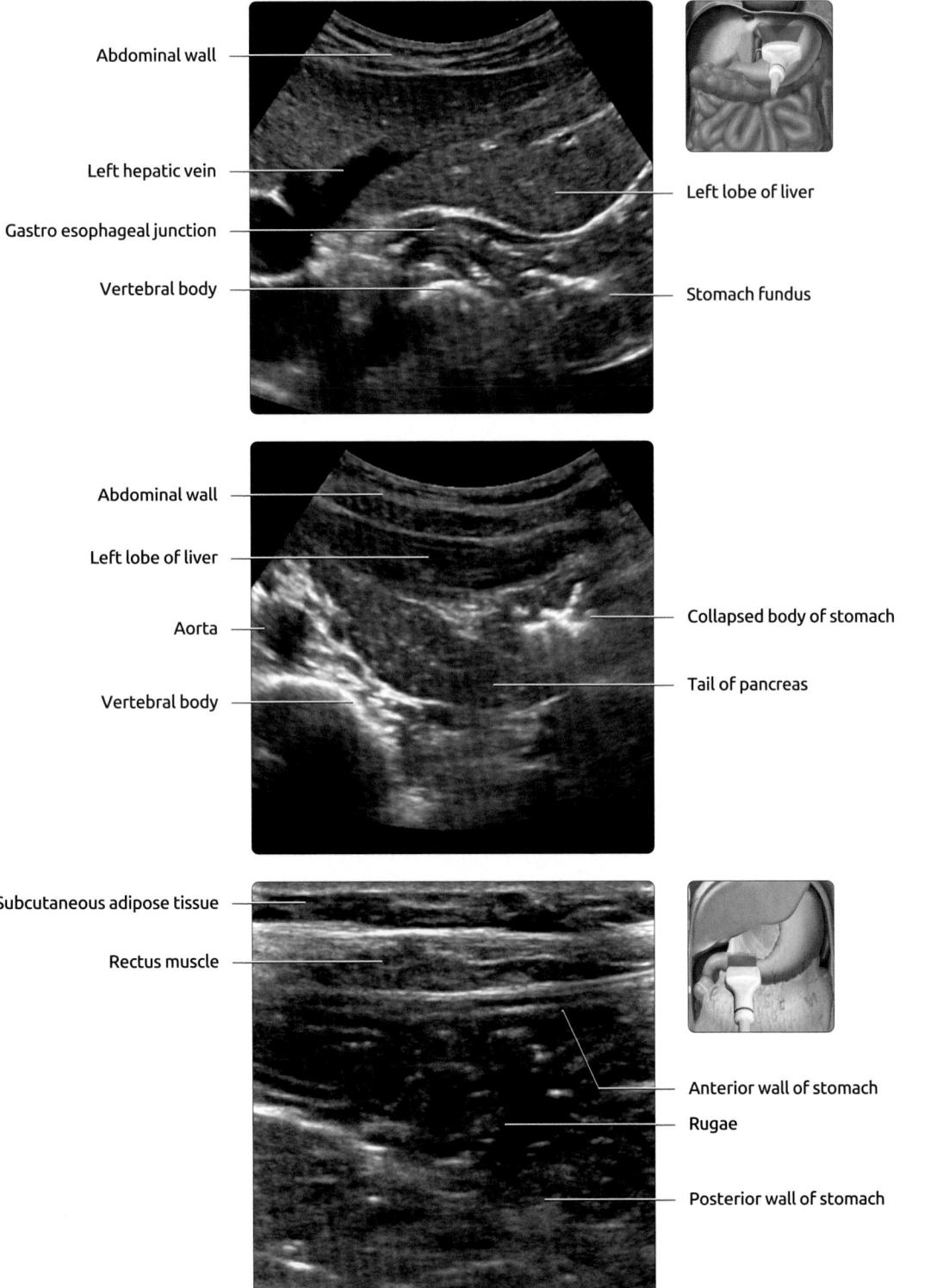

Top image labels:
- Abdominal wall
- Left hepatic vein
- Gastro esophageal junction
- Vertebral body
- Left lobe of liver
- Stomach fundus

Middle image labels:
- Abdominal wall
- Left lobe of liver
- Aorta
- Vertebral body
- Collapsed body of stomach
- Tail of pancreas

Bottom image labels:
- Subcutaneous adipose tissue
- Rectus muscle
- Anterior wall of stomach
- Rugae
- Posterior wall of stomach

(Top) *Transverse oblique ultrasound at the epigastric region shows the gastroesophageal (GE) junction, which can be traced to the fundus of the stomach. Note the relationship to the adjacent structures.* **(Middle)** *Transverse oblique ultrasound through the left upper quadrant shows the collapsed stomach body with the rugal folds. Echogenic gas is seen between the rugae. The tail of the pancreas is seen posterior to the stomach, and the left lobe of the liver is anterior to the stomach.* **(Bottom)** *High-resolution transverse ultrasound through the epigastric region shows the gastric body tapering to the gastric antrum. Note the gastric folds (rugae). The stomach wall shows the gut signature.*

GASTRODUODENAL REGION/DUODENUM

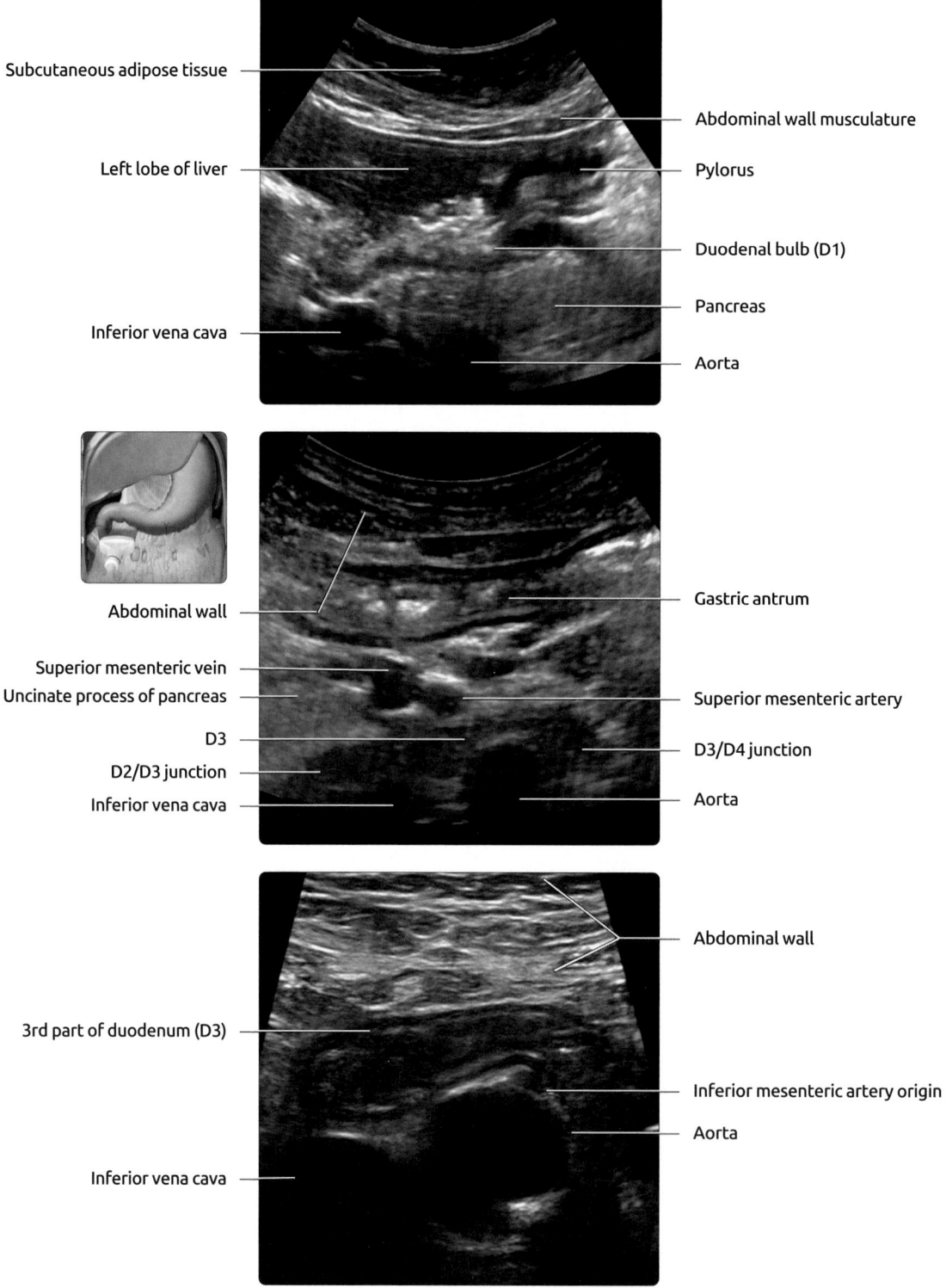

Subcutaneous adipose tissue

Left lobe of liver

Inferior vena cava

Abdominal wall musculature

Pylorus

Duodenal bulb (D1)

Pancreas

Aorta

Abdominal wall

Superior mesenteric vein

Uncinate process of pancreas

D3

D2/D3 junction

Inferior vena cava

Gastric antrum

Superior mesenteric artery

D3/D4 junction

Aorta

3rd part of duodenum (D3)

Inferior vena cava

Abdominal wall

Inferior mesenteric artery origin

Aorta

(Top) *Transverse oblique ultrasound through the epigastric region shows the pylorus with the hypoechoic prominent muscular wall leading to the duodenal bulb.* (Middle) *Transverse ultrasound through the upper abdomen shows the gastric antrum anteriorly compressed by the curvilinear probe and collapsed 3rd part of the duodenum (D3) posteriorly. The SMA and the superior mesenteric vein (SMV) are seen in the plane in between. The inferior vena cava (IVC) and aorta are seen posterior to the D3.* (Bottom) *Axial midline high-resolution ultrasound through the upper abdomen shows fluid distended in the D3 located across, in the upper retroperitoneum. Note the aorta and IVC posterior to the D3. Gut signature is seen in the wall of the D3.*

SMALL BOWEL

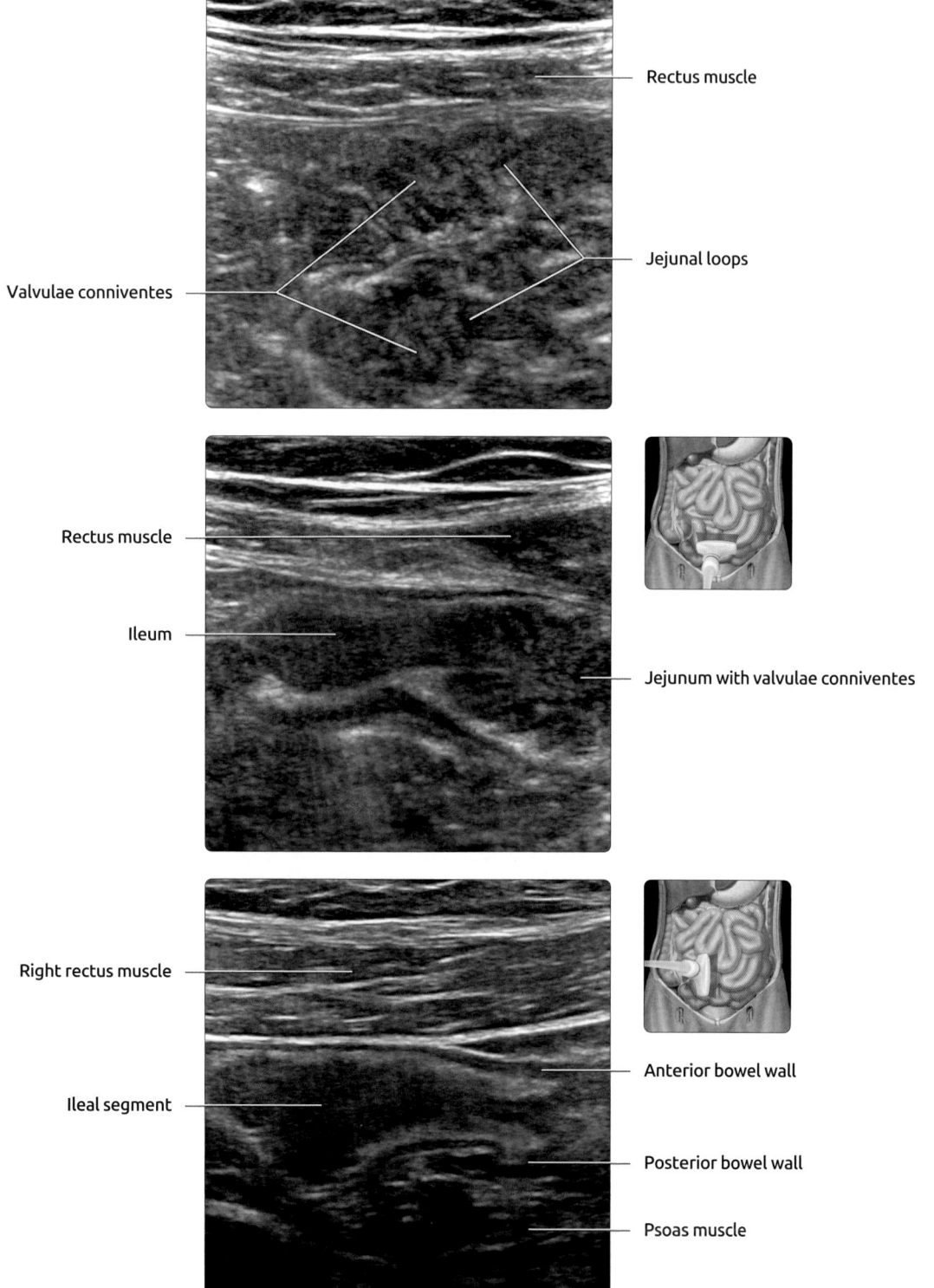

Rectus muscle

Jejunal loops

Valvulae conniventes

Rectus muscle

Ileum

Jejunum with valvulae conniventes

Right rectus muscle

Ileal segment

Anterior bowel wall

Posterior bowel wall

Psoas muscle

(Top) *Transverse oblique ultrasound through the left flank shows jejunal loops with mucosal folds, valvulae conniventes.* **(Middle)** *Transverse ultrasound through the lower abdomen close to midline shows jejunal ileal transition from a segment with folds to a segment with no folds.* **(Bottom)** *Sagittal oblique ultrasound through the right lower quadrant (RLQ) shows a normal ileal segment. Note the lack of folds and a normal gut signature in the wall.*

SMALL BOWEL AND LARGE BOWEL

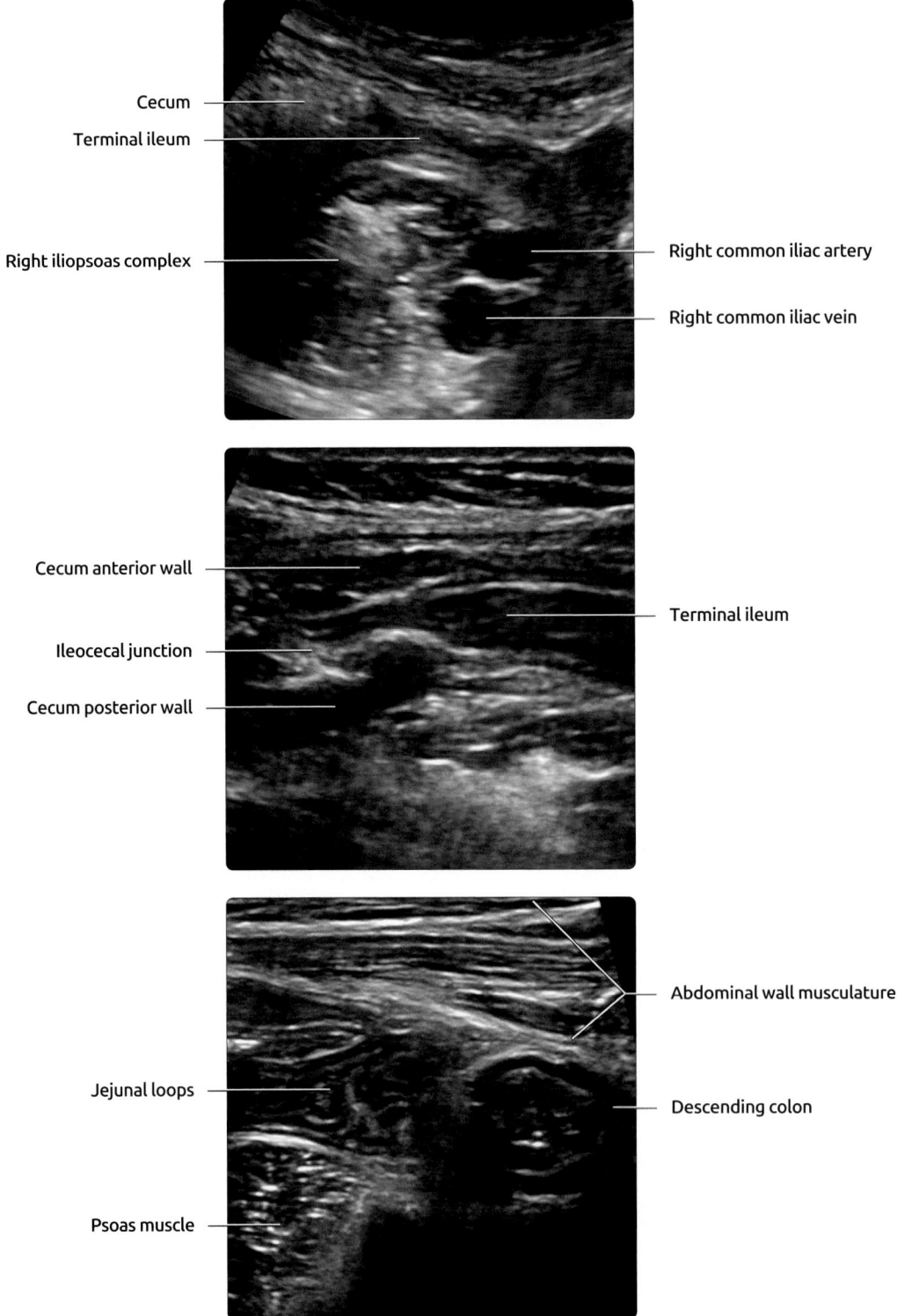

(Top) *Transverse oblique ultrasound through the right iliac fossa (RIF) with graded compression shows a compressed, normal terminal ileum (between the abdominal wall musculature anteriorly and psoas muscle posteriorly) leading to the cecum.* **(Middle)** *Transverse high-resolution ultrasound through the RIF in the same patient shows the ileocecal junction and the ileocecal valve.* **(Bottom)** *Transverse ultrasound through the left iliac fossa (LIF) shows a short-axis view of the descending colon with gut signature. Medial to the descending colon, normal jejunal loops can be seen with valvulae conniventes.*

ILEOCECAL JUNCTION

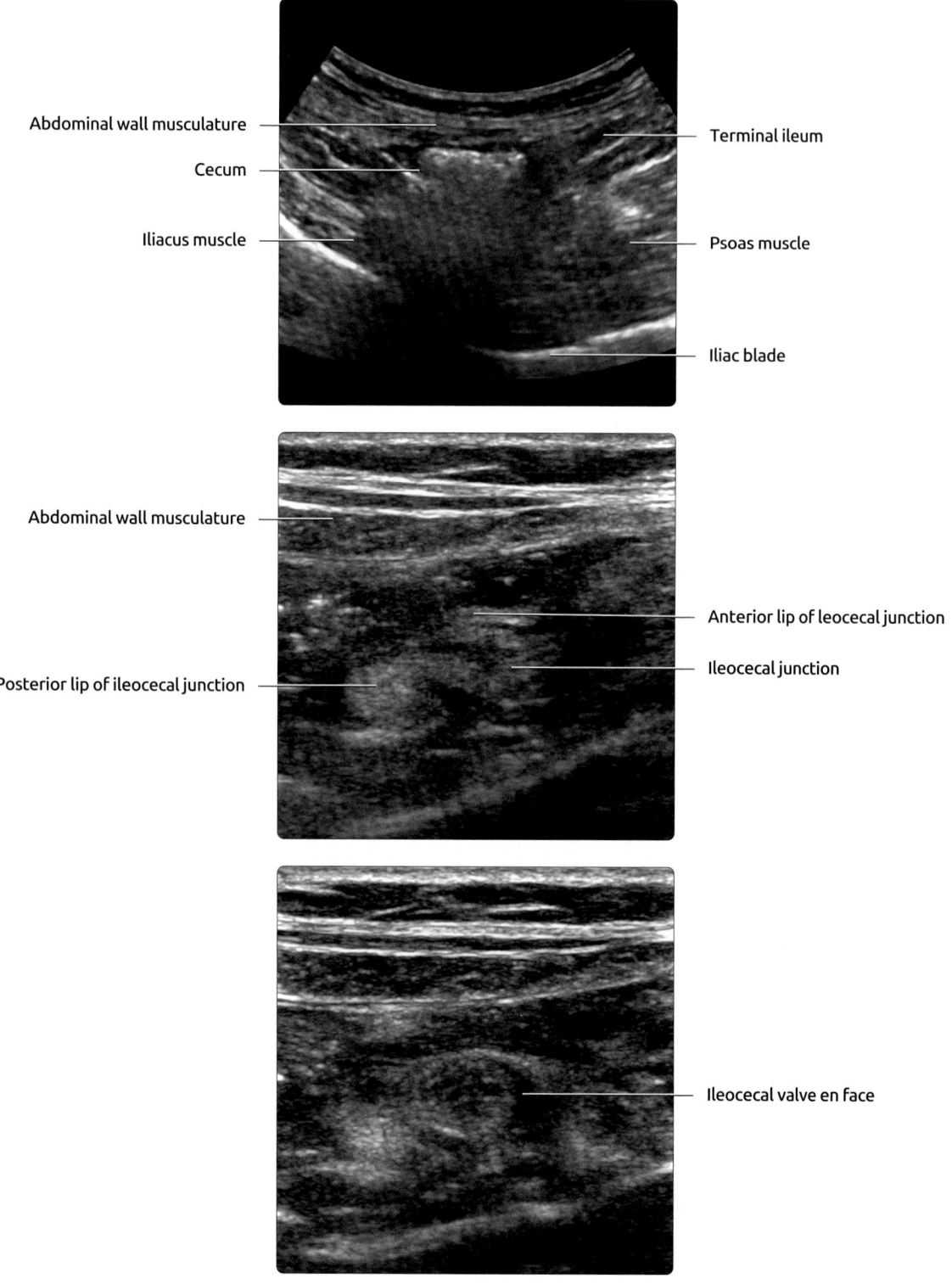

Abdominal wall musculature

Cecum

Iliacus muscle

Terminal ileum

Psoas muscle

Iliac blade

Abdominal wall musculature

Posterior lip of ileocecal junction

Anterior lip of leocecal junction

Ileocecal junction

Ileocecal valve en face

(Top) *Transverse ultrasound through the RIF shows the cecum, which is represented by curvicurvilinear echogenicity with posterior reverberation. Note the terminal ileum compressed by the curvicurvilinear probe between the abdominal wall musculature and the iliopsoas complex posteriorly.* (Middle) *High-resolution transverse ultrasound through the RIF shows echogenic (fatty) lips of a normal ileocecal valve.* (Bottom) *Oblique right sagittal ultrasound through the RIF in the same patient shows the ileocecal junction end on.*

APPENDIX

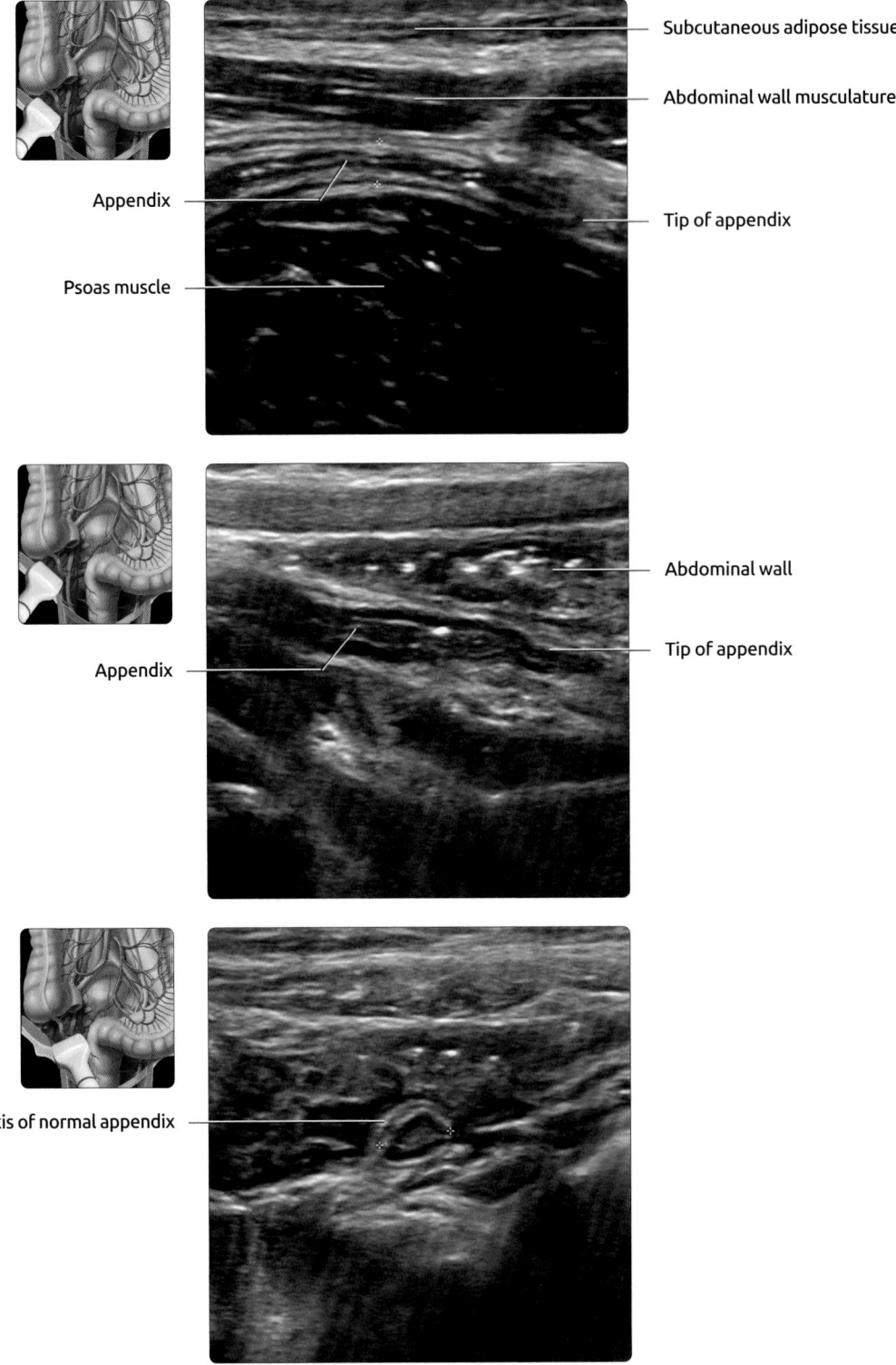

Subcutaneous adipose tissue

Abdominal wall musculature

Appendix

Tip of appendix

Psoas muscle

Abdominal wall

Appendix

Tip of appendix

Short axis of normal appendix

(Top) Coronal oblique ultrasound through the RIF shows a long-axis normal appendix with a stratified mural appearance. Note the absence of peri appendicular inflammatory changes. (Middle) Transverse oblique ultrasound through the RIF shows a blind-ending tubular structure with a gut signature representing the long-axis view of a normal appendix. (Courtesy A. Law, MD.) (Bottom) Transverse oblique ultrasound through the RIF shows the short-axis view of a normal appendix with preservation of gut signature. Note the normal appearance of peri appendicular fat. (Courtesy A. Law, MD.)

LARGE BOWEL

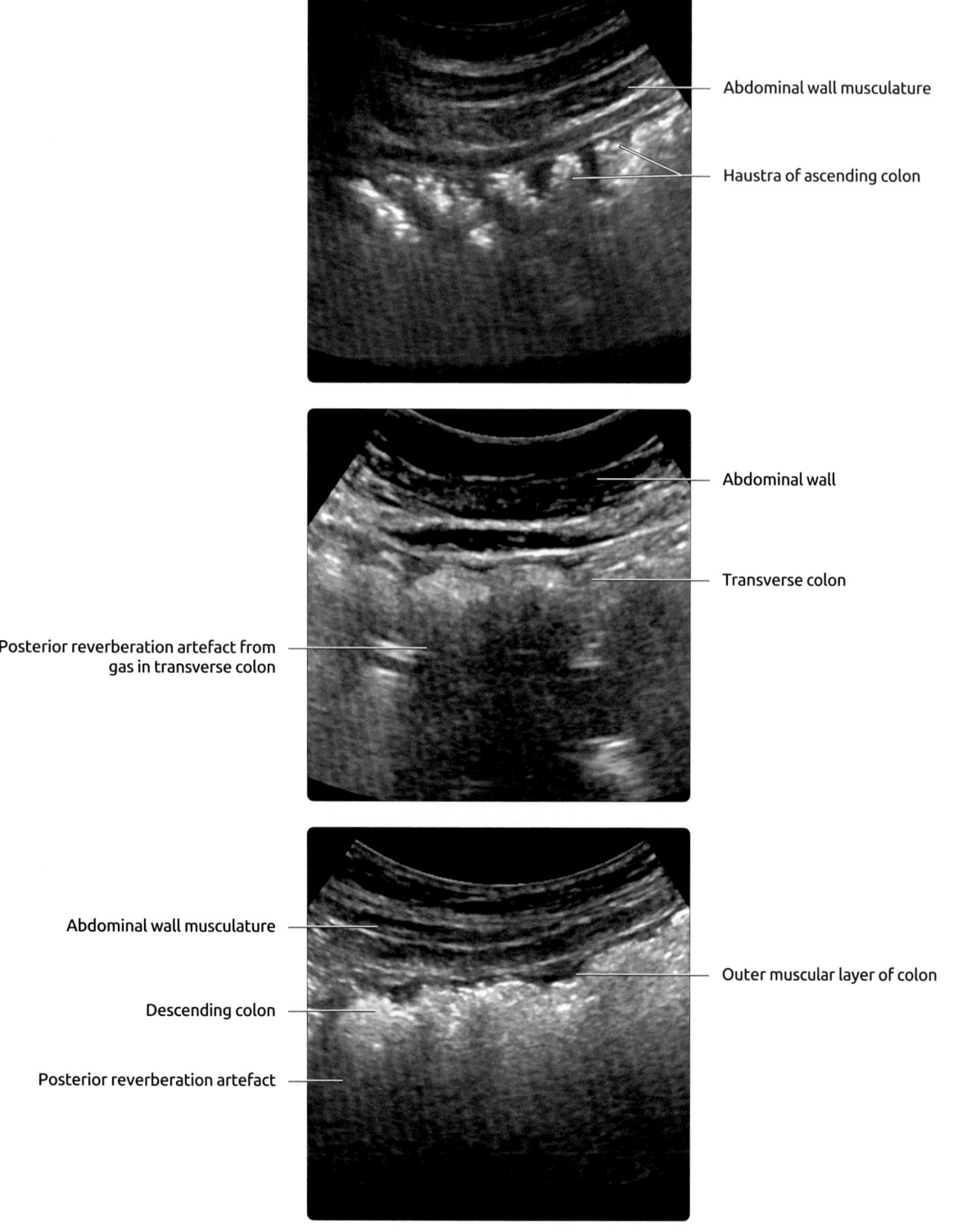

Abdominal wall musculature

Haustra of ascending colon

Abdominal wall

Transverse colon

Posterior reverberation artefact from gas in transverse colon

Abdominal wall musculature

Outer muscular layer of colon

Descending colon

Posterior reverberation artefact

(Top) *Right sagittal ultrasound shows a normal ascending colon with curvicurvilinear arcs of echogenicity from luminal gas/feces reflecting the normal haustra pattern.* **(Middle)** *Transverse ultrasound through the epigastric region close to the midline shows the normal haustral pattern of intraluminal gas/feces within the horizontally lying transverse colon. Note the posterior reverberation artifact from a gas-filled colon.* **(Bottom)** *Left sagittal ultrasound through the left side of the abdomen shows the descending colon represented by arcs of echogenicity with posterior reverberation artifacts due to gaseous contents of the colon. Note the normal haustral pattern. Images obtained with curvilinear probe or linear probe with virtual convex are better for orientation of anatomy within the peritoneal cavity.*

LARGE BOWEL

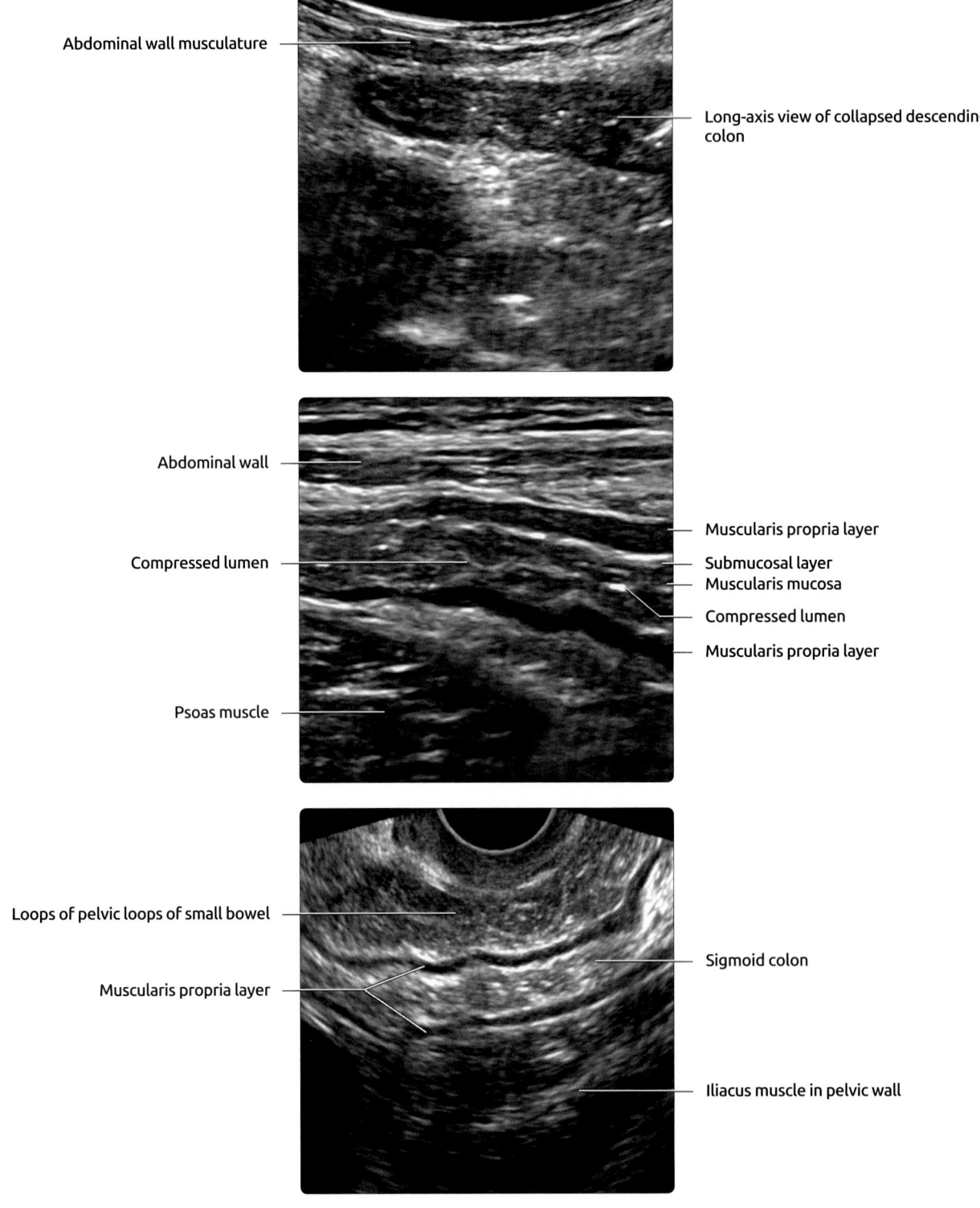

Abdominal wall musculature

Long-axis view of collapsed descending colon

Abdominal wall

Muscularis propria layer

Compressed lumen

Submucosal layer

Muscularis mucosa

Compressed lumen

Muscularis propria layer

Psoas muscle

Loops of pelvic loops of small bowel

Sigmoid colon

Muscularis propria layer

Iliacus muscle in pelvic wall

(**Top**) *Left sagittal ultrasound shows the normal descending colon in a collapsed state and compressed by the ultrasound probe. Note the gut signature. This is an alternative appearance to the descending colon when it is collapsed and empty.* (**Middle**) *High-resolution left sagittal ultrasound obtained with a higher frequency linear probe from the same patient shows the collapsed descending colon with gut signature. The hypoechoic outer layer represents the muscularis propria layer.* (**Bottom**) *Transvaginal ultrasound shows the sigmoid colon and pelvic loops of small bowel. Note the hypertrophied outer muscularis propria layer of the sigmoid colon, seen in patients with irritable bowel syndrome and early diverticular disease.*

RECTOSIGMOID REGION

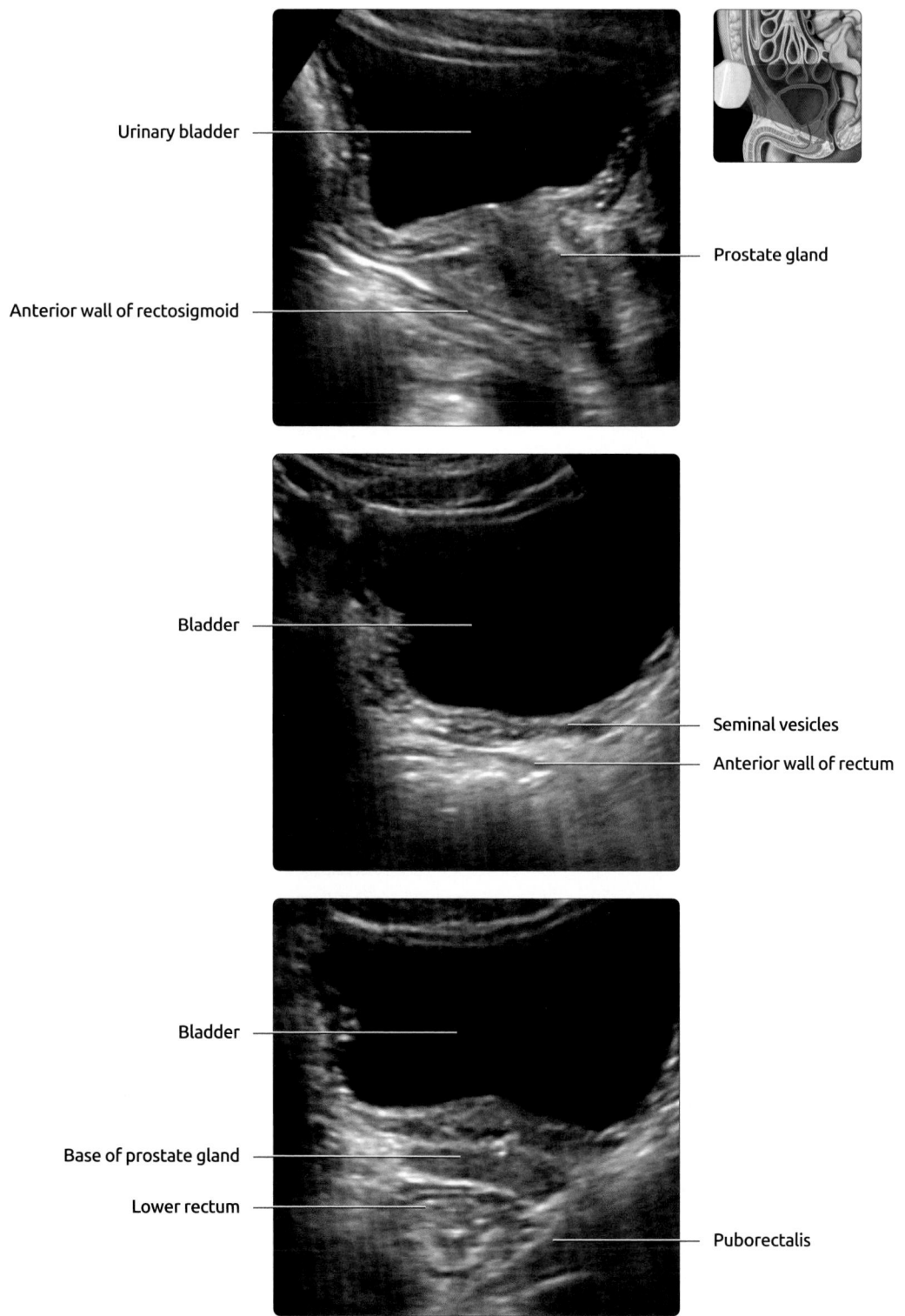

Urinary bladder

Prostate gland

Anterior wall of rectosigmoid

Bladder

Seminal vesicles

Anterior wall of rectum

Bladder

Base of prostate gland

Lower rectum

Puborectalis

(Top) *Midline sagittal ultrasound in a male patient shows the anterior wall of the rectosigmoid region and its relationship to the prostate gland anteriorly.* **(Middle)** *Transverse ultrasound through the pelvis in the same patient (with cystic fibrosis) shows the anterior wall of the rectosigmoid region and its relationship to the seminal vesicles anteriorly (note the small seminal vesicles seen here).* **(Bottom)** *Transverse ultrasound at a lower level in the same patient shows the lower rectum, pelvic floor, and anterior relationship to the prostate gland.*

GROSS ANATOMY

Overview

- Major lymphatic vessels and nodal chains lie along major blood vessels (aorta, IVC, iliac)
- Lymph nodes carry the same name as the vessel they accompany
- Lymph from alimentary tract, liver, spleen, and pancreas passes along celiac, superior mesenteric chains to nodes
  - Efferent vessels from alimentary nodes form intestinal lymphatic trunks
  - Cisterna chyli (chyle cistern)
    - Formed by confluence of intestinal lymphatic trunks and right and left lumbar lymphatic trunks, which receive lymph from nonalimentary viscera, abdominal wall and lower extremities
    - May be discrete sac or plexiform convergence
- Thoracic duct: Inferior extent is chyle cistern at the L1-2 level
  - Formed by convergence of main lymphatic ducts of abdomen
  - Ascends through aortic hiatus in diaphragm to enter posterior mediastinum
  - Ends by entering junction of left subclavian and internal jugular veins
- Lymphatic system drains surplus fluid from extracellular spaces and returns it to bloodstream
  - Important function in defense against infection, inflammation, and tumor via lymphoid tissue present in lymph nodes, gut wall, spleen and thymus
  - Absorbs and transports dietary lipids from intestine to thoracic duct and bloodstream
- Lymph nodes
  - Composed of cortex and medulla
  - Invested in fibrous capsule, which extends into the nodal parenchyma to form trabeculae
  - Internal honeycomb structure filled with lymphocytes that collect and destroy pathogens
  - Hilum: In concave side, with artery and vein, surrounded by fat

Abdominopelvic Nodes

- Preaortic nodes
  - Celiac nodes: Drainage from gastric nodes, hepatic nodes, and pancreaticosplenic nodes
  - Superior and inferior mesenteric nodes: Drainage from mesenteric nodes
- Lateral aortic nodes
  - Drainage from kidneys, adrenal glands, ureter, posterior abdominal wall, testes and ovary, uterus and fallopian tubes
- Retroaortic nodes
  - Drainage from posterior abdominal wall
- External iliac nodes
  - Primary drainage from inguinal nodes
  - Flow into common iliac nodes
- Internal iliac nodes
  - Drainage from inferior pelvic viscera, deep perineum, and gluteal region
  - Flow into common iliac nodes
- Common iliac nodes
  - Drainage from external iliac, internal iliac, and sacral nodes
  - Flow into lumbar (lateral aortic) chain of nodes
- Superficial inguinal nodes
  - In superficial fascia parallel to inguinal ligament, along cephalad portion of greater saphenous vein
  - Receive lymphatic drainage from superficial lower extremity, superficial abdominal wall, and perineum
  - Flow into deep inguinal and external iliac nodes
- Deep inguinal nodes
  - Along medial side of femoral vein, deep to fascia lata and inguinal ligament
  - Receive lymphatic drainage from superficial inguinal and popliteal nodes
  - Flow into external iliac nodes

IMAGING ANATOMY

Overview

- CT is test of choice for cancer staging
- May be supplemented by PET/CT in select cancers
- Ultrasound may be useful in children or thin adults
  - Normal nodes are elliptical with echogenic fatty hilum and uniform hypoechoic cortex
  - Normal lymph nodes rarely detected on abdominal ultrasound
- Normal diameter of lymph node varies depending on location
  - Short axis diameter
    - Abdominopelvic < 10 mm
    - Hepatogastric ligament < 8 mm
    - Retrocrural < 6 mm

ANATOMY IMAGING ISSUES

Imaging Recommendations

- Transducer: 2-5 MHz or 5-9 MHz for thinner patients
- Patient examined in supine position with < 4 hours of fasting to decrease bowel gas
- Graded compression technique to clear overlying bowel loops

CLINICAL IMPLICATIONS

Clinical Importance

- Nodal enlargement is nonspecific, may be neoplastic, inflammatory, or reactive
- Normal-sized lymph nodes may harbor metastatic malignancy
- Node morphology is more specific for pathology
  - Abnormal nodes have replacement or loss of fatty hilum
  - Look for central necrosis, cystic change, or calcification
- Lymphoma
  - Multiple enlarged hypoechoic or anechoic nodes
- Metastatic lymphadenopathy
  - More echogenic and heterogeneous nodes compared to lymphomatous nodes
- Infectious/reactive lymphadenopathy
  - Nonspecific sonographic features
  - May contain necrotic centers in mycobacterial infection

RETROPERITONEAL LYMPH NODES

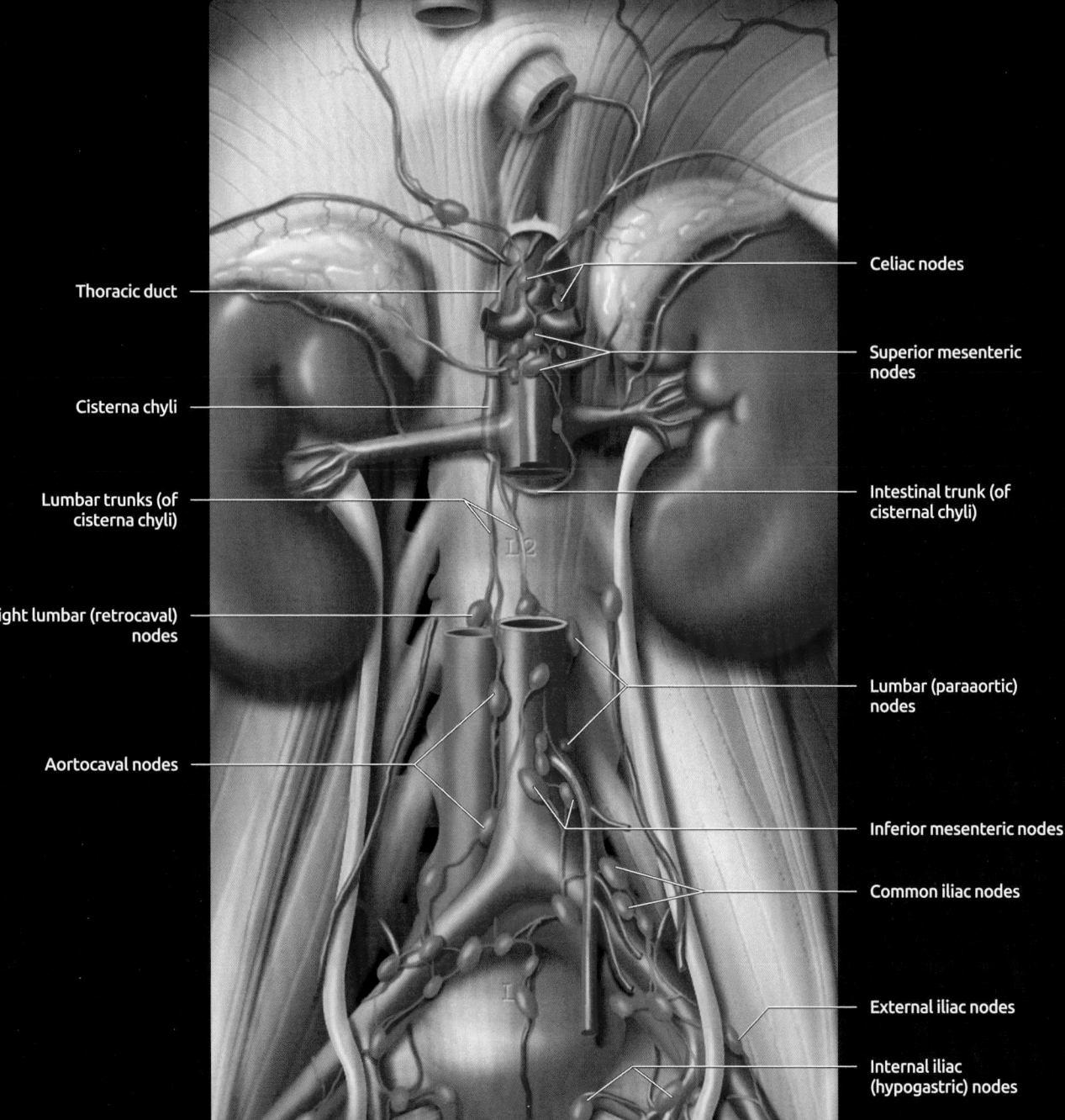

Thoracic duct

Cisterna chyli

Lumbar trunks (of cisterna chyli)

Right lumbar (retrocaval) nodes

Aortocaval nodes

Celiac nodes

Superior mesenteric nodes

Intestinal trunk (of cisternal chyli)

Lumbar (paraaortic) nodes

Inferior mesenteric nodes

Common iliac nodes

External iliac nodes

Internal iliac (hypogastric) nodes

Graphic shows that the major lymphatics and lymph nodes of the abdomen are located along, and share the same name as the major blood vessels, such as the external iliac nodes, celiac, and superior mesenteric nodes. The paraaortic and paracaval nodes are also referred to as the lumbar nodes and receive afferents from the lower abdominal viscera, abdominal wall, and lower extremities; they are frequently involved in inflammatory and neoplastic processes. The lumbar trunks join with an intestinal trunk (at about the L1 level) to form the cisterna chyli, which may be a discrete sac or a plexiform convergence. The cisterna chyli and other major lymphatic trunks join to form the thoracic duct, which passes through the aortic hiatus to enter the mediastinum. After picking up additional lymphatic trunks within the thorax, the thoracic duct empties into the left subclavian or innominate vein.

NONENLARGED NODES AND PATHOLOGIC NODES

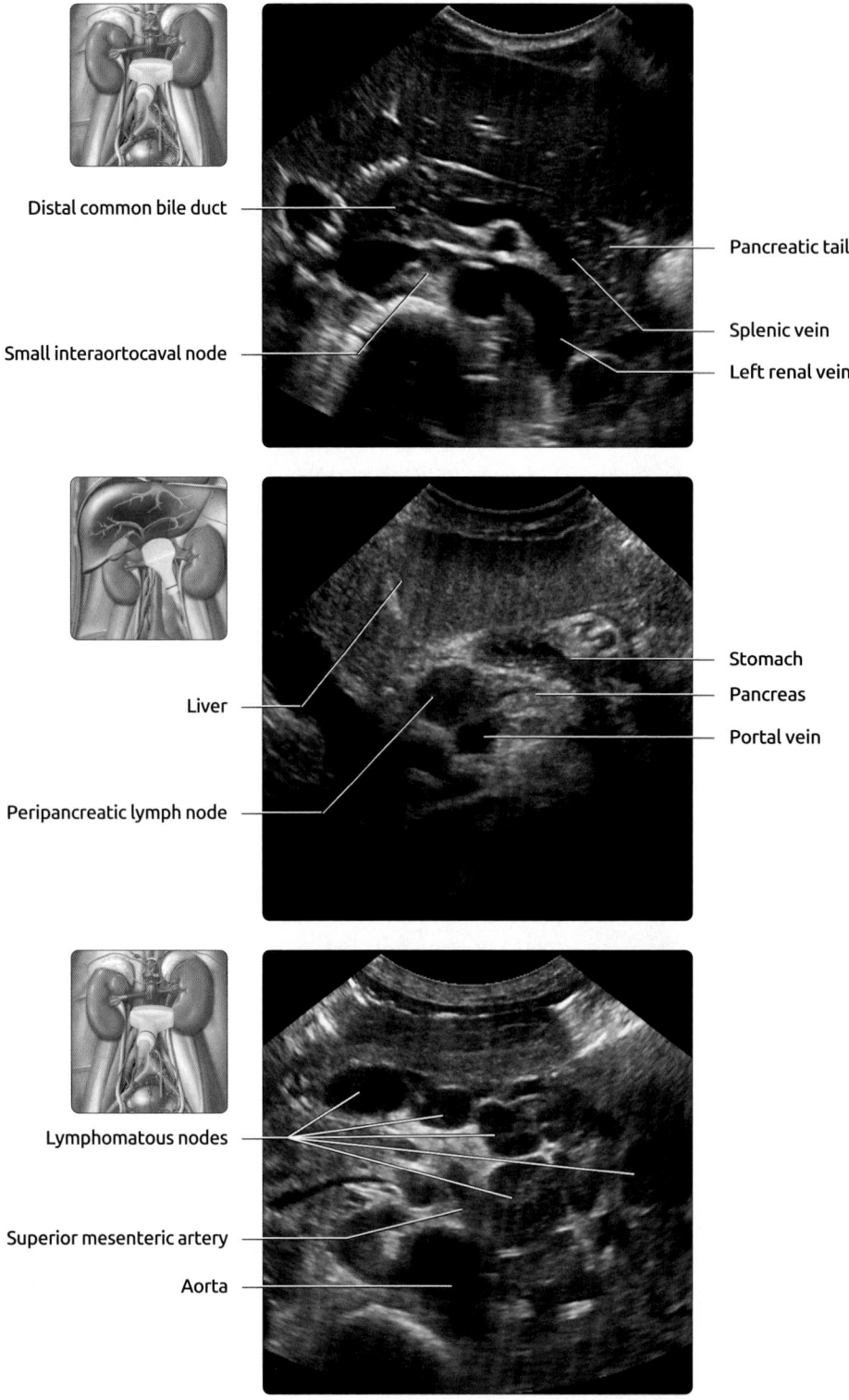

Distal common bile duct

Small interaortocaval node

Pancreatic tail

Splenic vein

Left renal vein

Liver

Peripancreatic lymph node

Stomach

Pancreas

Portal vein

Lymphomatous nodes

Superior mesenteric artery

Aorta

(Top) *Transverse ultrasound at the level of the pancreas and splenic vein shows a small interaortocaval node.* **(Middle)** *Transverse ultrasound of the epigastric region shows an enlarged hypoechoic peripancreatic lymph node anterior to the portal vein in a patient with hepatitis C. Normal-sized lymph nodes are rarely seen in adult abdominal ultrasound.* **(Bottom)** *Transverse ultrasound of the upper midline abdomen in a patient with lymphoma shows multiple abnormal enlarged hypoechoic lymph nodes around the superior mesenteric artery.*

LYMPHANGIOGRAM

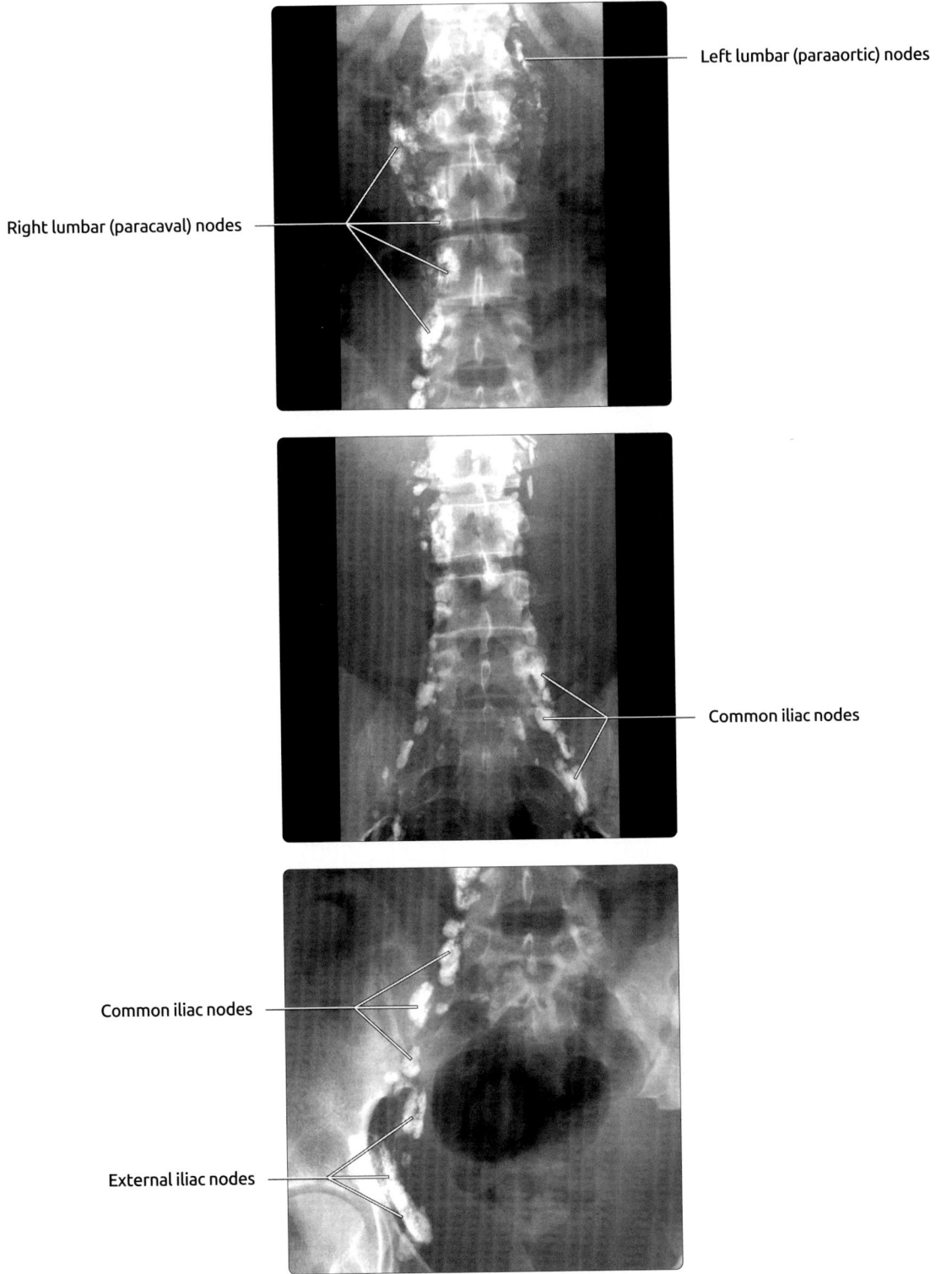

Left lumbar (paraaortic) nodes

Right lumbar (paracaval) nodes

Common iliac nodes

Common iliac nodes

External iliac nodes

(Top) *This is the 1st of 3 images from a lymphangiogram. Iodinated oil is slowly infused into the lymphatics of the foot to produce opacification of the lymph channels and nodes. Note the subcentimeter (short axis) diameter of these normal retroperitoneal lymph nodes.* (Middle) *Lymphatic channels and lymph nodes parallel the course of major blood vessels and share similar names, such as these common iliac nodes.* (Bottom) *With the availability of CT, MR, and PET/CT, lymphangiograms are rarely performed; however, they provide a unique depiction of the lymphatic system.*

TERMINOLOGY

Definitions

- Peritoneal cavity: Potential space in abdomen between visceral and parietal peritoneum, usually containing only small amount of peritoneal fluid (for lubrication)
- Abdominal cavity: Not synonymous with peritoneal cavity
  - Contains all of abdominal viscera (intra- and retroperitoneal)
  - Limited by abdominal wall muscles, diaphragm, and (arbitrarily) by pelvic brim

GROSS ANATOMY

Divisions

- Greater sac of peritoneal cavity
- Lesser sac (omental bursa)
  - Communicates with greater sac via epiploic foramen (of Winslow)
  - Bounded anteriorly by caudate lobe, stomach, and greater omentum; posteriorly by pancreas, left adrenal, and kidney; on left by splenorenal and gastrosplenic ligaments; on right by epiploic foramen and lesser omentum

Compartments

- Supramesocolic space
  - Divided into right and left supramesocolic spaces, which are separated by falciform ligament
    - Right supramesocolic space: Composed of right subphrenic space, right subhepatic space, and lesser sac
    - Left supramesocolic space: Divided into left perihepatic spaces (anterior and posterior) and left subphrenic (anterior perigastric and posterior perisplenic)
- Inframesocolic compartment
  - Divided into right inframesocolic space, left inframesocolic space, paracolic gutters, and pelvic cavity
  - Pelvic cavity is most dependent part of peritoneal cavity in erect and supine positions

Peritoneum

- Thin serous membrane consisting of single layer of squamous epithelium (mesothelium)
  - Parietal peritoneum lines abdominal wall
  - Visceral peritoneum (serosa) lines abdominal organs

Mesentery

- Double layer of peritoneum that encloses organ and connects it to abdominal wall
- Covered on both sides by mesothelium and has core of loose connective tissue containing fat, lymph nodes, blood vessels, and nerves passing to and from viscera
- Most mobile parts of intestine have mesentery, while ascending and descending colon are considered retroperitoneal (covered only by peritoneum on anterior surface)
- Root of mesentery is its attachment to posterior abdominal wall
- Root of small bowel mesentery is ~ 15 cm and passes from left side of L2 vertebra downward and to right; contains superior mesenteric vessels, nerves, and lymphatics

- Transverse mesocolon crosses almost horizontally in front of pancreas, duodenum, and right kidney

Omentum

- Multilayered fold of peritoneum that extends from stomach to adjacent organs
- Lesser omentum joins lesser curve of stomach and proximal duodenum to liver
  - Hepatogastric and hepatoduodenal ligament components contain common bile duct, hepatic and gastric vessels, and portal vein
- Greater omentum
  - 4-layered fold of peritoneum hanging from greater curve of stomach like an apron, covering transverse colon and much of small intestine
    - Contains variable amounts of fat and abundant lymph nodes
    - Mobile and can fill gaps between viscera
    - Acts as barrier to generalized spread of intraperitoneal infection or tumor

Ligaments

- All double layered folds of peritoneum, other than mesentery and omentum, are peritoneal ligaments
- Connect 1 viscus to another (e.g., splenorenal ligament) or viscus to abdominal wall (e.g., falciform ligament)
- Contain blood vessels or remnants of fetal vessels

Folds

- Reflections of peritoneum with defined borders, often lifting peritoneum off abdominal wall (e.g., median umbilical fold covers urachus and extends from dome of urinary bladder to umbilicus)

Peritoneal Recesses

- Dependent pouches formed by peritoneal reflections
- Many have eponyms (e.g., Morison pouch for posterior subhepatic [hepatorenal] recess; pouch of Douglas for rectouterine recess)

ANATOMY IMAGING ISSUES

Imaging Recommendations

- Transducer: Typically 2-5 MHz for abdominal survey and deep recesses, up to 9 MHz for thinner patients
- High frequency linear transducer 8-15 MHz may be used to evaluate anterior abdominal wall and parietal peritoneum
- Patient examined supine with additional decubitus positions to determine if fluid collection is free or loculated
- Peritoneal cavity and its various mesenteries and recesses are usually not apparent on imaging studies unless distended or outlined by intraperitoneal fluid or air

PERITONEAL CAVITY

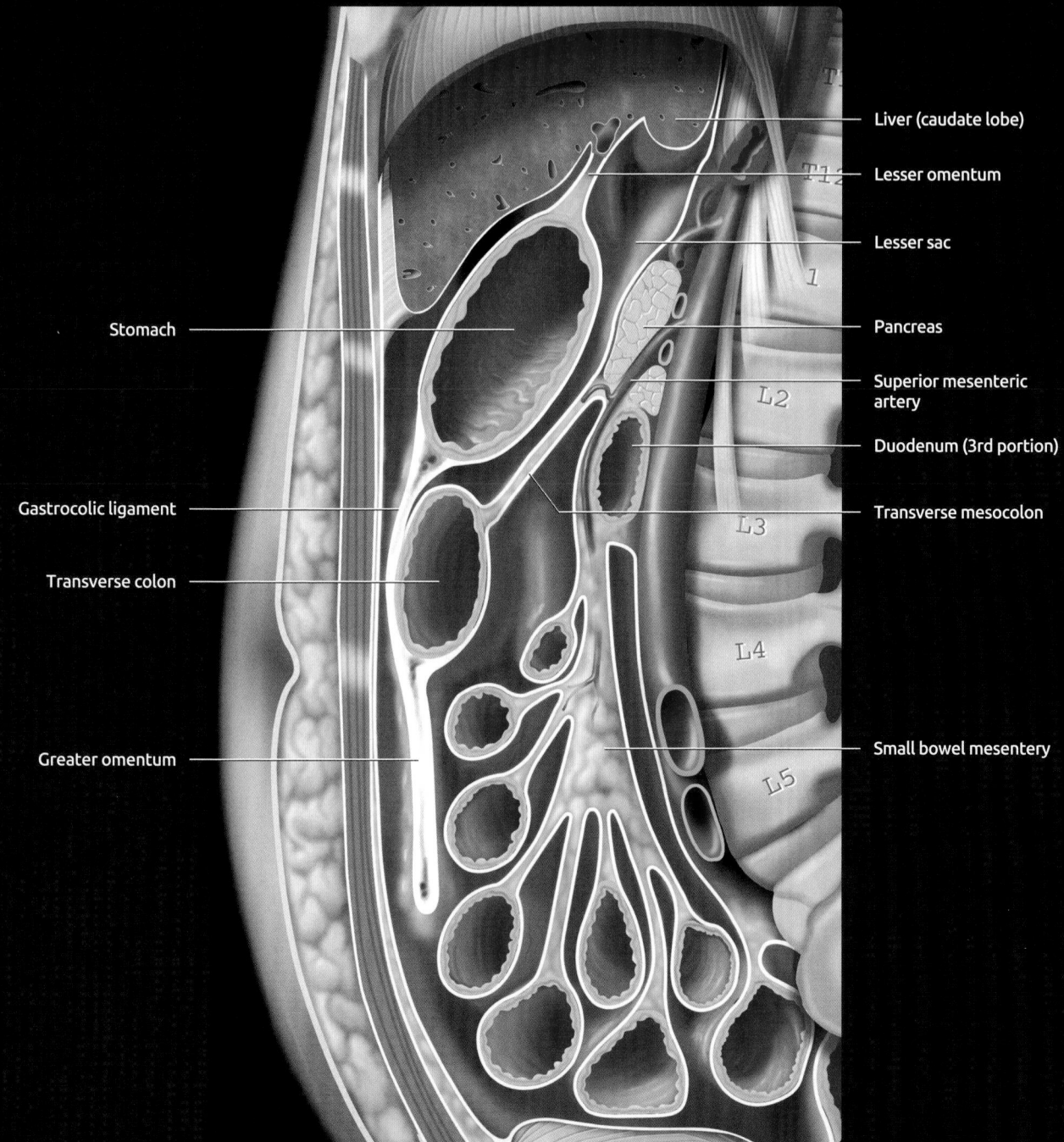

Liver (caudate lobe)

Lesser omentum

Lesser sac

Pancreas

Superior mesenteric artery

Duodenum (3rd portion)

Transverse mesocolon

Small bowel mesentery

Stomach

Gastrocolic ligament

Transverse colon

Greater omentum

Graphic of a sagittal section of the abdomen shows the peritoneal cavity artificially distended, as with air. Note the margins of the lesser sac in this plane, including the caudate lobe of the liver, stomach, and gastrocolic ligament anteriorly and pancreas posteriorly. The hepatogastric ligament is part of the lesser omentum and carries the hepatic artery and portal vein to the liver. The mesenteries are multilayered folds of the peritoneum that enclose a layer of fat and convey blood vessels, nerves, and lymphatics to the intraperitoneal abdominal viscera. The greater omentum is a 4-layered fold of the peritoneum that extends down from the stomach, covering much of the colon and small intestine. The layers are generally fused together caudal to the transverse colon. The gastrocolic ligament is part of the greater omentum.

PERITONEAL DIVISIONS AND COMPARTMENTS

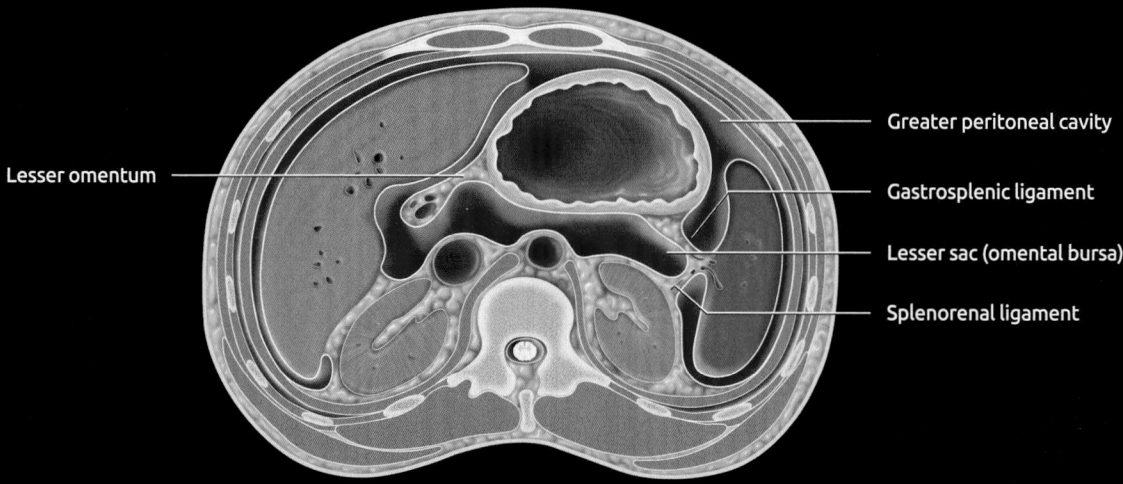

Lesser omentum

Greater peritoneal cavity

Gastrosplenic ligament

Lesser sac (omental bursa)

Splenorenal ligament

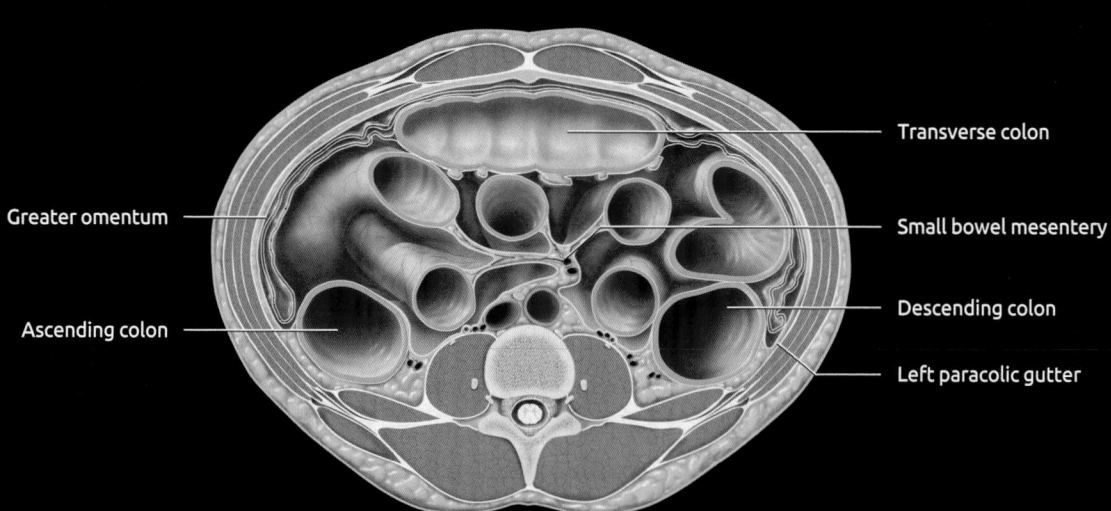

Greater omentum

Ascending colon

Transverse colon

Small bowel mesentery

Descending colon

Left paracolic gutter

(Top) *The borders of the lesser sac (omental bursa) include the lesser omentum, which contains the common bile duct and hepatic and gastric vessels. The left border includes the gastrosplenic ligament (with short gastric vessels) and the splenorenal ligament (with splenic vessels).* **(Bottom)** *The paracolic gutters are formed by reflections of the peritoneum covering the ascending and descending colon and the lateral abdominal wall. Note the innumerable potential peritoneal recesses lying between the bowel loops and their mesenteric leaves. The greater omentum covers much of the bowel like an apron.*

PERITONEAL DIVISIONS AND COMPARTMENTS

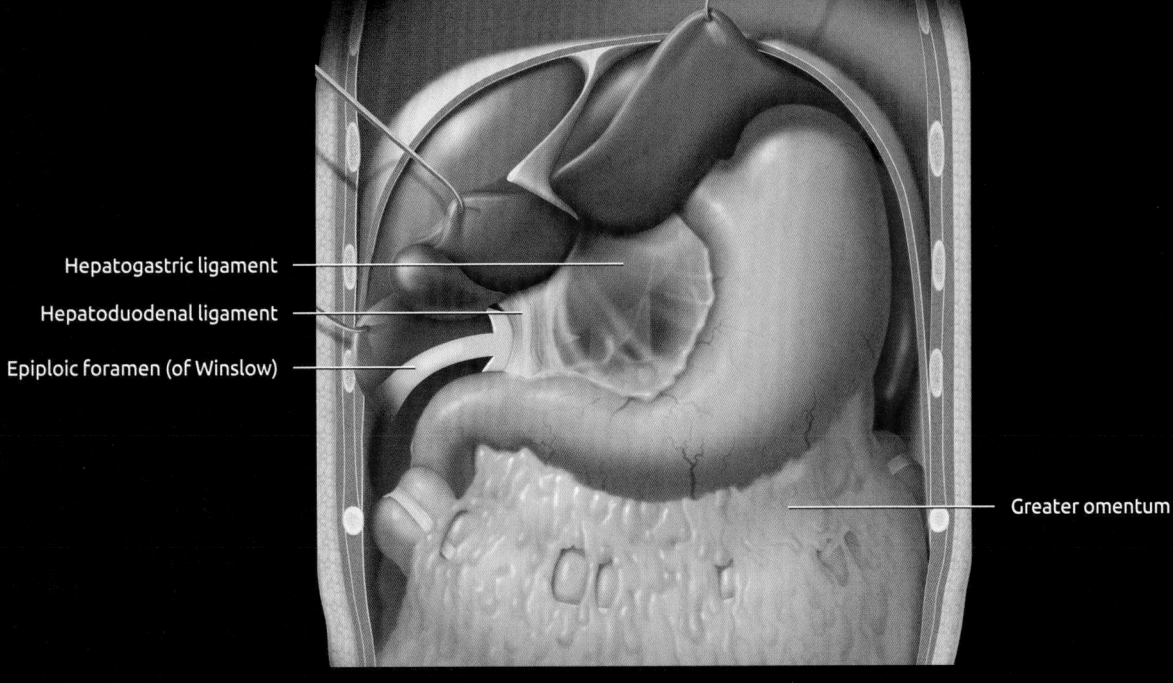

Hepatogastric ligament

Hepatoduodenal ligament

Epiploic foramen (of Winslow)

Greater omentum

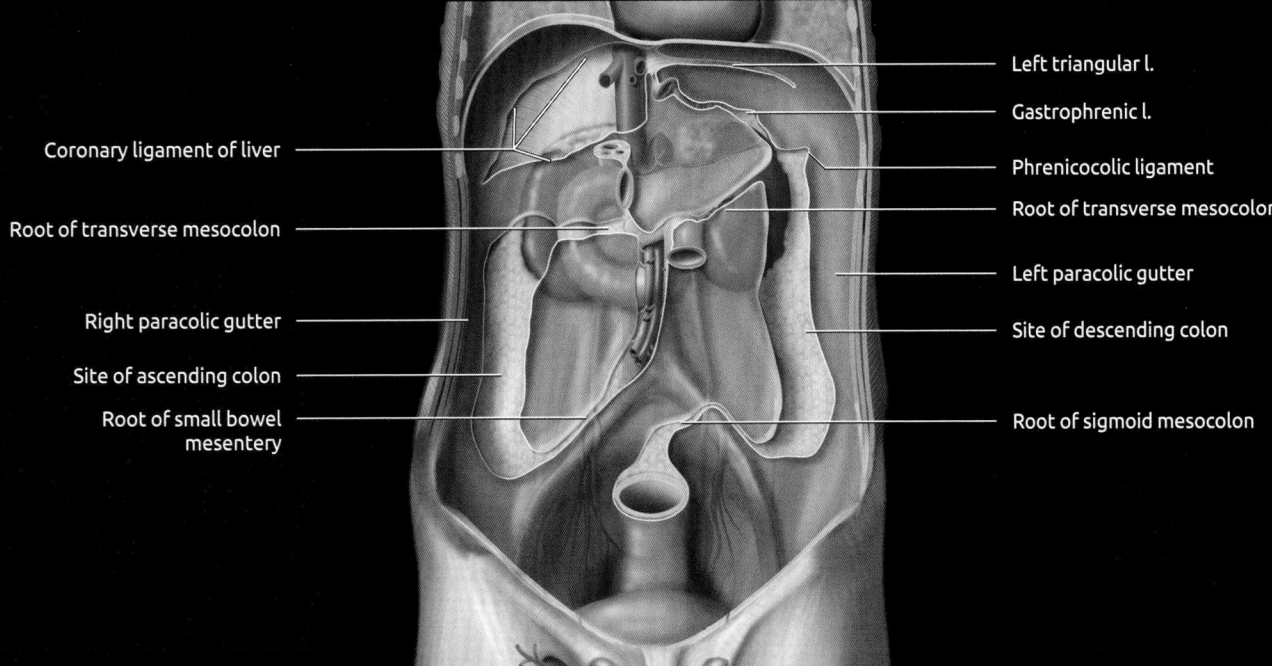

Left triangular l.

Gastrophrenic l.

Coronary ligament of liver

Phrenicocolic ligament

Root of transverse mesocolon

Root of transverse mesocolon

Left paracolic gutter

Right paracolic gutter

Site of descending colon

Site of ascending colon

Root of small bowel mesentery

Root of sigmoid mesocolon

(Top) *In this graphic, the liver has been retracted upward. The lesser omentum is comprised of the hepatoduodenal and hepatogastric ligaments. It forms part of the anterior wall of the lesser sac, and contains the common bile duct, hepatic and gastric vessels, and the portal vein. The aorta and celiac artery can be seen through the lesser omentum, as they lie just posterior to the lesser sac.* (Bottom) *Frontal view of the abdomen, with all of the intraperitoneal organs removed, shows that the root of the transverse mesocolon divides the peritoneal cavity into supramesocolic and inframesocolic spaces that communicate only along the paracolic gutters. The coronary and triangular ligaments suspend the liver from the diaphragm. The superior mesenteric vessels traverse the small bowel mesentery, whose root crosses obliquely from the upper left to the lower right posterior abdominal wall.*

RIGHT SUPRAMESOCOLIC SPACE

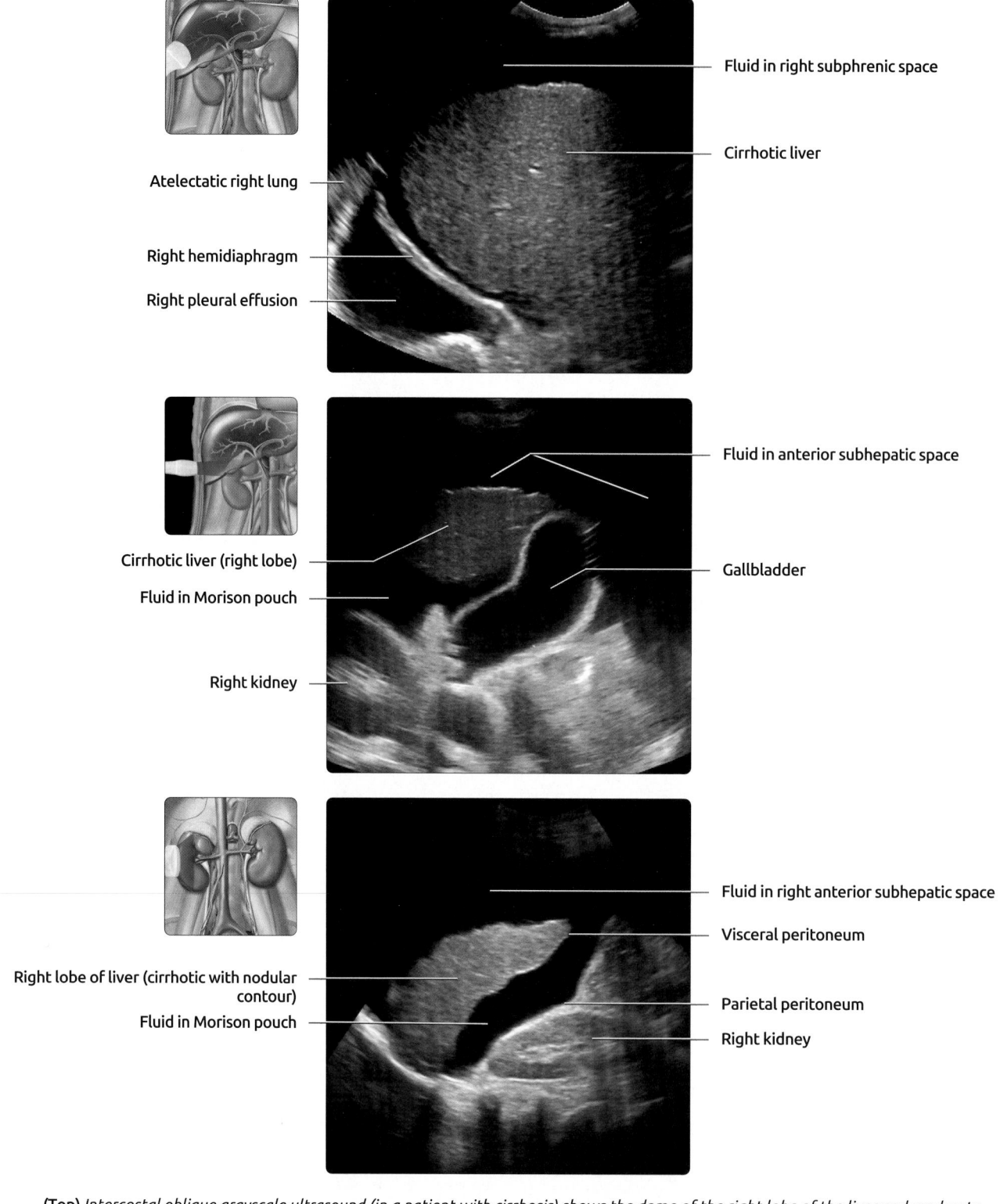

Atelectatic right lung

Right hemidiaphragm

Right pleural effusion

Fluid in right subphrenic space

Cirrhotic liver

Cirrhotic liver (right lobe)

Fluid in Morison pouch

Right kidney

Fluid in anterior subhepatic space

Gallbladder

Right lobe of liver (cirrhotic with nodular contour)

Fluid in Morison pouch

Fluid in right anterior subhepatic space

Visceral peritoneum

Parietal peritoneum

Right kidney

(Top) *Intercostal oblique grayscale ultrasound (in a patient with cirrhosis) shows the dome of the right lobe of the liver and moderate fluid in the right subphrenic region extending anterior to the liver. The fluid is separated from the right-sided pleural effusion by the right diaphragmatic leaf.* **(Middle)** *Subcostal oblique transverse ultrasound of the right upper quadrant shows fluid in the right anterior subhepatic space and in the hepatorenal space. The ascites are secondary to hepatic cirrhosis and the gallbladder is physiologically distended.* **(Bottom)** *Longitudinal transabdominal grayscale ultrasound shows fluid in the right posterior subhepatic space, also known as the Morison pouch, and hepatorenal fossa. This space is continuous with the right anterior subhepatic space and right paracolic gutter.*

RIGHT SUPRAMESOCOLIC SPACE: LESSER SAC

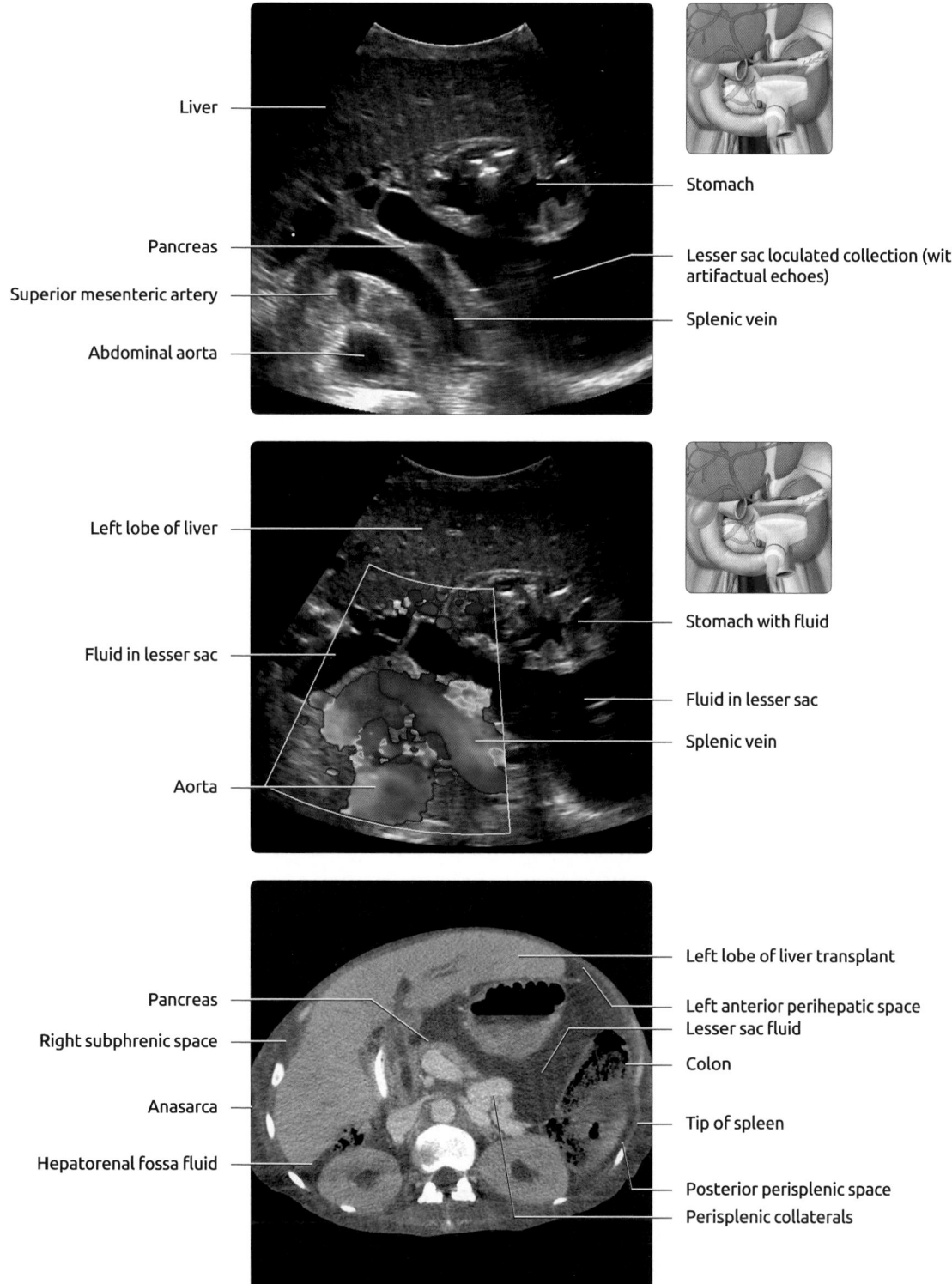

(Top) *Subxiphoid transverse grayscale ultrasound shows a fluid collection in the lesser sac, which extends to the left, behind the stomach and anterior to the pancreas. The lesser sac is part of the right supramesocolic space and communicates with the rest of the peritoneal cavity through the epiploic foramen (of Winslow).* **(Middle)** *Subxiphoid transverse color Doppler ultrasound of the same patient shows moderate fluid in the lesser sac posterior to the stomach. The splenic vein was dilated in this patient, with portal hypertension status post liver transplant.* **(Bottom)** *Axial CECT of the same patient shows fluid in the lesser sac and peritoneal cavity, as well as diffuse anasarca.*

LEFT SUPRAMESOCOLIC SPACE

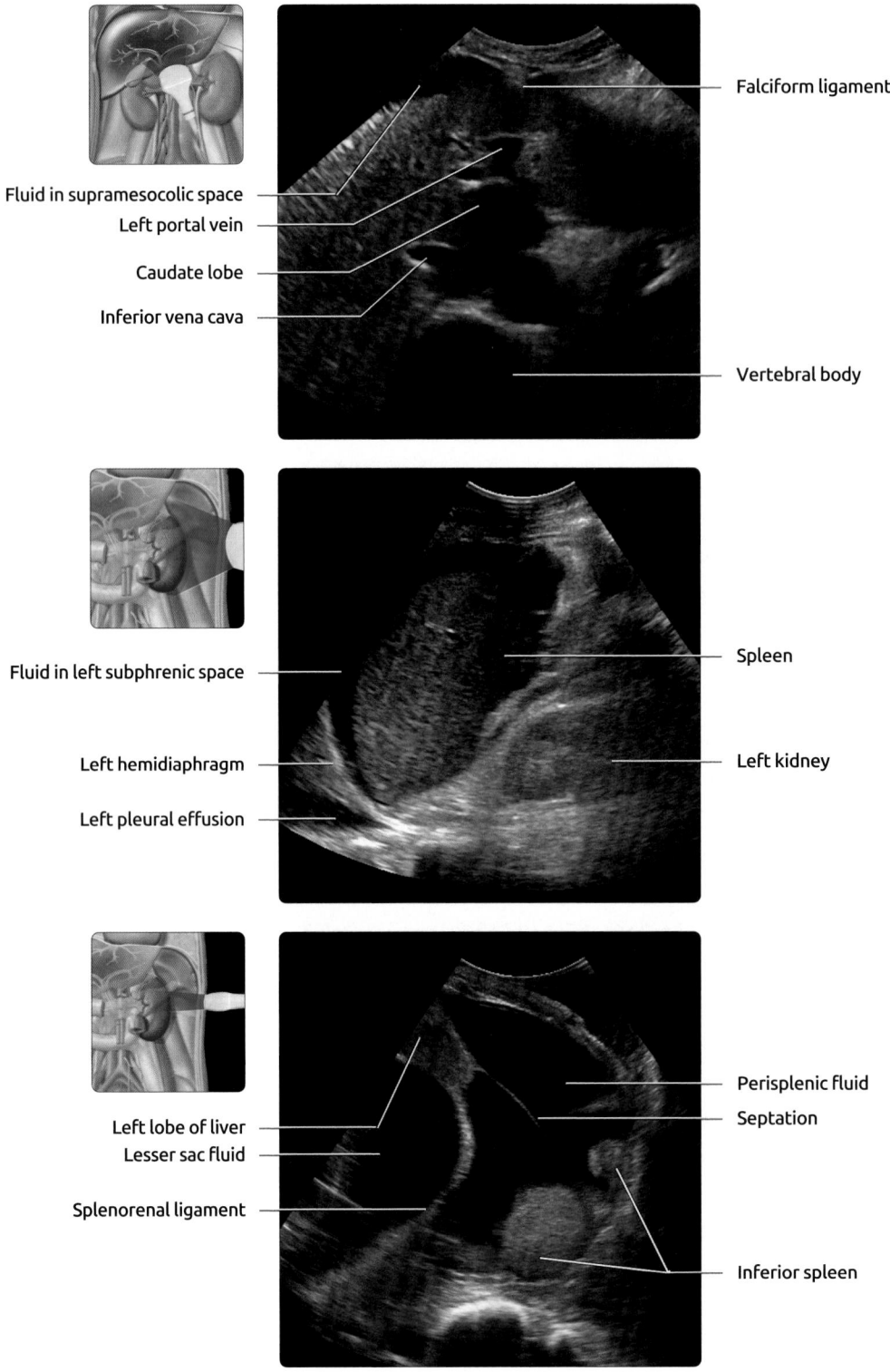

Fluid in supramesocolic space

Left portal vein

Caudate lobe

Inferior vena cava

Falciform ligament

Vertebral body

Fluid in left subphrenic space

Left hemidiaphragm

Left pleural effusion

Spleen

Left kidney

Left lobe of liver

Lesser sac fluid

Splenorenal ligament

Perisplenic fluid

Septation

Inferior spleen

(Top) *Subxiphoid transverse grayscale ultrasound shows fluid anterior to the left lobe of the liver that is localized to the left, posterior subhepatic space. Incidental calculi are seen within a dilated intrahepatic biliary duct.* **(Middle)** *Longitudinal grayscale ultrasound of the left upper quadrant shows a small amount of perisplenic fluid extending under the left hemidiaphragm. The left subphrenic space is separated from the right subphrenic space by the falciform ligament.* **(Bottom)** *Transverse grayscale ultrasound of the left upper quadrant reveals fluid in the perisplenic space and lesser sac.*

INFRAMESOCOLIC SPACE

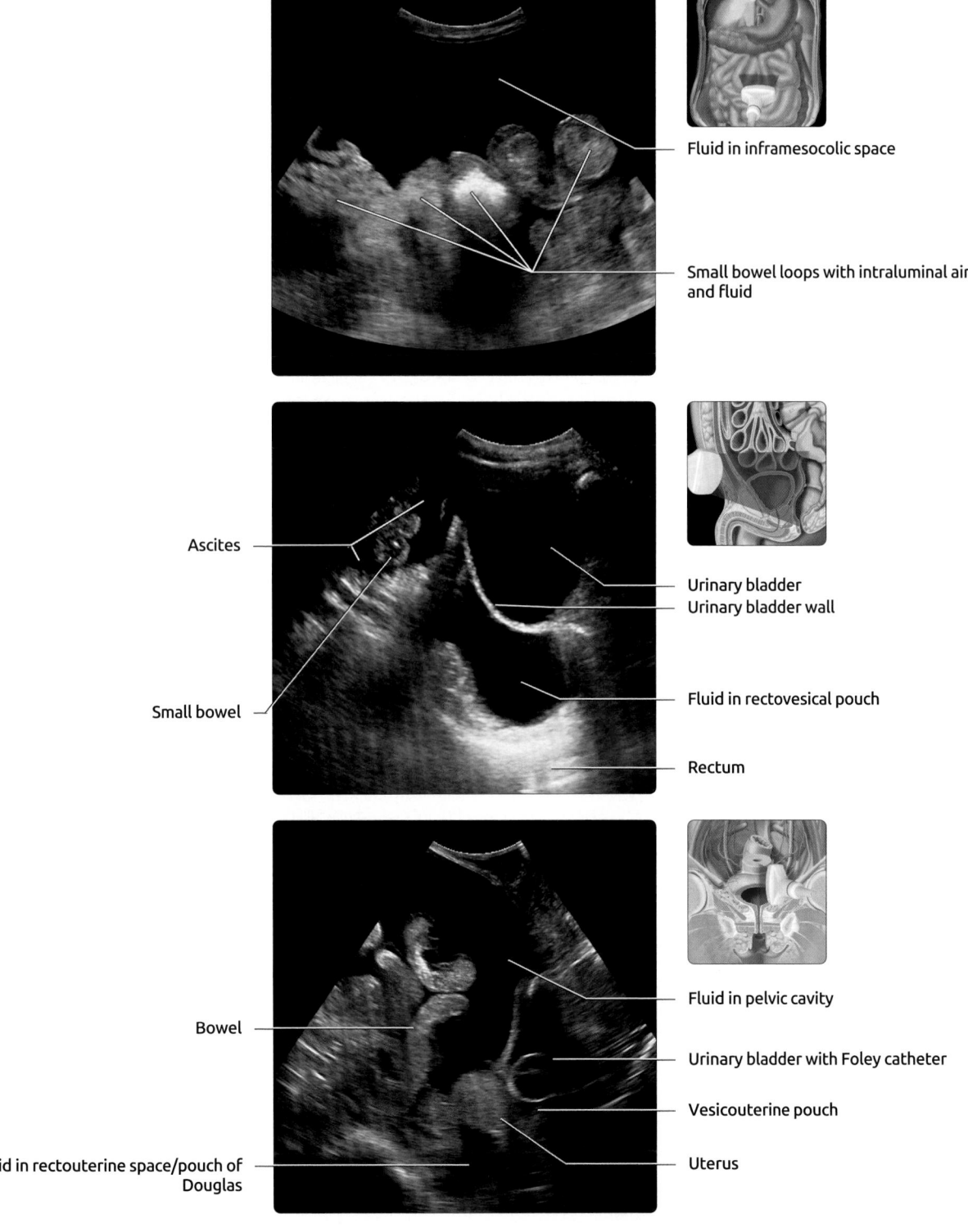

Fluid in inframesocolic space

Small bowel loops with intraluminal air and fluid

Ascites

Small bowel

Urinary bladder
Urinary bladder wall

Fluid in rectovesical pouch

Rectum

Bowel

Fluid in pelvic cavity

Urinary bladder with Foley catheter

Vesicouterine pouch

Fluid in rectouterine space/pouch of Douglas

Uterus

(Top) *Transverse transabdominal ultrasound of the central abdomen reveals moderate to large ascites with floating small bowel loops. The left inframesocolic space is larger compared to the right and communicates directly with the pelvic cavity.* **(Middle)** *Longitudinal ultrasound of the midline suprapubic region in a male patient demonstrates intraperitoneal fluid between bowel loops and extending into the dependent rectovesical pouch. There is a distended urinary bladder.* **(Bottom)** *Longitudinal grayscale ultrasound of the female pelvis shows free fluid. The uterus divides the pelvic cavity into the vesicouterine and rectouterine (pouch of Douglas) spaces. In this case the vesicouterine space contains minimal fluid.*

TERMINOLOGY

Definitions

- Abdomen is the region between diaphragm and pelvis

GROSS ANATOMY

Anatomic Boundaries

- Anterior abdominal wall bounded superiorly by xiphoid process and costal cartilages of 7th-10th ribs
- Anterior wall bounded inferiorly by iliac crest, iliac spine, inguinal ligament, and pubis
- Inguinal ligament is inferior edge of aponeurosis of external oblique muscle

Muscles of Anterior Abdominal Wall

- Consist of 3 flat muscles (external oblique, internal oblique, and transverse abdominal), and 1 strap-like muscle (rectus)
- Combination of muscles and aponeuroses (sheet-like tendons) act as a corset to confine and protect abdominal viscera
- Linea alba is a fibrous raphe stretching from xiphoid to pubis
    - Forms central anterior attachment for abdominal wall muscles
    - Formed by interlacing fibers of aponeuroses of the oblique and transverse abdominal muscles
    - Rectus sheath is also formed by these aponeuroses as they surround rectus muscle
- Linea semilunaris is a vertical fibrous band at lateral edge of rectus sheath bilaterally
    - Aponeuroses of internal and transversus abdominis join in linea semilunaris before forming rectus sheath
- External oblique muscle
    - Largest and most superficial of 3 flat abdominal muscles
    - Origin: External surfaces of ribs 5-12
    - Insertion: Linea alba, iliac crest, pubis via broad aponeurosis
- Internal oblique muscle
    - Middle of 3 flat abdominal muscles
    - Runs at right angles to external oblique
    - Origin: Posterior layer of thoracolumbar fascia, iliac crest, and inguinal ligament
    - Insertion: Ribs 10-12 posteriorly, linea alba via broad aponeurosis, pubis
- Transversus abdominis (transversalis) muscle
    - Innermost of 3 flat abdominal muscles
    - Origin: Lowest 6 costal cartilages, thoracolumbar fascia, iliac crest, inguinal ligament
    - Insertion: Linea alba via broad aponeurosis, pubis
- Rectus abdominis muscle
    - Origin: Pubic symphysis and pubic crest
    - Insertion: Xiphoid process and costal cartilages 5-7
    - Rectus sheath: Strong fibrous compartment that envelops each rectus muscle
        - Contains superior and inferior epigastric vessels
- Actions of anterior abdominal wall muscles
    - Support and protect abdominal viscera
    - Help flex and twist trunk, maintain posture
    - Increase intra-abdominal pressure for defecation, micturition, and childbirth
    - Stabilize pelvis during walking, sitting up
- Transversalis fascia
    - Lies deep to abdominal wall muscles and lines entire abdominal wall
    - Separated from parietal peritoneum by layer of extraperitoneal fat

Muscles of Posterior Abdominal Wall

- Consist of psoas (major and minor), iliacus, and quadratus lumborum
- Psoas: Long thick, fusiform muscle lying lateral to vertebral column
    - Origin: Transverse processes and bodies of vertebrae T12-L5
    - Insertion: Lesser trochanter of femur (passing behind inguinal ligament)
    - Action: Flexes thigh at hip joint; bends vertebral column laterally
- Iliacus: Large triangular sheet of muscle lying along lateral side of psoas
    - Origin: Superior part of iliac fossa
    - Insertion: Lesser trochanter of femur (after joining with psoas tendon)
    - Action: "Iliopsoas muscle" flexes thigh
- Quadratus lumborum: Thick sheet of muscle lying adjacent to transverse processes of lumbar vertebrae
    - Invested by lumbodorsal fascia
    - Origin: Iliac crest and transverse processes of lumbar vertebrae
    - Insertion: 12th rib
    - Actions: Stabilizes position of thorax and pelvis during respiration, walking, bends trunk to side

Paraspinal Muscles

- Also called erector spinae muscles
    - Invested by lumbodorsal fascia
- Composed of 3 columns: Iliocostalis: Lateral; longissimus: Intermediate; spinalis: Medial
- Origins: Sacrum, ilium, and spines of lumbar and 11th-12th thoracic vertebrae
- Insertions: Ribs and vertebrae with additional muscle slips joining columns at successively higher levels
- Action: Extends vertebral column

ANATOMY IMAGING ISSUES

Imaging Recommendations

- High-frequency (5-12 MHz) linear transducer for anterior abdominal wall and paraspinal muscles
- 3-5 MHz for posterior abdominal wall muscles
- Supine position for examination of anterior and lateral abdominal wall
    - Image during Valsalva maneuver and in standing position to increase abdominal pressure and elicit hernias
    - Prone position for ultrasound of paraspinal muscles
- Compare with contralateral side to check for symmetry

ANTERIOR ABDOMINAL WALL

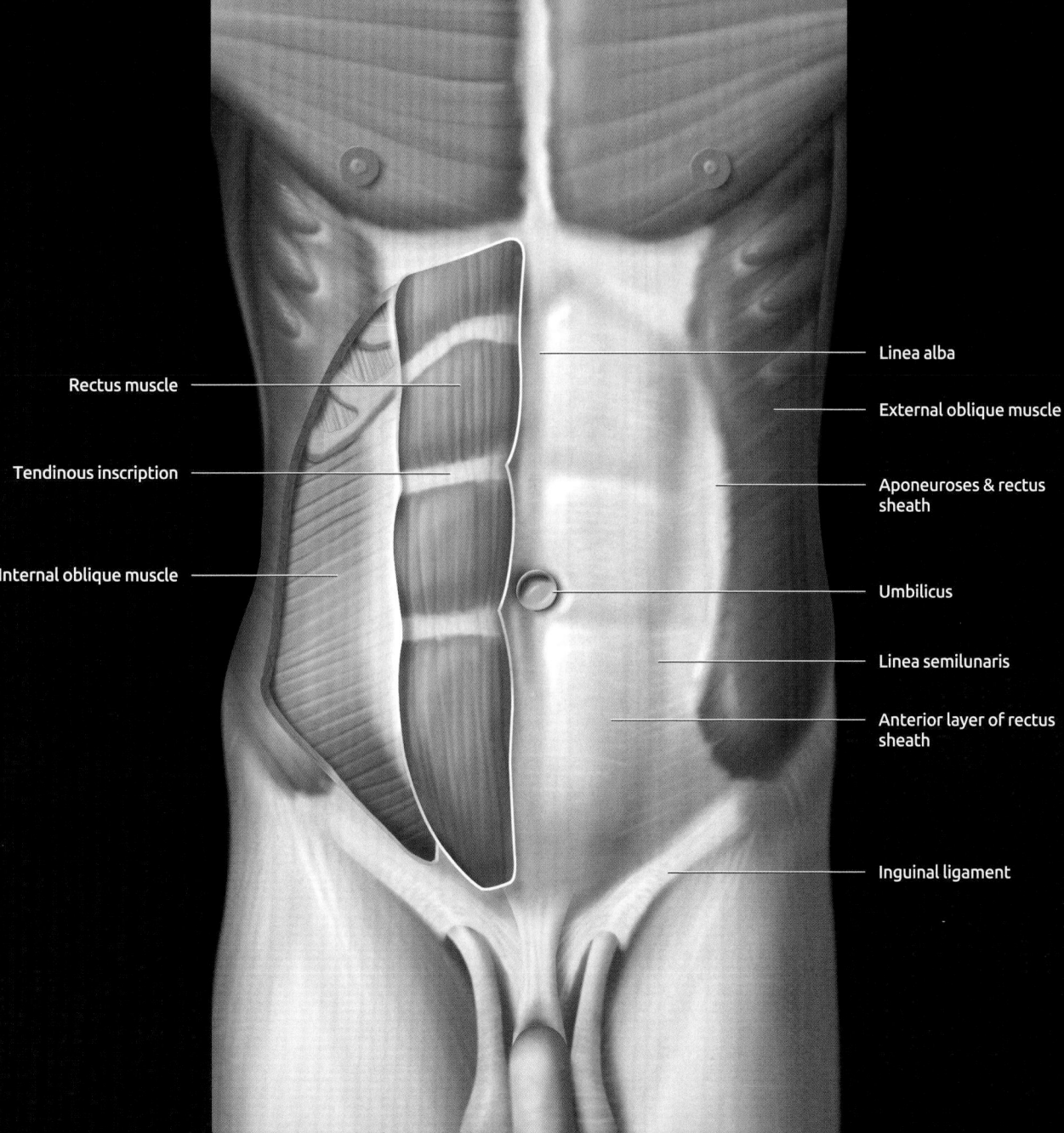

Rectus muscle

Tendinous inscription

Internal oblique muscle

Linea alba

External oblique muscle

Aponeuroses & rectus sheath

Umbilicus

Linea semilunaris

Anterior layer of rectus sheath

Inguinal ligament

Graphic shows the aponeuroses of the internal and external oblique and transverse abdominal muscles are 2-layered and interweave with each other, covering the rectus muscle, constituting the rectus sheath and linea alba. About midway between the umbilicus and symphysis, at the arcuate line, the posterior rectus sheath ends (arcuate line), and the transversalis fascia is the only structure between the rectus muscle and parietal peritoneum.

POSTERIOR ABDOMINAL WALL

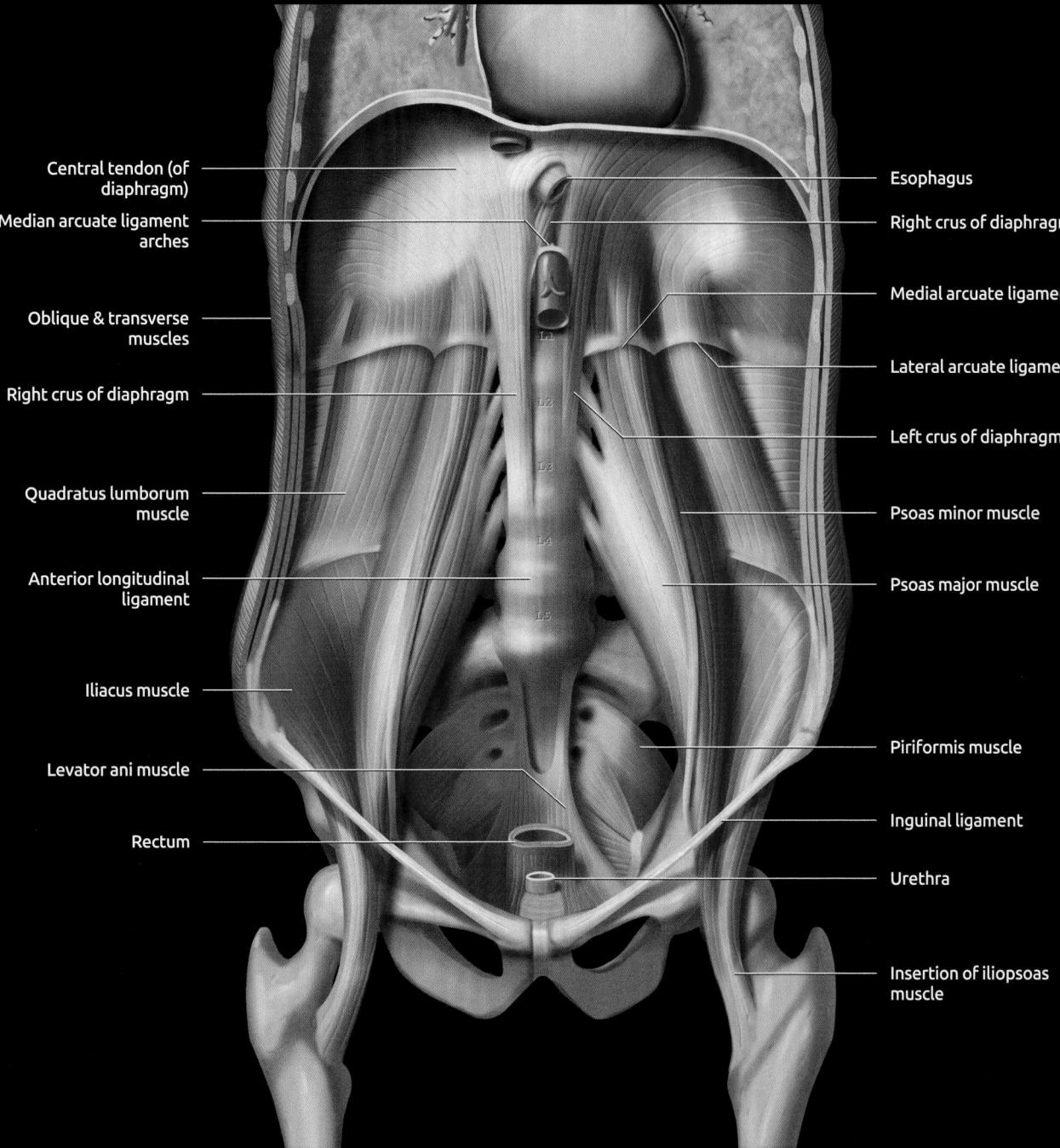

Central tendon (of diaphragm)

Median arcuate ligament arches

Oblique & transverse muscles

Right crus of diaphragm

Quadratus lumborum muscle

Anterior longitudinal ligament

Iliacus muscle

Levator ani muscle

Rectum

Esophagus

Right crus of diaphragm

Medial arcuate ligament

Lateral arcuate ligament

Left crus of diaphragm

Psoas minor muscle

Psoas major muscle

Piriformis muscle

Inguinal ligament

Urethra

Insertion of iliopsoas muscle

Graphic shows the lumbar vertebrae are covered and attached by the anterior longitudinal ligament, and the diaphragmatic crura are closely attached to it, as are the origins of the psoas muscles, which also arise from the transverse processes. Iliacus muscle arises from the iliac fossa of the pelvis and inserts into the tendon of the psoas major, constituting the iliopsoas muscle, which inserts onto the lesser trochanter. Quadratus lumborum arises from the iliac crest and inserts onto the 12th rib and transverse processes of the lumbar vertebrae. Diaphragmatic and transverse abdominal fibers interlace. Psoas and quadratus lumborum pass behind the diaphragm under medial and lateral arcuate ligaments.

MUSCLES OF BACK IN SITU

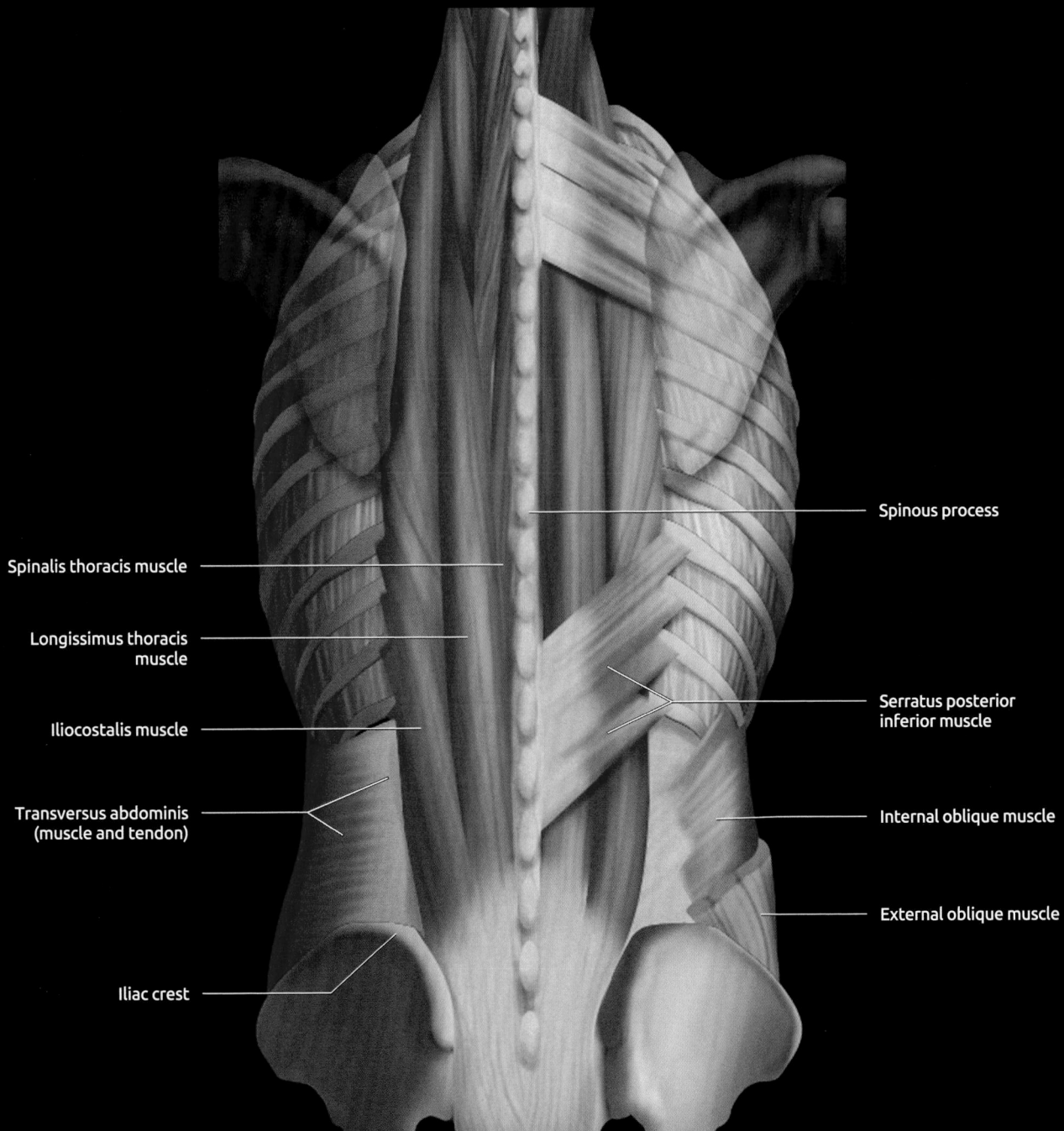

Spinalis thoracis muscle

Longissimus thoracis muscle

Iliocostalis muscle

Transversus abdominis (muscle and tendon)

Iliac crest

Spinous process

Serratus posterior inferior muscle

Internal oblique muscle

External oblique muscle

Graphic shows the paraspinal muscles and muscles of the back. The latissimus dorsi muscles are not included. The erector spinae have thick tendinous origins from the sacral and iliac crests and the lumbar and 11th to 12th thoracic spinous processes. Superiorly, the muscle becomes fleshy, and in the upper lumbar region subdivides to become the iliocostalis, longissimus, and spinalis muscles (from lateral to medial), tapering as they insert into the vertebrae and ribs. The erector muscles flank the spinous processes and span the length of the posterior thorax and abdomen. They are responsible for extension of the vertebral column.

ANTERIOR ABDOMINAL WALL

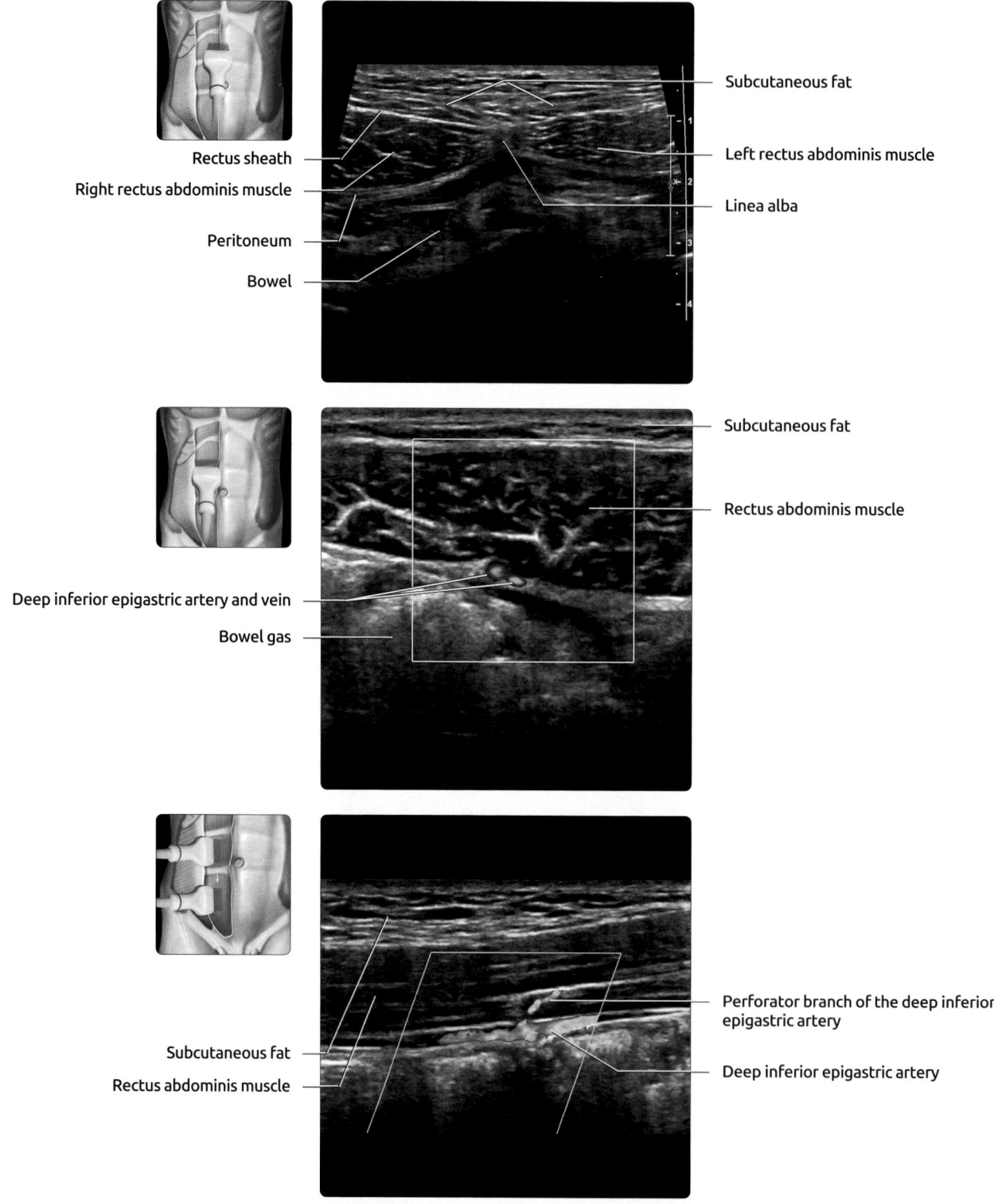

Rectus sheath

Right rectus abdominis muscle

Peritoneum

Bowel

Subcutaneous fat

Left rectus abdominis muscle

Linea alba

Subcutaneous fat

Rectus abdominis muscle

Deep inferior epigastric artery and vein

Bowel gas

Perforator branch of the deep inferior epigastric artery

Deep inferior epigastric artery

Subcutaneous fat

Rectus abdominis muscle

(Top) *Transverse grayscale ultrasound of the midline anterior abdominal wall shows the paired rectus abdominis muscles separated by the linea alba. The rectus abdominis muscles are comparable in echogenicity and thickness. The surrounding rectus sheath is seen as a fine, thin, echogenic structure around the muscles.* (Middle) *Transverse power Doppler ultrasound of a rectus abdominis muscle in the lower abdomen shows the deep inferior epigastric artery and vein. Branches of the superior epigastric artery that arise in the upper abdomen anastomose with branches of the inferior epigastric artery at the umbilicus.* (Bottom) *Longitudinal color Doppler ultrasound shows a perforating branch of the deep inferior epigastric artery extending into the rectus muscle. These perforators are important for breast reconstruction with abdominal wall flaps.*

ANTEROLATERAL ABDOMINAL WALL

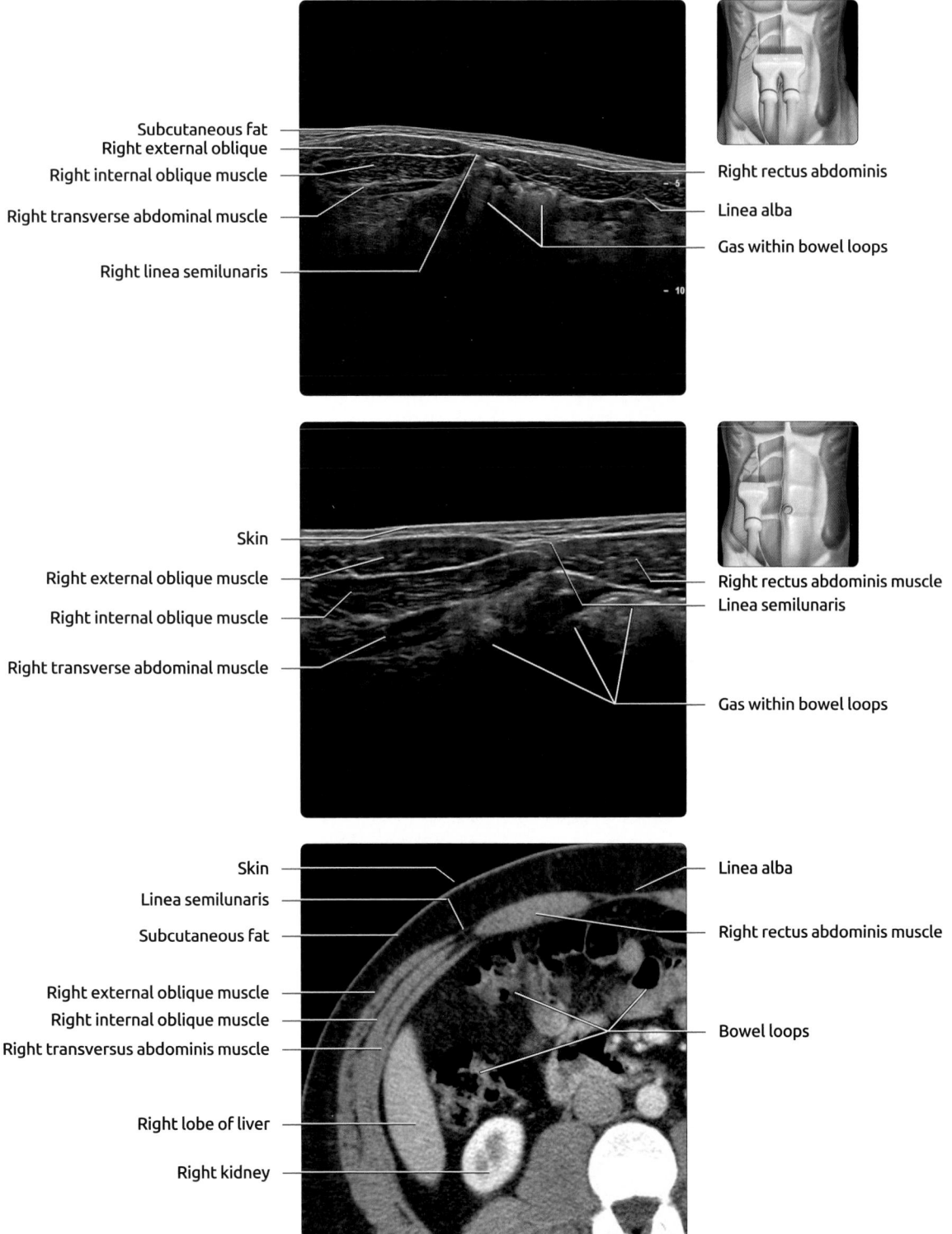

Subcutaneous fat
Right external oblique
Right internal oblique muscle
Right transverse abdominal muscle
Right linea semilunaris

Right rectus abdominis
Linea alba
Gas within bowel loops

Skin
Right external oblique muscle
Right internal oblique muscle
Right transverse abdominal muscle

Right rectus abdominis muscle
Linea semilunaris
Gas within bowel loops

Skin
Linea semilunaris
Subcutaneous fat
Right external oblique muscle
Right internal oblique muscle
Right transversus abdominis muscle
Right lobe of liver
Right kidney

Linea alba
Right rectus abdominis muscle
Bowel loops

(Top) *Transverse extended FOV, grayscale ultrasound shows the relationship of the medially located rectus abdominis and the laterally located oblique and transverse abdominal muscles. Medially the external and internal oblique and the transversus abdominal muscles form aponeuroses that comprise the rectus sheath, with the muscles thinning at the linea semilunaris. The linea alba is thin in the lower abdomen.* (Middle) *Transverse grayscale ultrasound at the right anterolateral abdominal wall shows the relationship of the lateral abdominal wall muscles in better detail. Note the oblique and transverse abdominal muscles taper medially as they become aponeuroses.* (Bottom) *Correlative, axial contrast-enhanced CT illustrates the muscles of the abdominal wall. The rectus abdominis muscle in the anterior abdominal wall, and the oblique and transverse abdominal muscles in the anterolateral abdominal wall and their aponeuroses are shown.*

POSTERIOR ABDOMINAL WALL

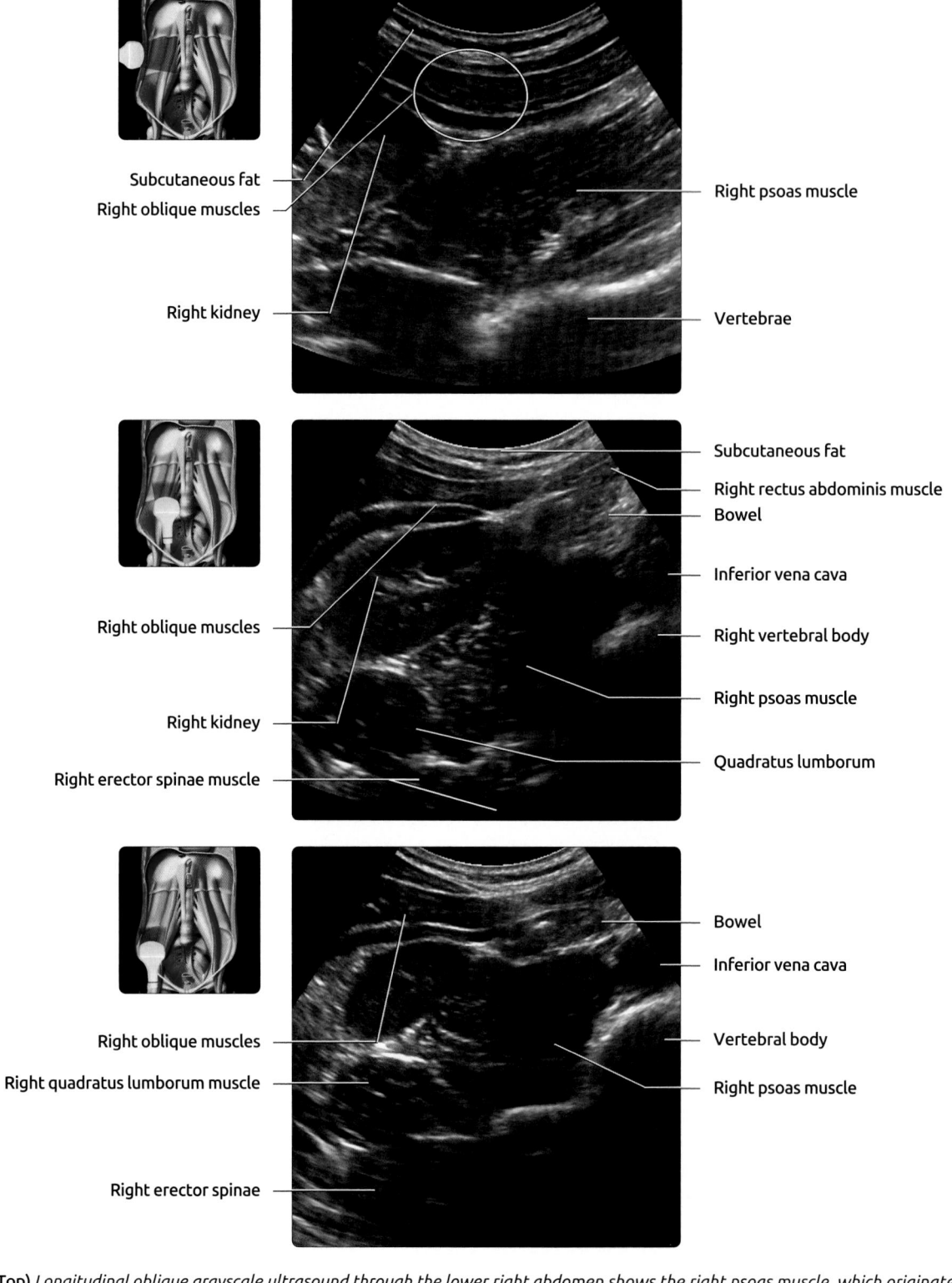

Subcutaneous fat
Right oblique muscles

Right kidney

Right psoas muscle

Vertebrae

Right oblique muscles

Right kidney

Right erector spinae muscle

Subcutaneous fat
Right rectus abdominis muscle
Bowel

Inferior vena cava

Right vertebral body

Right psoas muscle

Quadratus lumborum

Right oblique muscles

Right quadratus lumborum muscle

Right erector spinae

Bowel

Inferior vena cava

Vertebral body

Right psoas muscle

(Top) *Longitudinal oblique grayscale ultrasound through the lower right abdomen shows the right psoas muscle, which originates from the lumbar spine and inserts into the proximal femur.* **(Middle)** *Transverse grayscale ultrasound of right mid abdomen using the kidney as an acoustic window is shown. The kidney is anterior and lateral to the psoas and anterior to the quadratus lumborum. The psoas runs along the paravertebral region in its entire abdominal course. The quadratus lumborum originates from the iliolumbar ligament and iliac crest to insert into the last rib and lumbar transverse processes. It is easily identified as the muscle on which the kidney rests.* **(Bottom)** *Transverse grayscale ultrasound of the right upper abdomen, continuing the scan inferiorly shows the relationship of the posterior abdominal wall muscles are maintained.*

POSTERIOR ABDOMINAL WALL, CT CORRELATION

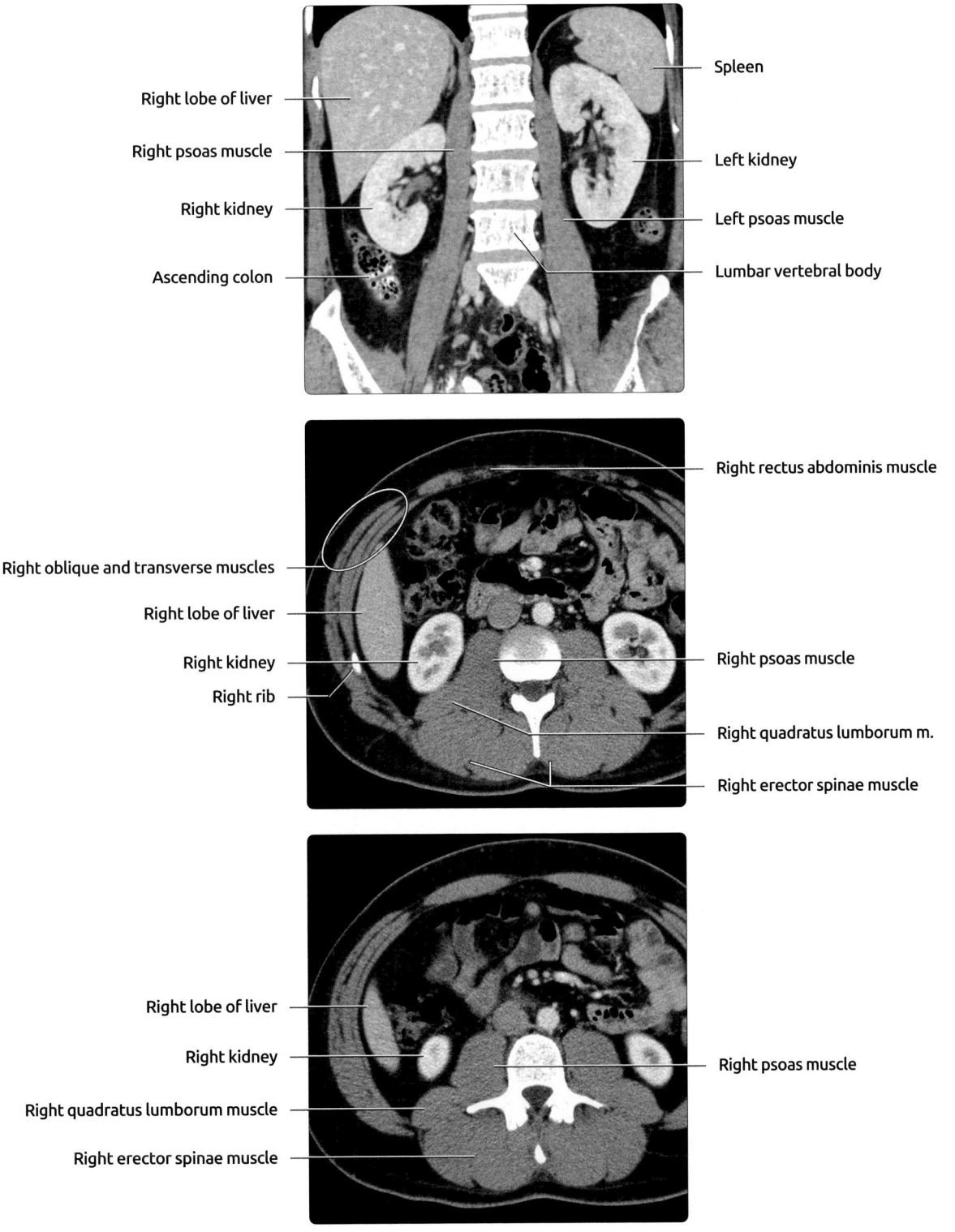

Right lobe of liver

Right psoas muscle

Right kidney

Ascending colon

Spleen

Left kidney

Left psoas muscle

Lumbar vertebral body

Right rectus abdominis muscle

Right oblique and transverse muscles

Right lobe of liver

Right kidney

Right rib

Right psoas muscle

Right quadratus lumborum m.

Right erector spinae muscle

Right lobe of liver

Right kidney

Right quadratus lumborum muscle

Right erector spinae muscle

Right psoas muscle

(Top) *Coronal correlative CECT shows the paralumbar location of the psoas muscles and their medial location relative to the kidneys. The psoas muscles originate from the lumbar and 12th thoracic vertebral bodies and their transverse processes and run past the pelvic brim where they course inferolaterally to be joined by the iliacus muscle.* **(Middle)** *Axial correlative CECT better illustrates the anatomic relationships of the kidney with the posterior abdominal wall muscles. The kidney is lateral to the psoas muscle and rests upon the quadratus lumborum muscle. The erector spinae muscles are immediately posterior to the quadratus lumborum, and the 2 muscles are invested by the lumbodorsal fascia.* **(Bottom)** *Axial correlative CECT at the level of the inferior pole of the right kidney. The psoas muscle and quadratus lumborum muscles, seen in their midsections, are now thicker.*

POSTERIOR ABDOMINAL WALL

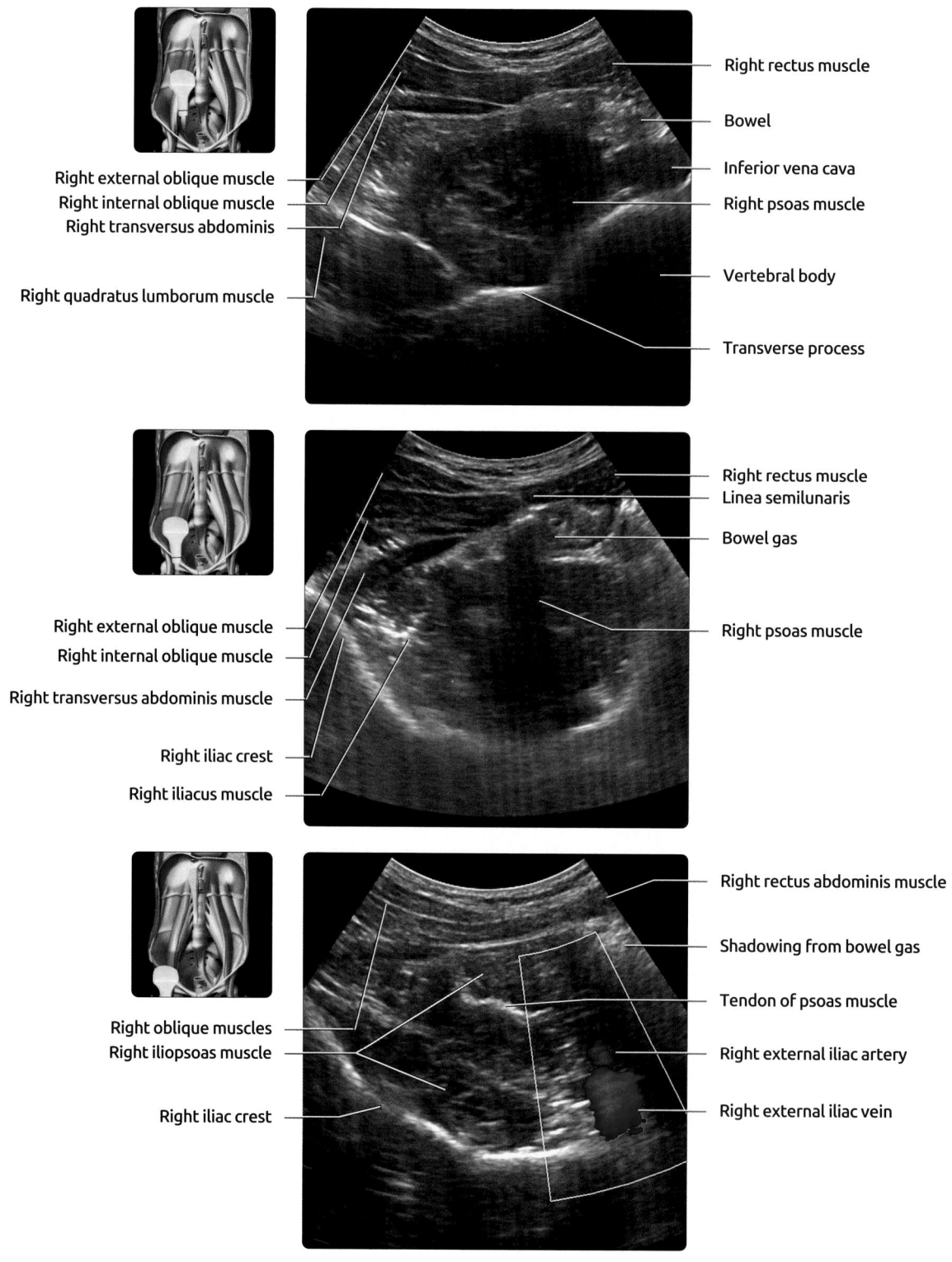

Right external oblique muscle
Right internal oblique muscle
Right transversus abdominis

Right quadratus lumborum muscle

Right rectus muscle
Bowel
Inferior vena cava
Right psoas muscle
Vertebral body
Transverse process

Right external oblique muscle
Right internal oblique muscle
Right transversus abdominis muscle
Right iliac crest
Right iliacus muscle

Right rectus muscle
Linea semilunaris
Bowel gas
Right psoas muscle

Right oblique muscles
Right iliopsoas muscle
Right iliac crest

Right rectus abdominis muscle
Shadowing from bowel gas
Tendon of psoas muscle
Right external iliac artery
Right external iliac vein

(**Top**) *Transverse grayscale ultrasound in the lower abdominal region shows the right psoas muscle, composed of the psoas minor which rests upon the psoas major. The 2 muscles cannot be separated clearly on ultrasound. Because of their depth, the paraspinal muscles cannot be demonstrated in detail.* (**Middle**) *Transverse grayscale ultrasound of the right lower abdomen, continued from the previous image, shows that the distal psoas muscle has diminished in size. It rests on the medial portion of the iliacus muscle; the latter is a flat muscle that fills the iliac fossa. Both continue inferiorly together.* (**Bottom**) *Distally, the fibers from the iliacus muscle converge and insert into the lateral side of the psoas muscle to form the iliopsoas muscle. Common iliac vessels can be seen medially.*

POSTERIOR ABDOMINAL WALL, CT CORRELATION

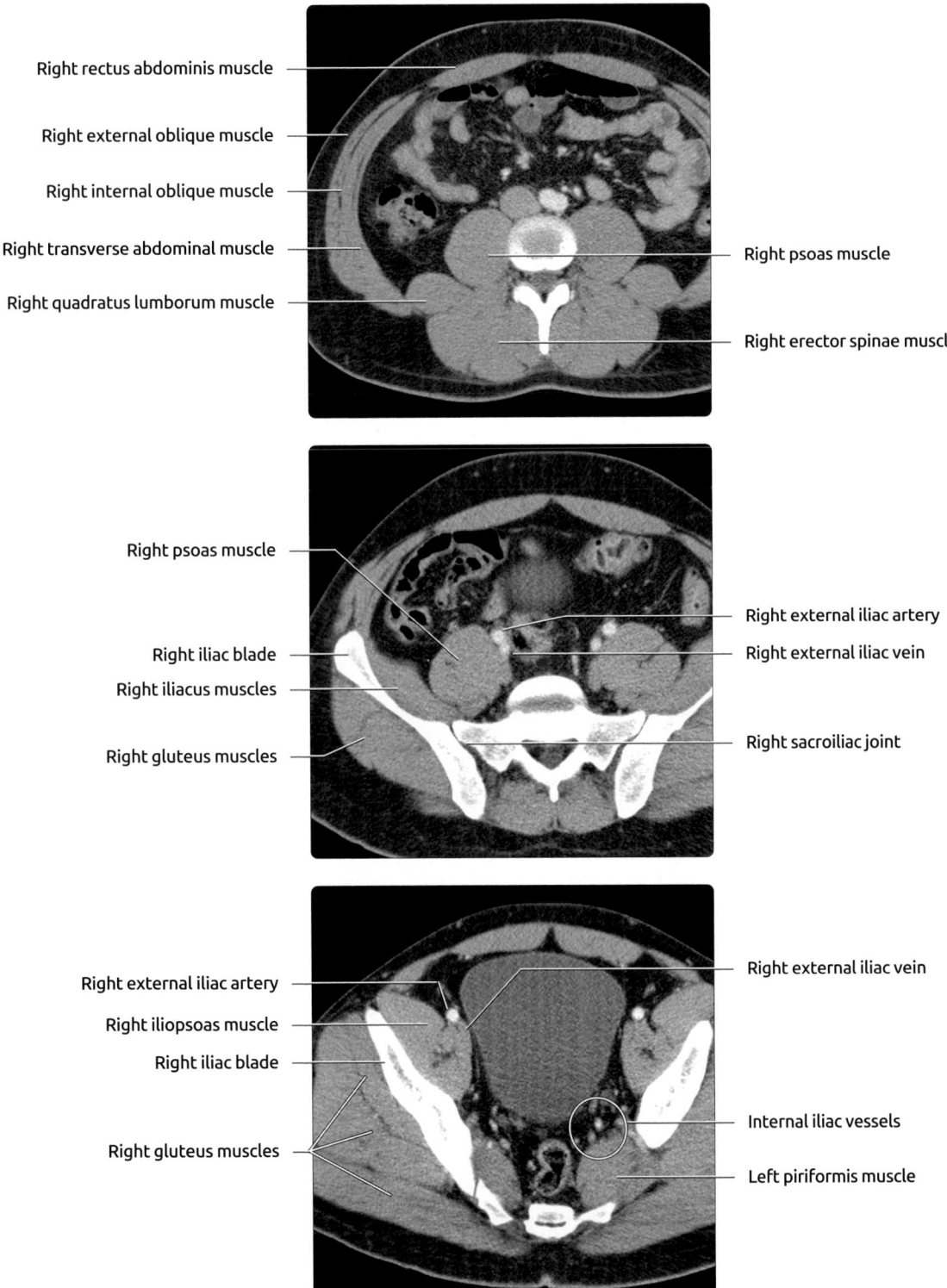

Right rectus abdominis muscle

Right external oblique muscle

Right internal oblique muscle

Right transverse abdominal muscle

Right quadratus lumborum muscle

Right psoas muscle

Right erector spinae muscle

Right psoas muscle

Right iliac blade

Right iliacus muscles

Right gluteus muscles

Right external iliac artery

Right external iliac vein

Right sacroiliac joint

Right external iliac artery

Right iliopsoas muscle

Right iliac blade

Right gluteus muscles

Right external iliac vein

Internal iliac vessels

Left piriformis muscle

(Top) *Axial correlative CECT below the kidneys shows the quadratus lumborum muscle is more laterally located and the psoas muscle is directly anterior to the erector spinae muscle.* (Middle) *Axial correlative CECT shows the psoas muscle has begun its dorsolateral course and is now anterior to the iliacus muscle. The iliacus muscle is easily identified as a flat muscle filling the iliac fossa, arising from the upper 2/3 of the iliac fossa, inner lip of the iliac crest, anterior sacroiliac and the iliolumbar ligaments, and base of the sacrum.* (Bottom) *Axial correlative CECT shows the psoas and iliacus muscles have converged and are now indistinguishable from one another. The resultant iliopsoas muscle passes beneath the inguinal ligament and becomes tendinous as it inserts into the lesser trochanter of the femur.*

PARASPINAL MUSCLES

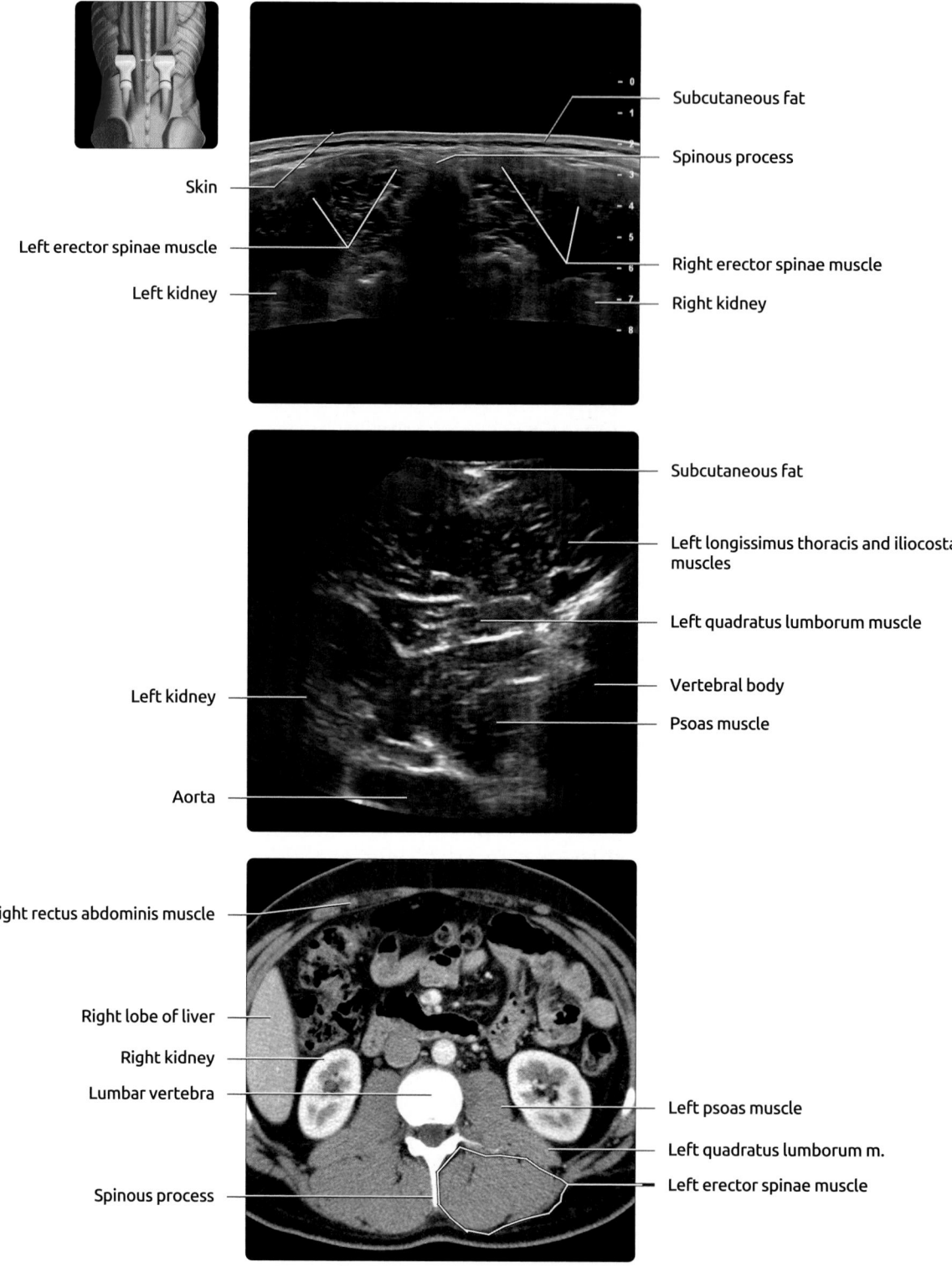

Skin

Left erector spinae muscle

Left kidney

Subcutaneous fat

Spinous process

Right erector spinae muscle

Right kidney

Left kidney

Aorta

Subcutaneous fat

Left longissimus thoracis and iliocostalis muscles

Left quadratus lumborum muscle

Vertebral body

Psoas muscle

Right rectus abdominis muscle

Right lobe of liver

Right kidney

Lumbar vertebra

Spinous process

Left psoas muscle

Left quadratus lumborum m.

Left erector spinae muscle

(Top) *Transverse extended FOV grayscale US of the back (with patient prone) shows the erector spinae muscles flanking the spinous process. They are invested by lumbodorsal fascia, which also invests the anteriorly located quadratus lumborum muscle. The kidneys are partially demonstrated.* **(Middle)** *Transverse oblique grayscale US of the left erector spinae muscle (with patient prone). The 3 columns (iliocostalis, longissimus, and spinalis muscles, from lateral to medial) comprising the erector spinae are not clearly separated from one another on ultrasound. They are identified collectively as a thick fleshy muscle lateral to the spinous process.* **(Bottom)** *Axial correlative CECT of the paraspinal muscles at the level of the kidneys shows the erector spinae muscles originate from a broad and thick tendon, which originates from the sacrum and iliac crest, lumbar, and 11th and 12th thoracic spinous processes.*

MR

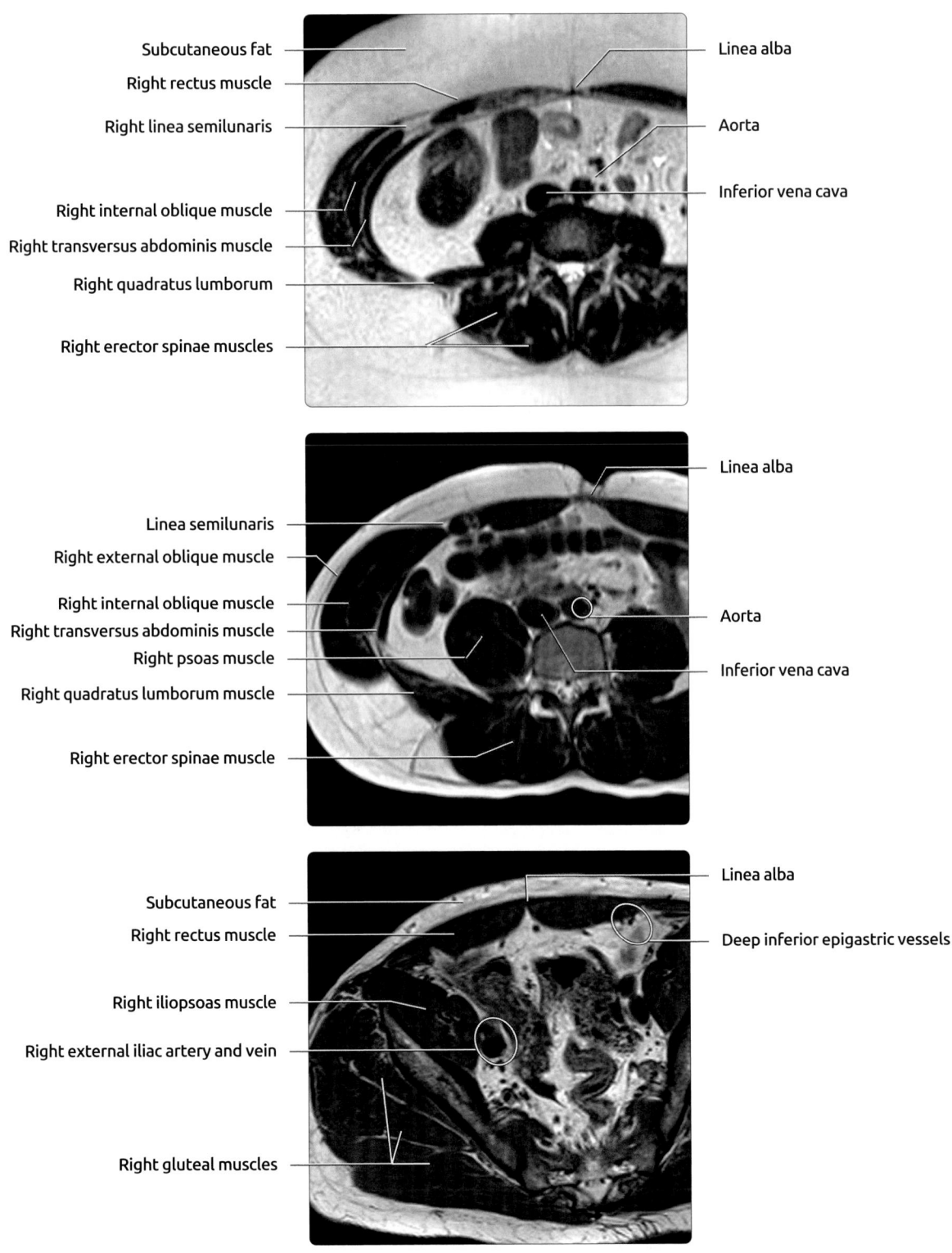

Subcutaneous fat
Right rectus muscle
Right linea semilunaris

Right internal oblique muscle
Right transversus abdominis muscle
Right quadratus lumborum

Right erector spinae muscles

Linea alba

Aorta

Inferior vena cava

Linea semilunaris
Right external oblique muscle

Right internal oblique muscle
Right transversus abdominis muscle
Right psoas muscle
Right quadratus lumborum muscle

Right erector spinae muscle

Linea alba

Aorta

Inferior vena cava

Subcutaneous fat
Right rectus muscle

Right iliopsoas muscle

Right external iliac artery and vein

Right gluteal muscles

Linea alba

Deep inferior epigastric vessels

(Top) *Axial T2 HASTE MR in an older patient with muscle atrophy shows fat in between the individual muscles of the anterior and posterior abdominal wall.* (Middle) *Axial T2 HASTE MR in a younger male patient shows more bulky abdominal wall musculature with little intermuscular fat.* (Bottom) *Axial T1 MR at a lower level shows the iliopsoas as 1 muscle bundle.*

PART I
SECTION 2
Pelvis

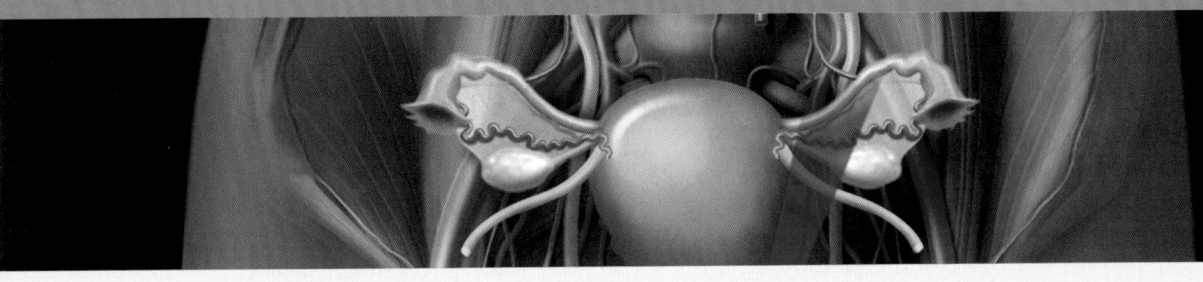

GROSS ANATOMY

Ureters

- Muscular tubes (25-30 cm long) that carry urine from kidneys to bladder
  - In abdomen, retroperitoneal location
    - Proximal ureters lie in perirenal space
    - Mid ureters lie over psoas muscles slightly medial to tips of L2-L5 transverse process
  - In pelvis, lie anterior to sacroiliac joints crossing common iliac artery bifurcation near pelvic brim
    - Lies anterior to internal iliac vessels, and course along pelvic sidewall
    - At level of ischial spines, ureters curve anteromedially to enter bladder at level of seminal vesicles (men) or cervix (women)
    - Ureterovesical junction: Ureters pass obliquely through muscular wall of bladder for ~ 2 cm, creating valve effect with bladder distension, preventing vesicoureteral reflux (VUR)
  - 3 points of physiological narrowing: Ureteropelvic junction, pelvic brim (crossing over the common iliac artery), and ureterovesical junction
- Vessels, nerves, and lymphatics
  - Arterial branches are numerous and variable, arising from aorta and renal, gonadal, internal iliac, vesical, and rectal arteries
  - Venous branches & lymphatics follow arteries with similar names
  - Innervation
    - Autonomic from adjacent sympathetic and parasympathetic plexuses, cause ureteral peristalsis
    - Also carry pain (stretch) receptors; "stone" in abdominal ureter perceived as back & flank pain; pain from stone in pelvic ureter may extend to scrotum or labia
  - Lymphatics to external & internal iliac nodes (pelvic ureter), aortocaval nodes (abdomen)

Bladder

- Hollow, distensible viscus with strong, muscular wall and normal adult capacity of 300-600 mL of urine
- Lies in extraperitoneal (retroperitoneal) pelvis
- Peritoneum covers dome of bladder
  - Reflections of peritoneum form deep recesses in pelvic peritoneal cavity
  - Rectovesical pouch (between rectum and bladder) is most dependent recess in men (and in women following hysterectomy)
  - Vesicouterine pouch (bladder and uterus) and rectouterine pouch (of Douglas; rectum and uterus) are most dependent in women
- Bladder is surrounded by extraperitoneal fat and loose connective tissue
  - Perivesical space (contains bladder and urachus)
  - Prevesical or retropubic space (of Retzius) between bladder and symphysis pubis
    - Communicates superiorly with infrarenal retroperitoneal compartment
    - Communicates posteriorly with presacral space
- Spaces can expand to contain large amounts of fluid (as in extraperitoneal rupture of bladder and hemorrhage from pelvic fractures)
- Wall of bladder composed mostly of detrusor muscle
  - Trigone of bladder: Triangular structure at base of bladder with apices marked by 2 ureteral orifices and internal urethral orifice
- Vessels, nerves, and lymphatics
  - Arteries from internal iliac
    - Superior vesical arteries and other branches of internal iliac arteries in both sexes
  - Venous drainage
    - Men: Vesical & prostatic venous plexuses → internal iliac and internal vertebral veins
    - Women: Vesical and uterovaginal plexuses → internal iliac vein
  - Autonomic innervation
    - Parasympathetic from pelvic splanchnic & inferior hypogastric nerves (causes contraction of detrusor muscle and relaxation of internal urethral sphincter to permit emptying of bladder)
    - Sensory fibers follow parasympathetic nerves

IMAGING ANATOMY

Overview

- Normal ureters are small in caliber (2-8 mm) and are nearly impossible to appreciate on ultrasound largely due to obscuration by overlying bowel gas
- Fluid-distended urinary bladder is anechoic with posterior acoustic enhancement
- Urinary bladder changes in shape and position depending on intraluminal volume of urine
  - In its nondistended state, urinary bladder is retropubic in location, lying anterior to uterus in females and rectum in males
  - In markedly distended state, urinary bladder may occupy abdominopelvic area
  - Urinary bladder wall changes in thickness depending on state of distension of urinary bladder, and is normally 3-5 mm in thickness

ANATOMY IMAGING ISSUES

Imaging Recommendations

- Transducer: Curvilinear 2-5 MHz
- Ureters
  - Ureters are normally not seen on ultrasound unless they are dilated; when dilated, overlying bowel gas may still limit ureteral evaluation in transabdominal approach
    - Proximal dilated ureters may be well seen using kidney as window in coronal oblique plane
    - Middle portion of dilated ureter may be identified in pediatric patients or thin adults using transabdominal approach
    - Dilated terminal ureter/ureterovesical junctions are seen best along posterolateral aspect of urinary bladder on transverse view
  - Ureteral caliber may slightly increase as result of overfilled urinary bladder

- Distended bladder may cause ureteral and pelvicalyceal dilation and rescanning post void is beneficial to exclude obstruction
  - Color Doppler evaluation of bladder helps assess normal ureteral jets and helps exclude complete ureteral obstruction
- Bladder
  - Recommend fluid intake prior to examination to ensure optimal distension of urinary bladder
    - In fully distended state, urinary bladder is easily visualized using transabdominal approach
  - Examine patient in supine position with transabdominal suprapubic approach
    - Perform scanning in sagittal and transverse planes
    - Patient may be placed in decubitus position, especially to determine mobility of intravesical masses or debris, if present
    - With smaller volumes, caudal angulation of transducer is needed to visualize urinary bladder in its retropubic location
  - Nature of cystic structure in pelvis may be ascertained by asking patient to void or by inserting Foley catheter
  - In some instances, transvaginal ultrasound may be used in women for evaluation of suspect bladder neck lesions, UVJ stone, or ureterocele
  - Advantages of ultrasound
    - Radiation-free, real-time assessment with high spatial resolution of bladder and bladder wall
    - Real-time assessment of intraluminal masses in bladder for mobility and vascularity
    - Real-time imaging guidance for bladder intervention, e.g., placement of percutaneous suprapubic catheters
    - Real-time assessment of ureteral jets using color Doppler imaging; particularly useful in pregnant patients with dilated collecting system
- Large midline ovarian or pelvic cystic mass may simulate bladder on transabdominal ultrasound
  - Attention to normal bladder shape, rescanning after voiding to confirm empty bladder, or transvaginal imaging is helpful to differentiate

Imaging Pitfalls

- Bladder
  - Reverberation artifacts are commonly encountered behind anterior wall of urinary bladder
    - Appear as regularly spaced lines at increasing depth as a result of repeated reflection of ultrasound signals between highly reflective interfaces close to transducer
    - May be reduced or avoided by changing scanning angle or by moving transducer or using spacer
  - Underdistended bladder may give false impression of wall thickening and limits intraluminal assessment

CLINICAL IMPLICATIONS

Clinical Importance

- Ureters are at high risk of inadvertent injury during abdominal or gynecological surgery due to close proximity to uterine (in uterosacral ligament) and gonadal arteries (at pelvic brim)
- Ectopic ureter

  - Usually (80%) associated with complete ureteral duplication; more common in females
  - Ectopic ureteral insertion in females can occur in urethra, vagina leading to urinary incontinence
  - In complete duplication, upper moeity inserts ectopically inferiorly and distally to lower moeity (Weigert-Meyer rule) and can be associated with ureterocele
  - In duplicated system, upper moiety has higher predisposition to obstruction from ureterocele, while lower moiety has predisposition to vesicoureteral reflux
- Ureterocele: Cystic dilation of intramural portion of ureter bulging into bladder
  - Orthotopic: Normal insertion of single ureter
  - Ectopic: Inserts below trigone, mostly in duplicated system
- Ureteral duplication
  - Bifid ureter drains a duplex kidney but ureters unite before entering bladder
- Extraperitoneal bladder rupture
  - Urine and blood distend prevesical space (Retzius)
  - Urine often tracks posteriorly into presacral space, superiorly into retroperitoneal abdomen
  - Usually caused by pelvic fractures
- Intraperitoneal bladder rupture
  - Urine flows up paracolic gutters into peritoneal recesses and surrounds bowel
  - Usually caused by blunt trauma to an overdistended bladder
  - Bladder ruptures along dome, which is in contact with intraperitoneal space
- Patent fetal urachus forms conduit between umbilicus and bladder
  - Urachus is normally obliterated to form median umbilical ligament
  - May persist as cyst, diverticulum, or rarely, fistula
  - May become infected or lead to carcinoma (adenocarcinoma)
- Bladder diverticula are common
  - Congenital: Hutch diverticulum (near ureterovesical junction)
  - Acquired (usually due to chronic bladder outlet obstruction), associated with trabeculated bladder wall
  - Can lead to infection, stones, tumor

SELECTED REFERENCES

1. Demir S et al: Value of sonographic anterior-posterior renal pelvis measurements before and after voiding for predicting vesicoureteral reflux in children. J Clin Ultrasound. ePub, 2014
2. Butler P, Mitchell A, Healy JC. Applied Radiological Anatomy. Cambridge University Press. 2012
3. Shimoya K et al: Diagnosis of ureterocele with transvaginal sonography. Gynecol Obstet Invest. 54(1):58-60, 2002
4. Djavan B et al: Bladder ultrasonography. Semin Urol. 12(4):306-19, 1994
5. Hayden CK Jr et al: Urinary tract infections in childhood: a current imaging approach. Radiographics. 6(6):1023-38, 1986
6. Glassberg KI et al: Suggested terminology for duplex systems, ectopic ureters and ureteroceles. J Urol. 132(6):1153-4, 1984

URETERS AND URINARY BLADDER IN SITU

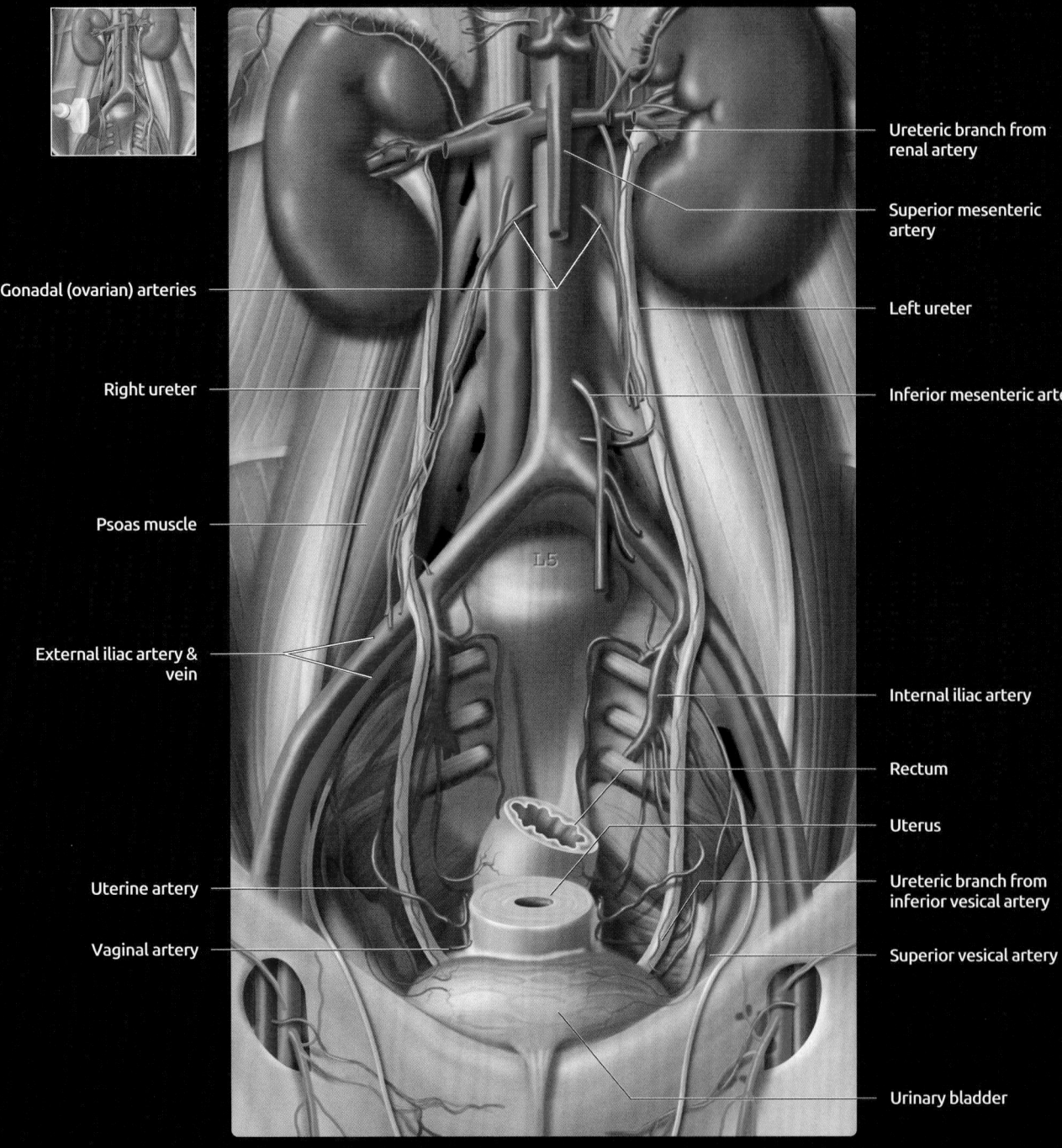

Ureteric branch from renal artery

Superior mesenteric artery

Gonadal (ovarian) arteries

Left ureter

Right ureter

Inferior mesenteric artery

Psoas muscle

External iliac artery & vein

Internal iliac artery

Rectum

Uterus

Uterine artery

Ureteric branch from inferior vesical artery

Vaginal artery

Superior vesical artery

Urinary bladder

The ureters receive numerous and highly variable arterial branches from the aorta, and the renal, gonadal, and internal iliac arteries. These vessels are short and can be easily ruptured by retraction of the ureter during surgical procedures. The arterial supply to the bladder is also quite variable. Both genders receive supply from the superior vesical arteries and from various branches of the internal iliac arteries. Branches to the prostate and seminal vesicles (men) also send branches to the inferior bladder wall. In women, branches to the vagina send arteries to the base of the bladder. Note how the ureters deviate anteriorly as they cross the external (or common) iliac vessels and pelvic brim. This may constitute a point of relative narrowing where the passage of ureteral calculi (stones) may be impeded. In the abdomen the ureters course along the psoas muscles.

URINARY BLADDER

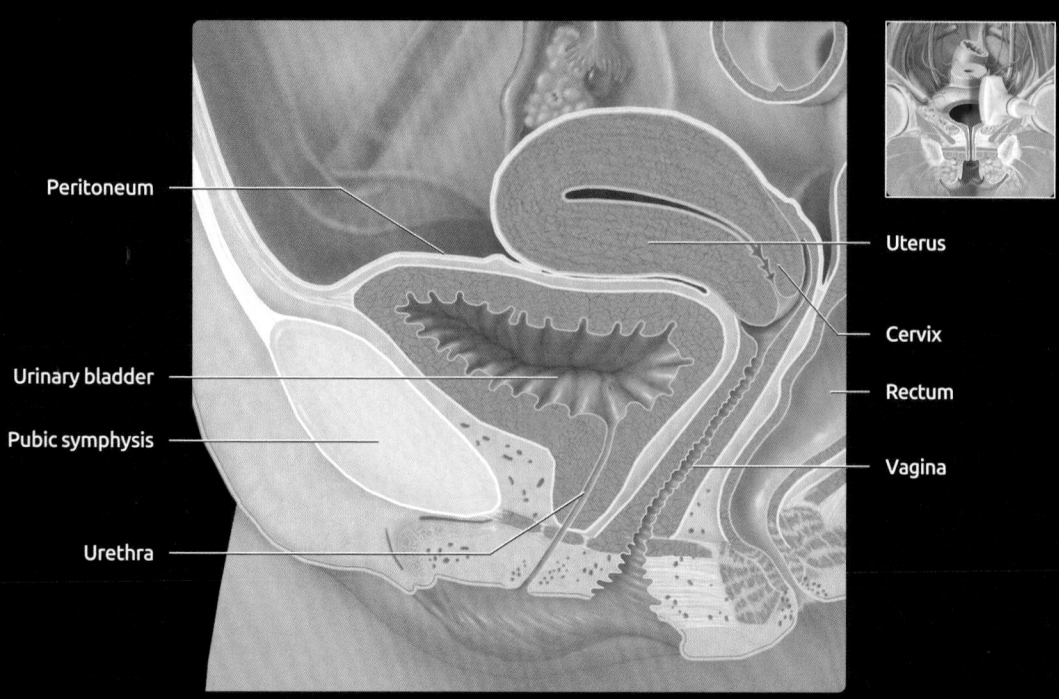

Peritoneum

Urinary bladder

Pubic symphysis

Urethra

Uterus

Cervix

Rectum

Vagina

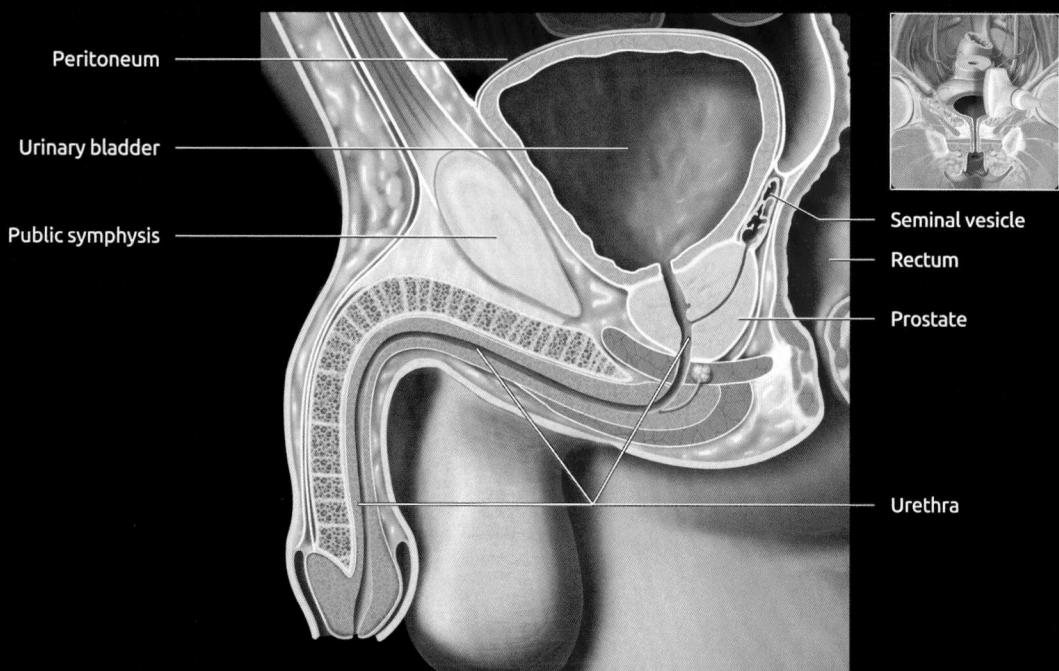

Peritoneum

Urinary bladder

Public symphysis

Seminal vesicle

Rectum

Prostate

Urethra

(Top) *Graphic of a sagittal section of the female bladder shows that it rests almost directly on the muscular floor of the pelvis. The dome of the bladder is covered with peritoneum. The bladder is surrounded by a layer of loose fat and connective tissue (the prevesical and perivesical spaces) that communicate superiorly with the retroperitoneum. Note the vagina/uterus in the female pelvis, which intervenes between the urinary bladder and rectum.* **(Bottom)** *Graphic of a sagittal section of the male bladder shows that it rests on the prostate, which separates it from the muscular pelvic floor. The bladder wall is muscular, strong, and very distensible. In males the urinary bladder is directly anterior to the rectum.*

URINARY BLADDER, ULTRASOUND

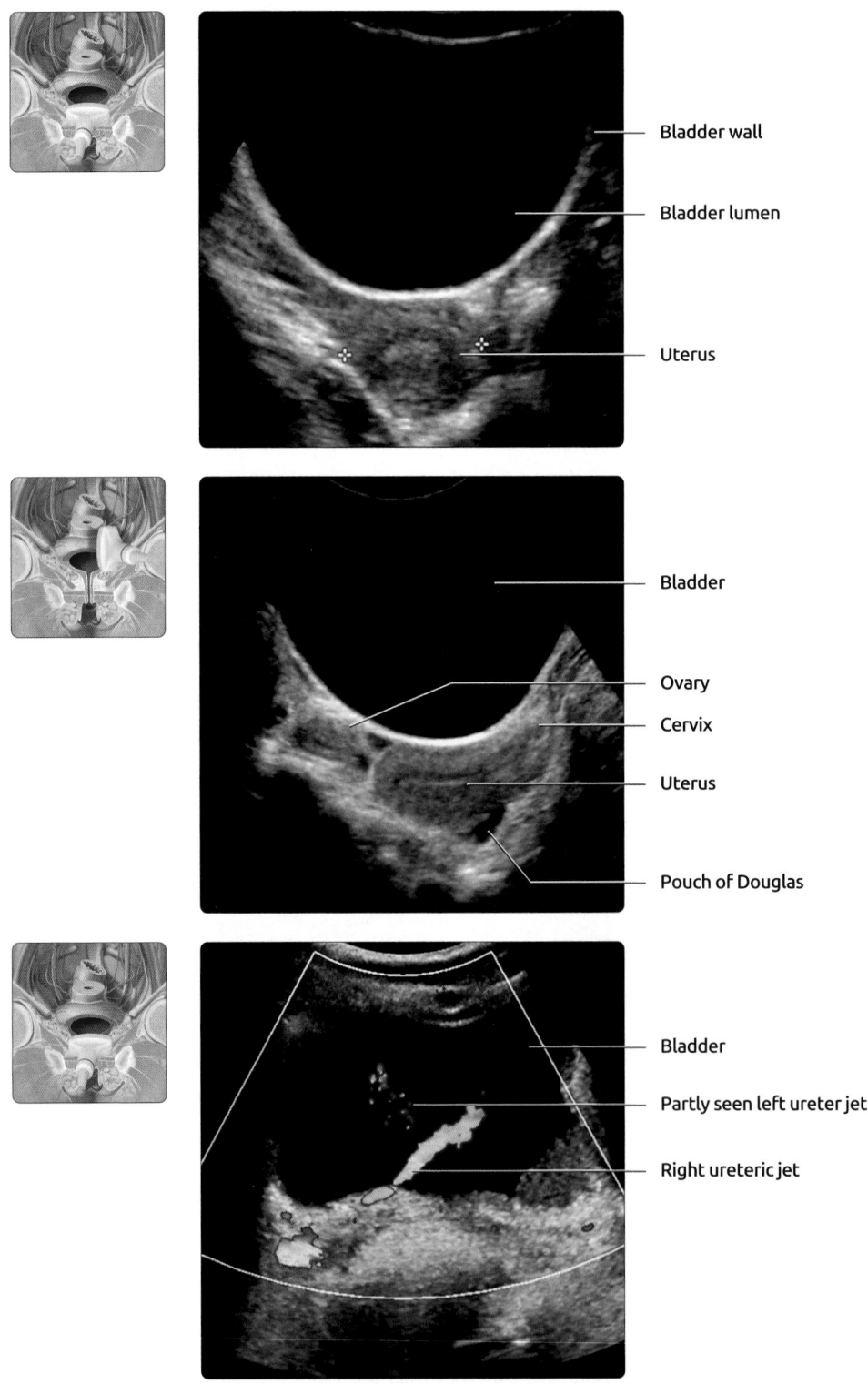

Bladder wall

Bladder lumen

Uterus

Bladder

Ovary

Cervix

Uterus

Pouch of Douglas

Bladder

Partly seen left ureter jet

Right ureteric jet

(Top) *Transverse transabdominal grayscale ultrasound shows the suprapubic region at the uterine body level. The transducer must be angled caudally to image the urinary bladder, especially when it is not well distended and assumes a retropubic location.* (Middle) *Longitudinal transabdominal grayscale ultrasound at the suprapubic region shows a well-distended urinary bladder with a posteriorly located uterus. Note the anechoic appearance of the urinary bladder due to its fluid-filled state, which acts as an acoustic window, permitting through transmission of the ultrasound beam and optimal visualization of posterior pelvic structures.* (Bottom) *Transverse color Doppler ultrasound of the bladder in the suprapubic region shows ureteral jets.*

CT UROGRAM CORRELATION, URETERS AND BLADDER

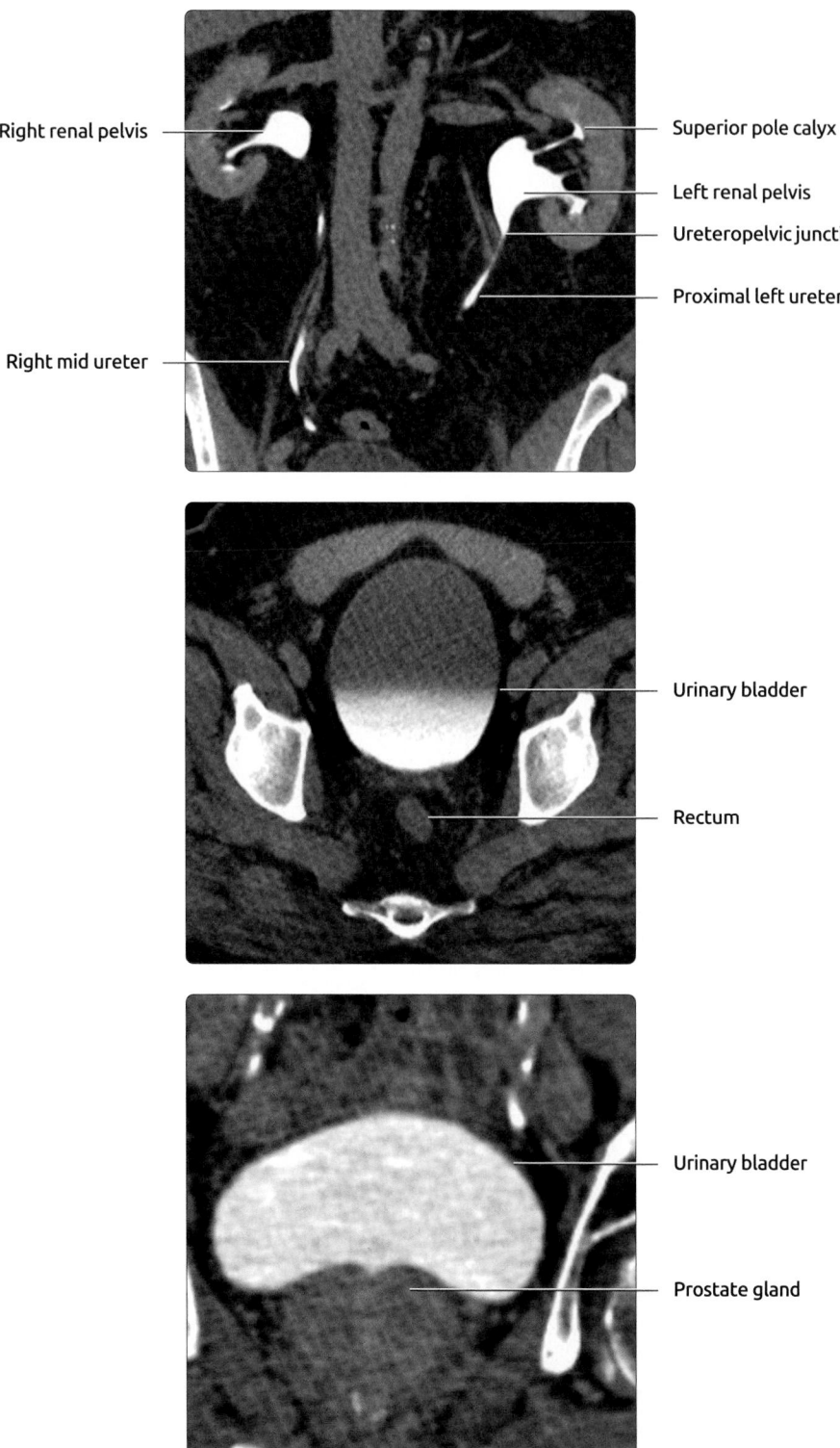

Right renal pelvis

Superior pole calyx

Left renal pelvis

Ureteropelvic junction

Proximal left ureter

Right mid ureter

Urinary bladder

Rectum

Urinary bladder

Prostate gland

(Top) *Coronal reformatted CT urogram (CTU) shows a normal, well-opacified pelvicalyceal system and proximal mid segments of the ureters.* **(Middle)** *Axial CTU through the pelvis shows an optimally distended urinary bladder with a uniform thin bladder wall and no intraluminal filling defect. Notice layering hyperdense excreted contrast with poorly opacified nondependent urine.* **(Bottom)** *Coronal reformatted CTU through the pelvis shows a well-distended and optimally opacified normal urinary bladder. Note the mildly enlarged prostate gland slightly indenting the bladder base.*

VOLUME-RENDERED 3D CT UROGRAM CORRELATION

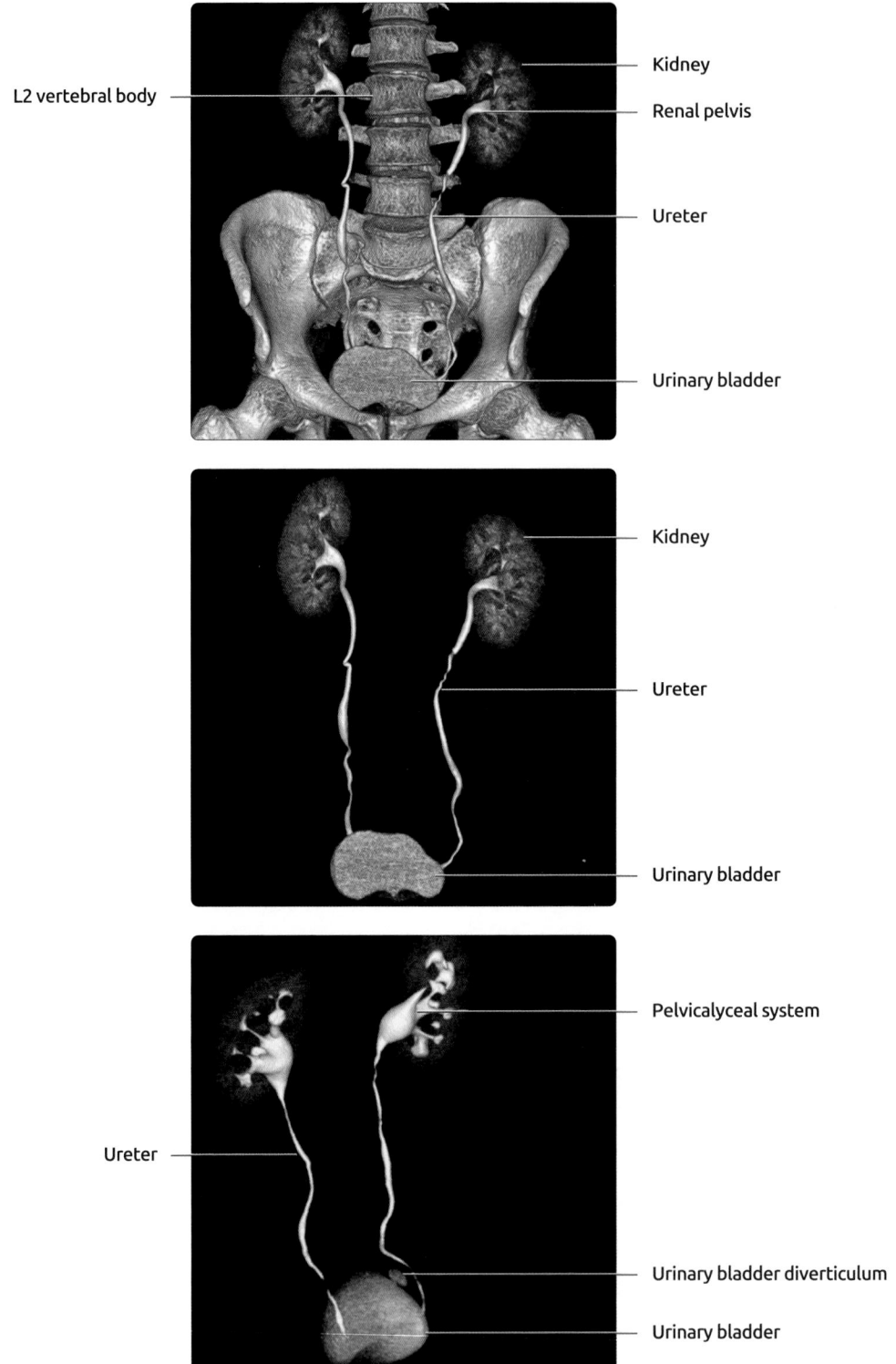

L2 vertebral body

Kidney

Renal pelvis

Ureter

Urinary bladder

Kidney

Ureter

Urinary bladder

Pelvicalyceal system

Ureter

Urinary bladder diverticulum

Urinary bladder

(Top) *Volume-rendered 3D reformatted image from a CTU shows the normal course of the ureters overlying L3-L5 transverse process.* (Middle) *Volume-rendered 3D reformatted image from a CTU shows normal kidneys, ureters, and bladder. Few normal nonobstructing smooth kinks may be observed.* (Bottom) *Volume-rendered 3D reformatted image from a CTU shows a small bladder diverticulum.*

URETER

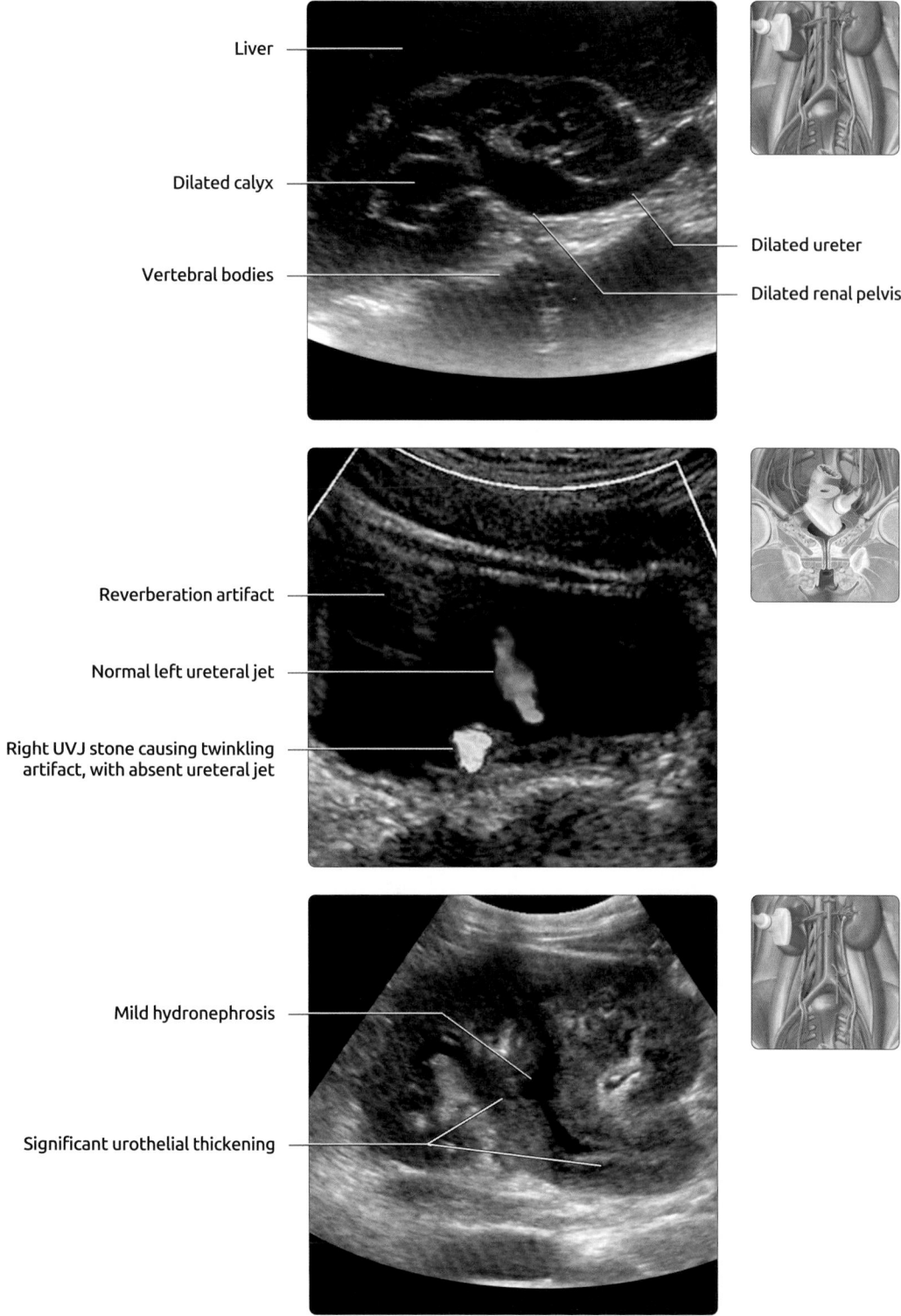

(Top) *Longitudinal transabdominal grayscale ultrasound of the right kidney shows a dilated pelvicalyceal system and proximal ureter. The ureter is normally not visible on ultrasound unless it is dilated as seen here.* **(Middle)** *Oblique color Doppler ultrasound of the suprapubic region shows calculus at the right ureterovesical junction (UVJ) causing twinkling artifact with absent ureteral jet. Normal left ureteric jet is seen.* **(Bottom)** *Longitudinal transabdominal ultrasound of the left kidney shows significant urothelial thickening of the pelvicalyceal system and proximal ureter in this patient with known extramedullary hematopoiesis.*

URINARY BLADDER

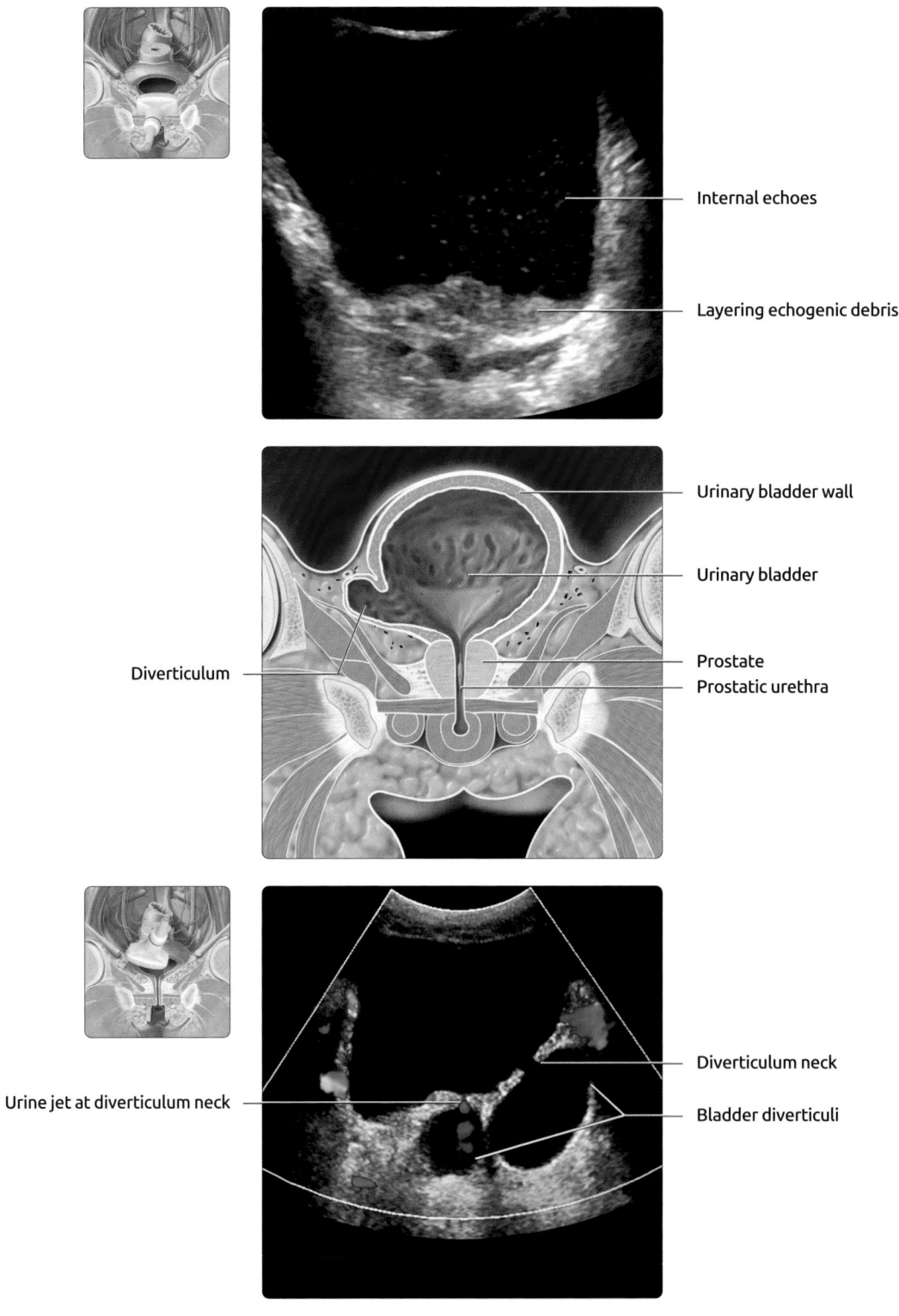

Internal echoes

Layering echogenic debris

Urinary bladder wall

Urinary bladder

Diverticulum

Prostate
Prostatic urethra

Urine jet at diverticulum neck

Diverticulum neck

Bladder diverticuli

(Top) *Transverse transabdominal ultrasound of the bladder shows floating internal echoes with layering echogenic debris in this patient with cystitis.* (Middle) *Graphic shows a diverticulum arising from the lateral urinary bladder wall due to herniation of the mucosa and submucosa through the muscular wall.* (Bottom) *Transverse oblique transabdominal color Doppler ultrasound through the bladder shows 2 well-distended bladder diverticuli along the left posterolateral bladder. Urine jet is identified in 1 of the diverticular necks.*

WEIGERT-MEYER LAW

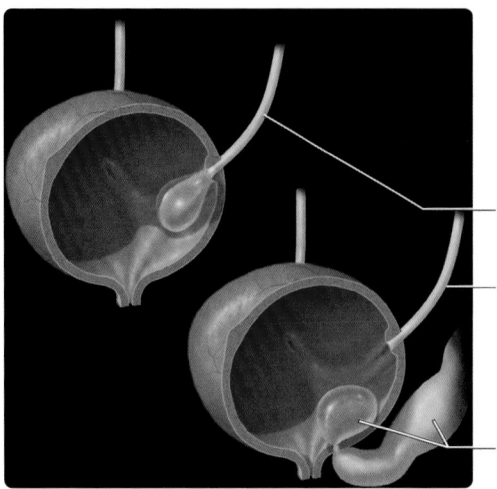

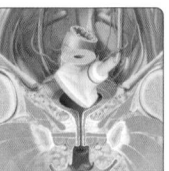

Orthotopic ureter with ureterocele

Orthotopic ureter

Dilated ectopic ureter and ureterocele

Bladder

Ureterocele

Dilated right distal ureter

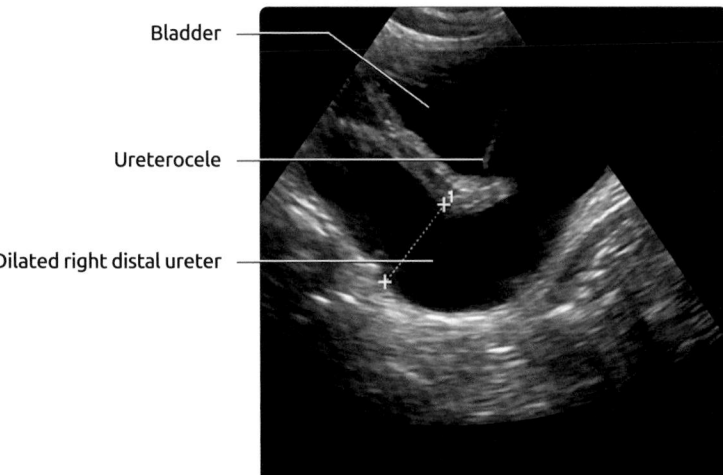

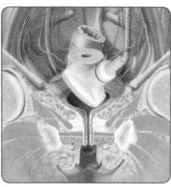

Nondilated lower pole collecting system

Dilated upper pole collecting system (moiety)

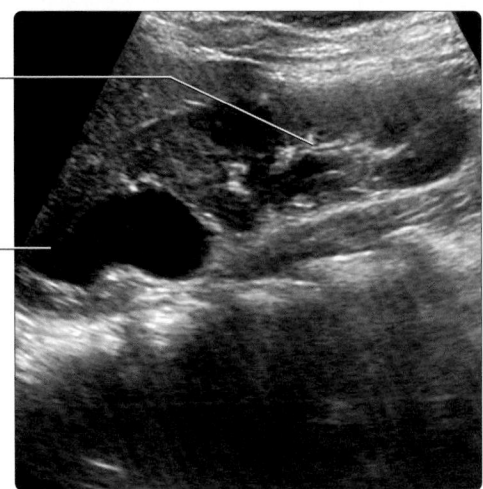

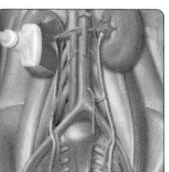

(Top) *Graphic illustrates orthotopic ureterocele in a single ureter system (left, upper) and ectopic ureterocele in a duplicated ureter system (right, lower). Note the hydroureter accompanying the ectopic ureterocele.* **(Middle)** *Longitudinal oblique transabdominal grayscale ultrasound at the suprapubic region shows a dilated ureter seen terminating in the ureterocele; the patient had complete duplication of the collecting system (Weigert-Meyer law).* **(Bottom)** *Longitudinal transabdominal grayscale ultrasound through the right kidney in the same patient shows a dilated upper pole moiety (the patient also had a dilated right ureter with ureterocele) with decompressed inferior moiety (Weigert-Meyer law).*

GROSS ANATOMY

Prostate

- Walnut-sized gland beneath bladder and in front of rectum
  - Normal prostate in young male ~ 3 cm length x 4 cm width x 2 cm depth
  - Normal weight ~ 20-30 grams
- Inverted conical shape
  - Base: Superior portion, continuous with bladder neck
  - Apex: Inferior portion, continuous with striated sphincter
- Capsule: Composed of condensed fibromuscular band, not true capsule
  - Does not completely envelop prostate: Absent at base and not clearly defined at apex
  - Capsular components are inseparable from prostatic stroma and periprostatic connective tissue
- Posteriorly, Denonvilliers fascia (thin layer of connective tissue) separates prostate and seminal vesicles from rectum
- Laterally, prostate is cradled by pubococcygeal portion of levator ani
- Toward apex, puboprostatic ligaments extend anteriorly to affix prostate to pubic bone
  - Apex is continuous with striated external urethral sphincter
- Ejaculatory ducts form at junction of vas deferens and seminal vesicles and to enter prostate base
- Prostatic urethra
  - Verumontanum (a.k.a. colliculus seminalis)
    - Midway between base and apex where urethra makes ~ 35° bend anteriorly
      - Openings of prostatic utricle and ejaculatory ducts
    - Divides prostatic urethra into proximal (preprostatic) and distal (prostatic) segments
      - **Preprostatic sphincter**: Thickened circular smooth muscle in proximal segment (a.k.a. involuntary internal urethral sphincter, periurethral zone)
      - Thought to function during ejaculation to prevent retrograde flow of seminal fluid; may also have resting tone, which maintains closure of preprostatic urethra, thereby aiding urinary continence
      - Contains small periurethral glands completely enclosed in sphincter; although these glands constitute < 1% of glandular prostate, they can contribute significantly to prostatic volume as 1 of the sites of origin of benign prostatic hyperplasia (BPH)
  - Urethral crest: Narrow longitudinal ridge on midline posterior wall
    - Prostatic sinuses: Grooves along either side of crest into which prostate fluid drain
  - Prostatic utricle
    - Small, superoposteriorly directed vestigial blind pouch with opening in verumontanum, ~ 6 mm long, müllerian remnant (homologous with uterus and vagina)
- Neurovascular bundles (NVB)
  - Lie posterolaterally to prostate
  - Carry nerves and vascular supply to corpora cavernosa
- Vascular supply

- Most commonly, arterial supply from inferior vesical artery; often divides into 2 main branches: Urethral arteries and capsular artery
  - Urethral arteries supply periurethral glands and transition zone (TZ) → main supply for BPH
  - Bulk of capsular artery runs posterolaterally with cavernous nerves in neurovascular bundles and ends at pelvic diaphragm
  - Venous drainage via periprostatic plexus; receives blood from dorsal vein of penis; drains into internal iliac veins
- Nerve supply: Pelvic plexuses arising from S2-4 (parasympathetic) and L1-2 (sympathetic) fibers
- Lymphatic drainage chiefly to obturator and internal iliac nodes; small portion may initially pass through presacral group or, less commonly, external iliac nodes

Lobar Anatomy (Lowsley)

- Based on studies on the human fetal prostate; distinct lobes do not exist in prepubertal and normal adult prostate
- Lobes: Anterior, median, posterior, and 2 lateral
  - Currently used in context of BPH
    - Lateral lobes: Hyperplasia of glands in TZ
    - Median lobe: Hyperplasia of periurethral glands in preprostatic sphincter vs. TZ may project into bladder
- Largely replaced by zonal anatomy

Zonal Anatomy (McNeal)

- Prostate is histologically composed of ~ 70% glandular and 30% nonglandular elements
- 2 nonglandular elements: Prostatic urethra and anterior fibromuscular stroma (AFS)
  - AFS is contiguous with bladder muscle and external urethral sphincter, up to 1/3 of prostatic mass
  - AFS runs anteriorly from bladder neck to striated urinary sphincter
- Peripheral zone (PZ): ~ 70% glandular tissue, covers posterolateral aspects of gland
  - Surrounds central zone and prostatic (distal) urethra; ducts drain into prostatic sinuses along urethra
  - Approximately 70-75% prostatic adenocarcinomas arise in this zone
- Central zone (CZ): ~ 25% glandular tissue; cone-shaped zone around ejaculatory ducts with widest portion making majority of prostatic base
  - Only 1-5% prostate adenocarcinoma originate in this zone; mainly involved by secondary invasion
- TZ: ~ 5-10% glandular tissue, 2 separate lobules surround preprostatic urethra (urethra proximal to verumontanum)
  - 1 site of origin of BPH, along with periurethral glands
  - Approximately 20-25% of prostate adenocarcinoma arise in this zone
- Periurethral glands in preprostatic sphincter: < 1% glandular tissue, a site of origin of BPH
- Prostate pseudocapsule ("surgical capsule"): Visible boundary between TZ and PZ representing compressed tissue
  - Frequently, calcified corpora amylacea (laminated bodies formed of secretions and degenerate cells) highlight plane between PZ and TZ

Seminal Vesicles and Ejaculatory Ducts

- Seminal vesicles

- Sac-like structures superolateral to prostate, lateral outpouchings of vas deferens
- Secrete fructose-rich fluid (energy source for sperm)
- Arterial supply: Vesiculodeferential artery (branch of superior vesical artery)
  - May have additional supply from inferior vesical artery
- Venous drainage into pelvic venous plexus
- Lymphatic drainage into external and internal iliac nodes
- Ejaculatory ducts
  - Located on either side of midline
  - Formed by union of seminal vesicle duct and vas deferens
  - Start at base of prostate and run forward and downward through gland in CZ

IMAGING ANATOMY

Prostate

- Transrectal ultrasound (TRUS)
  - Normal TZ is typically uniformly more echogenic than inner gland
  - Inner gland (TZ and CZ) is often distinguishable from PZ
    - Heterogeneous TZ in BPH
  - TRUS-guided biopsy generally recommended when patient's PSA level is elevated or abnormal digital rectal exam (DRE) (exception: When elevated PSA occurs with suspected prostatitis → repeat PSA 2-3 months later)
    - TRUS: Visual aid for systematic biopsy of entire prostate, estimate prostate volume
    - TRUS has become mainstay of many image-guided prostate interventions: Prostate biopsy, brachytherapy, cryotherapy, and high-intensity focused ultrasonography (HIFU) as well as BPH evaluation
- Prostate volume measurement
  - Prolate ellipse volume for 3 unequal axes: Width x height x length x 0.523
  - 1 cc of prostate tissue ~ 1 g; prostate weighs ~ 20 g in young men
  - Prostatic enlargement when gland is > 40 g

Seminal Vesicles and Vasa Deferentia

- Cystic appearance on TRUS, should be symmetric

ANATOMY IMAGING ISSUES

Imaging Recommendations

- Transducer
  - 7-10 MHz rectal transducer (end-firing or transverse panoramic)
  - 3.5-6 MHz curved linear transducer for transabdominal ultrasound
  - Perform in at least 2 orthogonal planes (axial and sagittal)
- Patient position
  - TRUS: Left lateral decubitus with flexed hips and knees or in lithotomy position
  - Transabdominal ultrasound: Supine, using urinary bladder as acoustic window (transvesical)
    - Fluid intake to ensure bladder distension

Imaging Pitfalls

- Abnormal vascularity on power Doppler ultrasound may be seen in hypertrophy, inflammation, and cancer
  - Useful for directing biopsy
- Transabdominal ultrasound of prostate is limited to evaluation of prostate size

Transrectal Biopsy of Prostate

- Most transrectal transducers have needle guidance system
- Periprostatic block with local anesthesia injected along neurovascular bundles; may also use anesthetic gel and intraprostatic injection of local anesthetic
- Complications
  - Common: Hematuria, hematochezia, and hematospermia
  - Other: Acute prostatitis, UTI, sepsis

CLINICAL IMPLICATIONS

Function

- Main function is to add nutritional secretions to sperm to form semen during ejaculation
- Also plays role in controlling flow of urine; prostate muscle fibers are under control of involuntary nervous system and contract to slow and stop urine

Zonal Distribution of Prostatic Disease

- Prostate adenocarcinomas
  - 75% in PZ
  - 20% in TZ
  - 5% in CZ
- BPH: Nodular stromal and epithelial hyperplasia in periurethral (preprostatic) glands and TZ
  - Compresses CZ and PZ
  - Can cause bladder outlet obstruction from urethral compression &/or increased smooth muscle tone along bladder neck, prostate, and urethra

Spread of Prostate Carcinoma

- Signs of extraprostatic extension of prostatic carcinoma
  - Asymmetry of NVB
  - Obliteration of rectoprostatic angle
  - Irregular bulge in prostatic contour
- Up to 80% of prostatic cancers in peripheral zone are hypoechoic

SELECTED REFERENCES

1. Chung B, et al: Anatomy of the lower urinary tract and male genitalia. In Campbell-Walsh Urology. 10th ed. Philadelphia: Saunders: 2012:33-70
2. Trabulsi E, et al: Ultrasonography and biopsy of the prostate. In Campbell-Walsh Urology. 10th ed. Philadelphia: Saunders: 2012: 2735-2747
3. Hammerich K, et al: Anatomy of the prostate gland and surgical pathology of prostate cancer. In Prostate Cancer. Cambridge, UK: Cambridge University Press: 2009: 1-14
4. Boczko J et al: Transrectal sonography in prostate evaluation. Radiol Clin North Am. 44(5):679-87, viii, 2006
5. McLaughlin PW et al: Functional anatomy of the prostate: implications for treatment planning. Int J Radiat Oncol Biol Phys. 63(2):479-91, 2005
6. McNeal JE. The zonal anatomy of the prostate. Prostate. 2(1):35-49, 1981

PROSTATE IN SITU

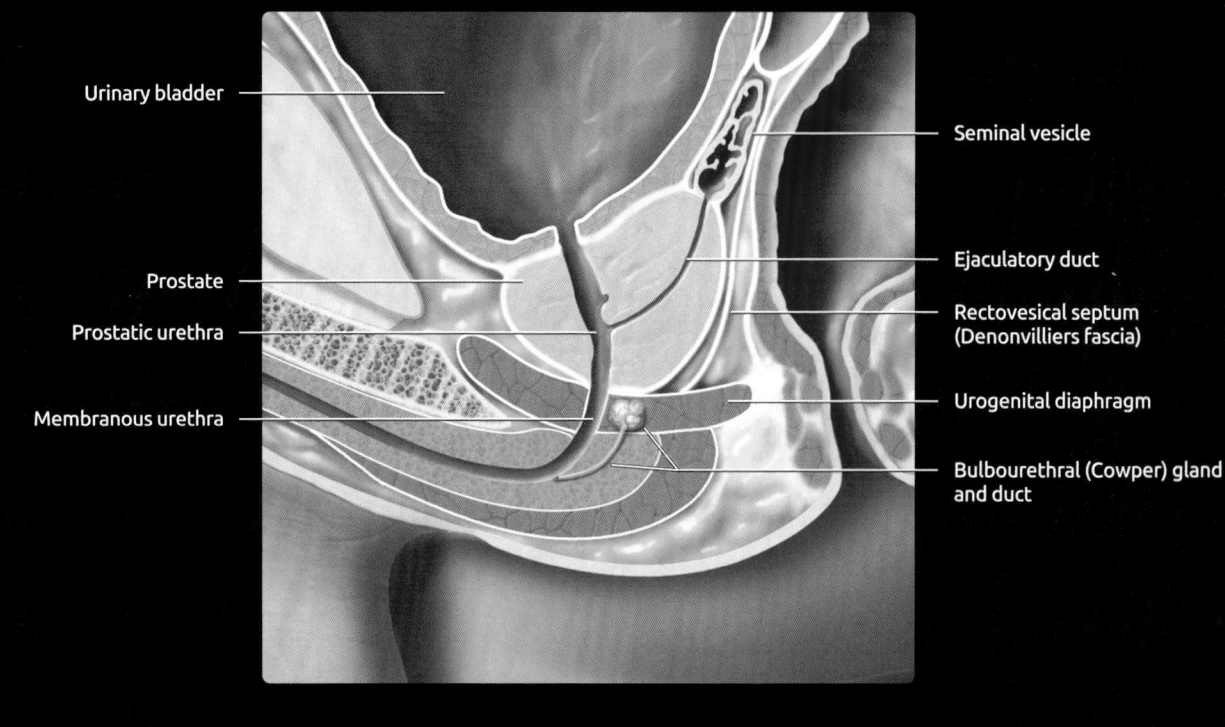

Urinary bladder

Prostate

Prostatic urethra

Membranous urethra

Seminal vesicle

Ejaculatory duct

Rectovesical septum
(Denonvilliers fascia)

Urogenital diaphragm

Bulbourethral (Cowper) gland
and duct

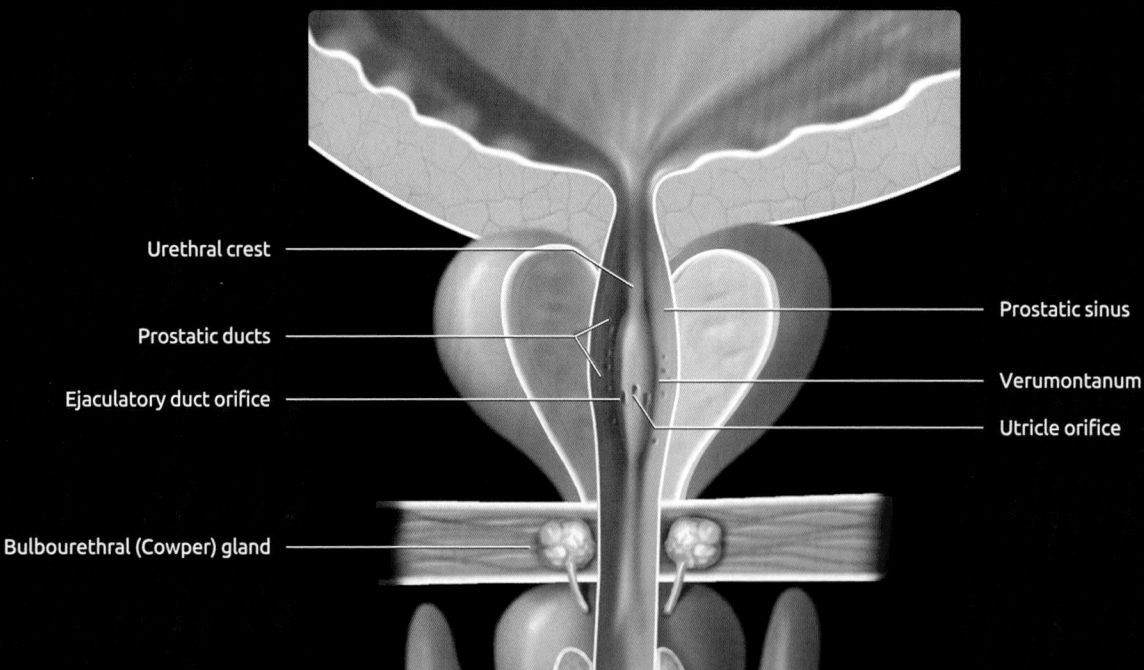

Urethral crest

Prostatic ducts

Ejaculatory duct orifice

Bulbourethral (Cowper) gland

Prostatic sinus

Verumontanum

Utricle orifice

(Top) *Graphic illustrates the relationship between the prostate and the male pelvic organs. The prostate surrounds the upper part of the urethra (prostatic urethra). The base of the prostate is continuous with the bladder neck and its apex is continuous with external sphincter. The posterior surface is separated from the rectum by the rectovesical septum (Denonvilliers fascia).* (Bottom) *Graphic shows the topography of the posterior wall of the prostatic urethra. The urethral crest is a mucosal elevation along the posterior wall, with the verumontanum being a mound-like elevation in the midportion of the crest. The utricle opens midline onto the verumontanum, with the ejaculatory ducts opening on either side. The prostatic ducts are clustered around the verumontanum and open into the prostatic sinuses, which are depressions along the sides of the urethral crest.*

ZONAL ANATOMY OF THE PROSTATE

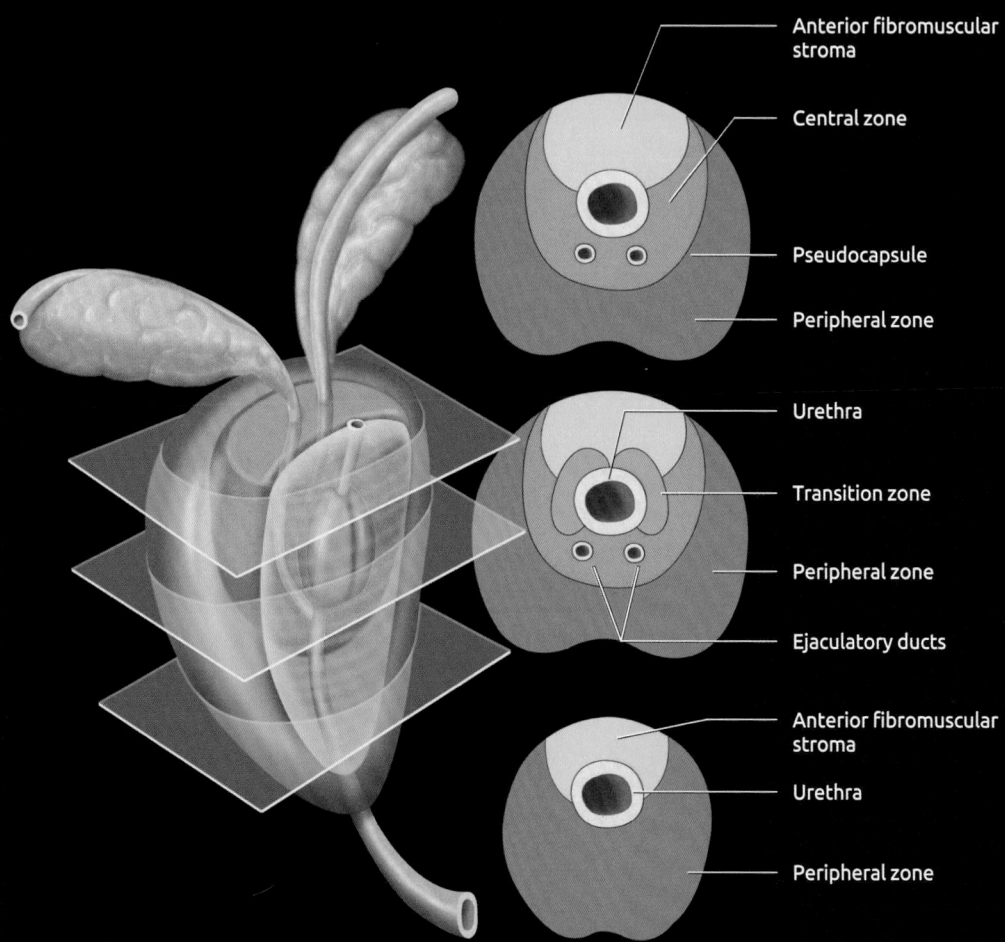

Anterior fibromuscular stroma

Central zone

Pseudocapsule

Peripheral zone

Urethra

Transition zone

Peripheral zone

Ejaculatory ducts

Anterior fibromuscular stroma

Urethra

Peripheral zone

Graphic depiction of the prostate with axial drawings of the zonal anatomy at 3 different levels is shown. The transition zone (in blue) is anterolateral to the verumontanum. The central zone (in orange) surrounds the ejaculatory ducts, and encloses the periurethral glands and the transition zone. It is conical in shape and extends downward to about the level of the verumontanum. The peripheral zone (in green) surrounds the posterior aspect of the central zone in the upper 1/2 of the gland and the urethra in the lower half, below the verumontanum. The prostatic pseudocapsule is a visible boundary between the central zone and peripheral zone. The anterior fibromuscular stroma (in yellow) covers the anterior part of the gland and is thicker superiorly and thins inferiorly in the prostatic apex.

ZONAL ANATOMY OF THE PROSTATE

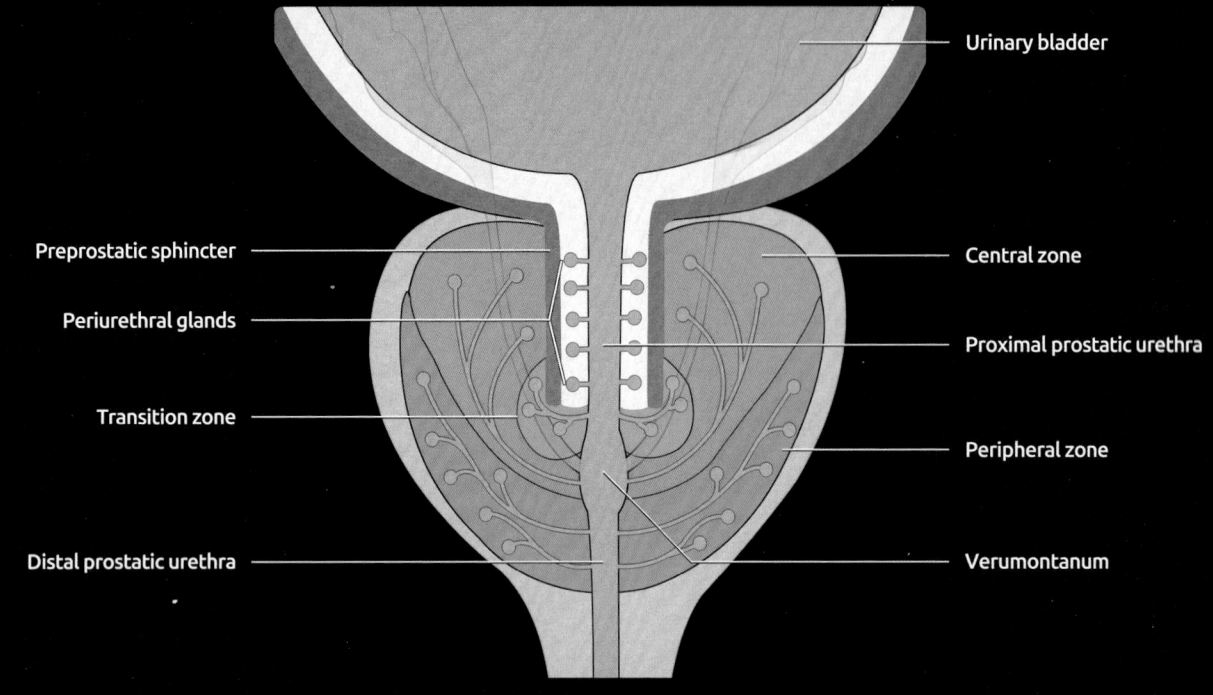

Preprostatic sphincter — Urinary bladder

Periurethral glands — Central zone

Transition zone — Proximal prostatic urethra

Peripheral zone

Distal prostatic urethra — Verumontanum

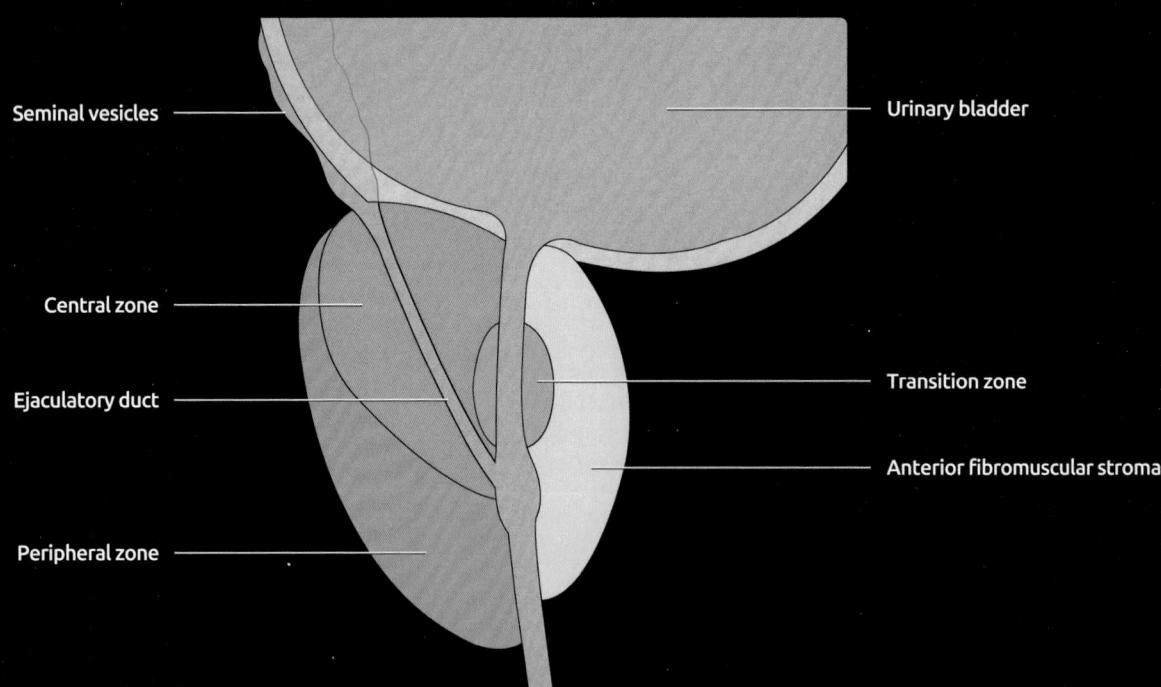

Seminal vesicles — Urinary bladder

Central zone

Ejaculatory duct — Transition zone

Anterior fibromuscular stroma

Peripheral zone

(Top) *Graphic illustrates the zonal anatomy of the prostate in the coronal plane. The proximal 1/2 of the prostatic urethra is surrounded by preprostatic sphincter, which extends inferiorly to the level of the verumontanum and encloses the periurethral glands. The transition zone is a downward extension of the periurethral glands around the verumontanum.* **(Bottom)** *Graphic illustrates the zonal anatomy of the prostate in the sagittal plane. The outer prostate is composed of the central zone and peripheral zone. The central zone surrounds the proximal urethra posterosuperiorly, enclosing both the periurethral glands and the transition zone. It forms most of the prostatic base. The peripheral zone surrounds both the central zone and the distal prostatic urethra.*

SEMINAL VESICLES AND VAS DEFERENS

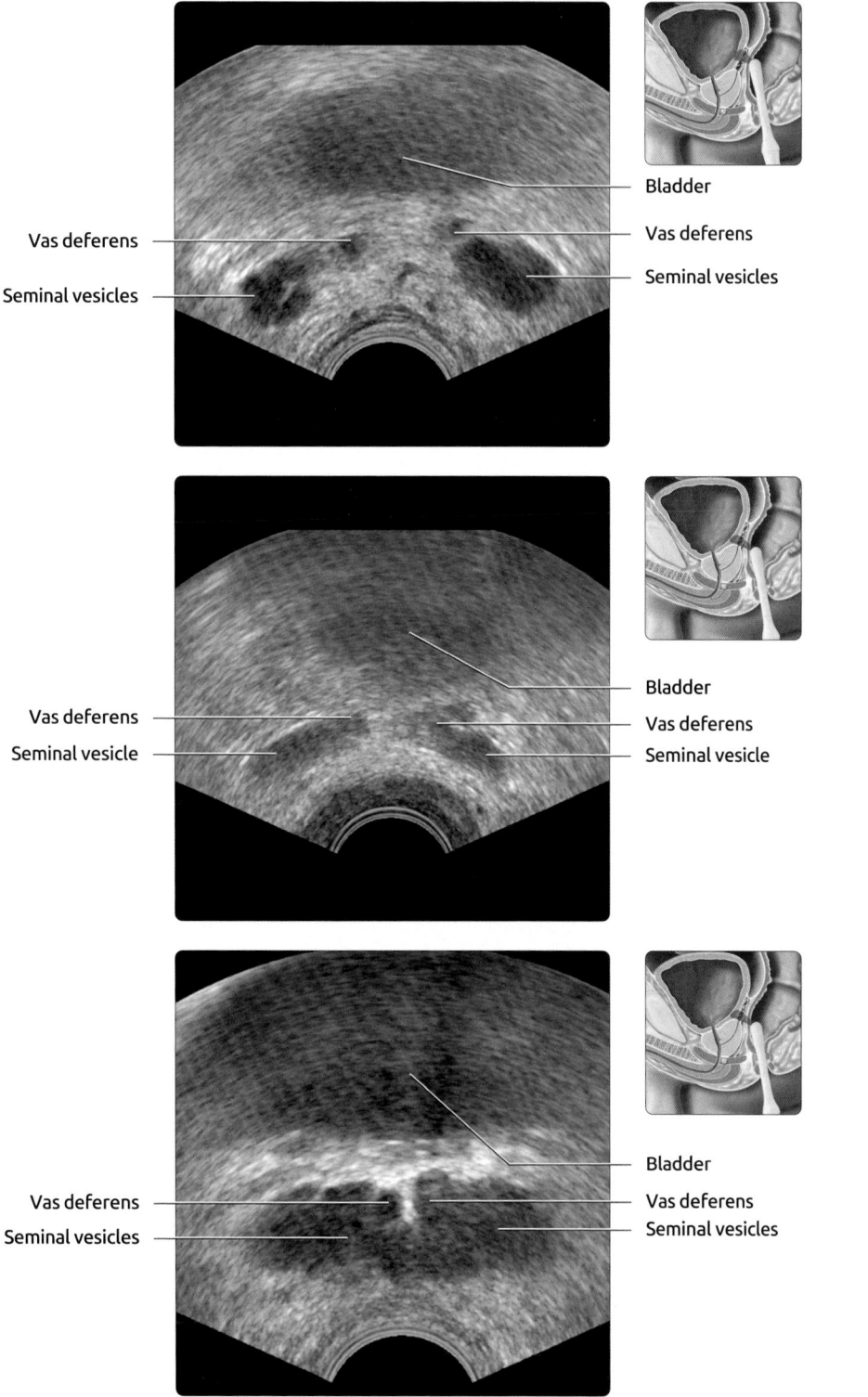

(Top) *Transverse transrectal ultrasound (TRUS) at the level of the seminal vesicles shows bilateral seminal vesicles and the vas deferens.* **(Middle)** *More inferior transverse TRUS shows convergence of the vas deferens and seminal vesicles just above the base of the prostate.* **(Bottom)** *Transverse TRUS shows the vas deferens converging with the seminal vesicles. Their union will form the ejaculatory ducts, which enter the prostate base and course within the prostate enclosed within the central zone. The ejaculatory ducts empty into the urethra at the verumontanum.*

PROSTATE, TRANSRECTAL ULTRASOUND

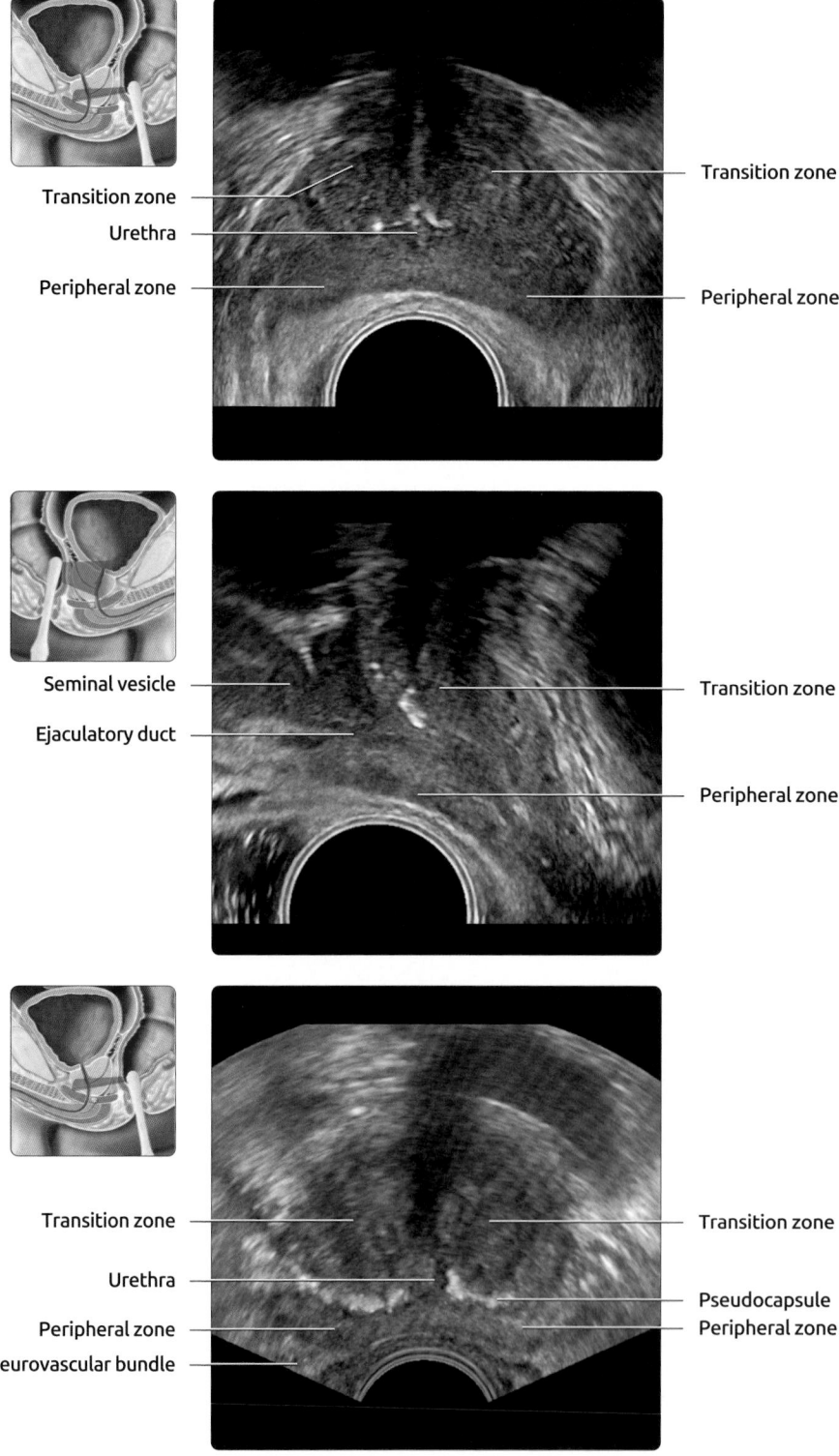

Transition zone
Urethra
Peripheral zone

Transition zone
Peripheral zone

Seminal vesicle
Ejaculatory duct

Transition zone
Peripheral zone

Transition zone
Urethra
Peripheral zone
Neurovascular bundle

Transition zone
Pseudocapsule
Peripheral zone

(Top) *Transverse TRUS at the level of the midprostate shows the 2 lobes of the transition zone on either side of the urethra. The more homogeneous peripheral zone is along the posterolateral aspects of the prostate. Note the periurethral calcifications.* (Middle) *Parasagittal TRUS shows the ejaculatory duct emerging after fusion of the vas deferens and seminal vesicle, entering the prostate base. The ejaculatory ducts are surrounded by the central zone, which is not readily distinguishable on TRUS. Calcifications are seen within the more anterior transition zone. The peripheral zone runs along the posterolateral aspect of the prostate.* (Bottom) *Transverse TRUS of the midprostate gland demonstrates an enlarged transition zone in a patient with benign prostatic hyperplasia (BPH). The pseudocapsule separates the transition zone from the peripheral zone. Frequently, the pseudocapsule will be outlined by calcifications, which represent calcified corpora amylacea (laminated bodies formed by secretions and degenerate cells).*

PROSTATE ANATOMY

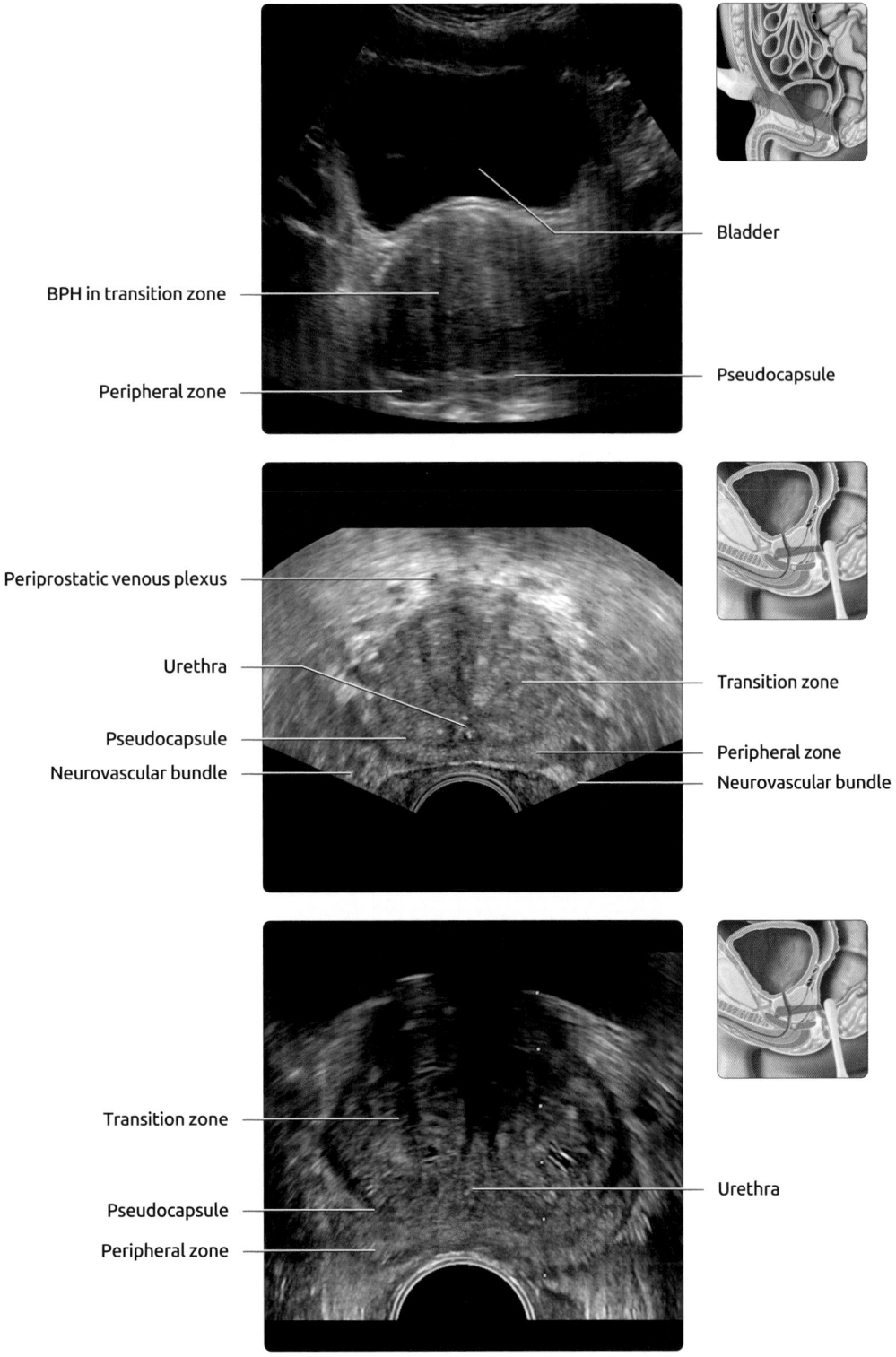

Bladder

BPH in transition zone

Peripheral zone

Pseudocapsule

Periprostatic venous plexus

Urethra

Pseudocapsule

Neurovascular bundle

Transition zone

Peripheral zone

Neurovascular bundle

Transition zone

Pseudocapsule

Peripheral zone

Urethra

(Top) *Transverse transabdominal ultrasound of the midprostate in a patient with BPH shows a markedly enlarged transition zone and hyperechoic pseudocapsule. The peripheral zone is compressed posterolaterally.* **(Middle)** *Transverse TRUS of the midprostate in a different patient with BPH. The heterogeneously enlarged transition zone expands the inner gland. The compressed central zone is not distinguishable. The peripheral zone is compressed posteriorly. Periurethral calcifications help identify the urethra. The neurovascular bundles course through the retroprostatic fat at the 5 and 7 o'clock positions.* **(Bottom)** *Transverse TRUS of the midprostate in a different patient with BPH shows heterogeneous enlargement of the 2 lobes of the transition zone, which flank the urethra. Tiny cystic spaces within the transition zone represent cystic BPH nodules vs. retention cysts, which are often indistinguishable by imaging. The more hyperechoic peripheral zone is along the posterolateral aspects of the prostate.*

GROSS ANATOMY

Testis

- Densely packed seminiferous tubules separated by thin fibrous septa
  o 200-300 lobules in adult testis
  o Each has 400-600 seminiferous tubules
  o Total length of seminiferous tubules 300-980 meters
- Seminiferous tubules converge posteriorly to form larger ducts (tubuli recti)
  o Drain into rete testis at testicular hilum
- Rete testis converges posteriorly to form 15-20 efferent ductules
  o Penetrate posterior tunica albuginea at mediastinum to form head of epididymis
- Tunica albuginea forms thick fibrous capsule around testis
- Mediastinum testis is thickened area of tunica albuginea where ducts, nerves, and vessels enter and exit testis
- Testicular appendage (appendix testis)
  o Small, nodular protuberance from surface of testis
  o Remnant of müllerian system

Epididymis

- Crescent-shaped structure running along posterior border of testis
- Efferent ductules form head (globus major)
  o Unite to form single, long, highly convoluted tubule in body of epididymis
- Tubule continues inferiorly to form epididymal tail (globus minor)
  o Attached to lower pole of testis by loose areolar tissue
- Tubule emerges at acute angle from tail as vas deferens (a.k.a. ductus deferens)
  o Continues cephalad within spermatic cord
  o Eventually merges with duct of seminal vesicle to form ejaculatory duct
- Epididymal appendage (appendix epididymis)
  o Small nodular protuberance from surface of epididymis
  o Remnant of wolffian system

Spermatic Cord

- Contains vas deferens, nerves, lymphatics, and connective tissue
- Begins at internal (deep) inguinal ring and exits through external (superficial) inguinal ring into scrotum
- Arteries
  o Testicular artery
    - Branch of aorta
    - Primary blood supply to testis
  o Deferential artery
    - Branch of inferior or superior vesicle artery
    - Arterial supply to vas deferens
  o Cremasteric artery
    - Branch of inferior epigastric artery
    - Supplies muscular components of cord and skin
- Venous drainage
  o Pampiniform plexus
    - Interconnected network of small veins
    - Merges to form testicular vein
    - Left testicular vein drains to left renal vein
    - Right testicular vein drains to inferior vena cava

- Lymphatic drainage
  o Testis follows venous drainage
    - Right side drains to interaortocaval chain
    - Left side drains to left paraaortic nodes near renal hilum
  o Epididymis may also drain to external iliac nodes
  o Scrotal skin drains to inguinal nodes

EMBRYOLOGY

Testis

- Testis develop from genital ridges, which extend from T6-S2 in embryo
- Composed of 3 cell lines (germ cells, Sertoli cells, Leydig cells)
- Germ cells
  o Form in wall of yolk sac and migrate along hindgut to genital ridges
  o Form spermatogenic cells in mature testes
- Sertoli cells
  o Supporting network for developing spermatozoa
  o Form tight junctions (blood-testis barrier)
  o Secrete müllerian inhibiting factor
    - Causes paramesonephric (müllerian) ducts to regress
    - Embryologic remnant may remain as appendix testis
- Leydig cells
  o Principal source of testosterone production
  o Lies within interstitium
  o Causes differentiation of mesonephric duct (wolffian) ducts
    - Each duct forms epididymis, vas deferens, seminal vesicle, ejaculatory duct
    - An embryologic remnant may remain as appendix epididymis
- Scrotum derived from labioscrotal folds
  o Folds swell under influence of testosterone to form twin scrotal sacs
    - Point of fusion is median raphe, which extends from anus, along perineum, to ventral surface of penis
  o Processus vaginalis, a sock-like evagination of peritoneum, elongates through abdominal wall into twin sacs
    - Aids in descent of testes, along with gubernaculum (ligamentous cord extending from testis to labioscrotal fold)
    - Results in component layers of adult scrotum
- Testicular descent
  o Between 7-12th week of gestation, testes descend into pelvis
    - Remain near internal inguinal ring until 7th month, when they begin descent through inguinal canal into twin scrotal sacs
    - Testes remain retroperitoneal throughout descent
    - Testes intimately associated with posterior wall of processus vaginalis
  o Component layers of spermatic cord and scrotum form during descent through abdominal wall
  o Transversalis fascia → internal spermatic fascia
    - Transversus abdominis muscle is discontinuous inferiorly and does not contribute to formation of scrotum

- o Internal oblique muscle → cremasteric muscle and fascia
- o External oblique muscle → external spermatic fascia
- o Dartos muscle and fascia embedded in loose areolar tissue below skin
- o Processus vaginalis closes and forms tunica vaginalis
  - – Mesothelial-lined sac around anterior and lateral sides of testis
  - – Visceral layer of tunica vaginalis blends imperceptibly with tunica albuginea

ANATOMY-BASED IMAGING ISSUES

Imaging Recommendations

- Palpation of scrotal contents and taking history prior to US examination
- High-frequency (10-15 MHz) linear transducer
- Patient in supine position
  - o Penis lies on anterior abdominal wall
  - o Towel draped over thighs to elevate scrotum
  - o Additional positions with patient upright or with patient performing Valsalva maneuver

IMAGING ANATOMY

Sonographic Anatomy

- Testes
  - o Ovoid, homogeneous, medium-level, granular echotexture
  - o Mediastinum testis may appear as prominent echogenic line emanating from posterior testis
  - o Blood flow
    - – Testicular artery pierces tunica albuginea and arborizes over periphery of testis
    - – Multiple, radially arranged vessels travel along septa
    - – May have prominent transmediastinal artery
    - – Low-velocity, low-resistance waveform on Doppler imaging, with continuous forward flow in diastole
- Epididymis
  - o Isoechoic to slightly hyperechoic compared with testis
  - o Best seen in longitudinal plane
  - o Head has rounded or triangular configuration
  - o Head 10-12 mm, body and tail often difficult to visualize
    - – May be helpful to follow course of epididymis in transverse plane if difficult to visualize in longitudinal plane
- Spermatic cord
  - o May be difficult to differentiate from surrounding soft tissues
  - o Evaluate for varicocele with color Doppler

CLINICAL IMPLICATIONS

Hydrocele

- Fluid between visceral and parietal layers of tunica vaginalis
- Small amount of fluid is normal
- Larger hydroceles may be either congenital (patent processus vaginalis) or acquired

Cryptorchidism

- Failure of testes to descend completely into scrotum
- Most lie near external inguinal ring
- Associated with decreased fertility and testicular carcinoma

- o Risk of carcinoma is increased for both testes, even if other side is normally descended

Varicocele

- Idiopathic or secondary to abdominal mass
  - o Idiopathic more common on left
- Vessel diameter > 3 mm abnormal
- Always evaluate with provocative maneuvers, such as Valsalva

Dilated Rete Testes

- Clusters of dilated tubules in mediastinum testis
- Empty into epididymis
- Often associated with epididymal cysts

Torsion

- Occurs most commonly when tunica vaginalis completely surrounds testis and epididymis
  - o Testis is suspended from spermatic cord (like bell-clapper) rather than being anchored posteriorly
- Normal grayscale appearance with early torsion
  - o Becomes heterogeneous and enlarged with infarction
- Color and spectral Doppler required for diagnosis
  - o Some flow may be seen even if torsed but will be decreased compared to normal side
  - o Venous flow compromised 1st, then diastolic flow, and finally systolic flow

Testicular Microlithiasis

- Calcifications in testicular parenchyma
- Association with testicular carcinoma
  - o Controversial whether risk factor

Testicular Carcinoma

- Most common malignancy in young men
  - o 95% are germ cell tumors
    - – Seminoma (most common pure tumor), embryonal, yolk sac tumor, choriocarcinoma, teratoma
    - – Mixed germ cell tumor (components of 2 or more cell lines) most common overall
  - o Remainder of primary tumors are sex cord (Sertoli cells) or stromal (Leydig cells)
  - o Lymphoma, leukemia, and metastases more common in older men
- Most metastasize via lymphatics in predictable fashion
  - o Right-sided 1st echelon nodes: Interaortocaval chain at 2nd vertebral body
  - o Left-sided 1st echelon nodes: Left paraaortic nodes in area bounded by renal vein, aorta, ureter, and inferior mesenteric artery

SELECTED REFERENCES

1. Appelbaum L et al: Scrotal ultrasound in adults. Semin Ultrasound CT MR. 34(3):257-73, 2013
2. American Institute of Ultrasound in Medicine et al: AIUM practice guideline for the performance of scrotal ultrasound examinations. J Ultrasound Med. 30(1):151-5, 2011
3. Dogra V et al: Acute painful scrotum. Radiol Clin North Am. 42 (2): 349-63, 2004
4. Dogra VS et al: Sonography of the scrotum. Radiology. 227(1):18-36, 2003
5. Dogra V et al: Ultrasonography of the scrotum. J Ultrasound Med. 21(8):848, 2002

TESTIS AND EPIDIDYMIS

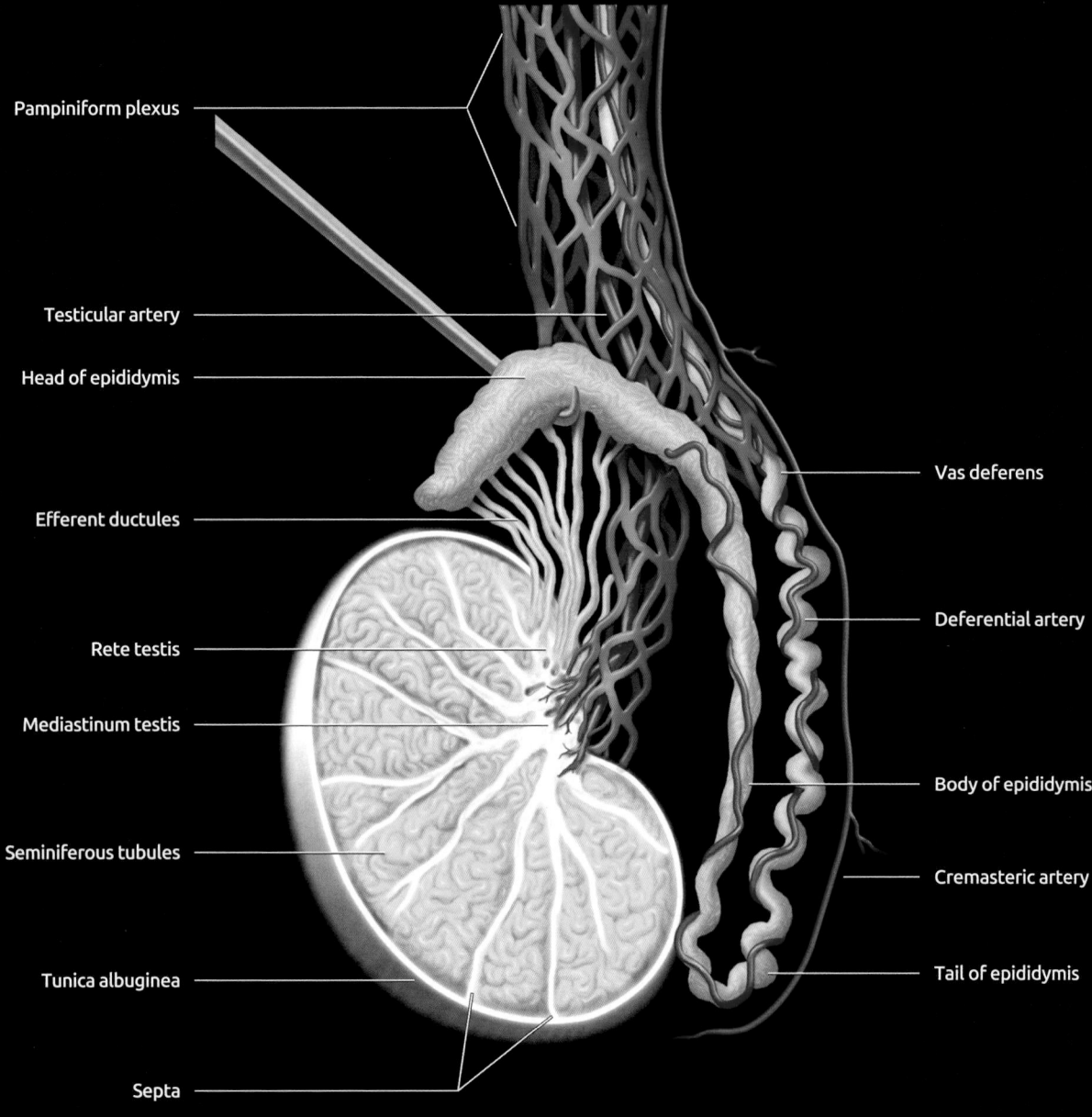

Pampiniform plexus

Testicular artery

Head of epididymis

Efferent ductules

Rete testis

Mediastinum testis

Seminiferous tubules

Tunica albuginea

Septa

Vas deferens

Deferential artery

Body of epididymis

Cremasteric artery

Tail of epididymis

Graphic shows the testis is composed of densely packed seminiferous tubules, which are separated by thin fibrous septa. These tubules converge posteriorly, eventually draining into the rete testis. The rete testis continues to converge to form the efferent ductules, which pierce through the tunica albuginea at the mediastinum testis and form the head of the epididymis. Within the epididymis these tubules unite to form a single, highly convoluted tubule in the body, which finally emerges from the tail as the vas deferens. In addition to the vas deferens, other components of the spermatic cord include the testicular artery, deferential artery, cremasteric artery, pampiniform plexus, lymphatics, and nerves.

EPIDIDYMIS AND SCROTAL WALL LAYERS IN SITU

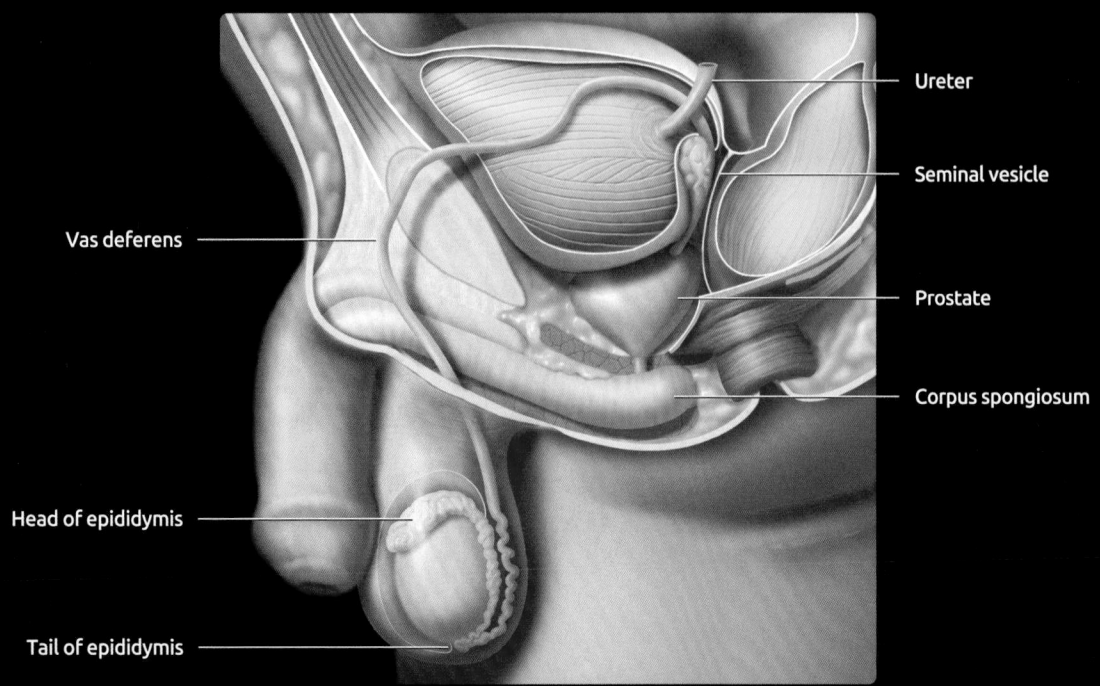

Vas deferens

Head of epididymis

Tail of epididymis

Ureter

Seminal vesicle

Prostate

Corpus spongiosum

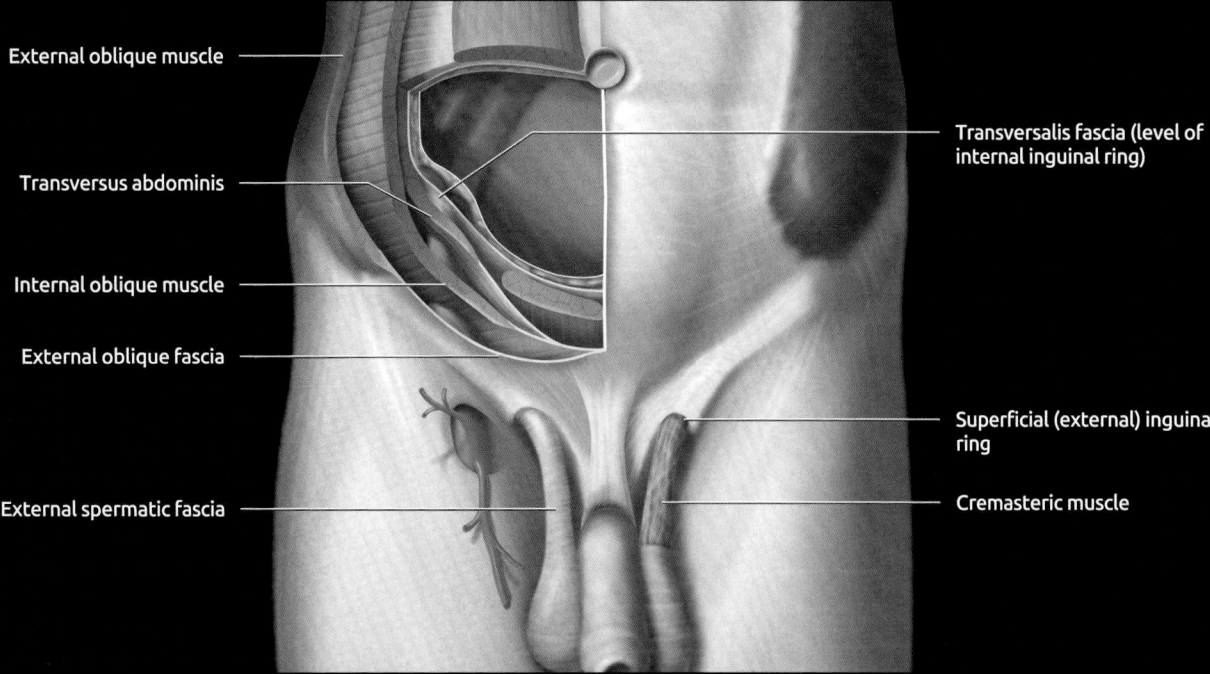

External oblique muscle

Transversus abdominis

Internal oblique muscle

External oblique fascia

External spermatic fascia

Transversalis fascia (level of internal inguinal ring)

Superficial (external) inguinal ring

Cremasteric muscle

(Top) *Graphic shows that the tail of the epididymis is loosely attached to the lower pole of the testis by areolar tissue. The vas deferens (also referred to as the ductus deferens) emerges from the tail at an acute angle and continues cephalad as part of the spermatic cord. After passing through the inguinal canal, the vas deferens courses posteriorly to unite with the duct of the seminal vesicle to form the ejaculatory duct. These narrow ducts have thick, muscular walls composed of smooth muscle, which reflexly contract during ejaculation and propel sperm forward.* **(Bottom)** *The muscle layers of the pelvic wall have been separated to show the spermatic cord as it passes through the inguinal canal. The cremasteric muscle is derived from the internal oblique muscle, while the external spermatic fascia is formed by the fascia of the external oblique muscle.*

TESTES, TRANSVERSE VIEW

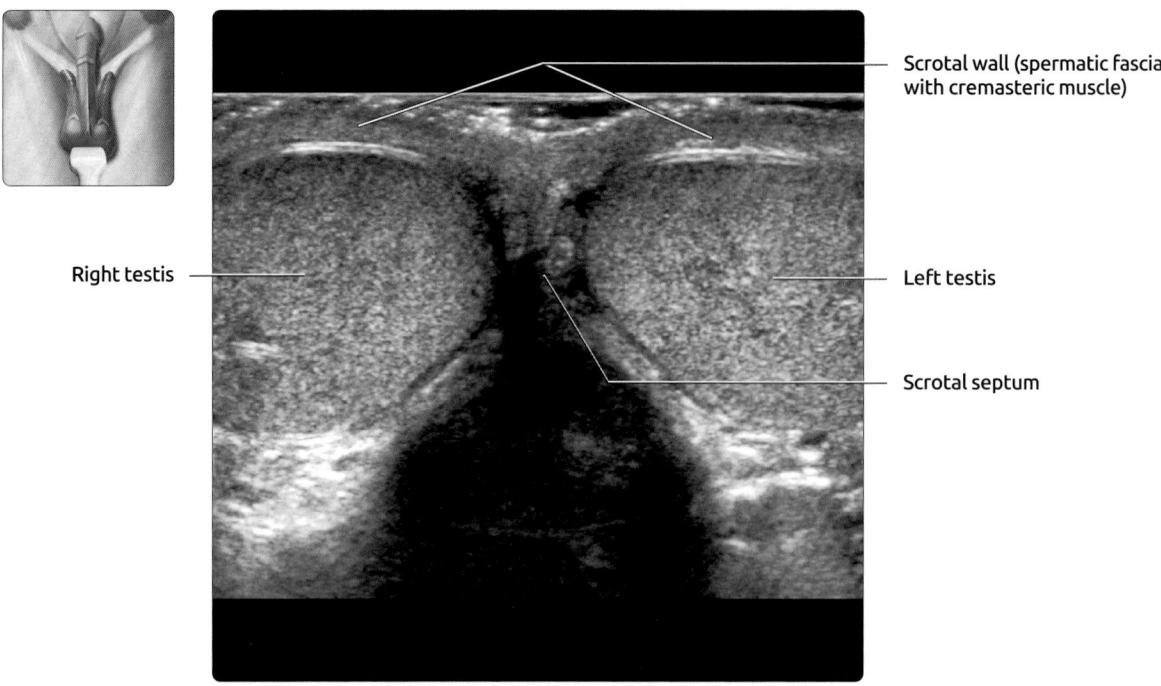

Right testis — Scrotal wall (spermatic fascia with cremasteric muscle)

Left testis

Scrotal septum

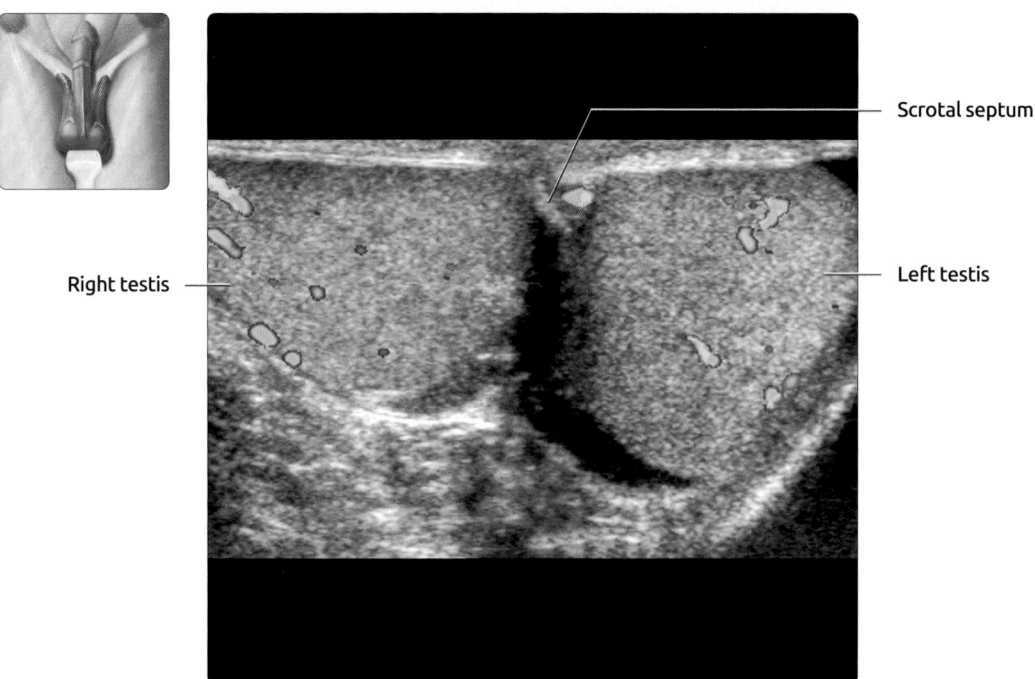

Scrotal septum

Right testis

Left testis

(Top) *Transverse grayscale ultrasound shows both testes. This is a useful approach for comparing the appearance of the testes, which should have similar, homogeneous, medium-level, granular echotexture.* **(Bottom)** *Transverse color Doppler ultrasound of the testes is shown. It is important to compare the flow between testes to determine if the symptomatic side has increased or decreased flow, when compared to the asymptomatic side. This approach also helps to globally evaluate edema, a hematoma, or an abnormality in the scrotal wall.*

TESTIS, SAGITTAL VIEW

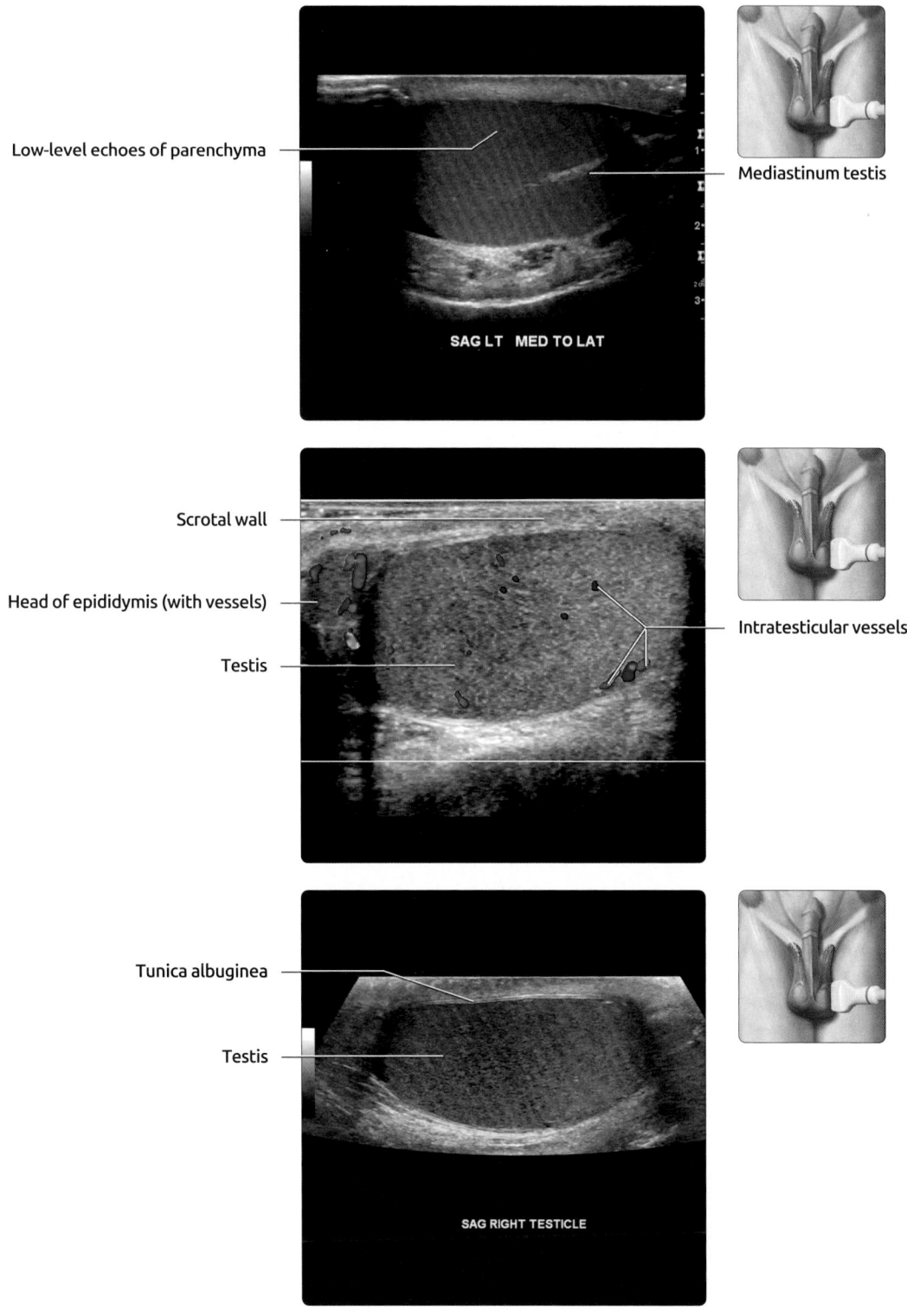

Low-level echoes of parenchyma

Mediastinum testis

SAG LT   MED TO LAT

Scrotal wall

Head of epididymis (with vessels)

Testis

Intratesticular vessels

Tunica albuginea

Testis

SAG RIGHT TESTICLE

(Top) *Sagittal grayscale ultrasound of the normal left testis shows homogeneous, low-level echoes and an echogenic linear structure representing the mediastinum testis.* (Middle) *Longitudinal color Doppler ultrasound shows normal vascularity of the testis.* (Bottom) *Sagittal grayscale ultrasound of the right testis shows 2 thin, echogenic layers covering the testis, representing the tunica albuginea, which is the fibrous covering of the testis.*

TESTIS, TRANSVERSE VIEW

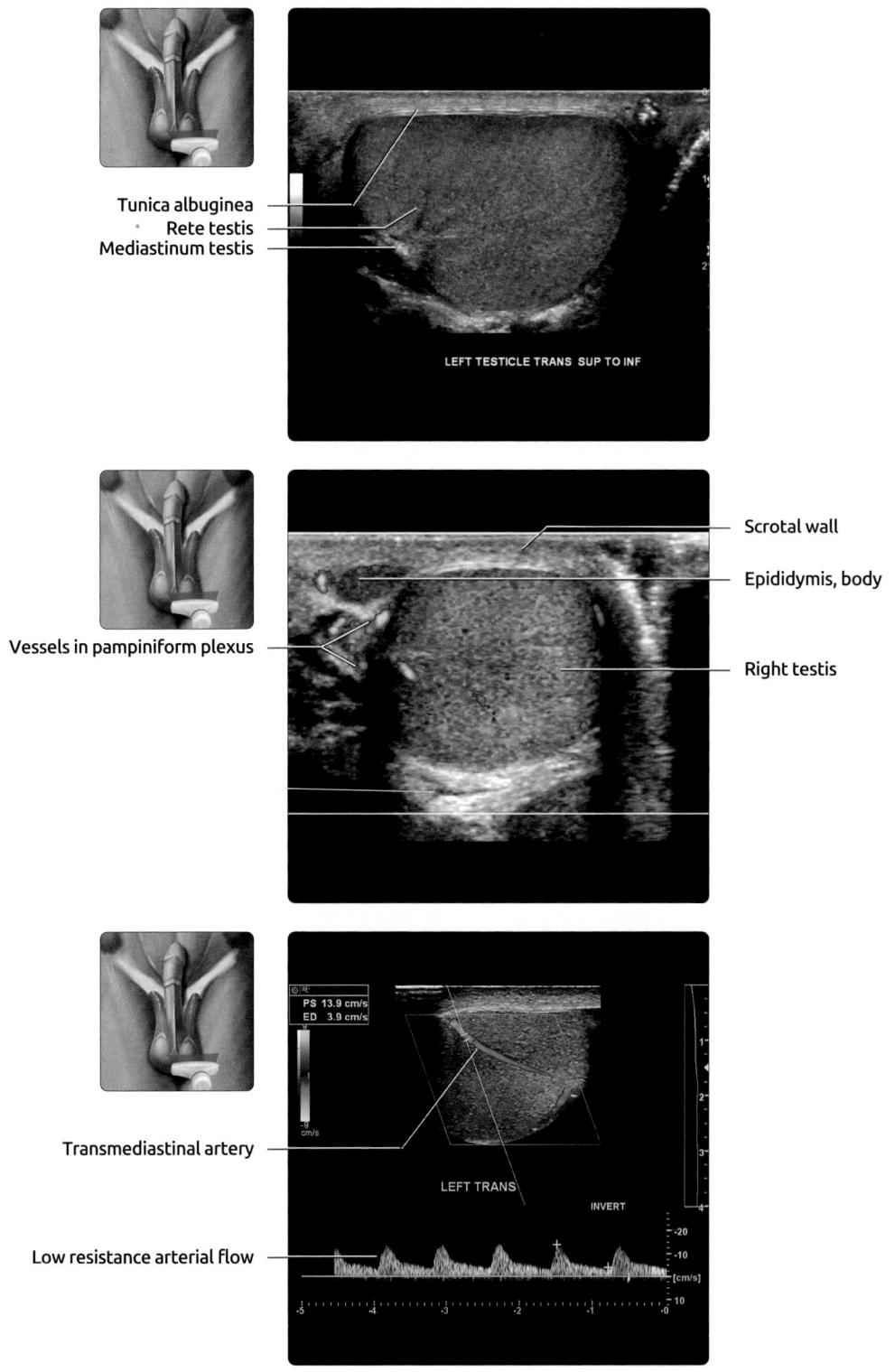

Tunica albuginea
Rete testis
Mediastinum testis

LEFT TESTICLE TRANS SUP TO INF

Scrotal wall

Epididymis, body

Vessels in pampiniform plexus

Right testis

Transmediastinal artery

PS 13.9 cm/s
ED 3.9 cm/s

cm/s

LEFT TRANS

INVERT

Low resistance arterial flow

(Top) *Transverse grayscale ultrasound of the normal testis shows diffuse low-level internal echoes in the parenchyma, mediastinum testis, and the striated pattern of rete testis. The testis is covered with 2 thin, echogenic layers of tunica albuginea.* (Middle) *Transverse color Doppler ultrasound again shows normal paucity of testicular vascularity. Some vessels are also identified in the epididymis. More vessels can be identified along the mediastinum testis.* (Bottom) *Pulsed Doppler ultrasound of an intratesticular artery and the transmediastinal artery shows low resistance with low systolic and end-diastolic flow velocities.*

EPIDIDYMIS, HEAD

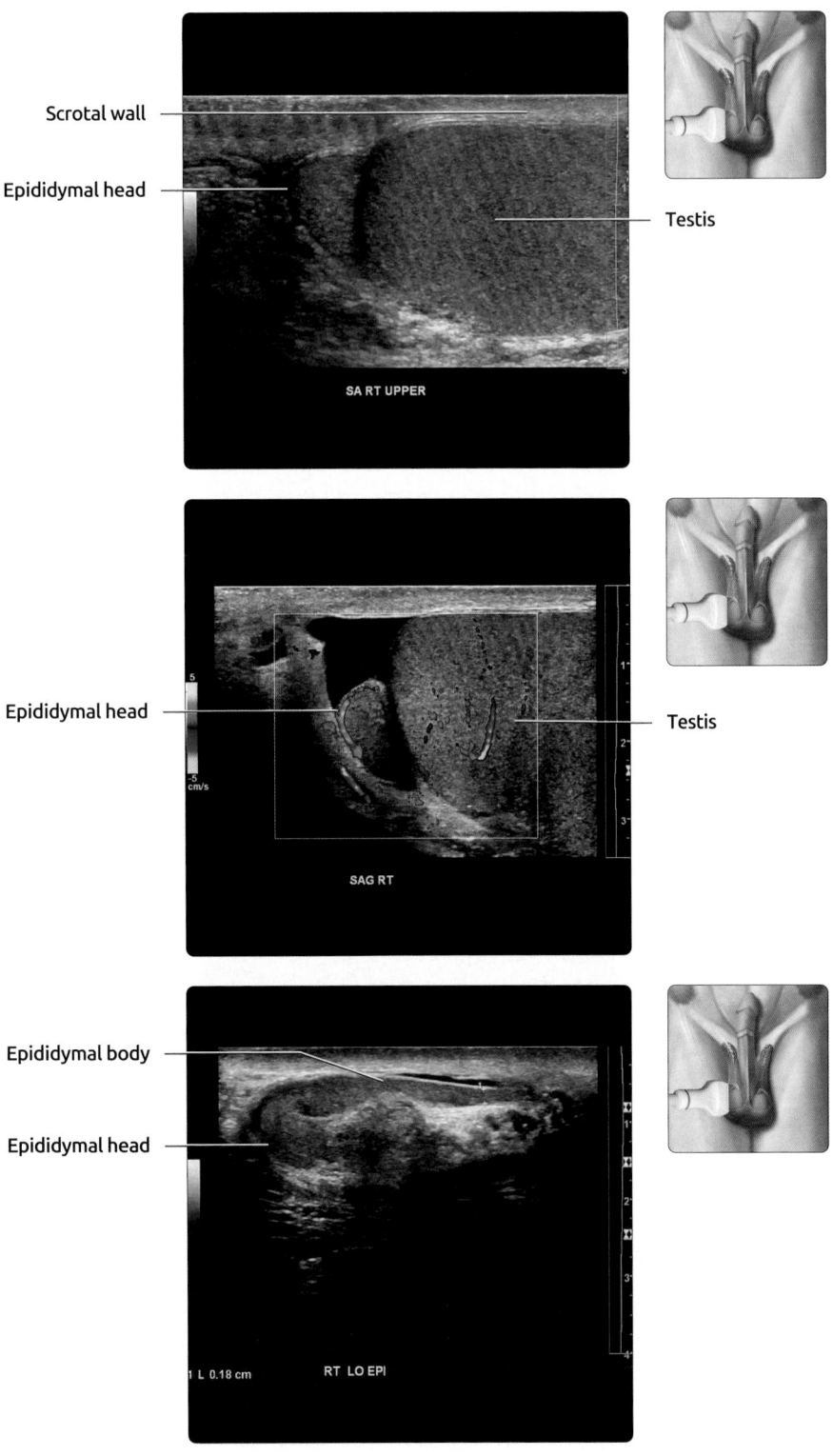

(Top) *Sagittal grayscale ultrasound of the epididymal head superior to the testis is shown.* **(Middle)** *Color Doppler ultrasound of the epididymal head shows normal vascularity compared with the testis.* **(Bottom)** *Sagittal grayscale ultrasound of the epididymis demonstrates a normal homogeneous epididymal head and body*

EPIDIDYMIS, BODY AND TAIL

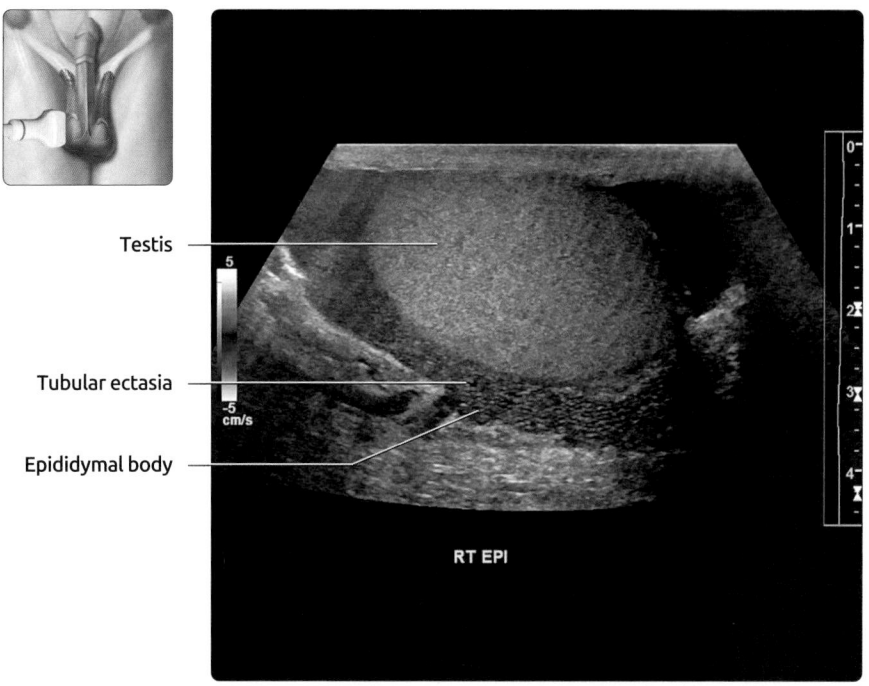

Testis

Tubular ectasia

Epididymal body

RT EPI

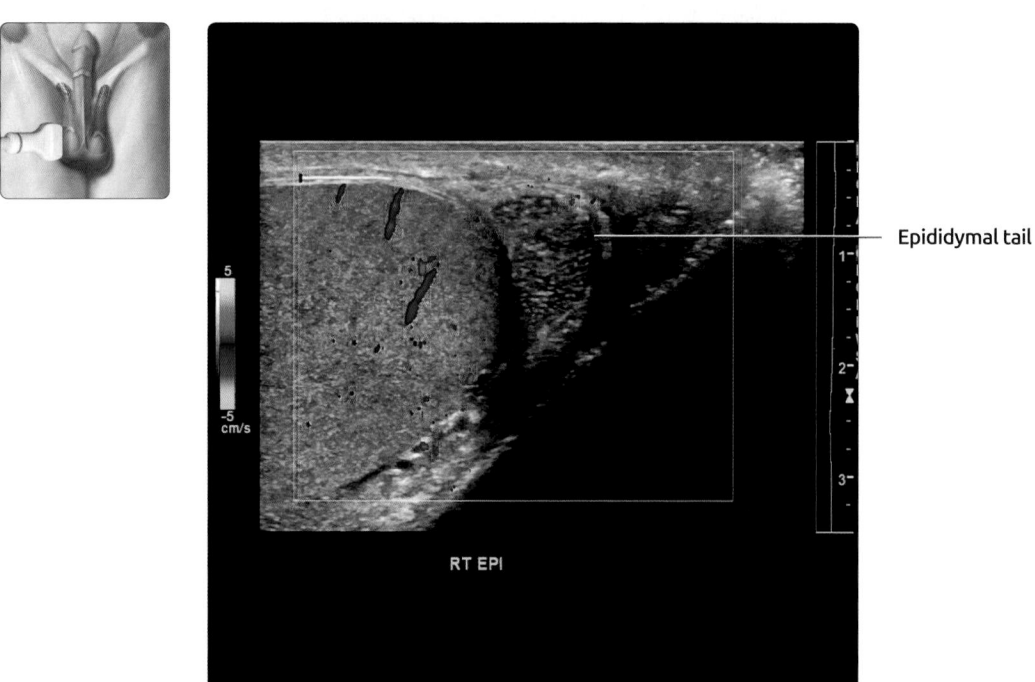

Epididymal tail

RT EPI

(Top) *Sagittal grayscale ultrasound of the epididymis demonstrates a normal heterogeneous epididymal body with mild tubular ectasia seen as tubular anechoic structures in the epididymis.* **(Bottom)** *Sagittal color Doppler ultrasound of the inferior testis demonstrates a normal epididymal tail with minimal internal vascularity.*

TESTICULAR AND EPIDIDYMAL APPENDAGE

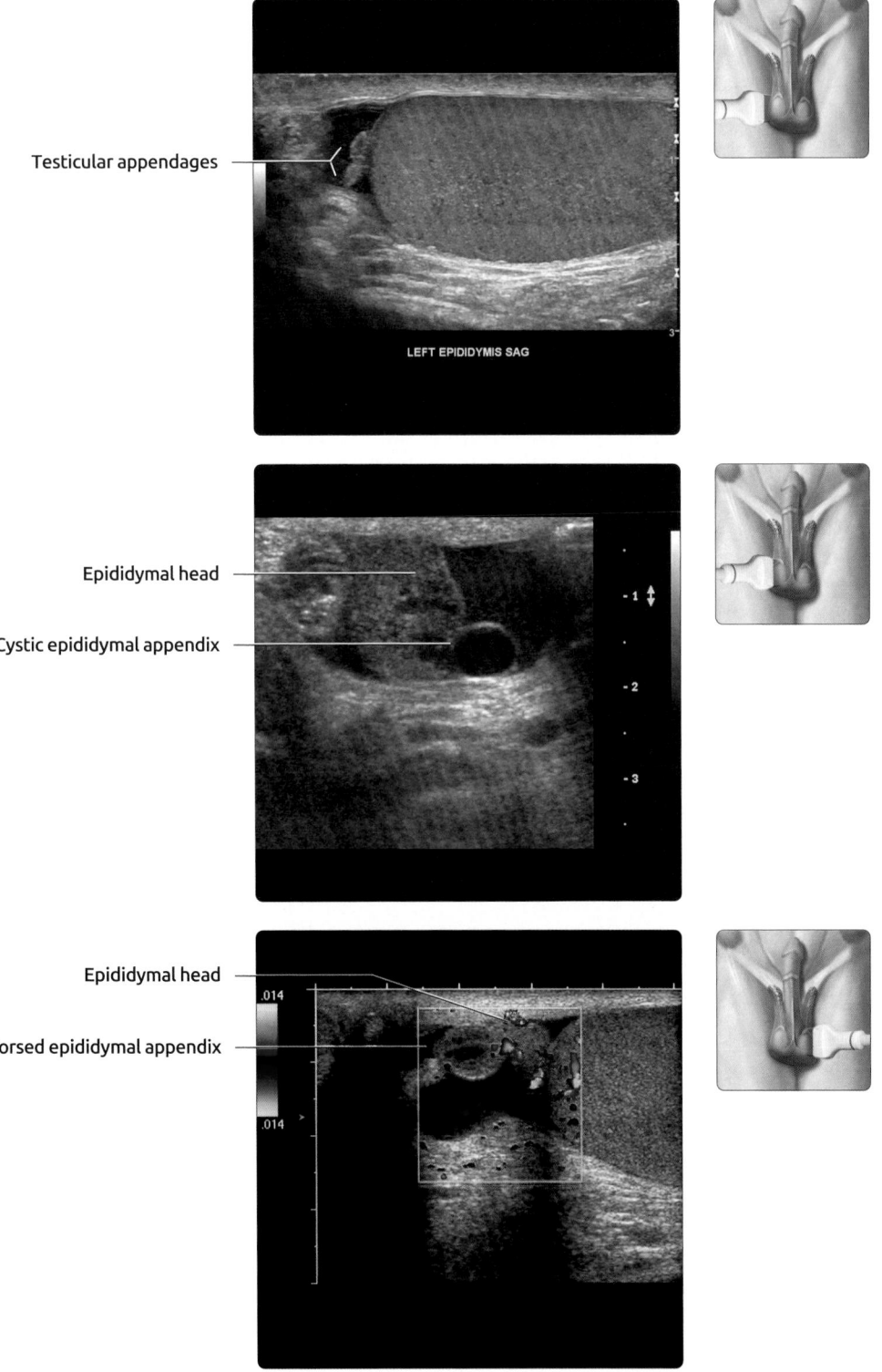

Testicular appendages

Epididymal head

Cystic epididymal appendix

Epididymal head

Torsed epididymal appendix

LEFT EPIDIDYMIS SAG

(Top) *Longitudinal grayscale ultrasound of the testis in a patient with a hydrocele shows 2 small nodular protuberances from the surface of the testis, isoechoic to normal testicular parenchyma. This is the appendix testis, which is a remnant of the müllerian system.* **(Middle)** *Transverse grayscale ultrasound of the epididymal head in a patient with a small hydrocele shows cystic protuberance from the surface of the epididymis. It is isoechoic to normal testicular parenchyma. This is the appendix testis, which is a remnant of the müllerian system.* **(Bottom)** *Sagittal color Doppler ultrasound of the left epididymal head shows an exophytically arising heterogeneous lesion without internal vascularity. The patient presented with acute scrotal pain. These findings are suggestive of a torsed epididymal appendix.*

TUNICA VAGINALIS, ALBUGINEA AND VASCULOSA

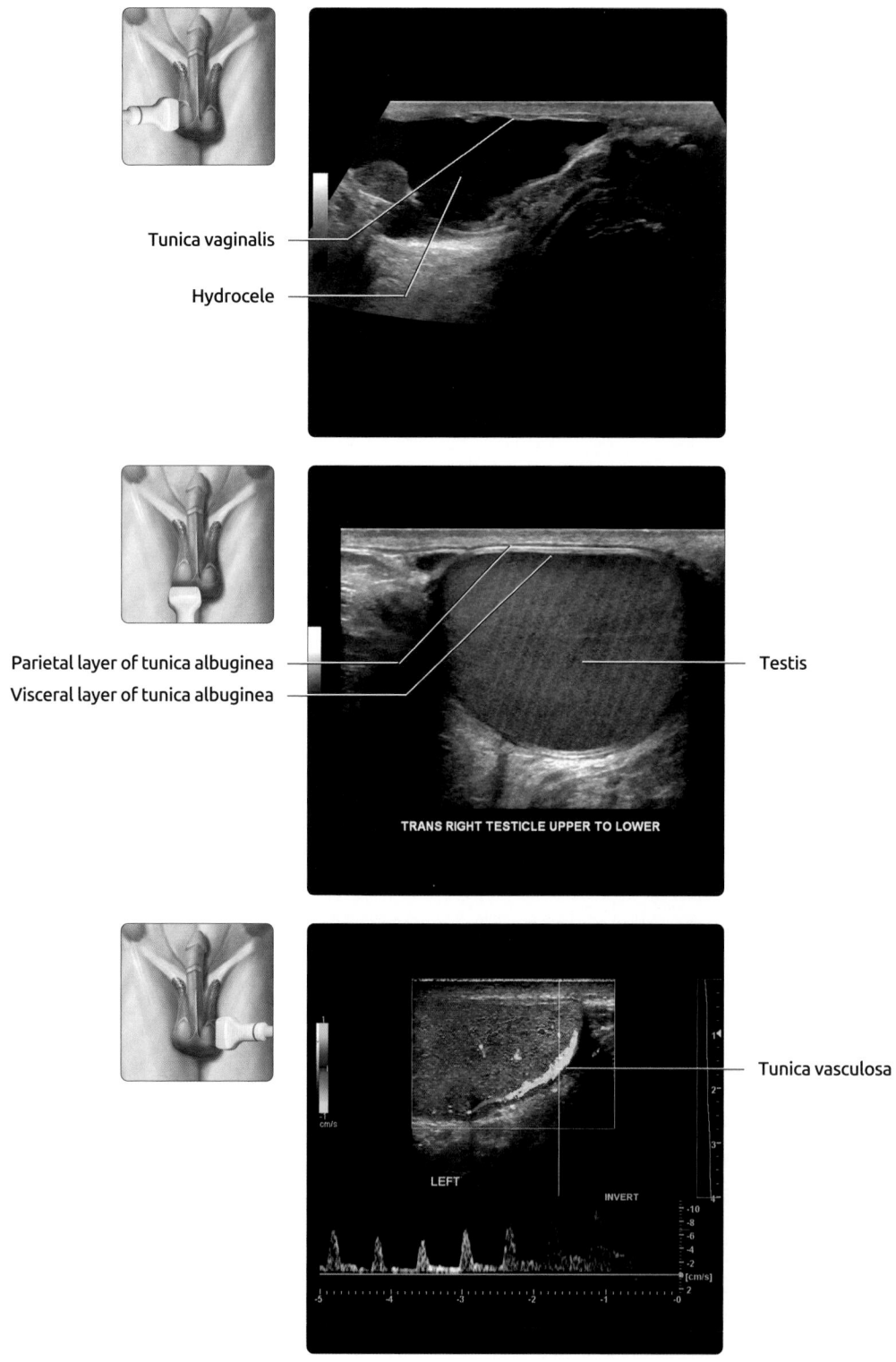

Tunica vaginalis

Hydrocele

Parietal layer of tunica albuginea

Visceral layer of tunica albuginea

Testis

TRANS RIGHT TESTICLE UPPER TO LOWER

Tunica vasculosa

LEFT   INVERT

(Top) *Sagittal grayscale ultrasound of the left scrotum shows the outermost serous membrane covering the testis and epididymis, the tunica vaginalis. There is small fluid within the tunica vaginalis (hydrocele). (Middle) Transverse grayscale ultrasound of the right testis shows 2 thin echogenic layers covering the testis, representing the parietal and visceral layers of tunica albuginea, which is the fibrous covering of the testis. (Bottom) Sagittal grayscale ultrasound of the left testis shows the innermost layer covering the outer aspect of the testis and inner aspect of the tunica albuginea, comprising the vascular plexus that is called the tunica vasculosa.*

ARTERIAL AND VENOUS SUPPLY

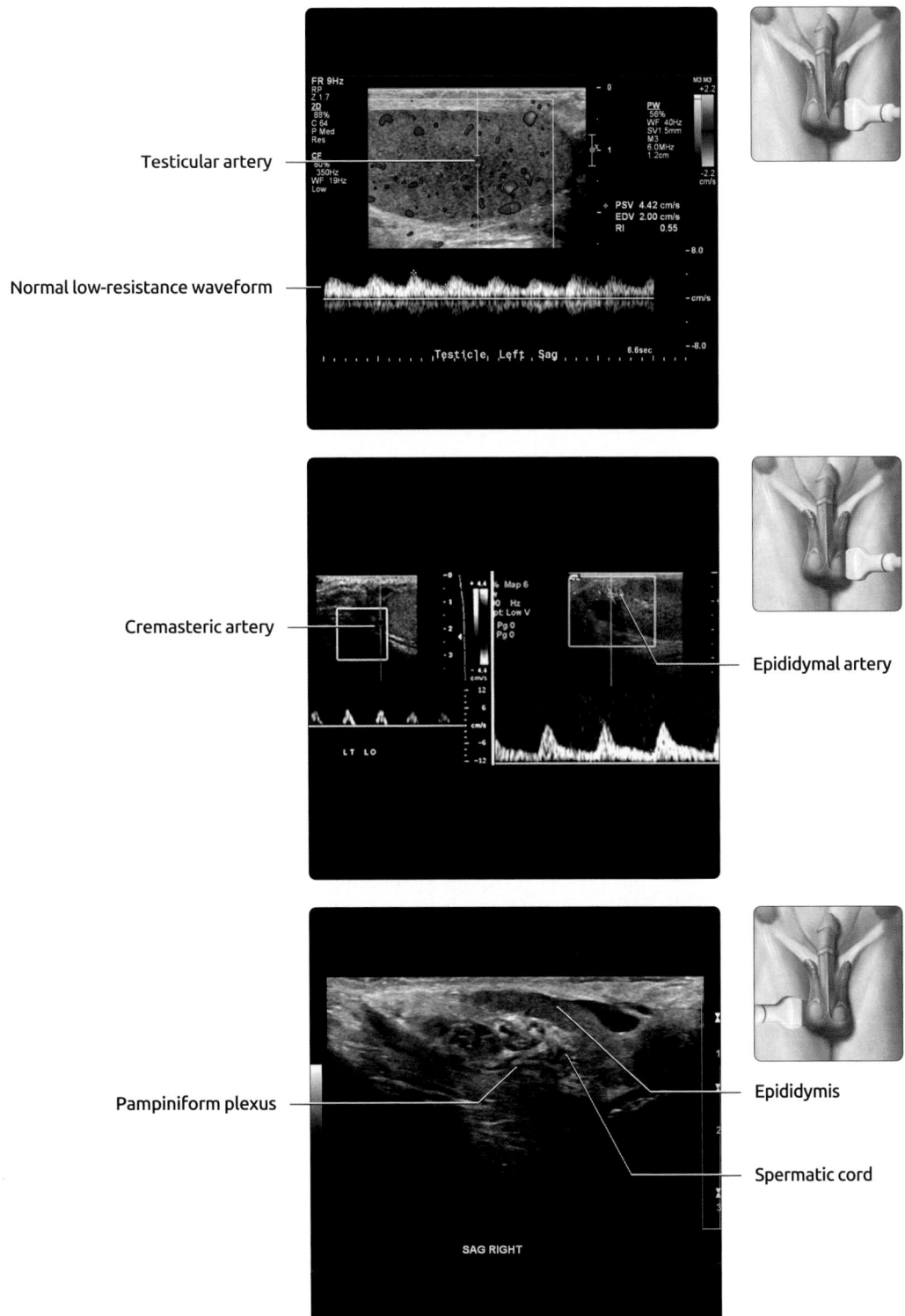

(Top) *Sagittal color Doppler ultrasound of a normal left testis shows normal blood flow with a normal spectral waveform of the testicular artery. The artery should have a low-resistance waveform and the resistive index (RI) should be between 0.48-0.75 (mean RI 0.62).* **(Middle)** *Two color Doppler ultrasounds show the epididymal arterial supply. The left image demonstrates the normal cremasteric artery with a low-flow high-resistance pattern. The right image shows the normal epididymal artery, a branch of the testicular artery with a low-resistance waveform.* **(Bottom)** *Sagittal grayscale ultrasound demonstrates a heterogeneous spermatic cord adjacent to the epididymis, with anechoic tubular structures representing normal pampiniform plexus.*

GROSS ANATOMY

Overview

- Anatomical divisions
  - Body (corpus): Upper 2/3 of uterus
    - Fundus: Uterine segment superior to ostia of fallopian tubes
  - Cervix: Lower 1/3 of uterus
    - Isthmus: Junction of body and cervix
- Parametrium: Outer layer, part of visceral peritoneum
- **Myometrium**: Middle layer
  - Smooth muscle; forms main bulk of uterus
  - Composed of 3 zones: Inner, middle, outer (outlined by arcuate arteries)
- **Endometrium**: Inner layer
  - Stratum functionalis (inner): Thicker, varies with cyclical changes
  - Stratum basalis (outer): Thin, does not change

Anatomic Relationships

- Extraperitoneal location in midline true pelvis
- Uterine position
  - **Flexion** is axis of uterine body relative to cervix
  - **Version** is axis of cervix relative to vagina
  - Anteversion with anteflexion is most common
- Peritoneum extends over bladder dome anteriorly and rectum posteriorly
  - Vesicouterine pouch: Anterior recess between uterus and bladder
  - Rectouterine pouch of Douglas: Posterior recess between vaginal fornix and rectum; most dependent portion of peritoneum in female pelvis
- Supporting broad ligaments
  - Paired, formed by double layer of peritoneum
  - Contain fallopian tubes superiorly, and round ligaments, ovaries, ovarian ligaments, and blood vessels inferiorly
- Fallopian tubes connect uterus to peritoneal cavity
  - 4 segments: Interstitial, isthmus, ampulla, infundibulum
- Arterial: Dual blood supply
  - Uterine artery (UA) arises from internal iliac artery (IIA), anastomoses with ovarian artery
  - Arcuate arteries arise from UAs; seen in outer 1/3 of myometrium
  - Radial arteries arise from arcuate arteries and penetrate vertically into myometrium
  - Basal and spiral arteries arise from radial arteries to supply stratum basalis and stratum functionalis, respectively
- Venous drainage mirrors arteries
  - Parametrial venous network prior to drainage into uterine or ovarian veins

Endometrial Variations With Menstrual Cycle

- Proliferative phase (follicular phase of ovary)
  - End of menstrual phase to ovulation (~ 14 days)
  - Estrogen induces proliferation of functionalis layer
- Secretory phase (luteal phase of ovary)
  - Ovulation to beginning of menstrual phase
  - Progesterone induces secretion of glycogen, mucus, and other substances
- Menstrual phase
  - Sloughing of functionalis layer

Uterine Variations With Age

- Neonatal: Prominent size secondary to effects of residual maternal hormone stimulation
- Infantile: Corpus < cervix (1:2)
- Prepubertal: Corpus = cervix (1:1)
- Reproductive: Corpus > cervix (2:1)
  - 7.5-9.0 cm (length)
  - 4.5-6.0 cm (breadth)
  - 2.5-4.0 cm (thickness)
- Postmenopausal: Overall reduction in size, similar to prepubertal uterus

IMAGING ANATOMY

Myometrium

- Inner layer (junctional zone): Thin and hypoechoic, < 12 mm
- Middle layer: Thick, homogeneously echogenic
- Outer layer: Thin, hypoechoic layer peripheral to arcuate vessels

Endometrium

- Proliferative phase
  - Early: Thin single echogenic line
  - Progressive hypoechoic thickening (4-8 mm), classic trilaminar appearance
- Secretory phase
  - Increased echogenicity and thickening up to 16 mm
- Menstrual phase
  - Early: Cystic areas within echogenic endometrium indicating endometrial breakdown
  - Progressive heterogeneity with mixed cystic (blood) and hyperechoic (clot or sloughed endometrium) regions

ANATOMY IMAGING ISSUES

Imaging Recommendations

- Sonohysterography (SHG) to evaluate endometrial pathology
- 3D ultrasound to evaluate müllerian duct anomalies

EMBRYOLOGY

Embryologic Events

- Organogenesis phase: Uterus formed from paired paramesonephric (müllerian) ducts
- Fusion phase: Paired ducts fuse in midline to form uterus and upper vagina
  - Unfused portions remain as fallopian tubes
- Resorption phase: Resorption of uterine septum

Practical Implications

- Müllerian duct anomalies occur during 1 of 3 phases of formation
  - Organogenesis: Uterine agenesis, hypoplasia, unicornuate
  - Fusion: Didelphys, bicornuate
  - Resorption: Septate, arcuate

ARTERIES OF UTERUS AND ADJACENT ORGANS

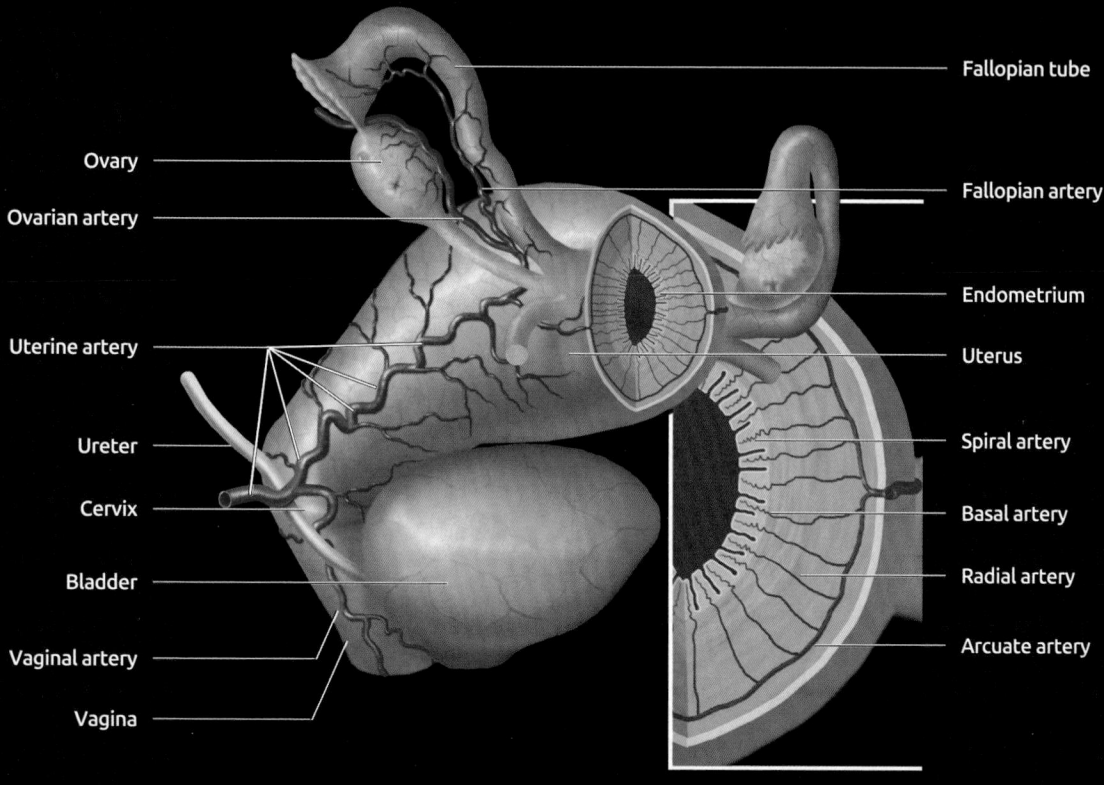

Ovary

Ovarian artery

Uterine artery

Ureter

Cervix

Bladder

Vaginal artery

Vagina

Fallopian tube

Fallopian artery

Endometrium

Uterus

Spiral artery

Basal artery

Radial artery

Arcuate artery

Graphic shows uterine vasculature. The descending segment of the uterine artery after branching off from the internal iliac artery runs medially toward the cervix. The ascending segment ascends laterally along the uterine wall to meet the ovarian and fallopian arteries. The transverse segments cross the cardinal ligament and anastomose extensively with each other to form the arcuate arteries, which give rise to the radial arteries penetrating the myometrium vertically. The arteries then branch into spiral and basal arteries in the functional and basal layers of the endometrium respectively.

NORMAL SAGITTAL IMAGES OF UTERUS

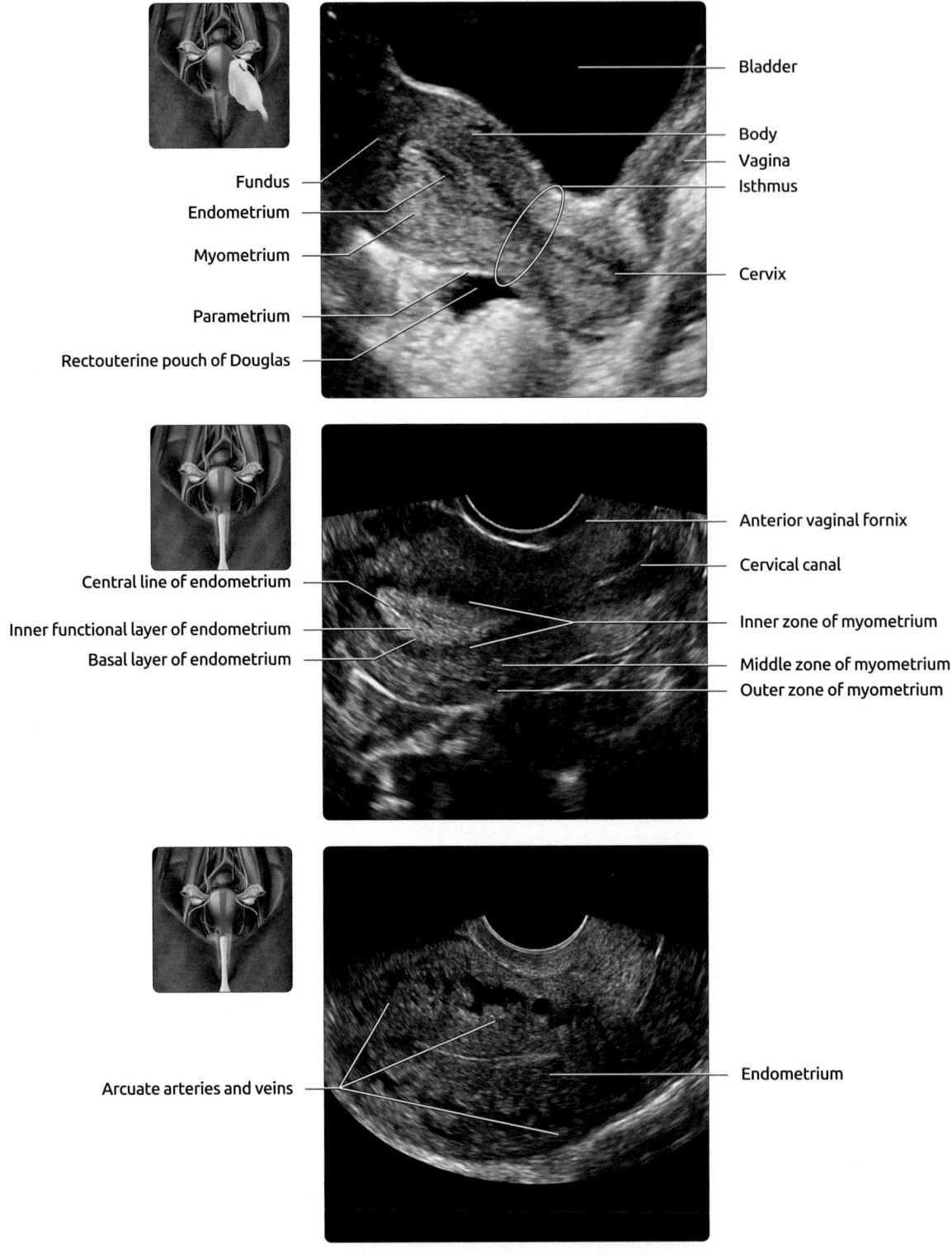

Bladder

Body
Vagina
Isthmus

Fundus
Endometrium
Myometrium

Cervix

Parametrium

Rectouterine pouch of Douglas

Anterior vaginal fornix

Cervical canal

Central line of endometrium

Inner functional layer of endometrium
Basal layer of endometrium

Inner zone of myometrium

Middle zone of myometrium
Outer zone of myometrium

Arcuate arteries and veins

Endometrium

(Top) *Longitudinal TA ultrasound shows a normal anteverted uterus. Version refers to the angle the cervix makes with the vagina. In this case, the cervix is angled anteriorly and the uterus continues in a straight line with the cervix. This is the most common position found in the female pelvis.* (Middle) *Longitudinal TV ultrasound obtained in the secretory phase demonstrates different zones. The smooth muscle within the inner zone of the myometrium is more compact, making it more hypoechoic (subendometrial halo). The majority of myometrium is homogeneously echogenic, with the outer zone being less echogenic.* (Bottom) *Longitudinal transvaginal scan obtained in the early proliferative phase shows prominent arcuate arteries and veins, which run in the outer 1/3 of the myometrium. These may become calcified following menopause.*

NORMAL VARIATIONS, UTERINE POSITION

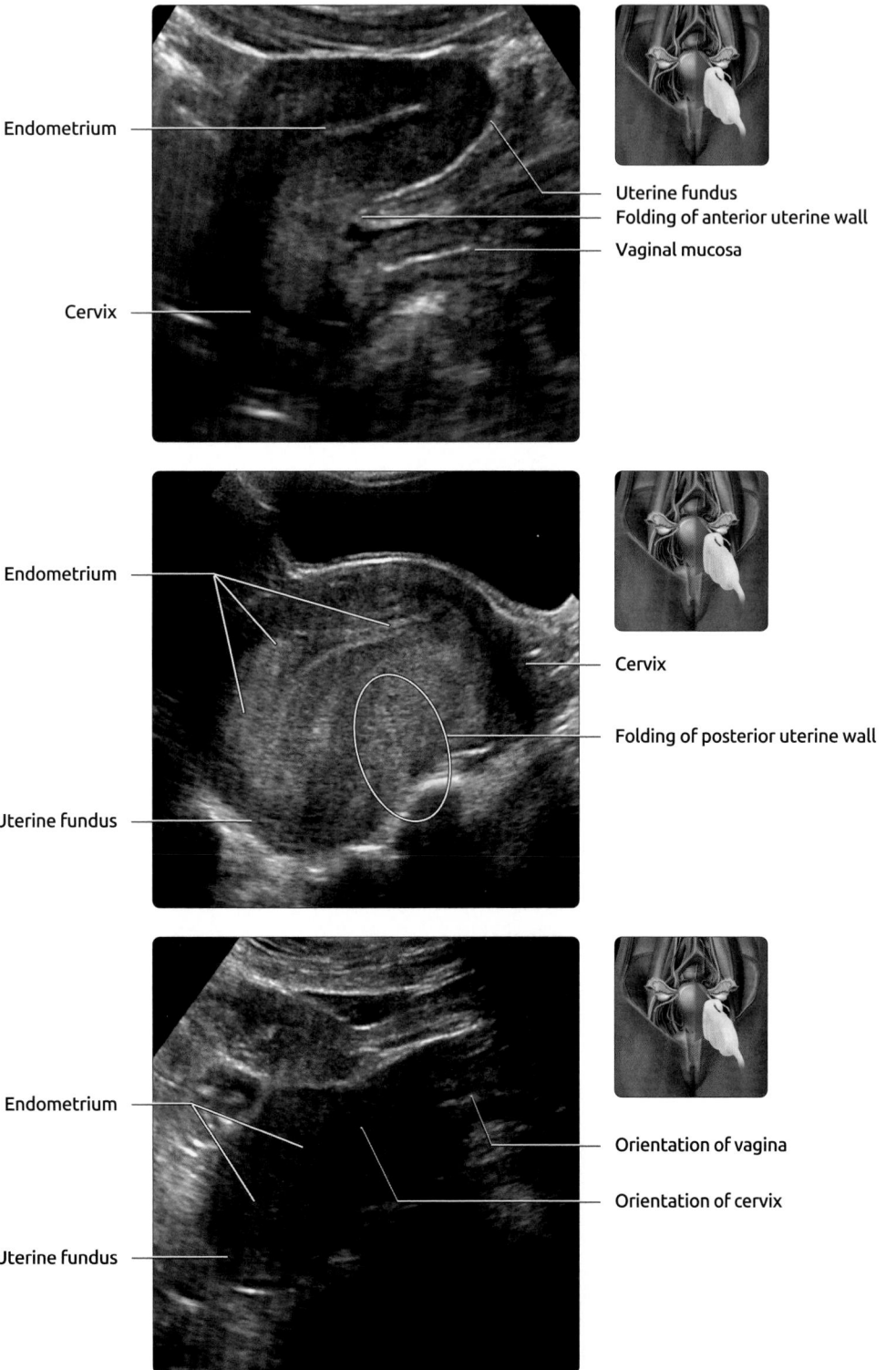

Endometrium

Cervix

Uterine fundus

Folding of anterior uterine wall

Vaginal mucosa

Cervix

Folding of posterior uterine wall

Orientation of vagina

Orientation of cervix

(Top) Longitudinal TA ultrasound of an anteverted, anteflexed uterus shows the uterine cervix is angled forward with respect to the vagina, and the uterine body is angled forward with respect to the cervix. Version refers to the angle of the cervix relative to the vagina. Flexion refers to the angle of the uterine body relative to the cervix, i.e., the uterus and the cervix are not in a straight line. (Middle) Uterine retroflexion. This is an anteverted uterus with exaggerated retroflexion in which the uterus resembles a boxing glove. Folding of the posterior uterine wall may be confused with an intramural fibroid. (Bottom) Uterine retroversion is shown. The orientation of the uterus and cervix is posterior with respect to the vagina. Retroversion frequently limits transabdominal evaluation of the uterus, as seen here.

UTERINE VARIATIONS WITH AGE

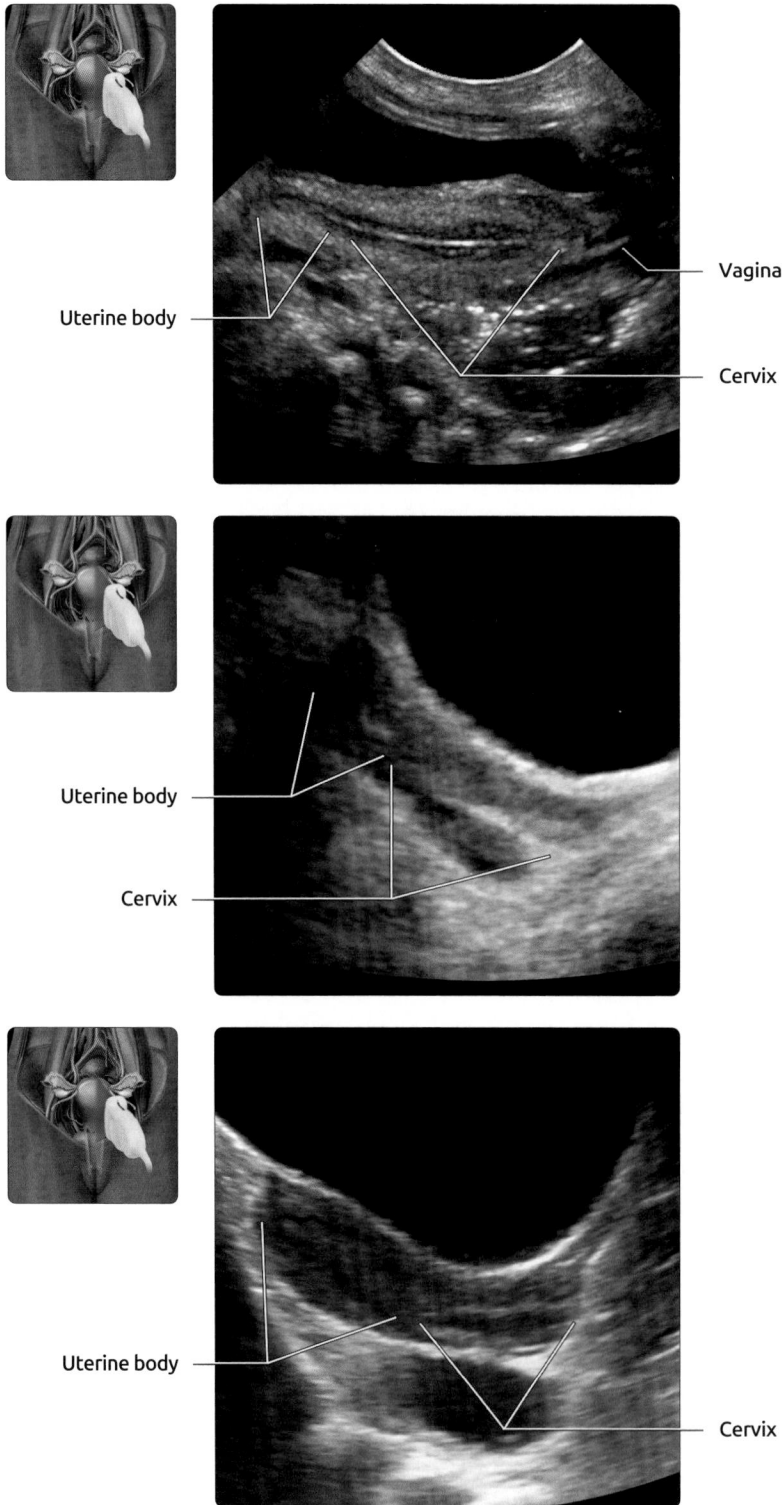

(Top) Longitudinal TA ultrasound shows an immediate neonatal uterus (day 2). The uterus is prominent with a bulbous cervix and a rudimentary body. The endometrium is seen as a thin, echogenic line, which may be due to stimulation by the residual maternal hormones. (Middle) Longitudinal TA ultrasound shows a prepubertal uterus in a patient 8 years old. The uterus demonstrates a tubular appearance with the length of the cervix nearly double that of the uterine body. (Bottom) Longitudinal TA ultrasound shows an early pubertal uterus in a patient 12 years old. The body length of the uterus approximates the cervical length with the endometrium, changing in appearance and thickness during the menstrual cycle. At this time, the uterine body grows dramatically until it reaches the adult size.

UTERINE VARIATIONS WITH AGE

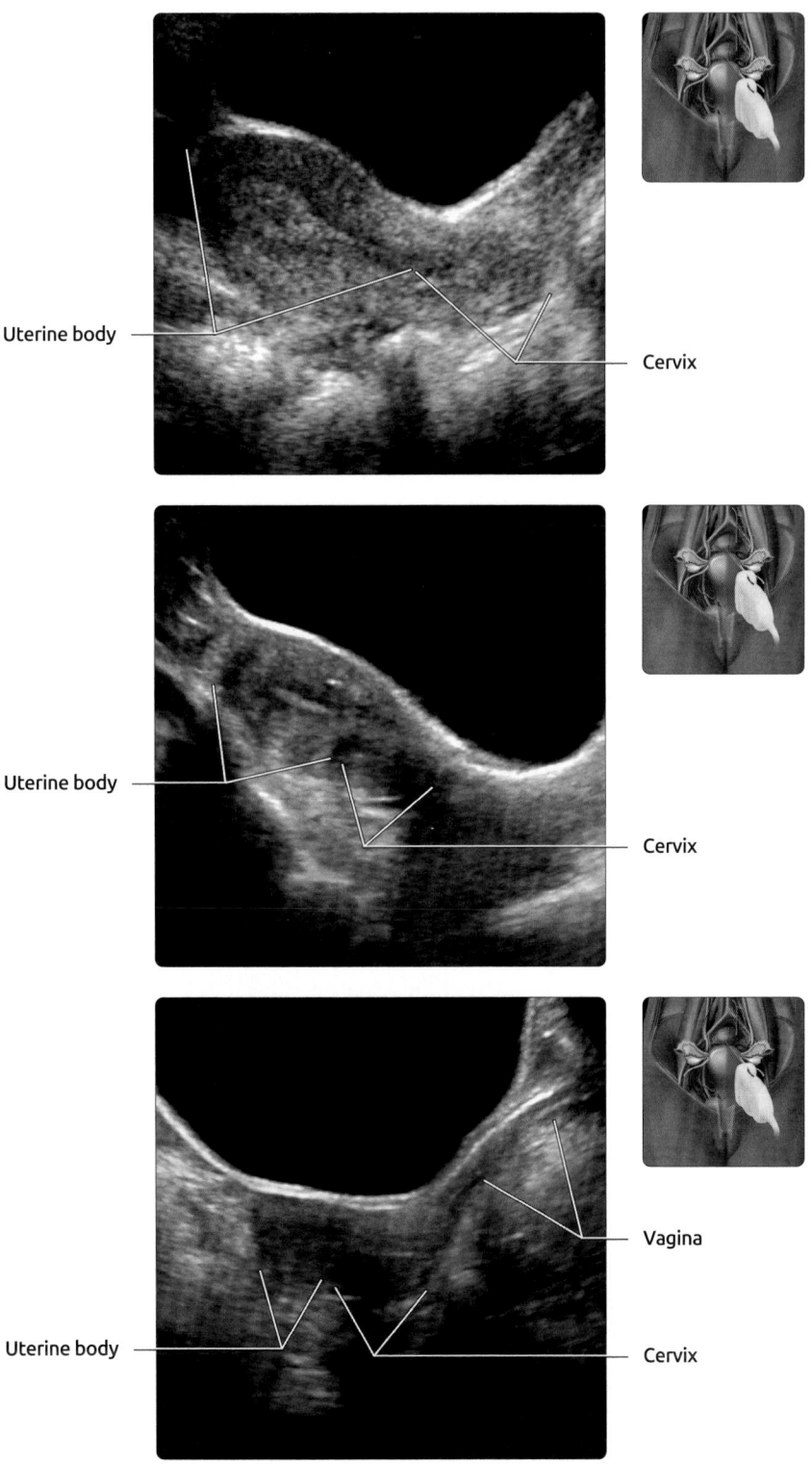

(Top) *Longitudinal TA ultrasound shows a nulliparous uterus. The normal adult uterus should attain a pear-shaped or hourglass appearance, with the length of the uterine body double that of the cervix. The size of a nulliparous uterus is usually smaller than that of a parous uterus.* **(Middle)** *Longitudinal TA ultrasound shows an early postmenopausal uterus, which is atrophic with prominent reduction in body size relative to the cervix.* **(Bottom)** *Longitudinal TA ultrasound shows a later postmenopausal uterus. Note that the cervix-to-body ratio is similar to that of a prepubertal uterus.*

CYCLIC CHANGES OF ENDOMETRIUM

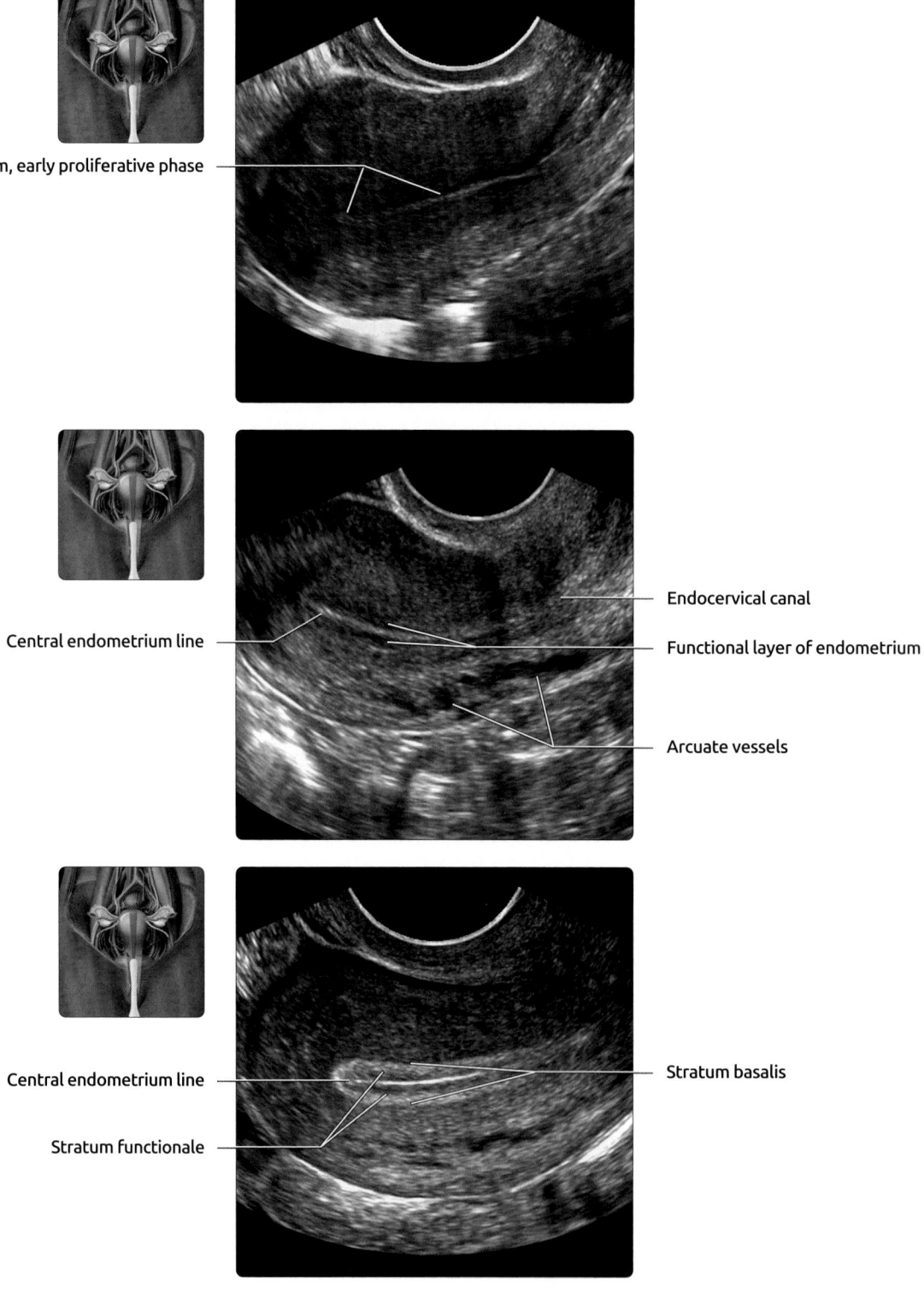

Endometrium, early proliferative phase

Central endometrium line

Endocervical canal

Functional layer of endometrium

Arcuate vessels

Central endometrium line

Stratum basalis

Stratum functionale

(Top) *Longitudinal TA ultrasound shows endometrium in the postmenstrual or early proliferative phase. Note the endometrium is thin and echogenic.* (Middle) *Longitudinal TA ultrasound of the endometrium during mid proliferative phase shows the endometrium progressively thickened and slightly more echogenic.* (Bottom) *Longitudinal TA ultrasound of endometrium in the periovulatory phase shows thickening of the stratum functionalis with an echogenic central line and a layered, trilaminar appearance.*

CYCLIC CHANGES OF ENDOMETRIUM

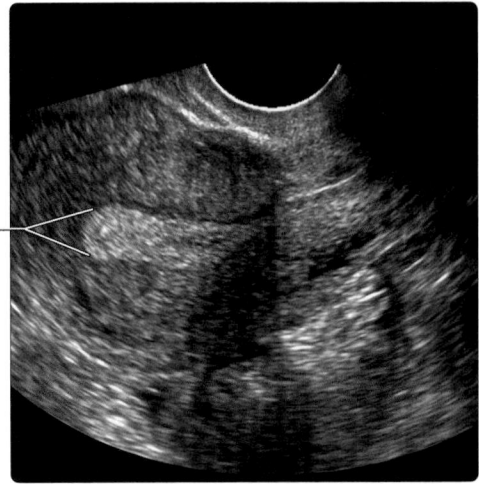
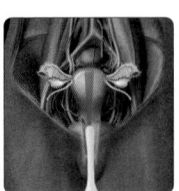

Endometrium, early secretory phase

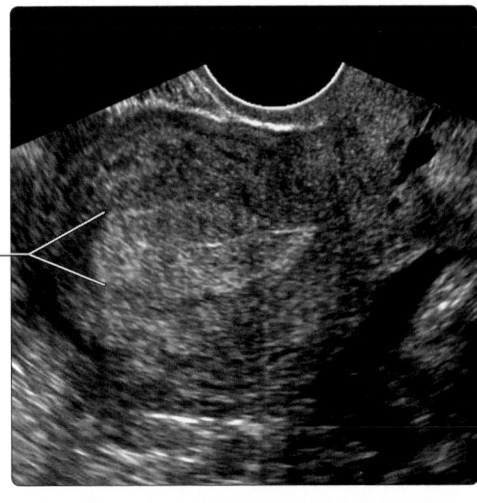
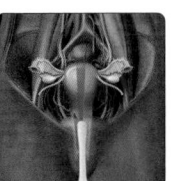

Endometrium, secretory phase

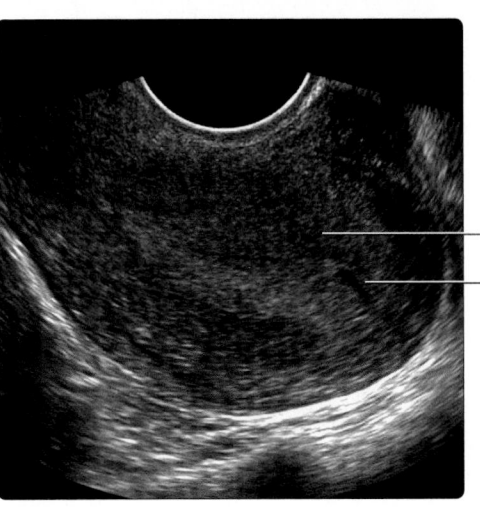
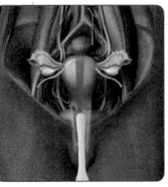

Shedding endometrium, onset of menstruation
Trace fluid in canal

(**Top**) *Longitudinal TV scan shows the endometrium during the early secretory phase. The endometrium becomes progressively thickened and more echogenic, with loss of the trilaminar appearance. These are cyclic endometrial changes in a neutral uterus.* (**Middle**) *Longitudinal TV ultrasound in the late secretory phase shows the endometrium is uniformly thickened and echogenic. The normal maximal endometrial thickness should not exceed 1.6 cm. Through transmission can sometimes be visualized secondary to the mucus-filled glands.* (**Bottom**) *Longitudinal TV ultrasound shows a thickened endometrium just prior to menstruation. Echogenicity has decreased and is more heterogeneous than in the secretory phase. A small amount of fluid can be seen within the endometrial cavity.*

Anatomy: Pelvis

INTRAUTERINE ARTERIES

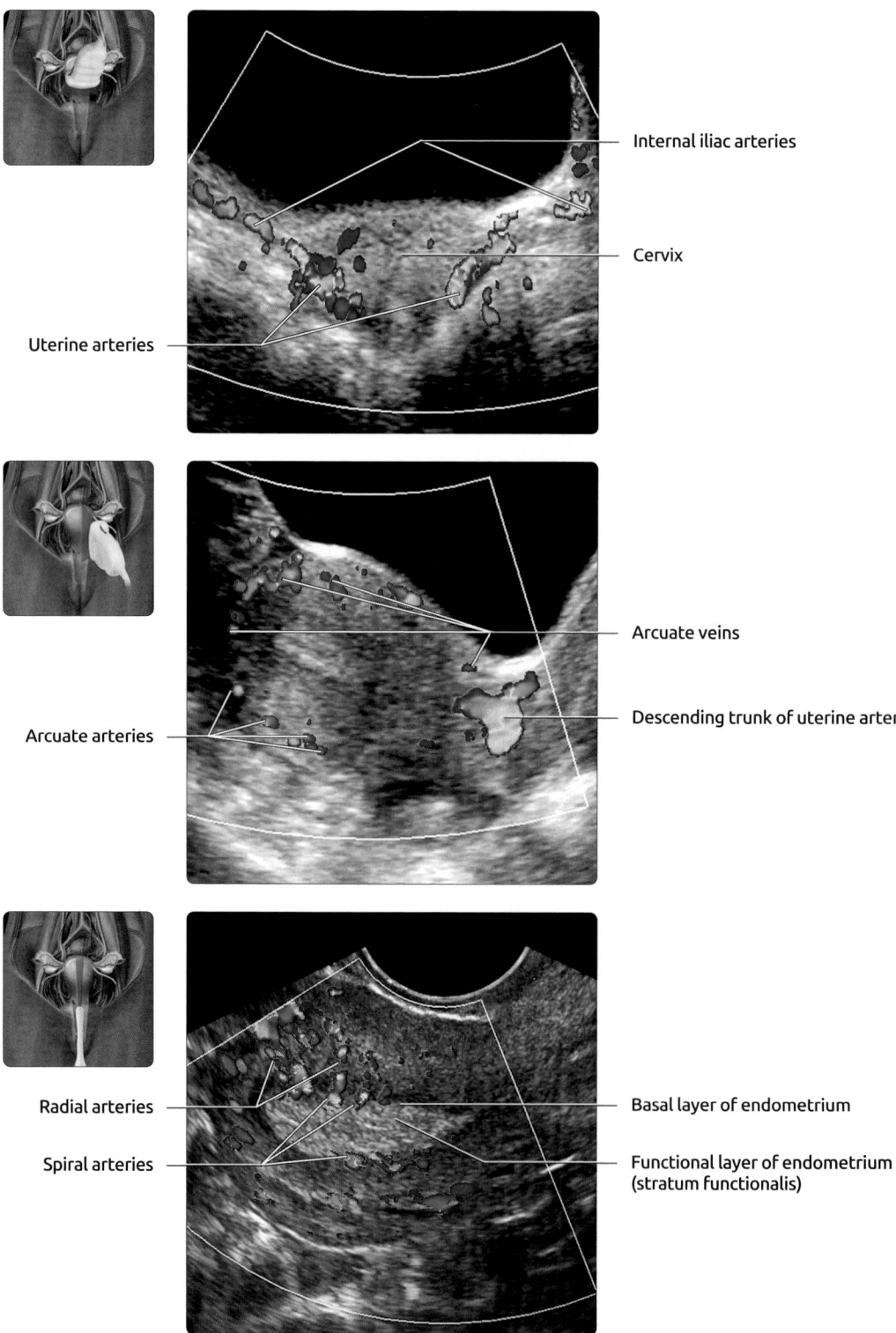

Internal iliac arteries

Cervix

Uterine arteries

Arcuate veins

Descending trunk of uterine artery

Arcuate arteries

Radial arteries

Spiral arteries

Basal layer of endometrium

Functional layer of endometrium (stratum functionalis)

(Top) *Transverse TA color Doppler ultrasound shows descending branches of both uterine arteries running medially at the level of the cervix. Care must be taken not to confuse these with the iliac arteries, which lie more laterally.* (Middle) *Longitudinal TA color Doppler ultrasound shows the arcuate arteries and veins located at the periphery of the uterus. The arcuate arteries commonly calcify with advancing age.* (Bottom) *Longitudinal TV color Doppler ultrasound shows arcuate arteries branching into radial arteries, which run vertically in the myometrium. These in turn give rise to the basal and spiral arteries, which supply the basal and functional layers of the endometrium, respectively. The spiral arteries penetrate deep into the stratum functionalis of the endometrium, which sheds during menstruation.*

FALLOPIAN TUBE

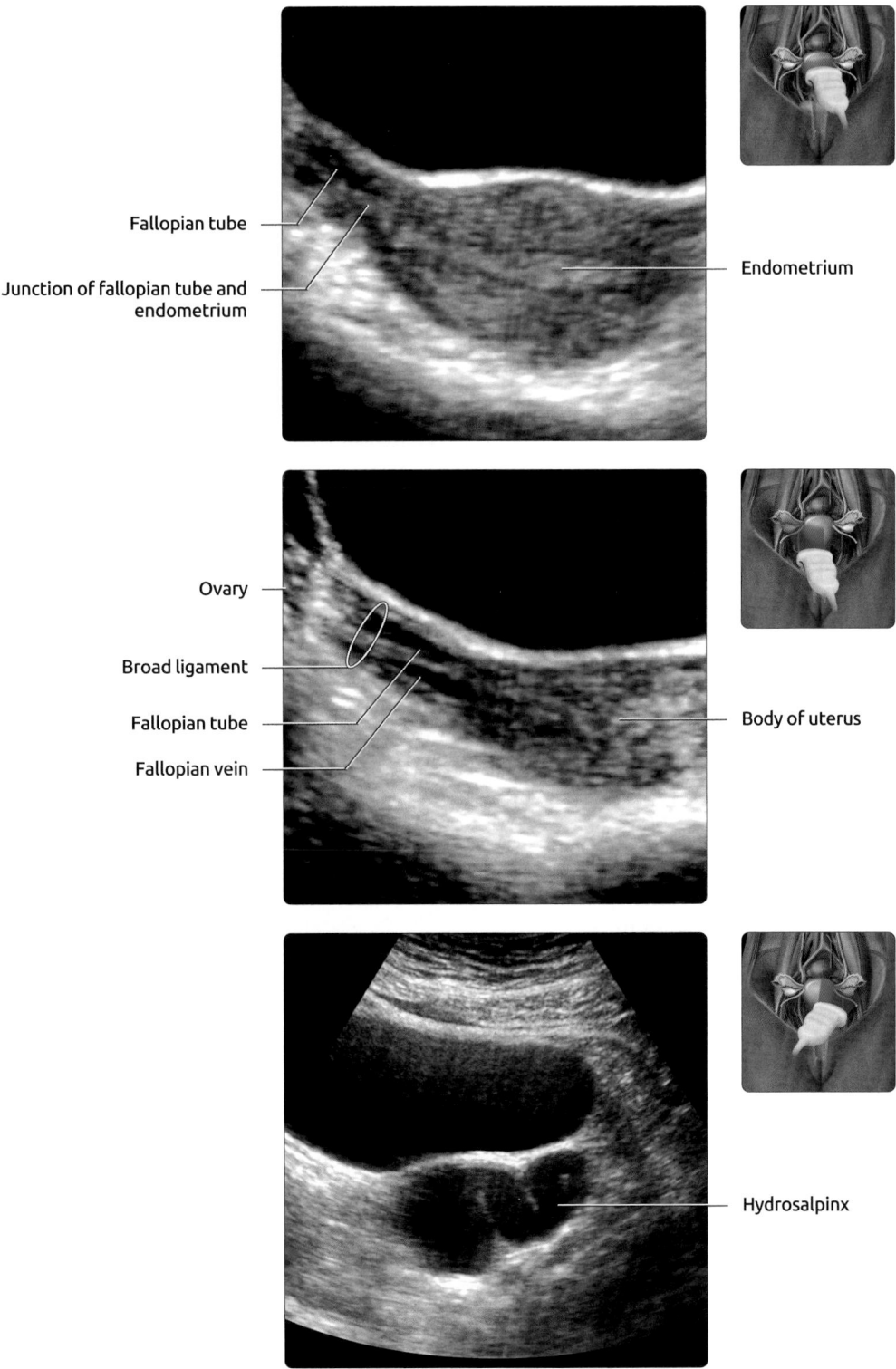

Fallopian tube

Junction of fallopian tube and endometrium

Endometrium

Ovary

Broad ligament

Fallopian tube

Fallopian vein

Body of uterus

Hydrosalpinx

(Top) *Transverse TA ultrasound of the uterus shows the level where the fallopian tube opens into the endometrial cavity. The fallopian tube has four segments including interstitial, isthmus, ampulla, and infundibulum. This image shows the interstitial portion of the tube traversing the myometrial wall at the cornu.* (Middle) *Normal appearance of broad ligament shows fallopian tube with peristaltic movement and a fallopian vessel running parallel to the tube, connecting uterus and ovary.* (Bottom) *Transverse TA ultrasound shows hydrosalpinx, which is a dilated, fluid-filled fallopian tube. It is important to elongate the tube during real-time scanning to differentiate it from a cystic ovarian mass.*

GROSS ANATOMY

Overview

- Begins at inferior narrowing of uterus (isthmus)
  - Supravaginal portion: Endocervix
  - Vaginal portion: Ectocervix
- Endocervical canal: Spindle-shaped cavity communicates with uterine body and vagina
- Internal os: Opening into uterine cavity
- External os: Opening into vagina
- Largely fibrous stroma with high proportion of elastic fibers interwoven with smooth muscle
- Endocervical canal lined by mucus-secreting columnar epithelium
  - Epithelium in a series of small V-shaped folds (plicae palmatae)
- Ectocervix lined by stratified squamous epithelium
- Squamocolumnar junction near external os but exact position variable
- Nabothian cysts are commonly seen
  - Represent obstructed mucus-secreting glands
- Entire cervix is extraperitoneal
  - Anterior: Peritoneum reflects over dome of bladder above level of internal os
  - Posterior: Peritoneum extends along posterior vaginal fornix, creating rectouterine pouch of Douglas (cul-de-sac)
- Arteries, veins, nerves and lymphatics
  - Arterial supply
    - Descending branch of uterine artery from internal iliac artery
  - Venous drainage
    - To uterine vein and drains into internal iliac vein
  - Lymphatics
    - Drain into internal and external iliac lymph nodes
  - Innervation
    - Sympathetic and parasympathetic nerves from branches of inferior hypogastric plexuses
- Variations with pregnancy
  - Nulliparous: Circular external os, arterial waveform shows high resistivity index (RI)
  - During pregnancy: Changes become apparent by ~ 6 weeks of gestation
    - Softened and enlarged cervix due to engorgement with blood with decreased RI of uterine artery
    - Hypertrophy of mucosa of cervical canal: Increased echogenicity of mucosal layer
    - Increased secretion of mucous glands: Increased volume of mucus ± mucus plug in cervical canal
  - Parous: Larger vaginal part of cervix, external os opens out transversely with an anterior and posterior lips
- Variations with age: Cervix grows less with age than uterus
  - Neonatal: Adult configuration due to residual maternal hormonal stimulation
  - Infantile: Cervix predominant with cervix to corpus length ratio ~ 2:1
  - Prepubertal: Cervix to corpus length ratio ~ 1:1
  - Reproductive: Uterus predominant, cervix to corpus length ratio ≥ 1:2
  - Postmenopausal: Overall reduction in size

Anatomy Relationships

- Anterior
  - Supravaginal cervix: Superior aspect of posterior bladder wall
  - Vaginal cervix: Anterior fornix of vagina
- Posterior
  - Supravaginal cervix: Rectouterine pouch of Douglas
  - Vaginal cervix: Posterior fornix of vagina
- Lateral
  - Supravaginal cervix: Bilateral ureters
  - Vaginal cervix: Lateral fornices of vagina
- Ligamentous support: Condensations of pelvic fascia attached to cervix and vaginal vault
  - Transverse cervical (cardinal) ligaments
    - Fibromuscular condensations of pelvic fascia
    - Pass to cervix and upper vagina from lateral walls of pelvis
  - Pubocervical ligaments
    - Two firm bands of connective tissue
    - Extend from posterior surface of pubis, position on either side of neck of bladder and then attach to anterior aspect of cervix
  - Sacrocervical ligaments
    - Fibromuscular condensations
    - Attach posterior aspect of cervix and upper vagina from lower end of sacrum
    - Form 2 ridges, one on either side of rectouterine pouch of Douglas

IMAGING ANATOMY

Ultrasound

- Transabdominal scan
  - Mucus within endocervical canal usually creates echogenic interface
  - In periovulatory phase, cervical mucus becomes hypoechoic due to high fluid content
  - Mucosal layer: Echogenic
    - Thickness and echogenicity shows cyclical changes similar to endometrium
  - Submucosal layer: Hypoechoic
  - Cervical stroma: Intermediate to echogenic
- Transvaginal scan
  - Angle of insonation should be optimized for best visualization
  - Imaging may be improved with withdrawal of probe into mid vagina

MR

- Important in local staging of cervical cancer
- Uniform intermediate signal on T1WI
- Zonal anatomy on T2WI
  - Endocervical canal: High signal
  - Cervical stroma: Predominately low signal, contiguous with junctional zone
  - Outer layer of smooth muscle (variably present): Intermediate signal
  - Parametrium: Variable signal intensity
    - Cardinal ligament and associated venous plexuses high signal
    - Sacrocervical ligament low signal

GRAPHICS OF CERVIX ANATOMY

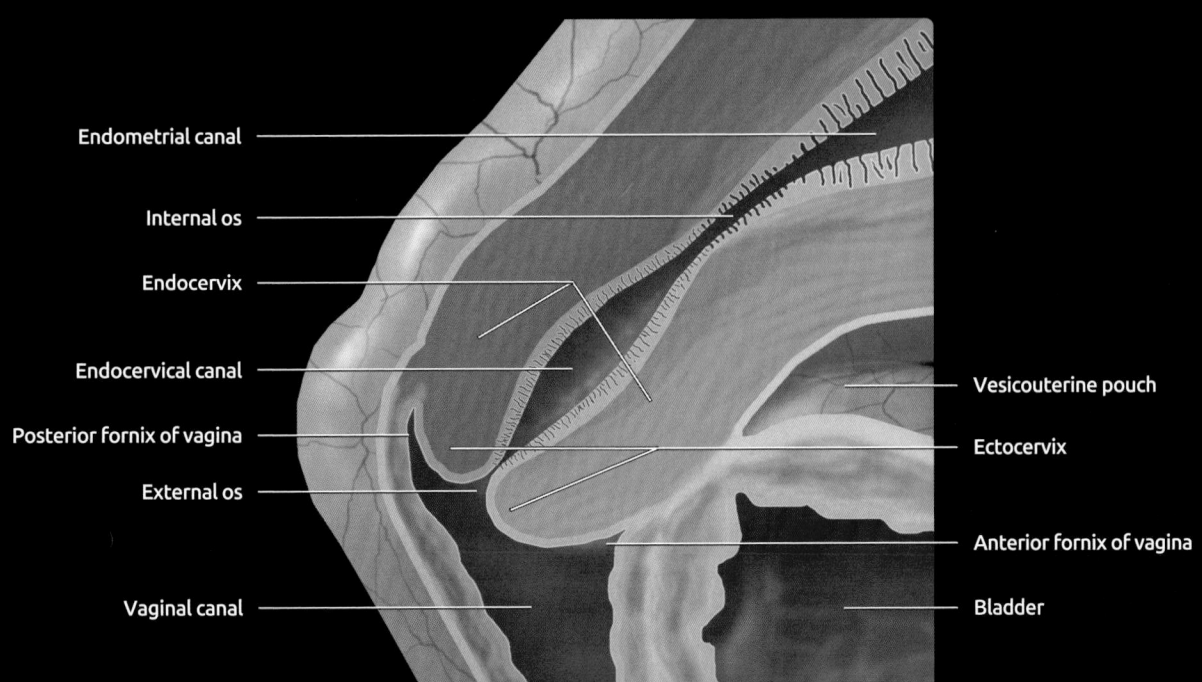

Endometrial canal

Internal os

Endocervix

Endocervical canal

Posterior fornix of vagina

External os

Vaginal canal

Vesicouterine pouch

Ectocervix

Anterior fornix of vagina

Bladder

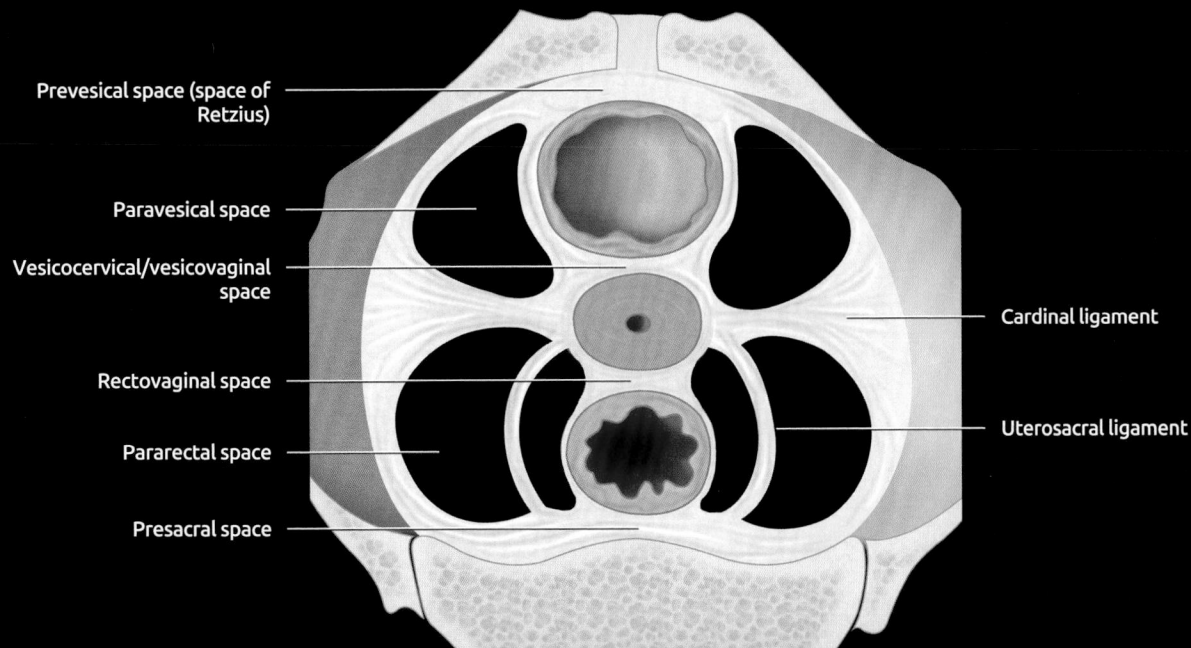

Prevesical space (space of Retzius)

Paravesical space

Vesicocervical/vesicovaginal space

Rectovaginal space

Pararectal space

Presacral space

Cardinal ligament

Uterosacral ligament

(Top) *Median sagittal graphic shows the cervix, which begins at the isthmus, the inferior narrowing portion of the uterus. It has a supravaginal portion (endocervix) and a vaginal portion (ectocervix), which divides the vagina into shallow anterior fornix, deep posterior, and lateral fornices.* **(Bottom)** *Graphic shows the female pelvic ligaments and spaces at the cervical/vaginal junction. The ligaments are visceral ligaments, which are composed of specialized endopelvic fascia and contain vessels, nerves, and lymphatics. Some of the main supporting ligaments for the uterus are attached to the cervix, which are cardinal and uterosacral ligaments. The spaces are largely filled with loose connective tissue and are used as dissection planes during surgery.*

TRANSVAGINAL ULTRASOUND OF CERVIX

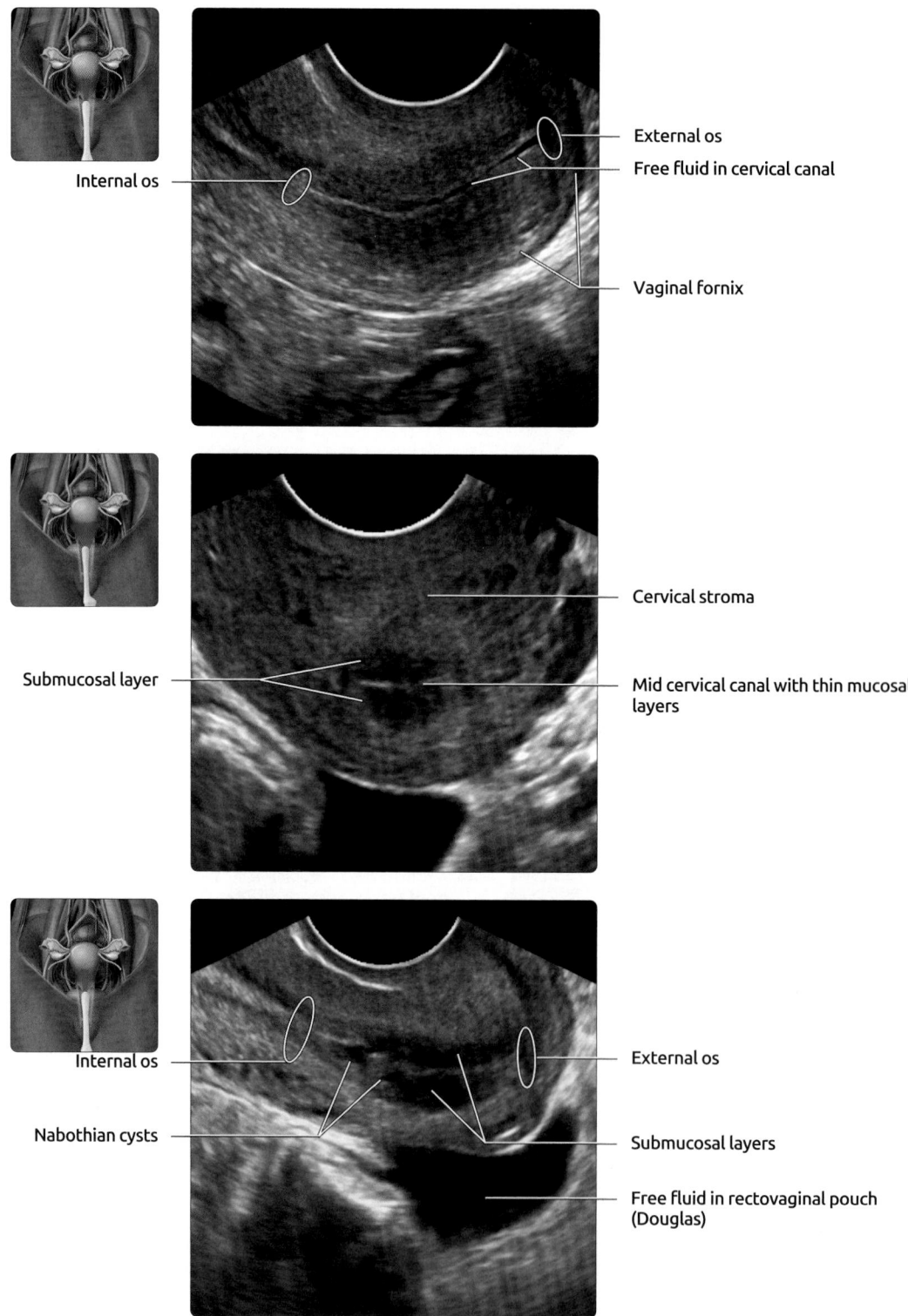

Internal os

External os
Free fluid in cervical canal

Vaginal fornix

Cervical stroma

Submucosal layer

Mid cervical canal with thin mucosal layers

Internal os

External os

Nabothian cysts

Submucosal layers

Free fluid in rectovaginal pouch (Douglas)

(Top) *Sagittal transvaginal ultrasound of the cervix shows hypoechoic fluid present in the endocervical canal. The endocervical canal is rich in mucus-secreting glands. The mucus secreted is usually slightly echogenic but becomes hypoechoic during periovulatory phase. As the transducer abuts the anterior lip of the cervix, the posterior wall of the vaginal fornix can be seen to cover the external os and extend along the posterior lip of the cervix.* (Middle) *Transverse transvaginal ultrasound of the cervix at the lower endocervical canal shows a typical appearance with an echogenic mucosal layer, a hypoechoic band of the submucosal layer, and intermediate echogenic stroma. The submucosal layer is filled with mucus-secreting glands leading to its hypoechoic appearance.* (Bottom) *Longitudinal transvaginal ultrasound shows the transducer abutting the anterior lip of the external os. The submucosal layer is thickened with typical low echogenicity.*

TRANSVAGINAL ULTRASOUND OF CERVIX

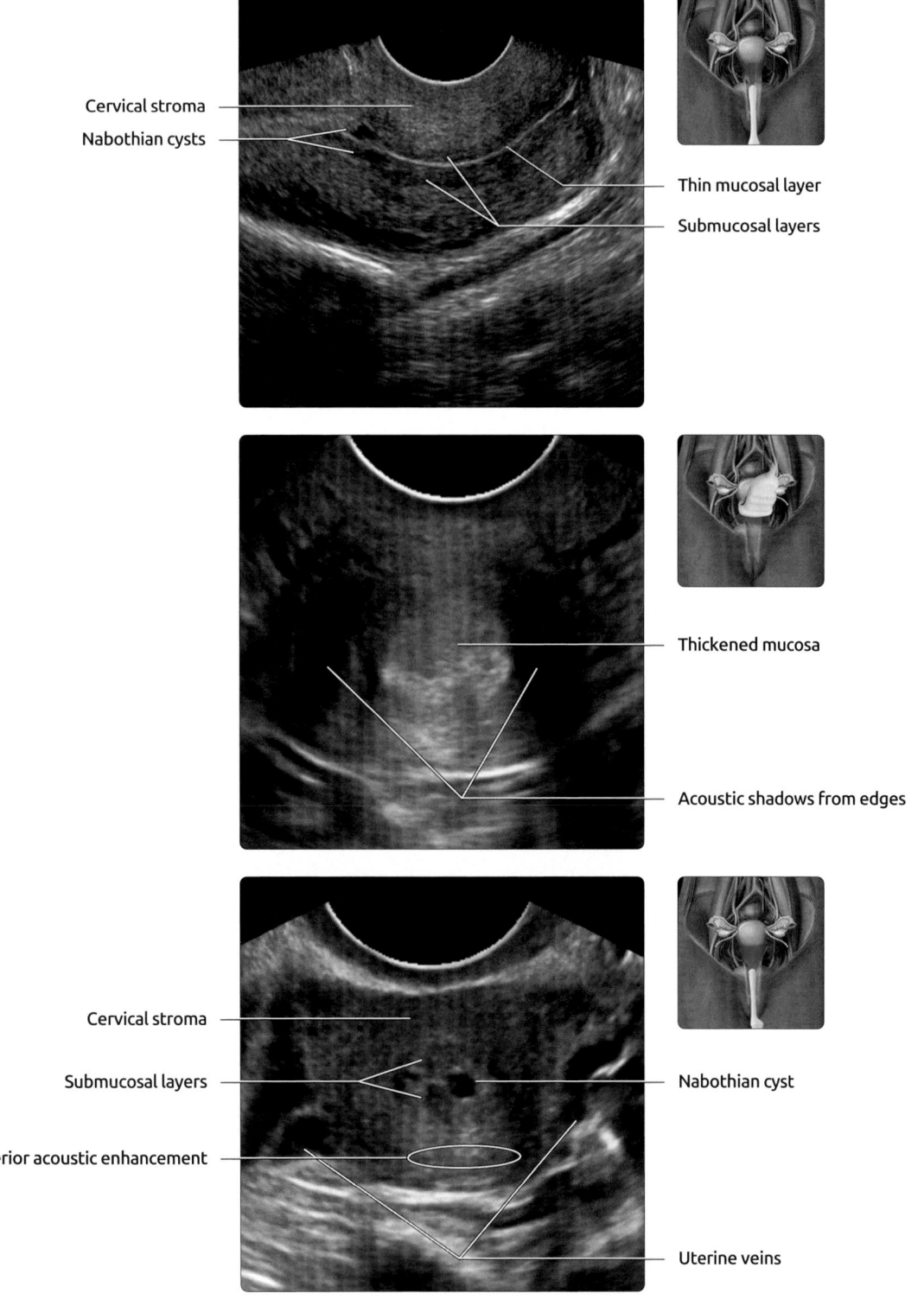

Cervical stroma

Nabothian cysts

Thin mucosal layer

Submucosal layers

Thickened mucosa

Acoustic shadows from edges

Cervical stroma

Submucosal layers

Nabothian cyst

Posterior acoustic enhancement

Uterine veins

(Top) *Longitudinal transvaginal ultrasound of cervix shows two small Nabothian cysts adjacent to the internal os. Nabothian cyst is a common sonographic finding in the cervix and is usually anechoic but sometimes can contain internal debris. It is generally of no clinical significance.* (Middle) *Transverse transabdominal ultrasound at the level of the cervix of a non-pregnant uterus commonly shows thickened mucosal layers. Note that, during the menstrual cycle, the thickness and echogenicity of the mucosal layer undergoes changes as the endometrium does. When thickened, it typically casts shadowing from its edges.* (Bottom) *Transverse transvaginal ultrasound of the cervix at the mid endocervical canal shows the echogenic mucosal layers and thickened submucosal layers. A simple Nabothian cyst is present with minimal posterior acoustic enhancement. The submucosal layer is filled with mucus-secreting glands leading to its hypoechoic appearance and posterior acoustic enhancement.*

TRANSABDOMINAL ULTRASOUND OF CERVIX

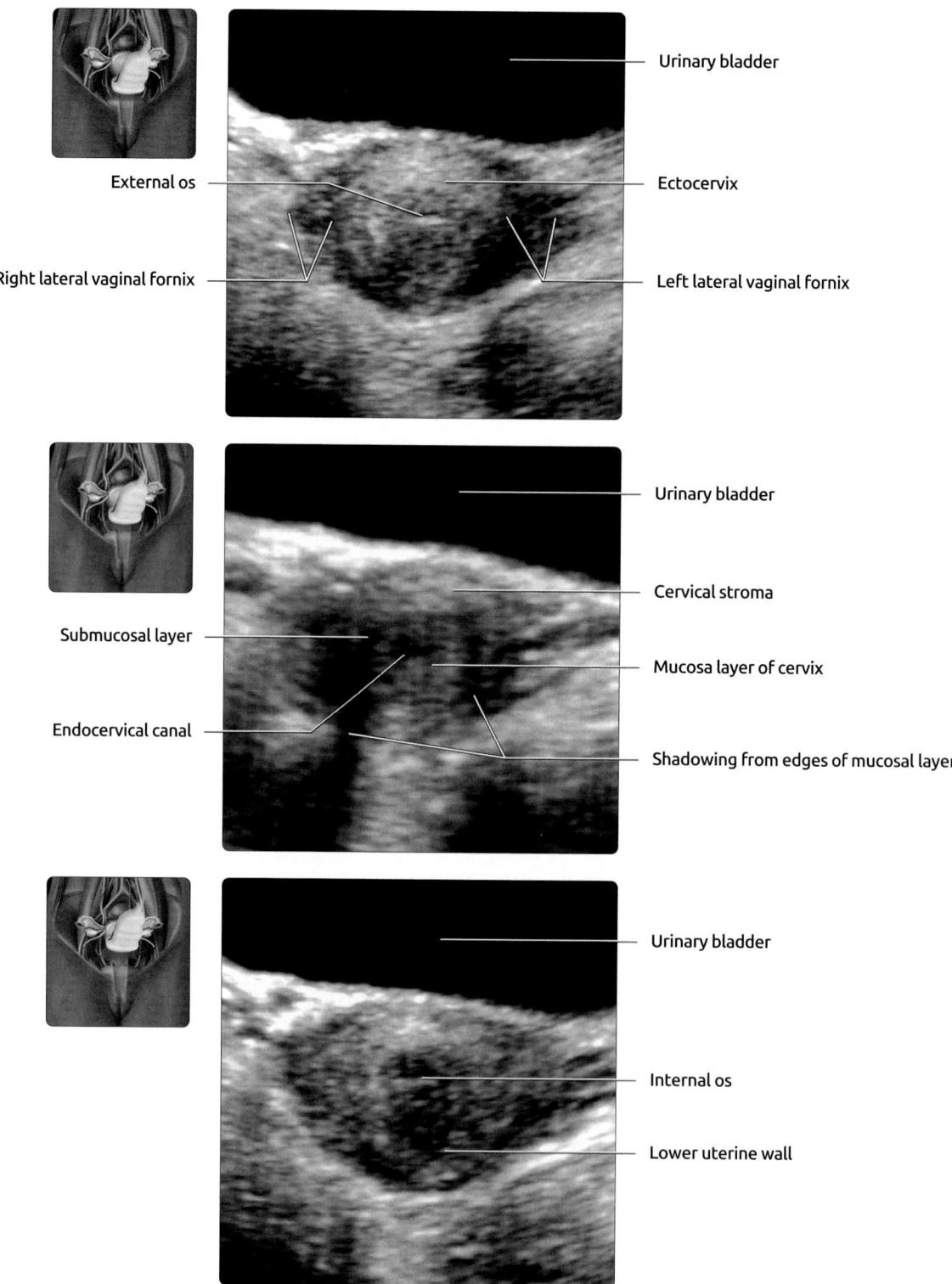

(Top) *Transverse transabdominal ultrasound shows the ectocervix at the level of external os. The lateral vaginal fornices are seen as relatively hypoechoic areas on each side of the ectocervix.* (Middle) *Transverse transabdominal ultrasound of the mid endocervix shows the mildly thickened and echogenic mucosal layer. Note that, during the menstrual cycle, the thickness and echogenicity of the mucosal layer undergoes changes as the endometrium does. When thickened, it typically casts shadowing from its edges.* (Bottom) *Transverse transabdominal ultrasound shows the upper cervix at the level of the internal os, which opens into the uterine cavity. Identification of the internal os is clinically significant in pregnancy for placental site localization.*

CHANGES OF CERVIX DURING PREGNANCY

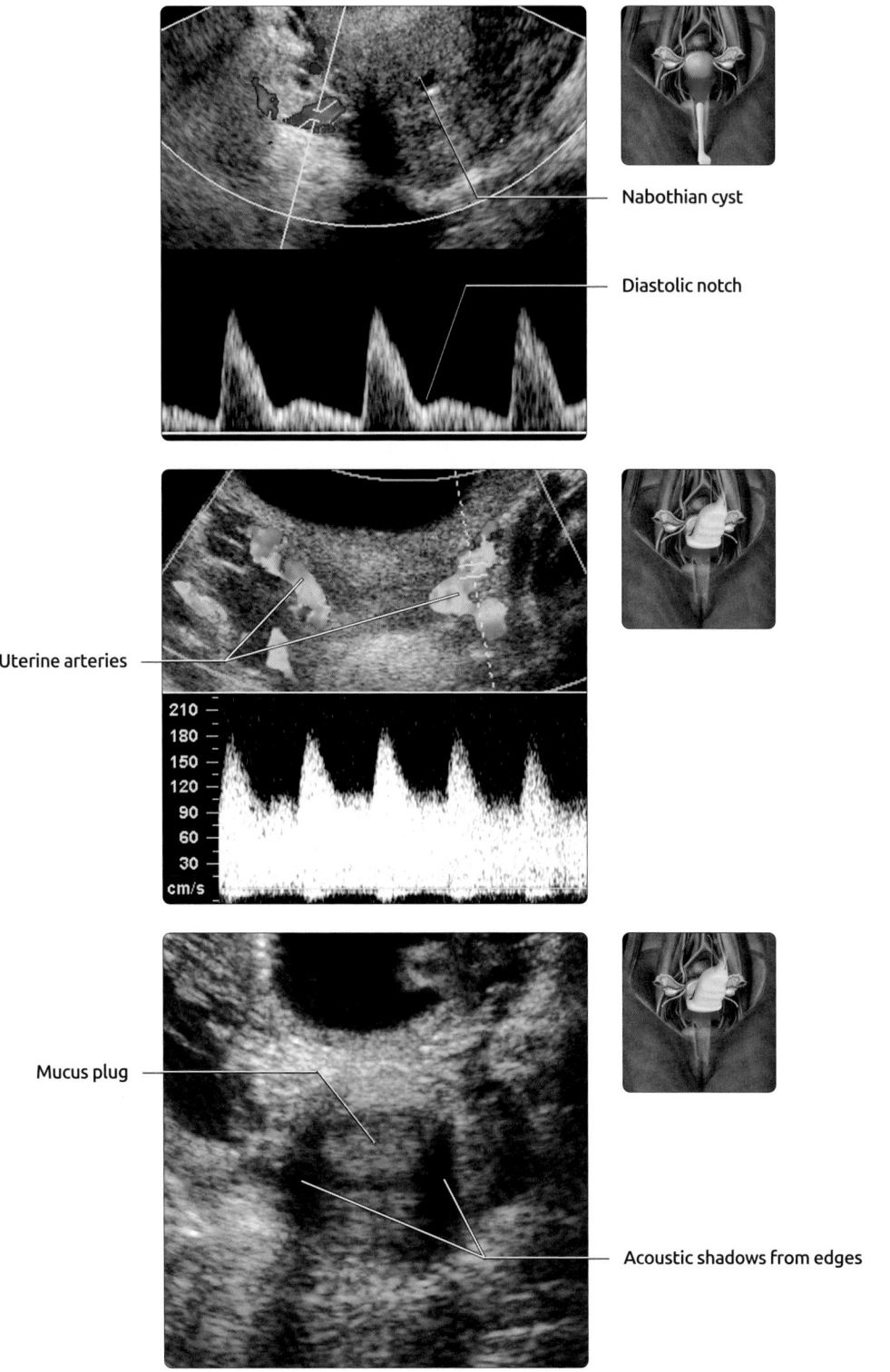

Nabothian cyst

Diastolic notch

Uterine arteries

210
180
150
120
90
60
30
cm/s

Mucus plug

Acoustic shadows from edges

(Top) *Transverse transvaginal ultrasound shows spectral waveform of the uterine artery at the lateral margin of a non-pregnant cervix. There is typical high-resistance flow with a diastolic notch. In normal women, the Doppler waveform usually demonstrates a high-resistance pattern except in late secretory phase.* (Middle) *As softening of the cervix due to engorgement with blood becomes apparent by 6 weeks after conception, the changes can be reflected in the uterine artery, with high-velocity, low-resistance flow seen on this transabdominal spectral Doppler examination.* (Bottom) *Transverse transabdominal ultrasound shows the typical thick and echogenic mucus plug in a pregnant cervix casting dense shadows from its edges.*

TERMINOLOGY

Abbreviations

- Ultrasound (US), vaginal artery (VA), uterine artery (UA)

GROSS ANATOMY

Overview

- Muscular tube formed by smooth muscle and elastic connective fibers
- Serves as excretory duct for uterus, female organ for copulation, and part of birth canal
- Extends up and back from vestibule of external genitalia to surround cervix of uterus
- Has anterior and posterior walls, normally in apposition, with longer posterior wall
- Superiorly, cervix projects downward and backward into vagina and divides vagina into shallow anterior, deep posterior, and lateral fornices
- Upper half of vagina lies above pelvic floor, lower half lies within perineum
- Lined with stratified squamous epithelium
- Inner mucosal surface of wall form rugae when collapsed
- Thin mucosal fold called hymen surrounds entrance to vaginal orifice
- Outer surface (adventitial coat) is thin fibrous layer continuous with surrounding endopelvic fascia
- Vasculature
  - Arterial supply
    - VA: Can branch directly from internal iliac artery (anterior trunk) or sometimes from inferior vesical artery or UA
    - Vaginal branches of UA
    - Branches of VA and UA anastomose to form 2 median longitudinal vessels: Azygos arteries, one in front and one behind vagina
  - Venous drainage
    - Form venous plexus around vagina
    - Eventually drains to internal iliac veins
- Variations with age
  - Menarche: 7-10 cm long
  - Postmenopausal: Shrinks in length and diameter; fornices virtually disappear

Anatomic Relationships

- Anterior
  - Superior: Bladder base
  - Inferior: Urethra
- Posterior
  - Upper 1/3: Rectouterine pouch of Douglas
  - Middle 1/3: Ampulla of rectum
  - Lower 1/3: Perineal body
- Lateral
  - Upper 1/3: Ureters
  - Middle 1/3: Levator ani and pelvic fascia
  - Lower 1/3: Bulb of vestibule, urogenital diaphragm, and bulbospongiosus muscles
- Ligamentous supports
  - Upper 1/3: Levator ani muscles, transverse cervical (cardinal), pubocervical, and sacrocervical ligaments
  - Middle 1/3: Urogenital diaphragm

- Lower 1/3: Perineal body

IMAGING ANATOMY

Ultrasound

- Transabdominal US with distended bladder is standard imaging technique
  - Caudal angulation on both longitudinal and transverse scans
  - Commonly found at/near sagittal midline of pelvis
  - Length and wall thickness vary in response to bladder and rectal filling
  - Combined thickness of anterior and posterior vaginal walls should not exceed 1 cm for transabdominal scan with distended bladder
  - Characteristic appearance of 3 parallel lines
    - Highly echogenic mucosa centrally, may be difficult to visualize if stretched by distended bladder
    - Moderately hypoechoic muscular walls
- Transperineal US with nondistended bladder for assessment of uterine prolapse or for difficult cases
  - Vagina, especially vaginal canal, is less well-defined

EMBRYOLOGY

Embryologic Events

- Uterus and upper vagina are formed from paired müllerian (paramesonephric) ducts
- Paired ducts meet in midline and fuse, forming uterovaginal canal
- Lower vagina is formed from urogenital sinus

CLINICAL IMPLICATIONS

Uterine Prolapse

- Ligamentous support of pelvic organs may be damaged or become lax, leading to uterine prolapse or prolapse of vaginal walls
- Cystocele: Sagging of bladder with bulging of anterior vaginal wall
- Rectocele: Sagging of ampulla of rectum with bulging of posterior vaginal wall
- Best to be investigated by transperineal US supplemented with 3D

Müllerian Duct Anomalies

- Failure of müllerian duct development ± fusion
- Vagina most commonly affected in uterus didelphys (class III anomaly); vaginal septum seen in ~ 75% of cases

Pelvic Abscess

- Common site: Rectouterine pouch of Douglas
- Feasible for transvaginal US-guided drainage of pelvic abscess without doing major operation

Persistent Sexual Arousal Syndrome

- Persistent sexual arousal during sleep in postmenopausal women
- VA blood flow as one diagnostic aid
- VA normally shows high-resistance flow
- During sexual arousal, increased blood flow to VA with low-resistance spectral waveform

GRAPHICS OF NORMAL VAGINAL ANATOMY

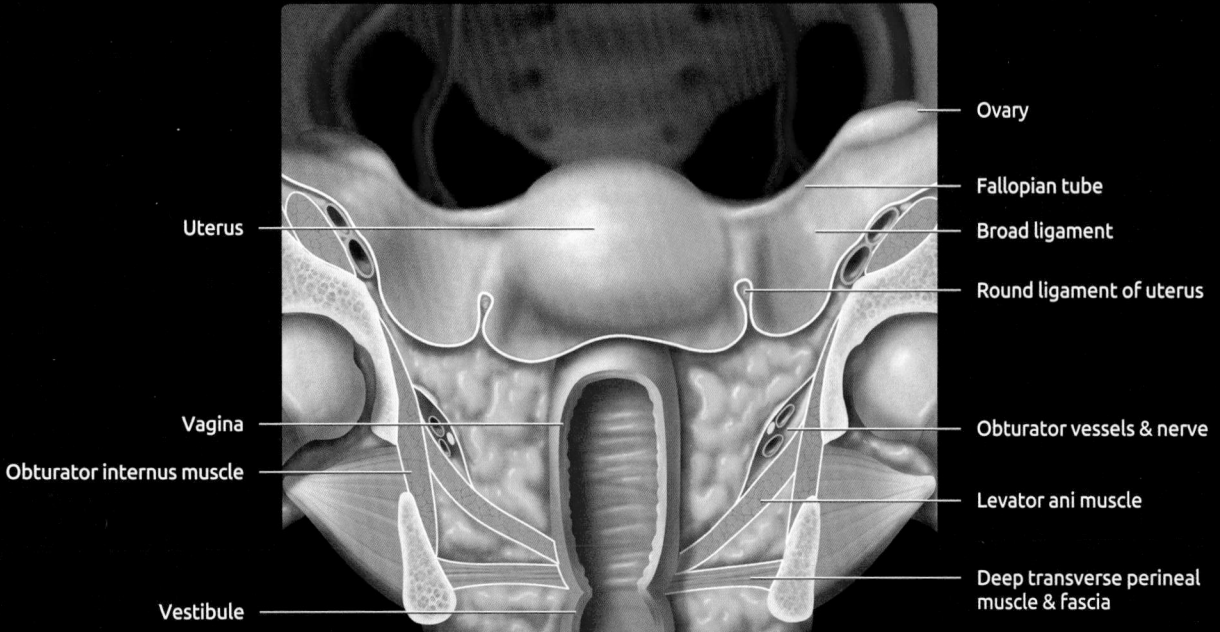

Uterus

Vagina

Obturator internus muscle

Vestibule

Ovary

Fallopian tube

Broad ligament

Round ligament of uterus

Obturator vessels & nerve

Levator ani muscle

Deep transverse perineal
muscle & fascia

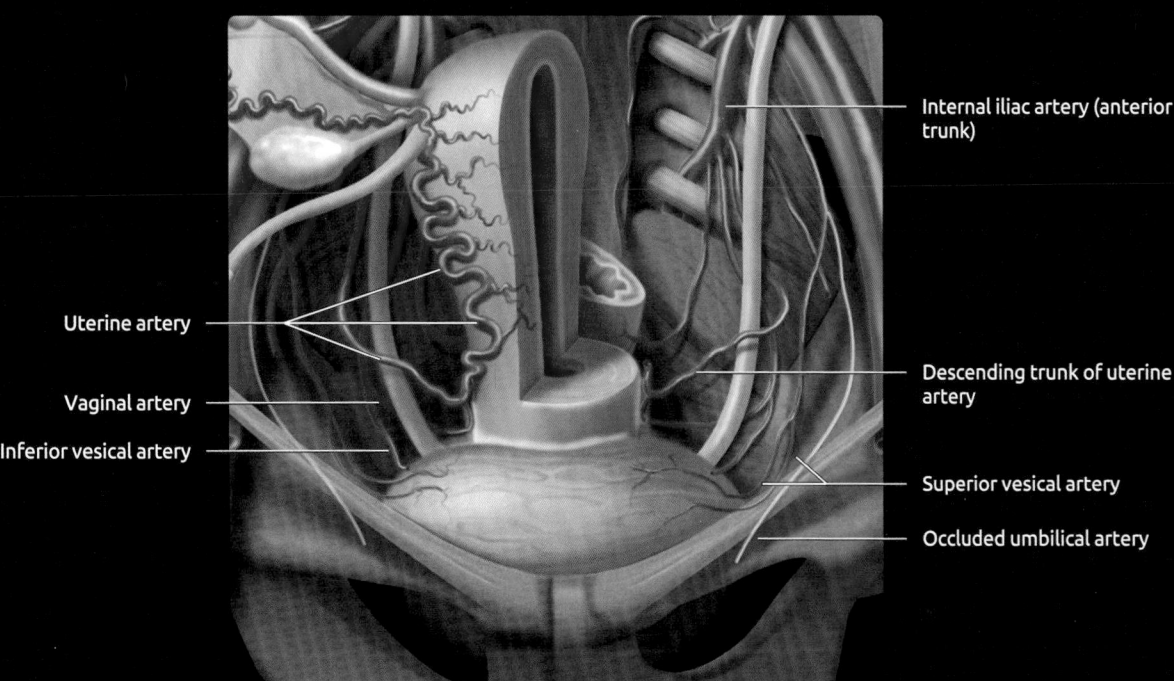

Uterine artery

Vaginal artery

Inferior vesical artery

Internal iliac artery (anterior
trunk)

Descending trunk of uterine
artery

Superior vesical artery

Occluded umbilical artery

(Top) *Coronal view shows the pelvic floor at the level of the vagina. The levator ani muscles form the pelvic floor through which the urethra, vagina, and rectum pass, and are the main support for the pelvic organs. The deep transverse perineal muscle and fascia, along with the urethral sphincter, form the urogenital diaphragm, which is the main support of the lower vagina.* (Bottom) *Frontal graphic shows the iliac vessels. The internal iliac artery divides into an anterior trunk and posterior trunk. The VA can branch off directly from the anterior trunk of the internal iliac artery or sometimes from the inferior vesical artery or UA. The arterial supply of the vagina includes the VA and vaginal branch of the descending trunk of UA.*

VAGINAL IMAGING BY VARIOUS TECHNIQUES

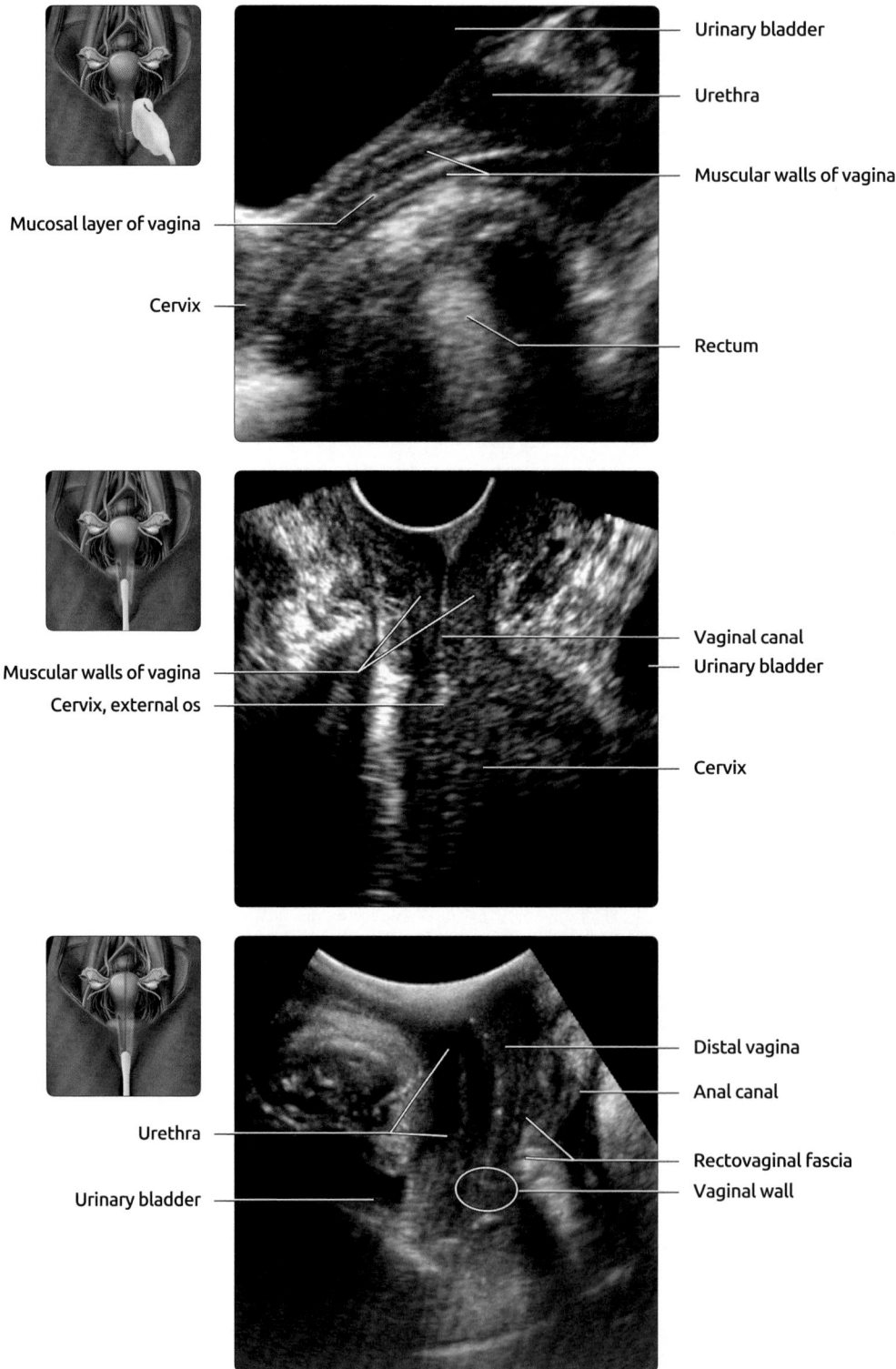

Urinary bladder

Urethra

Muscular walls of vagina

Mucosal layer of vagina

Cervix

Rectum

Muscular walls of vagina

Cervix, external os

Vaginal canal

Urinary bladder

Cervix

Urethra

Urinary bladder

Distal vagina

Anal canal

Rectovaginal fascia

Vaginal wall

(Top) *Transabdominal midline sagittal ultrasound of the vagina shows characteristic triple-line echoes, i.e., hypoechoic muscular walls interfaced by echogenic mucosa. When looking for the vagina using transabdominal US, it is best to view with a distended bladder, starting at midline near the cervical level and tilting the transducer further caudally.* **(Middle)** *Longitudinal transvaginal ultrasound of the vagina again shows characteristic triple-line echo pattern. Using transvaginal US, gradually withdraw the high-frequency vaginal transducer so as to outline the vaginal canal.* **(Bottom)** *Transperineal sagittal ultrasound shows the vagina sandwiched between the urethra anteriorly and the rectum posteriorly. Note that the vaginal canal is barely visible in the absence of intraluminal acoustic jelly or fluid.*

TRANSVERSE US OF VAGINA

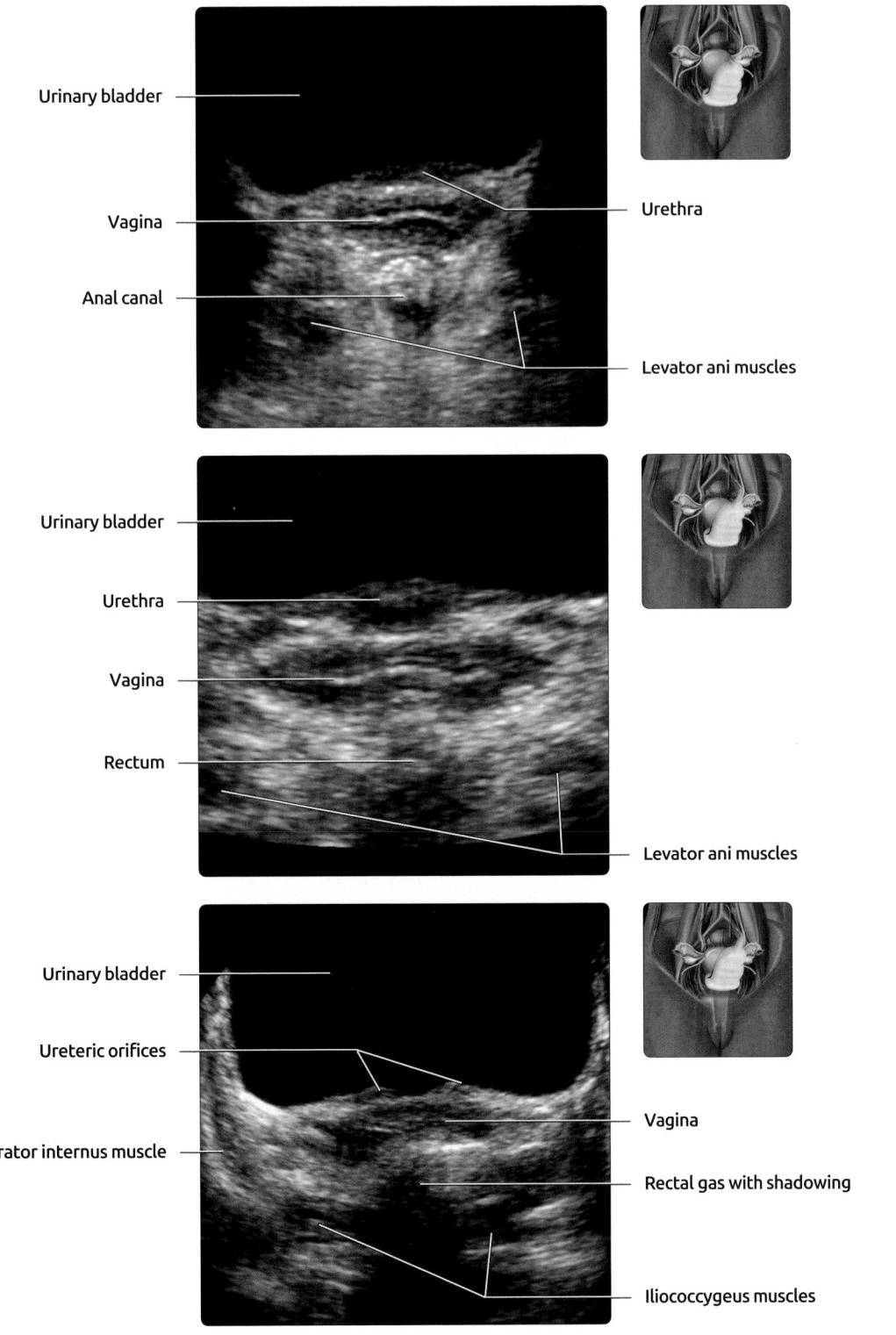

Urinary bladder

Vagina

Anal canal

Urethra

Levator ani muscles

Urinary bladder

Urethra

Vagina

Rectum

Levator ani muscles

Urinary bladder

Ureteric orifices

Obturator internus muscle

Vagina

Rectal gas with shadowing

Iliococcygeus muscles

(Top) *Transverse transabdominal ultrasound shows the mid to lower vagina at the level of anal canal. For transabdominal US of the vagina, caudal angulation of the US probe is needed on both longitudinal and transverse scans. Note that the vaginal canal is better demonstrated on transabdominal US because the angle of insonation is more favorable, approaching a right angle.* (Middle) *Transverse transabdominal ultrasound of the mid vagina shows the levator ani muscles adjacent to the posterolateral aspect of vagina.* (Bottom) *Upper vagina is shown at the level of the ureteric orifices. The ureters run lateral to the lateral fornices of the vagina, cross anteriorly, and then enter into the posterior wall of the bladder. This is a useful plane for investigation of the ureteric jets.*

COLOR DOPPLER US OF VAGINAL ARTERY

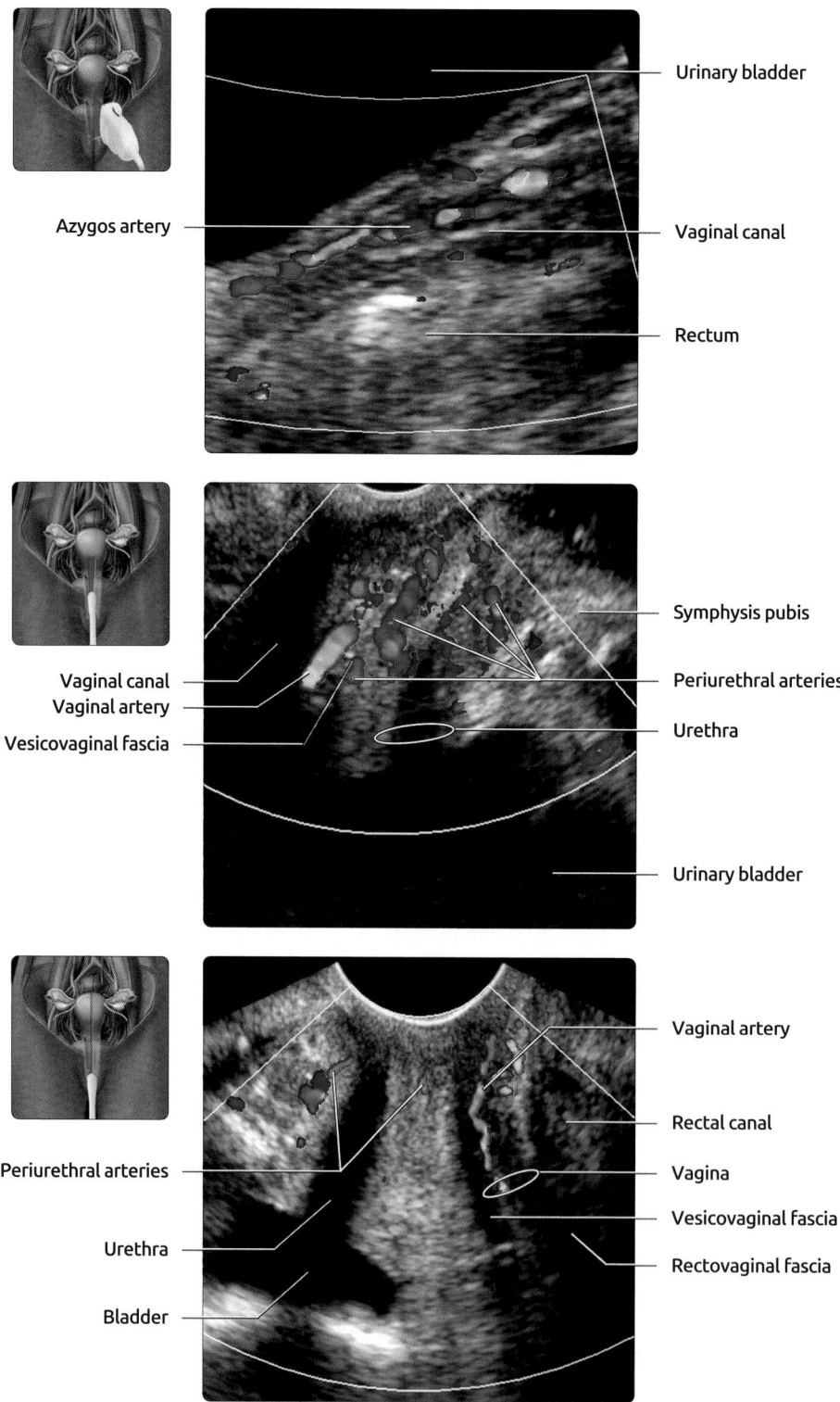

Urinary bladder

Azygos artery

Vaginal canal

Rectum

Symphysis pubis

Vaginal canal
Vaginal artery
Vesicovaginal fascia

Periurethral arteries

Urethra

Urinary bladder

Vaginal artery

Rectal canal

Periurethral arteries

Vagina

Urethra

Vesicovaginal fascia

Rectovaginal fascia

Bladder

(Top) *Longitudinal transabdominal color Doppler US of the vagina shows the longitudinally running azygos artery, which arises from the anastomosis of vaginal branches of the UA and branches of the VA.* (Middle) *Longitudinal transvaginal color Doppler US shows the highly vascularized vagina with multiple small branches of the VA running along the vesicovaginal fascia.* (Bottom) *Transperineal sagittal color Doppler US shows a tortuous branch of the vaginal artery running along the vesicovaginal fascia in the vagina.*

SPECTRAL WAVEFORM OF VAGINAL ARTERY

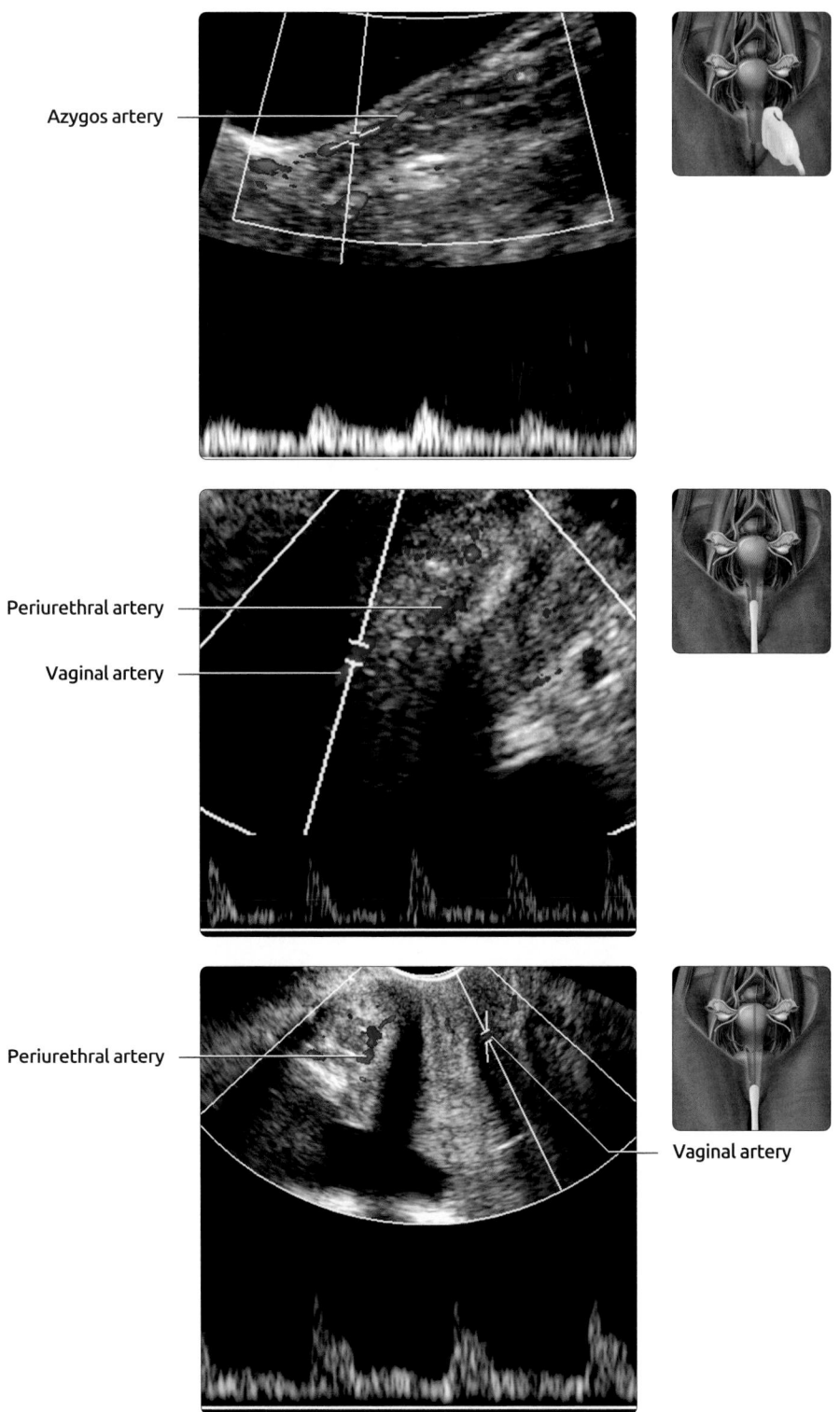

Azygos artery

Periurethral artery

Vaginal artery

Periurethral artery

Vaginal artery

(**Top**) *Transabdominal spectral Doppler US of the azygos artery shows low-resistance flow during mid cycle. The findings are most probably due to the influence of cyclical/hormonal change.* (**Middle**) *Spectral waveform of VA by transvaginal scan shows high-resistance flow, which is the most common pattern in normal females.* (**Bottom**) *Spectral Doppler ultrasound shows the VA by transperineal scan. The typical high flow resistance in the VA may decrease during sexual arousal, cyclically or related to hormonal changes. This phenomenon is useful for investigation and management of sexual dysfunction in postmenopausal women.*

GROSS ANATOMY

Overview

- Ovaries located in true pelvis, although exact position variable
  o Only pelvic organ entirely inside peritoneal sac
  o Laxity in ligaments allows some mobility
  o Location affected by parity, bladder filling, ovarian size, and uterine size/position
  o Located within ovarian fossa in nulliparous women
    – Lateral pelvic sidewall below bifurcation of common iliac vessels
    – Anterior to ureter
    – Posterior to broad ligament
  o Position more variable in parous women
    – Pregnancy displaces ovaries, seldom return to same spot
- Fallopian tube drapes over much of surface
  o Partially covered by fimbriated end
- Composed of medulla and cortex
  o Vessels enter and exit ovary through medulla
  o Cortex contains follicles in varying stages of development
  o Surface covered by specialized peritoneum called germinal epithelium
- Ligamentous supports
  o Suspensory ligament of ovary (infundibulopelvic ligament)
    – Attaches ovary to lateral pelvic wall
    – Contains ovarian vessels and lymphatics
    – Positions ovary in craniocaudal orientation
  o Mesovarium
    – Attaches ovary to broad ligament (posterior)
    – Transmits nerves and vessels to ovary
  o Proper ovarian ligament (utero-ovarian ligament)
    – Continuation of round ligament
    – Fibromuscular band extending from ovary to uterine cornu
  o Mesosalpinx
    – Extends between fallopian tube and proper ovarian ligament
  o Broad ligament
    – Below proper ovarian ligament
- Arterial supply: Dual blood supply
  o Ovarian artery is branch of aorta, arises at L1/L2 level
    – Descends to pelvis and enters suspensory ligament
    – Continues through mesovarium to ovarian hilum
    – Anastomoses with uterine artery
- Drainage via pampiniform plexus into ovarian veins
  o Right ovarian vein drains to inferior vena cava
  o Left ovarian vein drains to left renal vein
- Lymphatic drainage follows venous drainage to preaortic lymph nodes at L1 and L2 levels

Physiology

- ~ 400,000 follicles present at birth but only 0.1% (400) mature to ovulation
- Variations in menstrual cycle
  o Follicular phase (days 0-14)
    – Several follicles begin to develop

    – By days 8-12, dominant follicle develops, while remainder start to regress
  o Ovulation (day 14)
    – Dominant follicle, typically 2.0-2.5 cm, ruptures and releases ovum
  o Luteal phase (days 14-28)
    – Luteinizing hormone induces formation of corpus luteum from ruptured follicle
    – If fertilization occurs, corpus luteum maintains and enlarges to corpus luteum cyst of pregnancy

Variations With Age

- At birth: Large ovaries ± follicles due to influence of maternal hormones
- Childhood: Volume < 1 cm³, follicles < 2 mm diameter
- Above 8 year old: ≥ 6 follicles of > 4 mm diameter
- Adult, reproductive age: Mean volume ~ 10 ± 6 cm³, max 22 cm³
- Postmenopausal: Mean ~ 2-6 cm³, max 8 cm³ and may contain few follicle-like structures

IMAGING ANATOMY

Ultrasound

- Scan between uterus and pelvic sidewall
  o Ovaries often seen adjacent to internal iliac vessels
- Medulla mildly hyperechoic compared to hypoechoic cortex
- Dominant follicle around time of ovulation
  o Cumulus oophorus: Nodule or cyst along margin of dominant follicle represents mature ovum
- Corpus luteum may have thick, echogenic ring
  o Doppler: Vascular wall or "ring"
  o Hemorrhage common
- Echogenic foci common
  o Nonshadowing, 1-3 mm
  o Represent specular reflectors from walls of tiny unresolved cysts or small vessels in medulla
- Doppler: Low-velocity, low-resistance arterial waveform
- Volume (0.523 x length x width x height) more accurate than individual measurements

ANATOMY IMAGING ISSUES

Imaging Recommendations

- Transabdominal (TA) US with full bladder is good for overview of pelvic organs
  o Detects ovaries and masses superior to uterus that may be missed by TV US
- Transvaginal (TV) US is excellent in assessing detail of ovaries and characterizing lesions compared to TA US
  o Lesions higher in pelvis can be missed because of limited field of view
- Postmenopausal ovaries can be difficult to detect because of atrophy, paucity of follicles and surrounding bowel

LIGAMENTOUS SUPPORT AND ANATOMY OF OVARY

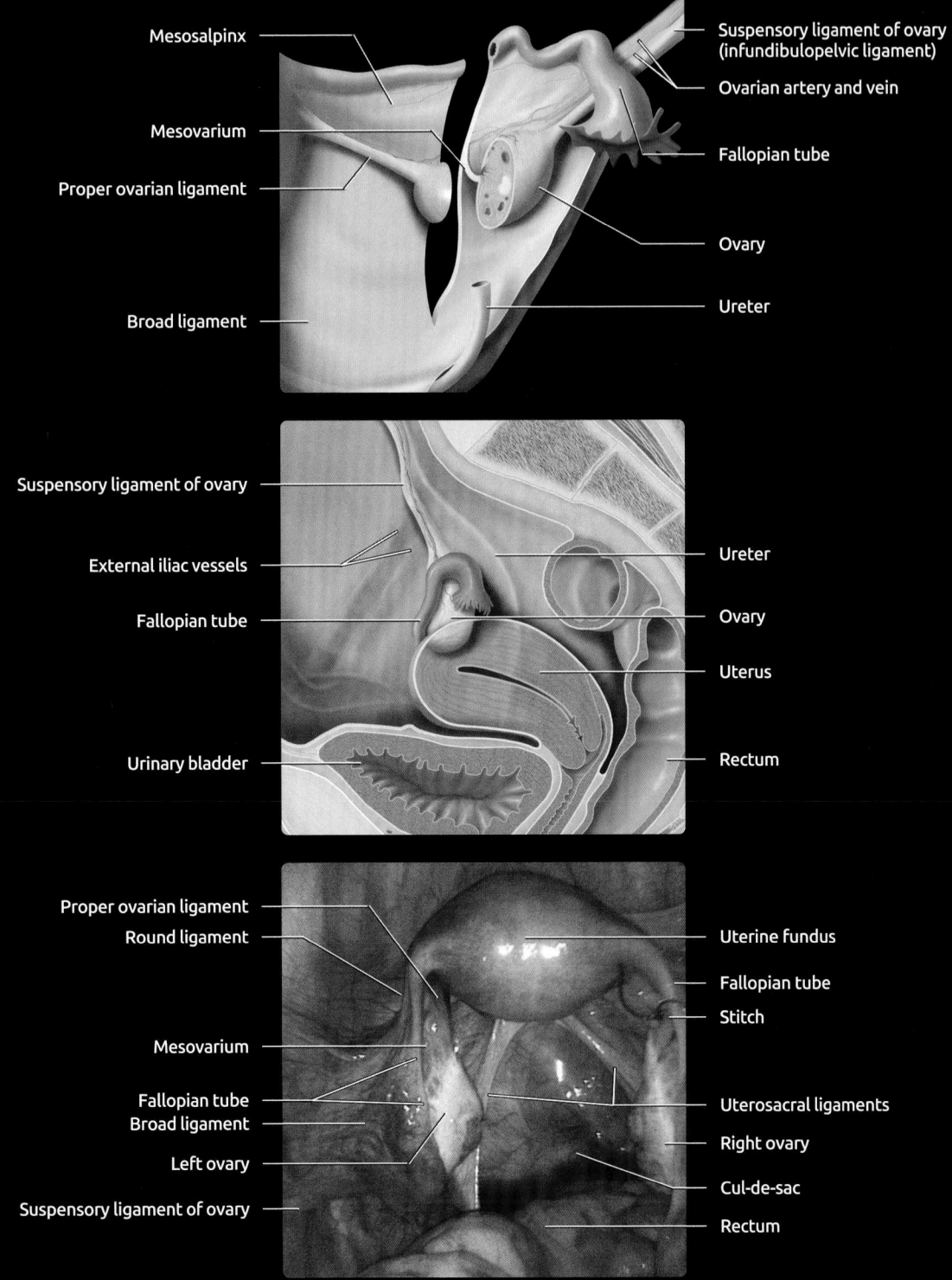

Top:
- Mesosalpinx
- Mesovarium
- Proper ovarian ligament
- Broad ligament
- Suspensory ligament of ovary (infundibulopelvic ligament)
- Ovarian artery and vein
- Fallopian tube
- Ovary
- Ureter

Middle:
- Suspensory ligament of ovary
- External iliac vessels
- Fallopian tube
- Urinary bladder
- Ureter
- Ovary
- Uterus
- Rectum

Bottom:
- Proper ovarian ligament
- Round ligament
- Mesovarium
- Fallopian tube
- Broad ligament
- Left ovary
- Suspensory ligament of ovary
- Uterine fundus
- Fallopian tube
- Stitch
- Uterosacral ligaments
- Right ovary
- Cul-de-sac
- Rectum

(Top) Posterior view of the ligamentous attachment of the ovary is shown. The ovary is attached to the pelvic sidewall by the suspensory ligament (infundibulopelvic ligament) of the ovary, which transmits the ovarian artery and vein. These vessels enter the ovary through the mesovarium, a specialized ligamentous attachment between the ovary and broad ligament. The ovary is attached to the uterus by the proper ovarian ligament, which divides the mesosalpinx above from the broad ligament below. (Middle) Sagittal graphic of the female pelvis shows the location of the ovary, which lies in the ovarian fossa, the area below the iliac bifurcation, posterior to the external iliac vessels, and anterior to the ureter. (Bottom) Photograph during laparoscopy viewing the uterine fundus from above demonstrates the ligamentous structures of the ovary and uterus.

NORMAL OVARY, VARIATIONS WITH AGE

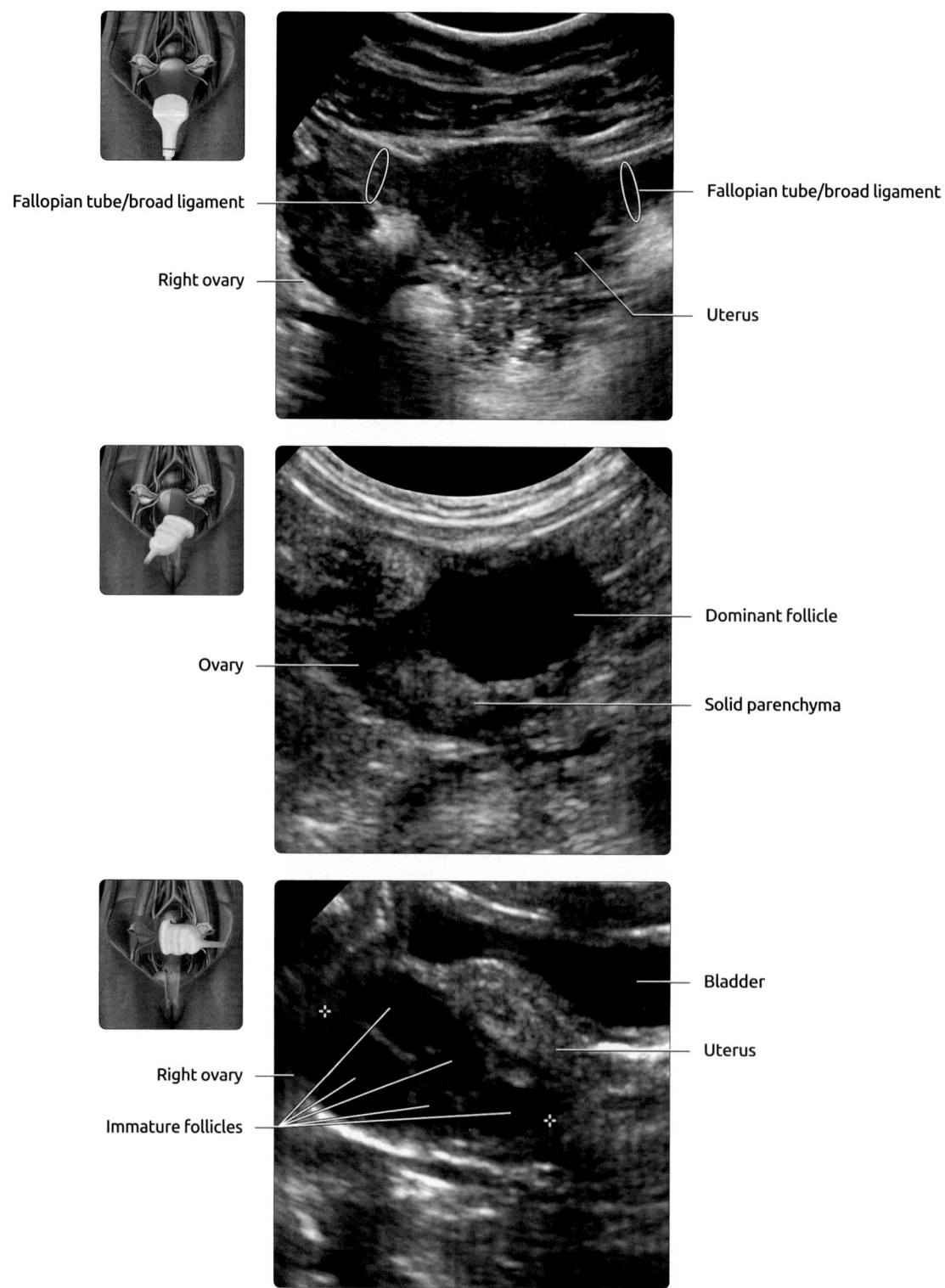

Fallopian tube/broad ligament

Right ovary

Fallopian tube/broad ligament

Uterus

Ovary

Dominant follicle

Solid parenchyma

Bladder

Uterus

Right ovary

Immature follicles

(Top) *Transverse TA ultrasound at the level of the uterine fundus in a 23-year-old woman shows the right ovary in the typical position of the ovarian fossa. The fallopian tube and broad ligament can sometimes be seen as a band of tissue connecting the ovary to the uterine horn. Ovarian ligaments can be lax making ovarian position quite variable from above the fundus to the posterior rectouterine pouch of Douglas.* **(Middle)** *Transverse TA ultrasound of the ovary in a neonate is shown. The size of the ovary is enlarged with a dominant follicle related to stimulation from residual maternal gonadotrophins. Visible follicles may persist until 9 months of age or longer.* **(Bottom)** *Longitudinal TA ultrasound of the ovary of a 5-month-old girl. The ovary is slightly prominent due to stimulation from maternal hormones. The ovary is small (total volume of 1.7 cc) with immature follicles of variable size (usually less than 0.9 cm). The size of the ovaries change very little in the first 6 years of life.*

NORMAL OVARY, VARIATIONS WITH AGE

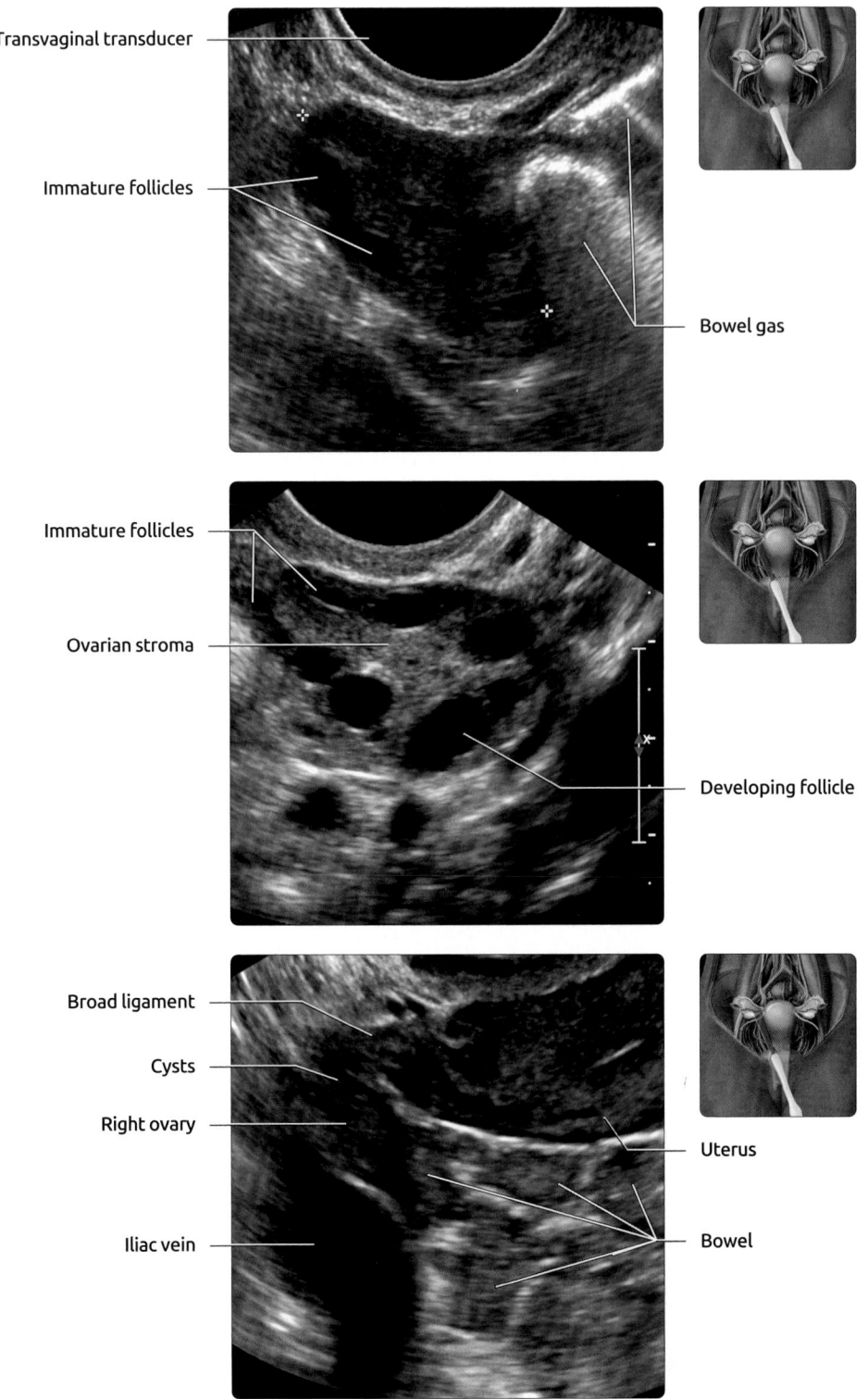

Transvaginal transducer

Immature follicles

Bowel gas

Immature follicles

Ovarian stroma

Developing follicle

Broad ligament

Cysts

Right ovary

Uterus

Iliac vein

Bowel

(Top) *Transverse TV ultrasound of the right ovary in a 18-year-old woman shows an oval ovary with immature follicles. This image also demonstrates the superior resolution of TV US from ability to bring the ovary to the near field as well as the higher frequencies used.* (Middle) *Transverse TV ultrasound of an adult ovary is shown. There are multiple developing follicles of variable size around the echogenic ovarian stroma (medulla) where the ovarian vessels and lymphatics enter and exit. Ovulation usually occurs when the follicle enlarges to between 2.0 and 2.5 cm.* (Bottom) *TV US in a 74-year-old postmenopausal woman demonstrates atrophic right ovary containing tiny cysts. Normal ovaries are variably detected in the postmenopausal woman because of their small size, lack of follicles, and surrounding bowel loops.*

COLOR DOPPLER IMAGING OF OVARIAN ARTERY

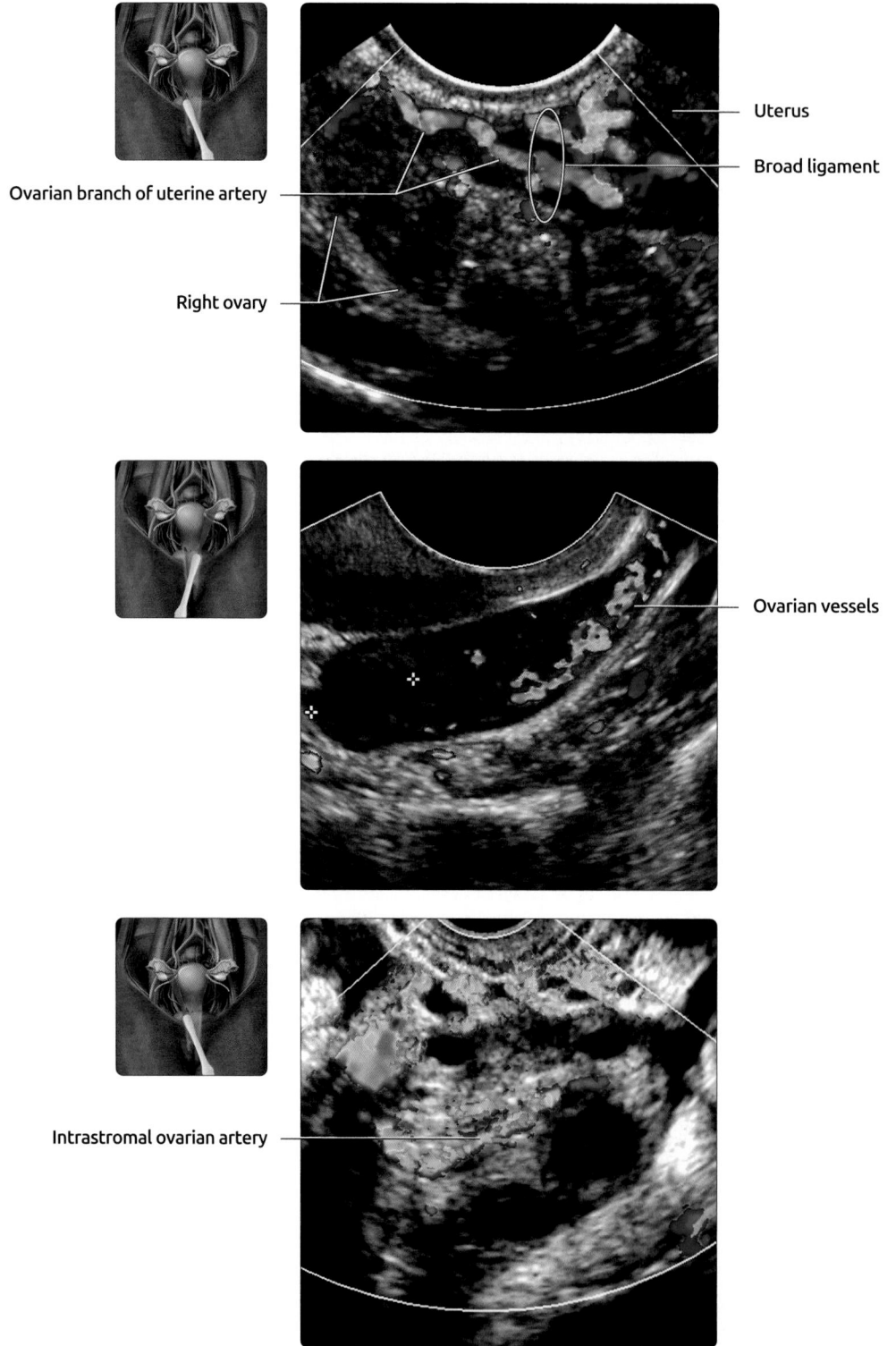

Ovarian branch of uterine artery

Right ovary

Uterus

Broad ligament

Ovarian vessels

Intrastromal ovarian artery

(Top) *Transverse TV ultrasound shows the ovarian branch of the uterine artery running in the broad ligament. It begins at the uterine horn and goes to the ovary through the proper ovarian ligament/mesovarium anastomosing with the ovarian artery.* **(Middle)** *Transverse TV ultrasound of the left ovary demonstrates involuting corpus luteum (calipers). The ovarian vessels are seen entering the ovary from the suspensory ligament of the ovary.* **(Bottom)** *Longitudinal color Doppler TV ultrasound shows an intrastromal ovarian artery running in the ovarian medulla. Note the ovarian vascularity will progressively increase after menstruation and approach a maximum in the luteal phase.*

SPECTRAL WAVEFORM OF OVARIAN ARTERY

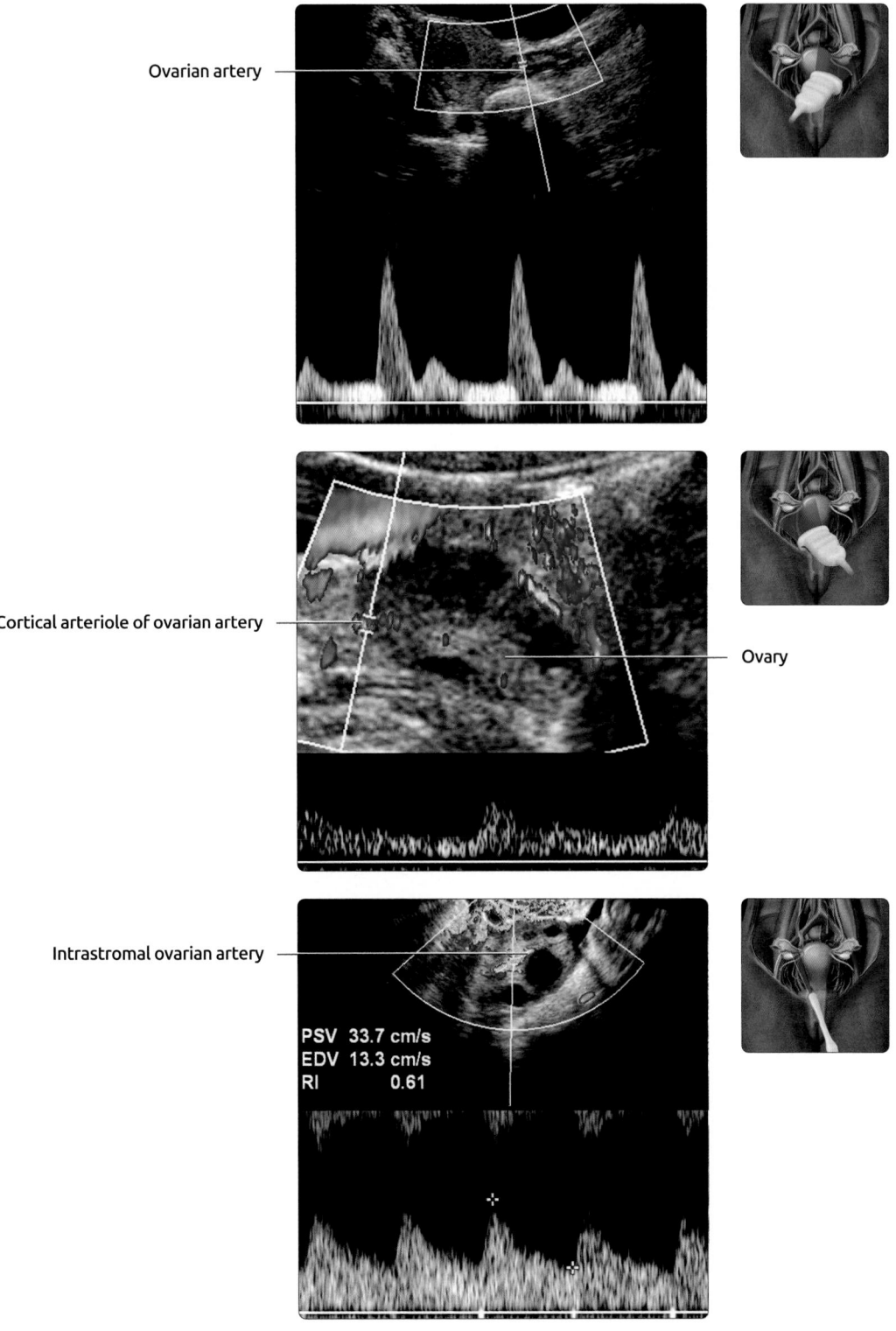

Ovarian artery

Cortical arteriole of ovarian artery

Ovary

Intrastromal ovarian artery

PSV 33.7 cm/s
EDV 13.3 cm/s
RI 0.61

(Top) *Transverse spectral Doppler TA ultrasound shows a normal ovarian artery with a high-resistance flow pattern suggestive of an inactive state of the ovary.* (Middle) *Transverse spectral Doppler TA ultrasound shows the waveform of the cortical arteriole of the ovarian artery.* (Bottom) *Transverse spectral Doppler TV ultrasound of the intrastromal ovarian artery as a continuation of the straight cortical arteriole shows a typical low-resistance, low-velocity waveform during the luteal phase.*

CYCLIC CHANGES OF OVARY

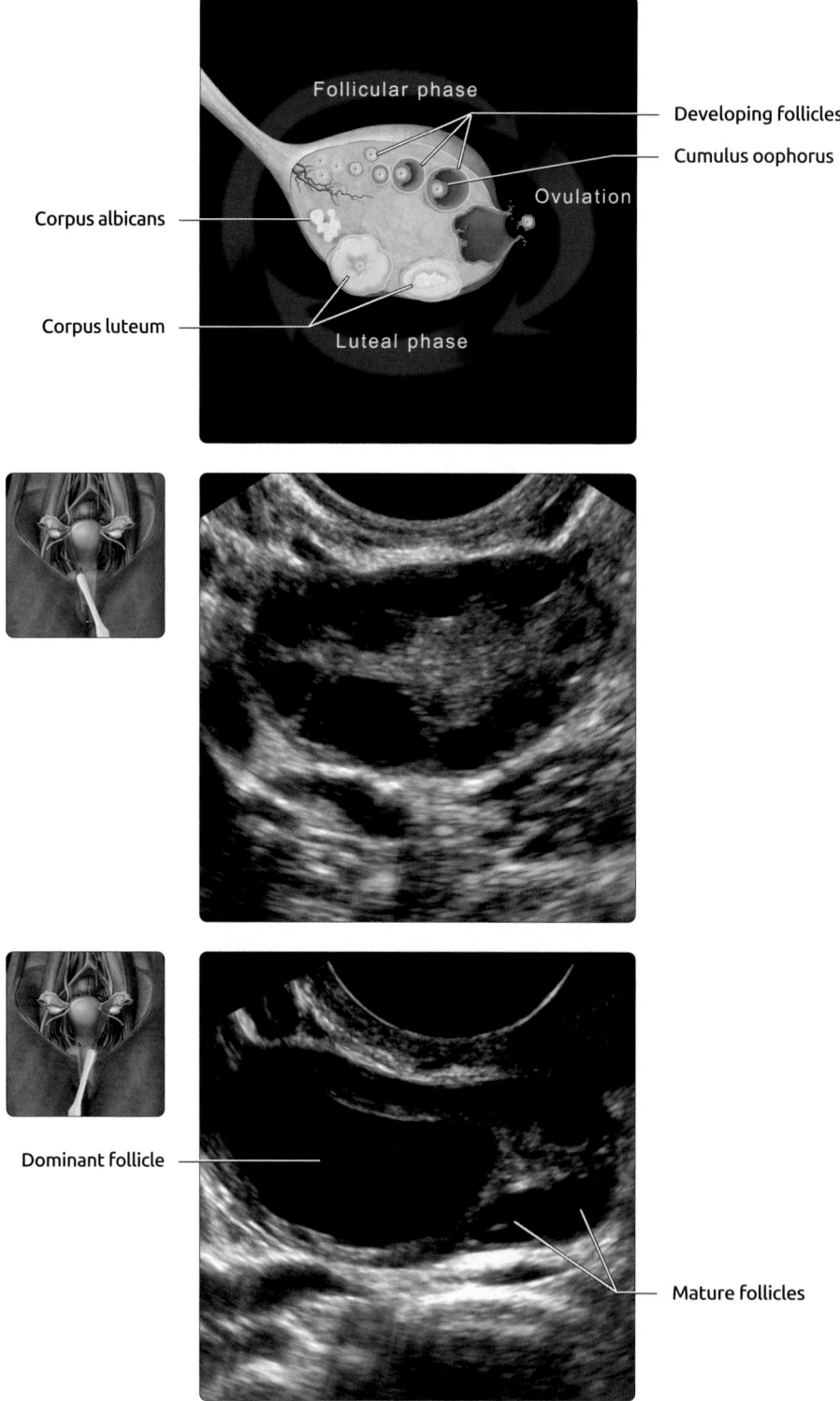

(Top) *During the follicular phase of the menstrual cycle, several follicles begin to develop, but by days 8-12, a dominant follicle has formed, and the remainder begin to regress. On day 14, the follicle ruptures and the egg is released. After ovulation, a corpus luteum forms, and if fertilization does not occur, the corpus luteum degenerates into a corpus albicans.* **(Middle)** *Longitudinal TV ultrasound of the ovary at the early follicular phase is shown. Note the developing follicles of variable size at the periphery of the ovary.* **(Bottom)** *TV ultrasound shows a dominant follicle developed in the late follicular phase days before ovulation. This should not be confused for a pathologic cyst.*

CYCLIC CHANGES OF OVARY

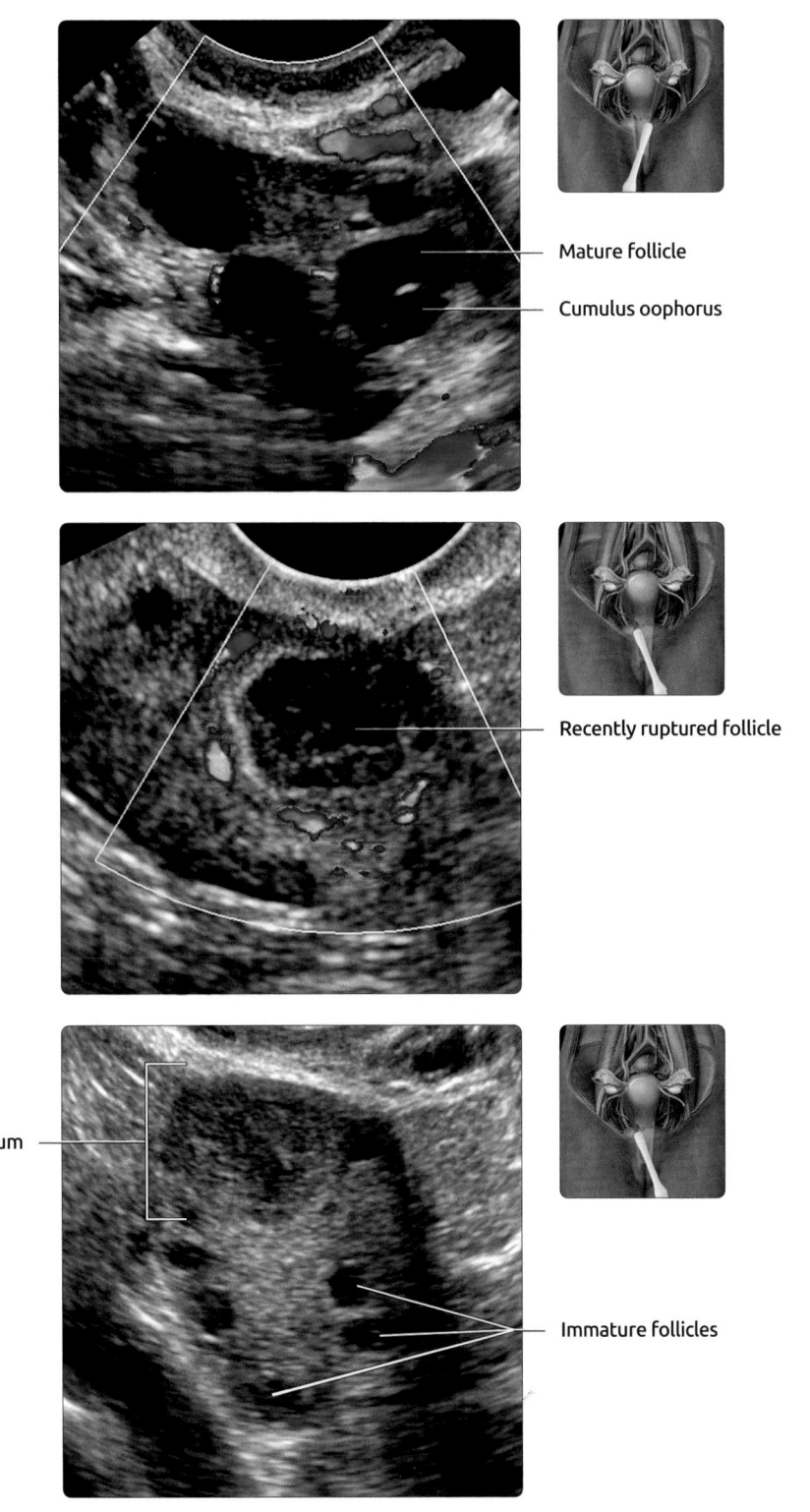

Mature follicle

Cumulus oophorus

Recently ruptured follicle

Regressing corpus luteum

Immature follicles

(Top) *Transverse TV color Doppler ultrasound of the ovary demonstrates a large mature follicle with a small cyst on its wall representing a cumulus oophorus. The size of a mature follicle can reach up to 25 mm before ovulation.* **(Middle)** *Longitudinal TV color Doppler ultrasound of the ovary shows a dominant follicle immediately after its rupture at ovulation. Note the partially collapsed wall resulting from loss of part of the liquor folliculi and the hypoechoic internal contents representing blood.* **(Bottom)** *Transverse TV ultrasound of the ovary shows a regressing corpus luteum with typical hypoechoic, thick, crenulated wall, and echogenic internal contents representing blood.*

CYCLIC CHANGES OF INTRAOVARIAN ARTERY

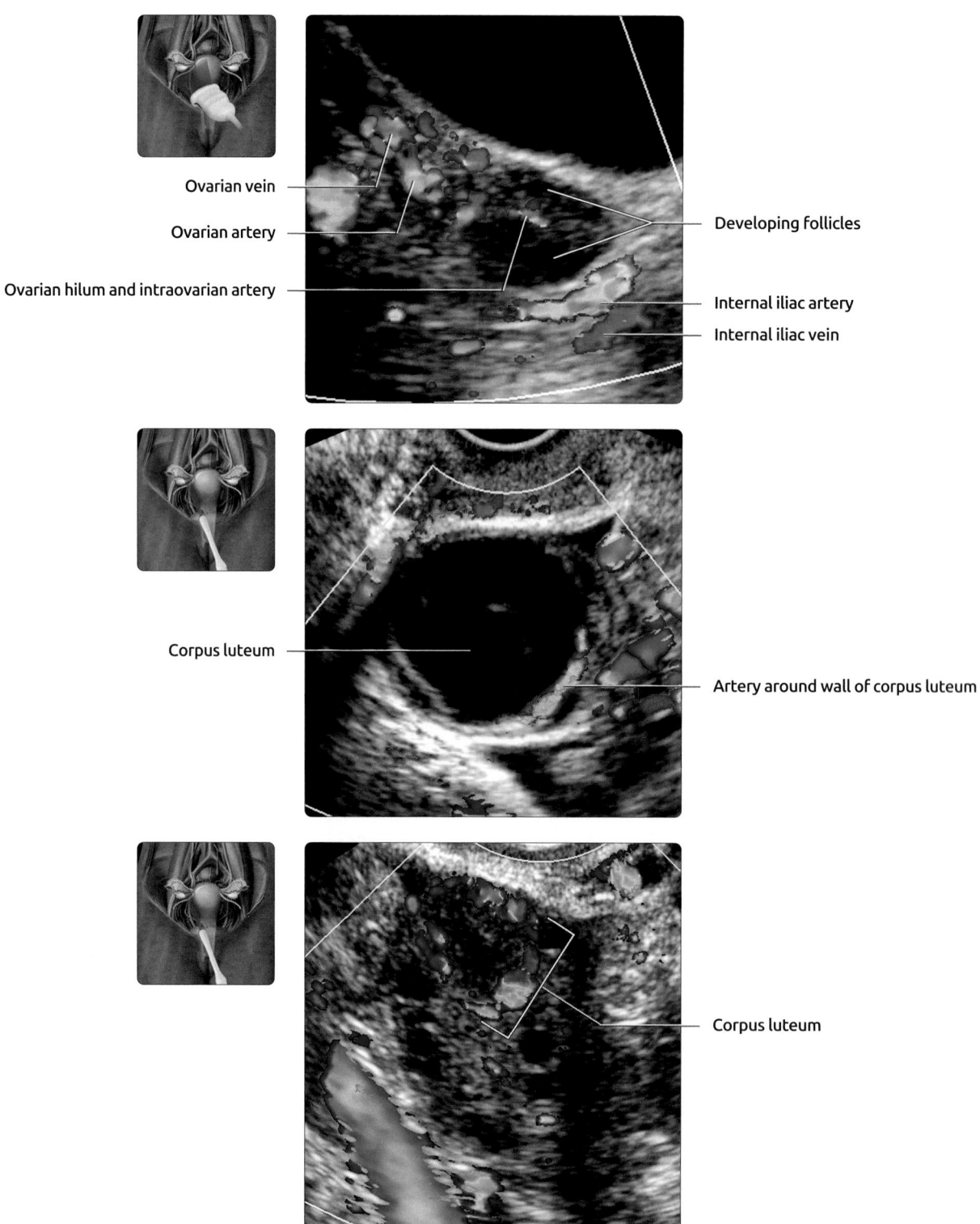

Ovarian vein

Ovarian artery

Ovarian hilum and intraovarian artery

Developing follicles

Internal iliac artery

Internal iliac vein

Corpus luteum

Artery around wall of corpus luteum

Corpus luteum

(Top) *Color Doppler TA ultrasound shows an inactive ovary. The ovary demonstrates a hilar artery surrounded by small developing follicles in the early follicular phase. Note the nondominant ovary may show similar appearance as an inactive ovary.* **(Middle)** *Longitudinal TV ultrasound of the ovary in the early luteal phase is shown. A corpus luteum with low-level internal echoes is seen following ovulation. The wall of the corpus luteum usually displays the most intense color pattern.* **(Bottom)** *Transverse TV ultrasound in midluteal phase is shown. The ovary shows a regressing corpus luteum with typical peripheral color Doppler vascularity.*

CYCLIC CHANGES OF INTRAOVARIAN ARTERY

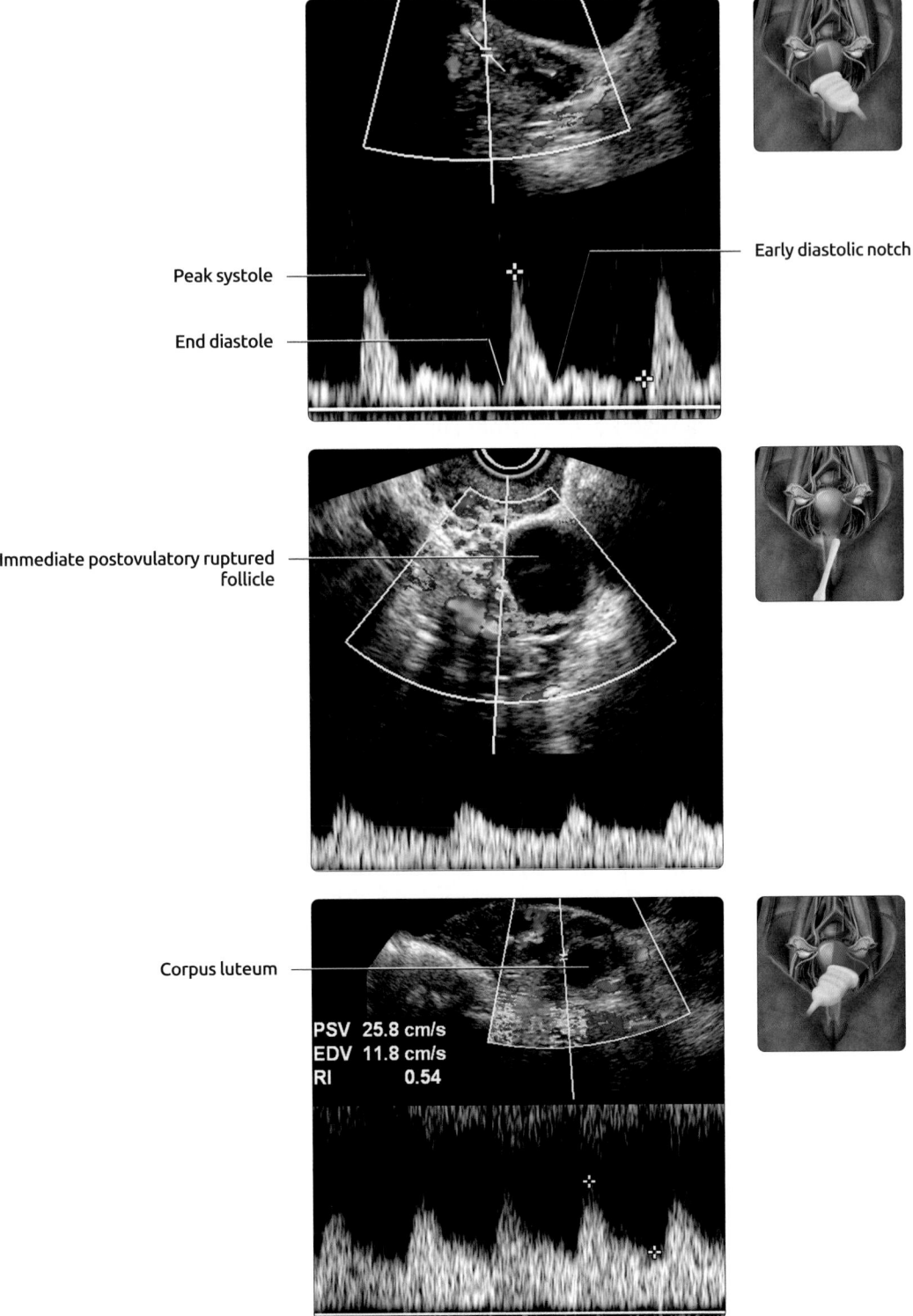

Peak systole

End diastole

Early diastolic notch

Immediate postovulatory ruptured follicle

Corpus luteum

PSV 25.8 cm/s
EDV 11.8 cm/s
RI 0.54

(Top) *Transverse spectral Doppler TA ultrasound of the ovarian artery is shown. The ovarian artery blood flow shows a high-resistance flow pattern with low end-diastolic velocity and an early diastolic notch. This notch indicates initial resistance to forward flow through the ovarian parenchyma. The flow resistance is maximum during the first 8 days of the cycle.* **(Middle)** *Spectral Doppler TV ultrasound of the intraovarian artery in early luteal phase is shown. The ovarian artery has a low-resistance flow, which reaches the lowest level in early luteal phase. At this time, the intraovarian vascularity is easily detectable.* **(Bottom)** *Spectral Doppler of TA ultrasound of the intraovarian artery in midluteal phase is shown. The ovarian arterial flow is of medium resistance and the flow resistance will gradually increase through to the regenerative phase.*

PART II
SECTION 1
Liver

Liver Transplants

Patient Preparation

Although no specific patient preparation is generally required to visualize the liver, the other organs of the hepatobiliary system, such as the gallbladder, are ordinarily examined as part of a complete sonographic liver assessment. Therefore, for a comprehensive hepatobiliary assessment, patients should be instructed to fast for 6-8 hours prior to the ultrasound examination. If dehydration is a concern, water may be given, but other activities that increase stomach and intestinal gas production should be limited.

Imaging Protocols

The liver is the largest organ in the abdomen and must be scanned systematically and carefully to ensure a thorough examination. The patient should be positioned supine initially, but a variety of positions, including decubitus scanning, may be needed depending on organ size and orientation and the presence of overlying bowel gas. Imaging from the subcostal approach with cranial angulation of the transducer in normal and deep suspended respiration typically provides optimal visualization. If the liver is high in position, or shrunken and cirrhotic, an intercostal approach may be necessary.

The scan protocol ordinarily begins by visualizing the left lobe in the mid sagittal plane beneath the sternum and xiphoid process and proceeds with the sonographer scanning laterally to visualize first the left lobe and then the right lobe. The transverse plane is scanned next, followed by oblique planes along the long and short axes of specific anatomic structures, such as the gallbladder and common bile duct. The sonographer must visualize the entire liver in real time from the most lateral portions of the left lobe through the right lobe, and then capture a series of standard sagittal and parasagittal views for documentation purposes. Similarly, in the transverse plane, the liver must be examined from the dome to the inferior tip. Standard views to be documented include the following:

- Longitudinal views: Lateral segments of left lobe, aorta, inferior vena cava, caudate lobe and ligamentum venosum, porta hepatis, gallbladder fossa, right lobe segments, right lobe with longitudinal view of right adrenal fossa and kidney
- Transverse views: Left lobe dome, left portal vein, caudate lobe and ligamentum venosum, right lobe dome, hepatic venous confluence and individual right, middle, and left hepatic veins, gallbladder, and liver with right kidney
- Oblique views: Common bile duct in long axis, main portal vein in long axis, gallbladder in long axis, short axis, and decubitus views

Transducer Selection and Technical Factors

The sonographer should select the highest frequency transducer that provides sufficient penetration to visualize the entire depth of the liver. As a visual check, in a normal liver the diaphragm should be clearly visible on longitudinal and transverse images of the right lobe. With modern ultrasound technology, this usually implies broad-bandwidth 3-5 MHz transducers capable of imaging in both harmonic and fundamental modes and with multiple focal zones. Curved linear transducers generally provide the best compromise between good near-field imaging and wide field of view. For images of the hepatic capsule, a high-frequency linear transducer should be used.

Time-gain compensation and the overall receiver gain settings should be set so that the liver has a homogeneous and uniform echo texture from the near field to the far field. Speckle reduction techniques, such as spatial and frequency compounding, and adaptive filtering techniques can work synergistically with harmonic imaging modes to reduce image noise.

Color, spectral, and power Doppler modes should be part of every dedicated assessment of the liver. Color Doppler mode should be used to document patency and direction of flow in the portal and hepatic veins as well as the hepatic artery. If flow appears absent on color Doppler, power Doppler should be used since it is less dependent on insonation angle. Power Doppler is also useful for minimizing artifacts resulting from background motion, and for distinguishing dilated bile ducts from vascular structures within the liver.

The Doppler signatures of the hepatic vessels obtained in spectral Doppler mode are often quite useful in the identification and characterization of hepatic pathology. The normal portal vein shows hepatopetal, minimally undulating flow. By contrast, the normal hepatic veins have a triphasic velocity waveform similar to the appearance of the central venous pressure waveforms. The hepatic artery interrogated in the hepatic hilum shows peak velocity ranging from 30-60 cm/sec, and a low-resistance waveform with continuous antegrade flow during diastole.

In liver transplants, careful evaluation of the hepatic artery, portal vein, and hepatic veins are important for detection of potential complications including stenosis or thrombosis. The hepatic duct should be carefully evaluated for developing strictures at the anastomosis.

Equipment parameters in Doppler modes, such as the wall filter and velocity scale (pulse repetition frequency), should be set so as to correctly display the expected range of velocities in the vessels being interrogated. For quantitative assessment of flow velocity, angle correction should be performed in spectral Doppler mode in order to calibrate the machine to calculate an accurate velocity from the frequency shift information that is detected at the transducer.

Anatomy-Based Imaging Issues

The normal liver should display relatively uniform, intermediate-level echogenicity slightly higher than that of the renal cortex. Its length should typically not extend below the inferior pole of the right kidney unless a Reidel lobe is present. Portal triads ramifying within the liver typically display echogenic walls, whereas the hepatic venous walls will not be echogenic unless insonated at exactly ninety degrees.

Certain normal hepatic structures can simulate pathology. For example, the fibrous ligamentum teres and ligamentum venosum may cause acoustic shadowing and create the appearance of mass lesions or abnormal echogenicity of the caudate lobe. Overlying ribs may also cause shadowing, particularly during intercostal scanning.

Selected References

1. Heller MT et al: The role of ultrasonography in the evaluation of diffuse liver disease. Radiol Clin North Am. 52(6):1163-75, 2014
2. McNaughton DA et al: Doppler US of the liver made simple. Radiographics. 31(1):161-88, 2011
3. Kruskal JB et al: Optimizing Doppler and color flow US: application to hepatic sonography. Radiographics. 24(3):657-75, 2004

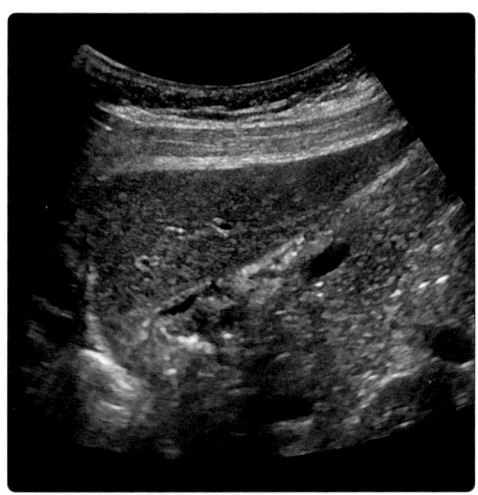

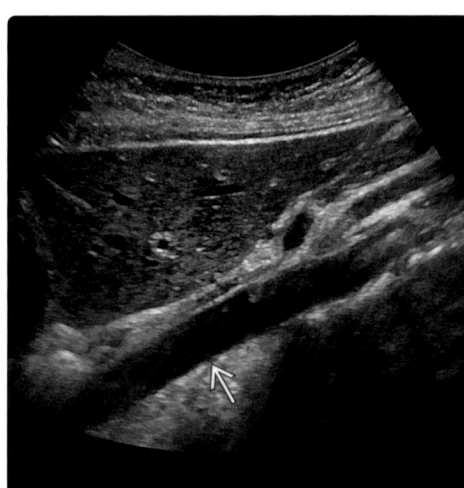

(Left) *Midline sagittal ultrasound shows the lateral segment of left lobe.* (Right) *Midline sagittal ultrasound shows the lateral segment of left lobe anterior to the aorta* ➡.

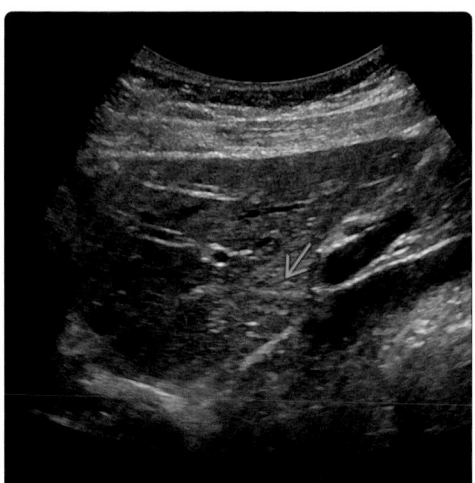

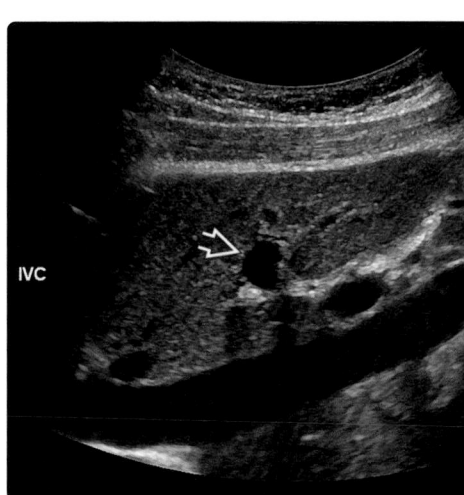

(Left) *Sagittal ultrasound shows the left lobe of the liver and the caudate lobe posterior to the fissure for the ligamentum venosum* ➡. (Right) *Right parasagittal ultrasound shows the left lobe with the left portal vein* ➡, *caudate lobe, and inferior vena cava.*

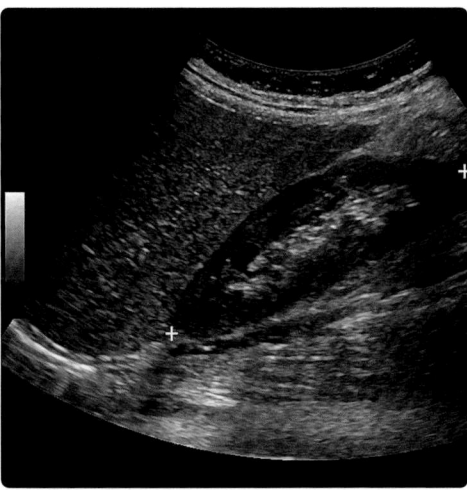

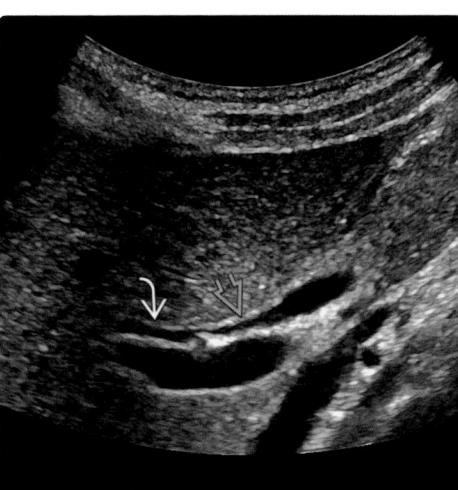

(Left) *Sagittal ultrasound shows the right lobe of the liver with the right kidney posteriorly (calipers). Note that the liver is normally more echogenic than the renal cortex.* (Right) *Oblique ultrasound along the plane of the porta hepatis shows the common hepatic duct* ➡ *and the common bile duct* ➡.

(Left) *Transverse ultrasound shows the liver dome.* **(Right)** *Transverse ultrasound shows the liver dome at the level of the hepatic venous confluence. The hepatic veins are labeled.*

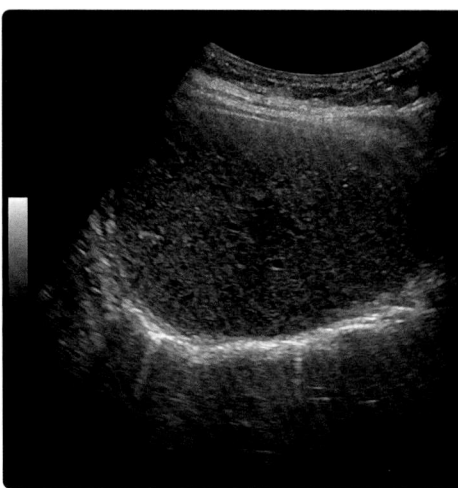
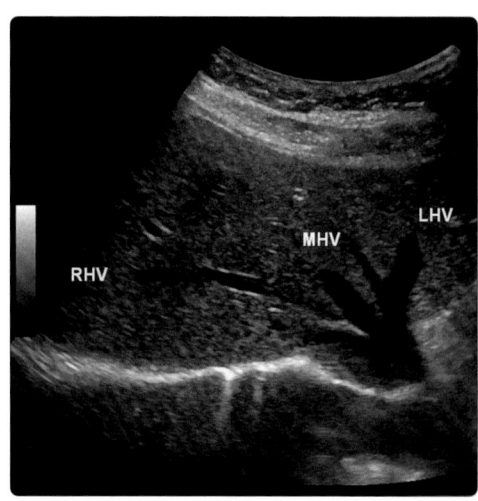

(Left) *Transverse ultrasound shows the right lobe of the liver at the level of the hepatic hilum. The right portal vein is shown* ⮕. **(Right)** *Inferior-most transverse ultrasound shows the right lobe of the liver at the level of the right kidney.*

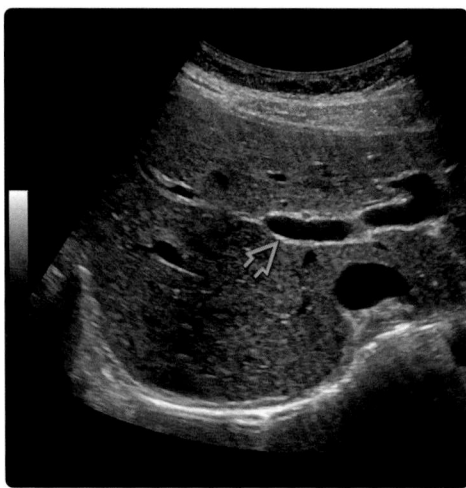
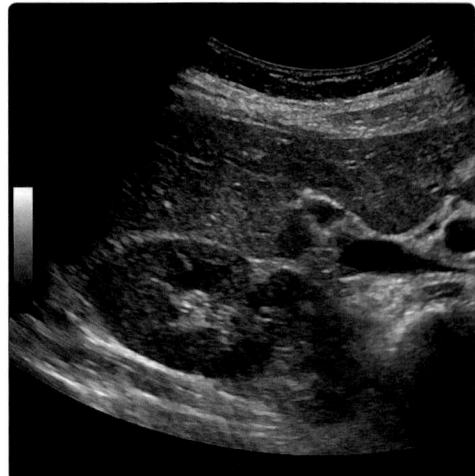

(Left) *Color Doppler ultrasound shows the hepatic venous confluence with the hepatic veins labeled.* **(Right)** *Color Doppler transverse oblique ultrasound through the plane of the right portal vein* ⮕ *is shown, with the anterior and posterior branches labeled.*

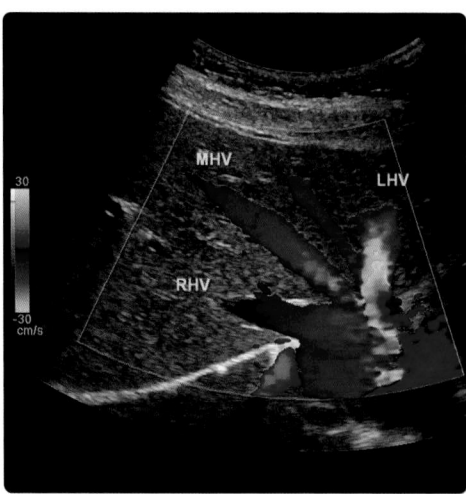
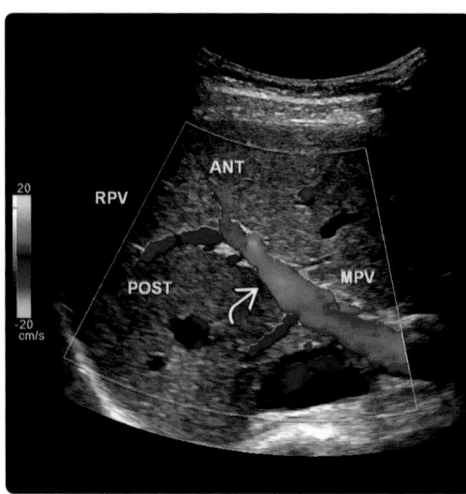

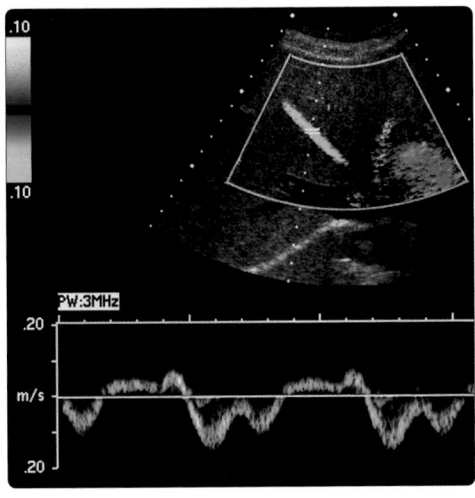

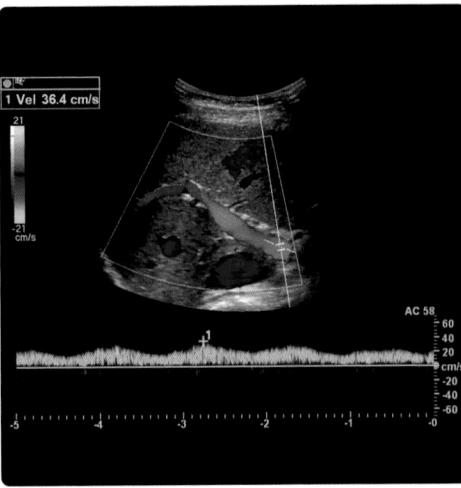

(Left) *Normal triphasic waveform shows the middle hepatic vein.* (Right) *Spectral Doppler tracing shows the normal portal vein. The normal waveform displays gently undulating low-velocity flow.*

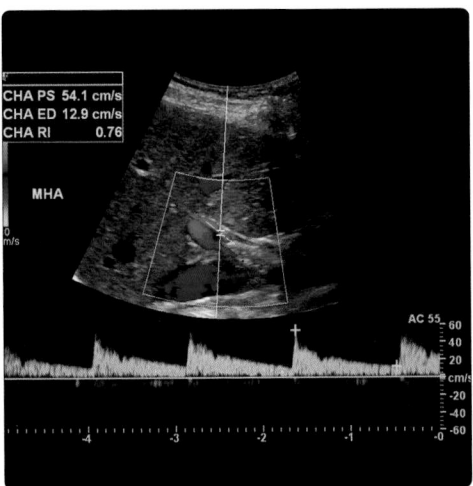

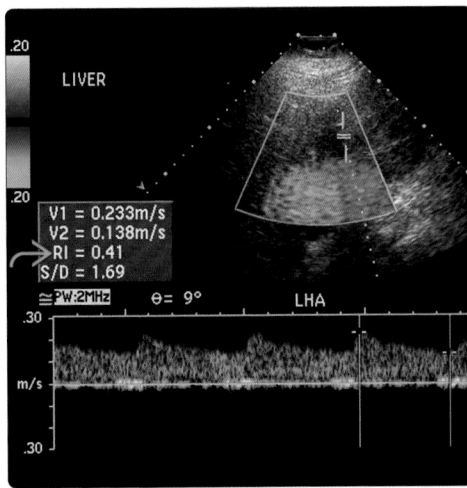

(Left) *Spectral Doppler tracing shows the normal hepatic artery, which has a low-resistance waveform, with continuous antegrade flow in diastole. The peak systolic velocity normally ranges from 30-60 cm/sec.* (Right) *Spectral Doppler waveform of a patient following liver transplantation shows a characteristic "tardus-parvus" waveform, indicating upstream stenosis at the hepatic arterial anastomosis. Note the low resistive index of 0.41 ⟹.*

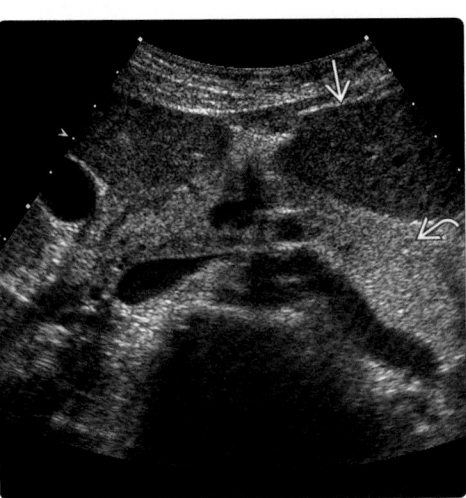

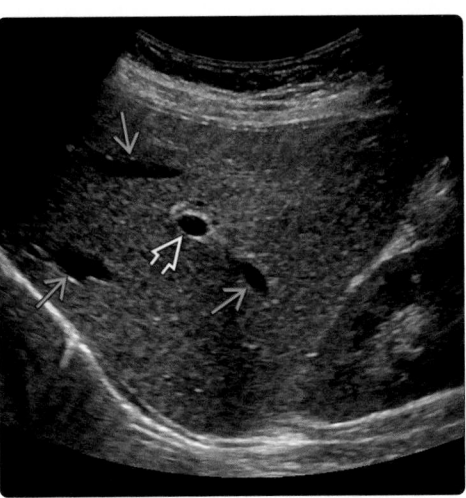

(Left) *The normal pancreas ⟹ is more echogenic than the normal liver ⟹.* (Right) *The portal veins in the liver typically have echogenic walls ⟹. By contrast, the hepatic veins lack echogenic walls ⟹.*

Acute Hepatitis

TERMINOLOGY

- Inflammation of liver due to viral infection or toxic agents

IMAGING

- Acute: Enlarged liver
- Chronic: Decrease in liver size
- Grayscale ultrasound
  - Acute hepatitis: Hepatomegaly and diffusely **hypoechoic** parenchyma
  - Steatohepatitis and acute alcoholic hepatitis: Hepatomegaly and diffusely **hyperechoic** liver parenchyma
  - Thickening of gallbladder wall
    - Most pronounced in acute hepatitis A
  - "Starry sky" appearance: Portal triads appear markedly echogenic against background hypoechoic liver (variably seen)
    - May be related to periportal edema
- Pulsed Doppler ultrasound
  - Elevated hepatic arterial velocity

TOP DIFFERENTIAL DIAGNOSES

- Infiltrative hepatocellular carcinoma (HCC)
- Lymphoma
- Steatosis (fatty liver)

PATHOLOGY

- Viral hepatitis: Caused by 1 of 5 viral agents
  - Hepatitis A (HAV), B (HBV), C (HCV), D (HDV), E (HEV) viruses
- Alcohol abuse
- Autoimmune reactions
- Metabolic disturbances
- Drug-induced injury
- Exposure to environmental agents
- Radiation therapy

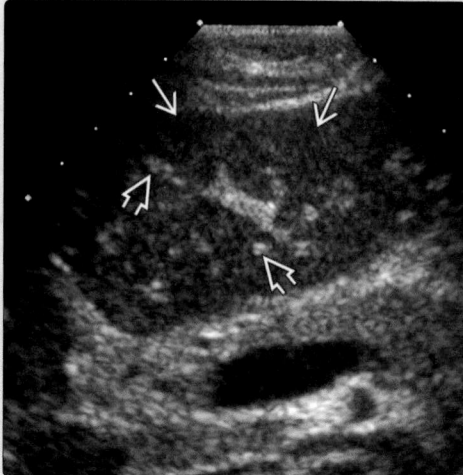
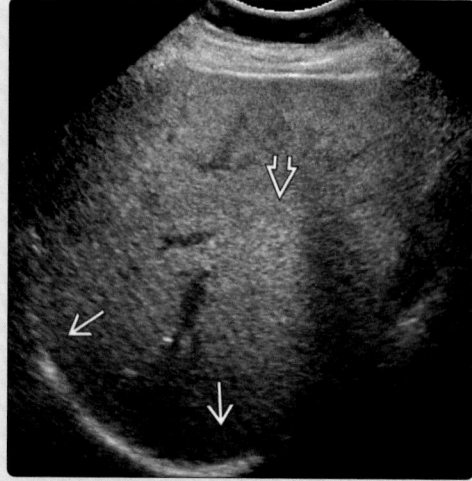

(Left) *Transverse transabdominal ultrasound in a patient with acute hepatitis shows diffusely hypoechoic liver parenchyma* ➡ *and hyperechoic portal triad walls* ⇉*, creating the "starry sky" appearance of acute hepatitis.* (Right) *Transverse transabdominal ultrasound in a patient with acute alcoholic hepatitis shows the rounded contour of hepatomegaly* ➡ *with diffusely increased echogenicity* ⇉ *throughout the liver, compatible with steatosis.*

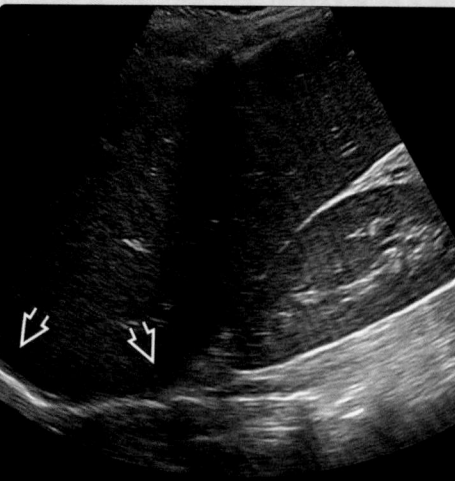
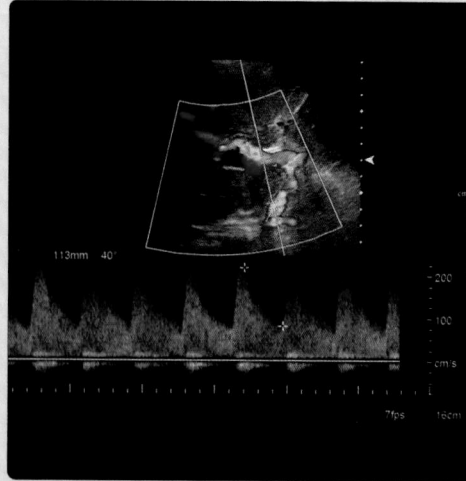

(Left) *Longitudinal oblique transabdominal ultrasound in a patient with acute alcoholic hepatitis shows a markedly enlarged liver with longitudinal extension much greater than the adjacent kidney. Rounded contour* ⇉ *is also compatible with hepatomegaly. Of note, the liver is not markedly steatotic.* (Right) *Anterior oblique transabdominal US in the same patient demonstrates elevated hepatic artery peak systolic velocity (PSV) of 220 cm/s in acute alcoholic hepatitis. The mean PSV in healthy patients is 66 cm/s.*

TERMINOLOGY

Definitions

- Inflammation of liver due to viral infection or toxic agents

IMAGING

General Features

- Best diagnostic clue
  - Acute viral hepatitis on US
    - Hepatomegaly and diffusely hypoechoic parenchyma
    - Steatohepatitis: Hepatomegaly and diffusely echogenic liver parenchyma
- Location
  - Diffusely; involving both lobes
- Size
  - Acute: Enlarged liver
  - Chronic: Decrease in liver size
- Nonalcoholic fatty liver disease (NAFLD)
  - Hepatic steatosis: Abnormal and excessive accumulation of lipids within hepatocytes
  - Important emerging cause of acute and progressive liver disease
  - Estimated prevalence 30% in USA
- Alcoholic hepatitis
  - Acute: Hepatomegaly with echogenic liver
  - Chronic: Variable size of liver, echogenic liver
- Viral hepatitis
  - Infection of liver by small group of hepatotropic viruses
  - Stages: Acute, chronic active hepatitis and chronic persistent hepatitis
  - Responsible for 60% of cases of fulminant hepatic failure in USA
  - Leading cause of hepatitis

Ultrasonographic Findings

- Grayscale ultrasound
  - **Acute viral hepatitis**
    - Hepatomegaly with diffusely hypoechoic parenchyma
    - "Starry sky" appearance: Portal triads appear markedly echogenic against background hypoechoic liver (variably seen)
      - May be related to periportal edema
      - Periportal hypo-/anechoic area (hydropic swelling of hepatocytes)
    - Thickening of gallbladder (GB) wall; most common in acute hepatitis A
  - **Chronic active viral hepatitis**
    - Increased echogenicity of liver
    - Loss of definition of portal vein walls
    - Heterogeneous parenchymal echotexture due to regenerating nodules
    - Adenopathy in hepatoduodenal ligament
  - **Acute alcoholic hepatitis**
    - Hepatomegaly with diffusely echogenic liver parenchyma
    - Increased hepatic artery diameter
      - Mean diameter in acute alcoholic hepatitis: 3.6 mm vs. 2.7 mm in healthy patients
  - **Late-stage alcoholic hepatitis**
    - Atrophic liver with micronodular cirrhosis

- Pulsed Doppler
  - Acute alcoholic hepatitis
    - High-velocity hepatic artery
    - Elevated hepatic artery peak systolic velocity (PSV) > 100 cm/s
      - Mean PSV: 187 cm/s vs. 66 cm/s in healthy patients
  - Acute or fulminant hepatotoxicity: May see markedly elevated resistive indices of hepatic artery

CT Findings

- NECT
  - Acute viral hepatitis
    - Hepatomegaly, GB wall thickening
  - Chronic active viral hepatitis
    - Lymphadenopathy in porta hepatis/gastrohepatic ligament and retroperitoneum (in 65% of cases)
    - Hyperdense regenerating nodules
  - Acute alcoholic hepatitis
    - Hepatomegaly
    - Steatosis: Diffuse low-attenuation liver
      - Liver-spleen attenuation difference < 10 HU
      - Normal liver is 60-65 HU; < 45 HU is 100% specific for steatosis
    - Steatosis may be focal, lobar, or segmental
    - Indistinguishable from nonalcoholic steatohepatitis (NASH)
  - Chronic alcoholic hepatitis
    - Mixture of steatosis and early cirrhotic changes depending on chronicity
- CECT
  - Acute and chronic viral hepatitis
    - ± heterogeneous parenchymal enhancement
  - Chronic hepatitis: Regenerating nodules may be isodense with liver

MR Findings

- Viral hepatitis
  - Increase in T1 and T2 relaxation times of liver
  - T2WI: High signal intensity bands paralleling portal vessels (periportal edema)
- Alcoholic steatohepatitis (fatty liver)
  - T1WI in-phase GRE: Increased signal intensity of liver; greater than spleen or muscle
  - T1WI out-phase GRE: Decreased signal intensity of liver (due to signal dropout from intravoxel lipid in liver)
    - % fat = (T1IP-T1OOP)/(2*T1IP)

Imaging Recommendations

- Best imaging tool
  - Ultrasound to rule out biliary obstruction or other hepatic pathology

DIFFERENTIAL DIAGNOSIS

Infiltrative Hepatocellular Carcinoma (HCC)

- Background cirrhosis
- Invasion of portal vein

Lymphoma

- Hepatomegaly due to diffuse infiltration
- Background vascular architecture may or may not be distorted

- Lymphoma more common in immune-suppressed patients

Steatosis (Fatty Liver)

- Hepatomegaly
- Diffuse, patchy or focal increase in echogenicity
- Normal vessels course through "lesion"

PATHOLOGY

General Features

- Etiology
  - Viral hepatitis: Caused by 1 of 5 viral agents
    - Hepatitis A (HAV), B (HBV), C (HCV), D (HDV), E (HEV) viruses
  - Other causes of hepatitis
    - Alcohol abuse
    - Autoimmune reactions
    - Metabolic disturbances
    - Drug-induced injury
    - Exposure to environmental agents
    - Radiation therapy
- Different stages of hepatitis
  - Cellular dysfunction, necrosis, fibrosis, cirrhosis
- HBV: Sensitized cytotoxic T cells → hepatocyte necrosis → tissue damage
- Alcoholic hepatitis: Inflammatory reaction leads to acute liver cell necrosis

Staging, Grading, & Classification

- Acute hepatitis
  - Often self-limiting
- Chronic hepatitis
  - Fibrosis and cirrhosis develop in 20% HCV and 10% HBV
- Staging liver fibrosis
  - Liver biopsy
    - Current gold standard to stage fibrosis
  - Shear-wave ultrasound and magnetic resonance elastography
    - Emerging noninvasive means of evaluating liver fibrosis

Gross Pathologic & Surgical Features

- Acute viral hepatitis: Enlarged liver + tense capsule
- Chronic fulminant hepatitis: Atrophic liver
- Alcoholic steatohepatitis: Enlarged, yellow, greasy liver

Microscopic Features

- Acute viral: Coagulative necrosis with ↑ eosinophilia
- Chronic viral: Lymphocytes, macrophages, plasma cells, or piecemeal necrosis
- Alcoholic hepatitis: Neutrophils/necrosis/Mallory bodies

CLINICAL ISSUES

Presentation

- Most common signs/symptoms
  - Acute hepatitis
    - Acute HAV: > 80% present with malaise, anorexia, fever, pain, hepatomegaly, or jaundice
    - Acute HCV: 75% asymptomatic at time of infection
      □ Fatigue, right upper quadrant pain in 25%
- Clinical profile

  - Teenage or middle-aged patient with history of fever, RUQ pain, hepatomegaly, and jaundice
- Lab data: ↑ serologic markers; ↑ liver function tests
- Diagnosis based on
  - Serologic markers; virological and clinical findings

Demographics

- Age
  - Any age group (particularly teen-/middle-age)
- Gender
  - M = F
- Epidemiology
  - Viral hepatitis in USA
    - HAV, HBC, and HCV account for 40%, 30%, and < 5% of acute viral hepatitis, respectively
    - HCV most common bloodborne infection in USA
      □ Leading cause of HCC and liver transplant

Natural History & Prognosis

- Hepatitis can be self-limited or progressive and chronic in nature
  - Chronic HCV infection: Occurs in 60-85%
  - Chronic HBV infection: Occurs in < 10% over age 5, 50% of children, 90% of neonates
    - HBV accounts for 15% of chronic viral hepatitis in USA
- Complications
  - Relapsing and fulminant hepatitis
  - Chronic viral (HBV, HCV) and alcoholic hepatitis
    - Cirrhosis: 10% of HBV and 20% of HCV
    - HCC: Particularly among carriers of HBsAg
- Prognosis
  - Acute viral and alcoholic: Good
  - Chronic persistent hepatitis: Good
  - Chronic active hepatitis: Not predictable
  - Fulminant hepatitis: Poor

Treatment

- Acute viral hepatitis (HAV): Supportive care; IG within 2 weeks of exposure, HBIG, vaccine
- Chronic HCV: Directly acting antiviral agents (DAAs)
  - Ledipasvir and sofosbuvir
  - Paritaprevir, ritonavir, ombitasvir, dasabuvir, ribavirin
  - Sofosbuvir and simeprevir, ± ribavirin
- Alcoholic hepatitis: Alcohol cessation and good diet

SELECTED REFERENCES

1. Firneisz G: Non-alcoholic fatty liver disease and type 2 diabetes mellitus: the liver disease of our age? World J Gastroenterol. 20(27):9072-89, 2014
2. Heller MT et al: The role of ultrasonography in the evaluation of diffuse liver disease. Radiol Clin North Am. 52(6):1163-75, 2014
3. Sudhamsu KC: Ultrasound findings in acute viral hepatitis. Kathmandu Univ Med J (KUMJ). 4(4):415-8, 2006
4. Cakir B et al: Unusual MDCT and sonography findings in fulminant hepatic failure resulting from hepatitis A infection. AJR Am J Roentgenol. 185(4):1033-5, 2005
5. Rubens DJ: Hepatobiliary imaging and its pitfalls. Radiol Clin North Am. 42(2):257-78, 2004
6. Han SH et al: Duplex Doppler ultrasound of the hepatic artery in patients with acute alcoholic hepatitis. J Clin Gastroenterol. 34(5):573-7, 2002

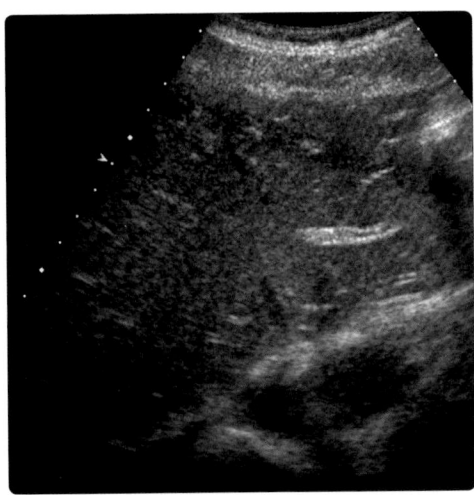

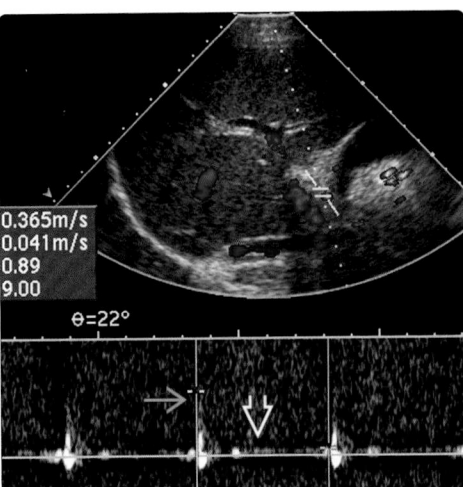

(Left) *Transverse grayscale ultrasound of the left lobe of the liver shows the liver parenchyma is only mildly hypoechoic in a patient with acute fulminant hepatic failure from acetaminophen toxicity.* (Right) *Transverse spectral Doppler evaluation of the hepatic artery in the same patient with acute fulminant hepatic toxicity from acetaminophen shows a markedly abnormal hepatic artery with weak systolic peak ⮕ and diminished diastolic flow ⮕.*

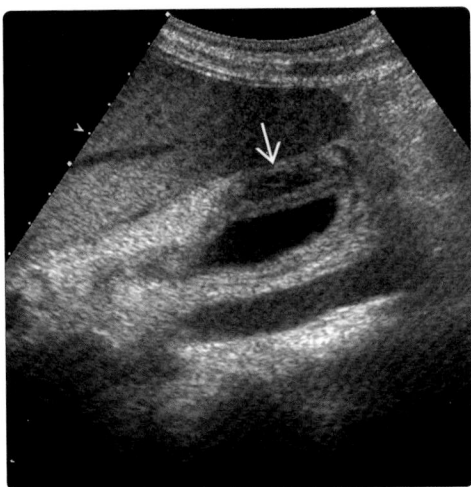

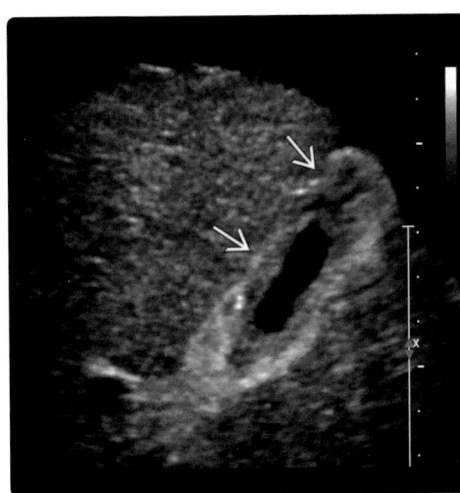

(Left) *Longitudinal view of the gallbladder in a patient with acute hepatitis shows a thickened gallbladder wall ⮕, a common finding in the setting of acute hepatitis.* (Right) *Transverse transabdominal ultrasound shows diffuse gallbladder wall thickening ⮕ in chronic hepatitis C. Liver surface nodularity and gallbladder fundus are outlined by ascites.*

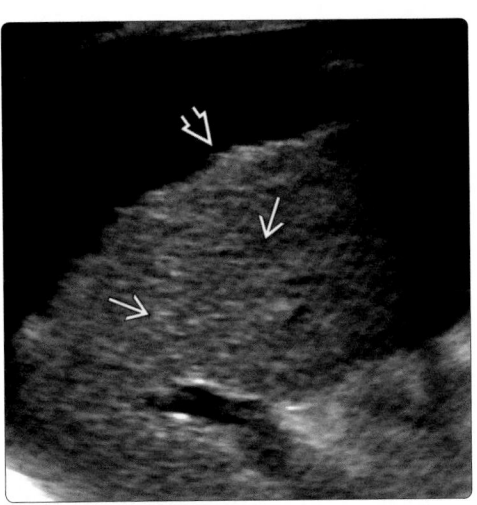

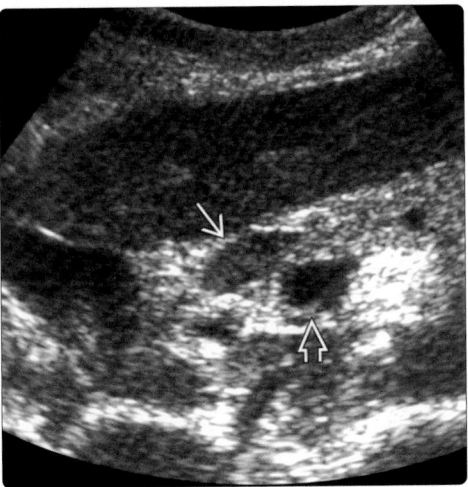

(Left) *Transverse ultrasound shows heterogeneous liver parenchyma ⮕ with a nodular surface ⮕ highlighted by ascites in chronic active viral hepatitis C.* (Right) *Transverse transabdominal ultrasound shows lymphadenopathy ⮕ adjacent to the portal vein ⮕ in a patient with viral hepatitis.*

Hepatic Cirrhosis

IMAGING

- Nodular contour, coarse or heterogeneous echotexture ± hypoechoic nodules
- General atrophy with enlargement of caudate/left lobes
- Atrophy of right lobe and medial segment of left lobe
- Coarsened echotexture, increase parenchymal echogenicity
- Regenerating nodules (siderotic)
- Signs of portal hypertension
  - Dilated hepatic and splenic arteries with increased flow
  - Splenomegaly
  - Varices
  - Ascites
- Signs of hypoalbuminemia
  - Edematous, thickened gallbladder wall and bowel wall (especially right colon)
  - Ascites

TOP DIFFERENTIAL DIAGNOSES

- Budd-Chiari syndrome

- Hepatocellular carcinoma
- Treated metastatic disease

PATHOLOGY

- Micronodular (Laennec) cirrhosis: Alcohol
- Macronodular (postnecrotic) cirrhosis: Viral
- Steatosis → hepatitis → cirrhosis
- USA: Alcohol (60-70%), chronic viral hepatitis B or C (10%)

CLINICAL ISSUES

- USA: Hepatitis C (cirrhosis) causes 30-50% of HCC cases
- Japan: Hepatitis C (cirrhosis) causes 70% of HCC cases
- Liver fibrosis staging
  - Determines prognosis and management
  - Liver biopsy is current reference standard
- Emerging noninvasive techniques to quantify liver fibrosis
  - US: Transient elastography and shear wave elastography
  - May replace liver biopsy

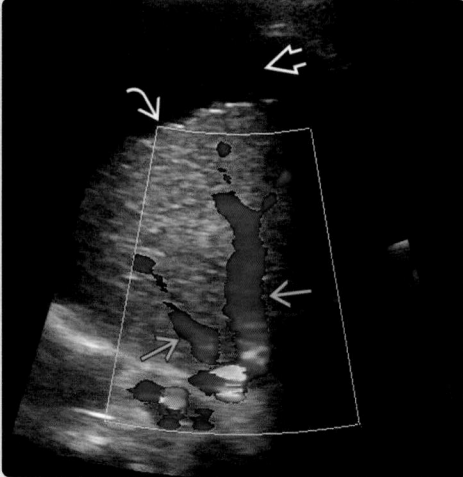 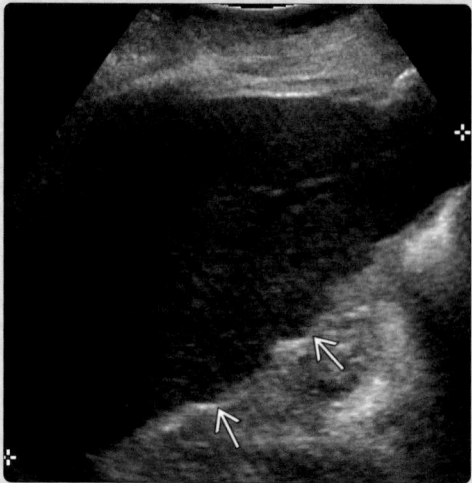

(Left) Transverse color Doppler ultrasound of a cirrhotic liver at the level of the hepatic veins ⇨ shows nodular liver capsule ⇗ and large-volume ascites ⇘. (Right) Longitudinal transabdominal ultrasound shows a nodular liver undersurface ➡ without ascites in a cirrhotic patient. Undersurface nodularity may be an early indicator of cirrhosis.

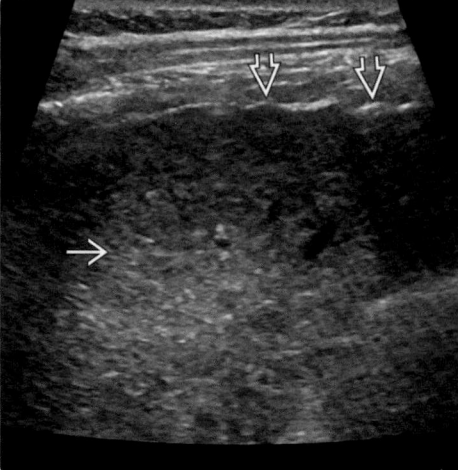 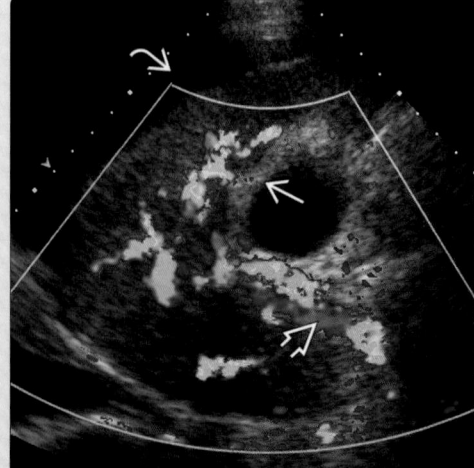

(Left) Longitudinal high-resolution view of the right liver surface shows a nodular liver capsule ⇗ and mildly heterogeneous liver parenchyma ➡ in a patient with liver cirrhosis. (Right) Longitudinal color Doppler ultrasound in a cirrhotic patient shows flow reversal (hepatofugal flow) in the main portal vein ⇗, thickened gallbladder wall ⇗, and moderate ascites ⇗.

TERMINOLOGY

Definitions

- Chronic liver disease characterized by diffuse parenchymal necrosis with extensive fibrosis and regenerative nodule formation
  - Common end response of liver to variety of insults and injuries

IMAGING

General Features

- Best diagnostic clue
  - Nodular contour, coarse echotexture ± hypoechoic nodules
- Location
  - Diffusely involving both lobes
- Size
  - General atrophy with relative enlargement of caudate/left lobes

Ultrasonographic Findings

- Grayscale ultrasound
  - Nodular liver surface contour
  - Hepatomegaly (early stage)/normal size/shrunken
  - Enlarged caudate lobe & lateral segment of left lobe
  - Atrophy of right lobe & medial segment of left lobe
  - Increased echogenicity of fissures & portal structures
  - Coarsened echotexture, increase parenchymal echogenicity
  - Steatosis
  - Regenerating nodules (siderotic)
    - Iso-/hypoechoic nodules
  - Dysplastic nodules (> 1 cm)
    - Considered to be premalignant
    - Difficult to differentiate from small hepatocellular carcinoma (HCC)
  - Compression of hepatic veins
  - Signs of portal hypertension
    - Splenomegaly
    - Portosystemic shunts, varices
    - Ascites
  - Signs of hypoalbuminemia
    - Ascites
    - Edematous gallbladder wall and bowel wall
- Color Doppler
  - Hepatic vein: Portalization of hepatic vein
    - Loss of normal triphasic/flattened hepatic vein
    - Turbulence if hepatic vein compressed
  - Portal vein: Increased pulsatility, decreased velocity
    - Hepatofugal flow (away from liver)
  - Hepatic artery: Dilatation of hepatic arteries with increased arterial flow
    - Hepatic artery hypertrophy often seen in setting of hepatofugal portal venous flow

CT Findings

- Nodular contour & widened fissures
- Atrophy of right lobe & medial segment of left lobe
- Enlarged caudate lobe & lateral segment of left lobe
- Regenerative nodules; fibrotic & fatty changes

- Portal hypertension: Varices, ascites, splenomegaly
- Siderotic regenerative nodules
  - NECT: Increased attenuation due to iron content
  - CECT: Nodules disappear after contrast
    - Nodules & parenchyma enhance to same level
- Dysplastic regenerative nodules
  - NECT: Large nodules are hyperdense (↑ iron + ↑ glycogen)
    - Small nodules are isodense with liver (undetected)
  - CECT: Iso-/hyperdense to normal liver

MR Findings

- Siderotic regenerative nodules: Paramagnetic effect of iron within nodules
  - T1WI: Hypointense
  - T2WI: Increased conspicuity of low signal intensity
  - T2 gradient-echo or FLASH: Markedly hypointense
  - Gamna-Gandy bodies (siderotic nodules in spleen)
    - Caused by hemorrhage (portal hypertension) into splenic follicles
    - T1 and T2WI: Hypointense
    - T2 GRE and FLASH images: Markedly hypointense
- Dysplastic regenerative nodules
  - T1WI: Hyperintense compared to liver parenchyma
  - T2WI: Hypointense relative to liver parenchyma
- Fibrotic and fatty changes
  - T1WI: Fibrosis: Hypointense; fat: Hyperintense
  - T2WI: Fibrosis: Hyperintense; fat: Hypointense

Elastographic Findings

- Transient elastography (FibroScan, Echosens; Paris, France)
  - Significant fibrosis ≥ 7.71 kPa (Metavir score F2)
  - Cirrhosis ≥ 15.08 kPa (Metavir score F4)
  - Morbid obesity and ascites preclude use of elastography
- Shear wave elastography
  - Cutoff values for fibrosis are device-specific, measured in m/s
    - F2 > 1.34 m/s
    - F3 > 1.55 m/s
    - F4 > 1.8 m/s

DIFFERENTIAL DIAGNOSIS

Budd-Chiari Syndrome

- Occluded or narrowed hepatic veins ± IVC, ascites
- Liver damaged, but no bridging fibrosis
- Ascites
- Acute phase: Hepatomegaly, hemorrhagic infarct
- Chronic phase: Fibrosis (post infarct), large regenerative nodules, collaterals
- Caudate lobe sparing (enlargement)

Hepatocellular Carcinoma

- Hypoechoic lesion within cirrhotic liver
- May see portal vein thrombosis/invasion

Treated Metastatic Disease

- Example: Breast cancer metastases to liver
  - May shrink and fibrose with treatment simulating nodular contour of cirrhotic liver

Hepatic Sarcoidosis

- Hypoattenuating nodules (size: Up to 2 cm)
- Hypointense nodules on T1- and T2WI MR

PATHOLOGY

General Features

- Etiology
  - Alcohol abuse is most common cause in West (1 of 10 leading causes of death [6th in USA]); hepatitis B in Asia
    - USA: Alcohol (60-70%), chronic viral hepatitis B/C (10%)
  - Primary biliary cirrhosis (5%), hemochromatosis (5%)
  - Primary sclerosing cholangitis, drugs, cardiac causes
  - In children: Biliary atresia, hepatitis, α-1 antitrypsin deficiency
- Micronodular (Laennec) cirrhosis: Alcohol
- Macronodular (postnecrotic) cirrhosis: Viral
- Catalase oxidation of ethanol → damage cellular membranes & proteins
- Steatosis → hepatitis → cirrhosis
- Regenerative (especially siderotic) nodules → dysplastic nodules → HCC
  - Dysplastic nodules considered premalignant

Staging, Grading, & Classification

- Based on morphology, histopathology, and etiology
  - Micronodular (Laennec) cirrhosis (< 1 cm diameter): Alcoholism (60-70% cases in USA)
  - Macronodular (postnecrotic) cirrhosis: Viral hepatitis (10% of cases in USA; majority of cases worldwide)

Gross Pathologic & Surgical Features

- Alcoholic cirrhosis
  - Early stage: Large, yellow, fatty, micronodular liver
  - Late stage: Shrunken, brown-yellow, hard organ with macronodules
- Postnecrotic cirrhosis
  - Macronodular (> 3 mm to 1 cm); fibrous scars

Microscopic Features

- Portal-central, portal-portal fibrous bands
- Micro- & macronodules; mononuclear cells
- Abnormal arteriovenous interconnections

CLINICAL ISSUES

Presentation

- Most common signs/symptoms
  - Alcoholic cirrhosis: May be clinically silent
  - Nodular liver, anorexia, malnutrition, weight loss
  - Portal hypertension: Splenomegaly, varices, caput medusae
  - Fatigue, jaundice, ascites, encephalopathy
  - Gynecomastia: Liver unable to metabolize estrogens
- Clinical profile
  - Patient with history of alcoholism, nodular liver, jaundice, ascites, and splenomegaly
- Lab data: Abnormal liver function tests; anemia
  - Alcoholic cirrhosis: Severe increase in AST (SGOT)
  - Viral: Severe increase in ALT (SGPT)

Demographics

- Epidemiology
  - Middle age and elderly; males > females
  - 3rd leading cause of death for men 34-54 years
  - Risk of HCC
    - USA: Hepatitis C (cirrhosis) causes 30-50% of HCC cases
    - Japan: Hepatitis C (cirrhosis) causes 70% of HCC cases
  - Mortality due to complication
    - Ascites (50%), variceal bleeding (25%), renal failure (10%), bacterial peritonitis (5%), complications of ascites therapy (10%)

Natural History & Prognosis

- Complications
  - Ascites, variceal hemorrhage, renal failure, coma
  - HCC: Due to hepatitis B & C, alcoholism
- Prognosis
  - Alcoholic cirrhosis: 5-year survival < 50%
  - Advanced disease: Poor prognosis
- Liver fibrosis staging
  - Determines prognosis and management
  - Liver biopsy is current reference standard
    - Metavir scoring system is specific to hepatitis C; provides grade and stage
      □ Grade (activity or inflammation) A0 = no activity to A3 = severe
      □ Stage (fibrosis) F0 = no fibrosis to F4 = cirrhosis
  - Emerging noninvasive techniques to quantify liver fibrosis
    - Ultrasound: Transient elastography and shear wave elastography
    - Magnetic resonance elastography (MRE)

Treatment

- Alcoholic cirrhosis
  - Abstinence; decreased protein diet; multivitamins
  - Prednisone; diuretics (for ascites)
- Management limited to treating complications & underlying cause
- Advanced stage: Liver transplantation

DIAGNOSTIC CHECKLIST

Consider

- Rule out other causes of nodular dysmorphic liver

Image Interpretation Pearls

- Nodular liver contour; lobar atrophy & hypertrophy
- Regenerative nodules, ascites, splenomegaly, varices

SELECTED REFERENCES

1. Beland MD et al: A pilot study estimating liver fibrosis with ultrasound shear-wave elastography: does the cause of liver disease or location of measurement affect performance? AJR Am J Roentgenol. 203(3):W267-73, 2014
2. Ferraioli G et al: Shear wave elastography for evaluation of liver fibrosis. J Ultrasound Med. 33(2):197-203, 2014
3. Buadu A et al: Small liver nodule detection with a high-frequency transducer in patients with chronic liver disease: report of 3 cases. J Ultrasound Med. 32(2):355-9, 2013
4. Irshad A et al: Current role of ultrasound in chronic liver disease: surveillance, diagnosis and management of hepatic neoplasms. Curr Probl Diagn Radiol. 41(2):43-51, 2012

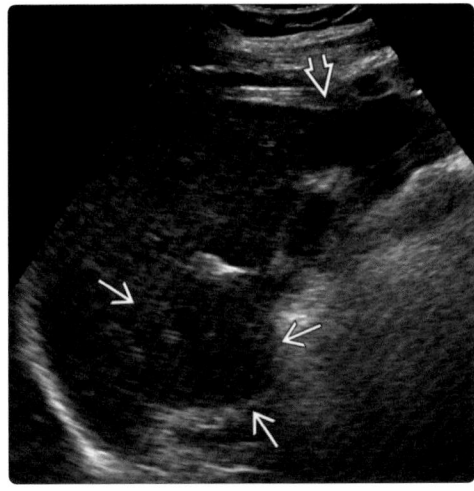

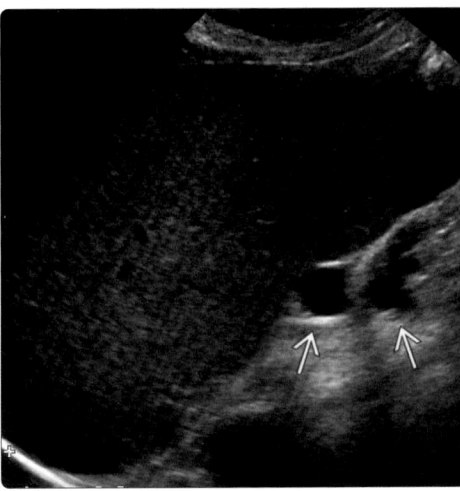

(Left) *Longitudinal transabdominal ultrasound in a cirrhotic patient shows heterogeneous liver echotexture with an enlarged caudate lobe ➡ compared to the atrophic medial segment of left lobe ➡. (Right) Oblique transabdominal ultrasound in the same patient shows splenomegaly (23 cm) and splenic varices ➡ due to portal hypertension and cirrhosis*

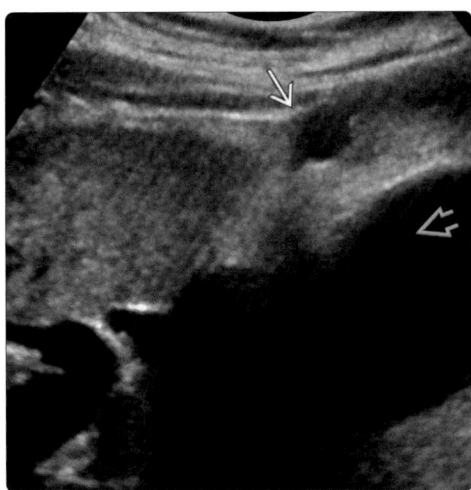

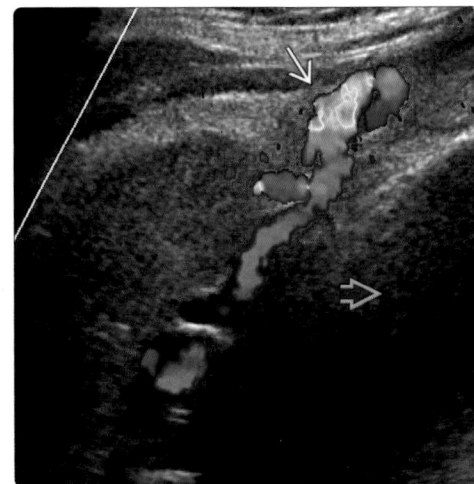

(Left) *Oblique transabdominal ultrasound shows recanalization of the paraumbilical vein ➡, which acts as a portosystemic collateral to compensate for portal hypertension. Large-volume ascites is partially visualized ➡. (Right) Longitudinal color Doppler ultrasound in the same patient shows portal venous flow in the recanalized paraumbilical veins ➡ as a result of portal hypertension. Large-volume ascites is again partially visualized ➡.*

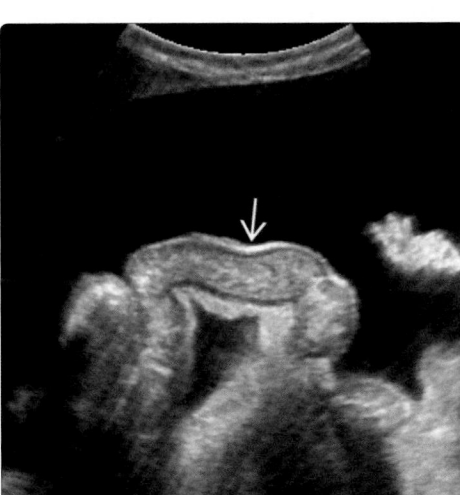

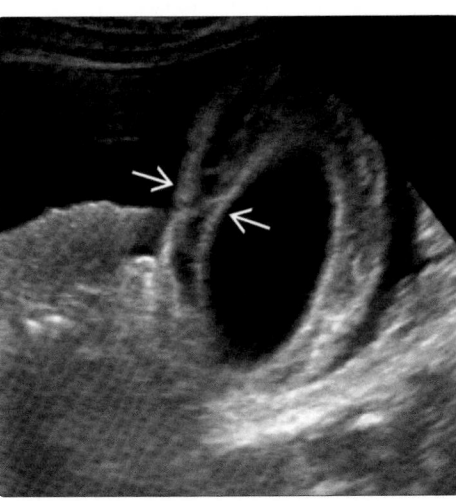

(Left) *Transverse transabdominal ultrasound shows thickened loops of bowel ➡ floating within ascites. Mural edema may be due to portal hypertension or hypoalbuminemia. (Right) Oblique transabdominal ultrasound shows diffuse gallbladder wall thickening ➡ in a cirrhotic patient, related to hypoalbuminemia or poor venous drainage.*

Hepatic Steatosis

TERMINOLOGY

- Accumulation of increasing amount of triglycerides within hepatocytes

IMAGING

- Diffuse fatty infiltration
  - Increased echogenicity with liver more echogenic than kidney
  - Attenuation of US beam results in poor visualization of diaphragm
  - Poor visualization of hepatic and portal veins
- Focal fatty infiltration
  - Hyperechoic nodule or multiple confluent hyperechoic lesions
  - No mass effect with vessels running undisplaced through lesion
  - Wedge-shaped/lobar/segmental distribution
- Focal fatty sparing
  - Direct drainage of hepatic blood into systemic circulation

- Gallbladder bed: Drained by cystic vein
- Segment 4 or anterior to portal bifurcation: Drained by aberrant gastric vein
- No mass effect with undisplaced vessel

TOP DIFFERENTIAL DIAGNOSES

- Steatohepatitis
- Fatty cirrhosis
- Hemangioma
- Metastasis or lymphoma

CLINICAL ISSUES

- Nonalcoholic steatohepatitis (NASH) may progress to cirrhosis and hepatocellular carcinoma

DIAGNOSTIC CHECKLIST

- Rule out other liver pathologies that may mimic focal or diffuse steatosis

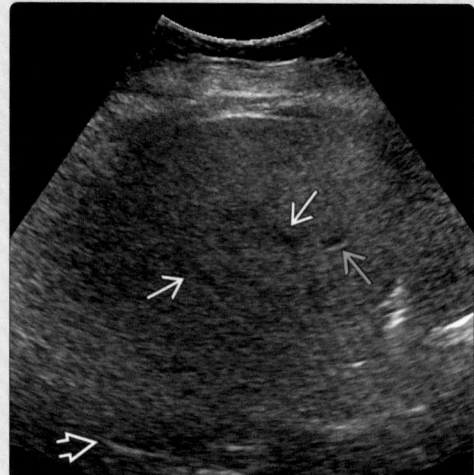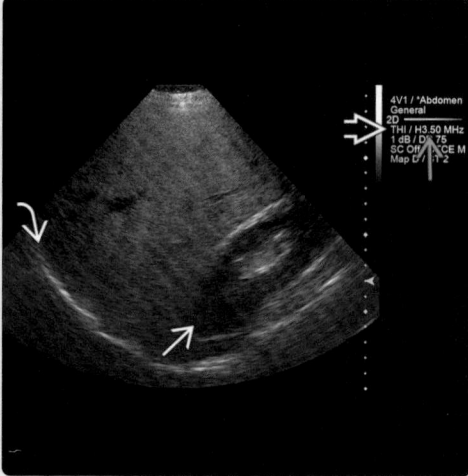

(Left) Abdominal US shows severe hepatic steatosis with a diffusely echogenic liver, poor visualization of the diaphragm ➡, and decreased visibility of hepatic vein ➡ and portal vein ➡ walls. (Right) Oblique US in a patient with severe steatosis shows diffusely increased liver parenchymal echogenicity in comparison with the right kidney ➡. Lower frequency ➡ vector transducer and harmonic imaging ➡ was applied to optimize penetration and diaphragm is well visualized ➡.

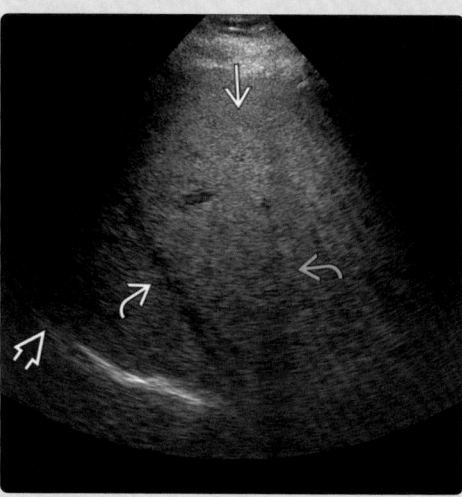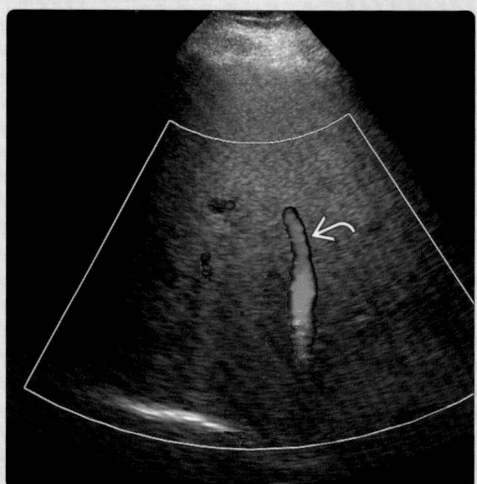

(Left) Transverse abdominal US in a patient with moderate hepatic steatosis shows diffusely increased parenchymal echogenicity ➡ with a poorly delineated right hepatic vein wall ➡ and a hardly visible middle hepatic vein ➡. Part of the diaphragm is not well visualized due to poor acoustic penetration ➡. (Right) Color Doppler US in the same patient depicts color flow in the middle hepatic vein ➡.

TERMINOLOGY

Synonyms
- Fatty liver, hepatic fatty metamorphosis

Definitions
- Accumulation of increasing amount of triglycerides within hepatocytes

IMAGING

General Features
- Best diagnostic clue
  - Preservation of normal hepatic architecture
  - Presence of normal vessels coursing through fatty infiltration
  - Decreased signal intensity of liver on T1W out of phase gradient-echo images
- Location
  - Focal, multifocal, or diffuse
  - Lobar, segmental, or wedge shaped
    - Common along hepatic vessels, ligaments, and fissures
- Morphology
  - Geographic/wedge shape
  - Multifocal spherical lesions may simulate metastasis or primary tumor
- Variable imaging features depend on
  - Amount of fat deposited in liver
  - Distribution of fat within liver: Focal vs. diffuse
  - Presence of associated hepatic disease

Ultrasonographic Findings
- Grayscale ultrasound
  - **Diffuse fatty infiltration**
    - Increased echogenicity of liver, becoming more echogenic than kidney
    - Attenuation of US beam by steatosis results in poor visualization of diaphragm
    - Margins of hepatic veins blurred due to increased refraction and scattering of sound
    - Loss of echogenic portal vein walls
    - Liver often enlarged and changes shape as volume of infiltration increases
    - US grading of steatosis is subjective and prone to interobserver variation
  - **Focal fatty infiltration**
    - Hyperechoic nodule/multiple confluent hyperechoic lesions
    - No mass effect, with vessels running undisplaced through lesion
    - Wedge-shaped lobar/segmental distribution
  - **Focal fatty sparing**
    - Hypoechoic area within echogenic liver
    - Due to direct drainage of hepatic flow into systemic circulation
      - Next to gallbladder bed (drained by cystic vein)
      - Segment 4, anterior to portal bifurcation (drained by aberrant gastric vein)
    - No mass effect

CT Findings
- NECT
  - Decreased attenuation of liver compared to spleen
    - Normal: Liver 8-10 HU more than spleen (50-65 HU)
    - Steatosis: Liver at least 10 HU less than spleen, or absolute liver attenuation < 40 HU
  - Focal nodular fatty infiltration: Low attenuation
    - Common location: Adjacent to falciform ligament
    - Due to nutritional ischemia at vascular watershed
- CECT
  - Attenuation measurements and comparisons are less reliable than NECT
    - Dependent on timing relative to contrast administration
    - On venous phase or delayed CECT, steatotic liver is usually > 35 HU less dense than spleen
  - Normal vessels course through fatty infiltration
  - Dual-energy CT: Steatosis accentuated on lower kVp sequence

MR Findings
- T1 in-phase GRE (chemical shift): Increased signal intensity of fatty liver vs. spleen
- T1 out of phase GRE: Decreased or loss of signal intensity of fatty liver
- T1 C+ out of phase GRE: Paradoxical decreased signal intensity of liver
- Short T1 inversion recovery (STIR): Fatty areas are low signal intensity

DIFFERENTIAL DIAGNOSIS

Steatohepatitis
- Diabetic fatty liver, alcoholic hepatitis, nonalcoholic steatohepatitis (NASH)
- Fatty liver + inflammatory change, fibrosis, and necrosis
- Smooth surface, decreased plasticity
- Hepatic veins show disjointed network-like appearance with blurred outline
- Increasing fibrosis and scarring

Fatty Cirrhosis
- Dense, firm liver
- Hypertrophied left caudate lobe/atrophy of right lobe
- Heterogeneous, hyperechoic parenchyma
- Rarefaction of hepatic veins

Hemangioma
- Typically well-defined, hyperechoic nodule
- Posterior acoustic enhancement

Metastases or Lymphoma
- Hyperechoic metastases may simulate focal steatosis
- Confluent or infiltrative tumor distorts vessels and bile ducts
- Diffuse lymphoma infiltration may be indistinguishable from normal liver or steatosis

PATHOLOGY

General Features
- Etiology

- o Metabolic derangement
  - Poorly controlled DM (50%), obesity, hyperlipidemia
  - Severe hepatitis and protein malnutrition
  - Parenteral hyperalimentation, malabsorption
  - Pregnancy, trauma, inflammatory bowel disease
  - Cystic fibrosis, Reye syndrome
- o Hepatotoxins: Alcohol (> 50%), carbon tetrachlorides, phosphorus
- o Drugs
  - Tetracycline, amiodarone, corticosteroids
  - Salicylates, tamoxifen, calcium channel blockers
- Associated abnormalities
- o NASH
  - Subset of nonalcoholic fatty liver disease: Strong association with metabolic syndrome
  - Seen in patients with hyperlipidemia and diabetes
  - May lead to "cryptogenic" cirrhosis
- Fat deposition in liver due to
- o Ethanol: Increased hepatic synthesis of fatty acids
- o Carbon tetrachloride/high-dose tetracycline: Decreases hepatic oxidation/utilization of fatty acids
- o Starvation, steroids, and alcohol
  - Excessively mobilizes fatty acids from adipose tissue
- o Segmental fatty infiltration: Where glycogen is depleted from liver
  - Decreased nutrients and insulin → decreased glycogen
  - Due to underlying mass, Budd-Chiari syndrome, or tumor thrombus
- o Focal steatosis or sparing: Due to variations in hepatic venous drainage

Staging, Grading, & Classification

- Sonographic grading for diffuse steatosis
- o Mild: Minimally increased parenchymal echogenicity and normal-appearing intrahepatic vessel walls
- o Moderate: Further increased parenchymal echogenicity causing decreased resolution of intrahepatic vessel walls
- o Severe: Markedly increased parenchymal echogenicity causing inability to resolve intrahepatic vessel walls
- Nonalcoholic fatty liver disease (NAFLD)
- o Includes nonalcoholic fatty liver (NAFL) and NASH
- o May progress to cirrhosis and hepatocellular carcinoma
- o Risk factors: Obesity, sedentary lifestyle, diet, type II diabetes, metabolic syndrome

Gross Pathologic & Surgical Features

- Enlarged, smooth capsule, rounded inferior contour
- Soft, yellow, greasy cut surface

Microscopic Features

- Triglyceride accumulation within hepatocyte cytoplasm
- Macrovesicular fatty liver (most common type)
- o Hepatocytes with large cytoplasmic fat vacuoles displacing nucleus peripherally
- o Alcohol and diabetes mellitus
- Microvesicular
- o Fat is present in many small vacuoles
- o Reye syndrome

CLINICAL ISSUES

Presentation

- Most common signs/symptoms
- o Asymptomatic, but often with abnormal liver function tests (LFTs)
- o Hepatomegaly in obese or diabetic patient
- o Alcoholics with acute injury: RUQ pain, tender hepatomegaly
- Lab data
- o Asymptomatic: Normal/mildly elevated LFTs
- o Alcoholic and NASH: May have markedly abnormal LFTs
- Diagnosis: Biopsy and histology
- o Distinguish simple steatosis from steatohepatitis
- o Sampling error
- o MR Elastography: Emerging noninvasive means for staging fibrosis and differentiating simple steatosis and NASH

Demographics

- Epidemiology
- o Most common cause of chronic liver disease in Western countries
- o 50% of patients with diabetes mellitus, > 50% of alcoholics; 80-90% of obesity
- o Seen in 25% of nonalcoholics
- o Increasing in prevalence with epidemic of obesity and metabolic syndrome

Natural History & Prognosis

- Alcoholics: Gradual disappearance of fat from liver after 4-8 weeks of adequate diet and abstinence from alcohol
- Resolves in 2 weeks after discontinuation of parenteral hyperalimentation
- Steatohepatitis may progress to acute/chronic liver failure
- Steatosis is synergistic with viral hepatitis

Treatment

- Removal of alcohol or offending toxins
- Correction of metabolic disorders
- Lipotropic agents (like choline) when indicated

DIAGNOSTIC CHECKLIST

Consider

- Rule out other liver pathologies that may mimic focal or diffuse steatosis

Image Interpretation Pearls

- Key on all imaging modalities is presence of normal vessels coursing through fatty infiltration

SELECTED REFERENCES

1. Loomba R et al: Magnetic resonance elastography predicts advanced fibrosis in patients with nonalcoholic fatty liver disease: a prospective study. Hepatology. 60(6):1920-8, 2014
2. Borges VF et al: Sonographic hepatorenal ratio: a noninvasive method to diagnose nonalcoholic steatosis. J Clin Ultrasound. 41(1):18-25, 2013
3. Kwon HJ et al: Value of the ultrasound attenuation index for noninvasive quantitative estimation of hepatic steatosis. J Ultrasound Med. 32(2):229-35, 2013

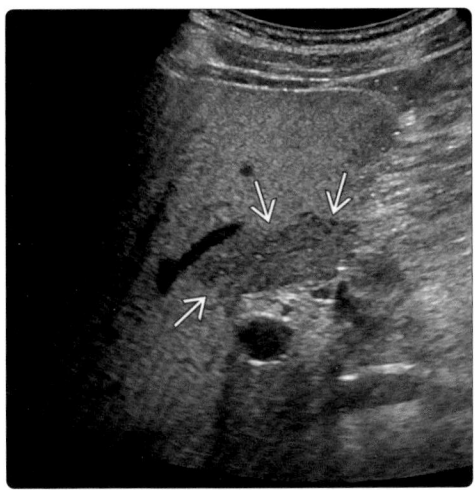
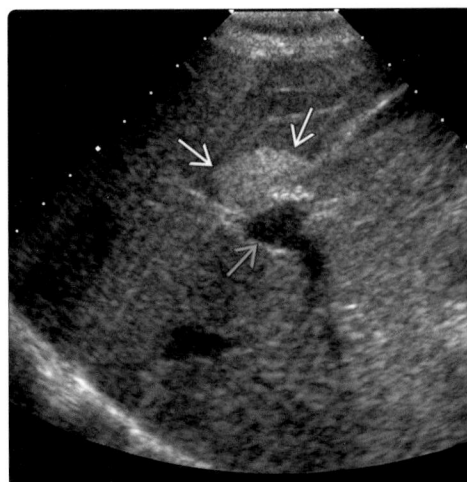

(Left) *Transverse abdominal US in a patient with hepatic steatosis shows a geographic area of decreased echogenicity, suggesting focal fatty sparing* ➡ *in the posterior subcapsular portion of segment 4 of liver, which is drained by an aberrant right gastric vein.* (Right) *Oblique abdominal US shows a fan-shaped area of focal fat deposition* ➡ *as increased echogenicity of the liver anterior to the porta hepatis* ⇨.

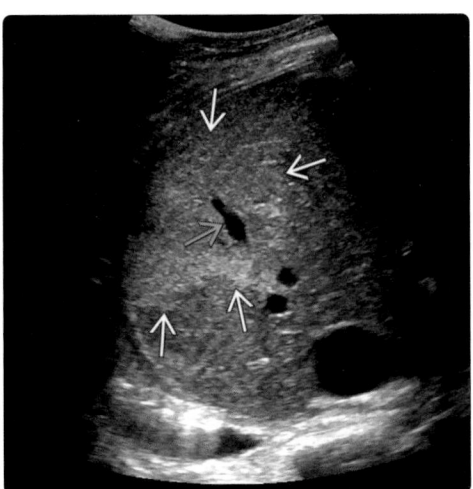
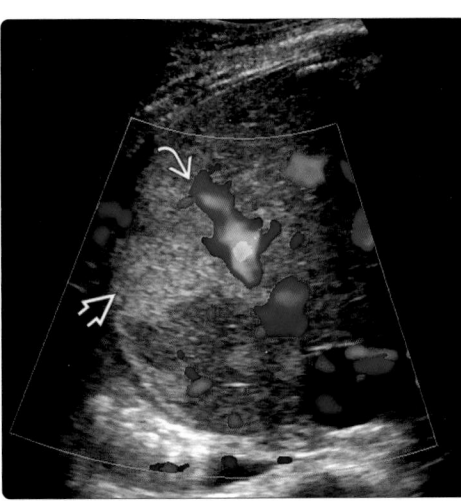

(Left) *Oblique abdominal grayscale US shows geographic focal fatty infiltration* ➡ *as a wedge-shaped area with increased echogenicity extending up to the subcapsular portion of right lobe of liver. Note the normal vessel* ⇨ *coursing through the area of fatty infiltration.* (Right) *Color Doppler US in the same patient shows focal fatty infiltration* ➡ *with a normal hepatic vein* ↗ *coursing through the area without displacement.*

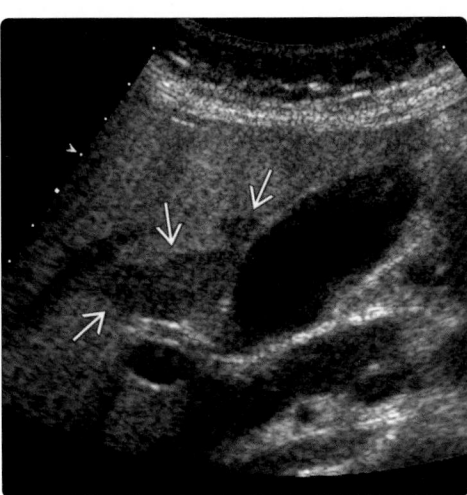
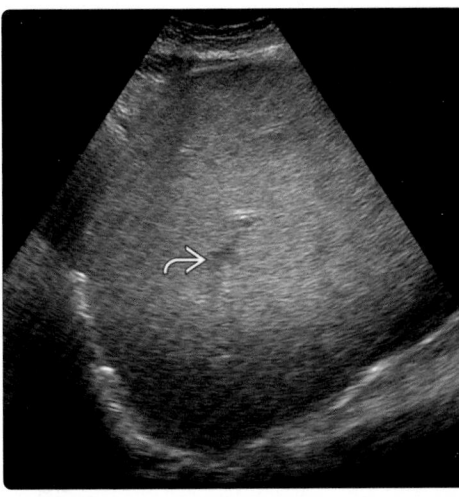

(Left) *Longitudinal abdominal US shows focal fatty sparing at the gallbladder fossa as a geographic area of decreased echogenicity* ➡. *Liver adjacent to the gallbladder fossa is a typical location for fatty sparing.* (Right) *Oblique abdominal US in a patient with acute alcoholic hepatitis shows moderate steatosis as diffusely increased echogenicity of hepatic parenchyma along with poorly delineated intrahepatic vascular margins* ↗.

Hepatic Schistosomiasis

TERMINOLOGY

- Hepatic parasitic infestation by *Schistosoma* species

IMAGING

- CT: "Tortoise shell" or "turtle back" appearance
  - Peripheral periportal fibrosis, widened fissures
  - Capsular calcification (parallel or perpendicular to liver surface)
- Portal hypertension in advanced disease
  - Splenomegaly and varices
- US: "Bull's-eye" lesion: Represents anechoic portal vein surrounded by echogenic mantle of fibrous tissue
  - Hyperechoic and thickened walls of portal venules
  - Network of echogenic septa outlining polygonal areas of normal-appearing liver

TOP DIFFERENTIAL DIAGNOSES

- Hepatic cirrhosis

- Often has widened fissures but periportal fibrosis is central in distribution (as opposed to peripheral in hepatic schistosomiasis)
- Both can be complicated by portal hypertension

CLINICAL ISSUES

- Most common cause of hepatic fibrosis in the world
  - Over 200 million persons, mostly in tropics
- Different *Schistosoma* species affect urinary tract more than liver
- Single dose of oral praziquantel cures > 85% of cases

DIAGNOSTIC CHECKLIST

- Exclude other causes of hepatic fibrosis or cirrhosis
- Hepatic mosaic "tortoise shell" pattern of fibrosis and calcification

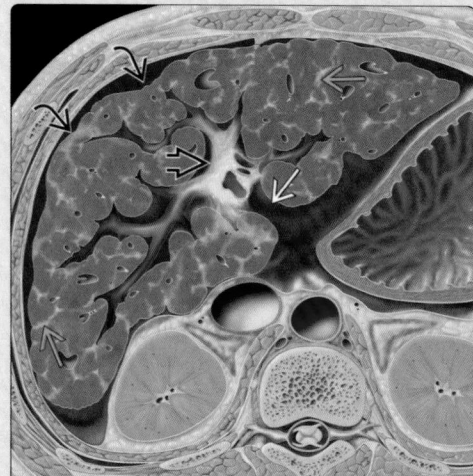
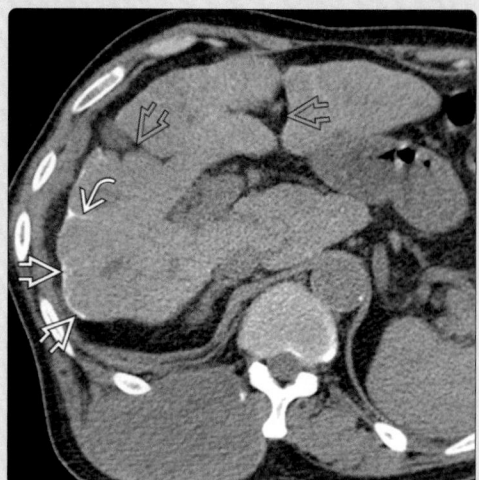

(Left) *Graphic of hepatic schistosomiasis shows striking periportal fibrosis ➘ with widened fissures ➡ between hepatic segments and lobulated liver contour ➶. Peripheral periportal fibrosis ➘ leads to a "turtle back" appearance of the liver.*
(Right) *Axial NECT of the liver in a patient with schistosomiasis shows predominantly peripheral calcifications ➘, with some calcifications perpendicular in orientation ➚ to the liver capsule. Note widened fissures ➘ and irregular hepatic surface.*

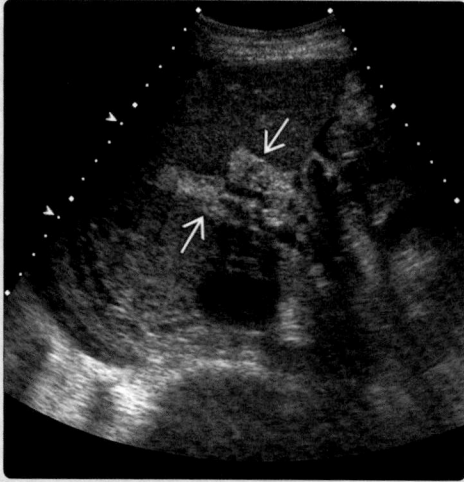
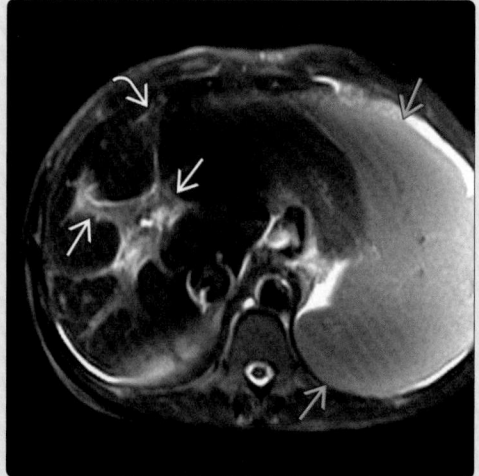

(Left) *Longitudinal ultrasound demonstrates thickening and hyperechogenicity at the porta hepatis ➡ consistent with periportal fibrosis in a patient with schistosomiasis. (Courtesy W. Chong, MD.)*
(Right) *Axial T2WI MR demonstrates T2-hyperintense subcapsular ➚ and periportal fibrotic bands ➡ consistent with periportal fibrosis in a patient with hepatic schistosomiasis. Additionally, splenomegaly ➘ indicates portal hypertension. (Courtesy W. Chong, MD.)*

TERMINOLOGY

Synonyms

- Bilharzia, blood fluke

Definitions

- Hepatic parasitic infestation by *Schistosoma* species

IMAGING

General Features

- Morphology
  - Distortion of liver architecture and surface contour by extension of periportal fibrosis
  - Most common cause of hepatic fibrosis worldwide
- Periportal fibrotic bands and widened fissures with calcification

Ultrasonographic Findings

- Grayscale ultrasound
  - Atrophic liver in late stage (fibrosis and portal hypertension)
  - Irregular/notched liver surface
  - Echogenic granulomata
    - Peripheral/subcapsular location
  - Periportal fibrosis
    - Most severe at porta hepatis
    - Widened portal tracts
    - Hyperechoic & thickened walls of portal veins
    - "Bull's-eye" lesion: Represents anechoic portal vein surrounded by echogenic mantle of fibrous tissue
  - Mosaic pattern
    - Network of echogenic septa outlining polygonal areas of normal-appearing liver
    - Represents complete septal fibrosis (inflammation and fibrosis as reaction to embolized eggs)

CT Findings

- CECT
  - "Tortoise shell" or "turtle back" appearance
    - Represents calcified septa, usually aligned perpendicular to liver capsule
  - Capsular calcification
  - Junctional notches or depressions, irregular hepatic contour
  - Dysmorphic liver with peripheral atrophy, caudate hypertrophy
  - Periportal edema, periportal fat, fibrosis, volume loss
  - Splenomegaly and varices

Imaging Recommendations

- Best imaging tool
  - Ultrasound &/or CT for diagnosis and follow-up

DIFFERENTIAL DIAGNOSIS

Hepatic Cirrhosis

- Hepatic schistosomiasis may cause or simulate cirrhosis from other causes
- Cirrhosis often has widened fissures but not as much periportal edema & fibrosis as with schistosomiasis

PATHOLOGY

General Features

- Etiology
  - Caused by parasites that live in certain freshwater snails
  - *S. japonicum*: North Asia
  - *S. mansoni*: Africa, Egypt, Caribbean, South America
    - Causes most severe disease in liver
  - *S. hematobium*: Mediterranean, Africa, Southeast Asia
    - Typically affects urinary tract
- Associated abnormalities
  - May involve urinary system
    - Thickened bladder wall ± calcification

Gross Pathologic & Surgical Features

- Adult worms live in pairs within portal veins for years
  - *S. japonicum* in superior mesenteric vein (SMV); *S. mansoni* in inferior mesenteric vein (IMV)
  - *S. hematobium*: Bladder and ureteric veins
- Female worm releases eggs, which travel in blood to become trapped in tissues of different organs
- Trapped eggs stimulate granulomatous reaction, which is reversible in early stages but becomes fibrotic later
- Fibrosis may lead to organ damage
  - Liver: Periportal fibrosis, portal hypertension, gastrointestinal hemorrhage
  - Urinary tract: Obstructive uropathy (renal failure), pyelonephritis, glomerulonephritis, amyloidosis

Microscopic Features

- Multiple tiny granulomas scattered in periphery of liver
- Granuloma consists of egg in center surrounded by macrophages, lymphocytes, neutrophils, and eosinophils

CLINICAL ISSUES

Presentation

- Most common signs/symptoms
  - Acute infection: Dermatitis, fever, hepatomegaly
- Clinical profile
  - Eosinophilia (may be absent in chronic disease)
  - Living eggs in stool/urine (need to perform egg viability test)
  - Antibody specific to *Schistosoma*

Treatment

- Single dose of oral praziquantel cures > 85% of cases
  - 2nd dose needed if viable eggs in stool or urine 6-12 weeks after initial treatment

SELECTED REFERENCES

1. Lambertucci JR: Revisiting the concept of hepatosplenic schistosomiasis and its challenges using traditional and new tools. Rev Soc Bras Med Trop. 47(2):130-6, 2014
2. Ma C et al: Histopathologic evaluation of liver biopsy for cirrhosis. Adv Anat Pathol. 19(4):220-30, 2012
3. MacConnachie A: Schistosomiasis. J R Coll Physicians Edinb. 42(1):47-9; quiz 50, 2012
4. Silva LC et al: Ultrasound and magnetic resonance imaging findings in Schistosomiasis mansoni: expanded gallbladder fossa and fatty hilum signs. Rev Soc Bras Med Trop. 45(4):500-4, 2012
5. Strahan R et al: Ultrasound study of liver disease caused by Schistosoma mansoni in rural Zambian schoolchildren. J Med Imaging Radiat Oncol. 56(4):390-7, 2012

TERMINOLOGY

- Hepatic venous outflow obstruction due to occlusion of terminal hepatic venules and sinusoids
- Synonym: Hepatic sinusoidal obstruction syndrome

IMAGING

- Hepatosplenomegaly, ascites, gallbladder wall thickening
- Narrowing of hepatic veins
- Color Doppler ultrasound
  - Elevated hepatic arterial velocity > 100 cm/s
  - Slow portal venous velocity (< 10 cm/s) or hepatofugal flow

TOP DIFFERENTIAL DIAGNOSES

- Graft-vs.-host disease
- Budd-Chiari syndrome
- Portal vein thrombosis
- Portal hypertension
- Opportunistic infection

PATHOLOGY

- Injury to hepatic venous endothelium
- Progresses to deposition of fibrinogen + factor VIII within venule and sinusoidal walls
- Progressive venular obstruction, centrilobular hemorrhagic necrosis
- Sclerosis of venular wall and intense collagen deposition in sinusoids and venules

CLINICAL ISSUES

- Occurs most frequently following hematopoietic cell transplantation
  - Responsible for 5-15% of deaths in population with VOD
- Signs and symptoms of liver failure with painful hepatomegaly, jaundice, peripheral edema, unexplained weight gain
- Clinical and laboratory features of VOD usually begin within 3 weeks of transplantation

(Left) Color Doppler US of the liver shows hepatofugal flow in the main portal vein ➡ in a patient with venoocclusive disease (VOD) after bone marrow transplant for AML. Note edematous appearance of the liver and hypertrophied hepatic artery ➡. (Right) On pulsed Doppler US in the same patient, peak systolic velocity measured at the common hepatic artery is elevated to 168 cm/s, confirming high flow state of the hepatic artery related to hepatic arterial buffer response to hepatofugal portal flow.

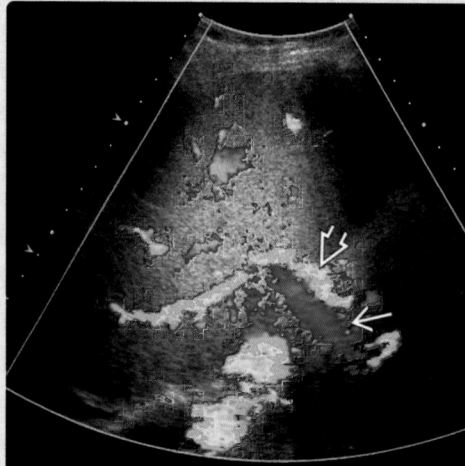
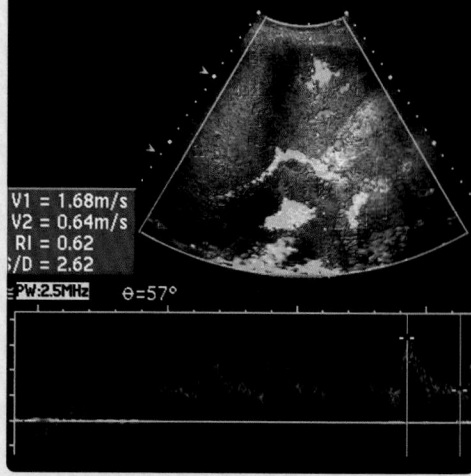

(Left) Grayscale ultrasound of liver shows markedly edematous and an enlarged liver resulting in narrowed hepatic veins ➡ and small-caliber inferior vena cava ➡ in this patient with VOD. A small right pleural effusion ➡ is also evident. (Right) Grayscale ultrasound shows diffuse gallbladder wall thickening ➡ and sludge ➡ in this patient with VOD. Gallbladder wall thickening in isolation is a nonspecific finding. However, in combination with other sonographic findings of VOD, is supportive of this diagnosis.

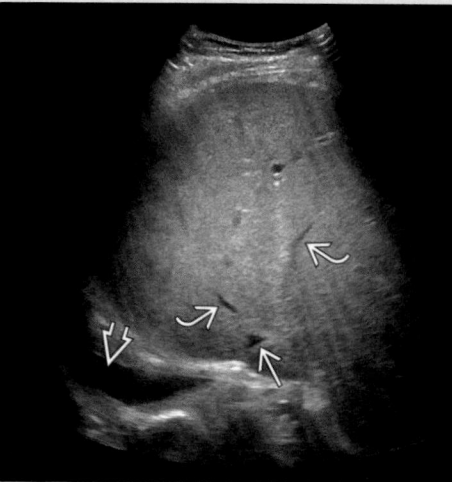
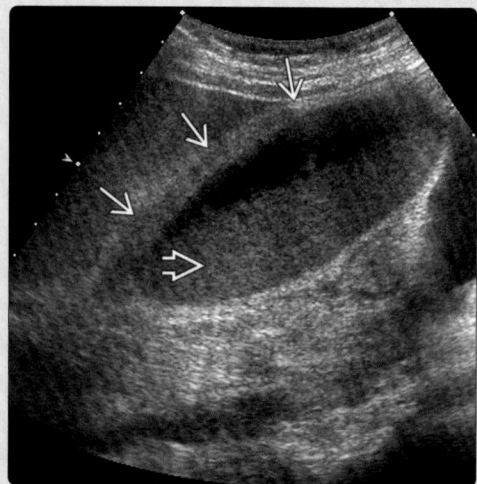

Venoocclusive Disease

TERMINOLOGY

Abbreviations

- Venoocclusive disease (VOD)

Synonyms

- Hepatic sinusoidal obstruction syndrome

Definitions

- Hepatic venous outflow obstruction due to occlusion of terminal hepatic venules and sinusoids

IMAGING

General Features

- Best diagnostic clue
  o Acute onset of painful hepatomegaly, jaundice, and ascites within 3 weeks following hematopoietic or stem cell transplantation
- Location
  o Diffuse process involving entire liver

Ultrasonographic Findings

- Grayscale ultrasound
  o Hepatomegaly
  o Splenomegaly
  o Gallbladder wall thickening
  o Ascites
  o Narrowing of hepatic veins due to hepatic edema
  o Rouleaux formation in portal veins due to slow flow
- Pulsed Doppler
  o Elevated hepatic arterial velocity > 100 cm/s
  o Abnormal hepatic arterial resistive index < 0.55 or > 0.75 (variably seen)
  o Slow portal venous velocity (< 10 cm/s) or hepatofugal flow
  o Monophasic waveforms in hepatic veins
- Color Doppler
  o Slow or reversed flow in portal vein
    – Flow may be so slow that it is undetectable on color Doppler
  o Prominent hepatic arteries
  o Narrowed hepatic veins

CT Findings

- Hepatomegaly
- Ascites
- Pleural effusion
- Hepatic vein narrowing
- Gallbladder edema and periportal edema
- Patchy hepatic parenchymal enhancement

MR Findings

- Same general findings as CT
- Hepatomegaly
- Ascites
- Pleural effusion
- Hepatic vein narrowing
- Periportal cuffing and gallbladder edema
  o High signal intensity of periportal area and gallbladder wall on T2WI
- Patchy hepatic parenchymal enhancement

Imaging Recommendations

- Best imaging tool
  o Ultrasound is imaging modality of choice
- Protocol advice
  o Doppler evaluation of hepatic vessels critical for appropriate diagnosis

DIFFERENTIAL DIAGNOSIS

Graft-vs.-Host Disease (GVHD)

- Primarily a clinical diagnosis
  o Characterized by acute hepatic injury, skin rash, and gastrointestinal disease
- Bowel wall thickening more frequently accompanies GVHD than VOD

Budd-Chiari Syndrome

- Thrombosis or obstruction at level of main hepatic veins or inferior vena cava (IVC)
- Not related to bone marrow transplantation

Portal Vein Thrombosis

- Bland thrombosis of portal vein
  o Variably echogenic clot
  o May be accompanied by cavernous transformation of portal vein
- Tumor thrombus of portal vein
  o Often seen in setting of hepatocellular carcinoma
  o Tumor vessels usually visible within tumor thrombus

Portal Hypertension

- Although some imaging features may overlap with VOD, typical history of chronic liver disease is key to diagnosis of portal hypertension
  o May see slow flow or reversed direction of flow in portal vein
  o Ascites suggests hepatic decompensation
  o Gallbladder wall thickening often seen

Opportunistic Infection

- Hematopoietic stem cell transplantation patients are at risk for hepatic infections
- Multifocal small hypoechoic lesions may suggest fungal or mycobacterial microabscesses

PATHOLOGY

General Features

- Liver biopsies are most striking for pronounced sinus congestion
- Injury to hepatic venous endothelium
- Progresses to deposition of fibrinogen + factor VIII within venule and sinusoidal walls
- Progressive venular obstruction and centrilobular hemorrhagic necrosis
- Sclerosis of venular wall and intense collagen deposition in sinusoids and venules
- Chronic VOD
  o Thickened collagen cuffs surrounding central veins

Staging, Grading, & Classification

- Disease severity (Seattle criteria)
  o Mild disease

- No adverse effects of liver disease, **and**
- No medications required for diuresis or hepatic pain, **and**
- All symptoms, signs, and laboratory features reversible
  - ○ Moderate disease (most common form of VOD)
    - Adverse effects of liver disease present, **and**
    - Sodium restriction or diuresis required, **or**
    - Medication for hepatic pain required, **and**
    - All symptoms, signs, and laboratory features reversible
  - ○ Severe disease
    - Adverse effects of liver disease present, **and**
    - Symptoms, signs, or laboratory features not resolved within 100 days of transplantation, **or**
    - Death

CLINICAL ISSUES

Presentation

- Most common signs/symptoms
  - ○ Painful hepatomegaly, jaundice, peripheral edema, unexplained weight gain
  - ○ Elevation of liver function tests
- Other signs/symptoms
  - ○ Signs and symptoms of liver failure such as ascites, encephalopathy, etc.

Demographics

- Gender
  - ○ Women affected more than men
- Risk factors
  - ○ Preexisting liver disease
  - ○ Specific types of conditioning therapy prior to transplantation
  - ○ Mismatched source of hematopoietic cells or marrow
  - ○ Use of specific antibiotics during transplantation

Natural History & Prognosis

- Clinical and laboratory features of VOD usually begin within 3 weeks of transplantation
- Occurs most frequently following hematopoietic cell transplantation
  - ○ Affects 50-80% of marrow transplant, stem cell, or umbilical cord blood recipients
  - ○ Responsible for 5-15% of deaths in population with VOD
  - ○ Fatality rate as high as 30% in VOD associated with hematopoietic cell transplantation
  - ○ Severe VOD seen in 15% of patients with hematopoietic cell transplantation
- Prognosis depends on extent of hepatic injury and dysfunctions
- VOD may occasionally be seen in setting of pyrrolizidine alkaloid ingestion in form of teas

Treatment

- Antithrombotic and thrombolytic medication
- Diuretics and sodium restriction
- Analgesia for right upper quadrant pain control

DIAGNOSTIC CHECKLIST

Consider

- Clinical history of recent prior hematopoietic or stem cell transplantation and high dose chemotherapy helpful in diagnosis
- Imaging can only suggest VOD; diagnosis based on clinical criteria ± biopsy
- Liver biopsy is usually diagnostic but is often hazardous due to coexisting coagulopathy
- Clinical diagnosis (modified Seattle criteria)
  - ○ At least 2 of the following occurring within 20 days of transplantation
    - Serum bilirubin > 34 µmol/L (> 2mg/dL)
    - Hepatomegaly with right upper quadrant pain
    - > 2% weight gain from baseline due to fluid retention

Image Interpretation Pearls

- Ultrasound is imaging modality of choice
- Doppler evaluation of hepatic vessels critical in appropriate diagnosis

SELECTED REFERENCES

1. Kambham N et al: Hematopoietic stem cell transplantation: graft versus host disease and pathology of gastrointestinal tract, liver, and lung. Adv Anat Pathol. 21(5):301-20, 2014
2. Zhou H et al: Hepatic sinusoidal obstruction syndrome caused by herbal medicine: CT and MRI features. Korean J Radiol. 15(2):218-25, 2014
3. Mahgerefteh SY et al: Radiologic imaging and intervention for gastrointestinal and hepatic complications of hematopoietic stem cell transplantation. Radiology. 258(3):660-71, 2011
4. Coppell JA et al: Hepatic veno-occlusive disease following stem cell transplantation: incidence, clinical course, and outcome. Biol Blood Marrow Transplant. 16(2):157-68, 2010
5. Rubbia-Brandt L: Sinusoidal obstruction syndrome. Clin Liver Dis. 14(4):651-68, 2010
6. Chung YE et al: Electronic clinical challenges and images in GI. Hepatic venoocclusive disease. Gastroenterology. 135(1):e3-4, 2008
7. Erturk SM et al: CT features of hepatic venoocclusive disease and hepatic graft-versus-host disease in patients after hematopoietic stem cell transplantation. AJR Am J Roentgenol. 186(6):1497-501, 2006
8. Lassau N et al: Prognostic value of doppler-ultrasonography in hepatic veno-occlusive disease. Transplantation. 74(1):60-6, 2002
9. McCarville MB et al: Hepatic veno-occlusive disease in children undergoing bone-marrow transplantation: usefulness of sonographic findings. Pediatr Radiol. 31(2):102-5, 2001
10. van den Bosch MA et al: MR imaging findings in two patients with hepatic veno-occlusive disease following bone marrow transplantation. Eur Radiol. 10(8):1290-3, 2000
11. Lassau N et al: Hepatic veno-occlusive disease after myeloablative treatment and bone marrow transplantation: value of gray-scale and Doppler US in 100 patients. Radiology. 204(2):545-52, 1997
12. McDonald GB et al: Veno-occlusive disease of the liver and multiorgan failure after bone marrow transplantation: a cohort study of 355 patients. Ann Intern Med. 118(4):255-67, 1993

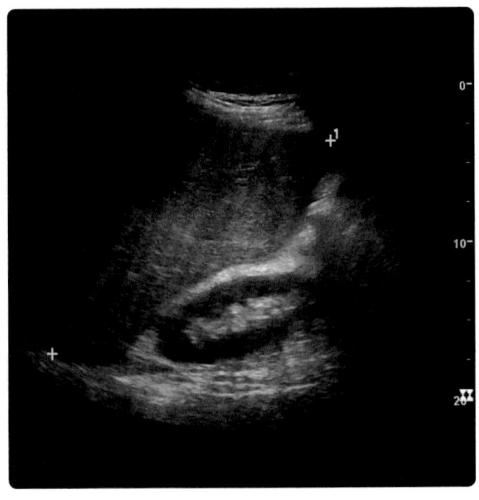

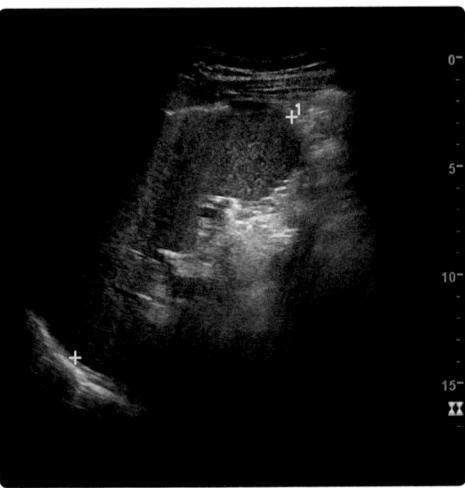

(Left) Grayscale ultrasound of the liver in a patient with VOD shows marked hepatomegaly with craniocaudal length measuring 22.6 cm. Liver extension beyond the edge of the kidney is indicative of hepatomegaly. (Right) Grayscale ultrasound of the spleen shows an enlarged spleen measuring 15 cm in length in this patient with venoocclusive disease.

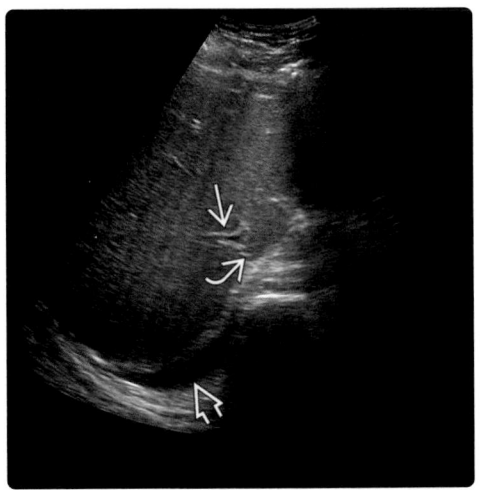

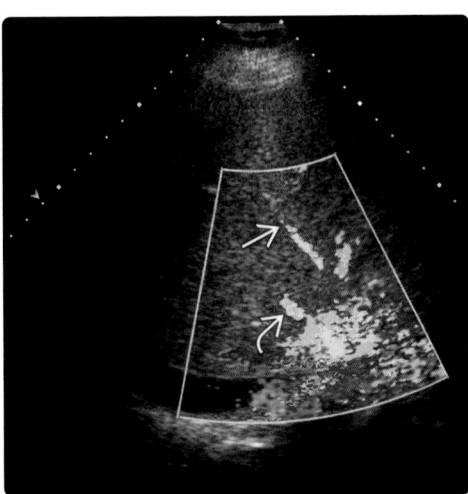

(Left) Grayscale ultrasound shows a small-caliber hepatic vein ➡ and inferior vena cava ➡ due to marked liver edema causing compression upon the compliant venous structures. Also note small right pleural effusion ➡ in this patient with VOD. (Right) Color Doppler ultrasound of the liver shows a narrowed middle ➡ and right ➡ hepatic veins due to diffuse edema of the liver in this patient with VOD.

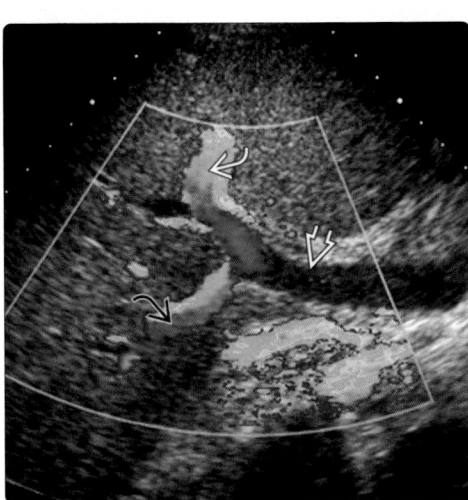

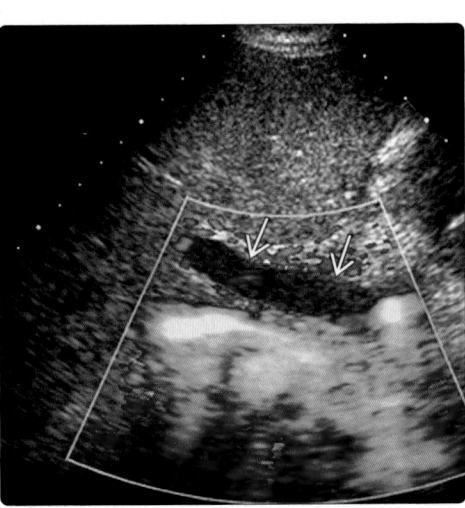

(Left) Color Doppler ultrasound of the liver shows undetectable flow in the main portal vein ➡. Portal flow is hepatofugal in the left portal vein ➡ and hepatopetal flow in the right portal vein ➡. (Right) Power Doppler ultrasound in the same patient shows the flow in the main portal vein is indeed so slow that it is not detectable ➡ even with power Doppler. Real-time grayscale imaging (not shown) was able to demonstrate slow flow in the portal vein with moving rouleaux formation.

TERMINOLOGY

- Benign, congenital or developmental, fluid-filled space with wall derived from biliary endothelium

IMAGING

- Anechoic lesion with posterior acoustic enhancement, well-defined back wall, and no internal vascularity
- May be unilocular or multilocular with barely perceptible septations
- Ultrasound
  - Often demonstrates septations to better advantage than CT or MR
- Current theory
  - True hepatic cysts arise from hamartomatous tissue
- When > 10 in number, consider fibropolycystic diseases
  - Autosomal dominant polycystic liver disease (ADPLD)
  - Autosomal dominant polycystic kidney disease (ADPKD)
  - Biliary hamartomas

TOP DIFFERENTIAL DIAGNOSES

- Biliary cystadenoma/cystadenocarcinoma
- Cystic metastases
- Pyogenic abscess
- Echinococcal/hydatid cyst
- Biloma

PATHOLOGY

- Lined by single layer of cuboidal bile duct epithelium
- Surrounding thin rim of fibrous stroma

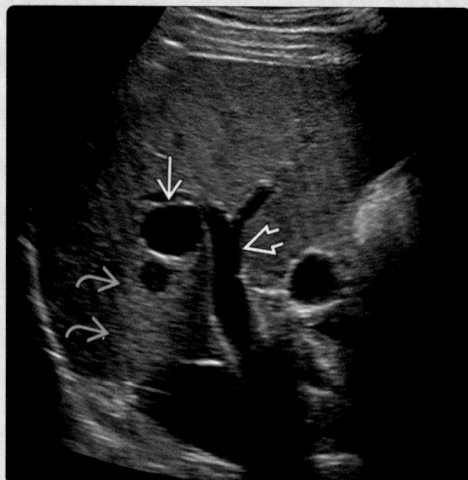
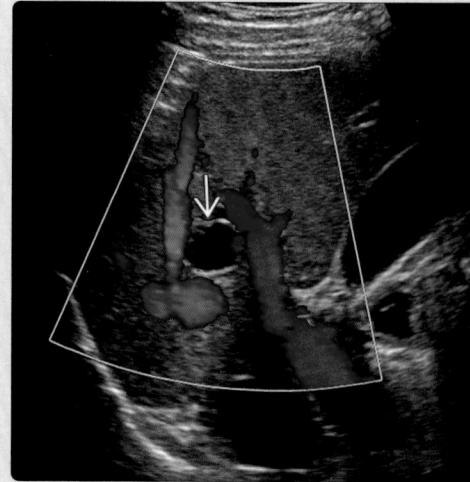

(Left) Transverse grayscale US of the liver shows a cyst ➡ adjacent to the portal vein ⊟. The cyst is anechoic with a well-defined back wall and posterior acoustic enhancement ➡. (Right) Transverse color Doppler US of the same patient shows no internal vascularity in the cyst ➡, confirming the cystic nature of the lesion.

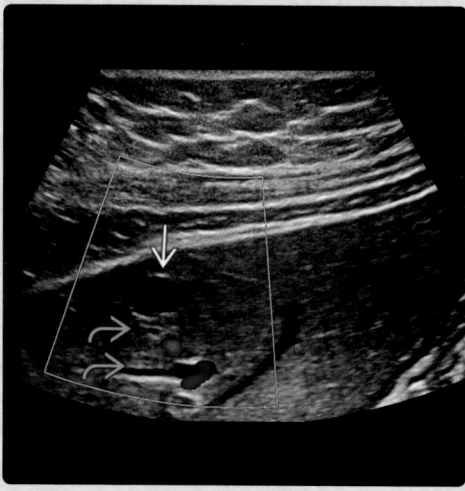
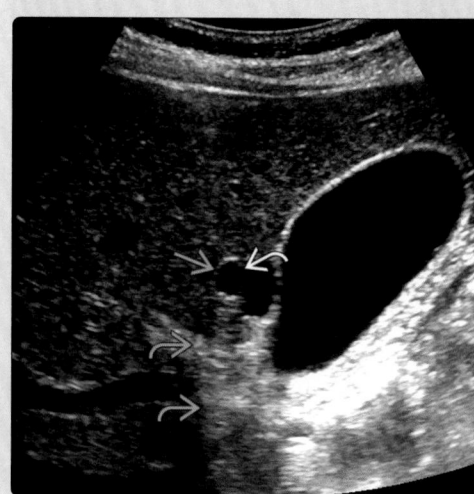

(Left) Longitudinal color Doppler US of the liver shows a cyst ➡ with an anechoic center, well-defined back wall, and posterior acoustic enhancement ➡. (Right) Longitudinal oblique grayscale US of the liver shows a bilobed cyst ➡ with barely perceptible septation ➡ and posterior acoustic enhancement ➡.

TERMINOLOGY

Synonyms

- Hepatic or bile duct cyst; liver cyst

Definitions

- Benign, congenital or developmental, fluid-filled lesion with cyst wall derived from biliary endothelium

IMAGING

General Features

- Best diagnostic clue
  - Anechoic lesion with posterior acoustic enhancement, well-defined back wall, and no internal vascularity
- Location
  - Occur throughout liver
- Size
  - Varies from few mm to 10 cm
- Morphology
  - May be unilocular or multilocular with barely perceptible septations
  - Anechoic fluid
  - Occasionally complicated by hemorrhage
- Key concepts
  - Current theory: True hepatic cysts arise from hamartomatous tissue
  - Common benign liver lesion in 2-7% of population
  - Congenital or developmental: Simple hepatic or bile duct cyst
    - Solitary or multiple
    - No communication with bile ducts
    - More prevalent in women
    - Usually asymptomatic
  - When > 10 in number, consider fibropolycystic diseases: Autosomal dominant polycystic liver disease (ADPLD) (> 20 cysts is diagnostic for ADPLD), autosomal dominant polycystic kidney disease (ADPKD), or biliary hamartomas
  - Acquired cyst-like hepatic lesions
    - Trauma (seroma or biloma)
    - Infection: Pyogenic or parasitic
    - Neoplasm: Primary or metastatic

Ultrasonographic Findings

- Grayscale ultrasound
  - Uncomplicated simple (bile duct) cyst
    - Anechoic rounded
    - Well-defined back wall
    - Posterior acoustic enhancement
    - Smooth or lobulated borders
    - Thin or nondetectable wall
    - No or few barely perceptible septations
    - No mural nodules or wall calcification
    - Do not cross segments
    - Normal adjacent liver parenchyma
  - Hemorrhagic or infected hepatic cyst
    - Internal debris (clots or fibrin strands) may layer or be dispersed within cyst
    - Septation/thickened wall
    - ± calcification
  - Autosomal dominant polycystic liver disease

- Multiple cysts (> 10) 1-10 cm in size
- Anechoic or with debris due to hemorrhage or infection
- Calcification of some cyst walls
- May have barely perceptible septations but no mural nodularity
- Liver often distorted by innumerable cysts
- In severe cases, little hepatic parenchyma is preserved; segmental liver anatomy and normal shape disappear
- Look at kidneys for presence of cysts (ADPKD)
- Color Doppler
  - Adjacent vessels may be distorted by large cysts
  - No internal or mural vascularity

CT Findings

- NECT
  - Simple liver or bile duct cyst
    - Well-defined margins with smooth, thin walls
    - Water density (-10 to +10 HU)
    - No septations or barely perceptible septations, typically up to 2 thin septa
    - No fluid-debris levels, mural nodularity, or wall calcification
  - When complicated by hemorrhage, layering debris may be hyperdense or lesion may mimic tumor
- CECT
  - Simple hepatic cyst or ADPLD
    - Uncomplicated or complicated (infected): No enhancement

MR Findings

- Simple hepatic cyst or ADPLD
  - T1WI: Hypointense
  - T2WI: Hyperintense
    - Markedly increased signal intensity due to pure fluid content
    - Sometimes indistinguishable from a typical hemangioma
  - MRCP: No communication with bile duct
- Complicated (hemorrhagic) cyst
  - T1WI & T2WI
    - Varied signal intensity (due to mixed blood products)
    - ± fluid level
- T1WI C+: No enhancement

Imaging Recommendations

- Best imaging tool
  - Ultrasonography
  - In some indeterminate lesions seen on CT or MR, ultrasound may help characterize lesions as cystic

DIFFERENTIAL DIAGNOSIS

Cystic or Necrotic Metastases

- No posterior acoustic enhancement
- Debris, mural nodularity, or thick septa
- Wall vascularity

Pyogenic Abscess

- Complex cystic mass with debris
- Thick or thin multiple septations
- Mural nodularity & vascularity

- Adjacent parenchyma may be coarse & hypoechoic

Echinococcal/Hydatid Cyst

- Large, well-defined cystic liver mass with numerous peripheral daughter cysts
- Cyst within cyst appearance
- Unilocular, multilocular, multiseptated, heterogeneous
- Floating membrane and daughter cysts within
- ± calcification & dilated bile ducts

Biliary Cystadenoma/Cystadenocarcinoma

- Multiseptated cystic mass; enhancing or vascular septations
- More common in women
- May show fine mural or septal calcification
- Mural nodule or papillary excrescence with vascularity suggests cystadenocarcinoma
- May be associated with dilated biliary ducts

Biloma

- Collection of bile usually associated with biliary tract injury
- Typically symptomatic

PATHOLOGY

General Features

- Etiology
  - Congenital simple hepatic cyst
    - Defective development of intrahepatic biliary duct (IHBD)
- Associated abnormalities
  - ADPLD
    - 50% have polycystic kidney disease; M:F = 1:2
    - Multiple hepatic cysts of varying size
  - Polycystic kidney disease: 83% have hepatic cysts
  - Tuberous sclerosis

Gross Pathologic & Surgical Features

- Cyst wall: ≤ 1 mm thick

Microscopic Features

- Single unilocular cyst with serous fluid
- Lined by single layer of cuboidal bile duct epithelium
- Surrounding thin rim of fibrous stroma

CLINICAL ISSUES

Presentation

- Most common signs/symptoms
  - Uncomplicated simple cysts & ADPLD
    - Usually asymptomatic, detected incidentally
  - Complicated cyst: Pain &/or fever
  - Large cysts may present with symptoms of mass effect
    - Abdominal pain (due to capsular distension), jaundice (due to biliary obstruction), palpable mass
  - Patients with advanced disease of ADPLD may present with
    - Hepatomegaly, liver failure, Budd-Chiari syndrome
- Clinical profile
  - Asymptomatic patient with incidental detection of simple hepatic cyst on imaging
  - Patients with large hepatic cyst & mass effect: ↑ direct bilirubin levels
  - Patients with advanced disease of ADPLD: ↑ LFTs

Demographics

- Age
  - Any age group (usually discovered incidentally in 5th-7th decades)
  - May slowly increase in size
- Gender
  - M:F = 1:5
- Epidemiology
  - Reported to occur in 2.5% of population
  - Incidence: 1-14% in autopsy series

Natural History & Prognosis

- Complications
  - Hemorrhage, infection, or rupture
  - Large cyst: Compression of IHBD & jaundice
- Prognosis
  - Small & large hepatic cysts: Good prognosis
  - Advanced disease of ADPLD: Good prognosis

Treatment

- Asymptomatic simple hepatic cyst & ADPLD
  - No treatment
- Large, symptomatic, infected hepatic cyst
  - Percutaneous aspiration & sclerotherapy with alcohol
  - Surgical resection or marsupialization
- Advanced disease of ADPLD
  - Partial liver resection, liver transplantation

DIAGNOSTIC CHECKLIST

Consider

- Rule out cyst-like hepatic lesions from infection, neoplasm, or trauma

Image Interpretation Pearls

- Anechoic, thin wall, posterior acoustic enhancement
- No internal or mural vascularity
- Internal debris may settle under gravity, visible at end of examination
- If multiple, evaluate kidneys to rule out ADPKD

SELECTED REFERENCES

1. Gevers TJ et al: Diagnosis and management of polycystic liver disease. Nat Rev Gastroenterol Hepatol. 10(2):101-8, 2013
2. Lantinga MA et al: Evaluation of hepatic cystic lesions. World J Gastroenterol. 19(23):3543-54, 2013
3. Jabłońska B: Biliary cysts: etiology, diagnosis and management. World J Gastroenterol. 18(35):4801-10, 2012
4. Anderson SW et al: Benign hepatic tumors and iatrogenic pseudotumors. Radiographics. 29(1):211-29, 2009
5. Mortelé KJ et al: Multimodality imaging of common and uncommon cystic focal liver lesions. Semin Ultrasound CT MR. 30(5):368-86, 2009
6. Liang P et al: Differential diagnosis of hepatic cystic lesions with gray-scale and color Doppler sonography. J Clin Ultrasound. 33(3):100-5, 2005
7. 1. Horton KM et al: CT and MR imaging of benign hepatic and biliary tumors. Radiographics. 19(2):431-51, 1999

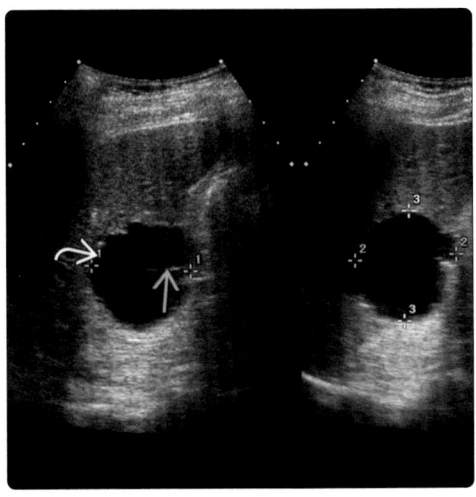
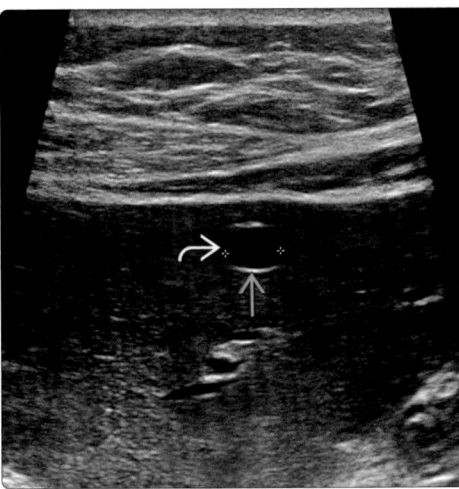

(Left) *Transverse and longitudinal grayscale views of the liver show a cyst ➡ with barely perceptible septation ➡.* (Right) *High-resolution transverse grayscale US of the liver shows a small cyst ➡ under the liver capsule with a well-defined back wall ➡.*

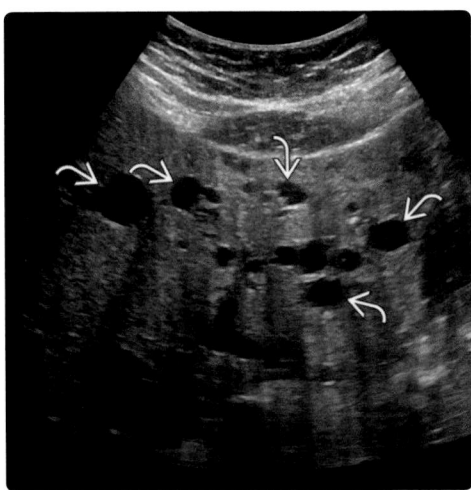
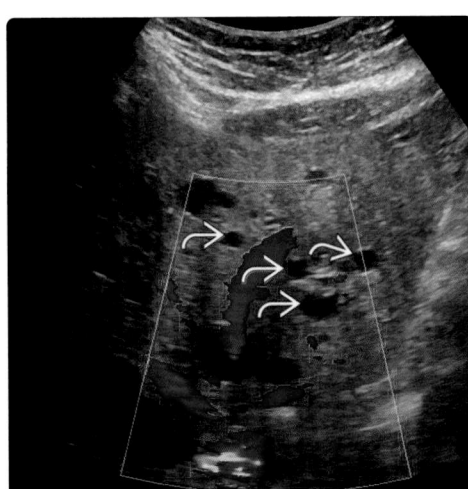

(Left) *Transverse grayscale US of the liver shows innumerable cysts ➡ throughout the liver in a patient with polycystic liver disease.* (Right) *Transverse color Doppler US of the liver confirms that multiple cysts ➡ in the liver do not have internal vascularity.*

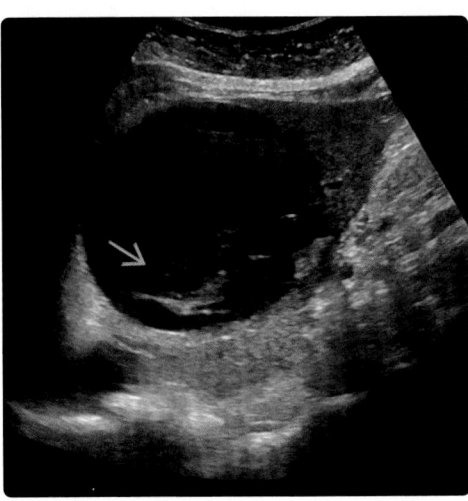
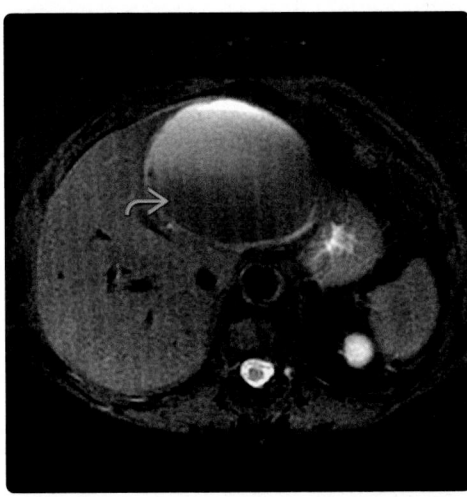

(Left) *Longitudinal oblique US of the liver shows a complicated liver cyst with internal layering debris ➡ from hemorrhage.* (Right) *Axial T2 FS MR in the same patient shows layering low signal ➡ in the complicated cyst reflecting internal blood components.*

Biliary Hamartoma

TERMINOLOGY

- Benign malformations of biliary tract
- Synonyms: von Meyenburg complex, bile duct hamartoma

IMAGING

- Ultrasound
  - Grayscale ultrasound
    - Numerous small, hypoechoic or hyperechoic foci uniformly distributed throughout liver
      - Leads to inhomogeneous and coarse appearance of liver echotexture
    - Multiple echogenic foci, often with associated "comet tail" artifacts
    - Typically smaller lesions appear as echogenic foci whereas larger lesions appear cystic
      - Often extent of echogenic foci on ultrasound is greater than anticipated, based on comparison CT or MR
  - Color Doppler ultrasound
    - Twinkling artifact may be seen
- MRCP
  - Numerous scattered, tiny cysts without communication between lesions and biliary tree

TOP DIFFERENTIAL DIAGNOSES

- Multiple simple hepatic cysts
- Multiple small hepatic metastasis
- Hepatic microabscesses
- Autosomal dominant polycystic liver disease
- Caroli disease

CLINICAL ISSUES

- May be misdiagnosed as multiple hepatic metastasis, microabscesses, cirrhosis, lymphoma, leukemia, etc. at initial imaging
- No further evaluation necessary when seen as isolated finding in healthy, nononcologic patient

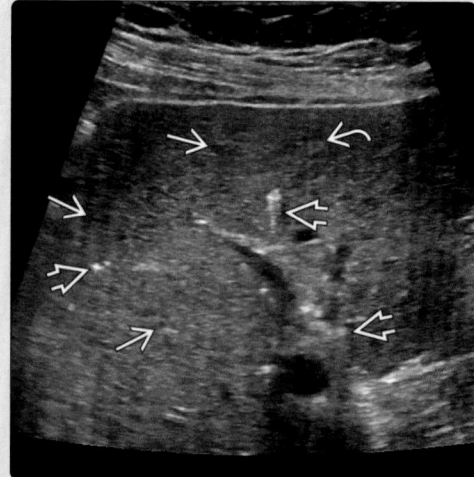
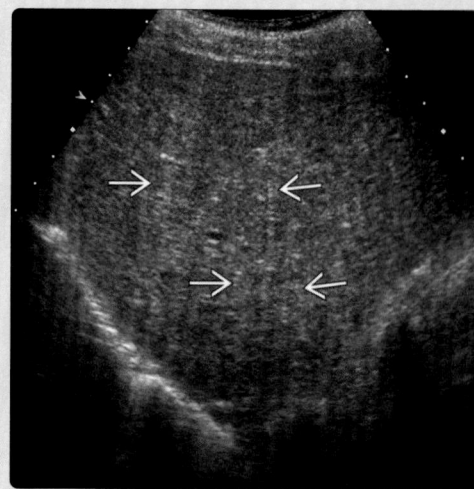

(Left) Grayscale ultrasound of liver with numerous biliary hamartomas shows diffuse inhomogeneous and coarse parenchymal echotexture with numerous small, hypoechoic ➡ and hyperechoic ➡ foci. Note some echogenic foci have associated "comet tail" artifacts ➡. (Right) Grayscale ultrasound of the liver shows diffuse, coarse, parenchymal echotexture with multiple echogenic foci, some with associated "comet tail" artifacts ➡ generated from the biliary hamartomas.

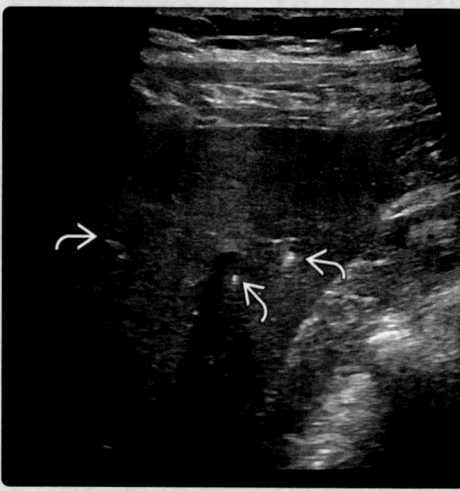
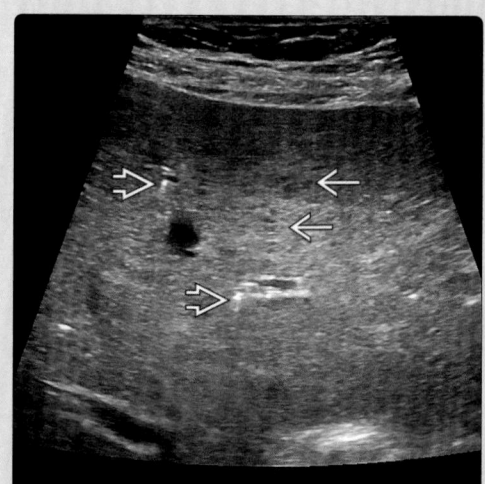

(Left) Grayscale ultrasound of the liver in a patient with multiple biliary hamartomas as evidenced by multiple tiny echogenic foci, some of which are associated with "comet tail" artifacts ➡. (Right) Grayscale ultrasound of liver shows heterogeneous echotexture of liver parenchyma due to numerous tiny, hypoechoic nodules ➡ representing biliary hamartomas. Note several "comet tail" artifacts emanating from several of the hamartomas ➡.

TERMINOLOGY

Synonyms
- von Meyenburg complex, bile duct hamartoma

Definitions
- Benign malformations of biliary tract

IMAGING

General Features
- Best diagnostic clue: Numerous small cystic lesions < 1.5 cm in diameter throughout whole liver
- Location: Subcapsular or intraparenchymal location
- Size: 0.2-1.5 cm (rarely larger)
- Morphology
  - Typically well circumscribed but not encapsulated
  - Multiple lesions much more common, rarely solitary

Ultrasonographic Findings
- Grayscale ultrasound
  - Numerous small, hypo-/hyperechoic foci uniformly distributed throughout liver
    - When small, appear hyperechoic due to inability to resolve tiny cysts
    - Appear cystic when > 2-3 mm
    - Leads to inhomogeneous and coarse appearance of liver echotexture
  - Multiple echogenic foci: May see associated "comet tail" artifacts
  - Liver often more echogenic with fewer cystic lesions than anticipated based on prior CT or MR due to cystic lesions being too small to resolve internal cystic space
- Color Doppler
  - May see twinkling artifact
    - Rapidly alternating red and blue color Doppler signal behind echogenic foci
    - Thought to be related to multiple reverberations from cholesterol crystals within cystic dilatation of bile ducts

CT Findings
- CECT
  - Solid components (fibrous stroma) can enhance and may become nearly isodense to liver
  - Multiple small, round, and well-defined nodules of low attenuation without enhancement

MR Findings
- T1WI: Low signal; T2WI: High signal due to fluid content
- T1WI C+: Usually no enhancement, but thin rim enhancement reported related to compressed liver parenchyma surrounding biliary hamartoma
- MRCP: Numerous tiny cysts without communication with biliary tree

Imaging Recommendations
- Best imaging tool
  - Ultrasound with grayscale and color Doppler
  - MRCP/heavily T2WI

DIFFERENTIAL DIAGNOSIS

Multiple Simple Hepatic Cysts
- Rarely as numerous as biliary hamartomas
- Regularly outlined and no contrast enhancement

Multiple Small Hepatic Metastasis
- More varied in size and distribution
- More mural nodularity and complexity, rim enhancement

Hepatic Microabscesses
- Enhancing wall, double target sign can be seen
- In immunosuppressed patient with fever

Autosomal Dominant Polycystic Liver Disease
- Usually larger cysts, and coexisting cysts in kidneys and other organs

Caroli Disease
- Small, round/saccular dilatations of intrahepatic ducts
- "Central dot" sign on US, CECT, and MR
  - Enhancing tiny dots (portal radicles) within dilated IHD

PATHOLOGY

General Features
- Etiology
  - Congenital ductal plate malformation due to failure of involution of embryonic bile ducts
  - May coexist with autosomal dominant polycystic kidney disease (APDKD), Caroli disease, congenital hepatic fibrosis, bile duct atresia, or choledochal cyst

Microscopic Features
- Noncommunicating bile ducts interspersed within hyalinized fibrocollagenous stroma; may contain proteinaceous debris or bile

CLINICAL ISSUES

Presentation
- Asymptomatic and of no clinical concern

Demographics
- Detected incidentally at autopsy in 0.6-5.6% of cases

DIAGNOSTIC CHECKLIST

Consider
- May be misdiagnosed as multiple hepatic metastases, microabscesses, cirrhosis, lymphoma, leukemia, etc. at initial imaging
- No further evaluation necessary when seen as isolated finding in healthy, nononcologic patient

Image Interpretation Pearls
- In setting of numerous small cysts in healthy patients
- Ultrasound: Numerous echogenic foci often with accompanying "comet tail" artifacts throughout whole liver; may see associated color Doppler twinkling artifact

SELECTED REFERENCES

1. Vachha B et al: Cystic lesions of the liver. AJR Am J Roentgenol. 196(4):W355-66, 2011

(Left) *Grayscale ultrasound of the liver shows inhomogeneous liver parenchymal echotexture due to multiple biliary hamartomas that are too small to resolve. Other small, cystic lesions* ➡ *represent slightly larger biliary hamartomas in which the internal cystic content can be resolved.* (Right) *On a color Doppler ultrasound, the cystic space is confirmed to be avascular* ➡ *in this patient with numerous biliary hamartomas.*

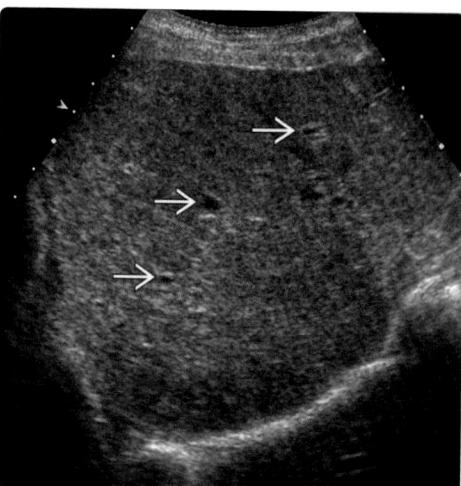 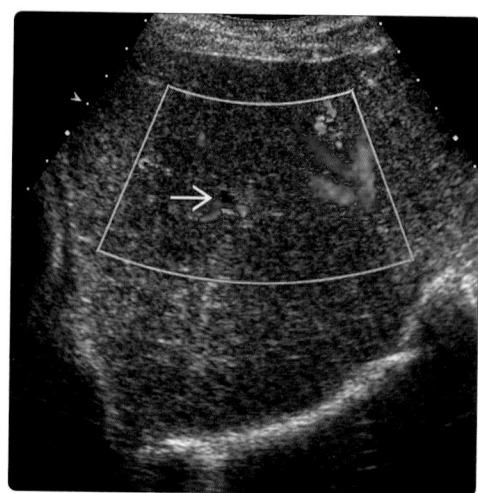

(Left) *Axial CECT in the same patient shows multiple tiny, low-density biliary hamartomas randomly distributed in the liver parenchyma* ➡. (Right) *Grayscale ultrasound of the liver shows multiple tiny, echogenic foci with associated "comet tail" artifacts* ➡ *in this patient with multiple biliary hamartomas.*

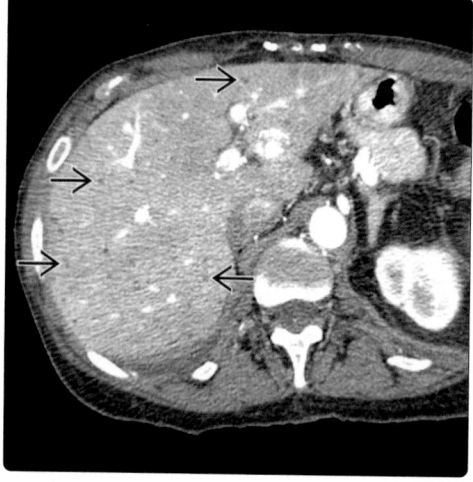 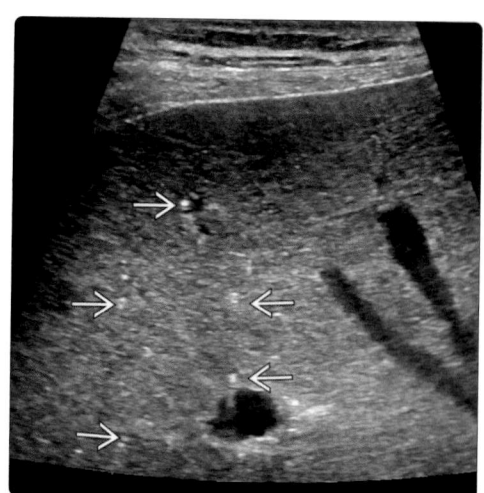

(Left) *Grayscale ultrasound of liver shows multiple tiny, echogenic foci* ➡ *with "comet tail" artifacts from biliary hamartomas.* (Right) *Axial T2 FS MR of the liver shows innumerable high signal intensity foci* ➡ *consistent with biliary hamartomas.*

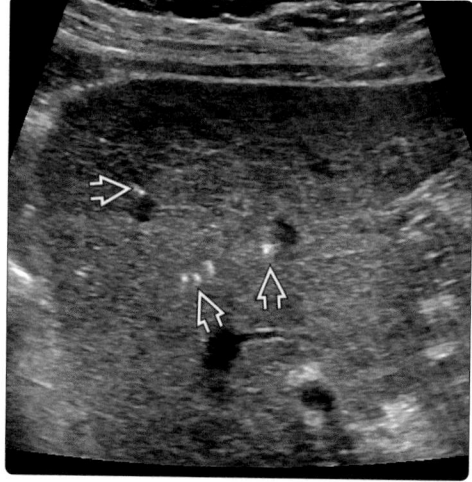 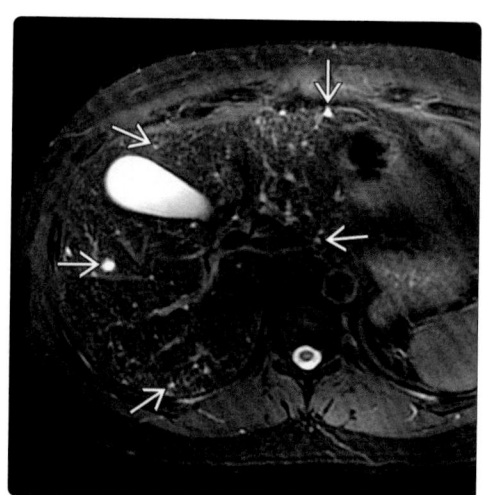

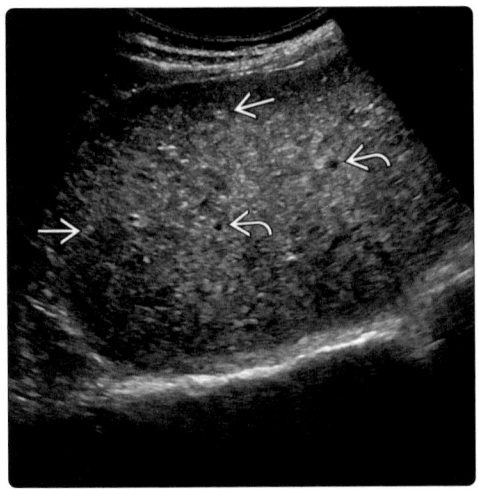
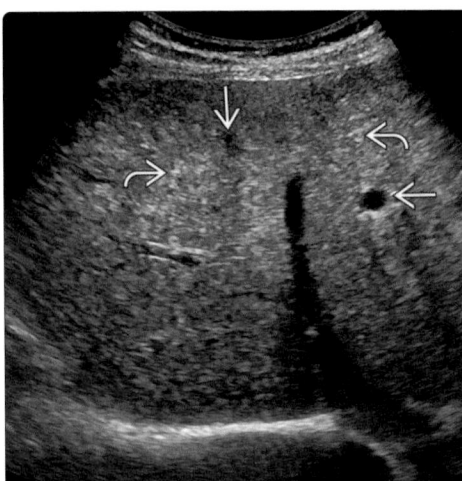

(Left) *Ultrasound of the liver shows numerous tiny echogenic foci* ➔ *and several cystic lesions* ➔, *corresponding to biliary hamartomas. Parenchymal echotexture is heterogeneous due to biliary hamartomas.* (Right) *Ultrasound shows heterogeneous liver echotexture due to multiple biliary hamartomas* ➔ *that are too small to resolve. Other slightly larger cystic lesions with posterior enhancement* ➔ *represent biliary hamartomas in which the internal content can be resolved.*

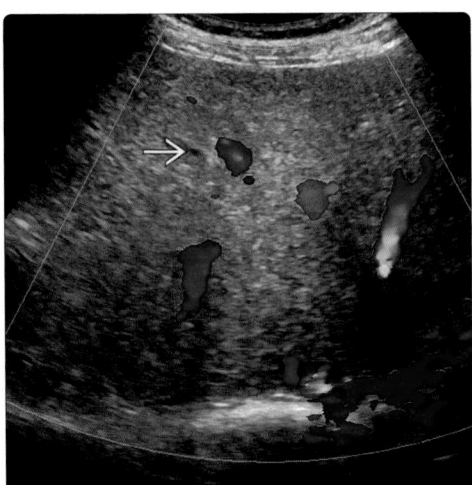
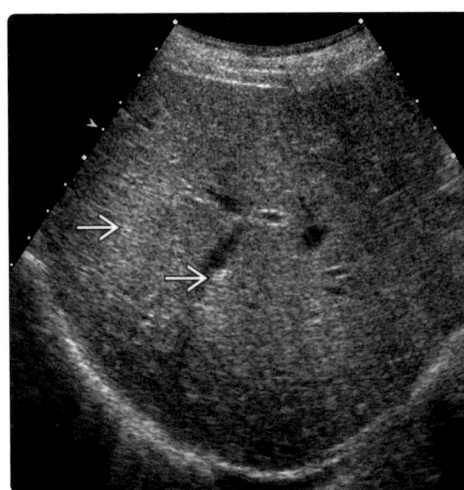

(Left) *Ultrasound shows heterogeneous liver parenchymal echotexture due to multiple biliary hamartomas that are too small to resolve. A small, cystic, slightly larger biliary hamartoma* ➔ *is seen in which the internal cystic content is resolved.* (Right) *Ultrasound of the liver shows coarse parenchymal echotexture with multiple tiny echogenic foci* ➔ *throughout the liver due to the presence of multiple small biliary hamartomas.*

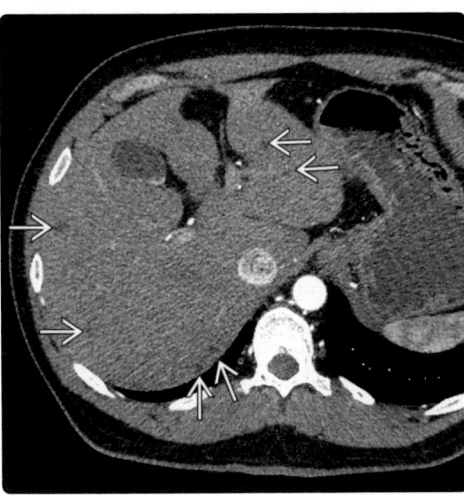
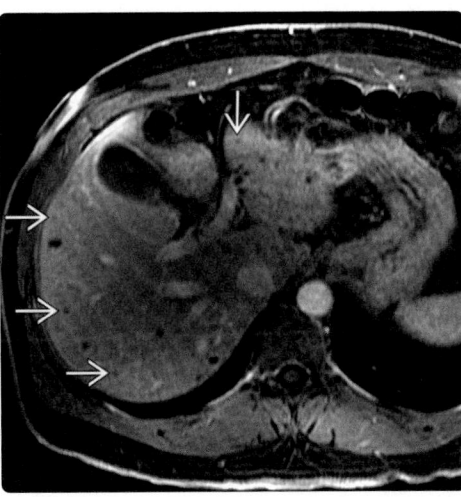

(Left) *Arterial phase of contrast-enhanced CT shows multiple tiny cystic lesions in the liver* ➔, *which represent biliary hamartomas.* (Right) *In the venous phase of a contrast-enhanced T1-weighted MR in the same patient, the same tiny biliary hamartomas* ➔ *are seen to a slightly better advantage as nonenhancing, tiny rounded foci throughout the liver.*

Caroli Disease

TERMINOLOGY

- Caroli disease: Congenital, multifocal, segmental, cystic dilatations of intrahepatic bile ducts
- Caroli syndrome: Cystic bile duct dilatation with hepatic fibrosis

IMAGING

- Segmental saccular dilatation of large intrahepatic bile ducts
- "Central dot" sign: Characteristic finding
  o Echogenic dots with color flow within cystic lesion on US/color Doppler US
  o Enhancing portal radicles within dilated intrahepatic bile ducts on CECT/MR

TOP DIFFERENTIAL DIAGNOSES

- AD polycystic liver disease
- Recurrent pyogenic cholangitis
- Primary sclerosing cholangitis

- Ascending cholangitis
- Biliary hamartoma

PATHOLOGY

- Etiology: Incomplete remodeling of ductal plate leading to persistence of embryonic biliary ductal structures
  o Caroli disease: Malformation of large-sized ducts (more common in adults)
  o Caroli syndrome: Malformation of large- and small-sized ducts (more common in children)
- Todani classification of congenital bile duct cysts: Type V

CLINICAL ISSUES

- Symptoms/signs: Related to cholangitis and hepatic fibrosis

DIAGNOSTIC CHECKLIST

- Rule out other liver diseases, which have hepatic cysts ± dilated bile ducts

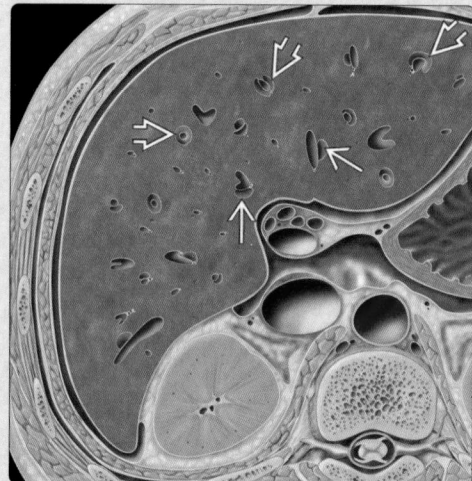
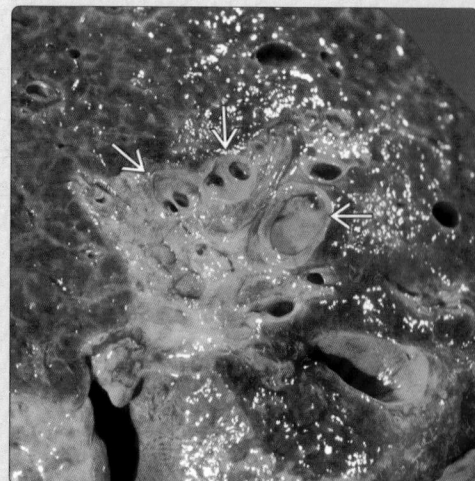

(Left) *Transverse graphic shows focally dilated intrahepatic ductules* ➡ *running adjacent to portal venules in Caroli disease. The dilated ductule may encircle* ➡ *the adjacent vein, creating a "central dot" sign appearance on cross-sectional imaging.* (Right) *Gross photograph of the liver shows clusters of dilated and cystic intrahepatic bile ducts* ➡. *(From: DP Nonneoplastic Pediatrics.)*

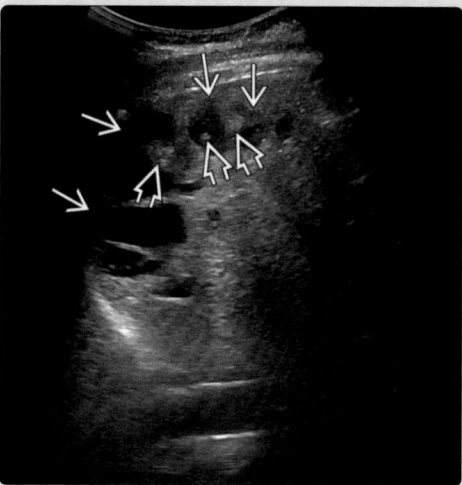
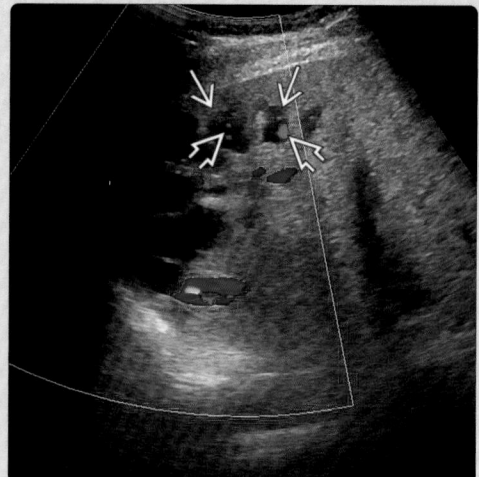

(Left) *Oblique abdominal ultrasound in a young patient with Caroli disease shows multiple dilated intrahepatic ducts* ➡. *Echogenic portal radicles* ➡ *are surrounded by dilated ducts.* (Right) *Oblique abdominal color Doppler ultrasound in the same patient shows color flow in portal radicles* ➡ *surrounded by dilated intrahepatic ducts* ➡, *which creates the "central dot" sign appearance.*

TERMINOLOGY

Synonyms

- Communicating cavernous biliary ectasia

Definitions

- Caroli disease: Congenital, multifocal, segmental, cystic dilatations of intrahepatic bile ducts (IHBD)
- Caroli syndrome: Caroli disease + congenital hepatic fibrosis

IMAGING

General Features

- Best diagnostic clue
  - "Central dot" sign: Portal radicles within dilated intrahepatic bile ducts on ultrasound, CECT/MR
  - Multiple intrahepatic cysts of varying size that communicate with biliary tree
- Location
  - Liver; diffuse, lobar, or segmental distribution
    - Caroli disease: Mostly diffuse, occasionally lobar
    - Caroli syndrome: Almost always diffuse
- Size
  - Varies from few millimeters to few centimeters
- Morphology
  - Segmental saccular dilatation of large intrahepatic bile ducts separated by normal or dilated bile ducts
  - Contiguous with biliary tree
  - Common bile duct is usually normal in caliber
    - If dilated, consider coexisting obstructing stone, cholangitis, concurrent choledochal cyst, or prior intervention
  - Todani classification of congenital bile duct cysts
    - Caroli disease is classified as type V: Cystic dilatation of intrahepatic bile ducts

Ultrasonographic Findings

- Grayscale ultrasound
  - Dilated intrahepatic bile ducts
    - Focal or diffuse involvement in liver
    - Saccular or fusiform configuration
    - Contains sludge due to biliary stasis
    - May contain calculi, which do not form casts of ducts
  - "Intraductal bridging" sign
    - Echogenic septa partially or completely traversing dilated lumen of bile ducts
  - "Central dot" sign
    - Small portal venous branches partially or completely surrounded by dilated IHBDs
  - Abscess formation if complicated by cholangitis
- Color Doppler
  - Color flow in portal radicles surrounded by dilated IHBDs: "Central dot" sign

Radiographic Findings

- Endoscopic retrograde cholangiopancreatogram (ERCP) findings
  - Saccular dilatations communicating with IHBDs
  - Sludge and hepatolithiasis, biliary stricture
  - May show communicating hepatic abscesses

CT Findings

- NECT
  - Multiple, rounded, hypodense areas inseparable from dilated IHBD
  - May see hyperdense biliary stones
  - Findings related to concurrent hepatic fibrosis
    - Hypertrophic left lobe, atrophic right lobe of liver
- CECT
  - Nonenhancing cysts of varying size communicating biliary tree
  - "Central dot" sign
    - Enhancing tiny dots (portal radicles) surrounded by dilated IHBD

MR Findings

- T1WI
  - Multiple hypointense, saccular dilatations of IHBDs
  - Hypointense in area of hepatic fibrosis
- T2WI
  - Hyperintense cystic spaces
- T1WI C+
  - "Central dot" sign: Enhancement of portal radicles within dilated IHBD
  - Cystic structures fill with contrast agent (gadoxetic acid) in hepatobiliary phase, contiguous with biliary tree
- MRCP
  - Multiple hyperintense, oval-shaped, cystic dilatations
  - Continuity with biliary tree
  - Luminal contents of bile ducts appear hyperintense in contrast to portal vein, which appears as signal void

Nuclear Medicine Findings

- Hepatobiliary scan: Unusual pattern of retained activity throughout liver
- Technetium sulfur colloid: Multiple cold defects

DIFFERENTIAL DIAGNOSIS

AD Polycystic Liver Disease

- Hepatic cysts
  - Numerous: > 10, usually hundreds
  - Do not communicate with each other or biliary tract
  - Not associated with biliary ductal dilatation
  - Do not demonstrate saccular configuration
- Often harbor renal cysts; not confined to medulla

Recurrent Pyogenic Cholangitis

- Intra- and extrahepatic biliary stones: Cast-like
- Dilatation of both intra- & extrahepatic bile ducts, usually of cylindrical and not saccular type
- Associated with parasitic and bacterial biliary infection (liver flukes)

Primary Sclerosing Cholangitis

- Strictures of both intra- and extrahepatic bile ducts
- Ductal dilatation not as great as Caroli disease; not saccular
- Often shows isolated obstructions of IHBDs
- Often progresses to cirrhosis and liver failure

Ascending Cholangitis

- Intrahepatic abscesses communicate with bile ducts: Irregular margin

- Bile duct wall thickening and enhancement
- Extrahepatic bile duct dilatation due to obstructing stones or tumor

Biliary Hamartoma

- Variant of fibropolycystic disease
- Ductal plate malformation: Involves small-sized IHBDs
- Innumerable subcentimeter cysts/nodules in liver
- Do not communicate with biliary tree
- Variable enhancement
  - Completely cystic: No enhancement
  - Solid elements in walls: Enhance and become isodense with liver

PATHOLOGY

General Features

- Etiology
  - Incomplete remodeling of ductal plate leading to persistence of embryonic biliary ductal structures
  - Varying spectrum of adult and juvenile manifestations of ductal malformations
    - Caroli disease: Malformation of large-sized ducts (more common in adults)
    - Caroli syndrome: Malformation of large- and small-sized ducts (more common in children)
      □ Ductal plate anomaly of small-sized ducts leads to hepatic fibrosis
- Genetics
  - Inherited as an autosomal recessive pattern
- Associated abnormalities
  - Medullary sponge kidney (renal tubular ectasia)
  - Autosomal recessive polycystic kidney disease (ARPKD); rarely autosomal dominant polycystic kidney disease (ADPKD)
  - Hepatic fibrosis, biliary hamartoma, choledochal cysts

Gross Pathologic & Surgical Features

- Saccular dilatations of large intrahepatic bile ducts
- Diffuse, lobar or segmental distribution

Microscopic Features

- Caroli disease
  - Segmental saccular dilatation of large IHBDs
  - Dilated ducts lined by hyperplastic or ulcerated biliary epithelium
  - Normal hepatic parenchyma
- Caroli syndrome
  - Segmental saccular dilatation of IHBDs
  - Proliferation of bile ductules and fibrosis
  - Hypoplastic portal vein branches

CLINICAL ISSUES

Presentation

- Most common signs/symptoms
  - Usually asymptomatic in early state
  - Symptoms/signs related to cholangitis
    - Fever, abdominal pain, jaundice
  - Symptoms/signs related to hepatic fibrosis
    - Hepatomegaly

- Portal hypertension and its sequelae (splenomegaly, varices, etc.)
- Other signs/symptoms
  - Enlarged kidneys due to associated ARPKD
- Lab data: May show elevated liver enzymes & bilirubin levels
- Diagnosis based on imaging; biopsy is rarely indicated

Demographics

- Age
  - Condition present at birth, but can be asymptomatic for years
    - 80% become symptomatic before age of 30
  - Caroli disease
    - Symptoms usually present in 2nd & 3rd decades
  - Caroli syndrome
    - Symptoms can present earlier during infancy or childhood
- Gender: M:F = 1:1
- Epidemiology: Rare disease

Natural History & Prognosis

- Complications
  - Recurrent cholangitis, biliary stone formation, hepatic abscesses
  - Secondary biliary cirrhosis; portal hypertension and its sequelae
  - Cholangiocarcinoma in 7% of patients
- Prognosis
  - Depends on severity of disease and coexisting renal disease
  - Long-term prognosis for Caroli disease is usually poor

Treatment

- Supportive therapy for cholangitis
- Decompression of biliary tract: External drainage or biliary-enteric anastomoses
- Surgery
  - Localized to lobe or segment: Hepatic lobectomy or segmentectomy
  - Diffuse disease: Liver transplantation

DIAGNOSTIC CHECKLIST

Consider

- Rule out other liver diseases, which have hepatic cysts ± dilated bile ducts

Image Interpretation Pearls

- US/CT/MR: "Central dot" sign
- ERCP/MRCP: Saccular dilatations show communication with IHBD, which differentiates Caroli from other variants of fibropolycystic disease

SELECTED REFERENCES

1. Venkatanarasimha N et al: Imaging features of ductal plate malformations in adults. Clin Radiol. 66(11):1086-93, 2011
2. Levy AD et al: Caroli's disease: radiologic spectrum with pathologic correlation. AJR Am J Roentgenol. 179(4):1053-7, 2002
3. Gorka W et al: Value of Doppler sonography in the assessment of patients with Caroli's disease. J Clin Ultrasound. 26(6):283-7, 1998

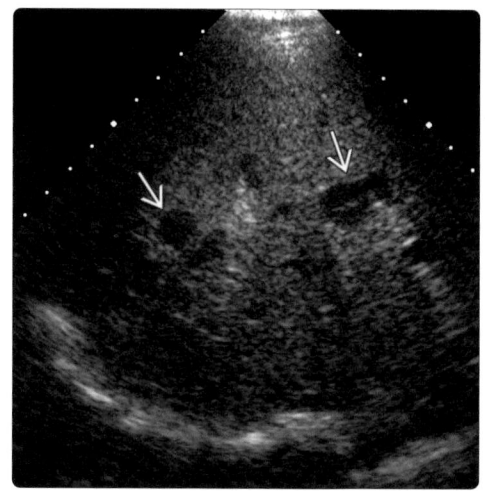
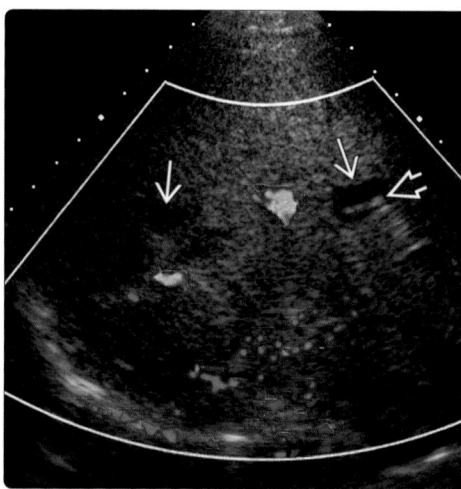

(Left) Oblique abdominal ultrasound in a patient with Caroli disease shows multiple dilated intrahepatic ducts ➡. (Right) Oblique abdominal color Doppler ultrasound in the same patient with Caroli disease shows dilated intrahepatic ducts ➡. The "intraductal bridging" sign is seen in 1 of the dilated ducts ➡ in which an echogenic septum traverses the dilated bile duct lumen. This is a finding often seen with Caroli disease.

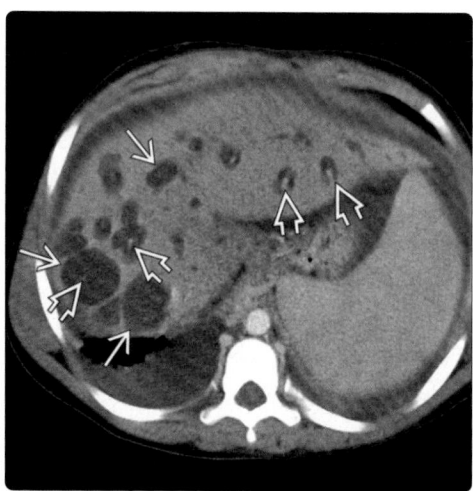
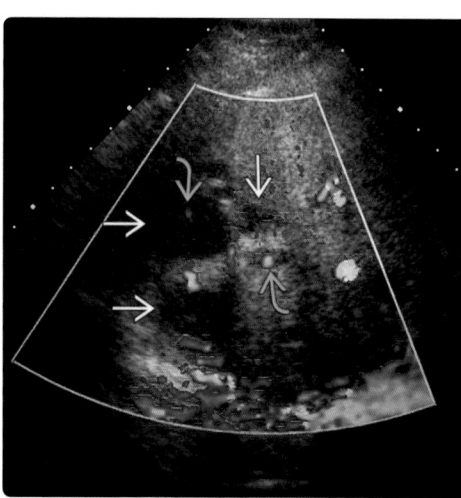

(Left) Axial CECT in a patient with Caroli disease shows massive dilatation of intrahepatic bile ducts ➡. Note the enhancing dots within many of the cystic structures representing portal radicles ➡ ("central dot" sign). (Right) Oblique abdominal color Doppler ultrasound in the same patient with Caroli disease shows multiple dilated intrahepatic ducts ➡ with central flow ➘, creating a "central dot" sign appearance.

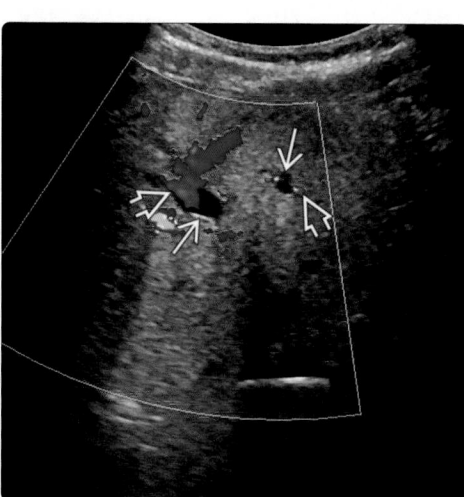
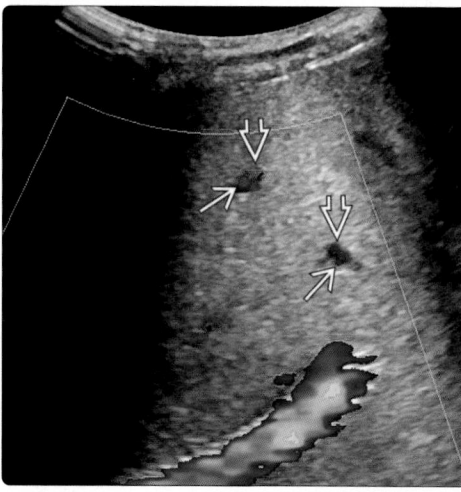

(Left) Oblique abdominal color Doppler ultrasound in a patient with Caroli disease shows several dilated intrahepatic ducts ➡ adjacent to portal veins ➡. (Right) Oblique abdominal color Doppler ultrasound in the same patient with Caroli disease shows color flow in the portal radicles ➡ that are surrounded by the dilated intrahepatic ducts ➡.

Biloma

TERMINOLOGY

- Encapsulated collection of bile outside biliary tree

IMAGING

- Ultrasound
  - Grayscale ultrasound
    - Focal collection of fluid within liver or close to biliary tree, or in gallbladder fossa in patients with recent cholecystectomy
    - Round or oval in shape, usually unilocular, usually no discernible thin capsule
    - Anechoic fluid content suggests fresh biloma
    - Debris or septa suggest infected biloma
    - May see echogenic foci at periphery related to dips from recent surgery
  - Color Doppler ultrasound
    - No vascularity within lesion
    - For infected biloma, there may be increased vascularity in adjacent tissue

- CECT: Well-defined or slightly irregular cystic lesion without identifiable wall

TOP DIFFERENTIAL DIAGNOSES

- Perihepatic collection/seroma/lymphocele
- Hepatic cyst
- Hepatic abscess
- Intrahepatic hematoma

PATHOLOGY

- Iatrogenic: Laparoscopic cholecystectomy, post liver transplantation, ERCP or other instrumentation of biliary tree, liver biopsy
- Post-traumatic: Blunt trauma, motor vehicle accident
- Spontaneous rupture of bile duct

DIAGNOSTIC CHECKLIST

- Consider underlying infection if low-level echoes within biloma on ultrasound

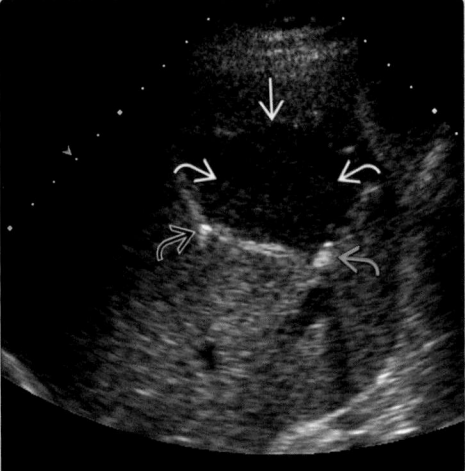
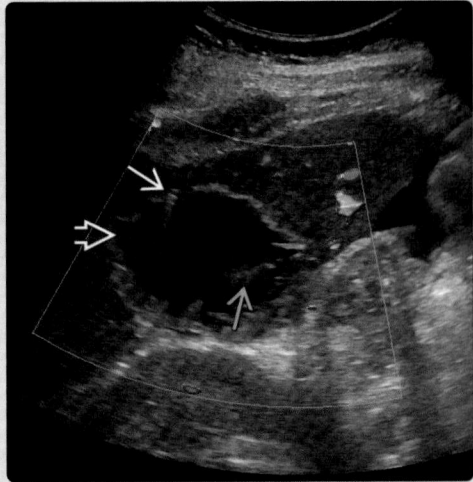

(Left) Grayscale US shows a biloma ➡ after surgical removal of a liver mass. Low-level internal echoes ➡ suggest infected bile. Peripheral surgical suture with a ring-down artifact ➡ and clip with posterior shadowing ➡ are seen. (Right) Transverse color Doppler US of the liver shows a biloma ➡ in a resection cavity with peripheral echogenic foci ➡ with posterior ring down, likely related to surgical clip. A small amount of internal debris is seen in the periphery of the biloma ➡.

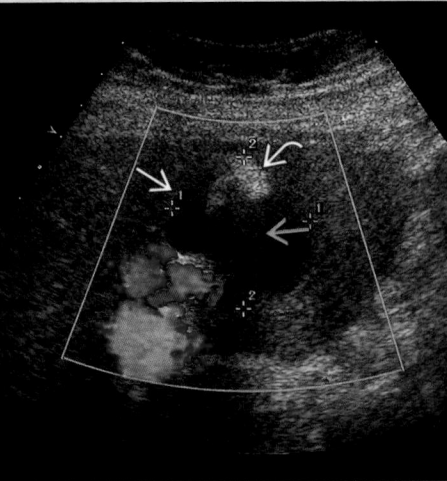
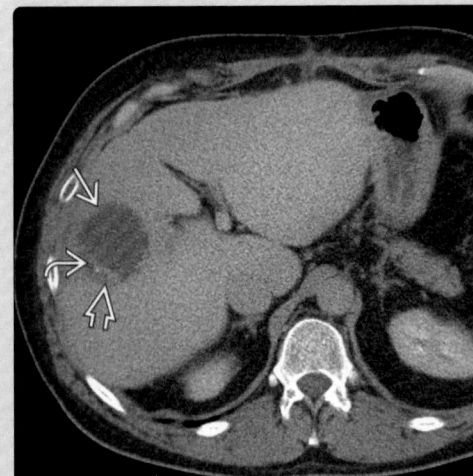

(Left) Transverse color Doppler US of the liver shows an infected biloma ➡. The lesion is avascular and contains gas ➡ that demonstrates posterior dirty shadowing ➡. (Right) Delayed phase CECT shows a round cystic mass without a discernible wall ➡ containing internal debris ➡ and layering debris ➡ in the dependent portion, which suggests infected biloma.

TERMINOLOGY

Definitions

- Encapsulated collection of bile outside biliary tree

IMAGING

General Features

- Location
  - Intrahepatic or extrahepatic, in gallbladder fossa in patients with recent cholecystectomy

Ultrasonographic Findings

- Grayscale ultrasound
  - Focal collection of fluid within liver or close to biliary tree, e.g. in gallbladder fossa in patient with recent cholecystectomy
  - Round or oval in shape and usually unilocular
  - Thin capsule wall usually not discernible
  - Anechoic fluid content suggests fresh biloma
  - Debris or internal septa suggest infected biloma
  - Posterior acoustic enhancement
  - May see echogenic foci at periphery related to clips from recent surgery
- Color Doppler
  - No vascularity within lesion
  - For infected biloma, there may be increased vascularity in adjacent tissue
- Needle aspiration under ultrasound guidance usually required to confirm diagnosis (detection of bilirubin in aspirate)

CT Findings

- Well defined or slightly irregular cystic lesion without identifiable wall
- High-attenuation internal debris may be seen
- Subcapsular or intrahepatic biloma may result in adjacent transient hepatic attenuation difference (THAD) on arterial phase imaging secondary to mass effect and diminished portal venous flow

MR Findings

- T1WI: Usually low but variable SI
- T2WI: High SI (same as gallbladder), internal debris can be seen as low SI
- Delayed phase MR using hepatobiliary contrast agent can determine bile leakage into biloma

Radiographic Findings

- Cholangiography may delineate leakage site: Extravasation of contrast outside biliary tree

Nuclear Medicine Findings

- Hepatobiliary scintigraphy may demonstrate continual bile leakage into biloma

Imaging Recommendations

- Best imaging tool
  - Ultrasound is good at lesion detection and provides information on site & size of lesion for progress monitoring or intervention

DIFFERENTIAL DIAGNOSIS

Perihepatic Collection/Seroma/Lymphocele

- May be anechoic or contain debris or loculations
- Thick, irregular wall may be present
- Difficult to distinguish from biloma; aspiration biopsy may be required

Hepatic Cyst

- Variable appearance depending on whether it is sterile, infected, or hemorrhagic

Hepatic Abscess

- Thick, irregular wall, surrounding vascularity

Intrahepatic Hematoma

- Echogenicity evolves over time: Echogenic initially, hypoechoic after 4-5 days, internal echoes and septations after 1-4 weeks

PATHOLOGY

General Features

- Etiology
  - Iatrogenic: laparoscopic cholecystectomy, post liver transplantation, ERCP or other instrumentation of biliary tree, liver biopsy
  - Post-traumatic: Blunt trauma, motor vehicle accident
  - Spontaneous rupture of bile duct

Gross Pathologic & Surgical Features

- Size of biloma depends on difference between leakage rate and reabsorption rate of bile by peritoneum/surroundings

CLINICAL ISSUES

Presentation

- Most common signs/symptoms
  - Vague abdominal pain, nausea and vomiting, fever, leukocytosis in case of infected biloma

Natural History & Prognosis

- Usually asymptomatic in simple biloma; most gradually decrease in size over weeks

Treatment

- Percutaneous drainage if large or infected
- ERCP stent placement to decrease biliary pressure and control leak
- Surgical resection and repair reserved for complicated cases unresponsive to drainage

DIAGNOSTIC CHECKLIST

Consider

- Other causes of fluid collection: Ascites, abscess, hematoma

SELECTED REFERENCES

1. Thompson CM et al: Management of iatrogenic bile duct injuries: role of the interventional radiologist. Radiographics. 33(1):117-34, 2013
2. Frydrychowicz A et al: Hepatobiliary MR imaging with gadolinium-based contrast agents. J Magn Reson Imaging. 35(3):492-511, 2012

Biliary Cystadenoma/Carcinoma

TERMINOLOGY

- Rare premalignant or malignant, unilocular or multilocular cystic tumor arising from biliary epithelium
- Synonyms: Hepatobiliary cystadenoma/carcinoma, biliary cystic tumor, biliary cystic neoplasm, mucinous cystic neoplasm of liver

IMAGING

- Solitary, large, well-defined, multiloculated and multilobulated hepatic cyst
  - Thick, irregular wall and enhancing internal septations
  - May show biliary dilation from mass effect
- Biliary cystadenoma
  - Thin and smooth septa
  - May have fine calcifications and subtle mural nodularity (< 1 cm)
  - Absence of mural nodularity makes cystadenoma more likely

- Biliary cystadenocarcinoma more commonly associated with
  - Thick and irregular septa
  - Mural and septal nodularity (> 1 cm) and papillary projections
  - Coarse calcifications
  - Hemorrhagic internal fluid
- Location
  - Intrahepatic biliary ducts (83%), extrahepatic biliary ducts (13%), gallbladder (0.02%)

TOP DIFFERENTIAL DIAGNOSES

- Simple/complex/complicated hepatic cyst
- Hepatic abscess
- Echinococcal (hydatid) cyst
- Cystic metastases

CLINICAL ISSUES

- Primarily occurs in middle-aged Caucasian women

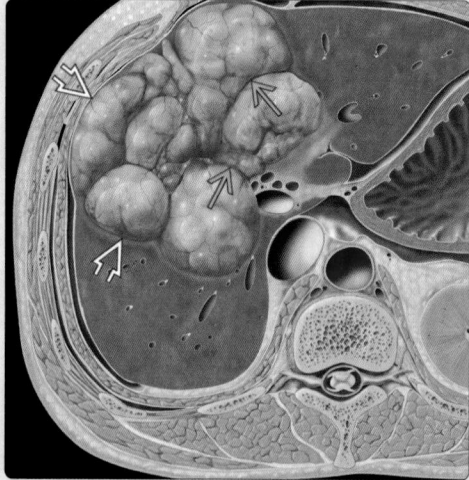
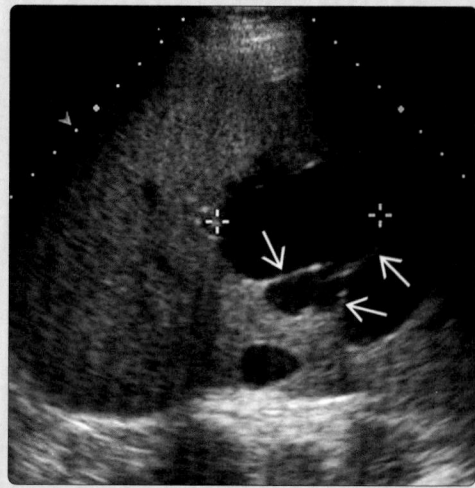

(Left) Axial graphic shows a biliary cystadenoma ⟹ with lobulated contour and multiple irregular, vascularized septations ⟶. (Right) Transverse grayscale ultrasound of the liver shows a biliary cystadenoma (with sonographic imaging appearance of a complex cyst) with multiple thickened septations ⟹. Most biliary cystadenomas are seen in middle-aged females.

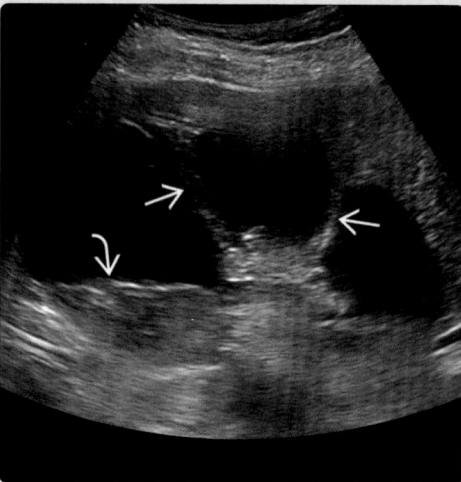
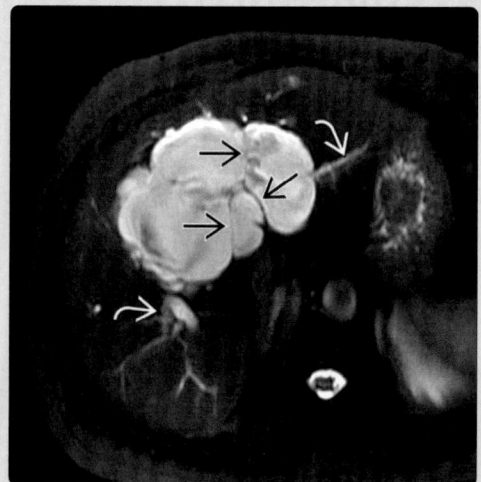

(Left) Transverse grayscale ultrasound of the liver shows a large, lobulated, multiseptated biliary cystadenoma with thick septations ⟹ and layering debris ⟹. (Right) Axial T2-weighted MR with fat saturation of the liver in the same patient shows the large biliary cystadenoma with lobulated contour, multiple thick septations ⟶, and associated mild peripheral biliary ductal dilatation ⟹ caused by central mass effect.

TERMINOLOGY

Synonyms

- Hepatobiliary cystadenoma/carcinoma, biliary cystic tumor, biliary cystic neoplasm
- Mucinous cystic neoplasm of liver

Definitions

- Rare premalignant or malignant, unilocular or multilocular cystic tumor arising from biliary epithelium

IMAGING

General Features

- Best diagnostic clue
  - Solitary, large, well-defined, multiloculated and multilobulated hepatic cyst
    - Thick, irregular wall and enhancing internal septations
    - May show biliary ductal dilation from mass effect
  - Biliary cystadenoma
    - Thin and smooth septa
    - May have fine calcifications and subtle mural nodularity (< 1 cm)
      - □ Absence of mural nodularity makes cystadenoma more likely
  - Biliary cystadenocarcinoma more commonly associated with
    - Thick and irregular septa
    - Mural and septal nodularity (> 1 cm) and papillary projections
    - Coarse calcifications
    - Hemorrhagic internal fluid
- Location
  - Intrahepatic biliary ducts (83%)
  - Extrahepatic biliary ducts (13%)
  - Gallbladder (0.02%)
- Size
  - 1-35 cm in diameter
    - Generally large at diagnosis if symptomatic (~ 10 cm)

Ultrasonographic Findings

- Well-defined, multiloculated, anechoic or hypoechoic mass
- Highly echogenic septa
- May see internal echoes with complex fluid, calcifications, mural/septal nodules, or papillary projections
- Color Doppler
  - Septal vascularity
- Contrast-enhanced ultrasound (CEUS)
  - Cystic wall, septa, and nodules display
    - Hyperenhancement in arterial phase after contrast injection
    - Hypoenhancement in portal and late phases (washout)

CT Findings

- NECT
  - Homogenous, hypodense, multiloculated cystic mass with internal septations
    - May be heterogeneous in attenuation if hemorrhage present
  - Calcifications, mural nodules, papillary projections, and intracystic debris, if present, may be visible
- CECT
  - Enhancement of capsule and septa

MR Findings

- T1WI
  - Typically hypointense to isointense
    - Variable signal intensity depending on protein content or blood products in cystic fluid
  - Septa are well delineated
- T2WI
  - Typically hyperintense due to cystic content
    - Variable signal depending on protein content or blood products
- T1WI C+
  - Enhancement of capsule and septa

Imaging Recommendations

- Best imaging tool
  - US depicts internal septations to better advantage
  - CECT or MR may be helpful

DIFFERENTIAL DIAGNOSIS

Simple/Complex/Complicated Hepatic Cyst

- Mostly unilocular homogenous or heterogenous cystic mass ± fluid level
- May have barely perceptible septations, no mural nodules

Hepatic Pyogenic Abscess

- Simple pyogenic abscess
  - Well-defined, round, hypodense mass (0-45 HU)
- "Cluster" sign: Small abscesses aggregate into single large septate cavity
  - Rim enhancement of locules
  - Intracystic contents > water density ± gas

Echinococcal (Hydatid) Cyst

- Large, well-defined, cystic hepatic mass
- Classically show peripheral daughter cysts of different density/intensity than mother cyst
- May have curvilinear or ring-like pericyst calcifications

Cystic Metastases

- Seen in mucin-producing adenocarcinomas (ovarian/colorectal carcinoma) or hypervascular metastases if outgrowing blood supply (sarcoma, melanoma, etc.)
- Ill-defined multilocular cystic mass with debris and mural nodularity

Biloma

- Encapsulated bile collection occurring after trauma or iatrogenic injury
- Well-defined unilocular cystic lesion ± enhancing rim
- Water density unless associated with hematoma

Rare

- Caroli disease
- Ciliated hepatic foregut cyst

PATHOLOGY

General Features

- Etiology

- o Considered to have congenital origin, but exact mechanism unknown
- o Theories: Ectopic rests of embryonal gallbladder tissue or ectopic ovarian stroma

Gross Pathologic & Surgical Features

- Solitary, multiloculated cystic tumor with thick, well-defined, fibrous capsule and septations
  - o Surface is shiny, smooth, or bosselated
  - o Large, polypoid excrescences in wall generally indicate malignant transformation

Microscopic Features

- Biliary cystadenoma
  - o Single layer of benign simple cuboidal or columnar epithelial cells
    - − Basally oriented nuclei with prominent nucleolus and thick chromatin
    - − Pale acidophil cytoplasm with mucin-filled vacuoles
- Biliary cystadenocarcinoma
  - o Multilayered epithelium with many papillary projections and invasion of stroma
  - o Lose epithelial nuclear stratification and tubulopapillary architecture, nuclear pleomorphism, atypia
- Stromal types
  - o Dense, hypercellular, spindle cell ovarian-like stroma (> 85% cases)
    - − Exclusively seen in women
    - − Estrogen receptor and progesterone receptor positive
  - o Nonovarian-type stroma
    - − Seen in both sexes
- Cystic fluid: Mucinous, serous, bilious, hemorrhagic, mixed fluid

CLINICAL ISSUES

Presentation

- Most common signs/symptoms
  - o Found incidentally if too small to be symptomatic
  - o Abdominal pain (most common), palpable mass, early satiety, anorexia, nausea
  - o May cause jaundice or cholangitis with compression of common bile duct
- Diagnosis: Mostly based on imaging and resection with final pathology
  - o Labs: Normal ALT/AST, bilirubin, and ALP (except with biliary obstruction)
    - − Generally normal Ca19-9 and CEA tumor markers (may be elevated)
  - o Fine-needle aspiration
    - − Generally avoided due to risk of peritoneal dissemination if malignant
    - − Cytology inconclusive (sensitivity 50%, specificity 97.6%)
      - □ Malignant cells not always recovered in cases of carcinoma
    - − Frequently show markedly ↑ Ca19-9 and mildly ↑ CEA
      - □ Unclear whether distinguishes it from simple cysts
  - o Intraoperative frozen section analysis
    - − Cannot exclude malignancy
      - □ May have undetectable malignant foci or synchronous carcinoma at borders

Demographics

- Age
  - o Predominantly occurs in middle-aged women (40-60 years old)
- Gender
  - o Biliary cystadenoma: > 85% of cases occur in women
  - o Biliary cystadenocarcinoma: ~ 63% of cases occur in women
    - − Higher suspicion for malignancy if detected in men
- Ethnicity
  - o Primarily seen in Caucasians
- Epidemiology
  - o Biliary cystic neoplasms account for < 5% of all reported intrahepatic cysts

Natural History & Prognosis

- Complications: Secondary infection, rupture into peritoneum or retroperitoneum, intracystic hemorrhage
- Recurrence: Inevitable if tumor is not completely resected
- Malignant transformation of biliary cystadenoma occurs in up to 20-30%
  - o Thought to be determined by presence of intestinal metaplasia, characterized by numerous goblet cells
- Prognosis of biliary cystadenocarcinoma
  - o Ovarian-type stromal tumors: Indolent course with favorable prognosis
  - o Nonovarian-type stromal tumors: More aggressive with poorer prognosis
    - − Rapid dissemination or distant metastasis

Treatment

- Complete surgical resection
  - o Liver resection with negative surgical margins preferred
  - o Enucleation: Maximizes preservation of hepatic parenchyma by using dissection plane between tumor and liver tissue
    - − Appropriate for benign lesions to prevent recurrence, but cannot definitively rule out malignancy

SELECTED REFERENCES

1. Arnaoutakis DJ et al: Management of Biliary Cystic Tumors: A Multi-institutional Analysis of a Rare Liver Tumor. Ann Surg. ePub, 2014
2. Cogley JR et al: MR imaging of benign focal liver lesions. Radiol Clin North Am. 52(4):657-82, 2014
3. Qian LJ et al: Spectrum of multilocular cystic hepatic lesions: CT and MR imaging findings with pathologic correlation. Radiographics. 33(5):1419-33, 2013
4. Xu HX et al: Imaging features of intrahepatic biliary cystadenoma and cystadenocarcinoma on B-mode and contrast-enhanced ultrasound. Ultraschall Med. 33(7):E241-9, 2012
5. Lewin M et al: Assessment of MRI and MRCP in diagnosis of biliary cystadenoma and cystadenocarcinoma. Eur Radiol. 16(2):407-13, 2006
6. Mortelé KJ et al: Cystic focal liver lesions in the adult: differential CT and MR imaging features. Radiographics. 21(4):895-910, 2001

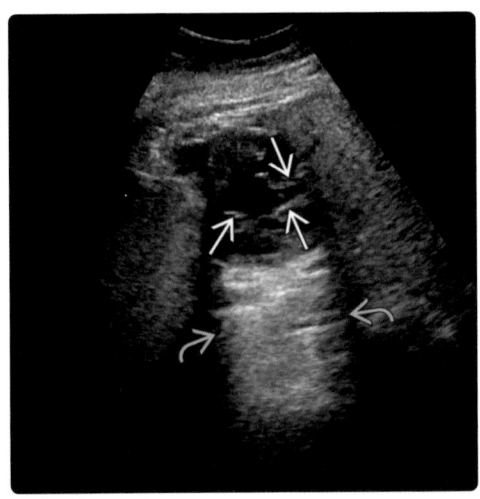

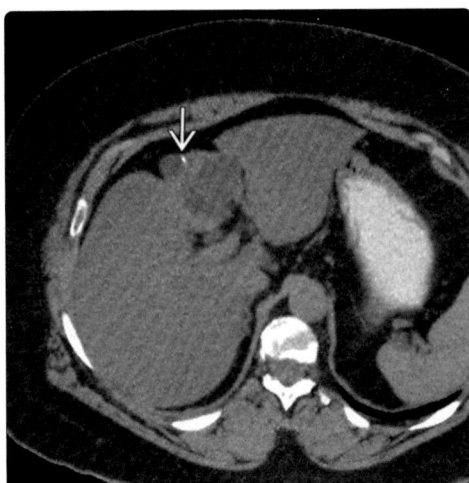

(Left) *Transverse grayscale ultrasound of the liver shows a biliary cystadenoma with complex cystic appearance. Multiple thick septations* ⮕ *are seen throughout the mass. Posterior acoustic enhancement* ⮕ *of the lesion confirms the cystic nature of the lesion.* **(Right)** *Axial CT in the same patient shows the biliary cystadenoma with lobulated contour, multiple septations, and tiny focus of calcification along the periphery* ⮕. *Note how septations are seen to better advantage on corresponding ultrasound.*

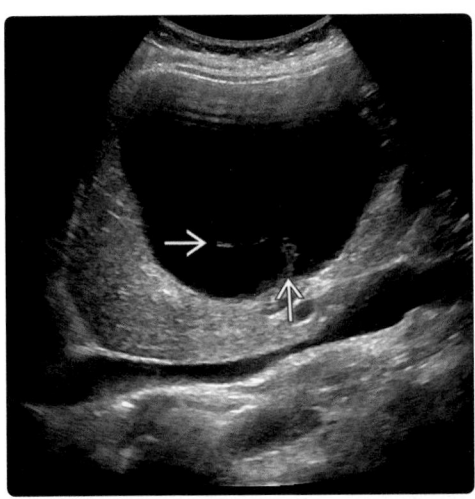

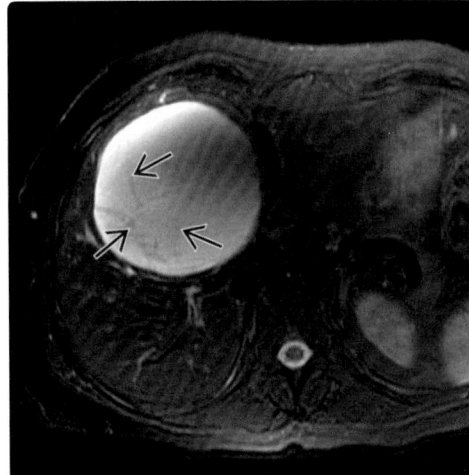

(Left) *Longitudinal grayscale ultrasound shows a large unilocular biliary cystadenoma in the liver with several thickened septations* ⮕. **(Right)** *Axial T2-weighted MR with fat saturation of the liver in the same patient shows unilocular biliary cystadenoma with multiple internal septations* ⮕. *Biliary cystadenomas are typically T2 hyperintense due to water content. However, variable hemorrhage or protein content may result in decreased T2 signal intensity (not seen in this case).*

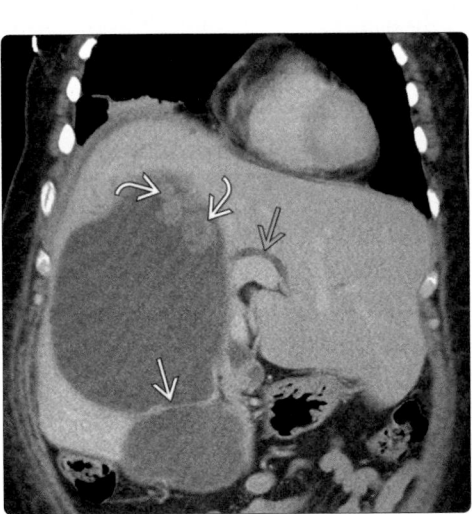

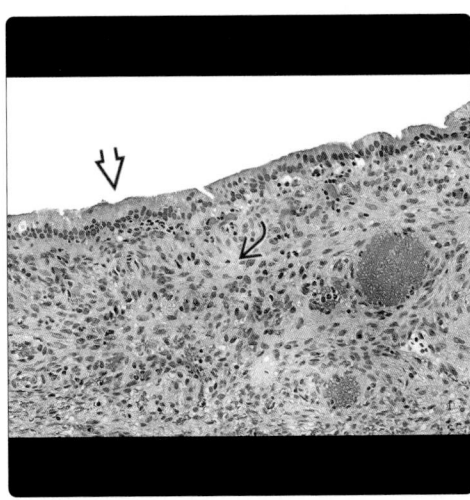

(Left) *Coronal CECT shows a biliary cystadenocarcinoma with rounded peripheral enhancing mural nodules* ⮕ *and thick septation* ⮕. *Associated biliary ductal dilatation is seen* ⮕. *The degree of complexity with enhancing mural nodules makes this lesion more suspicious for biliary cystadenocarcinoma.* **(Right)** *Histology of a biliary cystadenoma in a different patient displays bland cuboidal to columnar epithelium* ⮕ *associated with spindle cell stroma resembling ovarian-type stroma* ⮕.

Pyogenic Hepatic Abscess

TERMINOLOGY

- Localized collection of pus in liver due to bacterial infectious process with destruction of hepatic parenchyma and stroma

IMAGING

- Cluster sign: Cluster of small pyogenic abscesses that coalesce into single large cavity
- Ultrasound: Early lesions tend to be echogenic and poorly demarcated, evolve into well-demarcated anechoic lesions
- CECT: Double target sign
- May see central gas or fluid level

TOP DIFFERENTIAL DIAGNOSES

- Metastasis (post-treatment)
- Cholangiocarcinoma (peripheral mass-forming)
- Biliary cystadenocarcinoma
- Hepatocellular carcinoma (hypovascular)
- Amebic abscess

- Hemangioma (small)
- Hemorrhagic simple cyst
- Hydatid cyst (echinococcal cyst)
- Hepatic infarction in liver transplantation

PATHOLOGY

- Development via 5 major routes: Portal vein, biliary tract, hepatic artery, direct extension, trauma
- Common organisms: *Escherichia coli*, *Klebsiella pneumoniae* (adult), *Staphylococcus aureus* (children)

CLINICAL ISSUES

- Accounts for 88% of all liver abscesses
- Typical presentation: Middle-aged/elderly patient with history of fever, RUQ pain, tender hepatomegaly, leukocytosis

DIAGNOSTIC CHECKLIST

- Rule out amebic/fungal liver abscesses, cystic/hypovascular tumors

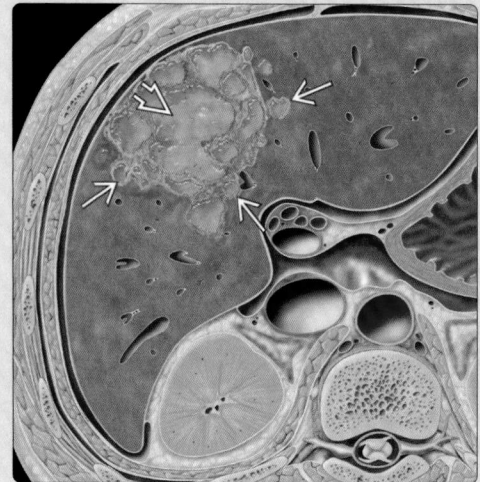
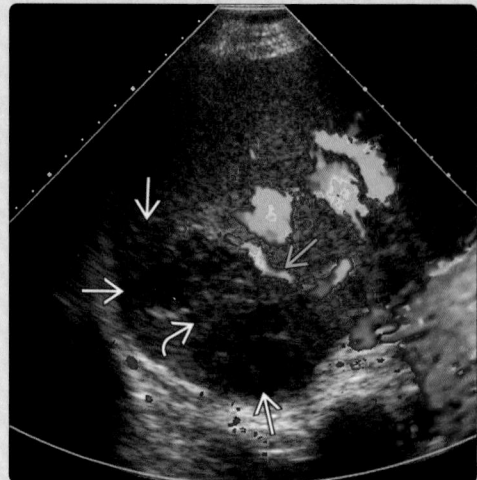

(Left) *Transverse graphic shows a cluster of multiple variable-sized pus collections in the right lobe of the liver* ➡ *coalescing to form a large abscess cavity* ➡. **(Right)** *Oblique transabdominal color Doppler ultrasound shows a cluster of coalescing abscesses* ➡ *in the right lobe of liver, representing a pyogenic hepatic abscess. The abscess has irregular walls, and contains low level internal echoes* ➡. *Adjacent hepatic parenchyma is edematous and hypervascular* ➡.

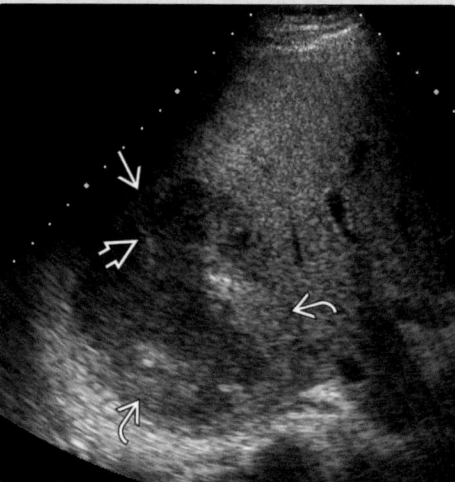
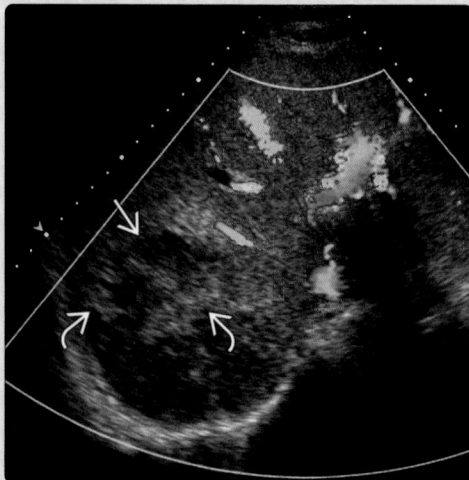

(Left) *Oblique transabdominal grayscale ultrasound shows an irregular-shaped hypoechoic pyogenic abscess* ➡ *in the right lobe of the liver. Several internal septations* ➡ *are seen, as well as peripheral echogenic components of the abscess* ➡. **(Right)** *Oblique transabdominal color Doppler ultrasound performed in the same patient shows no color flow within the abscess cavity* ➡. *Note irregular internal echogenic debris* ➡ *within the abscess cavity.*

TERMINOLOGY

Definitions

- Localized collection of pus in liver due to bacterial infectious process with destruction of hepatic parenchyma and stroma

IMAGING

General Features

- Best diagnostic clue
  - "Cluster" sign: Cluster of small pyogenic abscesses that coalesce into a single large cavity
- Location
  - Portal origin: Right lobe (65%); left lobe (12%); both lobes (23%)
  - Biliary origin: Both lobes (90%), near biliary ducts
  - If infection following an interventional procedure: In vicinity of procedure site
- Size
  - Varies from few mm to 10 cm; single or multiple
    - Portal origin: Usually solitary larger abscess
    - Biliary origin: Multiple small abscesses
    - Direct extension and trauma: Solitary large abscess
- Morphology
  - Spherical, multiseptated mass

Ultrasonographic Findings

- Grayscale ultrasound
  - Variable in shape and echogenicity
  - Usually spherical or ovoid in shape
  - Borders may be well-defined to irregular
  - Wall may be thin/thick, hypoechoic/mildly echogenic
  - Echogenicity of abscesses
    - Anechoic (50%), hyperechoic (25%), hypoechoic (25%)
  - Fluid level or debris, internal septa, and posterior acoustic enhancement
  - May see gas in an abscess: Bright echogenic foci with posterior reverberation artifact
  - Early lesions tend to be echogenic and poorly demarcated
  - May evolve into well-demarcated, nearly anechoic lesions
  - Hepatic parenchyma adjacent to abscess: Heterogeneous and hypoechoic due to edema
  - Associated right pleural effusion
- Color Doppler
  - Vascularity may be demonstrable in abscess wall
  - Edematous parenchyma adjacent to abscess may be hypervascular
- Contrast-enhanced ultrasound
  - Usually no internal enhancement
    - May be useful in differentiating abscess from hypovascular hepatic tumor, which shows diffuse or peripheral intratumoral enhancement

CT Findings

- NECT
  - Simple abscess: Well-defined, round, hypodense mass (0-45 HU)
  - "Cluster" sign
    - Small abscesses aggregate to coalesce into a single big cavity, usually septated
  - Complex pyogenic abscess: "Target" lesion
    - Hypodense center (pus), hyperdense capsule
  - Abscess with central gas (< 20% of cases)
    - Seen as air bubbles or an air-fluid level
  - Large air-fluid or fluid-debris level
    - Often associated with bowel communication or necrotic tissue
- CECT
  - "Double target" sign
    - Hypodense central abscess cavity surrounded by inner hyperdense ring/outer hypodense zone, enhancement of surrounding hepatic parenchyma
  - Well-defined, round or lobulated, hypodense mass
  - Rim/capsule enhancement and septal enhancement
  - Transient segmental hepatic parenchymal enhancement surrounding abscess
  - Right lower lobe atelectasis, pleural effusion

MR Findings

- T1WI
  - Hypointense
- T2WI
  - Variably hyperintense mass
  - Hyperintense perilesional edema
- T1WI C+
  - Hypointense pus in center
  - Rim or capsule enhancement
  - Small abscesses <1 cm: May show homogeneous enhancement (nonliquefied inflammation)
- MRCP
  - Highly specific in detecting obstructive biliary pathology

Nuclear Medicine Findings

- Hepatobiliary & sulfur colloid scans
  - Rounded, cold areas
  - Occasionally show communication between abscess cavity and biliary system
- Gallium scan (gallium citrate Ga-67)
  - Mixed lesions: Cold center & hot rim
- WBC scan
  - Hot lesions due to WBC accumulation
  - Highly specific for pyogenic abscesses compared to other nuclear or cross-sectional imaging

Imaging Recommendations

- Best imaging tool
  - CECT
  - Ultrasound finding is nonspecific, but useful in guiding aspiration and follow-up

DIFFERENTIAL DIAGNOSIS

Metastases (Post-Treatment)

- Usually not clustered or septate cystic mass
- Usually no atelectasis or elevation of diaphragm
- Treated necrotic metastases may be indistinguishable from abscess

Cholangiocarcinoma (Peripheral Mass-Forming Type)

- Delayed persistent enhancement of central portion

- More irregular and complex wall and septations
- Hepatic capsular retraction

Biliary Cystadenoma/Cystadenocarcinoma

- Rare, multiseptated cystic mass
- No surrounding inflammatory changes in liver parenchyma

Hepatocellular Carcinoma (Hypovascular)

- More heterogeneous; irregular infiltrating border
- Background liver cirrhosis

Amebic Abscess

- Peripheral location, abuts liver capsule
- Most often solitary (85%), rarely multiseptated
- Affects right lobe (72%) > left (13%)
- More common in recent immigrants or patient with travel history

Hemangioma (Small)

- Hyperechoic on US
- Often indistinguishable from small abscess on CECT/MR

Hemorrhagic Simple Cyst

- Hemorrhage may produce internal debris/septa/wall thickening within preexisting cyst
- Cyst may appear multiloculated

Hydatid Cyst (Echinococcal Cyst)

- Large cystic liver mass with peripheral daughter cysts
- ± curvilinear or ring-like pericyst calcification
- ± dilated intrahepatic bile ducts: Due to mass effect or rupture into bile ducts

Hepatic Infarction in Liver Transplantation

- Hepatic and biliary necrosis due to hepatic artery thrombosis
- Peripheral, wedge-shaped or geographic, segmental distribution
- No capsule or septal enhancement

PATHOLOGY

General Features

- Etiology
  - Portal vein route
    - Pylephlebitis from appendicitis, diverticulitis, proctitis, inflammatory bowel disease
    - Right colon infection spread: Superior mesenteric vein → portal vein → liver
    - Left colon infection spread: Inferior mesenteric vein → splenic vein → portal vein → liver
  - Biliary tract route
    - Ascending cholangitis from choledocholithiasis, benign or malignant biliary obstruction
  - Hepatic artery route
    - Septicemia from bacterial endocarditis, pneumonitis, osteomyelitis
  - Direct extension
    - Perforated gastric/duodenal ulcer, subphrenic abscess, pyelonephritis
  - Traumatic cause

- - Blunt or penetrating injuries or following interventional procedures
  - Most commonly bacterial organisms
    - Adult: *Escherichia coli*, *Klebsiella pneumoniae*
    - Children: Staphylococcus aureus

CLINICAL ISSUES

Presentation

- Most common signs/symptoms
  - Fever, RUQ pain, rigors, malaise
  - Nausea, vomiting, weight loss, tender hepatomegaly
  - If subphrenic then atelectasis & pleural effusion possible
- Clinical profile
  - Middle-aged/elderly patient with history of fever, RUQ pain, tender hepatomegaly, leukocytosis
- Lab data: Increased leukocytes & serum alkaline phosphatase
- Diagnosis by fine-needle aspiration cytology

Demographics

- Epidemiology
  - Accounts for 88% of all liver abscesses
  - Incidence increasing in Western countries due to ascending cholangitis & diverticulitis

Natural History & Prognosis

- Complications: Spread of infection to subphrenic space causes atelectasis & pleural effusion
- Prognosis: Good after medical therapy & aspiration

Treatment

- Antibiotics
- Percutaneous aspiration
- Catheter or surgical drainage

DIAGNOSTIC CHECKLIST

Consider

- Rule out amebic/fungal liver abscesses, cystic tumors
- Check for history of transplantation or ablation/chemotherapy for liver tumor

Image Interpretation Pearls

- "Cluster" sign: Small abscesses coalesce into big cavity
- Presence of central gas or fluid level
- Nonliquefied abscess may simulate solid tumor

SELECTED REFERENCES

1. Bonder A et al: Evaluation of liver lesions. Clin Liver Dis. 16(2):271-83, 2012
2. K C S et al: Long-term follow-up of pyogenic liver abscess by ultrasound. Eur J Radiol. 74(1):195-8, 2010
3. Benedetti NJ et al: Imaging of hepatic infections. Ultrasound Q. 24(4):267-78, 2008
4. Doyle DJ et al: Imaging of hepatic infections. Clin Radiol. 61(9):737-48, 2006
5. Kim KW et al: Pyogenic hepatic abscesses: distinctive features from hypovascular hepatic malignancies on contrast-enhanced ultrasound with SH U 508A; early experience. Ultrasound Med Biol. 30(6):725-33, 2004
6. Mortelé KJ et al: The infected liver: radiologic-pathologic correlation. Radiographics. 24(4):937-55, 2004

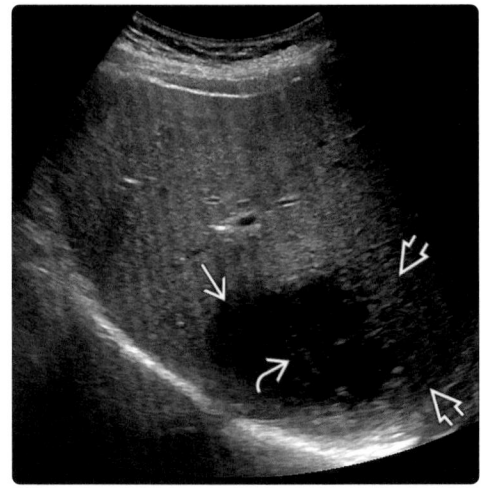

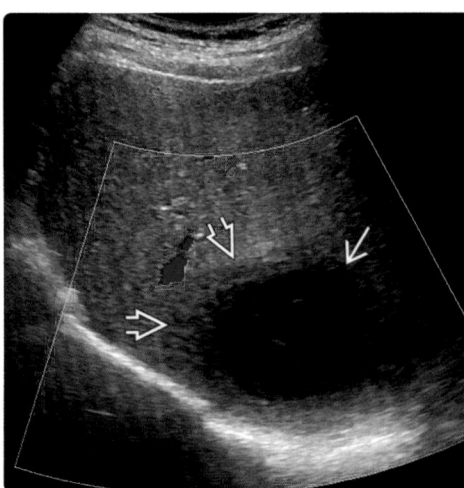

(Left) *Oblique transabdominal grayscale ultrasound shows an ovoid hypoechoic pyogenic abscess in the right lobe of the liver* ➔ *containing liquefied material as well as subtle irregular septations* ➔. *Note hypoechoic edematous adjacent hepatic parenchyma* ➔. **(Right)** *Oblique transabdominal color Doppler ultrasound performed in the same patient shows no color flow within the hepatic abscess* ➔. *Note the peripheral hypoechoic rim surrounding the abscess cavity* ➔ *due to edema of adjacent hepatic parenchyma.*

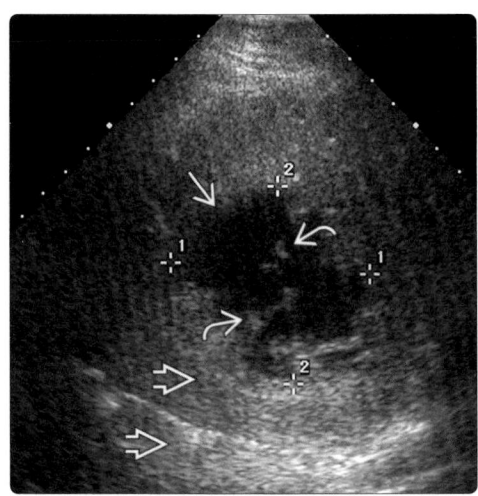

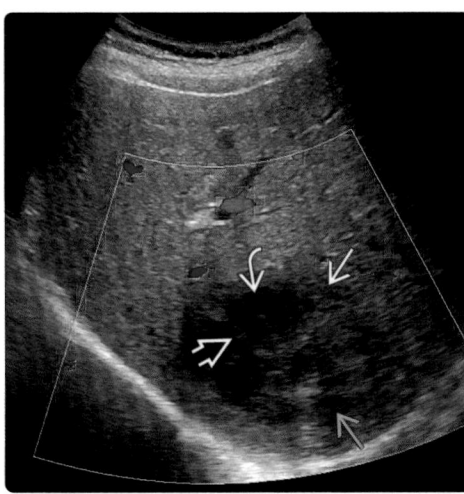

(Left) *Oblique transabdominal grayscale ultrasound shows an irregularly shaped, nearly anechoic abscess* ➔ *containing minimal internal echogenic debris* ➔. *Note posterior acoustic enhancement* ➔. **(Right)** *Oblique transabdominal color Doppler ultrasound shows a centrally cystic hepatic abscess* ➔ *with a surrounding hypoechoic hepatic parenchyma* ➔ *in the right lobe of the liver. Central internal septations* ➔ *and echogenic debris* ➔ *are seen within the hepatic abscess.*

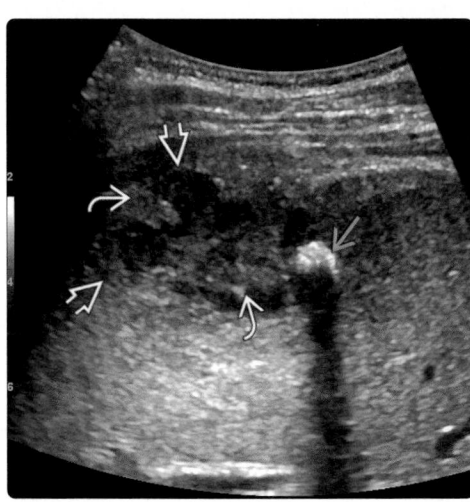

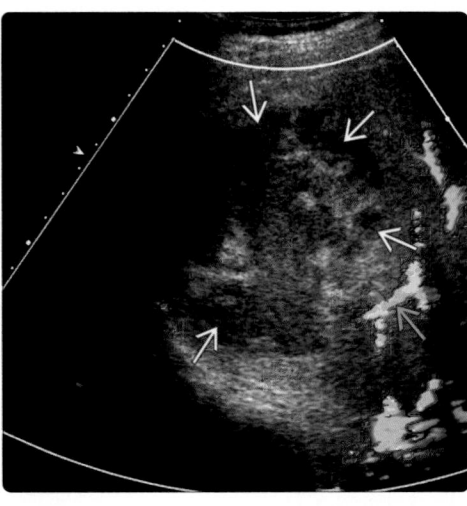

(Left) *Transverse ultrasound of the right lobe of the liver shows a hepatic abscess* ➔ *caused by a dropped appendicolith* ➔ *from remote appendectomy. The abscess cavity is hypoechoic and contains irregular internal echogenic debris* ➔. **(Right)** *Oblique abdominal color Doppler ultrasound shows a large pyogenic abscess in the right lobe of the liver composed of a cluster of multiple abscesses* ➔. *Note peripheral hepatic hypervascularity* ➔.

TERMINOLOGY

- Localized pus collection in liver due to Entamoeba histolytica with destruction of hepatic parenchyma

IMAGING

- General feature
  - Most often solitary (85%), peripherally located
- Ultrasound
  - Sharply demarcated, round or ovoid mass
  - Hypoechoic with low-level internal echoes
  - May see internal septa or wall nodularity
  - May see posterior acoustic enhancement
- CECT
  - Typically hypoattenuating unilocular lesion
  - Peripheral rim or capsule enhancement
  - May see hypodense halo due to edema

TOP DIFFERENTIAL DIAGNOSES

- Hepatic metastasis (post-treatment, cystic, or necrotic)

- Hepatic pyogenic abscess
- Hepatic hydatid cyst
- Biliary cystadenoma/cystadenocarcinoma
- Infarcted liver after transplantation

PATHOLOGY

- Entamoeba histolytica
- Primary source of infection: Human carriers passing amebic cysts into stool

CLINICAL ISSUES

- RUQ pain, tender hepatomegaly, diarrhea with mucus
- Indirect hemagglutination positive in 90% of cases

DIAGNOSTIC CHECKLIST

- Rule out pyogenic or fungal abscess, cystic lesions
- Check for history of transplantation, ablation, or chemotherapy for liver tumor or metastasis, which may simulate amebic abscess on imaging

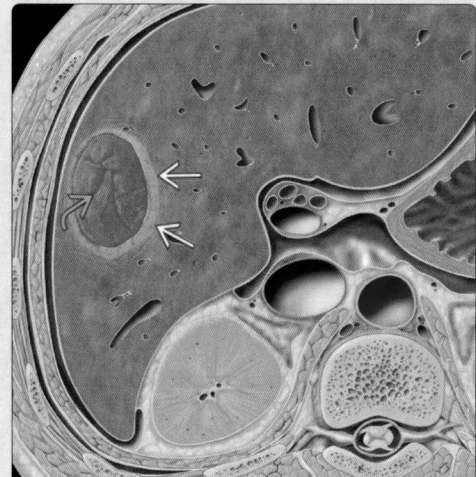 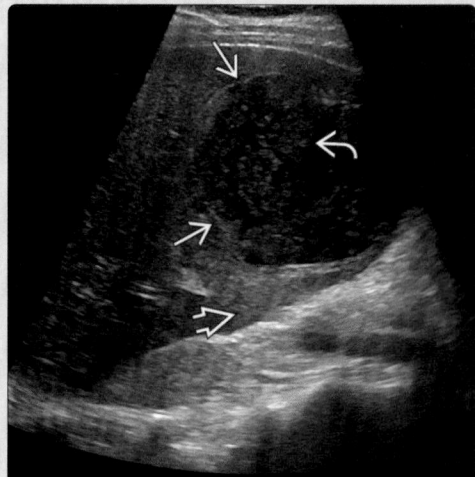

(Left) Graphic illustration demonstrates a unilocular encapsulated amebic abscess within the liver. Note the surrounding rim of edema ➡ and central anchovy paste consistency of contents ➡. (Right) Sagittal gray scale ultrasound of the liver shows a large, well-demarcated and encapsulated hypoechoic amebic abscess ➡. The contents are heterogeneous due to floating debris ➡. Also note the mild posterior acoustic enhancement ➡.

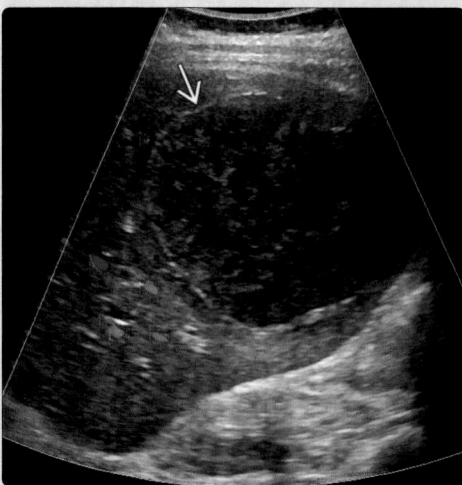 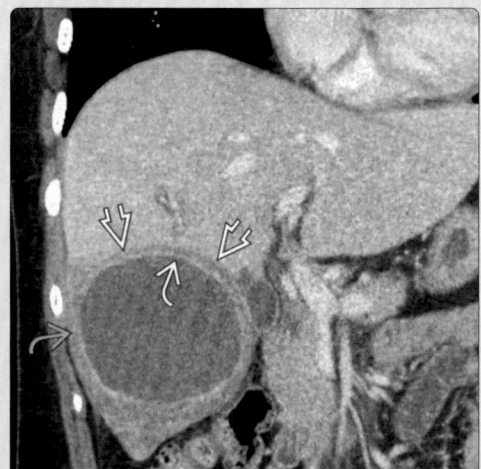

(Left) Color Doppler ultrasound in the same patient shows no detectable internal vascularity within the lesion ➡. (Right) Coronal contrast-enhanced CT in same patient shows a large unilocular amebic abscess in the right lobe of liver. The abscess is well defined with an enhancing capsule ➡ and hypodense halo of edema ➡. Note the abutment with liver capsule ➡.

TERMINOLOGY

Definitions

- Localized collection of pus in liver due to *Entamoeba histolytica* with destruction of hepatic parenchyma and stroma

IMAGING

General Features

- Best diagnostic clue
  - Well-defined hypo- or isoechoic mass, most often solitary and peripherally located
- Location
  - Right lobe (72%) > left lobe (13%)
  - Usually peripheral, near or abutting liver capsule
- Size
  - Varies from few millimeters to several centimeters
- Morphology
  - Most often solitary (85%)
- Other general features
  - Most common extraintestinal manifestation of amebic infestation

Ultrasonographic Findings

- Grayscale ultrasound
  - Peripheral location
    - Abuts liver capsule, often under diaphragm
  - Round or oval shape, sharply demarcated
    - Amebic abscess is more likely to have round or oval shape than pyogenic abscess
  - Hypoechoic with low-level internal echoes due to debris
  - Internal septa or wall nodularity may be present
  - May see hypoechoic halo
  - May see mild posterior acoustic enhancement
  - Often associated right pleural effusion

Radiographic Findings

- Radiography
  - Elevation of right hemidiaphragm
  - Right lower lobe atelectasis or infiltrate
  - Right pleural effusion
  - Ruptured amebic abscess into chest may cause
    - Lung abscess, cavity, hydropneumothorax
    - Pericardial effusion
  - Barium enema often shows changes of amebic colitis

CT Findings

- NECT
  - Peripheral, round or oval hypodense mass (10-20 HU)
- CECT
  - May appear unilocular (more common) or multilocular
  - Rim or capsule enhancement, wall nodularity
  - May demonstrate hypodense halo due to edema
  - Extrahepatic abnormalities
    - Right lower lobe atelectasis
    - Right pleural effusion
    - Usually colonic and rarely gastric changes

MR Findings

- T1WI
  - Hypointense
- T2WI
  - Hyperintense
  - Perilesional edema: High signal intensity
- T1WI C+
  - Abscess contents: No enhancement
  - Rim or capsule: Shows enhancement

Nuclear Medicine Findings

- Hepatobiliary scan (HIDA)
  - Cold lesion with hot periphery
- Technetium sulfur colloid
  - Cold defects
- WBC scan
  - Cold center and hot rim

Imaging Recommendations

- Best imaging tool
  - Ultrasound is ideal for detecting lesion and guiding biopsy
- Protocol advice
  - Abdominal scan to include lung bases through to pelvis

DIFFERENTIAL DIAGNOSIS

Hepatic Metastases

- More commonly multiple and smaller lesions, random distribution
- Post-treatment metastasis
  - Cystic or necrotic nature
  - May be indistinguishable from amebic abscess
- May have internal vascularity
- Usually no elevation of diaphragm or atelectasis
- No signs of infection

Hepatic Pyogenic Abscess

- Simple pyogenic abscess
  - Well-defined lobulated and irregular, hypo- or isoechoic mass, centrally located in liver
  - "Cluster" sign: Aggregation of small abscesses, sometimes coalesce into single septated cavity
- May contain gas within abscess
  - Seen as air bubbles or air-fluid level

Hepatic Hydatid Cyst

- Large well-defined cystic liver mass
- Numerous peripheral daughter cysts
- May show curvilinear or ring-like pericyst calcification
- Intrahepatic duct dilatation may be seen

Biliary Cystadenoma/Cystadenocarcinoma

- Multiseptated cystic mass
- Internal solid enhancing component may be present
- No surrounding inflammatory changes

Infarcted Liver After Transplantation

- Biliary and hepatic necrosis caused by hepatic artery thrombosis
- Less demarcated than abscess and follows vascular territory

PATHOLOGY

General Features

- Etiology
  - *Entamoeba histolytica*
  - Primary mode of infection: Human carriers pass amebic cysts into stool
  - May become secondarily infected with pyogenic bacteria
- Associated abnormalities
  - Amebic colitis
- Disease pathway
  - Cystic form of *Entamoeba histolytica* gains access to body via contaminated water
  - Mature cysts resistant to gastric acid, pass unchanged into intestine
  - Cyst wall is digested by trypsin and invasive trophozoites are released
  - Trophozoites enter mesenteric venules and lymphatics
  - Usually spread from colon to liver: Via portal vein (most common) and lymphatics
  - Rarely direct spread
    - Colonic wall to peritoneum
    - Peritoneum to liver capsule and finally liver

Gross Pathologic & Surgical Features

- Usually solitary abscess
- Predominantly in right lobe
- Fluid dark, reddish-brown
- Consistency of anchovy paste or chocolate sauce

Microscopic Features

- Blood, destroyed hepatocytes
- Necrotic tissue and rarely trophozoites

CLINICAL ISSUES

Presentation

- Most common signs/symptoms
  - RUQ pain, tender hepatomegaly
  - Diarrhea with mucus
- Clinical profile
  - Patient with history of diarrhea (mucus), RUQ pain, and tender hepatomegaly
- Laboratory data
  - Stool exam: Usually nonspecific or negative
  - Indirect hemagglutination positive in 90% cases

Demographics

- Age
  - More common in 3rd-5th decades
  - Can occur in any age group
- Gender
  - M:F = 4:1
- Epidemiology
  - Approximately 10% of world's population is infected with *Entamoeba histolytica*
  - Most common in India, Africa, Far East, Central and South America
  - In United States: Recent travel to endemic area

Natural History & Prognosis

- Complications

- Pleuropulmonary amebiasis (20-35%)
  - Pulmonary consolidation or abscess
  - Effusion, empyema, or hepatobronchial fistula
- Peritoneal amebiasis (2-7.5%)
- Pericardial or renal amebiasis
- Prognosis
  - Usually good after amebicidal therapy
  - Poor in individuals who develop complications
  - Mortality rate in USA: < 3%
    - < 1% when confined to liver
    - 6% with extension into chest
    - 30% with extension into pericardium

Treatment

- 90% respond to antimicrobial therapy
  - Metronidazole or chloroquine
  - Iodoquinol for luminal treatment
- 10% require aspiration and drainage

DIAGNOSTIC CHECKLIST

Consider

- Rule out other liver pathologies, which may simulate amebic abscess on imaging
  - Pyogenic or fungal abscess
  - Other cystic lesions
- Check for history of transplantation and ablation or chemotherapy for liver tumor or metastasis, which may simulate amebic abscess on imaging

Image Interpretation Pearls

- US: Solitary hypoechoic mass with internal low-level echo, peripherally located
- CT: Unilocular, round or ovoid hypodense mass with rim or capsule enhancement
- Diaphragmatic rupture in presence of adjacent hepatic abscess suggests amebic cause

SELECTED REFERENCES

1. Bammigatti C et al: Percutaneous needle aspiration in uncomplicated amebic liver abscess: a randomized trial. Trop Doct. 43(1):19-22, 2013
2. Debnath MR et al: Ultrasonographic evaluation of morphologic pattern of amoebic liver abscess. Mymensingh Med J. 21(4):583-7, 2012
3. Marn H, Ignatius R, Tannich E, Harms G, Schürmann M, Dieckmann S. Amoebic liver abscess with negative serologic markers for Entamoeba histolytica: mind the gap! Infection. 40(1):87-91, 2012
4. Sánchez-Aguilar M et al: Prognostic indications of the failure to treat amoebic liver abscesses. Pathog Glob Health. 106(4):232-7, 2012
5. Mishra K et al: Liver abscess in children: an overview. World J Pediatr. 6(3):210-6, 2010
6. Giorgio A et al: Amebic liver abscesses: a new epidemiological trend in a non-endemic area? In Vivo. 23(6):1027-30, 2009
7. Benedetti NJ et al: Imaging of hepatic infections. Ultrasound Q. 24(4):267-78, 2008
8. Salles JM et al: Invasive amebiasis: an update on diagnosis and management. Expert Rev Anti Infect Ther. 5(5):893-901, 2007
9. Mohan S et al: Liver abscess: a clinicopathological analysis of 82 cases. Int Surg. 91(4):228-33, 2006
10. Mortele KJ et al: The infected liver: radiologic-pathologic correlation. Radiographics. 24(4):937-55, 2004
11. Hughes MA et al: Amebic liver abscess. Infect Dis Clin North Am. 14(3):565-82, viii, 2000

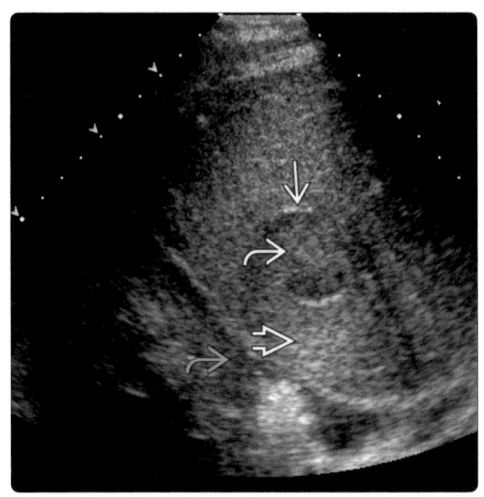
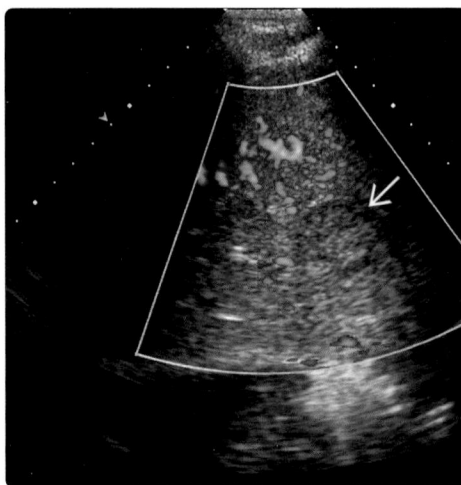

(Left) *Longitudinal ultrasound of the right lobe of the liver demonstrates a well-demarcated and capsulated hypoechoic amebic abscess* ➡️ *with internal echoes* ➡️ *indicating debris. Note the mild posterior acoustic enhancement* ➡️ *and small right pleural effusion* ➡️. (**Right**) *Power Doppler ultrasound performed in the same patient shows no detectable internal vascularity within the amebic abscess* ➡️.

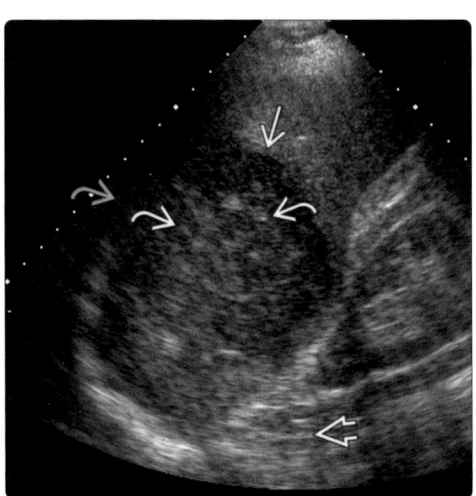
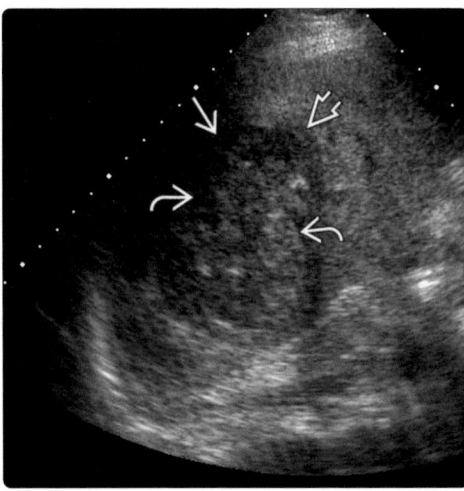

(Left) *Sagittal ultrasound shows a large, round hypoechoic amebic abscess in the right lobe of liver* ➡️ *abutting the liver capsule* ➡️. *Internal contents are hypoechoic with heterogeneously echogenic scattered foci* ➡️. *Also note the posterior acoustic enhancement* ➡️. (**Right**) *Transverse grayscale ultrasound in the same patient shows a hypoechoic mass* ➡️ *with internal heterogeneous echogenic contents* ➡️ *and hypoechoic halo* ➡️.

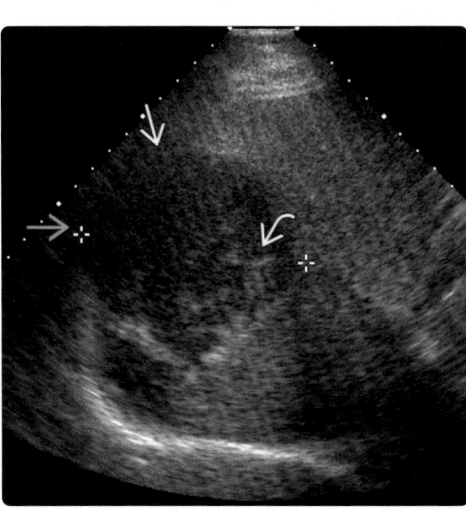
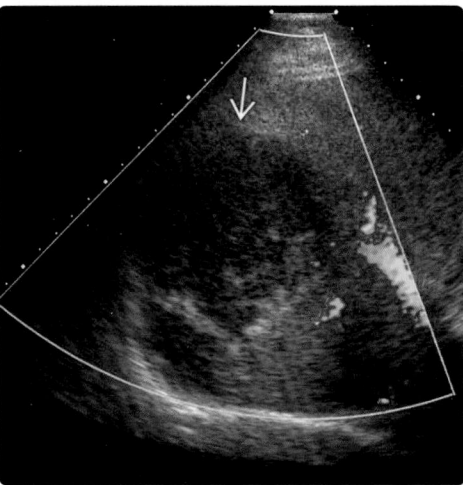

(Left) *Transverse grayscale ultrasound of the right lobe of the liver demonstrates a round, well-demarcated, hypoechoic amebic abscess* ➡️ *with low-level internal echoes* ➡️. *Note how the abscess abuts the liver capsule and diaphragm* ➡️ (**Right**) *Transverse color Doppler ultrasound performed in the same patient shows no detectable internal vascularity in the mass* ➡️.

Hepatic *Echinococcus* Cyst

TERMINOLOGY

- Infection of humans caused by larval stage of *Echinococcus granulosus* or *Echinococcus multilocularis*

IMAGING

- Best diagnostic clue: Membranes ± daughter cysts in complex heterogeneous mass
- *E. granulosus*
  - Anechoic cyst with double echogenic lines separated by hypoechoic layer
  - Honeycomb cyst, multiple septations
  - "Water lily" sign: Complete detachment of membrane
  - "Snowstorm pattern": Anechoic cyst with internal debris and hydatid sand
- *E. multilocularis*
  - Single/multiple echogenic lesions
  - Irregular necrotic lesions with microcalcifications
  - Ill-defined infiltrative solid masses

TOP DIFFERENTIAL DIAGNOSES

- Hemorrhagic or infected cyst
- Complex pyogenic abscess
- "Cystic" metastases
- Biliary cystadenocarcinoma

PATHOLOGY

- Caused by larval stage of *Echinococcus* tapeworm
  - *E. granulosus*: Most common form of hydatid disease, unilocular
  - *E. multilocularis*: Less common but aggressive

CLINICAL ISSUES

- Serologic test positive in more than 80% of cases

DIAGNOSTIC CHECKLIST

- Rule out other complex or septate cystic liver masses

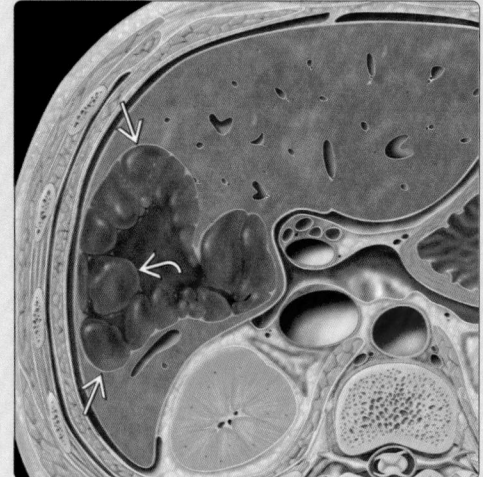
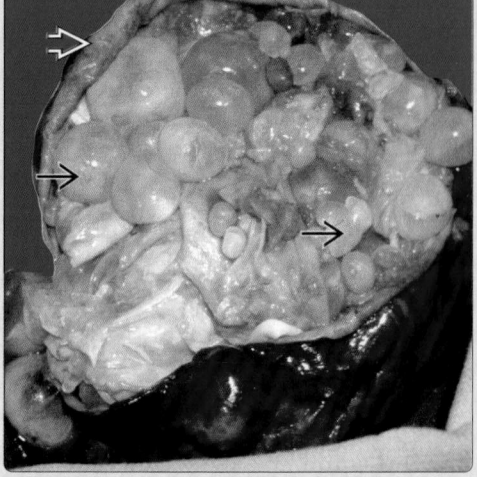

(Left) *This graphic shows an eccentric cystic mass (the pericyst or mother cyst)* ➡ *with numerous peripheral daughter cysts, or scolices,* ➡ *within in the right lobe of the liver.* (Right) *Gross photograph of the liver shows a hydatid cyst containing multiple daughter cysts* ➡. *The fibrous rim* ➡ *can be seen surrounding the cyst. (Courtesy G. Gray Jr., MD. From: DP: Spleen.)*

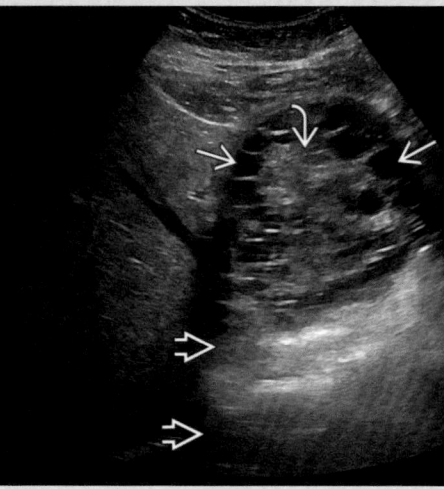
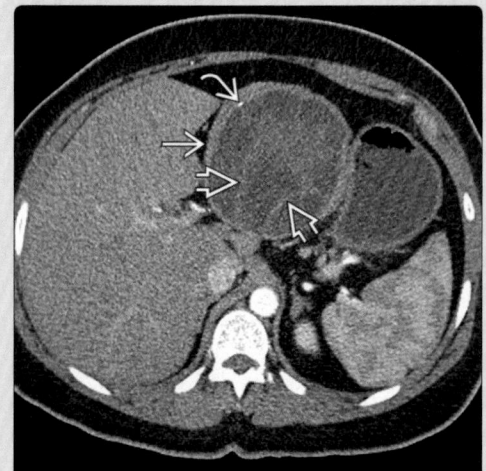

(Left) *Transverse abdominal US shows an echinococcal cyst containing multiple peripheral daughter cysts* ➡ *and central heterogeneous content* ➡ *in the left lobe of the liver. Note the posterior acoustic enhancement* ➡. (Right) *Axial contrast enhanced CT performed in the same patient shows a large multilocular well-defined cystic mass in the left lobe of the liver* ➡. *The cystic mass has thick wall with a tiny focus of calcification* ➡ *and multiple septations* ➡.

Hepatic *Echinococcus* Cyst

TERMINOLOGY

Synonyms
- Echinococcal or hydatid disease; echinococcosis

Definitions
- Infection of humans caused by larval stage of *Echinococcus granulosus* or *Echinococcus multilocularis*

IMAGING

General Features
- Best diagnostic clue
  - Membranes ± daughter cysts in complex heterogeneous mass
- **Location**: Right lobe > left lobe of liver
- **Size**: Variable, average 5 cm (max to 50 cm)
  - May contain up to 15 liters of fluid
- **Key concepts**
  - *E. granulosus*: Most common form of hydatid disease, unilocular form
    - Up to 60% of cysts are multiple
  - *E. multilocularis* (alveolaris): Less common but aggressive form
  - Most common sites: Liver and lungs

Ultrasonographic Findings
- Grayscale ultrasound
  - Variable manifestations based on stage of evolution and maturity
  - Lewall classification of hydatid lesions
    - Cyst with hydatid sand and no internal architecture
    - Ruptured cyst with detached endocyst
    - Cyst with matrix ± daughter cysts
    - Calcified mass
  - *E. granulosus*
    - Anechoic cyst with double echogenic lines separated by hypoechoic layer
    - Honeycombed cyst, multiple septations between daughter cysts in mother cyst
    - Detachment of endocyst from pericyst (partial or complete) results in varied appearances
    - Undulating floating membrane within cyst
    - "Water lily" sign: Complete detachment of membrane
    - "Snowstorm pattern": Anechoic cyst with internal debris, hydatid sand
    - Dilated IHDs due to compression by cysts
  - *E. multilocularis*
    - Single/multiple echogenic lesions
    - Irregular necrotic regions and microcalcifications
    - Ill-defined infiltrative solid masses
    - Tend to spread to liver hilum
    - Invasion of inferior vena cava and diaphragm
    - Evaluate lung, heart, and brain for deposits
  - US used to monitor efficacy of antihydatid therapy
    - Positive response findings include
      - Reduction in cyst size
      - Endocyst detachment
      - Progressive increase in cyst echogenicity
      - Mural calcification

Radiographic Findings
- Radiography
  - *E. granulosus*: Curvilinear or ring-like pericyst calcification
    - Seen in 20-30% of abdominal plain films
  - *E. multilocularis*: Microcalcifications in 50% of cases
- Endoscopic retrograde cholangiopancreatography (ERCP)
  - Hydatid cyst may communicate with biliary tree
    - Right hepatic duct 55%; left hepatic duct 29%, common hepatic duct 9%, gallbladder 6%, common bile duct 1%

CT Findings
- NECT
  - *E. granulosus*
    - Large unilocular/multilocular well-defined hypodense cysts
    - Contains multiple peripheral daughter cysts of less density than mother cyst
    - Curvilinear ring-like calcification
    - Calcified wall: Usually indicates no active infection if completely circumferential
    - Dilated intrahepatic bile duct: Due to compression/rupture of cyst into bile ducts
  - *E. multilocularis*
    - Extensive, infiltrative cystic and solid masses of low density (14-40 HU)
    - Margins are irregular/ill defined
    - Amorphous type of calcification
    - Can simulate primary or secondary tumor
- CECT
  - Enhancement of cyst wall and septations

MR Findings
- T1WI
  - Rim (pericyst): Hypointense (fibrous component)
  - Mother cyst (hydatid matrix)
    - Usually intermediate signal intensity
    - Rarely hyperintense: Due to reduction in water content
  - Daughter cysts: Less signal intensity than mother cyst (matrix)
  - Floating membrane: Low signal intensity
  - Calcifications: Difficult to identify on MR images
    - Display low signal on both T1- and T2WI
- T2WI
  - Rim (pericyst): Hypointense (fibrous component)
  - 1st echo T2WI: Increased signal intensity
    - Mother cysts more than daughter cysts
  - Strong T2WI: Hyperintense
    - Mother and daughter cysts have same intensity
  - Floating membrane
    - Low to intermediate signal intensity
- T1WI C+
  - Enhancement of cyst wall and septations
- MRCP
  - ± demonstrate communication with biliary tree

Imaging Recommendations
- Best imaging tool
  - US for diagnosis and follow-up

DIFFERENTIAL DIAGNOSIS

Hemorrhagic or Infected Cyst

- Complex cystic heterogeneous mass
- Septations, fluid-levels, and mural nodularity
- Calcification may or may not be seen

Complex Pyogenic Abscess

- "Cluster of grapes": Confluent complex cystic lesions

"Cystic" Metastases

- e.g., cystadenocarcinoma of pancreas or ovary
- May present with debris, mural nodularity, rim enhancement

Biliary Cystadenocarcinoma

- Rare, multiseptated water density cystic mass
- No surrounding inflammatory changes

PATHOLOGY

General Features

- Etiology
  - Caused by larval stage of *Echinococcus* tapeworm
    - *E. granulosus* and *E. multilocularis*
- Carried by sheep, transmitted to humans by dog or fox
  - Humans are incidental hosts
- Larvae → portal vein → liver (75%)
- *E. granulosus*
  - Develop into hydatid stage (4-5 days) within liver
  - Hydatid cysts grow to 1 cm during first 6 months, 2-3 cm annually
- *E. multilocularis*
  - Larvae proliferate and penetrate surrounding tissue
  - Cause diffuse and infiltrative granulomatous reaction, simulating malignancy
  - Necrosis → cavitation → calcification

Microscopic Features

- Cyst fluid content: Antigenic, pale yellow, neutral pH
- Endocyst: Gives rise to daughter vesicles/brood capsule, which may detach, form sediment, or produce daughter cysts
- Ectocyst: Acellular substance secreted by parasite
- Pericyst: Host response forming layer of granulation/fibrous tissue

CLINICAL ISSUES

Presentation

- Most common signs/symptoms
  - Cysts: Initially asymptomatic
    - Symptomatic when size ↑/infected/ruptured
  - Pain, fever, jaundice, hepatomegaly
  - Allergic reaction; portal hypertension
- Clinical profile
  - Middle-aged patient with right upper quadrant pain, palpable mass, jaundice
- Lab data
  - Eosinophilia; ↑ serologic titers
  - ± ↑ alkaline phosphatase/gamma-glutamyl transpeptidase (GGTP)

- Diagnosis
  - Serologic tests positive in more than 80% of cases
  - Percutaneous aspiration of cyst fluid
    - Danger of peritoneal spill and anaphylactic reaction

Demographics

- Age
  - Hydatid disease usually acquired in childhood
  - Not diagnosed until 30-40 years of age
- Gender: M = F
- Epidemiology
  - *E. granulosus*: Mediterranean region, Africa, South America, Australia, and New Zealand
  - *E. multilocularis*: France, Germany, Austria, USSR, Japan, Alaska, and Canada

Natural History & Prognosis

- Complications
  - Compression/infection or rupture into biliary tree
  - Rupture into peritoneal or pleural cavity
  - Spread of lesions to lungs, heart, brain, and bone
- Prognosis
  - *E. granulosus*: Good
  - *E. multilocularis*: Fatal in 10-15 years untreated

Treatment

- *E. granulosus*
  - Medical: Albendazole/mebendazole
  - Direct injection of scolicidal agents
  - PAIR procedure: Puncture, aspiration, injection, respiration
  - Surgical: Segmental or lobar hepatectomy
- *E. multilocularis*
  - Partial hepatectomy/hepatectomy + liver transplant

DIAGNOSTIC CHECKLIST

Consider

- Rule out other complex or septate cystic liver masses
  - Biliary cystadenoma, pyogenic liver abscess, cystic metastases, and hemorrhagic or infected cyst
  - *E. multilocularis* imaging and clinical behavior simulates solid malignant neoplasm

Image Interpretation Pearls

- Daughter cysts can float freely within mother cyst
  - Altering patient's position may change position of daughter cysts

SELECTED REFERENCES

1. Qian LJ et al: Spectrum of multilocular cystic hepatic lesions: CT and MR imaging findings with pathologic correlation. Radiographics. 33(5):1419-33, 2013
2. Li Q et al: Echinococcal cysts of the liver and spleen: complex hepatic and splenic cystic lesions. Ultrasound Q. 28(3):205-7, 2012
3. Marrone G et al: Multidisciplinary imaging of liver hydatidosis. World J Gastroenterol. 18(13):1438-47, 2012
4. Brunetti E et al: Expert consensus for the diagnosis and treatment of cystic and alveolar echinococcosis in humans. Acta Trop. 114(1):1-16, 2010
5. Pedrosa I et al: Hydatid disease: radiologic and pathologic features and complications. Radiographics. 20(3):795-817, 2000

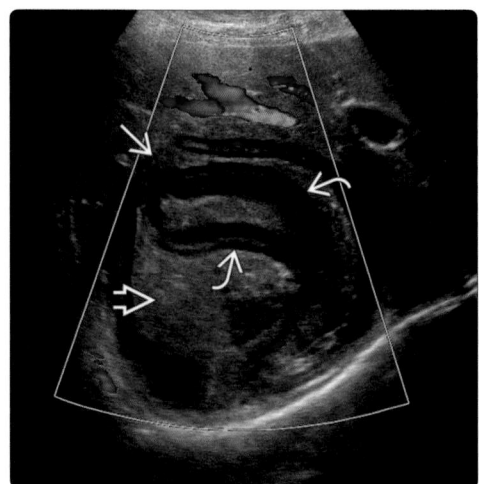

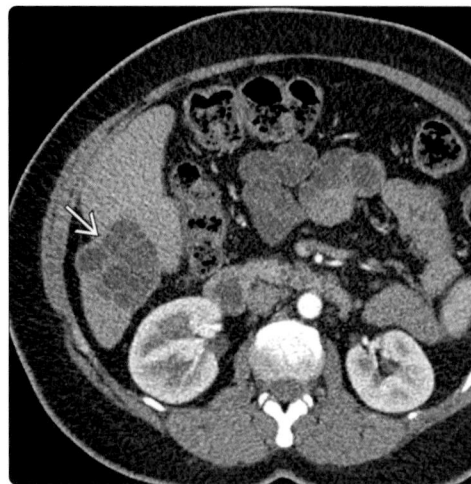

(Left) *Oblique abdominal color Doppler US shows a hepatic echinococcal cyst ➡ and fine echogenic debris (hydatid sand) ➡. Detachment of the endocyst membrane results in floating membranes within the pericyst ("water lily" sign) ➡. (Courtesy T. Morgan, MD.)* (Right) *Axial abdominal contrast-enhanced CT in a patient with an echinococcal cyst shows a multiloculated cystic mass in the right lobe of the liver ➡.*

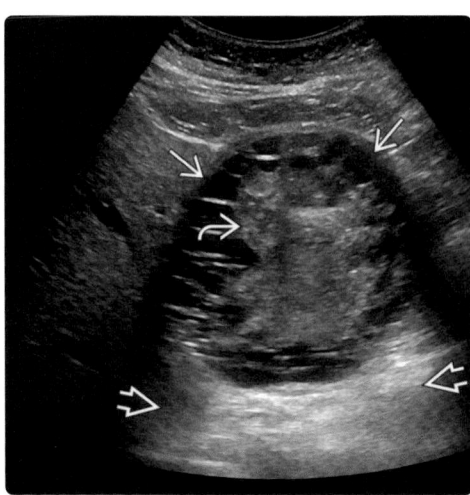

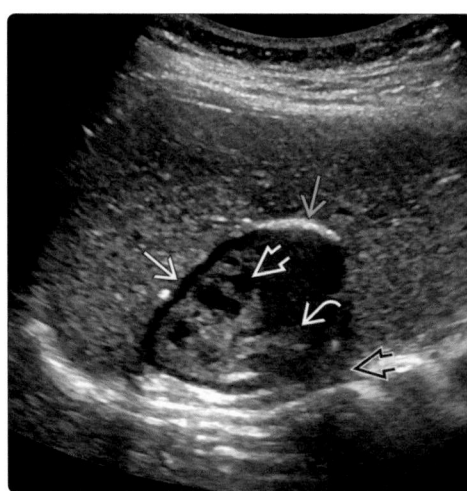

(Left) *Transverse abdominal ultrasound shows an echinococcal cyst containing multiple peripheral daughter cysts ➡ and heterogeneous material centrally ➡. Note the associated posterior acoustic enhancement ➡.* (Right) *Longitudinal abdominal grayscale US shows an ovoid hepatic echinococcal cyst ➡ containing daughter cysts ➡ and echogenic internal debris ➡. Note partial curvilinear rim calcification along the cyst wall ➡, which causes mild posterior acoustic shadowing ➡.*

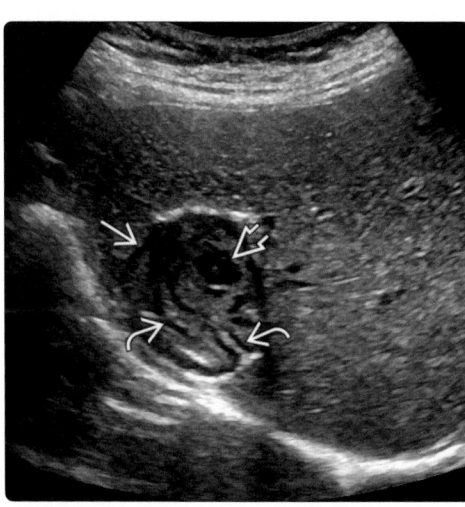

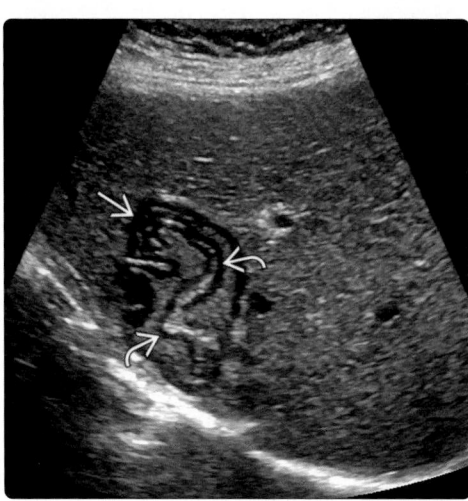

(Left) *Transverse abdominal grayscale US shows a hepatic echinococcal cyst ➡ containing a daughter cyst ➡, as well as detachment of the endocyst membrane, which results in floating membranes within the pericyst ("water lily" sign) ➡. (Right) Longitudinal abdominal grayscale US in the same patient shows a hepatic echinococcal cyst ➡ with multiple layers of floating endocyst membranes ➡ that have detached resulting in the "water lily" sign.*

Hepatic Diffuse Microabscesses

TERMINOLOGY

- Typically refers to hepatic candida abscesses in immunocompromised patients

IMAGING

- Multiple small hypoechoic lesions throughout liver (most common pattern)
- Target sign (hyperechoic center with hypoechoic halo) or bull's-eye configuration
- Wheel within a wheel pattern may be present in larger fungal lesions
- Multiple small, hyperchoic foci throughout liver (occurs in later stages)
- Lesions may resolve completely or calcify after successful treatment
- Similar lesions may be found in spleen

TOP DIFFERENTIAL DIAGNOSES

- Simple cysts

- Necrotic metastases
- Hepatic lymphoma
- Sarcoidosis
- Biliary hamartomas

PATHOLOGY

- Fungal infection: Most commonly *Candida albicans*, but may also include *Cryptococcus*, histoplasmosis, mucormycosis, *Aspergillus*
  - Occur more commonly in immunocompromised patients (leukemia, lymphoma, AIDS/post transplant)
- Pyogenic infections can appear similarly in patients with GI or biliary tract infection

DIAGNOSTIC CHECKLIST

- Rule out other causes of multiple liver lesions such as hepatic cysts, hepatic lymphoma, metastases, sarcoidosis
- Liver biopsy with culture often necessary to verify the lesions are due to fungal infection

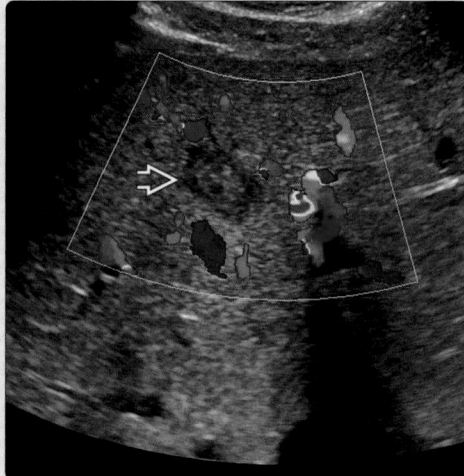
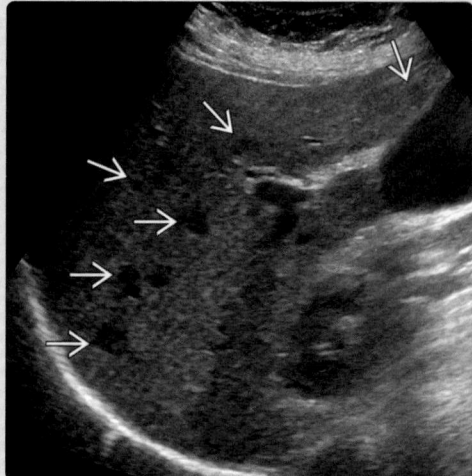

(Left) *Transverse color Doppler ultrasound of a hepatic fungal abscess* ➡ *shows characteristic wheel within a wheel or target appearance. Notice the fungal abscess is avascular in appearance.* (Right) *Longitudinal grayscale US shows multiple hypoechoic fungal abscesses* ➡ *throughout the liver in an immunocompromised patient.*

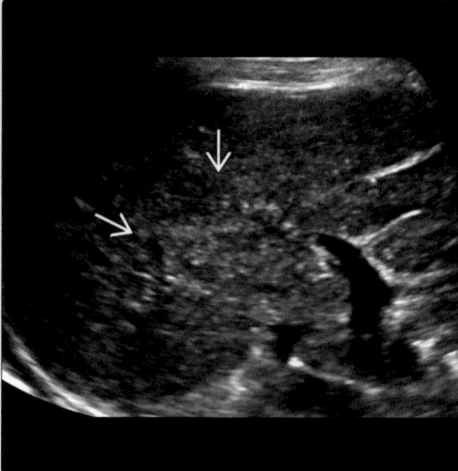
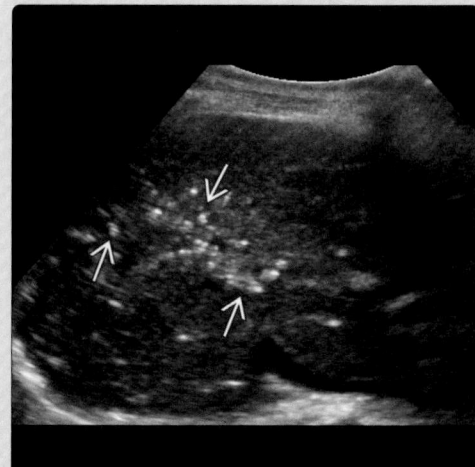

(Left) *Transverse transabdominal ultrasound shows a patchy heterogeneous echotexture due to diffuse involvement* ➡ *by Candida microabscesses.* (Right) *Longitudinal ultrasound in the same patient 2 years after treatment for disseminated candidiasis shows multiple hyperechoic, punctate parenchymal calcifications* ➡ *typical of treated Candida microabscesses.*

TERMINOLOGY

Definitions

- Hepatic parenchymal abscesses measuring ~ 1 cm in diameter
- Typically refers to hepatic candida abscesses in immunocompromised patients

IMAGING

General Features

- Best diagnostic clue
  - Multiple small liver lesions in patient with neutropenic fever (fungal abscesses)
  - Less commonly seen in setting of GI or biliary tract infection and positive blood culture (pyogenic microabscesses)
- Location
  - Diffusely distributed in liver ± spleen
- Size
  - ~ 1 cm
- Morphology
  - Usually rounded

Ultrasonographic Findings

- Grayscale ultrasound
  - Multiple small hypoechoic lesions throughout liver (most common pattern)
  - Target sign or bull's-eye configuration
    - Central hyperechoic inflammation surrounded by hypoechoic halo
  - Wheel within wheel pattern may be present in larger fungal lesions
    - Hyperechoic nodule of inflammatory cells with surrounding hypoechoic halo of fibrosis
    - Central hypoechoic area of necrosis within hyperechoic lesion
  - Multiple small, hyperchoic foci throughout liver (occurs in later stages)
    - Lesions may disappear or calcify after successful treatment
  - Similar lesions may be found in spleen

CT Findings

- CECT
  - Multiple small, hypodense lesions in liver ± spleen
  - Ill-defined margins
  - No contrast enhancement

DIFFERENTIAL DIAGNOSIS

Simple Cysts

- Typical uniformly hypoechoic/anechoic content

Necrotic Metastases

- May also demonstrate target sign (hypoechoic halo)
- Multiple
- Known primary tumor

Hepatic Lymphoma

- Often see coexisting lymphadenopathy
- Hepatosplenomegaly

Sarcoidosis

- Affects 5-15% of patients with sarcoidosis
- Coexists with pulmonary sarcoid ± splenic sarcoid nodules
- Asymptomatic

Biliary Hamartomas

- Small developmental malformations of intrahepatic bile ducts
- Hypoechoic or hyperechoic, < 1 cm, may have "comet tail" artifact
- Asymptomatic

PATHOLOGY

General Features

- Etiology
  - Fungal infection: Most commonly Candida albicans, but may also include *Cryptococcus*, histoplasmosis, mucormycosis, *Aspergillus*
  - Pyogenic infections can appear similarly in patients with GI or biliary tract infection

CLINICAL ISSUES

Presentation

- Most common signs/symptoms
  - Fever unresponsive to antibiotic treatment
  - Abdominal pain
  - Deranged liver function

Demographics

- Epidemiology
  - Mostly fungal: *Candida albicans*
  - Pyogenic: *Staphylococcus aureus*
  - Rare: *Escherichia coli*, CMV

Treatment

- Antifungal agents: Amphotericin B, fluconazole
- Liver biopsy with culture often necessary prior to treatment to verify infectious agent

SELECTED REFERENCES

1. Taşbakan MI et al: Isolated hepatic sarcoidosis mimicking liver microabscesses: a case report. Ir J Med Sci. 183(3):503-5, 2014
2. Krahn JF et al: Von Meyenburg complexes: a rare cause for multiple hepatic lesions on transabdominal ultrasound. J Clin Ultrasound. 40(3):174-5, 2012
3. Yellapu RK et al: Education and Imaging. Hepatobiliary and pancreatic: Candida liver abscesses associated with endocarditis. J Gastroenterol Hepatol. 25(5):1017, 2010
4. Koyama T et al: Radiologic manifestations of sarcoidosis in various organs. Radiographics. 24(1):87-104, 2004
5. Mortelé KJ et al: The infected liver: radiologic-pathologic correlation. Radiographics. 24(4):937-55, 2004
6. Verbanck J et al: Sonographic detection of multiple Staphylococcus aureus hepatic microabscesses mimicking Candida abscesses. J Clin Ultrasound. 27(8):478-81, 1999

Peribiliary Cyst

TERMINOLOGY

- Cystic dilatation of obstructed periductal glands of bile ducts
- Retention cyst of peribiliary gland

IMAGING

- Well-defined, cystic structures adjacent to portal triads
- Usually multiple; discrete, round/oval/tubular or confluent configuration
- Variable size, from 2 mm to 2 cm
- Smooth and thin walls without internal structures
- No enhancement of contents on CECT or MR
- Nonopacification with direct cholangiography or hepatobiliary phase MR using hepatocyte specific contrast agent
  - Due to lack of communication with biliary tree

TOP DIFFERENTIAL DIAGNOSES

- Biliary ductal dilatation
- Caroli disease
- Hepatic AD polycystic disease
- Periportal edema/inflammation

PATHOLOGY

- Disturbed portal venous flow, periductal fibrosis and inflammation → obliteration of neck of peribiliary glands → formation of retention cyst
- Associated with chronic hepatitis, cirrhosis, portal hypertension, portal vein thrombosis, liver transplantation

CLINICAL ISSUES

- Peribiliary cysts are typically asymptomatic; symptoms often related to underlying liver disease
- Obstructive jaundice may occur in end-stage liver cirrhosis or as complication of post-liver transplantation
- May increase in size and number of cysts as cirrhosis progresses

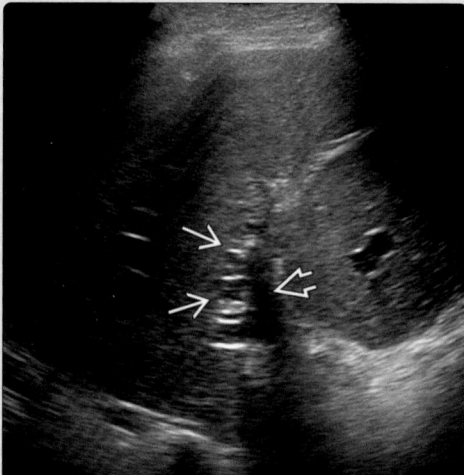
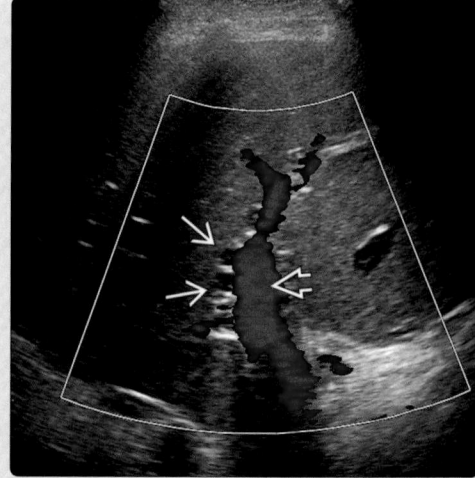

(Left) Grayscale ultrasound shows numerous small peribiliary cysts ➡ clustered in a linear configuration located along the portal vein ⏩. (Right) Color Doppler ultrasound in the same patient confirms the peribiliary cysts ➡ are located adjacent to the portal vein ⏩. Peribiliary cysts should not be confused with biliary ductal dilatation, which would have a more tubular and continuous appearance adjacent to the portal vein.

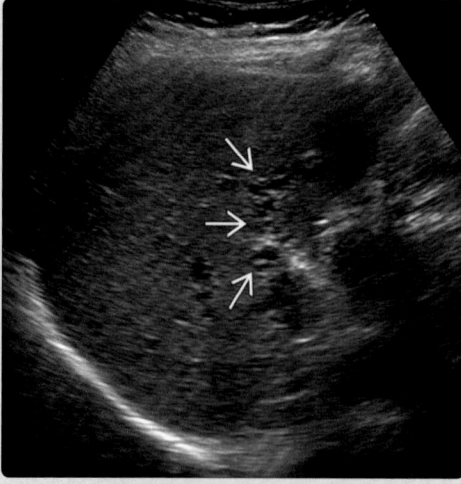
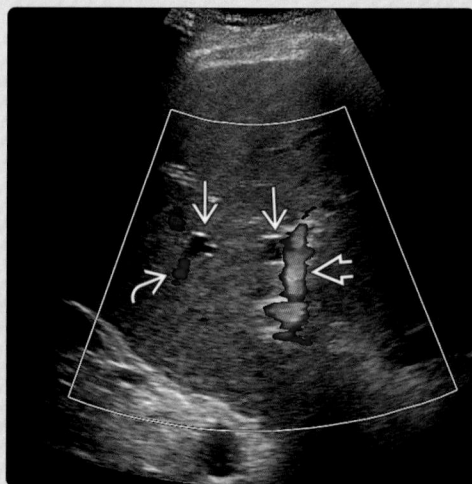

(Left) Longitudinal grayscale ultrasound shows numerous clustered small peribiliary cysts ➡ coursing along the hepatic hilum. (Right) Transverse color Doppler ultrasound shows small peribiliary cysts ➡ adjacent to the portal vein ⏩ and a proximal intrahepatic portal vein branch ➚.

TERMINOLOGY

Synonyms

- Retention cyst of peribiliary gland

Definitions

- Cystic dilation of obstructed periductal glands of bile ducts

IMAGING

General Features

- Best diagnostic clue
  - Well-defined cystic lesions of round/oval/tubular shape along portal triads
- Location
  - Along portal tracts in hepatic hilum
  - Adjacent to large intra- and extrahepatic ducts
  - Occasionally seen in peripheral liver
- Size
  - Variable, 2 mm to 2 cm
- Morphology
  - Usually multiple rounded cysts along portal triads

Ultrasonographic Findings

- Cluster of multiple small anechoic structures along portal triads most commonly at hepatic hilum

CT Findings

- Well-defined, water attenuation, round/oval/tubular structures
- Smooth, thin walls; no internal structures
- No enhancement on CECT
- Different configurations
  - Separate discrete cysts coursing along hilar/proximal intrahepatic portal vein
  - Linear cluster of cysts with "string of beads" appearance, mimicking sclerosing cholangitis
  - Confluent tubular cysts resembling dilated bile ducts

MR Findings

- T1WI: Iso- or hypointense compared to liver parenchyma
- T2WI: Markedly hyperintense due to fluid content
- T1WI C+: No enhancement
- Delayed phase: No contrast media filling cysts in hepatobiliary phase of MR using hepatocyte-specific contrast agent
  - Due to lack of communication with biliary system

Radiographic Findings

- Cholangiography: Nonopacification of cysts due to lack of communication with biliary system

DIFFERENTIAL DIAGNOSIS

Biliary Ductal Dilatation

- Dilated bile ducts along portal triads typically caused by downstream obstructive process
- Tubular in configuration

Caroli Disease

- Congenital, multifocal, segmental, saccular dilatation of intrahepatic bile ducts

- "Central dot" sign on CECT: Enhancement of portal radicles within cysts
- May coexist with peribiliary cysts

Periportal Edema/Inflammation

- CT: Circumferential zones of decreased attenuation around portal vein branches
- US: Echogenic appearance of portal triads; not typically confused with peribiliary cysts on US
- Seen in various conditions, including hypervolemia, cardiac congestion, hepatitis, etc.

PATHOLOGY

General Features

- Etiology
  - Disturbed portal venous flow, periductal fibrosis and inflammation → obliteration of neck of peribiliary glands → formation of retention cyst
  - Gene expression of autosomal dominant polycystic kidney disease (ADPKD) in peribiliary glands
  - Infrequent complications of liver transplantation
- Associated abnormalities
  - Chronic hepatitis, cirrhosis, portal hypertension, portal vein thrombosis
  - AD polycystic disease
  - Caroli disease

Gross Pathologic & Surgical Features

- Predominantly serous, rarely mucinous cysts

Microscopic Features

- Single layer of epithelial lining with thin fibrous tissue layer

CLINICAL ISSUES

Presentation

- Most common signs/symptoms
  - Generally asymptomatic from cysts
  - Obstructive jaundice may occur
    - Associated with end-stage liver cirrhosis
  - Symptoms related to underlying liver disease

Demographics

- Epidemiology
  - On pathology: 20% of normal population and 50% of patients with cirrhosis
  - On CT: 3% of normal population, 95% of patients with cirrhosis, and 20% of patients with AD polycystic disease

Natural History & Prognosis

- May increase in size and number of cysts in time with progression of cirrhosis

SELECTED REFERENCES

1. Kai K et al: An autopsy case of obstructive jaundice due to hepatic multiple peribiliary cysts accompanying hepatolithiasis. Hepatol Res. 38(2):211-6, 2008
2. Terayama N et al: Terada T, Nakanuma Y, Shinozaki K, et al. Peribiliary cysts in liver cirrhosis: US, CT, and MR findings. 19(3):419-23, 1995
3. Baron RL et al: liver disease: imaging-pathologic correlation. AJR Am J Roentgenol. 1994 Mar;162(3):631-6. 162(3):631-6, 1994
4. Itai Y et al: Hepatic peribiliary cysts: multiple tiny cysts within the larger portal tract, hepatic hilum, or both. Radiology. 191(1):107-10, 1994

Ciliated Hepatic Foregut Cyst

TERMINOLOGY
- Rare foregut developmental malformation in liver

IMAGING
- US
  - Single hypoechoic unilocular cyst
  - May have variable internal echoes
- CT
  - NECT: Hypoattenuating; sometimes iso- or hyperattenuating
  - CECT: No contrast enhancement
- MR
  - T1WI: Hyperintense due to mucin content
  - Brightly hyperintense on T2WI

TOP DIFFERENTIAL DIAGNOSES
- Complicated hepatic cyst
- Biliary cystadenoma/cystadenocarcinoma
- Biloma

- Hematoma

PATHOLOGY
- Detached outpouching of hepatic diverticulum or adjacent enteric foregut

CLINICAL ISSUES
- Mostly asymptomatic and incidentally found by imaging
- Clinical course usually benign
- 3% risk of malignant transformation: Squamous cell carcinoma, usually in setting of large cyst
- Treatment: Surgical excision or enucleation irrespective of size to eliminate subsequent cancer risk

DIAGNOSTIC CHECKLIST
- Rule out other cystic lesions and solid hypovascular tumorous lesions in liver
- Single unilocular cystic lesion in or close to hepatic segment IV in subcapsular portion with variable internal contents

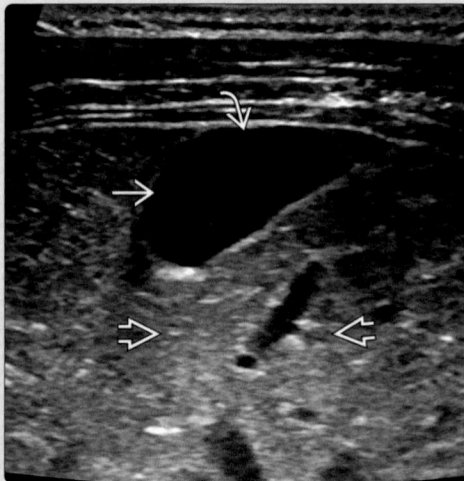
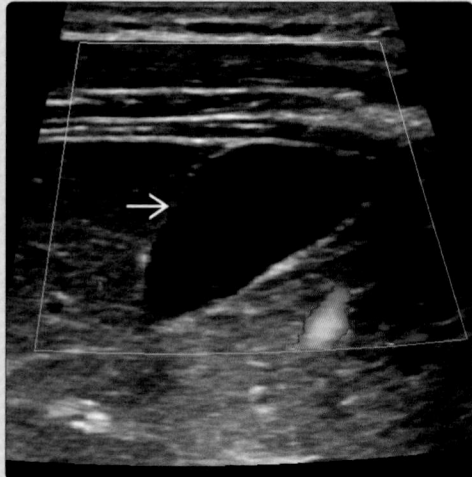

(Left) Oblique abdominal grayscale ultrasound in a patient with a ciliated hepatic foregut cyst shows a well-defined, ovoid, subcapsular cystic mass ➡ in segment IV of the liver ➡. Internal content of the cystic lesion is relatively homogeneous. Minimal posterior acoustic enhancement ➡ is visible. (Right) Color Doppler ultrasound in the same patient shows no detectable internal color flow within the cystic mass ➡.

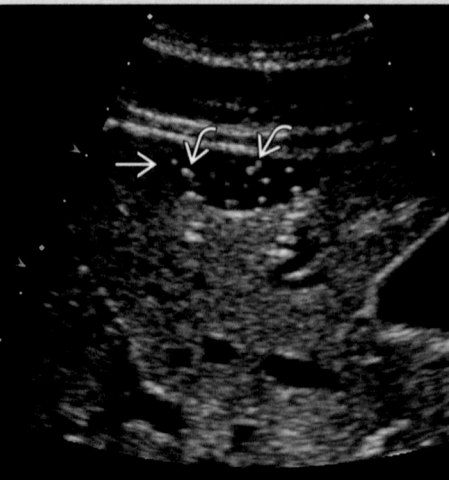
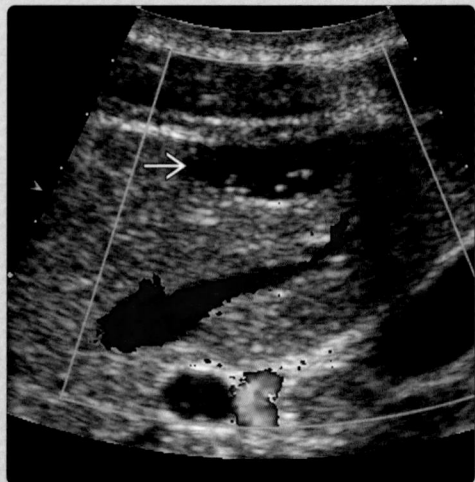

(Left) Transverse abdominal grayscale ultrasound in a patient with ciliated hepatic foregut cyst shows an ovoid subcapsular cystic mass in segment IV of the liver ➡. The lesion contains numerous tiny echogenic foci ➡ consistent with mucinous debris. (Courtesy R. Baxter, MD.) (Right) Color Doppler ultrasound in the same patient shows no detectable color flow within the cystic mass ➡. (Courtesy R. Baxter, MD.)

Ciliated Hepatic Foregut Cyst

TERMINOLOGY

Abbreviations

- Ciliated hepatic foregut cyst (CHFC)

Definitions

- Foregut developmental malformation in liver

IMAGING

General Features

- Best diagnostic clue
  - Subcapsular cystic lesion located within or close to segment IV of liver
- Location
  - Within or near medial segment of left lobe of liver (segment IV)
  - Either subcapsular or beneath Glisson capsule
- Size
  - Average: 3.6 cm (range: 1.1-13 cm)
- Morphology
  - Typically unilocular, rarely multilocular
  - Round or ovoid cystic lesion with smooth, well-defined walls

Ultrasonographic Findings

- Single unilocular cyst
- May contain internal echogenic foci
- Posterior acoustic enhancement

CT Findings

- NECT: Variable depending on fluid composition
  - Mostly hypoattenuating; sometimes iso- or hyperattenuating
- CECT: No enhancement

MR Findings

- T1WI: Frequently hyperintense due to mucin
  - Depends on viscosity, mucin density, presence or absence of cholesterol and calcium crystals
- T2WI: Brightly hyperintense

Imaging Recommendations

- Best imaging tool
  - Ultrasound is suggestive of diagnosis; correlation with CT or MR may be helpful

DIFFERENTIAL DIAGNOSIS

Complicated Hepatic Cyst

- May contain thin septa, internal debris, or fluid-debris level

Biliary Cystadenoma/Cystadenocarcinoma

- Usually multilocular or with complex septations or mural nodules
- Predominantly seen in women

Biloma

- Usually results from trauma, including prior surgery

Hematoma

- Due to hepatic trauma
- Echogenicity evolves over time

PATHOLOGY

General Features

- Etiology
  - Thought to arise from detached outpouching of hepatic diverticulum or adjacent enteric foregut
    - Share common embryological origin with bronchial cyst and esophageal cyst

Gross Pathologic & Surgical Features

- Cyst contents: Mostly viscous or mucinous
  - Infantile form: Bilious fluid with direct communication with bile ducts

Microscopic Features

- Similar to bronchogenic and esophageal cysts
- Lined, ciliated, pseudostratified, mucin-secreting columnar epithelium
- Cyst wall contains abundant smooth muscle fibers

CLINICAL ISSUES

Presentation

- Most common signs/symptoms
  - Asymptomatic and incidentally found by imaging
- Other signs/symptoms
  - Right upper quadrant pain
    - Small cyst: Subcapsular location may stretch Glisson capsule
  - Abdominal mass secondary to enlarged cystic swelling
  - Large cysts may cause obstructive jaundice or portal hypertension secondary to compression effects

Demographics

- Age: Middle-aged
- Gender: Slight male predominance (1.1:1)
- Prevalence: Very rare but increasingly diagnosed

Natural History & Prognosis

- Slowly growing congenital cyst
- Clinical course usually benign
- 3% risk of malignant transformation: Squamous cell carcinoma, usually in setting of large cyst

Treatment

- Surgical excision or enucleation irrespective of size so as to eliminate subsequent cancer risk
- Infantile CHFC: Liver resection and closure of biliary communication

DIAGNOSTIC CHECKLIST

Consider

- Rule out other cystic lesions and solid hypovascular tumorous lesions in liver

Image Interpretation Pearls

- Single subcapsular unilocular cystic lesion in or near hepatic segment IV with variable internal contents

SELECTED REFERENCES

1. Sharma S et al: Ciliated hepatic foregut cyst: an increasingly diagnosed condition. Hepatobiliary Pancreat Dis Int. 7(6):581-9, 2008

TERMINOLOGY

- Benign tumor composed of dilated vascular channels lined by single layer of endothelial cells and supported by thin fibrous stroma

IMAGING

- Well-defined, uniformly hyperechoic mass
- Internal vascularity often undetectable with color Doppler
- May see posterior acoustic enhancement
- "Typical atypical" hemangioma: Hyperechoic rim with hypoechoic center
- Contrast-enhanced imaging
  - Arterial hyperenhancement: "Flash fill" homogeneous hypervascularity or nodular discontinuous hyperenhancement
  - Centripetal fill-in on later images
  - Enhancement follows blood pool

TOP DIFFERENTIAL DIAGNOSES

- Focal steatosis
- Hepatocellular carcinoma
- Hypervascular metastases

PATHOLOGY

- Large vascular channels lined by single layer of endothelial cells supported by thin fibrous septa
- Most common benign tumor of liver

DIAGNOSTIC CHECKLIST

- Small hepatocellular carcinoma (HCC) or metastasis can mimic hemangioma
- Hemangioma may vary in echogenicity at different times of scanning due to rate of blood flow within lesion
- May see posterior acoustic enhancement

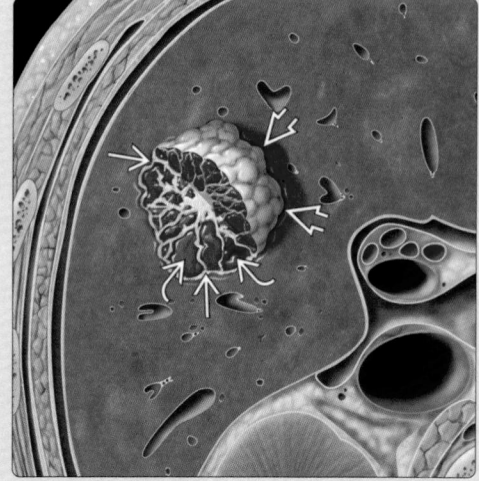
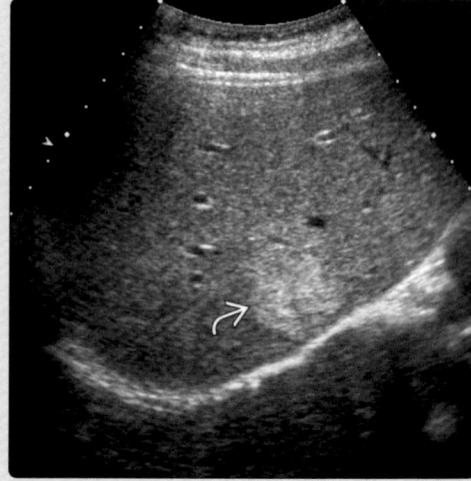

(Left) Transverse graphic shows a solitary hemangioma, illustrating the lobular contour ⇒ and multiple internal fibrous septa ➡, which are separating vascular channels ➘. (Right) Transverse US of the right lobe of the liver shows a homogeneously echogenic hemangioma ➘. This is a typical appearance of a hemangioma.

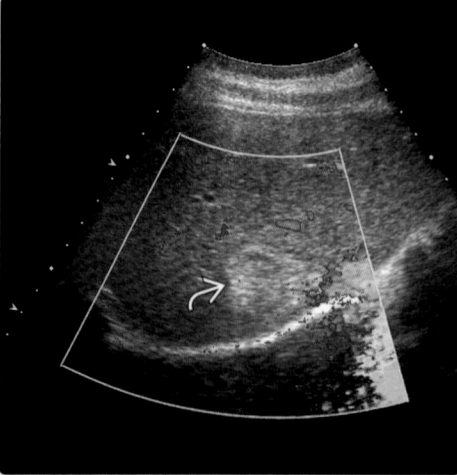
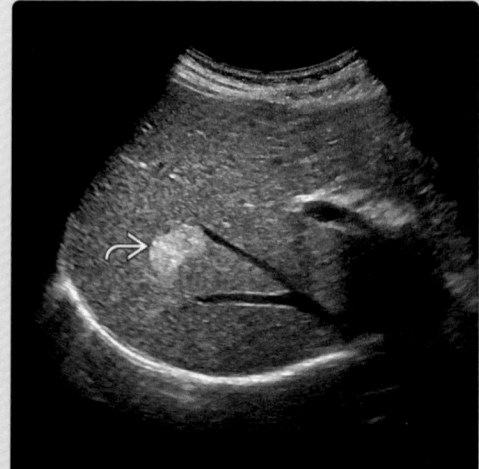

(Left) Color Doppler US of a hemangioma ➘ shows no detectable internal vascularity, likely related to flow that is too slow to be sonographically detected. (Right) Transverse US of the right lobe of the liver shows a typical hemangioma ➘, which is homogeneously echogenic with well-defined margins.

Hepatic Cavernous Hemangioma

TERMINOLOGY

Synonyms

- Liver hemangioma, capillary hemangioma, cavernous hemangioma

Definitions

- Benign tumor composed of dilated endothelial-lined vascular channels lined by single layer of endothelial cells supported by thin fibrous stroma

IMAGING

General Features

- Best diagnostic clue
  - Well-defined, uniformly hyperechoic mass
- Size
  - Small (capillary) hemangioma: < 2 cm
  - Typical hemangioma: 2-10 cm
  - Giant hemangioma: > 10 cm (arbitrary cutoff)
- Morphology
  - Most common benign tumor of liver
  - 2nd most common liver tumor after metastases
  - Usually solitary & grow minimally
  - May be multiple in up to 10% of cases
  - More commonly seen in postmenopausal women
  - May have central scar in giant hemangiomas
    - Calcification of scar is rare (< 10%)

Ultrasonographic Findings

- Grayscale ultrasound
  - Typically homogeneously hyperechoic (over 2/3 of patients)
    - Probably due to slow blood flow rather than multiple interfaces
    - Smooth or lobulated well-defined borders
    - Occasionally see posterior acoustic enhancement
  - Echogenicity may vary
    - Echogenicity may change over time during imaging
    - Direction & angle of insonation may alter echogenic appearance
    - In fatty livers, hemangiomas may appear hypoechoic
    - Heterogeneous in large lesions
      - Hypoechoic areas within large lesions may represent necrosis, hemorrhage, scar, or vessels
  - "Typical atypical" appearance
    - Hypoechoic center with thick or thin hyperechoic rim
- Pulsed Doppler
  - In "high-flow hemangioma" may see feeding artery and draining portal vein
- Color Doppler
  - May show vessels in periphery of tumor
    - Blood supply is from hepatic artery
  - Typically undetectable color Doppler flow in lesion, which is too slow to be sonographically detected
- Power Doppler
  - May detect slow flow within hemangiomas
- Contrast-enhanced US
  - Demonstrates same filling-in phenomenon as seen on CECT

CT Findings

- NECT
  - Same attenuation as blood pool (aorta)
  - Giant hemangioma (> 10 cm)
    - Heterogeneous hypodense mass
    - Central low-attenuation scar
- CECT
  - Small hemangioma: < 2 cm
    - Homogeneous "flash fill" enhancement in arterial and venous phases
  - Typical hemangioma: 2-10 cm
    - Arterial phase: Early peripheral, nodular, discontinuous enhancement
    - Venous: Progressive centripetal enhancement to uniform filling, isodense to blood vessels
    - Delayed: Persistent enhancement, similar to blood pool
  - Giant hemangioma: > 10 cm
    - Arterial: Peripheral nodular or globular discontiguous enhancement
    - Venous & delayed phases: Incomplete centripetal filling (scar does not enhance)
  - Hyalinized (sclerosed) hemangioma
    - Minimal enhancement
    - Cannot be diagnosed with confidence by imaging

MR Findings

- T1WI
  - Small & typical hemangiomas
    - Well marginated
    - Isointense to blood; hypointense to liver
  - Giant hemangioma
    - Hypointense to liver
    - Central cleft-like area of marked decreased intensity (scar or fibrous tissue)
- T2WI
  - Small & typical hemangiomas
    - Hyperintense, "light-bulb bright" similar to spinal CSF
  - Giant hemangioma
    - Hyperintense mass
    - Marked hyperintense center (scar or fibrosis)
    - Hypointense internal septa
- T1WI C+
  - Small hemangioma (< 2 cm)
    - Homogeneous "flash fill" enhancement in arterial and portal phases, similar to blood pool
  - Typical & giant hemangiomas
    - Arterial phase: Peripheral, nodular discontinuous enhancement
    - Venous phase: Progressive centripetal filling
    - Central scar: No enhancement & remains hypointense

Angiographic Findings

- Conventional
  - Dense opacification of lesion
  - "Cotton wool" appearance
    - Pooling of contrast within hemangioma
  - Normal-sized feeders
  - Typically retain contrast beyond venous phase

Nuclear Medicine Findings

- Tc-99m-labeled red blood cell scan with SPECT (95% accuracy)
  - Early dynamic scan: Focal defect or less uptake
  - Delayed scans (over 30-50 min): Persistent filling

Imaging Recommendations

- Best imaging tool
  - In absence of risk factors, US for diagnosis and follow-up (cost-effective plus radiation-free)
  - For definitive characterization, MR may be more diagnostic than CT
- Protocol advice
  - Atypical lesions or lesions in high-risk patients may require CT/MR or biopsy

DIFFERENTIAL DIAGNOSIS

Hepatocellular Carcinoma (HCC)

- Background cirrhosis or underlying liver disease
- Heterogeneous and usually hypoechoic
- Irregular or infiltrating borders

Hypervascular Metastases

- Usually multiple
- May have hypoechoic halo ("target" lesion)

Steatosis

- Geographic borders
- Vessels pass through lesion without distortion

Angiosarcoma

- Ill-defined and multicentric
- Highly aggressive, rapidly growing

PATHOLOGY

General Features

- Etiology
  - Hemangiomas occur sporadically without predisposing factors
- Associated abnormalities
  - Associated with focal nodular hyperplasia (FNH)
  - Kasabach-Merritt syndrome
    - Hemangioma with intravascular coagulation, clotting, and fibrinolysis resulting in thrombocytopenia

Gross Pathologic & Surgical Features

- Solitary, well-defined, blood-filled, soft nodule
  - Size ranges from 2-20 cm
- Cut section: Giant hemangioma
  - Areas of fibrosis, necrosis, and cystic spaces

Microscopic Features

- Large vascular channels lined by single layer of endothelial cells supported by thin fibrous septa
- No bile ducts or hepatocytes
- Thrombosis of vascular channels resulting in fibrosis and calcification

CLINICAL ISSUES

Presentation

- Most common signs/symptoms
  - Small and typical hemangioma
    - Usually asymptomatic
    - Commonly seen on routine examination & autopsy
  - Giant hemangioma
    - Asymptomatic or hepatomegaly/abdominal pain
- Lab data: Normal liver function tests
- Diagnosis
  - Multiphasic CECT, CEMR, or RBC scan with SPECT imaging are highly diagnostic

Demographics

- Age
  - All age groups (uncommon in children)
  - More common in postmenopausal age group
- Gender
  - M:F = 1:2-1:5
- Epidemiology
  - Incidence
    - 5-20% of population
    - Increases with multiparity
  - Prevalence: Uniform worldwide

Natural History & Prognosis

- Most often asymptomatic; complications are rare
  - Spontaneous rupture, coagulation, or inflammation
  - Compression of adjacent structures
- Often show slow growth

Treatment

- Asymptomatic: Usually ignore
- Symptomatic large lesions: Surgical resection

DIAGNOSTIC CHECKLIST

Consider

- Small HCC or metastasis can mimic hemangioma

Image Interpretation Pearls

- Hemangioma may vary in echogenicity at different times of scanning due to rate of blood flow within lesion
- May see posterior acoustic enhancement

SELECTED REFERENCES

1. Quaia E: The real capabilities of contrast-enhanced ultrasound in the characterization of solid focal liver lesions. Eur Radiol. 21(3):457-62, 2011
2. Wakui N et al: Diagnosis of hepatic hemangioma by parametric imaging using sonazoid-enhanced US. Hepatogastroenterology. 58(110-111):1431-5, 2011
3. Kamaya A et al: Hypervascular liver lesions. Semin Ultrasound CT MR. 30(5):387-407, 2009
4. Jang HJ et al: Hepatic hemangioma: atypical appearances on CT, MR imaging, and sonography. AJR Am J Roentgenol. 180(1):135-41, 2003
5. Perkins AB et al: Color and power Doppler sonography of liver hemangiomas: a dream unfulfilled? J Clin Ultrasound. 28(4):159-65, 2000
6. Vilgrain V et al: Imaging of atypical hemangiomas of the liver with pathologic correlation. RadioGraphics. 20: 379-97, 2000

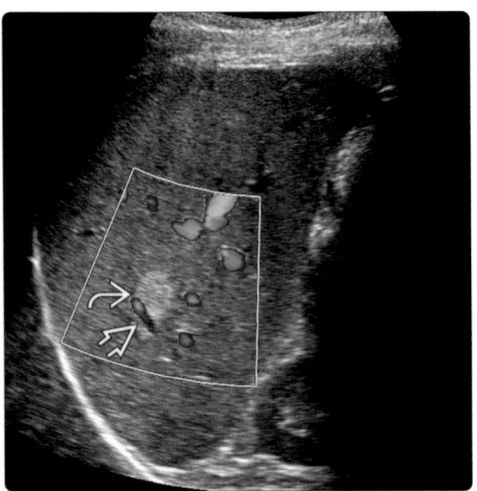
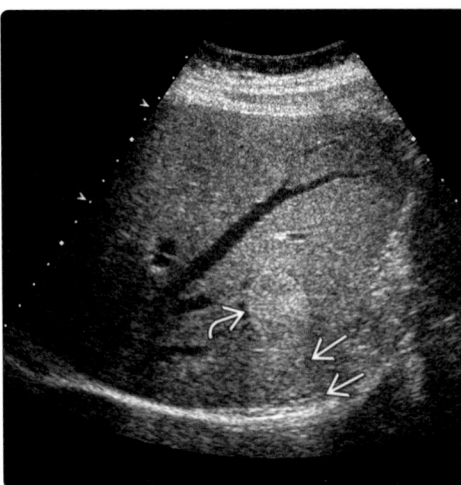

(Left) *Longitudinal color Doppler US of the right lobe of the liver shows a well-defined echogenic hemangioma ➜ with adjacent vessel ➜ but without detectable internal vascularity in the lesion itself.* (Right) *Longitudinal oblique US of the liver shows an echogenic, well-defined hemangioma ➜. Minimal posterior acoustic enhancement ➜ is seen, which is thought to be related to the homogeneous internal architecture of hemangiomas.*

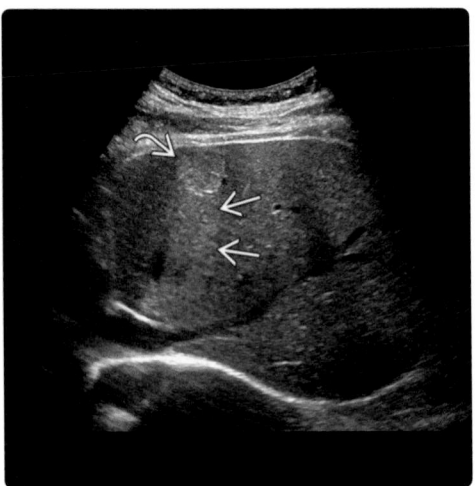
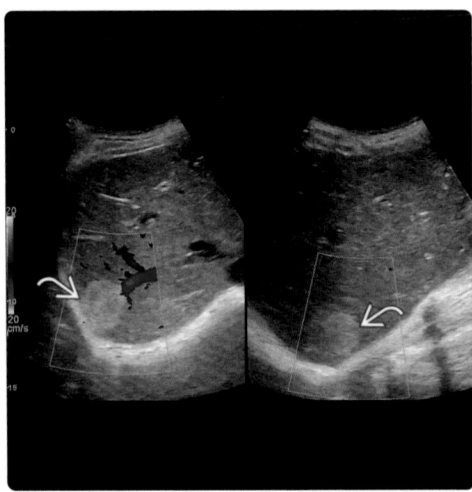

(Left) *Longitudinal view of the liver shows a well-defined echogenic hemangioma ➜ just below the liver capsule with minimal posterior acoustic enhancement ➜.* (Right) *Transverse and longitudinal color Doppler images show a well-defined echogenic hemangioma ➜ without detectable internal vascularity.*

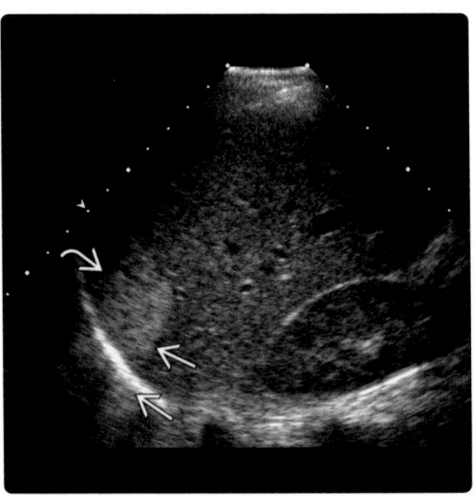
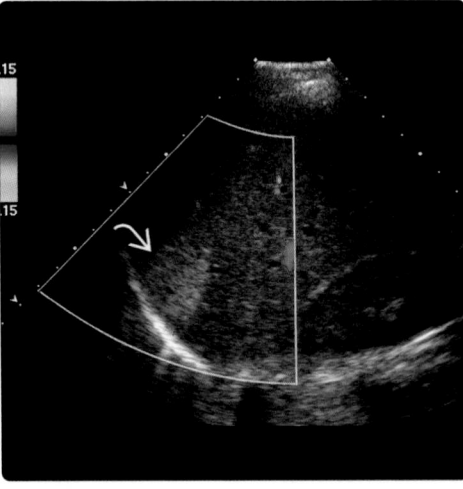

(Left) *Longitudinal grayscale US of the right lobe of the liver shows a homogeneously echogenic hemangioma ➜ with posterior acoustic enhancement ➜.* (Right) *Longitudinal color Doppler US of the same patient shows no detectable internal vascularity in the hemangioma ➜.*

(Left) *Transverse grayscale US of the liver using a high-frequency transducer shows a "typical atypical" appearance of a hemangioma in which the margins ⇒ are echogenic and the center ⇒ is hypoechoic.* **(Right)** *Transverse and longitudinal views show a "typical atypical" hemangioma ⇒ with an echogenic rim and a hypoechoic center.*

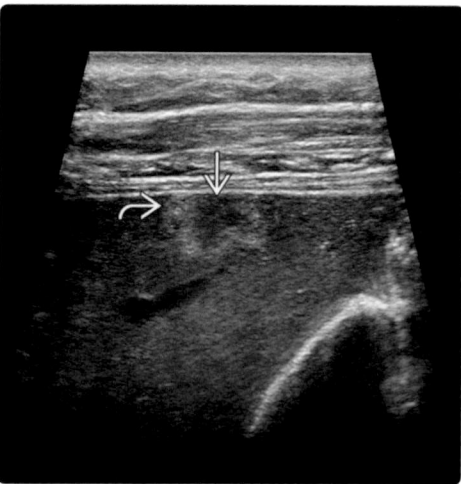
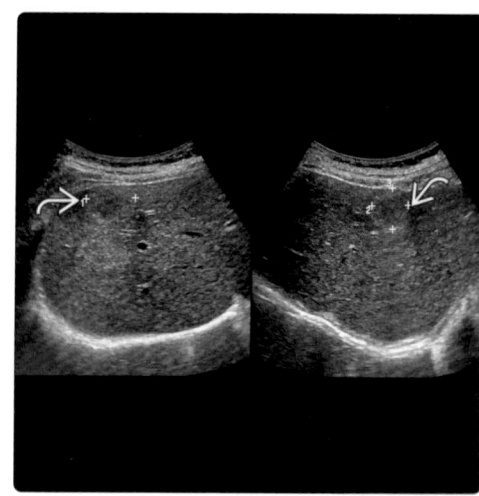

(Left) *Transverse grayscale ultrasound of the liver shows a "typical atypical" hemangioma with a well-defined echogenic periphery ⇒ and hypoechoic center ⇒. (Right) Transverse color Doppler ultrasound of the same hemangioma shows minimal, if any, detectable vascularity ⇒.*

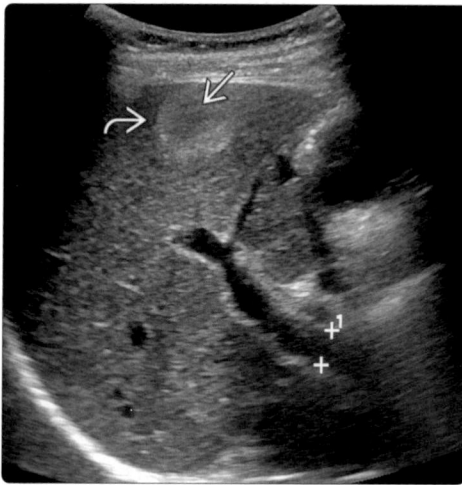
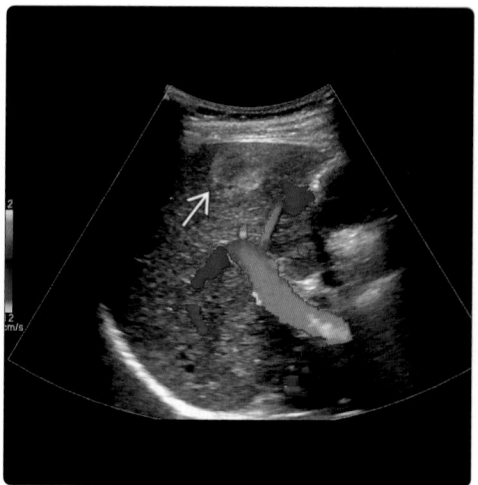

(Left) *Transverse and longitudinal views of the same lesion show a well-defined, echogenic hemangioma ⇒.* **(Right)** *Transverse high-frequency US of the liver shows a well-defined, homogeneously echogenic hemangioma ⇒.*

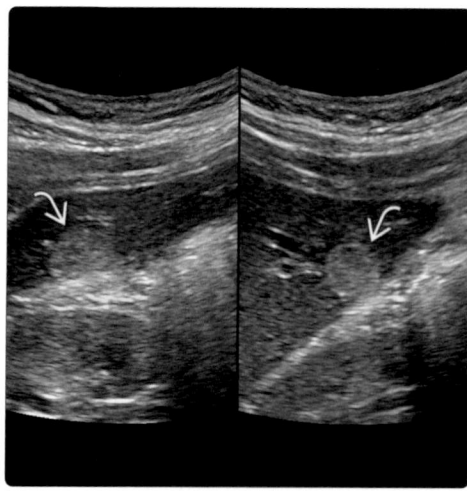
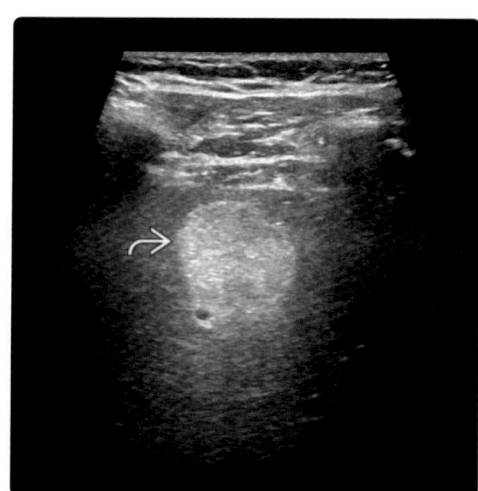

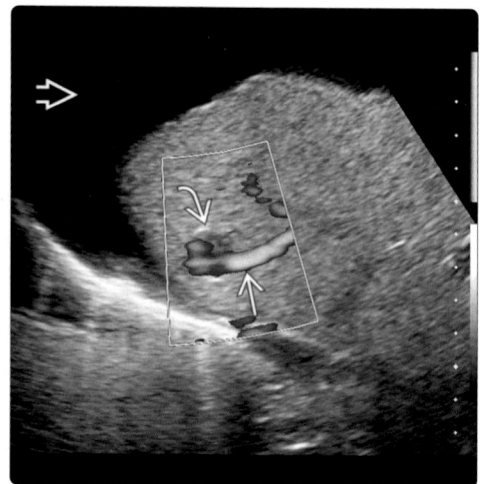

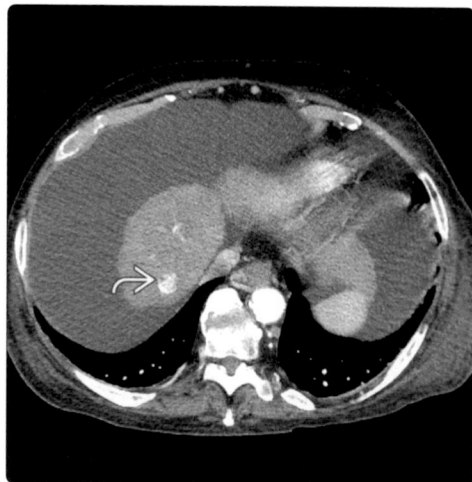

(Left) *Transverse US of the liver shows a high-flow hemangioma ⇨ with a large draining portal vein ➡. In the setting of ascites ⇉ and underlying cirrhosis, diagnosis of high-flow hemangioma is challenging by ultrasound alone.* (Right) *Contrast-enhanced CT in the same patient during late arterial phase shows the high-flow hemangioma ⇨ follows the blood pool. This lesion followed the blood pool on portal venous and delayed phase images as well as a draining portal vein (not shown).*

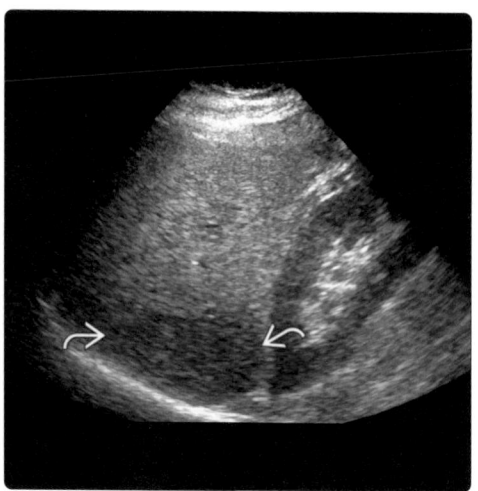

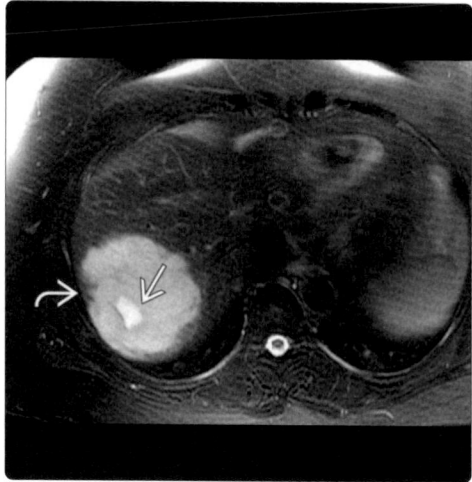

(Left) *Longitudinal grayscale US of the liver shows a hypoechoic hemangioma ⇨ in the setting of a fatty liver. In this case, the diagnosis of a hemangioma was confirmed with cross-sectional imaging with contrast (not shown).* (Right) *Axial T2-weighted MR of the liver shows a well-defined, lobulated, hyperintense hemangioma ⇨ with a markedly hyperintense central scar ➡.*

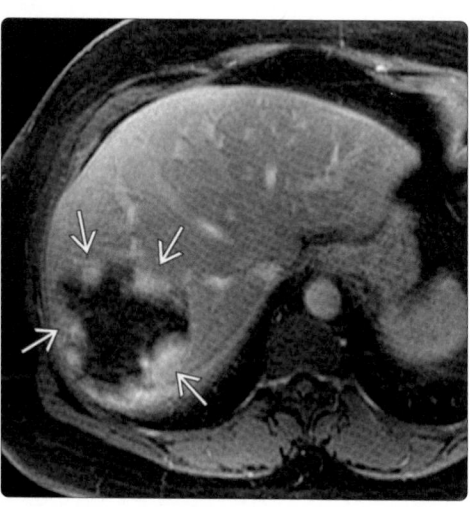

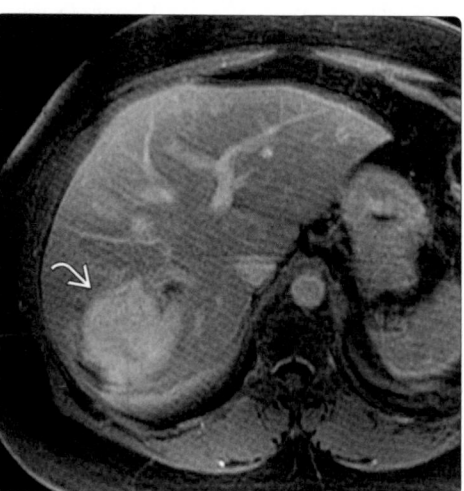

(Left) *Axial T1-weighted contrast-enhanced MR in the same patient during the portal venous phase shows peripheral nodular discontiguous enhancement ➡ of the hemangioma that follows the blood pool.* (Right) *Axial T1-weighted contrast-enhanced MR with fat saturation shows the same lesion fills-in ⇨ in a centripetal fashion with enhancement similar to blood pool.*

Focal Nodular Hyperplasia

TERMINOLOGY

- Focal nodular hyperplasia (FNH)
- Benign tumor of liver caused by hyperplastic response to localized vascular abnormality

IMAGING

- Ultrasound
  - Usually homogeneous and isoechoic
  - Spoke-wheel pattern on color Doppler US
    - Large central feeding artery with multiple small vessels radiating peripherally
- CEUS/CT/MR
  - Bright, homogeneously enhancing mass on arterial phase with delayed enhancement of central scar
- Gadoxetate-enhanced MR
  - Most specific test to diagnose FNH
  - Prolonged enhancement of entire FNH on hepatobiliary phase scan

TOP DIFFERENTIAL DIAGNOSES

- Hepatic adenoma
- Fibrolamellar hepatocellular carcinoma
- Hepatic cavernous hemangioma
- Hypervascular metastasis

PATHOLOGY

- Normal hepatocytes and malformed bile ductules
- Thick-walled arteries in fibrous septa radiating from center to periphery

CLINICAL ISSUES

- Common in young to middle-aged women
- Excellent prognosis

DIAGNOSTIC CHECKLIST

- Imaging is more reliable than histology in making diagnosis of FNH

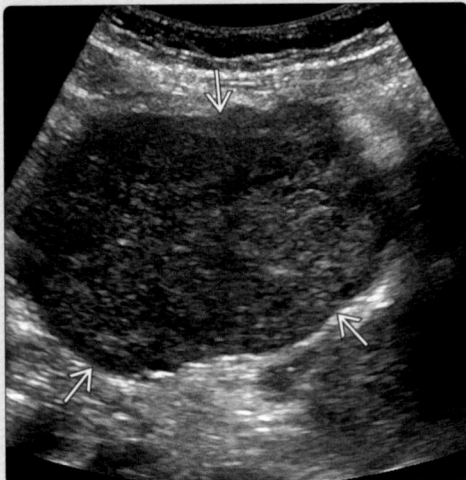
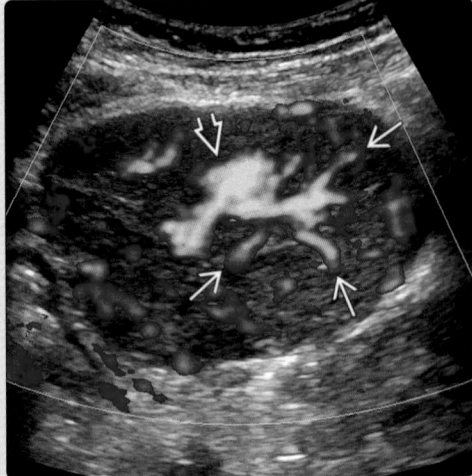

(Left) Transverse abdominal US shows a large FNH ➡ that appears as a homogeneously hypoechoic solid mass in the lateral segment of the left lobe of the liver. (Right) On power Doppler US in the same patient, the FNH shows a large central feeding artery ➡ with multiple small vessels radiating peripherally ➡, creating a "spoke wheel" vascularity pattern.

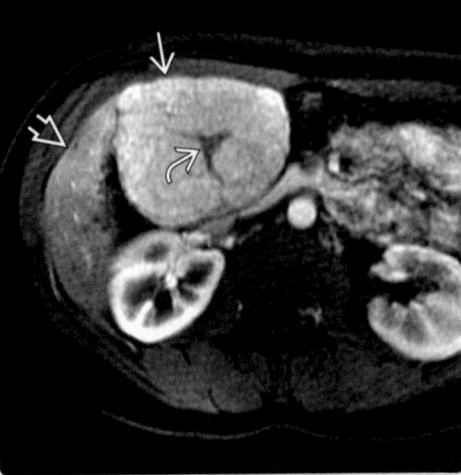
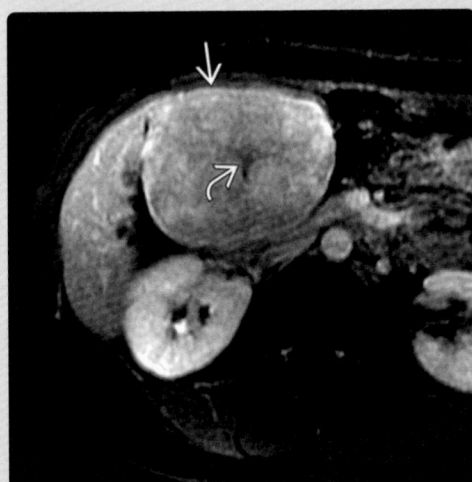

(Left) Axial arterial phase T1 contrast-enhanced MR in the same patient shows a slightly hyperenhancing FNH ➡ compared to adjacent liver parenchyma ➡. The FNH contains a hypointense stellate central scar ➡. (Right) Delayed phase T1 contrast-enhanced MR in the same patient shows that the FNH becomes isointense ➡ compared to background liver parenchyma. The central scar is hypointense ➡ but enhances slightly compared to the arterial phase image.

TERMINOLOGY

Abbreviations

- Focal nodular hyperplasia (FNH)

Definitions

- Benign tumor of liver caused by hyperplastic response to localized vascular abnormality

IMAGING

General Features

- Best diagnostic clue
  - Homogeneously isoechoic mass often with central scar
- Location
  - More common in right lobe
  - Usually subcapsular & rarely pedunculated
- Size
  - Majority are smaller than 5 cm (85%)
  - Mean diameter at time of diagnosis: 3 cm
- Key concepts
  - 2nd most common benign tumor of liver after hemangioma
  - Most frequent hepatic tumor in young women
  - Benign congenital hamartomatous malformation
  - Accounts for 8% of primary hepatic tumors in autopsy series
  - Usually solitary lesion (80%); multiple in 20%
  - Multiple FNHs associated with multiorgan vascular malformations and certain brain neoplasms

Ultrasonographic Findings

- Grayscale ultrasound
  - Mass: Mostly homogeneous and isoechoic to liver, occasionally hypoechoic or hyperechoic
  - Mass effect: Displacement of normal hepatic vessels and ducts
  - Central scar: Mostly hypoechoic, may be hyperechoic
  - Prominent draining veins seen as hypoechoic nodules around lesion
- Color Doppler
  - Spoke-wheel pattern
    - Large central feeding artery with multiple small vessels radiating peripherally
  - Large draining veins at tumor margins
  - Highly vascular tumor, but hemorrhage is rare
  - High-velocity Doppler signals
    - Due to increased blood flow or arteriovenous shunts
- Contrast-enhanced ultrasound
  - Arterial phase: Brisk enhancement with spoke-wheel pattern
    - Centrifugal enhancement: More common in small (≤ 3cm) FNH
  - Portal and delayed phase: No significant enhancement or washout

CT Findings

- NECT
  - Isodense or hypodense to normal liver
- CECT
  - Hepatic arterial phase
    - Transient, intense, and homogeneous enhancement

- Portal venous phase
  - Hypodense or isodense to normal liver
  - Large draining veins → hepatic veins
- Delayed phase
  - Mass: Isodense to liver
  - Central scar: Hyperdense due to fibrous tissue
  - Scar visible in 2/3 of large (> 3 cm) & 1/3 of small FNH

MR Findings

- T1WI
  - Mass: Isointense to slightly hypointense
  - Central scar: Hypointense
- T2WI
  - Mass: Slightly hyperintense to isointense
  - Central scar: Hyperintense
- T1WI C+
  - Arterial phase: Homogeneously hyperintense
  - Portal venous: Isointense
  - Delayed phase: Isointense mass with retention of contrast in central scar
- Specific hepatobiliary MR contrast agents
  - Gadoxetate (Eovist or Primovist)
    - Bright homogeneous enhancement on arterial phase
    - Delayed scan: Significant enhancement of scar
    - Prolonged enhancement on hepatobiliary phase (20 minutes) scan
      - □ Iso-/hyperintense mass with hypointense central scar
      - □ Due to functioning hepatocytes and malformed bile ductules
      - □ Most specific test to distinguish from all other hepatic masses

Angiographic Findings

- Conventional angiography
  - Arterial phase
    - Hypervascular mass with hypovascular central scar
    - Enlargement of main feeding artery with centripetal blood supply
    - Spoke-wheel pattern as on color Doppler
  - Venous phase: Large draining veins → hepatic veins
  - Capillary phase
    - Intense & nonhomogeneous stain
    - No avascular zones

Nuclear Medicine Findings

- Technetium sulfur colloid
  - Normal or increased uptake
  - Only FNH has both Kupffer cells & bile ductules
  - Almost pathognomonic in 60% of cases
- Tc-HIDA scan (hepatic iminodiacetic acid)
  - Normal or increased uptake
  - Prolonged enhancement (80%)
- Tc-99m tagged red blood cell scan (not useful)
  - Early isotope uptake and late defect

Imaging Recommendations

- Best imaging tool
  - CECT or contrast-enhanced MR for diagnosis
    - MR with gadoxetate hepatobiliary phase scans is most specific

o Color Doppler ultrasound/contrast enhanced ultrasound
  – Spoke-wheel pattern vessels, brisk centrifugal enhancement on arterial phase, especially in smaller lesions

DIFFERENTIAL DIAGNOSIS

Hepatic Adenoma

- Usually heterogeneous echogenicity due to hemorrhage, necrosis, or fat
- Rarely has central scar
- Washout on portal/delayed phase of CEUS/CT/MR

Fibrolamellar Carcinoma

- Usually Large (> 12 cm) heterogeneous mass
- Large fibrous central scar with calcification
  o Hypointense on T2WI
- Biliary, vascular, & nodal invasion may be present
- Metastases (70% of cases)

Cavernous Hemangioma

- Isoechoic or heterogeneous lesions may simulate FNH
- Nodular peripheral centripetal enhancement, no central scar

Hepatic Metastasis

- Multiple lesions, known primary tumor

PATHOLOGY

General Features

- Etiology
  o Ischemia caused by occult occlusion of intrahepatic vessels
    – Followed by hyperplastic response to abnormal vasculature
  o Localized arteriovenous shunting caused by anomalous arterial supply
  o Oral contraceptives do not cause FNH, but have trophic effect on growth
- Associated abnormalities
  o Hepatic hemangioma (23%)
  o Hepatic adenoma
  o Multiple lesions of FNH are associated with
    – Brain neoplasms: Meningioma, astrocytoma
    – Vascular malformations of various organs

Gross Pathologic & Surgical Features

- Localized, well-delineated, usually solitary (80%), subcapsular mass
- No true capsule, frequently central fibrous scar
- No intratumoral calcification, hemorrhage, or necrosis

Microscopic Features

- Normal hepatocytes with large amounts of fat, triglycerides, & glycogen
- Thick-walled arteries in fibrous septa radiating from center to periphery
- Proliferation & malformation of bile ducts lead to slowing of bile excretion
- Absent portal triads & central veins
- Difficult differentiation from regenerative cirrhotic nodule and liver adenoma by histology

CLINICAL ISSUES

Presentation

- Most common signs/symptoms
  o Often asymptomatic (in 50-90% incidental finding)
  o Vague abdominal pain (10-15%) due to mass effect
  o Hepatomegaly and abdominal mass: Very rare
  o Lab data: Usually normal liver function tests
  o Diagnosis
    – Characteristic imaging findings
    – Core needle biopsy (include central scar)

Demographics

- Age
  o Common in young to middle-aged women
    – 3rd-4th decades of life
- Gender
  o M:F = 1:8
- Epidemiology
  o 4% of all primary hepatic tumors in pediatric population
  o 3-8% in adult population

Natural History & Prognosis

- No risk of malignant transformation
- No hemorrhagic complication

Treatment

- Discontinuation of oral contraceptives
- FNH seldom requires surgery

DIAGNOSTIC CHECKLIST

Consider

- Imaging is more reliable than histology in making diagnosis of FNH

Image Interpretation Pearls

- Immediate, intense, homogeneously enhancing lesion on arterial phase followed rapidly by isodensity on venous phase with delayed enhancement of scar
- Classic FNH looks like cross section of orange (central "scar," radiating septa)

SELECTED REFERENCES

1. Kong WT et al: Contrast-enhanced ultrasound in combination with color Doppler ultrasound can improve the diagnostic performance of focal nodular hyperplasia and hepatocellular adenoma. Ultrasound Med Biol. 41(4):944-51, 2015
2. Li W et al: Differentiation of atypical hepatocellular carcinoma from focal nodular hyperplasia: diagnostic performance of contrast-enhanced US and microflow imaging. Radiology. 140911, 2015
3. Suh CH et al: The diagnostic value of Gd-EOB-DTPA-MRI for the diagnosis of focal nodular hyperplasia: a systematic review and meta-analysis. Eur Radiol. 25(4):950-60, 2015
4. Bertin C et al: Contrast-enhanced ultrasound of focal nodular hyperplasia: a matter of size. Eur Radiol. 24(10):2561-71, 2014
5. Pei XQ et al: Quantitative analysis of contrast-enhanced ultrasonography: differentiating focal nodular hyperplasia from hepatocellular carcinoma. Br J Radiol. 86(1023):20120536, 2013
6. Wang W et al: Contrast-enhanced ultrasound features of histologically proven focal nodular hyperplasia: diagnostic performance compared with contrast-enhanced CT. Eur Radiol. 23(9):2546-54, 2013
7. Kamaya A et al: Hypervascular liver lesions. Semin Ultrasound CT MR. 30(5):387-407, 2009

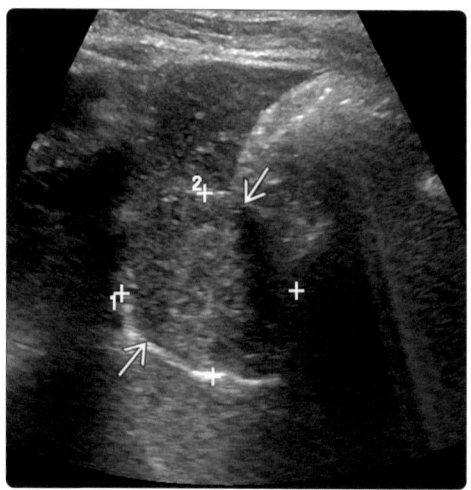
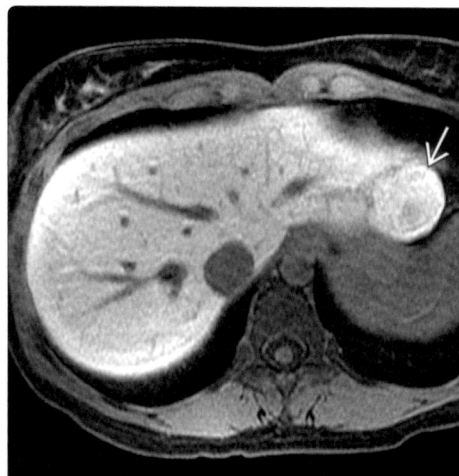

(Left) Transverse abdominal US shows an isoechoic FNH ➜ bulging from the lateral segment of the left lobe of the liver. (Right) Axial hepatobiliary phase MR image obtained 20 minutes after gadoxetate injection in the same patient shows an exophytic FNH in the lateral segment of left lobe of liver ➜. The lesion retains contrast to slightly greater degree than the background liver due to the presence of normal hepatocytes and abnormal bile ductules.

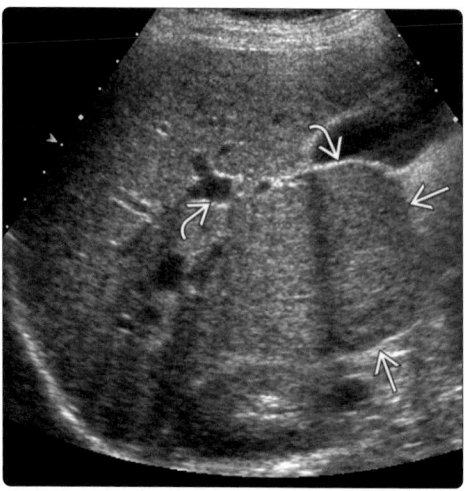
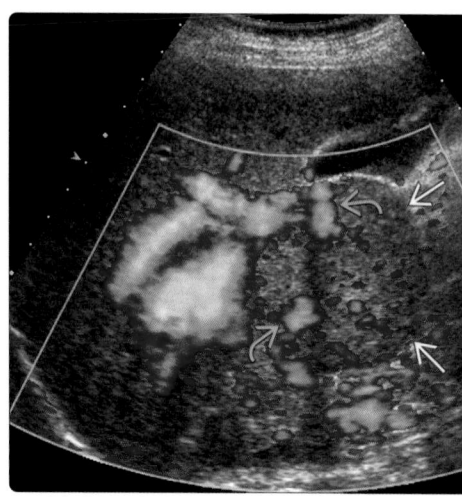

(Left) Longitudinal transabdominal US shows an isoechoic FNH in the caudate lobe of liver ➜. The mass causes contour deformity and mass effect upon the adjacent gallbladder and portal vein ➜. The lesion is difficult to distinguish from the surrounding liver, earning its moniker "stealth lesion." (Right) Power Doppler US in the same patient shows that the isoechoic FNH ➜ contains internal radiating vessels ➔ with a spoke-wheel configuration.

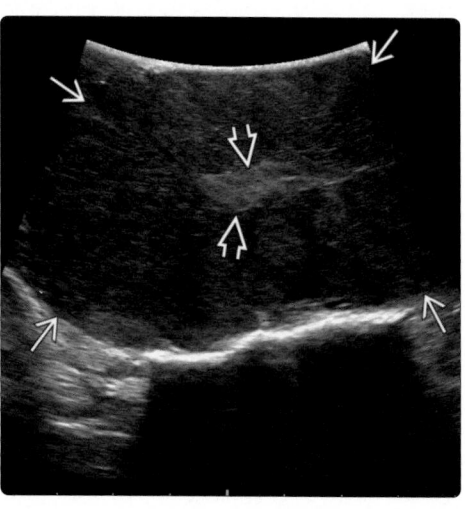
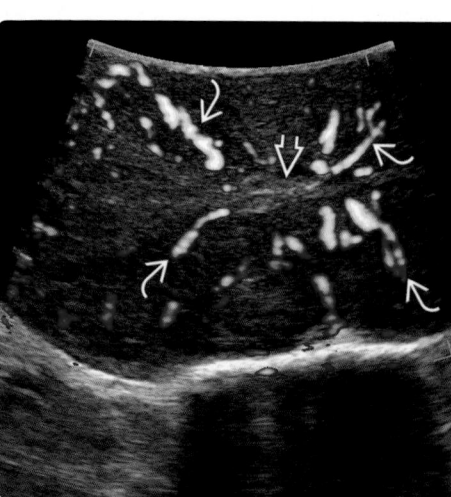

(Left) Transverse abdominal US shows a large hypoechoic FNH in the liver ➜ with a hyperechoic central scar ➜. (Right) Transverse power Doppler US in the same patient shows centrifugal blood flow away ➜ from the central scar ➜ of FNH, giving a spoke-wheel vascularity pattern.

Hepatic Adenoma

TERMINOLOGY

- Hepatocellular adenoma (HCA) or liver cell adenoma
- 2nd most frequent hepatic tumor in young women after focal nodular hyperplasia (FNH)

IMAGING

- Best diagnostic clue: Heterogeneous, hypervascular mass ± hemorrhage in young woman on oral contraceptives
- Subcapsular right hepatic lobe (75%)
- Round or mildly lobulated, well-defined borders
- Hypo-/iso-/hyperechoic mass
- Complex heterogeneous mixed echogenicity mass
- Hypoechoic halo of compressed liver tissue with multiple vessels
- Larger lesions prone to intratumoral hemorrhage or rupture with intraperitoneal hemorrhage
- Best imaging tool: Ultrasound for lesion detection, guiding biopsy, and monitoring size

- Liver-specific MR contrast agents have high accuracy in distinguishing HCA from other liver lesions

TOP DIFFERENTIAL DIAGNOSES

- Hemangioma
- Focal nodular hyperplasia (FNH)
- Hepatocellular carcinoma (HCC)

CLINICAL ISSUES

- Definitive diagnosis and subtype with biopsy
- Molecular classification (4 subtypes) helps determine prognosis and management
  - β-catenin-mutated subtype prone to malignant degeneration
- Lesions > 6 cm more prone to hemorrhage

DIAGNOSTIC CHECKLIST

- Rule out other liver tumors with similar imaging features, such as HCC or FNH

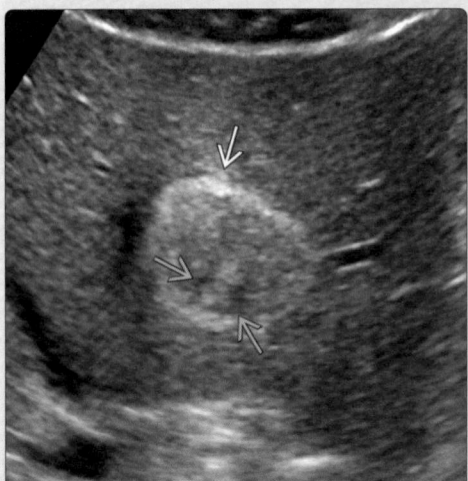
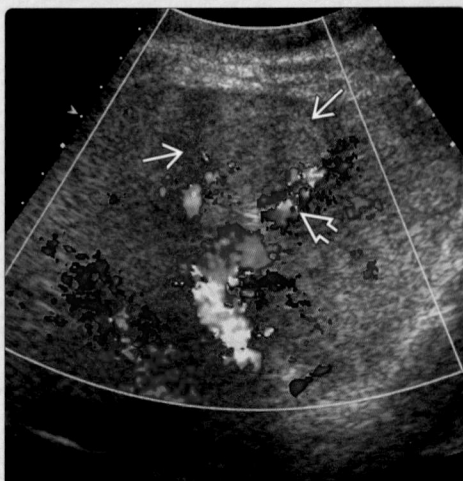

(Left) Transverse transabdominal ultrasound demonstrates a predominantly hyperechoic adenoma ➡ with hypoechoic central areas ➡, which could represent hemorrhage or necrosis. (Right) Transverse color Doppler ultrasound of the left lobe of the liver demonstrates a hyperechoic adenoma ➡ with large peripheral vessels ➡.

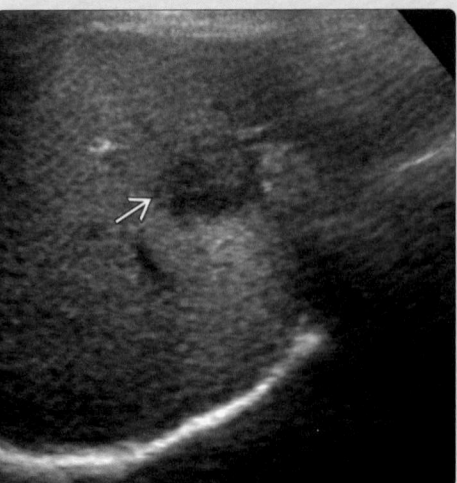
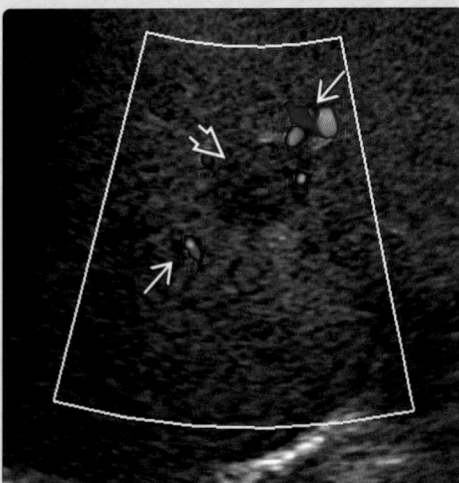

(Left) Transverse transabdominal grayscale ultrasound demonstrates a heterogeneously hypoechoic adenoma ➡. Heterogeneous areas likely represent necrosis from prior hemorrhage. (Right) Transverse color Doppler ultrasound in the same patient shows peripheral large vessels ➡ bordering the hypoechoic hepatic adenoma ➡.

TERMINOLOGY

Synonyms

- Hepatocellular adenoma (HCA) or liver cell adenoma

Definitions

- Benign tumor that arises from hepatocytes arranged in cords that occasionally form bile

IMAGING

General Features

- Best diagnostic clue
  - Heterogeneous, hypervascular mass with hemorrhage in a young woman, often with contraceptive use
- Location
  - Usually subcapsular right hepatic lobe (75%)
  - Intraparenchymal or pedunculated (10%)
- Size
  - Varies 1-30 cm, average 5-10 cm
- Key concepts
  - Rare benign neoplasm
  - 2nd most frequent hepatic tumor in young women after focal nodular hyperplasia (FNH)
  - Associated with oral contraceptive use
  - Usually single in 70-80% of cases (adenoma); rarely multiple (adenomatosis)

Ultrasonographic Findings

- Grayscale ultrasound
  - Well-defined borders
  - Round or mildly lobulated contour
  - 20-40% hypoechoic; 30% hyperechoic; 30% isoechoic
  - Complex hyper- and hypoechoic heterogeneous mass with anechoic/hypoechoic areas
    - Due to fat, hemorrhage, necrosis, and calcification
  - Hypoechoic halo of compressed liver tissue
  - Intratumoral or intraperitoneal hemorrhage from acute rupture (potential complication)
- Color Doppler
  - Hypervascular tumor, supplied by hepatic artery
  - Large peripheral arteries and veins
  - Intratumoral veins present
    - Absent in FNH
    - Useful discriminating feature for HCA

CT Findings

- NECT
  - Isodense to hypodense (due to lipid)
  - Hemorrhage: Intratumoral, parenchymal, or subcapsular
- CECT
  - Arterial phase
    - Heterogeneous, hyperenhancing
  - Portal venous phase
    - Less heterogeneous
    - Hyper-/iso-/hypodense to liver
  - Delayed phase (5-10 minutes)
    - Enhancement does not persist (due to arteriovenous shunting)
    - Pseudocapsule: Hyperattenuated to liver and adenoma

MR Findings

- T2WI
  - Mass: Heterogeneous signal intensity
    - Increased signal intensity (old hemorrhage/necrosis)
    - Decreased signal intensity (fat, recent hemorrhage)
  - Rim (fibrous pseudocapsule): Hypointense
- T1WI C+
  - Gadolinium arterial phase
    - Mass: Heterogeneous early arterial enhancement
  - Delayed phase
    - Mass: Becomes isointense to liver
    - Pseudocapsule: Hyperintense to liver and adenoma
  - Gadoxetate-enhanced MR (liver-specific contrast agent)
    - Mass: Hypointense on T1 hepatobiliary phase
- GRE in-/out-of-phase
  - Loss of signal on out-of-phase imaging due to intralesional lipid

Angiographic Findings

- Conventional
  - Hypervascular mass with centripetal flow
  - Enlarged hepatic artery with feeders at tumor periphery (50%)
  - Hypovascular; avascular regions due to hemorrhage, necrosis

Nuclear Medicine Findings

- Technetium sulfur colloid
  - Usually "cold" (photopenic): 80%
  - Uncommonly "warm": 20%
    - Due to uptake in sparse Kupffer cells

Imaging Recommendations

- Best imaging tool
  - Ultrasound is good for lesion detection, guiding biopsy, and monitoring size
- T2WI; T1WI with dynamic enhanced multiphasic; GRE in- and opposed-phase images
- Liver-specific MR contrast agents have high accuracy for differentiating HCA from other lesions

DIFFERENTIAL DIAGNOSIS

Hemangioma

- Hyperechoic mass ± posterior acoustic enhancement
- Large lesions may be heterogeneous

Focal Nodular Hyperplasia (FNH)

- No malignant degeneration or hemorrhage
- Central scar may be present
- When small (≤ 3 cm), FNH without scar may be indistinguishable from adenoma

Hepatocellular Carcinoma (HCC)

- May be difficult to distinguish from adenoma on imaging and histology
- Background cirrhosis usually present
- Biliary, vascular, nodal invasion, and metastases establish that lesion is malignant

Fibrolamellar Carcinoma

- Heterogeneous, large, lobulated mass with scar and septa

- Vascular, biliary, nodal invasion may be present

Metastases

- Usually multiple and look for primary tumors

PATHOLOGY

General Features

- Etiology
  - ↑ risk in oral contraceptives and anabolic steroid users
  - Pregnancy
    - Increased tumor growth rate and tumor rupture
  - Types I and III glycogen storage disease
    - Multiple adenomas: 60%
  - Diabetes mellitus
  - Klinefelter syndrome
  - Obesity
- High incidence of
  - Hemorrhage, necrosis, and fatty change

Staging, Grading, & Classification

- 4 molecular/pathological subtypes: Help determine prognosis and management
  - **β-catenin-mutated HCA** (10-15%): High risk of malignant transformation
    - Occurs more frequently in men
    - Steatosis is rare, inflammation is absent
    - Difficult to differentiate from well-differentiated HCC on pathology
  - **Inflammatory HCA** (50%): 10% risk of malignant transformation
    - Focal steatosis may be present
    - Previously classified as telangiectatic FNH
  - **Hepatocyte nuclear factor 1α-inactivated HCA** (30-35%)
    - Steatosis characteristically present
    - Absence of inflammatory infiltrate
  - **Unclassified** (< 10%)

Gross Pathologic & Surgical Features

- Well-circumscribed mass on external surface of liver
- Soft, pale, or yellow tan
- Large areas of hemorrhage or infarction
- "Pseudocapsule" and occasional "pseudopods"

CLINICAL ISSUES

Presentation

- Most common signs/symptoms
  - RUQ pain (40%): Due to hemorrhage
  - Asymptomatic (20%)
- Clinical profile
  - Usually normal liver function tests

Demographics

- Age
  - Young women of childbearing age group
- Gender
  - 98% seen in females (M:F = 1:10)
  - Males on anabolic steroids or with glycogen storage disease
- Epidemiology

  - Estimated incidence in oral contraceptive users
    - 4 adenomas per 100,000 users
  - Multiple adenomas in glycogen storage disease

Natural History & Prognosis

- Complications
  - Hemorrhage: Intrahepatic or intraperitoneal (40%)
  - Rupture: Increased risk in pregnancy
  - Malignant transformation
    - 4.3% risk in adenomas larger than 5 cm
    - High risk in β-catenin subtype
- Prognosis
  - Usually good
    - After discontinuation of oral contraceptives
    - After surgical resection of large/symptomatic
  - Poor
    - Intraperitoneal rupture
    - Rupture during pregnancy
    - Adenomatosis (> 10 adenomas)
    - Malignant transformation

Treatment

- Adenoma < 6 cm
  - Observation and discontinue oral contraceptives
- Adenoma > 6 cm and near surface
  - Surgical resection
- β-catenin mutated subtype
  - Resection due to increased risk of malignant transformation
- Avoid pregnancy due to increased risk of rupture

DIAGNOSTIC CHECKLIST

Consider

- Rule out other benign and malignant liver tumors, which have similar imaging features, particularly HCC or FNH
- Percutaneous biopsy is associated with high risk of bleeding
- Check for history of oral contraceptives and glycogen storage disease (in case of multiple adenomas)

SELECTED REFERENCES

1. Khanna M et al: Current updates on the molecular genetics and magnetic resonance imaging of focal nodular hyperplasia and hepatocellular adenoma. Insights Imaging. ePub, 2015
2. Dhingra S et al: Update on the new classification of hepatic adenomas: clinical, molecular, and pathologic characteristics. Arch Pathol Lab Med. 138(8):1090-7, 2014
3. Frulio N et al: Evaluation of liver tumors using acoustic radiation force impulse elastography and correlation with histologic data. J Ultrasound Med. 32(1):121-30, 2013
4. Bieze M et al: Diagnostic accuracy of MRI in differentiating hepatocellular adenoma from focal nodular hyperplasia: prospective study of the additional value of gadoxetate disodium. AJR Am J Roentgenol. 199(1):26-34, 2012
5. Purysko AS et al: Characteristics and distinguishing features of hepatocellular adenoma and focal nodular hyperplasia on gadoxetate disodium-enhanced MRI. AJR Am J Roentgenol. 198(1):115-23, 2012
6. Kamaya A et al: Hypervascular liver lesions. Semin Ultrasound CT MR. 30(5):387-407, 2009

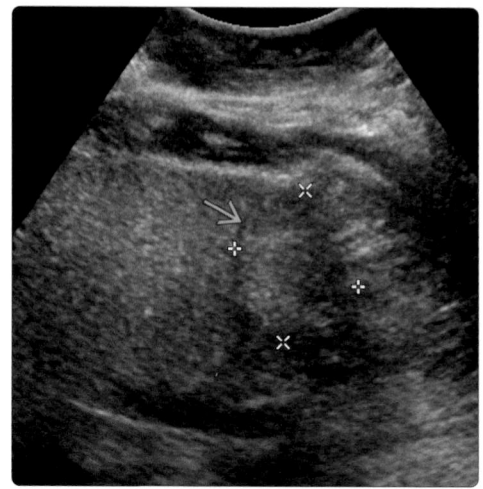
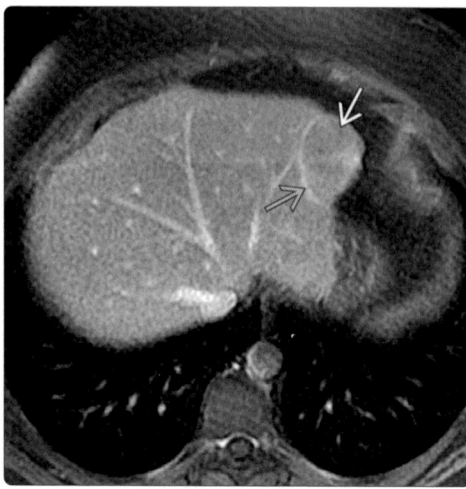

(Left) *Transverse transabdominal ultrasound demonstrates an isoechoic pedunculated adenoma ➡ in the left hepatic lobe.* (Right) *Axial post-contrast, delayed phase MR in the same patient demonstrates a typical appearance to the pseudocapsule ➡, which is hyperintense to the liver and the adenoma ➡.*

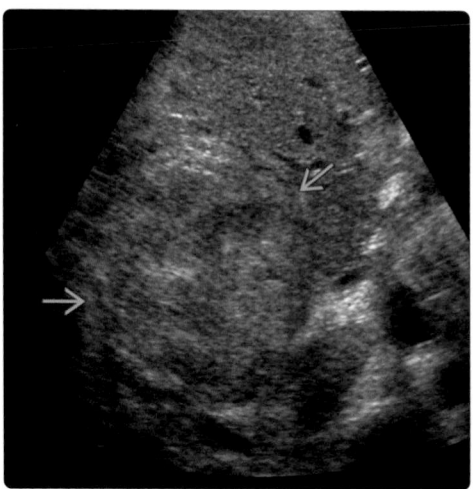
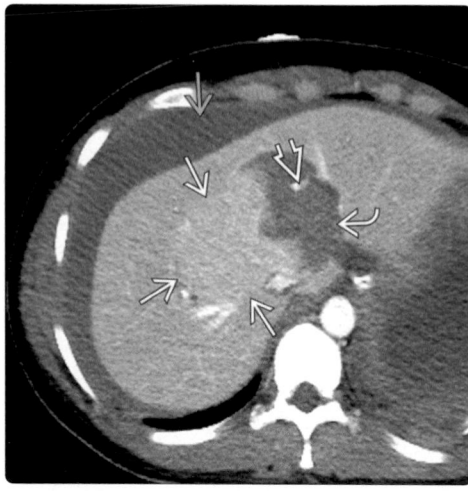

(Left) *Transverse intraoperative ultrasound of a heterogeneous adenoma ➡ in a patient in which hepatic adenoma ruptured and required surgical excision.* (Right) *Axial contrast-enhanced arterial phase CT scan demonstrates a large isodense adenoma ➡ complicated by acute rupture. Blush of active arterial contrast extravasation ➡ within intratumoral hemorrhage ➡ as well as hemoperitoneum ➡ are seen. Acute rupture is a known complication of hepatic adenomas.*

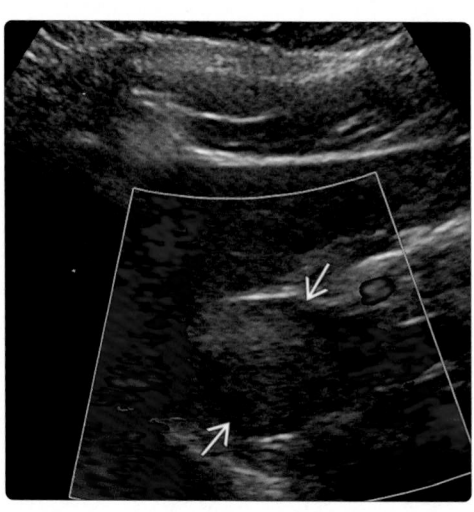
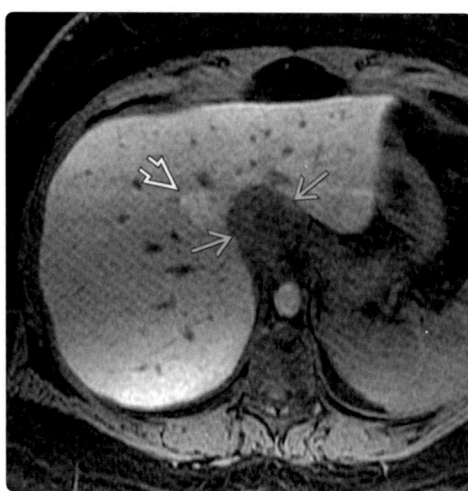

(Left) *Transverse color Doppler ultrasound shows an echogenic adenoma ➡ in the caudate lobe of the liver.* (Right) *Hepatobiliary phase MR with gadoxetate in the same patient shows the adenoma ➡ in the caudate lobe of the liver does not retain gadoxetate. In contrast, immediately adjacent to the adenoma is an incidental FNH ➡, which does retain gadoxetate. Hepatobiliary-specific MR can be very helpful in distinguishing adenoma from FNH.*

Hepatocellular Carcinoma

TERMINOLOGY

- Hepatocellular carcinoma (HCC)
- Synonyms: Hepatoma, primary liver cancer

IMAGING

- US: Solid, intrahepatic mass in patient with risk factors such as chronic hepatitis or cirrhosis
- Contrast-enhanced CT, MR, or US: Shows characteristic late arterial phase hyperenhancement and portal venous or delayed phase washout (hypoenhancement compared to adjacent liver parenchyma)
- Portal vein or hepatic vein tumor invasion highly suggestive of HCC

TOP DIFFERENTIAL DIAGNOSES

- Regenerative or dysplastic nodule
- Hepatic hemangioma
- Focal nodular hyperplasia
- Hepatic adenoma
- Metastases

PATHOLOGY

- Primary malignancy of liver arising from hepatocytes
- Risk factors
  - Cirrhosis (60-90%): Due to chronic viral hepatitis (HBV, HCV), alcoholic cirrhosis
  - HCV patients typically cirrhotic; HBV patients often not cirrhotic

CLINICAL ISSUES

- Treatment includes surgical resection, RF ablation, intra-arterial chemoembolization or radioembolization, liver transplant, sorafenib, or external beam radiation

DIAGNOSTIC CHECKLIST

- Any solid mass > 1 cm detected in cirrhotic liver is suspicious for HCC until proven otherwise

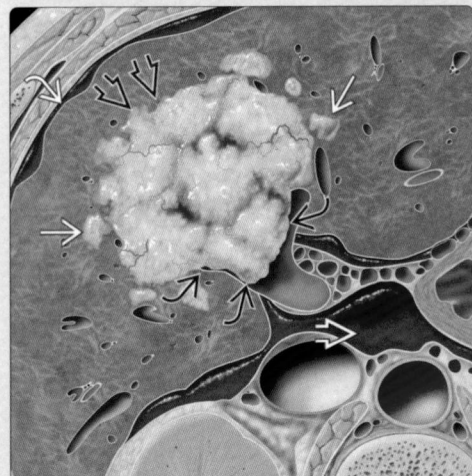
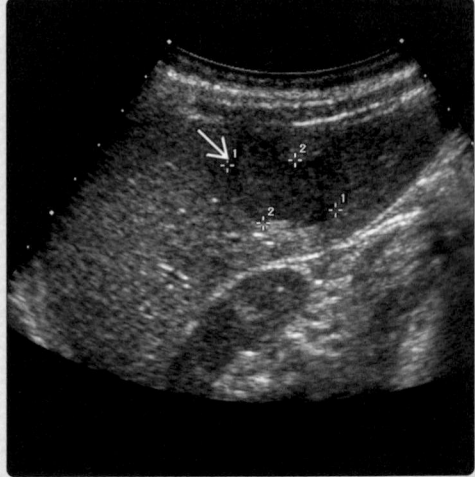

(Left) Graphic shows a heterogeneous, hypervascular hepatocellular carcinoma ⇗. Numerous adjacent satellite nodules ➡ as well as portal vein invasion ⬈ are depicted. Underlying liver disease is evident given the nodular liver capsule ⬈ and ascites ➡. (Right) Longitudinal grayscale ultrasound of the liver shows a hypoechoic, solid hepatocellular carcinoma ➡. In the setting of chronic hepatitis, this is highly suspicious for HCC and should be further characterized with contrast-enhanced CT or contrast-enhanced MR.

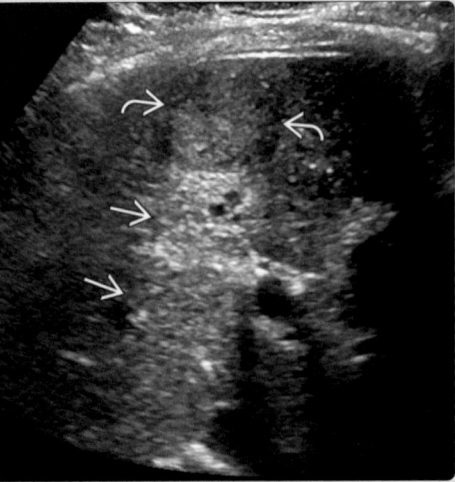
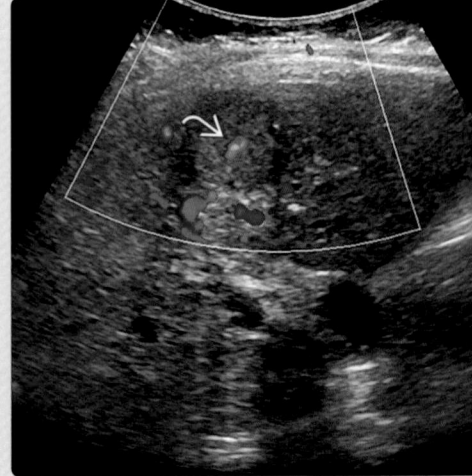

(Left) Transverse grayscale ultrasound of the liver shows a slightly hyperechoic, solid hepatocellular carcinoma ➡ with a hypoechoic halo and slight posterior acoustic enhancement ➡, occasionally seen with hepatocellular carcinoma. (Right) Color Doppler ultrasound of the same patient shows detectable internal vascularity ➡ in the hepatocellular carcinoma.

TERMINOLOGY

Abbreviations

- Hepatocellular carcinoma (HCC)

Definitions

- Malignant neoplasm originating from hepatocytes

IMAGING

General Features

- Best diagnostic clue
  - Solid, intrahepatic mass > 1 cm in patient with risk factors such as chronic hepatitis or cirrhosis
  - Portal vein or hepatic vein tumor invasion highly suggestive of HCC
- Size
  - Small or large: < 3 cm to > 5 cm
  - Diffuse or infiltrative: Subcentimeter to > 5 cm
- Key concepts
  - Most frequent primary visceral malignancy globally
    - Accounts for 80-90% of all adult primary liver malignancies
    - Usually arises in cirrhotic liver, due to chronic viral hepatitis (HBV, HCV) or alcoholism
  - 2nd most common malignant liver tumor after hepatoblastoma in children
  - Growth patterns of HCC: 3 major types
    - Solitary, often large mass
    - Multinodular or multifocal
    - Diffuse or infiltrative
  - Metastases to lung, bone, adrenal, lymph node

Ultrasonographic Findings

- Grayscale ultrasound
  - **Hypoechoic**: Most common sonographic appearance
    - Solid tumor
    - May be surrounded by thin, hypoechoic halo (capsule)
  - **Hyperechoic**
    - Indicates fatty metamorphosis/hypervascularity
    - Simulates hemangioma/focal steatosis
      - If risk factors are present and hyperechoic lesion > 1 cm detected, cannot assume hemangioma
  - **Mixed echogenicity**: More common in larger HCC
    - Indicates tumor necrosis/fibrosis
    - Focal fat in some HCCs appear echogenic
  - Background cirrhosis (except for fibrolamellar HCC and hepatitis B)
  - Calcification is rare unless treated
  - Invasion of portal vein & less commonly hepatic vein highly suggestive of HCC
  - Hemoperitoneum if subcapsular or exophytic HCC ruptures
  - Associated signs of portal hypertension: Ascites, splenomegaly, portosystemic collaterals
  - Fibrolamellar carcinoma
    - Rare, < 1% of all cases of primary liver cancer
    - Well-defined partially/completely encapsulated mass
    - Prominent central fibrous scar often with calcification
    - Intralesional necrosis/hemorrhage

- Regional adenopathy and metastases to lung and peritoneum
- Typically without chronic liver disease
- AFP usually negative or mildly elevated
- Pulsed Doppler
  - Arterial feeding vessels with low-resistance waveforms indicate tumor vessels
  - Tumor thrombus with arterial neovascularity
- Color Doppler
  - Irregular hypervascularity within neoplasm
  - Tumor thrombus, typically in portal vein, with neovascularity

CT Findings

- NECT
  - Iso- or hypodense liver mass, occasionally fat content detected
    - Characterization of lesion not possible on NECT
- CECT
  - Characterization and diagnosis of HCC can be made with triphasic CT: Late arterial, portal venous, delayed/equilibrium phase
    - Late arterial phase: Hyperenhancing compared to background liver
    - Portal venous phase: Variable enhancement, may be iso-, hypo-, or hyperdense compared to background liver
    - Delayed or equilibrium phase (3-5 min after contrast injection): "Washout" is characteristic of HCC; lesion hypodense compared to liver
      - May see delayed enhancing pseudocapsule

MR Findings

- T1WI
  - Typically hypointense compared to background liver but may be iso- or hyperintense depending on fat content or necrosis
- T2WI
  - Typically slightly hyperintense, similar intensity to spleen
- T1WI C+
  - Late arterial phase: Hyperenhancing compared to background liver
  - Portal venous phase: Variable but typically hypointense
  - Delayed or equilibrium phase: "Washout" is characteristic of HCC with lesion hypointense to background liver
    - Hyperintense pseudocapsule typically best seen on delayed or portal venous phase images
  - Hepatobiliary contrast (gadoxetate, Eovist, Primovist): Uptake in hepatocytes related to OATP8 receptor, down-regulated in most HCC, up-regulated in focal nodular hyperplasia (FNH)
    - Pitfall: Up to 10% of HCC can be isointense or hyperintense on hepatobiliary phase

Angiographic Findings

- Hypervascular tumor
  - Marked neovascularity and AV shunting
  - Large hepatic artery and vascular invasion
  - "Threads and streaks" sign in portal vein tumor thrombus

Nuclear Medicine Findings

- Hepatobiliary scan: Uptake in 50%

- Gallium scan: Gallium-avid in 90% of cases
- FDG PET/CT: Uptake in 55% of cases

Imaging Recommendations

- **Ultrasound:** Screening and surveillance in high-risk patients (chronic hepatitis or cirrhosis)
  - Current recommendation by American Association for the Study of Liver Disease (AASLD) is screening/surveillance US every 6 months
    - Nodule < 1 cm reimaged on US in 3 months to determine growth
    - Nodule > 1 cm further characterized by CECT or contrast-enhanced MR
- **CECT or CEMR**: Definitive lesion characterization
  - Use Liver Imaging Reporting and Database System (LI-RADS) or Organ Procurement and Transplantation Netwok (OPTN) imaging criteria
- **Contrast-enhanced US:** May be considered for lesion characterization if available

DIFFERENTIAL DIAGNOSIS

Regenerative or Dysplastic Nodule

- When < 1 cm, often not visible on US
- Regenerative and dysplastic nodules may be hypervascular on arterial phase but do not wash-out on portal or delayed phase

Focal Nodular Hyperplasia

- Homogeneous hypo-/iso-/hyperechoic mass with central scar and spoke-wheel vascularity
- Hypervascular on arterial phase but often isodense and isointense to liver on portal venous and delayed phase CECT & CEMR

Metastases

- Mimic nodular or multifocal HCC
- Lower incidence in cirrhotic livers

Cholangiocarcinoma

- Peripheral cholangiocarcinomas often obstruct bile ducts leading to ductal dilatation
- Capsular retraction; volume loss

Hepatic Hemangioma

- Unusual in cirrhotic liver
- Well-defined hyperechoic nodule
- Undetectable internal vascularity on color Doppler

PATHOLOGY

General Features

- Etiology
  - Cirrhosis (60-90%): Due to chronic viral hepatitis (HBV, HCV), alcoholic cirrhosis, primary biliary cirrhosis
    - HCV patients typically cirrhotic; HBV patients often not cirrhotic
  - Nonalcoholic steatohepatitis (NASH) increasing cause of HCC in North America
  - Carcinogens: Aflatoxins, siderosis, Thorotrast, androgens
  - α-1-antitrypsin deficiency, hemochromatosis, Wilson, hereditary tyrosinemia
- Genetics

  - HBV DNA integrated into host cell genome → genomic instability

Gross Pathologic & Surgical Features

- Soft tumor arising from hepatocytes; may contain necrosis, hemorrhage, calcification, fat, vascular invasion

Microscopic Features

- Sinusoidal vessels surround tumor cells
- Architectural growth patterns: Trabecular (most common), solid, tubular (acinar, duct-like, pseudo-glandular)
- HCC variants: Clear cell (may contain fat or glycogen), scirrhous, sarcomatoid, sclerosing, mixed hepatocellular-cholangiocarcinoma

CLINICAL ISSUES

Presentation

- Elderly patient with history of cirrhosis, ascites, weight loss, right upper quadrant pain, & ↑ α-fetoprotein (AFP)
- Lab data: Elevated serum AFP and liver function tests
  - Diagnosis: If imaging features characteristic, diagnosis made solely by CECT or MR; biopsy reserved for indeterminate cases

Demographics

- Age
  - Low incidence areas: 6th-7th decade
  - High incidence areas: 30-45 years
- Gender
  - Low incidence areas (M:F = 2.5:1)
  - High incidence areas (M:F = 8:1)
- Epidemiology
  - High incidence: Africa & Asia
  - HCC in cirrhosis due to hepatitis C virus
  - Up to 30% of noncirrhotic HBV may develop HCC

Natural History & Prognosis

- Complications: Spontaneous rupture & hemoperitoneum
- 30% 5-year survival

Treatment

- Surgical resection in patients with adequate hepatic reserve
- Radiofrequency/alcohol/microwave ablation for small, isolated tumors
- Liver transplant if Milan criteria met: Single tumor 2-5 cm or 3 tumors each < 3 cm, no vascular invasion or extrahepatic spread
- Intra-arterial chemoembolization or radioembolization (Yttrium-90) for multifocal unresectable tumor
- Sorafenib or external beam radiation in unresectable patients who failed other treatments

SELECTED REFERENCES

1. Davarpanah AH et al: The role of imaging in hepatocellular carcinoma: the present and future. J Clin Gastroenterol. 47 Suppl:S7-10, 2013
2. Liu YI et al: Quantitatively defining washout in hepatocellular carcinoma. AJR Am J Roentgenol. 200(1):84-9, 2013
3. Maturen KE et al: Posterior acoustic enhancement in hepatocellular carcinoma. J Ultrasound Med. 30(4):495-9, 2011
4. Management of Hepatocellular Carcinoma: An Update (AASLD)
5. Proposal for Improved Imaging Criteria for HCC Exceptions (OPTN)
6. Liver Imaging and Reporting Data System (LIRADS)

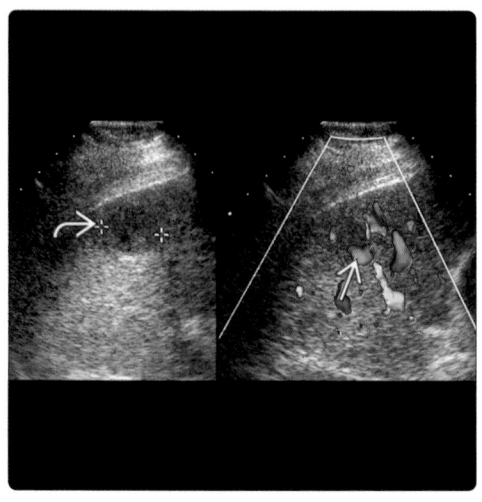
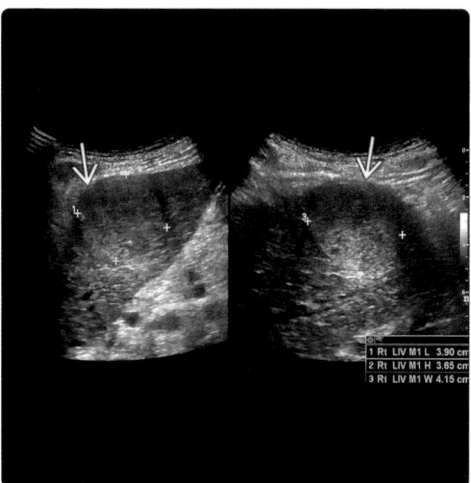

(Left) Transverse grayscale and color Doppler ultrasound of the liver show a solid, hypoechoic hepatocellular carcinoma ➡ with internal vascularity ➡. (Right) Longitudinal and transverse US of the left lobe of the liver show a relatively echogenic, solid hepatocellular carcinoma ➡ with a hypoechoic halo. Background liver is heterogeneous, indicating cirrhosis.

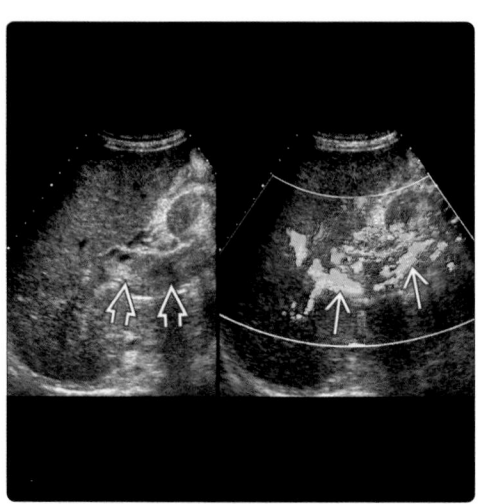
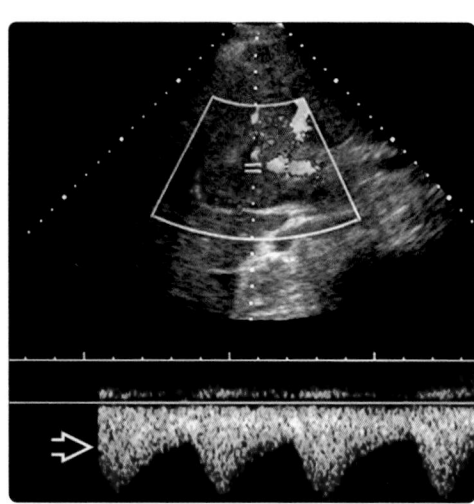

(Left) Transverse grayscale and color Doppler US of the main portal vein show a solid, intraluminal tumor thrombus ➡ with marked internal vascularity ➡. Presence of tumor thrombus almost always indicates infiltrative or extensive hepatocellular carcinoma. (Right) Spectral tracings of the vascular area in the tumor thrombus (same patient) show arterialized waveforms ➡ directed away from the liver, reflecting arterial neovascularity that feeds the tumor thrombus.

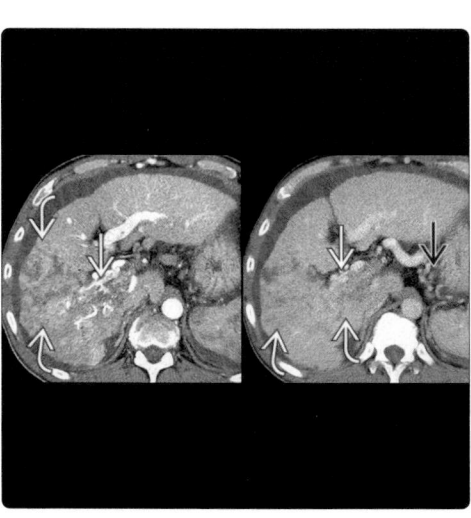
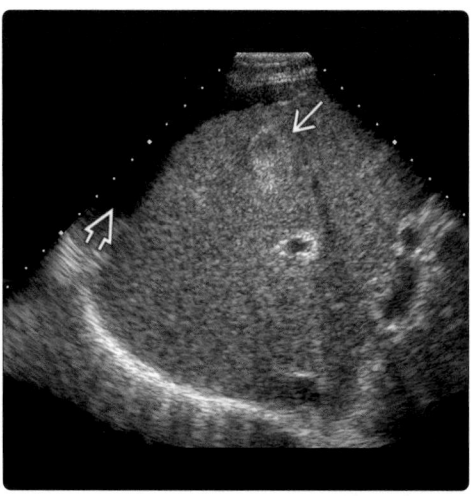

(Left) Contrast-enhanced CT in late arterial phase (left) and delayed phase (right) shows infiltrative hepatocellular carcinoma ➡ in the right lobe of the liver with tumor thrombus in the portal vein ➡. Underlying liver is cirrhotic, and gastric varices ➡ and moderate ascites are evident. (Right) Transverse grayscale US of the liver shows a mixed echogenicity hepatocellular carcinoma ➡. Background liver is mildly cirrhotic and ascites ➡ is present.

(Left) *Transverse and longitudinal grayscale ultrasound of the liver shows a solid, heterogeneous hepatocellular carcinoma ➡, which mildly bulges the liver contour ➡. **(Right)** Transverse grayscale ultrasound of the right lobe of the liver shows a large, echogenic, solid hepatocellular carcinoma ➡.*

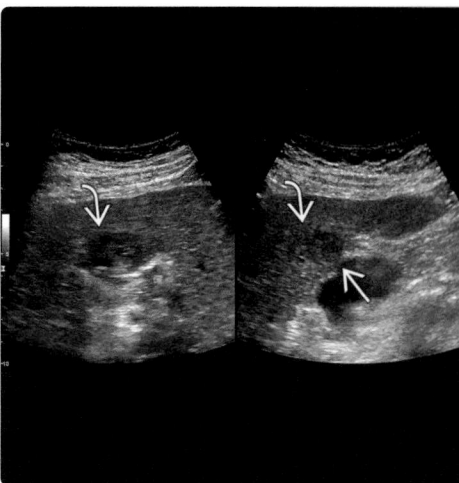 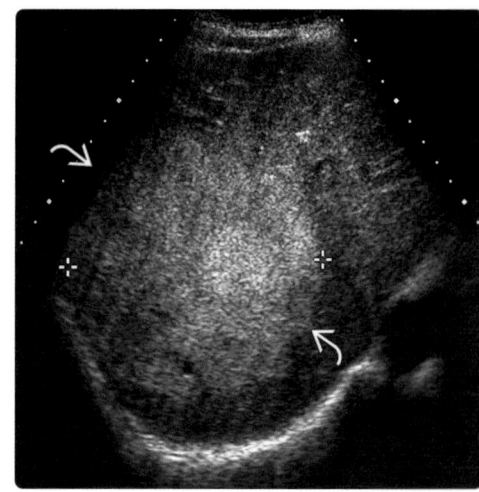

(Left) *Dual image contrast-enhanced ultrasound (left=contrast image, right=grayscale) of the liver during the arterial phase shows a hypervascular hepatocellular carcinoma ➡ clearly enhancing to greater extent compared to adjacent background parenchyma. **(Right)** Contrast-enhanced US of the same patient during the delayed phase shows the hepatocellular carcinoma has washed out ➡ compared to background liver, a characteristic imaging feature of hepatocellular carcinoma.*

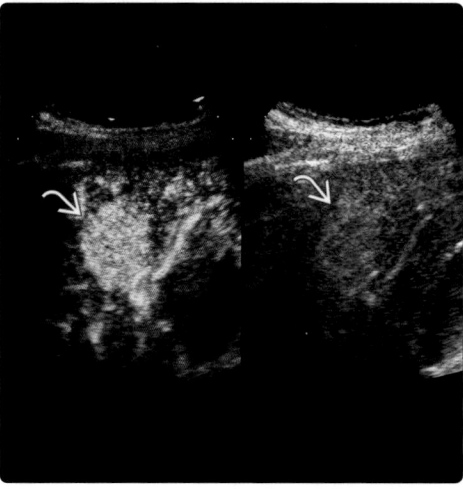 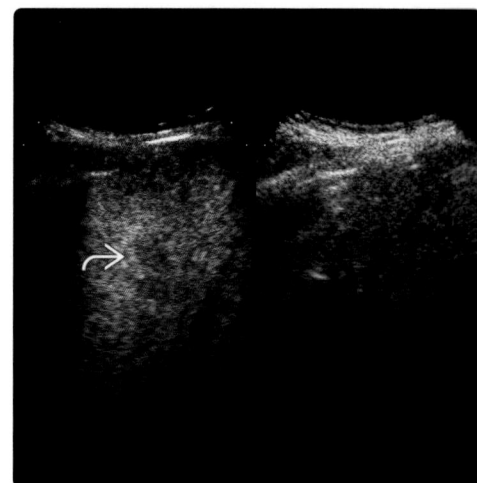

(Left) *Color Doppler US and contrast-enhanced CT show a large, infiltrative HCC ➡. Infiltrative tumor on US may be challenging to identify, but marked displacement of the hepatic vessels posteriorly ➡ is a helpful clue to the presence of the mass. Tumor thrombus ➡ is often seen with large, infiltrative HCC. **(Right)** Transverse grayscale US of the liver shows a large, predominantly echogenic mass ➡ with a thick, hypoechoic central scar ➡. Mass was proven to be a fibrolamellar carcinoma.*

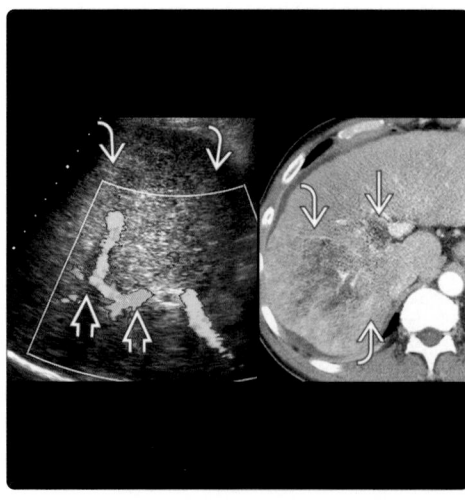 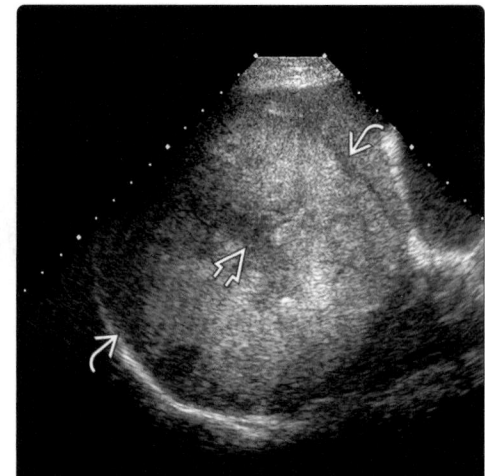

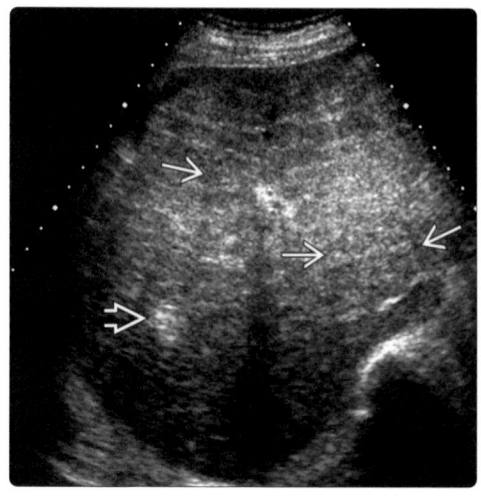

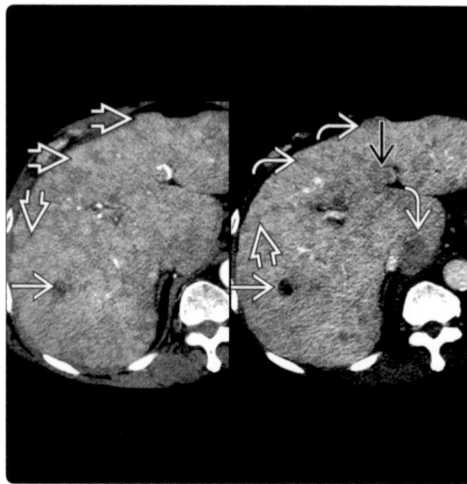

(Left) *Transverse grayscale US of the liver shows a markedly heterogeneous liver with multiple refractive shadows ➡ caused by diffuse, infiltrative hepatocellular carcinoma. Focal echogenic lesion ➡ was shown to be a fat-containing focus of HCC.* (Right) *Axial CECT in the same patient during the arterial phase (left) and delayed phase (right) shows innumerable hypervascular HCC ➡ that wash-out ➡. Focal fat-containing HCC ➡ is seen in the right lobe of the liver. Tumor thrombus is present in the left portal vein ➡.*

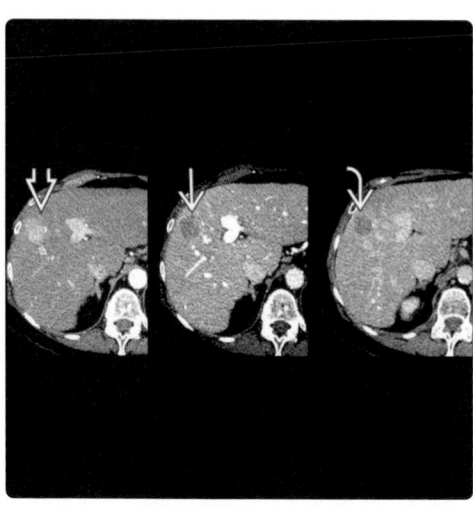

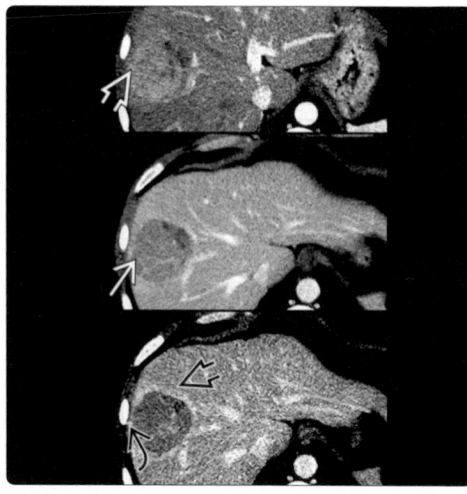

(Left) *Typical hepatocellular carcinoma on triphasic CT shows a hypervascular hepatocellular carcinoma ➡ on arterial phase that washes out on portal venous ➡ and delayed ➡ phase images.* (Right) *Axial CT images of the liver show a typical hepatocellular carcinoma that is hypervascular on arterial phase ➡ and washes out on portal venous ➡ and delayed ➡ phase. Delayed enhancing pseudocapsule ➡ is seen along the periphery of the lesion.*

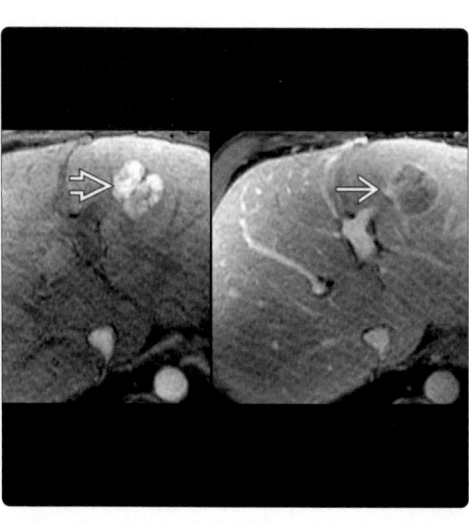

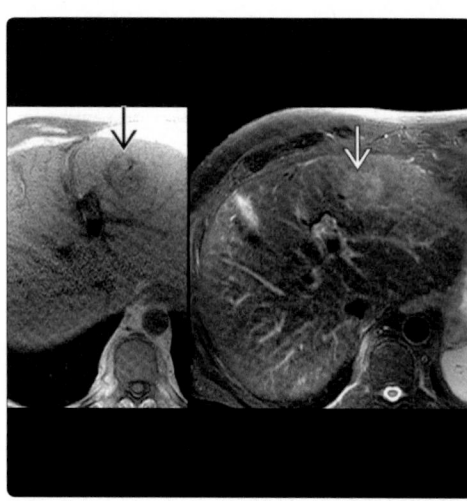

(Left) *Arterial phase CE T1 with FS MR (left) shows a hypervascular hepatocellular carcinoma ➡, which washes out on portal venous phase and has an enhancing pseudocapsule ➡.* (Right) *T1-weighted MR without contrast (left image) in the same patient shows typical low intrinsic T1 signal ➡ and mildly hyperintense T2 signal ➡ (right image).*

Hepatic Metastases

TERMINOLOGY

- Malignant spread of neoplasm to hepatic parenchyma

IMAGING

- Grayscale ultrasound
  - Hypoechoic metastasis: Usually from hypovascular tumors
  - Hyperechoic metastasis: Hypervascular metastasis
  - "Bull's-eye" or "target" metastatic lesions: Solid mass with hypoechoic rim or halo
  - Cystic/necrotic metastases: Mural nodules, thick walls, fluid-fluid levels, internal septa/debris
  - Calcified metastases: Mucinous or ossific primaries
  - Infiltrative/diffuse metastases: Lung or breast primary, may mimic cirrhosis
- Color Doppler ultrasound
  - Metastatic lesions follow vascularity of primary tumor
  - Contrast-enhanced US increases detectability of hepatic metastases

TOP DIFFERENTIAL DIAGNOSES

- Cysts (vs. hypoechoic or cystic metastases)
- Abscesses (vs. hypoechoic metastases)
- Hemangiomas (vs. hyperechoic metastases)
- Multifocal hepatocellular carcinomas or cholangiocarcinomas (vs. "target" lesion)
- Steatosis (vs. hypo-/hyperechoic metastasis)
- Hepatic adenomatosis

CLINICAL ISSUES

- Most common malignant tumor of liver

DIAGNOSTIC CHECKLIST

- Rule out other other causes of multiple liver lesions, e.g., hepatic cysts, abscesses, or hemangiomas
- Always correlate with clinical history and look for evidence of primary tumor

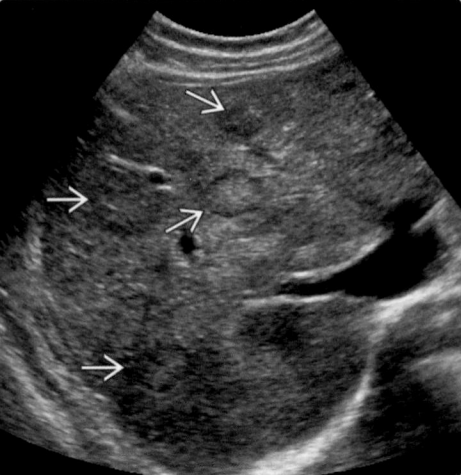
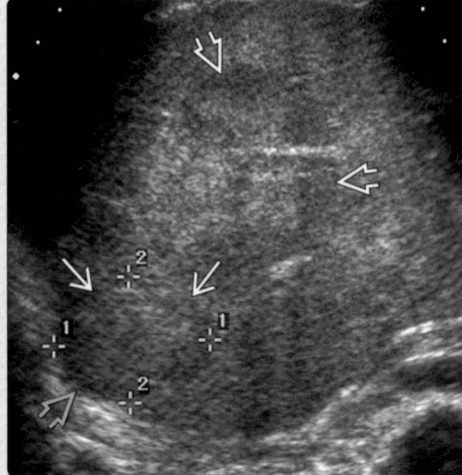

(Left) Transverse grayscale ultrasound in a patient with breast cancer metastases to the liver shows that the metastases have a classic target appearance ➡ in which rounded lesions are surrounded by a hypoechoic rim. (Right) Oblique transabdominal ultrasound in a different patient with breast cancer shows a minimally hypoechoic, solid metastasis ➡ in the right lobe of the liver, bulging its contour ➡, as well as other numerous, more subtle, hypoechoic solid masses ➡.

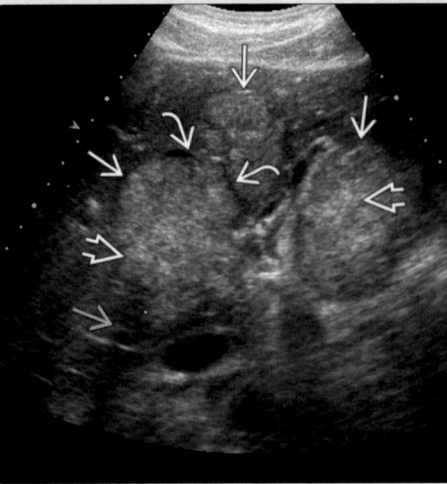
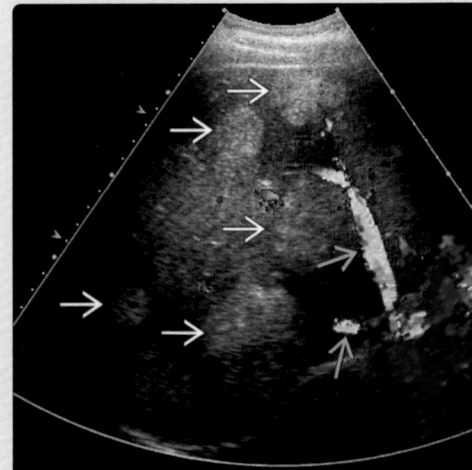

(Left) Transverse ultrasound in a patient with mucinous colon cancer metastases to the liver demonstrates multiple large, hyperechoic metastases ➡ containing diffuse echogenic foci ➡ related to subtle calcifications. Note posterior acoustic shadowing ➡ as well as distortion and compression of the right portal vein ➡ by metastases. (Right) Color Doppler ultrasound of the liver in the same patient with mucinous colon cancer shows multiple hyperechoic metastases ➡ throughout the liver, some of which abut and distort the hepatic veins ➡.

TERMINOLOGY

Definitions

- Malignant spread of neoplasm to hepatic parenchyma

IMAGING

General Features

- Best diagnostic clue
  - Multiple lesions scattered throughout liver in random distribution
- Location
  - Both lobes of liver
- Size
  - Variable from few mm to > 10 cm
- Key concepts
  - Most common malignant tumor of liver
  - Liver is 2nd only to regional lymph nodes as site of metastatic disease
  - Autopsy studies reveal up to 55% of oncology patients have liver metastases

Ultrasonographic Findings

- Grayscale ultrasound
  - Round or oval, with smooth or irregular borders
  - Causes architectural distortion if large or numerous
  - **Hypoechoic metastases**
    - Usually from hypovascular tumors
  - **Hyperechoic metastases**
    - Vascular metastases; from neuroendocrine tumors (classically carcinoid), choriocarcinoma, renal cell carcinoma, melanoma
  - **"Bull's-eye" or "target" metastatic lesions**
    - Alternating layers of hyper- & hypoechoic tissue
    - Solid mass with hypoechoic rim or halo
    - Usually from aggressive primary tumors
    - Classic example: Bronchogenic carcinoma
  - **Cystic/necrotic metastases**
    - May demonstrate posterior enhancement
    - Mural nodules, thick walls, fluid-fluid levels, internal septa/debris distinguish them from simple cysts
    - Necrotic center may be lined with irregular walls and contain debris
    - Cystic primaries: Cystadenocarcinoma of pancreas/ovary; colon
    - Necrosis/treated metastases: Sarcoma; squamous cell carcinoma
  - **Calcified metastases**
    - Markedly echogenic interface with acoustic shadowing or diffuse small echogenic foci
    - Mucinous primaries: Colon, ovary
    - Calcific/ossific primaries: Osteosarcoma, chondrosarcoma, neuroblastoma, malignant teratoma
    - Treated metastases
  - **Infiltrative/diffuse metastases**
    - Lung or breast primary
    - Refractive shadows often emanate from infiltrative tumor margins
    - May simulate cirrhosis
    - May distort or efface portal or hepatic veins
- Color Doppler

- Follows vascularity of primary tumor
- Contrast-enhanced US increases detectability of hepatic metastases
  - Vascularity in tumor bed
  - Kupffer phase defect after microbubble enhancement

CT Findings

- NECT
  - Calcified: Mucinous adenocarcinoma (colon), treated metastases (breast), malignant teratoma
  - Cystic metastases (less than 20 HU)
    - Fluid levels, debris, mural nodules
    - Thickened walls or septations may be seen
    - Usually cystadenocarcinoma or sarcoma (pancreatic, GI, or ovarian primaries)
- CECT
  - Hypovascular metastases
    - Low-attenuation center with peripheral rim enhancement (e.g., epithelial metastases)
    - Indicates vascularized viable tumor in periphery & hypovascular or necrotic center
    - Rim enhancement may also be due to compressed normal parenchyma
  - Hypervascular metastases
    - Hyperdense in late arterial phase images
    - May have internal necrosis without uniform hyperdense enhancement
    - Hypo- or isodense on NECT & portal venous phase; often washout becomes hypodense on delayed phase
    - e.g., neuroendocrine tumor, thyroid, breast, renal cell carcinomas, and pheochromocytoma

MR Findings

- T1WI
  - Melanoma metastasis: Hyperintense due to melanin
- T2WI
  - Moderate to high signal
  - "Light bulb" sign: Seen with cystic and neuroendocrine tumor metastases
    - Mimic cysts or hemangiomas, but usually with thick wall or fluid level
- T1WI C+
  - Hypovascular metastases
    - Same pattern of enhancement as CECT
    - Low signal in center and peripheral rim-enhancement
    - Perilesional enhancement may be tumor vascularity or hepatic parenchymal edema
  - Hypervascular metastases
    - Hyperintense enhancement on arterial phase
  - Hepatobiliary contrast agent (gadoxetic acid): Hepatobiliary phase (20 min)
    - Metastases are conspicuous as hypointense focal lesions, whereas normal liver parenchyma retains contrast
    - Sensitive imaging modality for determining presence and number of metastases (especially for neuroendocrine metastases to liver) but not specific

Imaging Recommendations

- Best imaging tool
  - CECT for tumor staging

Diagnoses: Liver

- o Intraoperative ultrasound for small lesions
- o PET/CT is useful for whole-body screening
- o Gadoxetic acid-enhanced MR for detection of subtle metastases
- o Abdominal ultrasound
  - For metastasis screening or surveillance
  - Readily accessible and radiation free, but low sensitivity

DIFFERENTIAL DIAGNOSIS

Cysts (vs. Hypoechoic or Cystic Metastases)

- May have internal debris due to prior hemorrhage or infection
- No peripheral rim or central vascularity/contrast enhancement
- No mural nodule, thick wall, internal septa
- Posterior acoustic enhancement

Abscesses (vs. Hypoechoic Metastases)

- May be solid or cystic (internal debris/septa, thick irregular wall)
- Typical systemic signs of infection
- "Cluster" sign on CT for pyogenic abscesses

Hemangiomas (vs. Hyperechoic Metastases)

- Classically uniformly hyperechoic on US
- Typical peripheral nodular discontinuous enhancement on CECT or CEMR
- Markedly hyperintense on T2WI

Multifocal Hepatocellular Carcinomas or Cholangiocarcinomas (vs. "Target" Lesion)

- Hepatocellular carcinoma (HCC): Cirrhotic liver, portal vein invasion/thrombosis
  - o In cirrhotic livers, metastases from non-hepatic primaries are rare due to decreased portal blood flow
    - Thus any mass in cirrhotic liver is highly suspicious for HCC rather than metastasis
- Cholangiocarcinoma: Capsular retraction, delayed enhancement

Steatosis (vs. Hypo- or Hyperechoic Metastasis)

- Focal fatty sparing: Hypoechoic area in hyperechoic liver
- Focal fatty infiltration: Hyperechoic area or areas
- Geometric borders, no architectural distortion, no mass effect
- Fat density on NECT
- Focal signal dropout on opposed-phase T1 GRE MR

Hepatic Adenomatosis

- Mimic hypervascular metastasis
- Fat-containing and hemorrhagic; better seen on MR
- History of OCP or anabolic steroid use

PATHOLOGY

General Features

- Etiology
  - o Hypovascular liver metastases
    - Lung, GI tract, pancreas, and most breast cancers
    - Lymphoma, bladder and uterine malignancy
  - o Hypervascular liver metastases
    - Neuroendocrine tumors, renal and thyroid cancers
    - Some breast cancers, sarcomas, and melanoma

Staging, Grading, & Classification

- Liver metastases indicate stage IV tumor

CLINICAL ISSUES

Presentation

- Most common signs/symptoms
  - o Asymptomatic, RUQ pain, tender hepatomegaly
  - o Weight loss, jaundice or ascites
- Lab data: Elevated LFTs; normal in 25-50% of patients

Natural History & Prognosis

- Depends on primary tumor site
- 20-40% have good 5-year survival rate if resectable
- In patients with metastatic colon cancer
  - o 3-year survival rate
    - 21% in patients with solitary lesions
    - 6% in patients with multiple lesions in 1 lobe
    - 4% in patients with widespread disease

Treatment

- Resection or ablation for colorectal liver metastases
- Chemo- or radioembolization: Hypervascular (neuroendocrine tumor) metastases
- Chemotherapy (oral or IV) for all others

DIAGNOSTIC CHECKLIST

Consider

- Rule out other causes of multiple liver lesions like hepatic cysts, abscesses, hemangiomas
- Correlate with clinical history and look for evidence of primary tumor

Image Interpretation Pearls

- In absence of other obvious metastasis
  - o Hepatic lesions that are "too small to characterize" rarely represent metastasis
  - o Lesions higher than blood density on NECT rarely represent metastasis

SELECTED REFERENCES

1. Westwood M et al: Contrast-enhanced ultrasound using SonoVue® (sulphur hexafluoride microbubbles) compared with contrast-enhanced computed tomography and contrast-enhanced magnetic resonance imaging for the characterisation of focal liver lesions and detection of liver metastases: a systematic review and cost-effectiveness analysis. Health Technol Assess. 17(16):1-243, 2013
2. Lefort T et al: Correlation and agreement between contrast-enhanced ultrasonography and perfusion computed tomography for assessment of liver metastases from endocrine tumors: normalization enhances correlation. Ultrasound Med Biol. 38(6):953-61, 2012

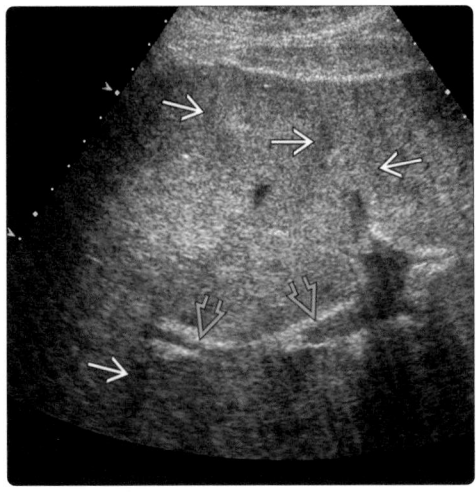

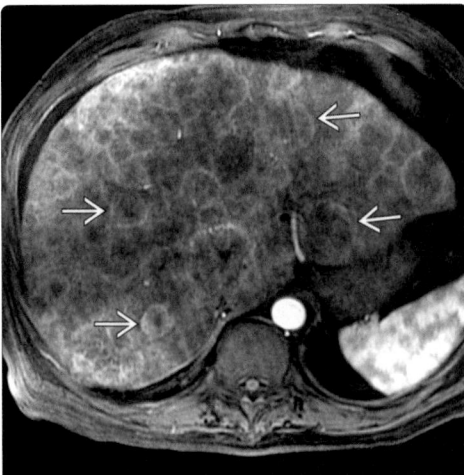

(Left) *Transverse abdominal grayscale ultrasound in a patient with diffuse hepatic metastases demonstrates a markedly heterogeneous appearance of the liver with numerous refractive shadows* ➡ *caused by underlying isoechoic metastases. Note distortion of the portal veins by mass effect* ➡. **(Right)** *T1WI C+ FS MR in the same patient demonstrates that a heterogeneous liver appearance on ultrasound is due to numerous masses* ➡ *virtually replacing the entire liver parenchyma.*

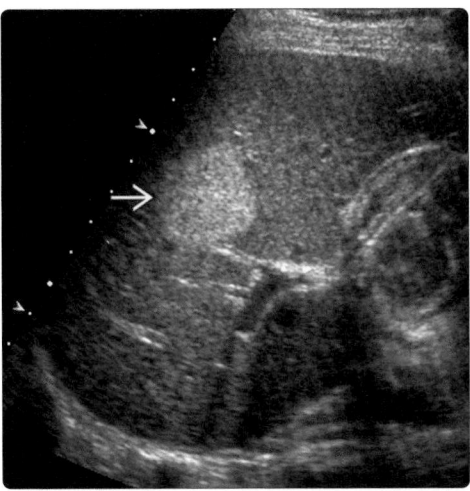

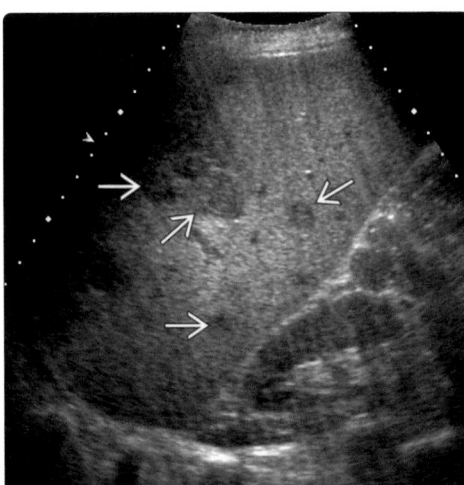

(Left) *Transverse abdominal grayscale ultrasound in a patient with carcinoid tumor shows a round, homogeneously hyperechoic metastasis in the right lobe of liver* ➡. **(Right)** *Longitudinal abdominal grayscale ultrasound in a patient with pancreatic cancer shows multiple small, hypoechoic metastases* ➡ *in a background of underlying hepatic steatosis.*

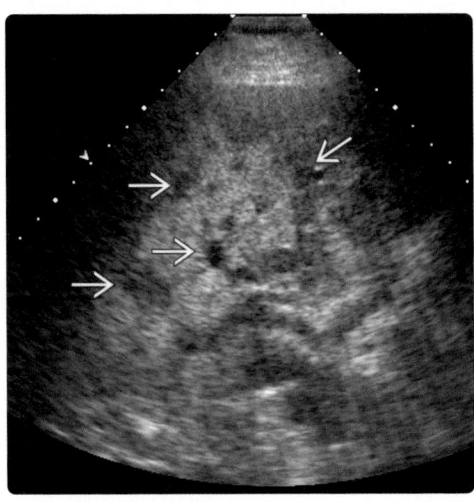

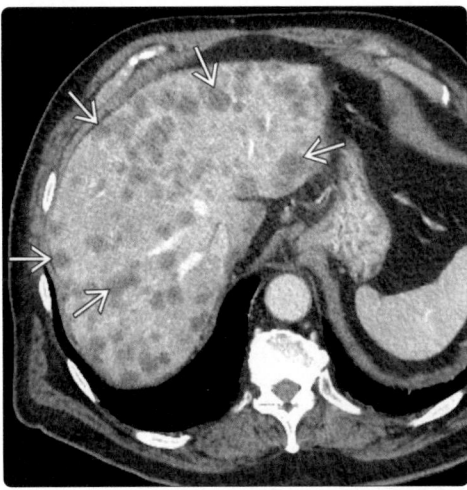

(Left) *Transverse abdominal grayscale ultrasound in a different patient with pancreatic cancer shows numerous small, hypoechoic metastases* ➡ *throughout the liver. Notice the background liver is echogenic from hepatic steatosis, a common finding in the setting of chemotherapy.* **(Right)** *Portal venous phase axial CECT in the same patient with pancreatic cancer shows numerous hypodense metastatic nodules* ➡ *scattered throughout the liver.*

Hepatic Lymphoma

TERMINOLOGY

- Neoplasm of lymphoid tissues in liver

IMAGING

- Hepatic lymphoma often favors periportal areas due to high content of lymphatic tissue
- Grayscale ultrasound
  - Discrete form: Multiple well-defined, hypoechoic masses
    - Hypoechogenicity due to high cellular density and lack of background stroma
  - Infiltrative form: Innumerable subcentimeter hypoechoic foci, miliary in pattern and periportal in location
    - May be indistinguishable from normal liver
- CECT
  - Solid lesions with poor contrast enhancement
  - Usually homogeneous density and rarely necrotic
  - May have thin rim enhancement
  - Diffuse infiltrative low-density areas

TOP DIFFERENTIAL DIAGNOSES

- Metastases
- Multifocal/diffuse hepatocellular carcinoma (HCC)
- Liver abscesses
- Hemangiomas
- Focal fat infiltration/sparing
- Hepatic cysts

CLINICAL ISSUES

- Primary hepatic lymphoma is rare
- Secondary hepatic involvement is more common

DIAGNOSTIC CHECKLIST

- Rule out other multiple liver lesions: Metastasis, HCCs, hepatic cysts, abscesses, hemangiomas
- Confirmation may require needle biopsy

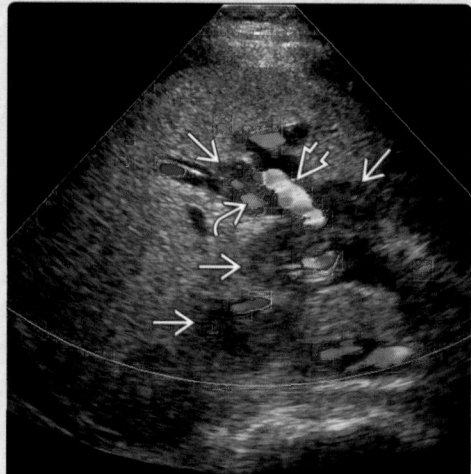
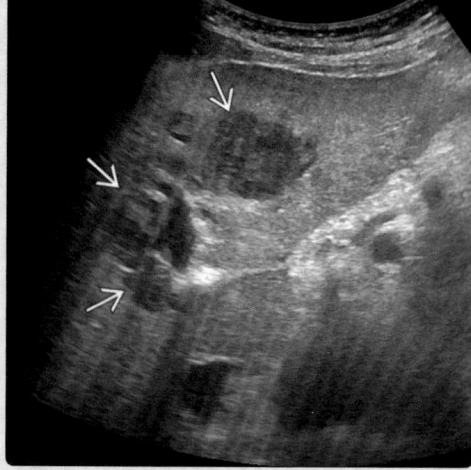

(Left) Transverse color Doppler ultrasound in a patient with lymphoma involving the liver shows multiple hypoechoic masses ➡ in a periportal distribution (right anterior portal vein) ➡ in the liver. Lesions are predominantly hypovascular with minimal vascularity seen along the periphery ➡. (Right) Transverse abdominal grayscale ultrasound in a patient with lymphoma shows several hypoechoic masses ➡ in a periportal distribution in the left lobe of the liver.

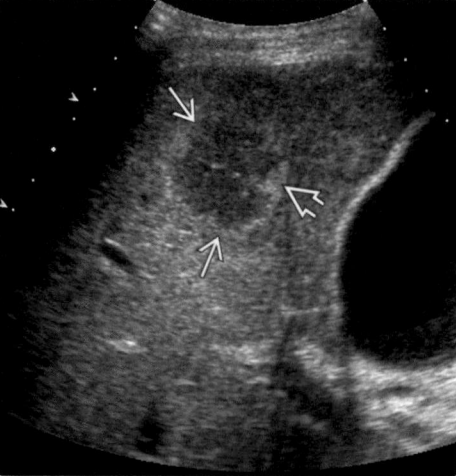
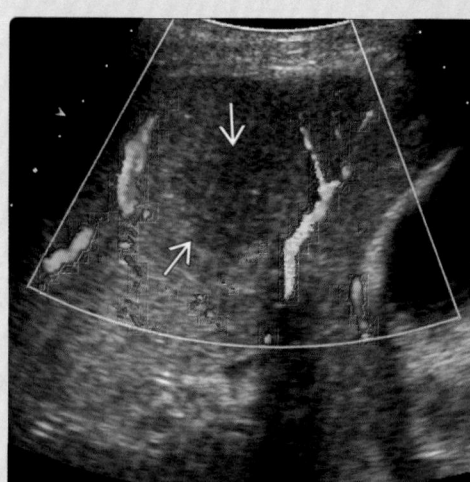

(Left) Transverse abdominal grayscale ultrasound in the same patient shows a well-defined, hypoechoic mass ➡ with a thin, hyperechoic rim ➡ in segment 5 of the liver. (Right) Transverse color Doppler ultrasound performed in the same patient shows no detectable vascular flow within the lymphomatous mass ➡.

TERMINOLOGY

Definitions

- Neoplasm of lymphoid tissues in liver

IMAGING

General Features

- Best diagnostic clue
  - No known specific imaging findings for diagnosis of hepatic lymphoma
  - Lobulated, hypoechoic/low-density, hypovascular masses
- Location
  - Favors periportal areas
    - Due to high content of lymphatic tissue
  - Liver is often secondary site for lymphoma
- Size
  - Variable; from few millimeters to centimeters
- Morphology
  - Discrete lesions
    - Solitary or multiple masses in liver
    - More likely to be primary non-Hodgkin lymphoma (NHL) or AIDS-associated lymphoma
  - Diffuse infiltration
    - Usually secondary site in Hodgkin disease (HD) or NHL
    - Often difficult to detect on imaging
- Key concepts
  - Hepatic lymphoma is detected in vivo in < 10% of cases
  - Primary hepatic lymphoma is rare
    - Mostly seen in immunocompromised patients
  - Secondary hepatic involvement is more common than primary
    - Seen in > 50% of patients with lymphoma on autopsy
  - Generally more common in immunosuppressed patients
    - Transplant recipients and AIDS patients are at high risk
  - Types of lymphoma: NHL > HD

Ultrasonographic Findings

- Grayscale ultrasound
  - **Discrete form**
    - Multiple, well-defined nodules or masses
    - Hypoechoic or anechoic lesions
      - Hypoechogenicity probably due to high cellular density and lack of background stroma
    - Large or conglomerate masses may appear to contain septa and mimic abscesses
  - **Diffuse/Infiltrative Form**
    - Innumerable subcentimeter hypoechoic foci, miliary in pattern and periportal in location
    - Infiltrative pattern may be indistinguishable from normal liver
    - Most are missed and only diagnosed on autopsy
  - Other signs of lymphoma
    - Hepatomegaly
    - Associated splenomegaly or splenic lesions
    - Lymphadenopathy (periportal, paraaortic, mesenteric)
    - Bowel wall thickening (infiltration)
    - Ascites

CT Findings

- NECT
  - May be normal
  - Primary lymphoma
    - Isodense or hypodense to liver
  - Secondary lymphoma
    - Multiple well-defined, large, homogeneous, lobulated, low-density masses
    - Diffuse infiltration: Indistinguishable from normal liver or steatosis
- CECT
  - Solid lesions with poor contrast enhancement
  - Usually homogeneous density and rarely necrotic
  - May have thin rim enhancement
  - Diffuse, infiltrative, low-density areas

MR Findings

- T1WI
  - Discrete lesion: Hypointense masses
  - Diffuse infiltration: Indistinguishable from normal liver
- T2WI
  - Discrete lesion: Hyperintense masses
  - Diffuse infiltration: Indistinguishable from normal liver
- T1WI C+
  - Poor gadolinium enhancement
  - May have rim enhancement

Nuclear Medicine Findings

- PET
  - F-18 FDG-avid lesions
    - Focal or diffuse hypermetabolic activity
    - Useful for staging disease
    - Background metabolic activity of liver may obscure some lesions

Imaging Recommendations

- Best imaging tool
  - Ultrasound for surveillance and monitoring lesion progress/treatment response
- Protocol advice
  - Ultrasound detection of lesion to be followed by CECT for disease staging

DIFFERENTIAL DIAGNOSIS

Metastases

- Peripheral rim enhancement, internal necrosis
- Often difficult to differentiate without history of primary lesion

Multifocal/Diffuse Hepatocellular Carcinoma (HCC)

- Background cirrhotic liver
- Hypovascular HCCs mimic discrete form of hepatic lymphoma
- Diffuse HCCs mimic infiltrative form of hepatic lymphoma
- Portal vein invasion/thrombosis

Liver Abscesses

- May see fluid content or internal debris or septations on US
- "Cluster" sign on CECT for pyogenic abscesses
- Often with atelectasis and right pleural effusion
- Typical systemic signs of infection

Hemangiomas

- Typically uniformly hyperechoic on US
- May be hypoechoic on underlying fatty liver
- CECT/CEMR: Typical peripheral, nodular, discontinuous enhancement
- Isodense with blood vessels on CT
- Strong hyperintensity on T2WI

Focal Fat Infiltration/Sparing

- Focal signal dropout on opposed-phase T1 GRE MR
- Vessels course through lesions without disruption
- Typical sites; periligamentous, perivascular distribution

Hepatic Cysts

- Homogeneous, anechoic lesion with posterior acoustic enhancement
- May have increased echogenicity or density due to prior bleed or infection (e.g., polycystic liver)
- No central or peripheral rim enhancement
- Imperceptible walls
- No mural nodules or debris

PATHOLOGY

General Features

- Etiology
  - Viral cause suggested
- Associated abnormalities
  - Immunocompromised patients are predisposed to lymphoma
    - Congenital immunodeficiency
    - Collagen vascular diseases
    - HIV infection/AIDS
    - Immunosuppressant therapy for organ transplant
  - Hepatitis B and C virus

Staging, Grading, & Classification

- Ann Arbor staging classification
- NHL classification
  - Revised European American Lymphoma (REAL) classification
  - World Health Organization (WHO) classification
  - International Working Formulation

Gross Pathologic & Surgical Features

- Miliary, nodular or diffuse form

Microscopic Features

- Hodgkin disease
  - Typical Reed-Sternberg cells
- Non-Hodgkin lymphoma
  - Follicular small cleaved cells (most common)
  - Small noncleaved cells (Burkitt lymphoma; rare)

CLINICAL ISSUES

Presentation

- Most common signs/symptoms
  - Hepatomegaly
  - Right upper quadrant pain
  - Fever, weight loss, night sweats
  - Jaundice

- Ascites or pleural effusion
- Lymphadenopathy: Periportal paraaortic, mesenteric
- Lab data: LFT abnormality, elevated serum lactate dehydrogenase (LDH)
- Diagnosis: Imaging, occasionally fine-needle aspiration biopsy

Demographics

- Age
  - Usually middle and older age group
- Gender
  - M > F
- Epidemiology
  - Approximately 60,000 new cases of lymphoma diagnosed per year in USA
  - Primary hepatic lymphoma is rare

Natural History & Prognosis

- Depends on histological classification and stage of disease
- Liver involvement may lead to fulminant hepatic failure with rapid progression of encephalopathy to coma and death

Treatment

- Chemotherapy
  - May be hampered by hepatic insufficiency
- Radiotherapy or surgery

DIAGNOSTIC CHECKLIST

Consider

- Rule out other multiple liver lesions
  - Metastasis, HCCs, hepatic cysts, abscesses, hemangiomas
- Often clue to diagnosis is abnormal hepatic parenchymal echo pattern associated with splenomegaly and lymphadenopathy
- Confirmation may require needle biopsy

SELECTED REFERENCES

1. Lu Q et al: Primary non-Hodgkin's lymphoma of the liver: sonographic and CT findings. Hepatobiliary Pancreat Dis Int. 14(1):75-81, 2015
2. Foschi FG et al: Role of contrast-enhanced ultrasonography in primary hepatic lymphoma. J Ultrasound Med. 29(9):1353-6, 2010
3. Elsayes KM et al: Primary hepatic lymphoma: imaging findings. J Med Imaging Radiat Oncol. 53(4):373-9, 2009
4. Stojković MV et al: Color Doppler sonography and angioscintigraphy in hepatic Hodgkin's lymphoma. World J Gastroenterol. 15(26):3269-75, 2009
5. Castroagudín JF et al: Sonographic features of liver involvement by lymphoma. J Ultrasound Med. 26(6):791-6, 2007
6. Low G et al: Diagnosis of periportal hepatic lymphoma with contrast-enhanced ultrasonography. J Ultrasound Med. 25(8):1059-62, 2006

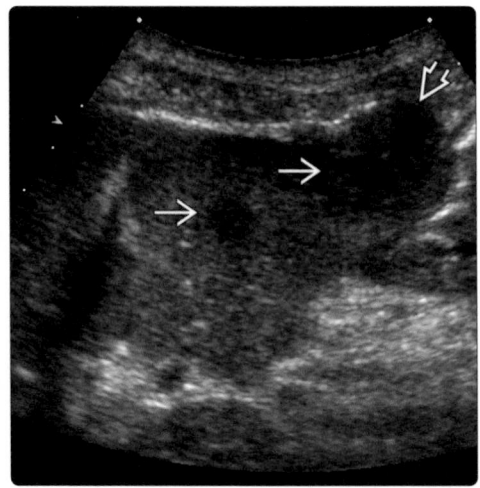
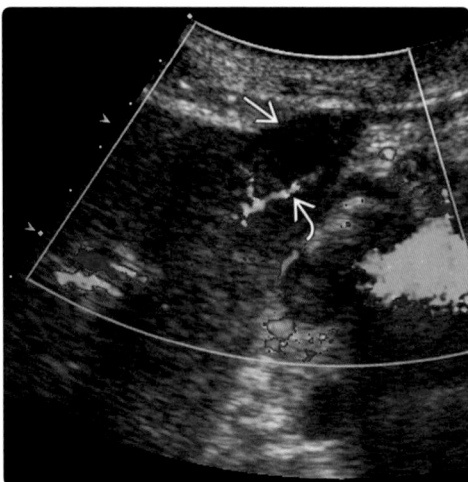

(Left) *Transverse abdominal ultrasound in a patient with lymphoma shows several hypoechoic masses in the lateral segment of the left lobe of the liver* ➡. *The more peripheral mass causes contour bulging of the liver capsule* ➡. **(Right)** *Longitudinal color Doppler ultrasound performed in the same patient shows some vascularity* ➡ *within the exophytic hypoechoic mass* ➡.

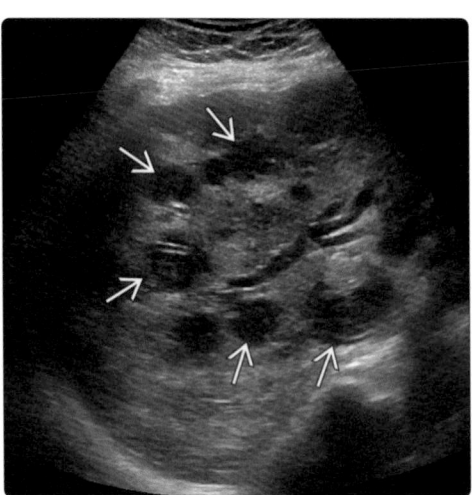
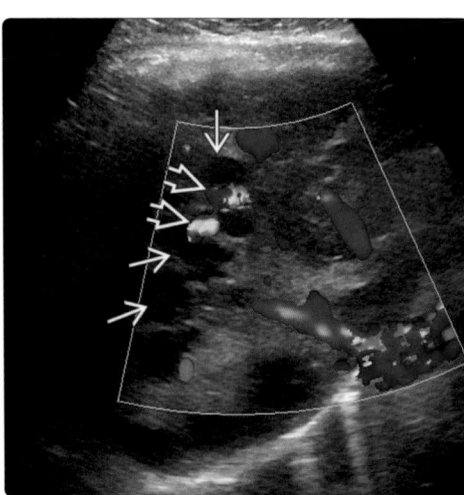

(Left) *Transverse abdominal ultrasound in a patient with lymphoma shows multiple hypoechoic nodules* ➡ *throughout the right lobe of the liver.* **(Right)** *Transverse color Doppler ultrasound in the same patient shows that the masses* ➡ *are predominantly hypovascular and abut the portal veins* ➡.

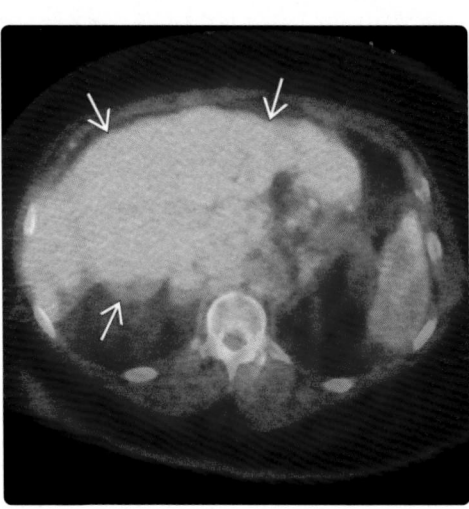
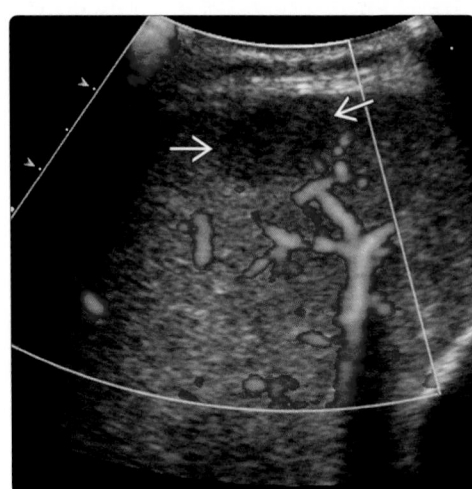

(Left) *F-18 FDG PET in the same patient shows marked diffusely hypermetabolic uptake within the entire liver parenchyma* ➡, *caused by hepatic lymphoma.* **(Right)** *Power Doppler ultrasound in a patient with lymphoma shows an ill-defined, hypoechoic mass in the subcapsular portion of the right lobe of the liver* ➡. *No vascularity is detected within the mass.*

TERMINOLOGY

- Shunt between main portal vein and hepatic vein created with balloon-expandable covered metallic stent

IMAGING

- Goal of US: Detection of stenosis before shunt occludes or symptoms recur
- Best imaging tool
  - US as primary TIPS surveillance tool
  - CTA/MRA indicated if US technically compromised or equivocal
- Doppler US findings of TIPS malfunction
  - PV
    - Hepatofugal flow
    - Peak velocity < 35 cm/sec
  - Within shunt
    - Peak velocity < 90 cm/sec or > 200 cm/sec at any point
    - Temporal change in peak velocity > 50 cm/sec

TOP DIFFERENTIAL DIAGNOSES

- Portal vein occlusion
- Hepatic vein occlusion
- Inferior vena cava occlusion

PATHOLOGY

- Stenosis usually secondary to intimal hyperplasia from hepatic venous side
- Hepatic encephalopathy if portal flow bypasses liver

CLINICAL ISSUES

- Most common symptoms/signs of stent malfunction
  - Variceal hemorrhage
  - Signs of worsening portal hypertension with increasing ascites

DIAGNOSTIC CHECKLIST

- Low flow may be difficult to detect with US
  - Confirm angiographically (CTA, MRA, shunt venography)

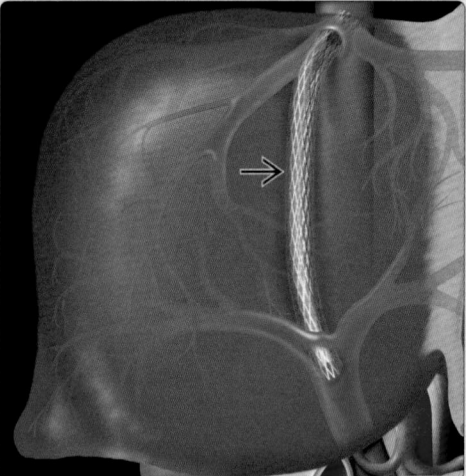

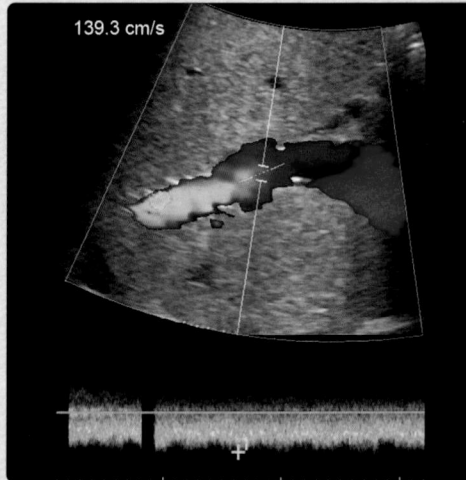

(Left) Graphic shows TIPS shunt creation. The hepatic vein is punctured within 2 cm of the inferior vena cava (IVC). A covered stent ⊡ is placed between the hepatic venous end and the right portal vein, adjacent to its junction with the main portal vein. (Right) Spectral Doppler ultrasound of a TIPS with interrogation at the proximal (portal venous) portion of the shunt shows appropriate flow direction and velocity of 139 cm/sec.

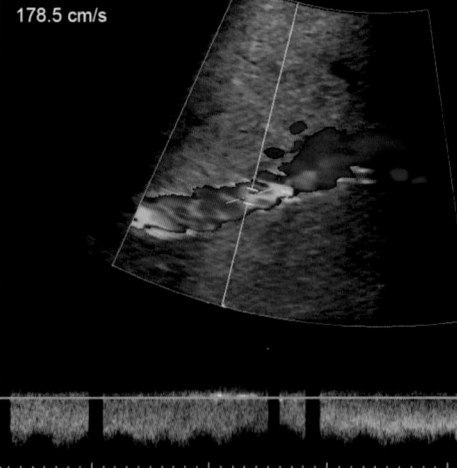

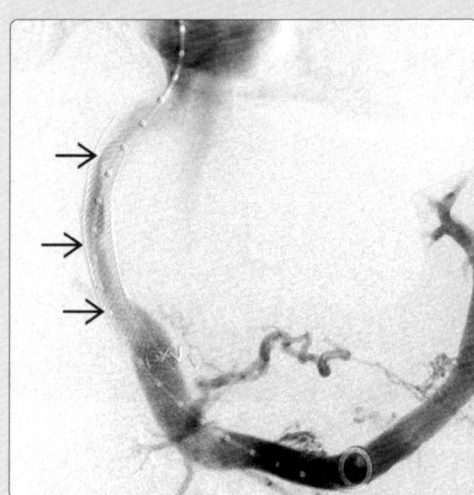

(Left) Spectral Doppler ultrasound (same patient) in the mid TIPS shows slight increase in velocity to 178 cm/sec, which is still within normal limits. Angle correction should always be used when evaluating TIPS for accurate velocity measurement. (Right) Anteroposterior supine portal angiogram in a 66-year-old man with a suspected TIPS stenosis based on Doppler ultrasound reveals multiple areas of intimal hyperplasia within the parenchymal portion of the shunt ⊡, consistent with stenosis.

Transjugular Intrahepatic Portosystemic Shunt (TIPS)

TERMINOLOGY

Abbreviations

- Transjugular intrahepatic portasystemic shunt (TIPS)

Definitions

- Shunt between portal vein (PV) and hepatic vein (HV) created typically with balloon-expandable polytetrafluoroethylene (PTFE)-covered stent graft
- Shunt dysfunction
  - Reduction > 50% of shunt lumen
  - Portosystemic gradient > 12-15 mmHg
  - Complete occlusion of shunt

IMAGING

General Features

- Location
  - Most common route: Right PV → right HV
- Size
  - 10-12 mm in diameter
- Morphology
  - Typically follows curved course through hepatic parenchyma
  - Portal end in right portal vein near main PV bifurcation
  - Hepatic end located near junction of HV/inferior vena cava (IVC)

Ultrasonographic Findings

- Grayscale ultrasound
  - Echogenic stent easily seen
  - Stent typically curved but should not be kinked
  - Hepatic and portal ends "squarely" within veins (best seen on grayscale US)
- Pulsed Doppler
  - PV, shunt malfunction
    - Peak velocity < 35 cm/sec
    - Change in direction of flow in left portal branch (i.e., change from hepatofugal to hepatopetal)
  - Within shunt, malfunction
    - Shunt velocity < 90 cm/sec or > 200 cm/sec at any point
    - Temporal change in velocity ≥ 50 cm/sec compared to prior studies
    - Focal severe turbulence or elevated velocity can suggest stenosis
    - Absence of flow: Occlusion
      - Always confirm angiographically
    - Loss of pulsatility or respiratory variation (less specific finding)
- Color Doppler
  - Within shunt, malfunction
    - Visible stenosis, focal or diffuse
    - Focal aliasing indicates high velocity and suggests stenosis
    - Absence of flow: Occlusion
      - Check with spectral Doppler (more sensitive); confirm angiographically
- Goal of US: Detection of stenosis before shunt occludes or symptoms recur

Angiographic Findings

- Shunt venography (gold standard)
  - Direct catheterization of shunt via peripheral vein approach
  - Detection and quantification of shunt patency or degree of stenosis
  - Simultaneous measurement of portosystemic gradient
  - Intervention if necessary
  - Limitation: Invasive nature

Other Modality Findings

- CTA, MRA
  - Anatomic depiction of stenosis, occlusion, and collateralization
  - Contrast enhancement essential for CTA, generally required for MRA
  - Obtain a global view

Imaging Recommendations

- Best imaging tool
  - US is primary TIPS surveillance tool
  - CTA/MRA indicated if US technically compromised or equivocal
- Protocol advice
  - Post-TIPS assessment (grayscale, color Doppler, spectral Doppler)
    - Stent configuration/position
    - Patency and flow direction in PV and its branches
      - Measure velocity mid-PV (not adjacent to shunt)
    - Assess shunt with color Doppler
      - Measure Doppler waveforms/peak velocities: Proximal, mid, distal shunt
      - Compare findings with prior results (velocities ideally within 50 cm/sec of prior measurement)
    - Presence of stenosis
      - If present, document peak stenosis velocity, usually at point of maximum turbulence
    - Patency, flow direction, Doppler waveforms in HV
    - Always check for coexisting hepatic masses, especially in cirrhotic patients
    - Evaluate presence/volume of ascites and pleural fluid

DIFFERENTIAL DIAGNOSIS

PV Occlusion

- Predisposing factors
  - Hypercoagulable states, pancreatitis, tumor invasion, dehydration, trauma, cirrhosis
- Acute
  - CECT may demonstrate transient hepatic attenuation difference (THAD) with affected lobe or segment on arterial phase
  - If main PV acutely thrombotic, central perihepatic low attenuation on arterial phase
- Chronic
  - Cavernous transformation
  - Innumerable periportal collaterals along hepatoduodenal ligament
  - "Cavernoma," i.e., mass-like tangle of collateral veins in porta hepatis

HV Occlusion

- Predisposing factors
  - Hypercoagulable states, Budd-Chiari syndrome, myeloproliferative states, birth control pills, tumor invasion (especially hepatocellular carcinoma)
- CECT
  - Arterial phase: Normal enhancing caudate lobe, mottled and reticular enhancement in liver periphery
    - Due to congestion and centrilobular necrosis
  - Venous phase: "Flip-flop" with lower attenuation of caudate lobe and increased density in liver periphery
  - Visualization of thrombi in HV and peridiaphragmatic collateral veins

IVC Occlusion

- Etiologies
  - Tumor infiltration, hepatocellular carcinoma most common; rarely metastases
  - Congenital web or band
  - Angiosarcoma of IVC

PATHOLOGY

General Features

- Etiology
  - Stenosis usually secondary to intimal fibroplasia within HV
    - Biliary leak or contamination of shunt may induce intimal hyperplasia
- Associated abnormalities
  - Hepatic encephalopathy as portal venous flow bypasses liver

Microscopic Features

- Intimal hyperplasia within areas of TIPS stenosis

CLINICAL ISSUES

Presentation

- Most common signs/symptoms
  - TIPS malfunction
    - Signs of worsening portal hypertension with increasing ascites
    - Variceal hemorrhage

Demographics

- Epidemiology
  - Maintaining TIPS shunt patency is major problem
    - Primary patency (no intervention): 1 year = 38-84%
    - Secondary (assisted) patency: 1 year = 96-100%

Natural History & Prognosis

- Causes of TIPS failure
  - Technical problems: Malposition, kinks, incomplete deployment, hepatic perforation with hemoperitoneum, or bile leak
  - Venous trauma during stent insertion: Usually HV progresses to fibrosis/stenosis, may result in acute occlusion of PV
  - Neointimal hyperplasia (ameliorated by covered stents)
  - Thrombosis: Coagulopathy, intercurrent illness due to above problems
  - Hepatic arterial injury and arteriovenous fistula

- Gallbladder injury
- Guarded prognosis
  - Maintaining shunt patency
  - Inevitable liver disease progression
  - High risk of cirrhosis-related hepatocellular carcinoma
  - 7-45% 30-day mortality

Indications for TIPS

- Variceal bleeding refractory to sclerosis/banding
- Refractory ascites
- Hepatic hydrothorax
- Budd-Chiari syndrome
- Bridge to liver transplantation

Relative Contraindications for TIPS

- Hepatobiliary or pancreatic malignancy
- Portal venous system thrombosis
- Polycystic liver disease
- Biliary obstruction
- Infectious cholangitis

DIAGNOSTIC CHECKLIST

Consider

- TIPS malfunction on Doppler US
  - If shunt velocity < 90 cm/sec or > 200 cm/sec or PV velocity < 35 cm/sec
- Low flow difficult to detect with US
  - Confirm occlusion angiographically (CTA, MRA, shunt venography)

SELECTED REFERENCES

1. Engstrom BI et al: Covered transjugular intrahepatic portosystemic shunts: accuracy of ultrasound in detecting shunt malfunction. AJR Am J Roentgenol. 200(4):904-8, 2013
2. Sajja KC et al: Long-term follow-up of TIPS created with expanded poly-tetrafluoroethylene covered stents. Dig Dis Sci. 58(7):2100-6, 2013
3. Wu Q et al: Transjugular intrahepatic portosystemic shunt using the FLUENCY expanded polytetrafluoroethylene-covered stent. Exp Ther Med. 5(1):263-266, 2013
4. Gazzera C et al: Fifteen years' experience with transjugular intrahepatic portosystemic shunt (TIPS) using bare stents: retrospective review of clinical and technical aspects. Radiol Med. 114(1):83-94, 2009
5. Kim MJ et al: Technical essentials of hepatic Doppler sonography. Curr Probl Diagn Radiol. 38(2):53-60, 2009
6. Bauer J et al: The role of TIPS for portal vein patency in liver transplant patients with portal vein thrombosis. Liver Transpl. 12(10):1544-51, 2006
7. Harrod-Kim P et al: Predictors of early mortality after transjugular intrahepatic portosystemic shunt creation for the treatment of refractory ascites. J Vasc Interv Radiol. 17(10):1605-10, 2006
8. Benito A et al: Doppler ultrasound for TIPS: does it work? Abdom Imaging. 29(1):45-52, 2004
9. Middleton WD et al: Doppler evaluation of transjugular intrahepatic portosystemic shunts. Ultrasound Q. 19(2):56-70; quiz 108 - 10, 2003
10. Bodner G et al: Color and pulsed Doppler ultrasound findings in normally functioning transjugular intrahepatic portosystemic shunts. Eur J Ultrasound. 12(2):131-6, 2000
11. Zizka J et al: Value of Doppler sonography in revealing transjugular intrahepatic portosystemic shunt malfunction: a 5-year experience in 216 patients. AJR Am J Roentgenol. 175(1):141-8, 2000

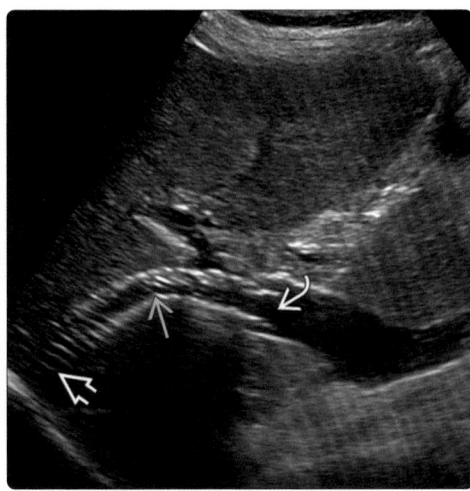

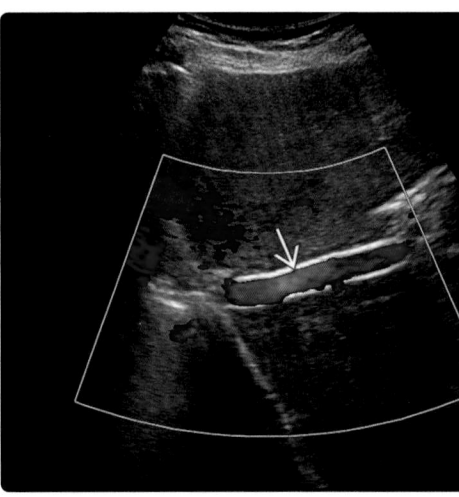

(Left) *Grayscale ultrasound of the liver shows a TIPS ⇨ extending from the main portal vein ⇲ to the right hepatic vein ⇶ near its confluence with the IVC. The proximal end of this patient's shunt is slightly more central than typically seen but was related to a shunt revision.* (Right) *Color Doppler image of a TIPS ⇶ shows appropriate direction of flow towards the IVC.*

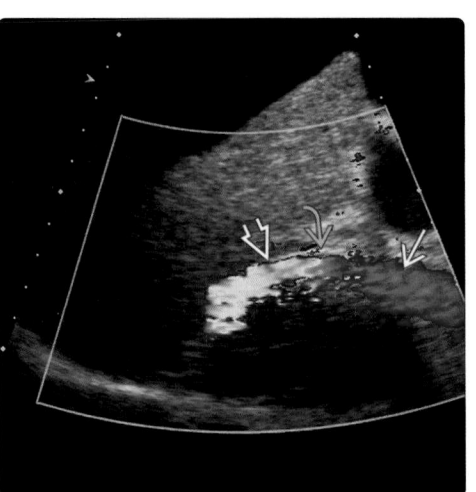

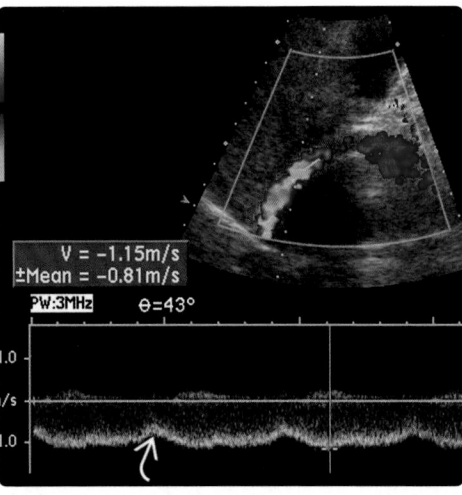

(Left) *In TIPS evaluation with color Doppler, the curvature of the stent in relation to the transducer may result in apparent flow towards the transducer (red) ⇶ before the bend ⇲, and flow away from the transducer (blue) distally ⇶. Flow within the TIPS however is uniformly directed towards the IVC.* (Right) *Longitudinal color Doppler ultrasound in a patient with a TIPS shows appropriate velocity of 115 cm/sec and gentle undulation of the waveform ⇲.*

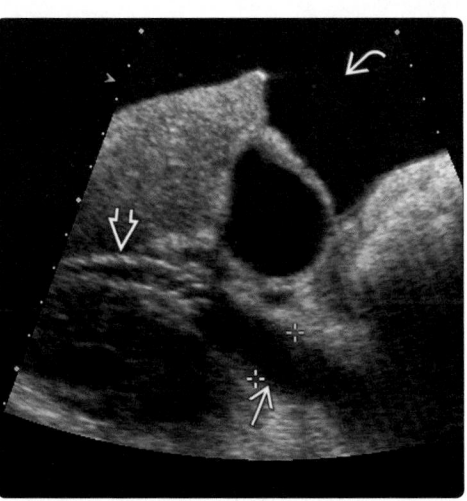

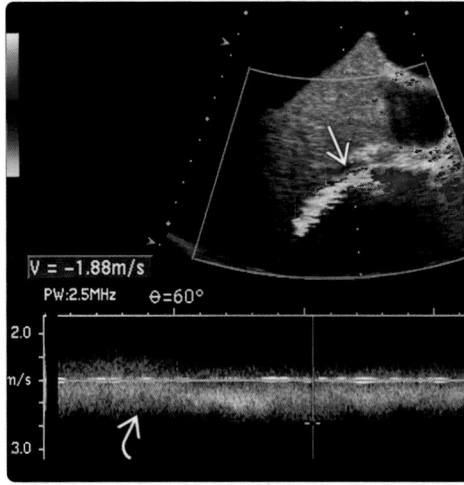

(Left) *Grayscale ultrasound of the liver shows the proximal portion of a TIPS ⇶ beginning at the distal portion of the main portal vein ⇶. Note large amount of ascites that suggests developing ⇲ shunt malfunction.* (Right) *Longitudinal spectral Doppler ultrasound in the same patient demonstrates borderline elevated velocity (188 cm/s) and loss of pulsatility ⇲ in the mid portion of shunt ⇶, suggestive of developing shunt stenosis.*

TERMINOLOGY

- Definition: Obstruction of portal vein due to thrombosis

IMAGING

- Color/spectral Doppler sonography
  - Surveillance and initial diagnosis
  - Absent blood flow within PV on color or spectral Doppler US
  - Cavernous transformation of PV
- CECT/MR
  - Comprehensive evaluation: Extent of occlusion and collateralization
  - Search for etiology and underlying condition

TOP DIFFERENTIAL DIAGNOSES

- Hepatic vein/IVC occlusion
- Splenic vein occlusion
- False-positive PV occlusion
- False-negative PV occlusion

- Nonocclusive thrombosis
- Dilated bile duct

PATHOLOGY

- Etiology
  - Thrombosis due to flow stasis, hypercoagulability, intraabdominal inflammation
  - Tumor thrombus or direct tumor invasion
- Acute thrombosis
  - Lumen filled with thrombus, diameter may be enlarged
- Chronic thrombosis
  - Lumen occlusion accompanied by cavernous transformation

DIAGNOSTIC CHECKLIST

- False-positive/-negative diagnoses are a problem
  - Appropriate Doppler ultrasound technique essential

(Left) Grayscale ultrasound of the liver shows mildly echogenic thrombus ➡ in the main portal vein. (Right) Power Doppler ultrasound in the same patient confirms absent flow within the thrombosed main portal vein ➡. Note the presence of ascites as well as underlying liver cirrhosis, which is a risk factor for development of portal vein thrombosis.

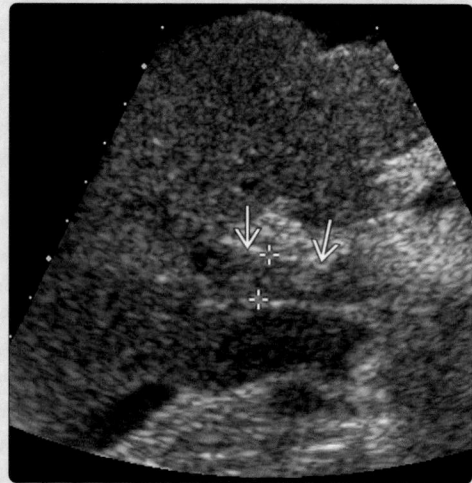
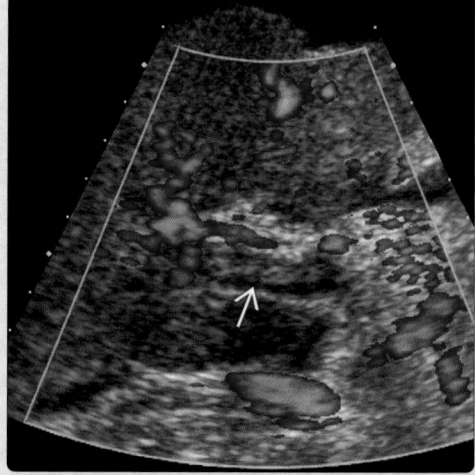

(Left) Grayscale ultrasound shows an echogenic, chronically thrombosed main portal vein ➔ and adjacent collateralized flow ➡ (cavernous transformation of the portal vein). (Right) Color Doppler ultrasound in the same patient shows collateralized flow ➡ in the porta hepatis in this patient with chronic portal vein thrombosis ➔. Color Doppler signal is heterogeneous because portal vein collaterals are tortuous, resulting in flow going both towards as well as away from the transducer.

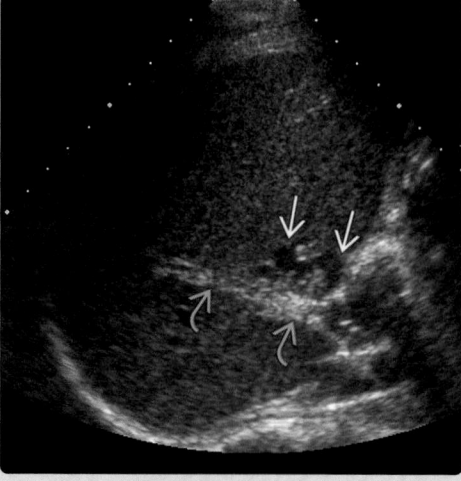
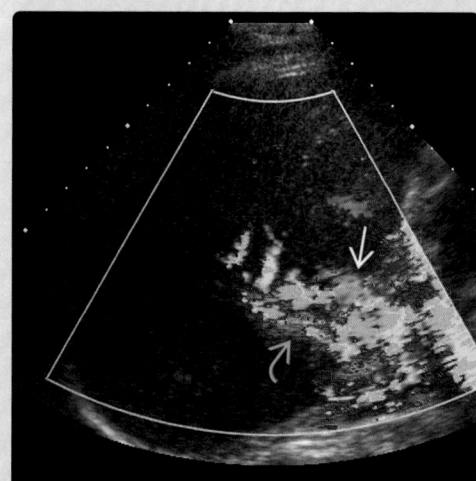

TERMINOLOGY

Abbreviations

- Portal vein (PV)

Definitions

- Obstruction of portal vein, most commonly due to thrombosis
- Cavernous transformation of PV: Portal venous collateralization

IMAGING

General Features

- Best diagnostic clue
  - Absent blood flow within PV on color or spectral Doppler US
  - Cavernous transformation of PV
- Location
  - Main portal vein &/or right and left branches
- Size
  - Acute thrombosis; PV diameter may be enlarged
  - Chronic occlusion; PV diameter small, echogenic, or not visible

Ultrasonographic Findings

- Grayscale ultrasound
  - Normal PV readily seen; nonvisualization suggests occlusion
  - Faintly echogenic material within PV lumen
  - Cavernous transformation of PV
    - Multiple tubular channels along usual course of thrombosed PV
    - Seen with subacute and especially chronic occlusion
  - Possible findings of pancreatitis if PV thrombosis due to this condition
  - If associated with tumor invasion of PV (tumor thrombus), may see heterogeneous, often expansile intraluminal soft tissue mass
- Pulsed Doppler
  - Absent Doppler signals in PV
  - Continuous flow in collaterals (no respiratory variation)
- Color Doppler
  - No color flow in PV
  - If associated with tumor invasion of PV (tumor thrombus)
    - May see tiny feeding vessels producing dot-dash pattern
    - Low-resistance arterial flow in feeding tumor vessels
    - Not consistently seen
  - Reversed flow in splenic vein; possibly superior mesenteric vein
  - Hepatopetal flow in cavernous transformation
  - Hepatofugal flow in portosystemic collaterals (due to portal hypertension)
  - Absent flow in hepatic vein or inferior vena cava (IVC) if PV occlusion secondary to these conditions

Imaging Recommendations

- Best imaging tool
  - Color/spectral Doppler sonography for surveillance and initial diagnosis
  - CECT/MR
    - Comprehensive evaluation: Extent of occlusion and collateralization
    - Evaluation of cause and underlying condition
- Protocol advice
  - Technical errors are major diagnostic impediment
    - Check to see if flow can be detected in other vessels at equivalent depth

DIFFERENTIAL DIAGNOSIS

Hepatic Vein/IVC Occlusion

- Causes slow flow in PV
- Possible secondary PV occlusion

Splenic Vein Occlusion

- No flow/nonvisualization of splenic vein
- Extensive left-sided collaterals
- Confirm that portal vein is patent

False-Positive PV Occlusion

- Poor ultrasound technique
  - Inadequate Doppler angle
  - Wrong velocity scale
  - Insufficient color/spectral Doppler gain
  - Wall filter too high
- Slow flow state
  - Very slow, or to-and-fro PV flow
  - No flow detected with color Doppler, sometimes spectral Doppler also
  - Usually due to cirrhosis/portal hypertension

False-Negative PV Occlusion

- Poor ultrasound technique
  - Nonocclusive thrombus
  - Too much color gain: "Blooming" of color beyond flow stream
    - Blooming overwrites grayscale image, obscuring thrombus
  - Less likely with tumor invasion, which typically is occlusive

Nonocclusive Thrombosis

- Variable degree of obstruction
- May be inapparent clinically

Dilated Bile Duct

- Patent adjacent PV seen with color Doppler

PATHOLOGY

General Features

- Etiology
  - Thrombosis
    - Combination of etiologic factors is common
    - Stasis: Sinusoidal obstruction as in cirrhosis; hepatic vein or IVC obstruction
    - Severe dehydration (especially in children)
    - Hypercoagulable states (genetic/neoplasm-related)
    - Pancreatitis: Portal/splenic vein inflammation (phlebitis) → thrombosis

- Abdominal sepsis → seeding of portal vein → phlebitis → thrombosis (e.g., appendicitis, diverticulitis, Crohn disease, etc.)
- Hepatic vein or IVC occlusion → secondary PV thrombosis
- Complication of surgery/liver transplantation
  ○ Tumor thrombus
    - Hepatocellular carcinoma (most common)
    - Cholangiocarcinoma
    - Metastatic disease
  ○ Direct neoplastic invasion
    - Usually pancreatic carcinoma
    - Rarely other neoplasms, usually metastatic
- Genetics
  ○ Inherited hypercoagulability may be causative factor in PV thrombosis
- Associated abnormalities
  ○ PV occlusion may be secondary to hepatic vein or IVC occlusion

Gross Pathologic & Surgical Features

- Acute thrombosis
  ○ Lumen partially filled with thrombus; flow maintained
  ○ Lumen entirely filled with thrombus; occlusion
  ○ Possible associated thrombosis of splenic vein/superior mesenteric vein
- Subacute/chronic thrombosis
  ○ PV replaced by tangle of collateral veins; cavernous transformation
    - Appearance 6-20 days after occlusion
    - Maturation gradual, most prominent chronically
  ○ 2 collateral routes
    - Portoportal along usual PV course
    - Portosystemic: Left gastric veins or splenogastric, splenorenal
- Tumor thrombus
  ○ Tumor grows within vein lumen
  ○ PV wall intact
- Tumor invasion
  ○ Tumor directly invades through vein wall
  ○ PV wall destroyed

Microscopic Features

- Vein wall inflammation is essential component of thrombosis (thrombophlebitis)

CLINICAL ISSUES

Presentation

- Most common signs/symptoms
  ○ Abdominal pain and distention
    - If phlebitis/inflammation → causes pain
    - Obstruction → bowel edema → pain
    - Bowel edema/congestion may cause ileus
    - Bowel edema possibly → ascites
  ○ Abnormal liver function tests
- Other signs/symptoms
  ○ Rare acute abdomen from venous bowel infarction
  ○ Asymptomatic incidental diagnosis (acute)
    - Nonocclusive thrombus
    - PV blood flow maintained

- Questionable clinical relevance
- Need for anticoagulation also questionable
  ○ Asymptomatic incidental diagnosis (chronic)
    - Cavernous transformation found on US, CT, MR
    - Possibly in otherwise healthy individual
    - Possibly in patient with cirrhosis
    - Remote disorder → PV thrombosis → effective collateralization
  ○ Gastrointestinal hemorrhage from portosystemic collaterals

Demographics

- Age
  ○ Usually adult, occasionally in children
- Gender
  ○ No gender predilection
- Epidemiology
  ○ Most cases of PV occlusion are related to cirrhosis or pancreatitis

Natural History & Prognosis

- Guarded
  ○ Usually related to underlying condition
  ○ Possible gastroesophageal varices → hemorrhage
- Good prognosis if asymptomatic or incidental

Treatment

- Anticoagulation
- Supportive
- TIPS plus PV thrombectomy/thrombolysis

DIAGNOSTIC CHECKLIST

Consider

- PV occlusion when PV is not readily seen with US

Image Interpretation Pearls

- PV readily seen; nonvisualization suggests occlusion
- False-positive/-negative diagnoses are a problem; good Doppler technique essential
- Tangle of veins in porta hepatis & absent portal vein suggest cavernous transformation

SELECTED REFERENCES

1. Manzano-Robleda Mdel C et al: Portal vein thrombosis: What is new? Ann Hepatol. 14(1):20-7, 2015
2. Handa P et al: Portal Vein Thrombosis: A Clinician-Oriented and Practical Review. Clin Appl Thromb Hemost. Epub ahead of print, 2013
3. Dănilă M et al: The value of contrast enhanced ultrasound in the evaluation of the nature of portal vein thrombosis. Med Ultrason. 13(2):102-7, 2011
4. Parikh S et al: Portal vein thrombosis. Am J Med. 123(2):111-9, 2010
5. Piscaglia F et al: Criteria for diagnosing benign portal vein thrombosis in the assessment of patients with cirrhosis and hepatocellular carcinoma for liver transplantation. Liver Transpl. 16(5):658-67, 2010
6. Rossi S et al: Contrast-enhanced ultrasonography and spiral computed tomography in the detection and characterization of portal vein thrombosis complicating hepatocellular carcinoma. Eur Radiol. 18(8):1749-56, 2008
7. Tarantino L et al: Diagnosis of benign and malignant portal vein thrombosis in cirrhotic patients with hepatocellular carcinoma: color Doppler US, contrast-enhanced US, and fine-needle biopsy. Abdom Imaging. 31(5):537-44, 2006

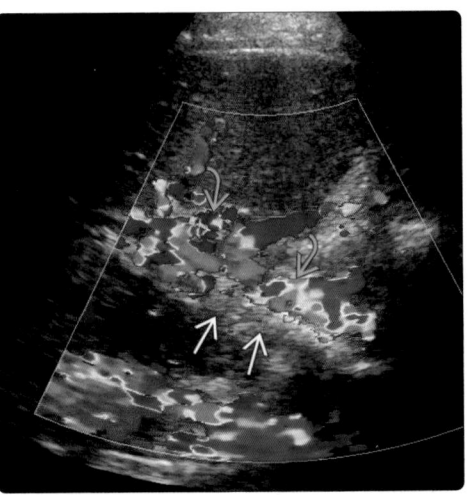

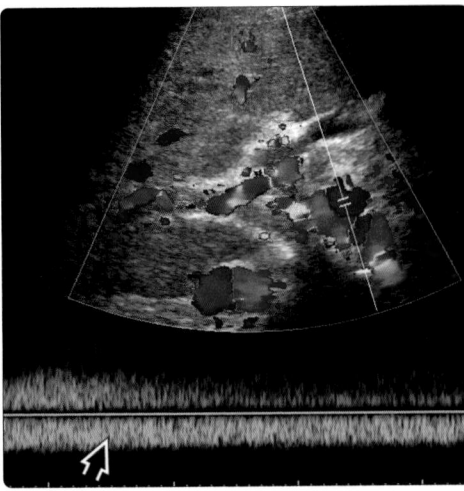

(Left) *Color Doppler ultrasound in patient with chronic portal vein thrombosis shows an echogenic thrombosed main portal vein* ➡ *and numerous tortuous collateral veins* ➱ *anterior to the thrombosed portal vein.* (Right) *Pulsed Doppler ultrasound shows flow within the collateral vessels is monophasic and without respiratory variation consistent with portal venous flow* ➡ *within collateral veins.*

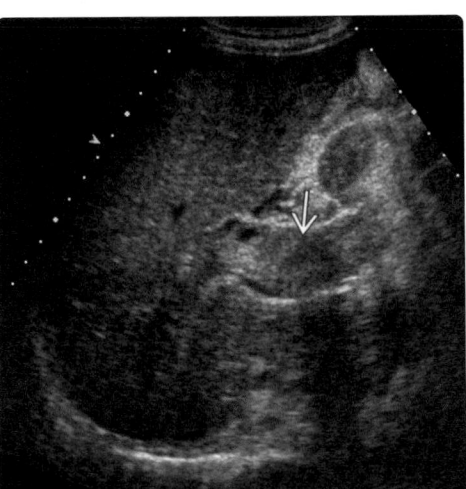

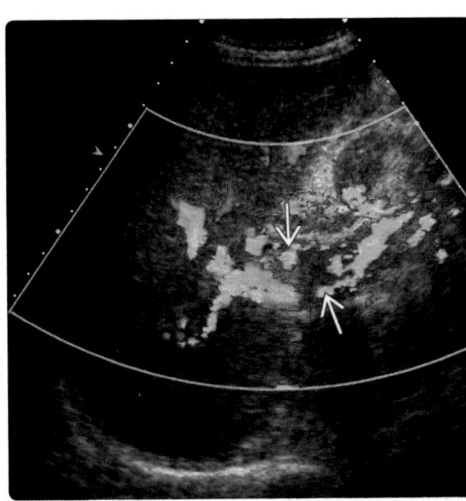

(Left) *Transverse grayscale ultrasound of the liver in a cirrhotic patient shows an expansile echogenic thrombus* ➡ *in the main portal vein.* (Right) *Color Doppler US in the same patient shows multiple small feeding vessels* ➡ *in the tumor thrombus with a dot-dash pattern. Tumor thrombus in the setting of hepatocellular carcinoma is almost always associated with infiltrative tumor and carries a poor prognosis.*

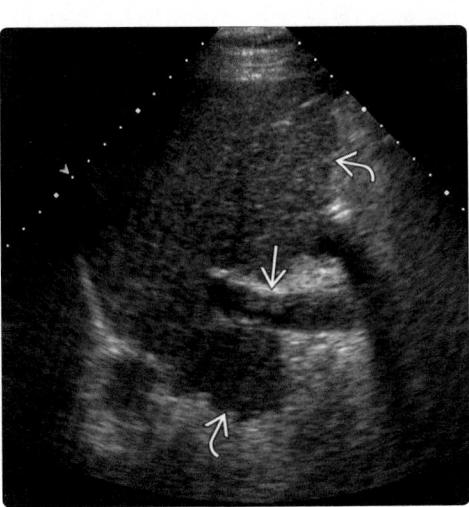

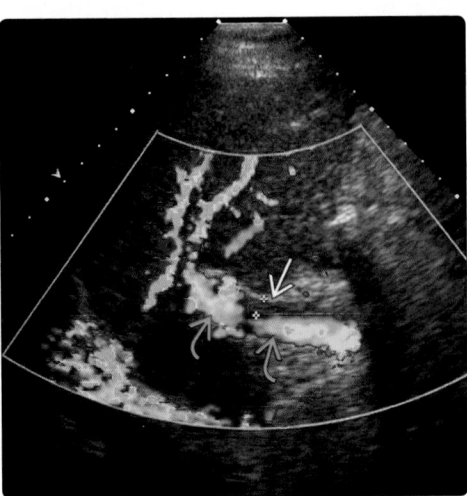

(Left) *Grayscale ultrasound shows mildly echogenic thrombus* ➡ *in the main portal vein. Note shrunken liver with irregular surface and parenchymal coarseness, indicating cirrhosis* ➱*.* (Right) *Color Doppler ultrasound in the same patient shows the thrombus* ➡ *is nonocclusive with flow seen along the posterior portion of the main portal vein* ➱*. In cases of nonocclusive portal vein thrombosis, care should be taken not to be fooled by "blooming artifact" on color Doppler, which can obscure thrombus visualization.*

Budd-Chiari Syndrome

TERMINOLOGY

- Budd-Chiari syndrome (BCS): Hepatic venous outflow obstruction
- Global or segmental obstruction of hepatic venous outflow or inferior vena cava (IVC)

IMAGING

- Ultrasound acute phase
  - Absent or restricted flow, possible thrombosis in hepatic veins (HVs)/IVC
  - Intrahepatic collateralization, bicolored HVs: Flow in opposite direction in HV branched with a common trunk
  - Reduced velocity, continuous flow in portal vein, possibly hepatofugal flow
- Ultrasound chronic phase
  - Hypertrophy of caudate lobe and unaffected segments, atrophy of involved segments, large regenerative nodules
  - Stenotic or occluded HVs/IVC

- Intrahepatic &/or extrahepatic collateralization
- CECT: "Flip-flop" enhancement pattern
  - Early enhancement of caudate lobe and central portion around IVC, decreased peripheral liver enhancement
  - Later decreased enhancement centrally and increased enhancement peripherally
  - Large regenerated nodules, hypertrophic caudate lobe

TOP DIFFERENTIAL DIAGNOSES

- Liver cirrhosis
- Portal vein thrombosis
- Acute, severe passive venous congestion
- Acute hepatitis

DIAGNOSTIC CHECKLIST

- Imaging interpretation pearls
  - Narrowed or obliterated HVs/IVC
  - Bicolored HVs due to intrahepatic collateralization on color Doppler ultrasound

(Left) *Grayscale US of the liver shows markedly narrowed right hepatic vein ➡, occluded more peripherally, and a narrow inferior vena cava (IVC) ➡ in a patient with acute Budd-Chiari syndrome. Associated ascites is present around the liver ➡.* (Right) *Color Doppler US reveals no detectable flow in the right hepatic vein ➡ with tortuous intrahepatic collateral vessels ➡ bypassing the occluded hepatic vein. Note the tortuous middle hepatic vein with bicolored appearance ➡ that cannot be seen communicating with the IVC.*

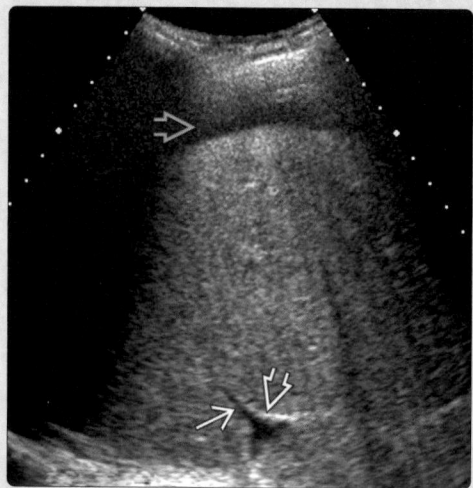
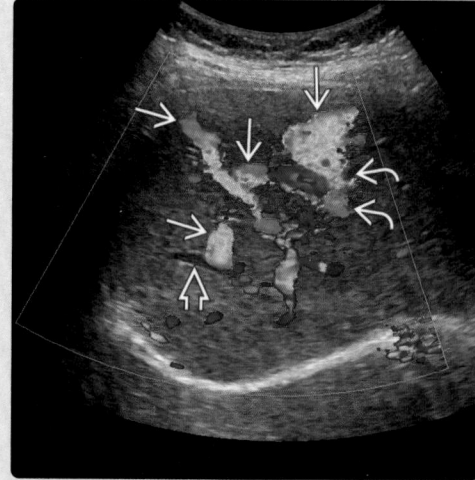

(Left) *Color Doppler US shows a thrombosed middle hepatic vein ➡. Note tortuous collateral flow around occluded hepatic vein ➡.* (Right) *Spectral Doppler ultrasound in the same patient demonstrates lack of detectable flow in middle hepatic vein ➡ on spectral tracing. Only noise ➡ is seen along the baseline of the tracing.*

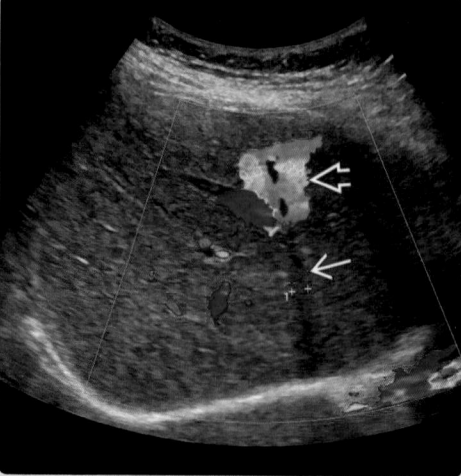
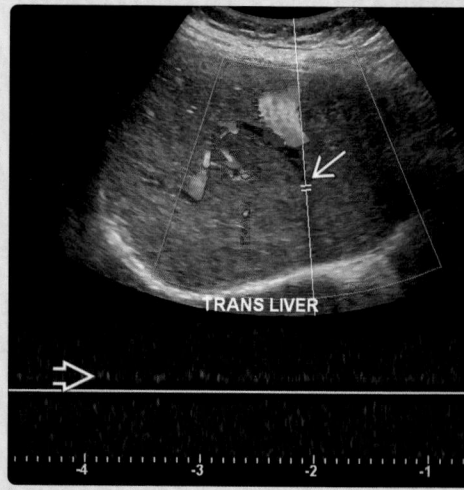

TERMINOLOGY

Abbreviations

- Budd-Chiari syndrome (BCS)

Synonyms

- Hepatic venous outflow obstruction

Definitions

- Global or segmental obstruction of hepatic venous outflow or inferior vena cava (IVC)
  o At level of large hepatic veins or suprahepatic segment of IVC

IMAGING

General Features

- Best diagnostic clue
  o Narrowing of obliteration of HVs and IVC
  o No flow in HVs/IVC on color Doppler ultrasound
  o Intrahepatic/extrahepatic venous collateralization
- Location
  o Obstruction may be in hepatic veins, IVC, sinusoidal (parenchymal) veins

Ultrasonographic Findings

- Grayscale ultrasound
  o **Acute stage**
    - HVs visualized, possibly distended
    - Partial or complete thrombosis in HVs/IVC
    - Involved parenchyma may be hypoechoic due to edema
  o **Chronic stage**
    - HVs narrowed, nonvisualized, or filled with thrombus
    - Compensatory hypertrophy of caudate lobe and unaffected segments/lobes
    - Atrophy of involved segments/lobes
    - Regenerative nodules, possibly large
- Color Doppler
  o **Acute stage**
    - Absent or severely restricted flow in HVs/IVC
    - Continuous (nonpulsatile) flow in patent portions of HVs proximal to obstruction
    - Intrahepatic collateralization, "bicolored HVs"
      □ Opposing flow directions seen in adjacent veins
    - HVs may appear tortuous, curvilinear, fragmented, stenotic, or as fibrous cord with slow, turbulent, or reversed flow
    - Reversed flow in patent portions of IVC
    - Reduced velocity, continuous flow in portal vein, possibly hepatofugal flow
  o **Chronic stage**
    - Stenotic or nonvisualized (occluded) HVs/IVC
    - Intrahepatic &/or extrahepatic collateralization

CT Findings

- Acute stage
  o NECT: Narrowed HVs/IVC; hyperdense thrombus; hypodense affected parenchyma, hepatomegaly, ascites
  o CECT: Classic "flip-flop" pattern

- Early enhancement of caudate lobe and central portion around IVC, decreased peripheral liver enhancement
- Later decreased enhancement centrally and increased enhancement peripherally
- Chronic stage
  o Total obliteration of IVC and HVs
  o Large regenerative nodules: Multiple 1-4 cm hyperdense and enhancing nodules
  o Atrophy of affected segments, hypertrophied caudate lobe, collateralization

MR Findings

- Narrowed or absent HVs and IVC, caudate lobe hypertrophy
- Regenerative nodules: High SI on T1WI, iso-/low SI on T2WI, delayed enhancement without washout
- Parenchymal enhancement pattern analogous to CT

Angiographic Findings

- Classic "spider web" pattern on wedged hepatic venography
- Thrombus in HVs or IVC, long segmental compression or stenosis of IVC
- Hepatic arteries: Narrowed and stretched in acute phase, dilated with arterioportal shunts in chronic phase

Imaging Recommendations

- Best imaging tool
  o Color Doppler sonography for initial diagnosis/exclusion of BCS
  o CECT or MR for comprehensive assessment

DIFFERENTIAL DIAGNOSIS

Liver Cirrhosis

- Patent HVs and IVC
- Hypertrophy of caudate lobe and lateral segment of left lobe
- Atrophy of right lobe and medial segment of left lobe
- Portosystemic collaterals, ascites, splenomegaly
- Regenerative nodules usually smaller in size

Portal Vein Thrombosis

- Liver dysfunction, ascites, portosystemic collaterals, splenomegaly
- Patent HVs/IVC

Acute, Severe Passive Venous Congestion

- Usually in congestive heart failure: Hepatic congestion/enlargement, ascites
- Dilated but patent HVs/IVC

Acute Hepatitis

- Hepatomegaly, liver dysfunction, ± ascites
- Patent HVs/IVC

PATHOLOGY

General Features

- Etiology
  o Thrombotic occlusion of HVs or IVC
    - Cirrhosis-related (immediate cause uncertain)
    - Hypercoagulable states dehydration/shock/sepsis

- o HV/IVC tumor propagation
  - Hepatocellular carcinoma (most common); also cholangiocarcinoma and rarely metastases, angiosarcoma of IVC
- o Extrinsic HV/IVC compression (stasis &/or thrombosis)
  - Hepatocellular carcinoma, hepatic metastasis, adrenal tumor, adenopathy
- o Centrilobular HV obstruction
  - Obstruction of tiny centrilobular veins (hepatic venoocclusive disease)
  - After bone marrow transplantation, antineoplastic drug use, radiation therapy
- o Congenital-membranous IVC obstruction
  - Etiology unclear: Congenital, injury, infection all hypothesized
  - Tapered or membrane-like IVC obstruction
  - May present in adulthood; "congenital" questioned
  - Japan, India, Israel, South Africa

Gross Pathologic & Surgical Features

- Acute phase
  - o Acute findings due to venous outflow obstruction > hepatic congestion
  - o Chronic findings due to ischemia, necrosis, regeneration
- Chronic phase
  - o Liver: Nodular, shrunken, may be cirrhotic
  - o Atrophy of affected lobes and hypertrophy of caudate lobe

Microscopic Features

- Acute: Centrilobular congestion, dilated sinusoids
- Chronic: Fibrosis, necrosis, and cell atrophy

CLINICAL ISSUES

Presentation

- Most common signs/symptoms
  - o Classical acute Budd-Chiari presentation
    - Rapid onset of abdominal pain, liver tenderness, hepatic dysfunction
    - Possible abdominal distention from ascites, hypotension
    - Acute signs/symptoms are variable: Depend on rapidity of obstructive process, extent of HV involvement, severity of obstruction, collateralization
  - o Chronic signs/symptoms
    - RUQ pain, hepatomegaly, hepatic dysfunction
    - Splenomegaly, ascites, varicosities
- Other signs/symptoms
  - o Acute or chronic lower extremity edema, if IVC obstructed

Demographics

- Age
  - o Any group, but usual onset in young adults
- Gender
  - o Females more than males

Natural History & Prognosis

- Complications
  - o Acute: Liver failure, shock, pulmonary embolization from IVC

- o Chronic: Regeneration/liver dysfunction/failure: Portal hypertension/variceal bleeding/cirrhosis
- o Congenital-membranous IVC obstruction: Complicated by hepatocellular carcinoma in 20-40% of cases in Japan & South Africa
- Prognosis
  - o Depends on degree of obstruction, etiology, extent of liver damage, or collateralization
  - o Neoplastic obstruction: Usually fatal
  - o Centrilobular obstruction: Variable prognosis ranging from complete recovery to fulminant hepatic failure and death

Treatment

- Medical management
  - o Anticoagulation, steroids, nutritional therapy
- Transjugular intrahepatic portosystemic shunt (TIPS)
  - o Ameliorates intractable ascites
  - o Controls intractable, recurrent gastrointestinal hemorrhage
- Congenital-membranous IVC occlusion
  - o Balloon angioplasty, stent insertion
- Liver transplantation; controversial

DIAGNOSTIC CHECKLIST

Image Interpretation Pearls

- Narrowed or obliterated HVs/IVC
- Bicolored HVs due to intrahepatic collateralization on color Doppler ultrasound

SELECTED REFERENCES

1. Patil P et al: Spectrum of imaging in Budd Chiari syndrome. J Med Imaging Radiat Oncol. 56(1):75-83, 2012
2. Raszeja-Wyszomirska J et al: Primary Budd-Chiari syndrome - a single center experience. Hepatogastroenterology. 59(118):1879-82, 2012
3. Jayanthi V et al: Budd-Chiari Syndrome. Changing epidemiology and clinical presentation. Minerva Gastroenterol Dietol. 56(1):71-80, 2010
4. Cura M et al: Diagnostic and interventional radiology for Budd-Chiari syndrome. Radiographics. 29(3):669-81, 2009
5. Boozari B et al: Ultrasonography in patients with Budd-Chiari syndrome: diagnostic signs and prognostic implications. J Hepatol. 49(4):572-80, 2008
6. Karaosmanoglu D et al: CT, MRI, and US findings of incidental segmental distal hepatic vein occlusion: a new form of Budd-Chiari syndrome? J Comput Assist Tomogr. 32(4):518-22, 2008
7. Aydinli M et al: Budd-Chiari syndrome: etiology, pathogenesis and diagnosis. World J Gastroenterol. 13(19):2693-6, 2007
8. Bozorgmanesh A et al: Budd-Chiari syndrome: hepatic venous web outflow obstruction treated by percutaneous placement of hepatic vein stent. Semin Intervent Radiol. 24(1):100-5, 2007
9. Brancatelli G et al: Budd-Chiari syndrome: spectrum of imaging findings. AJR Am J Roentgenol. 188(2):W168-76, 2007
10. Buckley O et al: Imaging of Budd-Chiari syndrome. Eur Radiol. 17(8):2071-8, 2007
11. Erden A: Budd-Chiari syndrome: a review of imaging findings. Eur J Radiol. 61(1):44-56, 2007
12. Bargallo X et al: Sonography of Budd-Chiari syndrome. AJR Am J Roentgenol. 187(1):W33-41, 2006
13. Chaubal N et al: Sonography in Budd-Chiari syndrome. J Ultrasound Med. 25(3):373-9, 2006
14. Brancatelli G et al: Benign regenerative nodules in Budd-Chiari syndrome and other vascular disorders of the liver: radiologic-pathologic and clinical correlation. Radiographics. 22(4):847-62, 2002

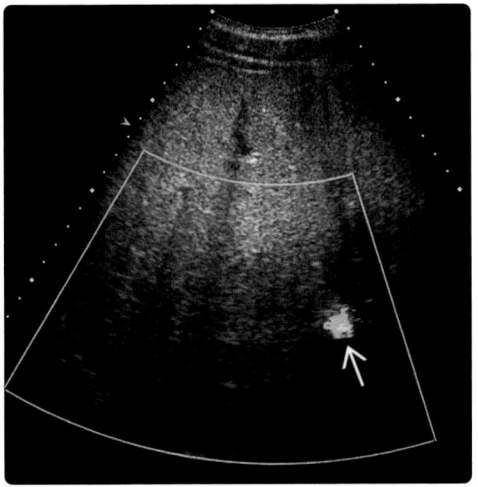
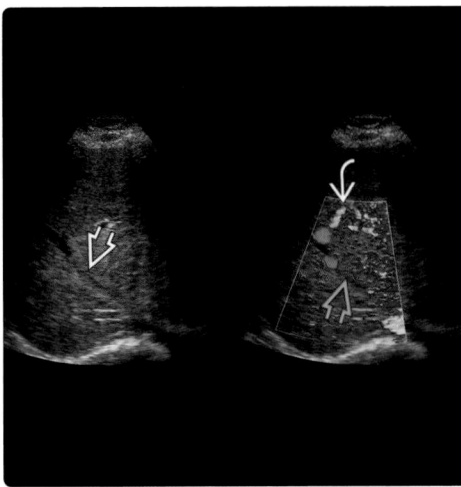

(Left) *Color Doppler ultrasound shows flow in the intrahepatic IVC ➡ but expected inflowing hepatic veins are not visualized, consistent with Budd-Chiari.* (Right) *Grayscale ultrasound of the liver (left) shows a somewhat narrowed and echogenic right hepatic vein ➡. On color Doppler ultrasound (right), no flow is detected in the right hepatic vein ➡, consistent with Budd-Chiari syndrome. Note intrahepatic collateral vessels ➡ bypassing the occluded hepatic vein.*

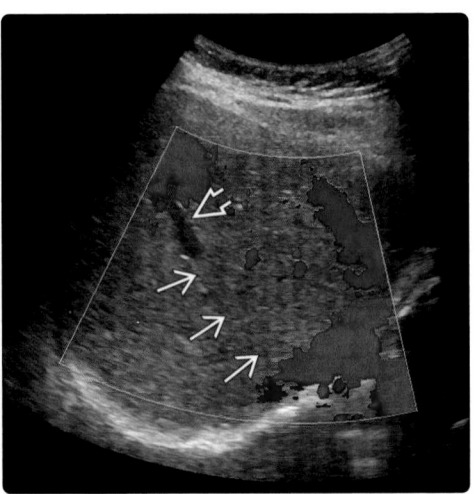
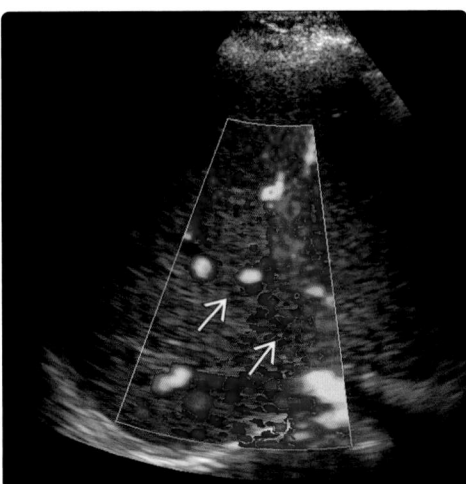

(Left) *Color Doppler US of the liver shows only the peripheral right hepatic vein ➡ is visible and is without detectable vascularity. The expected course of the more proximal right hepatic vein also has no detectable internal vascularity ➡ in this patient with Budd-Chiari.* (Right) *Power Doppler ultrasound in the same patient confirms no detectable flow in the right hepatic vein ➡. Power Doppler is often more sensitive for slow flow or minimal flow and should be employed for confirmation when color Doppler fails to detect vascularity.*

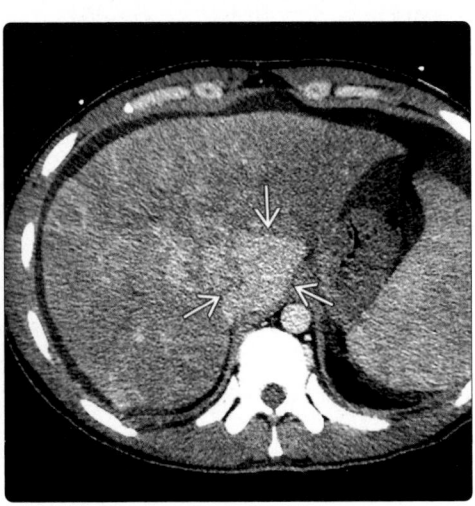
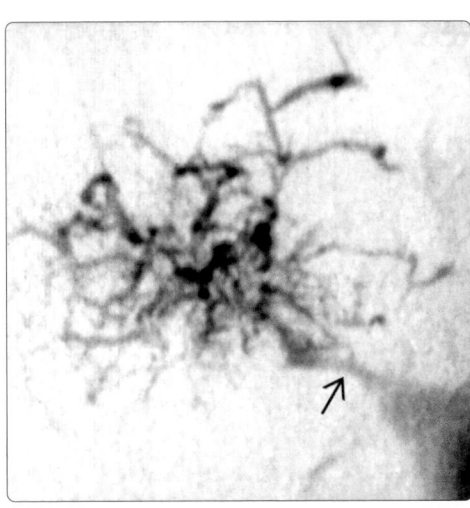

(Left) *Axial CECT shows a hyperdense and slightly hypertrophied caudate lobe ➡ in this patient with Budd-Chiari syndrome. The caudate is often spared in Budd-Chiari because of its separate venous drainage into the IVC.* (Right) *Oblique angiography shows "spider web" pattern of intrahepatic collateralization caused by hepatic vein obstruction. Note tight hepatic vein stenosis ➡.*

TERMINOLOGY

- Gas within portal venous system

IMAGING

- Grayscale ultrasound
  - Highly reflective foci in portal venous system
    - Move along with blood
  - Poorly defined, highly reflective parenchymal foci
    - Scattered small patches to numerous or large areas
- Pulsed Doppler ultrasound
  - High-intensity transient signals (HITS)
    - Strong transient spikes superimposed on portal venous flow pattern
- Color Doppler ultrasound
  - Bright reflectors in portal venous system

TOP DIFFERENTIAL DIAGNOSES

- Biliary tract gas
- Parenchymal abscess

- Biliary calculi/ parenchymal calcifications
- Echogenic hepatic metastases

PATHOLOGY

- Serious conditions
  - Necrotizing enterocolitis, bowel ischemia/infarction
- Benign conditions
  - Bowel distension, intervention-related, benign pneumatosis intestinalis

CLINICAL ISSUES

- Often sign of serious condition; sometimes inconsequential finding

DIAGNOSTIC CHECKLIST

- Rule out other conditions mimicking portal venous gas
  - Biliary tract gas, biliary calculi, or hepatic calcification
- Best imaging clue: Bright reflectors in portal veins on grayscale or color Doppler

(Left) *Oblique ultrasound of the liver shows several echogenic foci in the portal vein* ➡ *representing gas bubbles. Brightly echogenic patches* ➡ *in the liver more peripherally represent parenchymal gas.* (Right) *Oblique pulsed Doppler ultrasound in the same patient with portal venous gas shows strong, high-intensity transient signals (HITS)* ➡ *that appear as vertical spikes within the main portal vein interrogation. Spikes are in the same direction as the flow direction of the portal vein.*

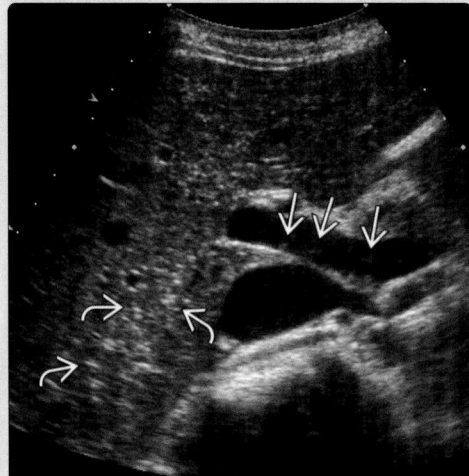
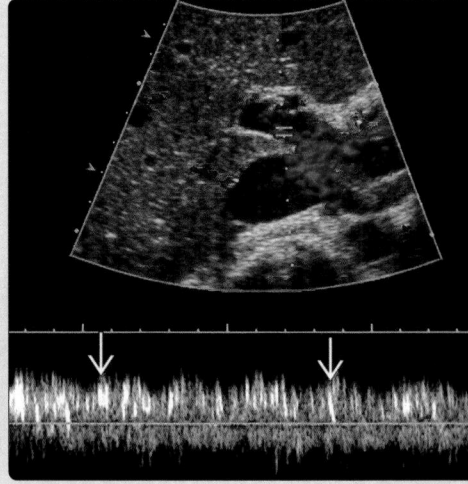

(Left) *Oblique abdominal pulsed Doppler ultrasound in a patient with portal venous gas secondary to small bowel ischemia and pneumatosis shows strong, high-intensity transient signals (HITS)* ➡ *superimposed upon the main portal vein waveform.* (Right) *Axial NECT shows extensive portal venous gas* ➡ *branching peripherally in the portal veins of the liver. Peripheral predominance of portal venous gas helps distinguish it from biliary gas, which tends to be more centrally located.*

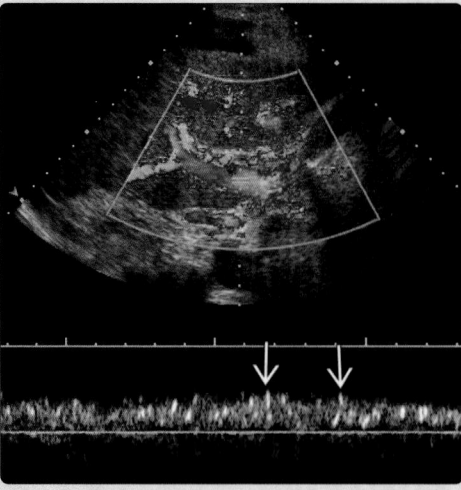
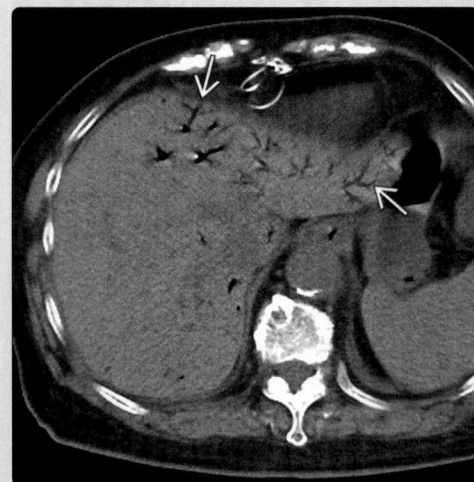

TERMINOLOGY

Abbreviations

- Portal vein (PV)

Definitions

- Gas within portal venous system

IMAGING

General Features

- Best diagnostic clue
  - Bright reflectors in portal veins on grayscale or color Doppler
- Location
  - Portal venous system, hepatic parenchyma

Ultrasonographic Findings

- Grayscale ultrasound
  - Highly reflective foci in portal venous system
    - Move with portal venous blood
    - Few to numerous, related to amount of gas
  - Poorly defined, highly reflective parenchymal foci
    - Scattered small patches to numerous or large areas
- Pulsed Doppler
  - High-intensity transient signals (HITS)
    - Strong spikes superimposed on portal venous flow pattern
    - Pinging sound from audible Doppler output
    - May be more sensitive than CT for detection of subtle portal venous gas
- Color Doppler
  - Bright reflectors in portal venous system
  - May be multicolored (twinkling artifact)

Imaging Recommendations

- Best imaging tool
  - Grayscale or color Doppler for initial detection
  - NECT/CECT to determine source of gas

DIFFERENTIAL DIAGNOSIS

Biliary Tract Gas

- Bright reflections in biliary tree, adjacent to portal vein branches
- Central concentration, near porta hepatis
- Stationary; move only with altered patient position

Biliary Calculi/Parenchymal Calcifications

- Not in portal venous system
- Sharply defined, immobile
- Strong posterior acoustic shadowing

Parenchymal Abscess

- May produce ill-defined echogenic patchy area in liver
- Localized, not multifocal

Echogenic Hepatic Metastases

- Well-defined margins

PATHOLOGY

General Features

- Etiology
  - 3 basic gas sources
    - Gas under pressure
    - Intravasation through injured mucosa
    - Gas-forming organisms
  - Serious, life-threatening causes
    - Necrotizing enterocolitis
    - Bowel ischemia/infarction
    - Peritoneal space abscess/infected gallbladder/liver abscess
    - Necrotizing pancreatitis
    - Malignancies involving bowel
  - Benign causes
    - Gastric or bowel distension, especially colon
    - Inflammatory bowel disease
    - Gastric ulcer
    - Interventions: Endoscopic biopsy, liver mass ablation, gastric tube, post surgery
    - Benign pneumatosis intestinalis: e.g., emphysema

CLINICAL ISSUES

Presentation

- Most common signs/symptoms
  - Related to underlying disorder

Demographics

- Age: Newborns to adults

Natural History & Prognosis

- Usually sign of serious condition
- Sometimes inconsequential finding

Treatment

- Related to underlying disorder

DIAGNOSTIC CHECKLIST

Consider

- Rule out other conditions mimicking portal venous gas
  - Biliary tract gas, biliary calculi or hepatic calcification
- Rule out potential life-threatening causes of portal venous gas such as necrotizing enterocolitis or bowel infarction

Image Interpretation Pearls

- Bright reflectors in portal veins on grayscale or color Doppler

SELECTED REFERENCES

1. Sadatomo A et al: Hepatic portal venous gas after endoscopy in a patient with anastomotic obstruction. World J Gastrointest Surg. 7(2):21-4, 2015
2. Bohnhorst B et al: Portal venous gas detected by ultrasound differentiates surgical NEC from other acquired neonatal intestinal diseases. Eur J Pediatr Surg. 21(1):12-7, 2011
3. Shah PA et al: Hepatic gas: widening spectrum of causes detected at CT and US in the interventional era. Radiographics. 31(5):1403-13, 2011
4. Franken JM et al: Hepatic portal venous gas. J Gastrointestin Liver Dis. 19(4):360, 2010
5. Abboud B et al: Hepatic portal venous gas: physiopathology, etiology, prognosis and treatment. World J Gastroenterol. 15(29):3585-90, 2009

IMAGING

- **Hepatic artery stenosis**
  - Elevated peak systolic velocity at anastomosis > 200 cm/sec
  - Parvus tardus waveforms in intrahepatic arteries
    - Acceleration time > 0.08 sec
    - Resistive index < 0.5
- **Hepatic artery thrombosis**
  - No detectable flow in hepatic artery with color or spectral Doppler
  - May see "collateral transformation of hepatic artery"
    - Tortuous collateral arteries in porta hepatis and parvus tardus intrahepatic arterial waveforms

PATHOLOGY

- **Hepatic artery stenosis**
  - Stenosis occurs at anastomosis
  - Usually occurs at > 3 months post transplant
- **Hepatic artery thrombosis**

- May occur < 15 days or years after transplant
- Risk factors: Difference in hepatic artery caliber between donor and recipient, prolonged graft ischemia time, ABO blood group incompatibility, CMV infection, acute or chronic rejection, hypercoagulable state, sepsis

CLINICAL ISSUES

- **Hepatic artery stenosis**
  - May be related to injury at time of surgery or disruption of vasa vasorum with ischemia of hepatic artery
- **Hepatic artery thrombosis**
  - Most common immediate vascular complication (2-12%)
  - Complete occlusion of hepatic artery in early transplant period leads to liver failure
    - Up to 75% of patients with hepatic artery thrombosis require retransplantation
  - Biliary ducts in liver transplants supplied only by artery
    - Hepatic artery thrombosis can result in biliary ischemia, bilomas, bile lakes

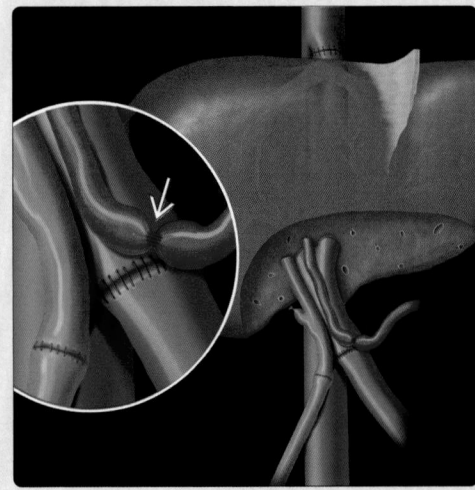
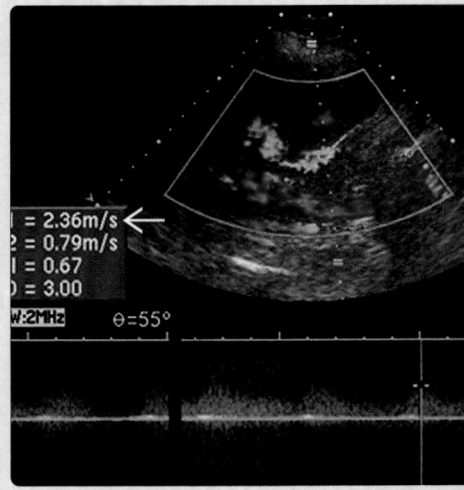

(Left) Graphic depicts focal stenosis ⇨ of the hepatic artery anastomosis in a liver transplant. (Right) Spectral Doppler evaluation of the main hepatic artery near the site of anastomosis shows an elevated hepatic artery velocity of 236 cm/sec ⇨, which is consistent with a stenosis.

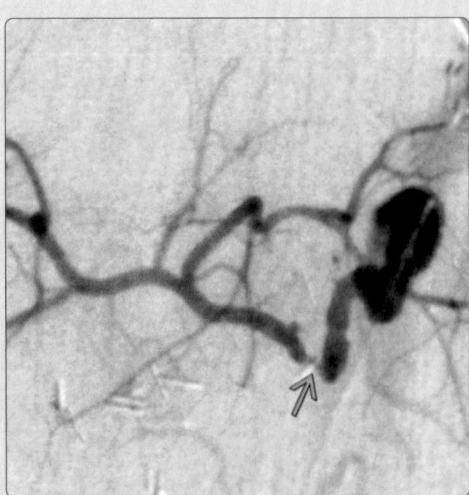
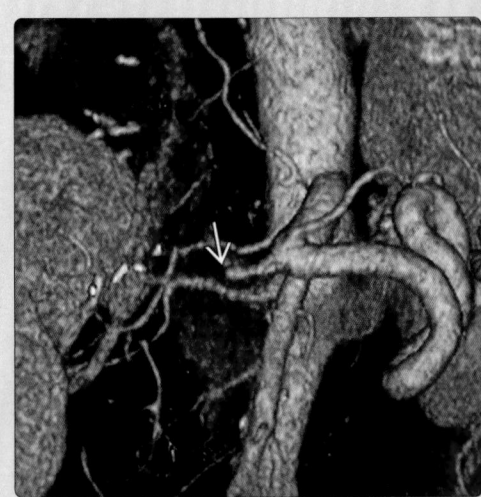

(Left) Angiographic image in the same patient confirms a focal stenosis ⇨ in the hepatic artery at the level of the anastomosis. (Right) Volume-rendered CT angiogram of the aorta and celiac artery shows an abrupt termination ⇨ of the hepatic artery, consistent with hepatic artery thrombosis in a patient with a liver transplant.

Liver Transplant Portal Vein Stenosis/Thrombosis

KEY FACTS

IMAGING

Portal vein stenosis

- Elevated portal vein velocity > 125 cm/sec at anastomosis
  - Portal vein velocity normally < 60 cm/sec
- Anastomotic to preanastomotic velocity ratio
  - Stenosis: > 3
  - Normal: ~ 1.5

Portal vein thrombosis

- No detectable flow in portal vein
- May see echogenic thrombus in portal vein, or portal vein may appear markedly hypoechoic or even anechoic
- May see enlarged hepatic arteries
  - Hepatic arteries compensate for portal vein thrombosis due to hepatic arterial buffer response
- Bidirectional low amplitude flow in portal vein may precede portal vein thrombosis

PATHOLOGY

- **Portal vein stenosis**
  - Occurs at site of anastomosis
- **Portal vein thrombosis**
  - Associated with surgical technique
  - Hypercoagulable state

CLINICAL ISSUES

- Portal vein stenosis typically occurs at the anastomosis
- Depending on degree of stenosis, may require balloon angioplasty
- In chronic or longstanding portal vein stenosis, may see portal vein aneurysm downstream from anastomosis
- Portal vein stenosis and thrombosis are relatively rare, occurring in 1-2.7% of liver transplants

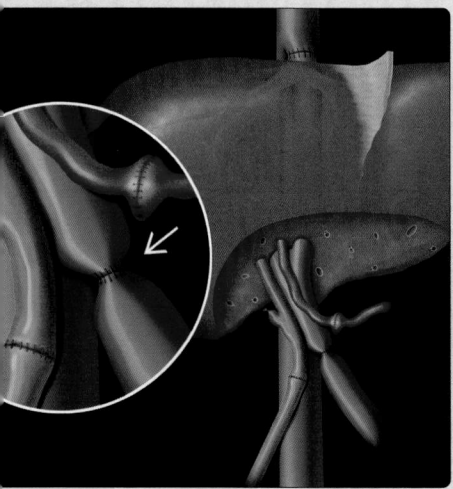

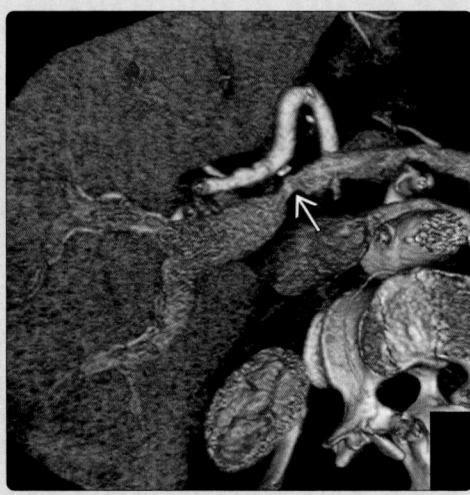

(Left) Graphic idepicts focal stenosis ➡ of the portal vein at the level of the anastomosis in a patient with a liver transplant. (Right) Volume-rendered CT angiogram in a patient with liver transplant shows a focal caliber change ➡ in the portal vein at the site of anastomosis, consistent with stenosis.

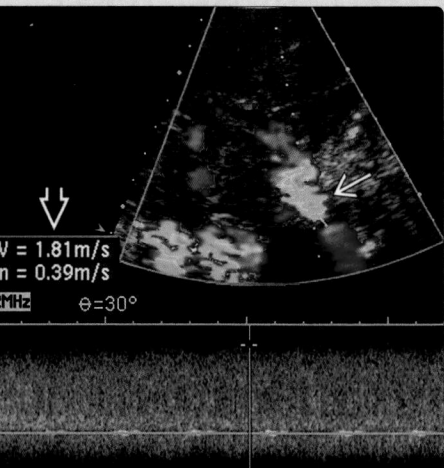

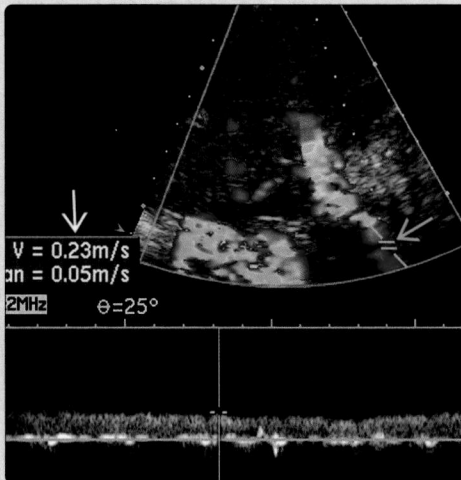

(Left) Pulsed Doppler evaluation of the main portal vein near the anastomosis shows a focal area of aliasing ➡ as well as corresponding elevated velocities measured to 181 cm/sec ➡. (Right) Pulsed Doppler interrogation in the same patient in the portal vein proximal ➡ to the area of aliasing shows velocity is in a normal range of 23 cm/sec ➡. Elevation of velocity at the anastomosis of > 3x the pre-anastomotic velocity is highly suggestive of stenosis in the portal vein.

IMAGING

- **Hepatic venous stenosis**
  - Color Doppler
    - May see focal turbulent flow at stenosis and stenotic jet
  - Spectral Doppler
    - Elevated velocity at site of stenosis or < 10 cm/sec away from site of stenosis
    - Loss of normal triphasic waveform
      - Most commonly monophasic in appearance
    - May see secondary slow portal vein velocity
  - Angiography
    - Pressure gradient > 5 mm Hg across stenosis
- **Hepatic venous thrombosis**
  - Direct visualization of thrombus in hepatic vein or lack of detectable flow with color, power, or spectral Doppler

PATHOLOGY

- Hepatic vein or IVC stenosis results in outflow obstruction of liver
- Immediate post-transplant period
  - Kinking of vessel
- Delayed presentation
  - Intimal hyperplasia

CLINICAL ISSUES

- Hepatic vein stenosis occurs in < 1% of liver transplants, 2-10% of liver transplants when piggy-back technique used
- Clinical presentation: Lower extremity edema, Budd-Chiari syndrome, ascites
- Treatment
  - Stenosis may be treated with balloon-expandable stents or angioplasty
  - Thrombosis may require surgery or retransplant

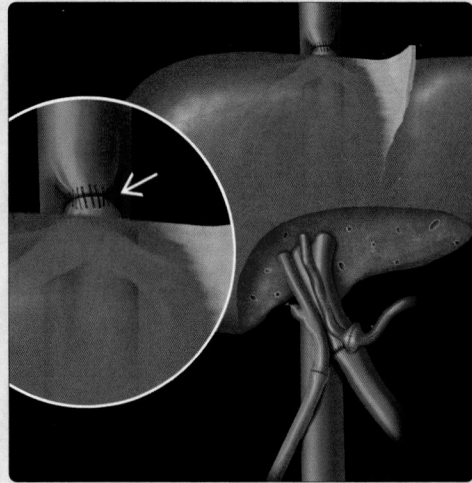
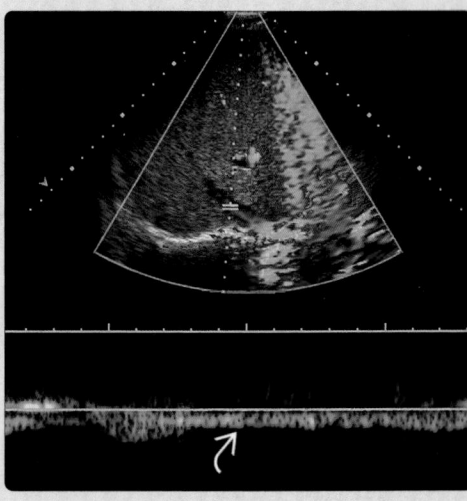

(Left) Graphic shows stenosis at the piggyback anastomosis ➡ in a liver transplant. In this technique, the donor suprahepatic IVC is anastomosed with the recipient common orifice of all three hepatic veins. (Right) Spectral Doppler in the right hepatic vein shows monophasic ➡ nonpulsatile waveform. When waveforms that were previously pulsatile become monophasic, a stenosis of the hepatic venous/IVC anastomosis should be suspected and warrants further evaluation.

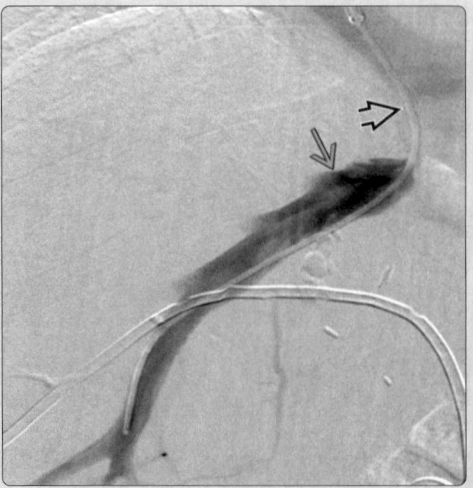
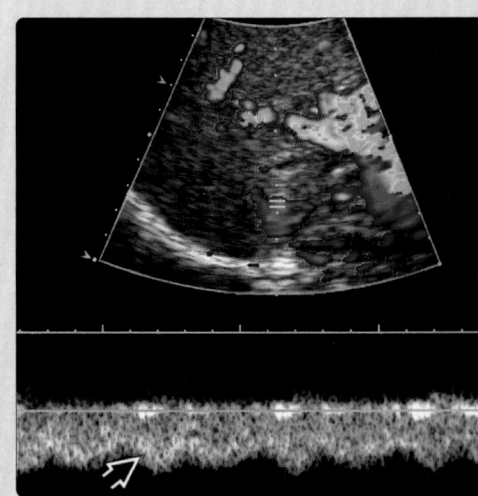

(Left) Catheter injection of the right hepatic vein (same patient) shows that contrast fills the hepatic vein ➡ but does not reflux readily into the IVC ➡, indicative of stenosis, which was subsequently balloon angioplastied. (Right) Spectral Doppler of the right hepatic vein in the same patient after balloon dilation shows increase in pulsatility as well as increased magnitude of flow ➡.

Liver Transplant Biliary Stricture

KEY FACTS

IMAGING
- Ultrasound
  - Initial imaging modality for evaluation of biliary system
  - Dilated biliary duct proximal to site of anastomosis
  - Focal area of narrowing may be seen in mid common hepatic duct or near hepatic hilum (latter in patients with hepaticojejunostomy)
- Magnetic resonance cholangiopancreatography (MRCP)
  - Heavily T2-weighted image of common hepatic duct shows upstream ductal dilatation and focal narrowing at anastomosis
- Cholangiogram
  - Performed in patients with hepaticojejunostomy in which access to anastomosis difficult with ERCP
- ERCP
  - May be diagnostic as well as therapeutic with balloon dilation and plastic stent placement

TOP DIFFERENTIAL DIAGNOSES
- Obstruction from other causes
  - Choledocholithiasis
  - Malignancy
  - Recurrent primary sclerosing cholangitis (PSC) (in patients with prior history of PSC)

PATHOLOGY
- Biliary stricture is most common type of complication after liver transplant, occurring in up to 60%
- In late stricture, > 1 month post-transplant, usually related to ischemic injury of bile duct anastomosis

CLINICAL ISSUES
- Early stricture
  - Usually responds well to a single endoscopic therapy
- Late stricture
  - Often require longer treatment regimens

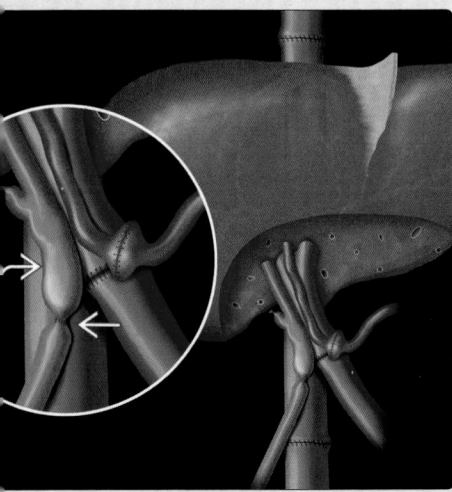
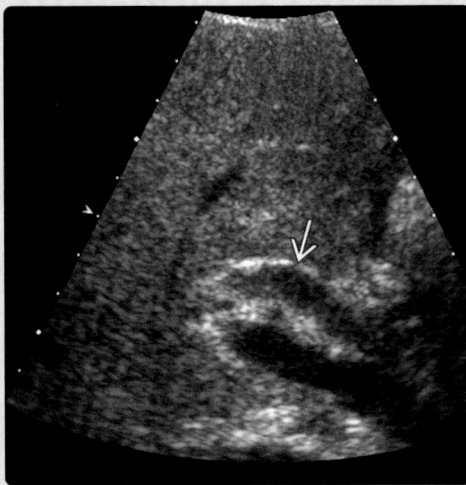

(Left) Graphic depicts a liver transplant with focal stricture in the common bile duct anastomosis ➡. Notice the mild upstream dilatation ➡, which may be seen with a biliary duct stenosis. (Right) Transverse grayscale ultrasound of the common bile duct in a patient status post liver transplant shows a moderately dilated common bile duct ➡, which was related to a biliary duct stricture at the anastomosis.

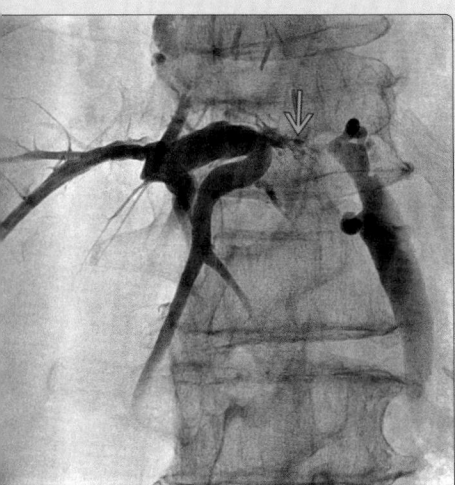
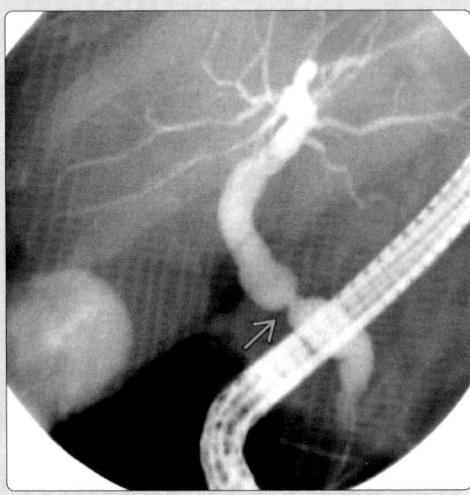

(Left) Percutaneous transhepatic cholangiogram in a patient with liver transplant and hepaticojejunostomy shows a severe stenosis of the right hepatic duct, at the junction ➡ of the right and common hepatic duct, near the hepaticojejunostomy site. (Right) ERCP in a patient after liver transplant shows a focal stenosis ➡ in the common bile duct at the level of the anastomosis.

PART II
SECTION 2
Biliary System

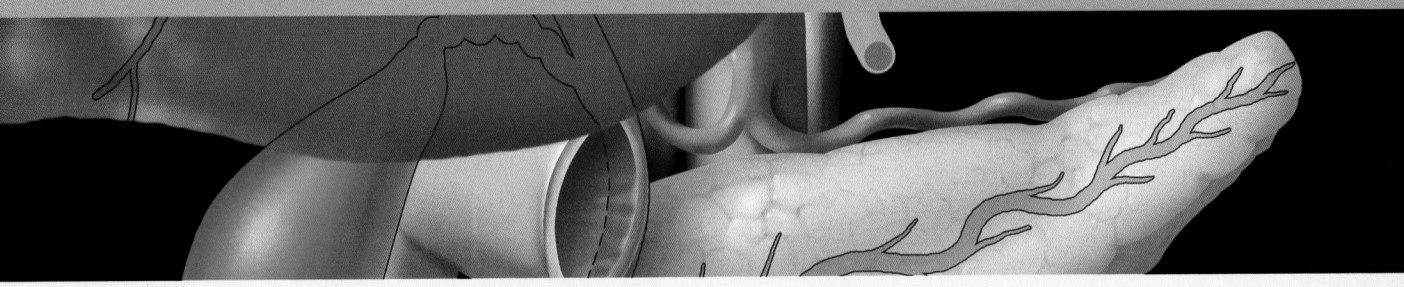

Introduction and Overview

Imaging Anatomy

The gallbladder is a fluid-filled, pear-shaped sac that lies in the vertical plane between the right and left hepatic lobes. The fundus is the most distal and distensible portion. The fundus is more mobile than the body and neck, which are attached to the liver. The neck drains into the cystic duct. The gallbladder is in contact with the duodenum, the posterior aspect of the liver, and the proximal transverse colon. The distended lumen is filled with anechoic bile. The wall is uniformly thin, typically 1-2 mm. When physiologically distended after fasting, the gallbladder can measure up to 5 x 5 x 10 cm. A fatty meal produces gallbladder emptying and apparent wall thickening.

Intrahepatic bile ducts drain toward the porta hepatis as the right and left hepatic ducts. These converge to form the common hepatic duct at the bifurcation of right and left portal veins. The cystic duct joins the common hepatic duct to form the common bile duct. The common bile duct runs through the pancreatic head and joins the pancreatic duct before draining into the duodenum at the major duodenal papilla. The normal common bile duct measures < 6 mm.

Anatomy-Based Imaging Issues

The bile-filled, distended gallbladder is easily and ideally evaluated with ultrasound. It is intimately related to the liver and is included during imaging of the liver. The gallbladder is located in the plane lying along the middle hepatic vein and interlobar fissure. If the gallbladder is contracted, look carefully along that plane in the transverse plane.

Due to their small caliber, the cystic duct and the second and third order intrahepatic ducts are only seen if dilated. The common hepatic duct is routinely visualized at the porta hepatis, but the common bile duct may be obscured by gastric or duodenal gas as it courses inferiorly toward the ampulla. After cholecystectomy, the common bile duct caliber may be slightly increased. There is debate as to whether biliary ductal caliber increases with age.

Pathologic Issues

The gallbladder and biliary tree are affected by a wide range of acute and chronic inflammatory conditions and benign and malignant neoplasms. The most common pathology is gallstone disease and its complications, such as acute and chronic cholecystitis. These are among the most common indications for ultrasound of the abdomen.

Imaging Protocols

Prior to elective right upper quadrant ultrasound, patients should fast for 6-8 hours. Tube feeds should be withheld for the same length of time; however, in an emergency, ultrasound can be performed in the non-fasted state and can still be diagnostic. Fasting is not necessary after cholecystectomy but may still improve diagnostic ability by reducing gas obscuring the common bile duct and pancreas.

Studies are performed with a curved array transducer at frequencies between 1-5 MHz for most adults and as high as 9 MHz in thin adults. Focal zone placement should be optimized to the lesion of interest, especially with gallstones. Use of harmonic techniques improves evaluation of the gallbladder lumen and increases tissue contrast with fewer artifacts. Compound imaging techniques are used to decrease speckle and increase lesion conspicuity.

Gallbladder

The gallbladder is evaluated in multiple planes and patient positions. The approach should include subcostal and intercostal windows with static images obtained in multiple longitudinal, transverse, and oblique planes. Patients are imaged in the supine position but the left lateral decubitus position is essential to ensure that small stones located in the gallbladder neck are not missed. Additionally, patient movement demonstrates mobility of intraluminal lesions and differentiates stones from polypoid mural lesions. Other useful positions include right lateral decubitus, semi-erect, erect, and prone. If the patient is immobile, elevation of the head of the bed or stretcher is an inferior substitute for decubitus or prone positioning. Deep inspiration can improve visualization of the gallbladder and determine the presence of the sonographic Murphy sign.

Gallbladder assessment includes evaluation of the wall for thickness and integrity, gallbladder volume, and intraluminal contents. Assessment of the sonographic Murphy sign is essential. Adjacent structures are also assessed.

Bile Ducts

Evaluation of the biliary tree is a key component of the study. The intrahepatic ducts, left and right hepatic ducts are evaluated during evaluation of the liver. The common hepatic duct is measured at the porta hepatis, anterior to the main portal vein with the proper hepatic artery in cross section. Decubitus positioning and deep inspiration can improve visualization. The bile duct should be followed distally through the head of the pancreas. A low insertion of the cystic duct is an important variant that should be conveyed to the surgeon considering surgery. Gastric or duodenal gas may obscure the distal common bile duct. Maneuvers such as turning the patient to their right side or having the patient drink water may allow a diagnostic study.

Color Doppler is used to identify and to confirm patency of vessels and differentiate vessels from intra- and extrahepatic dilated bile ducts. Color Doppler is helpful to evaluate potential masses and gallbladder or bile duct wall thickening. Color Doppler twinkling artifact can confirm stones or adenomyomatosis. Spectral Doppler is used to determine flow dynamics and direction.

Clinical Implications

Ruling Out Gallstones

In the majority of patients, gallstones are easy to diagnose by demonstrating mobile echogenic intraluminal lesions with acoustic shadowing. Shadowing from gallstones can be variable but can be enhanced with harmonic imaging. False-negatives include small nonshadowing stones mistaken for sludge or small stones hidden in the gallbladder neck with the patient supine. Other pitfalls include a contracted gallbladder packed with stones, misinterpreted as duodenum or a non-distended/non-visualized gallbladder. The contracted stone filled gallbladder can be diagnosed if the wall-echo-shadow (WES) sign is present. Suspected porcelain gallbladder is optimally confirmed with CT with a careful search for associated mass. Emphysematous cholecystitis or gas in the gallbladder from reflux can be difficult to evaluate with ultrasound, often requiring CT.

Intraluminal lesions to be differentiated from gallstones include sludge and polyps. Gallstones can be differentiated from polyps by demonstrating mobility, although rare stones may be embedded in the wall. Sludge is common in hospitalized patients and may be mass-like. It is important to distinguish tumefactive sludge from mass by using color Doppler to detect flow in a mass. Spectral Doppler can also distinguish twinkling artifact caused by microcalculi from true blood flow in a mass. The gallbladder wall should be evaluated for focal wall thickening and signs of malignancy such as adjacent wall thickening or retraction and invasion into liver. The majority of gallbladder polyps are small and have a characteristic appearance. Gallbladder adenomyomatosis is characterized by polypoid lesions with "comet tail" artifacts and diffuse or segmental wall thickening.

Right Upper Quadrant Pain
Ultrasound is the modality of choice for the evaluation of a patient with right upper quadrant pain, and is the highest rated modality in the ACR appropriateness criteria. The well known advantages of ultrasound include the high sensitivity and specificity for gallstones and acute cholecystitis as well as availability, lower cost, lack of ionizing radiation, repeatability, and short duration. The ability to derive a diagnosis in real time while interacting with the patient and determining the site of maximal tenderness is unrivaled.

The presence of the sonographic Murphy sign allows a definitive diagnosis of acute cholecystitis when added to other findings of gallstones, wall thickening, pericholecystic fluid and distension which may otherwise be secondary to other confounding factors. Diffuse gallbladder wall thickening in isolation is often caused by secondary causes such as hypoalbuminemia, cardiac, renal or hepatic failure, sepsis, pancreatitis, hepatitis, and trauma. When the Murphy sign cannot be elicited in obtunded or sedated patients or after opiate administration, the performance of ultrasound is inferior for the diagnosis of acute cholecystitis.

Cholescintigraphy has a higher accuracy, sensitivity, and specificity than ultrasound for acute cholecystitis, but the availability, ionizing radiation, length of study, and dependence on hepatic function promote ultrasound as the first-line modality. Ultrasound also has the advantage of determining alternative pathology, presence of gallstones, and status of the bile ducts; however, cholescintigraphy is extremely useful after equivocal or nondiagnostic ultrasound, especially in sick, septic patients at high risk for acalculous cholecystitis.

In patients with acute cholecystitis, detection of complications can influence the surgical approach. Gangrenous, perforated, or emphysematous cholecystitis may be diagnosed with ultrasound. However CT or MR should be considered given the wider field of view and fewer limitations regarding body habitus and acoustic window. The bile ducts should be carefully evaluated for bile duct stones; the biliary duct stones will definitely influence surgical management, requiring preoperative ERCP or intraoperative bile duct clearance.

In chronic cholecystitis, the gallbladder wall is thick but noninflamed and the gallbladder is not distended. Confirmation requires clinical correlation and HIDA scan.

Obstructive Jaundice, Elevated Liver Function Tests
The main role of ultrasound is to determine if there is biliary dilatation and the level and cause of biliary obstruction. The bile duct lumen, caliber, and walls should be evaluated in addition to the liver and gallbladder. Ultrasound may be sufficient for benign obstruction from bile duct stones but CT is used to confirm and stage malignant bile duct obstruction from cholangiocarcinoma, pancreatic carcinoma, gallbladder carcinoma, or extrinsic compression by lymphadenopathy. Bile duct caliber should be correlated with symptoms and biochemical tests, especially after cholecystectomy as dilated bile ducts are not necessarily obstructed.

Fever, Sepsis: Rule Out Biliary/Gallbladder Source
This is a common indication in septic, postoperative, intubated patients with multisystem failure. Ultrasound is less sensitive and specific for acute cholecystitis given the difficulty in detecting gallbladder tenderness and the fact that fasting, total parenteral nutrition, hypoalbuminemia, sepsis, and heart failure may contribute to gallbladder distension and wall thickening. Cholescintigraphy is often required to confirm acalculous cholecystitis.

The intrahepatic and extrahepatic bile ducts should be evaluated for dilatation or thickening secondary to cholangitis. Ascending cholangitis may be associated with biliary sludge or pus and obstructing stones. Rarely, there is pneumobilia. Cholangitis may be complicated by hepatic abscesses, typically clustered around the abnormal bile ducts.

The liver, pancreas, and other organs should also be screened for causes of sepsis during ultrasound.

Palpable Gallbladder
A palpable gallbladder could be secondary to gallbladder carcinoma or other tumors, mucocele, or benign obstruction. Gallbladder carcinoma has a poor prognosis and early diagnosis is difficult. Early carcinoma may present as a polypoid mass or wall thickening. More advanced tumors may obliterate the gallbladder lumen and extend into the nearby liver, making it difficult to determine the origin of the tumor. Gallstones are typically present, suggesting the origin of the tumor. Bile-filled obstructed noninflamed gallbladders typically result from non-stone disease such as pancreatic or distal bile duct carcinomas. Gallbladder mucoceles secondary to chronic stone obstruction are typically minimally tender with no wall thickening.

Selected References

1. Fagenholz PJ et al: Acute inflammatory surgical disease. Surg Clin North Am. 94(1):1-30, 2014
2. Yarmish GM et al: ACR appropriateness criteria right upper quadrant pain. J Am Coll Radiol. 11(3):316-22, 2014
3. McArthur TA et al: The common duct dilates after cholecystectomy and with advancing age: reality or myth? J Ultrasound Med. 32(8):1385-91, 2013
4. Kiewiet JJ et al: A systematic review and meta-analysis of diagnostic performance of imaging in acute cholecystitis. Radiology. 264(3):708-20, 2012
5. Brook OR et al: Lessons learned from quality assurance: errors in the diagnosis of acute cholecystitis on ultrasound and CT. AJR Am J Roentgenol. 196(3):597-604, 2011
6. Charalel RA et al: Complicated cholecystitis: the complementary roles of sonography and computed tomography. Ultrasound Q. 27(3):161-70, 2011
7. Gore RM et al: Gallbladder imaging. Gastroenterol Clin North Am. 39(2):265-87, ix, 2010
8. Horrow MM: Ultrasound of the extrahepatic bile duct: issues of size. Ultrasound Q. 26(2):67-74, 2010
9. Oktar SO et al: Comparison of conventional sonography, real-time compound sonography, tissue harmonic sonography, and tissue harmonic compound sonography of abdominal and pelvic lesions. AJR Am J Roentgenol. 181(5):1341-7, 2003

(Left) *Longitudinal ultrasound shows a normal gallbladder in the supine position. The lumen is anechoic and the wall ➡ is very thin or barely perceptible. The neck ➡ does not contain any stones.* **(Right)** *Longitudinal ultrasound shows a normal gallbladder in the left-side decubitus position. The neck ➡ and cystic duct are better evaluated.*

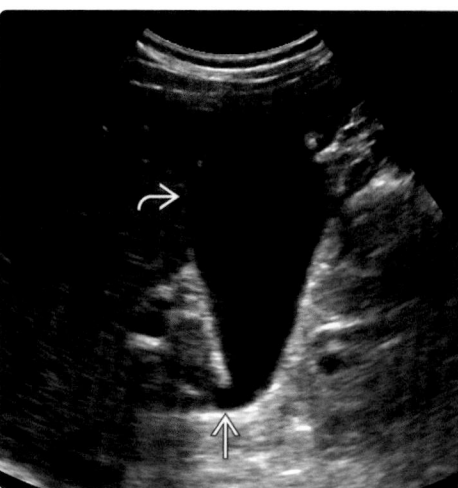
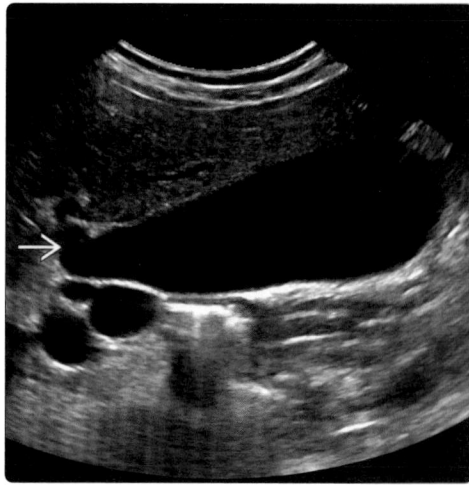

(Left) *Longitudinal oblique ultrasound of the porta hepatis shows a common bile duct ➡ measuring 6 mm (inner to inner measurement) proximally. Portal vein ➡ and inferior vena cava ➡ were normal.* **(Right)** *Longitudinal color Doppler ultrasound of the porta hepatis shows no flow in the common hepatic duct ➡. The portal vein ➡, inferior vena cava ➡, and proper hepatic artery ➡ were normal.*

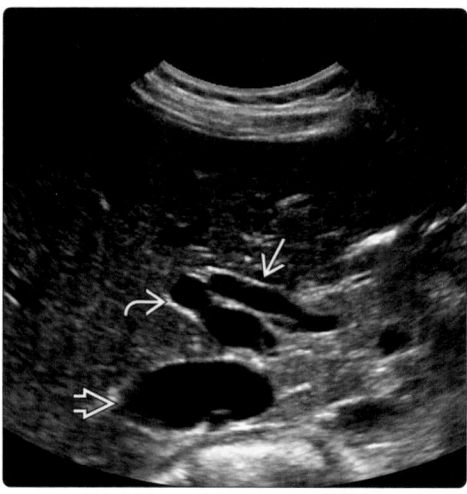
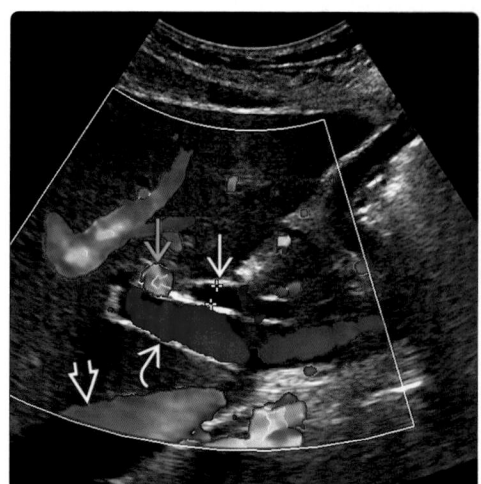

(Left) *Longitudinal oblique ultrasound of the distal common bile duct ➡ shows smooth tapering down to 3 mm with no stone or wall thickening. Main portal vein ➡ is noted.* **(Right)** *Transverse ultrasound through the head of the pancreas shows the normal distal common bile duct ➡. Adjacent vessels are splenic vein ➡, superior mesenteric artery ➡, aorta ➡, and inferior vena cava ➡.*

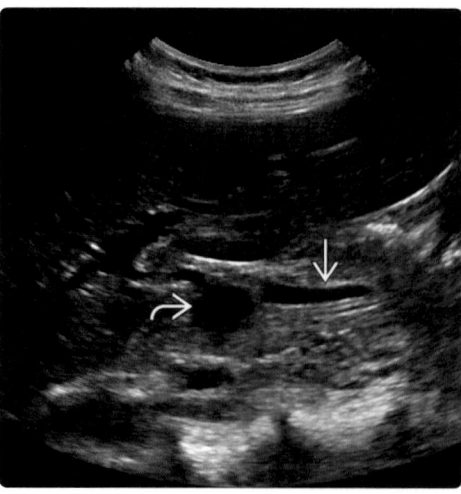
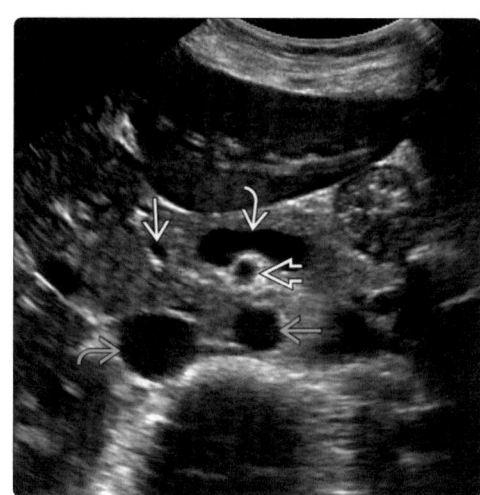

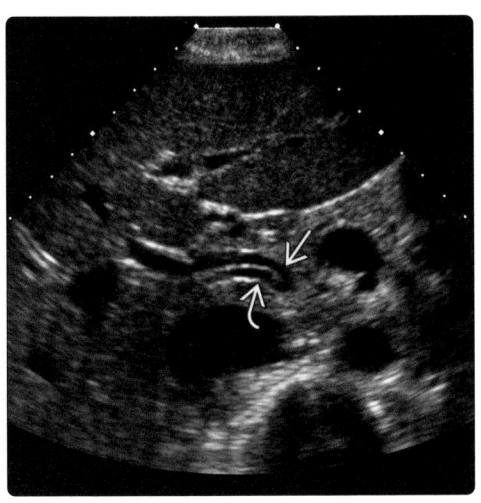

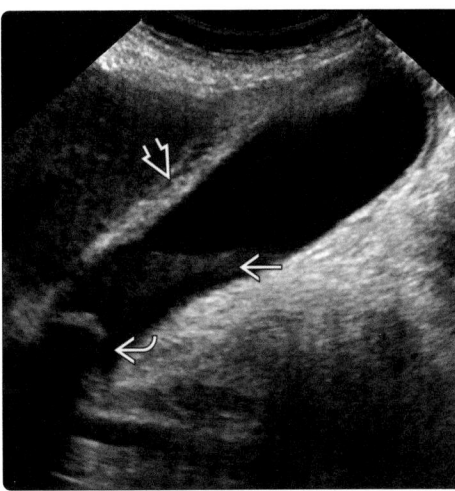

(Left) *Longitudinal oblique ultrasound through the distal bile duct shows a low union of the cystic duct* ➜ *and common hepatic duct* ➡. (Right) *Longitudinal oblique decubitus ultrasound of acute cholecystitis shows a non-mobile stone in the gallbladder neck* ➜ *with sludge* ➡ *and diffuse wall thickening* ➡. *Sonographic Murphy sign was present.*

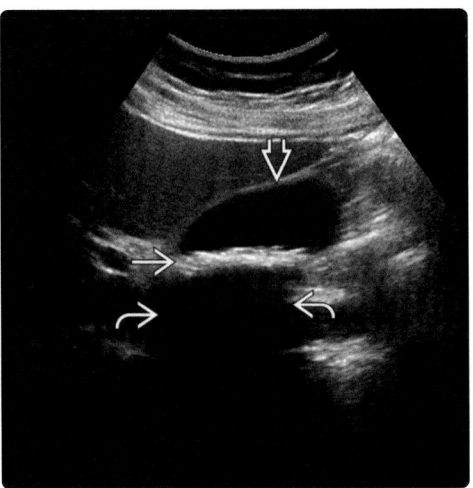

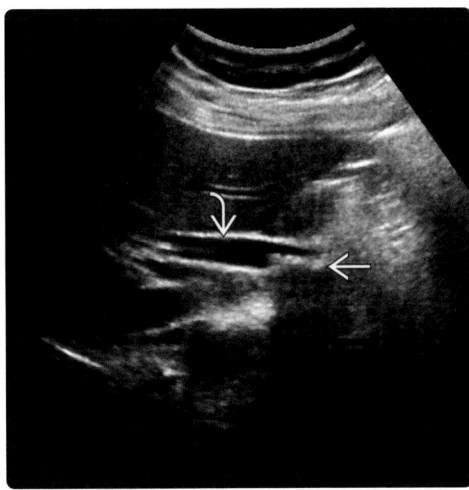

(Left) *Longitudinal oblique decubitus ultrasound shows a layer of stones* ➡ *producing a confluent shadow* ➜. *Note the normal wall* ➡. (Right) *Longitudinal oblique decubitus ultrasound in the same patient shows small shadowing stones* ➜ *present in the dilated common bile duct* ➜.

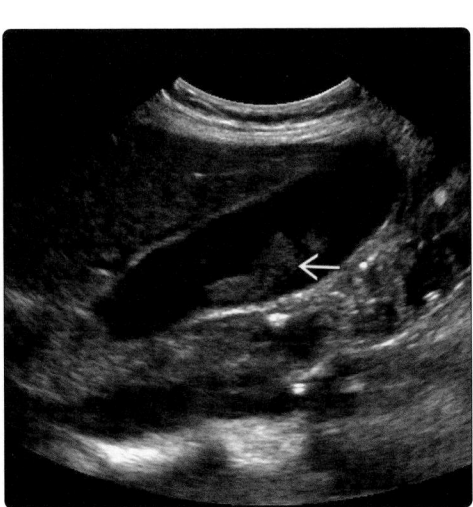

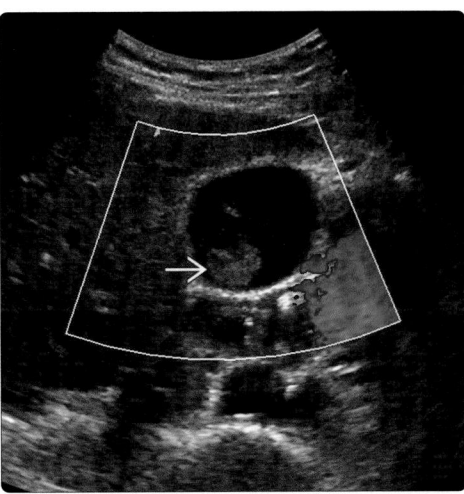

(Left) *Longitudinal oblique decubitus ultrasound shows gallbladder sludge* ➡. *The sludge is less echogenic than gallstones and nonshadowing. Unlike polyp or mass, sludge is not attached to the wall.* (Right) *Transverse color Doppler ultrasound shows no color flow in sludge balls* ➡.

(Left) *Longitudinal supine oblique ultrasound shows an empty gallbladder ➡. (Right) Longitudinal decubitus oblique ultrasound of the same patient now shows small nonshadowing stones ➡, which were symptomatic.*

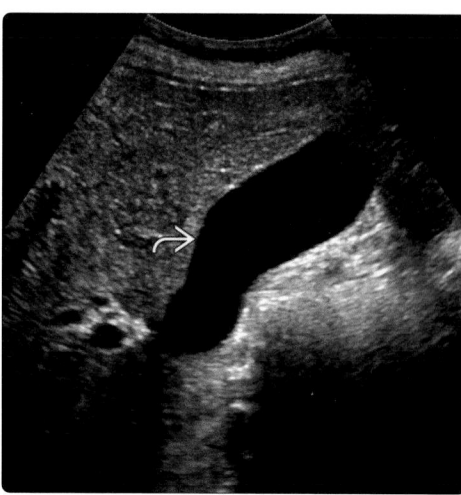
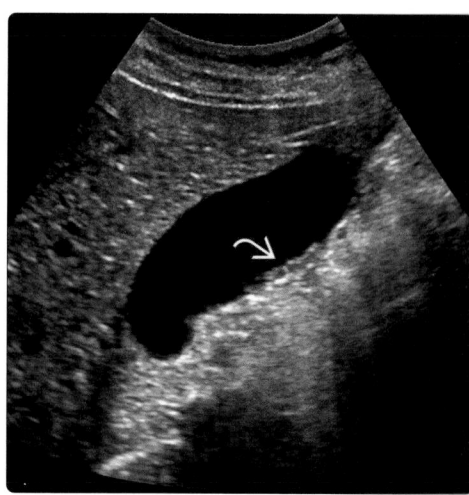

(Left) *Longitudinal decubitus shows multiple gallbladder stones with subtle shadowing ➡. (Right) Longitudinal decubitus ultrasound of the same patient with harmonic imaging shows improved acoustic shadowing ➡, increasing diagnostic confidence.*

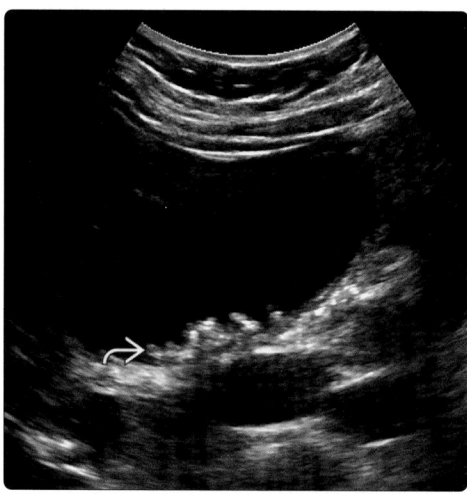
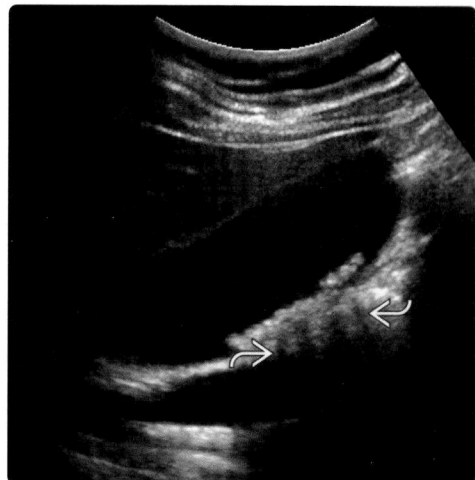

(Left) *Longitudinal decubitus of the gallbladder shows nondependent gas ➡ in the lumen, secondary to presence of a bile duct stent. This should be distinguished from emphysematous cholecystitis by demonstrating mobility and correlating with signs of wall inflammation. (Right) Transverse ultrasound shows multiple gallbladder stones with shadowing ➡. The gallbladder is distended with sludge ➡ and wall thickening ➡, findings indicating acute calculous cholecystitis in the correct clinical context.*

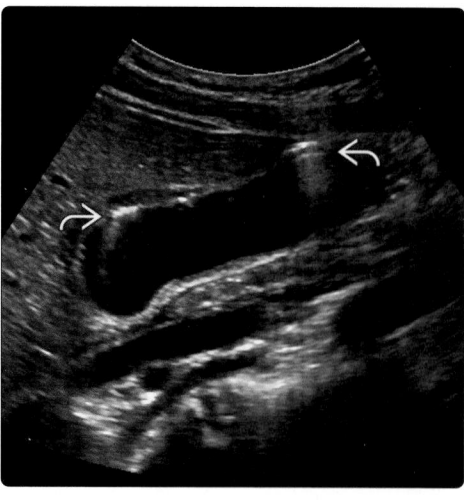
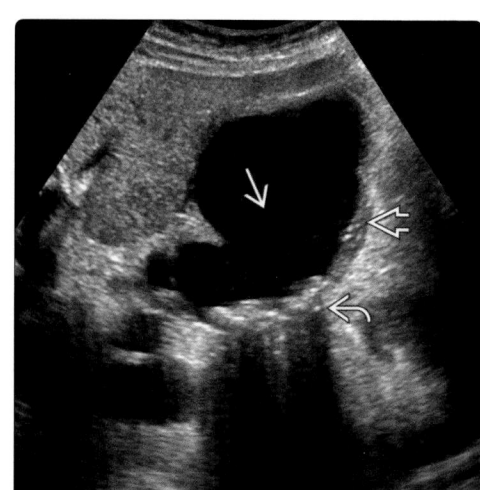

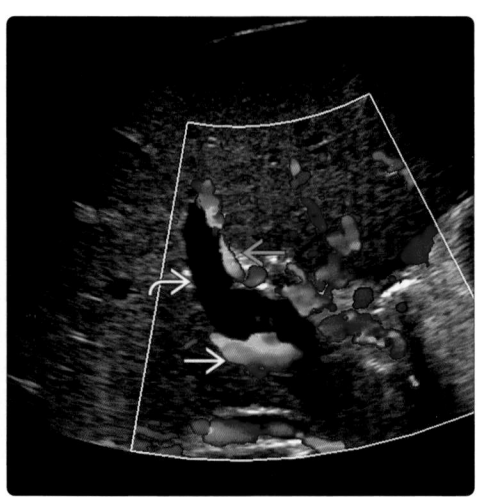
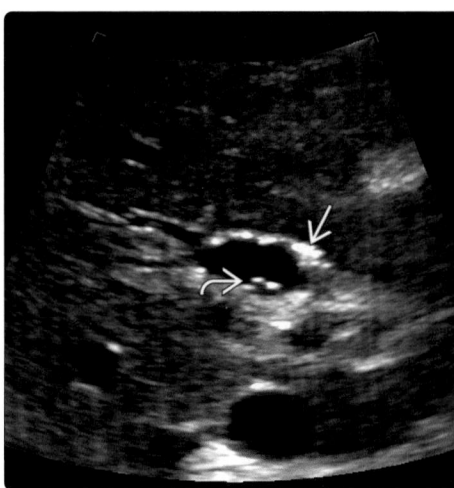

(Left) *Transverse oblique color Doppler ultrasound of the porta hepatis shows a dilated common hepatic duct ➡, differentiated from portal vein ➡ and left hepatic artery ➡.* (Right) *Transverse oblique ultrasound of the common hepatic duct post ERCP shows ductal dilatation with pneumobilia ➡ and debris ➡. Pneumobilia may obscure stones.*

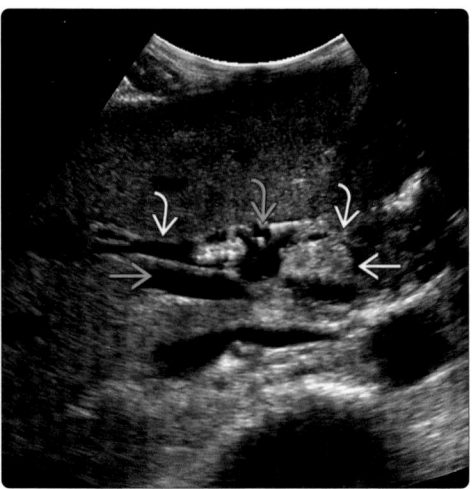
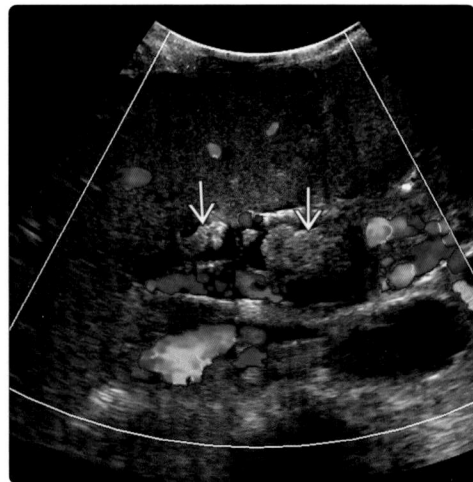

(Left) *Longitudinal oblique ultrasound of the porta hepatis in a patient with jaundice shows a dilated common hepatic duct ➡ with two echogenic nonshadowing stones ➡. The portal vein ➡ and proper hepatic artery ➡ are shown.* (Right) *Longitudinal oblique color Doppler ultrasound of the same patient shows no color flow in the bile duct stones ➡. Presence of flow in a bile duct lesion suggests mass.*

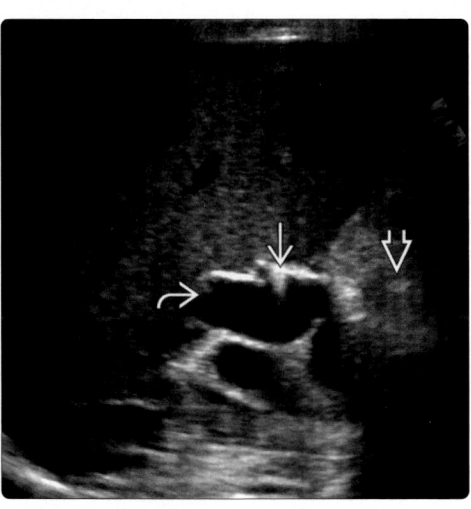
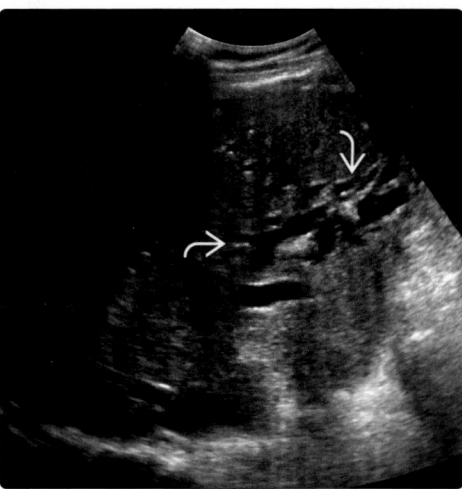

(Left) *Longitudinal oblique ultrasound of the porta hepatis in a patient with jaundice after cholecystectomy shows a dilated common hepatic duct ➡ measuring 16 mm. The distal bile duct was obscured by gas ➡. CT showed a pancreatic head carcinoma. Artifact from cholecystectomy clips was present ➡.* (Right) *Transverse ultrasound of the left lobe of the liver in the same patient shows diffuse ➡ intrahepatic biliary dilatation.*

Cholelithiasis

IMAGING

- US: Highly reflective intraluminal structures
- Gravity dependent and mobile
- Collection of bright echoes with acoustic shadowing in gallbladder (GB) representing GB packed with stones; may be mistaken for duodenal bulb
- Nonshadowing gallstone when < 5 mm
- Radiography: Radiopaque in 10-20%
- T2WI MR: Small focus of signal void or low signal outlined by markedly hyperintense bile within gallbladder
- Double-arc shadow sign or wall-echo-shadow (WES) sign: 2 echogenic curvilinear lines separated by sonolucent line (anterior GB wall, bile, curvilinear echo from stone and then shadow)

TOP DIFFERENTIAL DIAGNOSES

- Gallbladder polyp
- Gallbladder sludge
- Gallbladder carcinoma

- Focal adenomyomatosis

PATHOLOGY

- 80% cholesterol stones, containing > 50% cholesterol by definition
- 20% pigmented stones, containing cholesterol and calcium carbonate/bilirubinate

CLINICAL ISSUES

- Right upper quadrant pain/discomfort after fatty meal
- Asymptomatic, incidental finding on imaging
- Complications including acute or chronic cholecystitis, choledocholithiasis, cholangitis, pancreatitis, gallstone ileus, or cancer of gallbladder

DIAGNOSTIC CHECKLIST

- Ultrasound is best imaging tool for evaluation of patients with upper abdominal pain/discomfort
- Nonshadowing calculi may be mistaken for other lesions in GB such as polyp, sludge, carcinoma

(Left) Graphic shows multiple small, faceted stones in the gallbladder ➡ and distal bile duct ➡. (Right) Left lateral decubitus ultrasound in a patient with acute calculous cholecystitis shows an impacted shadowing stone ➡ in the gallbladder neck. Note acoustic shadowing ➡. There is mild gallbladder wall thickening ➡.

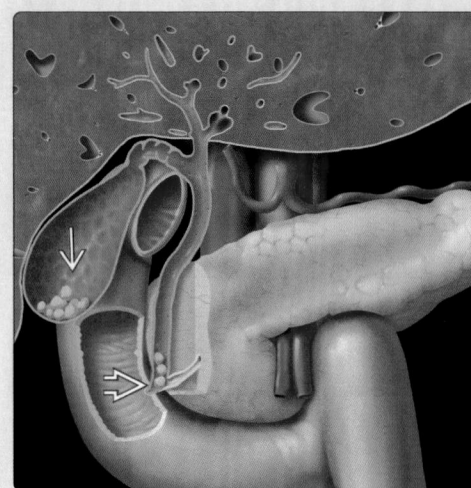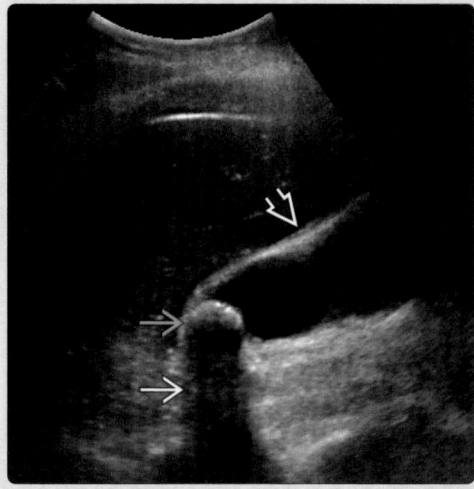

(Left) Left lateral decubitus ultrasound shows a cluster of large shadowing stones ➡ in the gallbladder. Note the acoustic shadowing ➡ and gallbladder wall thickening ➡. There was a positive Murphy sign. (Right) Oblique transabdominal ultrasound shows multiple shadowing stones in the gallbladder fundus ➡ with a layer of dependent sludge ➡.

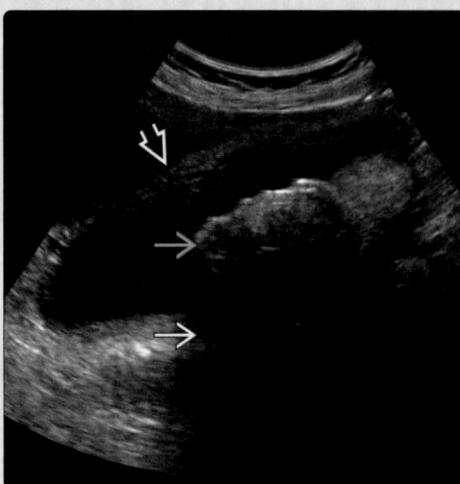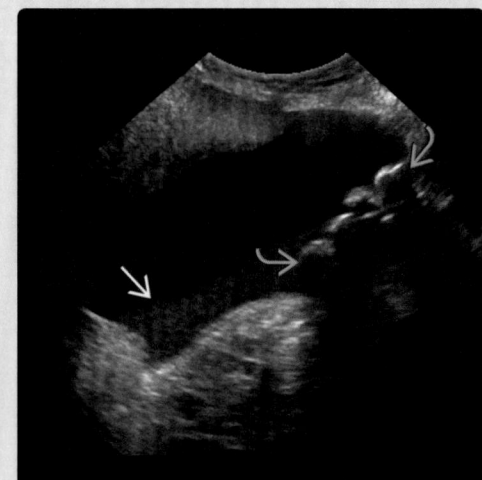

TERMINOLOGY

Synonyms

- Gallstone, cholecystolithiasis

IMAGING

General Features

- Best diagnostic clue
  - Ultrasound of gallbladder (GB)
    - Highly reflective intraluminal structures
    - Posterior acoustic shadowing
    - Mobile on changing patient's position
- Size
  - Variable
- Morphology
  - Laminated and faceted

Ultrasonographic Findings

- Grayscale ultrasound
  - Highly reflective intraluminal structures
  - Prominent posterior acoustic clean shadow
  - Gravity dependent and mobile
  - False-negative ultrasound: Small contracted GB full of stones, small gallstones, GB in ectopic/unusual position, obese/uncooperative patient
  - Variant ultrasound features
    - Collection of bright echoes with acoustic shadowing in gall bladder fossa representing GB packed with stones, may be mistaken for duodenal bulb
    - Double-arc shadow sign or wall-echo-shadow (WES) sign: 2 echogenic curvilinear lines separated by sonolucent line (anterior GB wall, bile, curvilinear echo from stone and then shadow)
    - Nonshadowing gallstone (stone < 5 mm)
    - Immobile adherent stone or nonmobile stones in GB neck
  - Associated findings if superimposed complications
    - Acute cholecystitis: Thick-walled and distended gallbladder, positive sonographic Murphy sign, pericholecystic fluid
    - Acute cholangitis: Obstructing common bile duct (CBD) stones, biliary dilatation
    - Acute pancreatitis: Ill-defined swelling of pancreatic parenchyma, inflammatory change in adjacent soft tissue
    - Biliary fistula/gallstone ileus
- Color Doppler
  - Twinkling artifact should not be mistaken for flow in GB mass; evaluate with spectral Doppler
  - Increased flow in pericholecystic region in cholelithiasis complicated by acute cholecystitis

Radiographic Findings

- Radiography
  - Radiopaque in 10-20%
    - Pigmented stone: 50% radiopaque
    - Cholesterol stone: 5% radiopaque

CT Findings

- NECT
  - Calcified gallstones are hyperdense to bile
  - Pure cholesterol stones are hypodense; inverse relationship between cholesterol content and CT attenuation
    - May be isodense to bile and will be missed by CT
  - Stones may contain nitrogen gas centrally: "Mercedes-Benz" sign

MR Findings

- T2WI
  - Small focus of signal void or low signal outlined by markedly hyperintense bile within gallbladder
- MRCP
  - Round foci of signal void inside gallbladder

Nonvascular Interventions

- ERCP
  - Mobile filling defects inside contrast-filled gallbladder
  - ± stones in extrahepatic bile ducts

Nuclear Medicine Findings

- Hepatobiliary scintigraphy
  - Not sensitive for gallstones
  - Used for diagnosis of acute or chronic cholecystitis
    - Nonfilling of gallbladder or decreased ejection fraction, respectively

Imaging Recommendations

- Best imaging tool
  - Ultrasound
- Protocol advice
  - Transabdominal ultrasound
    - Patients should fast for 6-8 hours
    - Examine patient in supine and left decubitus/oblique position to demonstrate mobility of gallstone, consider erect or semiprone positions
      - In supine position, stones are highly likely to be found in GB neck with gravitation to fundus in left decubitus position
    - Optimize parameters to maximize visualization of posterior acoustic shadowing from small stones
    - Always evaluate for biliary dilatation and signs of cholecystitis, cholangitis, or pancreatitis

DIFFERENTIAL DIAGNOSIS

Gallbladder Polyp

- Small, round nodule with smooth contour arising from gallbladder wall
- Low/medium echogenicity, usually multiple, no posterior acoustic shadowing
- Not mobile, may have short stalk or may be sessile

Gallbladder Sludge

- Sludge may aggregate into a mass or may layer
- Low/medium echogenicity; mobile
- Lack of posterior acoustic shadowing

Gallbladder Carcinoma

- Well- or poorly defined mass from gallbladder wall; nonmobile
- Infiltrates adjacent liver parenchyma, associated lymphadenopathy
- Increased vascularity within lesion on color Doppler

Focal Adenomyomatosis

- Focal polypoid lesion or wall thickening
- Gallbladder fundus or body; nonmobile
- Reverberation/"comet tail" artifacts due to cholesterol deposits within Rokitansky-Aschoff sinuses

Parasite Infestation in Gallbladder

- Tubular configuration, double parallel echogenic lines
- Active movement in viable worm, gravity-dependent movement in dead worm

Bowel Gas

- Echo with posterior reverberation

Emphysematous Cholecystitis

- Reverberation from gas in GB wall
- Wall thickening and other signs of cholecystitis

PATHOLOGY

General Features

- Etiology
  - Excessive biliary cholesterol, altered bile salts and phospholipids, stasis and infection are predisposing factors
    - Hemolytic diseases: Sickle cell disease, thalassemia, hereditary spherocytosis
    - Cholestasis: Biliary tree malformation such as choledochal cyst, Caroli disease, TPN, cirrhosis
    - Metabolic disorders: Obesity, cystic fibrosis, diabetes, pancreatic diseases, hyperlipidemia, pregnancy
    - Intestinal malabsorption: Crohn disease, bariatric surgery, ileal resection
- Genetics
  - Familial in some racial groups: Navajo, Pima, Chippewa Native Americans

Gross Pathologic & Surgical Features

- 80% cholesterol stones, containing > 50% cholesterol by definition
- 20% pigmented stones, containing cholesterol and calcium carbonate/bilirubinate
  - Black pigmented stones occur in hemolytic disorders and cirrhosis
  - Brown pigmented stones occur in chronic bacterial or parasitic infection, bile ducts more common than gallbladder

Microscopic Features

- Varied degree of acute/chronic inflammatory changes within gallbladder wall

CLINICAL ISSUES

Presentation

- Most common signs/symptoms
  - Right upper quadrant pain/discomfort after fatty meal
- Other signs/symptoms
  - Asymptomatic, incidental finding on imaging
  - Complications including acute or chronic cholecystitis, choledocholithiasis, cholangitis, pancreatitis, gallstone ileus, or cancer of gallbladder

Demographics

- Age
  - Peak: 5th to 6th decade, increases with age
- Gender
  - M:F = 1:3
- 10-15% of population, most common in obese female in their 5th decade
- Rare in neonates unless predisposing causes such as obstructive congenital biliary lesion, dehydration, infection, hemolytic anemia
- Older children associated with sickle cell disease, cystic fibrosis, hemolytic anemia, Crohn disease

Natural History & Prognosis

- Increasing cause of hospitalization, 20% symptomatic, 1-2% require cholecystectomy
- Excellent prognosis unless complications occur

Treatment

- Conservative management if asymptomatic
- If symptomatic, laparoscopic cholecystectomy, rarely open surgical reaction
- Nonsurgical management with dissolution therapy or extracorporeal shock wave lithotripsy prone to recur

DIAGNOSTIC CHECKLIST

Consider

- Ultrasound is best imaging tool for evaluation of patients with upper abdominal pain/discomfort
- Consider cholelithiasis in patients with RUQ pain/discomfort after fatty meal, especially in obese middle-age female

Image Interpretation Pearls

- Important to demonstrate posterior acoustic shadowing and mobility
- Nonshadowing calculi may be mistaken for other lesions in GB such as polyp, sludge, carcinoma
- Contracted stone filled GB: Look for WES sign or look in interlobar fissure

SELECTED REFERENCES

1. Knab LM et al: Cholecystitis. Surg Clin North Am. 94(2):455-70, 2014
2. O'Connell K et al: Bile metabolism and lithogenesis. Surg Clin North Am. 94(2):361-75, 2014
3. Duncan CB et al: Evidence-based current surgical practice: calculous gallbladder disease. J Gastrointest Surg. 16(11):2011-25, 2012
4. Gore RM et al: Gallbladder imaging. Gastroenterol Clin North Am. 39(2):265-87, ix, 2010
5. Gurusamy KS et al: Surgical treatment of gallstones. Gastroenterol Clin North Am. 39(2):229-44, viii, 2010
6. Stinton LM et al: Epidemiology of gallstones. Gastroenterol Clin North Am. 39(2):157-69, vii, 2010
7. Venneman NG et al: Pathogenesis of gallstones. Gastroenterol Clin North Am. 39(2):171-83, vii, 2010
8. Jüngst C et al: Gallstone disease: Microlithiasis and sludge. Best Pract Res Clin Gastroenterol. 20(6):1053-62, 2006
9. Hanbidge AE et al: From the RSNA refresher courses: imaging evaluation for acute pain in the right upper quadrant. Radiographics. 24(4):1117-35, 2004
10. Leung JW et al: Hepatolithiasis and biliary parasites. Baillieres Clin Gastroenterol. 11(4):681-706, 1997

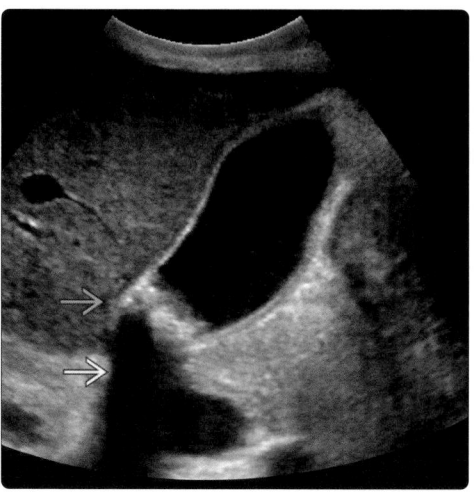

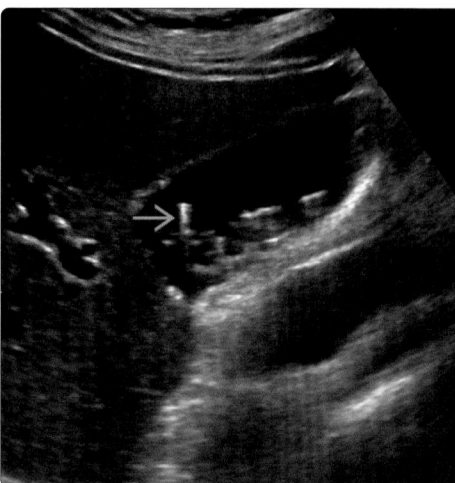

(Left) *Longitudinal supine ultrasound shows a cluster of stones ➡ in the gallbladder neck with acoustic shadowing ➡. There was also sludge but no cholecystitis.* (Right) *Left lateral decubitus ultrasound shows multiple floating gallbladder stones, which moved with repositioning. Reverberation artifact is noted ➡.*

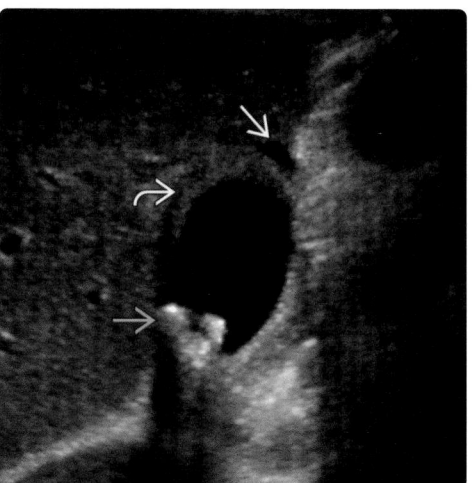

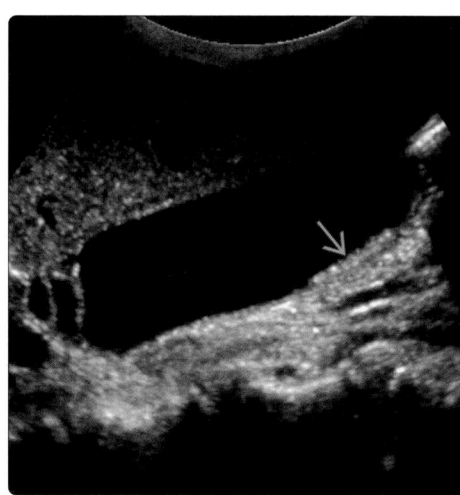

(Left) *Transverse ultrasound shows a cluster of small shadowing gallstones ➡ in the gallbladder. Mild wall thickening ➡ and pericholecystic ➡ fluid were secondary to pancreatitis.* (Right) *Left lateral decubitus ultrasound shows a layer of small, nonshadowing mobile gallstones ➡. The gallbladder wall was normal.*

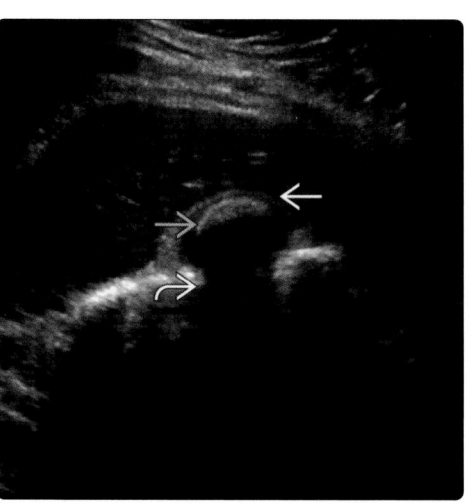

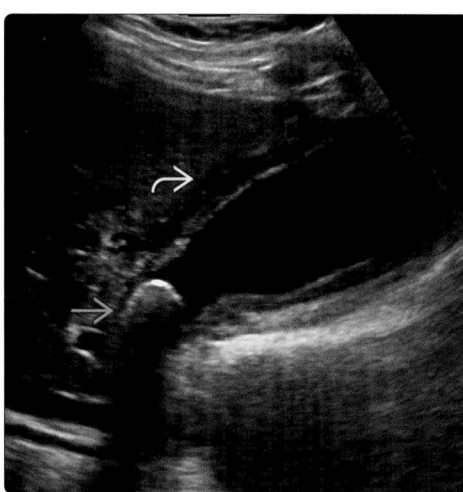

(Left) *Transverse ultrasound shows a gall stone filling the gallbladder. Note the wall ➡, echo ➡, and shadow ➡, which together form the WES sign.* (Right) *Longitudinal oblique ultrasound of acute calculous cholecystitis shows an impacted stone ➡ in the neck with an edematous, thick wall ➡. The Murphy sign was positive.*

(Left) *Longitudinal oblique ultrasound shows dependent gallstones ⮕. Acoustic shadowing is noted posterior to the largest stone ⮕. There is a "comet tail" artifact from focal adenomyomatosis ⮕.* (Right) *Oblique transabdominal ultrasound shows multiple small, nonshadowing stones ⮕ in a contracted gallbladder.*

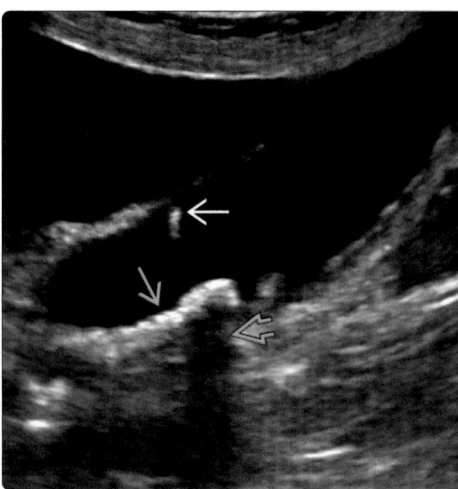
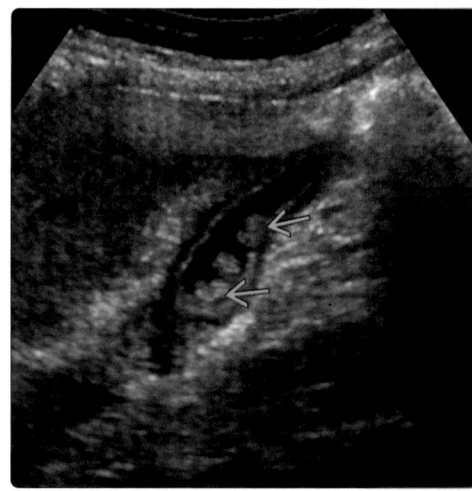

(Left) *Left lateral decubitus ultrasound of a poorly distended gallbladder shows a dependent layer of small stones ⮕ with an aggregate shadow ⮕.* (Right) *Axial T2 HASTE MR in the same patient shows multiple low-signal stones ⮕ in a mildly thickened gallbladder.*

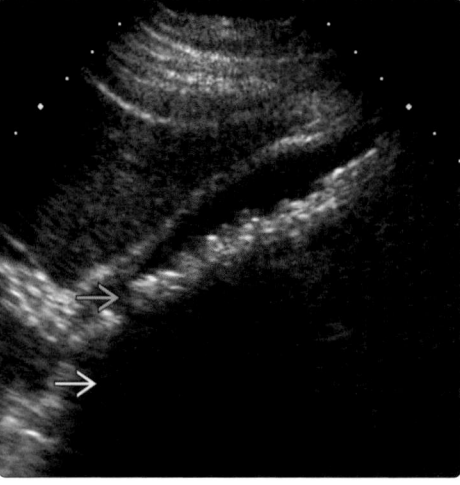
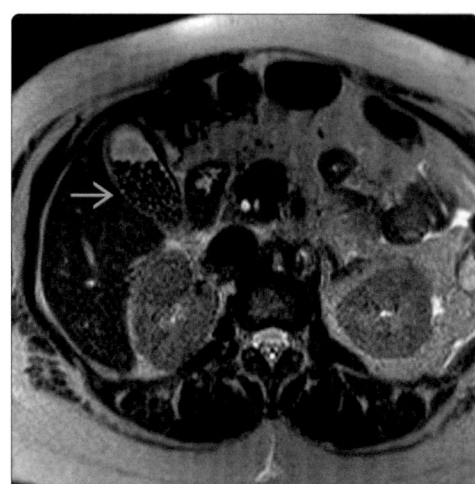

(Left) *Left lateral decubitus ultrasound shows a fundal gallstone ⮕ with acoustic shadowing ⮕. Note the sludge level ⮕ but no wall thickening.* (Right) *Left lateral decubitus ultrasound of the same patient shows twinkling artifact in the stone ⮕.*

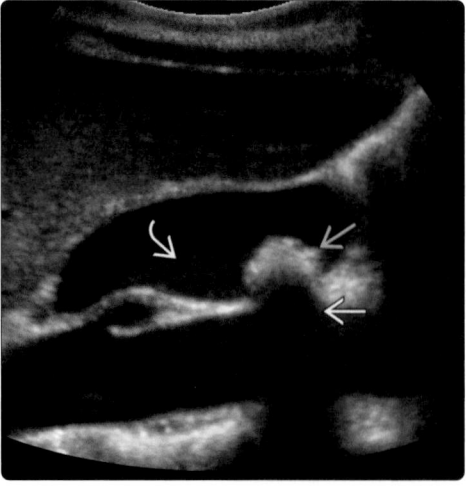
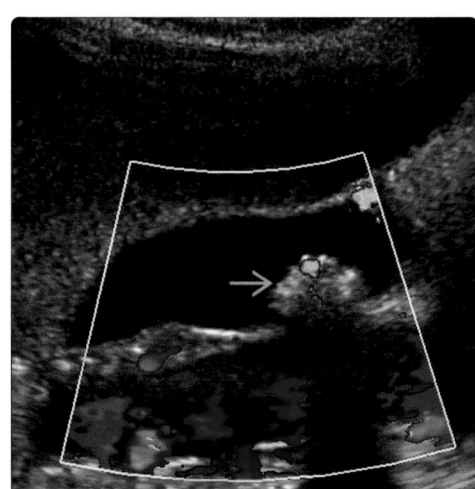

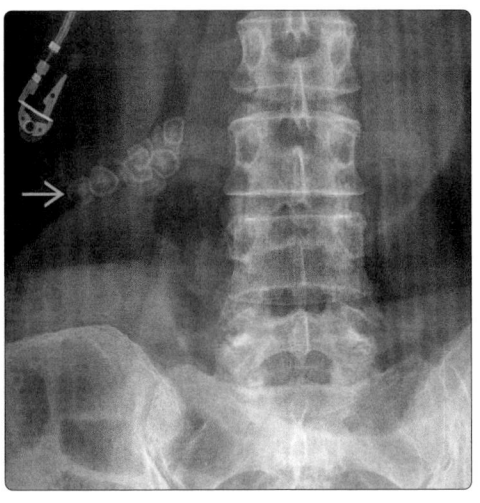

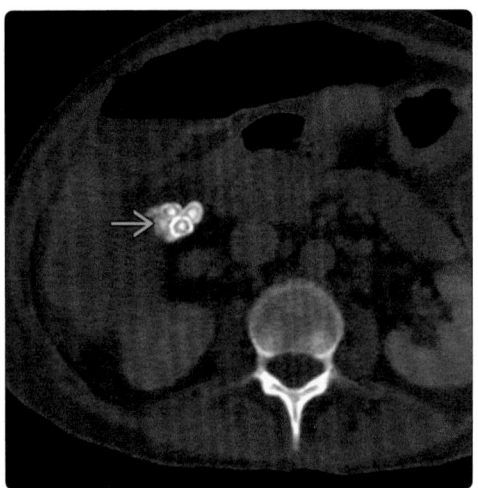

(Left) *Abdominal radiograph shows multiple laminated and faceted gallstones ➡. (Right) Axial NECT in the same patient shows a cluster of laminated and faceted gallstones ➡.*

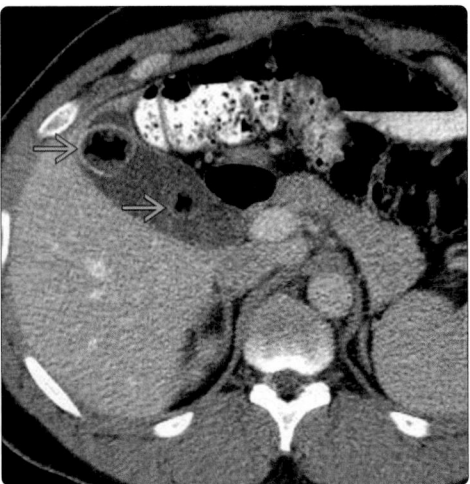

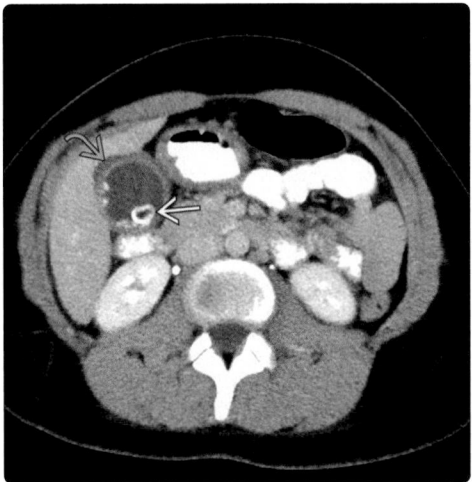

(Left) *Axial CECT through the gallbladder shows the "Mercedes-Benz" sign in 2 gas-containing stones ➡. There is no cholecystitis. (Right) Axial CECT of acute calculous cholecystitis shows calcified stones ➡ in a thick-walled gallbladder ➡.*

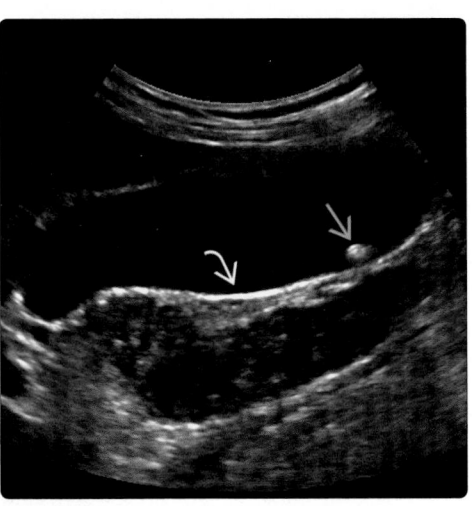

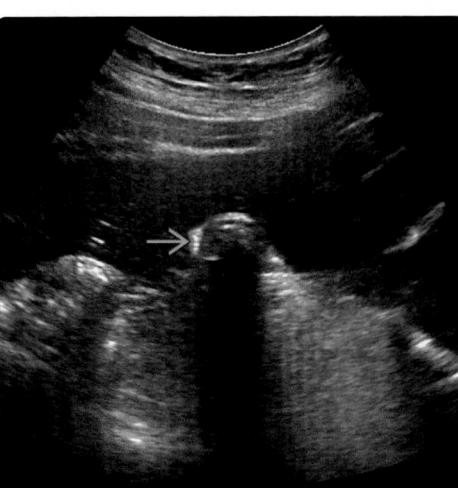

(Left) *Left lateral decubitus ultrasound shows a shadowing small stone in the gallbladder fundus ➡. The stone was mobile. Note the normal gallbladder wall ➡. (Right) Transverse ultrasound shows a markedly contracted gallbladder ➡ with a WES sign. This could be mistaken for gas filled duodenum.*

TERMINOLOGY

- Biliary sludge, tumefactive sludge, biliary sand, microlithiasis
- Presence of particulate material (calcium bilirubinate/phosphate or carbonate crystals with cholesterol monohydrate crystals) in bile
- Larger particles (1-3 mm) are microliths, which may become nidus for gallstones

IMAGING

- Amorphous, mid-/high-level echoes within gallbladder (GB)
- Sediment in dependent position
- Floating punctate echoes; may show ring-down artifact
- Lack of posterior acoustic shadowing
- Round, low to intermediate echogenicity mass-like "lesion"
- Note: Twinkling artifact may be mistaken for color flow
- Change patient position to demonstrate mobility of intraluminal material to dependent portion

TOP DIFFERENTIAL DIAGNOSES

- Cholelithiasis
- Focal adenomyomatosis
- Gallbladder polyp
- Gallbladder empyema
- Blood clot

CLINICAL ISSUES

- Mostly asymptomatic
- May have clinical symptoms when complications occur
- Stone formation
- Biliary colic
- Acute acalculous/calculous cholecystitis
- Pancreatitis

DIAGNOSTIC CHECKLIST

- Consider biliary sludge when mobile mid-/high-level echoes without acoustic shadowing are seen in GB

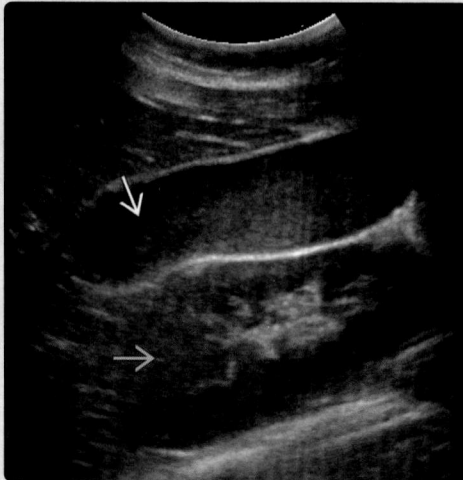
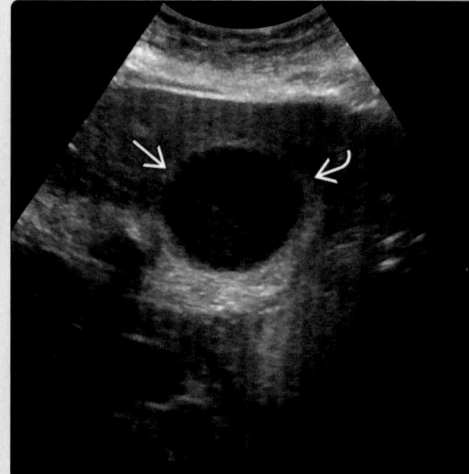

(Left) Longitudinal ultrasound in a decubitus position shows intraluminal sludge ➡ with a normal wall. The right kidney ⊟ is noted. (Right) Transverse ultrasound shows a dependent sludge layer in the gallbladder ➡. The gallbladder wall is asymmetrically mildly thickened ➡.

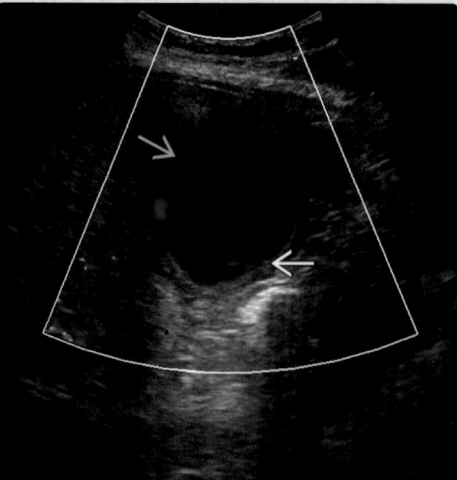
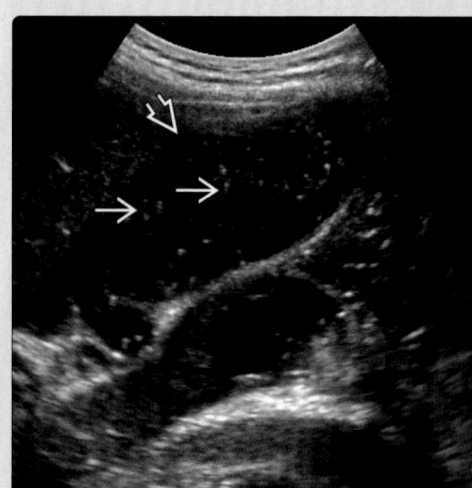

(Left) Transverse color Doppler ultrasound shows dependent echogenic sludge ➡ with no color flow. The gallbladder wall ⊟ is mildly thickened in this patient with liver disease. (Right) Longitudinal ultrasound in a decubitus position shows multiple bright intraluminal echoes, which were mobile on real-time imaging. Note the "comet tail" artifacts ➡. The gallbladder wall ➡ is normal.

TERMINOLOGY

Synonyms

- Biliary sludge, tumefactive sludge, biliary sand, microlithiasis

Definitions

- Presence of particulate material (calcium bilirubinate/phosphate or carbonate crystals with cholesterol monohydrate crystals) in bile
  - Larger particles (1-3 mm) are microliths, which may become nidus for gallstones

IMAGING

General Features

- Best diagnostic clue
  - Mobile, gravity-dependent nonshadowing echogenic layer within gallbladder (GB); mid-/high-level echoes
  - Echogenic, mobile "mass" within GB
- Location
  - Within gallbladder
- Size
  - Variable

Ultrasonographic Findings

- Grayscale ultrasound
  - Echogenic bile
    - Amorphous, mid-/high-level echoes within GB
    - Floating punctate echoes; may show ring-down artifact
    - Sediment in dependent position
    - Lack of posterior acoustic shadowing
    - "Hepatization" of gallbladder: Sludge-filled GB with same echotexture as liver
    - Lack of internal vascularity
  - Tumefactive sludge
    - Round, low to intermediate echogenicity mass-like "lesion"
    - No posterior acoustic shadowing
    - Gravitates slowly to dependent position on changing patient position
    - Lack of intralesional vascularity on color Doppler examination
      - □ Note that twinkling artifact may be mistaken for color flow
- Power Doppler
  - No internal vascularity in "mass-like" GB lesions

CT Findings

- NECT
  - Medium-density material within GB
  - No wall thickening or pericholecystic inflammatory change
- CECT
  - Lack of contrast enhancement
  - Intact GB wall without evidence of invasion in adjacent structures

MR Findings

- T1WI
  - High signal dependent layer
- T2WI
  - Lower signal dependent layer

Nonvascular Interventions

- ERCP
  - Filling defects within gallbladder
  - Gravitate to dependent position

Imaging Recommendations

- Best imaging tool
  - Transabdominal ultrasound
- Protocol advice
  - Use highest frequency transducer possible for better detail of intraluminal filling defect/echoes
  - Focal zone should be adjusted to level of gallbladder for optimal resolution
  - Change patient position to demonstrate mobility of intraluminal material to dependent portion
    - Distinguish from side lobe artifacts by scanning from different approaches
  - Interrogate areas of color flow with spectral Doppler to confirm twinkling artifact

DIFFERENTIAL DIAGNOSIS

Cholelithiasis

- Formed echogenic material within GB
- Marked posterior acoustic shadowing
  - Occasionally GB stone may be nonshadowing
- Mobile and gravitate to dependent position

Focal Adenomyomatosis

- Polypoid lesion arising from, and attached to, wall of GB
- Most common at GB fundus
- Not mobile on changing patient position
- May show "comet tail" artifact
- Lack of internal vascularity
- Other features of adenomyomatosis in rest of GB

Gallbladder Polyp

- Small (usually < 1 cm), smooth, polypoidal mass fixed to GB wall
- Smooth contour
- Single or multiple
- Usually avascular, occasionally with increased internal vascularity

Gallbladder Empyema

- Low-level echoes within GB lumen due to presence of pus/inflammatory exudate
- Distended GB
- Other features of acute cholecystitis
  - GB wall thickening, pericholecystic fluid collection, positive sonographic Murphy sign, impacted stone
- Clinically septic with localized peritoneal signs in right upper quadrant

Blood Clot

- Heterogeneous low-level echoes floating within GB, mobile
- Blood-fluid level within GB
- Retracting nonvascular clot; may conform to configuration of GB
- History of trauma, instrumentation, GI bleed
- May be associated with hemorrhagic cholecystitis

Gallbladder Carcinoma

- Infiltrative mass with early invasion of adjacent liver parenchyma
- Increased internal vascularity
- Regional nodal metastases
- Presence of gallstones

Parasitic Infection

- Ascariasis: Tubular or echogenic parallel lines within bile duct or gallbladder; sonolucent center; active movement of worm
- Hydatid: Daughter hydatid cysts are round and anechoic within bile duct/gallbladder; mother cyst seen in liver

PATHOLOGY

General Features

- Etiology
  - Altered composition of bile
  - Decreased gallbladder motility and bile stasis
  - Predisposing factors
    - Prolonged fasting/on total parenteral nutrition
    - Pregnancy
    - Rapid weight loss, post bariatric surgery
    - Presence of critical illness
    - Ceftriaxone or prolonged octreotide therapy
    - Post bone marrow transplantation
    - Liver transplantation

Gross Pathologic & Surgical Features

- Thick, crystallized bile sediment within normal-looking GB
- If longstanding disease ± superimposed inflammation
  - GB wall thickening with variable extent of chronic inflammatory infiltrate

CLINICAL ISSUES

Presentation

- Most common signs/symptoms
  - Mostly asymptomatic
  - May have clinical symptoms when complications occur
    - Stone formation
    - Biliary colic
    - Acute acalculous/calculous cholecystitis
    - Pancreatitis

Demographics

- Epidemiology
  - Biliary sludge
    - Similar epidemiology to cholelithiasis
    - M < F
    - More common in middle-aged, obese women

Natural History & Prognosis

- Biliary sludge
  - Approximately 50% of cases resolve spontaneously over 3-year period
  - 20% persist and remain asymptomatic
  - 5-15% develop gallstones
  - 10-15% become symptomatic

Treatment

- None required in vast majority of cases
- Elective cholecystectomy for complications

DIAGNOSTIC CHECKLIST

Consider

- Consider biliary sludge when mobile mid-/high-level echoes without acoustic shadowing are seen in GB

Image Interpretation Pearls

- Sludge is precursor to stones
  - May cause acute pancreatitis

SELECTED REFERENCES

1. Knab LM et al: Cholecystitis. Surg Clin North Am. 94(2):455-70, 2014
2. O'Connell K et al: Bile metabolism and lithogenesis. Surg Clin North Am. 94(2):361-75, 2014
3. Gore RM et al: Gallbladder imaging. Gastroenterol Clin North Am. 39(2):265-87, ix, 2010
4. Stinton LM et al: Epidemiology of gallstones. Gastroenterol Clin North Am. 39(2):157-69, vii, 2010
5. Venneman NG et al: Pathogenesis of gallstones. Gastroenterol Clin North Am. 39(2):171-83, vii, 2010
6. Smith EA et al: Cross-sectional imaging of acute and chronic gallbladder inflammatory disease. AJR Am J Roentgenol. 192(1):188-96, 2009
7. Pandya R et al: Hemorrhagic cholecystitis as a complication of anticoagulant therapy: role of CT in its diagnosis. Abdom Imaging. 33(6):652-3, 2008
8. Jüngst C et al: Gallstone disease: Microlithiasis and sludge. Best Pract Res Clin Gastroenterol. 20(6):1053-62, 2006
9. Choi D et al: Sonographic findings of active Clonorchis sinensis infection. J Clin Ultrasound. 32(1):17-23, 2004
10. Gremmels JM et al: Hemorrhagic cholecystitis simulating gallbladder carcinoma. J Ultrasound Med. 23(7):993-5, 2004
11. Green MH et al: Haemobilia. Br J Surg. 88(6):773-86, 2001
12. Nishiwaki M et al: Posttraumatic intra-gallbladder hemorrhage in a patient with liver cirrhosis. J Gastroenterol. 34(2):282-5, 1999
13. Schulman A: Ultrasound appearances of intra- and extrahepatic biliary ascariasis. Abdom Imaging. 23(1):60-6, 1998
14. Barton P et al: Biliary sludge after liver transplantation: 1. Imaging findings and efficacy of various imaging procedures. AJR Am J Roentgenol. 164(4):859-64, 1995
15. Khuroo MS et al: Sonographic findings in gallbladder ascariasis. J Clin Ultrasound. 20(9):587-91, 1992
16. Zargar SA et al: Intrabiliary rupture of hepatic hydatid cyst: sonographic and cholangiographic appearances. Gastrointest Radiol. 17(1):41-5, 1992

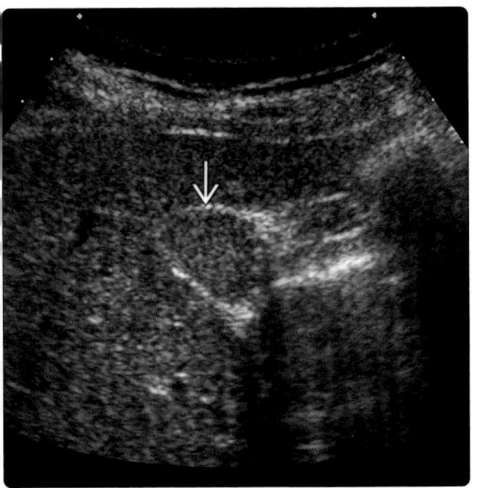

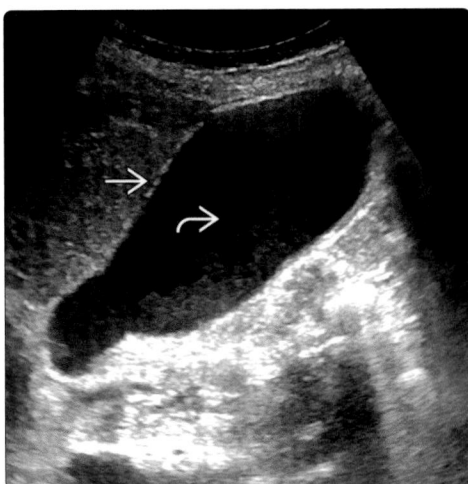

(Left) *Transverse ultrasound shows sludge filling the gallbladder ➡. The sludge is isoechoic to the liver, referred to as "hepatization."* (Right) *Longitudinal left lateral decubitus ultrasound shows dependent sludge with a polypoid appearance ➡. The gallbladder wall is normal ➡.*

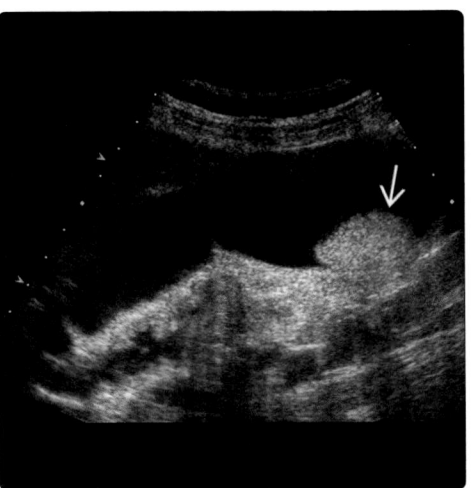

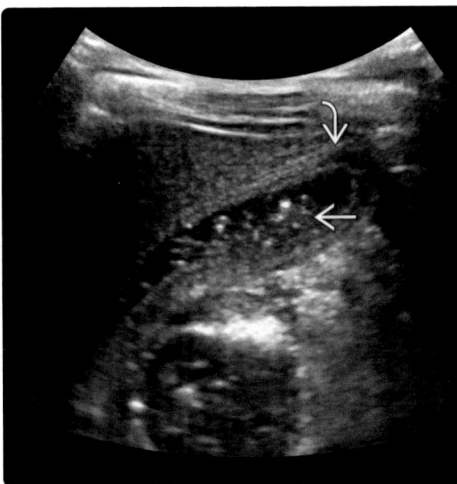

(Left) *Longitudinal ultrasound shows the gallbladder containing tumefactive sludge ➡, which does not shadow.* (Right) *Longitudinal ultrasound of the gallbladder in a decubitus position shows multiple bright, floating intraluminal echoes ➡, which were mobile. Note the poorly distended gallbladder with apparent wall thickening ➡.*

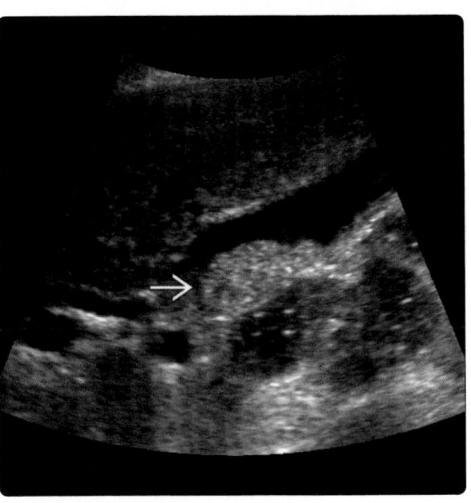

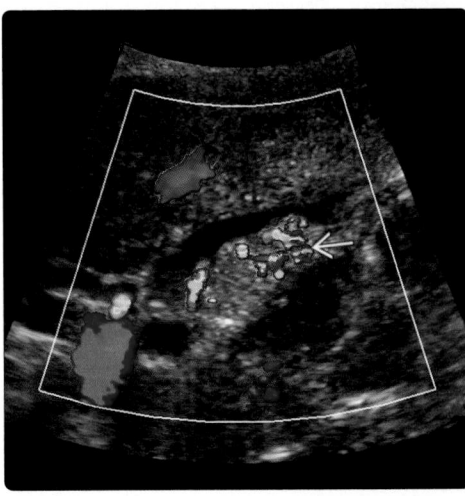

(Left) *Longitudinal ultrasound in a decubitus position shows dependent echogenic sludge ➡, which has aggregated into a clump.* (Right) *Longitudinal ultrasound of the same patient in decubitus position shows dependent echogenic sludge demonstrating twinkling artifact ➡.*

Gallbladder Cholesterol Polyp

TERMINOLOGY

- Focal gallbladder (GB) cholesterosis, polypoid cholesterosis
- Abnormal deposit of cholesterol ester producing villous-like structure covered with single layer of epithelium and attached via delicate stalk

IMAGING

- Transabdominal US is most sensitive technique for detecting small cholesterol polyps
- Optimize resolution and set focal zone to level of GB mass to improve accuracy of mass characterization
- Scan in supine, decubitus (left > right lateral) positions to demonstrate immobility of GB polyp
- Usually 2-10 mm in size
- Most commonly in middle 1/3 of gallbladder
- Intact GB wall
- Avascular or hypovascular on Doppler examination
- Larger lesions may have slight internal vascularity
- Variant US appearances
  - ○ Large size: Lesions up to 20 mm have been described
    - – Fine pattern of echogenic foci, best seen with endoscopic ultrasound
  - ○ Pedunculated with well-defined stalk from GB wall
- < 6 mm: No follow-up
- 7-9 mm: Yearly US follow-up to monitor size
- > 10 mm: Surgical consult

DIAGNOSTIC CHECKLIST

- Multiple small, round/ovoid masses attached to GB wall with no posterior acoustic shadowing
- Consider neoplastic GB polyp if size > 10 mm, irregular outline, sessile morphology with abnormality of GB wall and invasion of adjacent structures, growth on serial US examinations

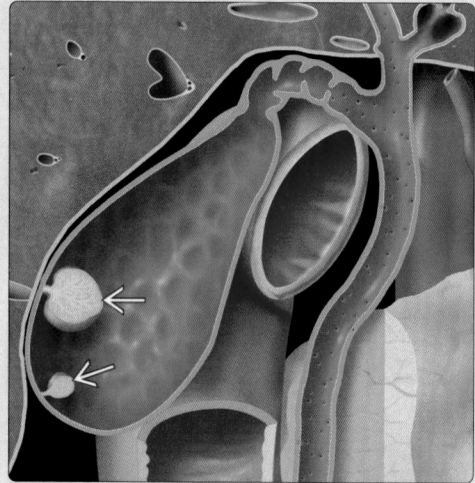
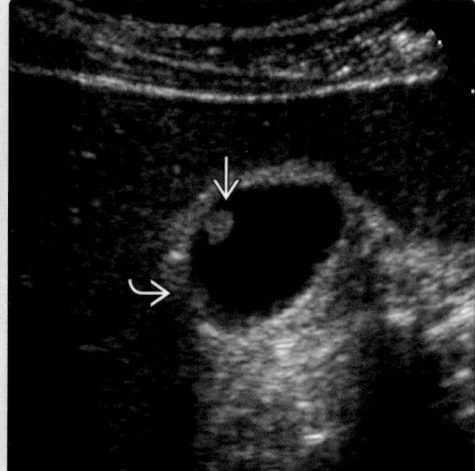

(Left) *Graphic shows well-circumscribed, pedunculated nodules* ➡ *arising from the gallbladder (GB) wall, suggestive of cholesterol polyps. Note the preserved GB wall without invasion to the adjacent liver parenchyma.* (Right) *Transverse ultrasound shows a small, lobulated polyp* ➡ *with diffuse mild wall thickening* ➡.

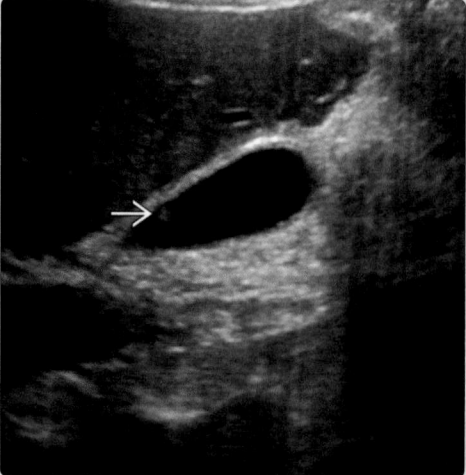
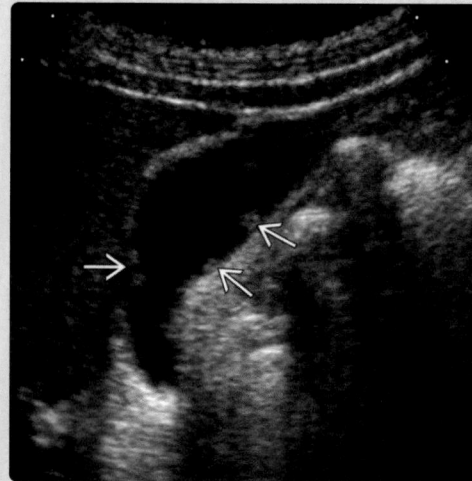

(Left) *Longitudinal ultrasound in the left lateral decubitus position shows a small polyp* ➡ *with no retraction of the adjacent wall.* (Right) *Longitudinal ultrasound in the left lateral decubitus position shows multiple small, smooth mural polyps* ➡.

Gallblabber Cholesterol Polyp

TERMINOLOGY

Synonyms

- Focal gallbladder (GB) cholesterosis, polypoid cholesterosis

Definitions

- Abnormal deposit of cholesterol ester producing villous-like structure covered with single layer of epithelium and attached via delicate stalk

IMAGING

General Features

- Best diagnostic clue
  - Multiple, small, nonshadowing lesions attached to gallbladder wall
- Location
  - Anywhere on GB wall
  - Most commonly in middle 1/3 of gallbladder
- Size
  - Usually 2-10 mm
- Morphology
  - Well-circumscribed, ovoid/round in configuration

Ultrasonographic Findings

- Grayscale ultrasound
  - Polypoidal mass arising from GB wall
    - Small, usually in range of 2-10 mm
    - Single or multiple
    - Medium- to high-level internal echoes
    - Smooth in contour, sometimes multilobulated outline
    - Round or ovoid shape, narrow base with gallbladder wall
    - Does not cast posterior acoustic shadow (vs. gallstone)
    - Not mobile on changing position (vs. biliary sludge)
    - Overlying GB wall is intact & normal
    - No invasion of adjacent liver parenchyma or regional nodal metastases
  - Variant US appearances
    - Large size: Lesions up to 20 mm have been described
      □ Fine pattern of echogenic foci, best seen with endoscopic ultrasound
    - Pedunculated with well-defined stalk from GB wall
- Power Doppler
  - Avascular or hypovascular on Doppler examination
  - Larger lesions may have slight internal vascularity

CT Findings

- NECT
  - Small, soft tissue density nodule on GB wall
  - Intact GB wall
  - No calcification or fat component
- CECT
  - Mild enhancement
  - Multiplicity usually better assessed after IV contrast administration

MR Findings

- T1WI
  - Small, round nodule in GB wall
  - Homogeneous, intermediate signal intensity
- T2WI
  - Homogeneous, intermediate to low signal intensity
- T1WI C+ FS
  - Mild enhancement with normal wall
- MRCP
  - Low signal intensity filling defect attached to GB wall
  - Contrast with markedly hyperintense bile within GB lumen

Imaging Recommendations

- Best imaging tool
  - Transabdominal US is most sensitive technique for detecting small cholesterol polyps
    - Endoscopic ultrasound may supplement transabdominal US
- Protocol advice
  - Adequate fasting prior to US is essential for optimal study
  - Optimize resolution and set focal zone to level of GB mass to improve accuracy of mass characterization
  - Scan in supine, decubitus (left > right lateral) positions to demonstrate immobility of GB polyp
  - Management algorithm for incidental polypoid GB mass
    - < 6 mm: No follow-up
    - 7-9 mm: Yearly US follow-up to monitor size
    - > 10 mm: Surgical consult
  - Further evaluation with CECT or enhanced MR for atypical features or proceed to surgery

DIFFERENTIAL DIAGNOSIS

Hyperplastic Cholecystosis/Adenomyomatosis

- Focal (fundal) form
  - Smooth, sessile mass in fundal region or mid body "waisting"
  - "Comet tail" artifacts from GB wall

Nonshadowing Cholelithiasis

- Highly echogenic
- Mobile and gravity dependent
- Note: Up to 20% of resected polyps represent stones stuck to gallbladder wall

Adenoma

- 4% of gallbladder polypoidal masses
- Solitary lesion
- Larger size (> 10 mm) but variable
- Usually pedunculated
- Color flow may be present; improved sensitivity using endoscopic ultrasound

Biliary Sludge

- Medium- to high-level echogenicity
- Mobile and gravity dependent
- Fluid sediment level
- No posterior acoustic shadowing

Inflammatory Polyp

- 5-10% of gallbladder polyps
- Multiple in 50% of cases
- Background of gallstone disease and chronic cholecystitis

Gallbladder Carcinoma

- Irregular soft tissue thickening of GB wall or mass
- Early noninvasive carcinoma may be homogeneous with broad base
- Evidence of invasion to adjacent liver parenchyma and regional nodal metastases
- Increased chaotic internal vascularity

GB Metastases

- Most common from melanoma and adenocarcinoma of GI origin
- Hyperechoic, broad-based polypoidal mass
- Usually > 10 mm in size
- Clinical history of known primary malignancy

PATHOLOGY

General Features

- Etiology
  - May be attributed to absorption of cholesterol from supersaturated bile
  - Does not predispose to cholecystitis or functional derangement
- Genetics
  - No documented genetic predisposition
- Associated abnormalities
  - Occasionally associated with cholelithiasis

Gross Pathologic & Surgical Features

- Multiple yellow nodules on cut sections
- Sessile/pedunculated smooth mucosal projections
- Intact mucosal surface
- GB wall is not thickened unless complicated or inflamed

Microscopic Features

- Focal accumulation of lipid-laden macrophages underneath normal columnar epithelium
- Fibrous stroma
- Infiltrated with variable degree of chronic inflammatory cells
- Intact mucosa with smooth projections
- No evidence of muscularis layers infiltration

CLINICAL ISSUES

Presentation

- Most common signs/symptoms
  - Asymptomatic, incidental finding on US for other purposes
- Other signs/symptoms
  - Mild nonspecific right upper abdominal discomfort

Demographics

- Age
  - More common in middle age
- Gender
  - M < F
- Epidemiology
  - 5% of population have polyps; 50% are cholesterol polyps
  - 6% of cholecystectomy specimens

Natural History & Prognosis

- No malignant potential
- No interval increase in size on serial follow-up US

Treatment

- Cholecystectomy only indicated if
  - Symptomatic
  - Associated with gallstones or cholecystitis
  - Risk factors for malignant polyp
    - Age > 50 years
    - Size > 10 mm (most malignant polyps > 10 mm)
    - Serial increase in size on follow-up US
    - Sessile morphology
    - Gallstones
    - Solitary lesion
    - Primary sclerosing cholangitis

DIAGNOSTIC CHECKLIST

Consider

- Consider neoplastic GB polyp if size > 10 mm, irregular outline, sessile morphology with abnormality of GB wall and invasion of adjacent structures, growth on serial US examinations
- Further evaluation with CECT or enhanced MR

Image Interpretation Pearls

- Multiple small, round/ovoid masses attached to GB wall with no posterior acoustic shadowing
- Easily differentiated from nonshadowing cholelithiasis or biliary sludge by demonstrating immobility of polyp

SELECTED REFERENCES

1. Sebastian S et al: Managing incidental findings on abdominal and pelvic CT and MRI, Part 4: white paper of the ACR Incidental Findings Committee II on gallbladder and biliary findings. J Am Coll Radiol. 10(12):953-6, 2013
2. Terada T: Histopathologic features and frequency of gall bladder lesions in consecutive 540 cholecystectomies. Int J Clin Exp Pathol. 6(1):91-6, 2013
3. Cairns V et al: Risk and Cost-effectiveness of Surveillance Followed by Cholecystectomy for Gallbladder Polyps. Arch Surg. 147(12):1078-83, 2012
4. Gallahan WC et al: Diagnosis and management of gallbladder polyps. Gastroenterol Clin North Am. 39(2):359-67, x, 2010
5. Chattopadhyay D et al: Outcome of gall bladder polypoidal lesions detected by transabdominal ultrasound scanning: a nine year experience. World J Gastroenterol. 11(14):2171-3, 2005
6. Sandri L et al: Gallbladder cholesterol polyps and cholesterolosis. Minerva Gastroenterol Dietol. 49(3):217-24, 2003
7. Sugiyama M et al: Endoscopic ultrasonography for differential diagnosis of polypoid gall bladder lesions: analysis in surgical and follow up series. Gut. 46(2):250-4, 2000

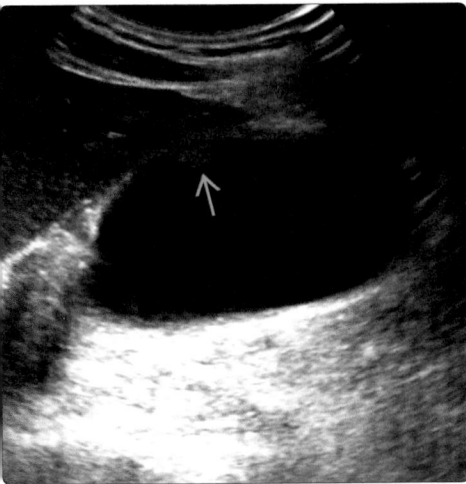

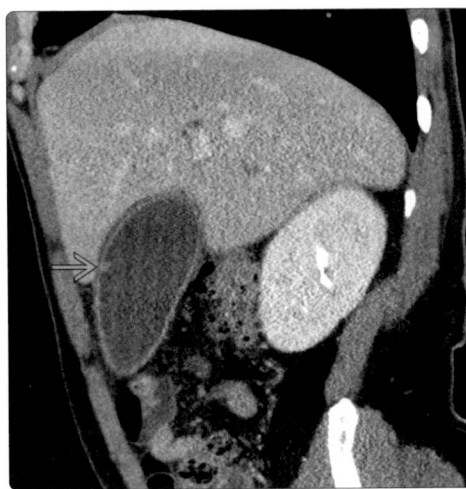

(Left) *Longitudinal left lateral decubitus ultrasound shows a cholesterol polyp with a normal gallbladder wall ➡.* (Right) *Sagittal CECT of the same patient at another time shows a cholesterol polyp ➡ with mild, nonspecific gallbladder wall thickening.*

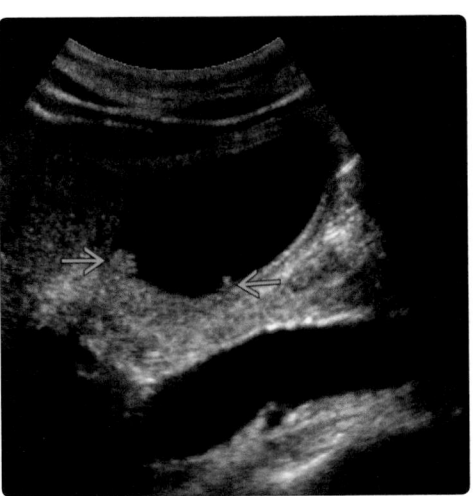

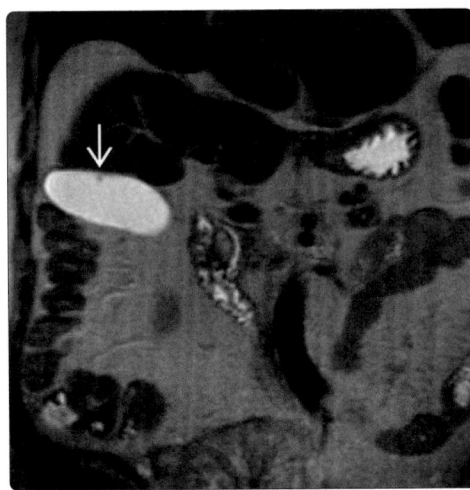

(Left) *Longitudinal ultrasound shows 2 small cholesterol polyps ➡. These were not mobile and did not shadow.* (Right) *Coronal T2 HASTE MR performed for a renal mass shows an incidental, tiny, low signal polyp ➡ with a normal gallbladder wall.*

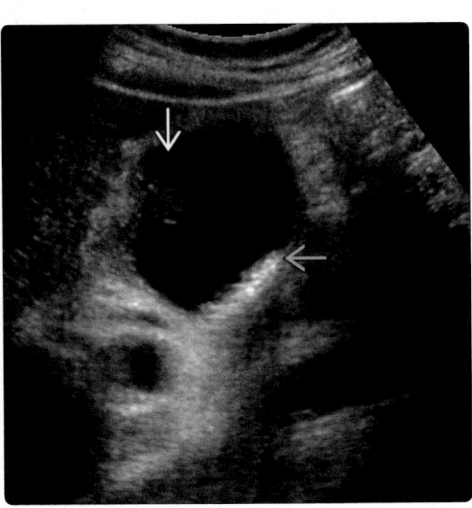

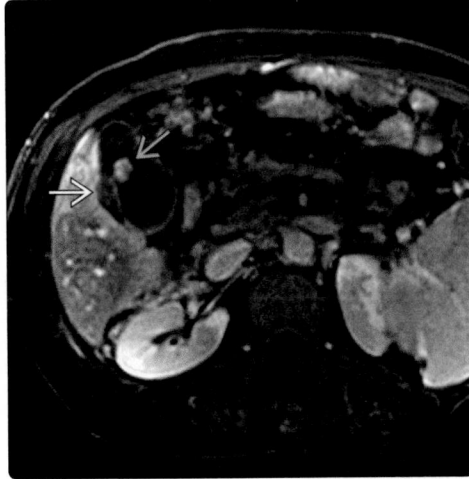

(Left) *Transverse ultrasound in a patient with cirrhosis shows a large, less echogenic polyp with a thin stalk ➡ and dependent shadowing gallstones ➡.* (Right) *Axial T1 C+ delayed phase MR of the same patient shows a smooth, enhancing gallbladder polyp ➡. The adjacent gallbladder wall was edematous ➡.*

TERMINOLOGY

- Acute inflammation of gallbladder (GB) secondary to calculus obstructing cystic duct

IMAGING

- Distended GB (> 5 cm transverse diameter)
- Gallstones ± impaction in GB neck or cystic duct
- Diffuse GB wall thickening (> 4-5 mm)
- Hazy delineation of GB wall with echogenic pericholecystic fat
- Positive sonographic Murphy sign: Pain and tenderness with transducer pressure directly over gallbladder
- US is first-line imaging tool
- HIDA after equivocal US, more sensitive than US
- CT and MR for complicated cholecystitis
- Gangrenous cholecystitis: Asymmetric wall thickening, marked wall irregularities, intraluminal membranes
- Gallbladder perforation: Defect in GB wall with pericholecystic abscess or extraluminal stones

- Emphysematous cholecystitis: Gas in GB wall/lumen
- Empyema of gallbladder: Highly reflective intraluminal echoes without shadowing, purulent exudate/debris
- Move patient to confirm impacted GB stone, assess Murphy sign and surrounding area

CLINICAL ISSUES

- May progress to gangrenous cholecystitis and perforation if untreated

DIAGNOSTIC CHECKLIST

- Combination of gallstones, wall thickening, and positive Murphy sign increase specificity
- Possibility of adjacent inflammatory disease such as perforated ulcer, acute hepatitis, or acute pancreatitis mimicking acute cholecystitis

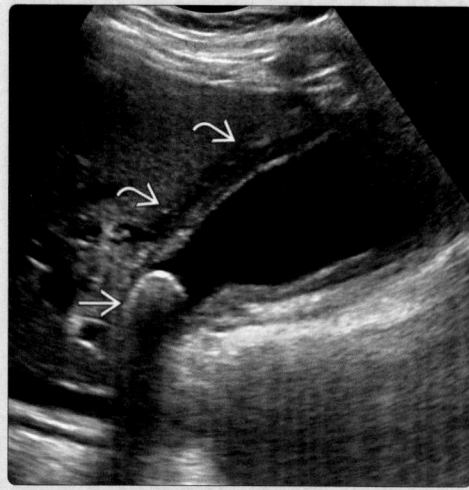 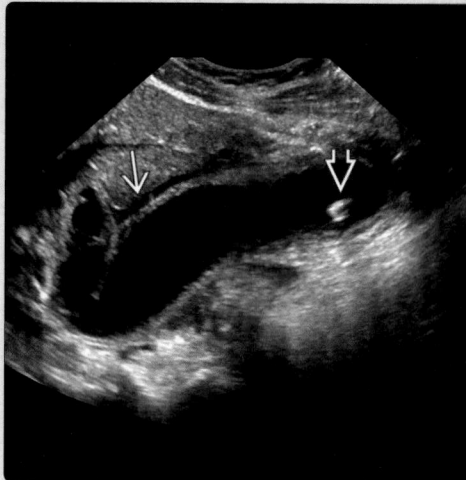

(Left) *Left lateral decubitus ultrasound shows a shadowing stone in the neck of the gallbladder* ➡. *Note the thick wall with subserosal edema* ➡. *Murphy sign was positive.* (Right) *Left lateral decubitus ultrasound shows a shadowing stone* ➡ *in the fundus of the gallbladder. Note the thick wall with subserosal edema* ➡.

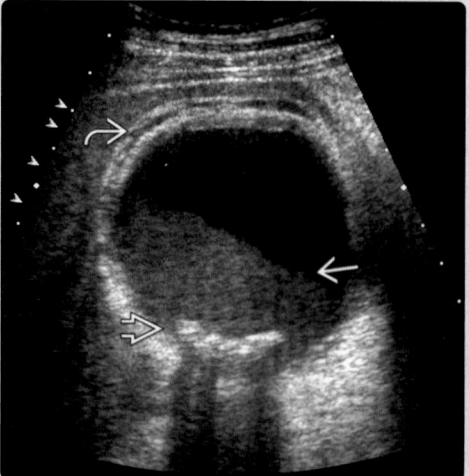 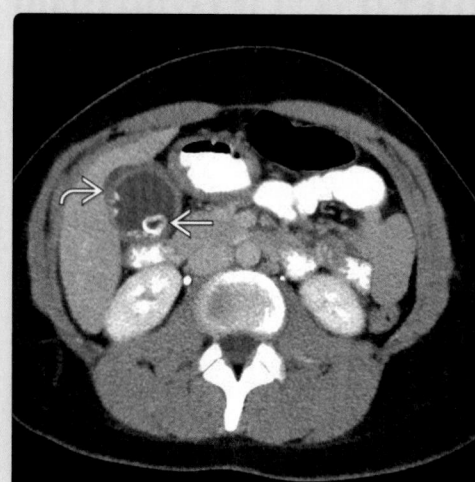

(Left) *Transverse ultrasound shows dependent shadowing gallstones* ➡ *with a sludge level* ➡. *Note the thickened gallbladder wall with a central hypoechoic halo* ➡. (Right) *Axial contrast-enhanced CT of acute calculous cholecystitis shows a thick-walled gallbladder* ➡ *containing calcified gallstones* ➡.

TERMINOLOGY

Abbreviations

- Acute cholecystitis

Definitions

- Acute inflammation of gallbladder (GB) secondary to calculus obstructing cystic duct

IMAGING

General Features

- Best diagnostic clue
  - Impacted gallstone in cystic duct
  - Gallbladder wall thickening
  - Positive sonographic Murphy sign
  - Pericholecystic collection
- Location
  - Stone impacted in GB neck or cystic duct
- Morphology
  - Distended GB is more rounded in shape than normal pear-shaped configuration

Ultrasonographic Findings

- Grayscale ultrasound
  - Uncomplicated cholecystitis
    - Gallstones ± impaction in GB neck or cystic duct
    - Diffuse GB wall thickening (> 4-5 mm)
      □ Variants: Uniform sonolucent middle layer (halo) or striated edema
    - Hazy delineation of GB wall with echogenic pericholecystic fat
    - Positive sonographic Murphy sign: Pain and tenderness with transducer pressure over gallbladder
    - GB distension with AP diameter > 5 cm
    - Sludge inside GB
  - Complicated cholecystitis
    - Gangrenous cholecystitis: Asymmetric wall thickening, marked wall irregularities, intraluminal membranes
    - Gallbladder perforation: Defect in GB wall with pericholecystic abscess or extraluminal stones
    - Emphysematous cholecystitis: Gas in GB wall/lumen
    - Empyema of gallbladder: Highly reflective intraluminal echoes without shadowing, purulent exudate/debris

Radiographic Findings

- Radiography
  - Insensitive for cholecystitis; 10-20% of stones are radiopaque
- ERCP
  - No filling of GB
  - Sharply defined filling defect in contrast-filled lumen of cystic duct

CT Findings

- CECT
  - Uncomplicated cholecystitis
    - Gallstones inside GB neck or cystic duct
    - GB wall thickening with subserosal edema
    - Increased mural enhancement
    - Pericholecystic fat stranding, pericholecystic fluid
    - Regional hepatic hyperemia
  - Complicated cholecystitis
    - Decreased or absent enhancement
    - Discontinuous wall thickening with intramural or pericholecystic abscesses
    - Gas in lumen &/or wall of GB
    - High attenuation in GB lumen from hemorrhage/pus or membranes

MR Findings

- T1WI
  - Hyperintense sludge or hemorrhage in GB
- T2WI
  - Uncomplicated cholecystitis
    - Distended GB
    - Lower signal stones and sludge
    - High signal in thickened wall and pericholecystic tissues
  - Complicated cholecystitis
    - Discontinuous wall thickening with intramural or pericholecystic abscesses
- T1WI C+
  - Decreased or absent enhancement in complicated cholecystitis
- MRCP
  - Low signal obstructing stone

Nuclear Medicine Findings

- Hepatobiliary scan
  - Tc-99m iminodiacetic acid derivatives
  - Nonvisualization of GB at 4 hours has 96% specificity
  - Increased uptake in gallbladder fossa during arterial phase due to hyperemia in 80% of patients
  - "Rim" sign seen in 34% of patients is due to increased uptake in gallbladder fossa

Imaging Recommendations

- Best imaging tool
  - US is first-line
  - HIDA after equivocal US, more sensitive than US
  - CT and MR for complicated cholecystitis
- Protocol advice
  - Move patient to confirm impacted GB stone, assess Murphy sign and surrounding area

DIFFERENTIAL DIAGNOSIS

Acute Acalculous Cholecystitis

- Signs of acute cholecystitis without gallstones
- Systemic illness, sepsis

Nonspecific Gallbladder Wall Thickening

- Negative sonographic Murphy sign
- Stones may be present
- Clinical evidence of underlying etiology: Congestive heart failure, hypoalbuminemia, cirrhosis, regional inflammation such as hepatitis, pancreatitis

Gallbladder Sludge/Echogenic Bile

- Nonshadowing
- No GB wall thickening or pericholecystic collection
- Negative sonographic Murphy sign

Gallbladder Carcinoma

- Wall thickening more irregular
- Soft tissue mass ± extension beyond GB
- Associated with gall stones

Hyperplastic Cholecystosis

- "Comet tail" artifacts from thick wall, no tenderness

PATHOLOGY

General Features

- Etiology
  - 85-95% of acute cholecystitis due to calculous cholecystitis (5-15% acalculous)
    - Obstructing stone in cystic duct
- Genetics
  - Increased incidence of gallstones in selected population
    - Hispanics, Pima Native Americans

Staging, Grading, & Classification

- Nonperforated
  - GB wall intact
- Gangrenous
  - Shaggy, irregular, asymmetric wall (mucosal ulcers, intraluminal hemorrhage, necrosis)
  - Intraluminal pseudomembranes
- Perforated
  - GB wall defect
  - Gallstone lying free in peritoneal cavity
  - Abscess surrounding GB or in liver

Gross Pathologic & Surgical Features

- Gallstones in gallbladder neck or cystic duct
- Thickened GB wall with hyperemia of wall
- Omental adhesions
- Vascular compromise from increased GB pressure leads to ischemia

Microscopic Features

- Lumen: Gallstones, sludge
- GB mucosa: Ulcerations
- GB wall: Acute polymorphonuclear infiltration
- Bacterial cultures positive in 40-70% of patients

CLINICAL ISSUES

Presentation

- Most common signs/symptoms
  - Acute RUQ pain
  - Fever, nausea, vomiting, anorexia
- Other signs/symptoms
  - Positive Murphy sign
- Clinical profile
  - Increased WBC
  - May have mild elevation in liver enzymes

Demographics

- Age
  - Typically > 25 years
- Gender
  - M:F = 1:3
- Epidemiology
  - Incidence parallels prevalence of gallstones

Natural History & Prognosis

- May progress to gangrenous cholecystitis and perforation if ischemia develops
- Excellent prognosis in uncomplicated cases or with prompt surgery
- Complications
  - Mirizzi syndrome: Stone in cystic duct causing common bile duct obstruction
  - Gallstone ileus: In chronic cholecystis, gallstone erodes into bowel and causes small bowel obstruction
  - Bouveret syndrome: Gallstone erodes into duodenum leading to duodenal obstruction

Treatment

- Prompt cholecystectomy
  - Laparoscopic surgery for uncomplicated cases
- Percutaneous cholecystostomy
  - Useful for poor operative risk patients with GB empyema
- Percutaneous drainage
  - For localized pericholecystic or intrahepatic abscesses

DIAGNOSTIC CHECKLIST

Consider

- Possibility of adjacent inflammatory disease such as perforated ulcer, acute hepatitis, or acute pancreatitis mimicking acute cholecystitis

Image Interpretation Pearls

- Stone impacted in cystic duct
- Diffuse GB wall thickening, distension, and pericholecystic fluid
- Combination of gallstones, wall thickening, and positive Murphy sign increase specificity
- Sonographic Murphy sign must be unequivocal to be considered positive

SELECTED REFERENCES

1. Knab LM et al: Cholecystitis. Surg Clin North Am. 94(2):455-70, 2014
2. Duncan CB et al: Evidence-based current surgical practice: calculous gallbladder disease. J Gastrointest Surg. 16(11):2011-25, 2012
3. Kiewiet JJ et al: A systematic review and meta-analysis of diagnostic performance of imaging in acute cholecystitis. Radiology. 264(3):708-20, 2012
4. Charalel RA et al: Complicated cholecystitis: the complementary roles of sonography and computed tomography. Ultrasound Q. 27(3):161-70, 2011
5. Gore RM et al: Gallbladder imaging. Gastroenterol Clin North Am. 39(2):265-87, ix, 2010
6. Smith EA et al: Cross-sectional imaging of acute and chronic gallbladder inflammatory disease. AJR Am J Roentgenol. 192(1):188-96, 2009
7. Catalano OA et al: MR imaging of the gallbladder: a pictorial essay. Radiographics. 28(1):135-55; quiz 324, 2008
8. Hanbidge AE et al: From the RSNA refresher courses: imaging evaluation for acute pain in the right upper quadrant. Radiographics. 24(4):1117-35, 2004

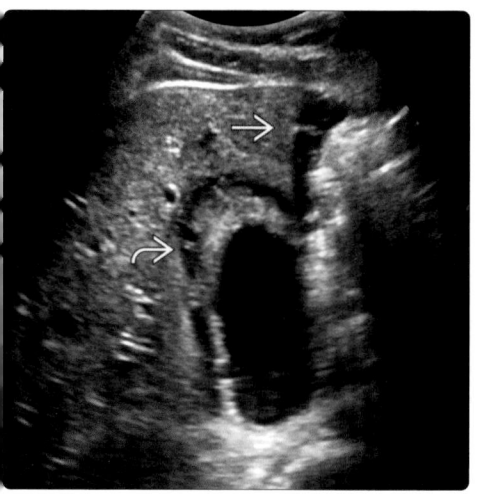
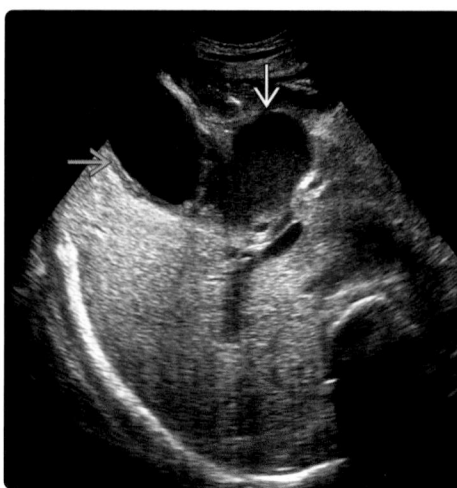

(Left) *Supine transverse ultrasound shows a thickened edematous gallbladder wall ➡ with dependent sludge (stones not shown). Note the complex fluid medial to the liver ➡.* (Right) *Transverse ultrasound of perforated acute cholecystitis. There is a collection with low-level echoes (abscess) ➡ medial to the thick-walled gallbladder ➡.*

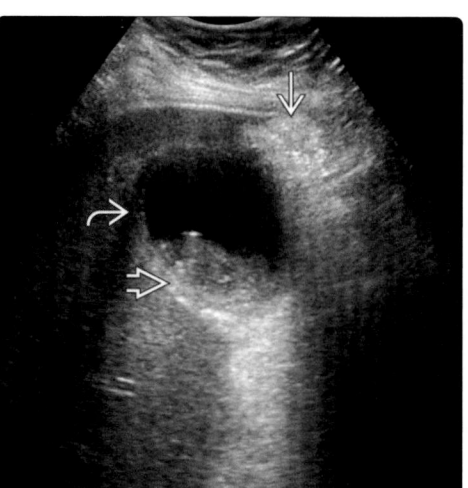
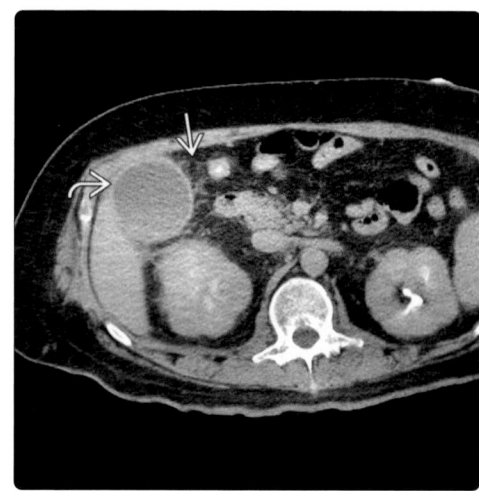

(Left) *Transverse ultrasound of acute cholecystitis shows dependent gallstones and sludge ➡. Note wall thickening ➡ and inflamed echogenic fat medially ➡.* (Right) *Axial CECT of the same patient shows a distended, thick-walled gallbladder ➡ with dependent stones and sludge. Note the inflammatory stranding in the pericholecystic fat ➡.*

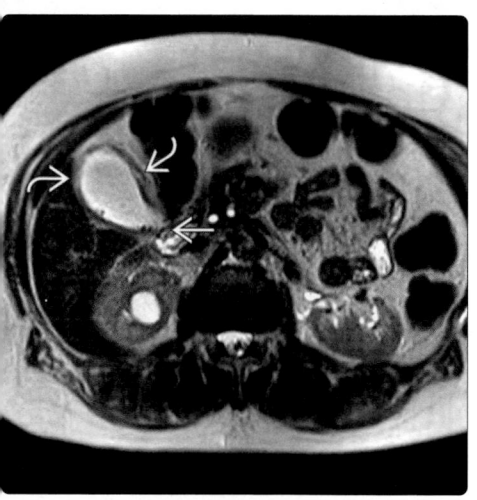
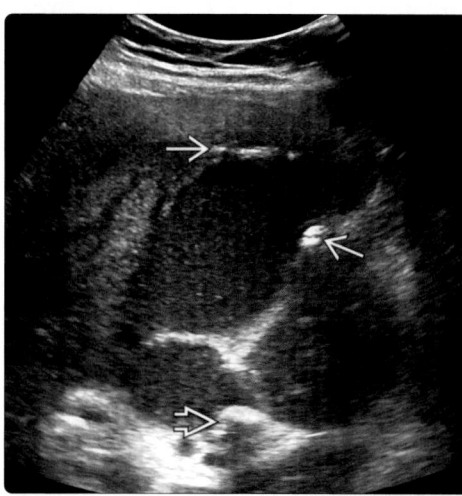

(Left) *Axial T2 HASTE MR in a patient with acute calculous cholecystitis shows multiple small gallstones ➡ and intramural edema ➡.* (Right) *Longitudinal oblique ultrasound in a patient with emphysematous acute cholecystitis shows that the gallbladder is distended and sludge-filled with an impacted gallstone ➡. Bright intramural echoes represent gas ➡.*

Acute Acalculous Cholecystitis

TERMINOLOGY

- Acute necroinflammatory disease of gallbladder (GB) not related to gallstone

IMAGING

- GB wall thickening (> 4 mm)
- Hypoechoic, layered/striated appearance
- GB distension
- Positive sonographic Murphy sign
- Critical illness with sepsis, shock, recent surgery, trauma, or burns
- Sonographic Murphy sign may not be elicited in patient who is obtunded, unconscious, or sedated
- US is first-line
- HIDA for indeterminate ultrasound
- CT for complications

TOP DIFFERENTIAL DIAGNOSES

- Acute calculous cholecystitis
- Sympathetic GB wall thickening
- Hyperplastic cholecystosis
- Gallbladder mucocele

PATHOLOGY

- More commonly seen in critically ill patients with multiple risk factors
- Acalculous cholecystitis constitutes ~ 10% of acute cholecystitis
- Pathogenesis is multifactorial
- Combination of Increased bile viscosity and wall Ischemia

CLINICAL ISSUES

- Worse prognosis than acute calculous cholecystitis
- 40% develop complications such as gangrene, perforation, and empyema
- Mortality rate up to 30%

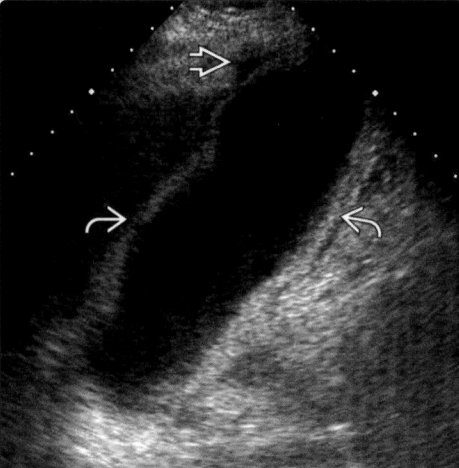
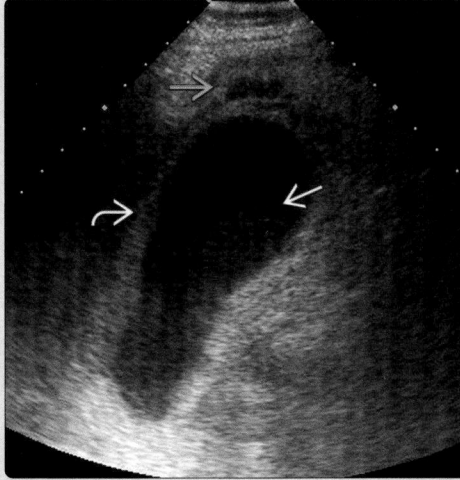

(Left) *Longitudinal oblique ultrasound of acalculous cholecystitis shows that the gallbladder is distended with sludge and wall thickening ➡. A small amount of pericholecystic fluid ➡ and no gallstones are noted.* (Right) *Left lateral decubitus ultrasound of acalculous cholecystitis shows sludge ➡, wall thickening ➡, and a pericholecystic collection ➡. No gallstones were found.*

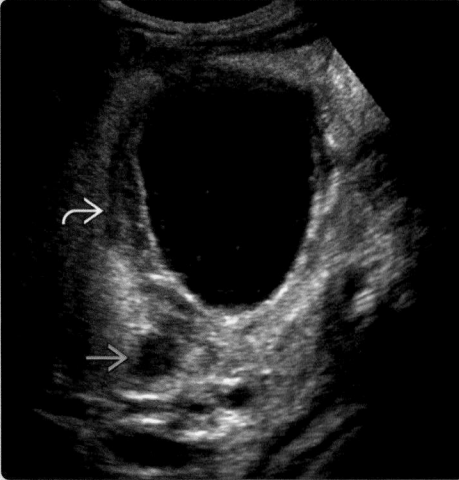
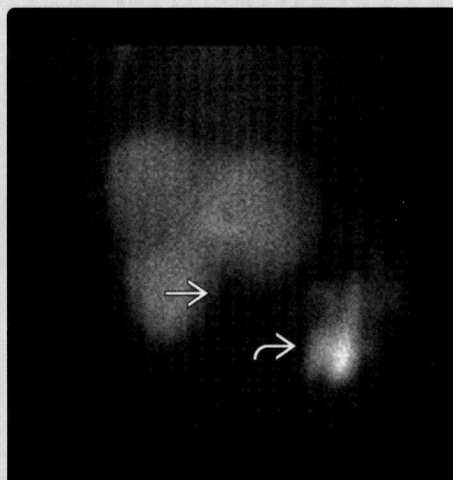

(Left) *Transverse ultrasound of perforated acalculous cholecystitis shows an irregularly thickened gallbladder wall ➡ with intramural edema. There is localized pericholecystic fluid ➡ with an abscess that is not shown.* (Right) *A 4-hour image from a HIDA scan in a patient with acalculous cholecystitis shows lack of activity in the gallbladder fossa ➡. Activity is seen in small bowel ➡.*

TERMINOLOGY

Definitions

- Acute necroinflammatory disease of gallbladder (GB) not related to gallstone
  - Usually secondary to stasis of bile and ischemia

IMAGING

General Features

- Best diagnostic clue
  - Gallbladder wall thickening without impacted gallstone
  - Positive sonographic Murphy sign
  - Critical illness with sepsis, shock, recent surgery, trauma, or burns

Ultrasonographic Findings

- Grayscale ultrasound
  - US features of acute acalculous cholecystitis are similar to acute calculous cholecystitis except for absence of impacted gallstone
  - GB wall thickening (> 4 mm)
    - Hypoechoic, layered/striated appearance
  - GB distension
    - Commonly filled with sludge
    - Hydrops; GB measuring > 8 cm longitudinally and > 5 cm transversely with anechoic bile
  - Pericholecystic fluid collection
  - Positive sonographic Murphy sign
    - Sonographic Murphy sign may not be elicited in patient who is obtunded, unconscious, or sedated
  - Complication
    - Gangrenous cholecystitis
      □ Irregular/asymmetric GB wall thickening
      □ Look for discontinuity of the wall and loss of echogenicity
      □ Intraluminal membranes and echogenic material due to sloughed mucosa
    - GB perforation
      □ Collapsed GB; wall defect with adjacent heterogeneous hypoechoic fluid collection
      □ Most common at fundus
- Color Doppler
  - Hyperemia within thickened/inflamed GB wall
    - Absent in gangrenous cholecystitis

CT Findings

- NECT
  - Distended GB with pericholecystic inflammation ± high-density sludge or hemorrhage
- CECT
  - Distended GB with hyperemic wall thickening and pericholecystic fat stranding
    - Wall may be discontinuous and poorly enhancing in setting of gangrene
  - Complications
    - Pericholecystic collection/abscess
    - Gas in gallbladder wall or lumen

MR Findings

- T1WI
  - High signal intensity luminal sludge
- T2WI
  - Distended GB
  - Intraluminal lower signal from sludge or pus
  - Thick wall with increased T2 signal
  - Complications
    - Pericholecystic collection/abscess
    - Irregular or asymmetric wall thickening
- T2WI FS
  - Increased signal in pericholecystic fat
  - Pericholecystic and perihepatic fluid
- T1WI C+
  - "Rim" sign of increased hepatic enhancement
  - Inhomogeneous or absent wall enhancement when gangrenous

Nonvascular Interventions

- Percutaneous cholecystostomy with bile aspiration and culture to confirm diagnosis in patients with no source for sepsis
- Bridge to cholecystectomy
- Catheter left in place for at least 3 weeks

Nuclear Medicine Findings

- Tc-99m iminodiacetic acid derivatives (HIDA) scan detects functional cystic duct obstruction
- Sensitivity 30-100%, specificity 89-100%
- Nonvisualized gallbladder at 4 hours or nonvisualized gallbladder at 90 minutes using morphine augmentation
- Less sensitive than in acute calculous cholecystitis, however useful adjunct to indeterminate ultrasound
- False-negatives: Infected nonobstructed gallbladder
- False-positives: Poor hepatic function, fasting, total parenteral nutrition

Imaging Recommendations

- Best imaging tool
  - US is first-line
  - HIDA for indeterminate ultrasound
  - CT for complications

DIFFERENTIAL DIAGNOSIS

Acute Calculous Cholecystitis

- US features similar to acalculous cholecystitis
- Presence of impacted gallstone

Sympathetic GB Wall Thickening

- Smooth wall thickening ± sludge
- Negative Murphy sign
- Clinically not septic
  - Multiple underlying causes such as hypoalbuminemia, cirrhosis, congestive heart failure, acute hepatitis or pancreatitis

Hyperplastic Cholecystosis

- Focal (fundal/mid body) or diffuse GB wall thickening
- "Comet tail" artifacts
- Intramural cystic spaces

Gallbladder Mucocele

- Distended gallbladder secondary to chronic obstructing stone
- Noninflammatory condition with minimal pain/tenderness

- Anechoic or low-level echoes in lumen from bile or mucus
- Nonthickened wall

PATHOLOGY

General Features

- Etiology
  - Acalculous cholecystitis constitutes ~ 10% of acute cholecystitis
  - Pathogenesis is multifactorial
    - Combination of increased bile viscosity and wall ischemia with reperfusion injury
      - Bile stasis secondary to fasting, obstruction, surgery, or procedures irritates gallbladder epithelium
      - Ischemia from systemic hypotension, shock, trauma, recent surgery, sepsis, burns, vasculitis
  - Occurs in critically ill patients with multiple risk factors
    - Post major surgery, severe trauma, sepsis, diabetes, atherosclerotic disease, TPN
    - Infection: Bacterial, viral, fungal, parasitic (opportunistic GB infection in AIDS)
    - Obstruction of cystic duct by extrinsic compression by metastases, lymphadenopathy

Gross Pathologic & Surgical Features

- Bile cultures positive in up to 78%, gram-negative bacilli most common

Microscopic Features

- Ischemia and reperfusion injury
- Increased and deeper bile infiltration into gallbladder wall
- Necrosis, leucocyte infiltration, lymphatic dilation

CLINICAL ISSUES

Presentation

- Most common signs/symptoms
  - Acute RUQ pain, fever, sepsis in critically ill patient
- Other signs/symptoms
  - Nonspecific leucocytosis, elevation of liver function tests
- Clinical profile
  - Raised WBC, abnormal liver function tests
- Diagnosis may be challenging in critically ill patient with multiple comorbidities

Demographics

- Age
  - More common in middle-aged and elderly
- Gender
  - M:F = 3:1
- Epidemiology
  - 0.2-0.4 % of critically ill patients

Natural History & Prognosis

- Worse prognosis than acute calculous cholecystitis
- 40% develop complications such as gangrene, perforation, and empyema
- Mortality rate up to 30%

Treatment

- Prompt cholecystectomy is standard if patient is surgical candidate
- Percutaneous cholecystostomy
  - Useful in poor operative risk patients, in combination with antibiotics
  - May be diagnostic (bile obtained for culture) and therapeutic
  - Not indicated for gangrenous gallbladders
  - Requires cholangiography to exclude bile duct stones and obstruction prior to removal of cholecystostomy tube
- Percutaneous drainage of pericholecystic fluid collections

DIAGNOSTIC CHECKLIST

Consider

- Ultrasound is first-line modality given portability, rapidity, and repeatability
- Consider diagnosis when US features of acute cholecystitis without impacted gallstone
  - High index of suspicion in critically ill patients
  - Repeat ultrasound for indeterminate cases
    - Or HIDA scan

Image Interpretation Pearls

- Confirm with HIDA scan
  - Limitations of HIDA: Lengthy, requires transportation of patient
- Assess for complications such as gangrene or perforation
  - CT more sensitive for complications or alternative diagnoses

SELECTED REFERENCES

1. Atar E et al: Percutaneous cholecystostomy in critically ill patients with acute cholecystitis: complications and late outcome. Clin Radiol. 69(6):e247-52, 2014
2. Charalel RA et al: Complicated cholecystitis: the complementary roles of sonography and computed tomography. Ultrasound Q. 27(3):161-70, 2011
3. Gore RM et al: Gallbladder imaging. Gastroenterol Clin North Am. 39(2):265-87, ix, 2010
4. Huffman JL et al: Acute acalculous cholecystitis: a review. Clin Gastroenterol Hepatol. 8(1):15-22, 2010
5. Ziessman HA: Nuclear medicine hepatobiliary imaging. Clin Gastroenterol Hepatol. 8(2):111-6, 2010
6. Smith EA et al: Cross-sectional imaging of acute and chronic gallbladder inflammatory disease. AJR Am J Roentgenol. 192(1):188-96, 2009
7. van Breda Vriesman AC et al: Diffuse gallbladder wall thickening: differential diagnosis. AJR Am J Roentgenol. 188(2):495-501, 2007
8. Hanbidge AE et al: From the RSNA refresher courses: imaging evaluation for acute pain in the right upper quadrant. Radiographics. 24(4):1117-35, 2004

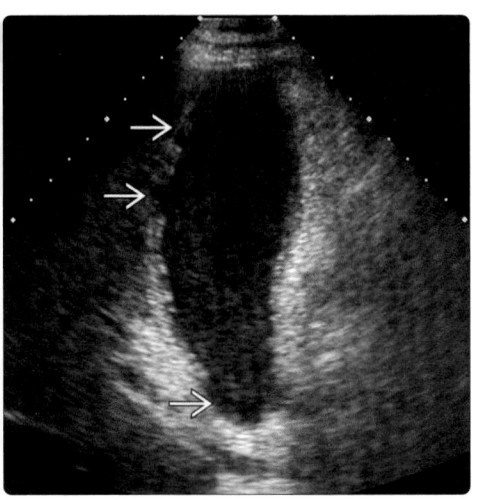

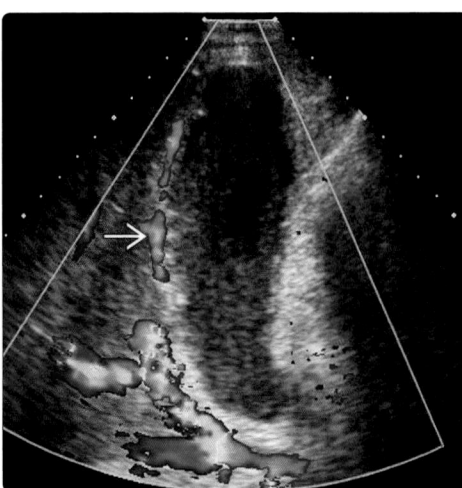

(Left) *Longitudinal oblique ultrasound of acute acalculous cholecystis with gangrene in a lung transplant recipient shows gallbladder distension with viscous sludge. The wall is thick and discontinuous* ➡. *(Right) Longitudinal oblique ultrasound of the same patient shows hyperemia around the gallbladder* ➡ *with no color flow in the necrotic wall.*

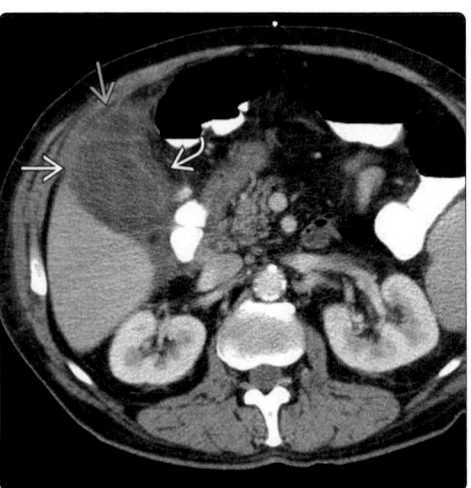

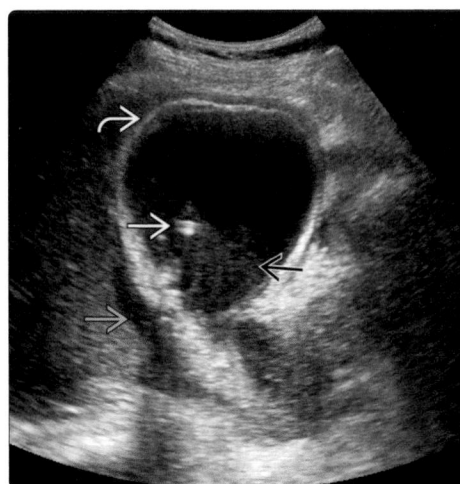

(Left) *Axial CECT of acute acalculous cholecystitis shows a distended, thick-walled gallbladder* ➡ *with fluid and inflammation in the pericholecystic fat* ➡. *Note the poor enhancement of the fundal wall* ➡. *(Right) Transverse ultrasound of acalculous cholecystitis shows sludge* ➡, *wall thickening* ➡, *and percutaneous cholecystostomy tube* ➡. *Pericholecystic fluid* ➡ *is noted.*

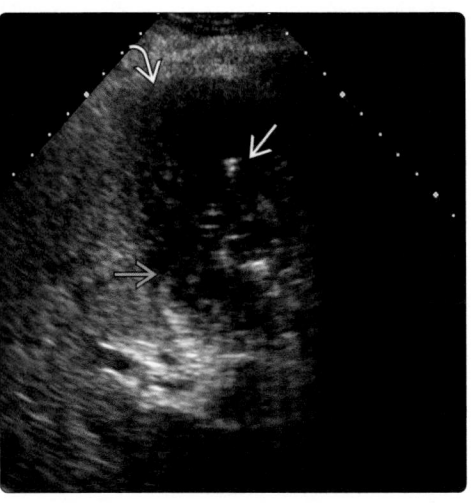

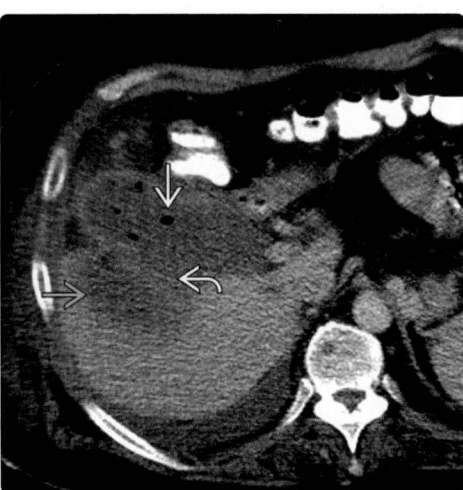

(Left) *Transverse ultrasound of acute emphysematous cholecystitis with perforation shows that the gallbladder wall* ➡ *is disrupted with loss of echogenic mucosal line. There is gas in the lumen* ➡ *and a pericholecystic collection* ➡. *(Right) Axial CECT of the same patient shows acute emphysematous cholecystitis with perforation. The gallbladder wall* ➡ *is focally disrupted. There is gas in the lumen* ➡ *and a pericholecystic collection containing gas* ➡.

Chronic Cholecystitis

TERMINOLOGY

- Chronic inflammation of (GB) gallbladder causing wall thickening and fibrosis

IMAGING

- Diffuse GB wall thickening, ± contraction
- Presence of gallstones in nearly all cases
- Pericholecystic inflammation usually absent
- No increased flow within thickened gallbladder wall
- US is initial imaging tool but is nonspecific
- Clinical history is critical

TOP DIFFERENTIAL DIAGNOSES

- Sympathetic/reactive GB wall thickening
- Adenomyomatosis of gallbladder
- Gallbladder carcinoma

PATHOLOGY

- Most common pathology of gallbladder

- 95% associated with gallstone disease
- Intermittent obstruction of cystic duct causes chronic inflammatory infiltration of wall, which can lead to fibrosis and contraction

CLINICAL ISSUES

- Seen in same population as gallstone disease (i.e., female < male, middle age, obesity, etc.)
- Good prognosis with minimal symptoms
- Complications include acute cholecystitis, gallbladder carcinoma, and rarely, biliary-enteric fistula

DIAGNOSTIC CHECKLIST

- Thick-walled gallbladder
- Gallstones
- No pericholecystic fluid
- Clinical history of recurrent biliary colic with typical US findings is diagnostic

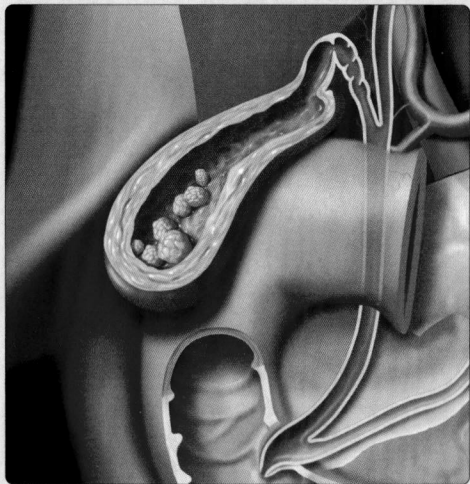

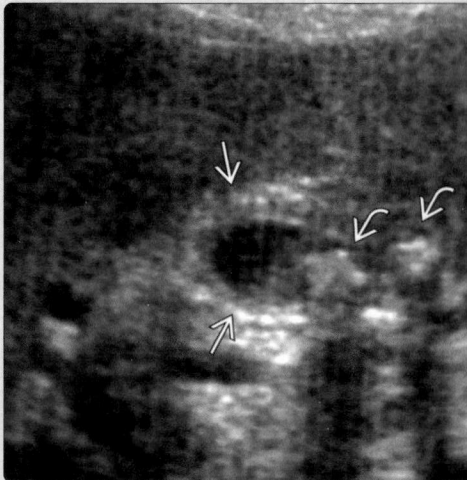

(Left) *Graphic shows multiple gallstones inside a contracted thick-walled gallbladder (GB), characteristic features of chronic cholecystitis.* (Right) *A contracted gallbladder is shown with diffuse wall thickening ➡ and shadowing gallstones ⬈. Note the absence of pericholecystic free fluid.*

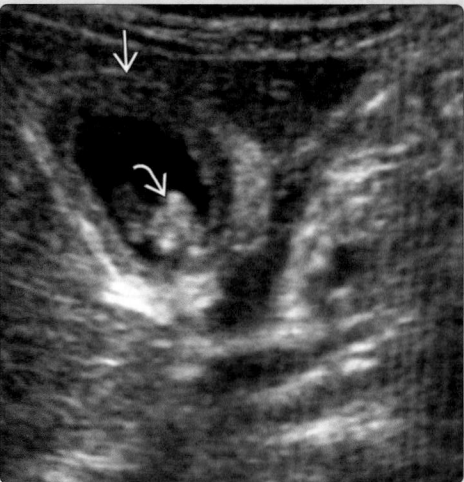

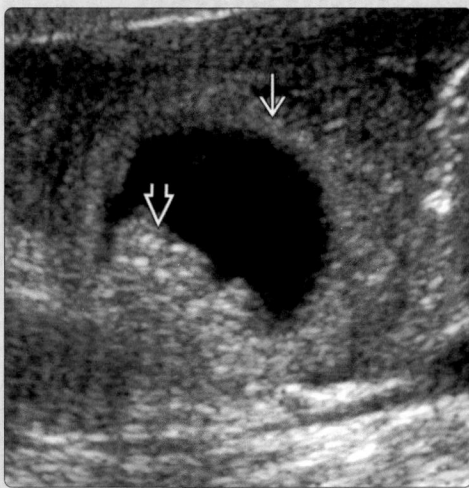

(Left) *Transverse transabdominal ultrasound shows a GB with diffuse wall thickening ➡ containing an echogenic sludge ball and nonshadowing gallstones ⬈.* (Right) *Transverse transabdominal ultrasound shows diffuse wall thickening ➡ within the contracted gallbladder. Note the presence of echogenic sludge and stones ➡ within the GB.*

TERMINOLOGY

Definitions

- Chronic inflammation of gallbladder (GB) causing wall thickening and fibrosis, following single or recurrent episodes of cystic duct obstruction

IMAGING

General Features

- Best diagnostic clue
  - Gallbladder wall thickening with gallstones, ± contraction
  - Absence of acute inflammation

Ultrasonographic Findings

- Grayscale ultrasound
  - Diffuse GB wall thickening, echogenic wall
  - Presence of gallstones in nearly all cases
  - Pericholecystic inflammation usually absent
  - Typically contracted but may be distended
    - When contracted, contraction persists in fasting state
- Power Doppler
  - No increased flow within thickened gallbladder wall

Nuclear Medicine Findings

- Hepatobiliary scintigraphy
  - Delayed GB visualization (up to 2-4 hours)
  - Visualization of bowel activity prior to GB activity
  - Dysmotility (ejection fraction < 35% after cholecystokinin)
  - Distinguishes acute from chronic cholecystitis

Imaging Recommendations

- Best imaging tool
  - US is initial imaging tool but is nonspecific
  - Clinical history is critical
- Protocol advice
  - Ensure adequate fasting (> 6 hours) prior to US examination to avoid false-positive contraction
  - Examine patient in multiple planes/positions to detect gallstone in severely contracted GB

DIFFERENTIAL DIAGNOSIS

Sympathetic/Reactive GB Wall Thickening

- Known underlying causes (e.g., hypoalbuminemia, cirrhosis, CHF) usually detected clinically
- Smooth hypoechoic wall thickening ± linear striations

Adenomyomatosis of Gallbladder

- "Comet tail" artifacts
- More commonly affects fundus or mid GB with focal thickening rather than diffuse involvement

Gallbladder Carcinoma

- Ill-defined infiltrative wall thickening/mass
- Invasion of adjacent liver parenchyma and regional nodal metastases

PATHOLOGY

General Features

- Etiology
  - Most common pathology of gallbladder
  - 95% associated with gallstone disease
  - Intermittent obstruction of cystic duct causes chronic low-grade inflammatory infiltration of wall, which can lead to fibrosis and contraction

Microscopic Features

- Often associated with acute cholecystitis

CLINICAL ISSUES

Presentation

- Most common signs/symptoms
  - Mostly asymptomatic
  - Mild RUQ pain/discomfort after meal
  - Recurrent acute cholecystitis or biliary colic

Demographics

- Epidemiology
  - Same as gallstone disease (i.e., female < male, age > 40, obesity, etc.)

Natural History & Prognosis

- Good prognosis with minimal symptoms
- Complications include acute cholecystitis, gallbladder carcinoma, and rarely, biliary-enteric fistula

Treatment

- Cholecystectomy in symptomatic cases or complication of acute cholecystitis

DIAGNOSTIC CHECKLIST

Image Interpretation Pearls

- Gallstones within thick-walled GB
- No pericholecystic fluid
- Lack of hyperemia in thickened gallbladder wall

SELECTED REFERENCES

1. Bennett GL. Cholelithiasis, cholecystitis, choledocholithiasis, and hyperplastic cholecystoses. In: Gore RM et al. Textbook of Gastrointestinal Radiology. 4th ed. Philadelphia: Saunders Elsevier, 2015
2. Knab LM et al: Cholecystitis. Surg Clin North Am. 94(2):455-70, 2014
3. Seretis C et al: Metaplastic changes in chronic cholecystitis: implications for early diagnosis and surgical intervention to prevent the gallbladder metaplasia-dysplasia-carcinoma sequence. J Clin Med Res. 6(1):26-9, 2014
4. O'Connor OJ et al: Imaging of cholecystitis. AJR Am J Roentgenol. 196(4):W367-74, 2011
5. Wang DQH et al. Gallstone disease. In: Feldman M et al. Sleisenger and Fordtran's Gastrointestinal and Liver Disease. 9th ed. Philadelphia: Saunders Elsevier, 2010
6. Smith EA et al: Cross-sectional imaging of acute and chronic gallbladder inflammatory disease. AJR Am J Roentgenol. 192(1):188-96, 2009
7. Catalano OA et al: MR imaging of the gallbladder: a pictorial essay. Radiographics. 28(1):135-55; quiz 324, 2008
8. van Breda Vriesman AC et al: Diffuse gallbladder wall thickening: differential diagnosis. AJR Am J Roentgenol. 188(2):495-501, 2007
9. Schiller VL et al: Color doppler imaging of the gallbladder wall in acute cholecystitis: sonographic-pathologic correlation. Abdom Imaging. 21(3):233-7, 1996
10. Lack EE. Cholecystitis, cholelithiasis, and unusual infections of the gallbladder. In: Lack EE. Pathology of the Pancreas, Gallbladder, Extrahepatic Biliary tract, and Ampullary Region. New York: Oxford University Press, 2003

Xanthogranulomatous Cholecystitis

TERMINOLOGY

- Uncommon destructive variant of chronic cholecystitis characterized by lipid-laden inflammation

IMAGING

- US findings
  - Marked GB wall thickening
  - Intramural hypoechoic nodules or bands
    - Nodular areas of foamy inflammatory cells or necrosis/abscess
  - Continuous mucosal line
  - Absence of hepatic invasion
  - Absence of biliary dilation
  - Gallstones
- When infiltrative with involvement of adjacent organs and surrounding fat/soft tissue obliterating the normal margins, preoperative differentiation from GB carcinoma nearly impossible

TOP DIFFERENTIAL DIAGNOSES

- Gallbladder carcinoma
- Gangrenous cholecystitis
- Hyperplastic cholecystoses

CLINICAL ISSUES

- Typical symptoms of acute cholecystitis
- Treatment: Open cholecystectomy
- Can coexist with gallbladder carcinoma (adenocarcinoma seen in up to 10% of resected specimens)

DIAGNOSTIC CHECKLIST

- Difficult to distinguish from GB carcinoma preoperatively but can be suggested based on imaging findings
- With preoperative awareness and heightened suspicion: Presence of marked wall thickening and dense fibrous adhesions should prompt intraoperative frozen section for diagnosis distinguishing XGC from nonoperable GB carcinoma

---

(Left) US in an 83-year-old woman with RUQ pain, anorexia, and weight loss shows multiple shadowing stones ➡ and diffuse wall thickening with hypoechoic intramural nodules ➡ and continuous mucosal line ➡. (Right) Sagittal MPR in the same orientation shows layering stones ➡ and intramural hypodense nodules ➡ within the markedly thickened GB wall. (Used with permission from the American Institute for Radiologic Pathology archives, Case ID #6173.)

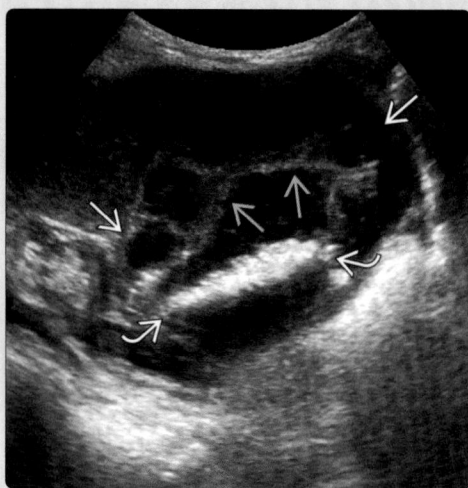
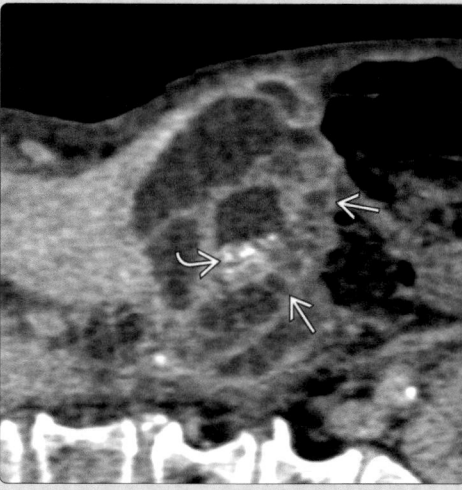

(Left) Longitudinal US shows asymmetric GB wall thickening with intramural hypoechoic nodules ➡ and a large shadowing stone ➡ in a 43-year-old woman who presented with 4-day history of intermittent RUQ pain. (Right) CT of the same patient shows wall thickening and a large stone ➡ with mass effect on the 2nd portion of the duodenum ➡. XGC with cholecystoduodenal fistula was confirmed at surgery. (Used with permission from the American Institute for Radiologic Pathology archives, Case ID #2129.)

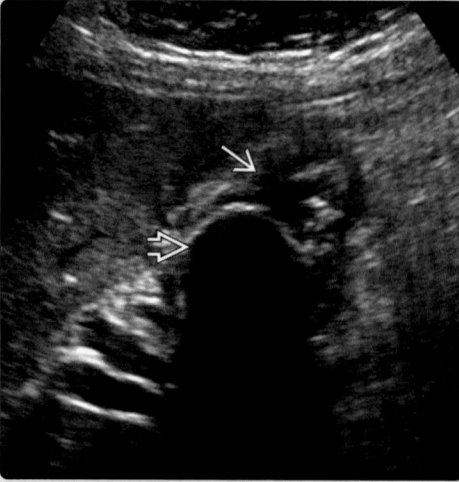
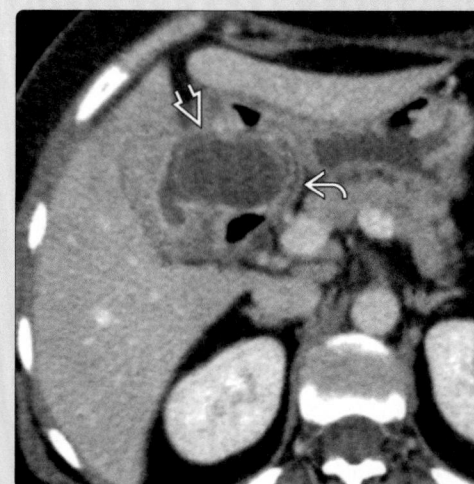

TERMINOLOGY

Abbreviations

- Xanthogranulomatous cholecystitis (XGC)

Synonyms

- Fibroxanthogranulomatous cholecystitis

Definitions

- Rare inflammatory process causing focal or diffuse destruction of gallbladder (GB) wall, with accumulation of lipid-laden macrophages, fibrous tissue, and acute and chronic inflammatory cells

IMAGING

General Features

- Diffuse wall thickening with intramural nodules (hypoechoic [US], hypodense [CT], slightly hyperintense [MR]) is characteristic
- Preoperative distinction between XGC and GB carcinoma difficult

Ultrasonographic Findings

- Gallbladder wall thickening, focal or diffuse
- Gallstones
- Intramural hypoechoic nodules or bands
- Gallbladder fossa mass, ± infiltrative, ± obscured margins between gallbladder and liver

CT Findings

- Diffuse GB wall thickening
- Hypodense intramural nodules/bands
- Continuous linear mucosal enhancement sign
- Infiltration into adjacent organs

Imaging Recommendations

- Presence of 3 of the following has > 80% sensitivity, 100% specificity, 91% accuracy in differentiating XGC from GB carcinoma
  - Diffuse wall thickening
  - Intramural nodules (hypoechoic, hypodense, slightly T2WI hyperintense)
  - Continuous mucosal line
  - Absence of hepatic invasion
  - Absence of biliary dilation

DIFFERENTIAL DIAGNOSIS

Gallbladder Carcinoma

- Many overlapping features (wall thickening/soft tissue mass, nodularity, infiltration of surrounding tissues)
- Periportal lymphadenopathy, biliary obstruction
- More likely associated with anorexia, weight loss, and palpable mass

Gangrenous Cholecystitis

- Asymmetric GB wall thickening
- Intraluminal membranes (sloughed mucosa or clot strands)

Hyperplastic Cholecystoses

- GB wall thickening
- Echogenic foci in Rokitansky-Aschoff (RA) sinuses, with reverberation "comet tail" artifact

PATHOLOGY

General Features

- Etiology
  - Gallstones (96-100%)
  - Pathogenesis
    - Extravasation of bile into GB wall from rupture of RA sinuses or by mucosal ulceration → inflammatory reaction in which macrophages and fibroblasts phagocytose biliary lipids → xanthomatous cells → fibrous reaction and scarring

CLINICAL ISSUES

Presentation

- Most common signs/symptoms
  - Typical symptoms of acute cholecystitis
    - Right upper quadrant pain associated with eating, nausea/vomiting, Murphy sign, leukocytosis
  - Obstructive jaundice
- Other signs/symptoms
  - Can present as acute pancreatitis, biliary colic

Demographics

- Age
  - Mean age at presentation: 44-63 years
- Epidemiology
  - Prevalence: 0.7% in USA patients with symptomatic gallbladder disease

Natural History & Prognosis

- Active and destructive inflammatory process with considerable morbidity
- Can coexist with gallbladder carcinoma

Treatment

- Surgical resection is definitive treatment
- Prognosis: Morbidity dependent on postoperative complications

DIAGNOSTIC CHECKLIST

Consider

- Difficult to distinguish from GB carcinoma preoperatively

Image Interpretation Pearls

- Presence of intramural (hypoechoic, hypodense, slightly T2WI hyperintense) nodules within thickened GB wall is highly suggestive

SELECTED REFERENCES

1. Bennett G et al: Cholelithiasis, cholecystitis, choledocholithiasis, and hyperplastic cholecystoses. In Gore RM et al: Textbook of Gastrointestinal Radiology. 4th ed. Philadelphia: Saunders Elsevier. Ch. 77, 2015
2. Revzin MV et al: The gallbladder: uncommon gallbladder conditions and unusual presentations of the common gallbladder pathological processes. Abdom Imaging. Epub ahead of print, 2014
3. Smith EA et al: Cross-sectional imaging of acute and chronic gallbladder inflammatory disease. AJR Am J Roentgenol. 192(1):188-96, 2009
4. Catalano OA et al: MR imaging of the gallbladder: a pictorial essay. Radiographics. 28(1):135-55; quiz 324, 2008
5. Levy AD et al: Benign tumors and tumorlike lesions of the gallbladder and extrahepatic bile ducts: Radiologic-pathologic correlation. RadioGraphics. 22: 387-413, 2002

Porcelain Gallbladder

TERMINOLOGY

- Intramural calcification of gallbladder wall, uncommon manifestation of chronic cholecystitis

IMAGING

- Type of calcification determines the ultrasound appearance
  - Thick diffuse GB wall calcification (complete)
  - Segmental GB wall calcification (incomplete)
- Set focus to maximize depiction of high-amplitude echoes and dense posterior acoustic shadowing
- Look for soft tissue mass in gallbladder or fossa, indicating presence of GB carcinoma

TOP DIFFERENTIAL DIAGNOSES

- Gallstone-filled gallbladder or large gallstone
  - Wall-echo-shadow (WES) complex appearance
  - Mobile stones may be positional
  - Dense, clean posterior acoustic shadowing (should not see posterior wall)

- Emphysematous cholecystitis
  - Echogenic crescent in gallbladder
  - Irregular (dirty) posterior acoustic shadowing
- Hyperplastic cholecystosis
  - Diffuse or focal GB wall thickening, echogenic foci with "comet tail" artifacts
  - No posterior acoustic shadowing

PATHOLOGY

- Associated with gallstones in 95%

CLINICAL ISSUES

- Risk of gallbladder cancer: 0-5%
  - Complete type: No risk, mucosa entirely denuded
  - Incomplete type: Mucosal metaplasia → dysplasia
- Prophylactic cholecystectomy is appropriate for healthy patients
- Nonoperative approach can be considered in patients with significant comorbidity

(Left) Grayscale US shows a thin, hyperechoic semilunar line ⟹ in the GB fossa with dense posterior acoustic shadowing ➡ in a 67-year-old woman who presented with chronic intermittent biliary pain as an example of complete calcification. (Right) Curvilinear diffuse, thin calcifications are shown in the RUQ of the same patient, in the expected location and shape of the gallbladder. (Courtesy American Institute for Radiologic Pathology archives, Case ID #2133052.)

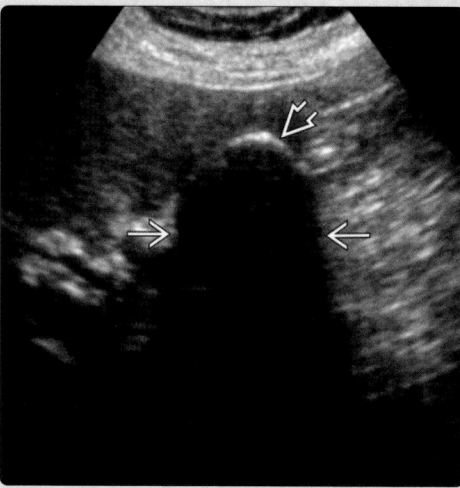
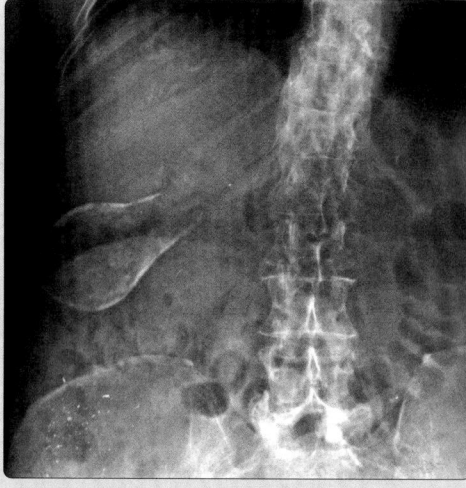

(Left) Discontinuous hyperechoic foci in the anterior ➡ and posterior ⟶ GB wall, with variable shadowing ⟹, in a 67-year-old woman with RUQ pain after eating; an example of incomplete calcification. (Right) Punctate mural calcifications ➡ in a 61-year-old obese man, an example of incomplete calcification. Gallstones found at pathology are not shown. (Courtesy American Institute for Radiologic Pathology archives, Case IDs #2674992, #642.)

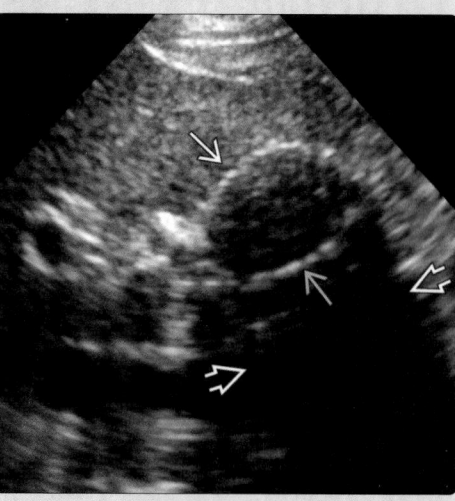
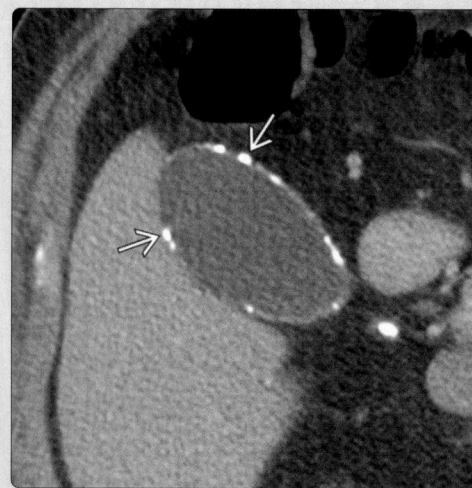

TERMINOLOGY

Abbreviations

- Porcelain gallbladder (PGB)

Synonyms

- Gallbladder calcifications, calcifying cholecystitis

Definitions

- Intramural calcification of gallbladder wall, uncommon manifestation of chronic cholecystitis

IMAGING

General Features

- Best diagnostic clue
  - Calcification in gallbladder (GB) wall
- Morphology
  - 2 patterns of mucosal calcification
  - Complete involvement: Diffuse calcification
  - Segmental involvement: Incomplete calcification

Ultrasonographic Findings

- Grayscale ultrasound
  - Type of calcification determines ultrasound appearance
  - Thick diffuse GB wall calcification (complete)
    - Hyperechoic semilunar line in GB fossa
    - Dense posterior acoustic shadowing
  - Segmental GB wall calcification (incomplete)
    - Biconvex curvilinear hyperechogenicity
    - Irregular (clumps) hyperechoic foci in GB wall
    - Variable posterior acoustic shadowing dependent on quantity of calcification

CT Findings

- NECT
  - Calcification in GB wall (diffuse or segmental)

Imaging Recommendations

- Best imaging tool
  - May be initially detected by US
  - CT is more sensitive, not limited by shadowing
- Protocol advice
  - Set focus at level of GB to maximize depiction of high-amplitude echoes and posterior acoustic shadowing
  - Look for soft tissue mass in gallbladder or fossa, indicating presence of GB carcinoma

DIFFERENTIAL DIAGNOSIS

Gallstone-Filled Gallbladder or Large Gallstone

- Wall-echo-shadow (WES) complex appearance
- Mobile stones may be positional
- Dense, clean posterior acoustic shadowing (should not see posterior wall)

Emphysematous Cholecystitis

- Echogenic crescent in gallbladder
- Irregular (dirty) posterior acoustic shadowing
- Clinical information of fulminant biliary sepsis

Hyperplastic Cholecystosis

- Diffuse or focal GB wall thickening

- Echogenic foci with "comet tail" artifacts
- No posterior acoustic shadowing

PATHOLOGY

General Features

- Etiology
  - Associated with gallstones in 95%
  - Chronic inflammation/irritation leads to scarring, hyalination, and dystrophic calcification
  - Complete type: Completely denuded mucosa
  - Incomplete type: Punctate glandular calcifications, mucosal metaplasia

CLINICAL ISSUES

Presentation

- Most common signs/symptoms
  - Usually asymptomatic
- Other signs/symptoms
  - Biliary-type pain
  - Palpable firm non-tender mass

Demographics

- Age
  - Usually occurs in 6th decade
- Gender
  - More common in women (5:1)
- Epidemiology
  - Rare (< 0.1% at autopsy)

Natural History & Prognosis

- Risk of gallbladder cancer: 0-5%
  - Complete type: No risk, mucosa entirely denuded
  - Incomplete type: Areas of mucosal metaplasia can lead to dysplasia

Treatment

- Prophylactic cholecystectomy is appropriate for healthy patients
- Nonoperative approach can be considered in patients with significant comorbidity

DIAGNOSTIC CHECKLIST

Consider

- Although association with GB carcinoma is weak, look for associated gallbladder mass

Image Interpretation Pearls

- WES sign on ultrasound helps to differentiate gallstones from porcelain GB
- Character of posterior acoustic shadowing can help differentiate gallstone (dense, clean) and emphysematous cholecystitis (dirty) from porcelain gallbladder

SELECTED REFERENCES

1. Schnelldorfer T: Porcelain gallbladder: a benign process or concern for malignancy? J Gastrointest Surg. 17(6):1161-8, 2013
2. O'Connor OJ et al: Imaging of cholecystitis. AJR Am J Roentgenol. 196(4):W367-74, 2011
3. Lack EE. Pathology of the Pancreas, Gallbladder, Extrahepatic Biliary Tract, and Ampullary Region. Oxford University Press, 2003

KEY FACTS

TERMINOLOGY

- Adenomyomatosis: Adenomyomatous hyperplasia, diverticular disease of gallbladder (GB)
- Although classified together, cholesterolosis and adenomyomatosis have different etiology and clinical features and should be considered separate entities
  - Cholesterolosis: Abnormal deposits of triglycerides and cholesterol esters in subepithelium of GB
  - Adenomyomatosis: Focal or segmental GB wall thickening due to mucosal proliferation and hypertrophy of muscularis with invagination of excess mucosa into thickened muscularis- forming Rokitansky-Aschoff (RA) sinuses; these sinuses can contain bile, cholesterol crystals, sludge, and calculi

IMAGING

- Cholesterolosis: May present as subtle mural nodules but usually occult

- Adenomyomatosis: Focal or segmental wall thickening with intramural hyperechoic foci and "comet tail" reverberation artifacts

TOP DIFFERENTIAL DIAGNOSES

- GB carcinoma
- Adenomatous polyp
- Diffuse GB wall thickening related to systemic illness
- Chronic cholecystitis
- Emphysematous cholecystitis

PATHOLOGY

- Gallstones in up to 90%

CLINICAL ISSUES

- When symptomatic, biliary pain (cystic duct obstructed by prolapsing or detached polyp) or dyspepsia (poor GB emptying)
- No conclusive evidence that presence of adenomyomatosis increases risk for GB cancer

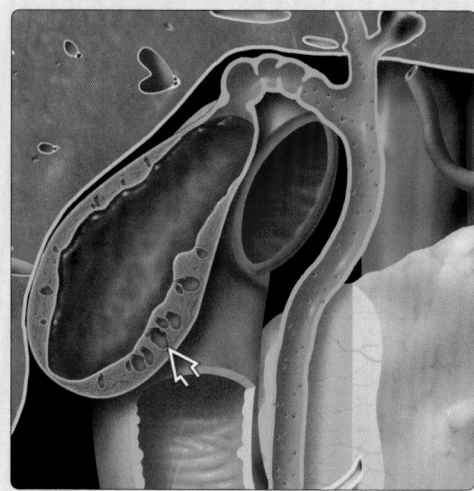
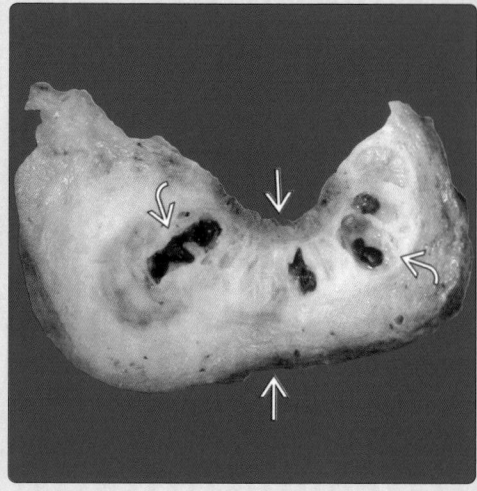

(Left) *Graphic shows characteristic features of adenomyomatosis. Note the thickened gallbladder (GB) wall with multiple intramural cystic spaces ➡. (Right) Gross image of sectioned gallbladder shows markedly thickened wall ➡ containing multiple cystic intramural cavities ➡ (Rokitansky-Aschoff [RA] sinuses), which are filled with bile and calculi. (Used with permission from the American Institute for Radiologic Pathology archives, Case ID # 2973667.)*

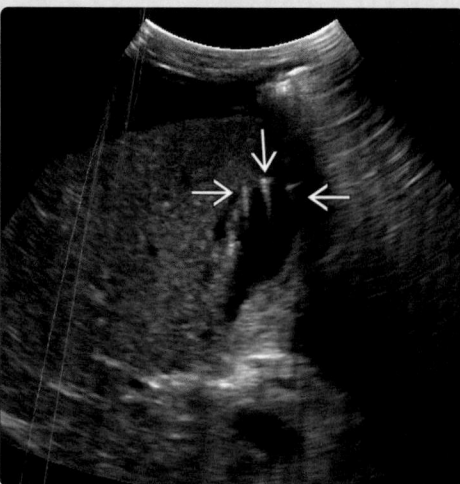
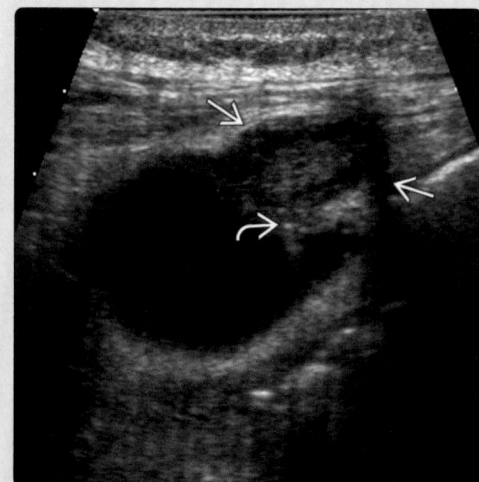

(Left) *Transverse oblique ultrasound demonstrates multiple anterior gallbladder wall "comet tail" artifacts ➡ emanating from debris in RA sinuses. The sinuses themselves are not visible. (Right) Longitudinal ultrasound through the gallbladder shows a focal soft tissue mass at the fundus ➡, with "comet tail" artifact associated with an echogenic focus ➡ (an example of fundal adenomyomatosis).*

Hyperplastic Cholecystosis (Adenomyomatosis)

TERMINOLOGY

Synonyms

- Adenomyomatous hyperplasia, diverticular disease of gallbladder (GB)

Definitions

- Generic term for nonneoplastic, noninflammatory proliferative disorders of GB wall
  - Cholesterolosis: Abnormal deposits of triglycerides and cholesterol esters in subepithelium of GB
  - Adenomyomatosis: Focal or segmental GB wall thickening due to mucosal proliferation and hypertrophy of muscularis with invagination of excess mucosa into thickened muscularis- forming Rokitansky-Aschoff (RA) sinuses
    - These sinuses can contain bile, cholesterol crystals, sludge, and calculi
- Although classified together, cholesterolosis and adenomyomatosis have different etiology and clinical features, and should be considered separate entities

IMAGING

General Features

- Best diagnostic clue
  - Cholesterolosis: Multiple tiny cholesterol flecks, usually occult on imaging, may cause wall nodularity
  - Adenomyomatosis: Focal or segmental wall thickening with intramural hyperechoic foci and "comet tail" reverberation artifacts
- Location
  - Gallbladder wall
    - Cholesterolosis: Subepithelial
    - Adenomyomatosis: Epithelial and muscularis mucosa
- Morphology
  - Adenomyomatosis: 3 morphological patterns
    - Diffuse
    - Focal
      - □ Fundal (adenomyoma): RA sinus forms nodule that projects into lumen
      - □ Segmental (hourglass): Circumferential ring divides GB into separate interconnected compartments

Ultrasonographic Findings

- Grayscale ultrasound
  - **Cholesterolosis**
    - Multiple tiny hyperechoic GB polyps may present as subtle mural nodules
    - Usually < 1 mm in size
    - No posterior acoustic shadowing or "comet tail" artifact
    - No evidence of invasion to adjacent liver parenchyma or regional lymphadenopathy
    - May coalesce into cholesterol polyps (4-10 mm in size)
  - **Adenomyomatosis**
    - Focal or diffuse GB wall thickening
    - Presence of intramural anechoic foci = dilated sinuses
    - Tiny echogenic intramural foci in GB wall, producing V-shaped or "comet tail" artifacts = debris in sinuses
    - Hourglass GB: Focal wall thickening forms ring around midbody
      - Fundal adenomyoma: Smooth intraluminal mass, usually fundal and solitary
- Color Doppler
  - No significant vascularity
  - "Twinkling" artifacts on Doppler examination associated with debris in RA sinuses

CT Findings

- CECT
  - Adenomyomatosis
    - Thickened GB wall (segmental, diffuse, fundal)
    - Cystic nonenhancing spaces within GB wall, corresponding to intramural diverticula
    - Hourglass configuration of GB (segmental type)
    - Low sensitivity for small (< 5 mm) polyps

MR Findings

- T2WI
  - "Pearl necklace" sign: Most specific sign of adenomyomatosis on MR, chain of fluid containing intramural diverticula
- T1WI C+
  - Sinuses: Nonenhancing, hypointense, within thickened GB wall

Imaging Recommendations

- Best imaging tool
  - US, MR
- Protocol advice
  - Use high frequency transducer for best visualization of "comet tail" artifacts and cystic spaces
  - Absence of cystic spaces, echogenic foci, or "twinkling" artifacts, or presence of internal vascularity should prompt further investigation to rule out neoplasm
    - Always examine adjacent liver for infiltration
    - Evaluate presence/absence of regional lymphadenopathy

DIFFERENTIAL DIAGNOSIS

Gallbladder Carcinoma

- Polypoid mass > 1 cm
- Infiltrative and ill-defined margin
- Increased internal vascularity
- Associated with gallstones in most cases
- Adjacent liver parenchymal invasion and regional metastatic lymphadenopathy

Adenomatous Polyp

- May mimic focal form of adenomyomatosis
- Usually solitary, 5-15 mm
- Nonmobile, nonshadowing polyp
- Usually avascular or hypovascular

Diffuse GB Wall Thickening

- Related to systemic illness (e.g., hepatitis, cirrhosis, congestive heart failure, etc.)
- Diffuse GB wall involvement
- Striated hypoechoic appearance
- Lack of "comet tail" artifacts or intramural cystic spaces

Chronic Cholecystitis

- Generalized GB wall thickening

- Contracted GB lumen
- Presence of gallstones within GB
- Lack of mural "comet tail" artifacts or intramural cystic space

Emphysematous Cholecystitis

- Intramural gas may mimic cholesterol deposits
- Dirty shadowing, no "comet tail" reverberation artifacts
- Clinically ill

PATHOLOGY

General Features

- Cholesterolosis: Mucosal villous hyperplasia with excessive accumulation of triglyceride and cholesterol esters within epithelial macrophages
  o Strawberry GB: Lipid accumulation is visible to naked eye; yellow cholesterol deposits on background of hyperemia mucosa ~ strawberry
- Adenomyomatosis: Excessive proliferation of surface epithelium with invaginations into thickened muscularis propria, forming diverticula known as RA sinuses
  o RA sinuses may be filled with bile, cholesterol crystals, sludge, or calculi
- Gallstones in up to 90% (cholesterol)

Gross Pathologic & Surgical Features

- Focal or diffuse GB wall thickening without inflammatory changes
- Adenomyomatosis: Diffuse or segmental GB wall thickening with multiple cystic spaces

Microscopic Features

- Cholesterolosis
  o Fat-laden foamy macrophages within elongated villi → small yellow subepithelial nodules → coalescent nodules = polyps
    – 2/3: Nodules < 1 mm in diameter → coarse and granular appearance of mucosa
    – 1/3: Nodules larger and polypoid
- Adenomyomatosis
  o Epithelium-lined cystic spaces in thickened muscular layer of GB wall = intramural diverticula or RA sinuses

CLINICAL ISSUES

Presentation

- Most common signs/symptoms
  o Most often asymptomatic
  o When symptomatic, biliary pain (cystic duct obstructed by prolapsing or detached polyp) or dyspepsia (poor GB emptying)

Demographics

- Age
  o > 35 years
- Gender
  o Cholesterolosis: F > M
  o Adenomyomatosis: F > M
- Epidemiology
  o Cholesterolosis more common, 12% prevalence
  o Adenomyomatosis relatively less common, 5% prevalence

Natural History & Prognosis

- Usually incidental finding
- No clinical significance in asymptomatic patients when diagnosed correctly
- No conclusive evidence that presence of adenomyomatosis increases risk for GB cancer

Treatment

- Cholecystectomy → symptomatic

DIAGNOSTIC CHECKLIST

Consider

- Consider chronic cholecystitis

Image Interpretation Pearls

- Cholesterolosis: Usually occult, multiple tiny polyps may produce irregular GB wall
- Adenomyomatosis
  o Focal or diffuse wall thickening with intramural cystic spaces
  o "Comet tail" reverberation artifacts
  o Hourglass appearances and fundal adenomyoma in focal form

SELECTED REFERENCES

1. Revzin MV et al: The gallbladder: uncommon gallbladder conditions and unusual presentations of the common gallbladder pathological processes. Abdom Imaging. Epub ahead of print, 2014
2. Runner GJ et al: Gallbladder wall thickening. AJR Am J Roentgenol. 202(1):W1-W12, 2014
3. Pellino G et al: Stepwise approach and surgery for gallbladder adenomyomatosis: a mini-review. Hepatobiliary Pancreat Dis Int. 12(2):136-42, 2013
4. Meacock LM et al: Evaluation of gallbladder and biliary duct disease using microbubble contrast-enhanced ultrasound. Br J Radiol. 83(991):615-27, 2010
5. Ash-Miles J et al: More than just stones: a pictorial review of common and less common gallbladder pathologies. Curr Probl Diagn Radiol. 37(5):189-202, 2008
6. Catalano OA et al: MR imaging of the gallbladder: a pictorial essay. Radiographics. 28(1):135-55; quiz 324, 2008
7. Stunell H et al: Imaging of adenomyomatosis of the gall bladder. J Med Imaging Radiat Oncol. 52(2):109-17, 2008
8. van Breda Vriesman AC et al: Diffuse gallbladder wall thickening: differential diagnosis. AJR Am J Roentgenol. 188(2):495-501, 2007
9. Boscak AR et al: Best cases from the AFIP: adenomyomatosis of the gallbladder. Radiographics. 26(3):941-6, 2006
10. Lack E et al: Pathology of the Pancreas, Gallbladder, Extrahepatic Biliary Tract, and Ampullary Region. Oxford New York: Oxford University Press. 427-9, 2003
11. Owen CC et al: Gallbladder polyps, cholesterolosis, adenomyomatosis, and acute acalculous cholecystitis. Semin Gastrointest Dis. 14(4):178-88, 2003
12. Gore RM et al: Imaging benign and malignant disease of the gallbladder. Radiol Clin North Am. 40(6):1307-23, vi, 2002
13. Levy AD et al: Benign tumors and tumorlike lesions of the gallbladder and extrahepatic bile ducts: Radiologic-pathologic correlation. RadioGraphics. 22: 387-413, 2002
14. Berk RN et al: The hyperplastic cholecystoses: cholesterolosis and adenomyomatosis. Radiology. 146(3):593-601, 1983

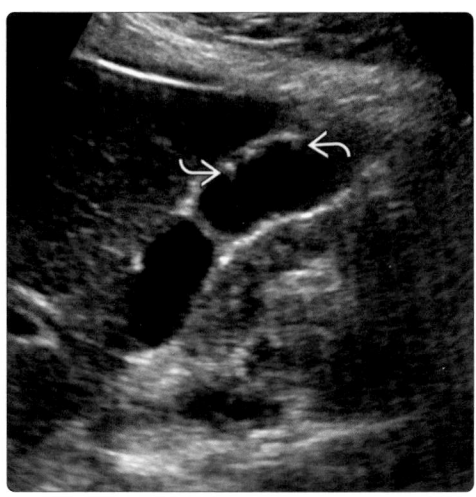

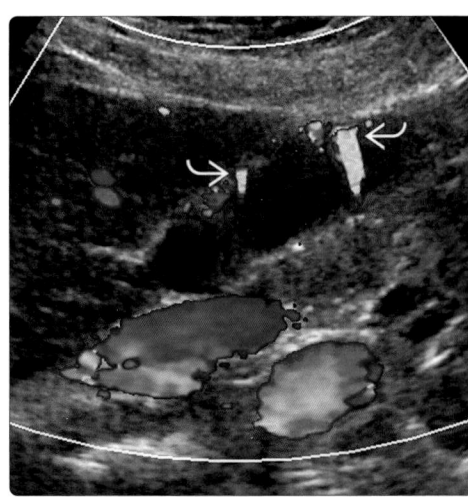

(Left) *Longitudinal ultrasound through the gallbladder shows multiple hyperechoic foci with V-shaped, "comet tail" reverberation artifact* ➡. (Right) *Longitudinal color Doppler ultrasound in the same patient shows characteristic color "comet tail," "twinkling" artifact* ➡ *with associated rough surfaces of contents (calculi) within the RA sinuses.*

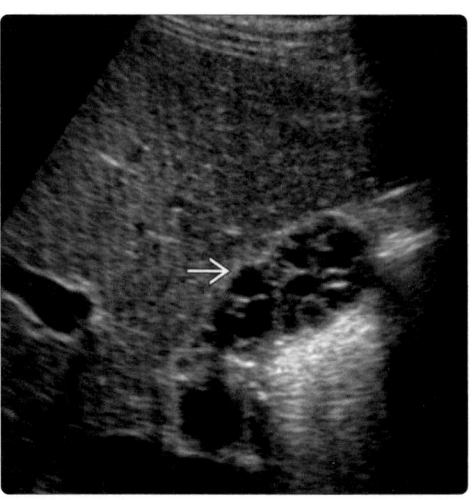

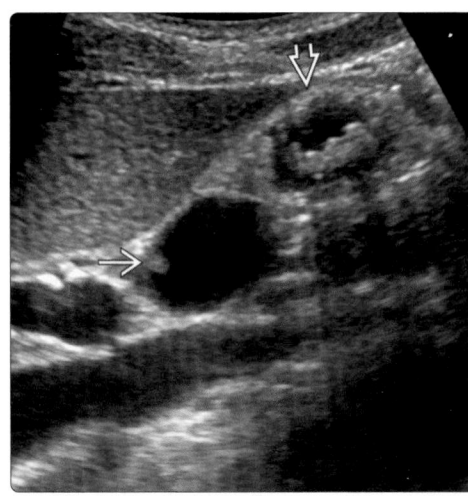

(Left) *Longitudinal ultrasound shows multiple cystic spaces* ➡ *in the thickened GB walls, pathologically shown to represent bile-filled RA sinuses in a patient with adenomyomatosis. (Used with permission from the American Institute for Radiologic Pathology archives, Case ID # 1794.)* (Right) *Longitudinal ultrasound shows both a solitary isoechoic polyp* ➡ *and fundal adenomyomatosis* ➡. *(Used with permission from the American Institute for Radiologic Pathology archives, Case ID # 728.)*

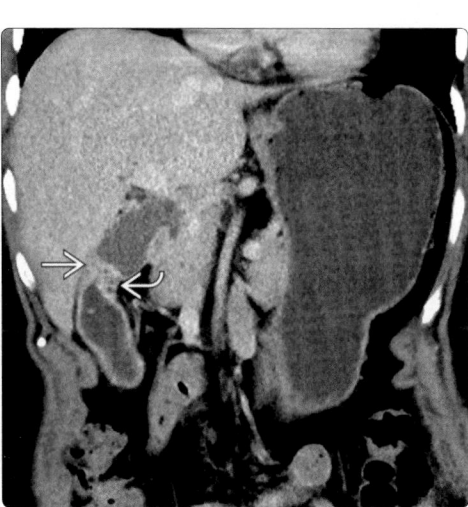

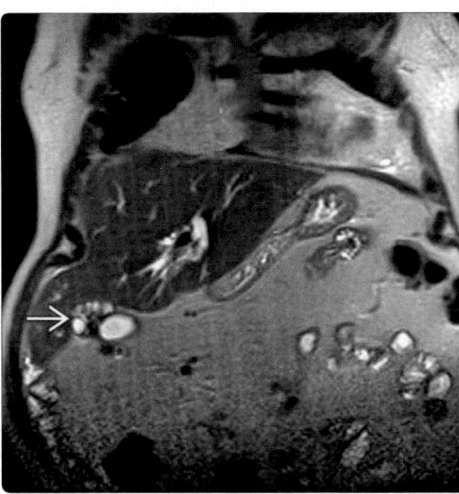

(Left) *Coronal CECT shows constriction of the midbody* ➡ *of the gallbladder, representing segmental adenomyomatosis. There are small cysts* ➡ *in the wall of the thick segment.* (Right) *Coronal T2 HASTE MR shows a cluster of fluid-filled intramural diverticula in the* ➡ *gallbladder fundus (the "pearl necklace" sign, characteristic of fundal adenomyomatosis).*

Gallbladder Carcinoma

TERMINOLOGY

- Most common malignancy of biliary tree, with worst prognosis
- Epithelial neoplasm arising from gallbladder (GB) mucosa with predilection for women and the elderly
- Characterized by early locoregional spread directly to liver and peritoneum and porta hepatic and paraaortic lymph nodes (LNs)

IMAGING

- 3 main morphological types
  - Large soft tissue mass infiltrating gallbladder fossa/replacing GB, ± invading liver (**most common**)
  - Diffuse or focal GB wall thickening: Asymmetric, irregular, extensive thickening
  - Polypoid intraluminal mass: > 1 cm, thickened base, irregular margins
- US for initial detection and characterization, CECT or MR for preoperative assessment and staging

TOP DIFFERENTIAL DIAGNOSES

- GB Polyp
  - Typically < 1 cm ± multiple = benign cholesterol polyp
- Focal or diffuse wall thickening
  - Hyperplastic cholecystoses
    - Tiny intramural echogenic foci with "comet tail" artifact
  - Chronic cholecystitis
    - Contracted GB (lumen may be obliterated)
  - Xanthogranulomatous cholecystitis
    - Infiltrative intramural inflammatory process resulting in ill-defined GB wall thickening
    - Nearly impossible to differentiate from gallbladder carcinoma preoperatively

CLINICAL ISSUES

- Most are adenocarcinoma, mean 5-year survival rate 5-10%
- Preoperative diagnosis occurs in < 20% of patients

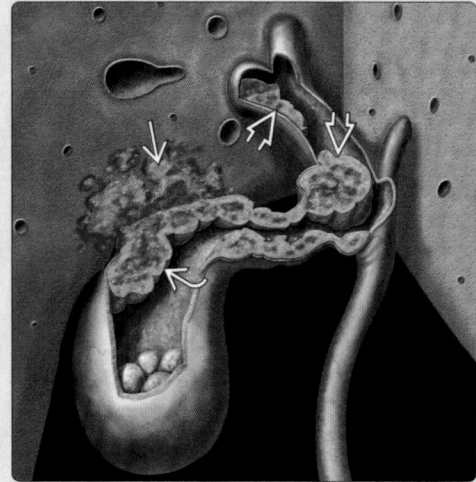
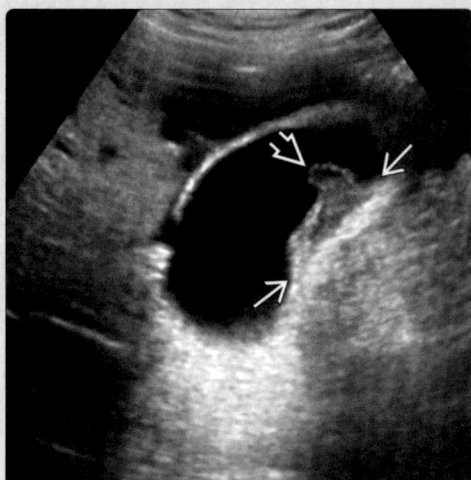

(Left) Graphic shows pathways of local tumor invasion from carcinoma of gallbladder ➡: Direct tumor infiltration to liver parenchyma ➡; retrograde spread along biliary tree ➡. (Right) Longitudinal US in a 67-year-old man shows a broad-based ➡, hypoechoic polypoid mass ➡ protruding into the gallbladder (GB) lumen. (Used with permission from the American Institute for Radiologic Pathology archives, Case ID #4067.)

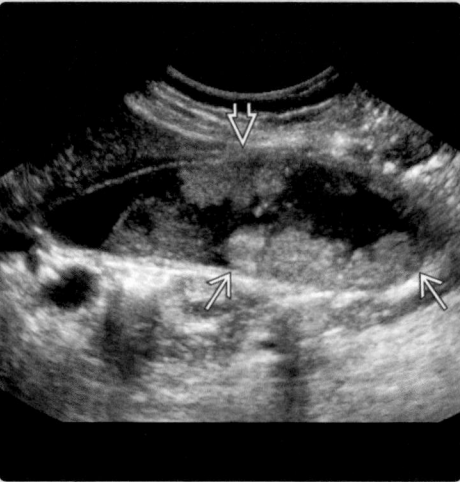
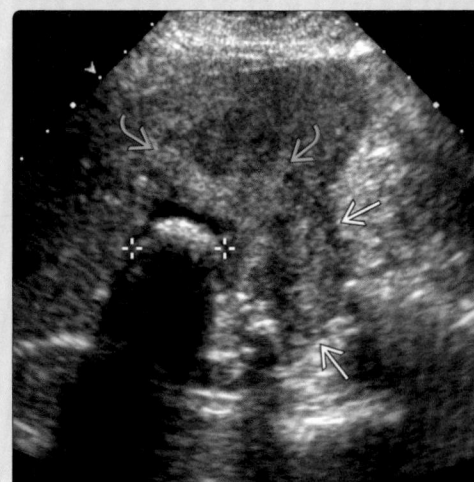

(Left) GBC can also appear as irregular, asymmetric, lobulated fundal wall thickening ➡ with mucosal disruption ➡, as in this 48-year-old woman. (Used with permission from the AIRP archives, Case ID # 422.) (Right) Most commonly, GBC appears as heterogeneous lobulated echogenic distension of the GB ➡, usually in presence of shadowing stones. Marginal obliteration and direct hepatic invasion ➡ are ominous signs. (Used with permission from the AIRP archives, Case ID # 923.)

Gallbladder Carcinoma

TERMINOLOGY

Abbreviations
- Gallbladder carcinoma (GBC)

Definitions
- Most common neoplasm of biliary tree, with worst prognosis

IMAGING

General Features
- Best diagnostic clue
  - Poorly defined mass in gallbladder (GB) fossa
  - Invasion into liver and adjacent organs
  - Regional metastatic lymphadenopathy (LAN)
- Morphology
  - 3 main morphological types
    - Polypoid intraluminal mass: > 1 cm, thickened base, irregular margins
    - Diffuse or focal GB wall thickening: Asymmetric, irregular, extensive thickening
    - Large soft tissue mass infiltrating gallbladder fossa/replacing GB, ± invading liver

Ultrasonographic Findings
- Grayscale ultrasound
  - Mass is usually hypoechoic relative to normal liver
  - Extraluminal mass infiltrating GB fossa, extending into liver
  - Heterogeneous irregular GB wall thickening
    - Malignant features include thickness > 5 mm, irregularity, and asymmetry
  - Intraluminal moderately echogenic polypoid mass
    - Size > 1 cm independent positive predictor
    - Lobulated surface
    - Hypoechoic internal echogenicity
  - Gallstones, ± GB wall calcification
  - Additional ominous findings include evidence of local invasion, LAN, and distant metastases
- Color Doppler
  - Areas of vascularity within the mass
  - Presence of vascular core in > 1 cm polyp
- Contrast-enhanced US
  - Features more likely associated with malignant wall thickening
    - Inner or outer wall discontinuity
    - Focal wall thickening > 10 mm
  - Better visualization of intraluminal polyp
  - Early phase hyperenhancement relative to liver, with washout within 35 seconds: Improved detection, characterization, and evaluation of invasion
  - Tortuous vasculature
- Newer US technologies under investigation
  - High-resolution US (HRUS): Combination of low- and high-frequency transducers may help in more accurate size assessment of intraluminal polyps

CT Findings
- May be useful adjunct when GB wall obscured by stones
- Preoperative evaluation for invasion, LAN, distant mets

MR Findings
- T1WI
  - Iso- or hypointense to normal liver
- T2WI
  - Heterogeneously hyperintense to liver
- T1WI C+
  - Ill-defined early arterial enhancement
  - Fibrous stromal portions of tumor may retain enhancement on delayed phases
- MRCP
  - Ductal obstruction or invasion, ± biliary dilation
- Primarily used for staging and assessing tumor invasion
  - T1WI C+ sequences (with fat suppression) most helpful for assessing invasion into adjacent organs and vascular structures (PV, HA), peritoneal implants

Nuclear Medicine Findings
- PET/CT
  - Avid accumulation of F-18 FDG
  - Difficult to distinguish from inflammation (wall thickening) or other malignancy

Imaging Recommendations
- Best imaging tool
  - US for initial detection and characterization, CECT or MR for preoperative assessment and staging

DIFFERENTIAL DIAGNOSIS

GB Polyp: Hyperplastic or Adenomatous
- Mucosal polypoid mass
  - Moderately echogenic without shadowing
  - Nonmobile, attached to wall
  - No vascularity detected on Doppler
- Typically < 1 cm ± multiple = benign cholesterol polyp

Hyperplastic Cholecystoses
- Focal or diffuse wall thickening
  - Focal thickening of the fundus
  - Focal thickening of the mid body ("hourglass GB")
- Intramural cholesterol crystals as tiny echogenic foci with "comet tail" artifact
  - "String of pearls" on MR
- No adjacent infiltration or lymph node metastases

Chronic Cholecystitis
- Diffuse wall thickening, smooth or irregular contour
- Contracted GB (lumen may be obliterated)
- Gallstones

Xanthogranulomatous Cholecystitis
- Infiltrative intramural inflammatory process resulting in ill-defined GB wall thickening
- Gallstones
- Distinguishing characteristics
  - Presence of intramural hypoechoic/hypodense nodules
  - Mucosal continuity
  - Lack of lymph node involvement and hepatic or biliary invasion
- Nearly impossible to differentiate from gallbladder carcinoma preoperatively

Metastatic Disease to GB Fossa

- Variable appearance (polypoid, mural infiltration, GB fossa mass)
- Metastases: Melanoma may directly metastasize to GB mucosa
- Direct invasion: Primary hepatic tumors may spread to GB via duct invasion
- Mimic: Porta hepatis lymphadenopathy
  - Lymphoma and GI tract carcinoma most common
- Require correlation with history of malignancy

PATHOLOGY

General Features

- Etiology
  - Pathogenesis
    - Most with gallstones → mucosal abrasion/ulceration → regeneration → metaplasia/dysplasia
    - Less commonly, malignant degeneration of adenomatous polyps
- Usually arises in fundus or neck
- Thin muscularis layer and close approximation to liver, lymphatics, and vasculature → early local, lymphatic, and hematogenous spread
  - Penetration of serosa → peritoneal dissemination (ascites, omental/peritoneal implants)

Staging, Grading, & Classification

- Stage I: Confined to mucosa
- Stage II: Involves mucosa and muscularis
- Stage III: Serosal extension
- Stage IV: Lymph node involvement
  - Nodal status most suggestive of overall prognosis
- Stage V: Direct extension to liver or distant metastases

Microscopic Features

- Adenocarcinoma (80-95%)

CLINICAL ISSUES

Presentation

- Most common signs/symptoms
  - Right upper quadrant (RUQ) pain, weight loss, anorexia, fever
  - Jaundice: When tumor invades common or right hepatic duct or CBD

Demographics

- Age
  - Mean: 65 years
- Gender
  - F:M 3:1; female gender is independent risk factor
- Epidemiology
  - Prevalence 3-7%
- Risk factors
  - Gallstones (GS)
  - Polyps
    - Up to 88% of adenomatous polyps > 10 mm in patients over 50, have been found to harbor malignancy
  - Chronic infection
    - *Salmonella typhi* and *S. paratyphi, Helicobacter pylori*

- Anomalous union of the pancreaticobiliary ducts (AUPBD)
- Porcelain gallbladder: Controversial
  - More likely, porcelain GB represents changes associated with chronic inflammation, harbinger of GBC
- Genetics: Marked geographic variability with genetic predisposition to GBC
  - Family history is strong risk factor
- Other chronic inflammatory states, including IBD (primary sclerosing cholangitis) and familial adenomatous polyposis, and toxic exposures (cigarette smoking; workers exposed to petroleum, rubber, paper mills)

Natural History & Prognosis

- Histologic type and stage at presentation are most important prognostic factors
- Spreads by local invasion to liver, nodal spread to porta hepatis and paraaortic nodes, hematogenous spread to liver

Treatment

- Early stage (Tis or T1a): Simple cholecystectomy
- Beyond muscularis: Radical cholecystectomy, ± partial hepatectomy, ± LN dissection
- Preventative treatment: Cholecystectomy recommended for polyps > 10 mm in patients > 50 years

DIAGNOSTIC CHECKLIST

Consider

- Most often, diagnosed incidentally after elective cholecystectomy for presumed benign disease

Image Interpretation Pearls

- Mass infiltrating GB fossa with liver invasion
- Large polypoid GB mucosal mass with flow
- Associated adjacent lymphadenopathy

SELECTED REFERENCES

1. Kim JH et al: High-resolution sonography for distinguishing neoplastic gallbladder polyps and staging gallbladder cancer. AJR Am J Roentgenol. 204(2):W150-9, 2015
2. Cariati A et al: Gallbladder cancers: associated conditions, histological types, prognosis, and prevention. Eur J Gastroenterol Hepatol. 26(5):562-9, 2014
3. Pitt SC et al: Incidental gallbladder cancer at cholecystectomy: when should the surgeon be suspicious? Ann Surg. 260(1):128-33, 2014
4. Runner GJ et al: Gallbladder wall thickening. AJR Am J Roentgenol. 202(1):W1-W12, 2014
5. Wernberg JA et al: Gallbladder cancer. Surg Clin North Am. 94(2):343-60, 2014
6. Xu JM et al: Differential diagnosis of gallbladder wall thickening: the usefulness of contrast-enhanced ultrasound. Ultrasound Med Biol. 40(12):2794-804, 2014
7. Zemour J et al: Gallbladder tumor and pseudotumor: Diagnosis and management. J Visc Surg. 151(4):289-300, 2014
8. Cairns V et al: Risk and Cost-effectiveness of Surveillance Followed by Cholecystectomy for Gallbladder Polyps. Arch Surg. 147(12):1078-83, 2012
9. Kai K et al: Clinicopathologic features of advanced gallbladder cancer associated with adenomyomatosis. Virchows Arch. 459(6):573-80, 2011
10. Edge SB et al: AJCC Cancer Staging Manual, 7th ed. New York: Springer, 2010
11. Meacock LM et al: Evaluation of gallbladder and biliary duct disease using microbubble contrast-enhanced ultrasound. Br J Radiol. 83(991):615-27, 2010
12. Catalano OA et al: MR imaging of the gallbladder: a pictorial essay. Radiographics. 28(1):135-55; quiz 324, 2008

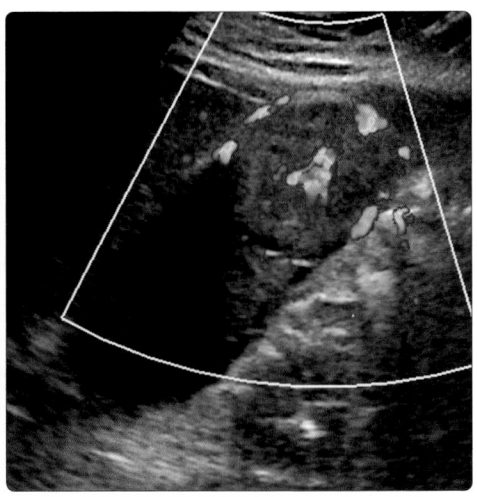
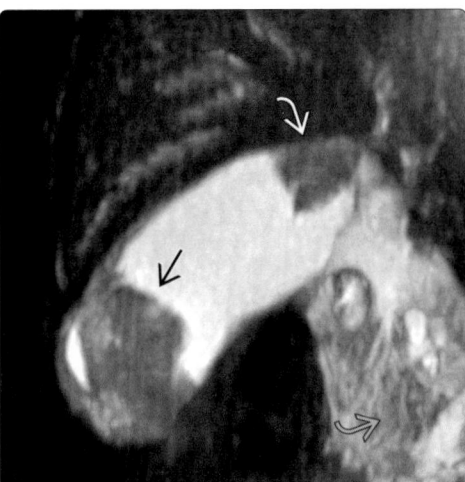

(Left) *Sagittal US in a 67-year-old woman with acute pancreatitis shows large polypoid mass in the GB fundus with internal vascularity. (Used with permission from the AIRP archives, Case ID # 6379.)* (Right) *Subsequent MR shows lobulated intraluminal polypoid mass ⮕ that is heterogeneously hyperintense to adjacent liver. Note the angulated stone ⮕ in the GB neck and edematous pancreas associated with acute interstitial edematous pancreatitis ⮕. (Used with permission from the AIRP.)*

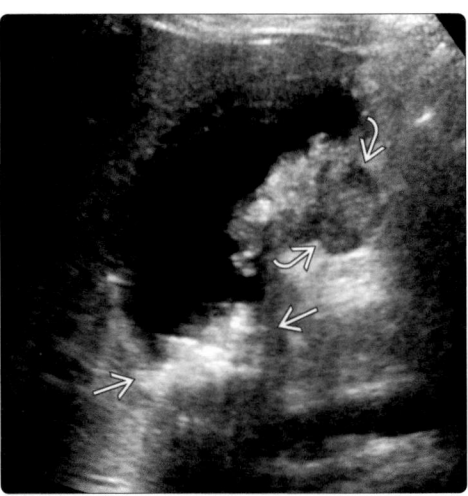
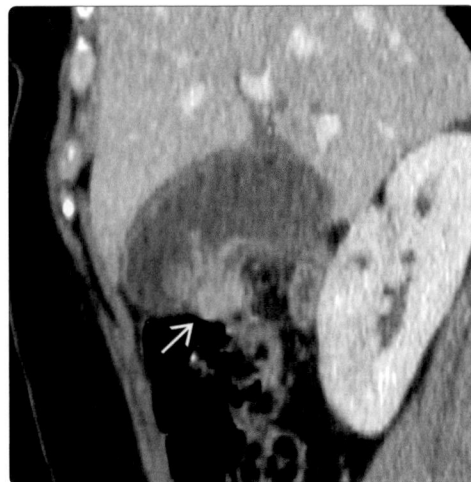

(Left) *Sagittal US of the GB in a 37-year-old woman who presented with acute RUQ pain shows shadowing gallstones and sludge ⮕ with a mass-like lobulated region of wall thickening, with transmural extension ⮕. (Used with permission from the AIRP archives, Case ID # 6379.)* (Right) *Sagittal CECT MPR in a similar plane shows the polypoid mass ⮕ enhances and arises from the GB wall. (Used with permission from the AIRP archives, Case ID # 6379.)*

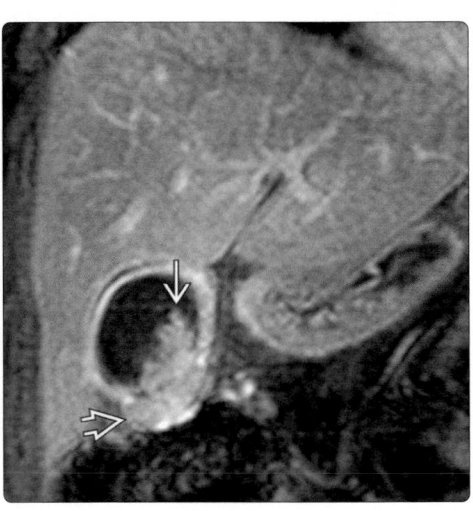
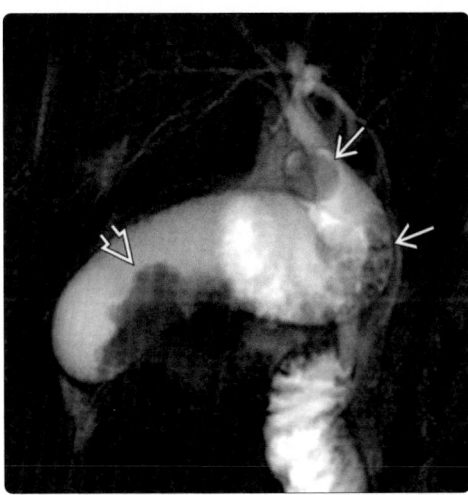

(Left) *Dynamic post-Gd MR in the coronal plane shows delayed progressive enhancement in the lobulated polypoid mass ⮕, with disruption of the enhancing wall ⮕. (Used with permission from the AIRP archives, Case ID # 6379.)* (Right) *MRCP in the same patient shows stones in the neck and body of the GB ⮕, with the lobulated polypoid mass protruding into the lumen ⮕. (Used with permission from the AIRP archives, Case ID # 6379.)*

Biliary Ductal Dilatation

TERMINOLOGY

- Biliary ductal dilatation, dilated ducts

IMAGING

- Tubular anechoic fluid-filled structures accompanying portal veins in extrahepatic and intrahepatic segments
- Intrahepatic ductal dilatation
  - Dilatation of ductal diameter > 2 mm
- Extrahepatic ductal dilatation
  - Dilatation of common hepatic/bile duct > 6-7 mm or more than 40% of diameter of adjacent portal vein

TOP DIFFERENTIAL DIAGNOSES

- Portal vein cavernoma
- Thrombosed portal vein branch
- Venovenous collaterals
- Peribiliary cysts
- Choledochal cyst

PATHOLOGY

- Obstructive causes
  - Intrahepatic: Calculus, recurrent pyogenic cholangitis, sclerosing/AIDS cholangitis, cholangiocarcinoma, etc.
  - Extrahepatic: Calculus, stricture, pancreatic head adenocarcinoma, cholangiocarcinoma, lymph node compression, etc.
- Nonobstructive causes
  - Advanced age
  - Previous cholecystectomy
  - Congenital disease (e.g., choledochal cyst)
  - Hepatic artery stenosis in liver transplant recipients

CLINICAL ISSUES

- Presentation
  - Often presents with obstructive jaundice: Painless or right upper quadrant pain

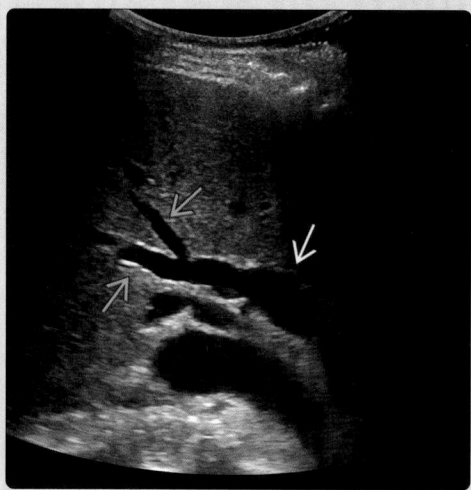
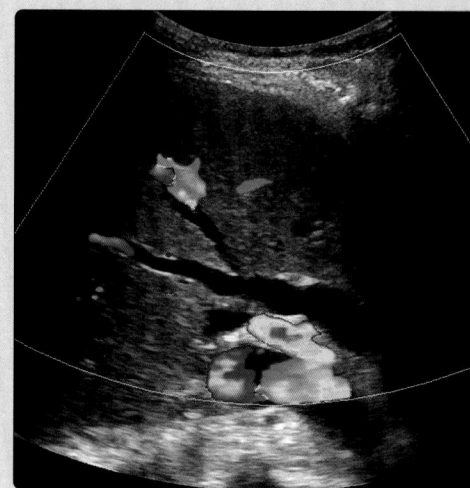

(Left) *Oblique transabdominal US through the liver shows moderate dilatation of the common bile duct ➡ and branching intrahepatic ducts ⇨ caused by an obstructing pancreatic head tumor (not shown).* **(Right)** *Lack of flow in the dilated tubular structures on this color Doppler ultrasound in the same patient confirms that these are indeed dilated biliary ducts. Color Doppler should be used routinely to confirm biliary ductal dilatation.*

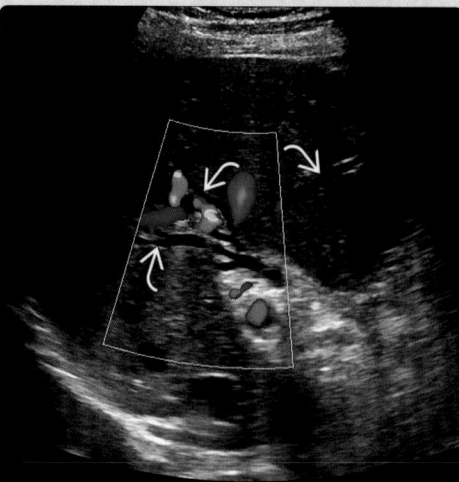
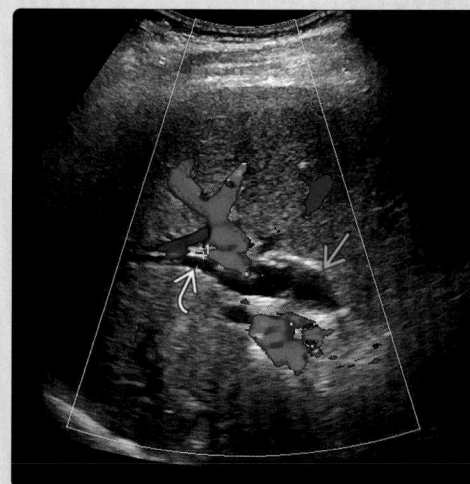

(Left) *Transverse color Doppler ultrasound of the liver shows mild biliary ductal dilatation in the intrahepatic ducts ➡, which measured just over 2 mm in diameter. The cause of mild biliary ductal dilatation was due to obstructing stone (not shown).* **(Right)** *Transverse color Doppler image of the liver shows mild biliary ductal dilatation in the intrahepatic ducts ➡, as well as extrahepatic ducts ⇨. Patient was found to have both ampullary stenosis, as well as cholangitis as cause of biliary ductal dilatation.*

IMAGING

General Features

- Best diagnostic clue
  - Tubular anechoic fluid-filled structures accompanying portal veins in extrahepatic and intrahepatic segments
- Location
  - Intrahepatic and extrahepatic bile ducts

Ultrasonographic Findings

- Grayscale ultrasound
  - Intrahepatic ductal dilatation
    - Ductal diameter > 2 mm
    - Tubular anechoic branching structures accompanying portal veins
      - "Parallel channel" sign
      - Earliest intrahepatic ducts to dilate are often in left hepatic lobe
    - Dilated ducts may be irregular and tortuous
    - Central stellate confluence of tubular structures proximally at liver hilum
  - Extrahepatic ductal dilatation
    - Diameter of common bile duct > 6-7 mm or more than 40% of diameter of adjacent portal vein
    - Anechoic tubular structure parallel to main portal vein and perpendicular to hepatic artery in porta hepatis
    - Can trace its communication with intrahepatic ducts
- Color Doppler
  - Helpful to distinguish dilated ducts (no color flow) from adjacent vascular branches of hepatic arteries and portal veins

CT Findings

- Near water attenuating tubular structures within liver parenchyma adjacent to intrahepatic portal veins
- Intrahepatic ducts communicate with near water attenuating tubular structure between the liver and duodenum

MR Findings

- T2 hyperintense tubular structures within liver parenchyma
- Intrahepatic ducts communicate with T2 hyperintense tubular structure between liver and duodenum

Imaging Recommendations

- Best imaging tool
  - Transabdominal US useful as initial investigative tool for assessment of degree, extent, and cause of biliary obstruction
  - Transabdominal US may help guide interventional procedures
  - For better anatomical evaluation of underlying pathology, CT or MR provides supplemental information
- Protocol advice
  - US scanning technique
    - Include comprehensive assessment on sagittal, transverse, and oblique planes, intercostal and subcostal approach
    - Intrahepatic ducts are better visualized on deep inspiration
    - Semierect right posterior oblique (RPO) or right lateral decubitus position helps minimize obscuration by overlying bowel gas
    - Harmonic imaging allows better visualization of dilated duct and its content

DIFFERENTIAL DIAGNOSIS

Portal Vein Cavernoma

- Cavernous transformation of portal vein; racemose conglomerate of collateral veins
- Color Doppler will show portal venous flow

Thrombosed Portal Vein Branch

- Hypoechoic (acute) or echogenic (chronic) filling defect within main portal vein and its branches
- Color Doppler: Patchy flow or complete absence of flow

Venovenous Collaterals

- Collateral between thrombosed/stenosed hepatic veins and normal hepatic veins/portal veins
- Color Doppler: Venous flow
- Seen in Budd-Chiari syndrome

Peribiliary Cysts

- Small cysts along biliary triads

Choledochal Cyst

- Congenital cystic dilatation of biliary tree

PATHOLOGY

General Features

- Etiology
  - Nonobstructive causes
    - Advanced age
    - Previous cholecystectomy
    - Congenital disease (e.g., choledochal cyst)
    - Hepatic artery stenosis in liver transplant recipients
  - Obstructive causes
    - Intrahepatic: Calculus, sclerosing/AIDS cholangitis, recurrent pyogenic cholangitis, ascending cholangitis, cholangiocarcinoma, trauma, etc.
    - Extrahepatic: Common duct calculus, pancreatic head adenocarcinoma, cholangiocarcinoma, lymph node compression, stricture, ampullary stenosis etc.

CLINICAL ISSUES

Presentation

- Depends on underlying cause (e.g., acute cholangitis: Right upper quadrant pain, fever and chills)
- Obstructive jaundice: Painless or right upper quadrant pain

SELECTED REFERENCES

1. Holm AN et al: What should be done with a dilated bile duct? Curr Gastroenterol Rep. 12(2):150-6, 2010
2. Rubens DJ. Ultrasound imaging of the biliary tract. Ultrasound Clinics. 2(3):391-413, 2007
3. Gandolfi L et al: The role of ultrasound in biliary and pancreatic diseases. Eur J Ultrasound. 16(3):141-59, 2003
4. von Herbay A et al: Color doppler sonography avoids misinterpretation of the "parallel channel sign" in the sonographic diagnosis of cholestasis. J Clin Ultrasound. 27(8):426-32, 1999

KEY FACTS

TERMINOLOGY

- Spectrum of extrahepatic and intrahepatic bile ducts malformations characterized by fusiform dilatation

IMAGING

- Todani Classification
  - Type I: Solitary fusiform or cystic dilatation of common duct
  - Type II: Extrahepatic supraduodenal diverticulum
  - Type III: Choledochocele
  - Type IVa: Both intrahepatic and extrahepatic cysts
  - Type IVb: Multiple extrahepatic cysts without intrahepatic cysts
  - Type V: Single or multiple intrahepatic cysts (Caroli disease)
- Ultrasound
  - Cystic extrahepatic mass separated from gallbladder and communicating with common hepatic or intrahepatic ducts
  - Intrahepatic ductal dilatation due to simultaneous involvement or secondary to stenosis
- MRCP and ERCP: Best depiction of choledochal cysts and anomalous pancreatobiliary junction union

TOP DIFFERENTIAL DIAGNOSES

- Biliary obstruction of various causes
- Pancreatic pseudocyst
- Primary sclerosing cholangitis
- Recurrent pyogenic cholangitis

CLINICAL ISSUES

- Usually diagnosed in childhood (80%)
- Triad: Recurrent RUQ pain, jaundice, palpable mass
- Complications: Biliary calculi, cholangitis, carcinoma
- Surgical excision and enterobiliary reconstruction

DIAGNOSTIC CHECKLIST

- Rule out other conditions that can cause marked biliary dilatation

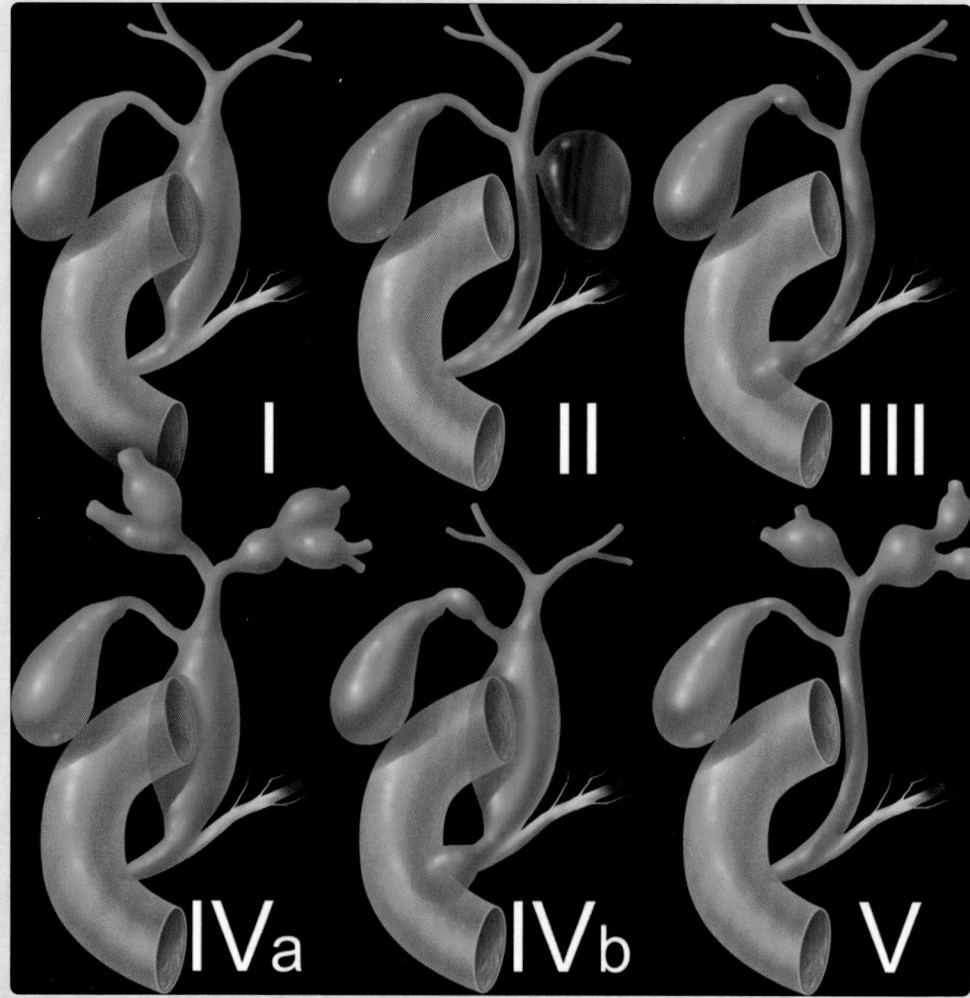

Graphic shows Todani classification of choledochal cyst. Type I: Solitary extrahepatic involvement; II: Diverticulum; III: Choledochocele; IVa: Multiple extrahepatic and intrahepatic involvement, IVb: Multiple extrahepatic involvement without intrahepatic involvement; V: Caroli disease.

Choledochal Cyst

TERMINOLOGY

Synonyms
- Choledochal malformation, biliary cyst, choledochocele

Definitions
- Congenital segmental dilatation of intrahepatic &/or extrahepatic bile ducts

IMAGING

General Features
- Best diagnostic clue
  - Nonobstructive, disproportional balloon-like dilatation of biliary tree
- Location
  - Involve extrahepatic ducts (more common), intrahepatic ducts, or both
- Size
  - Varies from 2-15 cm
- Morphology
  - Todani classification: Modified in 2003
    - Type I: Solitary cystic fusiform dilatation of common duct (CD) (50-85%)
      - Ia: Cystic dilatation of entire CD; associated with anomalous pancreatobiliary ductal union (APBDU)
      - Ib: Focal dilatation of entire CD; not associated with APBDU
      - Ic: Fusiform dilatation of entire CD; associated with APBDU
      - Mild dilatation of intrahepatic duct blurs distinction with type IVa
    - Type II: True diverticulum of supraduodenal CD (2%)
    - Type III: Choledochocele; dilatation limited to intraduodenal part of CD (1-5%)
      - IIIa: Cystic dilatation of intraduodenal CD
      - IIIb: Diverticulum of intraduodenal CD
    - Type IV: Presence of multiple cysts (15-35%)
      - IVa: Involvement of both intrahepatic and extrahepatic ducts
      - IVb: Multiple extrahepatic cysts without intrahepatic cysts
    - Type V: Single or multiple intrahepatic cysts (multiple intrahepatic cysts known as Caroli disease)

Ultrasonographic Findings
- Grayscale ultrasound
  - Best 1st test to demonstrate dilated biliary tree and extent of ductal involvement
  - Antenatal ultrasound (25 weeks): Right-sided cyst in fetal abdomen ± dilated hepatic ducts
  - Uncomplicated choledochal cyst
    - Cystic extrahepatic mass separate from gallbladder and communicating with common hepatic or intrahepatic ducts
    - Fusiform dilatation of extrahepatic bile duct
    - Abrupt change of caliber at junction of dilated segment to normal ducts
    - Intrahepatic ductal dilatation due to simultaneous involvement or secondary to stenosis
- Color Doppler
  - Useful for demonstrating position and displacement of adjacent vessels

CT Findings
- CECT
  - Cystic lesions contiguous with biliary tree
  - Multiplanar MIP images are ideal
  - Type V (Caroli disease): "Central dot" sign (enhancing portal vein radicles indenting cystic spaces)

MR Findings
- MRCP
  - Has replaced percutaneous cholangiogram in preoperative planning
  - Helpful to evaluate pancreatobiliary junction anatomy

Nuclear Medicine Findings
- Hepatobiliary scintigraphy
  - Large photopenic area in liver, showing late filling and prolonged stasis of isotope
  - Prominent intrahepatic ductal tracer activity
  - May be confused with other causes of biliary obstruction

Other Modality Findings
- ERCP and percutaneous cholangiogram
  - Usually reserved for difficult or complex cases
  - Best depiction of all types of choledochal cysts
  - Helpful to evaluate pancreatobiliary junction

Imaging Recommendations
- Best imaging tool
  - MRCP; ERCP if endoscopic intervention is being considered

DIFFERENTIAL DIAGNOSIS

Biliary Obstruction of Various Causes
- Proportional (rather than fusiform) dilatation
- Degree of dilatation less than choledochal cyst
- Primary lesion identifiable (e.g., choledocholithiasis, pancreatic ductal, ampullary, or distal common bile duct [CBD] cancer)

Pancreatic Pseudocyst
- No communication with bile ducts
- CECT: Enhancement of fibrous capsule
- MRCP: Hyperintense cyst contiguous with dilated pancreatic duct
- ERCP: Pseudocyst communicating with pancreatic duct seen in 70% of cases

Primary Sclerosing Cholangitis
- Idiopathic inflammatory process leading to progressive fibrosis and strictures of intra- and extrahepatic bile ducts
- Multifocal areas of alternating biliary strictures and dilatation
- Abnormal bile duct wall thickening and enhancement

Recurrent Pyogenic Cholangitis
- Dilatation of both intra- and extrahepatic bile ducts
- Cast-like biliary stones, sludge, pneumobilia, and abscess
- MRCP: Ductal rigidity and straightening, rapid tapering of peripheral intrahepatic duct
- More common in Asians

PATHOLOGY

General Features

- Etiology
  - 2 main hypotheses
    - Congenital ductal plate malformation
    - APBDU proximal to duodenal papilla forming long common channel, strongly associated with type I and IV
      - □ Higher pressure in pancreatic duct and absent ductal sphincter
      - □ Free reflux of pancreatic enzymes into CBD causes weakening of CBD wall and dilatation
  - Additional theories
    - Decrease in number of ganglion cells in narrow portion of bile duct causes increased intraluminal pressure, reovirus infection, failure of recanalization, familial pattern of inheritance, or duodenal duplication
- Associated abnormalities
  - Gallbladder: Aplasia or double gallbladder
  - Biliary anomalies
    - Biliary atresia or stenosis
    - Other forms of fibropolycystic disease (congenital hepatic fibrosis, biliary hamartomas)
  - Annular pancreas

Staging, Grading, & Classification

- Classification of choledochal cyst: Todani classification
- Classification of APBDU: Komi classification
  - Type P-B: Perpendicular insertion of pancreatic duct into CBD (acute-angled union, fusiform dilatation)
  - Type B-P: Perpendicular insertion of CBD into pancreatic duct (right-angled union, cystic dilatation)
  - 2 major duct unions are associated with type I choledochal cyst

Gross Pathologic & Surgical Features

- Cystic/fusiform dilated sac with bile, stones, or sludge
- Cyst wall is thickened, fibrotic, and occasionally calcified in adults
- Long ectatic common channel with pancreatic duct (normal length: 0.2-1.0 cm)

Microscopic Features

- Thickened ductal wall consists of chronic inflammation and fibrosis
- Widespread ulceration and denuded mucosa in dilated CBD
- Biliary epithelium lining the cyst is often intact in infants
- Goblet cell metaplasia and epithelial dysplasia may play role in subsequent development of carcinoma

CLINICAL ISSUES

Presentation

- Most common signs/symptoms
  - Triad: Recurrent RUQ pain, jaundice, palpable mass
  - Infant: Intermittent jaundice, acholic stools, hepatomegaly, palpable abdominal mass
  - Children and adult: Upper abdominal pain, jaundice, recurrent cholangitis/pancreatitis

Demographics

- Age
  - Usually diagnosed in infancy and childhood
  - 25% detected before age 1; 80% diagnosed in childhood (60% before age 10); 20% in adults
- Gender
  - M:F = 1:3-4 (more common in females)
- Epidemiology
  - Prevalence: 1:13,000 admissions
  - More common in Asians

Natural History & Prognosis

- Low-grade biliary obstruction may develop and can potentially result in cirrhosis and portal hypertension
- Prevalence of adenocarcinoma arising in choledochal cysts
  - Varies from 2-18%, corresponding to roughly 5-35x increased risk
- Other complications: Biliary calculi, cholangitis, pancreatitis
- Prognosis: Usually good after surgical repair, but poor if malignant degeneration occurs

Treatment

- Type I: Complete surgical excision + Roux-en-Y choledochojejunostomy
- Type II: Cysts can usually be surgically excised entirely
- Type III: Choledochocele < 3 cm: Endoscopic sphincterotomy; > 3 cm: Surgically excised via transduodenal approach
- Type IV: Dilatated extrahepatic duct completely excised with biliary-enteric drainage procedure, intrahepatic involvement left untreated
- Type V: If limited to single hepatic lobe, may be resected; diffuse disease + liver failure: Liver transplantation

DIAGNOSTIC CHECKLIST

Consider

- Rule out other causes of marked biliary dilatation

Image Interpretation Pearls

- MRCP or ERCP: Cystic or fusiform dilatation of bile ducts without obstructive lesion

SELECTED REFERENCES

1. Venkatanarasimha N et al: Imaging features of ductal plate malformations in adults. Clin Radiol. 66(11):1086-93, 2011
2. Lee HK et al: Imaging features of adult choledochal cysts: a pictorial review. Korean J Radiol. 10(1):71-80, 2009
3. Mortele KJ et al: Multimodality imaging of pancreatic and biliary congenital anomalies. Radiographics 26: 715-731; 2006
4. Sugiyama M et al: Anomalous pancreaticobiliary junction shown on multidetector CT. AJR Am J Roentgenol. 180(1):173-5, 2003
5. Todani T et al: Classification of congenital biliary cystic disease: special reference to type Ic and IVA cysts with primary ductal stricture. J Hepatobiliary Pancreat Surg. 10(5):340-4, 2003
6. Benya EC: Pancreas and biliary system: imaging of developmental anomalies and diseases unique to children. Radiol Clin North Am. 40(6):1355-62, 2002
7. de Vries JS et al: Choledochal cysts: age of presentation, symptoms, and late complications related to Todani's classification. J Pediatr Surg. 37(11):1568-73, 2002
8. Krause D et al: MRI for evaluating congenital bile duct abnormalities. J Comput Assist Tomogr. 26(4):541-52, 2002

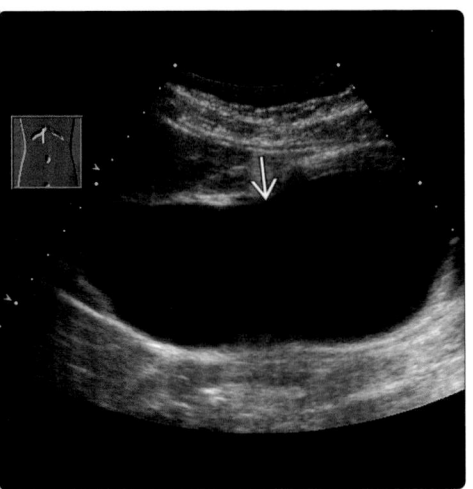

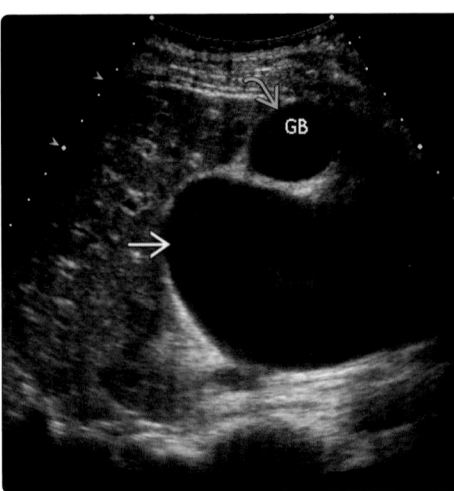

(Left) *Longitudinal transabdominal ultrasound shows marked fusiform dilatation of the extrahepatic bile duct* ➡ *in this patient with type I choledochal cyst.* (Right) *Transverse grayscale ultrasound in the same patient shows the markedly dilated common duct* ➡, *which has a cystic appearance in the hepatic hilum. The gallbladder (GB)* ➡ *is anterior and separate from the choledochal cyst (type I).*

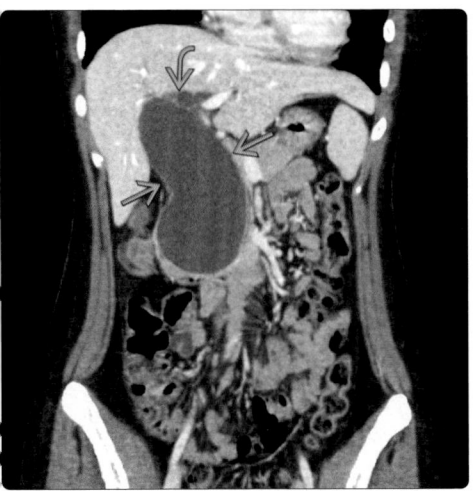

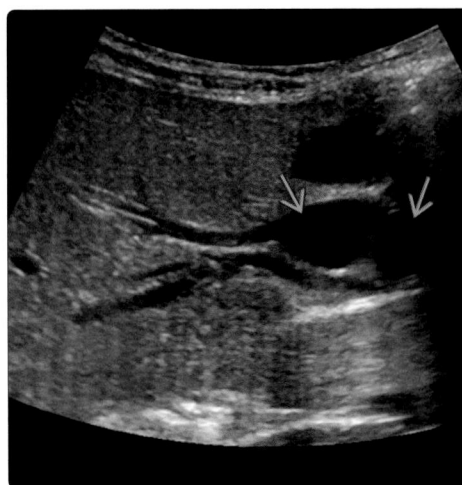

(Left) *Contrast-enhanced coronal CT in the same patient shows marked fusiform dilatation of the common duct* ➡ *communicating with intrahepatic ducts* ➡, *consistent with type I choledochal cyst.* (Right) *Longitudinal oblique grayscale ultrasound of the porta hepatis shows a multilobulated common duct with 2 distinct lobulations* ➡ *consistent with a type IVb choledochal cyst. (Courtesy S. Bhatt, MBBS.)*

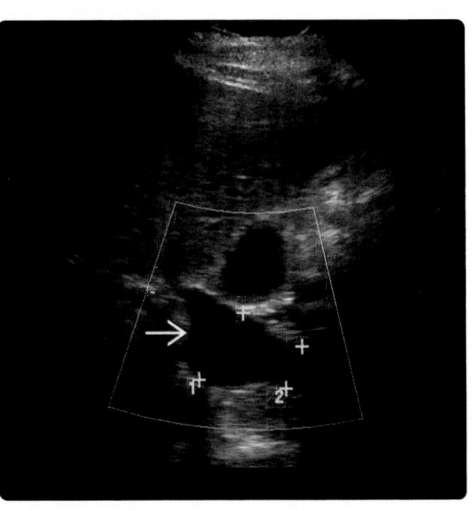

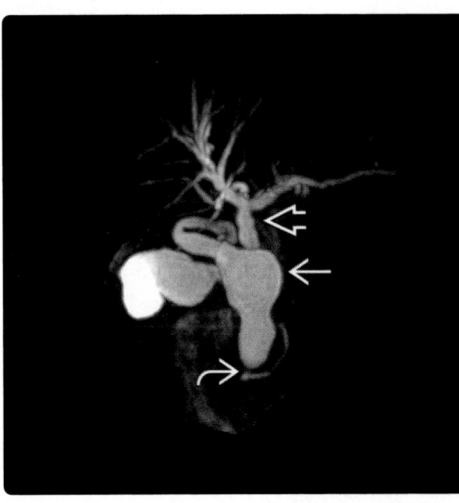

(Left) *Grayscale ultrasound shows marked fusiform dilatation of the common bile duct* ➡ *consistent with a type 1 choledochal cyst.* (Right) *MRCP in the same patient confirms the marked dilatation of the common duct* ➡ *with secondary mild dilatation of the intrahepatic duct* ➡, *consistent with a type 1 choledochal cyst. Note the common channel of the pancreas and common duct with an anomalous pancreatobiliary union* ➡.

Choledocholithiasis

TERMINOLOGY

- Cholangiolithiasis, hepatolithiasis, biliary calculi, common bile duct (CBD) stones

IMAGING

- Transabdominal ultrasound: Most stones appear as highly echogenic foci with posterior acoustic shadowing
  - First-line imaging modality
  - Most often found in periampullary region/distal portion of CBD, can be obscured by gas
- ERCP: Radiolucent, faceted, or angular filling defects within bile ducts
  - "Gold" standard, is diagnostic and potentially therapeutic
- MRCP: Low-intensity filling defects within increased signal intensity bile ducts
  - Very sensitive for detection of bile duct stones.
- NECT: Attenuation of stones varies from less than water density, through soft tissue, to dense calcification
  - Not very sensitive for detection of bile duct stones

TOP DIFFERENTIAL DIAGNOSES

- Cholangiocarcinoma, ampullary mass
- Biliary parasitic infection, ascending cholangitis, recurrent pyogenic cholangitis

PATHOLOGY

- Passage of gallstones into biliary ductal system (more common) vs. de novo stone formation within ducts
- Can cause obstruction with subsequent ductal dilation

CLINICAL ISSUES

- Presentation: RUQ pain, pruritus, jaundice; however, may be asymptomatic
- May present with acute complication: cholangitis, pancreatitis

DIAGNOSTIC CHECKLIST

- Rule out other causes of CBD obstruction

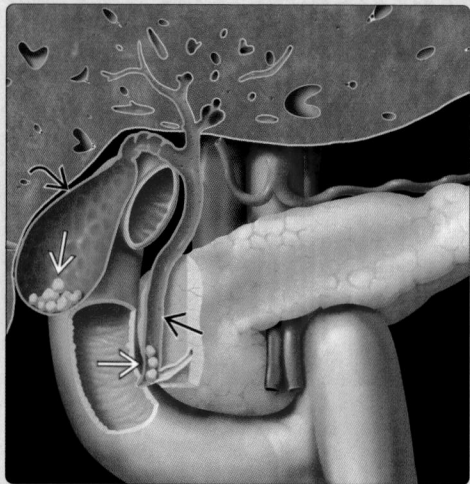
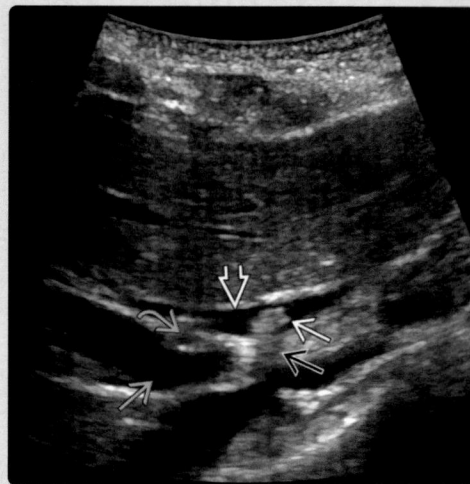

(Left) *Graphic shows multiple, nonobstructive stones ➡ in the distal common bile duct ➡ and gallbladder ➡.* (Right) *An echogenic focus ➡ with posterior shadowing ➡ that is compatible with a stone is present within the common bile duct (CBD) ➡ on this longitudinal US. The CBD is located anterior to the hepatic artery ➡ and the portal vein ➡. The hepatic artery crosses in between the portal vein and CBD.*

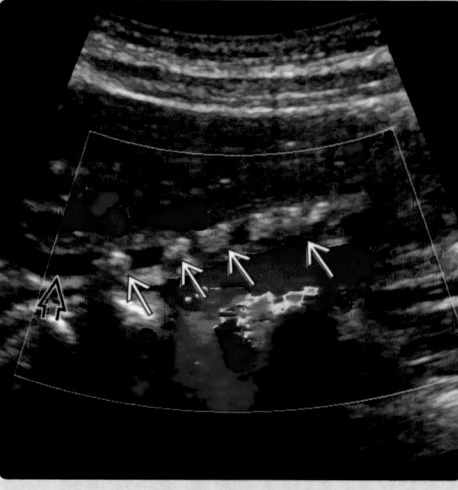
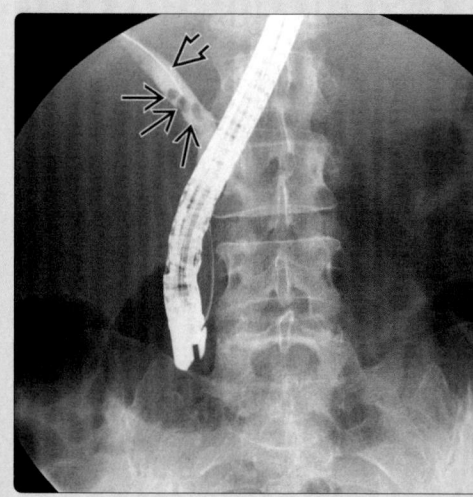

(Left) *More caudally, there are several more stones ➡, which are seen as echogenic shadowing foci, within the CBD ➡ extending to the level of the head of the pancreas. (Color Doppler ultrasound is helpful to distinguish the biliary ducts from the adjacent vasculature.)* (Right) *A spot fluoroscopic image from the subsequent endoscopic retrograde cholangiopancreatography (ERCP) procedure demonstrates several filling defects, compatible with stones ➡, within the CBD ➡.*

TERMINOLOGY

Abbreviations
- Cholangiolithiasis, hepatolithiasis, biliary calculi, common bile duct (CBD) stones

Definitions
- Choledocholithiasis: Extrahepatic ductal stones/calculi
- Hepatolithiasis: Intrahepatic stones/calculi

IMAGING

General Features
- Best diagnostic clue
  - Echogenic focus within bile duct, casting posterior acoustic shadowing
- Location
  - Intrahepatic and extrahepatic bile ducts
    - More common in CBD
- Size
  - Variable
- Morphology
  - Classified into 2 main types based on origin
    - Primary choledocholithiasis: De novo formation within bile duct
      - Calculi are composed predominantly of bilirubin (> 90% calcium bilirubinate composition)
      - Brown pigment stones are associated with bacterial infections
    - Secondary choledocholithiasis (more common): Gallstone migration from gallbladder to bile ducts
      - Calculi are composed primarily of cholesterol

Ultrasonographic Findings
- Grayscale ultrasound
  - Appearance depends on site, size, and composition of stones
  - Extrahepatic biliary stones
    - Most commonly seen within CBD
      - Most often within lumen of periampullary region/distal portion of CBD
    - Classic appearance: Rounded echogenic lesion with posterior acoustic shadowing
    - Can be associated with extrahepatic and intrahepatic ductal dilatation
  - Intrahepatic biliary stones
    - Majority appear as highly echogenic foci with posterior acoustic shadowing
    - Located in region of portal triads paralleling course of intrahepatic portal veins
    - Small (< 5 mm) or soft pigmented stones may not produce posterior shadowing
    - Larger stone may cause biliary obstruction with focal intrahepatic ductal dilatation
    - Duct is filled with stones, appears as linear echogenic structure with posterior acoustic shadowing
  - 10% stones: No posterior acoustic shadow
    - Small size, soft, and porous composition
  - CBD/intrahepatic bile duct dilatation (IHBD) based on stone size, degree, and duration of obstruction

- Transabdominal US sensitivity for choledocholithiasis reported between 20% and 78%, may be obscured distally by bowel gas
  - Endoscopic US sensitivity for choledocholithiasis reported between 94% and 98%
- Color Doppler
  - Echogenic focus is avascular, may show "twinkling" artifact
  - Aids definition of dilated biliary ducts against background intrahepatic parenchymal vessels

Radiographic Findings
- ERCP
  - Radiolucent filling defects within intrahepatic ± extrahepatic bile ducts
  - Potentially therapeutic: Portal for stone retrieval, sphincterotomy, or internal stent insertion
  - Sensitivity for choledocholithiasis reported between 90-95%, considered "gold standard"
- Intraoperative and postoperative (T tube) cholangiography
  - Direct test for detection of CBD stones
  - Meniscus of contrast material clearly outlines margins of stones

CT Findings
- NECT
  - Attenuation of calculi varies from less than water density, through soft tissue, to dense calcification
    - Typically high-density filling defect within biliary duct
  - Abrupt termination of CBD by obstructing stone
  - CBD &/or IHBD dilatation
    - Varies depending on stone size, degree, and duration of obstruction
  - Sensitivity for choledocholithiasis between 67-88%

MR Findings
- MRCP
  - Bile: T2 hyperintense signal
  - Ductal stones: T2 hypointense foci
  - Calculi manifest as low intensity filling defects within increased signal intensity bile ducts
  - Sensitivity for choledocholithiasis between 81-100%

Imaging Recommendations
- Best imaging tool
  - US, MRCP
- Protocol advice
  - CBD stones are most commonly located in region of ampulla of Vater
    - High chance of being obscured by bowel gas
  - Practical advice to optimize detection
    - Examine patient in different positions: Supine, left lateral oblique, sitting upright
    - Use firm probe pressure to collapse superficial bowel and its content
    - Perform detailed assessment of head region of pancreas
  - Postcholecystectomy patients with persistent RUQ pain
    - Image after fasting and 45 min to 1 hr after fatty meal
  - If gas obscures CBD; have patient drink 6-12 oz of water
    - Keep patient in right decubitus position for 2-3 minutes and rescan in semierect position

DIFFERENTIAL DIAGNOSIS

Cholangiocarcinoma

- Intrahepatic or extrahepatic infiltrative or irregular mass
- Soft tissue growth within ductal lumen
- Obstruction and dilatation of CBD and IHBD
- Regional nodal and liver metastases

Biliary Parasitic Infestation

- Most common infestation: *Ascaris*, *Clonorchis*
- Parallel echogenic tubular structures with sonolucent center within bile duct
- Active movement of parasite
- Lack of posterior acoustic shadowing

Ampullary Mass

- Hypodense mass in head of pancreas or ampulla
- Ill-defined infiltrative margin
- "Double duct" sign
  - o Obstruction and dilatation of pancreatic duct and CBD
- Vascular encasement
- Contiguous organ invasion/regional nodal metastases may be seen

Ascending Cholangitis

- Clinical information suggesting biliary sepsis
- Ductal wall thickening is hallmark in appropriate clinical setting
- Usually due to superinfection of biliary obstruction by CBD stone, less likely from strictures
- Can be associated with echogenic biliary sludge within ducts

Recurrent Pyogenic Cholangitis

- Historically in patients of East Asian demographic
- Recurrent bouts of cholangitis
- Strong association with parasites, such as *Ascaris lumbricoides* and *Clonorchis sinensis*
- Pigmented stones &/or sludge within dilated intrahepatic and extrahepatic bile ducts
- Disproportionate increased dilation of central and extrahepatic bile ducts with stricturing and stenosis of peripheral ducts

PATHOLOGY

General Features

- Etiology
  - o Primary choledocholithiasis: De novo formation of stones within bile ducts, precipitated by bile stasis and infection
  - o Secondary choledocholithiasis: Gallstones migrate into CBD, most common
- Associated abnormalities
  - o Gallstones
    - − 5-20% of patients with gallstones will have choledocholithiasis at time of cholecystectomy
  - o Dilated ducts

CLINICAL ISSUES

Presentation

- Most common signs/symptoms

- o RUQ pain, pruritus, jaundice
- o May be asymptomatic
- Other signs/symptoms
  - o May present with complication: Acute cholangitis, acute pancreatitis
- Clinical profile
  - o "Fat, fertile, 40, female": Overweight, middle-aged female with history of acute or intermittent RUQ pain and jaundice
- Lab data
  - o Increased alkaline phosphatase and direct bilirubin

Demographics

- Age
  - o Usually adults; can be seen in any age group
- Gender
  - o F > M

Natural History & Prognosis

- Small stones may pass spontaneously without causing any symptoms
- Complications: Cholangitis, obstructive jaundice, pancreatitis, secondary biliary cirrhosis

Treatment

- ERCP: Preoperative, intraoperative, or postoperative
- Intraoperative common bile duct exploration: Open versus laparoscopic
- Other lithotripsy: Extracorporeal shock wave, electrohydraulic, laser

DIAGNOSTIC CHECKLIST

Consider

- Rule out other causes of "CBD obstruction"

Image Interpretation Pearls

- Echogenic filling defects casting posterior acoustic shadowing associated with dilatation of CBD/intrahepatic bile ducts

SELECTED REFERENCES

1. Costi R et al: Diagnosis and management of choledocholithiasis in the golden age of imaging, endoscopy and laparoscopy. World J Gastroenterol. 20(37):13382-401, 2014
2. Stinton LM et al: Epidemiology of gallbladder disease: cholelithiasis and cancer. Gut Liver. 6(2):172-87, 2012
3. O'Connor OJ et al: Imaging of biliary tract disease. AJR Am J Roentgenol. 197(4):W551-8, 2011
4. Yeh BM et al: MR imaging and CT of the biliary tract. Radiographics. 29(6):1669-88, 2009
5. Rubens DJ. Ultrasound imaging of the biliary tract. Ultrasound Clinics. 2(3):391–413, 2007
6. Caddy GR et al: Gallstone disease: Symptoms, diagnosis and endoscopic management of common bile duct stones. Best Pract Res Clin Gastroenterol. 20(6):1085-101, 2006
7. Freitas ML et al: Choledocholithiasis: evolving standards for diagnosis and management. World J Gastroenterol. 12(20):3162-7, 2006
8. Tazuma S: Gallstone disease: Epidemiology, pathogenesis, and classification of biliary stones (common bile duct and intrahepatic). Best Pract Res Clin Gastroenterol. 20(6):1075-83, 2006
9. Hanbidge AE et al: From the RSNA refresher courses: imaging evaluation for acute pain in the right upper quadrant. Radiographics. 24(4):1117-35, 2004

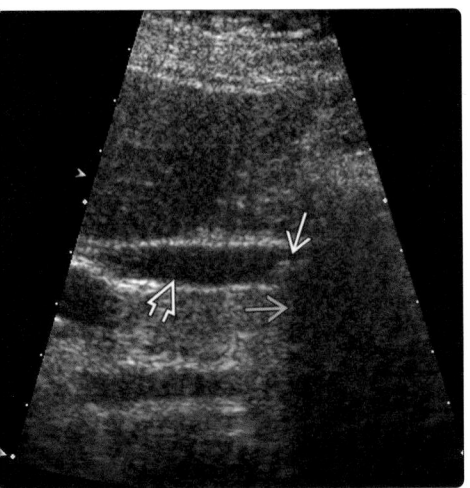

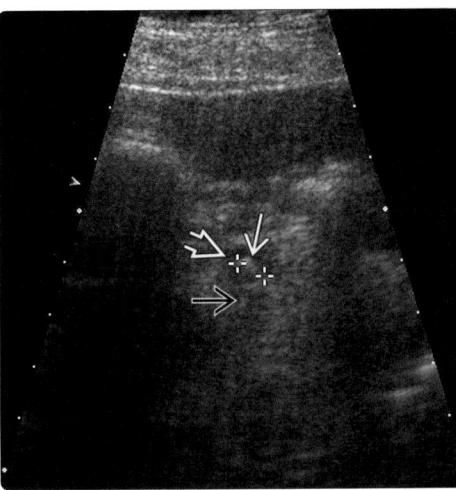

(Left) *A single echogenic focus ⇨ with dense posterior acoustic shadowing ⇨ compatible with a stone is seen in the CBD ⇨ on this longitudinal ultrasound. The CBD is mildly dilated, likely secondary to obstruction from the stone.* **(Right)** *Transverse oblique ultrasound in the same patient confirms the calculus ⇨ within the common bile duct ⇨. There is shadowing ⇨ noted posteriorly.*

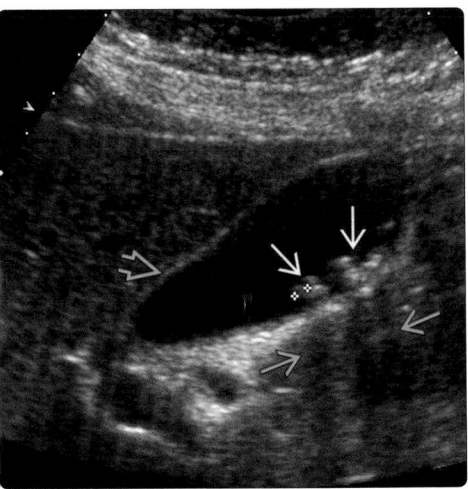

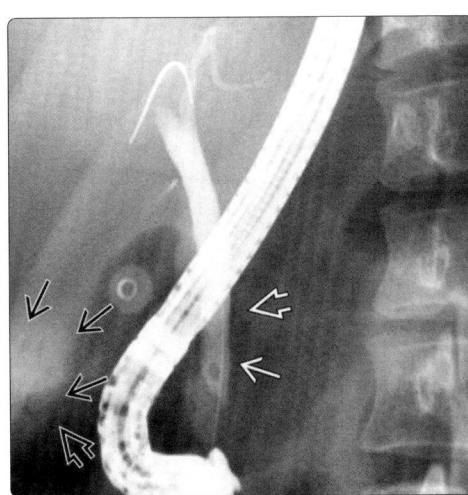

(Left) *Longitudinal ultrasound of the gallbladder ⇨ in the same patient demonstrates several stones ⇨ within its lumen. The calculi are echogenic and demonstrate posterior acoustic shadowing ⇨.* **(Right)** *A spot fluoroscopic image from the ERCP procedure demonstrates a filling defect near the distal end of the dilated CBD ⇨, consistent with choledocholithiasis ⇨. Contrast also has refluxed into the gallbladder ⇨, where multiple other gallstones ⇨ appear as filling defects in the lumen of the gallbladder.*

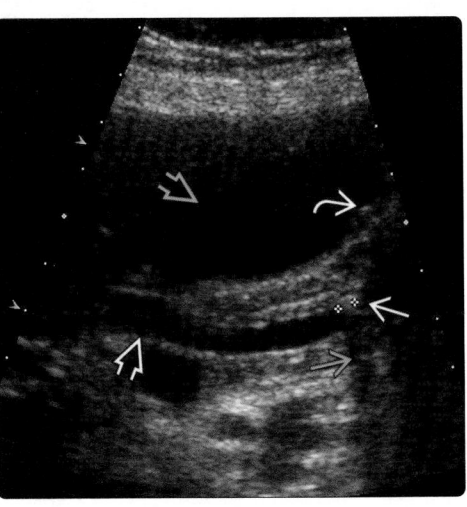

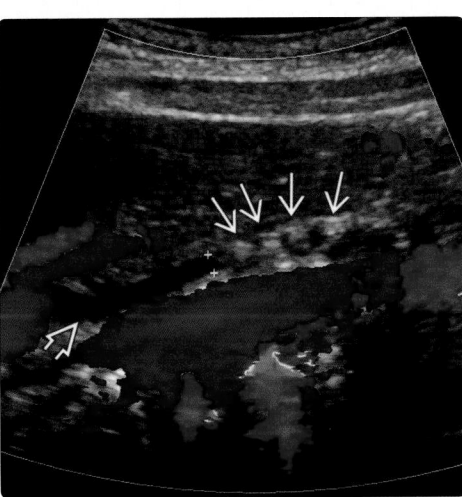

(Left) *Longitudinal ultrasound shows a hyperechoic stone ⇨ with dense posterior shadowing ⇨ present in the CBD ⇨. The gallbladder ⇨ contains an additional stone ⇨ within its lumen.* **(Right)** *Several stones ⇨ are present in the CBD ⇨, causing mild extrahepatic biliary ductal dilation. Color Doppler is helpful to distinguish the CBD (which does not fill in with color) from the adjacent vasculature.*

KEY FACTS

TERMINOLOGY

- Definition: Gas within biliary tree including bile ducts or gallbladder
- Synonyms: Pneumobilia, aerobilia

IMAGING

- Bright echogenic foci in linear/branching configuration following portal triads associated with "dirty" shadowing/reverberation artifact
- Most commonly seen within intrahepatic bile ducts, though may also involve extrahepatic bile ducts and gallbladder
- Movement of gas, best demonstrated following change in patient's position

TOP DIFFERENTIAL DIAGNOSES

- Portal venous gas
  - Branching echogenic foci in periphery of liver parenchyma within portal venous radicle
- Intrahepatic ductal stones/sludge

- Echogenic foci casting dense posterior acoustic shadowing ± dilated duct
- Hepatic arterial calcifications
  - Hyperechoic lines accompanying portal veins

PATHOLOGY

- Etiology
  - Previous biliary intervention, classically papillotomy
  - Cholecysto-enteric/choledocho-enteric fistula
  - Biliary infection with gas-forming organism
  - Recurrent pyogenic cholangitis

CLINICAL ISSUES

- Majority will resolve spontaneously
- Prognosis depends on underlying etiology

DIAGNOSTIC CHECKLIST

- Examine patient in supine and oblique positions to demonstrate movement of gas
- Consider CT for improved delineation

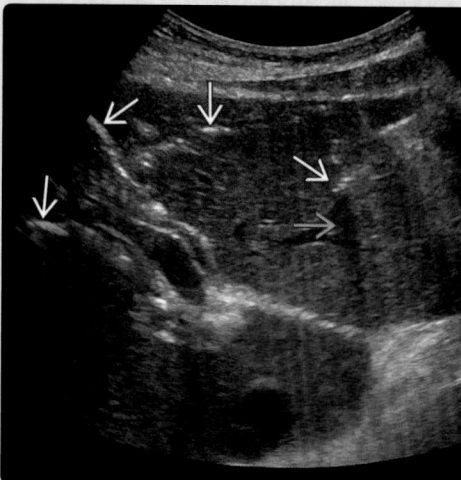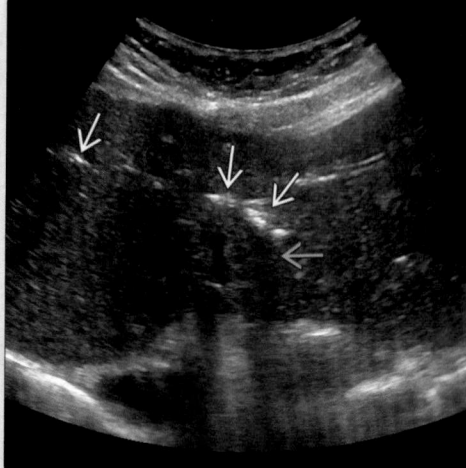

(Left) Transverse US through the left hepatic lobe demonstrates multiple linear echogenic areas along the expected course of the biliary tree ➡, some with associated with posterior shadowing ⇨, compatible with intrahepatic biliary gas. (Right) Transverse US through the left hepatic lobe demonstrates linear echogenic foci ➡ associated with "dirty" posterior shadowing ⇨, compatible with intrahepatic biliary ductal gas.

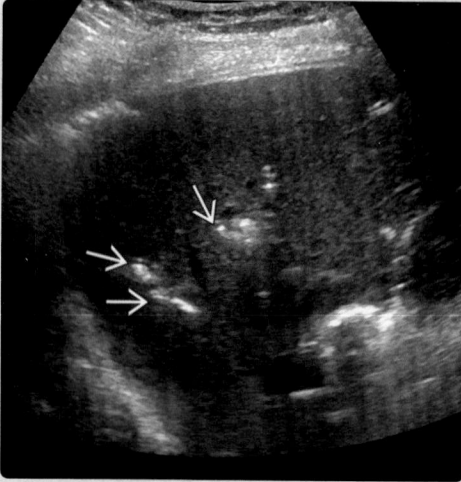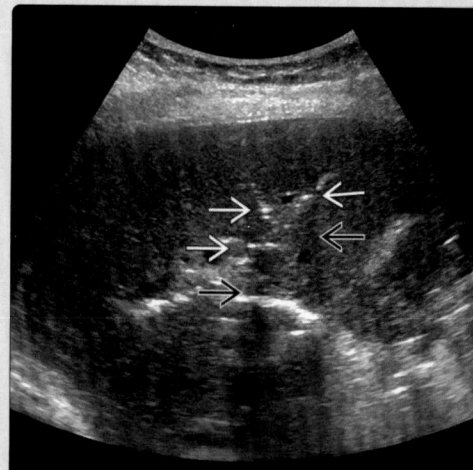

(Left) Transverse US through the right hepatic lobe demonstrates several echogenic foci ➡ in linear configurations, with "dirty" posterior shadowing, compatible with biliary ductal gas. (Right) Transverse US through the right hepatic lobe demonstrates several echogenic foci ➡ in linear configurations which are associated with "dirty" posterior shadowing ⇨, compatible with biliary ductal gas.

TERMINOLOGY

Synonyms

- Pneumobilia, aerobilia

Definitions

- Gas within biliary tree including bile ducts or gallbladder

IMAGING

General Features

- Best diagnostic clue
  - Bright echogenic foci in linear/branching configuration following portal triads associated with reverberation artifact/dirty shadowing
- Location
  - Most commonly seen within intrahepatic bile ducts, though may also involve extrahepatic bile ducts and gallbladder

Ultrasonographic Findings

- Grayscale ultrasound
  - Gas within intrahepatic bile duct
    - Bright echogenic foci in linear configuration following portal triads
    - In nondependent position: Left > right lobe biliary ducts with patient in supine position
    - Associated with "dirty" shadowing: Shadows filled with acoustic noise caused by sound-reflecting objects (gas)
    - Reverberation artifacts with large quantities of gas
    - Movement of gas, best demonstrated following change in patient's position
  - Gas within extrahepatic bile duct
    - Linear echogenic foci with "dirty" shadowing
    - Within extrahepatic bile ducts adjacent to major structures in porta hepatis
  - Gas within gallbladder
    - Band-like echogenic layer in nondependent portion of gallbladder
    - Prominent reverberation artifacts obscures lumen

CT Findings

- CECT
  - Linear/tubular gas density adjacent to well-opacified portal venous radicles and portal veins
    - May be found within bile ducts (intrahepatic &/or extrahepatic) or within gallbladder
  - Biliary ductal gas tends to be more central in location as opposed to portal venous gas, which tends to be more peripheral

Radiographic Findings

- "Saber" sign: Sword-shaped lucency in right paraspinal region

Fluoroscopic Findings

- Filling defects: May be rounded, whereas calculi may be angular/faceted

MR Findings

- Hypointense filling defect on T2-weighted MRCP (similar to stones)
- Signal void structures producing susceptibility artifact on T1-weighted dual echo gradient sequence

Imaging Recommendations

- Best imaging tool
  - Ultrasound, CT
- Protocol advice
  - Examine patient in supine and oblique positions to demonstrate movement of gas
  - Set appropriate focus level to optimize visualization of reverberation artifacts or posterior acoustic shadowing

DIFFERENTIAL DIAGNOSIS

Portal Venous Gas

- Branching echogenic foci in periphery of liver parenchyma within portal venous radicle
- Sharp bidirectional spikes on Color Doppler, superimposed upon usual Doppler tracing of portal vein

Intrahepatic Ductal Stones/Sludge

- Echogenic foci casting dense posterior acoustic shadowing
- In region of portal triad or within dilated intrahepatic ducts

Hepatic Arterial Calcification

- Hyperechoic double lines representing calcified arterial wall accompanying portal veins
- Acoustic shadows of various sizes throughout liver

PATHOLOGY

General Features

- Etiology
  - Previous biliary intervention, iatrogenic causes
    - ERCP ± sphincterotomy
    - Biliary-enteric anastomosis
    - Presence of internal biliary stent or external biliary drainage catheter
  - Cholecysto-enteric/choledocho-enteric fistula
    - Prolonged acute cholecystitis ± superimposed gallstone ileus
    - Perforated duodenal ulcer
    - Erosion by biliary malignancy (e.g., carcinoma of gallbladder)
  - Biliary infection with gas-forming organism
    - Emphysematous cholecystitis
    - Acute bacterial cholangitis
  - Recurrent pyogenic cholangitis

CLINICAL ISSUES

Natural History & Prognosis

- Majority will resolve spontaneously
- Prognosis depends on underlying etiology

SELECTED REFERENCES

1. Shah PA et al: Hepatic gas: widening spectrum of causes detected at CT and US in the interventional era. Radiographics. 31(5):1403-13, 2011
2. Sherman SC et al: Pneumobilia: benign or life-threatening. J Emerg Med. 30(2):147-53, 2006
3. Okuda K et al: Sonographic features of hepatic artery calcification in chronic renal failure. Acta Radiol. 44(2):151-3, 2003
4. Rubin JM et al: Clean and dirty shadowing at US: a reappraisal. Radiology. 181(1):231-6, 1991

Cholangiocarcinoma

TERMINOLOGY

- Malignancy that arises from intrahepatic bile duct (IHBD) or extrahepatic bile duct epithelium

IMAGING

- Best diagnostic clue: Intra- or extrahepatic bile duct mass with upstream bile duct dilatation
- Intrahepatic cholangiocarcinoma
  - Mass with ill-defined margin, heterogeneous echotexture
  - Isolated thickening of IHBD or intraductal mass, with upstream ductal dilatation
- Hilar cholangiocarcinoma
  - Nonunion of right and left hepatic ducts
  - Primary tumor may not be discernible, or appears as small, infiltrative iso-/hyperechoic mass in hilar region
- Extrahepatic cholangiocarcinoma
  - Proportional bile duct dilatation

- Primary tumor often undetectable due to its deep location
  - Ill-defined, solid, heterogeneous mass within or surrounding duct at point of obstruction
  - Polypoidal intraluminal tumor visible as iso-/hyperechoic mass within bile duct

TOP DIFFERENTIAL DIAGNOSES

- Pancreatic head adenocarcinoma
- Choledocholithiasis
- Recurrent pyogenic cholangitis
- Primary sclerosing cholangitis
- Porta hepatis tumor

PATHOLOGY

- Pathogenesis: Biliary intraepithelial neoplasm is considered premalignant lesion

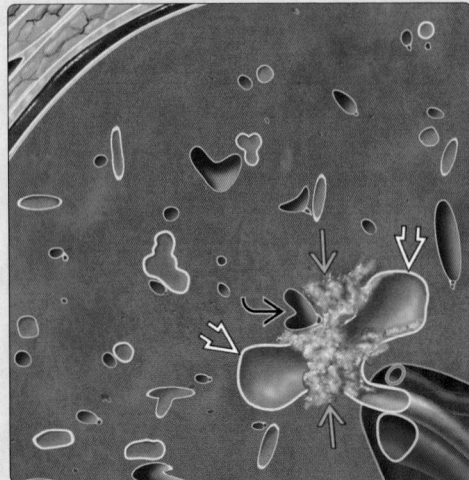

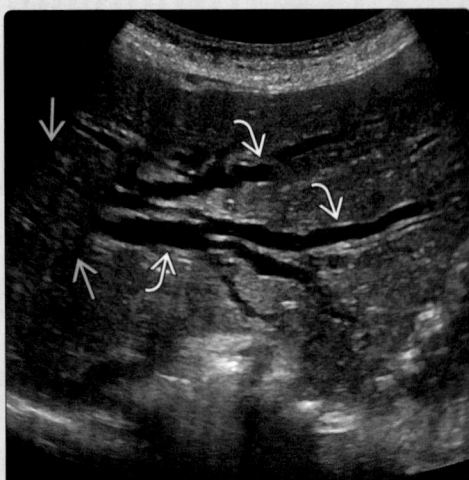

(Left) Graphic shows an infiltrative mass ⇨ at the confluence of the right and left hepatic ducts (Klatskin tumor). The mass invades adjacent liver parenchyma and hepatic veins ⬈, a common finding with cholangiocarcinoma. Note upstream dilatation of intrahepatic bile ducts ⇛. (Right) Transverse abdominal grayscale ultrasound shows an ill-defined isoechoic cholangiocarcinoma ⇨ at the hepatic confluence associated with marked left intrahepatic ductal dilatation ⬂.

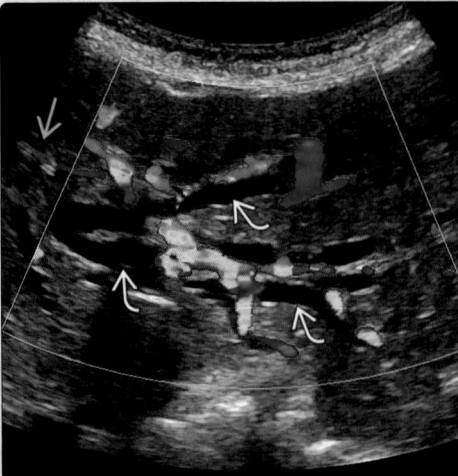

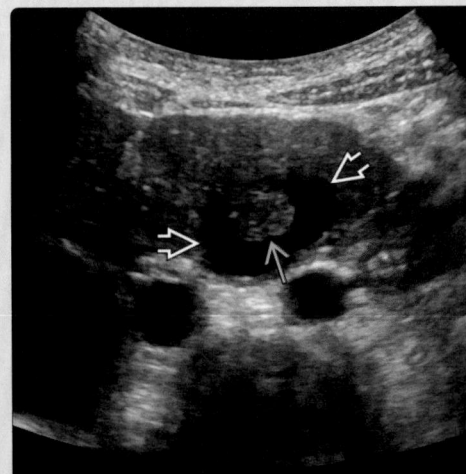

(Left) Color Doppler ultrasound performed in the same patient confirms tubular structures are indeed dilated intrahepatic bile ducts ⬂ caused by an isoechoic cholangiocarcinoma involving the hepatic confluence ⇨. (Right) Isoechoic polypoid intraluminal cholangiocarcinoma ⇨ in the distal common bile duct ⇛ is seen on this transverse view of the common bile duct at the level of the pancreatic head.

Cholangiocarcinoma

TERMINOLOGY

Synonyms
- Cholangiocellular carcinoma or bile duct adenocarcinoma

Definitions
- Malignancy that arises from intrahepatic bile duct (IHBD) or extrahepatic bile duct epithelium

IMAGING

General Features
- Best diagnostic clue
  - Intra- or extrahepatic bile duct mass with upstream bile duct dilatation
- Location
  - Distribution in different segments of biliary tree
    - Distal common bile duct (CBD): 30-50%, most common extrahepatic location
    - Proximal CBD: 15-30%
    - Common hepatic duct (CHD): 14-37%
    - Confluence of hepatic ducts (Klatskin tumor): 10-26%
    - Isolated right or left IHBD: 8-13%
    - Cystic duct: 6%
  - Classification based on anatomy or radiography
    - Peripheral (10%): Intrahepatic; proximal to secondary biliary radicles
    - Hilar (50%): Klatskin tumor; confluence of hepatic ducts
    - Distal (40%): Extrahepatic; distal CBD
- Size
  - Intrahepatic mass: A few cm up to 20 cm
  - Extrahepatic: Typically present when smaller
- Morphology
  - Classification by Liver Cancer Study Group of Japan
    - Mass-forming type
    - Periductal-infiltrating type
    - Intraductal-growing type

Ultrasonographic Findings
- Grayscale ultrasound
  - **Intrahepatic cholangiocarcinoma**
    - Mass with ill-defined margin, mixed and heterogeneous echotexture
    - Isolated thickening of IHBD or intraductal mass, with upstream ductal dilatation
  - **Hilar cholangiocarcinoma (Klatskin tumor)**
    - Dilatation of intrahepatic ducts without extrahepatic ductal dilatation
    - Apparent nonunion of dilated right and left IHBDs
    - Primary tumor may not be discernible, or appears as small infiltrative iso-/hyperechoic mass in hilar region
    - Nodular or polypoid mass in bile ducts
    - Mass effect, invasion of portal vein and hepatic artery
  - **Extrahepatic cholangiocarcinoma**
    - Dilatation of intrahepatic and proximal extrahepatic bile duct
      - Primary tumor often undetectable due to its deep location
    - Ill-defined, solid, heterogeneous mass within or surrounding duct at point of obstruction
      - May be exophytic: Heterogeneous mass arising from bile duct
      - May be intraluminal: Polypoid iso-/hyperechoic mass within bile duct
  - Other signs of malignancy
    - Infiltration of liver parenchyma
    - Lymphatic spread; commonly to porta hepatis, paraceliac and peripancreatic lymph nodes
    - Liver metastases

Radiographic Findings
- Cholangiography (PTC/ERCP)
  - Intraductal filling defect with upstream ductal dilatation
  - Ductal wall irregularity and shouldering
  - "Missing duct" sign: Unopacified segmental IHBDs upstream to tumor (ERCP)
  - Infiltrating type: Frequently long, rarely short concentric focal stricture
  - Klatskin tumor: Nonunion of left and right IHBDs

CT Findings
- NECT
  - Intrahepatic/hilar: Peripheral hypodense lesions with IHBD proximal to obstruction
  - Extrahepatic: Large growth (seen as hypodense mass) and IHBD dilatation
- CECT
  - Arterial phase: Peripheral enhancement with progressive, central patchy enhancement and IHBD dilatation
  - Portal venous phase: Moderate enhancement of thickened bile duct wall, vascular invasion, lymphadenopathy
  - Delayed phase (10-15 min): Persistent enhancing tumor due to fibrous stroma

MR Findings
- T1WI: Iso-/hypointense
- T2WI: Hyperintense periphery (viable) and hypointense center (fibrosis)
- T1WI C+: Superior to CT in detecting small hilar tumors, intrahepatic and periductal tumor infiltration
- T1WI FS: Tumor of intrapancreatic portion of CBD seen as hypointense against hyperintense pancreatic head
- MRCP: Reveals site of obstruction and extension of tumor growth

Imaging Recommendations
- Best imaging tool
  - US: Detection and initial assessment of level and cause of biliary obstruction
  - ERCP/MRCP: Extent of biliary ductal involvement
  - CECT/CEMR: More detailed tumor extent (liver invasion, porta hepatis involvement, regional nodal metastases)

DIFFERENTIAL DIAGNOSIS

Pancreatic Head Adenocarcinoma
- Irregular hypoechoic mass in pancreatic head on US
- Abrupt obstruction of pancreatic duct &/or distal CBD
- Early invasion of celiac axis and superior mesenteric vessels common
- Obliteration of retropancreatic fat

Choledocholithiasis

- Intra- and extrahepatic bile duct stones with ductal dilatation
- Echogenic filling defects with posterior acoustic shadowing
- Biliary sludge of medium echoes mimic intraluminal form of extrahepatic tumor
- May see ductal wall thickening due to superimposed cholangitis

Recurrent Pyogenic Cholangitis

- Ductal wall thickening due to repeated and longstanding cholangitis
- Intrahepatic biliary stones and echogenic biliary sludge
- Accompanies atrophy of involved hepatic segment &/or biliary cirrhosis
- Present clinically with repeated episodes of acute ascending cholangitis

Primary Sclerosing Cholangitis (PSC)

- Multiple strictures associated with beading and peripheral pruning of bile ducts
- Bile duct wall thickening
- Risk for cholangiocarcinoma: 10% of PSC patients

Porta Hepatis Tumor

- Bulky primary tumor (e.g., hepatocellular carcinoma [HCC]), lymph node metastasis, metastasis
- May invade or obstruct IHBDs and cause dilatation

PATHOLOGY

General Features

- Etiology
  - Biliary intraepithelial neoplasm is considered premalignant lesion
  - Risk factors
    - Primary sclerosing cholangitis
    - Choledochal cyst
    - Biliary papillomatosis
    - Parasites (clonorchiasis, *Opisthorchis*)
    - Recurrent pyogenic cholangitis
    - Ulcerative colitis
    - Chronic liver disease
    - Thorotrast exposure
- Patterns of disease progression
  - Local extension along bile duct
  - Local infiltration of liver parenchyma
  - Spread to regional lymph nodes; porta hepatis, paraceliac and peripancreatic lymph node (LN)
  - Perineural spread
  - Intraperitoneal seeding (peritoneal carcinomatosis)
  - Hematogenous spread

Gross Pathologic & Surgical Features

- Bismuth-Corlette classification of Klatskin tumor
  - I: Tumor involving CHD below confluence
  - II: Tumor involving CHD reaching confluence
  - IIIa: Tumor involving right 2nd-order branch
  - IIIb: Tumor involving left 2nd-order branch
  - IV: Tumor involving both 2nd-order branches

Microscopic Features

- Sclerosing type: Stricture, most common type, worst prognosis
- Nodular type: Exophytic intrahepatic masses
- Papillary type: Intraluminal polypoid lesions, least common type, best prognosis

CLINICAL ISSUES

Presentation

- Most common signs/symptoms
  - Painless obstructive jaundice, pain, palpable mass, weight loss
- Lab data: ↑ bilirubin/alkaline phosphatase, ↑ CEA/CA19-9

Demographics

- Age: Peak at 6th-7th decade
- Gender: M:F = 3:2
- Epidemiology
  - More common in Asia
  - Causes 15-33% of primary hepatobiliary cancers
  - 2nd most common primary hepatic tumor (after HCC)

Natural History & Prognosis

- 5-year survival rate: 5-10%
- Resectability rate: Distal 91%, hilar 56%, peripheral 60%

Treatment

- Surgical resection (only potentially curative method) + adjuvant chemoradiation
- Palliative treatment: Chemotherapy, radiation; laser therapy; biliary stenting

DIAGNOSTIC CHECKLIST

Consider

- Rule out other biliary & pancreatic pathologies that can mimic cholangiocarcinoma by obstructing extrahepatic bile duct

Image Interpretation Pearls

- Long and rarely short focal extrahepatic biliary stricture, irregular ductal wall, stenosis and prestenotic biliary ductal dilatation
- Klatskin tumor: Small tumor at confluence of right/left hepatic and proximal common hepatic ducts

SELECTED REFERENCES

1. Chung YE et al: Varying appearances of cholangiocarcinoma: radiologic-pathologic correlation. Radiographics. 29(3):683-700, 2009
2. Vilgrain V: Staging cholangiocarcinoma by imaging studies. HPB (Oxford). 10(2):106-9, 2008
3. Han JK et al: Cholangiocarcinoma: pictorial essay of CT and cholangiographic findings. Radiographics. 22(1):173-87, 2002

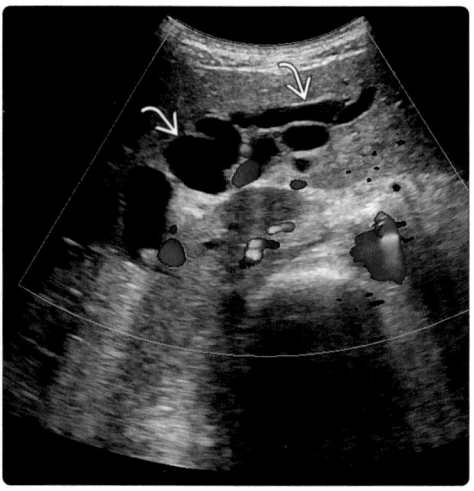
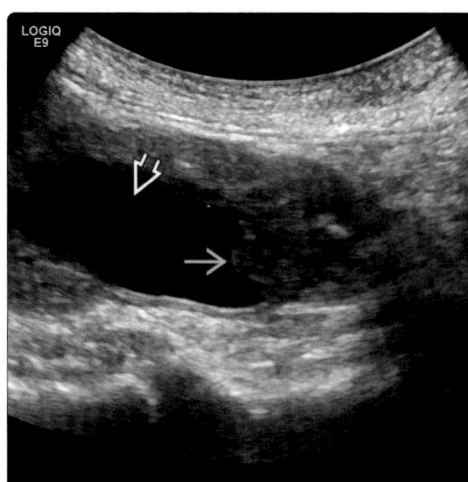

(Left) *Ultrasound in a different patient shows marked intrahepatic biliary ductal dilatation* ⇗ *caused by an extrahepatic common bile duct cholangiocarcinoma (not shown in this image).* (Right) *Longitudinal view of the common bile duct in the same patient shows the obstructing cholangiocarcinoma* ⇒ *causes proximal marked biliary ductal dilatation* ⇛.

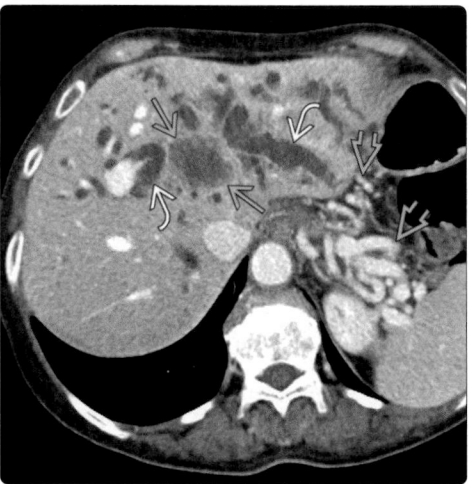
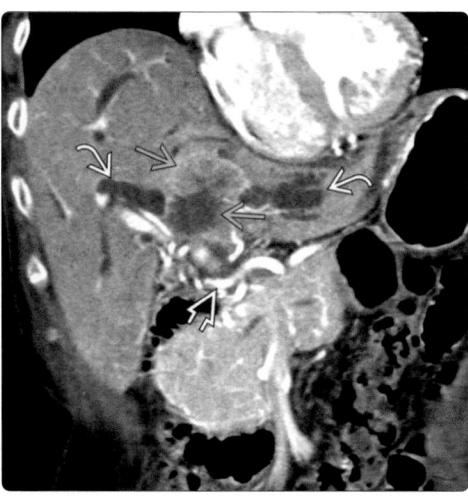

(Left) *Axial CECT shows a hypodense cholangiocarcinoma at the hepatic hilar level invading liver parenchyma* ⇒ *with marked intrahepatic duct dilatation* ⇗ *in right and left lobes. Note gastric/splenic varices* ⇒ *caused by portal vein obliteration (not shown) by the tumor.* (Right) *Coronal CT in the same patient shows a cholangiocarcinoma at the hepatic hilum* ⇒ *with marked intrahepatic duct dilatation* ⇗*. Note collateral vessels at the porta hepatis* ⇛ *caused by portal vein obliteration.*

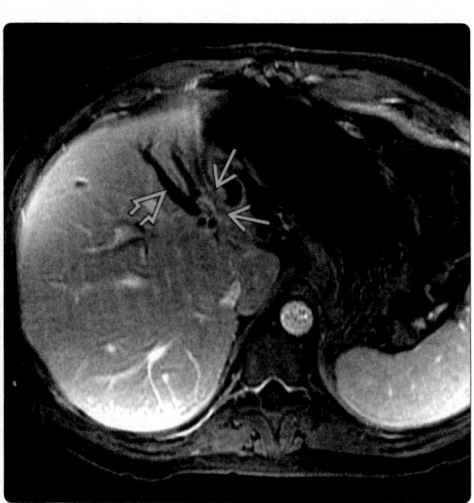
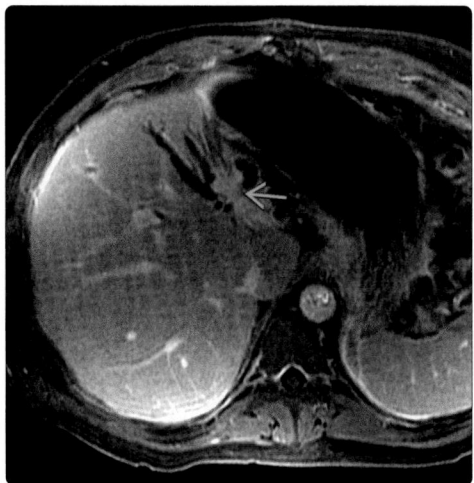

(Left) *Axial contrast-enhanced MR shows a cholangiocarcinoma that appears as an ill-defined isointense soft tissue mass* ⇒ *near the hepatic hilum. Dilatated intrahepatic ducts* ⇒ *in segment 4 abruptly terminate at the level of the mass.* (Right) *Delayed phase contrast-enhanced MR in the same patient shows the cholangiocarcinoma* ⇒ *to better advantage due to retention of contrast, which causes the tumor to appear slightly hyperintense compared to background liver parenchyma.*

Diagnoses: Biliary System

TERMINOLOGY

- Inflammation of intra-/extrahepatic bile duct walls due to ductal obstruction and infection

IMAGING

- Dilatation of intra- and extrahepatic bile ducts
  - In cases of early cholangitis or intermittent CBD obstruction, bile ducts may not be dilated
- Circumferential thickening of bile duct wall
- Presence of obstructing choledocholithiasis
- Periportal hypo-/hyperechogenicity adjacent to dilated intrahepatic ducts
- Presence of purulent bile/sludge
- Multiple small hepatic cholangitic abscesses

TOP DIFFERENTIAL DIAGNOSES

- Cholangiocarcinoma
- Pancreatic ductal carcinoma
- Primary sclerosing cholangitis (PSC)

- Recurrent pyogenic cholangitis (RPC)
- Other forms of secondary cholangitis

PATHOLOGY

- Risk factors
  - Choledocholithiasis: Most common
  - Biliary stricture, biliary stent, choledochal surgery, recent biliary manipulation, sphincter of Oddi dysfunction

CLINICAL ISSUES

- Charcot triad: RUQ pain, fever, jaundice
- Complications: Cholangitic liver abscesses & septicemia, portal vein thrombosis
- Treatment: Antibiotics + biliary decompression

DIAGNOSTIC CHECKLIST

- Correlate with clinical & laboratory data to achieve accurate imaging interpretation

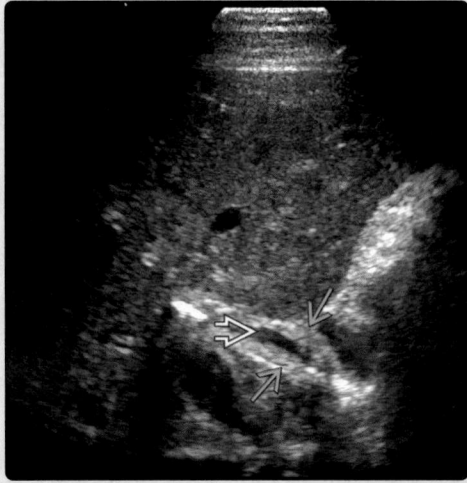
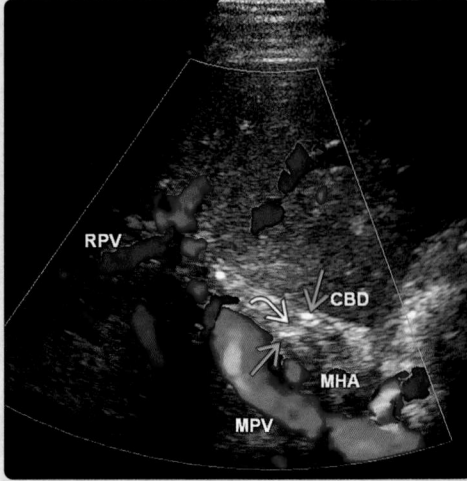

(Left) Transverse abdominal ultrasound in a patient with ascending cholangitis shows circumferential markedly thickened common bile duct wall ➡ with only minimal luminal ⬦ distension. (Right) Transverse color Doppler ultrasound in the same patient with ascending cholangitis shows lack of detectable vascularity in the thickened common bile duct wall ➡. In addition, echogenic debris ⬦ within the CBD is evident on this image.

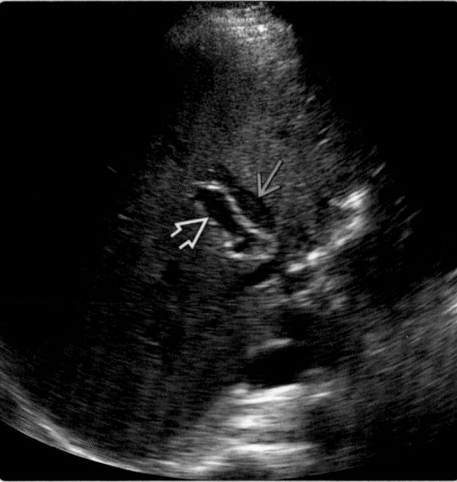
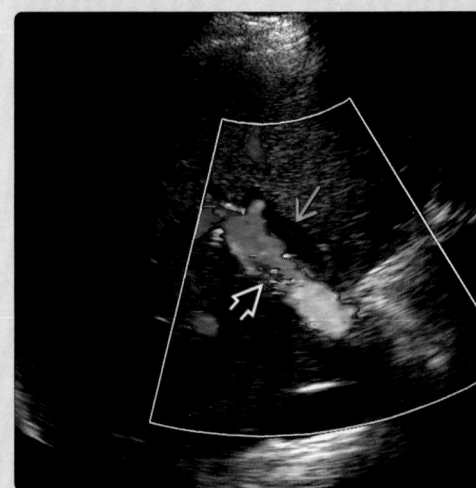

(Left) Transverse abdominal grayscale US in a patient with ascending cholangitis shows mildly dilated proximal intrahepatic duct ➡ anterior to right portal vein ⬦, consistent with mild degree of biliary obstruction. (Right) Transverse abdominal color Doppler US in the same patient imaged closer to the porta hepatis confirms the tubular structure is a dilated common bile duct ➡, which lies anterior to main portal vein ⬦.

TERMINOLOGY

Synonyms

- Bacterial cholangitis, acute obstructive cholangitis, suppurative cholangitis, biliary infection

Definitions

- Inflammation of intra-/extrahepatic bile duct walls due to ductal obstruction and infection

IMAGING

General Features

- Best diagnostic clue
  - Biliary ductal dilatation due to obstructing CBD stone associated with biliary ductal wall thickening
- Location
  - Usually obstruction in extrahepatic bile duct (most common in CBD)
  - Inflammation affecting both intra-/extrahepatic bile ducts
- Morphology
  - May involve entire biliary system, lobar or segmental in distribution

Ultrasonographic Findings

- Grayscale ultrasound
  - Dilatation of intra- and extrahepatic bile ducts (in 75% of cases)
    - Diameter of common bile duct > 6 mm is considered abnormal in most adult patients without prior cholecystectomy
    - Intrahepatic duct dilatation: > 1-2 mm
    - In cases of early cholangitis or intermittent CBD obstruction, bile ducts may not be dilated
  - Circumferential thickening of bile duct wall
    - Thick hypoechoic layer of inner wall of bile duct
    - May extend to gallbladder causing GB wall thickening
  - Periportal hypo-/hyperechogenicity along dilated intrahepatic ducts
    - Due to presence of periductal inflammatory change/edema
  - Presence of obstructing choledocholithiasis
    - Echogenic focus within dilated CBD casting posterior acoustic shadowing
    - Mobile with patient position changes
  - Presence of purulent bile/sludge
    - Intraluminal echogenic material, usually within dilated intrahepatic ducts
    - Usually does not cast acoustic shadow
  - Multiple small hepatic cholangitic abscesses
    - Anatomically clustered in lobe or segment of liver
    - Represent liquefaction of biliary inflammation, late finding
    - Hypoechoic cystic lesions with floating internal echoes and debris
  - Pneumobilia: Rare finding
    - Due to ascending infection by gas-forming organisms or presence of choledochoenteric fistula
    - Echogenic foci in linear configuration along portal triad
    - Presence of reverberation artifacts

- Color Doppler
  - May show increased periportal vascularity related to reactive hyperemia

Radiographic Findings

- Cholangiography
  - Irregular bile duct lumen/wall
  - Ductal stricture, obstruction, & proximal dilatation
  - Stone: Radiolucent filling defect
  - IHBD may show communication with hepatic abscesses

CT Findings

- NECT
  - Dilatation of intra-/extrahepatic bile ducts
  - Obstructing stone: May be calcific, soft tissue, or water density
  - Bull's-eye sign: Rim of bile surrounding a stone
  - High-density intraductal material (purulent bile)
  - Multiple small, rim-enhancing cystic lesions indicate development of cholangitic abscesses
- CECT
  - Concentric biliary wall thickening and enhancement
  - Hepatic parenchymal enhancement: Wedge-shaped, peribiliary, patchy
  - Can be associated with liver abscess or portal vein thrombosis

MR Findings

- T2WI
  - Hypointense stones within hyperintense bile
  - Hepatic parenchymal hyperintensity
    - Wedge shaped, peribiliary or patchy distribution
- MRCP
  - Intrahepatic biliary ductal dilatation
  - Irregular strictures, proximal dilatation of bile ducts
  - Hypointense stones within hyperintense bile
  - Cholangitic abscesses: Multiple small hyperintense hepatic lesions

Imaging Recommendations

- Best imaging tool
  - US is ideal tool for initial evaluation
  - In difficult or equivocal cases, MRCP or contrast cholangiography (ERCP, PTC) may be indicated
  - ERCP/PTC serve as portal for biliary drainage (internal/external biliary drainage)
- Protocol advice
  - Subtle US features (such as ductal dilatation, ductal wall thickening) may be difficult to appreciate
  - Scan patient in different positions (supine, oblique, lateral) using multiple acoustic windows (intercostal, oblique subcostal) to detect subtle ductal change

DIFFERENTIAL DIAGNOSIS

Cholangiocarcinoma

- Ill-defined infiltrative mass
- Commonly at hepatic confluence
- Dilated intrahepatic ducts with nondilated extrahepatic ducts distal to site of tumor
- Regional metastatic lymph node and liver metastases

Pancreatic Ductal Carcinoma

- Infiltrative hypoechoic mass in pancreatic head
- Dilatation of intra- and extrahepatic bile ducts and pancreatic ducts
- Vascular encasement
- Regional nodal and liver metastases

Primary Sclerosing Cholangitis (PSC)

- Segmental strictures, beaded and pruned ducts
- Involves both intrahepatic & extrahepatic ducts
- End-stage: Lobular liver, hypertrophy, and atrophy

Recurrent Pyogenic Cholangitis (RPC)

- Intra-/ and extrahepatic biliary pigmented stones
- Lateral segment of left lobe and posterior segment of right lobe are more commonly involved
- Presence of multifocal intrahepatic ductal strictures with segmental dilatation
- Clinical information of ethnic origin and recurrent attacks of cholangitis help in suggesting etiology

Other Forms of Secondary Cholangitis

- AIDS-related cholangitis
- Chemotherapy-induced cholangitis
- Ischemic cholangitis

PATHOLOGY

General Features

- Etiology
  - Pathogenesis: Stone/stricture → obstruction → bile stasis → increased biliary pressure → infection
  - Source of infection: Usually ascending from duodenum; rarely hematogenous
  - Risk factors
    - Choledocholithiasis and hepatolithiasis (most common)
    - Biliary stricture: In setting of PSC or malignancy
    - Biliary stents: Can act as nidus of infection
    - Choledochal surgery
    - Recent manipulation: ERCP, PTC
    - Sphincter of Oddi dysfunction or stenosis
  - Bacteriology
    - *Escherichia coli*, *Klebsiella*, *Enterococcus* species, *Enterobacter* species
    - Anaerobes in mixed infections
- Associated abnormalities
  - Gallstone disease

Staging, Grading, & Classification

- Severity of disease
  - Mild: Responsive to antibiotics and supportive therapy
  - Moderate: Not responsive to medical therapy, but no organ dysfunction
  - Severe: Organ dysfunction

Microscopic Features

- Acute inflammatory infiltrates involving ductal mucosa/submucosa
- Periductal aggregates of leukocytes with edema
- Liquefied necrosis in cholangitic abscesses

CLINICAL ISSUES

Presentation

- Most common signs/symptoms
  - **Charcot triad**: RUQ pain, fever, jaundice
- Other signs/symptoms
  - Septicemia, septic shock
  - Lethargy, mental confusion
    - Especially in elderly patients
- Lab data
  - Increased WBC count & bilirubin levels
  - Increased alkaline phosphatase and GGT
  - Transaminitis
  - Positive blood cultures in toxic phase

Demographics

- Age: More common in middle age or elderly
- Epidemiology: Most common type of cholangitis in Western countries

Natural History & Prognosis

- Complications: Cholangitic liver abscesses & septicemia, portal vein thrombosis
- Majority improve with antibiotic treatment
- High mortality if not decompressed
- Overall mortality significantly improved with antibiotic treatment and biliary decompression

Treatment

- Antibiotics to cover gram-negative organisms
- Biliary decompression for uncontrolled sepsis and failed medical therapy
  - ERCP: Sphincterotomy + stone extraction, internal stent
  - PTC: External biliary drainage via percutaneous transhepatic biliary drainage (PTBD)
  - Surgical decompression: Fulminant cases and failed nonoperative decompression

DIAGNOSTIC CHECKLIST

Consider

- Correlate with clinical & laboratory data to achieve accurate imaging interpretation
  - Due to overlap in US features of various cholangitis

Image Interpretation Pearls

- Biliary ductal dilatation and thickening related to obstructing choledocholithiasis in appropriate clinical setting

SELECTED REFERENCES

1. Spârchez Z et al: Role of contrast enhanced ultrasound in the assessment of biliary duct disease. Med Ultrason. 16(1):41-7, 2014
2. Kiriyama S et al: TG13 guidelines for diagnosis and severity grading of acute cholangitis (with videos). J Hepatobiliary Pancreat Sci. 20(1):24-34, 2013
3. Patel NB et al: Multidetector CT of emergent biliary pathologic conditions. Radiographics. 33(7):1867-88, 2013
4. Eun HW et al: Assessment of acute cholangitis by MR imaging. Eur J Radiol. 81(10):2476-80, 2012
5. Kim SW et al: Diagnostic performance of multidetector CT for acute cholangitis: evaluation of a CT scoring method. Br J Radiol. 85(1014):770-7, 2012

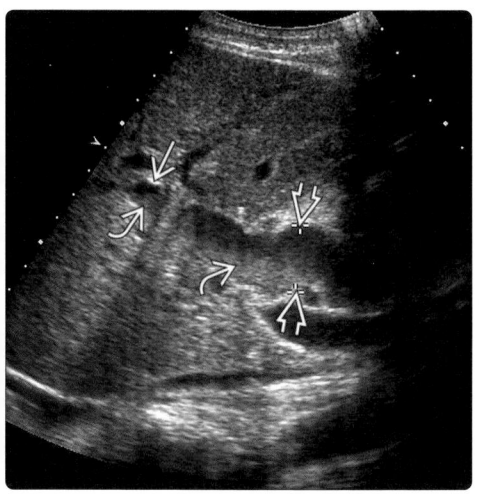
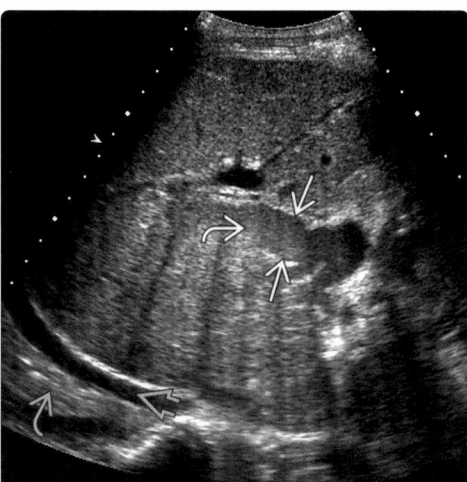

(Left) *Longitudinal abdominal US in a patient with severe cholangitis shows a markedly dilated common bile duct ⇒ and right intrahepatic duct ➜, containing layering debris ⇒ due to biliary stasis.* **(Right)** *Transverse abdominal US in the same patient with cholangitis shows amorphous echogenic material ➜ within the dilated common hepatic duct ➜, which represents a combination of sludge and pus. Small right pleural effusion ⇒ and atelectatic lung ⇒ is likely reactive.*

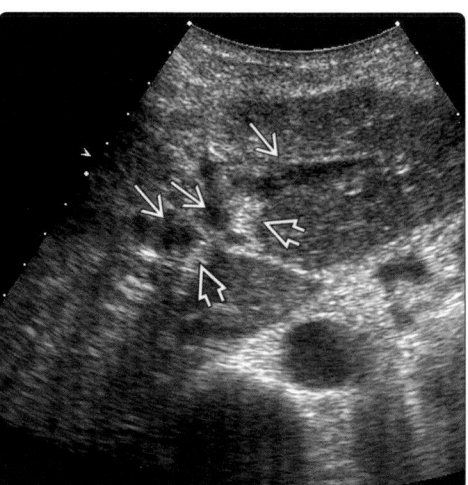
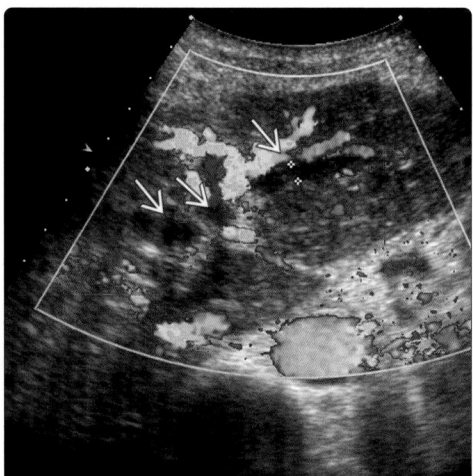

(Left) *Transverse abdominal US in a patient with cholangitis shows mild to moderate ductal dilatation ➜ and duct wall thickening ⇒ of the left intrahepatic ducts.* **(Right)** *Transverse abdominal color Doppler US in the same patient with cholangitis shows no color flow in the dilatated left intrahepatic ducts ➜. Color Doppler US confirms that these lesions are dilated bile ducts rather than hepatic vessels.*

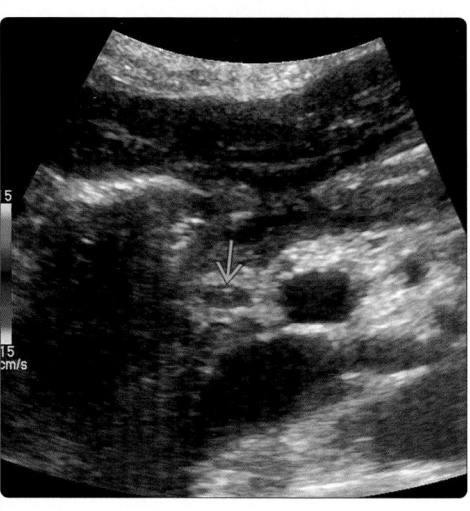
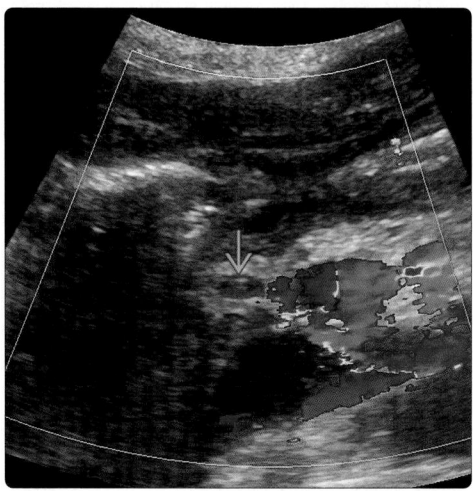

(Left) *Transverse abdominal US in a patient with cholangitis shows wall thickening of the common bile duct ⇒ without luminal distension.* **(Right)** *Transverse abdominal color Doppler US in the same patient with cholangitis shows wall thickening of the common bile duct without luminal dilatation ⇒. Color Doppler US confirms that this lesion is the bile duct rather than a hepatic vessel.*

Recurrent Pyogenic Cholangitis

TERMINOLOGY

- Recurrent episodes of acute pyogenic cholangitis with intra- and extrahepatic biliary pigment stones
- Synonyms: Hepatolithiasis, oriental cholangiohepatitis

IMAGING

- Intra- and extrahepatic biliary ductal dilatations with stones
- Lateral segment of left lobe and posterior segment of right lobe more commonly involved
- Biliary ductal thickening due to repeated inflammation
- Severe atrophy of affected lobe/segment, biliary cirrhosis
- Grayscale ultrasound
  - Presence of echogenic sludge/stones ± posterior acoustic shadowing in intrahepatic and extrahepatic duct
  - Periportal hypo-/hyperechogenicity due to periductal inflammation
  - Ductal rigidity and straightening, rapid tapering of peripheral intrahepatic duct
- Cholangiography and MRCP
  - Intra- and extrahepatic duct dilatation with stones as filling defects

TOP DIFFERENTIAL DIAGNOSES

- Ascending cholangitis
- Sclerosing cholangitis
- Cholangiocarcinoma
- Intrahepatic stones secondary to biliary stricture
- Caroli disease

CLINICAL ISSUES

- Common symptoms/signs: Recurrent episodes of RUQ pain, fever and jaundice
- Risk of developing cholangiocarcinoma (5-6%)

DIAGNOSTIC CHECKLIST

- Consider RPC in southeast Asian patients with recurrent episodes of acute bacterial cholangitis

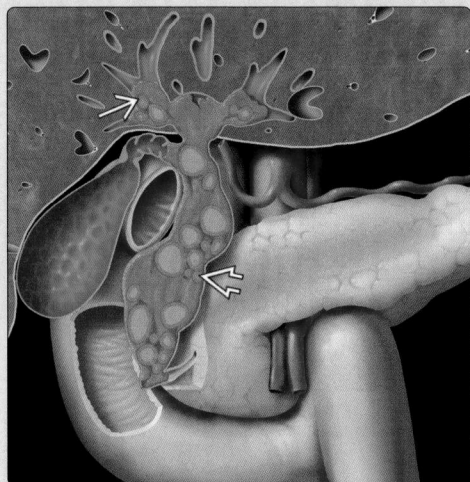
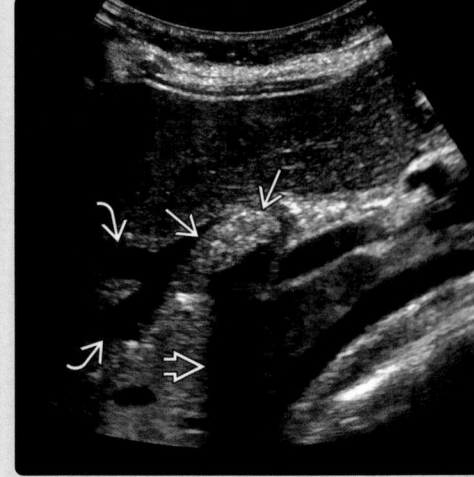

(Left) *Graphic shows recurrent pyogenic cholangitis with marked dilation of intrahepatic ➡ and extrahepatic ➡ bile ducts with multiple common bile duct and intrahepatic duct stones. The peripheral intrahepatic duct shows rapid tapering and decreased arborization.* **(Right)** *Grayscale ultrasound shows an ovoid intrahepatic stone ➡ with posterior acoustic shadowing ➡ in the right hepatic duct causing upstream intrahepatic bile duct dilatation ➡.*

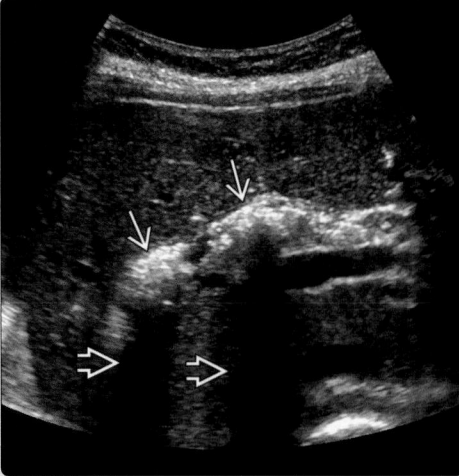
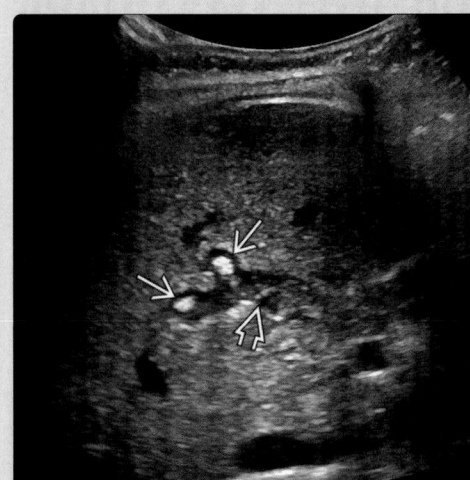

(Left) *Grayscale ultrasound of the liver shows multiple echogenic regions ➡ with posterior acoustic shadowing ➡ in the intrahepatic biliary system, consistent with intrahepatic stones in this patient with recurrent pyogenic cholangitis.* **(Right)** *Transverse grayscale ultrasound of the liver shows echogenic stones ➡ and sludge ➡ filling moderately dilated intrahepatic ducts.*

Recurrent Pyogenic Cholangitis

TERMINOLOGY

Abbreviations
- Recurrent pyogenic cholangitis (RPC)

Synonyms
- Hepatolithiasis, oriental cholangiohepatitis

Definitions
- Recurrent episodes of acute pyogenic cholangitis with intra- and extrahepatic biliary pigment stones

IMAGING

General Features
- Best diagnostic clue
  - Intra- and extrahepatic biliary pigmented stones within dilated biliary ducts
- Location
  - Lateral segment of left lobe and posterior segment of right lobe are more commonly involved

Ultrasonographic Findings
- Grayscale ultrasound
  - Commonly used for screening and monitoring disease
  - Findings depend on stage of disease and presence of any associated complication
  - Early disease without biliary sepsis
    - Dilated intrahepatic and extrahepatic bile ducts
    - Presence of echogenic sludge/stones ± posterior acoustic shadowing
    - May appear as multiple echogenic masses in serpiginous configuration along portal triads if stones/sludge fills dilated ducts
  - Early disease with active biliary sepsis
    - Periportal hypo-/hyperechogenicity due to periductal inflammation
    - Biliary ductal thickening related to edematous inflammation
    - Floating echoes within dilated ducts due to inflammatory debris
    - Multiple cholangitic abscesses appear as small cystic cavities with internal debris
  - Late-stage disease
    - Severe atrophy of affected lobe/segment
    - Crowded, stone-filled ducts may appear as single heterogeneous mass
    - Development of biliary cirrhosis with portal hypertension
- Color Doppler
  - No flow within dilated bile ducts

Radiographic Findings
- Cholangiography
  - Intrahepatic or extrahepatic duct stones as filling defects
  - Dilatation of extrahepatic and central intrahepatic ducts
  - Ductal rigidity and straightening, right-angle branching pattern
  - Decreased arborization and rapid tapering of peripheral intrahepatic duct
  - Ductal luminal irregularity and focal strictures

CT Findings
- CECT
  - Dilated intra- and extrahepatic biliary ducts within involved segments
  - Biliary stones may be high attenuation or isodense to liver
  - May be associated with low-attenuation pyogenic liver abscesses, fatty liver atrophy of segments with chronic biliary obstruction

MR Findings
- T1WI
  - Intrahepatic stones may be hyperintense
- T2WI
  - Hyperintense bile within obstructed ducts and hypointense ductal stones
- MRCP
  - Dilated intra- and extrahepatic ducts with filling defects representing stones
  - Ductal rigidity and straightening, rapid tapering of peripheral intrahepatic duct
  - Findings similar to direct cholangiography but advantageous in case of missing duct by severe stricture

Nuclear Medicine Findings
- Hepatobiliary scintigraphy
  - Delay in tracer excretion and drainage into biliary tree
  - Tracer retention within dilated intrahepatic ducts of affected lobe/segment

Imaging Recommendations
- Best imaging tool
  - Ultrasound is best initial imaging modality for disease detection, assessment of complication, and as guidance for percutaneous drainage
  - CECT/MRCP may help anatomical delineation in
    - Patients with small, atrophic liver, which is suboptimally assessed by US
    - Patients contemplating surgical treatment
- Protocol advice
  - Scan patient in different positions & imaging planes to detect subtle ductal changes & small, intrahepatic stones in early disease
  - Assessment of small atrophic liver may be technically difficult; CT/MRCP may allow better delineation

DIFFERENTIAL DIAGNOSIS

Ascending Cholangitis
- Obstruction of common bile duct (CBD) with proportional dilatation of intra- and extrahepatic ducts
- Enhanced wall thickening of inflamed bile ducts
- Periportal hypo- or hyperechogenicity due to periductal inflammation

Primary Sclerosing Cholangitis
- Multiple areas of intrahepatic strictures alternating with biliary dilatation resulting in beaded appearance
- Ductal dilatation is usually mild due to periductal fibrosis
- Associated with inflammatory bowel disease (particularly ulcerative colitis)

Cholangiocarcinoma

- May have a periductal soft tissue density appearance
- Prominent enhanced ductal wall thickening
- Often associated with hepatic or lymph node metastases
- Portal vein of affected segment may be obliterated

Intrahepatic Stones Secondary to Biliary Stricture

- Stricture may be due to prior surgery, trauma or chemotherapy
- Non-Asian patient
- Similar clinical presentation as RPC with RUQ pain, fever and chills

Caroli Disease

- Congenital, multifocal, segmental, saccular dilatation of intrahepatic bile ducts
- May have intraductal stones

PATHOLOGY

General Features

- Etiology
  - Associated with biliary parasitic infection with *Clonorchis sinensis* &/or *Ascaris lumbricoides*
  - Associated with *E. coli* infection of bile ducts
    - Bacterial production of beta-glucuronidase
    - Leads to hydrolysis of bilirubin, development of calcium bilirubinate stones within intra- and extrahepatic bile ducts
  - Associated with poor general nutrition
- Genetics
  - No known genetic predisposition

Staging, Grading, & Classification

- Classification based on distribution of affected biliary segment
  - May be isolated to left lobe, particularly lateral segment
  - May involve all biliary segments, as well as CBD

Gross Pathologic & Surgical Features

- Dilated bile ducts with brown, mud-like pigment stones, pus
- May have parasitic infection in biliary ducts with *Clonorchis* or *Ascaris*

Microscopic Features

- Periductal inflammatory changes with infiltration of periportal spaces with inflammatory cells leading to periductal fibrosis and ultimately biliary cirrhosis
- Localized segmental hepatic atrophy
- Fatty changes in liver

CLINICAL ISSUES

Presentation

- Most common signs/symptoms
  - Recurrent episodes of RUQ pain, fever and jaundice
  - Other signs/symptoms
    - Hypotension, septic shock
    - Related to gram-negative septicemia
- Clinical profile
  - Leukocytosis, elevated alkaline phosphatase and bilirubin

Demographics

- Age: Over 40
- No gender predilection
- Epidemiology: Primarily within southeast Asia and immigrants from southeast Asia

Natural History & Prognosis

- Repeated episodes of acute bacterial cholangitis
- May be life-threatening due to uncontrolled fulminant biliary sepsis
  - Treated with urgent surgical or percutaneous biliary drainage
- Complications
  - Biliary strictures, cholangitic liver abscesses
  - Repeated episodes of cholangitis & stricture formation lead to biliary cirrhosis
  - Cholangiocarcinoma (5-6%)

Treatment

- Options, risks, complications
  - Most mild cases respond to broad-spectrum intravenous antibiotics
  - In severe biliary sepsis, prompt biliary drainage is mandatory
  - Endoscopic sphincterotomy
  - Surgical drainage
    - Biliary drainage with hepaticojejunostomy
    - Left hepatic lobe resection if isolated left lobe disease
  - Interventional radiology
    - Percutaneous biliary drainage of affected segments
    - Basket removal of pigment stones
    - Balloon dilation of biliary strictures
    - Repeated percutaneous procedures to clear pigment stones & mud-like biliary debris
  - Medical therapy
    - Long-term suppressive antibiotic therapy

DIAGNOSTIC CHECKLIST

Consider

- Consider RPC in southeast Asian patient with recurrent episodes of acute bacterial cholangitis

Image Interpretation Pearls

- Intra- and extrahepatic bile duct dilatation with pigmented stones and ductal inflammation

SELECTED REFERENCES

1. Katabathina VS et al: Adult bile duct strictures: role of MR imaging and MR cholangiopancreatography in characterization. Radiographics. 34(3):565-86, 2014
2. Park HS et al: CT Differentiation of cholangiocarcinoma from periductal fibrosis in patients with hepatolithiasis. AJR Am J Roentgenol. 187(2):445-53, 2006
3. Jeyarajah DR: Recurrent Pyogenic Cholangitis. Curr Treat Options Gastroenterol. 7(2):91-98, 2004
4. Chan FL et al: Modern imaging in the evaluation of hepatolithiasis. Hepatogastroenterology. 44(14):358-69, 1997
5. Lim JH: Oriental cholangiohepatitis: pathologic, clinical, and radiologic features. AJR Am J Roentgenol. 157(1):1-8, 1991

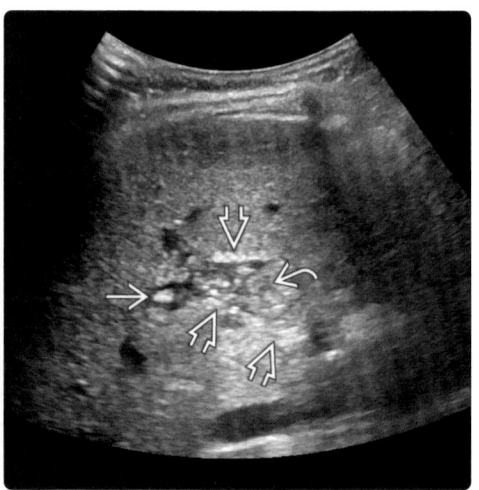

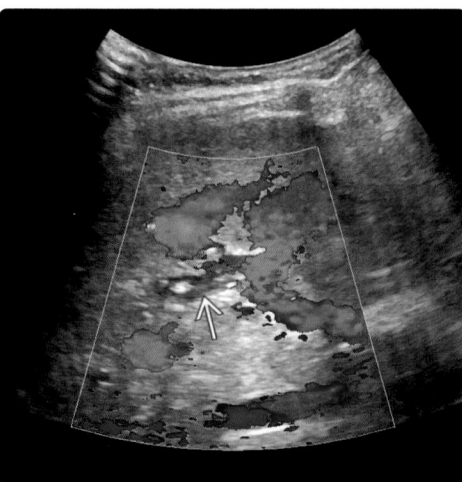

(Left) *Grayscale ultrasound of the liver shows echogenic intrahepatic duct stones ➡ and sludge ➡ within moderately dilated intrahepatic biliary ducts. Note periductal hyperechogenicity ➡, related to periductal inflammation in this patient with RPC.* (Right) *Color Doppler ultrasound in the same patient demonstrates no flow within the dilated intrahepatic duct ➡, confirming the findings are indeed in the biliary tree rather than the portal or hepatic arterial system.*

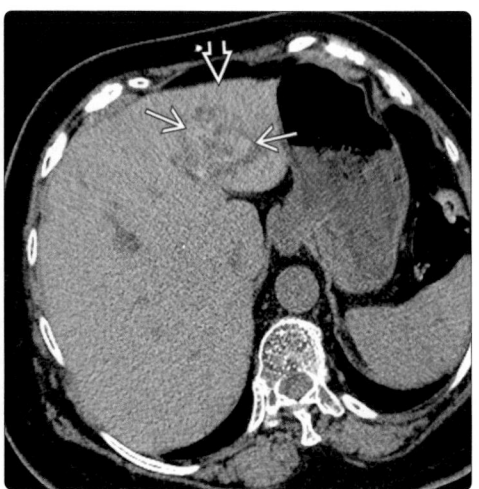

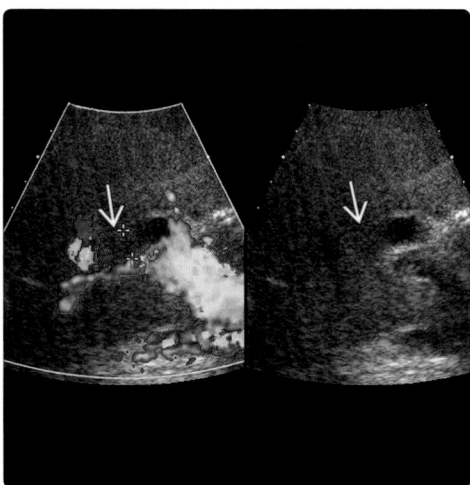

(Left) *Axial noncontrast CT shows hyperdense stones ➡ filling dilated intrahepatic ducts predominantly affecting the left lateral segment of the liver. Also note mild atrophy of left lateral segment ➡, often seen in affected segments of the liver.* (Right) *Color Doppler and grayscale ultrasound of the liver show a dilated right intrahepatic duct filled with hypoechoic material ➡ consistent with intrahepatic biliary sludge. No color signal is detectable in the dilated duct, confirming this is the biliary system in this patient with RPC.*

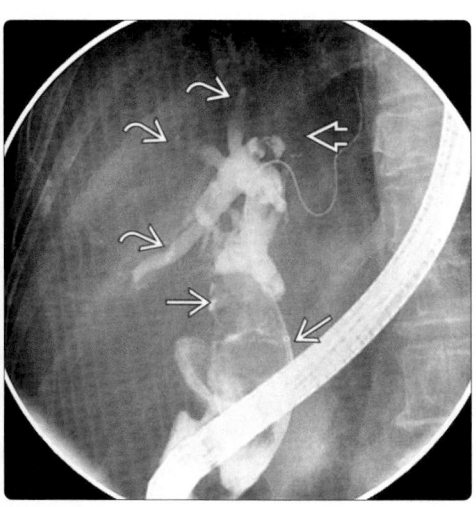

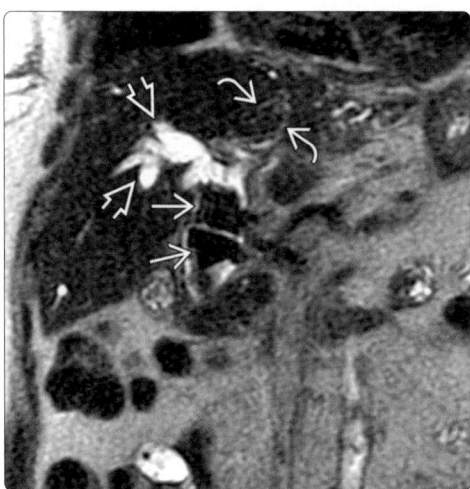

(Left) *ERCP shows multiple stones ➡ in a dilated common bile duct (CBD). Upstream intrahepatic biliary ductal dilatation with rapid tapering and decreased arborization ➡ is characteristic of RPC. Also notice the left main biliary duct is "missing" due to obstruction by an intrahepatic biliary stone ➡.* (Right) *Coronal T2-weighted MR in the same patient shows impacted stones ➡ in the CBD and left intrahepatic duct ➡ with associated biliary ductal dilatation. Right intrahepatic ducts are dilated and taper abruptly ➡.*

AIDS-Related Cholangiopathy

TERMINOLOGY

- Secondary sclerosing cholangitis usually resulting from opportunistic infection of biliary tract in AIDS patients with CD4 count < 100/mm³

IMAGING

- AIDS patient with papillary stenosis, intrahepatic strictures, thickened bile ducts and gallbladder (GB) walls
- Normal US essentially rules out diagnosis
- Combination of sclerosing cholangitis and papillary stenosis are unique to AIDS cholangiopathy

TOP DIFFERENTIAL DIAGNOSES

- Primary sclerosing cholangitis
- Autoimmune cholangitis
- Ascending cholangitis
- Cholangiocarcinoma

PATHOLOGY

- Chronic inflammation of biliary tract from opportunistic pathogens
- Most common pathogens: Cryptosporidium, CMV

CLINICAL ISSUES

- Epigastric/RUQ pain, diarrhea
- Fever and jaundice, less common

DIAGNOSTIC CHECKLIST

- Late-stage AIDS patient (CD4 < 100/mm³)
- Papillary stenosis, intrahepatic strictures, or acalculous cholecystitis

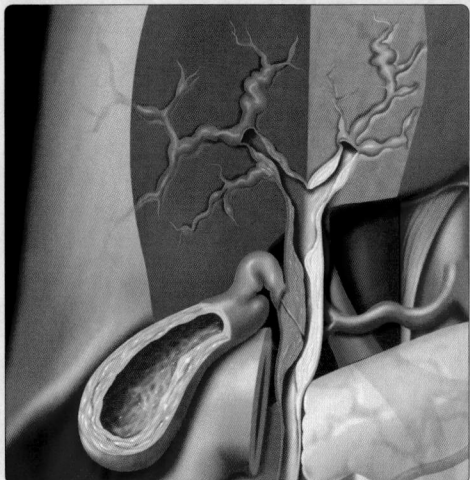
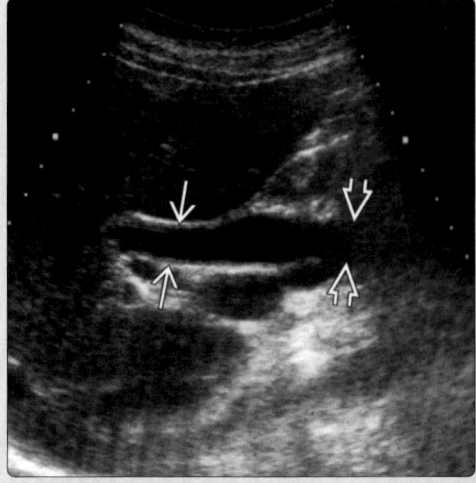

(Left) Graphic of AIDS-related cholangiopathy shows multiple segments of biliary wall thickening with stenosis involving both the intrahepatic and extrahepatic bile ducts. Also note gallbladder wall thickening. (Right) Ultrasound of the porta hepatis shows mild wall thickening of the dilated common bile duct (CBD) ➡, with abrupt tapering distally ➡. (Courtesy American Institute for Radiologic Pathology archives, case ID# 2447987, US2.)

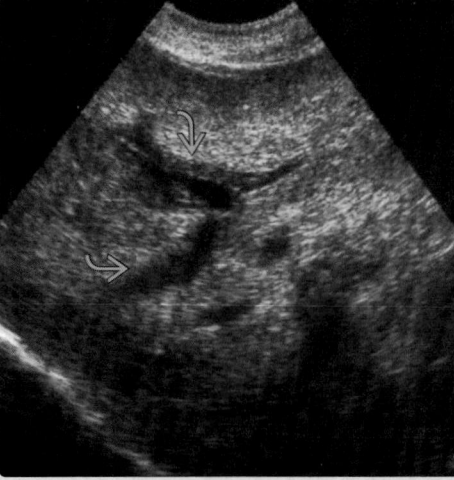
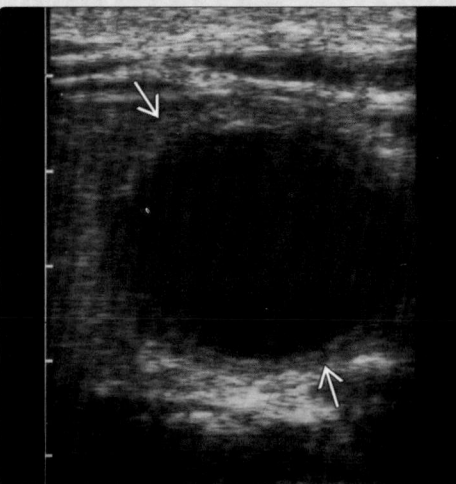

(Left) Longitudinal ultrasound through the right lobe shows dilated intrahepatic ducts with wall thickening ➡. (Courtesy American Institute for Radiologic Pathology archives, case ID# 2383220, US1.) (Right) Transverse ultrasound through the gallbladder shows mild circumferential wall thickening ➡ without visible stones. (Courtesy American Institute for Radiologic Pathology archives, case ID# 2383220, US3.)

TERMINOLOGY

Abbreviations

- AIDS cholangitis, AIDS-related sclerosing cholangitis, AIDS cholangiopathy, HIV cholangiopathy

Definitions

- Secondary sclerosing cholangitis usually resulting from opportunistic infection of biliary tract in AIDS patients with CD4 count < 100/mm^3

IMAGING

General Features

- Best diagnostic clue
  - AIDS patient with papillary stenosis, intrahepatic strictures, thickened bile ducts and gallbladder (GB)

Ultrasonographic Findings

- Grayscale ultrasound
  - Focal biliary duct strictures and associated dilatation
  - Bile duct wall thickening
  - Dilatation and wall thickening of common bile duct (CBD) with papillary stenosis
  - Diffuse GB wall thickening without gallstones

Radiographic Findings

- ERCP
  - Sclerosing cholangitis and papillary stenosis
    - Unique to AIDS cholangiopathy
  - Long extrahepatic bile duct strictures, ± intrahepatic sclerosing cholangitis

MR Findings

- MRCP
  - Multiple intra- and extrahepatic biliary strictures, with associated dilation
  - Papillary stenosis with CBD dilation
  - Isolated intermediate to long segment CBD stricture
  - GB wall and bile duct thickening

Imaging Recommendations

- Best imaging tool
  - US: Initial imaging test
    - Normal US essentially rules out diagnosis
  - MRCP
  - ERCP: Diagnostic and therapeutic

DIFFERENTIAL DIAGNOSIS

Primary Sclerosing Cholangitis

- Multifocal irregular ductal strictures with alternating ductal ectasia
- Affects intrahepatic and extrahepatic ducts

Autoimmune Cholangitis

- Bile duct wall thickening and strictures
- Most commonly affects distal CBD, can affect intrahepatic ducts
- Seen in setting of autoimmune pancreatitis

Ascending Cholangitis (Acute Bacterial Cholangitis)

- Ductal stricture and biliary wall thickening
- Usually secondary to choledocholithiasis

Cholangiocarcinoma

- Infiltrative mass along ductal epithelium
- Invades hepatic parenchyma and regional lymph node metastases

PATHOLOGY

General Features

- Chronic inflammation of biliary tract from opportunistic pathogens
- Most common pathogens: Cryptosporidium, CMV

CLINICAL ISSUES

Presentation

- Most common signs/symptoms
  - Epigastric/RUQ pain, diarrhea
  - Fever and jaundice, less common
- Clinical profile
  - ↑ ↑ cholestatic enzymes (Alk Phos and GGT)
  - Mild ↑ AST/ALT, bilirubin normal or ↑

Demographics

- Epidemiology
  - Late-stage AIDS patients (CD4 < 100/mm^3)
  - ↓ ↓ incidence 2° highly active retroviral therapy (HAART)

Natural History & Prognosis

- Survival not affected by cholangiopathy
- Mortality rate determined by natural history of AIDS

Treatment

- Papillary stenosis with symptoms: Sphincterotomy for pain relief, does not alter intrahepatic disease
- Dominant CBD stricture: Stenting
- Intra- or extrahepatic sclerosing cholangitis: Options limited, mainstay is restoration of immune system with HAART

DIAGNOSTIC CHECKLIST

Image Interpretation Pearls

- AIDS patient with papillary stenosis, intrahepatic strictures, or acalculous cholecystitis

SELECTED REFERENCES

1. Katabathina VS et al: Adult bile duct strictures: role of MR imaging and MR cholangiopancreatography in characterization. Radiographics. 34(3):565-86, 2014
2. Datta J et al: Extrahepatic cholangiocarcinoma developing in the setting of AIDS cholangiopathy. Am Surg. 79(3):321-2, 2013
3. Imam MH et al: Secondary sclerosing cholangitis: pathogenesis, diagnosis, and management. Clin Liver Dis. 17(2):269-77, 2013
4. Tonolini M et al: HIV-related/AIDS cholangiopathy: pictorial review with emphasis on MRCP findings and differential diagnosis. Clin Imaging. 37(2):219-26, 2013
5. Shanbhogue AK et al: Benign biliary strictures: a current comprehensive clinical and imaging review. AJR Am J Roentgenol. 197(2):W295-306, 2011
6. Catalano OA et al: Biliary infections: spectrum of imaging findings and management. Radiographics. 29(7):2059-80, 2009
7. Daly CA et al: Sonographic prediction of a normal or abnormal ERCP in suspected AIDS related sclerosing cholangitis. Clin Radiol. 51(9):618-21, 1996
8. Lack, E. E. Pathology of the Pancreas, Gallbladder, Extrahepatic Biliary Tract, and Ampullary Region. Oxford University Press. 2003

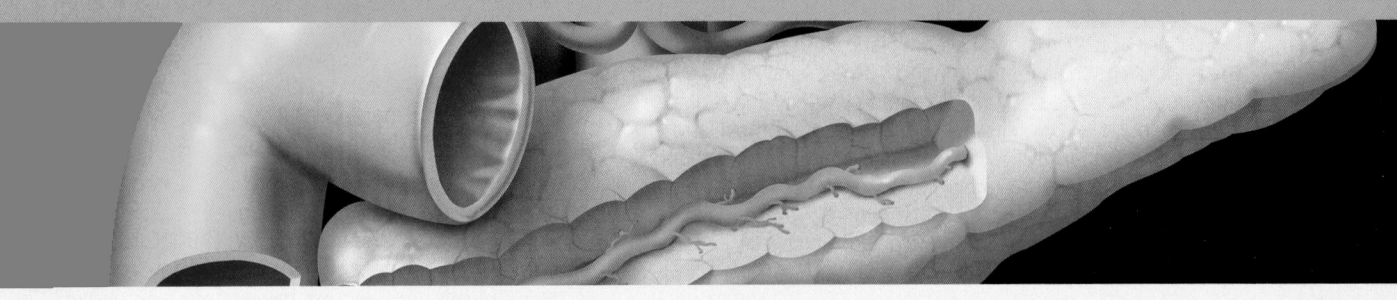

PART II
SECTION 3

Pancreas

Imaging Anatomy

The pancreas resides in the anterior pararenal space of the retroperitoneum, which also includes the second-fourth segments of the duodenum and the ascending and descending segments of the colon. The gland is an elongated structure situated in the transverse plane, with the head to the right of the midline, surrounded by the c-loop of the duodenum, and the body/tail extending laterally and slightly cranially to the splenic hilum. The head, neck (isthmus), and body are almost always visible via transabdominal ultrasound; the tail and uncinate are variably obscured by bowel gas. The gland is typically isoechoic or slightly hyperechoic to the liver, often increasing in echogenicity with age, which may in part be secondary to increasing lipomatosis.

In patients with good sonographic visualization, the pancreatic duct can be identified as a thin curvilinear structure situated within the center of the gland, oriented along the long axis, although when normal in caliber it may not always be visible. It can be seen as two thin echogenic lines, representing the epithelial walls of the duct, separated by a thin hypoechoic layer of fluid within the duct itself. Other readily visible anatomic landmarks include the superior mesenteric vein between the uncinate and pancreatic neck; in the head, the gastroduodenal artery anteriorly and common bile duct posteriorly; and in the body, the splenic vein along the posterior margin.

Anatomy-Based Imaging Issues

Frequently, the pancreatic tail, and often parts of the distal body, are not visible secondary to the presence of gas within the stomach, colon, and small bowel. Obesity is another common limitation in scanning of the pancreas. Related fatty infiltration of the liver may alter the relative echogenicity of the pancreas, which may then appear as hypoechoic relative to the steatotic liver, potentially mimicking a pathologic process such as pancreatitis.

Pathologic Issues

The pancreas can be affected by acute and chronic inflammatory processes, benign and malignant cystic and solid neoplasms, and autoimmune processes.

Imaging Protocols

Transabdominal ultrasound imaging can be facilitated by fasting prior to the exam, preferentially for at least six hours or overnight, in order to reduce the amount of gas within the stomach and bowel. Imaging is obtained with a curved transducer with the highest possible frequency, typically up to five MHz, although technological advances on modern scanners may allow for imaging at up to nine MHz without loss of acoustic penetration. Tissue harmonic imaging is used to improve image quality, particularly of fluid-filled structures such as cystic lesions, pancreatic duct, and the vasculature system. Compound imaging is used to improve tissue contrast and spatial resolution. Doppler ultrasound is essential to evaluate the vascular structures, as well as internal vascularity of tumors.

The gland should be evaluated in both the transverse and longitudinal planes. Imaging in different orientations such as in decubitus or erect positions, or with suspended respiration (inspiration or expiration), may improve visualization of structures not visible in the usual supine position. Graded continual transducer pressure on the abdomen can improve

visualization by collapsing and mobilizing bowel; however, this may be limited by focal tenderness depending upon the clinical setting. Although not routinely utilized, a moderate amount (100-300 mL) of degassed water or oral contrast administered prior to imaging can improve visualization of the tail; however, this can also introduce air bubbles leading to additional artifacts. Overdistention of the stomach should be avoided, as it is less compressible and may make the exam uncomfortable for the patient. The spleen can be used as an acoustic window to visualize the pancreatic tail.

Contrast-enhanced ultrasound can be obtained using second generation microbubble contrast agents, following a conventional ultrasound in which focal or diffuse pancreatic pathology has been detected. As microbubble contrast remains entirely intravascular, the distinction between solid and cystic masses is improved. Parenchymal enhancement can also be evaluated, which can potentially aid in distinguishing focal pancreatitis from neoplasm. Imaging requires specialized software, most commonly pulse inversion, to suppress background tissues and allow visualization of only vascularized structures. Imaging acquisition occurs immediately after intravenous administration in order to evaluate the arterial inflow to the pancreas and early parenchymal enhancement. Usage is limited in the United States, as there are no contrast agents approved by the Food and Drug Administration for noncardiac use.

Clinical Implications

The major role of sonography in imaging of the pancreas is in the evaluation of acute pancreatitis and pancreatic malignancy.

Acute Pancreatitis

Acute pancreatitis is diagnosed by a combination of clinical presentation and laboratory abnormalities, with imaging acquired to evaluate atypical presentations and for complications. Ultrasound is the primary imaging test obtained within the first 48-72 hours in a patient presenting for the first time with classic pancreatitis, in order to assess for the presence of gallstones. Transabdominal ultrasound is limited in evaluating the pancreas in the acute inflammatory phase, and findings may be subtle or absent in mild cases.

Grayscale assessment includes evaluation of the pancreatic parenchyma for signs of hemorrhage or necrosis, and peripancreatic tissues for the presence of fluid and fluid collections. The duct is visualized for signs of obstruction, either from stones in the common bile duct or secondary to pancreatic edema. Color Doppler can demonstrate the presence of splenic vein thrombosis.

Chronic Pancreatitis

Chronic pancreatitis results from progressive destruction of the gland secondary to multiple episodes of mild or even subclinical pancreatitis, with development of fibrosis and atrophy. Ultrasound is not sensitive for the diagnosis; however, the presence of ductal dilatation with ductal and parenchymal calcifications is highly suggestive. The location of stones, i.e., intraductal vs. parenchymal, may be better demonstrated with ultrasound than with CT.

Diffuse or focal enlargement of the gland is common, and the appearance can mimic neoplasm, particularly when focal in the pancreatic head. Contrast-enhanced MR and endoscopic ultrasound (EUS) are useful for distinguishing the two.

Cystic Pancreatic Lesions

Cystic lesions of the pancreas are common, and include pseudocysts, simple cysts, and cystic neoplasms such as serous and mucinous cystadenomas, intraductal papillary mucinous neoplasm (IPMN), and solid pseudopapillary neoplasm. Ultrasound can demonstrate the presence of thickened septations, soft tissue nodules, calcifications, or associated ductal dilatation, when present. In conjunction with the clinical history and the patient age and gender, these ultrasound findings are suggestive of the diagnosis. Ultimately, endoscopic ultrasound or contrast-enhanced CT or MR is required for definitive characterization.

Solid Pancreatic Lesions

Pancreatic ductal adenocarcinoma is the most common solid pancreatic neoplasm. Ultrasound is frequently an initial imaging study obtained to evaluate associated obstructive jaundice or abdominal pain. The appearance is typically that of a hypoechoic, poorly defined mass with limited acoustic penetration. Secondary pancreatic and biliary ductal dilatation is well visualized but not specific, as chronic pancreatitis can have this finding as well. Although ultrasound is relatively sensitive and specific for ductal adenocarcinoma, contrast-enhanced CT is required for complete characterization and staging.

Transabdominal ultrasound is limited in evaluating for neuroendocrine tumors, most of which are functional and detected clinically when still small in size. Nonfunctioning neuroendocrine tumors tend to be large and may be detected when ultrasound is obtained to evaluate for associated upper abdominal symptoms. In contrast to ductal adenocarcinomas, they appear well circumscribed.

Differential Diagnosis

Pancreatic Duct Dilatation

- Chronic pancreatitis
- Pancreatic ductal carcinoma
- Obstructing distal common bile duct stone
- Intraductal papillary mucinous neoplasm (IPMN)

Diffuse Pancreatic Enlargement

- Acute pancreatitis
- Autoimmune pancreatitis

- Lymphoma

Cystic Pancreatic Mass

- Pancreatic pseudocyst
- Serous cystadenoma of pancreas
- Mucinous cystic neoplasm (MCN)
- Intraductal papillary mucinous neoplasm (IPMN)
- Necrotic pancreatic ductal carcinoma
- Cystic pancreatic neuroendocrine tumor
- Congenital cyst
- Lymphoepithelial cyst
- Cystic metastasis

Solid Pancreatic Mass

- Pancreatic ductal carcinoma
- Focal acute pancreatitis
- Chronic pancreatitis
- Pancreatic neuroendocrine tumor
- Metastasis
- Lymphoma
- Solid pseudopapillary neoplasm
- Intrapancreatic splenule

Selected References

1. D'Onofrio M. Ultrasonography of the Pancreas. Milan: Springer, 2012
2. O'Connor OJ et al: Imaging of acute pancreatitis. AJR Am J Roentgenol. 197(2):W221-5, 2011
3. D'Onofrio M et al: Ultrasonography of the pancreas. Contrast-enhanced imaging. Abdom Imaging. 32(2):171-81, 2007
4. Martínez-Noguera A et al: Ultrasonography of the pancreas. Conventional imaging. Abdom Imaging. 32(2):136-49, 2007
5. Oktar SO et al: Comparison of conventional sonography, real-time compound sonography, tissue harmonic sonography, and tissue harmonic compound sonography of abdominal and pelvic lesions. AJR Am J Roentgenol. 181(5):1341-7, 2003
6. Abu-Yousef MM et al: Improved US visualization of the pancreatic tail with simethicone, water, and patient rotation. Radiology. 217(3):780-5, 2000

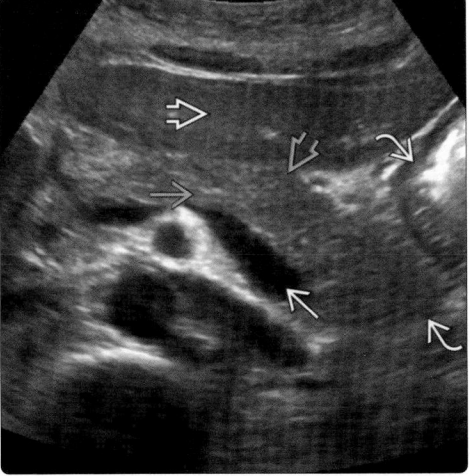
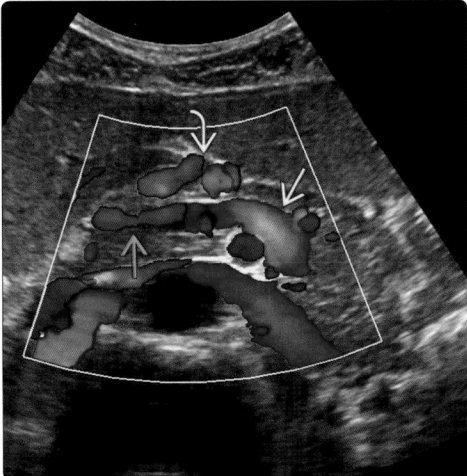

(Left) Transverse ultrasound utilizing left lobe of the liver as an acoustic window shows the pancreatic neck and body ⇗ are hyperechoic relative to the liver ⇗. Gas from the stomach partially obscures the tail ⇗. The splenic vein is posterior ⇗. The normal caliber duct is partially visible ⇗. (Right) Color Doppler US at the same level in a different patient shows red flow in the splenic vein towards the transducer ⇗, and blue flow in the superior mesenteric vein away from the transducer ⇗. The common hepatic artery is anterior ⇗.

(Left) *Transverse supine ultrasound of the pancreatic head, neck, and proximal body shows that portions of the head* ➡ *and distal body* ➡ *are not well visualized in this position.* (Right) *Ultrasound obtained in the same patient in a semierect position shows improved visualization of the pancreatic head margin* ➡*, and more of the body is now visible* ➡*.*

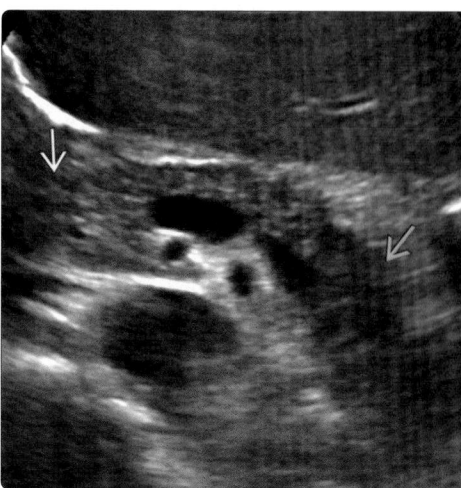
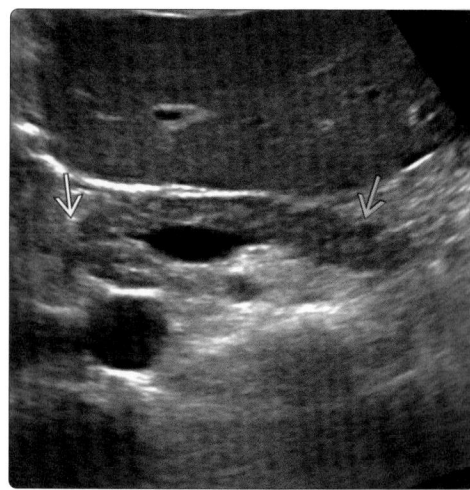

(Left) *Transverse US of the uncinate, head, neck, and body shows the superior mesenteric vein* ➡ *situated between the neck* ➡ *and uncinate process* ➡*. The pancreatic duct* ➡ *and distal common bile duct* ➡ *are visible just proximal to the major papilla.* (Right) *Transverse US shows a normal pancreatic duct* ➡ *as a thin, echogenic line partially visible in the body/neck region. Other structures typically visible at this level include the common bile duct* ➡*, IVC* ➡*, aorta* ➡*, SMA* ➡*, splenic vein* ➡*, and left renal vein* ➡*.*

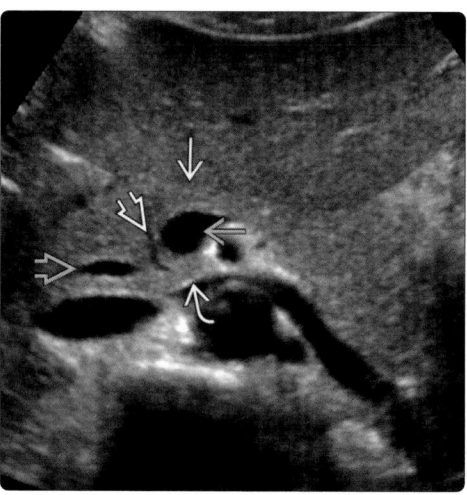
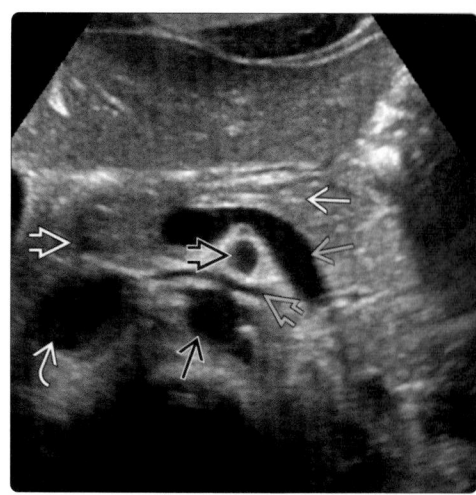

(Left) *Longitudinal midline ultrasound shows the separation of the pancreatic neck* ➡ *and uncinate* ➡ *by the superior mesenteric vein* ➡*. The aorta is visible posteriorly* ➡*.* (Right) *Longitudinal US obtained in the left paramidline upper abdomen shows the midpancreatic body* ➡*, hyperechoic to the adjacent liver* ➡*. The splenic vein* ➡ *is an easily recognizable landmark along the posterior margin of the gland.*

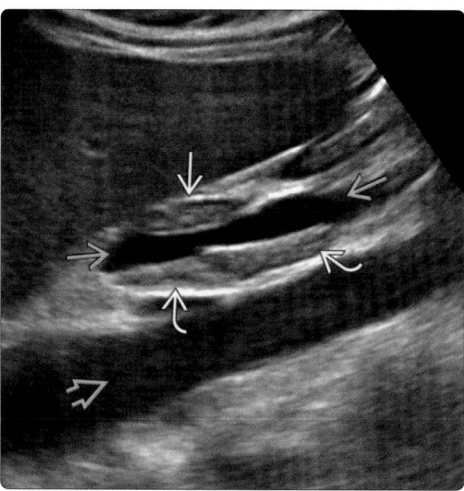
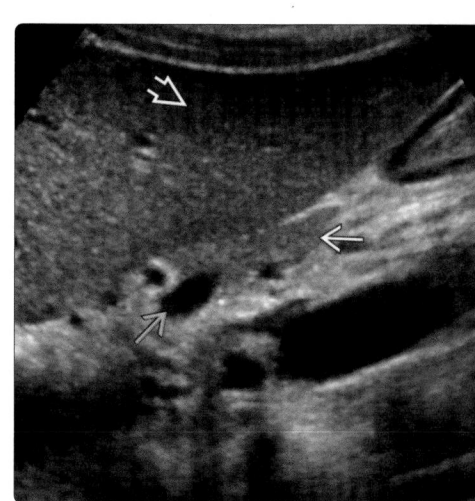

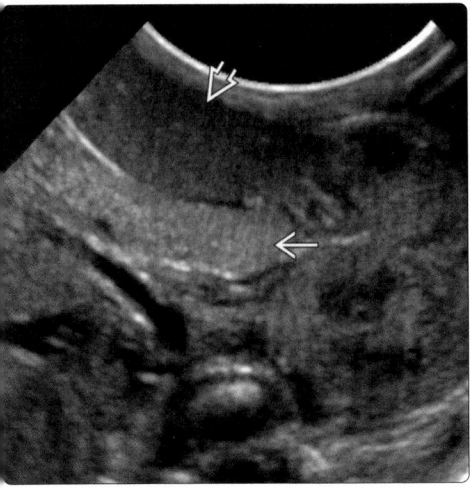

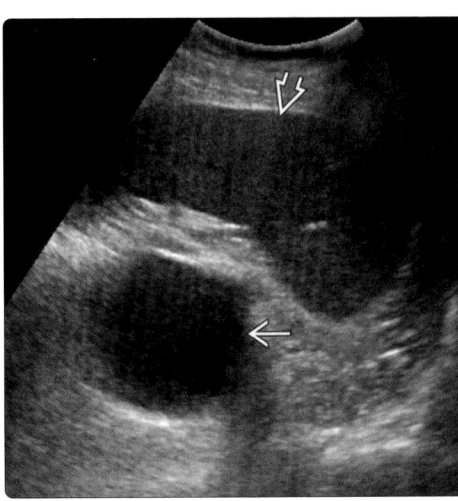

(Left) *Transverse ultrasound in a pediatric patient demonstrates the use of the spleen ⮕ as an acoustic window to visualize the tail of the pancreas ⮕.* (Right) *Transverse ultrasound in an adult with acute pancreatitis demonstrates the use of the spleen ⮕ to visualize, in this case, a pseudocyst at the tail of the pancreas ⮕.*

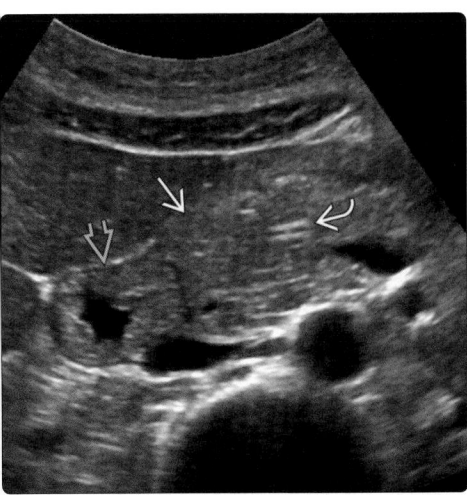

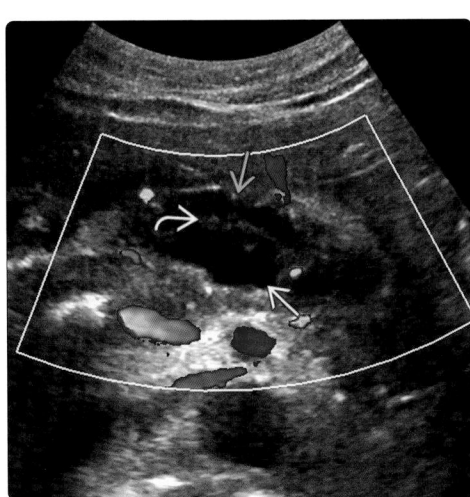

(Left) *Transverse ultrasound shows the relationship of the head of the pancreas ⮕ to the duodenum ⮕. An endoscopically placed stent accentuates the main pancreatic duct ⮕.* (Right) *Transverse ultrasound of the midbody of the pancreas shows a lobular cystic lesion ⮕ in the pancreatic head, separated from the adjacent dilated pancreatic duct ⮕ by a thin septation ⮕. Color Doppler confirms the absence of vascularity, helpful in confirming this as a pseudocyst.*

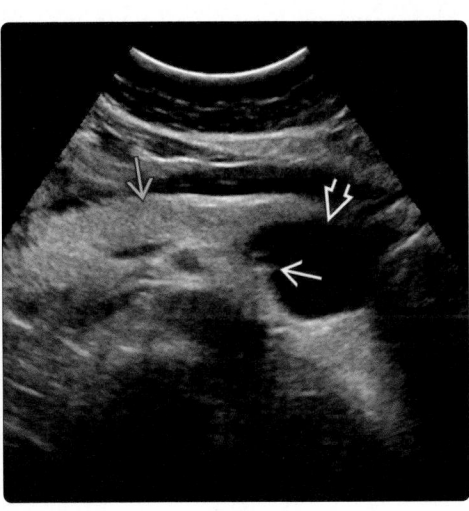

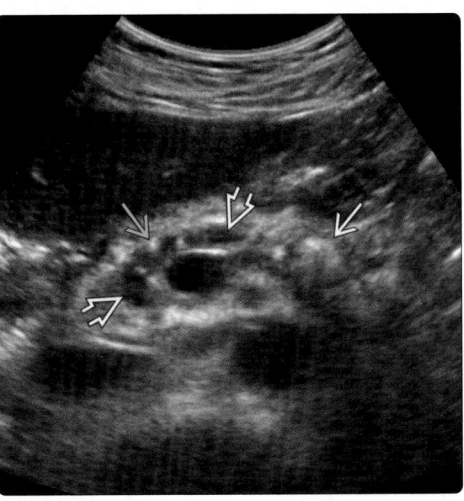

(Left) *Transverse US shows a well-defined anechoic cystic lesion ⮕ in the body of the pancreas with hyperechoic peripheral foci ⮕. The appearance is nonspecific, and this was proven to be a mucinous cystic neoplasm. A normal pancreatic parenchyma ⮕ is seen.* (Right) *Transverse ultrasound shows an atrophic, echogenic gland with a dilated pancreatic duct ⮕ containing calculi ⮕. Scattered parenchymal calcifications ⮕ are also visible. The findings are highly specific for chronic pancreatitis.*

TERMINOLOGY

- Acute inflammatory process of pancreas with variable involvement of other local tissues and remote organ systems
- Types
  - Interstitial edematous pancreatitis (IEP), necrotizing pancreatitis (NP)
  - Acute pancreatic fluid collection (APFC), ± infection
  - Acute necrotic collection (ANC), ± infection

IMAGING

- Focal or diffuse enlargement of pancreas with ill-defined margins, infiltration of peripancreatic fat
- Blurred pancreatic outline/margin: Due to pancreatic edema and peripancreatic exudate
- Heterogeneous echotexture in patients with intrapancreatic necrosis or hemorrhage
- Collections: Anechoic peripancreatic fluid = APFC; fluid within pancreatic parenchyma or containing debris = ANC

- US best to evaluate for cholelithiasis in acute pancreatitis of unknown etiology
  - In mild pancreatitis, sonographic signs may be subtle or normal
- CECT best in late phase to delineate extent of inflammation and detect necrosis and complications
- MR best to detect choledocholithiasis (MRCP) or in patients who cannot undergo CECT

TOP DIFFERENTIAL DIAGNOSES

- Infiltrating pancreatic carcinoma
- Lymphoma & metastases
- Autoimmune pancreatitis
- Perforated duodenal ulcer
- "Shock" pancreas

CLINICAL ISSUES

- Revised Atlanta Classification of Acute Pancreatitis: Early phase < 1 week, late phase > 1 week

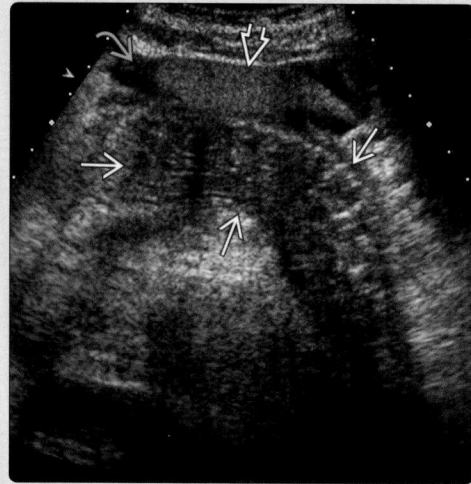
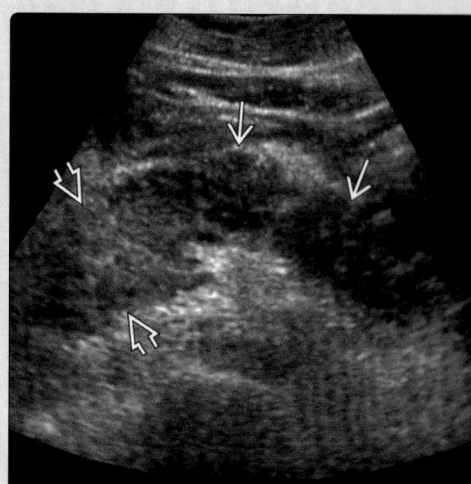

(Left) *Transverse ultrasound shows a markedly heterogeneous, enlarged pancreas ➡ consistent with acute interstitial edematous pancreatitis (IEP). There is a small amount of free fluid ⊿ surrounding segment III of the liver ⊠ anteriorly.* (Right) *Transverse ultrasound shows a markedly hypoechoic pancreatic body ➡ suggestive of focal necrosis, relative to the normal echogenicity in the head ⊠. This was confirmed with CECT.*

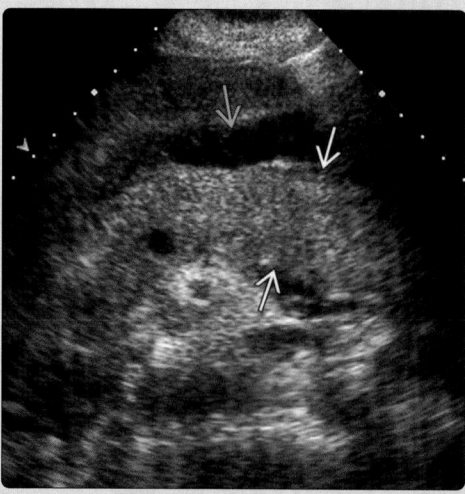
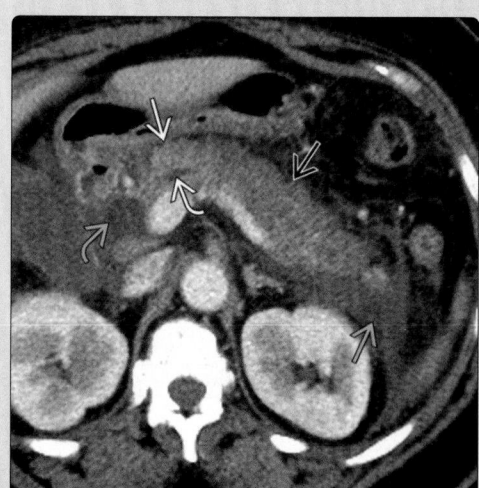

(Left) *Transverse ultrasound shows an enlarged pancreas ➡ consistent with IEP, with an anterior fluid collection ⊿ consistent with APFC.* (Right) *Transverse CECT demonstrates heterogeneous decreased enhancement of the pancreatic body ➡ relative to the head ⊠, consistent with acute IEP. There is an APFC ⊿ adjacent to the tail. The common bile duct ⊠ is dilated secondary to a distal obstructing calculus (not visible on CT), with associated minimal pancreatic ductal dilatation ➡.*

Acute Pancreatitis

TERMINOLOGY

Abbreviations

- Interstitial edematous pancreatitis (IEP), necrotizing pancreatitis (NP)
- Acute pancreatic fluid collection (APFC), ± infection
- Acute necrotic collection (ANC), ± infection

Definitions

- Acute inflammatory process of pancreas with variable involvement of local tissues and remote organ systems

IMAGING

General Features

- Best diagnostic clue
  - Enlarged pancreas with peripancreatic fluid, edema, and obliteration of fat planes
- Size
  - Focal or diffuse enlargement

Ultrasonographic Findings

- Grayscale ultrasound
  - In mild pancreatitis, US signs may be subtle or absent
  - Enlarged, hypoechoic pancreas: Interstitial edema
  - Blurred pancreatic margin: Pancreatic edema and peripancreatic exudate
  - Heterogeneous echotexture: Intrapancreatic necrosis or hemorrhage
  - Pancreatic abscess or infected collections: Difficult to confirm with US; thick walled, mostly anechoic with internal echoes and debris
  - Gallstones or biliary intraductal calculi
- Color Doppler
  - Helpful to detect pseudoaneurysm formation and portosplenic venous thrombosis

CT Findings

- Focal or diffuse enlargement of pancreas with ill-defined margins, infiltration of peripancreatic fat
- Homogeneous or mildly heterogeneous enhancement (IEP); focal or diffuse nonenhancement (necrosis)
- Complications
  - Peripancreatic collections (APFC and ANC) do not have defined wall < 4 weeks after onset
  - Late collections have defined wall with enhancement: Pseudocyst following APFC; WON (walled-off necrosis) following ANC
  - Pseudoaneurysm: Cystic vascular lesion, enhances like adjacent blood vessels
  - Portal/splenic venous thrombosis: Nonenhancement of thrombosed vein
  - Infection: Presence of gas, unless secondary to fistula to colon or interventional procedure

MR Findings

- T2WI FS
  - Collections, necrotic areas: Hyperintense
  - Peripancreatic edema, infiltrating fluid: Hyperintense
- T1WI C+
  - Enhancement: Homogeneous or mildly heterogeneous (IEP) vs. focal or diffuse nonenhancement (necrosis)

- Vascular occlusions: Filling defects or nonenhancement of vessel
- MRCP
  - Dilated or normal main pancreatic duct (MPD)
  - Gallstones, choledocholithiasis: Filling defects in gallbladder or common bile duct

Imaging Recommendations

- Best imaging tool
  - CECT
- Protocol advice
  - US best to evaluate for cholelithiasis in acute pancreatitis of unknown etiology
  - CECT best in late phase to delineate extent of inflammation, detect necrosis and complications
  - MR best to detect choledocholithiasis (MRCP) or in patients unable to undergo CECT

DIFFERENTIAL DIAGNOSIS

Infiltrating Pancreatic Carcinoma

- Irregular, heterogeneous, hypoechoic mass
- Abrupt obstruction & dilatation of pancreatic duct
- Regional nodal metastases: Splenic hilum & porta hepatis
- Contiguous organ invasion: Duodenum, stomach, liver, mesentery

Lymphoma & Metastases

- Nodular, bulky, enlarged pancreas due to infiltration
- Retroperitoneal adenopathy
- Peripancreatic infiltration (obliteration of fat planes)

Autoimmune Pancreatitis

- Focal or diffuse enlargement
- Narrowed pancreatic duct
- Lack of calcifications or fluid collections

Perforated Duodenal Ulcer

- Penetrating ulcers may infiltrate anterior pararenal space, simulating pancreatitis
- < 50% of cases have evidence of extraluminal gas or contrast medium collections
- Pancreatic head may be involved

"Shock" Pancreas

- Infiltration of peripancreatic & mesenteric fat planes following hypotensive episode (e.g., blunt trauma)
- Pancreas itself looks normal or diffusely enlarged

PATHOLOGY

General Features

- Etiology
  - Alcohol/gallstones/metabolic/infection/trauma/drugs/ERCP
  - Pathogenesis: Due to reflux of pancreatic enzymes, bile, duodenal contents, and increased ductal pressure
    - MPD or terminal duct blockage
    - Edema, spasm; incompetence of sphincter of Oddi
- Genetics
  - Hereditary pancreatitis: Autosomal dominant, incomplete penetrance
- Associated abnormalities

CT Severity Index

Grade	CT Findings
A	Normal pancreas
B	Focal or diffuse enlargement of gland, contour irregularities & heterogeneous attenuation; no peripancreatic inflammation
C	Intrinsic pancreatic abnormalities & associated inflammation in peripancreatic fat
D	Small and usually single, small ill-defined fluid collection
E	2 or more large fluid collections, presence of gas in pancreas or retroperitoneum

- o Embryology-anatomy
  - – Annular pancreas: Failure of migration of ventral bud to contact dorsal
  - – Pancreas divisum: Ventral & dorsal pancreatic buds fail to fuse; relative obstruction at minor papilla

Gross Pathologic & Surgical Features

- Bulky pancreas, necrosis, fluid collection

Microscopic Features

- Interstitial edematous pancreatitis
  - o Edema, congestion, leukocytic infiltrates
- Acute hemorrhagic pancreatitis
  - o Tissue destruction, fat necrosis, and hemorrhage

CLINICAL ISSUES

Presentation

- Most common signs/symptoms
  - o Acute-onset epigastric pain, often radiating to back
  - o Tenderness, fever, nausea, vomiting
- Clinical profile
  - o Diagnosis based on presence of at least 2 out of 3 of the following
    - – Abdominal pain consistent with pancreatitis
    - – Lipase or amylase level > 3x upper limit of normal
    - – CECT, MR, or US findings consistent with acute pancreatitis
  - o Other: Hyperglycemia, increased lactate dehydrogenase (LDH), leukocytosis, hypocalcemia, fall in hematocrit, rise in blood urea nitrogen (BUN)

Demographics

- Age
  - o Usually young and middle-aged groups
- Gender
  - o Males > females

Natural History & Prognosis

- Revised Atlanta Classification of Acute Pancreatitis: Early phase < 1 week, late phase > 1 week
  - o Early phase: Severity based entirely on clinical parameters (APACHE II, Ranson, Marshall scoring system for organ failure, presence of SIRS)
  - o Late phase: Severity based on imaging/morphologic criteria, in addition to clinical parameters
- Clinical: Presence of organ failure is main determinant of severity; 3 grades
  - o Mild: Absence of local or systemic complications, absence of organ failure; usually resolves in early phase; mortality very rare

- o Moderately severe: Transient organ failure (< 48 hours duration); local or systemic complications; may resolve spontaneously; fluid collections, necrosis may require prolonged intervention
- o Severe: Persistent organ failure (> 48 hours duration)
- Imaging: CT severity index (CTSI): Point system based on 1 of 5 grades (A-E) and extent of necrosis
- Complications
  - o APFCs develop into pseudocysts, ANCs develop into walled-off necrosis (WON); either can become infected
  - o GI: Hemorrhage, infarction, obstruction, ileus
  - o Biliary: Obstructive jaundice
  - o Vascular: Pseudoaneurysm, portosplenic vein thrombosis, hemorrhage
  - o Disseminated intravascular coagulation (DIC), shock, renal failure

Treatment

- IEP: Conservative management; nothing by mouth (NPO); gastric tube decompression; analgesics, antibiotics
- IEP with complications: Infected or obstructing fluid collections require drainage (surgical, endoscopic, or percutaneous routes)
- NP: Need for intervention based on CT severity index; infected necrosis needs surgery/catheter drainage

DIAGNOSTIC CHECKLIST

Consider

- Rule out other pathologies that can cause "peripancreatic infiltration"

Image Interpretation Pearls

- Bulky, irregularly enlarged pancreas with obliteration of peripancreatic fat planes, peripancreatic collections, abscess formation

SELECTED REFERENCES

1. Banks PA et al: Classification of acute pancreatitis–2012: revision of the Atlanta classification and definitions by international consensus. Gut. 62(1):102-11, 2013
2. Thoeni RF: The revised atlanta classification of acute pancreatitis: its importance for the radiologist and its effect on treatment. Radiology. 262(3):751-64, 2012
3. O'Connor OJ et al: Imaging of acute pancreatitis. AJR Am J Roentgenol. 197(2):W221-5, 2011
4. Balthazar EJ: Acute pancreatitis: assessment of severity with clinical and CT evaluation. Radiology. 223(3):603-13, 2002

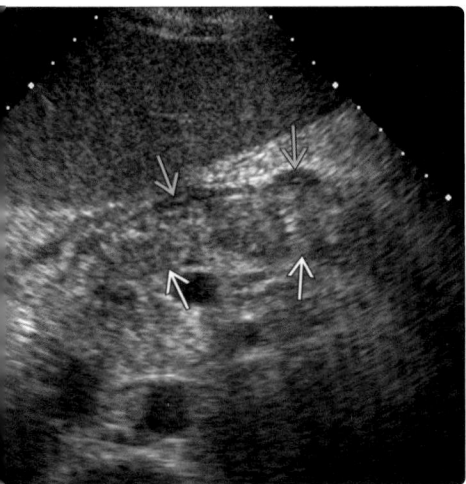
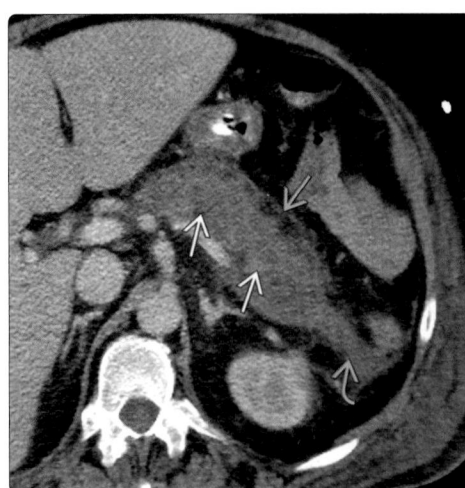

(Left) Transverse abdominal ultrasound demonstrates a heterogeneous, hypoechoic pancreas ➡ consistent with IEP. Peripancreatic hypoechoic fluid ⇥ consistent with APFC is present anterior to the pancreatic body. (Right) Transverse CECT in the same patient demonstrates a heterogeneous, hypoenhancing pancreas ➡ consistent with acute IEP. Peripancreatic edema ⇥ surrounds the pancreatic body, and there is an APFC at the tail ⇥.

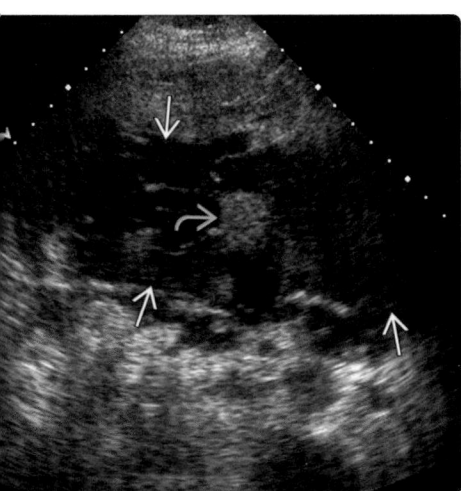
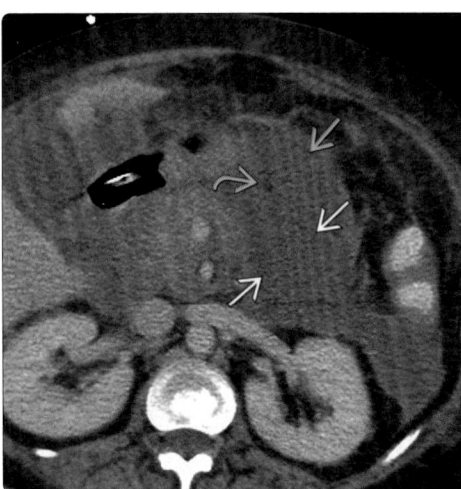

(Left) Transverse midline ultrasound shows a heterogeneous collection in the pancreatic bed ➡ containing nonliquefied components ⇥, indicating pancreatic and peripancreatic necrosis. (Right) Transverse CECT in the same patient shows complete lack of enhancement of the body and tail ➡ of the pancreas, consistent with NP. There is peripancreatic fluid ⇥ with nonliquefied components ⇥, consistent with peripancreatic necrosis and acute necrotic collection (ANC).

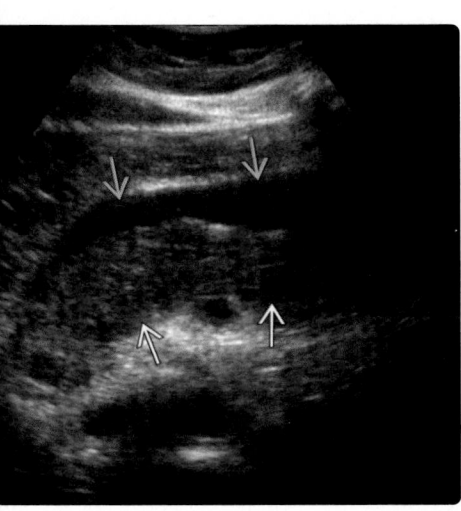
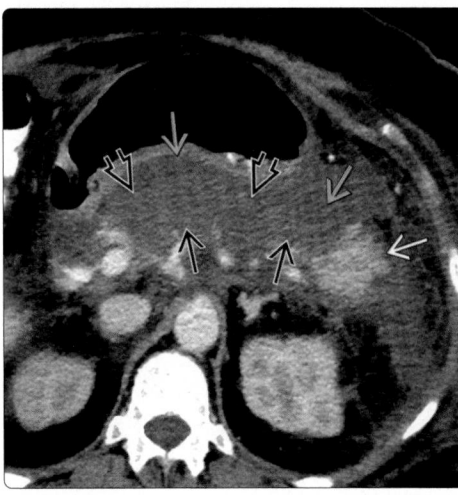

(Left) Transverse ultrasound shows an enlarged, hypoechoic pancreas ➡ consistent with acute pancreatitis. There is a fluid collection ⇥ anterior to the gland. The presence and extent of necrosis is not readily evident. (Right) Transverse CECT in the same patient reveals absence of enhancement in the majority of the gland ⇥, consistent with necrosis, with residual viable tissue in the tail ➡. The anterior border of the pancreas ⇥ is barely distinguishable from the anterior ANC ⇥.

Pancreatic Pseudocyst

TERMINOLOGY

- Collection of pancreatic fluid and inflammatory exudate encapsulated by nonepithelial fibrous tissue developing > 4 weeks after acute pancreatic fluid collection (APFC)

IMAGING

- Well-defined unilocular peripancreatic cystic mass in setting of prior pancreatitis
  - 2/3 are peripancreatic: Body and tail (85%)
- US demonstrates well-circumscribed, smooth-walled, unilocular anechoic mass with posterior acoustic enhancement
  - Complex pseudocysts may have fluid-debris level, internal echoes, or septations (due to hemorrhage/infection)
- CT best to evaluate extent of pseudocyst and complications
  - Gas within pseudocyst: Infection vs. decompression into stomach or bowel

- MRCP helpful to visualize communication with pancreatic duct

TOP DIFFERENTIAL DIAGNOSES

- Mucinous cystic neoplasm
- Serous cystadenoma
- Intraductal papillary mucinous neoplasm (IPMN) of pancreas
- Cystic islet cell tumor
- True epithelial cysts

CLINICAL ISSUES

- Clinical significance is related to size and complications
- Percutaneous drainage required when symptomatic or enlarging

DIAGNOSTIC CHECKLIST

- Rule out other cystic lesions of pancreas, particularly mucinous neoplasms
- Cyst aspiration may be required for definitive diagnosis

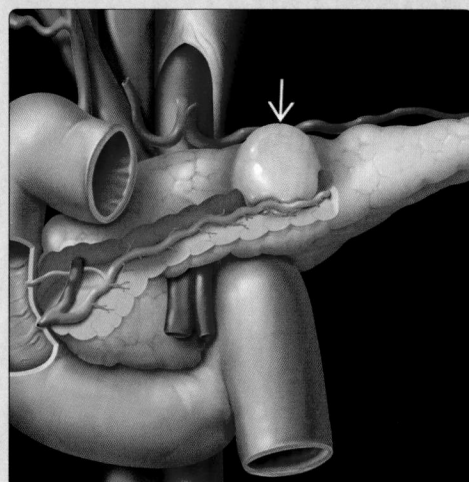
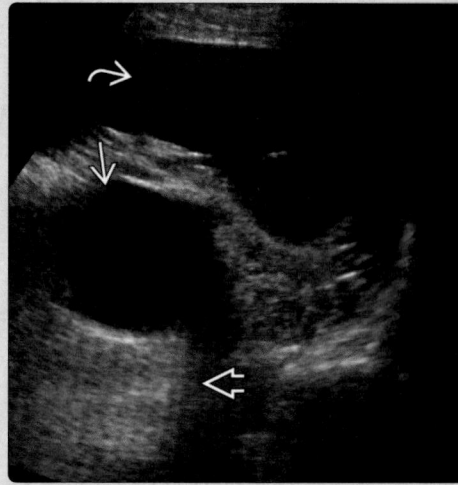

(Left) Graphic shows a well-circumscribed cystic lesion ➡ in the pancreatic body consistent with a pancreatic pseudocyst. The adjacent pancreatic duct is not compressed or displaced. (Right) Transverse ultrasound through the left upper quadrant shows a well-circumscribed, unilocular pseudocyst in the pancreatic tail ➡. Posterior acoustic enhancement ➡ is noted. The spleen ➡ provides an acoustic window.

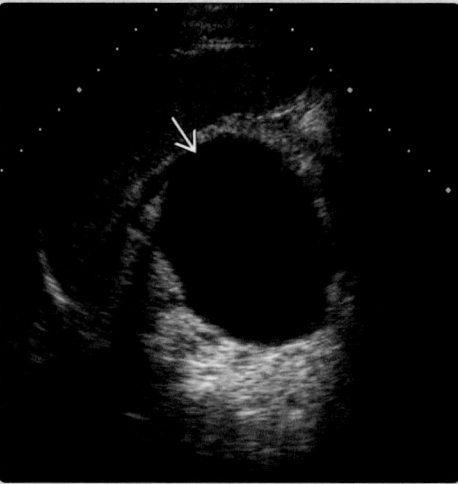
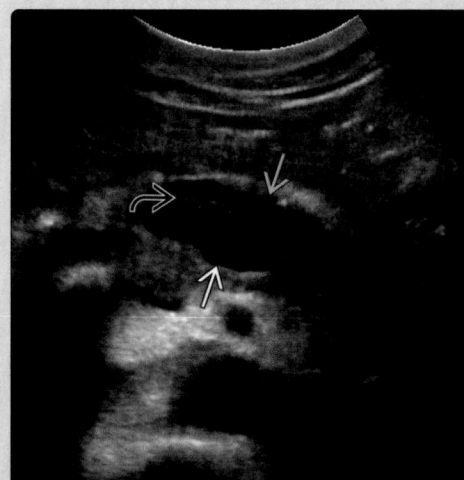

(Left) Transverse ultrasound via left posterolateral approach shows a well-circumscribed, unilocular simple cyst ➡ at the pancreatic tail, consistent with pseudocyst. (Right) Transverse ultrasound of the midbody of the pancreas shows a lobular pseudocyst ➡ in the pancreatic head, separated from the adjacent dilated pancreatic duct ➡ by a thin septation ➡.

TERMINOLOGY

Definitions

- Collection of pancreatic fluid and inflammatory exudate encapsulated by nonepithelial fibrous tissue developing > 4 weeks after acute pancreatic fluid collection (APFC)

IMAGING

General Features

- Best diagnostic clue
  - Well-defined unilocular peripancreatic cystic mass in setting of prior pancreatitis
- Location
  - 2/3 peripancreatic
    - Body and tail (85%); head (15%)
  - 1/3 extrapancreatic
    - Juxtasplenic, retroperitoneum, intraperitoneal, and mediastinum
    - Intraparenchymal: Left lobe of liver, spleen, kidney
- Size
  - 2-10 cm
- Morphology
  - Spherical or ovoid fluid collection
  - Pancreatic secretions encapsulated by granulation tissue and fibrous capsule
  - In contrast to true cysts, pseudocysts lack true epithelial lining

Ultrasonographic Findings

- Grayscale ultrasound
  - Uncomplicated pseudocyst
    - Well-circumscribed, smooth-walled, unilocular anechoic mass with posterior acoustic enhancement
  - Variant/complicated pseudocyst
    - Multilocular (approximately 6% of cases)
    - Fluid-debris level, internal echoes and septations (due to hemorrhage/infection)
    - Solid or complex in morphology (during initial phase of cyst formation)
    - Wall calcification: May make it difficult to assess details of pseudocyst
  - Dilated pancreatic duct and common bile duct (CBD)
    - Compression by pseudocyst
    - Fibrosis/stricture related to chronic pancreatitis
- Color Doppler
  - Absence of internal blood flow
- Endoscopic ultrasound (EUS) may be required for aspiration and histologic diagnosis

CT Findings

- Round or oval, homogeneous, hypodense lesion with near water density ("mature" pseudocyst)
- Hemorrhagic, infected pseudocyst: Lobulated, heterogeneous, mixed density lesion
- Gas within pseudocyst: Infection vs. decompression into stomach or bowel
- May have imperceptible thin fibrous capsule vs. thick enhancing wall
- No enhancement of internal contents
- Pseudoaneurysm: Arterial enhancement in cyst wall

MR Findings

- T2WI
  - Hyperintense (fluid)
  - Mixed intensity (fluid + layering debris)
- T1WI C+
  - May show enhancement of fibrous capsule
- MRCP
  - Hyperintense cyst contiguous with dilated pancreatic duct

Fluoroscopic Findings

- ERCP: Communication of pseudocyst with pancreatic duct seen in 70% of cases (decreases over time)

Imaging Recommendations

- Best imaging tool
  - CECT, US
- Protocol advice
  - Pseudocyst formation usually requires 6-8 weeks to mature, which is best time for detection
  - In addition to peripancreatic space, other locations such as peritoneal space, intraabdominal parenchyma, and intrathoracic cavity should also be evaluated
  - Follow-up US helps to monitor serial change in size and to select patients requiring decompression

DIFFERENTIAL DIAGNOSIS

Mucinous Cystic Neoplasm

- Location: Tail of pancreas (more common)
- Multiloculated, thick-walled cystic mass
- Internal solid component/echogenic septa
- May be indistinguishable from pseudocyst by imaging alone

Serous Cystadenoma

- Benign pancreatic tumor (arises from acinar cells)
- Location: Head of pancreas (most common)
- Solid mass with small cystic areas (< 20 mm), usually in periphery
- Central echogenic scar with calcifications
- Increased vascularity on Doppler examination

Intraductal Papillary Mucinous Neoplasm (IPMN) of Pancreas

- Low-grade malignancy arising from main pancreatic duct (MPD) or side branches
- Cystic lesion contiguous with dilated MPD may be indistinguishable from pseudocyst
- Side branch type usually arises in pancreatic head/uncinate, resembling cluster of grapes or small tubular cysts
- Main duct type causes dilatation of MPD ± cystic spaces

Cystic Islet Cell Tumor

- Usually nonfunctioning
- Thick-walled cystic mass with minor solid component
  - No pancreatic ductal dilatation
- Angiography/CECT: Hypervascular primary and secondary

True Epithelial Cysts

- Associated with von Hippel-Lindau (VHL) and
- Adult polycystic kidney disease (ADPKD)
- Rare, usually small and multiple nonenhancing cysts

- No pancreatic ductal dilatation

PATHOLOGY

General Features

- Etiology
  - Pseudocysts develop in 10-20% of patients with APFC
  - Pathogenesis
    - Release of enzymes and pancreatic juice
      □ Rupture of pancreatic duct
      □ Exudation of fluid from surface of pancreas due to activation of enzymes within gland
    - Unabsorbed APFC organize and develop fibrous capsule within 4-6 weeks
    - Develop due to post-traumatic/inflammatory autodigestion of pancreas
    - Walls arise from reaction of surrounding tissue to inflammatory exudate
- Associated abnormalities
  - Acute or chronic pancreatitis

Gross Pathologic & Surgical Features

- Collection of fluid, tissue, debris, pancreatic enzymes, and blood covered by thin rim of fibrous capsule

Microscopic Features

- Inflammatory cells, necrosis, hemorrhage
- Absence of epithelial lining
- Wall consists of granulation tissue and fibrosis

CLINICAL ISSUES

Presentation

- Most common signs/symptoms
  - Clinical significance is related to size and complications
    - Abdominal pain, typically radiating to back
    - Palpable, tender mass in middle or left upper abdomen
- Other signs/symptoms
  - May be asymptomatic throughout clinical course
- Clinical profile
  - Patient with history of chronic alcoholism, abdominal pain, and palpable tender mass
- Lab data
  - Cyst aspiration: Elevated amylase and lipase
  - Acute pancreatitis
    - Increased serum amylase and lipase
  - Chronic pancreatitis
    - Serum markers, exocrine function tests not helpful nor readily available

Demographics

- Age
  - More common in young and middle-aged group
- Gender
  - M > F
- Epidemiology
  - Rarely form during initial attack of pancreatitis (1-3% of patients)
  - Develop after several episodes of alcoholic pancreatitis in 12% of patients

- Present in up to 40% of patients with chronic pancreatitis

Natural History & Prognosis

- May persist, resolve, or continue to grow
- Spontaneous resolution can occur in 25-40%
- Complications: More common in pseudocysts > 4-5 cm in size
  - Compression of adjacent bowel or bile duct
    - Obstruction, severe pain, jaundice
  - Spontaneous rupture into peritoneal cavity
    - Ascites, peritonitis
  - Fistula to bowel
  - Secondary infection
  - Erosion into adjacent vessel
    - Hemorrhage or pseudoaneurysm formation
- Rupture and hemorrhage are prime causes of death from pseudocyst

Treatment

- Conservative therapy
  - If asymptomatic or decrease in size on serial scans
- Drainage
  - If symptomatic or continued increase in size
    - Size alone not indication for drainage
  - Drainage routes
    - Percutaneous: Retroperitoneal, transperitoneal, transhepatic
    - Endoscopic: EUS-guided cystogastrostomy
    - Surgical: Internal (usually into stomach) or external drainage
  - Requires long-term catheter if pseudocyst still communicates with pancreatic duct
  - Curative in up to 90% of cases

DIAGNOSTIC CHECKLIST

Consider

- Rule out other cystic lesions of pancreas, particularly mucinous neoplasms

Image Interpretation Pearls

- Correlate with ancillary imaging findings and clinical evidence of prior pancreatitis to confirm diagnosis
- Cyst aspiration may be required for definitive diagnosis

SELECTED REFERENCES

1. Banks PA et al: Classification of acute pancreatitis--2012: revision of the Atlanta classification and definitions by international consensus. Gut. 62(1):102-11, 2013
2. Kucera JN et al: Cystic lesions of the pancreas: radiologic-endosonographic correlation. Radiographics. 32(7):E283-301, 2012
3. Thoeni RF: The revised atlanta classification of acute pancreatitis: its importance for the radiologist and its effect on treatment. Radiology. 262(3):751-64, 2012
4. Khan A et al: Cystic lesions of the pancreas. AJR Am J Roentgenol. 196(6):W668-77, 2011
5. Kim YH et al: Imaging diagnosis of cystic pancreatic lesions: pseudocyst versus nonpseudocyst. Radiographics. 25(3):671-85, 2005

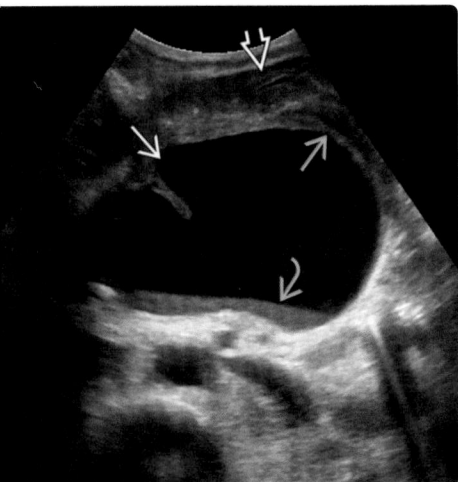

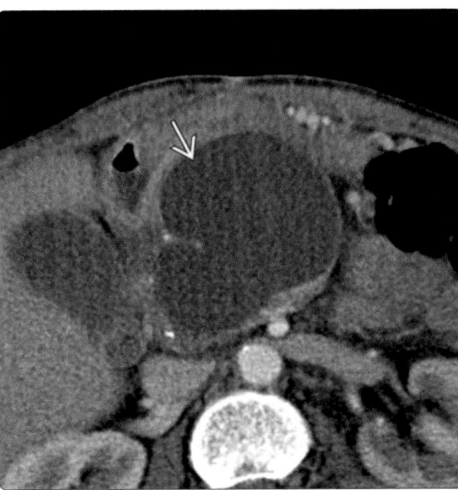

(Left) *Transverse ultrasound shows a slightly lobular pseudocyst ➡ within the pancreatic body with a well-defined ➡ capsule and layering sediment dependently ➡. Note the mass effect on the stomach ➡ which is displaced anteriorly.* (Right) *Axial CECT in the same patient shows the pseudocyst ➡ in the pancreatic body. The layering debris is not readily evident on this image, and is much better demonstrated on the ultrasound.*

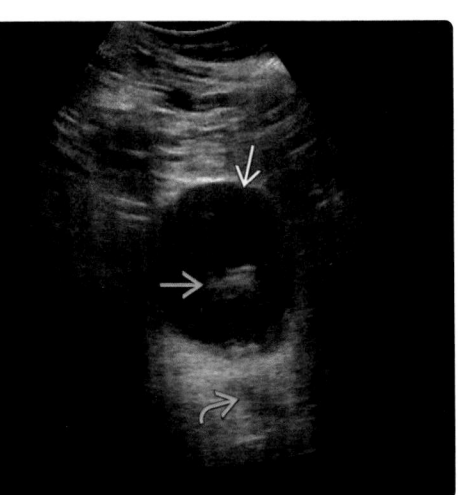

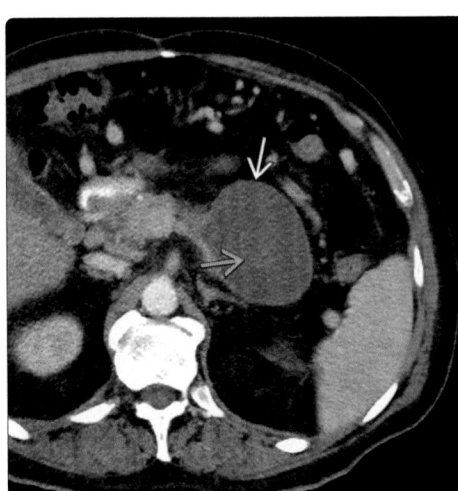

(Left) *Transverse ultrasound at the pancreatic tail shows a complex unilocular pseudocyst ➡ with internal echogenic debris ➡, likely hemorrhage. Note the faint posterior shadowing ➡.* (Right) *Axial CECT in the same patient is shown. Although the pseudocyst ➡ is well delineated, the internal debris ➡ is barely visible, and much better depicted with ultrasound.*

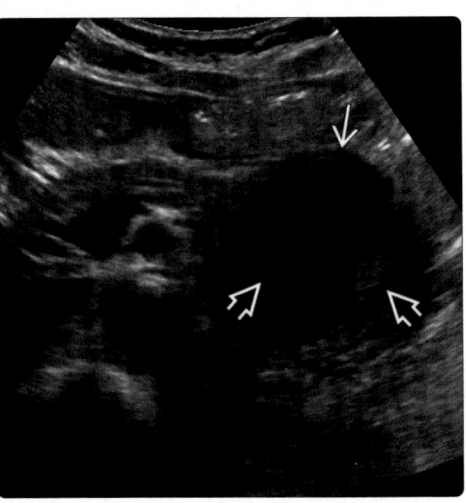

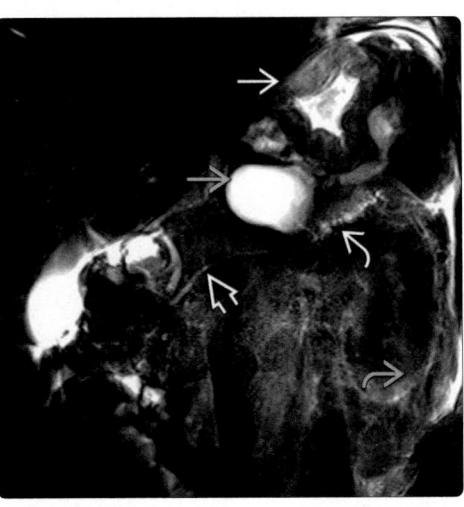

(Left) *Transverse transabdominal ultrasound shows a large pseudocyst ➡ at the pancreatic tail. Internal echoes ➡ are the result of hemorrhage within the pseudocyst.* (Right) *Thick-slab MRCP shows a pseudocyst ➡ superior to the tail of the pancreas in a patient with acute on chronic pancreatitis. The pseudocyst communicated with the dilated irregular duct in the tail of pancreas ➡. Note undilated irregular duct in the head and body ➡, edematous stomach ➡, and inflammatory fluid in the left retroperitoneum ➡.*

TERMINOLOGY

- Progressive, irreversible inflammatory and fibrosing disease of pancreas

IMAGING

- Dilated main pancreatic duct (MPD) with intraductal calculi is highly specific for chronic pancreatitis
- Diffuse or focal involvement of pancreatic parenchyma with inflammation and fibrosis
- Gland is usually atrophic, but can have focal enlargement, especially in head
- Parenchymal calcifications associated with alcohol abuse
- US can demonstrate dilated MPD, atrophy, and calcifications
- MRCP best to visualize dilated MPD and side branches
  - Assess for ductal disruption: Continuity of MPD with pseudocyst, bowel, or pleural space
- MR with contrast helpful to distinguish tumor from enlargement related to inflammation

- CT best to evaluate extent of calcifications and inflammation related to acute on chronic pancreatitis

TOP DIFFERENTIAL DIAGNOSES

- Infiltrating pancreatic carcinoma
- Acute pancreatitis
- Groove pancreatitis
- Autoimmune pancreatitis
- IPMN (intraductal papillary mucinous neoplasm) of pancreas

DIAGNOSTIC CHECKLIST

- Glandular atrophy, dilated MPD, and intraductal calculi/parenchymal calcifications are best signs for chronic pancreatitis
- May be very difficult to distinguish chronic pancreatitis with focal fibrotic enlargement of head from pancreatic adenocarcinoma

(Left) Transverse ultrasound demonstrates marked pancreatic ductal dilatation ⇒, intraductal stones ⇒, and parenchymal calcifications ⇒ within the atrophic parenchyma. (Right) Transverse ultrasound demonstrates a dilated main pancreatic duct (MPD) ⇒ with intraductal calculus ⇒ and parenchymal calcifications ⇒, consistent with chronic pancreatitis. A bilobed fluid collection in the head ⇒ is consistent with a small pseudocyst. The parenchyma ⇒ has normal size and echogenicity.

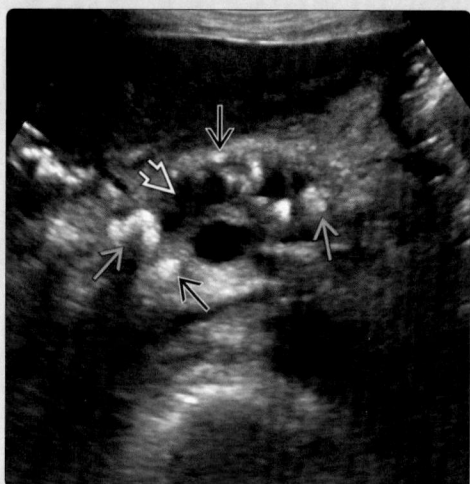
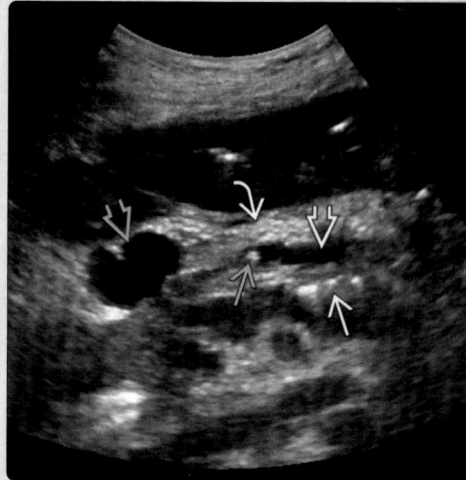

(Left) Transverse ultrasound shows predominantly parenchymal calcifications ⇒ without intraductal calculi. The gland is normal in size in this example. (Right) Transverse ultrasound demonstrates a dilated pancreatic duct ⇒ with intraductal calcifications in the head/neck region ⇒.

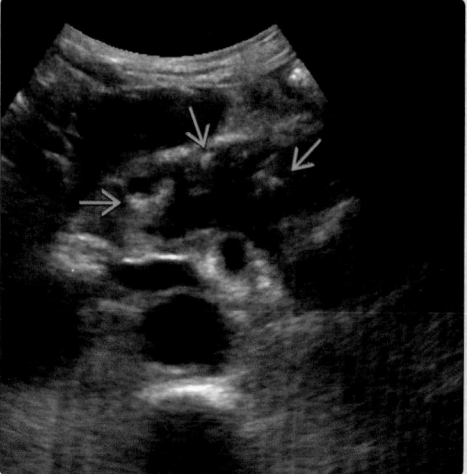
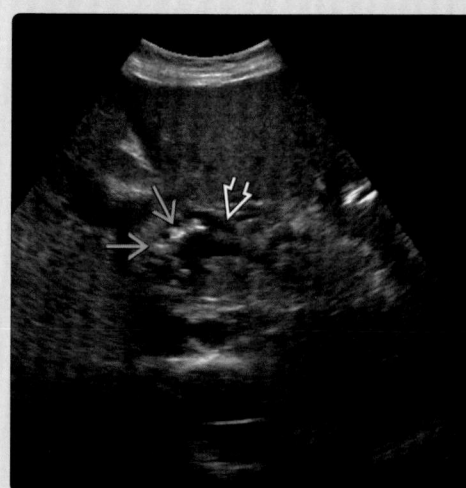

TERMINOLOGY

Abbreviations

- Main pancreatic duct (MPD)
- Common bile duct (CBD)

Definitions

- Progressive, irreversible inflammatory and fibrosing disease of pancreas

IMAGING

General Features

- Best diagnostic clue
  - Dilated MPD with intraductal calculi
- Location
  - Diffuse or focal involvement of pancreatic parenchyma
- Size
  - Usually atrophic
  - Focal enlargement in 30-40%, especially head; can mimic adenocarcinoma
- Morphology
  - Inflammatory disease of pancreas characterized by irreversible damage to morphology & function
  - Pancreatic calcifications
    - In 40-60% of patients with alcoholic pancreatitis
    - ~ 90% of calcific pancreatitis caused by alcoholism
  - Pseudocyst formation in up to 40%

Ultrasonographic Findings

- Grayscale ultrasound
  - Evaluation by ultrasound alone can be limited
    - Calcification/calculi: Posterior shadowing obscures portions of pancreas and adjacent structures
    - Margins are ill-defined and difficult to delineate
  - Gland may be enlarged in early stage of chronic pancreatitis or during acute on chronic episode; enlargement may be focal or diffuse
  - Heterogeneous echo pattern
    - Hypoechoic: Inflammation
    - Hyperechoic: Fibrosis and calcification
  - Dilated MPD (irregular, smooth, or beaded) in up to 90%
  - Pancreatic calcifications
    - Intraductal calculi: Deposition of calcium carbonate on intraductal protein plugs
    - Parenchymal calcifications
  - Irregular pancreatic contour
  - Pseudocyst: Unilocular, anechoic & sharply defined
  - Dilatation of common bile duct: 5-10%
    - Smooth gradual tapering; distinguish from adenocarcinoma (abrupt cutoff)
- Color Doppler
  - Portosplenic venous thrombosis: 5%
  - Arterial pseudoaneurysm formation

Radiographic Findings

- Small, irregular calcifications (local or diffuse)
- Gastric distention secondary to duodenal obstruction

Fluoroscopic Findings

- Upper GI
  - Duodenum with thickened irregular mucosal folds
  - Duodenal stricture and proximal dilatation
  - Enlarged papilla of Vater (Poppel papillary sign)
- ERCP
  - Dilated & beaded MPD plus radicals (side branches)
  - MPD filling defects: Intraductal calculi
  - CBD may appear dilated with distal narrowing

CT Findings

- Glandular atrophy, parenchymal calcifications
- Dilated MPD with intraductal calculi
- Intra- and peripancreatic cysts
- Heterogeneous enhancement
- Hypodense focal mass (fibrosis and fat necrosis) with varied enhancement

MR Findings

- T1WI
  - Decreased signal intensity due to loss of proteinaceous material
- T2WI FS
  - Pseudocyst, necrotic areas: Hyperintense
  - Gallstones, intraductal calculi: Signal void within ducts
- T1WI C+ FS
  - Heterogeneous enhancement pattern due to inflammation and fibrosis
  - Vascular thrombosis: Filling defect or occlusion
- MRCP
  - Dilated MPD, usually with smooth tapering
  - Dilated side branch ducts in severe cases
  - Ductal disruption: MPD in continuity with pseudocyst, bowel, or pleural space
  - CBD may be dilated with smooth distal tapering

Imaging Recommendations

- Best imaging tool
  - EUS for detecting early disease; MRCP, CECT for morphologic changes
- Protocol advice
  - MRCP best to evaluate dilated MPD and side branches
  - MR with contrast helpful to distinguish tumor from enlargement related to inflammation
  - CT best to evaluate extent of calcifications and inflammation related to acute on chronic pancreatitis

DIFFERENTIAL DIAGNOSIS

Infiltrating Pancreatic Carcinoma

- Irregular, heterogeneous, hypoechoic mass
- Abrupt obstruction & dilatation of pancreatic duct
- Regional nodal metastases: Splenic hilum & porta hepatis
- Contiguous organ invasion: Duodenum, stomach, liver, mesentery

Acute Pancreatitis

- Diffuse/focal parenchymal enlargement
- Hypoechoic echogenicity in inflamed parenchyma
- Pancreatic ductal dilatation uncommon
- Lack of pancreatic calcification
- Peripancreatic edema and fluid collection

Intraductal Papillary Mucinous Neoplasm (IPMN) of Pancreas

- Low-grade malignancy arising from main pancreatic duct or side branches
- Involvement of main pancreatic duct may simulate chronic pancreatitis
- Dilated MPD and parenchymal atrophy

Groove Pancreatitis

- Focal chronic pancreatitis in pancreatoduodenal groove
- Sheet-like fibrotic mass between pancreas and thickened duodenal wall
- Smooth tapering of distal CBD

Autoimmune Pancreatitis

- Focal or diffuse enlargement
- Narrowed pancreatic duct
- Lack of calcifications or fluid collections

PATHOLOGY

General Features

- Etiology
  o Alcohol abuse is most common cause in USA
  o Hyperlipidemia, hyperparathyroidism (hypercalcemia), trauma
  o Idiopathic in up to 40%
  o Gallstones not considered risk factor
  o Pathogenesis: Chronic reflux of pancreatic enzymes, bile, duodenal contents & increased ductal pressure
    – MPD or terminal duct blockage
    – Edema, spasm, or incompetent sphincter of Oddi
    – Periduodenal diverticulum or tumor causing obstruction
- Genetics
  o Cystic fibrosis
  o Hereditary pancreatitis: Autosomal dominant with incomplete penetrance
- Embryological consideration
  o Pancreas divisum: Minor papilla too small to adequately drain pancreatic secretions, leading to chronic stasis
  o Annular pancreas: Pancreatic ductal obstruction and stasis of secretions

Gross Pathologic & Surgical Features

- Hard atrophic pancreas with intraductal calculi & dilated MPD
- Areas of multiple parenchymal calcifications
- Pseudocysts may be seen

Microscopic Features

- Atrophy & fibrosis of acini with dilated ducts
- Mononuclear inflammatory reaction
- Occasionally squamous metaplasia of ductal epithelium

CLINICAL ISSUES

Presentation

- Most common signs/symptoms
  o Recurrent attacks of epigastric pain, occasionally radiating to back
  o Diarrhea secondary to exocrine deficiency

  o Weight loss from exocrine dysfunction, pain, or duodenal obstruction
- Clinical profile
  o Patient with history of chronic alcoholism, recurrent attacks of epigastric pain, diarrhea, and weight loss
  o Diagnosis usually not made until years following initial onset of symptoms
- Labs
  o Serum and fecal markers not sensitive or specific; helpful only in advanced disease
  o Pancreatic exocrine function hormone stimulation tests are helpful in early disease but not widely available

Demographics

- Age
  o Mean: 5th decade
- Gender
  o Males > females
- Epidemiology
  o More common in developing countries

Natural History & Prognosis

- Pseudocyst formation
- Diabetes mellitus in ~ 1/3 of patients
- Splenic vein thrombosis, portal hypertension
- Increased incidence of pancreatic cancer: ~ 4% at 20 years
- Increased mortality: 30% at 10 years, 55% at 20 years

Treatment

- Surgical or endoscopic intervention
  o Ductal & GI obstruction
  o GI bleeding
  o Large pseudocyst or persistently symptomatic
- Conservative treatment if no major complication (e.g., pain control, medical therapy for diabetes mellitus, etc.)

DIAGNOSTIC CHECKLIST

Consider

- Differentiate from other conditions that can cause MPD dilatation & glandular atrophy
- May be very difficult to distinguish chronic pancreatitis with focal fibrotic enlargement of head from pancreatic adenocarcinoma

Image Interpretation Pearls

- Glandular atrophy, dilated MPD, and intraductal calculi/parenchymal calcifications are best signs for chronic pancreatitis

SELECTED REFERENCES

1. Choueiri NE et al: Advanced imaging of chronic pancreatitis. Curr Gastroenterol Rep. 12(2):114-20, 2010
2. Siddiqi AJ et al: Chronic pancreatitis: ultrasound, computed tomography, and magnetic resonance imaging features. Semin Ultrasound CT MR. 28(5):384-94, 2007
3. Bruno MJ: Chronic pancreatitis. Gastrointest Endosc Clin N Am. 15(1):55-62, viii, 2005
4. Lankisch PG: The problem of diagnosing chronic pancreatitis. Dig Liver Dis. 35(3):131-4, 2003
5. Varghese JC et al: Value of MR pancreatography in the evaluation of patients with chronic pancreatitis. Clin Radiol. 57(5):393-401, 2002

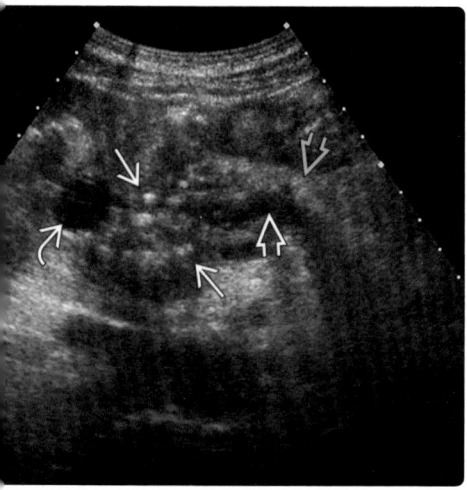

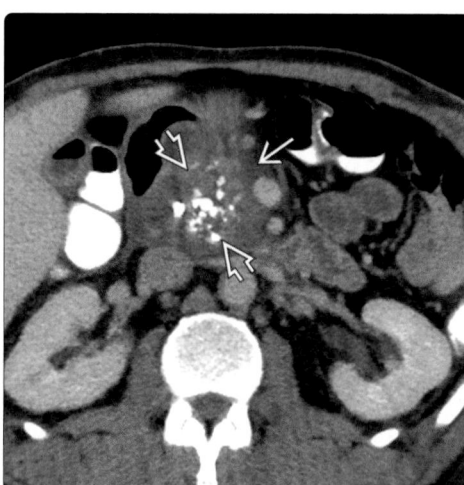

(Left) *Transverse ultrasound shows parenchymal calcifications in the enlarged pancreatic head ➡. There is pancreatic ductal dilatation ➡ in the atrophic body and tail ➡. Also note the dilated common bile duct ➡. Pancreatic margins are indistinct.* (Right) *CT in the same patient demonstrates the enlarged pancreatic head with numerous parenchymal calcifications ➡. Peripancreatic edema ➡ and loss of distinct margins are suggestive of acute on chronic pancreatitis.*

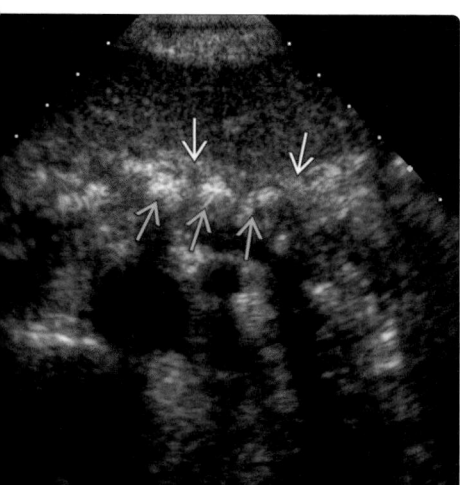

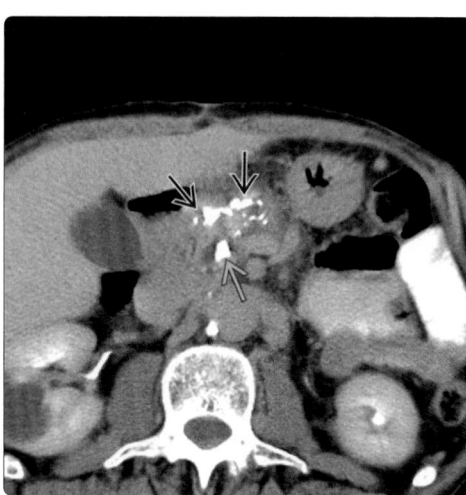

(Left) *Transverse ultrasound demonstrates multiple enlarged parenchymal calcifications ➡ in the body of the pancreas. The parenchyma ➡ is atrophic and heterogeneous, with indistinct margins.* (Right) *CT scan in the same patient shows calcifications ➡ in the pancreatic head and neck, as well as a large intraductal calculus in the distal MPD ➡. Enlargement of the pancreatic head can mimic neoplasm.*

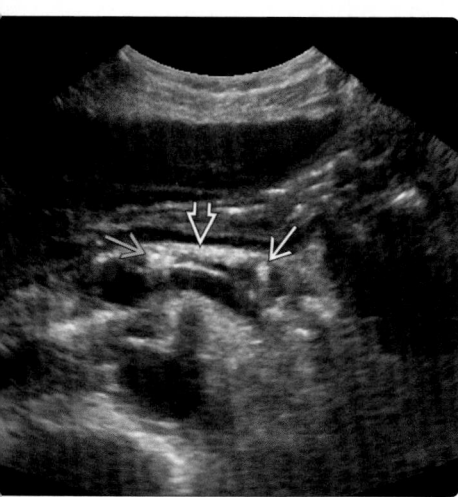

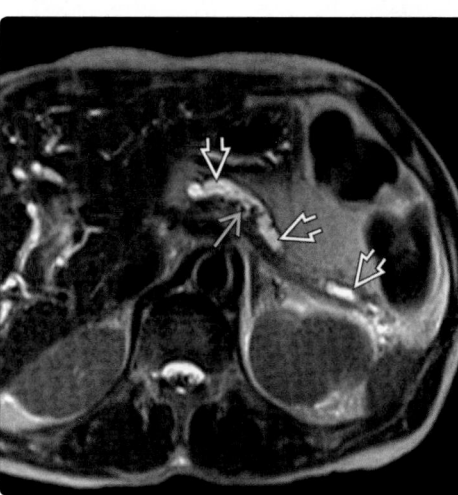

(Left) *Transverse ultrasound demonstrates an atrophic, echogenic gland ➡ with intraductal ➡ and parenchymal ➡ calcifications. The distal body/tail are obscured by bowel gas.* (Right) *Transverse T2-weighted MR in the same patient shows ductal dilatation in the body and tail ➡ better than on the US. Intraductal stones ➡ are visible as signal voids.*

Mucinous Cystic Pancreatic Tumor

TERMINOLOGY

- Synonyms: Mucinous cystic neoplasm, macrocystic cystadenoma/carcinoma, mucinous cystadenoma/carcinoma

IMAGING

- US: Not modality of choice: Difficult to visualize entire pancreas due to overlying bowel or fat
  - Nonspecific hypovascular cystic mass
  - Cyst contents may be anechoic, echogenic with debris or septations, ± solid component
- Contrast enhanced CT or MR used to accurately characterize morphology and guide treatment
  - Solitary, uni- or multilocular cystic lesion in body or tail of the pancreas
  - Typically fewer than 6 cystic components, which are each > 2 cm in size
  - May contain peripheral calcification
  - No communication with pancreatic duct

- Endoscopic ultrasound (EUS): Invasive technique reserved for when FNA is being considered

TOP DIFFERENTIAL DIAGNOSES

- Pseudocyst
- Intraductal papillary mucinous neoplasm
- Macrocystic variant of serous cystadenoma
- Solid pseudopapillary tumor
- Cystic pancreatic neuroendocrine tumor

CLINICAL ISSUES

- Seen almost exclusively in middle-aged women; termed "mother lesion"
- Excellent prognosis without invasive carcinoma
- Worse prognosis when invasive carcinoma is present; however better than with typical ductal-type adenocarcinoma (75% vs. 5%)

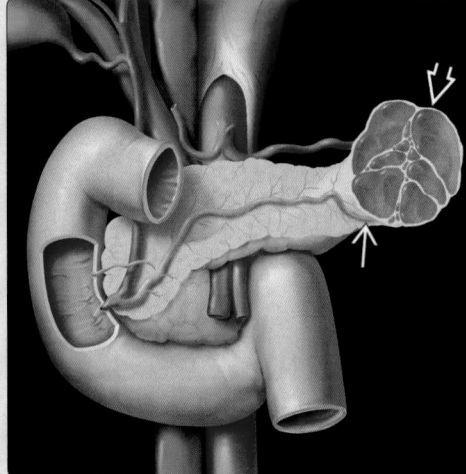
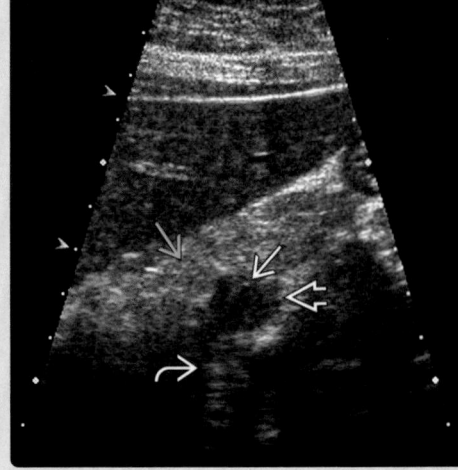

(Left) Graphic shows a multiseptated, cystic mass ⇥ in the tail of the pancreas. Note that the pancreatic duct ⇥ is displaced but not obstructed. (Right) Transverse oblique transabdominal ultrasound shows a well-defined cystic lesion ⇥ arising from the posterior body of the pancreas ⇥ with a thin internal septation ⇥ and posterior acoustic enhancement ⇥.

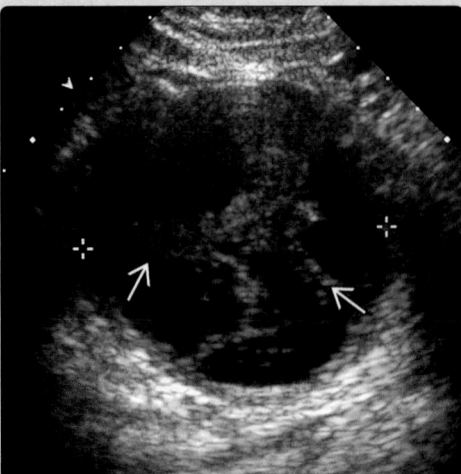
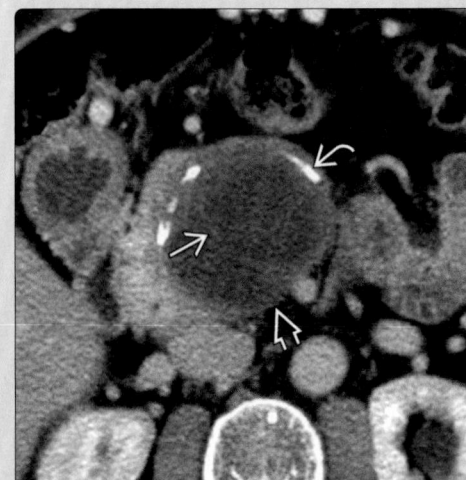

(Left) Transverse transabdominal ultrasound shows a well-defined, complex cystic pancreatic mass (calipers) with thick internal septations ⇥. (Right) Axial CECT of the same lesion, shows an encapsulated, complex cystic mass ⇥ with internal septations ⇥ and peripheral calcification ⇥. Note the few, relatively larger cysts and unusual location in the head of the pancreas.

TERMINOLOGY

Abbreviations

- Mucinous cystic pancreatic tumor (MCN)

Synonyms

- Mucinous cystic neoplasm of pancreas
- Mucinous cystadenoma/cystadenocarcinoma
- Macrocystic cystadenoma/cystadenocarcinoma
- Macrocystic adenoma

Definitions

- Septated cystic neoplasm composed of mucin-producing epithelium and distinctive ovarian-type stroma, ranging in grade from potentially malignant to invasive carcinoma

IMAGING

General Features

- Best diagnostic clue
  - Thick-walled, multilocular cystic mass with internal septations and possibly mural nodularity
- Location
  - Body and tail of pancreas (more common)
- Size
  - Range from 2 cm to > 10 cm in diameter
  - Mean size 8.7 cm

Ultrasonographic Findings

- Grayscale ultrasound
  - Well-circumscribed, anechoic, or hypoechoic mass, commonly in pancreatic body or tail
  - Unilocular or multilocular with echogenic septations
    - Cyst contents may be anechoic, echogenic with debris, ± solid component
  - No communication with pancreatic ductal system
  - May contain calcification
  - Mural nodularity suggests malignancy
    - When malignant: Possible adenopathy ± thick-walled cystic liver lesions
- Color Doppler
  - Hypovascular mass
  - May encase splenic vein or displace surrounding vessels
- Findings on US are nonspecific and further evaluation with CT or MR is necessary

CT Findings

- CECT
  - Well circumscribed and smoothly marginated
  - Unilocular or multilocular low-attenuation cystic lesion
    - When multiloculated, typically contains fewer than 6 cystic components
    - Each > 2 cm in size
  - May show peripheral curvilinear or septal calcification
  - Enhancement of cyst wall, internal septations and any mural nodules
  - Features favoring malignancy
    - Solid mural nodules
    - Thick septations
    - Wall thickening

MR Findings

- T1WI
  - Variable signal intensity based on cyst content
    - May be hypointense, isointense, or hyperintense on FS T1, depending on proteinaceous content
  - Hypointense focal calcifications
- T2WI
  - T2 hyperintense cysts with mixed signal of internal septa
  - T2 hypointense capsule and calcifications
- T1WI C+
  - Enhancement of fibrous cyst wall on more delayed post-contrast sequences
  - Features suggesting malignancy
    - Enhancing septations and solid components
- MRCP
  - Pancreatic duct may be displaced or narrowed by mass
  - Confirms absence of communication with pancreatic duct

Other Modality Findings

- Endoscopic ultrasound (EUS)
  - High spatial resolution; can depict internal septations, mural nodules, wall thickness
  - Can guide aspiration of fluid and biopsy of solid components, increasing overall accuracy for diagnosis over CT and MR
    - Cyst contents
      - High CEA (< 5 ng/mL virtually excludes mucinous lesion)
      - Low amylase (though can be increased)
      - When malignant high CA 19.9 level
      - Positive mucin stain

Imaging Recommendations

- Best imaging tool
  - CT or MR
    - Provides accurate characterization of cyst morphology
  - EUS
    - Invasive technique
    - Often performed in conjunction with cyst fluid aspiration for definitive diagnosis
- Protocol advice
  - CT or MR should be performed with contrast enhancement
    - Dual-phase pancreatic protocol (late arterial and portal venous phases)
    - Improves sensitivity for depicting morphological features, including internal septation and mural nodularity
  - MRCP
    - To characterize relationship between lesion and pancreatic duct

DIFFERENTIAL DIAGNOSIS

Pseudocyst

- Unilocular anechoic or hypoechoic cyst with no septations or solid components
- May show communication to pancreatic duct
- Peripancreatic fat plane infiltration
- Clinical history of pancreatitis

Intraductal Papillary Mucinous Neoplasm

- Branch duct type: Grape-like clusters of small cysts
- Communicates with pancreatic duct
- Typically in head of pancreas or uncinate process

Macrocystic Variant of Serous Cystadenoma

- Unilocular cystic lesion usually in pancreatic head
- Typically shows thinner, nonenhancing imperceptible wall

Solid Pseudopapillary Tumor (SPN)

- Large solid and heterogeneously cystic mass commonly in tail of pancreas
- Intratumoral hemorrhage is more typical of SPN; rarely seen with MCN
- Typically in young women

Cystic Pancreatic Neuroendocrine Tumor

- Hypervascular mass with nonenhancing cystic/necrotic components
- May be multiple
- May see metastatic disease in liver

PATHOLOGY

Staging, Grading, & Classification

- Tumors in this group include
  - Benign mucinous cystadenoma (72%)
  - Borderline mucinous cystic tumor (10.5%)
  - Mucinous cystic tumor with carcinoma in situ (5.5%)
  - Mucinous cystadenocarcinoma (12%)
- Any tumor in this group has potential to transform into invasive carcinoma

Gross Pathologic & Surgical Features

- Large mass with thick fibrous capsule
- Mucin-containing cystic cavity
  - May be filled with thick mucoid material/clear/green/blood-tinged fluid
- No communication with pancreatic duct
- Solid papillary projections may protrude into tumor

Microscopic Features

- Cysts lined by columnar mucin-producing epithelium supported by ovarian-type stroma
  - Ovarian-type stroma distinguishes MCN from intraductal papillary mucinous neoplasm (IPMN) with stroma ductal in origin
- Epithelium ranges in grade from benign to carcinoma
  - Can have benign configurations adjacent to areas of invasive carcinoma in same lesion
  - Biopsy to determine benign vs. malignant disease is therefore unreliable

CLINICAL ISSUES

Presentation

- Most common signs/symptoms
  - Often asymptomatic
  - May present with epigastric pain, palpable mass, or fullness

Demographics

- Age
  - Mean age: 50 years
  - Range: 20-82 years
- Gender
  - M:F = 1:20
- Epidemiology
  - 10% of cystic pancreatic tumors
  - 1% of pancreatic neoplasms

Natural History & Prognosis

- Invariably transforms into cystadenocarcinoma
- Resection in absence of invasive carcinoma usually curative
- 0% risk of recurrence
- 5-year survival rate for invasive MCN 75%

Treatment

- All tumors in this class are considered surgical lesions
  - Typically seen in younger patient population and nonoperative management would require years of high-cost, high-resolution imaging
  - Additionally, imaging and biopsy are unreliable in excluding invasive elements
  - Even benign lesions have future potential for malignant conversion
- Tumors < 4 cm without mural nodule
  - May perform laparoscopic procedure
  - Parenchyma-sparing resections (e.g., middle pancreatectomy) and distal pancreatectomy with spleen preservation should be considered
- Observation may be considered in elderly frail patients if unfit for surgery

DIAGNOSTIC CHECKLIST

Consider

- Differentiate from other cystic pancreatic lesions
- EUS and cyst aspiration for further evaluation

Image Interpretation Pearls

- Large, round, solitary, encapsulated uni- or multiloculated cystic mass with enhancing wall and internal septations

SELECTED REFERENCES

1. Khashab MA et al: Should we do EUS/FNA on patients with pancreatic cysts? The incremental diagnostic yield of EUS over CT/MRI for prediction of cystic neoplasms. Pancreas. 42(4):717-21, 2013
2. Sahani DV et al: Diagnosis and management of cystic pancreatic lesions. AJR Am J Roentgenol. 200(2):343-54, 2013
3. Dewhurst CE et al: Cystic tumors of the pancreas: imaging and management. Radiol Clin North Am. 50(3):467-86, 2012
4. Tanaka M et al: International consensus guidelines 2012 for the management of IPMN and MCN of the pancreas. Pancreatology. 12(3):183-97, 2012
5. Sakorafas GH et al: Primary pancreatic cystic neoplasms revisited: part II. Mucinous cystic neoplasms. Surg Oncol. 20(2):e93-101, 2011
6. Reddy RP et al: Pancreatic mucinous cystic neoplasm defined by ovarian stroma: demographics, clinical features, and prevalence of cancer. Clin Gastroenterol Hepatol. 2(11):1026-31, 2004

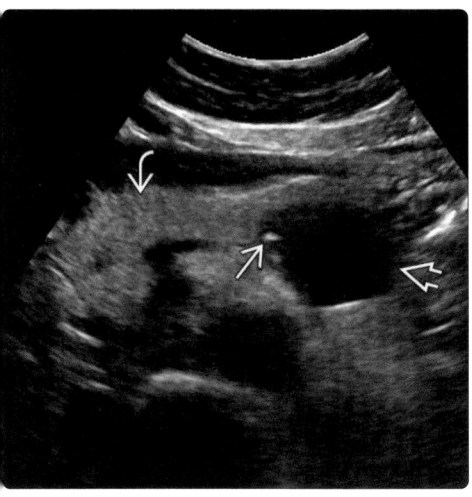

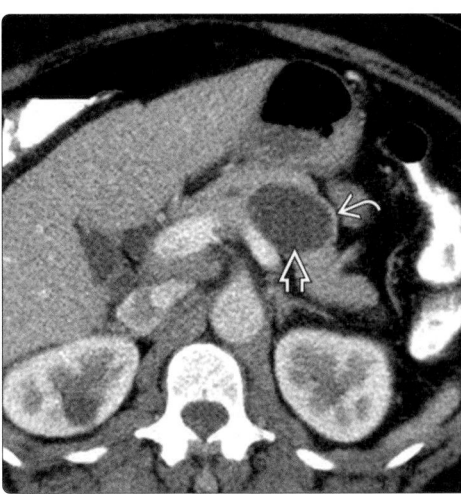

(Left) *Transverse transabdominal ultrasound shows a well-defined, anechoic, cystic lesion ⇉ in the body of the pancreas with a few hyperechoic peripheral foci ⇉. Note the normal pancreas ⇉.* (Right) *Corresponding axial CECT shows an oval, cystic mass ⇉ in the body of the pancreas with an enhancing capsule ⇉. The lesion contained internal septations not seen on CT.*

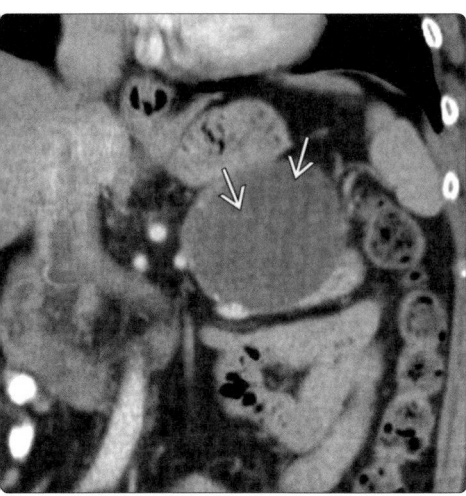

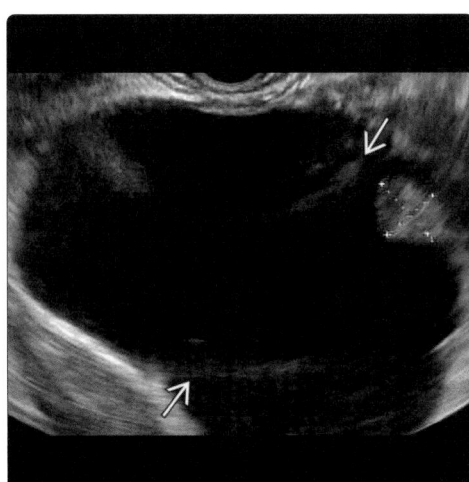

(Left) *Coronal CECT demonstrates a well-circumscribed, round cystic mass in the tail of the pancreas with subtle internal septations ⇉.* (Right) *Corresponding endoscopic ultrasound demonstrates a large cystic mass with internal septations ⇉ and a small mural nodule (calipers), which was not well seen on CT.*

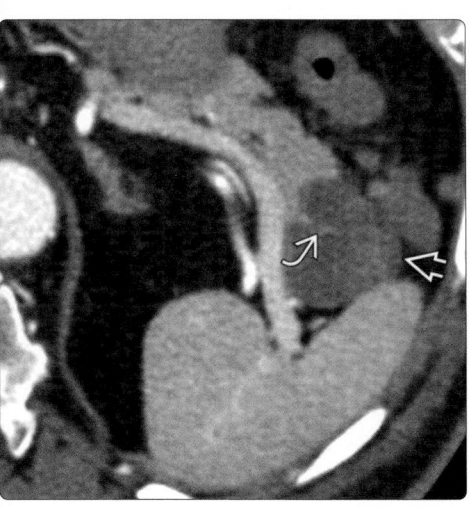

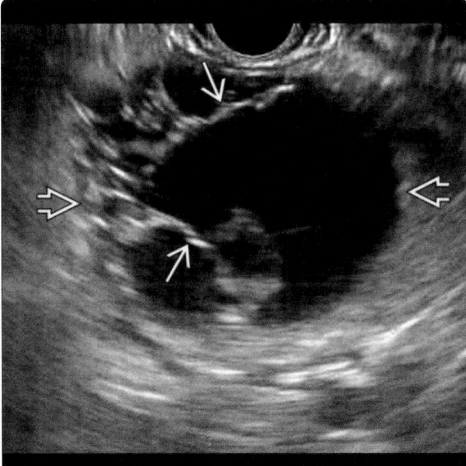

(Left) *Axial CECT shows a well-circumscribed, rounded, cystic mass ⇉ in the tail of the pancreas with subtle enhancing internal septations ⇉.* (Right) *Endoscopic ultrasound demonstrates a well-defined, multilocular cystic lesion ⇉ in the tail of the pancreas with internal septations ⇉.*

Serous Cystadenoma of Pancreas

TERMINOLOGY

- Synonyms: Pancreatic serous cystic neoplasm (SCN), microcystic adenoma of pancreas

IMAGING

- 2 morphologic types based on WHO subclassification
  - Serous microcystic adenoma: sponge-like/ honeycomb or polycystic mass with central scar
  - Serous oligocystic adenoma / macrocystic variant: unilocular or with a few large cysts (less common)
- US: Nonspecific, solid echogenic appearance due to numerous interfaces between small cysts
- CT: Better characterization of classic honeycomb pattern
  - Cluster of > 6 cysts; each typically < 1-2 cm
  - Coalescing enhancing septa → central scar ± calcification
  - May mimic solid mass
- MR: Can better identify T2-hyperintense cysts separated by T2-hypointense septa

- EUS: May allow for presumptive diagnosis based on typical features

TOP DIFFERENTIAL DIAGNOSES

- Pancreatic pseudocyst
- Mucinous cystadenoma of pancreas
- Intraductal papillary mucinous neoplasm (IPMN)
- Cystic neuroendocrine tumor
- Ductal pancreatic carcinoma

CLINICAL ISSUES

- Commonly seen in elderly women, termed "grandmother lesion"
- Typically benign and slow-growing; (nearly) no malignant potential

DIAGNOSTIC CHECKLIST

- Well-demarcated, microcystic lesion with a central scar in an asymptomatic elderly woman

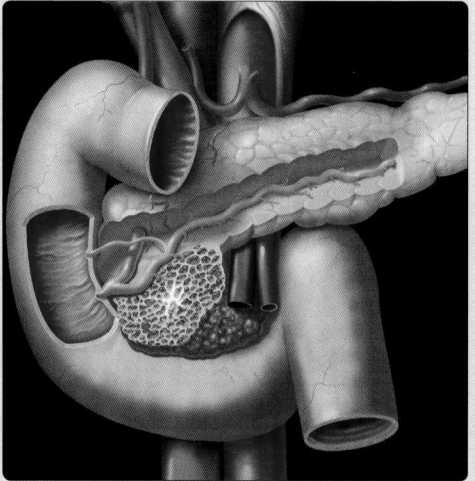

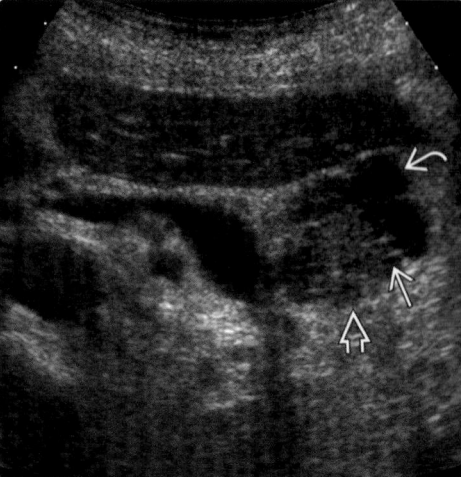

(Left) Graphic shows a sponge-like or honeycombed mass in the pancreatic head. Note presence of innumerable small cysts and central scar. The pancreatic duct (PD) is not obstructed. (Right) Transverse transabdominal ultrasound shows a well-circumscribed, solid-appearing mass ➡ in the body of the pancreas, containing tiny microcysts ➡ and larger peripheral cystic components ➡. (Courtesy A. Kamaya, MD.)

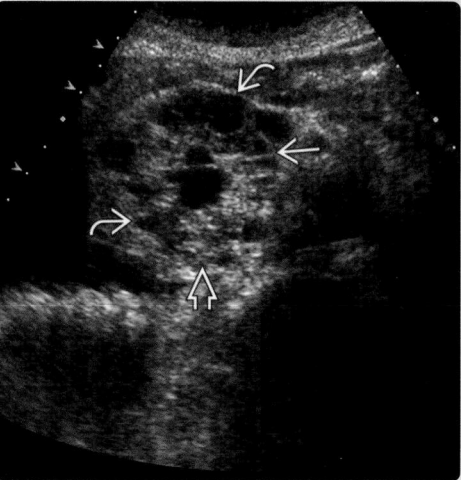

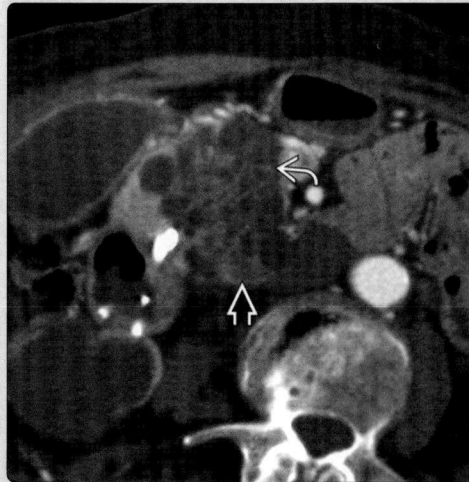

(Left) Transverse transabdominal ultrasound shows a hyperechoic, solid-appearing mass in the head of the pancreas ➡ with small cystic components ➡ of varying sizes and thin intervening septa ➡. (Right) Corresponding axial CECT image in the same patient better demonstrates the mass composed of numerous clustered small cysts ➡ separated by thin enhancing septa ➡.

Serous Cystadenoma of Pancreas

TERMINOLOGY

Abbreviations

- Serous cystadenoma (SCA)

Synonyms

- Pancreatic serous cystic neoplasm (SCN), glycogen-rich cystadenoma, microcystic adenoma of pancreas

Definitions

- Benign epithelial neoplasm arising from centroacinar cells of the exocrine pancreas, and composed of small cysts containing proteinaceous fluid separated by fibrovascular connective tissue septa.

IMAGING

General Features

- Best diagnostic clue
  - Solitary, honeycomb or sponge-like mass with central radiating scar
- Location
  - Commonly in the body and tail; 30% in pancreatic head
- Size
  - Variable sizes; mean: 4.9 cm
  - Giant SCA (>10 cm) are rare
- Morphology
  - Lobulated, well-demarcated, cystic mass
  - 2 morphologic types based on WHO subclassification:
    - Serous microcystic adenomas: Honeycomb (20-40% of cases) or polycystic
    - Serous oligocystic adenoma/macrocystic variant (< 10% of cases): Usually unilocular or fewer larger cysts (> 2cm)

Ultrasonographic Findings

- Grayscale ultrasound
  - Well-demarcated, lobulated, heterogeneous mass with posterior acoustic enhancement
  - Generally → solid echogenic appearance due to interfaces between cysts
    - Slightly echogenic, solid-appearing mass (many interfaces between numerous small cysts)
    - Multicystic mass with septa and solid-appearing component
      - □ Anechoic cystic areas usually in periphery
      - □ Central echogenic area = central scar (present in 30% of cases); ± calcification
    - Macrocystic variant: Anechoic cyst ± a few septa
  - Pancreatic and common bile duct dilatation not typical
- Color Doppler
  - Increased vascularity within septa

CT Findings

- Microcystic form: Classic honeycomb pattern
  - Thin wall with enhancing septa delineating small cysts
    - Cluster of > 6 cysts; each typically < 1 cm
    - Coalescing septa may form characteristic central stellate scar ± calcification
    - May mimic solid mass if cystic locules are small and enhancing septa predominate

- Polycystic pattern: Multiple cysts ≤2 cm separated by enhancing fibrous septa ± calcification
- Macrocystic serous cystadenoma: Usually unilocular
  - One/ few locules; thin nonenhancing imperceptible wall

MR Findings

- Can help identify cystic locules in tumors that appear solid on US and CT
- T1WI: Hypointense tumor, central scar and calcification
  - Rarely may see intratumoral hemorrhage → varied signal intensity
- T2WI: Hyperintense cystic components, hypointense septa, central scar, and calcification
- T1WI C+: Delayed enhancement of septa and central scar
- MRCP: No communication to the pancreatic duct

Other Modality Findings

- Endoscopic ultrasound (EUS)
  - Higher spatial resolution than transabdominal ultrasound → often diagnostic for microcystic form:
    - Well-delineated honeycomb appearance with central stellate scar (microcystic type)
    - Poorly developed cyst wall
    - Thin internal septa; hypervascular on Doppler
  - Can be used to guide fine needle aspiration (FNA) of cyst fluid for indeterminate cases eg macrocystic variant
    - Low viscosity, amylase, and CEA levels (< 5ng/mL)

Imaging Recommendations

- Best imaging tool
  - Contrast enhanced CT or MR
  - EUS: Improves characterization of lesion morphology and can guide cyst aspiration/biopsy
    - Invasive technique
    - Presumptive diagnosis based on typical microcystic features
    - EUS-FNA when EUS appearance is nonspecific
- Protocol advice
  - In patients with thin body habitus, higher frequency transabdominal US transducer help to depict small cysts within the mass
  - Careful examination for subtle pancreatic calcification

DIFFERENTIAL DIAGNOSIS

Pancreatic Pseudocyst

- Most common cystic pancreatic lesion
- Collection of pancreatic fluid encapsulated by fibrous tissue
- Shows well-defined capsule vs. imperceptible wall of SCA
- Usually unilocular, no septa, solid component, or central calcification
- Pancreatitis present or history of previous pancreatitis

Mucinous Cystadenoma of Pancreas

- Multiloculated cystic mass with echogenic internal septa
- May be indistinguishable from macrocystic SCA by imaging
- Most commonly located in tail of pancreas
- Thicker wall with calcification that tends to be peripheral
- Internal solid component suggests malignant tumor

Intraductal Papillary Mucinous Neoplasm (IPMN)

- Low grade malignancy arises from main pancreatic duct (MPD) or side branch pancreatic duct (SBD)

- SBD type lesion simulates serous microcystic adenoma due to presence of dilated small branch ducts
  - Grape-like cluster of small cysts
  - Communicates with the MPD
  - May be multiple
- Can show pancreatic ductal dilatation

Cystic Neuroendocrine Tumor

- Solid mass with no pancreatic ductal dilatation
- May show cystic components due to degeneration or central necrosis which can contain hemorrhagic debris
- Intratumoral hemorrhage rare with SCA

Ductal Pancreatic Carcinoma

- More common tumor than serous cystadenoma
- Rarely shows necrosis, or appears cystic due to fibrosis
- Lack of tumoral calcification
- Shows pancreatic &/or common bile ductal dilatation; vascular encasement ± regional/distant metastases

Solid Pseudopapillary Neoplasm

- Rare solid and cystic tumor with thick capsule and areas of necrosis and hemorrhage
- Intratumoral hemorrhage rare with SCA
- Typically in young women

PATHOLOGY

General Features

- Associated abnormalities
  - von Hippel-Lindau disease: May have multiple SCAs
- In general no malignant potential

Gross Pathologic & Surgical Features

- Well-circumscribed, round/ovoid, cystic mass with lobulated margin due to bulging cysts
- Macroscopic cut section
  - Spongy appearance due to many small cysts (1-20 mm)
  - Fluid in cysts : Typically clear with no mucoid plugs
    – Rarely hemorrhagic in nature
  - Thin septa radiating from central scar ± dystrophic calcification

Microscopic Features

- Cysts lined by small cuboidal epithelial cells with clear cytoplasm and minimal mucin
  - Glycogen-rich; no cytologic atypia nor mitotic figures
- Positive staining for epithelial membrane antigen & cytokeratin of low and high molecular weights
- Fibrovascular septa
- Adjacent pancreatic tissue: Normal or focally atrophic

CLINICAL ISSUES

Presentation

- Most common signs/symptoms
  - Typically asymptomatic or vague epigastric pain
  - May present with nausea, vomiting, weight loss, palpable mass, jaundice
  - Other signs/symptoms of mass effect on adjacent structures (stomach & bowel)

Demographics

- Age
  - Middle & elderly age group (more common)
  - Mean age 61.5 years
- Gender
  - M:F = 1:4
- Epidemiology
  - Cystic pancreatic neoplasms are rare
  - Accounts for 20% of all cystic pancreatic lesions; only 1% of all pancreatic neoplasms

Natural History & Prognosis

- Clinical practice assumes benign, slow-growing course
  - Most remain static over time with slow growth rate (~ 0.12 cm/year) and no complications
- Rare tumors may behave aggressively or become symptomatic (usually large lesions and location in the head of the pancreas)
  - Tumors > 4cm grow faster (~ 2 cm/year)
  - Potential complications: CBD obstruction or obstructive chronic pancreatitis, bowel obstruction; invasion of surrounding structures or vessels
  - Very rarely metastases to lymph nodes or distant organs
- Prognosis
  - Excellent: Classically thought to have no malignant potential
  - However, rare aggressive subtypes can be locally aggressive or malignant (0.8%)
  - Good prognosis after complete excision with negative surgical margins, in symptomatic or aggressive cases
  - May recur after incomplete resection

Treatment

- Nonoperative management if asymptomatic, small, and confidently diagnosed
  - Imaging surveillance at 6-12 month intervals until stability demonstrated over 2 year period
- Symptomatic & large tumors → complete surgical excision
  - No imaging surveillance necessary if negative surgical margins

DIAGNOSTIC CHECKLIST

Consider

- Differentiate from other cystic pancreatic lesions such as pseudocysts or cystic neoplasms that have malignant potential

Image Interpretation Pearls

- Well-demarcated, lobulated cystic lesion composed of innumerable small cysts (1-20 mm) separated by thin hypervascular septa

SELECTED REFERENCES

1. But DY et al: To fine needle aspiration or not? An endosonographer's approach to pancreatic cystic lesions. Endosc Ultrasound. 3(2):82-90, 2014
2. Dewhurst CE et al: Cystic tumors of the pancreas: imaging and management. Radiol Clin North Am. 50(3):467-86, 2012
3. Kucera JN et al: Cystic lesions of the pancreas: radiologic-endosonographic correlation. Radiographics. 32(7):E283-301, 2012
4. Choi JY et al: Typical and atypical manifestations of serous cystadenoma of the pancreas: imaging findings with pathologic correlation. AJR Am J Roentgenol. 193(1):136-42, 2009

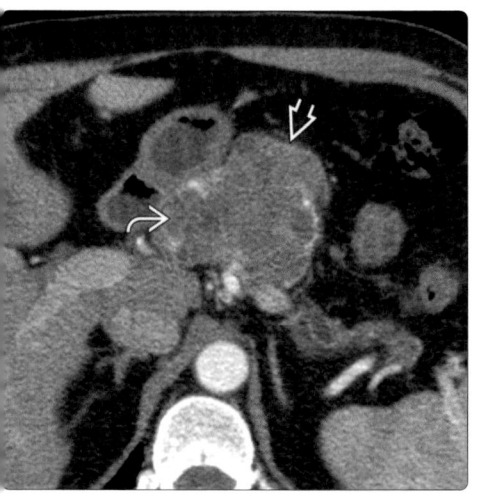

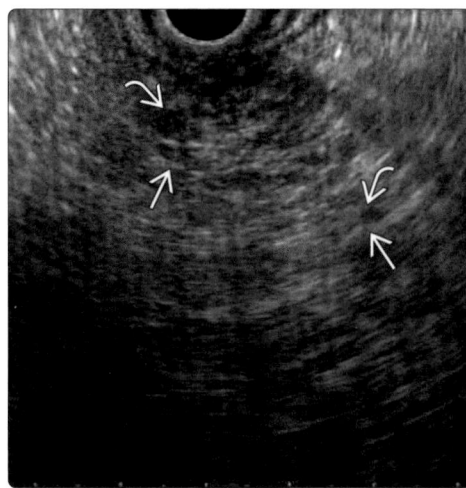

(Left) *Axial CECT shows a well-circumscribed, lobulated pancreatic mass ➡ containing clusters of tiny cysts ➘ resulting in the characteristic honeycomb appearance of a serous cystadenoma.* (Right) *Endoscopic ultrasound image in the same patient shows a predominantly echogenic mass due to the numerous acoustic interfaces between the innumerable tiny cysts ➘ and intervening fibrous stroma ➡. Surgical resection confirmed this lesion to be a serous cystadenoma of the pancreas.*

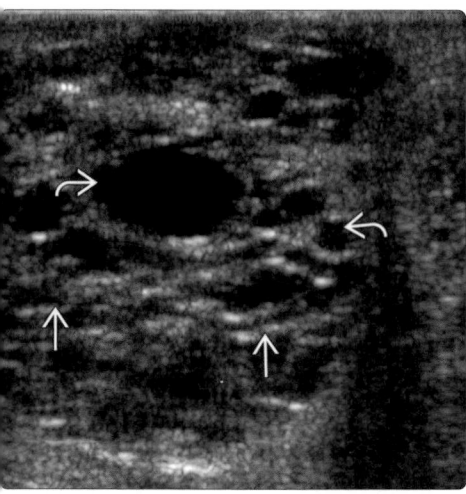

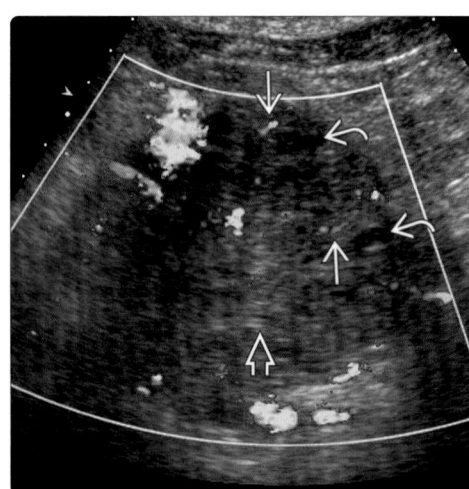

(Left) *Transverse intraoperative ultrasound of a pancreatic mass shows innumerable small cysts ➘ with intervening linear septations ➡. (Courtesy A. Kamaya, MD.)* (Right) *Transverse color Doppler ultrasound of a pancreatic mass shows central echogenicity ➡ with peripherally-oriented small cysts ➘ and color Doppler flow within intervening septa ➡. (Courtesy A. Kamaya, MD.)*

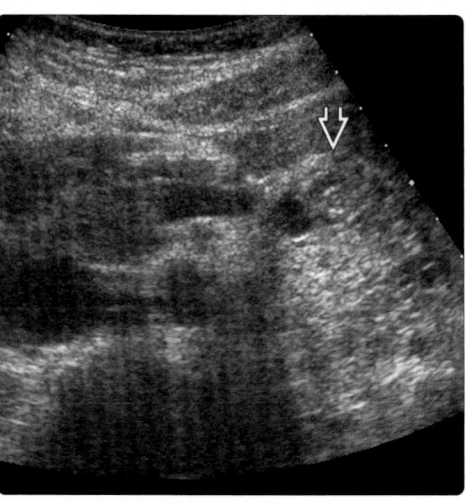

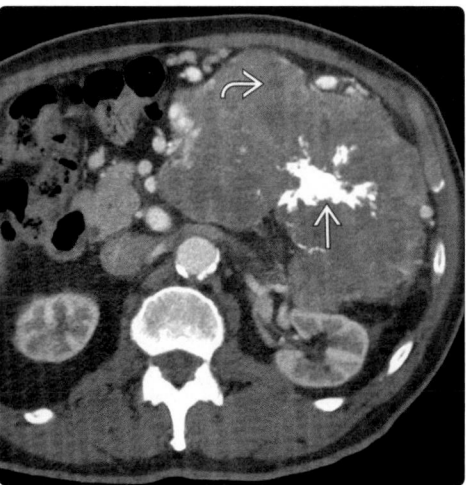

(Left) *Transverse transabdominal ultrasound shows an ill-defined, heterogeneous hyperechoic mass ➡ in the tail of pancreas with highly reflective acoustic interfaces resulting from innumerable tiny cysts which are difficult to resolve. (Courtesy A. Kamaya, MD.)* (Right) *Axial contrast enhanced CT shows a large lobulated, low-attenuation mass in the body and tail of the pancreas with small cystic spaces ➘ and dense stellate calcification ➡ within the central scar of a serous cystadenoma.*

Intraductal Papillary Mucinous Neoplasm (IPMN)

TERMINOLOGY

- Cystic neoplasm of pancreas arising from mucin-producing epithelium of main pancreatic duct (MPD) &/or side branch pancreatic ducts (SBD) with variable malignant potential

IMAGING

- Main pancreatic duct type: > 5 mm; no obstructive cause
- Side branch duct type: Multicystic, grape-like cluster of cysts contiguous with the MPD
- US: Not modality of choice: Difficult to evaluate entire pancreas due to bowel gas and limited characterization
  - Nonspecific anechoic or hypoechoic mass ± PD dilatation
- Endoscopic ultrasound (EUS): Provides best morphologic evaluation and opportunity for cyst aspiration &/or biopsy
- CT or MR: Important in identifying features associated with increased risk of malignancy
- MRCP: Best noninvasive imaging modality for identification of ductal communication
- Follow-up surveillance imaging with CEMR/MRCP

TOP DIFFERENTIAL DIAGNOSES

- Mucinous cystic pancreatic neoplasm
- Pancreatic serous cystadenoma
- Chronic pancreatitis
- Pancreatic pseudocyst
- Pancreatic ductal adenocarcinoma

CLINICAL ISSUES

- If high-risk stigmata present based on Tanaka criteria → surgical resection
- If worrisome features present → EUS for biopsy/aspiration
- If no worrisome features present → follow-up interval determined by cyst size

DIAGNOSTIC CHECKLIST

- Look for communication between cystic lesion and pancreatic duct, which may be dilated

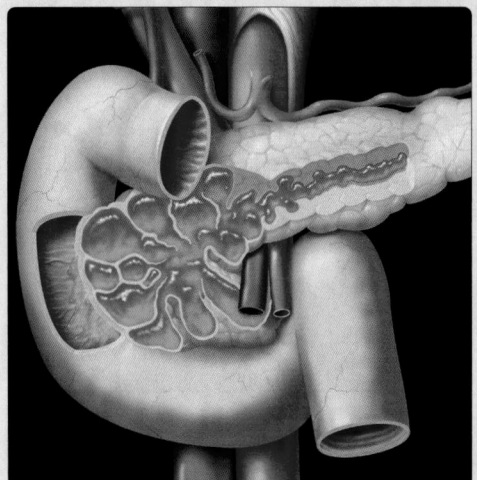
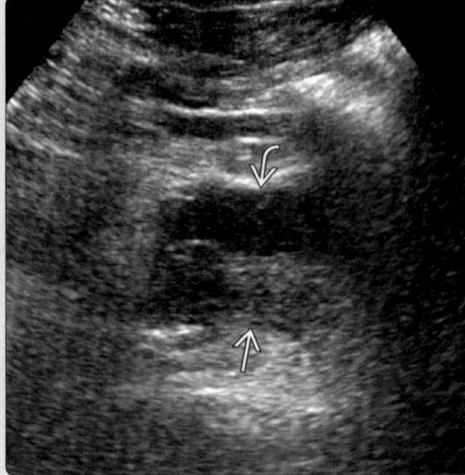

(Left) Graphic demonstrates irregular, dilated main and branch pancreatic ducts within the head and uncinate process of the pancreas, typical of intraductal papillary mucinous neoplasm (IPMN). (Right) Transverse transabdominal ultrasound shows marked dilatation of the pancreatic duct ➡ that measures > 10 mm in the body of the pancreas. Note the associated ill-defined hypoechoic mass posteriorly ➡.

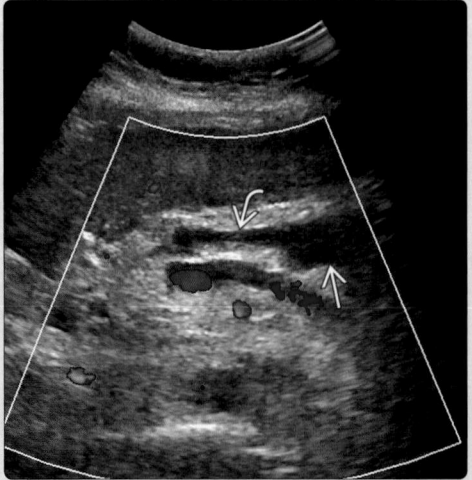
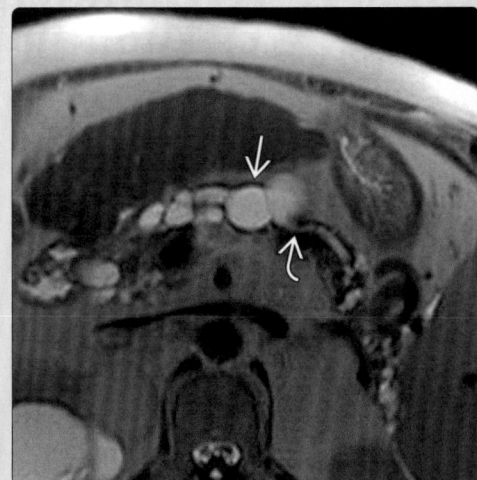

(Left) Color Doppler transabdominal ultrasound demonstrates an anechoic cystic lesion ➡ communicating with a dilated main pancreatic duct ➡. (Right) Axial T2WI in the same patient better characterizes the presence of multiple cystic lesions ➡ some of which show communication with the mildly dilated main pancreatic duct ➡.

TERMINOLOGY

Abbreviations

- Intraductal papillary mucinous neoplasm (IPMN)

Synonyms

- Intraductal papillary mucinous tumor, duct ectatic mucinous cystadenoma, mucinous hypersecretory neoplasm, mucin-producing tumor

Definitions

- Cystic neoplasm of pancreas arising from mucin-producing epithelium of main pancreatic duct (MPD) &/or side branch pancreatic ducts (SBD) with variable malignant potential

IMAGING

General Features

- Best diagnostic clue
  - Grossly dilated MPD without obstructive mass
  - Cystic lesion in pancreatic head or uncinate process with small cystic loculations and communication to MPD
- Location
  - Typically in head/uncinate
  - May be multiple (21-40%); can involve entire pancreas in up to 20% of cases
- Size
  - Side branch cysts typically 0.5-2.0 cm; can grow > 3 cm
- Morphology
  - MPD type: Dilated MPD (> 5 mm); no obstructive cause
  - SBD type: Multicystic lesion contiguous with the MPD
  - Mixed type: Findings of both types

Ultrasonographic Findings

- MPD type: Dilated MPD, may contain low-level internal echoes (mucin vs. mural nodule)
- SBD type: Anechoic or hypoechoic cystic mass ± septations; may see communication with PD if it is dilated

Other Modality Findings

- Endoscopic ultrasound (EUS)
  - Higher spatial resolution than transabdominal US; can depict internal septations, mural nodules, wall thickening
  - Used to guide aspiration of cyst contents and biopsy of soft tissue components
    - Cyst contents: High CEA levels with malignancy; < 5 ng/mL excludes mucinous lesion

Radiographic Findings

- Endoscopic retrograde cholangiopancreatography (ERCP)
  - Bulging "fish eye" ampulla of Vater, pathognomonic for IPMN
  - Dilated MPD with filling defects due to excessive mucin production; cystic dilatation of branch ducts
  - Traditionally used to show communication with MPD

CT Findings

- MPD type: > 5 mm, tortuous; segmental or diffuse
- SBD-type: Multilocular cystic lesion with possible communication to MPD
  - Grape-like clusters of small cysts or tubes and arcs; may be multifocal

- CECT may show enhancing soft tissue thickening or mural nodularity

MR Findings

- T1WI: Hypointense
- T2WI: Hyperintense for both SBD and BPD-types
  - SBD: Focal or multifocal, lobulated, cystic lesion with thin internal septations
    - Clustered small T2-bright cysts; ± curvilinear T2-hyperintense connection to MPD
- MRCP
  - T2-hyperintense ductal communication best depicted with thin slice and thick slab techniques
  - May show intraductal nodules as filling defects → raising concern for malignant conversion
  - Can assess for biliary obstruction in setting of malignancy
- T1WI C+
  - Typically shows lack of enhancing components
  - Enhancing soft tissue thickening or nodularity within duct or cystic mass suggests malignant conversion

Imaging Recommendations

- Best imaging tool
  - CT or MR important in identifying features associated with increased risk of malignancy
  - EUS: ↑ overall accuracy for diagnosis over CT and MR
    - Invasive technique
    - Best morphologic evaluation and can guide cyst aspiration/biopsy
  - MRCP
    - Best noninvasive imaging modality for identification of ductal communication
- Protocol advice
  - Initial evaluation and morphologic characterization of pancreatic cystic lesions > 1 cm
    - CECT with curved planar reconstructions; or CE MR with MRCP (angled to MPD)
    - To assess for high-risk stigmata or worrisome features
  - Follow-up surveillance imaging with CE MR/MRCP

DIFFERENTIAL DIAGNOSIS

Mucinous Cystic Pancreatic Neoplasm

- Solitary; no communication with MPD; may contain peripheral calcification
- Typically in body/tail of pancreas in middle-aged women

Pancreatic Serous Cystadenoma

- Solitary; no communication with MPD; may contain spoke wheel calcification
- Commonly in body/tail of pancreas in elderly women

Chronic Pancreatitis

- Atrophic pancreas, dilated ducts, parenchymal calcifications

Pancreatic Pseudocyst

- Possible communication with MPD or SBD
- Findings &/or history of acute or chronic pancreatitis

Pancreatic Ductal Adenocarcinoma

- Solid, infiltrative mass obstructing the MPD

PATHOLOGY

General Features

- Cystically dilated segment of pancreatic duct due to intraluminal protrusion of papillary neoplastic epithelial growth

Staging, Grading, & Classification

- Main duct type: Considered precursor to invasive pancreatic ductal carcinoma
- Branch duct type: Generally benign with low malignancy risk
- Mixed type: Behaves similar to main duct type
- Tanaka criteria (update to Sendai classification): Classifies IPMN as high risk, worrisome, or low risk based on imaging features in order to guide treatment decisions
  - High-risk stigmata: Obstructive jaundice with cystic lesion at head of pancreas, enhancing solid component within cyst, or MPD > 10 mm
  - Worrisome features: Largest cyst ≥ 3 cm, thickened/enhancing cyst walls, MPD 5-9 mm, nonenhancing mural nodule, or abrupt change in diameter of MPD with parenchymal atrophy
  - Low risk: No worrisome features and largest cyst < 3 cm
  - Imaging findings direct towards interval follow-up, EUS, or surgical resection

Gross Pathologic & Surgical Features

- MPD type: Mass or nodule in dilated mucin-filled duct
- SBD type: May be multifocal, lack of nodule formation, contains inspissated mucin; may not see connection of branch duct IPMN to MPD on gross specimen

Microscopic Features

- Histologically similar mucinous-type epithelium as seen with mucinous cystic neoplasms but without ovarian-type stroma
- Variable grades of dysplasia to gross invasion
  - MPD type: ~ 40% contain invasive carcinoma
  - SBD type: Most show no or low-grade dysplasia
- May see fibrotic atrophy of surrounding parenchyma due to ductal obstruction
  - Can result in calcifying obstructive pancreatitis; however, calcification does not usually involve tumor itself

CLINICAL ISSUES

Presentation

- Most common signs/symptoms
  - > 60% cystic pancreatic lesions found incidentally
  - May present with nonspecific symptoms of nausea/vomiting, abdominal pain, weight loss, anorexia
- Other signs/symptoms
  - MPD type may result in pancreatitis from obstruction secondary to excess mucin production
- Associations
  - Extrapancreatic malignancies, most commonly gastric or colorectal carcinoma
  - Possibly greater prevalence of extensive SBD-type IPMN after transplantation and immunosuppression

Demographics

- Age

  - Mean at diagnosis: 68 years; range: 60-80 years
- Gender
  - M > F

Natural History & Prognosis

- Overall 5-year survival for all patients with IPMN: ~ 60%
- Up to 70% of MPD type progress to invasive carcinoma
- SBD type often quiescent with low overall risk of malignancy if < 3 cm
- Mixed type tends to behave similar to MPD type
- Long-term surveillance warranted even after resection because of risk for multifocal disease: Synchronous and metachronous

Treatment

- Imaging findings direct need for surgical resection, EUS, or interval follow-up according to Tanaka criteria
- Surgical resection for all IPMN with high-risk features
  - Excellent 5-year survival in absence of invasive component (94-100% vs. 40-60%)
  - Recurrence rate with invasive disease: 50-65% vs. < 8% without
- If worrisome features present, EUS should be performed for biopsy &/or aspiration
- If largest cyst > 3 cm with no other worrisome features should also consider EUS
- If no associated concerning features, cyst size determines follow-up intervals
  - < 1 cm: CT/MR in 2-3 years
  - 1-2 cm: CT/MR yearly for 2 years, then lengthen interval if no change
  - 2-3 cm: Endoscopic ultrasound in 3-6 months, then lengthen interval if no change, alternating MR and endoscopic ultrasound

DIAGNOSTIC CHECKLIST

Image Interpretation Pearls

- Main duct type: Dilation of main pancreatic duct (> 5 mm) without obstructive mass
- Branch duct type: Grape-like cluster of small cysts, with communication to MPD

Reporting Tips

- Describe high-risk and worrisome features, including cyst size, enhancing walls, MPD dilation, mural nodule, or abrupt change in duct size with parenchymal atrophy
- Will require interval follow-up, EUS, or possible resection based on associated features

SELECTED REFERENCES

1. Freeny PC et al: Moving beyond morphology: new insights into the characterization and management of cystic pancreatic lesions. Radiology. 272(2):345-63, 2014
2. Kim JH et al: Intraductal papillary mucinous neoplasms with associated invasive carcinoma of the pancreas: imaging findings and diagnostic performance of MDCT for prediction of prognostic factors. AJR Am J Roentgenol. 201(3):565-72, 2013
3. Tanaka M et al: International consensus guidelines 2012 for the management of IPMN and MCN of the pancreas. Pancreatology. 12(3):183-97, 2012
4. Gore RM et al: The incidental cystic pancreas mass: a practical approach. Cancer Imaging. 12:414-21, 2012
5. Remotti HE et al: Intraductal papillary mucinous neoplasms of the pancreas: clinical surveillance and malignant progression, multifocality and implications of a field-defect. JOP. 13(2):135-8, 2012

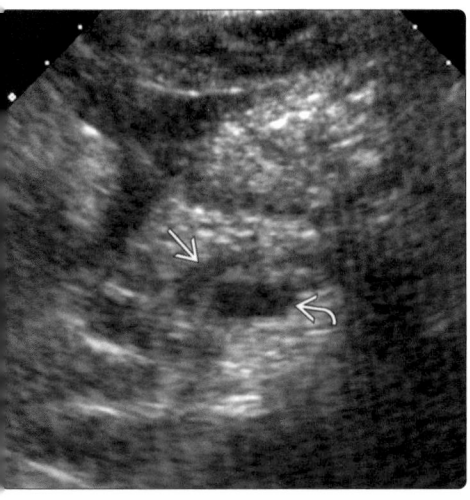
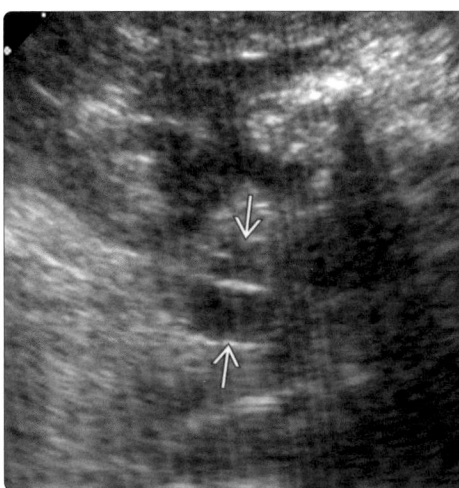

(Left) *Transverse oblique transabdominal ultrasound demonstrates a prominent main pancreatic duct* ➡. *Superior mesenteric vein* ➡ *is noted.* (Right) *Transabdominal ultrasound in the same patient demonstrates a septated cystic lesion* ➡ *just caudal to the dilated main pancreatic duct in the head of the pancreas.*

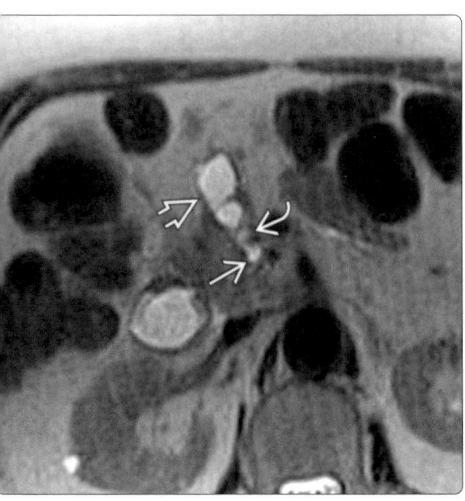
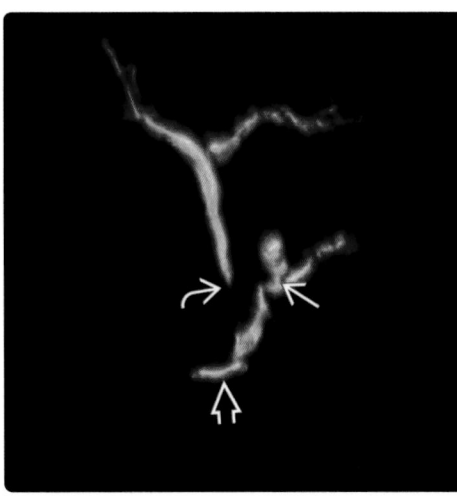

(Left) *Corresponding axial T2WI MR in the same patient demonstrates a thin-walled, tubular cystic lesion* ➡ *with curvilinear connection* ➡ *to the main pancreatic duct* ➡ *consistent with side-branch-type IPMN.* (Right) *Corresponding 3D volume-rendered MRCP better demonstrates the communication* ➡ *between the cystic lesion and the main pancreatic duct* ➡ *consistent with a side-branch-type IPMN. A long segment of stricturing* ➡ *is incidentally noted in the common bile duct.*

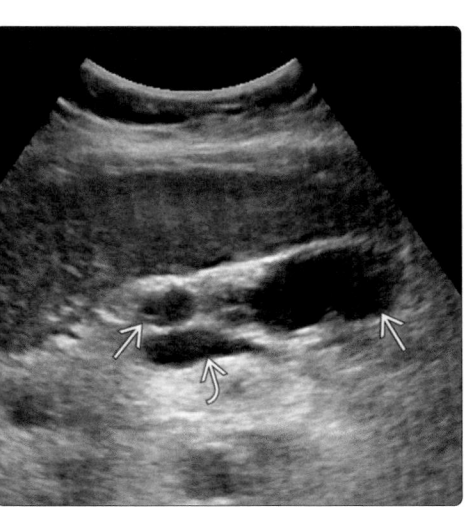
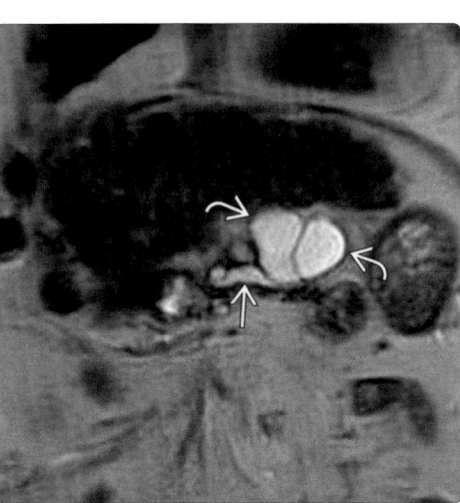

(Left) *Transabdominal ultrasound demonstrates multiple oval and elongated cystic lesions in the pancreatic head/body* ➡. *Splenic vein* ➡ *is also noted.* (Right) *Coronal T2 HASTE MR better demonstrates the elongated, cystic dilatation of side branches* ➡ *in the body of the pancreas with curvilinear communication to the dilated main pancreatic duct* ➡.

(Left) *Axial T2WI MR demonstrates grape-like cystic lesions* ⇨ *throughout the pancreatic body and tail with a multiloculated cystic lesion* ⇨ *in the neck of the pancreas. Note the mildly dilated pancreas duct* ⇨, *which appeared to communicate with some of the lesions (not shown).* **(Right)** *Endoscopic ultrasound in the same patient demonstrates multiple clustered, thin-walled, cystic lesions* ⇨ *involving the entire pancreas, consistent with extensive side-branch-type IPMN.*

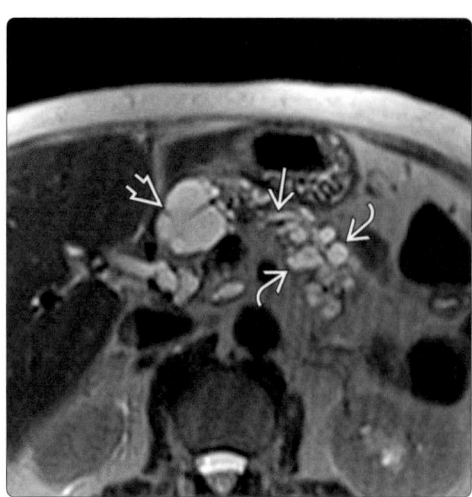
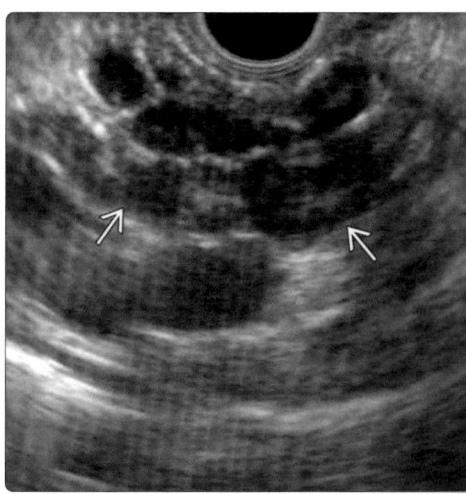

(Left) *Axial CT demonstrates a thin-walled, elongated, nonenhancing, cystic lesion* ⇨ *in the head of the pancreas.* **(Right)** *Axial T2WI MR in the same patient better demonstrates curvilinear communication* ⇨ *between the cystic lesion and the mildly dilated main pancreatic duct* ⇨ *consistent with a side-branch-type IPMN.*

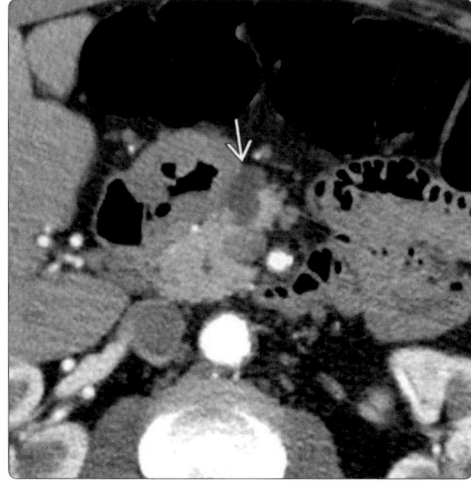
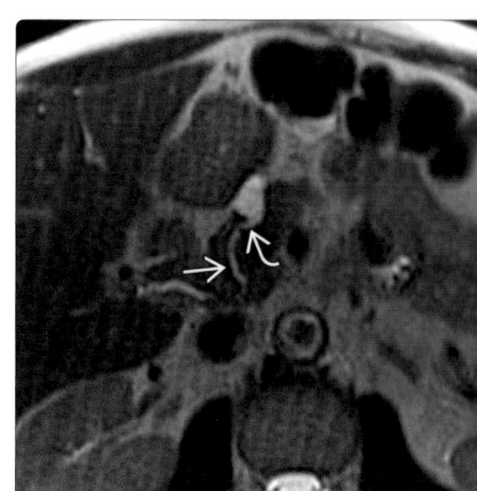

(Left) *Direct endoscopic visualization shows a classic bulging "fish eye" papilla extruding mucin, pathognomonic for IPMN.* **(Right)** *Endoscopic ultrasound demonstrates a large cystic mass* ⇨ *in the head of the pancreas, in continuity with a very dilated pancreatic duct (not shown). Note the mural nodularity* ⇨, *a worrisome finding for malignancy.*

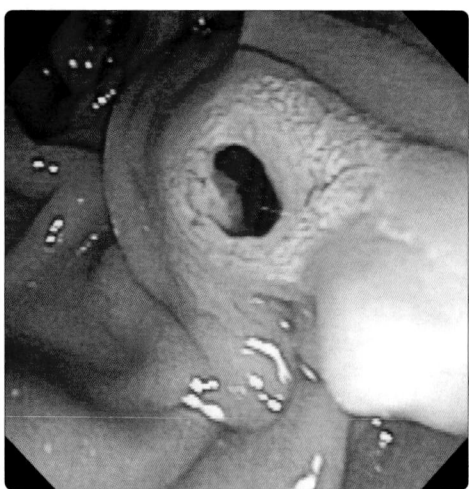
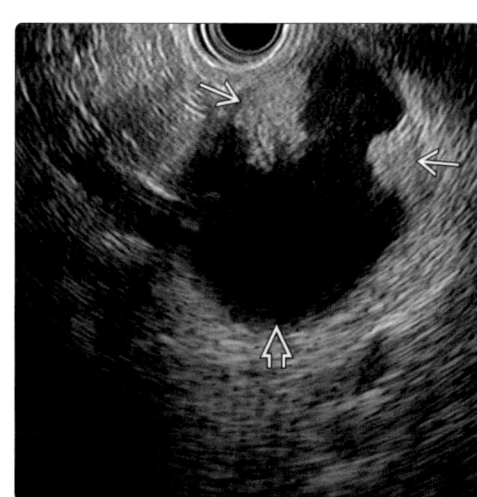

Intraductal Papillary Mucinous Neoplasm (IPMN)

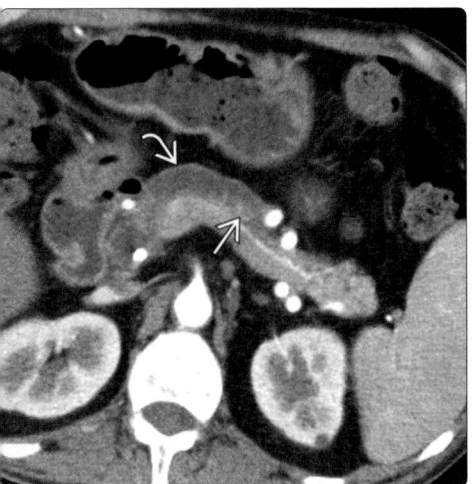
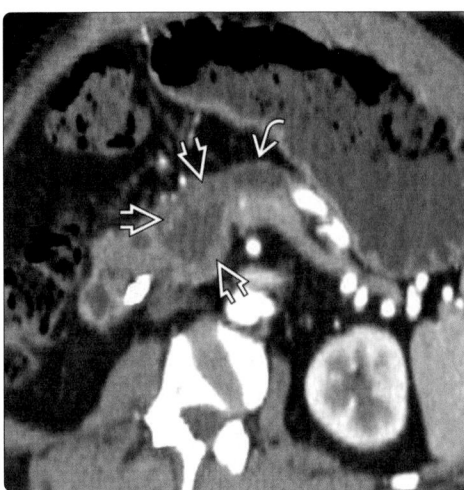

(Left) Axial CT demonstrates marked diffuse dilation of the main pancreatic duct ⟹ with intraluminal soft tissue nodularity ⟹. (Right) Curved planar reconstruction in the same patient demonstrates the diffusely dilated main pancreatic duct ⟹ communicating with a cystic mass in the head of the pancreas. Note the irregular peripheral soft tissue thickening and nodularity ⟹.

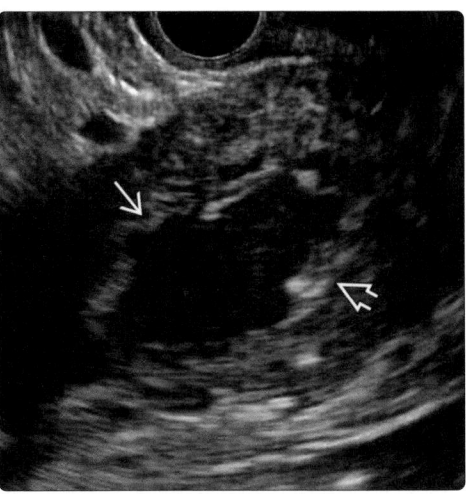
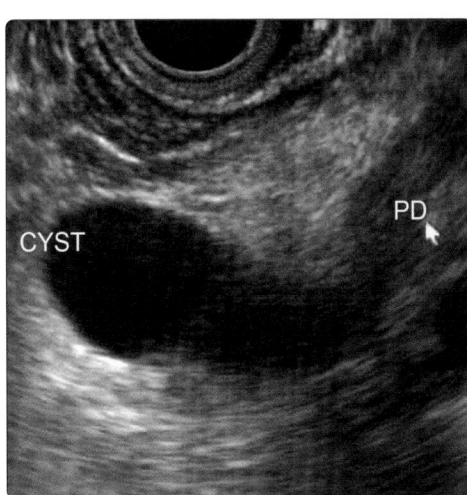

(Left) Endoscopic ultrasound in the same patient better demonstrates mural nodularity ⟹ associated with the cystic lesion ⟹ in the pancreatic head, contiguous with a dilated main pancreatic duct (not shown). (Right) Endoscopic ultrasound in a different patient demonstrates a diffusely dilated pancreatic duct (labeled PD) communicating with a focal cystic lesion (labeled cyst), consistent with a main duct IPMN.

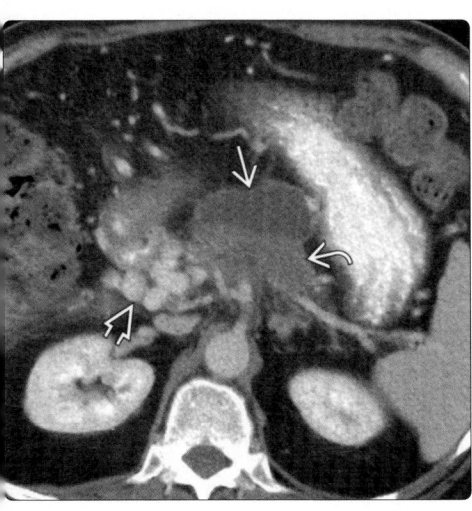
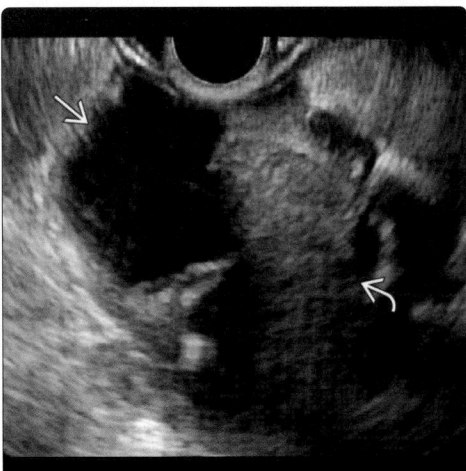

(Left) Axial CECT shows very marked dilatation of the pancreatic duct ⟹ and a large infiltrative soft tissue mass ⟹ compatible with malignant transformation of a main duct IPMN. Note the cavernous transformation of the portal vein ⟹ due to venous occlusion from the mass. (Right) Corresponding endoscopic ultrasound shows the very dilated, mucin-filled duct ⟹ with low-level echoes and the large soft tissue mass ⟹ arising posteriorly.

Pancreatic Ductal Carcinoma

TERMINOLOGY

- Solid epithelial neoplasm from ductal epithelium of exocrine pancreas

IMAGING

- Ill-defined pancreatic mass obstructing pancreatic and possibly common bile duct (producing "double duct" sign)
- Best imaging tool: CECT for demonstrating mass and evaluating resectability
- Without metastatic disease, resectability determined by vascular involvement
  - Best assessed on CTA using NCCN criteria
- US often first-line imaging to evaluate obstructive jaundice
  - Often shows level of obstruction
  - Not as sensitive as CT or MR for demonstrating mass or assessing resectability

TOP DIFFERENTIAL DIAGNOSES

- Chronic pancreatitis

- Mucinous cystic pancreatic neoplasm
- Lymphoma
- Neuroendocrine tumor of pancreas
- Metastases

CLINICAL ISSUES

- Poor overall prognosis; 5-year survival rate of ~ 5%
- Usually presents late with unresectable disease
- Better long-term survival through complete resection

DIAGNOSTIC CHECKLIST

- Heterogeneous pancreatic head mass with ductal dilatation, upstream atrophy, and often extensive local extension around vessels, &/or regional metastases

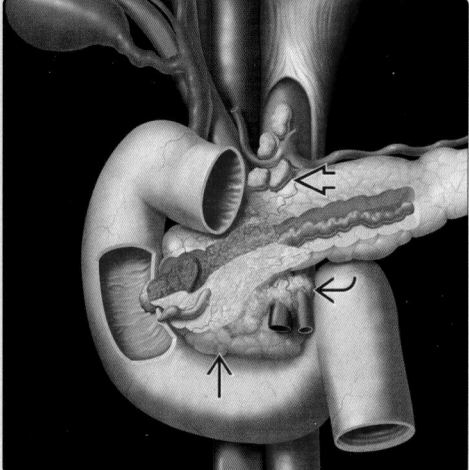
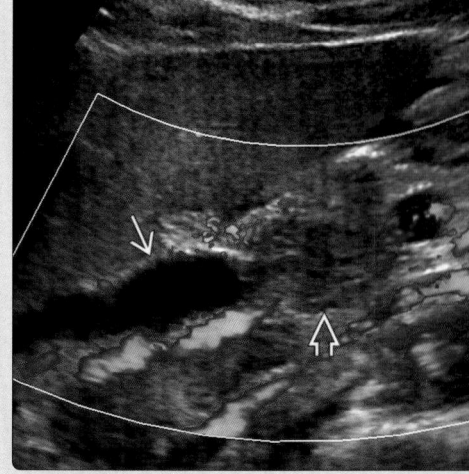

(Left) Graphic shows an infiltrative mass ⮕ in the pancreatic head partially obstructing the common bile duct and pancreatic duct. Superior mesenteric vessels are encased ⮕. Celiac nodes ⮕ are present. (Right) Longitudinal oblique color Doppler ultrasound shows an ill-defined, solid, hypoechoic mass ⮕ in the pancreatic head obstructing the terminal portion of the common bile duct with proximal dilatation ⮕.

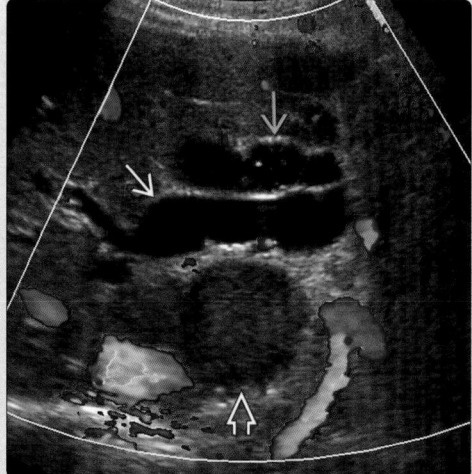
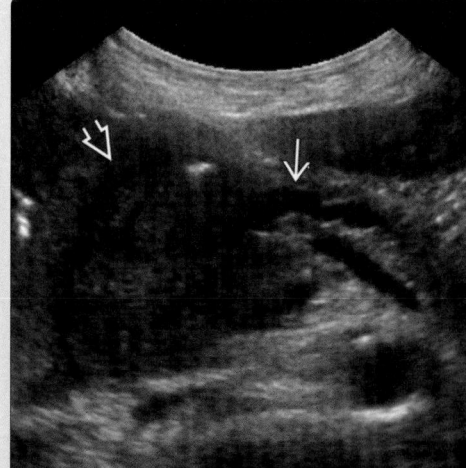

(Left) Longitudinal oblique color Doppler ultrasound shows dilatation of the common bile duct in the porta hepatis ⮕ and a solid, hypoechoic hepatic metastasis ⮕. Note the sludge-filled gallbladder ⮕. (Right) Transverse transabdominal ultrasound in the same patient shows a large, ill-defined, solid, hypoechoic mass ⮕ in the pancreatic head, with pancreatic duct dilatation ⮕ in the atrophic pancreatic body and tail.

TERMINOLOGY

Synonyms

- Pancreatic ductal adenocarcinoma (PDA), pancreatic cancer

Definitions

- Solid epithelial neoplasm from ductal exocrine pancreas

IMAGING

General Features

- Best diagnostic clue
  - Ill-defined pancreatic mass obstructing pancreatic and possibly common bile duct (producing "double duct" sign)
- Location
  - Head (60-70%), body (5-10%), tail (10-15%), multiple regions or diffuse (22%)
- Size
  - Average diameter: 2-3 cm
- Morphology
  - Accounts for 85-90% of all pancreatic tumors
  - Encases intrapancreatic blood vessels and usually not resectable for cure at time of presentation
  - Local infiltrative invasion
  - Metastatic involvement of liver, portal hilar nodes, peritoneum, lungs, pleura, bone

Ultrasonographic Findings

- Grayscale ultrasound
  - Hypoechoic, infiltrative mass
    - Pancreatic ductal dilatation
      - > 3 mm upstream from tumor with tortuous configuration and loss of parallel nature
    - Bile duct dilatation
      - Common in pancreatic head carcinoma
      - Obstruction at level of pancreatic head or porta hepatis, depending on tumor size and regional adenopathy
      - ± dilatation of cystic duct and gallbladder (Courvoisier sign)
    - Calcification or necrosis/cystic change: Rarely seen
  - Can be small, isoechoic mass, with subtle focal contour deformity (e.g., in uncinate process)
  - Diffuse glandular tumor involvement can be difficult to differentiate from acute pancreatitis
  - Secondary findings
    - Displacement/encasement of adjacent vascular structures
    - Atrophy or pancreatitis proximal to pancreatic ductal obstruction
    - Ascites due to peritoneal metastasis
    - Liver and regional lymph node metastases
- Color Doppler
  - May be helpful in assessing vascular encasement or venous obstruction
- Endoscopic ultrasound (EUS): Most sensitive test for small hypoechoic mass in pancreatic head
- Can guide fine-needle aspiration biopsy

Radiographic Findings

- ERCP

  - Pancreatic stricture with upstream dilatation
  - Combined with endoscopic ultrasound for biopsy
  - Allows drainage of obstructed ducts

CT Findings

- CECT
  - Hypoenhancing, poorly defined, infiltrating mass with secondary signs of
    - Obstruction of pancreatic duct and common bile duct when located in head of pancreas
    - Upstream atrophy of pancreas
  - Isodense masses (10-15%) and tumors < 2 cm are more difficult to detect
    - May only see secondary signs with subtle parenchymal fullness
  - Can detect contiguous organ invasion (duodenum, stomach, splenic hilum, porta hepatis, mesentery)
  - Distant metastases to liver, peritoneum, regional nodes
- CTA
  - More accurate for detecting vascular involvement
    - Abutment (< 180° vessel circumference), encasement (> 180° vessel circumference), narrowing, or occlusion
    - Teardrop-shaped superior mesenteric vein (SMV) suggests venous invasion

MR Findings

- T1WI
  - Hypointense relative to normal parenchyma due to fibrous nature of tumor
  - Fat-saturation increases conspicuity
- T2WI
  - Improves detection of ductal dilatation
- T1WI C+
  - Best sequence for delineating mass, which shows limited enhancement
  - Shows imaging features of vascular encasement and tumor extension similar to CECT
- MRCP
  - Dilated ducts proximal to obstructing mass

Imaging Recommendations

- Best imaging tool
  - CECT overall accuracy: 86-99%
- Protocol advice
  - CECT should follow pancreas-specific protocol with CT arteriography
- US often first-line imaging for painless obstructive jaundice to show level of obstruction
  - Less sensitive than CT or MR for detection of pancreatic mass or for determining resectability
- EUS used to guide biopsy in setting of ductal obstruction without mass
  - Increased sensitivity for small lesions < 2 cm that can be missed on CT

DIFFERENTIAL DIAGNOSIS

Chronic Pancreatitis

- Focal or diffuse atrophy of gland with dilated main pancreatic duct and bulky calcifications
- May have long segment distal common bile duct stricture with prestenotic dilatation

- Thickening of peripancreatic fascia and fat necrosis
- Focal pancreatitis may be mass-like and difficult to distinguish from carcinoma

Mucinous Cystic Pancreatic Tumor

- Septated cystic mass, more commonly in pancreatic tail; may have peripheral calcification; no pancreatic duct dilation

Lymphoma

- Focal or diffuse glandular enlargement of pancreas, rarely obstructs pancreatic or biliary ducts
- Associated intraabdominal lymphadenopathy, splenic involvement

Neuroendocrine Tumor of Pancreas

- Hypervascular primary and secondary tumors without pancreatic duct dilation

Metastases

- Solitary/multiple pancreatic masses, usually with disease elsewhere (e.g., liver, adrenals, lymph nodes)
- Rarely obstruct pancreatic or biliary ducts

Serous Cystadenoma

- Mixed cystic/solid pancreatic head lesion; may have central stellate calcification; no pancreatic duct dilation

PATHOLOGY

General Features

- Etiology
  - Risk factors: Cigarette smoking, obesity, diabetes mellitus, chronic pancreatitis, family history

Staging, Grading, & Classification

- Staging based on tumor size, location, vessel involvement, and presence of metastatic disease (TMN staging system)
- NCCN criteria: Describes resectability
  - Resectable (stage I, II): Clear fat planes around celiac artery (CA), SMA, HA (hepatic artery); no superior mesenteric vein (SMV), portal vein (PV) distortion

Gross Pathologic & Surgical Features

- Poorly defined, firm, solid, infiltrative soft tissue mass

Microscopic Features

- Densely cellular neoplastic cells from ductal epithelium, with nuclear atypia
- Vascular and perineural invasion commonly seen, associated with desmoplastic stroma

CLINICAL ISSUES

Presentation

- Most common signs/symptoms
  - Usually asymptomatic until late in course
  - Clinical presentation depends on site of primary tumor
    - Pancreatic head: Obstructive jaundice
    - Body or tail: Weight loss, likely metastases to liver
  - Most commonly presents with distant metastases (~ 65%); least likely to present with tumor confined to pancreas (~ 15%)
  - Serum biomarker: CA 19-9

Demographics

- Age
  - Mean at onset: 55 years; peak: 7th decade
- Gender
  - M:F = 2:1
- Epidemiology
  - 2nd most common gastrointestinal malignancy after colorectal cancer

Natural History & Prognosis

- Generally poor prognosis due to advanced stage at presentation
  - Without surgery: 5-year survival rate ~ 5%
  - With surgery: 5-year survival rate 15-20%

Treatment

- Pancreaticoduodenectomy (Whipple procedure) followed by adjuvant therapy, for resectable tumor (< 15%)
- Neoadjuvant therapy for stage III borderline resectable cancers, to downstage prior to resection
- Stage III locally advanced disease treated with chemotherapy &/or chemoradiation
  - Palliative therapy including biliary stent placement, gastric bypass (for duodenal obstruction), celiac nerve block (for chronic abdominal pain)

DIAGNOSTIC CHECKLIST

Consider

- Differentiate from other solid pancreatic masses by presence of main pancreatic duct dilatation

Image Interpretation Pearls

- Infiltrative mass in head of pancreas with ductal obstruction/dilation and often extensive local invasion and regional metastases at time of presentation

Reporting Tips

- Follow NCCN criteria to assess resectability

SELECTED REFERENCES

1. Al-Hawary MM et al: Pancreatic ductal adenocarcinoma radiology reporting template: consensus statement of the Society of Abdominal Radiology and the American Pancreatic Association. Radiology. 270(1):248-60, 2014
2. Wolfgang CL et al: Recent progress in pancreatic cancer. CA Cancer J Clin. 63(5):318-48, 2013
3. Estrella JS et al: Post-therapy pathologic stage and survival in patients with pancreatic ductal adenocarcinoma treated with neoadjuvant chemoradiation. Cancer. 118(1):268-77, 2012
4. Săftoiu A et al: Role of endoscopic ultrasound in the diagnosis and staging of pancreatic cancer. J Clin Ultrasound. 37(1):1-17, 2009

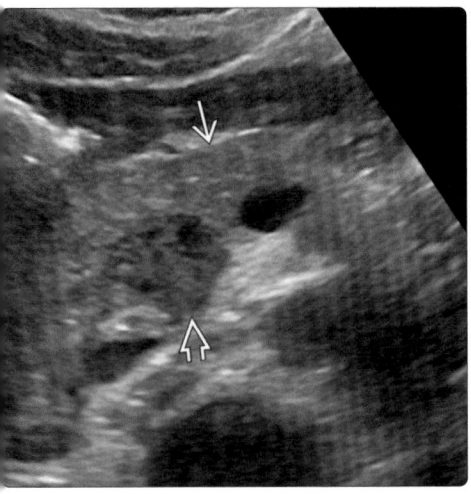

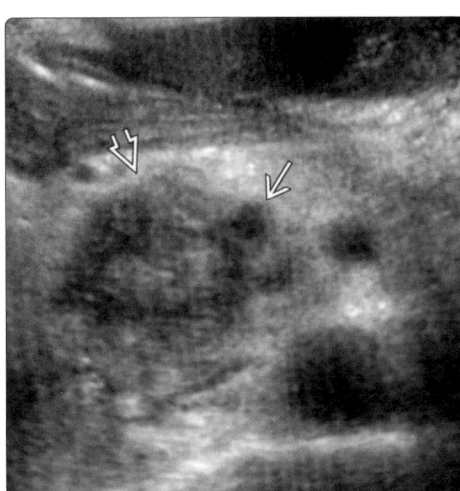

(Left) *Transverse transabdominal ultrasound shows a rounded mass ⇒ in the pancreatic head, which is hypoechoic relative to the normal pancreas ➡. (Right) Transverse transabdominal ultrasound shows an infiltrative, heterogenous, hypoechoic mass ⇒ in the pancreatic head with vascular encasement of the superior mesenteric vein ➡.*

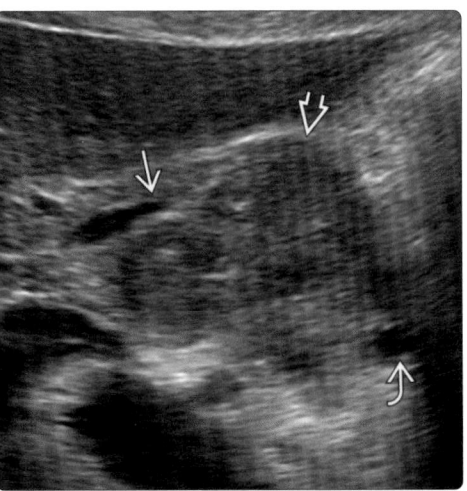

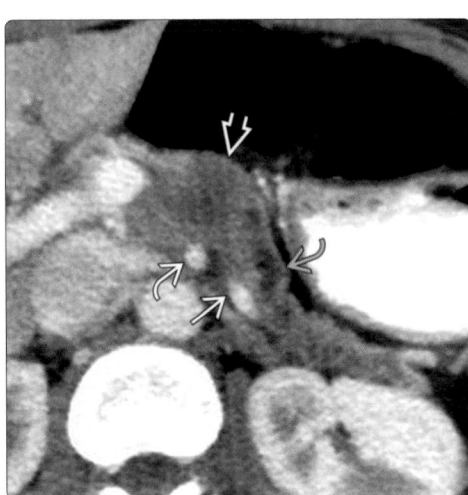

(Left) *Transverse transabdominal ultrasound shows a large, hypoechoic mass in the pancreatic body ➡, narrowing the splenic vein as it approaches the portal confluence ➡. The distal body is obscured; however, the pancreatic duct appears dilated ➡. (Right) Axial CECT also demonstrates the infiltrative pancreatic body mass ➡ encasing the splenic vein ➡ to the portal confluence and abutting the superior mesenteric artery ➡. Note the upstream pancreatic ductal dilatation and parenchymal atrophy ➡.*

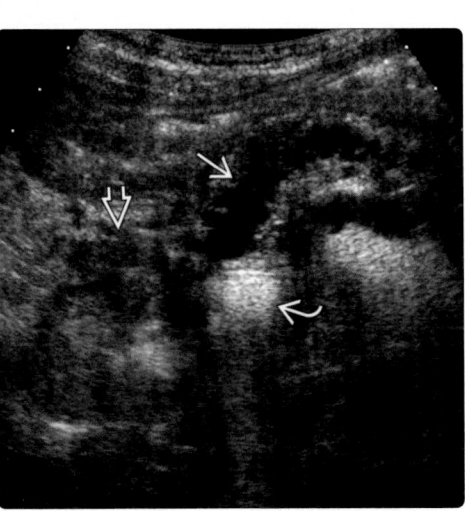

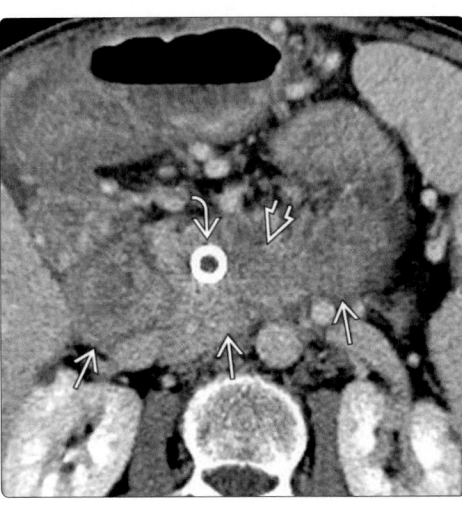

(Left) *Transverse transabdominal ultrasound shows a tortuous dilated pancreatic duct ➡. The pancreatic head is obscured by gas in the common bile duct stent ➡. Note the mass-like enlargement of the duodenum ➡. (Right) Axial CECT better shows the ill-defined hypodense mass ➡ infiltrating the peripancreatic fat and invading the duodenum ➡. There is a common bile duct stent in place ➡.*

Pancreatic Neuroendocrine Tumor

TERMINOLOGY

- Historical terms: Islet cell tumor; carcinoid

IMAGING

- Well-differentiated, circumscribed mass(es) in pancreas without pancreatic ductal dilation
- Functioning tumors: Small, round, hypervascular mass
- Nonfunctioning: Large, well-demarcated, lobulated mass with heterogeneous enhancement pattern
  - Small areas of cystic change/necrosis and calcification
  - Displaces, rather than invades, adjacent structures

TOP DIFFERENTIAL DIAGNOSES

- Mucinous cystic pancreatic neoplasm
- Solid pseudopapillary neoplasm
- Pancreatic ductal carcinoma
- Pancreatic metastases or lymphoma
- Serous cystadenoma of pancreas

PATHOLOGY

- All pETs have malignant potential
- ↑ serum **chromogranin A** is 70% sensitive for pETs

CLINICAL ISSUES

- Most occur sporadically
- Familial syndromes: Multiple endocrine neoplasia type I; von Hippel-Lindau , neurofibromatosis type I, tuberous sclerosis
- **Nonfunctional tumors**: Usually asymptomatic but large size at time of diagnosis may cause mass effect and abdominal pain
- **Functional tumors** present with syndromes, commonly
  - Whipple triad, Zollinger-Ellison
- **Prognosis**: Best for insulinomas
  - 50-80% noninsulinomas recur or metastasize
  - Poor prognostic features: size > 2-4 cm; cystic change, calcification, necrosis
- Surgical resection is only curative treatment for pETs

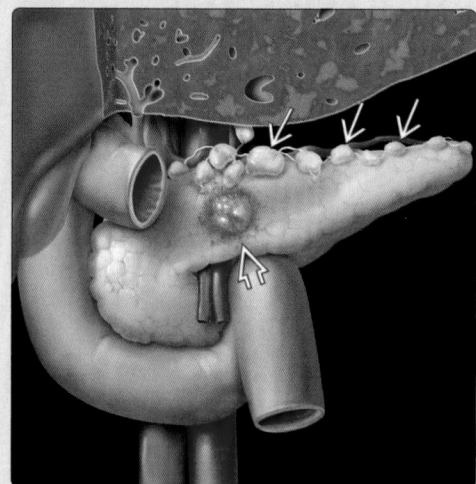
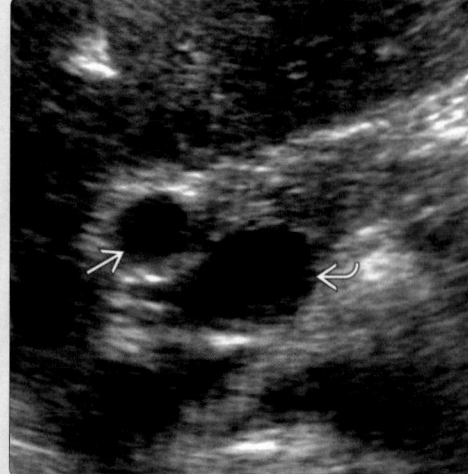

(Left) *Graphic demonstrates a well-circumscribed, round, solid mass ➡ in the pancreatic body with regional metastatic lymphadenopathy ➡. (Right) Transabdominal ultrasound demonstrates a well-defined, hypoechoic pancreatic mass ➡ to the right of the superior mesenteric vein ➡.*

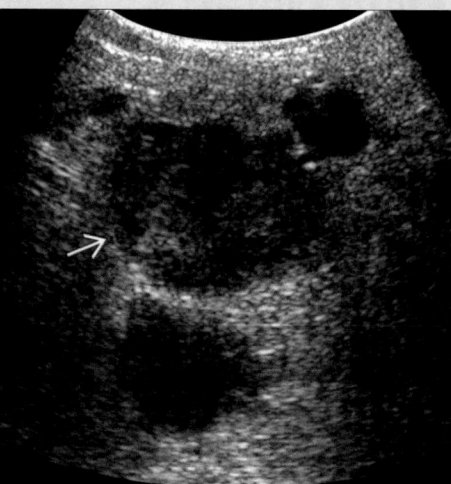
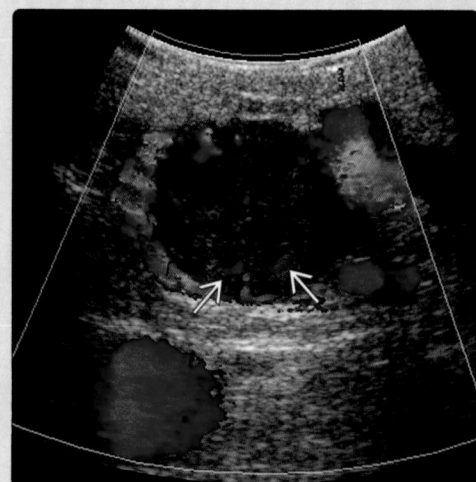

(Left) *Transverse intraoperative ultrasound demonstrates a round, hypoechoic, solid-appearing mass with through transmission ➡ in the body of the pancreas. (Courtesy A. Kamaya, MD.) (Right) Corresponding intraoperative color Doppler ultrasound demonstrates internal flow ➡ within the solid mass. (Courtesy A. Kamaya, MD.)*

TERMINOLOGY

Synonyms

- Pancreatic/gastroenteropancreatic neuroendocrine tumor (NET); pancreatic endocrine tumor (pET)
- Historical terms: Islet cell tumor; carcinoid

Definitions

- Solid epithelial neoplasm believed to arise from pluripotent pancreatic ductal cells with capacity to differentiate along neuroendocrine lines

IMAGING

General Features

- Best diagnostic clue
  - Well-circumscribed, round hypervascular mass(es); no pancreatic ductal dilation
  - Calcification, necrosis, and cystic change in larger tumors
- Location
  - 85% within pancreas: Usually body/tail; 15% ectopic
    - Duodenum, stomach, lymph nodes, ovaries
  - May be multiple
- Size
  - Variable: Range from < 1 cm to > 20 cm; typically 1-5 cm
    - Functioning tumors: Smaller at time of presentation
    - Nonfunctioning tumors: Usually larger at diagnosis
- Morphology: Functioning vs. nonfunctioning subtypes
  - Functioning tumors: Small, round, enhancing mass
    - May be subtle
  - Nonfunctioning: Large, well-demarcated, lobulated mass with heterogeneous enhancement pattern
    - Areas of cystic change/necrosis and calcification
    - Displaces, rather than invades, adjacent structures

Transabdominal Ultrasound (TA US)

- Well-defined, round, hypoechoic mass; can appear isoechoic (focal contour asymmetry)
- Large tumors may be echogenic ± calcification &/or central hypoechogenicity (necrosis)
  - Intratumoral calcification suggests malignancy
  - 60-90% have adenopathy and liver metastases at clinical presentation
    - Hyperechoic, hypoechoic, or target lesions
- Color Doppler: Demonstrates intratumoral flow
- Reported sensitivity for detection of small tumors ~ 25-60%
  - Limited role in detection for functional NETs given typical small tumor size and body habitus limitations

Endoscopic Ultrasound (EUS)

- ↑ sensitivity for detection of small tumors (up to 94%)
- Can guide biopsy and sample cyst fluid

Intraoperative Ultrasound (IOUS)

- Highest sensitivity for small lesions (75-100%)

CT Findings

- CECT
  - Smoothly marginated and hypervascular (arterial/PV phases)
  - Large lesions: Heterogeneous due to nonenhancing cystic/necrotic areas ± calcification
  - Cystic variant: Hypervascular rim, central necrosis (distinguishing feature vs. other cystic pancreatic lesions)
  - Rarely appears infiltrative (poorly differentiated NET)
  - Liver and nodal metastases: Hypervascular, often with ring-like enhancement in liver lesions

MR Findings

- T1WI ± FS: Hypointense to normal pancreas
  - Unenhanced, FS T1WI has highest sensitivity (75%)
- T2WI ± FS: Usually hyperintense to normal pancreas
- T1 C+: Hypervascular
  - Small tumors: Homogeneous enhancement pattern
  - Large tumors: More heterogeneous with nonenhancing cystic, necrotic/hemorrhagic areas and hyperenhancing tumor
  - Liver and nodal metastases: Prominent enhancement, ring like in liver

Nuclear Medicine Findings

- Octreotide scintigraphy
  - Limitations: Uptake by nontarget sites, ↑ image acquisition time, poor image resolution
- PET/CT with Ga-68-(DFO)-octreotide
  - Advantages: Rapid excretion from nontarget sites, ↓ acquisition time, CT localization → ↑ precision
- Useful for metastatic disease or if primary lesion undetected by other imaging modalities
  - Low sensitivity for insulinomas (↓ expression of somatostatin receptors)

Imaging Recommendations

- Best imaging tool
  - Contrast-enhanced CT or MR
  - Endoscopic US: ↑ detection rate for small tumors compared to transabdominal US
    - Invasive technique
    - Performed for localization if CT/MR is negative with high clinical suspicion or to guide biopsy
  - Even if initial CECT/MR/US are negative, if positive biochemical evidence exists, further imaging studies are essential
    - Consider somatostatin receptor functional imaging
  - Intraoperative ultrasound helps ensure complete detection/resection of small tumors
- Protocol advice
  - **CT**: Dual phase pancreatic protocol should be performed (late arterial and portal venous phases)
    - Arterial phase increases conspicuity of small lesions
  - **MR**: Include T1/T2 ± FS and C+ T1W FS dynamic imaging

DIFFERENTIAL DIAGNOSIS

Mucinous Cystic Pancreatic Tumor

- Multiloculated cystic mass with septations
- Can appear similar to cystic NET variant
- Usually with larger cystic component and no thick enhancing rind

Solid Pseudopapillary Neoplasm

- Rare solid and cystic mass than can appear similar to a nonfunctioning NET
- Occurs in overlapping younger age demographic

- Encapsulated lesion that more typically shows necrotic and hemorrhagic features

Pancreatic Ductal Carcinoma (PDC)

- Infiltrative, solid mass, with ductal obstruction
- Poorly differentiated NET can be infiltrative
- PDC rarely shows necrotic change or calcification

Pancreatic Metastases

- Single/multiple small, well-defined, hypervascular lesion(s)
- Common primaries: Renal cell carcinoma and melanoma

Pancreatic Lymphoma

- Solid hypoechoic mass with intraabdominal lymphadenopathy

Serous Cystadenoma of Pancreas

- Honeycomb lesion that can have heterogeneous echogenic appearance on US
- Cystic components tend to be peripherally located with enhancing septa and central scar
  - As opposed to central cystic area and solid enhancing peripheral tissue with cystic NET

PATHOLOGY

General Features

- Etiology
  - Most are sporadic
- Genetics
  - 1-2% associated with familial syndromes: **Multiple endocrine neoplasia, type I** (*MEN1*); **von Hippel-Lindau syndrome** (*VHL*), **neurofibromatosis, type I** (*NF1*); **tuberous sclerosis complex** (*TSC1* and *TSC2*)
    - Typically multiple, and present at younger age

Staging, Grading, & Classification

- **Classification**: Nonfunctional (60-80%) vs. functional
  - Nonfunctional tumors tend to be larger with poor prognosis
- **Functional tumors**: Most commonly insulinomas
  - **Insulinoma**: Typically solitary and benign (90%)
  - **Gastrinoma**: ~ 60% demonstrate malignant behavior
  - **Glucagonoma, vipoma, somatostatinoma**: Rare and most are malignant
- **WHO grading of pETs (2010)**: Based on mitotic rate and cell proliferation
  - **Well-differentiated endocrine tumor**
    - Low and Intermediate grades
  - **Poorly differentiated endocrine carcinoma**
    - High grade
  - Majority are well differentiated (97%)
  - No histologic criteria differentiates benign and malignant tumors (except metastases)
    - All tumors > 5 mm considered malignant
- **TNM staging**: Size (2 cm); extrapancreatic extension; invasion of adjacent structure

Gross Pathologic & Surgical Features

- Round, well differentiated without capsule
- Large lesions: Small areas of degenerative necrosis/hemorrhage are common
  - Usually central uniloculated area ± calcifications in 20%

- 5-10% have extensive degeneration

Microscopic Features

- Sheets of small round cells, uniform nuclei/cytoplasm resemble normal islet cells (uniform polygonal cells)
- Stippled salt and pepper chromatin; Eosinophilic granular cytoplasm
- Electron microscopy: Positive neuron specific enolase
- ↑ serum **chromogranin A** (regardless of functional status)
  - 70% sensitive for detection of pETs

CLINICAL ISSUES

Presentation

- Most common signs/symptoms
  - May be incidentally detected if < 2 cm
  - **Nonfunctional tumor**: Usually asymptomatic; may present with abdominal pain or mass effect
  - **Insulinoma** (Whipple triad)
    - Hypoglycemia, palpitations, sweating, tremors, headache, coma → IV glucose relief
  - **Gastrinoma** (Zollinger-Ellison syndrome)
    - Peptic ulcer, esophagitis, and diarrhea
  - **Glucagonoma** (4D syndrome)
    - **D**ermatitis, **d**iabetes, **D**VT, and **d**epression

Demographics

- Age
  - Peak: 4th-6th decades, younger in familial cases
- Gender
  - Overall no gender predilection, but subtypes do
    - Insulinoma (F > M); gastrinoma (M > F)
- Epidemiology
  - Prevalence of 1/100,000 people
  - Account for 2-3% of all pancreatic neoplasms

Natural History & Prognosis

- All tumors > 5 mm considered malignant
- Cystic change/necrosis and calcification → poorer prognosis
- Indolent growth; metastasizes to nodes, liver, bone
- Insulinomas: Best prognosis, survival rate similar to general population
  - Usually small and nonmetastatic at time of presentation
- Noninsulinoma NETs recur or metastasize in 50-80% cases
  - 5-year survival rate of 50-65%

Treatment

- Surgical resection is only curative treatment for NETs
  - Enucleation vs. partial pancreatectomy
- Chemotherapy: Poorly differentiated tumors
- Radionuclide therapy: Tumors with somatostatin receptors
- Transarterial chemoembolization or radiofrequency ablation for liver metastases

SELECTED REFERENCES

1. Sahani DV et al: Gastroenteropancreatic neuroendocrine tumors: role of imaging in diagnosis and management. Radiology. 266(1):38-61, 2013
2. Klimstra DS et al: The pathologic classification of neuroendocrine tumors: a review of nomenclature, grading, and staging systems. Pancreas. 39(6):707-12, 2010
3. Lewis RB et al: Pancreatic endocrine tumors: radiologic-clinicopathologic correlation. Radiographics. 30(6):1445-64, 2010

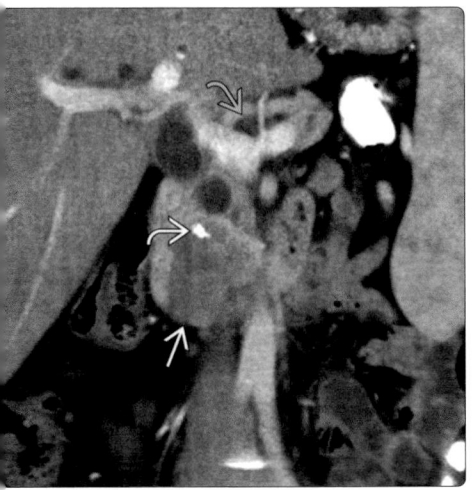

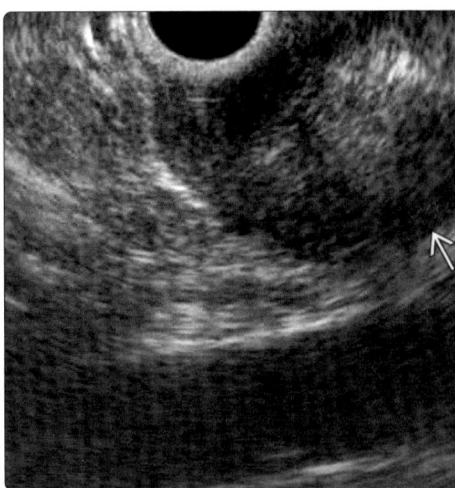

(Left) *Coronal CECT shows a large heterogeneous, hypodense mass ➡ in the pancreatic head with intratumoral calcification ➡, which is suggestive of malignancy. Note the pancreatic ductal dilatation due to mass effect in the head of the pancreas ➡.* (Right) *Corresponding endoscopic ultrasound shows a well-circumscribed, hypoechoic, solid mass ➡ in the pancreas.*

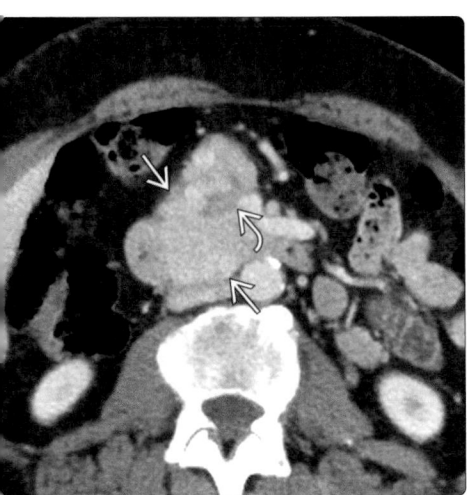

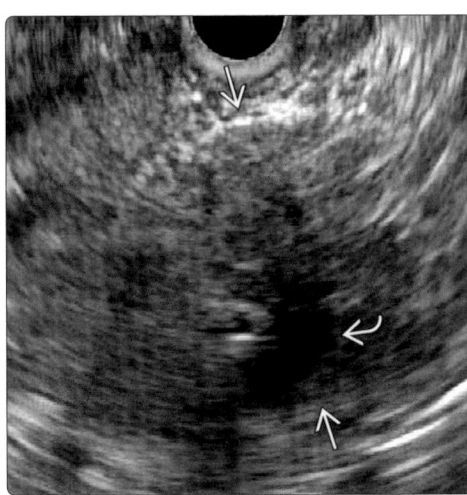

(Left) *Axial CECT demonstrates a large hypervascular mass ➡ in the pancreatic head with a small, focal hypoattenuating area of central necrosis ➡.* (Right) *Corresponding endoscopic ultrasound demonstrates a lobulated, well-circumscribed isoechoic solid mass ➡ containing a focal hypoechoic area of cystic change ➡.*

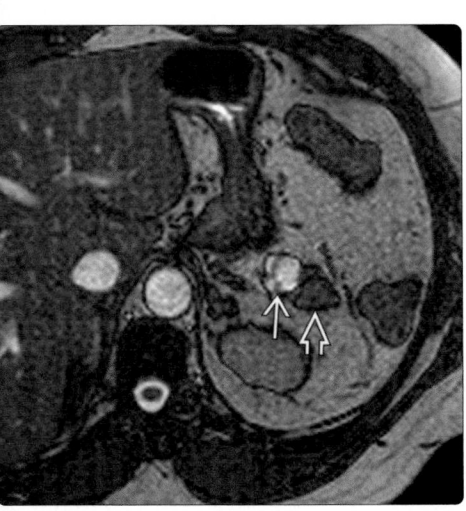

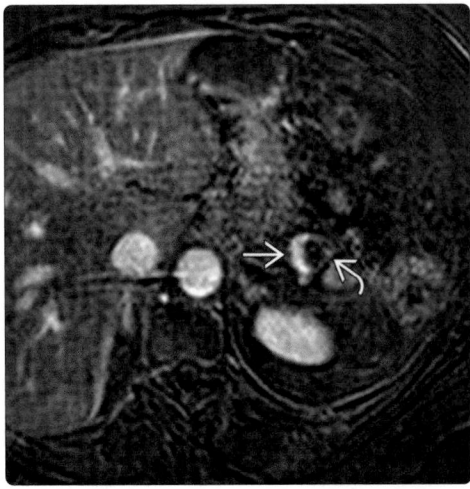

(Left) *Axial T2 true FISP MR demonstrates a well-circumscribed mass ➡ in the body of the pancreas with 2 T2 bright components. Note the lack of pancreatic ductal dilatation in the normal-appearing pancreatic parenchyma distal to the mass ➡.* (Right) *Axial T1 C+ FS MR in the same patient shows peripheral enhancing tumor in the medial aspect of the mass ➡, while the cystic/necrotic lateral component is nonenhancing ➡.*

Solid Pseudopapillary Neoplasm

TERMINOLOGY

- Epithelial tumor of exocrine pancreas with low-grade malignant potential and solid and cystic features

IMAGING

- Large, well-demarcated mass with solid and heterogeneous cystic areas due to hemorrhage and necrosis; typically in pancreatic tail
- **US:** Heterogeneous mass due to mixture of isoechoic soft tissue and hypoechoic central necrosis/hemorrhage
- **Best imaging tool:** CT and MR for demonstrating intratumoral hemorrhage and enhancing capsule/solid components

TOP DIFFERENTIAL DIAGNOSES

- Mucinous cystic pancreatic tumor
- Pancreatic neuroendocrine tumor
- Pancreatic serous cystadenoma
- Pancreatic ductal carcinoma

PATHOLOGY

- Fibrous, hypervascular capsule with solid and pseudopapillary tissue surrounding hemorrhagic and necrotic center
- Low malignant potential

CLINICAL ISSUES

- Very rare, < 3% of all pancreatic tumors
- Typically in asymptomatic, young, non-Caucasian women; termed "daughter lesion"
- Excellent prognosis after surgical excision
- < 10% metastasize or recur

DIAGNOSTIC CHECKLIST

- Consider diagnosis if encapsulated pancreatic tail mass with solid, cystic, and hemorrhagic components is found in young non-Caucasian female and there is no pancreatic ductal dilation

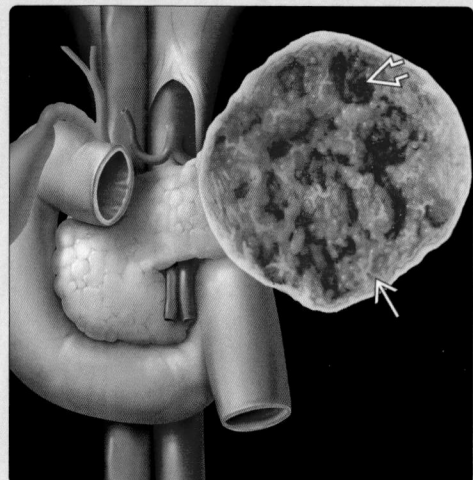
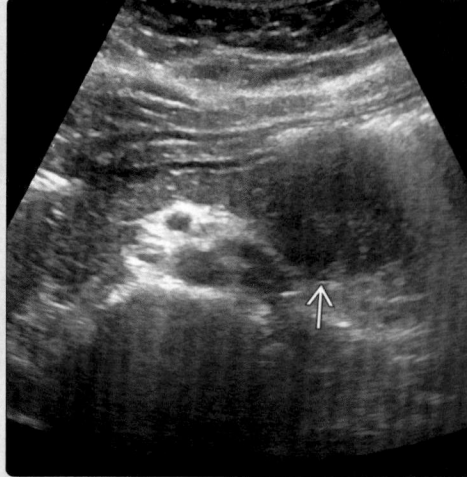

(Left) Graphic shows a large encapsulated mass in the pancreatic tail with solid ➡ and cystic or hemorrhagic ➡ components. (Right) Transverse transabdominal ultrasound demonstrates a large, well-defined, heterogeneous cystic mass ➡ in the pancreatic tail. (Courtesy A. Kamaya, MD.)

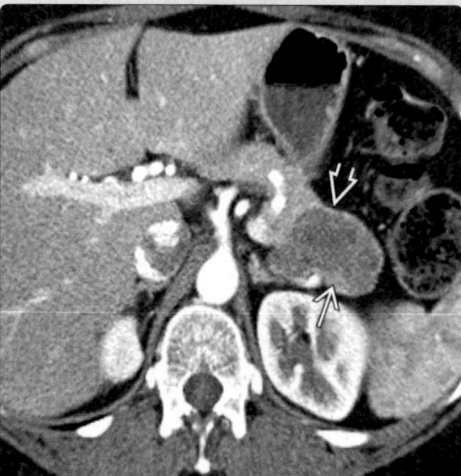
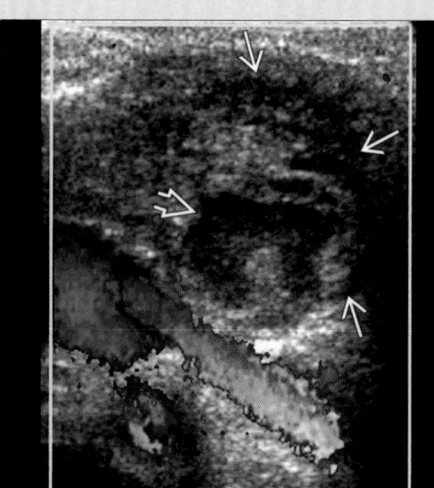

(Left) Axial CECT demonstrates an encapsulated, complex cystic mass ➡ in the pancreatic tail with enhancing peripheral components ➡. (Courtesy A. Kamaya, MD.) (Right) Intraoperative US shows a mass with peripheral soft tissue ➡ surrounding a complex cystic ➡ center with internal echoes reflecting hemorrhage and necrosis. (Courtesy A. Kamaya, MD.)

TERMINOLOGY

Abbreviations

Solid pseudopapillary neoplasm (SPN)

Synonyms

Solid and papillary epithelial neoplasm (SPEN); papillary cystic epithelial neoplasm; papillary cystic tumor; solid and cystic tumor of pancreas, Franz or Hamoudi tumor

Definitions

Epithelial tumor of exocrine pancreas with low-grade malignant potential and solid and cystic features

IMAGING

General Features

Best diagnostic clue
- Large, encapsulated, round, complex cystic pancreatic mass with no associated ductal dilatation

Location
- Commonly in pancreatic tail

Size
- Usually large (average: 10 cm; range: 2.5-20 cm)

Morphology
- Typically well-defined, large, solid and cystic mass
- Lesions < 3 cm show solid, homogeneous appearance
- May contain dystrophic calcifications
- Aggressive features are uncommon, but can be seen
  - Perivascular invasion, ductal dilation; metastases usually to liver, but also lymph nodes and peritoneum

Ultrasonographic Findings

Well-defined, heterogeneous mass with solid and cystic components
- Hypoechoic center due to tumor necrosis/hemorrhage
- Cystic portion may show fluid-debris level

Color Doppler: Hypovascular, due to areas of necrosis

Endoscopic ultrasound (EUS): More sensitive for small mass
- Can guide fine-needle aspiration biopsy

CT Findings

Heterogeneous density with mixed solid/cystic areas

Enhancing capsule and soft tissue projections

Hyperdensity on unenhanced CT from hemorrhage; low attenuation from nonenhancing areas of necrosis

MR Findings

Well-demarcated mass with central areas of heterogeneously bright T1 and T2 signal
- Low T1 SI: Capsule and solid components that enhance on post-contrast T1WI
- High T1 SI: Intratumoral hemorrhage
- High T2 signal: Necrosis and hemorrhage
- Low T2 signal: Thick fibrous capsule

Imaging Recommendations

Best imaging tool
- Multiplanar CECT or MR

Protocol advice
- Unenhanced CT and MR can best demonstrate intratumoral hemorrhage
- Post-contrast imaging should include arterial phase

DIFFERENTIAL DIAGNOSIS

Mucinous Cystic Pancreatic Tumor

- No hemorrhage; commonly seen in middle-aged women

Nonfunctioning Neuroendocrine Tumor

- Cystic components typically do not show T1 hyperintensity; peripheral portions are more hypervascular

Pancreatic Serous Cystadenoma

- No large solid component; usually located in head of pancreas; more common in elderly women

Pancreatic Ductal Carcinoma

- Rarely necrotic or hemorrhagic; typically shows pancreatic &/or common bile duct obstruction; older adults

PATHOLOGY

General Features

- Large solitary tumor with variable mixture of solid, hemorrhagic, and necrotic components
- Low malignant potential

Gross Pathologic & Surgical Features

- Thick, fibrous, hypervascular capsule surrounding soft tumor, usually with no mass effect/ductal obstruction

Microscopic Features

- Solid nests of homogeneous, epithelioid cells with areas of separation into pseudopapillary aggregates due to degeneration

CLINICAL ISSUES

Presentation

- Usually asymptomatic or nonspecific abdominal pain
- May have palpable abdominal mass

Demographics

- ~ 90% female; < 35 years of age
- African Americans or non-Caucasian groups

Natural History & Prognosis

- Usually benign, but with low malignant potential
- Prognosis: Excellent after surgical resection; usually curative (95% 5-year survival)
- < 10% metastasize (usually to liver) or recur

Treatment

- Complete surgical excision

DIAGNOSTIC CHECKLIST

Image Interpretation Pearls

- Encapsulated pancreatic tail mass with solid, cystic, and hemorrhagic components in young non-Caucasian female

SELECTED REFERENCES

1. Ganeshan DM et al: Solid pseudo-papillary tumors of the pancreas: current update. Abdom Imaging. 38(6):1373-82, 2013
2. Reddy S et al: Surgical management of solid-pseudopapillary neoplasms of the pancreas (Franz or Hamoudi tumors): a large single-institutional series. J Am Coll Surg. 208(5):950-7; discussion 957-9, 2009
3. Choi JY et al: Solid pseudopapillary tumor of the pancreas: typical and atypical manifestations. AJR Am J Roentgenol. 187(2):W178-86, 2006

(Left) *Axial T2 MR shows a small, well-defined T2-bright lesion in the pancreatic body* ⇒. *Notice that the signal is less intense than that of fluid* ⇒ *in the gallbladder and spinal canal* ⇒. **(Right)** *Corresponding axial T1 C+ FS MR shows a small hypoenhancing mass in the body of the pancreas mimicking, pancreatic adenocarcinoma except for the notable lack of pancreatic ductal dilation or surrounding infiltration* ⇒.

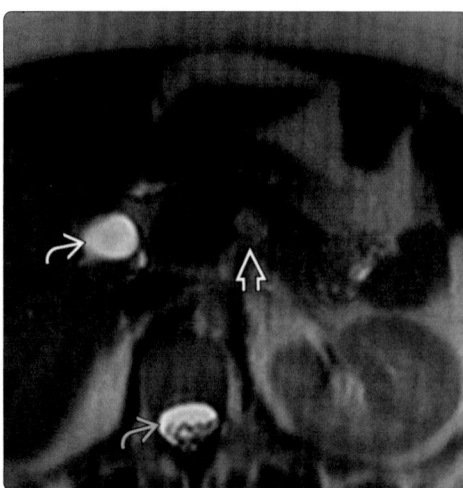
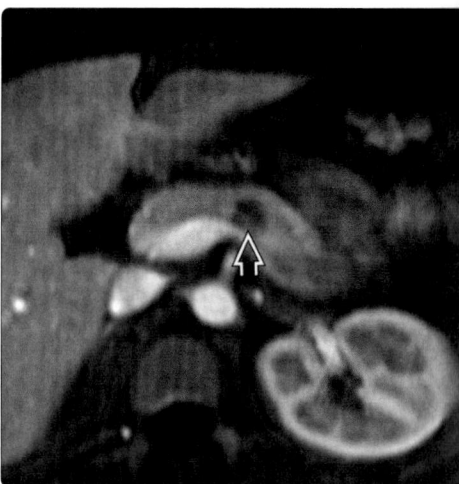

(Left) *Axial CECT shows a heterogeneous mass* ⇒ *with solid* ⇒ *and cystic* ⇒ *components in the pancreatic body in a 19-year-old woman.* **(Right)** *Corresponding coronal CECT shows the large, predominantly cystic* ⇒ *mass with an enhancing rim* ⇒ *and peripheral soft tissue* ⇒.

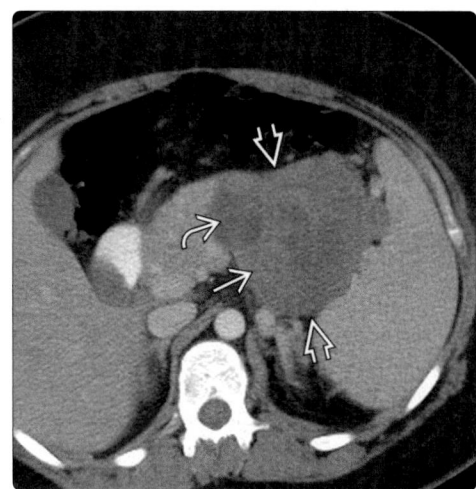
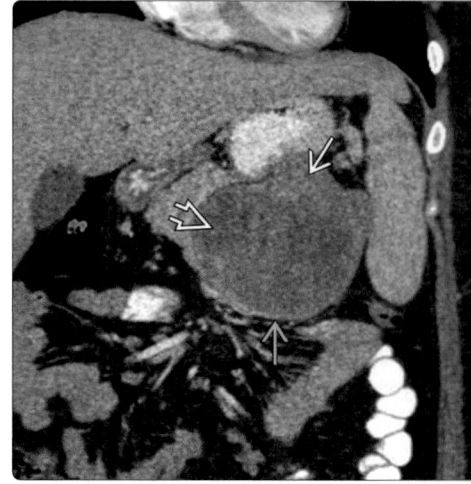

(Left) *Corresponding endoscopic US in the same patient shows a heterogeneous appearance with solid* ⇒ *and small anechoic cystic* ⇒ *areas and a larger complex cystic component* ⇒. **(Right)** *Endoscopic ultrasound-guided biopsy shows the needle* ⇒ *within a peripheral soft tissue nodular component* ⇒ *of the large solid and cystic pancreatic mass* ⇒, *which was a proven SPN.*

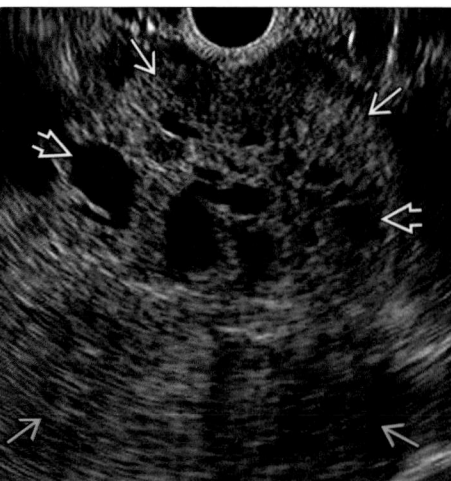
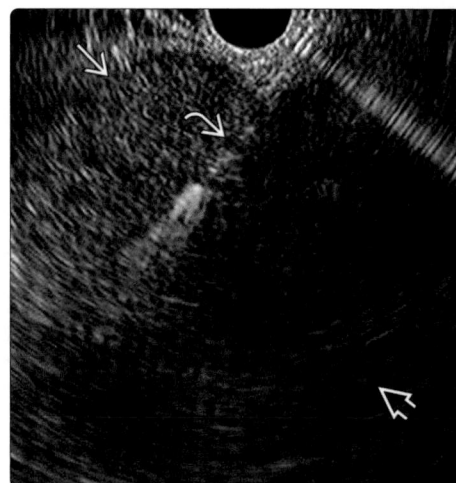

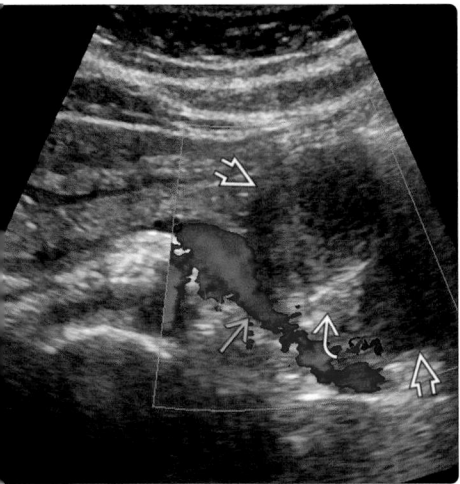
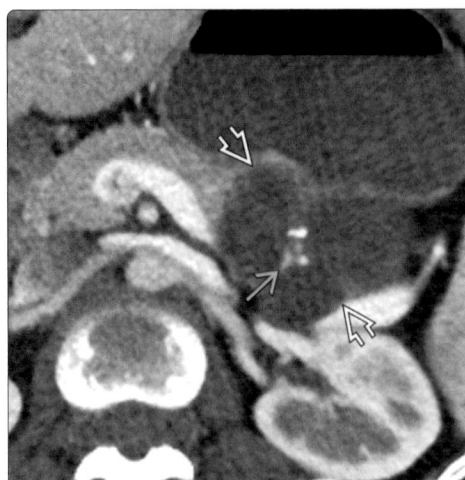

(Left) Transverse color Doppler ultrasound demonstrates a lobulated, cystic mass ➡️ with central hyperechogenicity ➡️. Note the adjacent, patent splenic vein ➡️. (Courtesy A. Kamaya, MD.) (Right) Corresponding axial CECT shows a large, lobulated hypodense mass ➡️ with calcifications within the central portion of the mass ➡️. (Courtesy A. Kamaya, MD.)

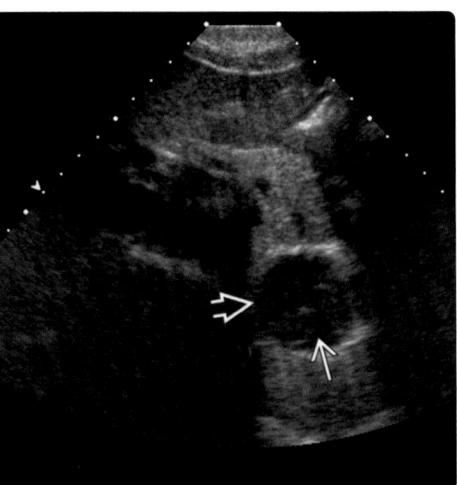
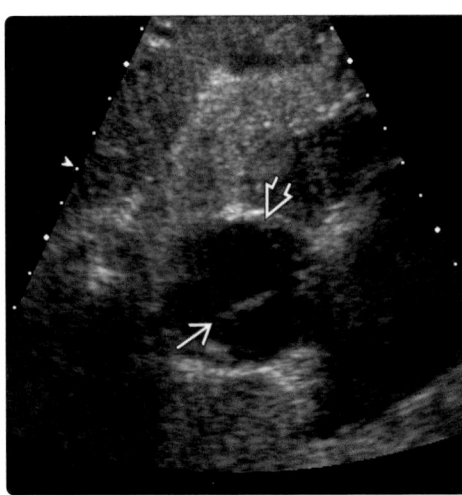

(Left) Transabdominal ultrasound demonstrates a well-defined complex cystic pancreatic mass ➡️ in the tail of the pancreas with layering internal echogenic material ➡️. (Right) Corresponding sagittal zoomed-in transabdominal ultrasound demonstrates a well-defined complex cystic pancreatic mass ➡️ with central echogenic material ➡️.

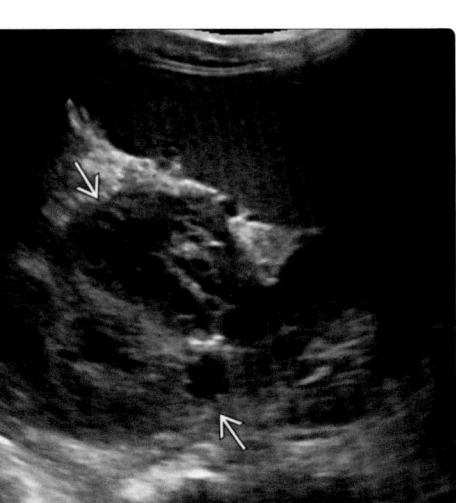
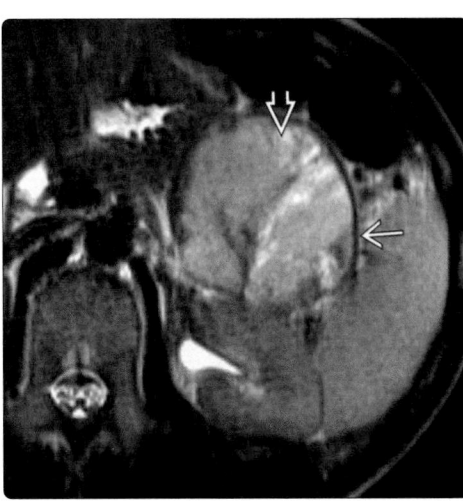

(Left) Transverse transabdominal ultrasound shows a complex solid and cystic mass in the tail of the pancreas ➡️. (Right) Corresponding axial T2 FS MR shows a large complex cystic mass with heterogeneously hyperintense T2 signal intensity ➡️ and a T2-dark, thick, and fibrous capsule ➡️.

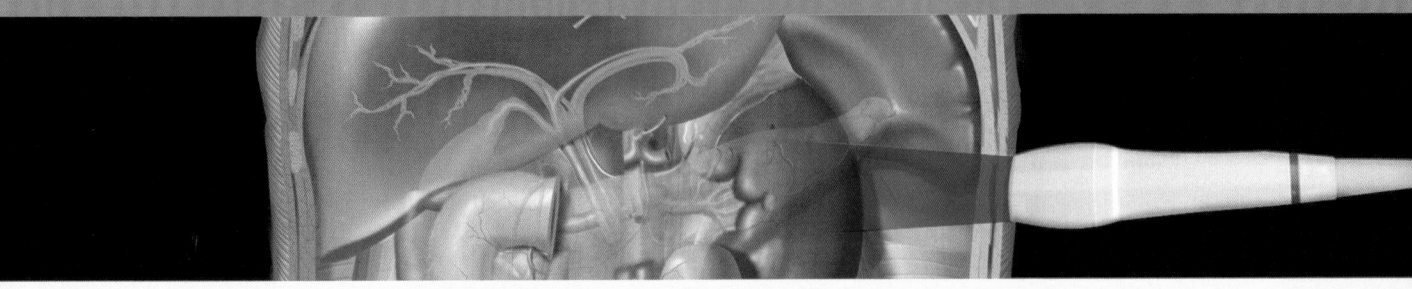

PART II
SECTION 4
Spleen

Introduction and Overview

Splenic Lesions

Transducer Selection

Similar to other intraabdominal organs, the spleen is best imaged using a 3-5 MHz curvilinear transducer. A curvilinear (or curved) transducer is preferred due to its larger area of coverage (suitable to include the entire span of the spleen), as compared to a sector (vector) transducer or linear array transducer.

Finding an Acoustic Window

The spleen is an intraperitoneal organ of variable size and morphology that occupies the left upper quadrant. The anatomy of the spleen and its relationships to adjacent organs are discussed in a separate chapter. Visualization of the spleen in the left upper quadrant is challenged by several anatomic factors, chiefly artifacts caused by the ribs, the left lung, the splenic flexure of the colon, and the stomach. The positioning of both the transducer and the patient will play a role in optimizing the acoustic window.

An anterior subcostal approach may be attempted in the supine position, though such an approach is often limited due to bowel gas artifact from the colon &/or the stomach. When this view can be successfully achieved, it will often require an anterolateral oblique positioning of the transducer. Occasionally, patients may have variant liver anatomy in which the left hepatic lobe extends far across midline to the left upper quadrant. In this setting, the left hepatic lobe may serve as an acoustic window to visualize the spleen. A posterior approach is of little utility, limited by the anatomy of the lungs and diaphragm, which extend most caudally at this site.

A lateral or posterolateral intercostal approach, with transducer parallel to the ribs and the patient in the supine or right lateral decubitus (i.e., left-side up) position, provides the best acoustic window for the spleen. The 10th to 11th rib intercostal space is an ideal place to start. The 9th to 10th rib intercostal space may also yield a satisfactory window.

Several other techniques may aid in visualization of the spleen. Positioning the patient in the supine or right lateral decubitus positions has already been discussed. Note, however, the right lateral decubitus position may cause the spleen to fall away from the chest and abdominal wall, reducing visualization of the organ from an intercostal approach. Having the patient fast prior to the ultrasound examination may reduce gaseous distension of the stomach in the left upper quadrant. This may not be possible in the emergency setting, but can be feasible in the outpatient setting. During the ultrasound examination, asking the patient to perform deep inspiration (to bring the spleen down into the field of view) is a useful technique. Experimenting with different degrees of inspiration or expiration (partial or complete) with breath hold may improve visualization.

Anatomic Orientation and Imaging Planes

The posterolateral intercostal approach is the favored acoustic window of most sonographers and radiologists. Because of the orientation of the ribs, an intercostal approach effectively provides an oblique plane with respect to the standard x, y, and z anatomical planes of the body (i.e., the axial, coronal, and sagittal planes). Fortunately, because the anatomic orientation of the spleen is variable and may itself lie obliquely compared to the standard anatomical planes, this posterolateral oblique view is well-suited to identify the long axis of the spleen. By standard convention, this anatomically oblique plane is referred to as the "longitudinal" plane of the spleen (often abbreviated "long"). When the transducer orientation is flipped by 180°, this is, by convention, referred to as the "transverse" plane of the spleen (often abbreviated "trans").

Note that the conventional "longitudinal" and "transverse" planes of the spleen via the posterolateral intercostal approach are not perpendicular views; rather, they are mirror images of each other. The true transverse cross section of the spleen would be pie- or oval-shaped, rather than crescent-shaped (as is seen in the longitudinal cross section). A true transverse image of the spleen could be obtained either by a 90° rotation of the transducer in the intercostal approach (a view that is limited by the orientation of the ribs) or from an oblique anterior subcostal approach (which is often limited by bowel gas artifact).

Because of both the transducer orientation and the spleen's anatomic orientation, the conventional "longitudinal spleen" view (truly a longitudinal oblique) does not correspond directly to the traditional coronal or sagittal planes of CT or MR. Likewise, the conventional "transverse spleen" view does not correspond directly to the axial plane of CT or MR. In a similar regard, the "longitudinal spleen" view and the "longitudinal left kidney" view will not represent the same anatomic plane in the same patient, as these planes are "longitudinal" to the organs of interest, not the patient's body.

Understanding the difference between imaging planes and anatomic planes also has important implications for the measurement of spleen size. By convention, the splenic length is measured as the greatest dimension in the "longitudinal" view. Splenic thickness is measured from the hilum to outer capsule on the "transverse" view (though it would be the same measurement on the "longitudinal" view). Splenic width is generally considered the greatest dimension on the "transverse" view, but because of the discrepancies in imaging and anatomic planes, the sonographic splenic width based on the conventional transverse view and the true splenic width (most accurately measured by CT or MR) are not synonymous. The maximum splenic dimension on the conventional longitudinal and transverse views are, in actuality, the same measurement.

Routine Evaluation of Spleen

The standard evaluation of the spleen involves both grayscale and color Doppler interrogation. On grayscale ultrasound, the size, echotexture, and overall morphology of the spleen should be documented. As previously described, the size may be documented in terms of the length and thickness (and less accurately, the width, as described previously). The presence or absence of perisplenic fluid should also be noted.

Routine evaluation of the splenic vein is an important component of a thorough sonographic exam of the spleen. The splenic vein can be assessed in two locations: at the splenic hilum and at midline, posterior to the pancreas. Proper interrogation of the splenic vein involves evaluating for vessel patency and ensuring flow is appropriately directed away from the spleen, toward the liver (hepatopetal flow). Splenic vein flow may be reversed, for example, in the setting of chronic portal hypertension.

The splenic artery is often not part of routine splenic evaluation, but should be included when assessing for causes of splenic infarction or other vascular abnormalities of the spleen. Like the vein, the splenic artery can be assessed at the splenic hilum or at midline, arising from the celiac axis. Intrasplenic vascularity may also be assessed.

In the event that a focal splenic abnormality is identified, it is critical to document the cystic or solid nature of the lesion, the echogenicity relative to normal parenchyma, singularity or multiplicity, and the presence or absence of vascularity (by color &/or power Doppler techniques).

Supplemental Findings

The spleen may serve as an acoustic window to visualize the pancreatic tail. Masses of the pancreatic tail may be intimately associated with the splenic hilum, and the origin of masses in this location may be difficult to distinguish by ultrasound alone. Accessory spleens (splenules) may also be located at the splenic hilum or be closely associated to the pancreatic tail.

In certain scenarios, a thorough ultrasound exam should assess for supplemental findings that can add diagnostic value. Take, for example, a scenario in which diffuse splenomegaly is incidentally detected. The presence of enlarged lymph nodes when scanning the upper abdomen or retroperitoneum in the setting of splenomegaly could help make the diagnosis of lymphoma. If cirrhosis were suspected as the cause of splenomegaly, it would be important to evaluate the patency and flow direction of the splenic vein and assess for other stigmata of portal hypertension, such as splenorenal varices or ascites.

Sonographic Work-Up

Ultrasound is a cost-effective and safe initial imaging test to evaluate the spleen, particularly for splenic size and the presence of focal splenic lesions. However, because there is significant overlap in the sonographic appearance of both benign and malignant splenic lesions, further imaging work-up with CT, MR, or PET may often be needed. Even with these imaging tests, the findings may remain nonspecific and additional work up with tissue sampling could be necessary to arrive at a diagnosis. It is important to make use of all available demographic, historical, and laboratory data when developing a differential diagnosis for splenic abnormalities.

Ultrasound is also useful in the rapid assessment of splenic injury (focused assessment with sonography for trauma [FAST] exam) in the setting of blunt abdominal trauma. Bedside ultrasound is particularly adept in assessing for subcapsular, perisplenic, or other intraperitoneal hemorrhage. Hemodynamically unstable patients with a positive FAST exam are typically taken directly to the operating room for emergent laparotomy. However, contrast-enhanced CT remains the imaging gold standard in the grading of splenic laceration and a negative bedside ultrasound does not exclude intraparenchymal splenic injury.

Differential Diagnosis

Most lesions that are incidentally seen in the spleen are benign, with the vast majority representing either cysts or benign tumors (including hemangiomas, lymphangiomas, or hamartomas.) The most common splenic malignancy is lymphoma, followed by metastasis. Primary non-hematologic splenic malignancies are very rare and may arise from vascular or other mesenchymal elements; the most common of these is angiosarcoma.

Benign Splenic Lesions

Benign splenic lesions are very common. Depending on imaging appearance, the following may be considered as potential etiologies.
- Acquired cyst: Most common splenic cyst
- Congenital (epidermoid) cyst
- Abscess (pyogenic, fungal, parasitic, granulomatous)
- Infarct
- Hematoma/laceration
- Granuloma (tuberculosis, histoplasmosis, sarcoidosis)
- Gamna-Gandy bodies
- Hamartoma
- Littoral cell angioma(s)
- Peliosis

Malignant Splenic Lesions

Compared to benign lesions, malignant splenic lesions are relatively uncommon. In the proper clinical setting, however, malignant entities should be considered.
- Lymphoma: Most common malignant splenic tumor
- Metastasis
- Rare primary splenic neoplasms: Angiosarcoma, fibrosarcoma, malignant fibrous histiocytoma, leiomyosarcoma

Diffuse Splenic Enlargement

The spleen is considered to be enlarged when it measures > 13 cm in length. The following may be considered as possible etiologies for splenomegaly.
- Congestive: Cirrhosis with portal hypertension, heart failure, splenic vein thrombosis, sickle cell sequestration
- Neoplasm: Leukemia, lymphoma, metastases, primary neoplasm, Kaposi sarcoma
- Storage disease: Gaucher, Niemann-Pick, amyloidosis, hemosiderosis, histiocytosis
- Infection: HIV, mononucleosis (Ebstein-Barr virus), Cytomegalovirus (CMV), hepatitis, malaria, tuberculosis, typhoid, kala-azar, schistosomiasis, brucellosis
- Hematologic: Hemoglobinopathy, hereditary spherocytosis, thrombocytopenic purpura, polycythemia
- Extramedullary hematopoiesis: Osteopetrosis, myelofibrosis
- Collagen vascular disease: Systemic lupus erythematosus, rheumatoid arthritis (Felty syndrome)

Selected References

1. Nishijima DK et al: Does this adult patient have a blunt intra-abdominal injury? JAMA. 307(14):1517-27, 2012
2. Benter T et al: Sonography of the spleen. J Ultrasound Med. 30(9):1281-93, 2011
3. Parulekar SG et al. Ultrasound Measurements of the Spleen. In Goldberg BB et al. Atlas of Ultrasound Measurement. Philadelphia: Mosby, Inc. 439-442, 2006
4. Giovagnoni A et al: Tumours of the spleen. Cancer Imaging. 5:73-7, 2005
5. Middleton WD et al. Ultrasound: The Requisites. Philadelphia: Mosby, Inc. 209-219, 2004

(Left) *Axial CECT through the left upper quadrant shows the anatomic factors which may limit visualization of the spleen: Posteriorly, the left lung base; anteriorly, the stomach ➡; and from all directions, the ribs ➡. Note also the simple cyst in the posterior, superior spleen ➡.* **(Right)** *A few centimeters more caudally (same case), note the optimal acoustic window that can be obtained from lateral intercostal approach, between ribs 9 and 10 ➡, or posterolateral intercostal approach, between ribs 10 and 11 ➡.*

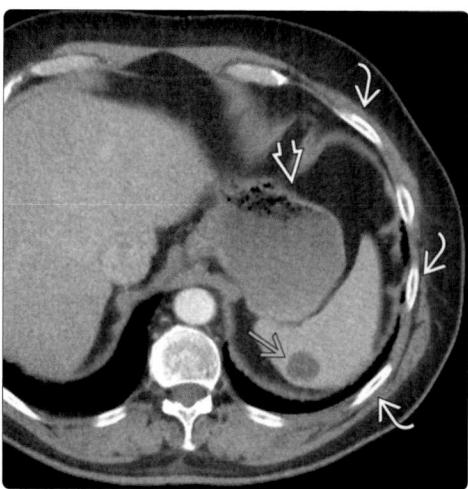
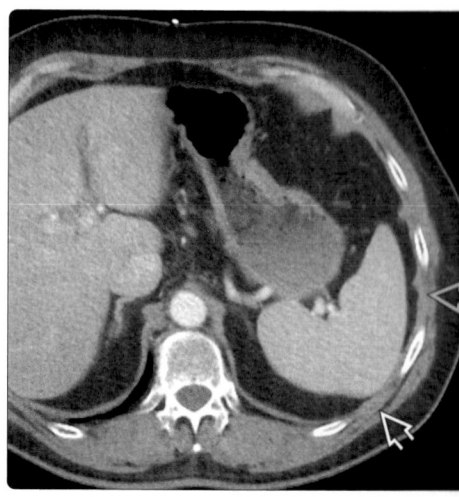

(Left) *Conventional "longitudinal spleen" US from lateral intercostal approach is shown. In actuality, this is a longitudinal oblique view. Note superior position of the cyst ➡, left hemidiaphragm ➡, and stomach ➡. Calipers measure spleen length.* **(Right)** *Conventional "transverse spleen" US is shown in the same patient. In actuality, this is almost a mirror image of the longitudinal oblique view. Note the position of the cyst ➡, left hemidiaphragm ➡, and stomach ➡. Calipers measure spleen thickness.*

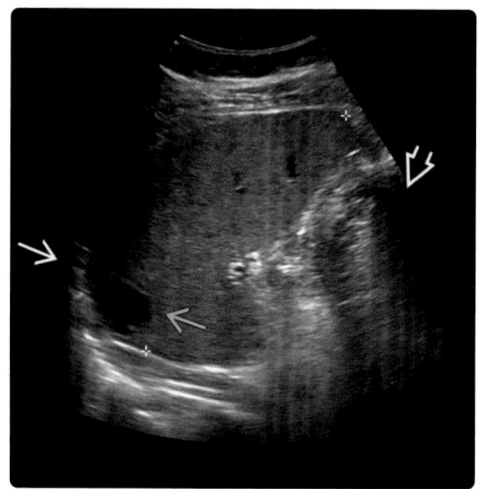
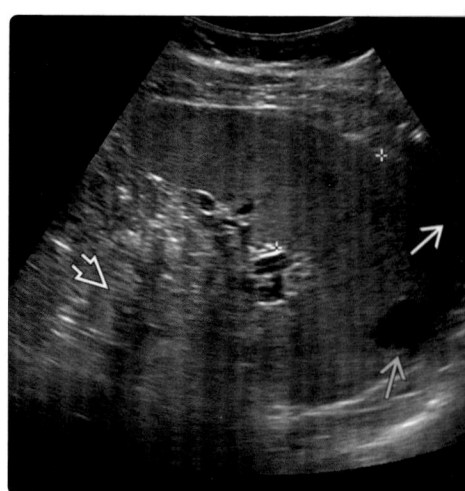

(Left) *Oblique reformatted CT corresponding to the conventional "longitudinal spleen" US is shown. Note the position of the cyst ➡, the left lung base ➡, and the stomach ➡. A transducer would be positioned here ➡.* **(Right)** *For comparison, sagittal CT through the spleen shows the oblique orientation of the organ with respect to the longitudinal (sagittal) axis of the body. Note the superior position of the splenic cyst ➡ and the positions of the stomach ➡ and left diaphragm ➡.*

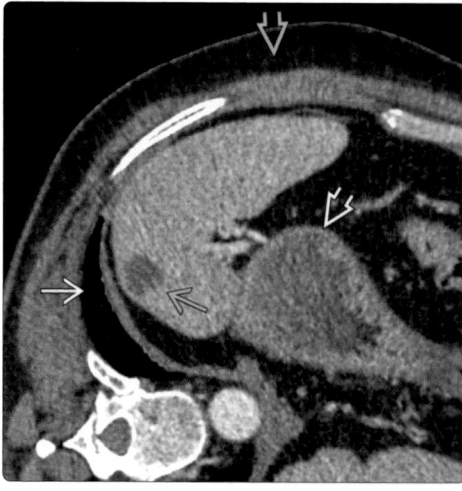
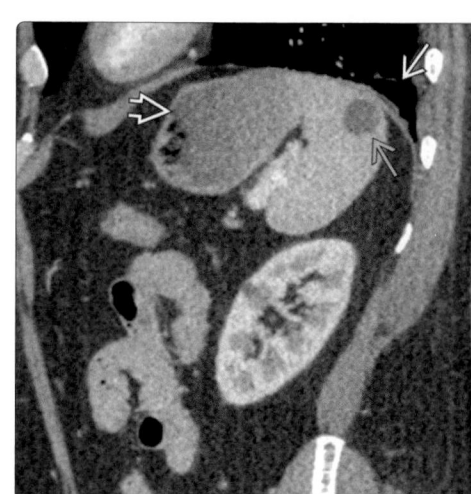

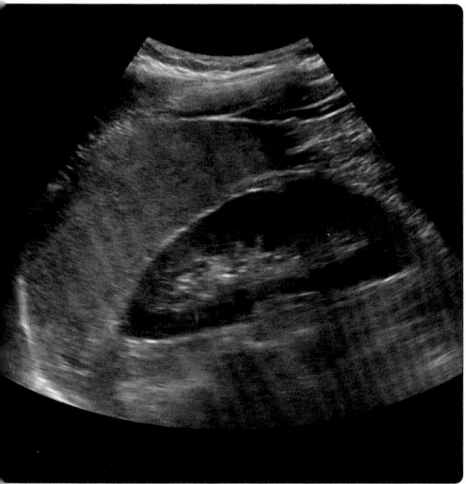
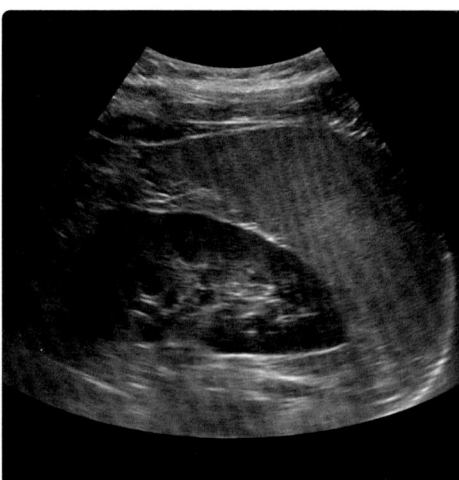

(Left) Longitudinal oblique US in a patient with splenomegaly shows the spleen from a lateral intercostal approach (a conventional "long" plane). (Right) Conventional transverse US in the same patient shows the spleen from the lateral intercostal approach.

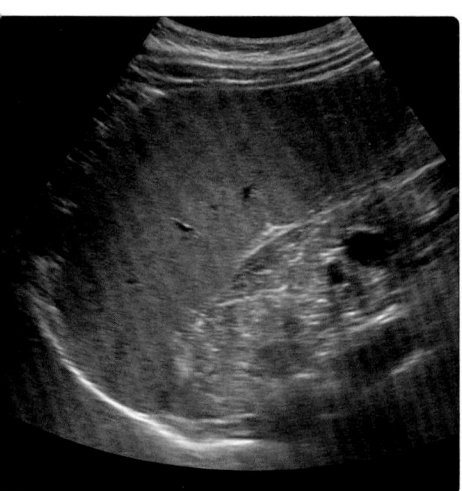
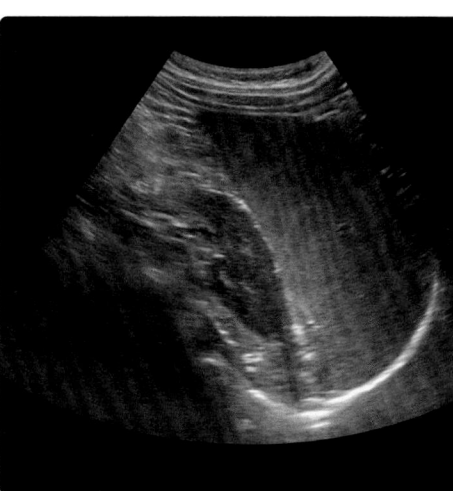

(Left) For comparison, a conventional "long" (longitudinal oblique) US in the same patient shows the spleen from an anterior/anterolateral oblique subcostal approach. This view is often limited by bowel gas, but was possible in this patient due to splenomegaly. (Right) Corresponding conventional transverse US in the same patient shows the spleen from an anterior oblique subcostal approach.

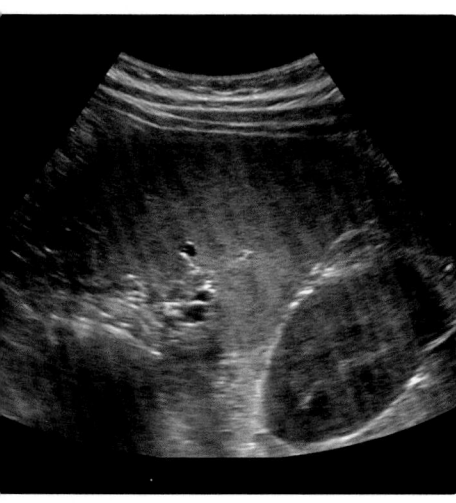
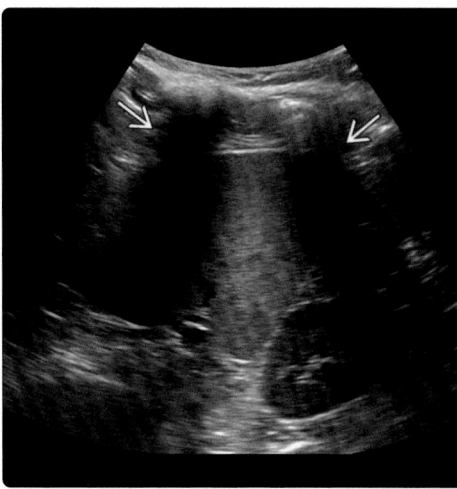

(Left) True transverse plane (anatomic transverse slice through hilum) in the same patient, from anterior oblique subcostal approach, shows a triangular splenic shape rather than the crescent shape seen in the conventional transverse plane. (Right) True transverse US of the spleen from the intercostal approach (90° turn of the transducer rather than usual 180°) in the same patient is shown. Note the limitations caused by the ribs, resulting in posterior acoustic shadowing ➡, one reason why the true transverse plane is not traditionally used.

(Left) *Midline color Doppler US shows a normal splenic vein* ⇶*, deep to the pancreas* ➡*, with flow directed toward the liver. Note the left renal vein* ➡*, draining into the IVC.* (Right) *Color Doppler US in a 52-year-old man shows reversal of flow in the splenic vein (SV)* ➡*. Flow is directed toward the spleen rather than the liver.*

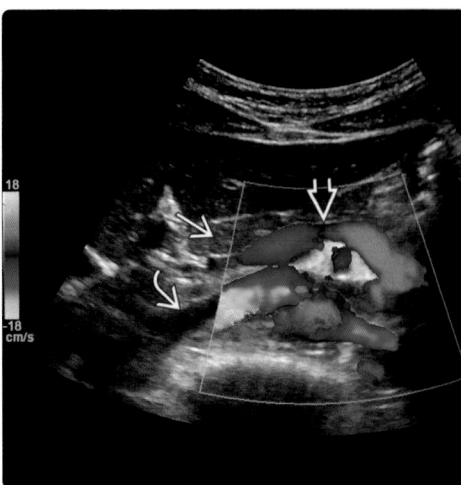
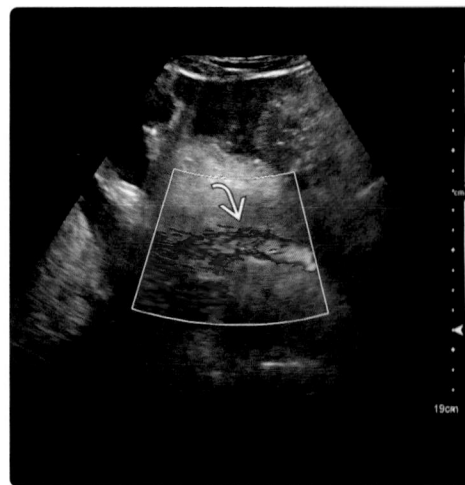

(Left) *US evaluation of the SV at the hilum* ⇶ *in the same patient also shows reversal of flow (directed toward the spleen). In addition, the spleen is enlarged.* (Right) *It is important to assess for potential causes of splenomegaly and SV flow reversal. Evaluation of the liver shows nodular contour* ⇨ *and heterogeneous parenchymal echogenicity. Ascites is also present* ➡*. The overall picture is that of cirrhosis with portal hypertension.*

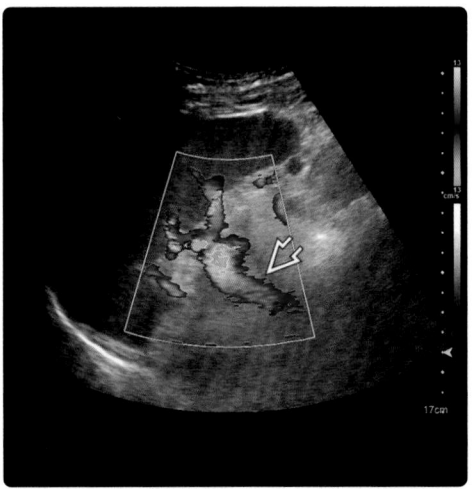
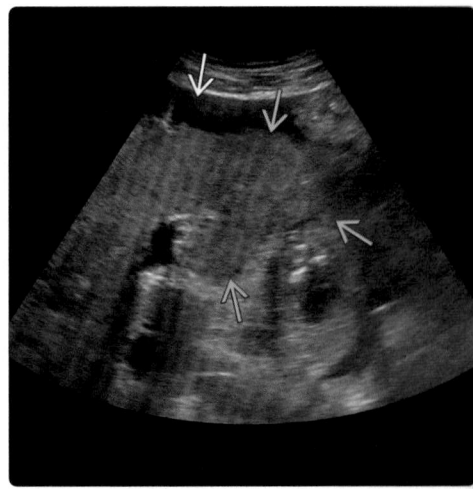

(Left) *Portal hypertension may also manifest by the presence of varices* ⇶ *in and around the splenic hilum, as seen in this patient with cirrhosis. Note the flow reversal, predominantly directed away from the spleen.* (Right) *Corresponding axial CT through the left upper quadrant shows the abundant dilated varices along the splenic hilum* ➡*. In addition, there are scattered calcified granulomas in the spleen.*

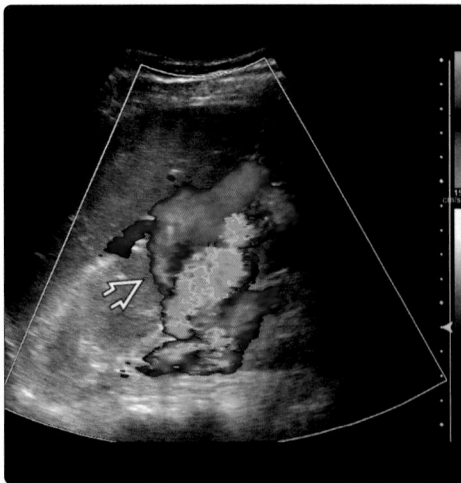
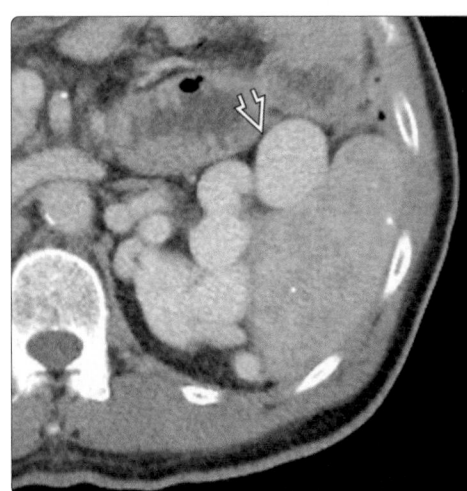

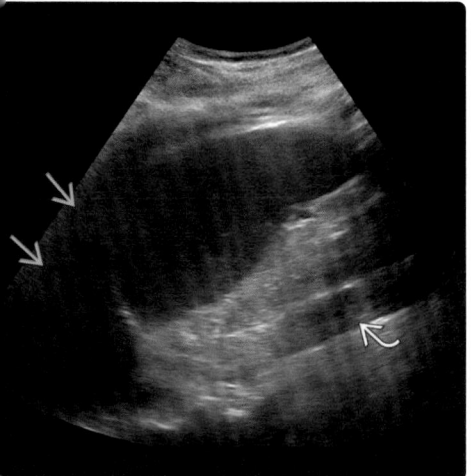

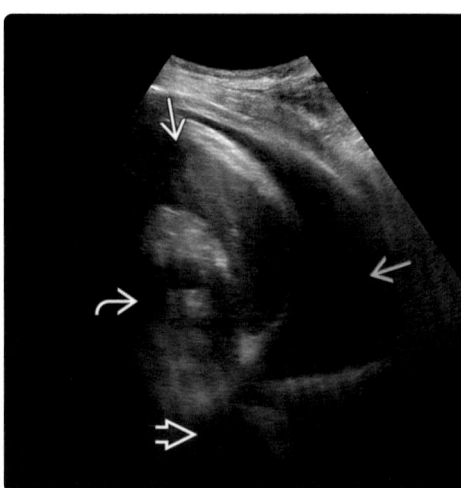

(Left) *A large left pleural effusion* ⮕ *is shown in conventional longitudinal view from an intercostal approach, nicely delineating the relationship between the spleen and the left hemidiaphragm. The aorta is partially visualized* ⮕. **(Right)** *A large left pleural effusion* ⮕ *is shown in conventional transverse view from an intercostal approach, in right lateral decubitus position. Note the spleen* ⮕, *left kidney* ⮕, *and vertebral body* ⮕.

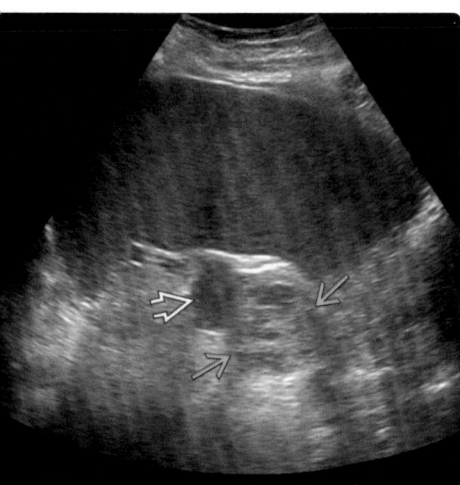

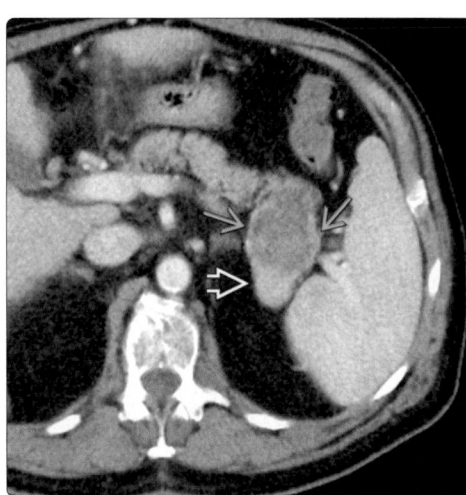

(Left) *Here, the spleen is used as an acoustic window to visualize the pancreatic tail. At the splenic hilum, there is a splenule* ⮕ *as well as a heterogeneous pancreatic tail mass immediately adjacent* ⮕. **(Right)** *Corresponding axial CT through the spleen also shows the splenule* ⮕ *adjacent to a large pancreatic tail mass* ⮕, *proven to represent a neuroendocrine tumor.*

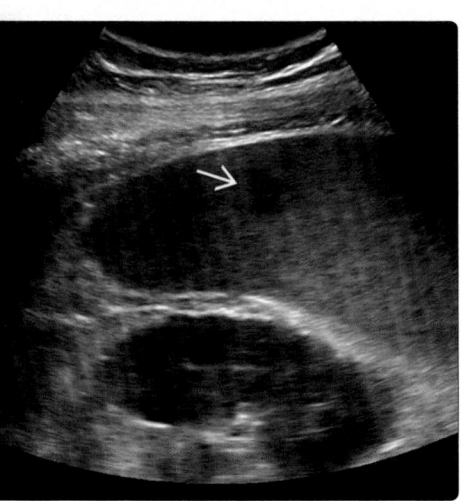

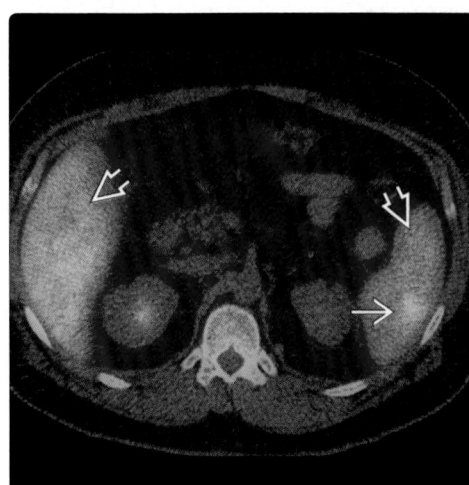

(Left) *Transverse US in a 44-year-old man with fever and pancytopenia is shown. The spleen is enlarged with a focal, ill-defined hypoechoic lesion* ⮕, *a nonspecific US finding with a broad differential diagnosis.* **(Right)** *PET/CT showed ↑ avidity of the focal splenic lesion* ⮕ *and ↑ background uptake in the spleen and liver* ⮕. *Final diagnosis was hemophagocytic lymphohistiocytosis, a rare entity. Splenic US is a good initial test, but abnormal findings may often require further imaging or histologic work-up.*

Splenomegaly

IMAGING

- No universal consensus on SMG cut off due to variability in normal adult spleen size
- SMG is diagnosed when length > 13 cm; additional measurements of thickness > 5 cm or width > 8 cm may also be used
- Splenic index (product of length, thickness, and width): Normally 120-480 cm³; SMG considered index > 500 cm³

TOP DIFFERENTIAL DIAGNOSES

- Splenomegaly without focal mass
  - Portal hypertension (cirrhosis)
  - Infection (mononucleosis, *Salmonella typhi*)
  - Lymphoma (Hodgkin or non-Hodgkin lymphoma)
  - Leukemia and myeloproliferative disorders
  - Hematologic disorders (hemoglobinopathy, TTP)
  - Storage diseases (Gaucher, hemosiderosis)
- Solitary splenic masses
  - Large splenic abscess

- Hemangioma
- Lymphangioma
- Primary malignancy (e.g., lymphoma, angiosarcoma)
- Metastasis

PATHOLOGY

- Myriad etiologies of SMG; systemic vs. primary splenic, focal lesion(s) vs. diffuse enlargement

DIAGNOSTIC CHECKLIST

- Is SMG present by size measurements?
- Is SMG diffuse or related to space-occupying lesions?
- Any other clues to underlying cause?
- SMG usually manifestation of systemic disease, rather than primary splenic pathology
- US best initial test; very useful for estimating spleen size; can distinguish between diffuse SMG or focal abnormality, can assess SV patency and flow direction

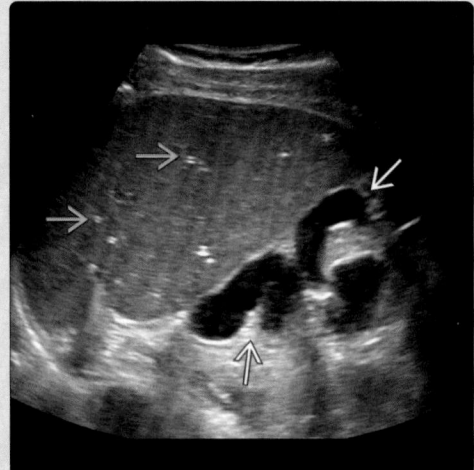
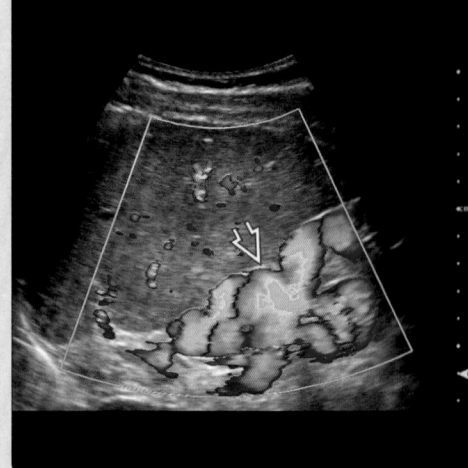

(Left) *US in a 47-year-old man with hepatitis C cirrhosis and splenomegaly (length 13.5 cm, thickness 6.5 cm) shows the dilated, tubular anechoic structures at the splenic hilum, consistent with splenic varices* ➡. *Echogenic foci without posterior acoustic shadowing throughout the spleen represent Gamna-Gandy bodies* ➡. (Right) *Color Doppler in the same patient confirms dilated splenic hilar varices* ➡ *in this patient with portal hypertension.*

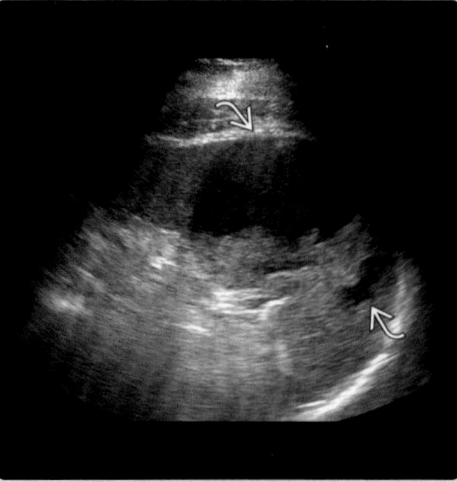
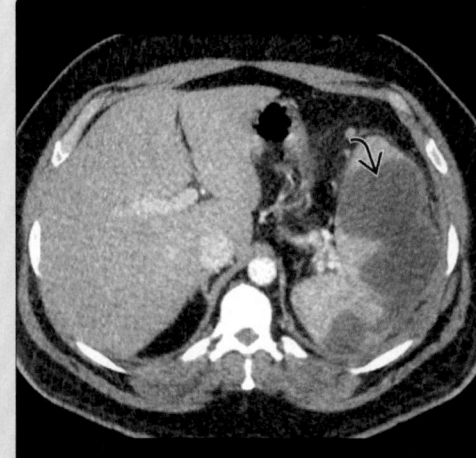

(Left) *US in a 47-year-old man shows splenomegaly (length 19.5 cm) due to space-occupying hypoechoic masses* ➡, *without internal vascularity (not pictured). These represented splenic abscesses.* (Right) *Axial CECT in the same patient demonstrates large, lobulated, hypodense splenic lesions* ➡ *resulting in splenomegaly. Pus was revealed on percutaneous drain placement, consistent with splenic abscess.*

TERMINOLOGY

Abbreviations

- Splenomegaly (SMG), hypersplenism (HS)

Definitions

- SMG: Increased splenic size, length > 13 cm in adults, weight > 250 g
- HS: Clinical syndrome consisting of SMG and pancytopenia

IMAGING

General Features

- Best diagnostic clue
  - Increased size of spleen
- Location
  - Spleen occupies left upper quadrant (LUQ) with tip extending inferiorly below 12th rib
- Size
  - No universal consensus on SMG cutoff due to variability in normal spleen size
    - Generally, normal adult spleen considered 12 cm in length (longest diameter in longitudinal plane), 4 cm in thickness (transverse from hilum), and 7 cm in width (longest diameter in transverse plane)
  - SMG is diagnosed when length > 13 cm; additional measurements of thickness > 5 cm or width > 8 cm can be used
  - Splenic index (product of length, thickness, and width): Normally 120-480 cm³; SMG considered index > 500 cm³
  - Splenic size correlates with height and can exceed normal size in tall, healthy people
  - SMG can be subjectively characterized as mild, moderate, or severe
    - Mild: Mononucleosis, febrile/bacterial infections, CHF
    - Moderate: Portal HTN, acute leukemias, thalassemia, TB, amyloidosis, sarcoidosis
    - Severe: Chronic leukemias, chronic myeloproliferative disorders, lymphoma, malaria, Gaucher disease
- Morphology
  - Enlarged spleen tends to have bulging shape and rounded poles

Ultrasonographic Findings

- Grayscale ultrasound
  - Normal splenic parenchyma is homogeneous; hyperechoic compared to liver and kidney
  - SMG with altered parenchymal echogenicity can be seen in different etiologies (some overlap)
  - **SMG with normal echogenicity**
    - Infection (mononucleosis, *Salmonella typhi*), congestion (portal HTN), early sickle cell disease
    - Hereditary spherocytosis, hemolysis, Felty syndrome
    - Wilson disease, polycythemia, myelofibrosis, leukemia
  - **SMG with hyperechoic pattern**
    - Leukemia, lymphoma, sarcoidosis, metastasis
    - Infections (malaria, tuberculosis, brucellosis), hematoma
    - Hereditary spherocytosis, polycythemia, myelofibrosis
  - **SMG with hypoechoic pattern**
    - Leukemia, lymphoma, metastasis, multiple myeloma

  - Congestion (portal HTN), noncaseating granulomatous infection
  - Sickle cell sequestration crisis: Peripheral hypoechoic areas
  - Gaucher disease: Multiple well-defined, discrete, hypoechoic lesions; fibrosis or infarction
  - **SMG with mixed echogenic pattern**
    - Abscesses, metastases, infarction, hemorrhage/hematoma in different stages of evolution
- Color Doppler
  - Portal hypertension: Dilated splenic vein (SV); direction of flow may be reversed; SV thrombus, splenic hilar collaterals, splenorenal shunt, recanalized umbilical vein

Radiographic Findings

- Radiography
  - Unreliable for determination of SMG
  - Splenic tip extending below 12th rib
  - Severe SMG may displace stomach and splenic flexure of colon

CT Findings

- Congestive SMG
  - Portal hypertension: SMG with varices, nodular shrunken liver, ascites
  - SV occlusion or thrombosis (i.e., secondary to pancreatitis or pancreatic tumors)
  - Sickle cell sequestration crisis: Peripheral low- & high-attenuation areas (areas of infarct & hemorrhage)
- Space-occupying lesions: Cysts, abscess, tumor
  - Cysts: Hypodense on NECT, no enhancement on CECT
  - Abscess: Hypodense on NECT with irregular, shaggy margin enhancing on CECT
  - Tumor: Hyperdense/hypodense on NECT and variable enhancement on CECT
- Storage disorders
  - Amyloidosis
    - NECT & CECT: Generalized or focal ↓ attenuation
  - Hemochromatosis
    - Primary: Spleen size normal or enlarged; normal attenuation compared to liver
    - Secondary (hemosiderosis): SMG with ↑↑ attenuation
- Splenic trauma
  - Splenic laceration or subcapsular hematoma, surrounding perisplenic hematoma (> 30 HU)

MR Findings

- Congestive SMG
  - Portal hypertension: Multiple tiny (3-8 mm) foci of decreased signal, hemosiderin deposits (siderotic nodules, a.k.a. Gamna-Gandy bodies)
  - Sickle cell sequestration crisis: Areas of abnormal signal intensity, hyperintense with dark rim on T1WI (subacute hemorrhage)
- Infarction: Peripheral, wedge-shaped areas of hypointensity resulting from iron deposition
- Secondary hemochromatosis (hemosiderosis): ↓ signal intensity on T1- and T2WI, GRE

Nuclear Medicine Findings

- Chromium 51-labeled RBCs or platelets

o Hypersplenism: Injected RBCs exhibit shortened half-life (average of 25-35 days)
- Tc-99m sulfur colloid scan: Measure of splenic function

Imaging Recommendations

- Best imaging tool
  o Ultrasound fast, safe, and reliable for confirmation of SMG; can detect focal lesions, assess SV patency, and direction of flow
  o CT most accurately determines spleen size/volume, allows for characterization of some lesions; MR preferred for siderosis
- Protocol advice
  o Best visualized following deep inspiration with patient in right lateral decubitus position
  o Splenic vein assessed at splenic hilum or at midline, posterior to pancreatic body

DIFFERENTIAL DIAGNOSIS

Splenomegaly Without Focal Mass

- Portal hypertension (cirrhosis)
- Infection (mononucleosis, *Salmonella typhi*)
- Lymphoma
- Leukemia and myeloproliferative disorders

Solitary Splenic Masses

- Large splenic abscess
  o Irregular wall, well defined, hypoechoic to anechoic depending on degree of liquefaction and necrosis
- Benign primary tumor
  o Hemangioma
    – Solid, echogenic mass ± cystic component; central punctate or peripheral calcification
  o Lymphangioma
    – Thin-walled & hypoechoic; variable vascularity; usually subcapsular in location; ± calcification
- Malignant primary tumor
  o Lymphoma (Hodgkin or non-Hodgkin lymphoma)
    – 1% of all lymphomas; can invade capsule and extend beyond spleen
    – Pattern: Diffuse SMG or focal hypoechoic lesions (no posterior acoustic enhancement)
  o Primary vascular tumors
    – All rare; angiosarcoma most common; littoral cell angioma
- Secondary malignancy
  o Large, solitary metastasis or lymphoma deposit

PATHOLOGY

General Features

- Etiology
  o Congestive SMG: Cirrhosis with portal hypertension, heart failure, SV thrombosis, sickle cell sequestration
  o Neoplasm: Leukemia, lymphoma, metastases, primary neoplasm, Kaposi sarcoma
  o Storage disease: Gaucher, Niemann-Pick, amyloidosis, hemosiderosis, histiocytosis
  o Infection: HIV, mononucleosis (EBV), CMV, hepatitis, malaria, TB, typhoid, kala-azar, schistosomiasis, brucellosis

o Hematologic: Hemoglobinopathy, hereditary spherocytosis, thrombocytopenic purpura, polycythemia
o Extramedullary hematopoiesis: Osteopetrosis, myelofibrosis
o Collagen vascular disease: Systemic lupus erythematosus, RA (Felty syndrome)

CLINICAL ISSUES

Presentation

- Most common signs/symptoms
  o Enlarged spleen by physical exam; unreliable compared to imaging
  o Signs & symptoms related to underlying cause
  o Variable presentation: Asymptomatic, abdominal fullness and discomfort, dragging pain
- Lab data: Abnormal complete blood count, liver function tests, antibody titers, cultures, or bone marrow biopsy

Natural History & Prognosis

- Complications
  o Splenic rupture can occur spontaneously or following minor trauma (as in athletes)
- Hypersplenism: Usually develops as a result of SMG
  o Hyperfunctioning spleen removes normal RBC, WBC, and platelets from circulation
- Prognosis
  o Depends on underlying disease

Treatment

- Treatment directed at underlying condition
- Splenectomy in symptomatic & complicated cases

DIAGNOSTIC CHECKLIST

Consider

- SMG most common cause of LUQ mass
- Usually manifestation of systemic disease, rather than primary splenic pathology

Image Interpretation Pearls

- Is SMG present by size measurements?
- Is SMG diffuse or related to space-occupying lesions?
- Any other clues to underlying cause?
- US great for spleen size; can distinguish between diffuse SMG or focal abnormality, can assess SV patency and flow direction
- CT & MR can further characterize abnormalities

SELECTED REFERENCES

1. Chiorean L et al: Ultrasonography of the spleen. Pictorial essay. Med Ultrason. 16(1):48-59, 2014
2. Benter T et al: Sonography of the spleen. J Ultrasound Med. 30(9):1281-93, 2011
3. Spielmann AL et al: Sonographic evaluation of spleen size in tall healthy athletes. AJR Am J Roentgenol. 184(1):45-9, 2005

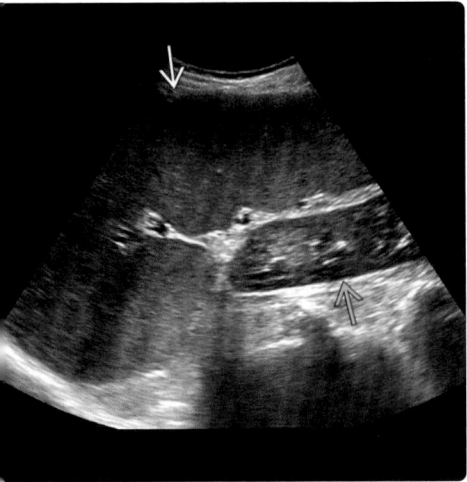

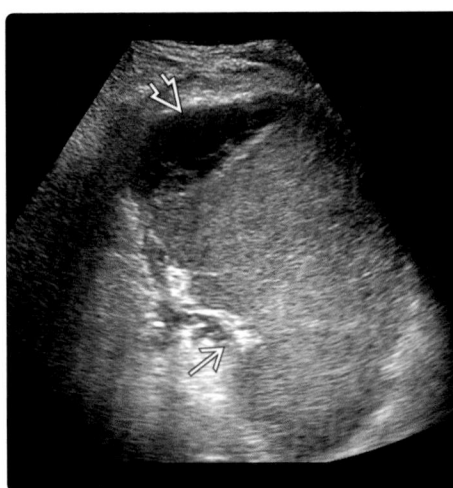

(Left) *US in a 92-year-old man with clinical syndrome of hypersplenism (pancytopenia and splenomegaly ➡) is shown. The spleen measured 20 x 8 x 21 cm (width x thickness x length). Note left kidney for comparison ➡.* (Right) *US in a 81-year-old man with splenomegaly ➡ due to chronic myelomonocytic leukemia (CMML) is shown. The spleen length measured 16.7 cm, thickness 9.7 cm. Note a geographic hypoechoic region at the pole with linear echogenic bands ➡, compatible with an infarct.*

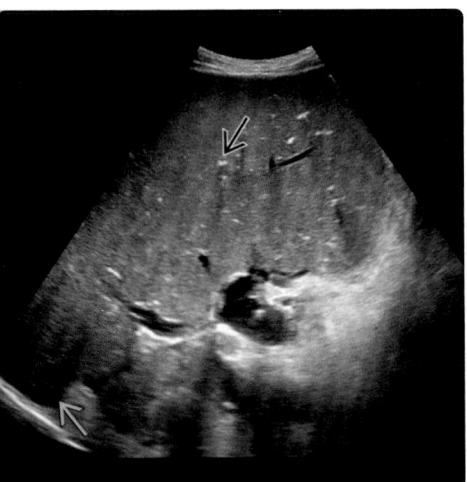

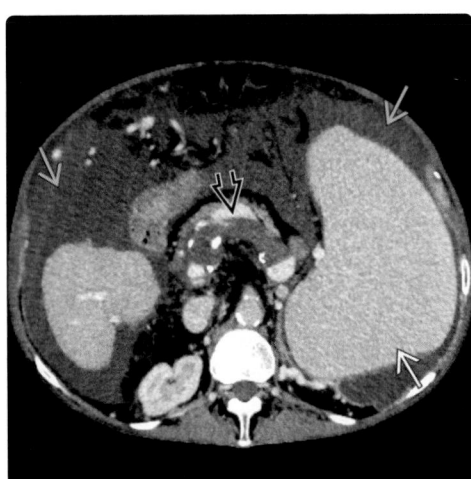

(Left) *US in a 64-year-old man with alcoholic cirrhosis shows severe splenomegaly (length of 22.8 cm). Multiple tiny echogenic foci ➡ with mild posterior acoustic shadowing represent sequelae of old granulomatous disease. Note the presence of perisplenic ascites ➡.* (Right) *Corresponding CT shows severe splenomegaly ➡, ascites ➡, and chronic (partially calcified) splenic vein and portal confluence thrombus ➡.*

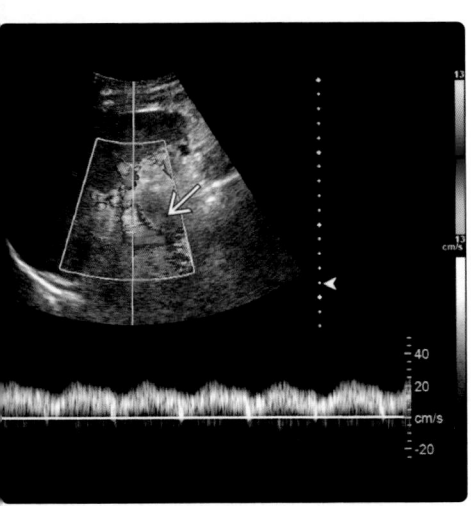

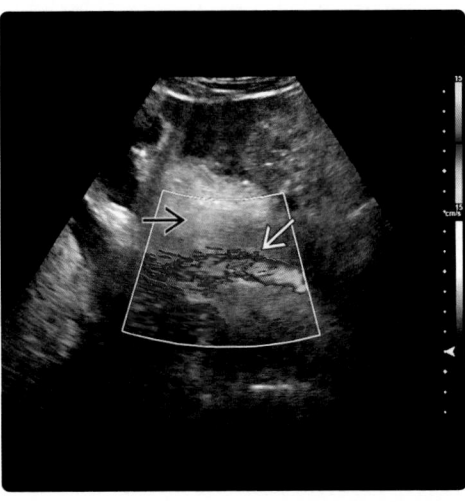

(Left) *Color Doppler US in a 52-year-old man with alcoholic cirrhosis and splenomegaly (14.9 cm in length) shows the reversal of flow in the splenic vein by color ➡ and spectral waveform (abnormally directed towards the spleen), consistent with severe portal hypertension.* (Right) *Assessment of the splenic vein ➡ at the midline (deep to the pancreatic body ➡) in the same patient shows reversal of the normal direction of flow.*

Splenic Cyst

IMAGING

- Can be classified as primary (congenital) vs. secondary (acquired) **or** true (epithelial lined) vs. false (no epithelial lining)
  - Secondary more common than primary (80% vs. 20%)
  - Hydatid cyst is an example of acquired true cyst
- Classically, anechoic to hypoechoic, avascular, sharply defined spherical lesion with posterior acoustic enhancement
  - Variable presence of internal debris/septation, wall calcification depending on type and etiology

TOP DIFFERENTIAL DIAGNOSES

- Inflammatory or infection
  - Pyogenic, fungal, or granulomatous abscess
- Neoplastic
  - Benign (hemangioma, lymphangioma) or malignant (cystic metastasis, lymphoma)
- Vascular
  - Hematoma, infarction, peliosis, intrasplenic pseudoaneurysm
- Intrasplenic pancreatic pseudocyst

DIAGNOSTIC CHECKLIST

- Rule out infectious, vascular, and neoplastic cystic lesions
- Consider if congenital or acquired cyst
  - Congenital (epidermoid): Typically larger, anechoic, with thin wall; ± calcification or debris (less common)
  - Acquired: Most commonly post-traumatic; usually smaller, often anechoic, but may have debris; thicker wall ± calcification
- Often impossible to distinguish primary vs. secondary (or true vs. false) cysts by imaging

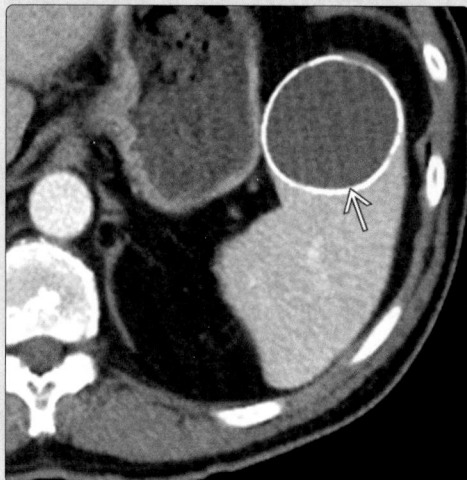
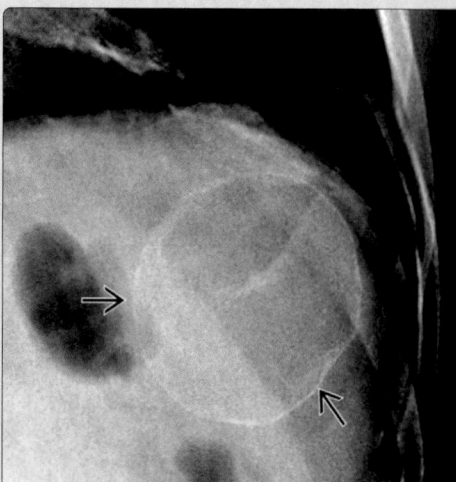

(Left) *Axial CECT of the left upper quadrant shows a large, rim-calcified, post-traumatic pseudocyst in the anterior spleen ➡. (Right) Zoomed-in view of the left subdiaphragmatic space on frontal chest radiograph in the same patient shows the cyst delineated by thin rim calcification ➡.*

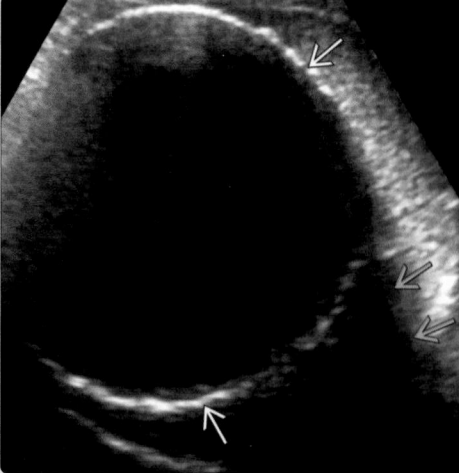
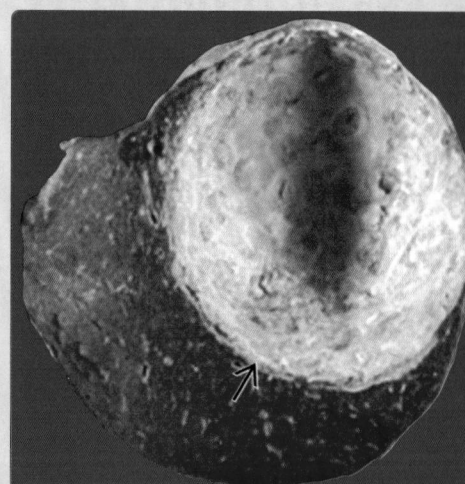

(Left) *Grayscale US shows an anechoic splenic pseudocyst with curvilinear rim calcification ➡, which causes posterior acoustic shadowing ➡. (Right) Gross pathology of an acquired pseudocyst in the spleen shows a calcified, fibrous wall ➡.*

Splenic Cyst

TERMINOLOGY

Definitions

Cystic parenchymal lesions of spleen

IMAGING

General Features

- Best diagnostic clue
  - Anechoic to hypoechoic, avascular, sharply defined spherical lesion with posterior acoustic enhancement
- Location
  - Usually subcapsular (65%)
- Size
  - Variable
- Key concepts
  - 2 classification schemes of splenic cysts
    - **Primary (congenital) vs. secondary (acquired)**
      - □ **Primary:** Epidermoid cyst
      - □ **Secondary:** Due to trauma (hematoma), infarction, infection, pancreatitis
    - **True vs. false/pseudocyst**
      - □ **True:** Epithelial lined; includes epidermoid and parasitic (e.g., hydatid) cysts
      - □ **False:** No epithelial lining; may have fibrous wall; includes post-traumatic, infectious (nonparasitic), or degenerative
    - "Primary" & "true" or "secondary" & "false/pseudo" often treated as synonymous
      - □ However, not all secondary cysts are pseudocysts; hydatid cyst is an example of a secondary (acquired) true cyst
  - Congenital cysts comprise about 20% of splenic cysts
    - Epidermoid cyst most common
    - Splenic cysts related to autosomal dominant polycystic kidney disease (ADPKD) are rare (> 5% of ADPKD)
    - More commonly encountered in children and young adults
  - Acquired cysts are more common (about 80%)
    - Wall calcification more common (38-50%) than in primary cysts (10-15%)
    - Generally, higher incidence of debris and smaller size than primary cysts, though can be large
  - Often impossible to distinguish primary vs. secondary (or true vs. false) cysts by imaging

Ultrasonographic Findings

- Grayscale ultrasound
  - Well-defined anechoic or hypoechoic lesion ± posterior acoustic enhancement
  - Congenital cysts
    - Anechoic, smooth borders, nondetectable walls ± trabeculation (36%), posterior acoustic enhancement
    - If complicated: Septations, internal echoes (hemorrhage, inflammatory debris); floating debris within cyst may produce mobile, uniform internal echoes ("snowstorm" or "pseudosolid" appearance), thick wall ± calcification
  - Acquired cysts

- Post-traumatic: Anechoic or mixed with internal echoes, echogenic wall, ± calcification, ± trabeculation of cyst wall (15%)
    - Parasitic (hydatid cyst): ± internal small daughter cysts and floating membranes ± calcification, hydatid sand
- Color Doppler
  - Avascular on color or power Doppler

Radiographic Findings

- May see curvilinear or plaque-like wall calcification

CT Findings

- Congenital cyst
  - Solitary, well-defined, spherical, unilocular cystic lesion (water or near water HU)
  - If hemorrhagic, infected, proteinaceous: ↑ attenuation or septation
  - No rim or intracystic enhancement, may have calcified wall (uncommon)
- Acquired cyst
  - Nonparasitic/post-traumatic: Usually small, solitary, sharply defined, water HU, ± wall calcification (may resemble eggshell)
  - Hydatid cyst: Peripheral calcification, ± daughter cysts; liver involvement far more common

MR Findings

- Congenital cyst
  - T1WI: ↓ signal, variable intensity if infected or hemorrhagic; T2WI: ↑ signal
- Acquired cyst
  - T1WI: ↓ signal, variable intensity (blood); T2WI: ↑ signal
  - Calcification or hemosiderin deposited in wall
    - T1WI & T2WI: ↓ signal
  - Hematoma: Varied intensity based on age & evolution of blood products
    - After 3 weeks, appears cystic: T1WI ↓; T2WI ↑

Imaging Recommendations

- Best imaging tool
  - Ultrasound for initial evaluation; if needed, CT or MR for further characterization
- Protocol advice
  - Patient is best scanned in supine or right lateral decubitus position following deep inspiration with US transducer along long axis of spleen

DIFFERENTIAL DIAGNOSIS

Inflammatory or Infection

- Pyogenic abscess
  - Solitary or multiple, well defined, ± irregular shape, hypoechoic to anechoic depending on stage of liquefaction/necrosis, ± gas within abscess
- Fungal abscess
  - e.g., *Candida, Aspergillus, Cryptococcus*
  - Usually microabscesses: Multiple, small, well-defined, hypoechoic to echogenic, throughout parenchyma
- Granulomatous abscesses
  - e.g., TB, atypical mycobacterium (MAC); cat-scratch
  - Multiple small, well-defined, hypoechoic lesions

Neoplastic

- Benign: e.g., hemangioma & lymphangioma
  - Hemangioma
    - Variable size and echogenicity, solid ± cystic areas, rarely solitary large lesion involving entire spleen
  - Lymphangioma
    - Heterogeneous/multicystic appearance, intracystic echoes: Proteinaceous material
- Malignant: e.g., lymphoma & metastases
  - Lymphoma
    - Hypoechoic/anechoic type of lymphomatous nodules: May resemble cysts, however reveal "indistinct boundary" echo pattern
    - Posterior acoustic enhancement absent
  - Metastases: Necrotic/cystic
    - Relatively common; e.g., malignant melanoma, adenocarcinoma of breast, pancreas, ovaries, and endometrium may cause "cystic" splenic metastases
    - Multiple focal, cystic lesions of variable size

Vascular

- Hematoma or laceration
  - Hypo-/iso-/hyperechoic, blood-filled cleft; nonspherical shape
  - Hematoma echogenicity depends on stage of bleed; fresh blood echo-free initially, later becomes echogenic
  - End stage: Cystic degeneration → pseudocyst
- Infarction (arterial or venous)
  - Acute phase: Well-defined, wedge-shaped areas of decreased echogenicity
  - Subacute & chronic phases: Anechoic (due to liquefactive necrosis)
- Peliosis
  - Rare; usually with liver findings; multiple indistinct areas of hypo-/hyperechogenicity that may involve entire spleen
- Intrasplenic pseudoaneurysm
  - Post-traumatic; anechoic on grayscale, fills with color Doppler

Intrasplenic Pancreatic Pseudocyst

- In 1-5% of patients with pancreatitis
- Direct extension of pancreatic pseudocyst; pancreatic secretions extend along splenic vessels to hilum, pancreatic enzymes cause erosion into spleen
- Well-defined, rounded, cystic splenic lesion; associated inflammatory changes of pancreas

PATHOLOGY

General Features

- Etiology
  - Congenital: Genetic defect of mesothelial migration
  - Acquired: Most often post-traumatic, end-stage of splenic hematoma/infarction
    - Pathogenesis: Liquefactive necrosis, cystic change

Gross Pathologic & Surgical Features

- Congenital cyst
  - Usually large, glistening, smooth walls
- Acquired cyst
  - Smaller than true cysts, debris, wall calcification

  - Parasitic: Hydatid (*Echinococcus granulosus* most common form to affect spleen), *Taenia solium*

Microscopic Features

- True cyst: Epithelial lining present
  - Epidermoid (stratified, nonkeratinizing squamous epithelium), mesothelial (low cuboidal to low columnar), dermoid (squamous lining with dermal structures)
  - Epidermoid most common
- False cyst: No epithelial lining, may have fibrous capsule

CLINICAL ISSUES

Presentation

- Most common signs/symptoms
  - Depends on etiology, acuity
  - Often asymptomatic
  - Mild pain or tenderness, palpable mass in LUQ, splenomegaly

Demographics

- Age
  - 2/3 < 40 years old
- Gender
  - M:F = 2:3

Natural History & Prognosis

- Complications: Hemorrhage, rupture, infection
- Prognosis
  - Good: Uncomplicated cases; after surgical removal
  - Poor: Complicated cases

Treatment

- Symptomatic: Surgery (total cystectomy, marsupialization, cyst decapsulation, or partial/total splenectomy)
- Asymptomatic
  - Small: No treatment
  - Large (> 5-6 cm): Surgical removal (controversial)
- Ultrasound-guided drainage ± injection of sclerosing agent is alternative option

DIAGNOSTIC CHECKLIST

Consider

- Rule out infectious, vascular, and neoplastic cystic lesions

Image Interpretation Pearls

- Congenital: Larger, well defined, anechoic, thin wall; ± calcification and debris (less common)
- Acquired: Usually smaller, well defined; often anechoic with thicker wall; ± calcification, ± debris
- Often impossible to distinguish primary vs. secondary (or true vs. false) cysts by imaging

SELECTED REFERENCES

1. Gaetke-Udager K et al: Multimodality imaging of splenic lesions and the role of non-vascular, image-guided intervention. Abdom Imaging. 39(3):570-87, 2014
2. Li W et al: Real-time contrast enhanced ultrasound imaging of focal splenic lesions. Eur J Radiol. 83(4):646-53, 2014
3. Caremani M et al: Focal splenic lesions: US findings. J Ultrasound. 16(2):65-74, 2013

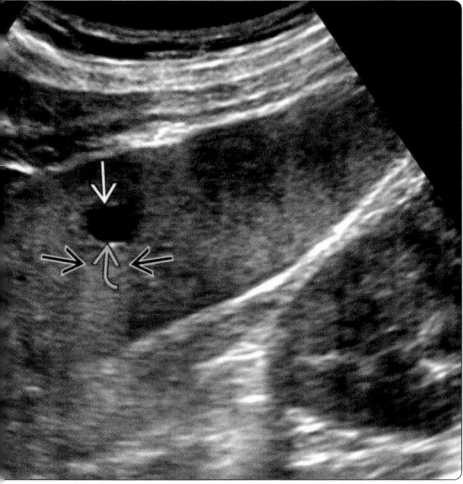

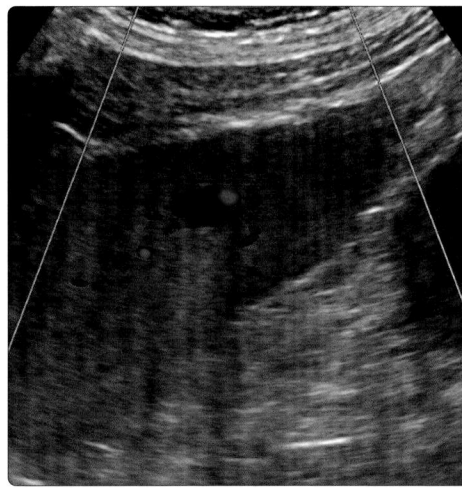

(Left) *Grayscale US of the spleen shows an incidental 8 mm, anechoic splenic cyst ⇥. Note the posterior acoustic enhancement ⇥ and well-defined back wall ⇥, confirming the cystic nature of this lesion.* (Right) *Color Doppler US in the same patient confirms that this lesion is avascular and indeed a splenic cyst. Rarely, splenic pseudoaneurysms may mimic a splenic cyst on grayscale imaging; color Doppler imaging is therefore important to distinguish the 2 entities.*

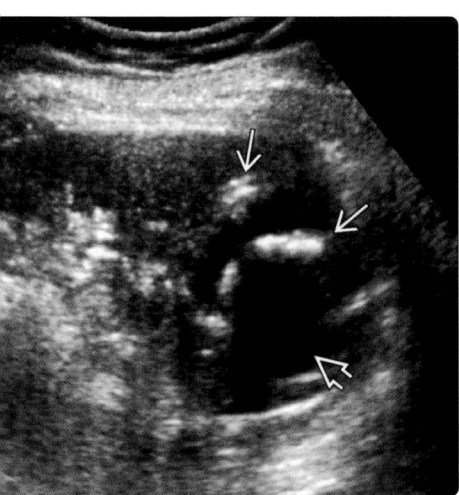

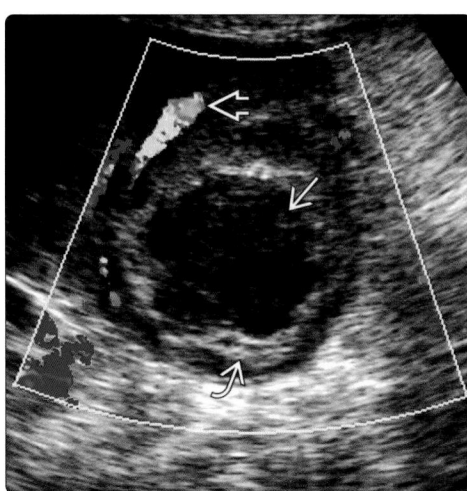

(Left) *Transverse grayscale US of the spleen shows a multiloculated cyst with a cyst-within-cyst appearance. The contents of the cyst are anechoic ⇥. Partial curvilinear calcification ⇥ is seen in the cyst wall. This represents a chronic, healed hydatid cyst.* (Right) *Color Doppler US shows a pyogenic splenic abscess, seen as a well-defined solitary avascular lesion with a hypoechoic necrotic center ⇥ and a thick irregular wall ⇥. Note surrounding splenic parenchymal vessels displaced by the abscess ⇥.*

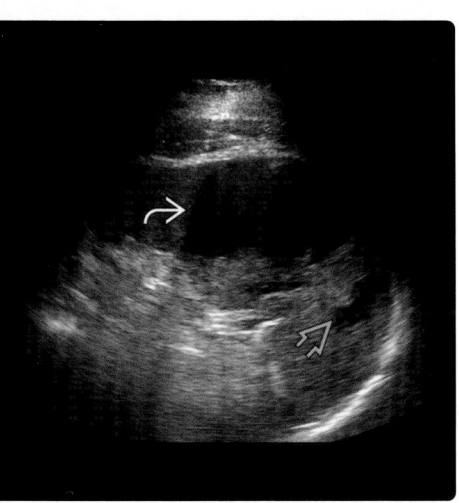

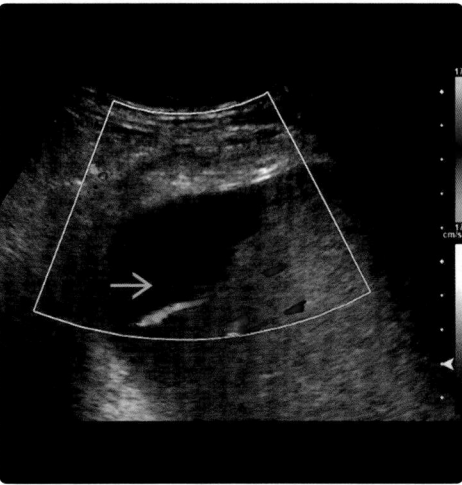

(Left) *Grayscale US shows a large, hypoechoic, splenic complex cystic lesion ⇥, proven to be a pyogenic abscess by percutaneous drainage. Note the irregular shape and multiplicity ⇥, which may help differentiate this from a simple cyst.* (Right) *Color Doppler US in a patient with leukemia shows a splenic infarct, which may mimic a cyst. Note the avascularity, peripheral wedge-shaped (rather than spherical) configuration, and echogenic fine internal bands ⇥, characteristic of splenic infarct.*

IMAGING

- All tumors (benign and malignant) can have variable appearances, a lot of overlap by US
- Benign tumors
  - Hemangioma: #1 benign splenic tumor; classic = echogenic
  - Hamartoma: Classic = echogenic, homogenous
  - Lymphangioma: Classic = hypoechoic, loculated, avascular; younger age
  - Littoral cell angioma: Rare; variable appearance, splenomegaly
- Malignant tumors
  - Lymphoma (HD, NHL, primary splenic, AIDS-related), leukemia, myeloproliferative disorders
    - Classic: Diffuse SMG; if focal: Hypoechoic, indistinct margins
  - Metastasis (breast, lung, ovary, stomach, melanoma)
    - Cystic, solid, or mixed; can be targetoid lesions

- Primary splenic malignancies very rare (angiosarcoma most common of these)
- Color Doppler vascularity may be helpful if present (to conclude not cyst), but absent color flow does not entirely exclude benign or malignant tumor

TOP DIFFERENTIAL DIAGNOSES

- Splenic infarct
- Splenic infection/abscess
- Splenic cyst
- Splenic hematoma
- Hepatosplenic sarcoidosis

DIAGNOSTIC CHECKLIST

- Primary splenic malignancies are rare; biggest diagnostic dilemma is usually an indeterminate splenic lesion in patients with extrasplenic malignancy (i.e., is it metastasis or not)
- Considerable overlap in US findings; reliable differentiation on imaging is not always possible, requires histology

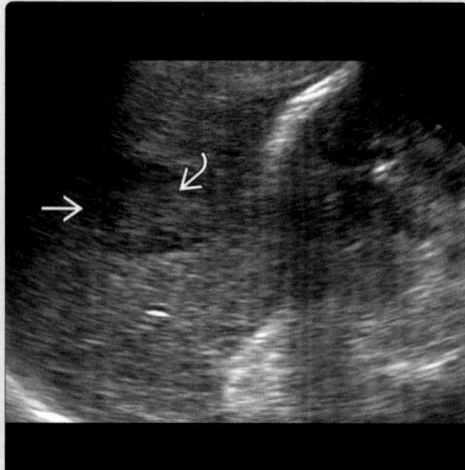 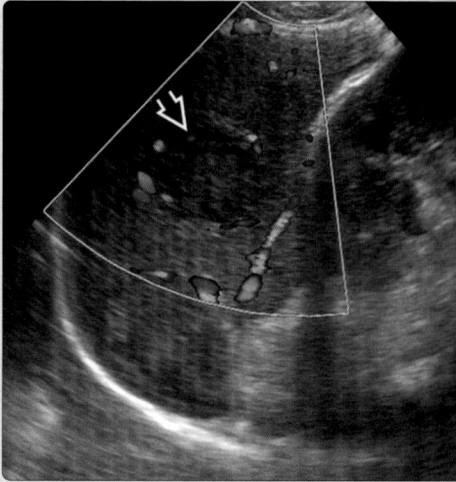

(Left) *Grayscale ultrasound image of the spleen in a patient with hepatitis C (HCV) and previously treated hepatocellular carcinoma (HCC) shows a solitary solid mass in the spleen with central hyper-echogenicity* ➘ *and peripheral hypo-echogenicity* ➘ *(target-like pattern).* (Right) *Color Doppler evaluation of the lesion demonstrates a small amount of flow within the lesion* ➘, *confirming its solid (not-cystic) nature.*

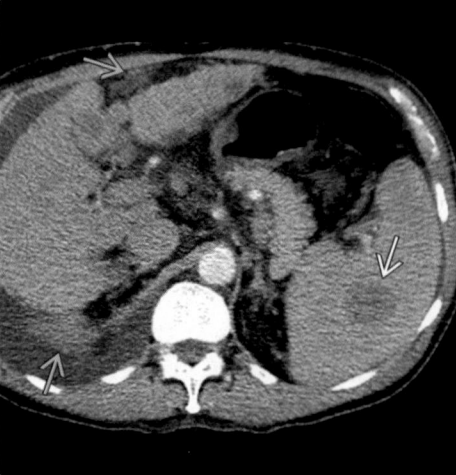 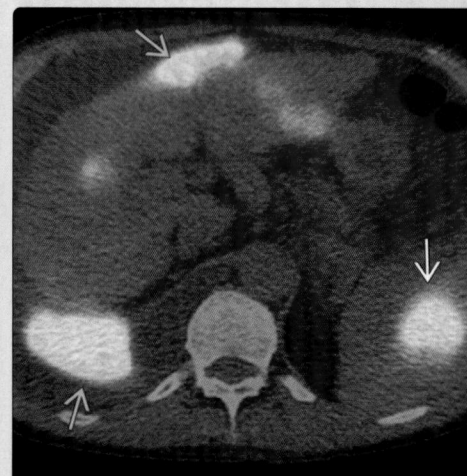

(Left) *Corresponding axial contrast-enhanced CT image shows the solitary, solid hypoattenuating splenic lesion* ➘. *Also, note the presence of peritoneal soft tissue implants along the surface of the liver* ➚. (Right) *¹⁸F FDG PET/CT fusion image in the same patient shows intense metabolic activity of the splenic lesion* ➘, *peritoneal implants* ➚, *and sites of hepatic involvement. Histology revealed large B-cell lymphoma. Note that HCC metastasis to the spleen is rare; HCV infection has been linked to B-cell lymphomas.*

TERMINOLOGY

Definitions

- Space occupying benign or malignant tumor(s) of spleen

IMAGING

General Features

- Best diagnostic clue
  - Solitary or multiple, solid or cystic splenic masses
- Key concepts
  - Classification based on pathology and histology; overlap of imaging appearances
  - Benign tumors
    - Hemangioma, hamartoma, lymphangioma, littoral cell angioma
  - Hemangioma
    - #1 primary benign neoplasm of spleen (up to 14%)
    - Typically small, incidental, asymptomatic
    - Multiple in diffuse splenic hemangiomatosis or syndromes (Klippel-Trenaunay-Weber and Beckwith-Wiedemann syndrome)
  - Hamartoma
    - Rare; incidentally detected at autopsy or imaging; no age/gender predilection
    - Contains anomalous mixture of normal elements of splenic tissue
    - Syndromic associations: Tuberous sclerosis and Wiskott-Aldrich syndrome
  - Lymphangioma
    - Rare; most occur in childhood; variable size
    - Uni- or multilocular; typically subcapsular in location
    - Solitary or multiple (as in systemic lymphangiomatosis)
  - Littoral cell angioma (LCA)
    - Rare 1° vascular tumor; commonly considered benign, though malignant LCAs have been reported
    - Solitary or multiple; usually presents with splenomegaly, hypersplenism
  - Malignant tumors
    - Lymphoma, leukemia, myeloproliferative disorders
    - Metastases
    - Rare 1° splenic malignancies: Angiosarcoma, leiomyosarcoma, malignant fibrous histiocytoma
  - Lymphoma
    - #1 malignant tumor of spleen: Hodgkin disease (HD) and non-Hodgkin lymphoma (NHL)
    - Spleen: Nodal organ in HD and extranodal organ in NHL
    - Manifest: Focal lesions (> 1 cm) or diffuse (typical)
    - Primary splenic lymphoma: Typically NHL (B-cell origin)
  - Metastases
    - Relatively uncommon; may be multiple (60%), solitary (31%), nodular, and diffuse (9%)
    - Common route: Hematogenous spread (splenic artery)
      - Retrograde (less common): Via splenic vein and lymphatics
      - Direct extension (uncommon): From gastric, renal, pancreatic, colonic

- Common primary sites for splenic metastases: Breast (21%), lung (18%), ovary (8%), stomach (7%), melanoma (6%), prostate (6%)
- "Cystic" splenic metastases: Melanoma; adenocarcinoma of breast, ovary, and endometrium
  - Angiosarcoma
    - Very rare malignant tumor of spleen; seen in patients with previous exposure to Thorotrast
    - Poor prognosis with early, widespread metastases

Ultrasonographic Findings

- Grayscale ultrasound
  - Benign tumors
  - Hemangioma
    - Typically well defined, hyperechoic
    - Echogenicity can be variable (range from solid to cystic to mixed); ± calc when complex
    - Rarely, can be large and involve entire spleen with atypical features: Heterogeneous echotexture, areas of necrosis and hemorrhage
  - Hamartoma
    - Typically well defined, homogeneous, hyperechoic
    - Depending on histologic subtype, echogenicity and vascularity can be variable; can have cystic component or calc
  - Lymphangioma
    - Normal or enlarged spleen depending on number, size, loculations
    - Well-defined hypoechoic mass ± internal septations and intralocular debris; ± wall calc
    - Avascular on color Doppler, unless along cyst walls
  - Littoral cell angioma
    - Variable echogenicity and vascularity; solitary or multiple; splenomegaly
  - Malignant tumors
  - Lymphoma
    - US pattern corresponds to 3 macroscopic patterns; diffuse/infiltrative, miliary/nodular, focal hypoechoic
    - "Indistinct boundary" echo pattern
    - Anechoic/mixed echoic, small or large nodules; hyperechoic lesion uncommon (< 10%)
    - Lymphadenopathy: Abdominal or retroperitoneal
  - Leukemia and myeloproliferative disorders
    - Diffuse enlargement of spleen with variable echogenicity, very rarely focal hypoechoic nodular lesions
  - Metastases
    - Multiple focal lesions with variable size and appearance; iso-/hypo-/hyperechoic
    - "Target" lesions with hypoechoic "halo"
  - Angiosarcoma: Very rare, solid, mixed echogenicity mass; associated metastasis in liver (70%)

CT Findings

- Benign tumors
  - Hemangioma
    - Homogeneous, hypodense, solid or cystic masses
    - Concentric rim of C+ with uniform delayed fill-in; classic "peripheral nodular C+" associated with liver hemangioma is less common in spleen
  - Hamartoma

– Isodense (typically) or hypodense; variable early C+; uniform C+ on delayed scans
  - **Lymphangioma**
    – Low-attenuation lesion(s); sharp margins; typically subcapsular; no enhancement; ± wall calcification
- Malignant tumors
  - **Lymphoma**
    – Solitary, multifocal or diffuse; Hypodense lesions with minimal enhancement
  - **Metastases**
    – Multiple, solid (common) or cystic, hypodense, central or peripheral enhancement
  - **Angiosarcoma**
    – Solitary or multiple, irregular margins, heterogeneous density; variable enhancement; ± calcification
    – Usually liver or distant metastases

MR Findings
- Benign tumors
  - **Hemangioma**: T1 ↓, T2 ↑; C+: uniform or heterogeneous centripetal
  - **Hamartoma**: T1 iso; T2 hetero; C+: similar to CT
  - **Lymphangioma**: T1 ↓ or ↑ (depending on protein/blood content), T2 ↑↑; No C+
- Malignant tumors
  - **Lymphoma**
    – MR not reliable due to similar T1, T2 relaxation times and proton densities of spleen/lymphoma
  - **Metastases**
    – T1WI: Isointense to hypointense, T2WI: Hyperintense
    – T1 C+: Enhancement depends on type of primary

Nuclear Medicine Findings
- PET/CT
  - 18F-FDG avidity can be a helpful feature to distinguish between benign and malignant solid splenic lesions
    – In patients with known malignancy, SUV > 2.3 can differentiate benign and malignant with 100% sens/spec
    – High NPV in patients without known malignancy
    – False-positives can be due to granulomatous diseases

Image-Guided Biopsy
- Splenic biopsy is gaining increased acceptance
  - Risks include hemorrhage (leading to hypotensive shock), pneumothorax, or colonic injury
- Ultrasound or CT used; US may be preferred due to real time assessment of the vessels with color Doppler
- Splenic FNA: Low complication rate but lower success rate
- Splenic core biopsy: Higher diagnostic success rate (> 88%) but higher complication rate (up to 12% reported)

Imaging Recommendations
- Best imaging tool
  - US initially, CT/MR for further characterization
- Protocol advice
  - Patient is best scanned in supine or right decubitus position for intercostal acoustic window

DIFFERENTIAL DIAGNOSIS

Splenic Infarct
- Wedge-shaped, well-defined, hyperechoic/hypoechoic area (depending on the age of infarct), avascular

Splenic Infection/Abscess
- Pyogenic abscess: Solitary or multiple, small or large, hypoechoic lesions with ± thick irregular walls
- Fungal microabscesses; mycobacterial (TB, MAC) granulomas: Multiple hypoechoic avascular lesions

Splenic Cyst
- Anechoic/hypoechoic, sharp margins, posterior acoustic enhancement, ± peripheral rim calcification, avascular

Splenic Hematoma
- Subcapsular of intrasplenic; hyper/hypoechoic (depending on stage of liquefaction) fluid collection/lesion

Hepatosplenic Sarcoidosis
- Splenic involvement uncommon; SMG; multiple hypoechoic nodules (or iso/hyper)

CLINICAL ISSUES

Presentation
- Most common signs/symptoms
  - Varies from asymptomatic incidental finding to symptomatic depending on size, type of tumor
  - Left upper quadrant pain, palpable mass, splenomegaly, weight loss

Natural History & Prognosis
- Complications: Hemorrhage, rupture
- Prognosis: Good (benign tumors); poor (malignant)

Treatment
- Splenectomy depending on type (can also be diagnostic if image guided biopsy not possible)

DIAGNOSTIC CHECKLIST

Consider
- 1° splenic malignancies are rare; biggest diagnostic dilemma is usually an indeterminate splenic lesion in patients with extrasplenic malignancy (i.e., is it metastasis)

Image Interpretation Pearls
- Considerable overlap in US findings; reliable differentiation on imaging is not always possible, requires histology

SELECTED REFERENCES

1. Gaetke-Udager K et al: Multimodality imaging of splenic lesions and the role of non-vascular, image-guided intervention. Abdom Imaging. 39(3):570-87, 2014
2. Thipphavong S et al: Nonneoplastic, benign, and malignant splenic diseases: cross-sectional imaging findings and rare disease entities. AJR Am J Roentgenol. 203(2):315-22, 2014
3. Kamaya A et al: Multiple lesions of the spleen: differential diagnosis of cystic and solid lesions. Semin Ultrasound CT MR. 27(5):389-403, 2006
4. Bachmann C et al: Color Doppler sonographic findings in focal spleen lesions. Eur J Radiol. 56(3):386-90, 2005

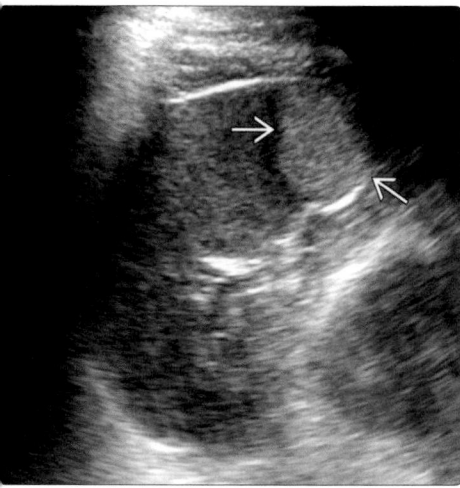
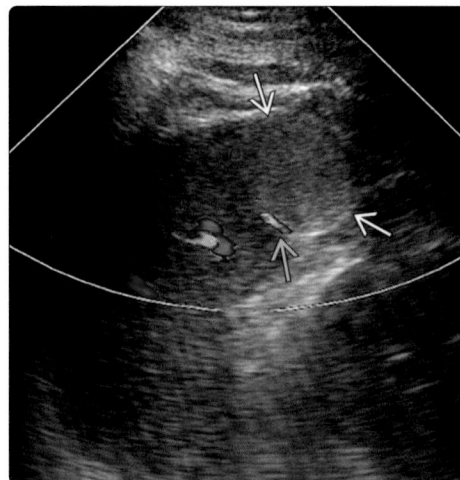

(Left) *Longitudinal grayscale ultrasound image demonstrates a splenic hemangioma, which appears as a well-circumscribed, homogenously hyperechoic mass in the inferior spleen ➡.* (Right) *Corresponding color Doppler image of the lesion ➡ shows a scant amount of flow along its periphery ➡.*

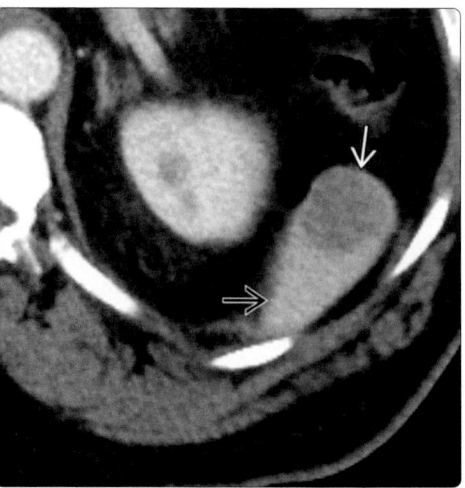
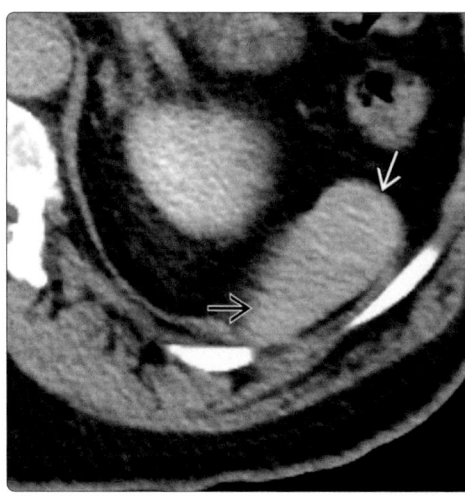

(Left) *Axial CT image through the inferior spleen during portal venous phase shows a well-circumscribed lesion ➡, which is hypoattenuating compared to spleen parenchyma ➡.* (Right) *Axial CT image at the same level during the 3-minute delayed phase shows retention of contrast within the lesion ➡, now nearly isodense to spleen parenchyma ➡. This represents a hemangioma, though a hamartoma could have a similar appearance.*

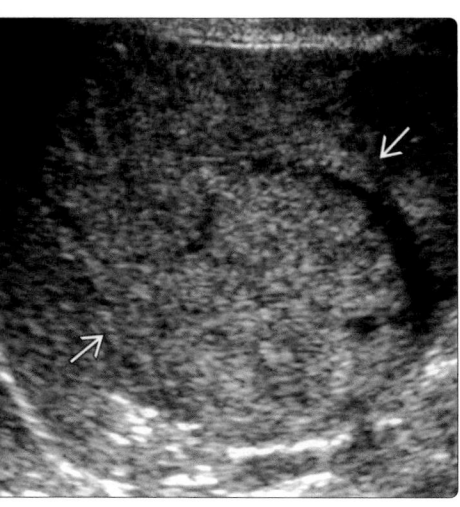
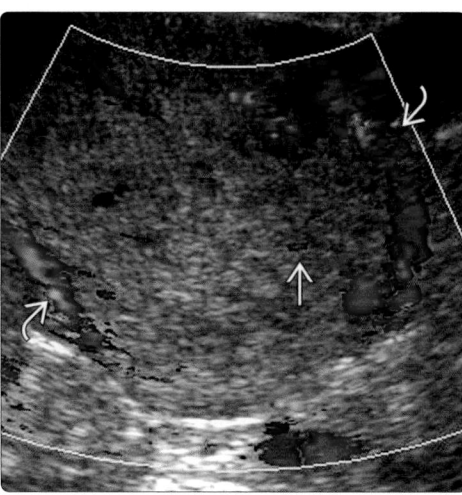

(Left) *Transverse transabdominal ultrasound shows a large, ill-defined hemangioma ➡ occupying almost the entire spleen. Note it is isoechoic to the spleen and the displaced vessel is the clue.* (Right) *Transverse color Doppler ultrasound in the same patient shows minimal internal vascularity ➡ within the mass. Note the displacement of surrounding parenchymal vessels ➡.*

(Left) *Transverse transabdominal ultrasound shows an ill-defined splenic lymphangioma* ➡ *with a cystic component* ⬈. **(Right)** *Corresponding color Doppler ultrasound shows the splenic lymphangioma* ⬈ *has peripheral vascularity* ⬈ *and avascular central cystic area.*

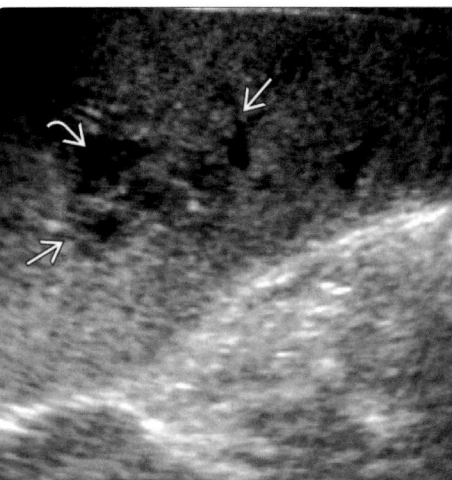
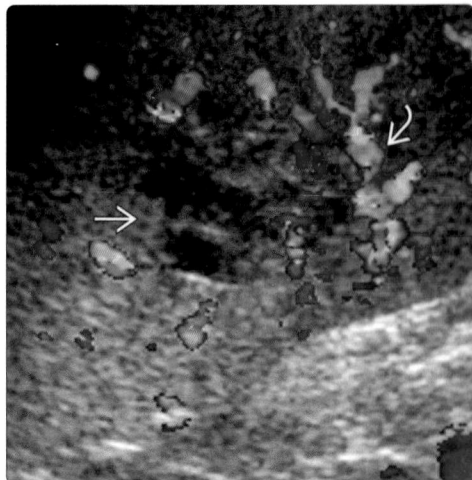

(Left) *Grayscale US shows a large, ill-defined, heterogeneous echogenicity, cystic and solid mass replacing the spleen. There are areas of shadowing calcification* ➡. *Histology revealed angiosarcoma. Evaluation of the liver can be helpful as the majority (> 70%) of splenic angiosarcomas have hepatic metastases on presentation.* **(Right)** *Grayscale US of a cystic mass* ➡ *in the anterior aspect of the spleen in a 45-year-old woman is shown. Note the solid internal components* ➡. *This was further worked-up with MR and PET/CT.*

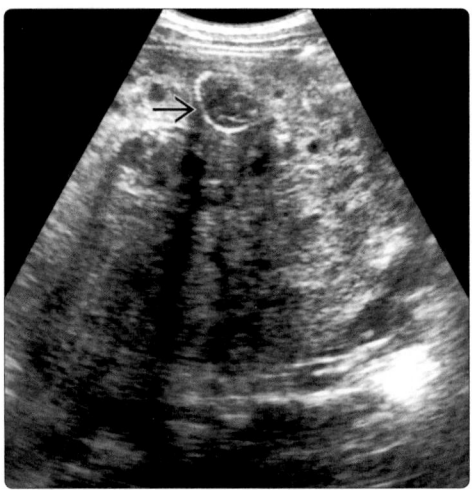
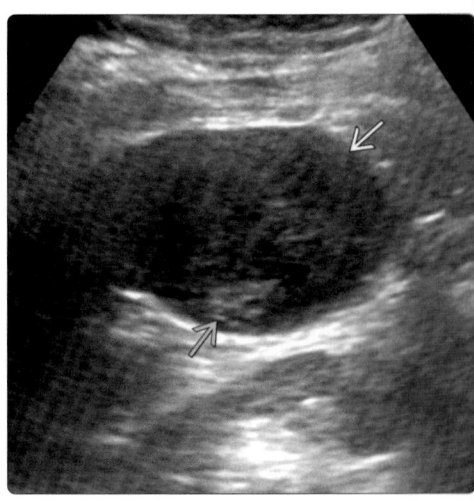

(Left) *Axial contrast-enhanced MR image shows enhancement of the solid components* ➡ *along the anteromedial aspect of the cystic mass. At this stage, both benign and malignant etiologies can be considered.* **(Right)** *Fused axial PET/CT in the same patient shows intense FDG avidity of the solid components* ➡ *(SUV max > 11). This lesion is suspicious for malignancy (particularly lymphoma or metastasis) and will require tissue sampling for final diagnosis.*

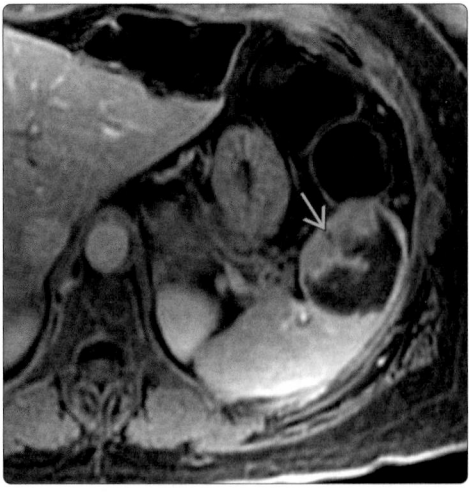
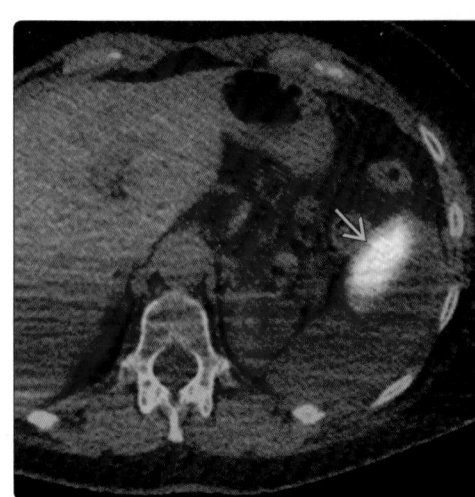

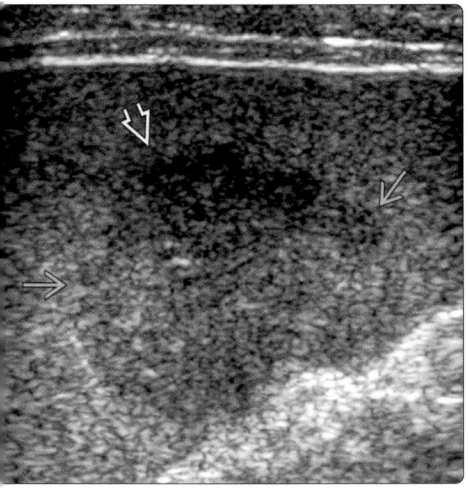

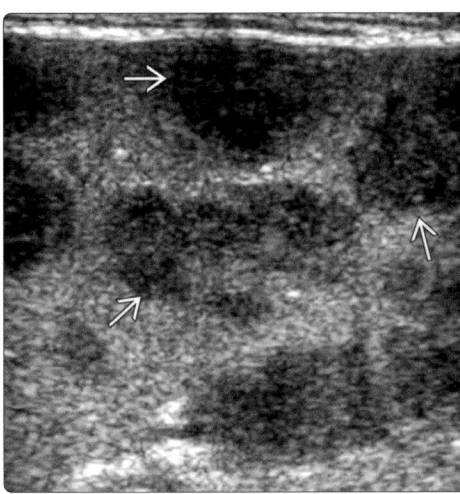

(Left) *A solid, hypoechoic mass ➡️ in the spleen consistent with a solitary lymphomatous deposit is shown. Note the indistinct margins ➡️, characteristic of this entity. Lymphoma can present with diffuse involvement, solitary focal lesion, or multifocal lesions.* (Right) *Longitudinal transabdominal ultrasound shows multiple hypoechoic lesions ➡️ in a patient with multifocal lymphomatous involvement of the spleen.*

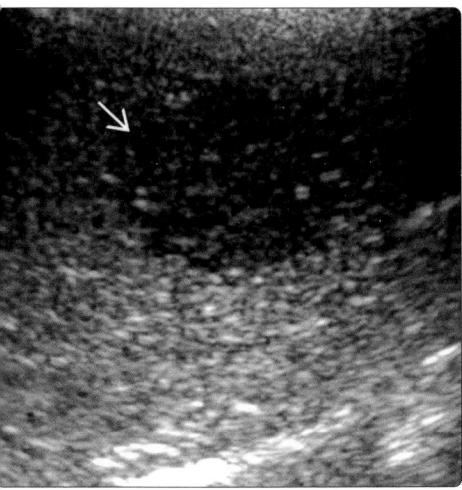

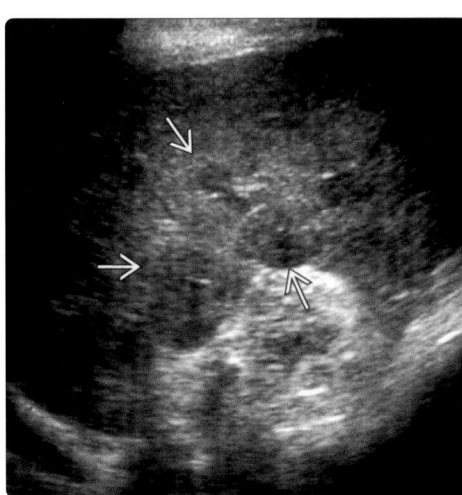

(Left) *Transverse transabdominal US shows a solitary, hypoechoic splenic metastasis ➡️. Metastases may vary from a target appearance to a uniform iso-/hypo-/hyperechoic lesion or heterogeneous mass. This may be difficult to differentiate from entities such as lymphoma; clinical history is helpful.* (Right) *Multifocal hypoechoic spleen lesions ➡️, of varying sizes and some with indistinct margins, representing melanoma metastases, are shown. Note: Melanoma metastases can also present as cystic masses.*

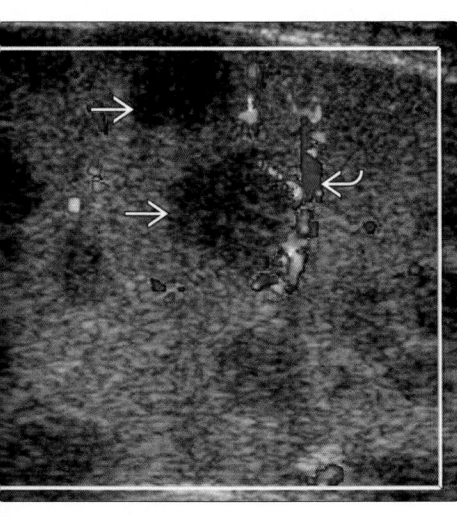

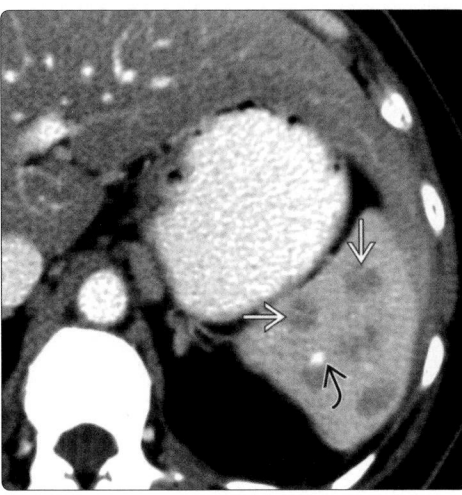

(Left) *Color Doppler US image shows multiple hypoechoic granulomas ➡️, without internal vascularity. Note the normal splenic parenchymal vascularity ➡️. On US, splenic granulomas (TB, MAC, sarcoid) appear as multiple small, well-defined, hypoechoic lesions, which may mimic lymphoma or metastasis.* (Right) *Axial CECT in the same patient shows no enhancement within the hypodense splenic granulomas ➡️. Focal calcification ➡️ is noted as well, which can be seen with granulomatous disease.*

Splenic Infarct

IMAGING

- Variable sonographic appearance of acute splenic infarction
  - Classic
    - Hypoechoic, peripheral, wedge shaped, and avascular
  - Non-classic
    - Rounded or peripheral band morphology
    - Global infarction
    - Isoechoic to hyperechoic
  - Bright band sign
    - Thin, parallel echogenic lines within the hypoechoic infarcted area
    - Thought to represent preserved fibrous trabeculae within infarcted tissue
- Chronic infarction
  - Atrophic, scarred spleen, ± calcification
- Associated findings
  - Splenomegaly, splenic vein occlusion (with large perisplenic varices), splenic artery thrombosis

TOP DIFFERENTIAL DIAGNOSES

- Splenic laceration
- Splenic hematoma
- Splenic cyst
- Splenic mass
- Splenic metastases
- Splenic lymphoma

DIAGNOSTIC CHECKLIST

- Color and power Doppler are critical components of ultrasound evaluation of splenic infarct
- Grayscale appearance can be variable depending on morphology, evolution of the infarct
- Clinical history is very helpful
  - Multitude of underlying disorders can predispose to splenic infarction

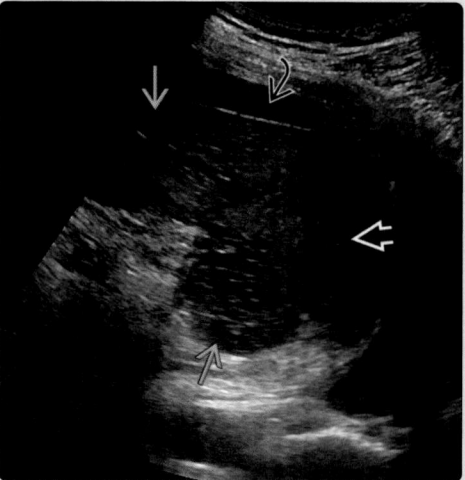
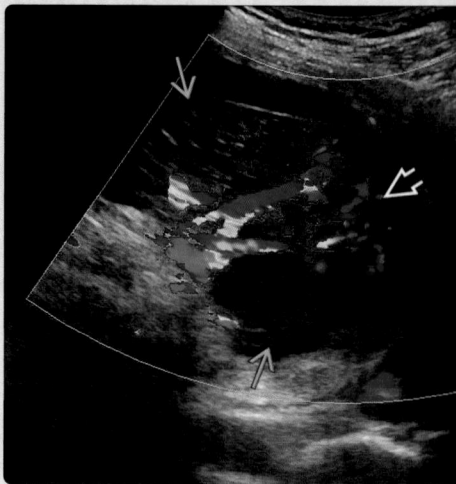

(Left) *Transverse US of the spleen demonstrates inhomogeneity of the splenic echotexture, with geographic areas of hypoechogenicity ➡ containing parallel echogenic bands; these regions represent infarct. Compare this to normal parenchyma ➡. Note also the presence of perisplenic fluid ➡.* (Right) *Corresponding color Doppler US shows absent vascularity in the infarcted parenchyma ➡ and normal vascularity within the uninvolved parenchyma ➡.*

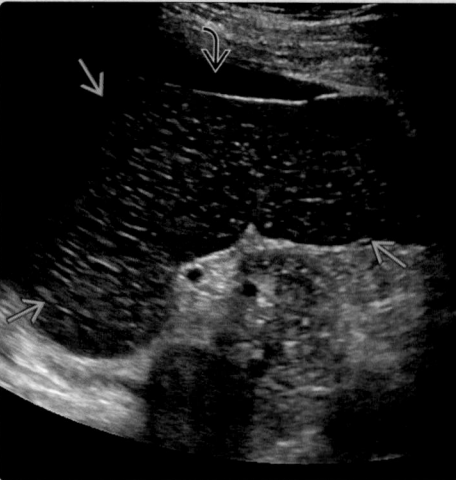
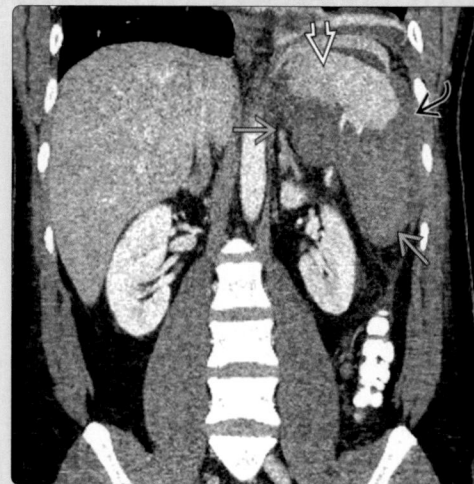

(Left) *Longitudinal splenic view is shown in the same patient. In this plane of view, the extent of the infarct can be appreciated. The infarcted tissue ➡ is hypoechoic with numerous thin, parallel echogenic bands (the bright band sign). Note again the free fluid ➡.* (Right) *Corresponding coronal CECT image clearly shows areas of nonenhancement ➡ within the inferior 2/3 of the enlarged spleen (splenomegaly). Normal tissue shows enhancement ➡. Fluid ➡ surrounding the spleen indicates rupture.*

TERMINOLOGY

Abbreviations

- Splenic artery (SA); splenic vein (SV)

Definitions

Global or segmental parenchymal splenic ischemia and necrosis caused by vascular occlusion

IMAGING

General Features

- Best diagnostic clue
  - Hypoechoic region within splenic parenchyma on grayscale US that is avascular on Color Doppler
  - Key concepts
    - Acute infarction: Hypo- to anechoic (depending on stage), avascular; different patterns, size, morphology
      □ Bright band sign
    - Chronic infarction: Atrophic, scarred spleen
    - Assess for underlying cause
      □ Presence of splenomegaly
      □ Evaluate splenic artery and vein for occlusion or thrombosis
- Location
  - Infarction: Classically in peripheral location (i.e., abutting splenic capsule), but may be nonperipheral
  - SA occlusion: Usually entire artery; or distal only
  - SV thrombosis: Entire vein or distal only (near hilum)
- Size
  - Focal (polar or central location) vs. global (entire spleen)
- Morphology
  - Classic acute infarct: Peripheral wedge-shaped
  - Other appearances: Rounded/spherical or peripheral band

Ultrasonographic Findings

- Grayscale ultrasound
  - **Acute infarct**
    - Classic: Hypoechoic, peripheral, wedge-shaped region
    - Grayscale findings may not appear for 24-48 hours after loss of blood flow
    - Over time, may become iso- to hyperechoic
    - **Bright band sign**: Parallel thin specular reflectors perpendicular to US beam within hypoechoic parenchymal lesions
  - **Chronic infarct**: Atrophy, scarring/indentation of splenic contour, ± calcification
  - **Acute SA occlusion**: Grayscale diagnosis unlikely
  - **Chronic SA occlusion**: Absence of SA (scarred)
  - **SV thrombosis (SVT)**: Echogenic material in SV (with good visualization)
    - Look for neoplastic mass surrounding/invading SV
- Color Doppler
  - **Acute infarct**: Classically avascular or hypovascular; power Doppler helpful to confirm
  - **Acute SA occlusion**: SA visible but no blood flow in part or all of lumen
  - **Chronic SA occlusion**: Nonvisualization of all or part of SA, with possible visualization of collaterals

  - **Acute SV thrombosis**: SV visualized but no flow on color Doppler
    - Tumor invasion: Mass adjacent to/surrounding SV; low-resistance arterial flow in tumor vessels
    - Note: Visualization of blood flow in splenic hilar branches does not exclude SV thrombosis
  - **Chronic SV thrombosis**: Nonvisualization of part or all of SV (scarred)
    - Classic findings: Massive left-sided venous collaterals (splenogastric or splenorenal) **without** findings indicative of portal hypertension

CT Findings

- Acute segmental: Wedge-shaped or rounded low-attenuation/hypovascular area
- Acute global: Complete nonenhancement of spleen ± cortical rim sign
- Chronic: Atrophy, ± calcification; absence (complete autoinfarction)

MR Findings

- T1: Acute, ↑ signal in areas of hemorrhagic infarction; Chronic, ↓ signal; no C+
- T2: ↑ signal in area of infarct

Imaging Recommendations

- Best imaging tool
  - Contrast-enhanced CT or MR more accurate than US for most splenic vascular disorders
- Protocol advice
  - Color and power Doppler US are essential for US diagnosis; grayscale value alone is limited

DIFFERENTIAL DIAGNOSIS

Splenic Laceration/Hematoma

- Hematoma may be indistinguishable by imaging alone depending on stage
- History of trauma is crucial

Splenic Cyst/Mass

- Abscess or complex splenic cysts may mimic infarct if contents are echogenic
- May be consequence of infarction (i.e., superinfection or pseudocyst)

Splenic Metastases

- May see blood flow in lesion(s)
- Metastases to spleen are not common due to lack of afferent lymphatics and contractile motion of the spleen which may squeeze tumor emboli out
- If spleen involved with metastases, typically liver involved as well

Splenic Lymphoma

- May appear as marked splenomegaly, multiple hypoechoic masses, or single large mass in spleen

PATHOLOGY

General Features

- Etiology
  - Infarction due to embolization

– Emboli to small intraparenchymal arteries → small infarcts, often multiple, may be asymptomatic
– Emboli to splenic artery/major branches → large or massive infarcts, acute symptoms
– Cardioembolic: Myocardial infarction, atrial fibrillation
– Atheroembolic: Aorta, celiac artery
– Emboli from aneurysm: Aortic, celiac, SA
○ Infarction due to severe splenomegaly
– Chronic myelogenous leukemia, myelofibrosis (extramedullary hematopoiesis), lymphoma, hemoglobinopathies, infections (EBV, CMV, malaria)
– Infiltrative disorders → splenomegaly and increased oxygen requirement; congestion from intrasplenic microcirculatory obstruction and possibly anemia; result: Ischemia that may become critical → infarction
– Hemoglobinopathies → splenomegaly/increased oxygen demand and direct microcirculatory obstruction (e.g., sickle cell crisis)
○ Infarction due to splenic artery occlusion
– Atherosclerosis, vasculitis, fibromuscular dysplasia, complication of liver transplantation/other surgery, torsion (wandering spleen)
○ Infarction due to SVT or parenchymal small vessel thrombosis
– Pancreatitis-related SVT
□ Chronic pancreatitis: 10-40% SV thromboses
□ Associated with pseudocysts: (1) edema, cellular infiltration, fibroinflammatory reaction in vein wall; (2) direct compression of SV
□ Acute pancreatitis: Less frequent cause than chronic pancreatitis
– Other etiologies: Hypercoagulable states, direct neoplastic invasion/compression (usually pancreatic carcinoma), portal vein thrombosis > SV extension, abdominal sepsis (SV thrombophlebitis), blunt trauma, complication of variceal sclerotherapy or surgery

Gross Pathologic & Surgical Features

- Infarction
  ○ Necrosis/hemorrhage within splenic parenchyma; possibly splenic pseudocyst chronically

Microscopic Features

- Bright band sign thought to reflect preserved fibrous trabeculae surrounded by intervening coagulative necrosis
- Infarction may be accompanied by microscopic features of an underlying infiltrative disorder

CLINICAL ISSUES

Presentation

- Most common signs/symptoms
  ○ Often asymptomatic, found incidentally by imaging
    – Only ~ 10% of infarcts are recognized clinically
    – Asymptomatic infarcts are small but may be sequential and multiple
  ○ Left upper quadrant abdominal pain; nausea/vomiting/malaise
  ○ Splenomegaly, due to congestion, inflammation, hemorrhage, or underlying disorder
  ○ If related to chronic SV thrombosis, may see secondary signs related to varices (such as upper GI bleeding)

Demographics

- Age
  ○ Related to underlying disorders
- Gender
  ○ Related to underlying disorders
- Epidemiology
  ○ Governed by underlying disorders

Natural History & Prognosis

- Small infarcts → parenchymal scarring
  ○ Multiple infarcts may reduce splenic function
- Large infarcts
  ○ Resorption of necrotic tissue/hematoma → scar
  ○ Encapsulation of necrotic tissue/hematoma → pseudocyst
  ○ Splenic abscess: Potential complication especially when infarct caused by septic embolization
  ○ Splenic rupture
- Acute SA or SV thrombosis
  ○ May cause infarction and associated pathology, but collateralization may prevent this outcome
- Chronic SV thrombosis
  ○ Possible gastroesophageal hemorrhage, depending on route of major collaterals
  ○ Can be recurrent, intractable, life threatening

Treatment

- **Infarction**: Treatment governed by size
  ○ Small: Self-limiting, no treatment
  ○ Large: Observation or splenectomy; rupture risk with massive infarcts
- **SA or SV thrombosis**: Treatment governed by extent of infarction and gastroesophageal hemorrhage
  ○ Gastroesophageal hemorrhage: Endoscopic sclerotherapy, splenectomy if recurrent/intractable

DIAGNOSTIC CHECKLIST

Image Interpretation Pearls

- Classic appearance of acute splenic infarct: Hypoechoic, peripheral, wedge shaped, and avascular
  ○ Non-classic: Rounded or peripheral band morphology; global infarction; hyperechoic
  ○ Bright band sign
- Chronic infarction: Atrophic, scarred spleen, ± calcification
- Associated findings: Splenomegaly, SV occlusion (with large perisplenic varices), SA thrombosis

SELECTED REFERENCES

1. Llewellyn ME et al: The sonographic "bright band sign" of splenic infarction. J Ultrasound Med. 33(6):929-38, 2014
2. Mackenzie DC et al: Identification of splenic infarction by emergency department ultrasound. J Emerg Med. 44(2):450-2, 2013
3. Benter T et al: Sonography of the spleen. J Ultrasound Med. 30(9):1281-93, 2011
4. Kamaya A et al: Multiple lesions of the spleen: differential diagnosis of cystic and solid lesions. Semin Ultrasound CT MR. 27(5):389-403, 2006
5. Madoff DC et al: Splenic arterial interventions: anatomy, indications, technical considerations, and potential complications. Radiographics. 25 Suppl 1:S191-211, 2005
6. Goerg C et al: Splenic infarction: sonographic patterns, diagnosis, follow-up, and complications. Radiology. 174(3 Pt 1):803-7, 1990

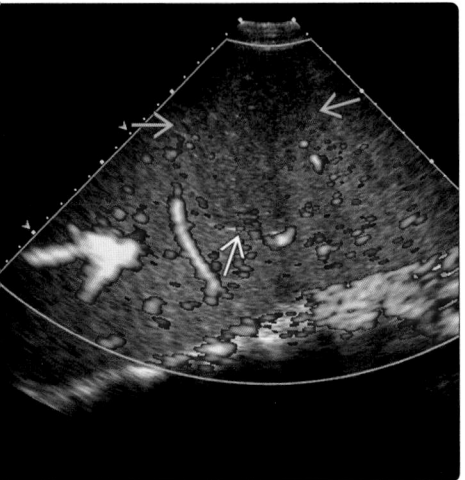

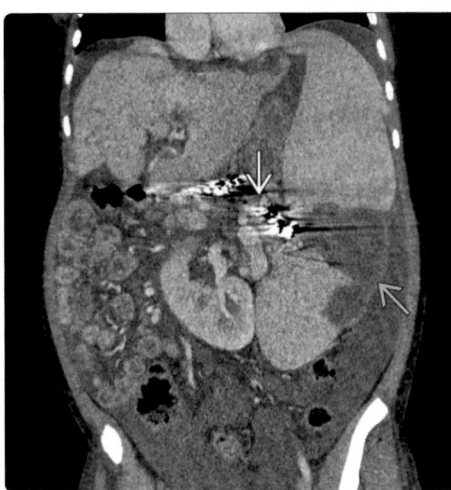

(Left) Power Doppler US of the spleen in longitudinal plane shows a central, well-demarcated, wedge-shaped area of relative hypoechogenicity ➡. There is diminished (but not absent) power Doppler signal within the area of infarct ➡. (Right) Corresponding coronal CECT in a patient with end-stage liver disease with portal hypertension marked by massive ascites and splenomegaly with central infarct ➡. Streak artifact from metallic embolization coils present ➡ (therapeutic splenic artery emobilization).

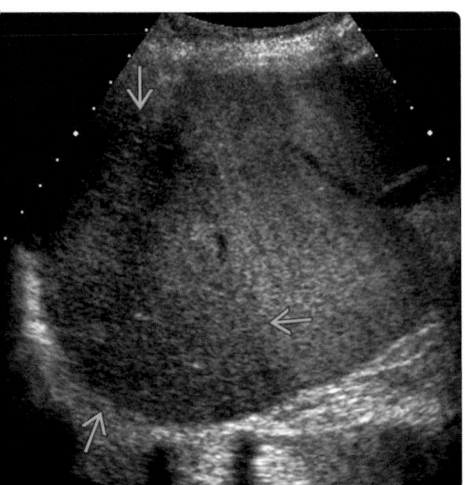

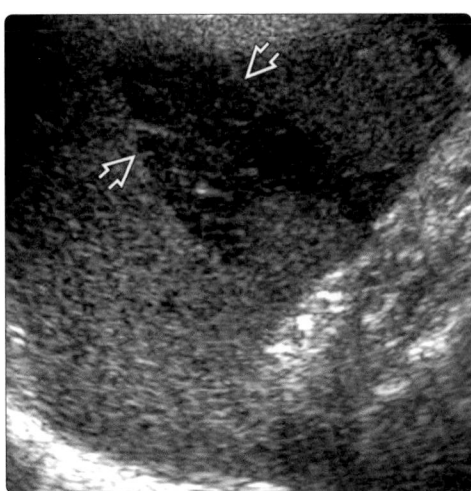

(Left) Rounded polar splenic infarct is shown on grayscale US. The infarcted area is hypoechoic and well-demarcated ➡. Color Doppler (not shown) demonstrated absent flow. (Right) A mimic of splenic infarction is splenic laceration, shown here as a well-defined, hypoechoic, band-like area ➡ extending to the subcapsular region. The history of trauma is an important differentiating factor. The spleen is the most frequently injured intraperitoneal organ in patients with blunt abdominal trauma.

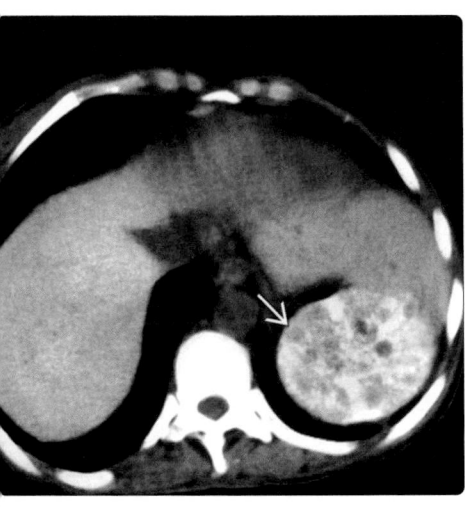

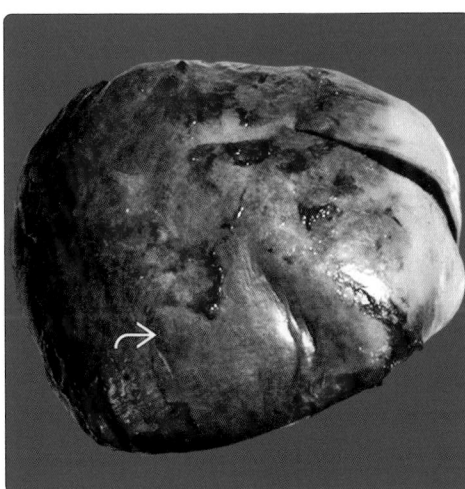

(Left) Axial NECT shows a heavily calcified and heterogeneous spleen ➡, indicating chronic, and possibly acute, infarction. (Right) The splenectomy specimen shows a mottled spleen with capsular discoloration ➡ that was heavily calcified on microscopy.

PART II
SECTION 5
Urinary Tract

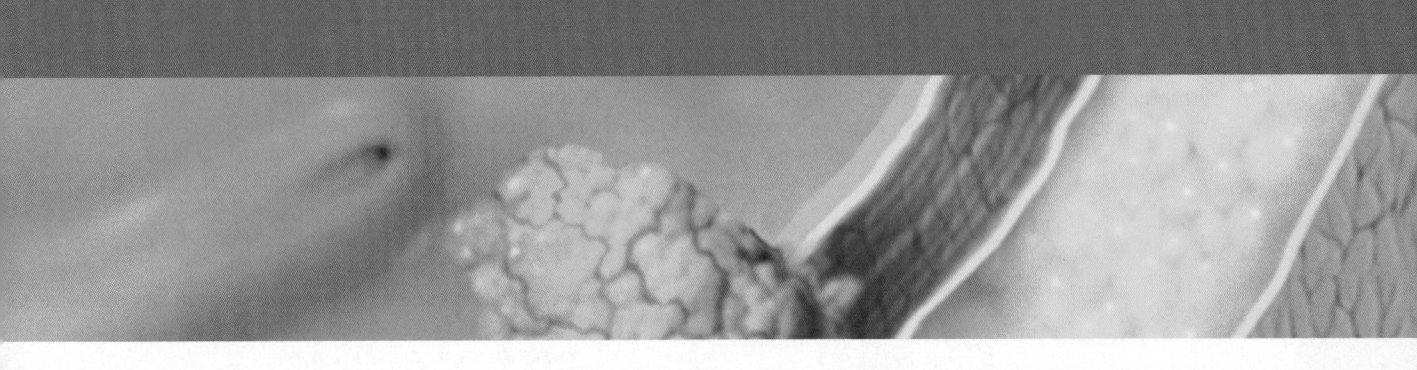

Imaging Anatomy

Standard retroperitoneal ultrasound includes transabdominal scanning of the kidneys and bladder. The adrenal glands and ureters are usually not visible unless they are enlarged or dilated, respectively. The prostate gland is sometimes well seen through the sonographic window of the bladder, but dedicated prostate sonography requires a transrectal approach.

Kidneys

- Bean-shaped parenchymal organs oriented obliquely in upper retroperitoneum
- Perinephric space is filled with fat, invested by Gerota fascia
- Serosal surface of kidney is covered by capsule; not sonographically visible unless thickened
- Renal cortex is outer rind of parenchyma; may be lobulated in infancy and generally thins with advancing age
- Medullary pyramids extend from cortex into central kidney, usually less echogenic than cortex
- Renal calyces converge on renal pelvis
- Renal sinus fat surrounds pelvis

Ureters

- Muscular tubes draining urine from kidneys to bladder
- Peristalsis occurs at regular intervals, increasing with greater urine volume
- Rarely seen unless dilated

Bladder

- Hollow organ in central pelvis with muscular wall
- Ureteral orifices are posterior, at approximately 5 and 7 o'clock positions in supine patient
- Trigone is specialized muscular segment posteriorly that connects internal urethral orifice and ureteral orifices

Imaging Protocols

Abdominal sonography should be performed with the highest frequency technique that the patient body habitus allows, to maximize resolution. Typically, this is a curved 3-8 MHz transducer. As with other abdominal organs, visualization of the urinary tract structures is quite dependent upon patient body habitus and clinical status, as well as sonographer experience and tenacity.

Kidneys

- May be imaged using liver or spleen as sonographic window respectively, or posteriorly
- Multiple transverse and longitudinal images should be obtained
- Correct obliquity is needed for accurate measurement of length
- Harmonics often useful for deeply positioned organs or to "clear" cyst; commonly used for best imaging and to reduce artifact, for example in evaluating renal cyst content
- Color Doppler evaluation needed to assess vascularity of any indeterminate lesions
- Most institutions proceed to spectral Doppler assessment of renal arteries, veins, and arcuate artery resistive indices when collecting system dilation is present
- Spatial compounding improves image quality but can obscure posterior acoustic effects like shadowing and enhancement; consider turning off to preserve these features when needed for diagnosis
- Color Doppler with high-PRF settings (machine maximum) may be useful to demonstrate "twinkling" artifact on surface of stones

Bladder

- Bladder distension allows more accurate assessment of wall thickness
- Post void residual volume may be measured in 3 dimensions and calculated when clinically requested
- Mobility and vascularity of any masses should be evaluated
- Color Doppler can be used to evaluate for ureteral jets if obstruction suspected; can also be performed transvaginally in women

Clinical Implications

Top 4 Urinary Tract Issues Resolved With Ultrasound

For renal failure, rule out hydronephrosis

- Assessment of renal pelvis and calyceal dilation
- Evaluate renal cortical thickness and echogenicity; renal insufficiency is usually chronic and nonmechanical in origin in hospitalized patients
- Evaluate intrarenal resistive indices: Symmetric?
- Check ureteral jets if asymmetric collecting system dilation

For pain, rule out stones

- Tiny stones often occult by sonography
- Echogenic shadowing focus with twinkling artifact has highest positive predictive value
- Presence or absence of hydronephrosis governs management

For lesion, rule out mass

- Differentiate cysts from masses
- Use harmonics to "clear" cyst
- Document septations, nodules, calcifications or layering density in lesion
- Color Doppler to demonstrate vascularity in solid lesion

For infection, rule out structural abnormality

- Evaluate collecting systems for dilation or duplication
- Urothelial thickening or abscess may be seen in acute infection
- Bladder imaging for jets, ureteroceles, trabeculations, diverticula, debris, or masses

Selected References

1. Rahbari-Oskoui F et al: Renal relevant radiology: radiologic imaging in autosomal dominant polycystic kidney disease. Clin J Am Soc Nephrol. 9(2):406-15, 2014
2. Remer EM et al: ACR Appropriateness Criteria(®) on renal failure. Am J Med. 127(11):1041-8.e1, 2014
3. Wagstaff PG et al: The role of imaging in the active surveillance of small renal masses. Curr Urol Rep. 15(3):386, 2014
4. Kang SK et al: Contemporary imaging of the renal mass. Urol Clin North Am. 39(2):161-70, vi, 2012
5. Dillman JR et al: Sonographic twinkling artifact for renal calculus detection: correlation with CT. Radiology. 259(3):911-6, 2011
6. Kim HC et al: Color Doppler twinkling artifacts in various conditions during abdominal and pelvic sonography. J Ultrasound Med. 29(4):621-32, 2010
7. Kamaya A et al: Twinkling artifact on color Doppler sonography: dependence on machine parameters and underlying cause. AJR Am J Roentgenol. 180(1):215-22, 2003
8. Diagnostic Ultrasound, 4th Ed. Rumack CM, Wilson SR, Charboneau JW, Levine D, eds. Elsevier Mosby 2011

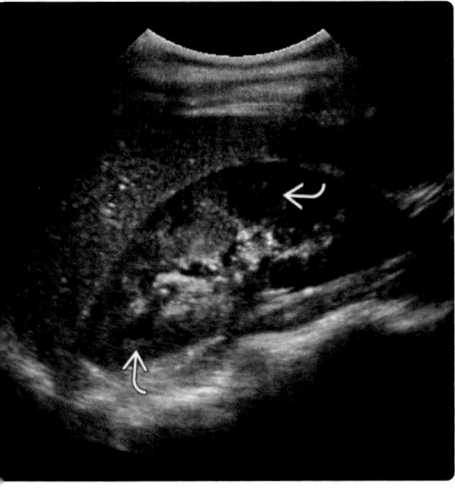
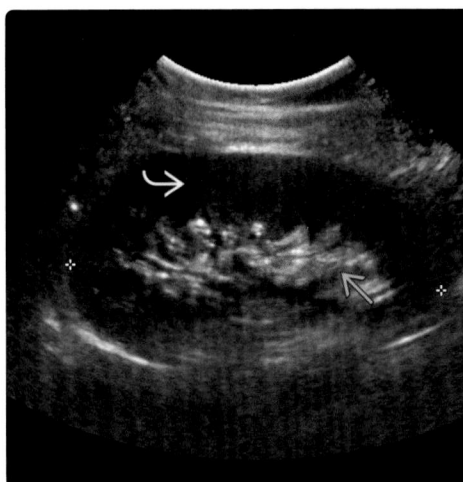

(Left) *Normal kidney in longitudinal oblique view through the liver shows relatively hypoechoic medullary pyramids ⮕.* (Right) *Corticomedullary differentiation may not always be sonographically apparent, even in normal kidneys. Patient habitus and technical factors may create a relatively homogeneous cortex and medulla ⮕, as in this normal kidney. The echogenic material centrally ⮕ is renal sinus fat and collapsed renal pelvis.*

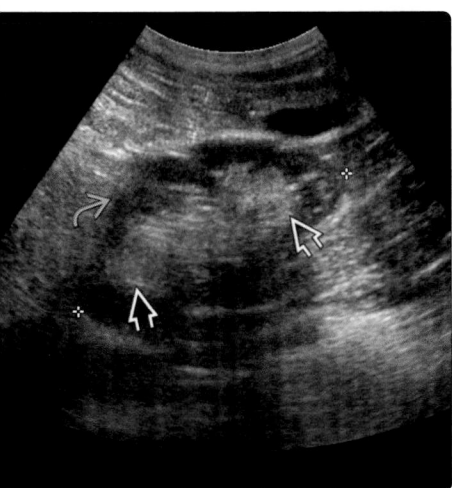
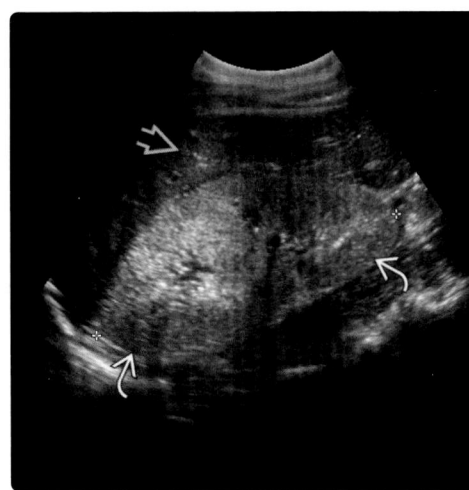

(Left) *This kidney in an elderly patient exhibits renal atrophy and cortical thinning ⮕. Note that the kidney is small in size and the echogenic renal sinus fat appears expanded ⮕, replacing the lost parenchyma.* (Right) *The renal cortex ⮕ is markedly echogenic compared with the adjacent liver ⮕ in this patient with lupus nephritis.*

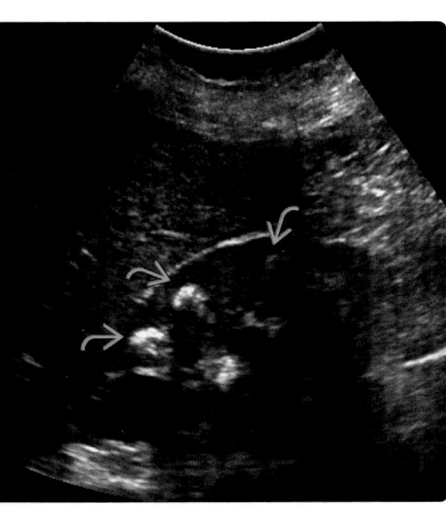
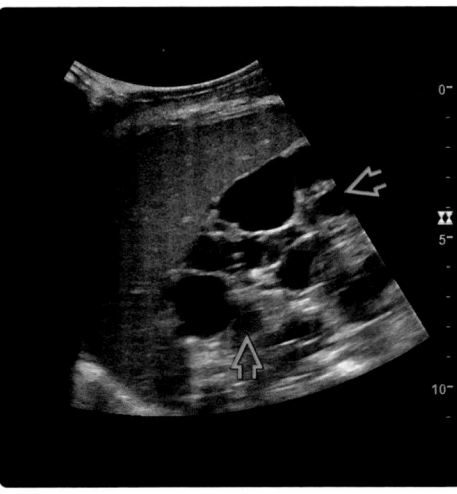

(Left) *The renal pyramids ⮕ are highly echogenic in this patient with medullary nephrocalcinosis.* (Right) *The kidney ⮕ is massively enlarged and the parenchyma replaced by cysts in this patient with polycystic kidney disease.*

(Left) *Echogenic, shadowing foci* ➡ *in the renal pelvis with associated twinkling artifact* ➡ *are diagnostic of nephrolithiasis.* (Right) *The left renal collecting system* ➡ *is dilated, but the cortex is normal thickness, compatible with an acute process in this patient with flank pain.*

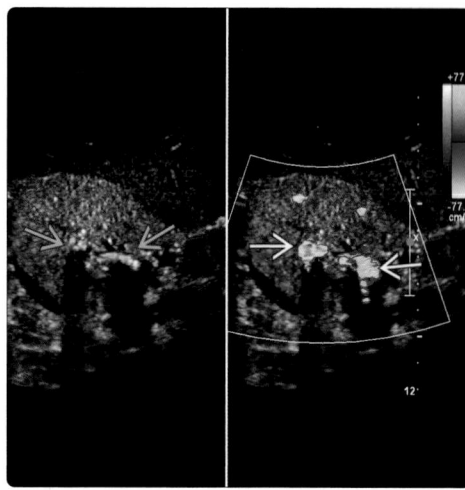
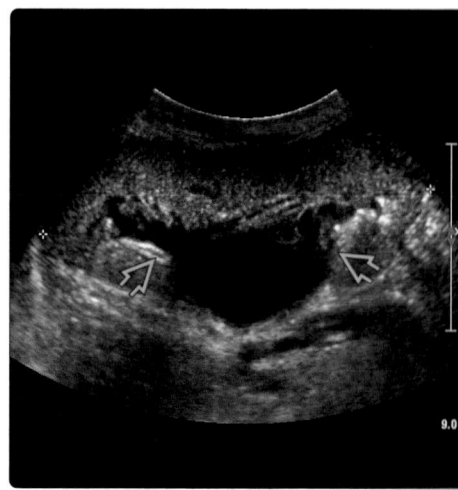

(Left) *The left ureter is dilated throughout its imaged length* ➡. (Right) *The ureteral obstruction is due to an echogenic shadowing calculus* ➡ *with associated twinkling artifact* ➡ *at the left ureterovesical junction.*

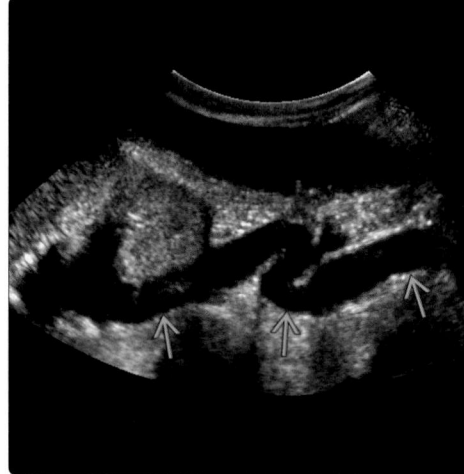
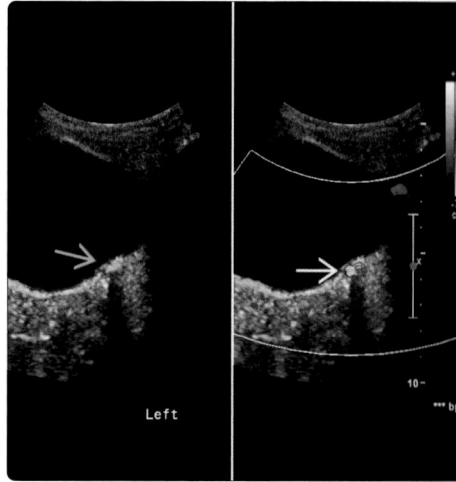

(Left) *A large stone (calipers) is noted in the right ureter in another patient. Note posterior acoustic shadowing* ➡. (Right) *Coronal CT in the same patient confirms a dilated right ureter* ➡ *due to a mid-ureteral stone* ➡.

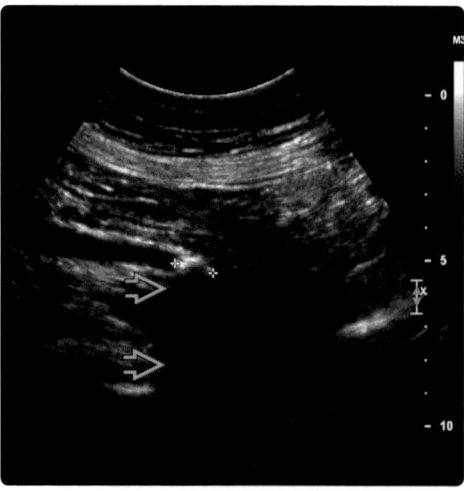
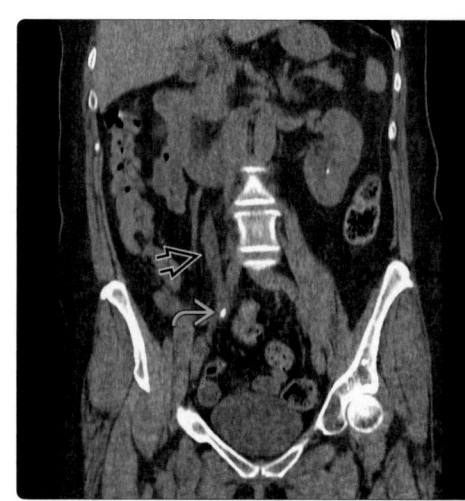

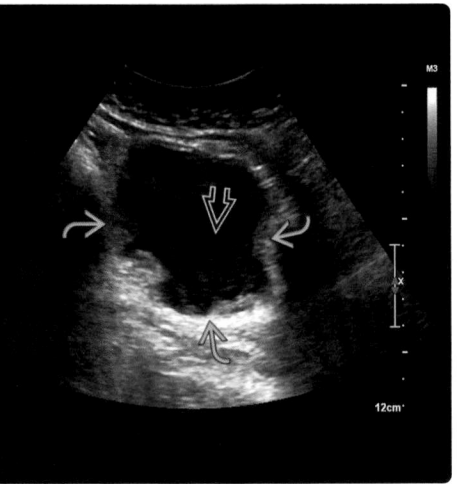

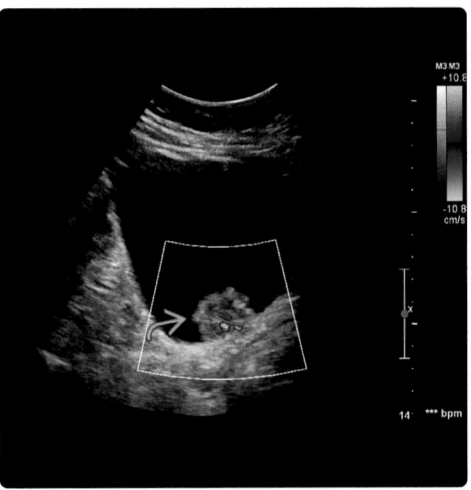

(Left) *The urinary bladder wall is thickened and trabeculated* ⊿ *and there is intraluminal debris* ⇉ *in this patient with neurogenic bladder.* (Right) *This polypoid mass with internal vascularity* ⊿ *was an incidental finding in a 62-year-old woman. Cystoscopy confirmed papillary urothelial carcinoma.*

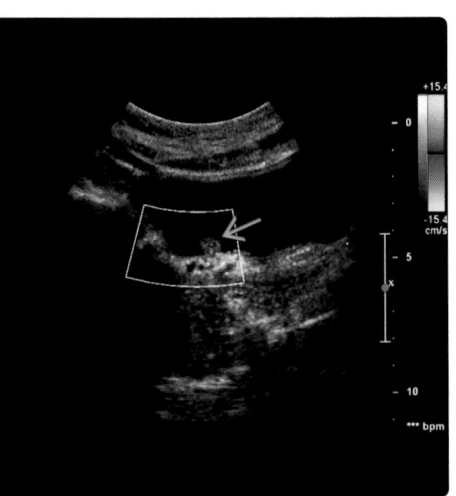

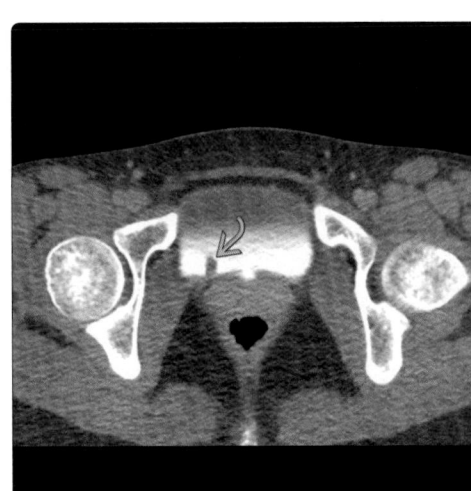

(Left) *This tiny bladder mass* ⇉ *caused hematuria in a 25 year old.* (Right) *Excretory phase CT shows a small polypoid mass* ⊿ *near the right ureteral orifice. The mass was excised and the diagnosis was papillary urothelial neoplasm of low malignant potential (PUNLMP).*

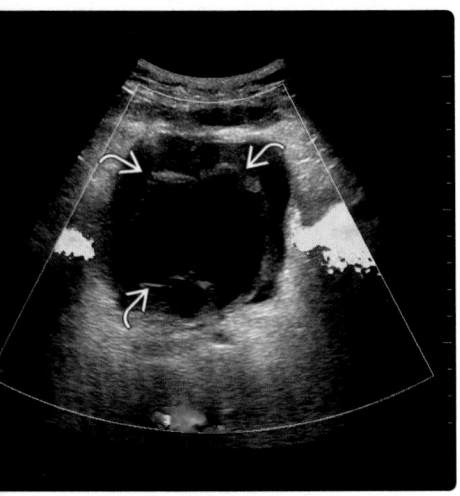

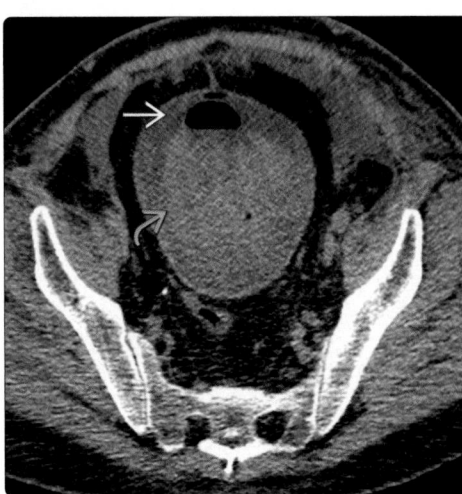

(Left) *Color Doppler US shows thick and irregular but avascular septations* ⇉ *within the bladder lumen in a patient with hemorrhagic cystitis.* (Right) *Coronal CT in the same patient a few days later shows a large hematoma in the bladder lumen* ⊿*, as well as gas* ⇉ *introduced at the time of Foley catheter placement.*

Column of Bertin, Kidney

TERMINOLOGY

- Hypertrophic band of normal cortical tissue that separate pyramids of renal medulla

IMAGING

- Isoechoic and continuous with renal cortex, indenting renal sinus laterally
- Echogenicity may be increased because of anisotropy
- At junction of upper and middle 1/3 of kidney
- Left side > right side
- Extends between renal pyramids
- Normal renal contour
- No vascular distortion with preserved arcuate arteries surrounding pyramids
- Similar enhancement as normal renal cortex on corticomedullary and excretory phases on CECT
- Similar signal intensity to renal cortex on T1W, T2W and contrast-enhanced sequences

TOP DIFFERENTIAL DIAGNOSES

- Renal tumor
- Renal scarring
- Renal duplication
- Dromedary hump

PATHOLOGY

- Embryology: Incomplete resorption of polar parenchyma or subkidneys that fuse to form normal kidney

CLINICAL ISSUES

- Most commonly asymptomatic (presents as imaging finding)
- Normal variant
- Most likely to simulate mass on sonography

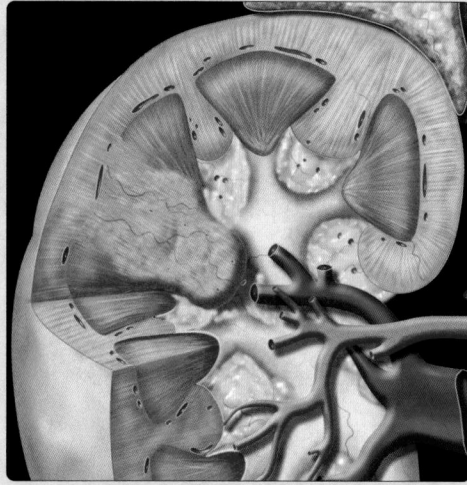
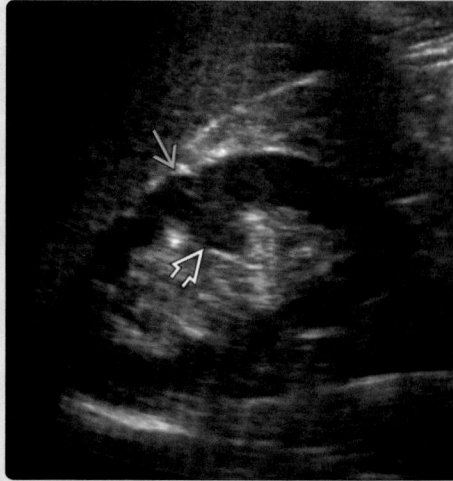

(Left) *Graphic shows a column of Bertin, which is not a real mass but an extension of renal cortical tissue between the pyramids.* (Right) *Longitudinal ultrasound of the right kidney demonstrates a hypertrophied column of Bertin* ➡ *indenting the sinus fat in the mid kidney. Note its isoechogenicity relative to the cortex and the smooth external contour* ➡.

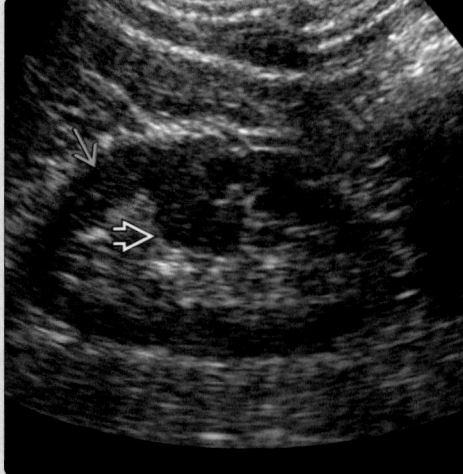
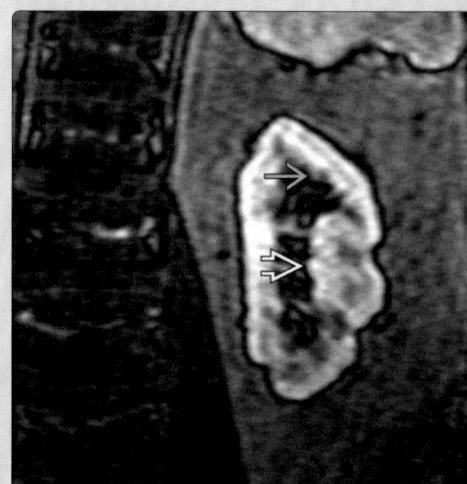

(Left) *Longitudinal ultrasound of the left kidney demonstrates a hypertrophied column of Bertin* ➡, *which is isoechoic to renal cortex* ➡. (Right) *Enhanced MR of the same patient (performed for another renal lesion, not shown) shows that the lesion* ➡ *has the same signal intensity as the renal cortex* ➡, *compatible with a hypertrophied column of Bertin.*

TERMINOLOGY

Synonyms

Hypertrophic or enlarged column of Bertin, junctional parenchyma, lobar dysmorphism, renal pseudotumor, renal septum, septal cortex, focal cortical hyperplasia, benign cortical rest

Definitions

Hypertrophic band of normal cortical tissue that separates pyramids of renal medulla

IMAGING

General Features

Best diagnostic clue
- Isoechoic and continuous with renal cortex, indenting renal sinus laterally
- No abnormal vascularity

Location
- At junction of upper and middle 1/3 of kidney
- Left side > right side
- Unilateral > bilateral (18% of cases)

Size
- Less than 3 cm

Ultrasonographic Findings

Grayscale ultrasound
- Homogenous round lesion isoechoic to renal cortex
- Extends between renal pyramids
- Normal renal contour
- Bordered by echogenic junctional parenchymal line and echogenic triangular junctional parenchymal defect
- Indentation of renal sinus laterally
- Echogenicity may be increased because of anisotropy

Color Doppler
- Normal perfusion indicating normal renal tissue
- No vascular distortion with preserved arcuate arteries surrounding pyramids
- No abnormal vessels

Contrast-enhanced ultrasound
- Enhancement of column of Bertin is identical to normal renal cortex on all phases

CT Findings

CECT
- Similar enhancement as normal renal cortex on corticomedullary and excretory phases

MR Findings

Similar signal intensity to renal cortex on T1WI, T2WI, and contrast-enhanced sequences

DIFFERENTIAL DIAGNOSIS

Renal Tumor

Renal cell carcinoma

Lymphoma

Angiomyolipoma

Metastases
- Masses usually differ in echogenicity from renal cortex and may be heterogeneous
- Doppler: Masses may be hypervascular or displace arcuate arteries

Renal Scarring

- Cortical loss at site of scarring
- Adjacent compensatory hypertrophy of unaffected tissue

Renal Duplication

- 2 central echogenic renal sinuses separated by intervening bridging renal parenchyma

Dromedary Hump

- Hypoechoic pseudotumor composed of normal renal tissue
- External bulge on renal contour
- Left sided
- Secondary to moulding of kidney by spleen

PATHOLOGY

General Features

- Embryology: Incomplete resorption of polar parenchyma of subkidneys that fuse to form normal kidney
  - Normal renal development: Superior and inferior subkidneys corresponding to upper and lower calyces fuse, with upper pole of inferior subkidney overlapping lower pole of superior subkidney

CLINICAL ISSUES

Presentation

- Most common signs/symptoms
  - Asymptomatic, normal variant
- Diagnosis
  - Usually found incidentally on imaging
  - Most likely to simulate mass on sonography
  - Optimize ultrasound by focusing on lesion and placing it in center of FOV

DIAGNOSTIC CHECKLIST

Consider

- Normal variant, but can mimic solid tumor

Image Interpretation Pearls

- Isoechoic to, and continuous with, renal cortex
- Normal perfusion, no vascular distortion
- No mass on CECT or T1WI C+
- In duplication, bridging parenchyma separates collecting systems; in column of Bertin, there is no bridging

SELECTED REFERENCES

1. McArthur C et al: Current and potential renal applications of contrast-enhanced ultrasound. Clin Radiol. 67(9):909-22, 2012
2. Fretzayas A et al: Differential diagnosis of renal mass. Columns of Bertin. Pediatr Nephrol. 25(3):441-4, 2010
3. Yeh HC: Some misconceptions and pitfalls in ultrasonography. Ultrasound Q. 17(3):129-55, 2001
4. Yeh HC et al: Junctional parenchyma: revised definition of hypertrophic column of Bertin. Radiology. 185(3):725-32, 1992
5. Lafortune M et al: Sonography of the hypertrophied column of Bertin. AJR Am J Roentgenol. 146(1):53-6, 1986

KEY FACTS

TERMINOLOGY

- Defect or line representing incomplete embryologic fusion of 2 primary renal lobes: Upper and lower poles of kidney

IMAGING

- Wedge-shaped hyperechoic defect or echogenic line at upper to middle 1/3 of kidney
- No associated loss of parenchyma
- Characteristic location at anterosuperior aspect of kidney
- More commonly seen on right
- Variable size of defect
- Overlays column of Bertin

TOP DIFFERENTIAL DIAGNOSES

- Scar
- Fetal lobulation
- Angiomyolipoma

PATHOLOGY

- Layer of connective tissue trapped from fusion of 2 metanephric elements in formation of kidney
- Deep diagonal groove extending from anterior surface of upper pole of kidney into hilum

CLINICAL ISSUES

- Normal variant

DIAGNOSTIC CHECKLIST

- Absence of parenchymal loss useful to differentiate it from cortical scar
- Characteristic location
- Increased echogenicity on ultrasound
- Fat density on CT
- Fat signal intensity on MR

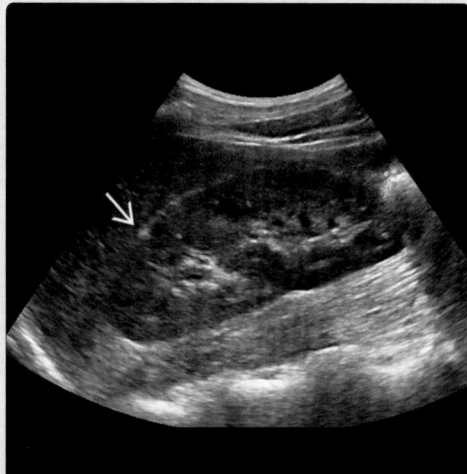
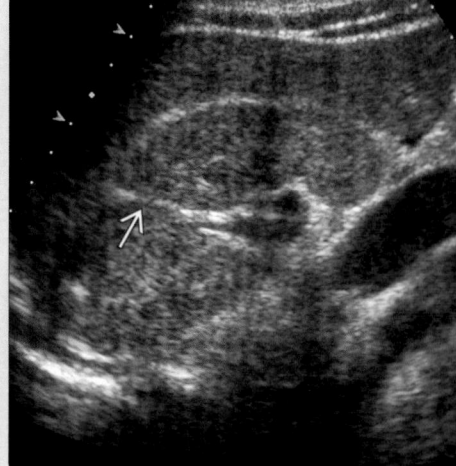

(Left) Longitudinal transabdominal ultrasound demonstrates a junctional parenchymal defect ➡ as a small triangular echogenic focus between the upper and middle 1/3 of the kidney. (Right) Longitudinal transabdominal ultrasound demonstrates an interrenuncular septum ➡ as a thin echogenic line communicating with the renal sinus.

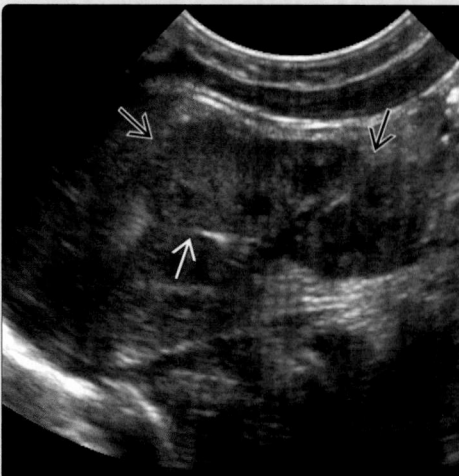
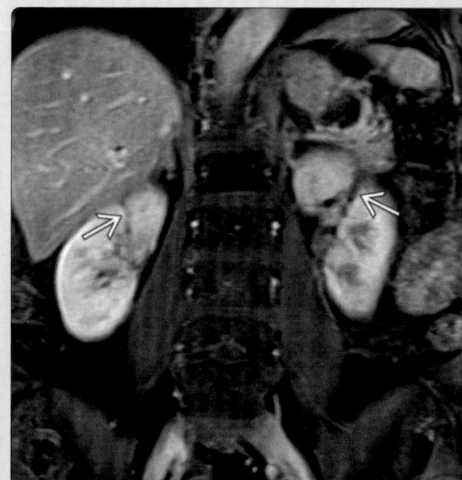

(Left) Longitudinal transabdominal ultrasound demonstrates an interrenuncular septum ➡ as a thin echogenic line at the upper to middle 1/3 of the kidney. Note the fetal lobulation ➡ as indentations between the medullary pyramids in this infant. (Right) Coronal T1 C+ FS MR of the kidneys shows bilateral interrenuncular septa ➡ as complete clefts extending into the renal sinus.

TERMINOLOGY

Synonyms

Junctional parenchymal defect

Interrenuncular septum

Oddono sulcus
- Named after Oddono, who described this in 1899

Definitions

Defect or line representing incomplete embryologic fusion of 2 primary renal lobes: Upper and lower poles of kidney

IMAGING

General Features

Best diagnostic clue
- Wedge-shaped hyperechoic defect or echogenic line at upper to middle 1/3 of kidney
- No associated loss of parenchyma
- Characteristic location at anterosuperior aspect of kidney

Location
- Upper to middle 1/3 in anterior aspect of kidney
- More commonly seen on right
- Uncommonly at posteroinferior surface via posterior approach

Size
- Variable size of defect
  - Superficial small linear indentation or sulcus
  - Deep fissure of varying depth
  - Complete cleft with lobar sulcus extending in continuity into renal sinus

Ultrasonographic Findings

Grayscale ultrasound
- Junctional parenchymal defect
  - Triangular hyperechoic defect containing fat
  - Upper to middle 1/3 of kidney
- Interrenuncular septum
  - Echogenic line at upper to middle 1/3 of kidney
  - Connects perirenal space to renal sinus
  - Occasionally may indent cortex

CT Findings

Superficial notch containing fat at anterosuperior aspect of kidney

Complete cleft crossing entire thickness of renal parenchyma into renal sinus

Overlays column of Bertin

MR Findings

T1WI
- Isointense to fat

T2WI
- Isointense to fat

T1WI C+ FS
- Nonenhancing

DIFFERENTIAL DIAGNOSIS

Scar

Associated with parenchymal thinning

Focal indentation directly over calyces

- Calyces may be dilated
- Different location from renal junction line

Fetal Lobulation

- Indentations lie between renal pyramids or calyces
- No cortical loss

Angiomyolipoma

- Discrete, round echogenic mass
- Intraparenchymal in location

PATHOLOGY

General Features

- Layer of connective tissue trapped from fusion of 2 metanephric elements in formation of kidney

Gross Pathologic & Surgical Features

- Deep diagonal groove extending from anterior surface of upper pole of kidney into hilum

CLINICAL ISSUES

Natural History & Prognosis

- Normal variant

Treatment

- None

DIAGNOSTIC CHECKLIST

Image Interpretation Pearls

- Absence of parenchymal loss useful to differentiate it from cortical scar
- Characteristic location
- Increased echogenicity on ultrasound
- Fat density on CT
- Fat signal intensity on MR

SELECTED REFERENCES

1. Siegel, Marilyn J. "Urinary Tract." In Pediatric Sonography. 4th ed. Philadelphia: Lippincott Williams & Wilkins, 2011
2. Hiromura T et al: Lobar dysmorphism of the kidney: reevaluation of junctional parenchyma using helical CT. Abdom Imaging. Mar-Apr; 24(2):196-9, 1999
3. Currarino G et al: The Oddono's sulcus and its relation to the renal "junctional parenchymal defect" and the "interrenicular septum". Pediatr Radiol. 27(1):6-10, 1997
4. Yeh HC et al: Junctional parenchyma: revised definition of hypertrophic column of Bertin. Radiology. 185(3):725-32, 1992
5. Kenney IJ et al: The renal parenchymal junctional line in children: ultrasonic frequency and appearances. Br J Radiol. 60(717):865-8, 1987
6. Carter AR et al: The junctional parenchymal defect: a sonographic variant of renal anatomy. Radiology. 154(2):499-502, 1985
7. Hoffer FA et al: The interrenicular junction: a mimic of renal scarring on normal pediatric sonograms. AJR Am J Roentgenol. 145(5):1075-8, 1985

TERMINOLOGY

- Renal ectopia (RE), crossed fused ectopia (CFE)
- Separated into multiple categories, of which simple RE and CFE represent most common forms

IMAGING

- Best diagnostic clue: Absence of kidney in expected renal fossa
- RE can range in location from pelvic (most common) to thoracic (rare)
- Simple RE: Kidney located ipsilateral to its ureteral insertion
- CFE: Ectopic kidney is malrotated; usually fusion of upper pole of ectopic kidney to lower pole of normally positioned kidney
  - Kidney located contralateral to its ureteral insertion
  - Left kidney more commonly ectopic than right
- CECT and CEMR with urography can better delineate ureteral course and presence of crossing vessels

TOP DIFFERENTIAL DIAGNOSES

- Renal transplant (iatrogenic ectopia)
- Horseshoe kidney
- Ptotic kidney
- Acquired renal displacement

PATHOLOGY

- Most common coincident urological abnormality in RE is vesicoureteral reflux
- Contralateral renal abnormalities in RE up to 50%
- Abnormalities in other organ systems in up to 1/3

CLINICAL ISSUES

- Treat complications
- No need to separate fused components

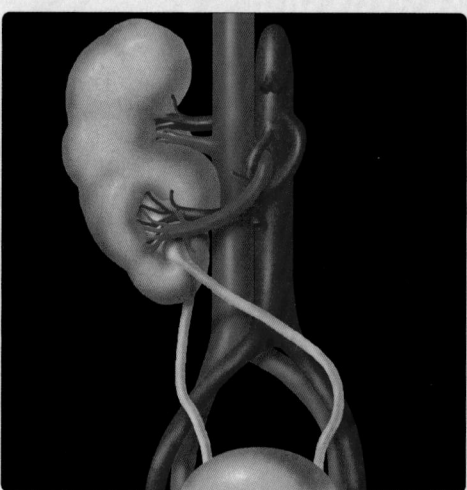
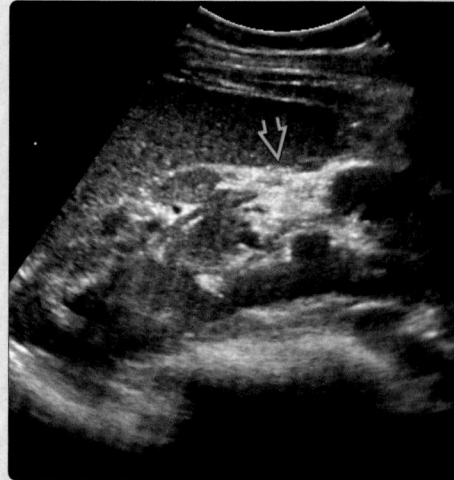

(Left) Graphic shows inferior crossed fused renal ectopia. Note the left ureter inserts on the opposite side, in its normal location. (Right) Grayscale ultrasound image demonstrates crossed fused renal ectopia on the right. Note the anterior orientation of the renal pelvis ➡.

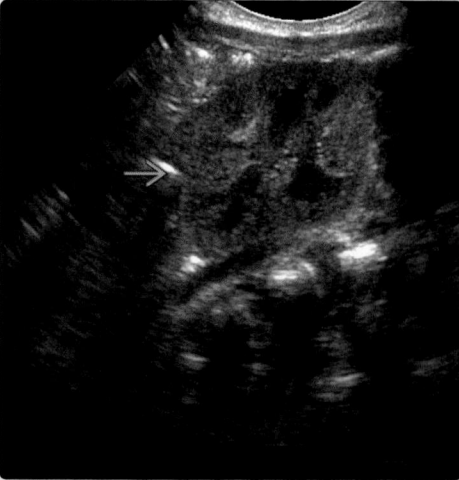
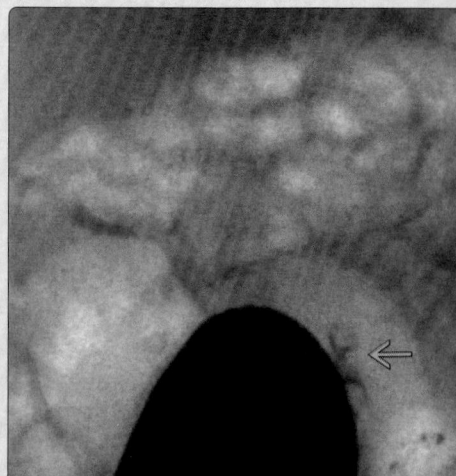

(Left) Grayscale ultrasound image demonstrates ectopic location of the left kidney ➡, which is situated within the pelvis. (Right) Voiding cystourethrogram performed in the same patient demonstrates grade 2 reflux into the ectopic left kidney ➡.

TERMINOLOGY

Abbreviations

- Renal ectopia (RE), crossed fused ectopia (CFE)

Definitions

- Aberrant location of kidney
- Separated into multiple categories, of which simple RE and CFE represent most common forms
  - Crossed nonfused RE, solitary crossed RE, and bilateral crossed RE represent rare variants

IMAGING

General Features

- Best diagnostic clue
  - Absence of kidney in expected renal fossa
  - In both CFE and RE, affected kidney noted in abnormal location
- Location
  - Normal renal position: Between transverse processes of T12-L3
  - RE can range in location from pelvic (most common) to thoracic (rare)
  - Simple RE: Kidney located ipsilateral to its ureteral insertion
  - CFE: Kidney located contralateral to its ureteral insertion
- Size
  - Ectopic kidneys vary in size

Ultrasonographic Findings

- Grayscale ultrasound
  - Simple RE
    - Aberrant location of kidney, from thorax to pelvis, with kidneys on contralateral sides
    - Ectopic kidney small and malrotated, often with dysmorphic features
    - Morphology described as "pancake," "disc," or "lump"
    - Collecting system located near surface of kidney (anterior orientation)
      - □ Normal sinus echo complex absent or eccentrically positioned
    - Intrathoracic RE
      - □ Mediastinal location
      - □ Note intact diaphragm below kidney
  - CFE
    - Both kidneys located on same side of spine
    - Empty contralateral renal fossa
    - 90% of crossed ectopia involves fusion to normally located kidney
      - □ Crossed nonfused RE rare
    - Left kidney more often ectopic than right
    - Ectopic kidney is malrotated
      - □ Usually fusion of upper pole of ectopic kidney to lower pole of normally positioned kidney
      - □ S-shaped mass with 2 renal sinuses
      - □ While normal ipsilateral ureter enters ipsilateral trigone, ureter of ectopic kidney crosses midline and enters at contralateral trigone
- Color Doppler
  - RE: Arterial supply from regional arteries

    - For example, pelvic kidney supplied by common or internal iliac arteries
    - Often with multiple arterial supply
  - CFE
    - Separate vascular supply to each kidney, with aberrant supply to ectopic kidney
      - □ Aberrant arteries may cross ureter and cause obstruction
    - Ureteric jets from ureterovesical junctions located in their normal position
    - Color Doppler may aid in prenatal diagnosis

Nuclear Medicine Findings

- Can confirm location and assess function of ectopic kidney

CT Findings

- CECT
  - Arterial phase for optimal delineation of vascular supply in both CFE and RE
  - Excretory phase for ureteral course and number

MR Findings

- MR arteriography/urography
  - Can appreciate course of ureters without use of ionizing radiation or intravenous contrast
  - Dilated ureters easier to follow
  - Contrast-enhanced sequences can delineate vascular anatomy and allow for assessment of crossing vessels

DIFFERENTIAL DIAGNOSIS

Renal Transplant (Iatrogenic Ectopia)

- Most common location for transplant is right lower quadrant
- Atrophic echogenic kidneys appreciated in bilateral renal fossae
- Renal vessels anastomosed to ipsilateral external iliac artery and vein

Horseshoe Kidney

- Fusion of lower poles of kidneys in low mid-abdomen
- Isthmus connecting kidneys in midline: Fibrous or renal tissue

Ptotic Kidney

- Mobile, low-lying kidney
- May mimic pelvic kidney
- Low position due to poor fascial reinforcement

Abdominal, Pelvic, or Thoracic Mass

- Do not have characteristic renal morphology or function

Acquired Renal Displacement

- Secondary to mass effect from hepatomegaly, splenomegaly, or abdominal mass lesion
- Autotransplantation for vascular diseases such as renal artery stenosis
- Diaphragmatic hernia can result in acquired intrathoracic kidney

PATHOLOGY

General Features

- Etiology

- o Arrested migration during embryologic development
- o RE inherited as autosomal recessive trait; reported in monozygotic twins
- o CFE related to abnormal development of ureteric bud and metanephric blastema during 4th-8th weeks of development
- Associated abnormalities
  - o Other genitourinary abnormalities in ~ 1/2 of cases
    - – RE
      - □ Vesicoureteral reflux (most common associated abnormality)
      - □ Contralateral renal abnormalities in up to 50% of RE such as renal agenesis
      - □ Absent or hypoplastic vagina
    - – CFE
      - □ Megaureter, cryptorchidism, urethral valves, multicystic dysplasia
  - o Occur in conjunction with anomalies in other organs in ~ 1/3 of cases
    - – Skeletal (up to 50%)
      - □ Rib and vertebral anomalies; scoliosis may impact renal ascent
      - □ Absence of radius
    - – Cardiovascular (40%)
    - – Gastrointestinal (33%)
      - □ Anorectal malformations such as imperforate anus
    - – Ears, lips, palate (33%)
      - □ Low-set or absent ears
      - □ External canal atresia
      - □ Cleft palate

CLINICAL ISSUES

Presentation

- Most common signs/symptoms
  - o Commonly asymptomatic, incidental finding
  - o May present with signs and symptoms of obstruction, urolithiasis, reflux, and infection

Demographics

- Epidemiology
  - o RE: Pelvic ectopia, most common
    - – Noted in 1:500 to 1:1,200
  - o CFE represents 2nd most common fusion abnormality after horseshoe kidney
    - – Male predominance, with incidence reported as M:F = 3:2
    - – Incidence reported ranging from 1:1,000 to 1:7,500 on autopsy studies
  - o Crossed nonfused RE: Very rare, reported as 1:75,000

Natural History & Prognosis

- Complications
  - o ~ 50% have complications related to vesicoureteral reflux, hydronephrosis, stones, and infection
    - – Repeated infections can lead to scarring
  - o May have increased susceptibility to trauma
  - o Increased incidence of multicystic dysplasia

Treatment

- Treat complications
- No need to separate fused components

DIAGNOSTIC CHECKLIST

Image Interpretation Pearls

- Do not confuse RE with mass in pelvis or thorax
- Do not confuse CFE with renal mass

SELECTED REFERENCES

1. Solanki S et al: Crossed fused renal ectopia: challenges in diagnosis and management. J Indian Assoc Pediatr Surg. 18(1):7-10, 2013
2. Chang PL et al: Prenatal diagnosis of cross-fused renal ectopia: does color Doppler and 3-dimensional sonography help? J Ultrasound Med. 30(4):578-80, 2011
3. Siegel MJ, ed. Pediatric Sonography. 4th edition. Baltimore: Lippincott Williams & Wilkins, 2011
4. Singer A et al: Spectrum of congenital renal anomalies presenting in adulthood. Clin Imaging. 32(3):183-91, 2008
5. Guarino N et al: The incidence of associated urological abnormalities in children with renal ectopia. J Urol. 172(4 Pt 2):1757-9; discussion 1759, 2004
6. Goodman JD et al: Crossed fused renal ectopia: sonographic diagnosis. Urol Radiol. 8(1):13-6, 1986
7. McCarthy S et al: Ultrasonography in crossed renal ectopia. J Ultrasound Med. 3(3):107-12, 1984

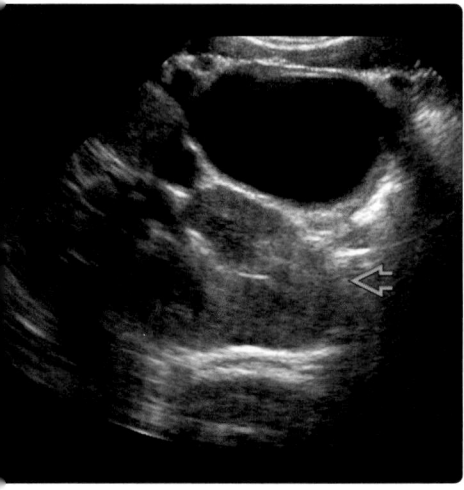
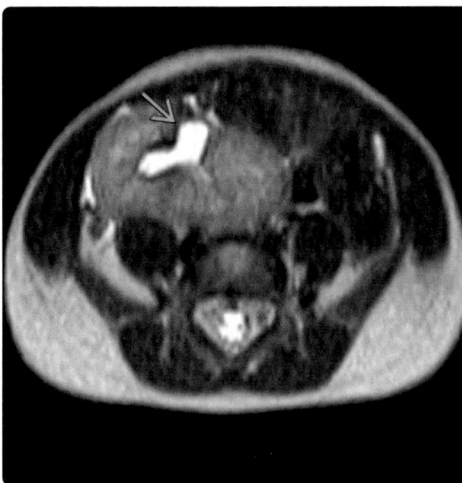

(Left) *Grayscale ultrasound image demonstrates ectopic location of the right kidney ⇨, which is located within the pelvis posterior to the bladder.* (Right) *Axial T2 HASTE image obtained in the same patient better delineates the ectopic right kidney. Note the anterior orientation of the renal collecting system ⇨.*

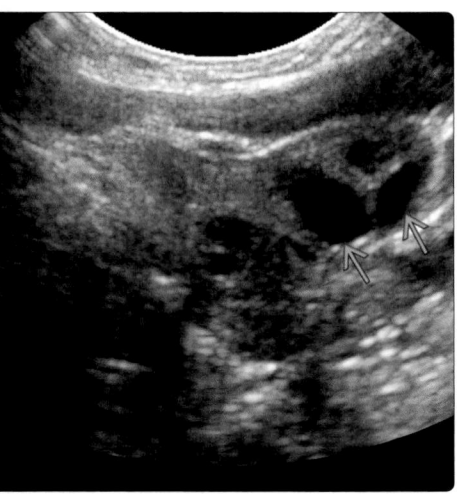
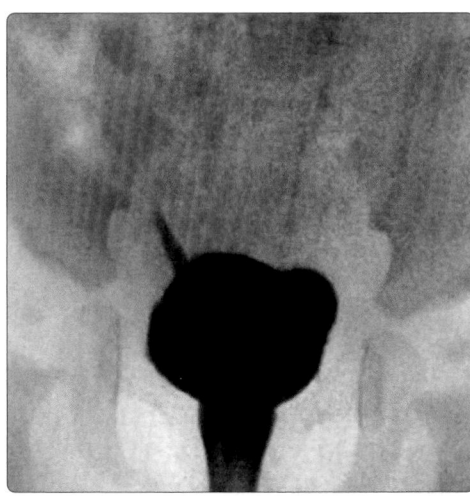

(Left) *Grayscale ultrasound image demonstrates an ectopic left kidney, located in the pelvis. Multiple discrete cysts are noted ⇨.* (Right) *Voiding cystourethrogram image in the same patient demonstrates contralateral reflux into the ureter of the normally located right kidney.*

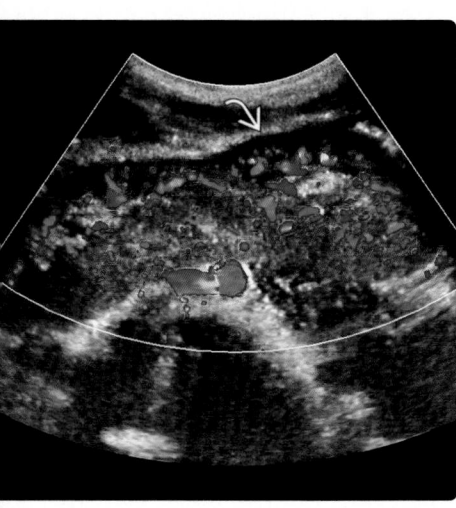
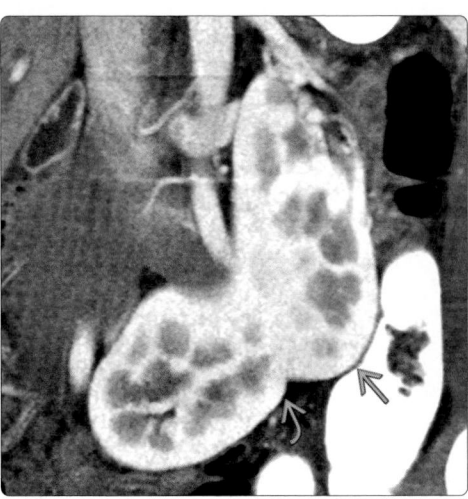

(Left) *Color Doppler ultrasound image demonstrates crossed fused ectopia ⇨ in the left lower quadrant.* (Right) *Coronal CECT in the same patient demonstrates fusion of the upper pole of the malrotated ectopic right kidney ⇨ to the lower pole of the left kidney ⇨, which is slightly lower than normal.*

Horseshoe Kidney

TERMINOLOGY

- Congenital anomaly in which kidneys are fused at their lower poles in midline
  - In contradistinction to crossed fused ectopia, where both kidneys are located on 1 side

IMAGING

- Kidneys on opposite sides with lower poles fused in midline
- Presence of isthmus is defining feature; crosses midline anterior to spine and aorta, but posterior to inferior mesenteric artery
- Cross-sectional imaging (CT or MR) to define vascular anatomy and can be used to visualize associated complications such as malignancy

TOP DIFFERENTIAL DIAGNOSES

- Renal ectopia
- Paraaortic lymphadenopathy/retroperitoneal mass

PATHOLOGY

- Proposed theory of fusion of nephrogenic blastomas at 4 weeks gestational age when still located in pelvis, preventing appropriate ascent
- Numerous associated abnormalities and congenital disorders

CLINICAL ISSUES

- Complications include obstruction, infection, nephrolithiasis, and malignancy
- Prognosis is good in absence of associated abnormalities

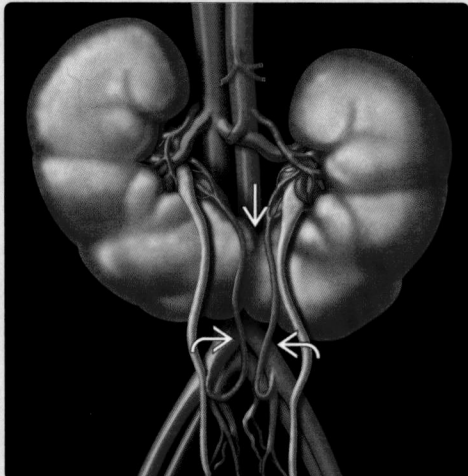 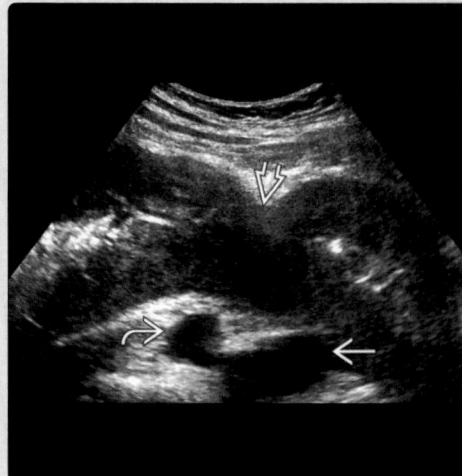

(Left) *Graphic shows a horseshoe kidney with the isthmus* ➡ *anterior to the aorta and inferior vena cava. Note the additional renal arteries arising from the common iliac arteries* ➡. (Right) *Transverse ultrasound in the midline shows a horseshoe kidney. The isthmus* ➡ *of the horseshoe kidney lies anterior to the aorta* ➡ *and inferior vena cava* ➡. *The isthmus is composed of functioning renal tissue.*

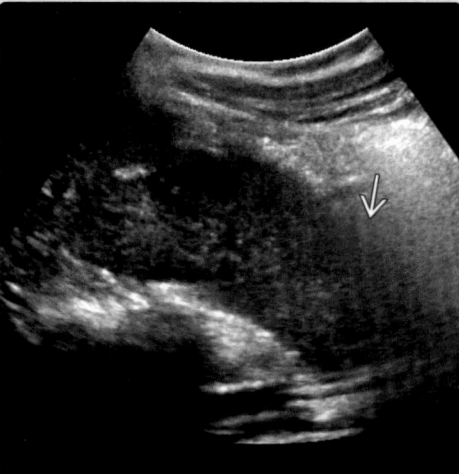 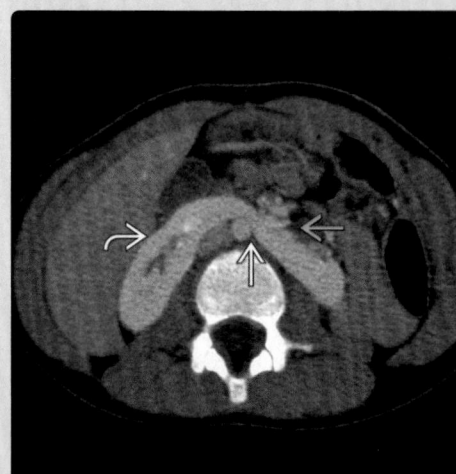

(Left) *In this longitudinal ultrasound, note the boomerang configuration of the left kidney, with the lower pole* ➡ *obscured as it bends away from the transducer.* (Right) *Axial CECT in the same patient demonstrates horseshoe kidney* ➡ *draped over the aorta* ➡ *in the lower abdomen. The inferior mesenteric artery* ➡ *prevents ascent of the kidney in utero.*

TERMINOLOGY

Definitions

- Congenital anomaly in which kidneys are fused at their lower poles in midline
  - In contradistinction to crossed fused ectopia (CFE), where both kidneys are located on 1 side

IMAGING

General Features

- Best diagnostic clue
  - Kidneys on opposite sides with lower poles fused in midline
- Location
  - Ectopic, lies lower than normal kidneys
    - Isthmus caudally positioned at L3-L5
    - Isthmus most often anterior to great vessels
      - □ Rarely, can be posterior, or less commonly in between aorta and inferior vena cava (IVC)
- Morphology
  - 2 types of fusion
    - Midline or symmetric fusion (90% of cases)
    - Uncommonly can have lateral or asymmetric fusion

Ultrasonographic Findings

- Grayscale ultrasound
  - Kidneys often low-lying
    - Renal pelvis frequently anteriorly oriented
  - Boomerang shape: Bent on sagittal imaging, with lower poles pointed away from transducer
  - Presence of isthmus is defining feature
    - Crosses midline anterior to spine and aorta, but posterior to inferior mesenteric artery
    - Can be difficult to visualize isthmus in subjects with large body habitus, or if isthmus is composed of fibrous tissue
    - Transverse midline view of aorta for best visualization
  - Look for associated collecting system dilatation (ureteropelvic junction obstruction), calculi, or signs of infection

CT Findings

- CECT
  - Often incidentally detected
  - Define structural abnormalities
    - Degree and site of fusion: Midline or lateral fusion
    - Renal malrotation
    - Collecting system abnormalities (e.g., hydronephrosis secondary to ureteropelvic junction [UPJ] obstruction)
    - Complication
      - □ Calculi
      - □ infection
      - □ Malignancy
  - Presence of enhancing tissue distinguishes functional renal tissue in isthmus vs. fibrous tissue
- CTA
  - Useful in demonstrating variant arterial supply
  - Multiple renal arteries, including arteries arising from vessels other than abdominal aorta

- e.g., common, external or internal iliac arteries, inferior mesenteric artery
  - Isthmus located posterior to inferior mesenteric artery

MR Findings

- Similar utility as CT in defining structure as well as associated abnormalities and complications, without ionizing radiation
- MRA can be utilized to define arterial supply

Nuclear Medicine Findings

- Tc-labeled radiotracers are taken up by functional renal tissue and thus can demonstrate horseshoe kidney

Imaging Recommendations

- Best imaging tool
  - US often sufficient but can be difficult to appreciate isthmus
  - CT or MR best demonstrates horseshoe kidney in its entirety

DIFFERENTIAL DIAGNOSIS

Renal Ectopia

- Kidney congenitally abnormal in position
- Crossed renal ectopia: 2 kidneys on same side of the body (left kidney more often ectopic than right)
  - Fused CFE: 90%
    - Kidneys on same side of spine; ureter of crossed kidney crosses midline to insert into bladder at contralateral trigone
  - Nonfused
    - Kidneys on same side of spine, although without fusion
    - As in CFE, ureter of crossed kidney inserts at contralateral trigone
  - Bilateral: Left and right kidneys arise on wrong side, both ureters cross midline to insert into bladder
- Ipsilateral or simple ectopia
  - Kidney on same side of body as its ureter; most often located in pelvis

Paraaortic Lymphadenopathy/Retroperitoneal Mass

- Soft tissue mass at midline anterior to spine
- Note normal appearance and location of bilateral kidneys, as well as absence of typical reniform shape of retroperitoneal tissue

PATHOLOGY

General Features

- Etiology
  - Proposed theory of fusion of nephrogenic blastomas at 4 weeks gestational age when still located in pelvis, preventing appropriate ascent
    - Abnormal flexion or growth of developing spine brings nephrogenic elements together
    - Isthmus cannot ascend due to inferior mesenteric artery
  - Alternate theory that horseshoe kidney develops due to abnormal migration of posterior nephrogenic precursors, creating an isthmus
- Genetics

○ Reported in identical twins and siblings, but no genetic component yet known
- Associated abnormalities
  ○ Congenital disorders
    – Chromosomal abnormalities: Turner syndrome (60%), trisomy 21, trisomy 18, trisomy 13, Gardner syndrome
    – Hematological abnormalities: Fanconi anemia, dyskeratosis congenita with pancytopenia
    – Laurence-Biedl-Moon syndrome
    – Thalidomide embryopathy
  ○ Genitourinary
    – UPJ obstruction
      □ May be bilateral and noted in up to 35%
    – Vesicoureteral reflux
    – Cystic dysplasia
    – Unilateral or bilateral duplication
      □ Less common: Megaureter, ectopic ureter, retrocaval ureter
    – Hypospadias
    – Septate vagina
    – Undescended testes
  ○ Gastrointestinal
    – Anorectal malformation
    – Esophageal atresia
    – Rectovaginal fistula
    – Omphalocele
  ○ Vascular: Few reports of duplicated IVC, duplicated superior vena cava (SVC), persistent left SVC
  ○ Skeletal: Kyphosis, scoliosis, macrognathia
  ○ Neurological: Encephalocele, myelomeningocele, spina bifida

Gross Pathologic & Surgical Features
- Isthmus composed most commonly of fibrous tissue, but can consist of normal parenchyma

CLINICAL ISSUES

Presentation
- Most common signs/symptoms
  ○ Commonly asymptomatic but may be identified due to associated abnormalities
  ○ May present with symptoms related to infection, stones, or obstruction, such as abdominal pain, fever, nausea/vomiting

Demographics
- Age
  ○ Any age, but decreased incidence with age as more proportionally detected earlier in life due to coincident anomalies
- Gender
  ○ M:F = 2:1
- Epidemiology
  ○ 1:400 people

Natural History & Prognosis
- Complications
  ○ Increased susceptibility to blunt trauma
    – Low position prevents protection by ribs
  ○ UPJ obstruction

– Secondary to abnormal high insertion of ureter, resulting in high UPJ
  ○ Recurrent infections
    – Due to reflux and UPJ obstruction
  ○ Nephrolithiasis
    – Increased due to stasis and infections; higher incidence of staghorn calculi
  ○ Malignancy
    – Increased risk of renal cell carcinoma: Most common neoplasm associated with horseshoe kidney
    – Wilms tumors in children: At least 2x more common
      □ Wilms tumor accounts for 28% of malignancy associated with horseshoe kidney (1/2 located within isthmus)
    – Transitional cell carcinoma: 3-4x higher incidence
    – Markedly increased incidence of primary carcinoid tumor (62x higher risk)
- Prognosis
  ○ Good, in absence of other significant abnormalities
  ○ Poor, with associated abnormalities causing significant morbidity and mortality

Treatment
- Usually none
- Surgical separation in symptomatic patients

DIAGNOSTIC CHECKLIST

Consider
- Associated abnormalities and other complications in imaging, treatment, and prognosis

Image Interpretation Pearls
- Kidney low in position, appears U-shaped with isthmus in midline
- Look for isthmus in midline anterior to aorta
- Assess for associated complications, including obstruction, infection, nephrolithiasis, malignancy

SELECTED REFERENCES

1. Natsis K et al: Horseshoe kidney: a review of anatomy and pathology. Surg Radiol Anat. 36(6):517-26, 2014
2. O'Brien J et al: Imaging of horseshoe kidneys and their complications. J Med Imaging Radiat Oncol. 52(3):216-26, 2008
3. Strauss S et al: Sonographic features of horseshoe kidney: review of 34 patients. J Ultrasound Med. 19(1):27-31, 2000
4. Banerjee B et al: Ultrasound diagnosis of horseshoe kidney. Br J Radiol. 64(766):898-900, 1991
5. Grainger R et al: Horseshoe kidney—a review of the presentation, associated congenital anomalies and complications in 73 patients. Ir Med J. 76(7):315-7, 1983
6. Mindell HJ et al: Horseshoe kidney: ultrasonic demonstration. AJR Am J Roentgenol. 129(3):526-7, 1977

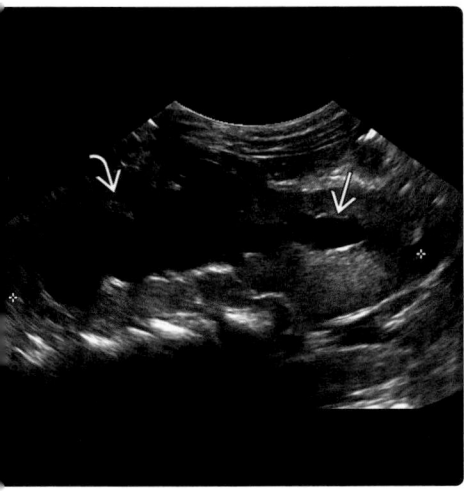

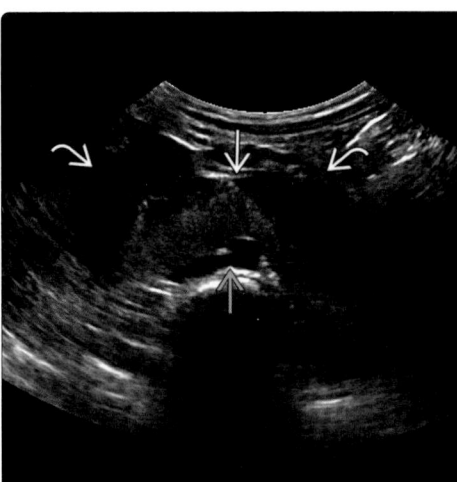

(Left) *Longitudinal oblique ultrasound through the right lower abdomen in a child shows a horseshoe kidney with hydronephrosis of both moieties. The right hydronephrosis ➡ was more severe than the left ➡. Both pelves are malrotated.* (Right) *Transverse ultrasound of the same patient shows the thick parenchymal isthmus ➡ and bilateral collecting system dilatation ➡. Aorta and inferior vena cava ➡ are also seen.*

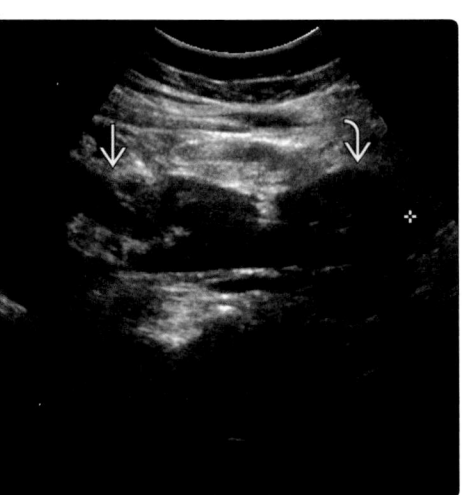

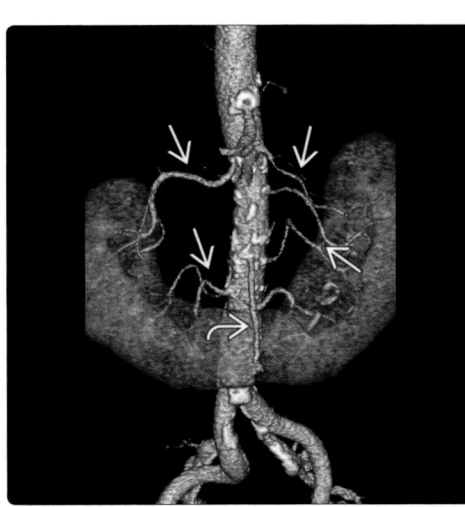

(Left) *Longitudinal oblique ultrasound of an adult with a horseshoe kidney shows the malrotated right moiety ➡ fused to the left moiety ➡.* (Right) *Volume rendered CT arteriogram of a horseshoe kidney in a 73 year old. There are multiple renal arteries ➡ supplying the kidneys. The inferior mesenteric artery ➡ runs anterior and superior to the isthmus which consists of renal tissue.*

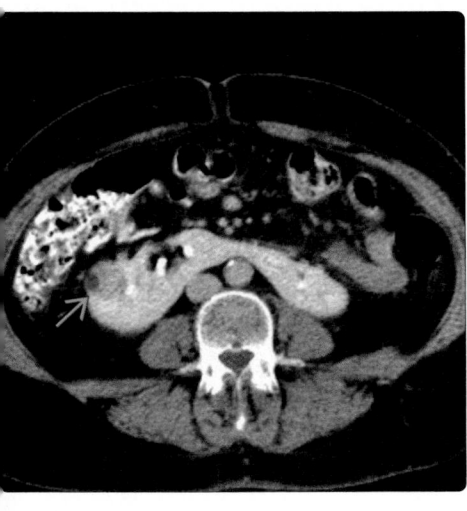

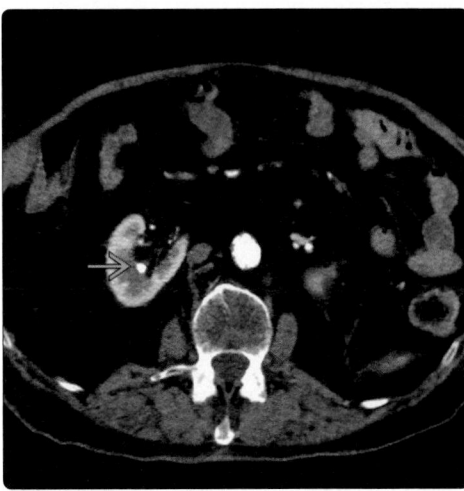

(Left) *In the right moiety of the horseshoe kidney, a hypoenhancing slightly heterogeneous mass is appreciated ➡ on this axial CECT. Because of coexisting gynecologic cancer, percutaneous ultrasound-guided biopsy was performed, revealing renal cell carcinoma.* (Right) *On this axial CECT, incidental note is made of nephrolithiasis ➡ within the right moiety of a horseshoe kidney, without obstruction.*

Ureteral Duplication

TERMINOLOGY

- Presence of 2 separate pelvicalyceal collecting systems draining 1 kidney, which may join above bladder (partial), drain into bladder separately (complete), or beyond bladder

IMAGING

- 2 distinct renal pelves or 2 exiting ureters in single kidney
- 2 central echogenic renal sinuses with intervening bridging renal parenchyma
- Weigert-Meyer rule: Upper moiety ureter inserts inferior and medial to lower moiety ureter (85%)
- Result of Weigert-Meyer rule
  - Upper pole tends to obstruct
  - Lower pole tends to have vesicoureteral reflux

TOP DIFFERENTIAL DIAGNOSES

- Column of Bertin
- Segmental multicystic dysplastic kidney

PATHOLOGY

- Abnormal bifurcation of ureteral bud arising from mesonephric duct

CLINICAL ISSUES

- Most often diagnosed on antenatal ultrasound or incidentally
- Longstanding obstruction, reflux and infection can lead to secondary hypertension and renal insufficiency/failure

DIAGNOSTIC CHECKLIST

- Young females with recurrent urinary tract infections
- US, IVP or CT/MR urography are imaging modalities of choice
- VCUG to exclude reflux

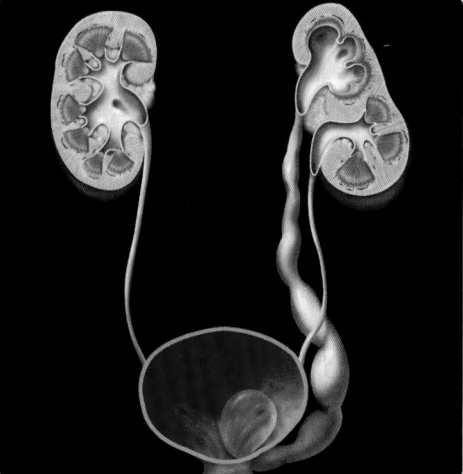 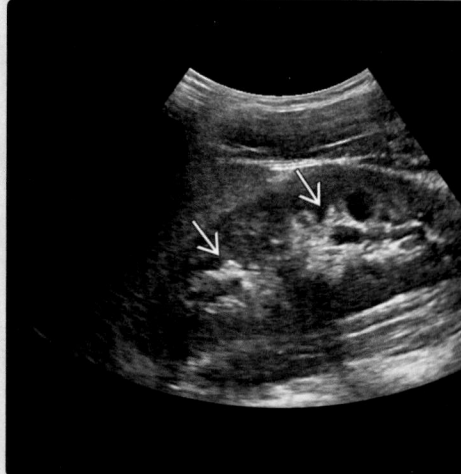

(Left) *Graphic shows a left duplex kidney. Upper moiety is hydronephrotic with hydroureter draining into a ureterocele. Note the upper moiety ureter inserts inferior and medial to lower moiety ureter.* (Right) *Longitudinal US demonstrates an intervening bridge of renal tissue, with two separate renal pelves ➡, without collecting system dilatation.*

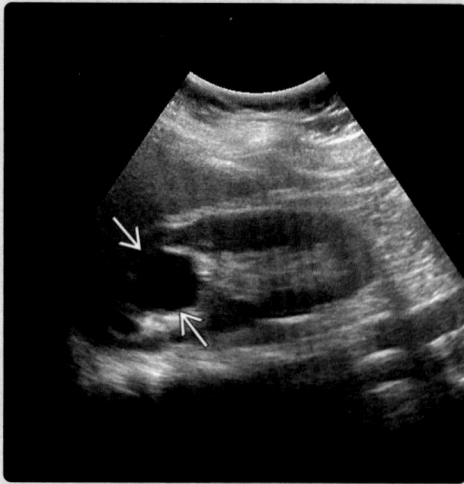 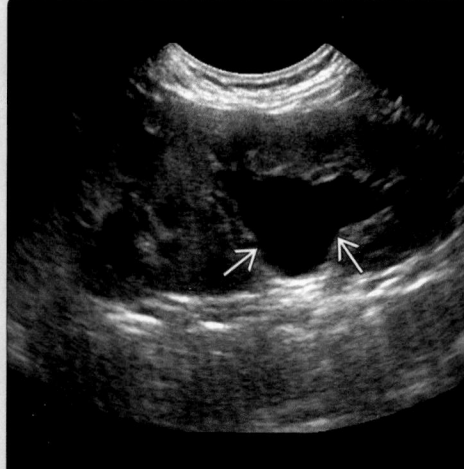

(Left) *Longitudinal US demonstrates a round anechoic structure in the upper pole ➡, reflecting a dilated upper moiety of a duplex kidney.* (Right) *Longitudinal US demonstrates a dividing prominent band of renal tissue with dilatation of the lower moiety ➡, secondary to reflux.*

TERMINOLOGY

Synonyms

- Ureteropelvic duplication, duplicated kidney, duplex or bifid collecting system

Definitions

- Presence of 2 separate pelvicalyceal collecting systems draining 1 kidney, which may join above bladder (partial), drain into bladder separately (complete), or beyond bladder

IMAGING

General Features

- Best diagnostic clue
  - 2 distinct renal pelves or 2 exiting ureters in single kidney
  - 2 central echogenic renal sinuses with intervening bridging renal parenchyma
- Other general features
  - Weigert-Meyer rule: Upper moiety ureter inserts inferior and medial to lower moiety ureter (85%)
  - Result of Weigert-Meyer rule
    - Upper pole tends to obstruct
    - Lower pole tends to have vesicoureteral reflux
  - Upper moiety ureteral insertion is by definition ectopic, and often associated with ureterocele
  - Lower moiety subjected to reflux due to its shortened ureteric tunnel at bladder insertion
  - Kidney and ureter may be normal, except duplicated
  - 20% are bilateral
  - 40% have complete duplication
  - 60% have bifid ureter

Ultrasonographic Findings

- Grayscale ultrasound
  - Asymmetric renal enlargement
  - 2 central echogenic renal sinuses with intervening bridging renal parenchyma
  - 2 distinct renal pelves or 2 exiting proximal ureters
  - Upper moiety commonly hydronephrotic due to obstruction
  - Lower moiety collecting system may also be dilated due to vesicoureteral reflux
  - With longstanding obstruction and reflux, cortical thinning/scarring with dysplastic cystic change
  - Look for presence of ureterocele (cystic structure) in bladder
- Color Doppler
  - Can be useful to distinguish collecting system from vessel in renal pelvis
  - Ureteral jets can be helpful to identify vesicoureteral junction of both upper and lower moieties

Fluoroscopic Findings

- Voiding cystourethrogram
  - Early filling defect in bladder may reflect presence of ureterocele
  - Look for reflux, usually occurring more often in lower pole than upper pole
  - Drooping lily sign: Hydronephrotic upper moiety exerts mass effect and can inferiorly displace lower pole

Nuclear Medicine Findings

- Assess relative function, drainage, and scarring, which is important for surgical planning

Radiographic Findings

- IVP (or CT/MR urography)
  - Presence of two ureters in single kidney
    - Fewer calyces & infundibula of lower pole collecting system; shortened upper pole infundibulum
  - Poor or no excretion by upper pole moiety when obstructed
  - Drooping lily sign: hydronephrotic upper moiety exerts mass effect and can inferiorly displace lower pole
  - Calyceal clubbing, thin overlying parenchyma ± scarring in lower pole

CT Findings

- "Faceless kidney": Absence of the renal sinus between upper & lower pole
- Contrast enhancement useful to detect course of ureters

MR Findings

- T2WI
  - High signal intensity fluid within collecting system
  - Maximum-intensity projection (MIP) image and coronal thick slab series helpful to demonstrate relative positions of upper and lower moiety ureters
- T1 C+
  - Poor or little excretion of upper moiety when obstructed
  - Delayed images can demonstrate whole course of non-dilated ureter

Imaging Recommendations

- Best imaging tool
  - Ultrasound, IVP, or CT/MR urography
  - VCUG to exclude vesicoureteral reflux

DIFFERENTIAL DIAGNOSIS

Column of Bertin

- Prominent band of tissue does not completely divide kidney
- Only 1 exiting ureter

Segmental Multicystic Dysplastic Kidney

- May mimic obstructed upper pole

Upper Pole Mass

- Can mimic drooping lily sign due to mass effect

Ureterocele

- Can be isolated finding

PATHOLOGY

General Features

- Etiology
  - Abnormal bifurcation of ureteral bud or 2 separate ureteral buds arising from mesonephric duct
  - Not inherited although some familial tendency reported
- Associated abnormalities
  - Increased incidence of ureteropelvic obstruction
  - Genital anomalies found in 50% of affected females

CLINICAL ISSUES

Presentation

- Most common signs/symptoms
  - Most often diagnosed on antenatal ultrasound or incidentally
  - Usually asymptomatic
  - Urinary tract infection including pyelonephritis
  - Hematuria, abdominal/flank pain due to obstruction or formation of calculi
  - Voiding dysfunction, urinary retention
  - Ectopic insertion
    - Females: Incontinence due to insertion below bladder sphincter
    - Males: Prostatitis, epididymitis
- Other signs/symptoms
  - Transitional cell carcinoma of duplicated ureter occurs in elderly population

Demographics

- Gender
  - More common in females
- Epidemiology
  - 1 per 125-250 persons

Natural History & Prognosis

- Longstanding obstruction, reflux and infection can lead to secondary hypertension and renal insufficiency/failure

Treatment

- Lower grades of reflux: Medical treatment
- Higher grades of reflux, upper pole obstruction, ectopy, poor renal function: Surgical treatment

DIAGNOSTIC CHECKLIST

Consider

- Young females with recurrent urinary tract infections
- Young females with continuous dribbling urinary incontinence

Image Interpretation Pearls

- 2 distinct renal pelves or ureters
- US, IVP, or CT/MR urography are imaging modalities of choice
- VCUG to exclude reflux

SELECTED REFERENCES

1. Lipson JA et al: Subtle renal duplication as an unrecognized cause of childhood incontinence: diagnosis by magnetic resonance urography. J Pediatr Urol. 4(5):398-400, 2008
2. Wah TM et al: Lower moiety pelvic-ureteric junction obstruction (PUJO) of the duplex kidney presenting with pyonephrosis in adults. Br J Radiol. 76(912):909-12, 2003
3. Callahan MJ: The drooping lily sign. Radiology. 219(1):226-8, 2001
4. Zissin R et al: Renal duplication with associated complications in adults: CT findings in 26 cases. Clin Radiol. 56(1):58-63, 2001
5. Fernbach SK et al: Ureteral duplication and its complications. Radiographics. 17(1):109-27, 1997
6. Ulchaker J et al: The spectrum of ureteropelvic junction obstructions occurring in duplicated collecting systems. J Pediatr Surg. 31(9):1221-4, 1996
7. Bellah RD et al: Ureterocele eversion with vesicoureteral reflux in duplex kidneys: findings at voiding cystourethrography. AJR Am J Roentgenol. 165(2):409-13, 1995
8. Fernbach SK et al: Complete duplication of the ureter with ureteropelvic junction obstruction of the lower pole of the kidney: imaging findings. AJR Am J Roentgenol. 164(3):701-4, 1995
9. Husmann DA et al: Ureterocele associated with ureteral duplication and a nonfunctioning upper pole segment: management by partial nephroureterectomy alone. J Urol. 154(2 Pt 2):723-6, 1995
10. Share JC et al: The unsuspected double collecting system on imaging studies and at cystoscopy. AJR Am J Roentgenol. 155(3):561-4, 1990
11. Winters WD et al: Importance of prenatal detection of hydronephrosis of the upper pole. AJR Am J Roentgenol. 155(1):125-9, 1990
12. Share JC et al: Ectopic ureterocele without ureteral and calyceal dilatation (ureterocele disproportion): findings on urography and sonography. AJR Am J Roentgenol. 152(3):567-71, 1989
13. Ahmed S et al: Vesicoureteral reflux in complete ureteral duplication: surgical options. J Urol. 140(5 Pt 2):1092-4, 1988
14. Bisset GS 3rd et al: The duplex collecting system in girls with urinary tract infection: prevalence and significance. AJR Am J Roentgenol. 148(3):497-500, 1987
15. Mesrobian HG: Ureteropelvic junction obstruction of the upper pole moiety in complete ureteral duplication. J Urol. 136(2):452-3, 1986
16. Nussbaum AR et al: Ectopic ureter and ureterocele: their varied sonographic manifestations. Radiology. 159(1):227-35, 1986
17. Amis ES Jr et al: Lower moiety hydronephrosis in duplicated kidneys. Urology. 26(1):82-8, 1985
18. Lavallee G et al: Obstructed duplex kidney in an adult: ultrasonic evaluation. J Clin Ultrasound. 13(4):281-3, 1985
19. Gartell PC et al: Renal dysplasia and duplex kidneys. Eur Urol. 9(2):65-8, 1983
20. Inamoto K et al: Duplication of the renal pelvis and ureter: associated anomalies and pathological conditions. Radiat Med. 1(1):55-64, 1983
21. Gates GF: Ultrasonography of the urinary tract in children. Urol Clin North Am. 7(2):215-22, 1980
22. Morgan CL et al: Ultrasonic diagnosis of obstructed renal duplication and ureterocele. South Med J. 73(8):1016-9, 1980
23. Rose JS et al: Ultrasound diagnosis of ectopic ureterocele. Pediatr Radiol. 8(1):17-20, 1979
24. Mascatello VJ et al: Ultrasonic evaluation of the obstructed duplex kidney. AJR Am J Roentgenol. 129(1):113-20, 1977

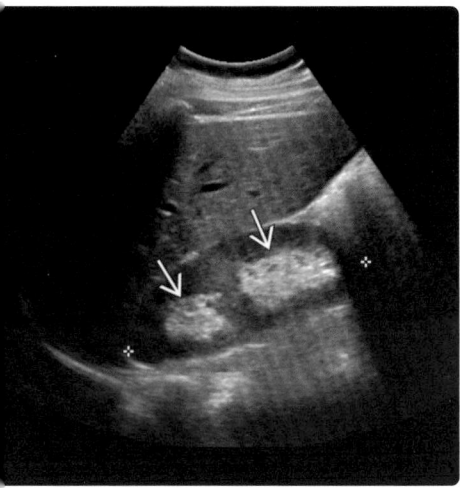

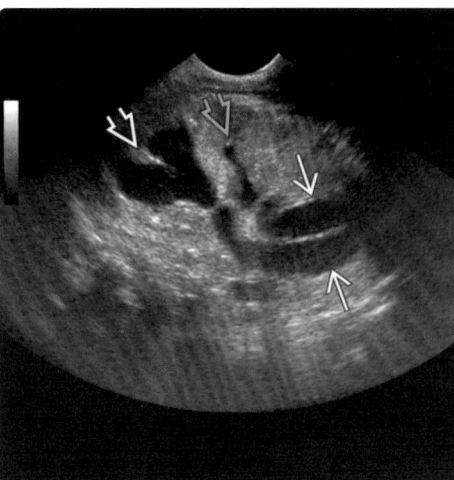

(Left) Longitudinal US demonstrates 2 renal pelves ➔, separated by intervening bridging renal tissue. (Right) Longitudinal US demonstrates 2 exiting ureters ➔ compatible with duplication. The upper moiety is hydronephrotic ➔ and the lower moiety is also mildly dilated ➪, secondary to vesicoureteral reflux.

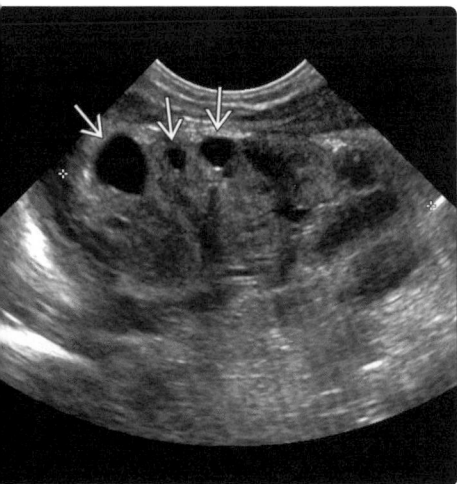

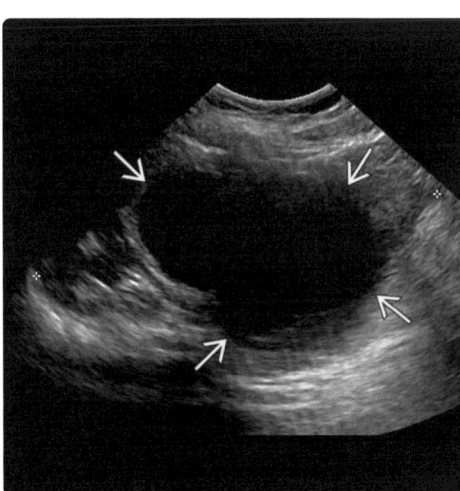

(Left) Longitudinal US demonstrates dysplastic cystic changes ➔ of an obstructed upper moiety with loss of the normal corticomedullary differentiation and cortical thinning. (Right) Longitudinal US demonstrates marked dilatation ➔ of a lower moiety renal pelvis, shown to be ureteropelvic junction obstruction.

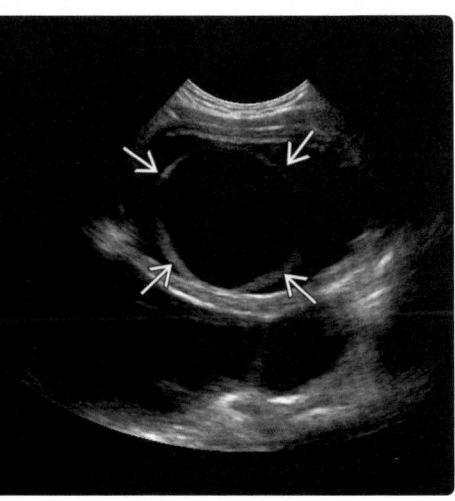

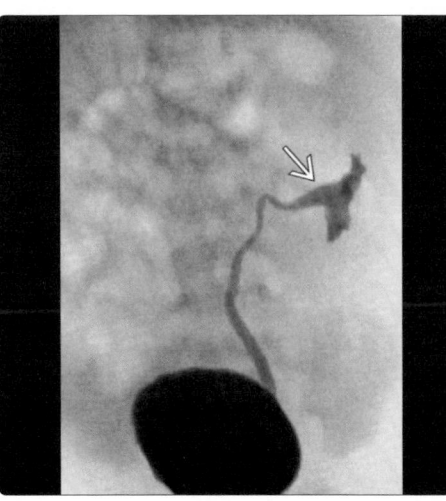

(Left) Transverse US demonstrates a round, thin-walled, anechoic structure ➔ within the bladder compatible with an ureterocele. (Right) Voiding cystourethrogram demonstrates the drooping lily sign, with opacification of a lower moiety ureter and renal pelvis, with displacement of the normal axis ➔ by an obstructed upper moiety.

TERMINOLOGY

- Strict definition: Ureter that does not terminate at bladder trigone
- Common usage: Ureter that terminates outside bladder

IMAGING

- Best diagnostic clue
  - 70-80% associated with complete ureteral duplication
  - Dilated ureter that extends beyond bladder
- Extravesicular insertion
  - Males: Prostatic urethra most common insertion site
  - Females: Vestibule or urethra most common insertion site
- Orifice commonly stenotic, leading to obstruction of renal moiety

TOP DIFFERENTIAL DIAGNOSES

- Bladder diverticulum
- Hydrosalpinx

PATHOLOGY

- Failure of separation of ureteral bud from wolffian duct results in caudal ectopia

CLINICAL ISSUES

- Recurrent or chronic urinary tract infections (UTIs)
- Females: Continuous dribbling urinary incontinence (50%) due to insertion below external sphincter
- Males: Chronic or recurrent epididymitis
  - No incontinence due to insertion above external sphincter
- M:F = 1:6
- Females: 80% of ectopic ureters are duplicated systems
- Males: Majority associated with single system ectopic ureter (SSEU)

DIAGNOSTIC CHECKLIST

- Consider diagnosis in female with continuous dribbling urinary incontinence

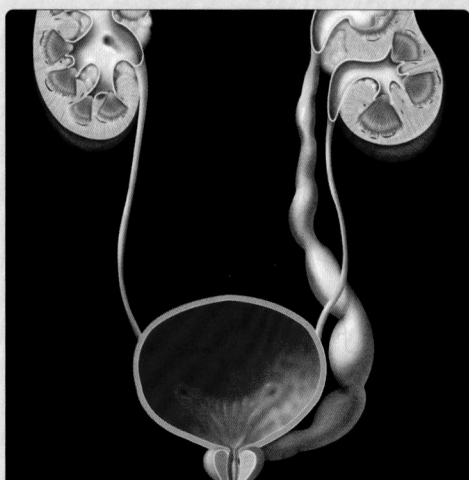
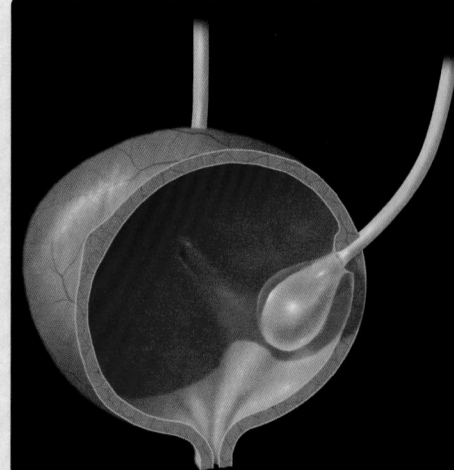

(Left) Graphic shows a dilated upper moiety ureter of a left duplex kidney with extravesicular ectopic insertion into the prostatic urethra. (Right) Graphic shows intravesicular insertion of a ureter from a duplex left kidney with an associated ureterocele.

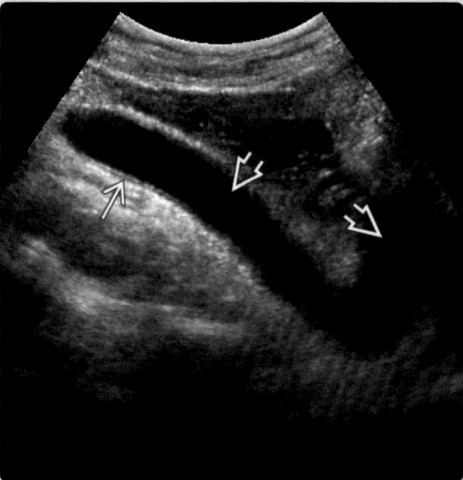
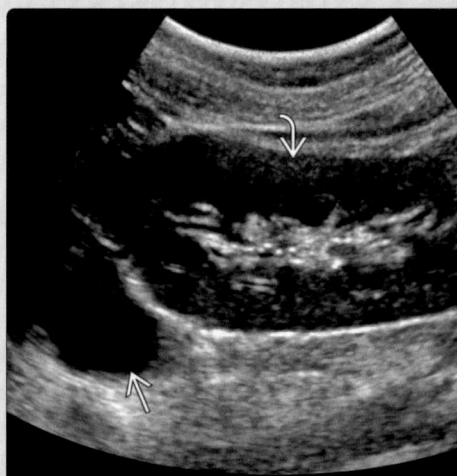

(Left) Longitudinal oblique ultrasound of the left pelvis shows a dilated ureter ➡. There is mild urothelial thickening ➡. (Right) Longitudinal ultrasound of the left kidney shows a fluid-filled thin-walled structure ➡ representing the atrophic upper pole moiety of a duplicated system. The lower pole moiety appears normal ➡.

Ureteral Ectopia

TERMINOLOGY

Abbreviations

- Ectopic ureter (EU)

Definitions

- Ureter that does not terminate at bladder trigone
- Common usage: Ureter that terminates outside bladder (extravesicular)

IMAGING

General Features

- Best diagnostic clue
  - 70-80% associated with complete ureteral duplication
  - Dilated ureter that extends beyond bladder
- Location
  - Intravesicular insertion with complete ureteral duplication
    - Weigert-Meyer rule: Upper moiety ureter inserts inferior and medial to lower moiety ureter
    - Results of Weigert-Meyer rule
      - □ Upper pole tends to obstruct
      - □ Lower pole tends to have vesicoureteral reflux
  - Extravesicular insertion
    - Males: Prostatic urethra most common insertion site
      - □ Prostatic urethra: 54%, seminal vesicle: 28%, vas deferens: 10%, ejaculatory duct: 8%
    - Females: Vestibule or urethra most common insertion site
      - □ Vestibule: 38%, urethra: 32%, vagina: 27%, uterus or cervix: 3%
  - 5-17% of EUs are bilateral
- Morphology
  - Orifice commonly stenotic, leading to obstruction of renal moiety

Ultrasonographic Findings

- Grayscale ultrasound
  - Dilated ureter extends beyond bladder trigone
    - Transrectal/transvaginal US may delineate site of insertion
  - Ureterocele may be present if ectopic vesicular insertion
  - Hydronephrotic or dysplastic renal moiety
  - Detection of fetal hydronephrosis may be earliest sign
- Color Doppler
  - Ureteral jet can be used to identify ectopic intravesicular insertion
  - Compare normal position of contralateral ureteral jet at interureteric bar

Radiographic Findings

- IVP
  - Complete ureteral duplication
    - Dilated upper pole collecting system
    - Nonvisualization of upper pole moiety with severe obstruction/dysplasia
      - □ Visualized lower pole moiety: Fewer calyces than normal for entire kidney
      - □ Lower pole displaced inferolaterally by obstructed upper pole ("drooping lily" sign)

- Single-system ectopic ureter (SSEU): Usually small, dysplastic, and nonfunctioning kidney

Fluoroscopic Findings

- Voiding cystourethrogram
  - Early filling defect in bladder may reflect presence of ureterocele
  - Look for reflux into either moiety, most commonly, lower
  - May locate insertion of EU if within urinary tract (bladder neck or posterior urethra)

CT Findings

- CECT
  - Hydronephrotic upper moiety with variable function
  - Dilated, tortuous ureter to level of insertion
  - Males with SSEUs: Dilated ipsilateral seminal vesicle
  - May be used occasionally to locate small, poorly functioning, dysplastic kidney

MR Findings

- T2WI
  - High signal intensity fluid within collecting system
  - With obstruction, tortuous dilated ureter can be followed to level of ectopic insertion
  - High signal cystic dysplasia of upper pole moiety
- T1WI C+
  - Poor or little excretion when upper moiety is obstructed
  - Delayed images can demonstrate whole course of ureter to level of ectopic insertion

Nuclear Medicine Findings

- Renal scintigraphy
  - Assess relative function, drainage, and scarring, which is important for surgical planning

Imaging Recommendations

- Best imaging tool
  - Ultrasound and CT/MR urography
    - MR urography can display ectopic ureteral insertions, even those outside urinary tract
  - CT may be useful to locate small, poorly functioning, dysplastic kidney with single EU
  - VCUG to exclude reflux in complete ureteral duplication
- Protocol advice
  - Trace dilated ureter on US to its termination below bladder

DIFFERENTIAL DIAGNOSIS

Bladder Diverticulum

- Fluid-filled round or ovoid outpouching from bladder, with neck

Hydrosalpinx

- Also tubular but has incomplete septa and tiny mural folds
- Anechoic and thin walled when chronic
- Thick walled with internal debris and thicker folds when acutely infected in pelvic inflammatory disease
- Does not course in craniocaudal direction

Dilated Pelvic Vessels

- Typically more numerous

- Evidence of color Doppler flow

Fluid-Filled Bowel Loop

- Active peristalsis and change in configuration during real-time scanning

Seminal Vesical Cyst

- Lateral to bladder base, superior to prostate
- Associated with ipsilateral renal agenesis
- May contain internal echoes from debris or hemorrhage
- EU may drain into seminal vesicle

Urachal Cyst or Diverticulum

- Midline and supravesical
- Tubular or spherical and fluid filled

Müllerian, Ejaculatory Duct, and Utricular Cysts

- Midline, posterior and inferior to bladder, not tubular

PATHOLOGY

General Features

- Etiology
  - Congenital: Abnormal ureteral bud migration
    - Failure of separation of ureteral bud from wolffian duct
    - EU is situated along path of wolffian duct
    - Caudal to normal ureteral insertion
- Associated abnormalities
  - Hypoplasia or dysplasia of renal moiety drained by EU
    - Degree of ureteral ectopia correlates with degree of renal abnormality
  - Urethral duplication, hypospadias, cloacal abnormalities
  - VACTERL spectrum including imperforate anus, tracheoesophageal fistula

Gross Pathologic & Surgical Features

- SSEU: Absent ipsilateral hemitrigone
- Distance from trigone correlates with degree of renal dysplasia

Microscopic Features

- Muscularis of ectopic ureteral wall may have ultrastructural abnormalities

CLINICAL ISSUES

Presentation

- Most common signs/symptoms
  - Recurrent or chronic urinary tract infections (UTIs)
  - Females: Continuous dribbling urinary incontinence (50%) due to insertion below external sphincter
  - Males: Chronic or recurrent epididymitis
    - No incontinence due to insertion above external sphincter
  - May be asymptomatic

Demographics

- Age
  - Age at diagnosis varies widely
  - Some cases not detected during life
  - Many cases diagnosed with prenatal ultrasound
- Gender

  - M:F = 1:6
  - Females: 80% of EUs are duplicated systems
  - Males: Majority associated with SSEU
  - SSEUs more common in males
- Epidemiology
  - Incidence: At least 1 in 1,900
  - True incidence uncertain since many cases asymptomatic

Natural History & Prognosis

- Most EUs drain single kidneys, which tend to be hypoplastic or dysplastic or upper pole moieties with minimal function

Treatment

- Surgery depends on function and whether system is duplicated
- EU with duplicated system: Partial upper pole nephrectomy
- SSEU: Nephrectomy if minimal function
- If renal function preserved or if diagnosis is made prenatally: Ureteropyelostomy or common sheath ureteral implantation

DIAGNOSTIC CHECKLIST

Consider

- EU in female with continuous dribbling urinary incontinence

Image Interpretation Pearls

- Dilated ureter extends beyond bladder trigone
- 70-80% associated with complete ureteral duplication

SELECTED REFERENCES

1. Figueroa VH et al: Utility of MR urography in children suspected of having ectopic ureter. Pediatr Radiol. 44(8):956-62, 2014
2. Ehammer T et al: High resolution MR for evaluation of lower urogenital tract malformations in infants and children: feasibility and preliminary experiences. Eur J Radiol. 78(3):388-93, 2011
3. Roy Choudhury S et al: Spectrum of ectopic ureters in children. Pediatr Surg Int. 24(7):819-23, 2008
4. Wille S et al: Magnetic resonance urography in pediatric urology. Scand J Urol Nephrol. 37(1):16-21, 2003
5. Berrocal T et al: Anomalies of the distal ureter, bladder, and urethra in children: embryologic, radiologic, and pathologic features. Radiographics. 22(5):1139-64, 2002
6. Damry N et al: Ectopic vaginal insertion of a duplicated ureter: demonstration by magnetic resonance imaging (MRI). JBR-BTR. 84(6):270, 2001
7. Staatz G et al: Magnetic resonance urography in children: evaluation of suspected ureteral ectopia in duplex systems. J Urol. 166(6):2346-50, 2001
8. Engin G et al: MR urography findings of a duplicated ectopic ureter in an adult man. Eur Radiol. 10(8):1253-6, 2000
9. Gylys-Morin VM et al: Magnetic resonance imaging of the dysplastic renal moiety and ectopic ureter. J Urol. 164(6):2034-9, 2000
10. Livingston L et al: Seminal vesicle cyst with ipsilateral renal agenesis. AJR Am J Roentgenol. 175(1):177-80, 2000
11. Cabay JE et al: Ectopic ureter associated with renal dysplasia. JBR-BTR. 82(5):228-30, 1999

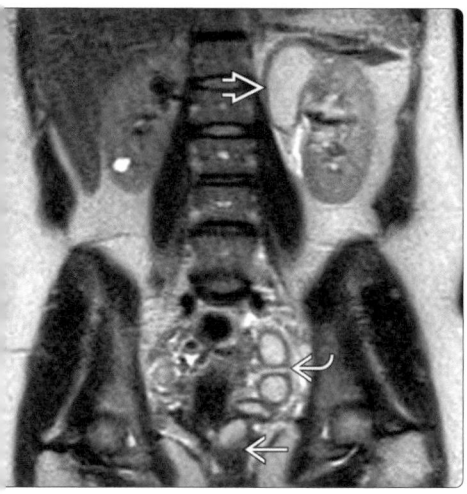

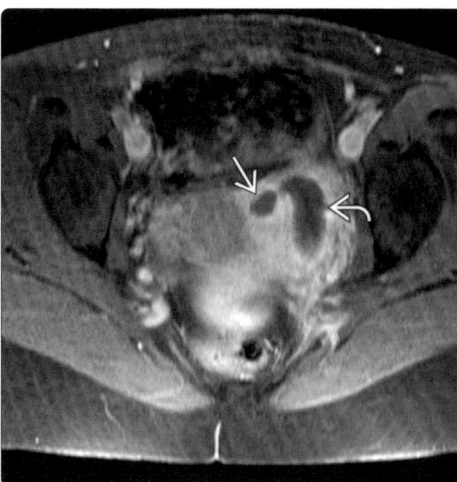

(Left) *Coronal T2 HASTE MR provides a more comprehensive overview of the duplicated left kidney with an obstructed atrophic upper pole moiety* ⬦. *The tortuous dilated ureter* ⬦ *inserts into the vagina* ⬦. *The ureter was thick, secondary to infection.* (Right) *Axial T1 C+ FS shows the ectopic insertion of the left upper ureter* ⬦ *into the vagina* ⬦. *Increased enhancement of the ureteral wall and surrounding tissue are secondary to infection.*

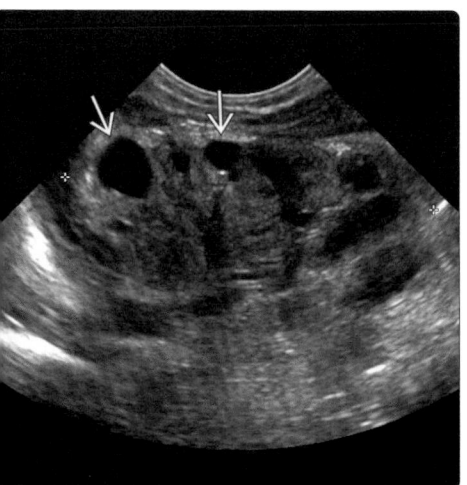

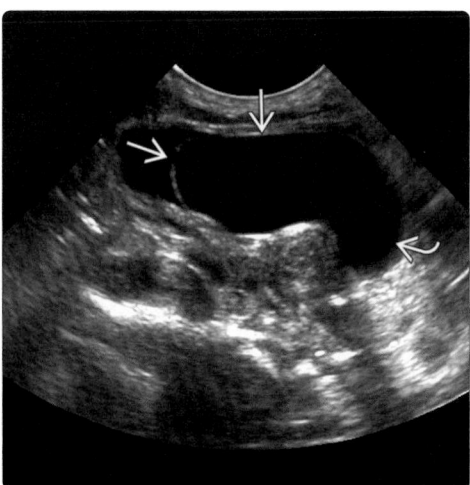

(Left) *Longitudinal ultrasound of a duplex left kidney shows dysplastic cystic change in the upper moiety* ⬦. (Right) *Transverse ultrasound of the bladder shows a dilated left ureter* ⬦ *from a duplex left kidney that is terminating as a large ureterocele* ⬦.

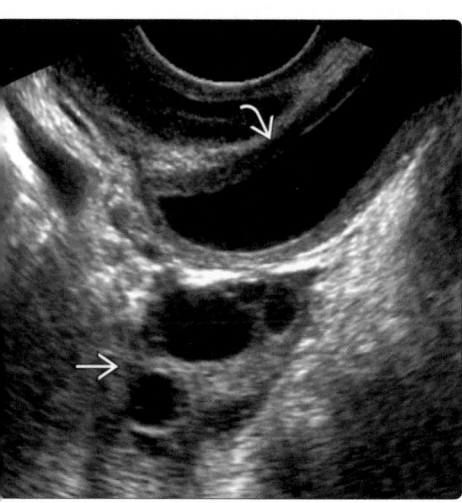

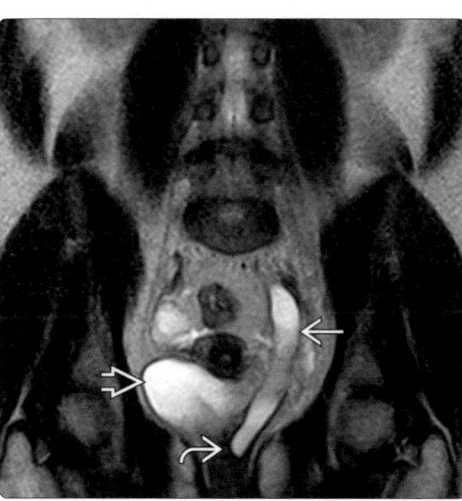

(Left) *Transvaginal ultrasound shows a thick-walled infected ectopic ureter* ⬦ *with internal debris next to a normal left ovary* ⬦. *This may be mistaken for a pyosalpinx, but the configuration and course of the ureter are different.* (Right) *Coronal T2 HASTE MR shows a dilated left ureter* ⬦ *inserting below the bladder neck into the vagina* ⬦. *The upper pole moiety of this duplicated system was severely dilated. The bladder* ⬦ *was normal.*

Ureteropelvic Junction Obstruction

TERMINOLOGY

- Ureteropelvic junction (UPJ) obstruction, pelviureteric junction obstruction (PUJO)
- Obstruction of urine flow at level of ureteropelvic junction

IMAGING

- Marked hydronephrosis to level of UPJ without dilatation of ureter
- Renal pelvis disproportionately enlarged compared to calyces
- Presence of crossing vessel
- Nuclear renal scan: Hydronephrosis with poor drainage, suggesting obstruction
- Imaging recommendations
  - Ultrasound in both prenatal and postnatal evaluation
  - Nuclear renal scan to determine whether hydronephrosis is obstructive and degree of obstruction
  - CT or MR to detect crossing vessel

TOP DIFFERENTIAL DIAGNOSES

- Multicystic dysplastic kidney
- Hydronephrosis of other etiology

PATHOLOGY

- Intrinsic vs. extrinsic causes
  - Abnormal peristalsis at UPJ secondary to abnormal muscle or nerve fibers
  - Crossing vessels near UPJ (50% of older children)

CLINICAL ISSUES

- M > F
- Most common cause of antenatal and neonatal hydronephrosis
- Prognosis generally good, depends on degree of preserved renal function
- Treatment: Pyeloplasty (open, laparoscopic, or robotic-assisted laparoscopic)

(Left) Graphic shows a markedly dilated renal pelvis ➡ and calyces ➡ in a ureteropelvic junction obstruction. The ureter ➡ is not dilated. (Right) Longitudinal image of the left kidney demonstrates marked dilatation of the renal pelvis ➡ as well as the renal calyces ➡. Note the severe cortical thinning ➡.

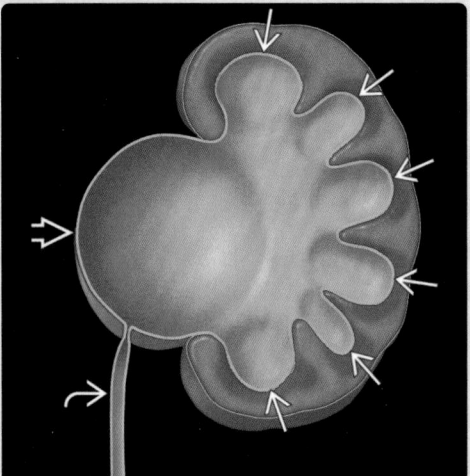
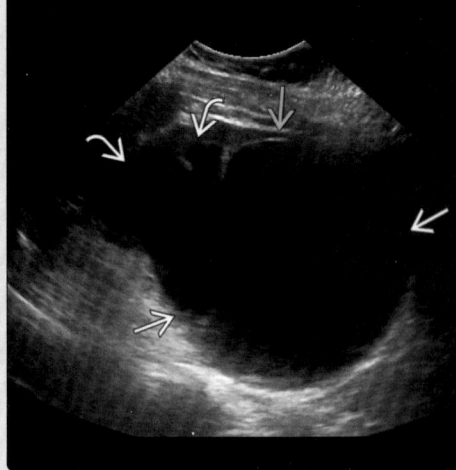

(Left) Longitudinal image of the left kidney demonstrates moderate dilatation of the renal pelvis ➡ and the calyces ➡. (Right) Delayed static image of a diuresis MAG 3 radioisotope scan shows stasis of the tracer within a dilated collecting system above the UPJ ➡ in both 1 hour (left) and 3 hour (right) delayed scan.

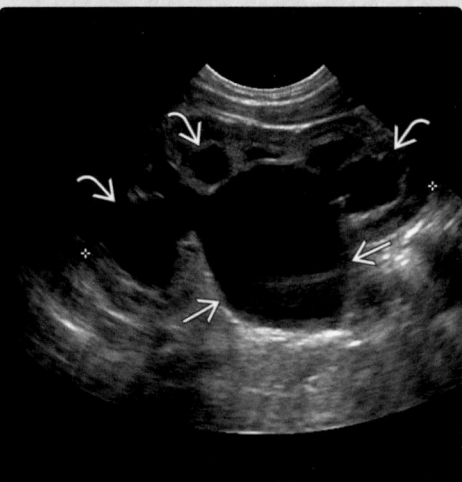
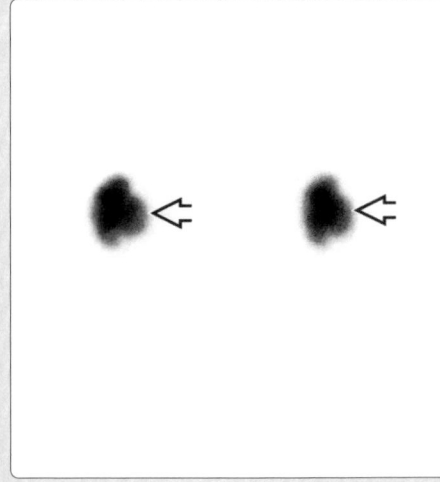

TERMINOLOGY

Abbreviations

Ureteropelvic junction (UPJ) obstruction, pelviureteric junction obstruction (PUJO)

Definitions

Obstruction of urine flow at level of UPJ

IMAGING

General Features

- Best diagnostic clue
  - Marked hydronephrosis to level of UPJ without dilatation of ureter
  - Renal pelvis disproportionately enlarged compared to calyces
- Location
  - Left kidney 2x as commonly affected
  - 10-30% are bilateral
- Morphology
  - Likened to Hirschsprung disease of ureter with focal transitional point and aperistaltic segment

Ultrasonographic Findings

- Grayscale ultrasound
  - Prenatal findings
    - Pyelectasis or fetal hydronephrosis
    - Anteroposterior diameter > 10 mm in 3rd trimester fetus or newborn suggests obstruction
    - Large urinoma or urine ascites in severe cases
    - Oligo-, poly-, or euhydramnios
  - Postnatal findings
    - Dilatation of renal pelvis and calyces to level of ureteropelvic junction
    - Marked ballooning of renal pelvis, out of proportion to calyces
    - Normal caliber ureter
    - Normal bladder size and contour
    - If longstanding, renal parenchymal atrophy with hypertrophy of normal contralateral kidney
    - Associated contralateral renal anomalies: Multicystic dysplastic kidney, renal duplication, and agenesis
- Pulsed Doppler
  - Elevated resistive indices (RI) may correlate with degree of obstruction when contralateral kidney normal
  - Strict cut off values do not pertain to pediatric population due to changing RI values with age
- Color Doppler
  - Can be used to detect crossing vessel
  - Ureteral jets can be used to exclude complete obstruction
- Endoureteral US
  - Demonstrate crossing vessels in more than 50% of UPJ obstruction, most commonly anteromedial in location
  - Demonstrate septum between ureteral and renal pelvic lumen in UPJ obstruction secondary to high insertion of ureter
  - Useful to guide site of endopyelotomy to avoid damage to adjacent vessels

Radiographic Findings

- IVP
  - Delayed nephrogram depending on degree of obstruction
  - Contrast opacification of a markedly dilated renal pelvis, with abrupt tapering into a normal caliber ureter
  - "Linear band" sign: Linear oblique crossing defect in proximal end of ureter
- Retrograde ureteropyelography
  - Assess ureter if not visualized in other studies

CT Findings

- CECT
  - Marked dilatation of renal pelvis with nonvisualized or normal caliber ureter
  - Delayed nephrogram and contrast excretion
  - ± acquired etiologies (e.g., crossing vessels, neoplasm, retroperitoneal inflammatory conditions) and associated abnormalities (e.g., renal malformation)
- CTA
  - Detect crossing vessels

MR Findings

- T2WI
  - Marked dilatation of T2 hyperintense renal pelvis with nonvisualized or normal caliber ureter
- T1WI C+
  - Delayed nephrogram and contrast excretion
- MRA
  - Detect crossing vessels

Nuclear Medicine Findings

- Diuresis renography
  - Hydronephrosis with poor drainage, suggesting obstruction
  - Assess differential renal function and degree of obstruction, often preoperatively
  - "Homsy" sign: Delayed double-peak pattern; suggests intermittent UPJ obstruction

Imaging Recommendations

- Best imaging tool
  - Ultrasound in both prenatal and postnatal evaluation
  - Nuclear renal scan to determine whether hydronephrosis is obstructive and degree of obstruction
  - CT or MR to detect crossing vessel
- Protocol advice
  - Postnatal US should be done several days after birth due to relative neonatal oliguria
  - CTA or MRA: Define vessels and their relation to UPJ

DIFFERENTIAL DIAGNOSIS

Multicystic Dysplastic Kidney

- Multiple cysts of varying sizes that do not communicate
- Largest cyst is not central as in UPJ obstruction

Hydronephrosis of Other Etiology

- Determine level of obstruction with associated findings
- Can also be secondary to vesicoureteral reflux

Extrarenal Pelvis

- Prominent renal pelvis beyond contour of kidney

- Calyces not dilated
- Much smaller in size than UPJ obstruction

Pararenal Cyst

- Lymphatic in origin or develops from embryologic rests
- Well-defined anechoic renal sinus mass not communicating with calyces

PATHOLOGY

General Features

- Etiology
  - Intrinsic
    - Abnormal peristalsis at UPJ, secondary to abnormal muscle or nerve fibers
    - Stenosis from scarring of ureteral valves
    - Intraluminal lesions
      - Tumors: Benign polyps, urothelial carcinoma, squamous carcinoma, metastases
      - Others: Stone, clot, papilla, fungus ball
  - Extrinsic
    - High insertion of ureter at renal pelvis
    - Crossing vessels near UPJ (50% of older children)
    - Abnormal rotation of kidney
    - Secondary UPJO: Prior surgery, inflammation, trauma, or stone disease
- Associated abnormalities
  - Higher incidence in multicystic dysplastic kidneys
  - Can be present in upper or lower moiety of duplex kidney
  - Renal ectopia and fusion anomalies
  - VACTERL spectrum

Microscopic Features

- Decreased number of nerve and muscular fibers with abnormal increased collagen deposition within ureteric wall

CLINICAL ISSUES

Presentation

- Most common signs/symptoms
  - Neonates
    - Often diagnosed by prenatal screening
    - Palpable, sometimes visible abdominal mass
  - Children and adults
    - Intermittent abdominal or flank pain, nausea, vomiting, failure to thrive
    - Hematuria, renovascular hypertension (rare)
    - Can present after minor trauma, possibly with rupture

Demographics

- Age
  - Can present at any age; more common in pediatric population
- Gender
  - Overall, M:F = 2:1
  - In infants, M:F = 5:1
- Epidemiology
  - 1 in 1,000 to 1,500 newborns
  - Most common cause of antenatal and neonatal hydronephrosis
    - 50% of all patients with antenatal hydronephrosis

Natural History & Prognosis

- May improve or worsen spontaneously
- Prognosis generally good, depends on degree of preserved renal function
- After successful surgery, dilatation of renal pelvis and calyces may persist for years on US
  - Evaluate interval renal growth and good drainage on postsurgical imaging

Treatment

- Pyeloplasty (open, laparoscopic, or robotic-assisted laparoscopic)
  - Resection of narrowed segment at UPJ
  - Crossing vessel is rerouted
  - Ureteral stents often left in place for several weeks postoperatively
  - Preferred approach when crossing or aberrant vessels are present; hemorrhage as complication of endoscopic approach
- Endopyelotomy: Endoscopic incision
- Endopyeloplasty: Horizontal percutaneous suturing of conventional longitudinal endopyelotomy incision
- Percutaneous nephrostomy, as temporary measure, especially if infected

DIAGNOSTIC CHECKLIST

Consider

- CT or MR to evaluate potential acquired etiologies of UPJ obstruction
- CTA or MRA to look for crossing vessel

Image Interpretation Pearls

- Look for presence of crossing vessel on all modalities

SELECTED REFERENCES

1. Arora S et al: Predictors for the need of surgery in antenatally detected hydronephrosis due to UPJ obstruction - A prospective multivariate analysis. J Pediatr Urol. ePub, 2015
2. Lin L et al: Role of endoluminal sonography in evaluation of obstruction of the ureteropelvic junction. AJR Am J Roentgenol. 191(4):1250-4, 2008
3. Calder AD et al: Contrast-enhanced magnetic resonance angiography for the detection of crossing renal vessels in children with symptomatic ureteropelvic junction obstruction: comparison with operative findings. Pediatr Radiol. 37(4):356-61, 2007
4. Williams B et al: Pathophysiology and treatment of ureteropelvic junction obstruction. Curr Urol Rep. 8(2):111-7, 2007
5. Jones RA et al: Dynamic contrast-enhanced MR urography in the evaluation of pediatric hydronephrosis: Part 1, functional assessment. AJR Am J Roentgenol. 185(6):1598-607, 2005
6. McDaniel BB et al: Dynamic contrast-enhanced MR urography in the evaluation of pediatric hydronephrosis: part 2, anatomic and functional assessment of uteropelvic junction obstruction. AJR Am J Roentgenol. 185(6):1608-14, 2005
7. Khaira HS et al: Helical computed tomography for identification of crossing vessels in ureteropelvic junction obstruction-comparison with operative findings. Urology. 62(1):35-9, 2003
8. Rooks VJ et al: Extrinsic ureteropelvic junction obstruction from a crossing renal vessel: demography and imaging. Pediatr Radiol. 31(2):120-4, 2001
9. Keeley FX Jr et al: A prospective study of endoluminal ultrasound versus computerized tomography angiography for detecting crossing vessels at the ureteropelvic junction. J Urol. 162(6):1938-41, 1999

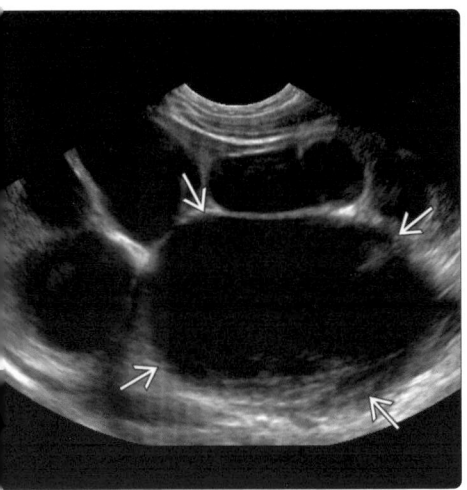
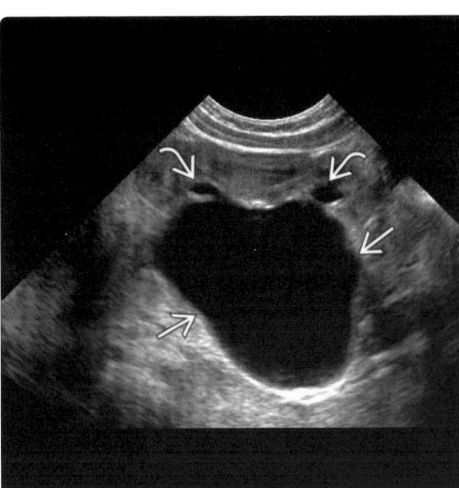

(Left) *Longitudinal image of the left kidney demonstrates multiple cystic structures with the largest centrally ➡, suggestive of UPJ obstruction rather than multicystic dysplastic kidney. Note the severe cortical thinning.* **(Right)** *Longitudinal image of the left kidney demonstrates marked dilatation of the renal pelvis ➡ with only mild dilatation of the renal calyces ⤵.*

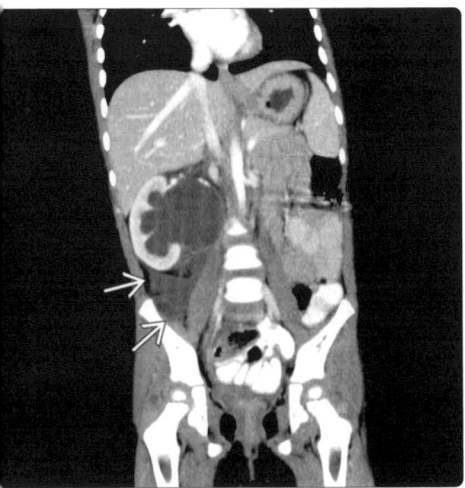
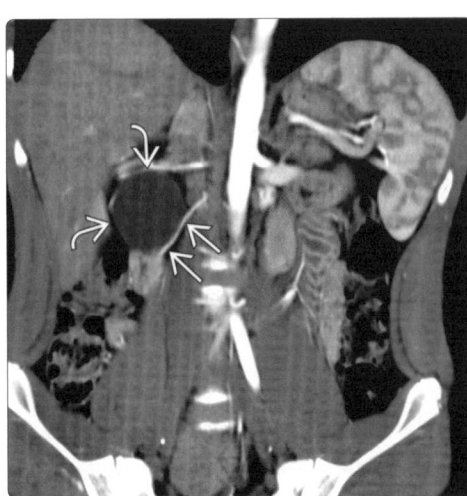

(Left) *Post-contrast coronal CT abdomen demonstrates right UPJ obstruction in a boy who presented after minor trauma. Note the fluid in the right retroperitoneum ➡, suggestive of rupture.* **(Right)** *Coronal CT angiogram demonstrates the presence of a crossing arterial vessel ➡ in the region of the right UPJ, with a dilated renal pelvis ⤵.*

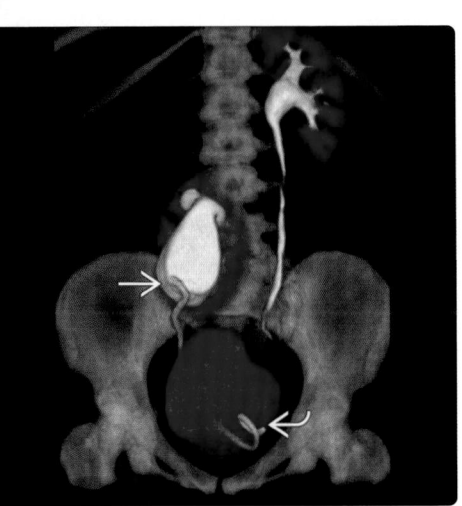
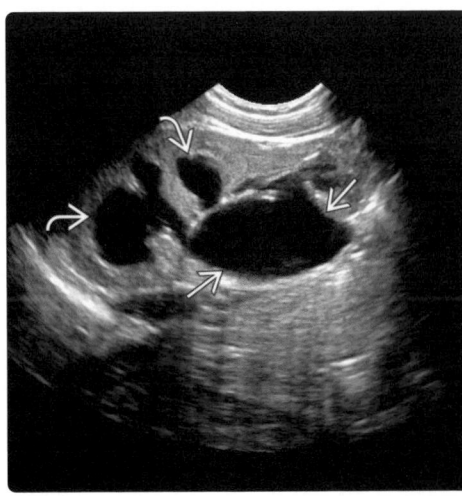

(Left) *Coronal reformatted 3D image from a CT urogram demonstrates a malrotated right pelvic kidney with UPJ obstruction ➡, with a normal caliber ureter. There is a double "J" ureteral stent ⤵ terminating in the bladder.* **(Right)** *Longitudinal ultrasound shows a right kidney with UPJ obstruction obtained after pyeloplasty. Note the residual dilatation of the renal pelvis ➡ and calyces ⤵, which may persist for years.*

Urolithiasis

TERMINOLOGY

- Urinary tract stone, urinary calculous disease, nephrolithiasis, ureterolithiasis, vesicolithiasis
- Macroscopic concretions of crystals in urinary system, sometimes mixed with proteins

IMAGING

- US has 96% sensitivity, nearly 100% specificity for renal stones > 5 mm
- US is valuable for follow-up imaging, particularly in patients with renal colic & known renal stones or patients not improving on treatment for known stone
- Virtually all stones are visible (including those radiolucent on KUB) on CT except pure matrix stones & protease inhibitor stones (e.g. indinavir, treatment of HIV)
- NECT is preferred imaging modality to confirm stone in adult patients with acute flank pain

TOP DIFFERENTIAL DIAGNOSES

- Nephrocalcinosis
- Papillary necrosis
- Emphysematous pyelonephritis (EP)

CLINICAL ISSUES

- Size, number, location, evidence of obstruction or infection & relevant anatomic findings (aberrant vasculature, distorted pelvicalyceal architecture, infundibular orientation) are all imaging findings that impact treatment

DIAGNOSTIC CHECKLIST

- US protocol should include fasting (↓ bowel gas) & bladder filling, if possible
- Always include bladder with special attention to UVJ
- Twinkling artifact on color Doppler is useful to identify otherwise occult stone; more sensitive than acoustic shadowing but higher false-positive rate

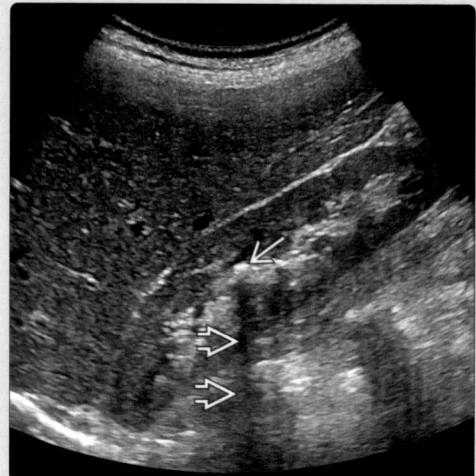
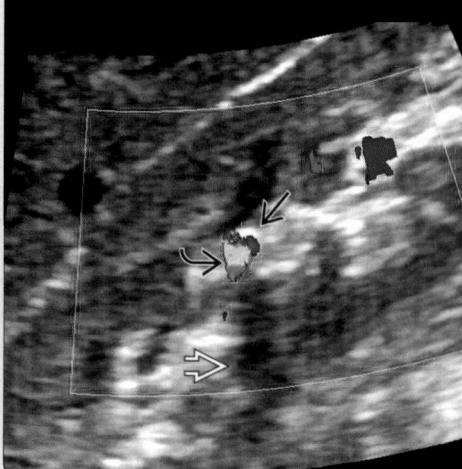

(Left) Longitudinal US of the right kidney shows an echogenic stone ➡ within the mid right kidney. Posterior acoustic shadowing ➡ helps differentiate this stone from the surrounding sinus fat. (Right) Zoomed-in longitudinal color Doppler US of the right kidney in the same patient shows the echogenic stone ➡ with twinkling artifact ➡ and posterior acoustic shadowing ➡.

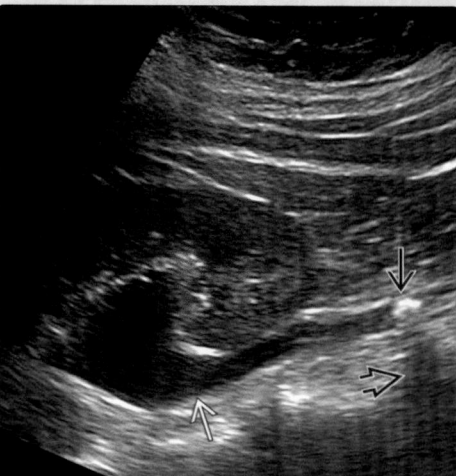
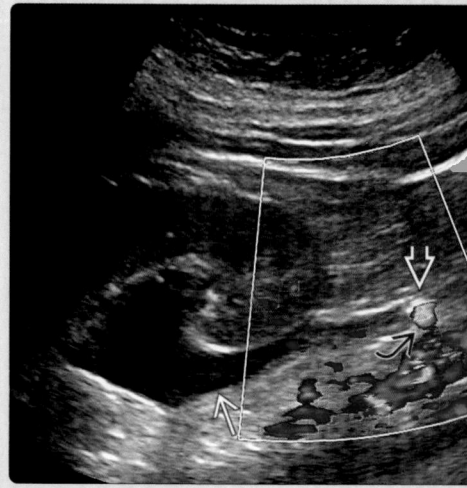

(Left) Longitudinal US of the inferior pole of the left kidney shows an obstructing proximal ureteral calculus ➡ with posterior acoustic shadowing ➡ and hydroureteronephrosis ➡. (Right) Longitudinal color Doppler US of the inferior pole of the left kidney in the same patient now shows twinkling artifact ➡ posterior to the proximal ureteral calculus ➡ causing hydroureteronephrosis ➡.

TERMINOLOGY

Abbreviations
Ureterovesicular junction (UVJ); ureteropelvic junction (UPJ); intravenous pyelogram (IVP)

Synonyms
Urinary tract stone, urinary calculous disease, nephrolithiasis, ureterolithiasis, vesicolithiasis

Definitions
Macroscopic concretions of crystals in urinary system, sometimes mixed with proteins

IMAGING

General Features
Location
- Renal stones: Upper pole, mid kidney (interpolar region), lower pole
- Ureter stones: Can divide ureter into UPJ, proximal, mid, distal, and UVJ
  - Iliac vessels are an important landmark for treatment planning: Divide ureter into UPJ, proximal (UPJ to iliac vessels), distal (iliac vessels to UVJ), and UVJ
- Bladder stones

Ultrasonographic Findings
Grayscale ultrasound
- Advantages: No ionizing radiation, inexpensive, accessible
- Disadvantages: Operator dependent, deep ureter difficult to visualize, limited sensitivity for < 5 mm stone, overestimates stone size relative to CT, limited in obese patients
- Calculi = echogenic foci with sharp posterior acoustic shadowing
- For renal stones > 5 mm: 96% sensitivity, nearly 100% specificity
- May be difficult to detect small, nonshadowing renal and ureteral calculi, unless there is obstruction
  - Most calculi missed by US are < 3 mm, which are more likely to pass spontaneously without intervention
- Optimize technique
  - Fast for 4 hours to decrease bowel gas and hydrate to fill bladder
  - Maximize shadowing by placing single focal zone at or slightly deep to stone
  - Always include bladder with attention to UVJ
    - Roll patient to show mobility of bladder calculus
- Valuable for follow-up imaging, especially in patients with stones & renal colic or those not improving on treatment
Color Doppler
- Twinkling artifact: Focus of alternating colors on color Doppler behind rough, reflective object
  - Helps ID otherwise occult stone that blends with renal sinus fat; more sensitive than acoustic shadowing
  - ↑ sensitivity compared with grayscale alone, but also ↑ false-positives (up to 51%)
- Should see ureteral jets intermittently and bilaterally

- High-grade obstruction: Ureteral jet almost always absent
- Low-grade obstruction: May (~ 1/3) or may not have absent ureteral jet
  - Asymmetric decrease or continuous low-amplitude jet on affected side

Radiographic Findings
- Radiography
  - ~ 90% of calculi are radiopaque; calcium stones > struvite & cystine stones
    - More sensitive than CT scout image (63% vs. 47%)
    - Valuable for planning treatment (e.g., ESWL) & monitoring stone burden
    - Disadvantages: Limited sensitivity (~ 60%); limiting factors: Bowel gas, extrarenal calcification, obesity
  - Radiolucent: Uric acid, xanthine, pure matrix, drug stones, 2,8-dihydroxyadenine
- IVP
  - Formerly study of choice; has been replaced by CT
  - Fails to detect calculi in 31-48% of cases

CT Findings
- NECT
  - Preferred imaging modality to confirm stone in adult patients with acute flank pain
  - Virtually all stones are visible (including those radiolucent on KUB) except pure matrix stones and protease inhibitor stones (e.g., indinavir)
  - Advantages: Fast, no IV contrast, high sensitivity (nearly 100%), allows detection of unsuspected abnormalities, useful for treatment planning
  - CT attenuation measurements (highest to lowest) for evaluating stone composition
    - Calcium oxalate monohydrate and brushite (1700-2800 HU)
    - Calcium phosphate (1200-1600 HU)
    - Cystine (600-1100 HU)
    - Struvite (600-900 HU)
    - Uric acid (200-450 HU)
    - 35-65% of stones are of mixed composition; CT attenuation measurements most valuable in differentiating 100% uric acid stones from others
  - Ureterolithiasis
    - Direct sign: Visualization of calculus within ureteral lumen; ureteral dilation may be absent
    - Secondary signs: Most reliable: Hydroureter/hydronephrosis, perinephric stranding, periureteral edema, and unilateral renal enlargement
    - "Soft tissue rim" sign = ureteral stone: Soft tissue halo around calcific focus = ureteral wall edema around stone; highly specific (≥ 90%) for ureteral stone
    - "Comet tail" sign = phlebolith: Eccentric, tapering soft tissue density adjacent to calcification = noncalcified portion of pelvic vein and phlebolith; specificity nearly 100% for phlebolith
    - Phlebolith: Central lucency, calculus, nearly all are centrally dense
  - Best way to measure stone size is with bone windows and magnification
  - Randall plaque = stone precursor; subepithelial calcification seen as whitish build-up in papillary tips

- CECT
  - CT lucent stones → filling defects
  - In select cases, CT IVP may help differentiate distal ureteral stone from phlebolith
- Dual-energy CT (DECT): Scanning at different energies (80 and 140 kVp) allows better stone characterization
  - Can differentiate: Urate stones from other stones; struvite from cystine stones → both relevant for treatment planning

MR Findings

- Virtually all stones = signal voids
- Ureteral calculi: Abrupt change in ureter caliber indicates obstruction level; secondary signs

DIFFERENTIAL DIAGNOSIS

Nephrocalcinosis (NC)

- Calcification within parenchyma: Medullary NC (most common) & cortical NC
- Often associated with urolithiasis

Papillary Necrosis

- Calcified sloughed papilla
- Nonshadowing echoes within medullary cavities; empty medullary cavities after passed sloughed papilla

Emphysematous Pyelonephritis (EP), Pyelitis

- Gas within renal parenchyma (pyelonephritis) or renal collecting system (pyelitis) with dirty shadowing

PATHOLOGY

General Features

- Etiology
  - Exact mechanism is unknown, but concept of urinary supersaturation is essential
  - Low urine volume/dehydration (most common)
  - Metabolic: Commonly hypercalciuria, hyperuricosuria, hypocitraturia, hyperoxaluria
  - Urine composition: pH, crystal inhibitors, stone-forming substances
  - Disease states: Obesity, RTA type 1, IBD, medullary sponge kidney, sarcoid, etc.
  - UTI, including urease-producing bacteria (*Klebsiella, Proteus, Pseudomonas*, some *Staphylococci*)
  - Sedentary lifestyle, immobilization
  - Anatomic: Urinary obstruction or stasis
  - Medications: Protease inhibitors (Indinavir), supplements (e.g., ephedrine), triamterene, sulfonamides
- Types of stones
  - Calcium-based stones (70-80%): Calcium oxalate monohydrate and dihydrate, calcium phosphate
  - Struvite (5-15%): Magnesium ammonium phosphate
  - Uric acid (5-10%)
  - Cystine (1-2.5%)
  - Other (< 5%): Xanthine, matrix, drugs, 2,8-dihydroxyadenine

CLINICAL ISSUES

Presentation

- Most common signs/symptoms

  - Acute flank pain, renal colic
  - Associated symptoms: Microscopic or gross hematuria, nausea, and vomiting

Demographics

- Gender
  - M > F
- Epidemiology
  - Up to 14% of men and 6% of women develop stones

Natural History & Prognosis

- Spontaneous ureteral stone passage based on size
  - > 8 mm rarely pass without intervention
  - 95% of stones up to 4 mm pass within 40 days
- Complications: Obstruction, infection, and renal insufficiency
- Recurrence rate is ~ 75% over 20 years

Treatment

- Options for upper tract urolithiasis
  - Surveillance (trial of passage): Hydration & pain relief; medical expulsive therapy (MET)
  - Extracorporeal shock wave lithotripsy (ESWL)
  - Ureteroscopy and endoscopic lithotripsy (URS)
  - Percutaneous nephrolithotomy (PCNL)
  - Dissolution (chemolysis)
  - Open or laparoscopic surgery
- Size, number, location, obstruction or infection, and anatomic findings (aberrant vasculature, distorted pelvicalyceal architecture) all impact treatment
  - Urate stones (< 450 HU): Only stones efficiently treated with oral chemolysis (alkalinization)
  - CT findings that ↓ success of ESWL: Lower pole stone location, larger stone size, high-attenuation (> 1000 HU) and cystine stones, larger stone-to-skin distance
  - > 1000 HU → URS or PCNL
- For renal stones: 0.5-1.5 cm stones → increasing popularity of URS due to high stone-free rates
  - < 1 cm: Asymptomatic → observation; symptomatic → SWL or URS
  - 1-2 cm → SWL or PCNL
  - > 2 cm or staghorn → PCNL
    - Staghorn calculi → progressive renal damage and persistent infection; treatment goal: Complete stone removal
- For ureteral stones: < 10 mm → MET or SWL, URS; > 10 mm → SWL or URS

SELECTED REFERENCES

1. Spettel S et al: Using Hounsfield unit measurement and urine parameters to predict uric acid stones. Urology. 82(1):22-6, 2013
2. Cheng PM et al: What the radiologist needs to know about urolithiasis: part 2--CT findings, reporting, and treatment. AJR Am J Roentgenol. 198(6):W548-54, 2012
3. Cheng PM et al: What the radiologist needs to know about urolithiasis: part 1--pathogenesis, types, assessment, and variant anatomy. AJR Am J Roentgenol. 198(6):W540-7, 2012

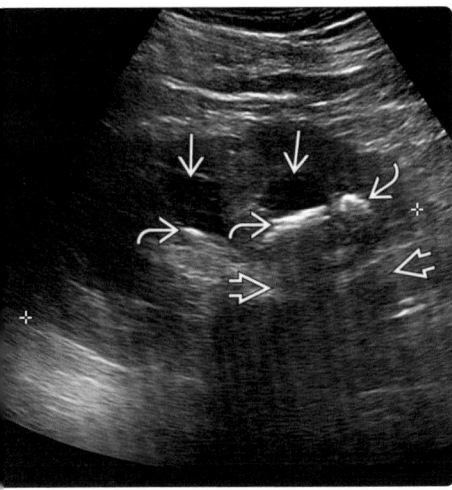
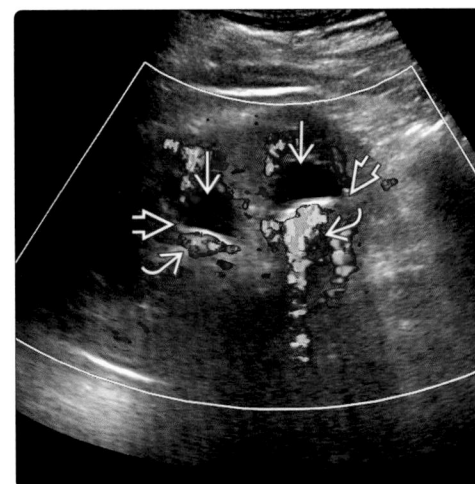

(Left) *Longitudinal US of the left kidney shows dilated calyces* ➡ *containing multiple echogenic stones* ➡ *causing posterior acoustic shadowing* ➡. **(Right)** *Transverse color Doppler US of the left kidney in the same patient demonstrates twinkling artifact* ➡ *posterior to multiple echogenic stones* ➡ *in dilated calyces* ➡.

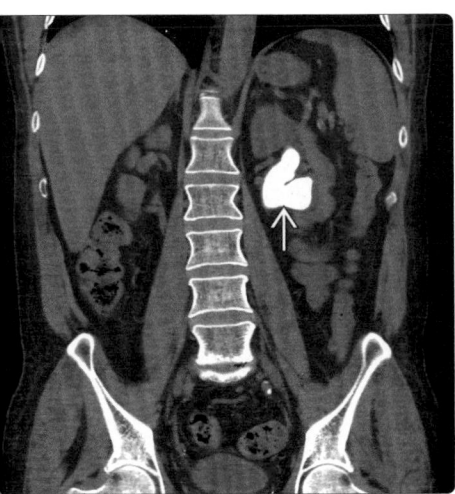
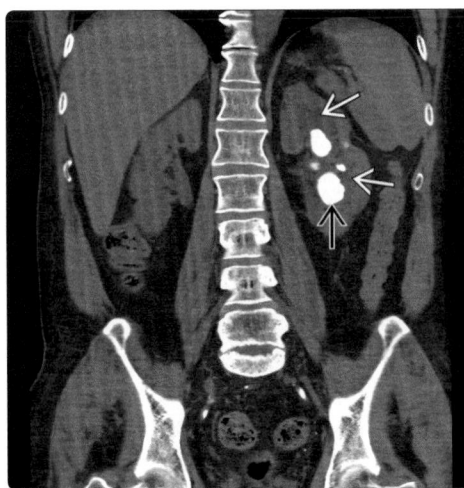

(Left) *Coronal NECT in the same patient shows a large staghorn calculus* ➡ *within the left renal collecting system.* **(Right)** *Another coronal NECT in the same patient partially shows the large staghorn calculus* ➡, *which is causing obstruction (dilated calyces)* ➡.

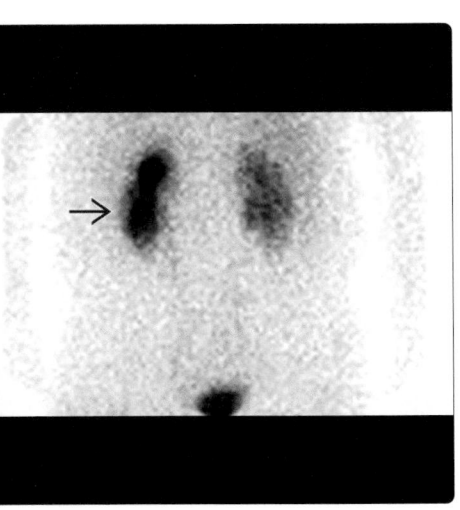
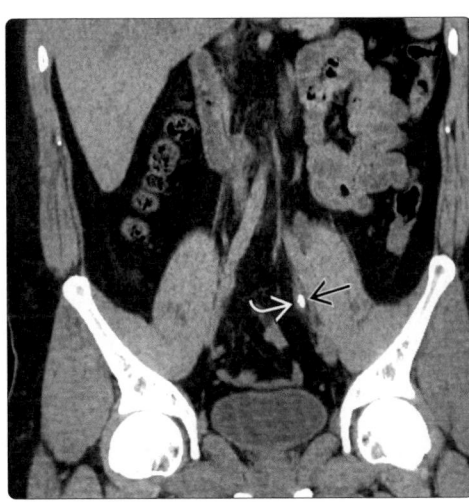

(Left) *Coronal Tc-99m MAG3 (posterior) in the same patient shows delayed clearance from the left kidney* ➡. *No clearance of radiotracer after Lasix administration indicated complete obstruction.* **(Right)** *Coronal NECT of the abdomen and pelvis in a different patient reveals a calculus within the proximal left ureter* ➡. *Soft tissue attenuation surrounding the calcification ("soft tissue rim" sign)* ➡ *represents ureteral wall edema.*

(Left) *Longitudinal US of the left kidney shows a calculus within the proximal ureter* ➡ *causing obstruction with severe dilation of the extrarenal pelvis* ➡. (Right) *Longitudinal US of the left ureter shows an obstructing distal ureteral calculus* ➡ *causing hydroureter* ➡.

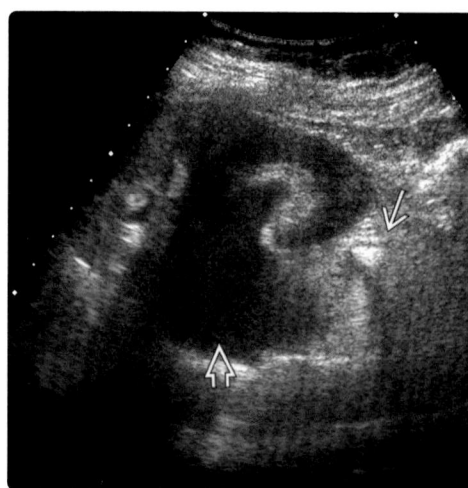
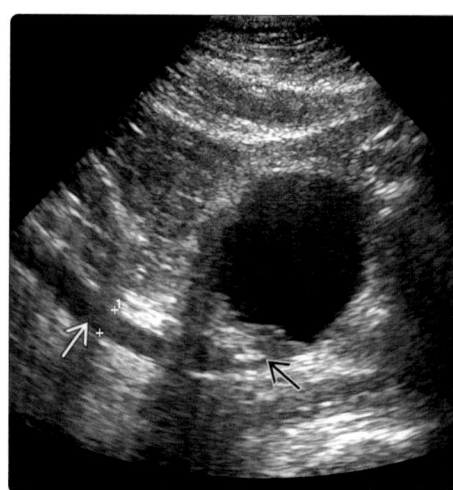

(Left) *Transverse color Doppler US of the bladder in the same patient reveals only a right ureteral jet* ➡. *Absence of a left ureteral jet in association with a distal left ureteral stone* ➡ *indicates high-grade/complete obstruction. Interestingly, this stone does not demonstrate twinkling artifact; visibility of twinkling artifact is highly dependent on machine settings and stone composition.* (Right) *Transverse US of the bladder shows a stone at the right UVJ* ➡ *with posterior acoustic shadowing* ➡.

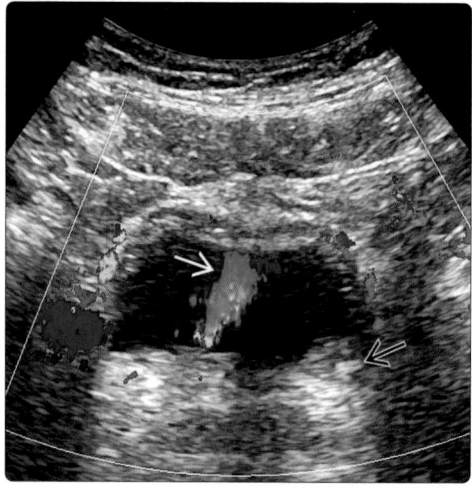
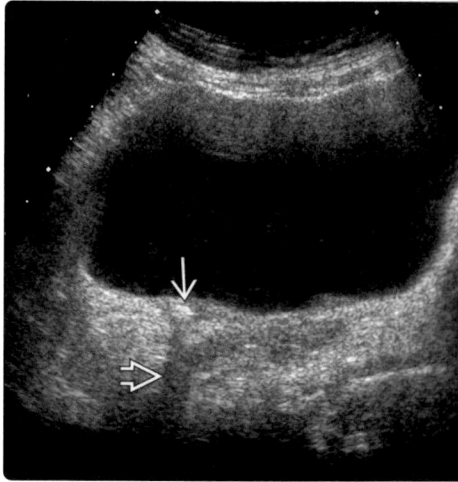

(Left) *In the same patient, zoomed-in transverse color Doppler US of the right UVJ stone demonstrates twinkling artifact* ➡ *and posterior acoustic shadowing* ➡. (Right) *Longitudinal US of the distal right ureter in the same patient shows the right UVJ calculus* ➡ *with posterior acoustic shadowing* ➡ *and proximal hydroureter* ➡.

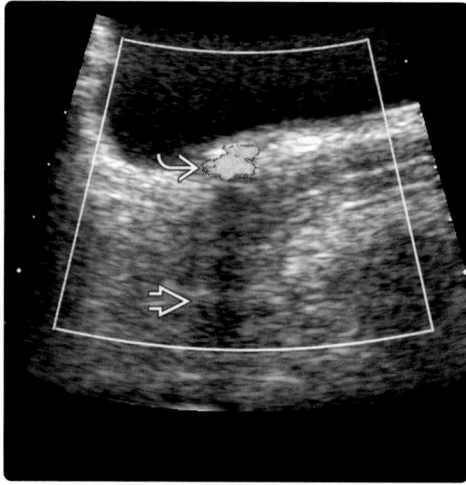
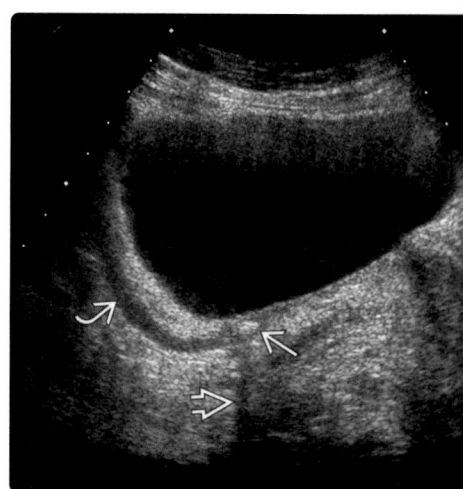

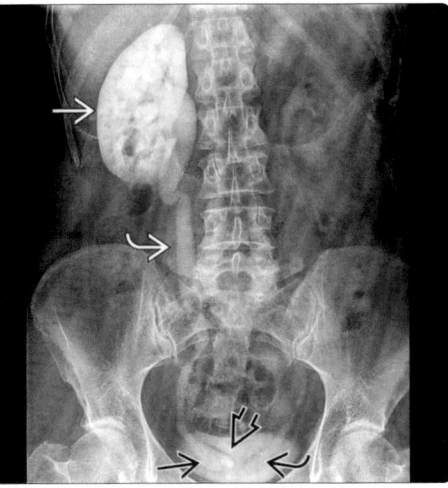

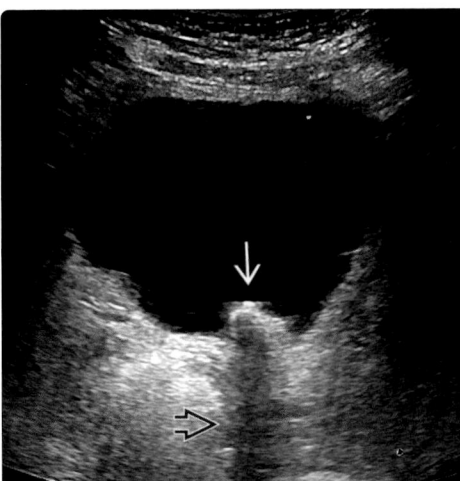

(Left) *Intravenous pyelogram (IVP) shows markedly delayed right nephrogram ➡ and right hydroureteronephrosis ➡ caused by an obstructing distal ureteral stone ➡ within a ureterocele ➡ (outpouching of distal ureter into bladder). In addition, a contralateral ureterocele is present ➡.* (Right) *Transverse US of the bladder shows a bladder stone ➡ with posterior acoustic shadowing ➡.*

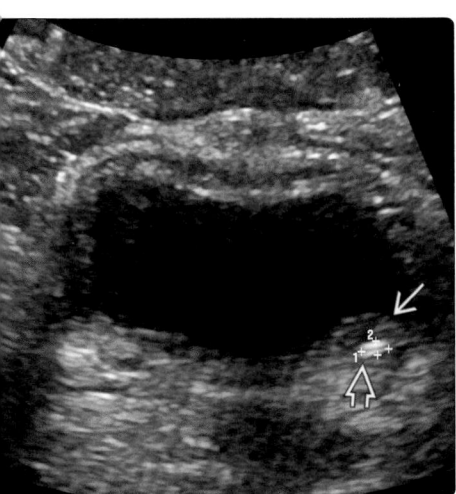

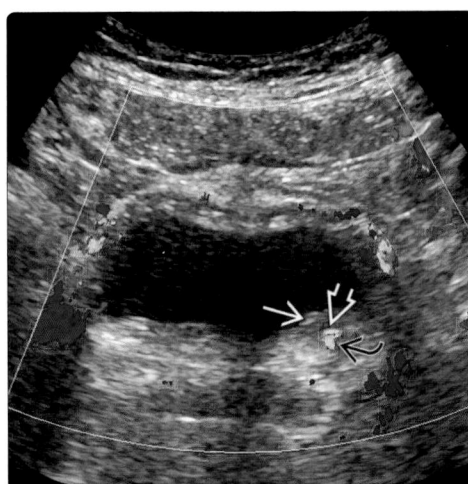

(Left) *Transverse US of the bladder shows a hyperechoic stone ➡ in the left UVJ. Notice the surrounding halo of edema ➡, which can yield a pseudoureterocele appearance on IVP.* (Right) *Transverse color Doppler US of the bladder in the same patient shows a left UVJ stone ➡ with halo of edema ➡ and twinkling artifact ➡.*

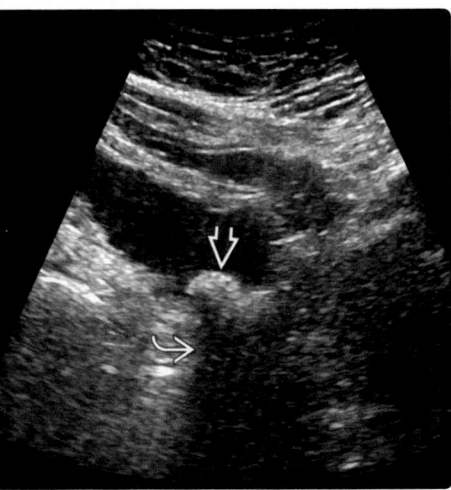

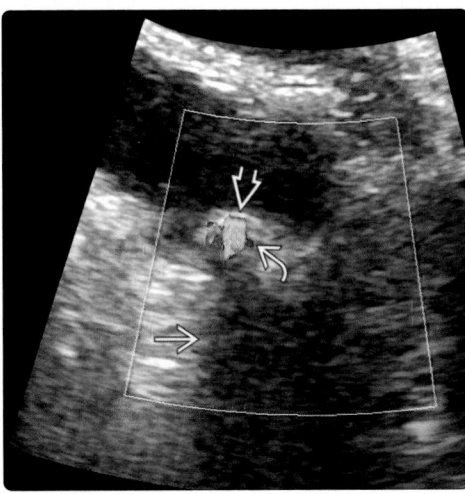

(Left) *Longitudinal US of the bladder shows a shadowing ➡ bladder calculus ➡.* (Right) *Longitudinal color Doppler US in the same patient shows twinkling artifact ➡ and acoustic shadowing ➡ posterior to the bladder stone ➡.*

TERMINOLOGY

- Medullary nephrocalcinosis (NC), cortical nephrocalcinosis
- Calcification of renal parenchyma

IMAGING

- Medullary NC: Generalized increased echogenicity of renal pyramids with reversal of normal corticomedullary differentiation ± shadowing
- Cortical NC: Increased cortical echogenicity ± acoustic shadowing
- Noncontrast CT is best imaging modality in adults
  - Exception: CT intravenous pyelogram (IVP) may be best for medullary sponge kidney given high sensitivity for stones and collecting tubule dilation
- US is 1st diagnostic imaging option in infants and children with suspected nephrocalcinosis

TOP DIFFERENTIAL DIAGNOSES

- Renal calculus

- Emphysematous pyelonephritis
- Other causes of hyperechoic medulla: Metabolic and protein deposition disorders, autosomal recessive polycystic kidney disease

PATHOLOGY

- Most common causes of medullary NC are hyperparathyroidism, renal tubular acidosis (RTA) type 1 (distal), and medullary sponge kidney
- Most common causes of cortical NC are acute cortical necrosis, chronic glomerulonephritis, and oxalosis
- Medullary and cortical NC is rare and seen in oxalosis

DIAGNOSTIC CHECKLIST

- Medullary sponge kidney → asymmetrical, segmental, or unilateral medullary NC
- Hyperparathyroidism and RTA type 1 → usually diffuse or uniform calcification
- Oxalosis typically causes both medullary and cortical NC
- Nephrocalcinosis is often associated with urolithiasis

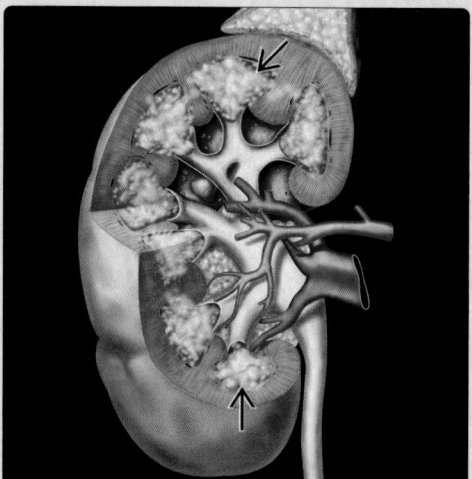
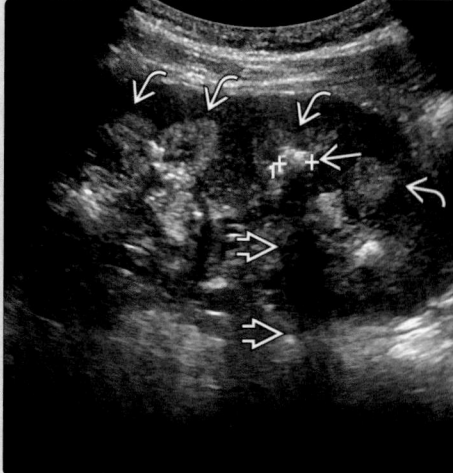

(Left) Graphic shows diffuse calcification ⊟ in renal the pyramids, representing medullary nephrocalcinosis. (Right) Longitudinal US of the left kidney shows echogenic pyramids with reversal of the normal corticomedullary differentiation. Note the medullary ring ⊟ of hyperechoic rim outlining the pyramid. Posterior acoustic shadowing ⊟ helps identify a stone ⊟.

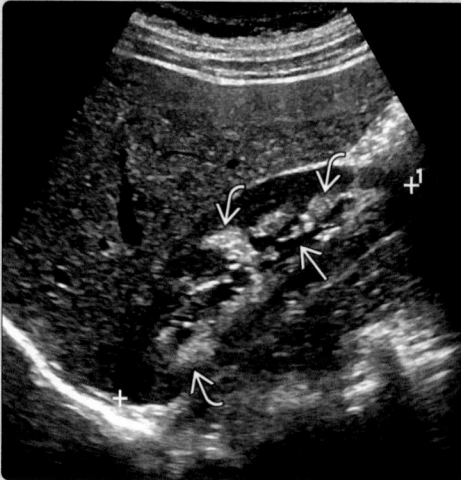
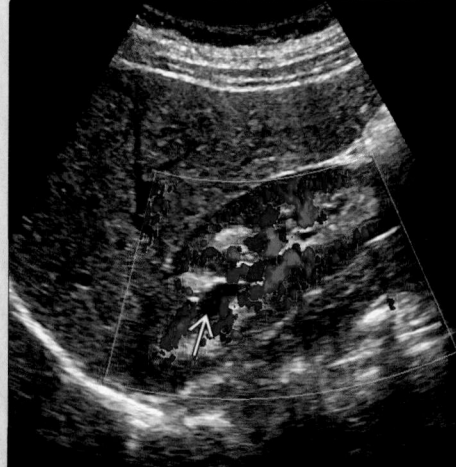

(Left) Longitudinal US of the right kidney shows hyperechoic pyramids ⊟ with reversal of the normal corticomedullary differentiation. Mild fullness of the right renal collecting system ⊟ is present. (Right) Longitudinal color Doppler US of the right kidney in the same patient confirms the hypoechoic spaces represents caliectasis ⊟.

TERMINOLOGY

Abbreviations
Nephrocalcinosis (NC)

Synonyms
Medullary nephrocalcinosis, cortical nephrocalcinosis

Definitions
Calcification of renal parenchyma

IMAGING

General Features
Best diagnostic clue
- Calcification within renal parenchyma

Location
- Medullary NC (95%): Calcification in medullary pyramids
- Cortical NC (5%): Cortical calcification and along central septa of Bertin
- Both cortical and medullary: Rare

Size
- Kidneys often have normal size and contour

Ultrasonographic Findings
Grayscale ultrasound
- **Medullary nephrocalcinosis**
  - Generalized increased echogenicity of renal pyramids ± acoustic shadowing
  - Reversal of normal corticomedullary differentiation
  - Medullary rings: Hyperechoic rim outlining medullary pyramids
  - Medullary sponge kidney: Echogenic medullary pyramids regardless of whether or not medullary nephrocalcinosis is present
  - Papillary necrosis → sloughed papilla seen as echogenic nonshadowing structure at pyramids
    - Calcified sloughed papilla with distal acoustic shadowing
    - Clubbing of adjacent calyces
    - Cystic collections within medullary pyramids
- **Cortical nephrocalcinosis**
  - Increased cortical echogenicity ± acoustic shadowing
- Comparison of US and CT in induced nephrocalcinosis in rabbits showed higher sensitivity for US (96% vs. 64%) but better specificity for CT (96% vs. 85%)

Radiographic Findings
Radiography
- Medullary NC: Stippled, coarse, or confluent calcification in pyramids
- Cortical NC
  - Diffusely dense renal shadows
  - Thin, peripheral band of calcification, often with extension into septal cortex
  - 2 thin, parallel calcified tracks (tram lines)
  - Punctate calcifications representing necrotic cortical tubules (least common)

IVP
- Medullary sponge kidney (MSK)
  - Mild → "paintbrush" appearance of linear striations in pyramids from contrast in ectatic tubules

- Moderate to severe → "bouquet of flowers" and "bunch of grapes" appearances of contrast pooling in cystic dilations of collecting tubules
- Pros: Highly sensitive for collecting tubule dilation
- Cons: Contrast and radiation exposure; low sensitivity for small stones and nephrocalcinosis; not routinely used

CT Findings
- NECT
  - Medullary NC: Stippled, coarse, or confluent calcifications in medulla
    - Hyperparathyroidism and renal tubular acidosis (RTA) type 1 → usually diffuse, uniform calcification
      - Dense, confluent medullary calcification: Common in renal tubular acidosis
    - Medullary sponge kidney → often asymmetrical, segmental, or unilateral calcifications
      - Cluster of calcifications in papillae is characteristic
      - Highly sensitive for stones but low sensitivity for tubular ectasia
      - Medullary NC is often present but not mandatory for diagnosis of MSK
    - Papillary necrosis → coarsely calcified necrotic papillae (commonly in analgesic nephropathy)
  - Cortical NC: Thin band or tram line cortical calcification with small perpendicular extensions in Bertin columns
- CECT
  - MSK on CT intravenous pyelogram (IVP) = "paintbrush" appearance in mild cases; "bouquet of flowers" or "bunch of grapes" appearances in more severe cases
    - CT IVP: Highly sensitive for stones, medullary cysts, and collecting tubule dilation; contrast and radiation exposure
    - Advanced → deformed papillae and distorted calyces

Imaging Recommendations
- Best imaging tool
  - US is 1st diagnostic imaging option in infants and children with suspected nephrocalcinosis
  - Noncontrast CT in adults except for MSK where CT IVP may be best (sensitive for stones and collecting tubule dilation)
- Protocol advice
  - US is sensitive for screening of early nephrocalcinosis in children with known predisposing metabolic conditions, such as RTA and hyperoxaluria
  - Detection of nephrocalcinosis on plain films is improved by low kV technique

DIFFERENTIAL DIAGNOSIS

Renal Calculus
- Discrete echogenic focus with sharp posterior acoustic shadowing

Emphysematous Pyelonephritis
- Gas within renal parenchyma associated with "dirty shadowing"

Other Causes of Hyperechoic Medulla
- Autosomal recessive polycystic kidney disease

- Hyperuricemia: Gout, Lesch-Nyhan, glycogen storage disease (hyperechoic medulla and cortex)
- Hypokalemia: Primary aldosteronism, pseudo-Bartter syndrome
- Renal medullary fibrosis
- Abnormal protein deposition

PATHOLOGY

General Features

- Etiology
  - 3 primary mechanisms for calcium deposition
    - Metastatic: Metabolic abnormality → calcium deposition in medulla of morphologically normal kidneys
    - Urinary stasis: Calcium salts precipitate in dilated collecting ducts containing static urine
    - Dystrophic: Calcium deposition in damaged tissue
  - Causes of hypercalciuria
    - Bone resorption: Hyperparathyroidism, bone metastases, immobilization, multiple myeloma, hyperthyroidism, Cushing syndrome
    - Increased intestinal absorption of calcium: Sarcoidosis, milk-alkali syndrome, hypervitaminosis D, idiopathic hypercalciuria
    - Decreased tubular reabsorption
  - Medullary nephrocalcinosis
    - Hyperparathyroidism = most common cause; 5% of patients with hyperparathyroidism have medullary NC
    - Renal tubular acidosis type 1 (distal) = 2nd most common cause
      □ May be 1° or 2° to other systemic disease (Sjögren, lupus, etc.)
      □ Type 2 (proximal) RTA does not cause NC
    - MSK: Common cause; congenitally abnormal dilation of collecting ducts
      □ Calcium in ectatic collecting ducts rather than renal substance
      □ Calcium deposits are larger and more sharply defined
      □ May be unilateral
    - Renal papillary necrosis: Especially analgesic nephropathy with calcified papillae; sickle cell disease
    - Furosemide therapy in newborns; long-term furosemide use in adults
    - Tuberculosis
  - Cortical nephrocalcinosis
    - Acute cortical necrosis (e.g., septic or hemorrhagic shock, commonly in obstetrical complication)
    - Chronic glomerulonephritis
    - Alport syndrome: Hereditary nephritis and deafness
    - Nephrotoxic drugs and poisoning: Amphotericin B, methoxyflurane anesthesia, ethylene glycol
    - Hemolytic uremic syndrome
    - Chronic rejection of renal transplant
    - Sickle cell disease
  - Combined medullary and cortical nephrocalcinosis
    - Hyperoxaluria: Hereditary (altered bile metabolism) and acquired (intestinal over absorption of oxalate; small bowel pathology, e.g., IBD, surgery, or too much oxalate in diet)

      □ Hyperoxaluria → NC and urolithiasis → eventual renal failure → oxalosis
      □ Oxalosis = calcium oxalate crystal deposits in vessels, bones, and organs
    - AIDS-related infections: Described with *Mycobacterium avium-intracellulare, pneumocystis carinii, Histoplasma*, and cytomegalovirus

Microscopic Features

- Calcium deposition in interstitium, tubule epithelial cells, along basement membranes
- Calcium deposition within lumen of tubules

CLINICAL ISSUES

Presentation

- Most common signs/symptoms
  - Most often asymptomatic
  - MSK may present with complication: UTI, hematuria, urolithiasis

Demographics

- Age
  - Any
- Gender
  - M > F
- Epidemiology
  - Incidence: 0.1-6%
  - MSK: 0.5-1% general population
    - ~ 18% female and 12% male calcium stone formers

DIAGNOSTIC CHECKLIST

Image Interpretation Pearls

- Unilateral, asymmetric, or segmental medullary nephrocalcinosis → MSK

SELECTED REFERENCES

1. Koraishy FM et al: CT urography for the diagnosis of medullary sponge kidney. Am J Nephrol. 39(2):165-70, 2014
2. Lee H: Nephrocalcinosis. In Kim S: Radiology Illustrated: Uroradiology. 2nd ed. Berlin: Springer. 528-49, 2012
3. Aziz S et al: Rapidly developing nephrocalcinosis in a patient with end-stage liver disease who received a domino liver transplant from a patient with known congenital oxalosis. J Ultrasound Med. 24(10):1449-52, 2005
4. Kim YG et al: Medullary nephrocalcinosis associated with long-term furosemide abuse in adults. Nephrol Dial Transplant. 16(12):2303-9, 2001
5. Schepens D et al: Images in nephrology. Renal cortical nephrocalcinosis. Nephrol Dial Transplant. 15(7):1080-2, 2000
6. Dyer RB et al: Abnormal calcifications in the urinary tract. Radiographics. 18(6):1405-24, 1998
7. Toyoda K et al: Hyperechoic medulla of the kidneys. Radiology. 173(2):431-1989

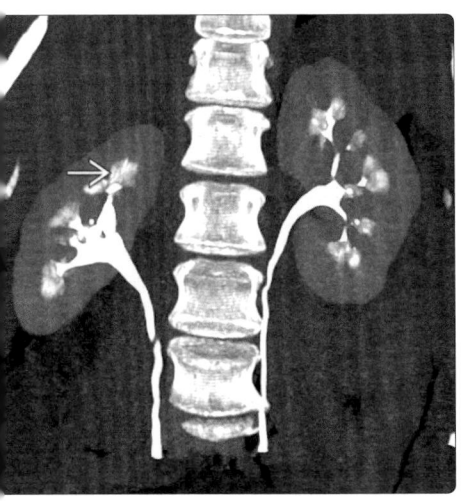

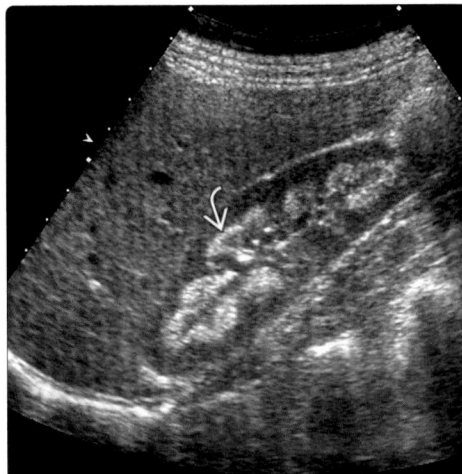

(Left) Coronal MIP from CT urogram shows "paintbrush" appearance ➡ of the renal pyramids consistent with medullary sponge kidney. (Right) Longitudinal US of the right kidney shows echogenic pyramids with reversal of the normal corticomedullary differentiation. Note medullary ring ➡ of the hyperechoic rim outlining the pyramid.

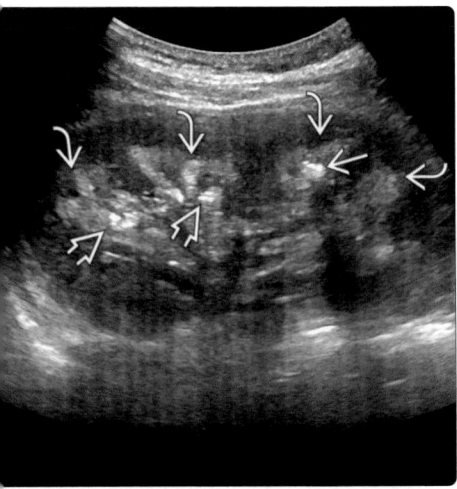

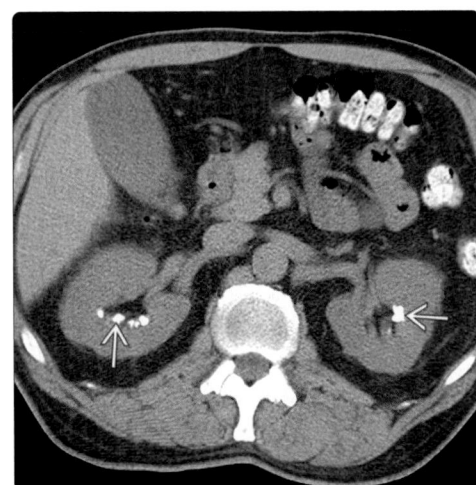

(Left) Longitudinal US of the left kidney shows echogenic pyramids ➡. A shadowing stone ➡ is identified in the lower pole. Other echogenic regions ➡ represent additional nonshadowing calculi. (Right) Axial NECT through the kidneys shows multiple calculi within the tips of bilateral medullary pyramids ➡. Larger calcium deposits within renal papillae and uneven, asymmetric distribution indicate medullary sponge kidney as cause of medullary nephrocalcinosis.

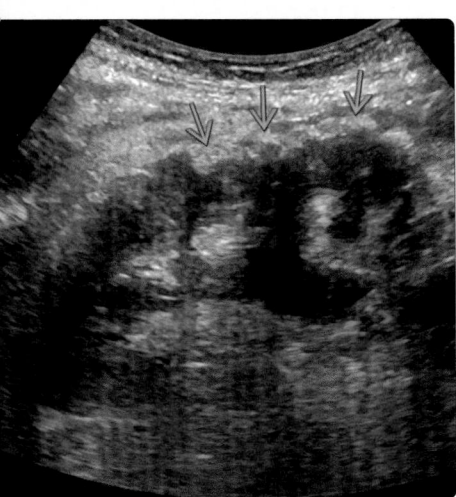

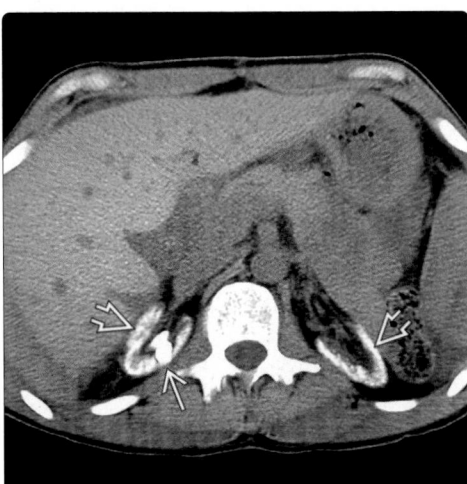

(Left) Longitudinal grayscale ultrasound shows a transplant kidney with cortical nephrocalcinosis ➡ related to cortical necrosis from ischemic injury after renal vein thrombosis and subsequent revascularization. (Right) Axial NECT through the kidney shows hyperdense, atrophic bilateral kidneys ➡ with cortical nephrocalcinosis related to underlying oxalosis. Large, dense right renal calculi ➡ are also identified.

KEY FACTS

TERMINOLOGY

- Dilation of renal collecting (pelvicalyceal) system ± ureteral dilation from intrinsic or extrinsic cause
- Renal collecting system dilation, pelvicalyceal dilatation, pelvocaliectasis

IMAGING

- Dilated intercommunicating fluid-filled anechoic channels (renal calyces and pelvis) in kidney
- Severity of hydronephrosis depends on degree and duration of obstruction
- Presence of internal echoes within dilated collecting system may represent underlying infection/pyonephrosis
- Antenatal US: Renal pelvis AP diameter ≥ 4 mm prior to 20-week gestation
- Fetal renal pelvis diameter ≥ 7 mm at 20-28 weeks or ≥ 10 mm beyond 28-week gestation requires postnatal follow-up

- CT has high sensitivity in evaluating site and etiology of obstruction (intrinsic [stone] or extrinsic)
- CT may show striated nephrogram &/or urothelial enhancement in superadded infection (pyelonephritis)
- CT urogram: Useful in nonstone etiology (urothelial neoplasm, necrosed/sloughed papillae, clot)
- MAG 3/DTPA scan: Central photopenic area at vascular phase, tracer accumulation within hydronephrotic collecting system with delayed drainage

TOP DIFFERENTIAL DIAGNOSES

- Parapelvic cyst
- Extrarenal pelvis
- Prominent renal vasculature
- Autosomal dominant polycystic kidney

PATHOLOGY

- Chronic obstruction: Loss of renal parenchyma and functio

(Left) Axial transabdominal renal ultrasound shows an echogenic stone ⏎ in the renal pelvis with mild hydronephrosis ➡. (Right) Pulsed Doppler ultrasound in the same patient with ureteral stone ⏎ shows elevated resistive indices (RI) (1.0) ➡, which indicates obstruction is acute in nature. The contralateral normal kidney had a normal RI of 0.7 (not shown), which is another finding indicative of acute obstruction in this kidney.

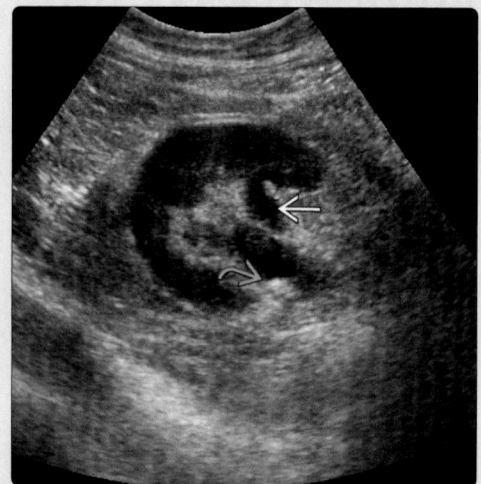
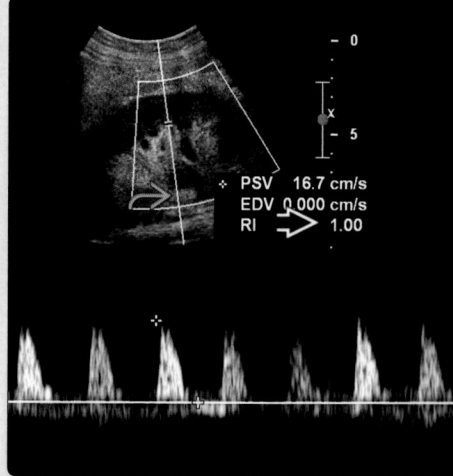

(Left) Longitudinal transabdominal ultrasound of the right kidney shows moderate hydronephrosis as evidenced by the presence of caliectasis ➡ as well as pelviectasis ⏎. (Right) Longitudinal transabdominal ultrasound in a different patient shows a moderately dilated renal pelvis ➡ with echogenic debris ⏎, which raises concern for pyonephrosis in the proper clinical setting of superimposed infection. Additional finding of a few echogenic intracalyceal stones ➡ may be nidus for infection.

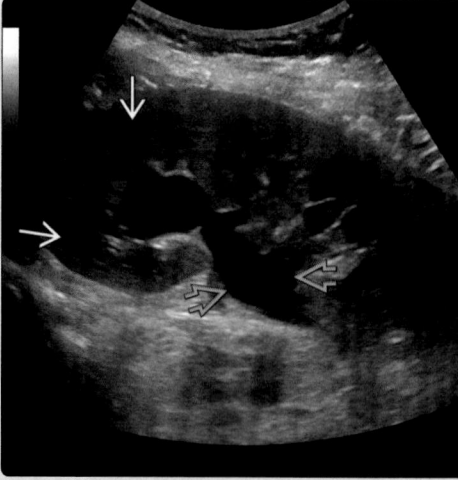
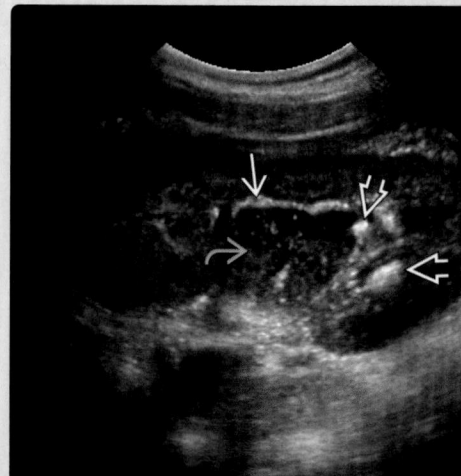

TERMINOLOGY

Synonyms

Renal collecting system dilation, pelvicalyceal dilatation, pelvocaliectasis

Definitions

Dilation of renal collecting (pelvicalyceal) system ± ureteral dilation

IMAGING

General Features

- Best diagnostic clue
  - Dilated intercommunicating fluid-filled anechoic channels (renal calyces and pelvis) on ultrasound
- Size
  - Severity of hydronephrosis depends on
    - Degree of obstruction (partial or complete)
    - Duration of obstruction
    - Renal function and urine output

Radiographic Findings

- IVP
  - Radiologic technique more commonly replaced with CT urogram (CTU/CT IVP)
    - Many findings seen on traditional IVP also seen on CT urogram
    - Increasingly dense nephrogram in acute obstruction
    - Site of obstruction seen as abrupt or gradual cut-off ± filling defect of contrast opacified column in urinary tract

CT Findings

- NECT
  - Dilated hypodense renal collecting system ± hydroureter
  - High sensitivity in evaluating site and etiology of obstruction (intrinsic [stone] or extrinsic)
  - Perinephric or periureteral fat stranding suggest reactive inflammation
  - Ureteral rim sign: Thickening of ureteral wall secondary to edema from stone impaction
- CECT
  - May show striated nephrogram &/or urothelial enhancement in superimposed infection (pyelonephritis)
  - CTU/CT IVP useful in nonstone etiology (urothelial neoplasm, necrosed/sloughed papillae, clot)
    - Delayed contrast opacification of collecting system
    - May see urine leak from forniceal rupture in high-grade obstruction
    - Useful in evaluation of parapelvic cysts, ureteropelvic junction (UPJ) obstruction
    - Diminished nephrogram with reduced parenchymal thickness in chronic hydronephrosis
    - Dilated renal collecting system ± ureter, widening of forniceal angles, renal enlargement

MR Findings

Utilized in pediatric population due to lack of ionizing radiation to define site of obstruction, parenchymal loss

Ultrasonographic Findings

- Grayscale ultrasound
  - Anechoic intercommunicating fluid-filled spaces (calyces) and pelvis ± hydroureter
    - Presence of internal echoes within dilated collecting system may represent underlying infection/pyonephrosis
  - Renal enlargement based on degree of obstruction
    - Mild hydronephrosis: Small separation of calyceal pattern (splaying), normal bright sinus echoes, normal parenchymal thickness
    - Moderate hydronephrosis: Ballooning of major and minor calyces, diminished sinus echoes, normal or thinned parenchymal thickness
    - Severe hydronephrosis: Massive dilatation of renal pelvis and calyces, associated with cortical thinning and loss of normal renal sinus echogenicity
  - Antenatal US: Renal pelvis AP diameter ≥ 4 mm prior to 20-week gestation
    - Fetal renal pelvis diameter ≥ 7 mm at 20-28 weeks or ≥ 10 mm beyond 28-week gestation requires postnatal follow-up
  - Hydronephrosis secondary to UPJ obstruction
    - Etiology for up to 48% of fetal hydronephrosis
    - Dilated renal pelvicalyceal system with stenosed UPJ
  - Focal hydrocalyx/caliectasis: Congenital, infectious stricture
    - Anechoic cystic focus with smooth margin; may be difficult to differentiate on ultrasound from renal cyst
- Pulsed Doppler
  - Resistive indices (RI) may be useful in differentiating acute from chronic (atony, gravid uterus, vesicoureteral reflux) obstruction
  - Obstructive hydronephrosis: RI > 0.7 or RI 0.08-0.1 higher than normal contralateral side in unilateral obstruction
  - Arteriolar vasoconstriction in obstruction, hence reduces diastolic arterial flow velocity
- Color Doppler
  - Presence of ureteral jets in bladder help exclude complete ureteral obstruction on affected side
    - Useful in pregnant patients

Nuclear Medicine Findings

- DMSA scan: Central photopenic area ± cortical scar
- MAG 3/DTPA scan: Central photopenic area at vascular phase, tracer accumulation within hydronephrotic collecting system with delayed drainage

Imaging Recommendations

- Best imaging tool
  - Early evaluation: Ultrasound
  - CT ± contrast (CTU): Helps to confirm and identify etiology
- Protocol advice
  - Work-up of prenatal diagnosed hydronephrosis
    - Post natal US for serial monitoring
    - Voiding cystourethrogram to evaluate vesicoureteric reflux or posterior urethral valves in severe cases
  - Postnatal US to be performed 4-7 days after birth because of relative dehydration in 1st days of life: False-negative sign of hydronephrosis

DIFFERENTIAL DIAGNOSIS

Parapelvic Cyst
- Lymphatic in origin or develop from embryologic rests
- Well-defined anechoic renal sinus mass
- No communication with pelvicalyceal system
- CT urogram for confirmation

Extrarenal Pelvis
- No dilation of renal calyces or ureter
- Focal ballooning of renal pelvis beyond contour of renal sinus

Multicystic Dysplastic (MCD) Kidney
- Developmental anomaly, a.k.a. renal dysplasia, renal dysgenesis, multicystic kidney usually unilateral
- Small kidney with multiple noncommunicating cysts
- Absence of both normal parenchyma and normal renal sinus complex

Prominent Renal Vasculature
- Mimics dilated renal pelvis on transverse scans
- Vascular flow demonstrated on color Doppler

Autosomal Dominant Polycystic Kidney
- Bilateral enlarged kidneys with multiple asymmetrical cysts of varying size
- Cysts with internal echoes if hemorrhage or infected

Multilocular Cystic Nephroma
- Uncommon benign cystic neoplasm
- Seen as focal multilocular noncommunicating cysts

PATHOLOGY

General Features
- Etiology
  - Obstruction: Stone, blood clot, sloughed papilla, crossing of iliac vessels, stricture (benign or malignant)
    - ± ureteric dilatation, depending on level of obstruction
    - Confirmation: CT urogram, antegrade/retrograde pyelography, isotope renogram
    - Chronic obstruction: Loss of renal parenchyma and function
  - Relieved obstruction
    - If obstruction is severe or prolonged, dilatation may not return to normal secondary to atony
    - Pulsed Doppler: Normal RIs
  - Reflux nephropathy
    - Usually focal caliectasis, associated with renal cortical scarring
  - Pregnancy
    - More marked on right side (from gravid uterus, sigmoid protective of left side) may become permanent after multiple pregnancies
    - Doppler: Normal ureteral jets in bladder; pulsed Doppler: Normal RIs
  - Congenital hydronephrosis: Isolated abnormality
    - Ureteropelvic obstruction, posterior urethral valve, ectopic ureterocele, prune belly syndrome, vesicoureteric junction obstruction

- Papillary necrosis: Calyces with sloughed papillae become clubbed
- Pyelonephritis: Calyceal clubbing, focal caliectasis, and cortical scar

CLINICAL ISSUES

Presentation
- Most common signs/symptoms
  - Adults: Flank pain/hematuria for renal or ureteric stone
  - Pediatric: Abdominal mass
  - Neonate: Diagnosed on antenatal ultrasound

Natural History & Prognosis
- Urine leak from forniceal/renal pelvic tear if acute significant obstruction
- Superimposed infection + obstruction, consider pyonephrosis, a surgical emergency
- Parenchymal atrophy if chronic obstruction, leading to renal impairment

DIAGNOSTIC CHECKLIST

Consider
- Communicating anechoic tubular spaces in kidney with altered renal sinus fat

Image Interpretation Pearls
- False-positive sign of hydronephrosis
  - Full bladder may cause distension of calyces, normal when bladder empty
  - Increased urine flow: Overhydration, medication, following urography

SELECTED REFERENCES

1. Liu DB et al: Hydronephrosis: prenatal and postnatal evaluation and management. Clin Perinatol. 41(3):661-78, 2014
2. Jandaghi AB et al: Assessment of ureterovesical jet dynamics in obstructed ureter by urinary stone with color Doppler and duplex Doppler examinations. Urolithiasis. 41(2):159-63, 2013
3. Piazzese EM et al: The renal resistive index as a predictor of acute hydronephrosis in patients with renal colic. J Ultrasound. 15(4):239-46, 201.
4. Estrada CR Jr: Prenatal hydronephrosis: early evaluation. Curr Opin Urol. 18(4):401-3, 2008
5. Becker A et al: Obstructive uropathy. Early Hum Dev. 82(1):15-22, 2006
6. Sidhu G et al: Outcome of isolated antenatal hydronephrosis: a systematic review and meta-analysis. Pediatr Nephrol. 21(2):218-24, 2006
7. Moon DH et al: Value of supranormal function and renogram patterns on 99mTc-mercaptoacetyltriglycine scintigraphy in relation to the extent of hydronephrosis for predicting ureteropelvic junction obstruction in the newborn. J Nucl Med. 44(5):725-31, 2003
8. Perez-Brayfield MR et al: A prospective study comparing ultrasound, nuclear scintigraphy and dynamic contrast enhanced magnetic resonance imaging the evaluation of hydronephrosis. J Urol. 170(4 Pt 1):1330-4, 2003
9. Grenier N et al: Dilatation of the collecting system during pregnancy: physiologic vs obstructive dilatation. Eur Radiol. 10(2):271-9, 2000

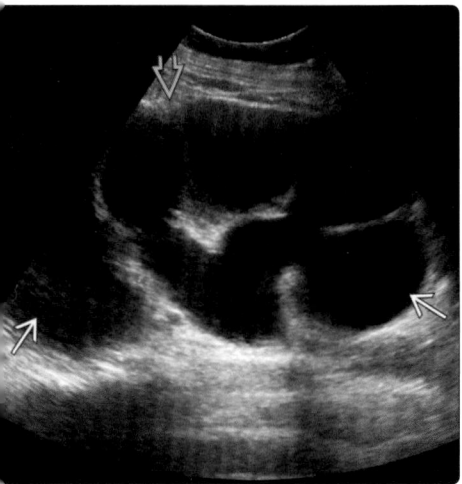

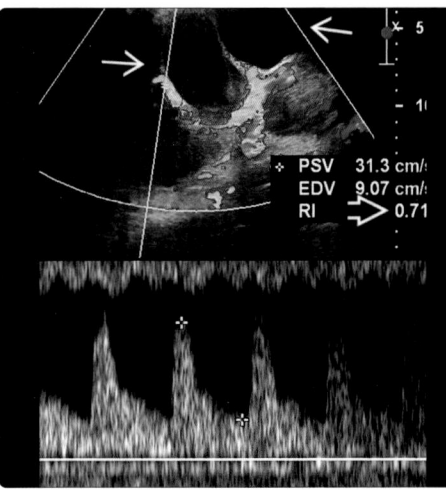

(Left) *Longitudinal transabdominal ultrasound of the kidney shows significant dilation of the renal collecting system* ➡️. *The degree of marked parenchymal thinning* ⇒ *indicates this is a longstanding process.* (Right) *Color Doppler ultrasound in the same patient shows that the RI = 0.7* ➡️ *is in the normal range, consistent with the chronic nature of this patient's significant hydronephrosis* ➡️.

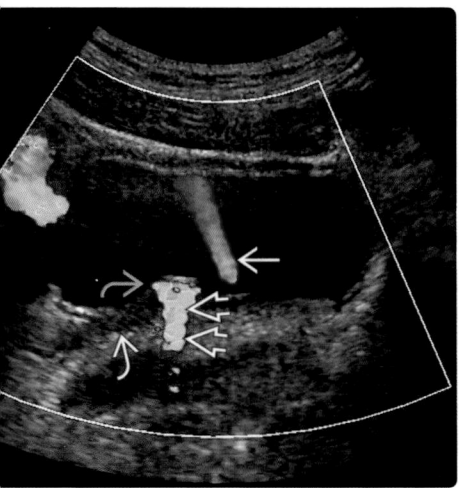

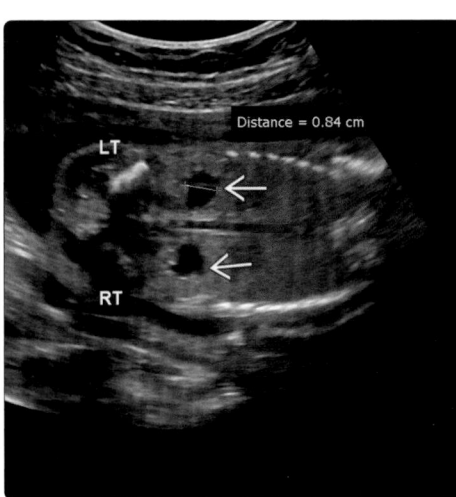

(Left) *Transverse transabdominal color Doppler ultrasound of the urinary bladder shows an obstructing stone* ⇗ *at right UVJ. Twinkling artifact* ➡️ *is seen distal to the stone, which can be useful to identify stones in the urinary system. The ureter proximal to the obstructing stone is moderately dilated* ➡️. *A normal left ureteral jet* ➡️ *is seen on the contralateral side.* (Right) *Coronal antenatal fetal US shows a bilateral dilated renal collecting system* ➡️ *(pelvis = 8 mm, normally measured in the AP dimension on a transverse image).*

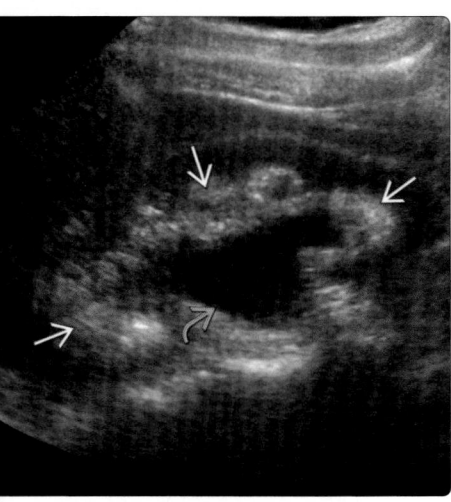

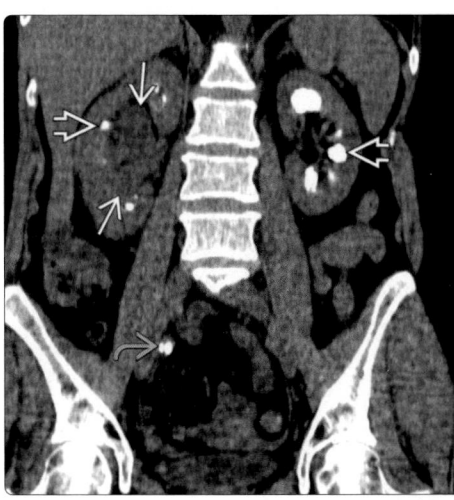

(Left) *Longitudinal ultrasound of a kidney with moderate hydronephrosis* ⇗ *shows increased echogenicity of the medulla* ➡️, *which is a finding consistent with medullary nephrocalcinosis, a condition that can predispose patients to development of renal calculi.* (Right) *Coronal reformat NECT of the abdomen in the same patient confirms nephrocalcinosis with bilateral multiple stones* ➡️ *and right moderate hydronephrosis* ➡️, *caused by an obstructing right ureteral stone* ⇗.

KEY FACTS

TERMINOLOGY

- Benign, fluid-filled, nonneoplastic renal lesion
- Most common renal lesion, usually detected incidentally on imaging

IMAGING

- Unilocular, thin-walled, round/oval renal lesion
- Anechoic: No internal echoes, septations, or solid components
- Increased sound transmission gives rise to characteristic posterior acoustic enhancement (increased through transmission)
- Ultrasound is ideal for characterizing simple or complex renal cysts in nonobese patients
- Once diagnosis of simple renal cyst is established, no further imaging or monitoring of cyst is warranted

TOP DIFFERENTIAL DIAGNOSES

- Complex renal cyst

- Peripelvic cysts
- Prominent pyramids
- Cystic disease of dialysis
- Perinephric collections
- Pyelogenic cyst/pyelocalyceal diverticulum
- Multilocular cystic nephroma

CLINICAL ISSUES

- Present in 20-30% of middle-aged adults
- Present in 50% of patients > 50 years of age

DIAGNOSTIC CHECKLIST

- Well-defined round or ovoid renal lesion with posterior acoustic enhancement, distinct echogenic posterior wall, and complete lack of internal echoes (anechoic)
- Important to distinguish simple renal cysts from complex cystic renal lesions

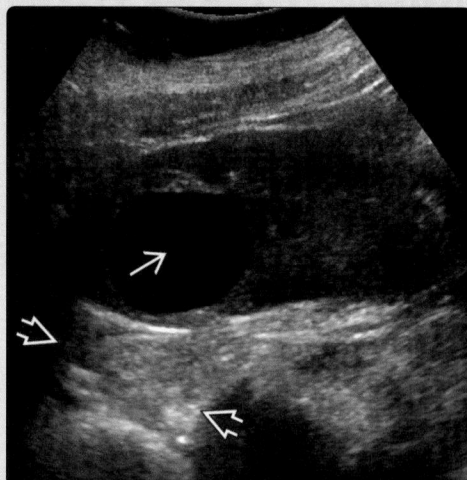
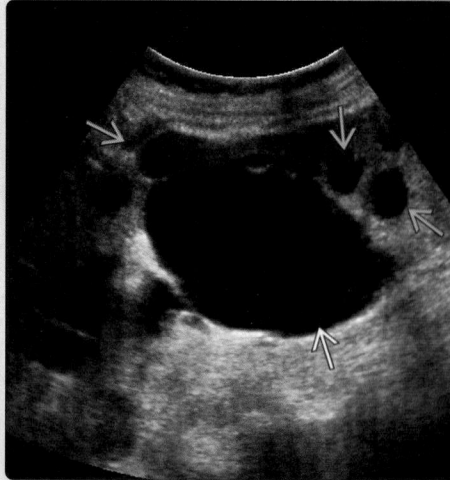

(Left) Longitudinal ultrasound shows a typical simple cortical cyst, with complete lack of internal echoes ➡️, imperceptible walls, and posterior acoustic enhancement ➡️. (Right) Longitudinal transabdominal ultrasound shows a large parapelvic renal cyst ➡️ in addition to multiple smaller cortical cysts ➡️. Large cysts may produce distension, pain, or spontaneous hemorrhage.

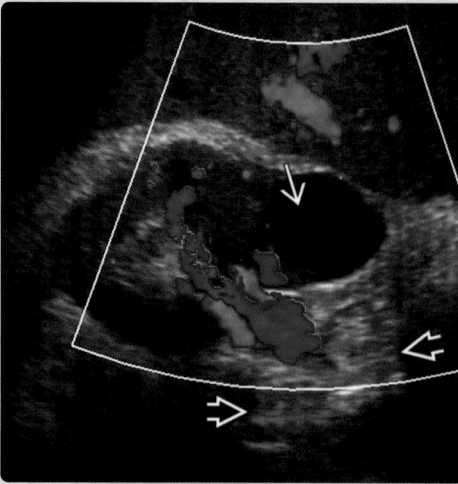
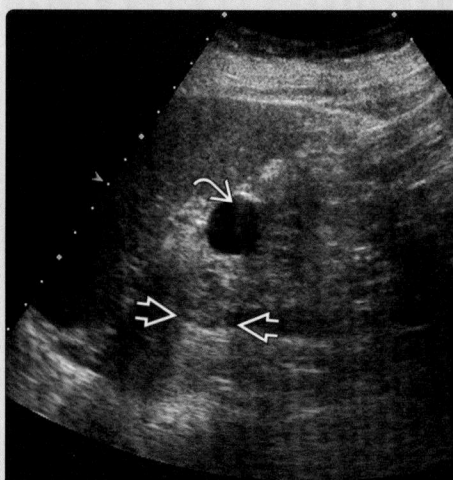

(Left) Transverse color Doppler ultrasound shows a simple cortical renal cyst with complete lack of internal flow ➡️. Posterior acoustic enhancement ➡️ remains visible. (Right) Longitudinal US shows a small simple cyst in an echogenic kidney. Minimal echoes within the peripheral aspect of the cyst ➡️ are artifactual and confounding. Posterior acoustic enhancement remains evident ➡️. In the setting of underlying renal disease, the possibility of acquired cystic disease should be considered.

TERMINOLOGY

Definitions

- Benign, fluid-filled, nonneoplastic renal lesion
- Parapelvic cyst: Simple cyst that indents the renal sinus
- Peripelvic cysts: Lymphatic origin, multiple small cystic lesions in renal sinus

Associated Syndromes

- Associated with tuberous sclerosis, von Hippel-Lindau disease, neurofibromatosis, or Caroli disease

IMAGING

General Features

- Best diagnostic clue
  - Well-defined round or ovoid renal lesion with posterior acoustic enhancement, distinct echogenic posterior wall, and complete lack of internal echoes (anechoic)
- Location
  - Renal cortex (deep or superficial/exophytic)
  - Renal sinus (parapelvic/peripelvic cysts)
- Size
  - Subcentimeter to > 10 cm
- Morphology
  - Round, fluid-filled lesion with imperceptible walls
  - Single or multiple; when multiple, rarely unilateral

Ultrasonographic Findings

- Grayscale ultrasound
  - Unilocular, thin-walled, round/oval renal lesion
  - Anechoic: No internal echoes, septations, or solid components
  - Increased sound transmission gives rise to characteristic posterior acoustic enhancement (increased through transmission)
    - May be absent in small cysts (< 3 mm)
      - Tiny cysts may appear as echogenic nonshadowing foci
  - US is more accurate than CT or MR in demonstrating internal cyst morphology
  - In at-risk patients, criteria for polycystic kidney disease
    - 3 renal cysts from age 15-39
    - At least 2 cysts in each kidney if age 40-59
    - At least 4 cysts in each kidney if age > 60
- Color Doppler
  - Lack of intracystic color signal
  - Adjacent blood vessels may be displaced
- Contrast-enhanced ultrasound (CEUS)
  - Most useful for further characterization of nonsimple cysts: Internal echoes, septations, wall thickening
  - Provides information analogous to the Bosniak classification, good concordance with CECT
  - Contrast uptake within cystic lesion suspicious for malignancy (other than thin, smooth septa)

CT Findings

- Categorized as Bosniak class I cyst
  - Well-defined, round, homogeneous, low-density mass (< 20 HU, near water density) with thin or imperceptible nonenhancing wall
  - No septations or calcifications

- Small (< 1 cm) cysts may be too small to accurately measure density; if less than blood density on NECT, likely cyst
- No enhancement on CECT: Change of <10 HU between imaging phases

MR Findings

- T1WI: Round/oval, homogeneous, hypointense
- T2WI: Homogeneous, hyperintense (water signal) with imperceptible wall; smooth & distinct inner margin
- CEMR: No enhancement

Imaging Recommendations

- Best imaging tool
  - Ultrasound is ideal for characterizing simple or complex renal cysts in nonobese patients
  - Contrast-enhanced CT is highly sensitive and specific
  - Consider CEUS in patients with impaired renal function
- Protocol advice
  - Once diagnosis of simple renal cyst is established, no further imaging or monitoring of cyst is warranted

DIFFERENTIAL DIAGNOSIS

Complex Renal Cyst

- Fluid-filled nonneoplastic renal lesion not meeting imaging criteria of simple renal cyst
- Distinguish from simple cyst by presence of internal septations, debris, calcifications

Peripelvic Cysts

- Likely to be lymphatic in origin
- Medially located cystic lesion, may compress collecting system or vessels
- Benign; distinction from parapelvic cysts is not clinically relevant

Prominent Pyramids

- Prominent pyramids may be observed in normal pediatric kidneys, acute glomerulonephritis, transplant acute rejection, acute tubular necrosis, and chronic kidney disease
- Multiple, typical location, not anechoic

Cystic Disease of Dialysis

- Small kidneys with multiple small cysts (< 3 cm) bilaterally
- Patients with chronic kidney disease on long-time dialysis
- Increased risk of renal cell carcinoma (RCC)

Perinephric Collections

- Loculated perinephric fluid collections may indent or distort renal contour
- Seromas or urinomas invariably simulate simple renal cysts

Pyelogenic Cyst/Pyelocalyceal Diverticulum

- Urine-containing eventration of upper collecting system
- Appears as cystic lesion, sometimes thick-walled arising from renal parenchyma
- Intracystic milk of calcium or mobile calculi suggest diagnosis; contrast filling confirms diagnosis

Multilocular Cystic Nephroma

- Unilateral, large multilocular cystic renal mass
- Well-circumscribed cystic mass with thick fibrous capsule ± herniation into renal pelvis

Bosniak Classification of Renal Cysts (CT-Based)

Class	Definition	Imaging Features
Bosniak I	Benign simple cyst	Homogeneous, water density (< 20 HU), thin walls, no septations or calcifications, no enhancement
Bosniak II	MInimally complex benign cyst	Hyperdense, thin septa, minimal thin septal or wall calcifications, no enhancement
Bosniak IIF	Indeterminate complex cyst, requires follow-up	Hyperdense, minimally thickened walls or septations, thickened calcifications, no enhancement or questionable
Bosniak III	Indeterminate complex cystic mass, surgery or ablation recommended	Smooth walls or septations with measurable enhancement
Bosniak IV	Malignant cystic lesion, surgery required	Clearly malignant lesions with enhancing solid components

PATHOLOGY

General Features

- Etiology
  - Believed to be caused by obstruction of ducts or tubules, or may arise in embryonic rests

Gross Pathologic & Surgical Features

- Unilocular, arises in cortex and bulges from renal surface, less commonly into renal sinus
- Clear or straw-colored fluid
- Smooth, yellow-white, thin translucent wall
- No communication with renal pelvis

Microscopic Features

- Cyst wall is composed of fibrous tissue and is lined by flattened cuboidal epithelium
- Cyst fluid contains plasma transudate

CLINICAL ISSUES

Presentation

- Most common signs/symptoms
  - Mostly asymptomatic
- Other signs/symptoms
  - May present with palpable mass
  - Local pain due to wall distention of large cyst or spontaneous intracystic hemorrhage
  - Flank pain, malaise, and fever if infected
  - Occasionally, severe abdominal pain and hematuria caused by spontaneous, iatrogenic, or traumatic rupture
  - Rarely, hypertension may occur secondary to renal segmental ischemia as result of cyst obstruction

Demographics

- Age
  - Present in 20-30% of middle-aged adults
  - 50% of patients > 50 years of age
  - Rare in individuals < 30 years of age
- Gender
  - Most reports show no gender predilections but some suggest incidence M > F

Natural History & Prognosis

- Slow-growing; increase in size by 5% annually
- Rare complications include hydronephrosis, hemorrhage, infection, or rupture
  - Following rupture, cyst may regress or disappear completely
- Spontaneous cyst rupture into collecting system or perinephric space may occur due to build-up of pressure within cyst secondary to either intracystic hemorrhage or change in cyst fluid content

Treatment

- Cyst rupture is managed conservatively
- Indications for surgical intervention reserved solely for symptomatic cysts or those that affect renal function
  - Percutaneous needle aspiration of cyst ± injection of sclerosing agent
  - Ureteroscopic or laparoscopic marsupialization
  - Laparoscopic excision

DIAGNOSTIC CHECKLIST

Consider

- Imaging findings more reliable than clinical correlation (except for abscess)
- Multiple simple cysts may indicate polycystic kidney disease in at-risk patients; may require clinical follow-up

Image Interpretation Pearls

- Anechoic intracystic content with posterior acoustic enhancement
- Important to distinguish simple renal cysts from complex cystic renal lesions

SELECTED REFERENCES

1. Wood CG 3rd et al: CT and MR Imaging for Evaluation of Cystic Renal Lesions and Diseases. Radiographics. 35(1):125-41, 2015
2. Di Salvo DN et al: Lithium nephropathy: unique sonographic findings. J Ultrasound Med. 31(4):637-44, 2012
3. McArthur C et al: Current and potential renal applications of contrast-enhanced ultrasound. Clin Radiol. 67(9):909-22, 2012
4. Whelan TF: Guidelines on the management of renal cyst disease. Can Urol Assoc J. 4(2):98-9, 2010
5. Israel GM et al: An update of the Bosniak renal cyst classification system. Urology. 66(3):484-8, 2005
6. Terada N et al: The natural history of simple renal cysts. J Urol. 167(1):21-3, 2002
7. Rathaus V et al: Pyelocalyceal diverticulum: the imaging spectrum with emphasis on the ultrasound features. Br J Radiol. 74(883):595-601, 2001

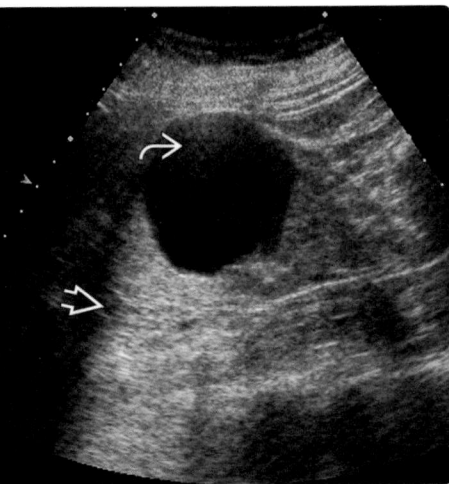

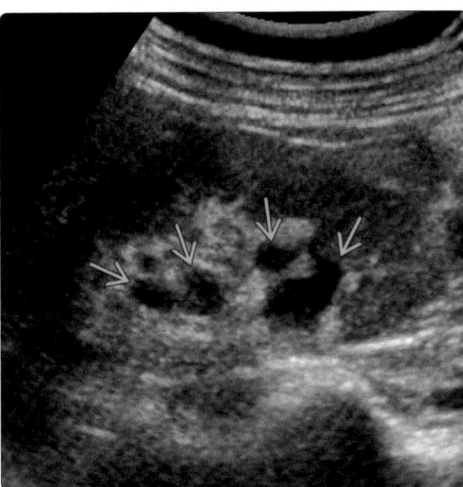

(Left) *Longitudinal ultrasound shows a simple cyst. Artifactual echoes are present in the peripheral aspect ➦, which should not be confused with internal debris or nodularity. Strong posterior acoustic enhancement is visible ➡.* **(Right)** *As seen on this longitudinal ultrasound, multiple small peripelvic cysts ➡ can mimic hydronephrosis; CT may be required to distinguish between them. Small cysts may not demonstrate clear posterior acoustic enhancement, as in this case.*

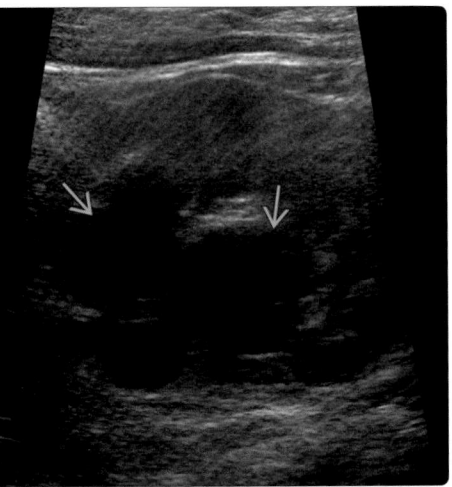

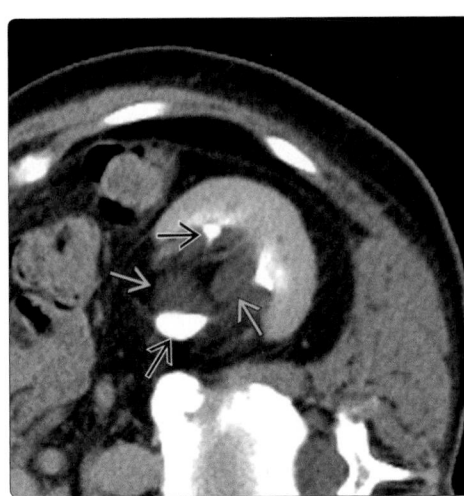

(Left) *Transverse ultrasound of the left kidney shows multiple large peripelvic cysts ➡, mimicking hydronephrosis. The renal pelvis cannot be distinguished from the cysts.* **(Right)** *Delayed-phase CECT in the same patient, rotated 90° to match the ultrasound, confirms the presence of peripelvic cysts ➡, which surround the contrast-filled collecting system ➡ but do not communicate with it.*

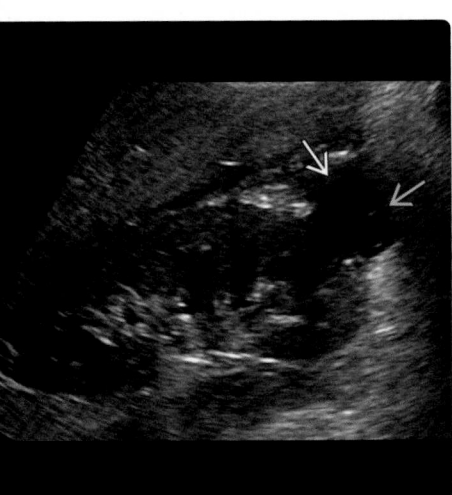

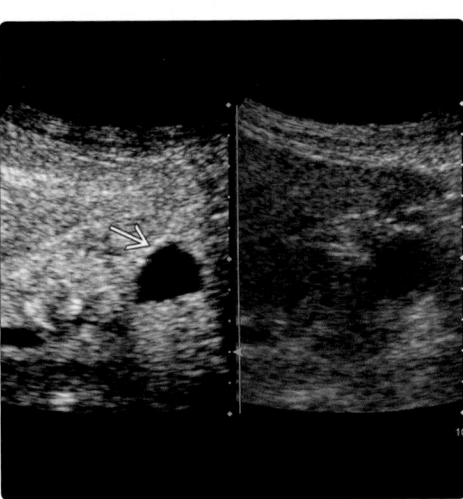

(Left) *Longitudinal ultrasound of the right kidney shows an exophytic lower pole cystic lesion ➡ with thin internal septa ➡. (Courtesy P. Sidhu, MD.)* **(Right)** *Contrast-enhanced ultrasound (left) and corresponding grayscale ultrasound (right) of the same cystic right renal lesion ➡ show no internal enhancement, confirming a benign minimally complex cyst. (Courtesy P. Sidhu, MD.)*

TERMINOLOGY

- Benign, fluid-filled nonneoplastic renal lesion not meeting criteria of simple renal cyst
- Bosniak classes II, IIF, and III

IMAGING

- Round, oval, or irregular-shaped anechoic lesion
- Hemorrhagic cyst: Appearance varies with age of blood
- Proteinaceous cyst: May contain low-level echoes, with bright reflectors or even layers of echoes
- Infected cyst: Thick wall with scattered internal echoes ± debris-fluid level
- Calcified cyst: Wall or septal calcification ± shadowing
- Neoplastic features: Solid mural or septal nodules, irregular wall, or irregular septal thickening
- Complex cysts should be evaluated with CEUS, CECT, or CEMR for decision of surgical intervention
- CEUS: Increased sensitivity for detecting malignancy compared with unenhanced US and CECT

- Contrast uptake within cystic lesion on CEUS is suspicious for malignancy (other than a few bubbles in thin smooth septa or wall)

TOP DIFFERENTIAL DIAGNOSES

- Renal cell carcinoma
- Multilocular cystic nephroma
- Localized cystic disease
- Renal abscess
- Renal metastasis
- Renal lymphoma

DIAGNOSTIC CHECKLIST

- Correct imaging classification of cystic masses is key to management

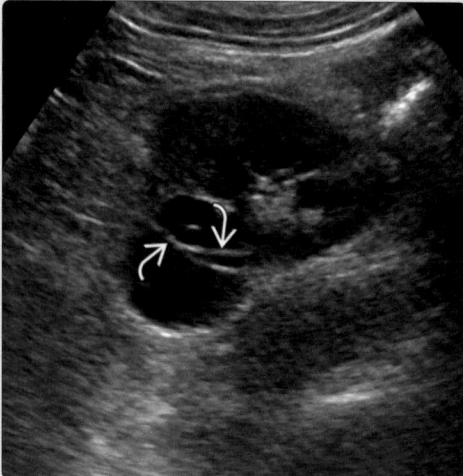 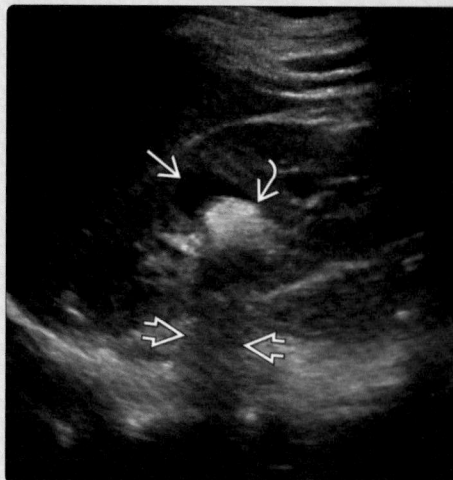

(Left) Transverse US shows a near anechoic lesion other than thin internal septations ➡, which did not have flow on color Doppler. There are no internal nodules, wall, or septal thickening; this corresponds to a Bosniak II lesion. (Right) Longitudinal US shows a cyst ➡ with dependent, layering echogenic material ➡ with posterior shadowing ➡, consistent with milk of calcium. In the absence of internal septations or nodularity, this is consistent with a minimally complex cyst (Bosniak II).

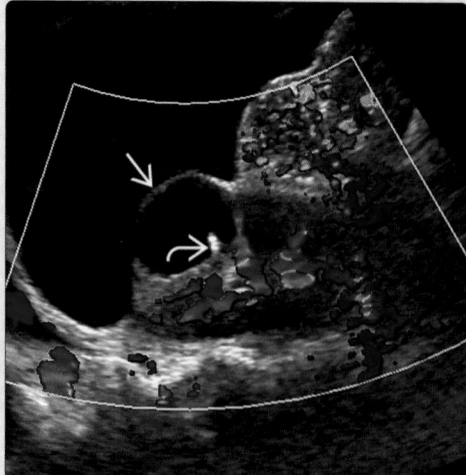 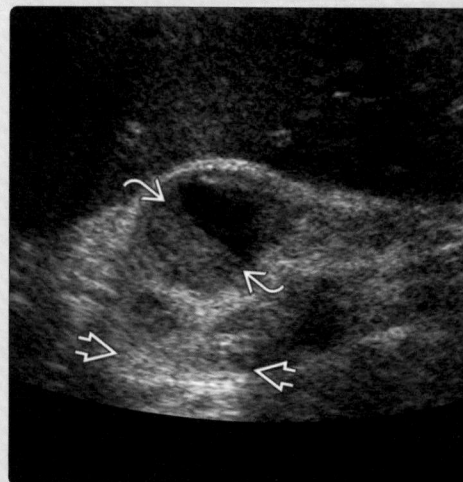

(Left) Longitudinal US of the right kidney shows an upper pole cyst ➡ with a small echogenic peripheral nodule ➡. Color Doppler does not show internal flow; however, the presence of a nodule warrants follow-up (Bosniak IIF). (Right) Longitudinal US shows a mixed echogenicity cystic lesion with layering echogenic material ➡ and posterior acoustic enhancement ➡. The findings are consistent with a hemorrhagic cyst although contrast-enhanced imaging is suggested to confirm the absence of malignancy.

TERMINOLOGY

Definitions

Benign, fluid-filled nonneoplastic renal lesion not meeting criteria of simple renal cyst
- Bosniak classes II, IIF, and III

IMAGING

General Features

Best diagnostic clue
- Well-defined fluid-filled renal lesion with internal features: Calcifications, septations, turbid content; wall thickening, absent or equivocal enhancement

Size
- Usually 2-5 cm in diameter (up to 10 cm)

Morphology
- Depends on histology

Ultrasonographic Findings

Grayscale ultrasound
- Round, oval, or irregular-shaped anechoic lesion
- Hemorrhagic cyst: Appearance varies with age of blood
  - Acute: Hyperechoic, hypoechoic, or isoechoic, containing fluid-debris level or solid avascular clot, later septated lesion
  - Chronic: Thick calcified wall ± multiloculated
- Proteinaceous cyst: May contain low-level echoes, with bright reflectors or even layers of echoes
- Infected cyst: Thick wall with scattered internal echoes ± debris-fluid level
- Calcified cyst: Wall or septal calcification ± shadowing
  - Milk of calcium cyst: "Comet tail" artifact + line of calcium intracystic debris
  - Wall nodularity may be obscured by wall or diffuse calcification of cystic mass
- Neoplastic features: Solid mural or septal nodules, irregular wall, or irregular septal thickening

Color Doppler
- Lack of intracystic color signal
- Low sensitivity for detecting vascularity

Contrast-enhanced US (CEUS)
- Provides information analogous to Bosniak classification
- Increased sensitivity for detecting color flow (and malignancy) compared with unenhanced US and CECT
- Contrast uptake within cystic lesion is suspicious for malignancy (other than a few bubbles in thin smooth septa or wall)

CT Findings

Denser than simple fluid on NECT (> 20 HU)
- Lack of enhancement on CECT: Change of < 10 HU from pre- to postcontrast images
- Hemorrhagic cyst
  - NECT: Hyperdense; CECT: Hypodense relative to enhancing parenchyma
  - Homogeneous density 60-90 HU (acute)
  - Heterogeneous (clot or debris), ↑ wall thickness and ↓ attenuation ± calcification (chronic)
- Infected cyst: Thick wall, septated, heterogeneous fluid, debris- or gas-fluid level; ± calcification (chronic)
- Ruptured cyst: Retroperitoneal or perinephric fluid collection, blood (varied density)
- Septations: 1 or more thin partial or complete septa
- Milk of calcium cyst: Dependent, fluid-calcium layer
- Neoplastic wall: Focal thickening or enhancing nodule

MR Findings

- Contrast-enhanced MR is useful to detect intracystic enhancement
- MR superior to CECT for detection of internal septa within cyst
- Hemorrhagic cyst: Variable signal intensity dependent on age of hemorrhage
  - T1WI: Highest intensity in subacute (< 72 hr)
  - T2WI: Hyperintense but less than simple cyst; fluid-debris level; ± heterogeneous mass and lobulation of contour
- Proteinaceous cyst: ↑ protein simulates hemorrhage: T1 hyperintense
- Infected cyst: T1WI: ↑ intensity, less homogeneous than simple cyst; ↓ intensity than subacute hemorrhage (similar to chronic); ± thickened wall
- Calcified cyst: MR is insensitive to detect calcification but is superior to CT to detect enhancement within calcified cyst
- Neoplastic wall: Focal thickening or enhancing nodule mass or wall thickening

Imaging Recommendations

- Best imaging tool
  - US, as initial investigation for characterizing simple or minimally complex renal cysts + monitoring of complex renal cysts (Bosniak class IIF)
  - CEUS or MR best to evaluate for internal cyst enhancement, further characterize Bosniak II and III lesions
- Protocol advice
  - Complex cysts should be evaluated with CEUS, CECT, or CEMR for decision of surgical intervention
  - CT evaluation must include NECT and CECT on same scanner, same time, same technique

DIFFERENTIAL DIAGNOSIS

Renal Cell Carcinoma (RCC)

- Cystic RCC: Thick septa, septal or peripheral calcification, enhancing wall, or septal nodularity
- Papillary RCCs are homogeneous with minimal enhancement, can mimic complex cysts on CT/MR

Localized Cystic Disease

- Conglomerate of simple cysts simulating a multilocular cystic mass, usually unilateral
- Lacks well-defined pseudocapsule around aggregate of cysts
- Renal parenchyma is present between cysts
- Can simulate multilocular cystic nephroma, cystic neoplasm, or autosomal dominant polycystic kidney disease

Multilocular Cystic Nephroma

- Multilocular cystic lesion with thick and thin septa
- Propensity to herniate into renal pelvis

Renal Abscess

- May extend into calyces and perinephric space

Bosniak Classification of Renal Cysts (CT-Based)

Class	Definition	Imaging Features
Bosniak I	Benign simple cyst	Homogeneous, water density (< 20 HU), thin walls, no septations or calcifications, no enhancement
Bosniak II	MInimally complex benign cyst	Hyperdense, thin septa, minimal thin septal or wall calcifications, no enhancement
Bosniak IIF	Indeterminate complex cyst, requires follow-up	Hyperdense, minimally thickened walls or septations, thickened calcifications, no enhancement or is questionable
Bosniak III	Indeterminate complex cystic mass, surgery, or ablation recommended	Smooth walls or septations with measurable enhancement
Bosniak IV	Malignant cystic lesion, surgery required	Clearly malignant lesions with enhancing solid components

- Appears as thick-walled, complex cystic mass with internal debris and septations
- Clinical features point to diagnosis

Renal Metastasis

- Common in patients with advanced malignancy
- Primary sites include lung, breast, melanoma, stomach, cervix, colon, pancreas, prostate, and contralateral kidney
- May appear as isoechoic, hypoechoic, or hyperechoic masses

Renal Lymphoma

- Secondary renal lymphoma more common than primary
- Diffuse renal enlargement, bilateral multiple hypoechoic renal masses, direct infiltration from retroperitoneum and perirenal space
- Perinephric extension with vascular and ureteral encasement is common

PATHOLOGY

General Features

- Hemorrhagic cyst (6%): Unknown, trauma, bleeding diathesis or varicosities in simple cyst
- Calcified cyst (1-3%): Hemorrhage, infection, or ischemia
- Infected cyst: Hematogenous spread, vesicoureteric reflux, surgery, or cyst puncture

Gross Pathologic & Surgical Features

- Hemorrhagic cyst: Rust-colored putty-like material surrounded by thick fibrosis and plates of calcification
- Infected cyst: Markedly thickened wall ± calcification; varying pus, fluid, and calcified or noncalcified debris
- Neoplastic wall: Discrete nodule at base of cyst

Microscopic Features

- Hemorrhagic cyst: Uni- or multilocular, thickened wall
- Neoplastic wall: Well-differentiated clear/granular cell
- Septated cyst: Compressed normal parenchyma or nonneoplastic connective tissue

CLINICAL ISSUES

Presentation

- Most common signs/symptoms
  - Asymptomatic or palpable mass and flank pain
  - Infected cyst: Pain in flank, malaise, and fever
  - Hemorrhagic cyst: Abrupt and severe pain
  - Ruptured cyst: Severe abdominal pain, hematuria

Demographics

- Age
  - Present in 20-30% of middle-aged adults
    - > 50% of patients > 50 years of age
    - Rare in patients < 30 years of age
- Gender
  - M > F

Natural History & Prognosis

- Complications: Hydronephrosis, hemorrhage, infection, cyst rupture, or carcinoma
- Follow-up: Increase in size, change in configuration, and internal consistency suggest carcinoma
- Prognosis: Very good

Treatment

- Bosniak class II: No treatment unless symptomatic
- Bosniak class IIF: Follow-up by imaging
- Bosniak class III and IV: Surgical excision (partial or radical nephrectomy) or ablation

DIAGNOSTIC CHECKLIST

Consider

- CEUS when CECT or CEMR not feasible

Image Interpretation Pearls

- Correct imaging classification of cystic masses is key to management

SELECTED REFERENCES

1. Nicolau C et al: Prospective evaluation of CT indeterminate renal masses using US and contrast-enhanced ultrasound. Abdom Imaging. 40(3):542-51, 2015
2. Wood CG 3rd et al: CT and MR imaging for evaluation of cystic renal lesions and diseases. Radiographics. 35(1):125-41, 2015
3. Barr RG et al: Evaluation of indeterminate renal masses with contrast-enhanced US: a diagnostic performance study. Radiology. 271(1):133-42, 2014
4. Quaia E et al: Comparison of contrast-enhanced sonography with unenhanced sonography and contrast-enhanced CT in the diagnosis of malignancy in complex cystic renal masses. AJR Am J Roentgenol. 191(4):1239-49, 2008

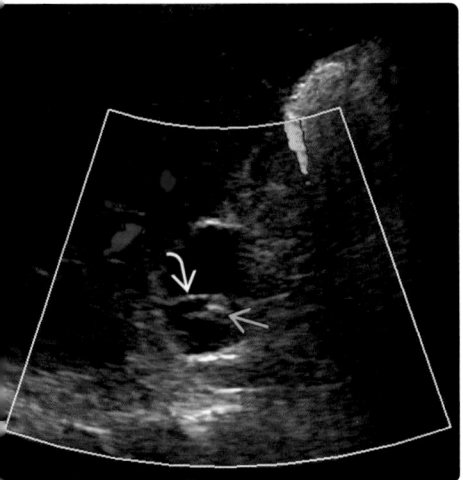

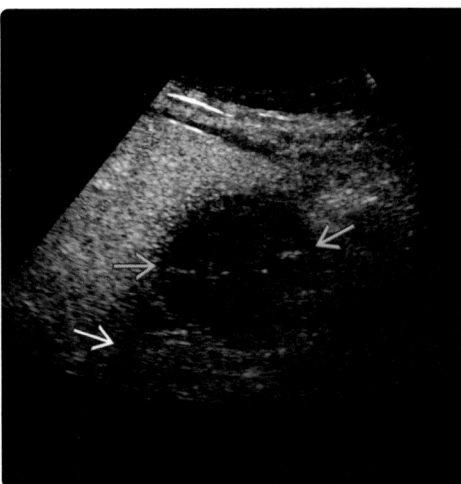

(Left) Transverse Doppler US shows a complex cyst with a thin internal septation ⬈ and potential nodule ➡. Although there is no color Doppler flow, contrast-enhanced imaging is more sensitive for detecting internal flow. (Right) Longitudinal contrast-enhanced US of the right kidney ➡ shows an exophytic cyst with a thin, smooth internal septation ➡. A few microbubbles are seen in the septation with no other enhancement, confirming a benign complex cyst. (Courtesy P. Sidhu, MD.)

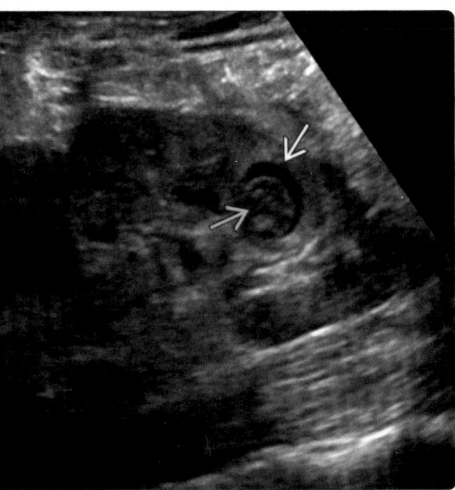

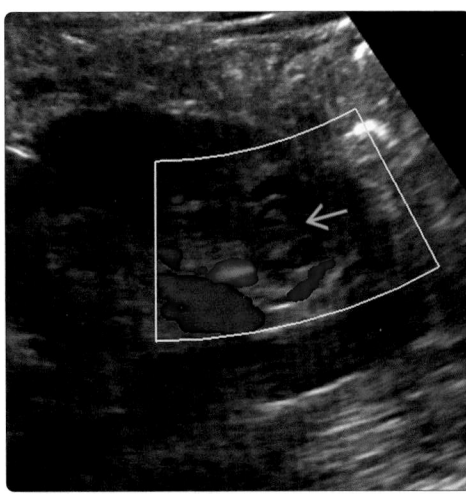

(Left) Longitudinal US shows a suspicious lower pole cystic lesion ➡ with an internal mass-like nodule ➡, which is suspicious for a malignant lesion. (Right) Color Doppler US in the same patient does not demonstrate internal color flow ➡, which is most consistent with a hemorrhagic cyst with retracting clot. However, Doppler imaging is insensitive for detecting subtle vascularity, and contrast-enhanced imaging is recommended.

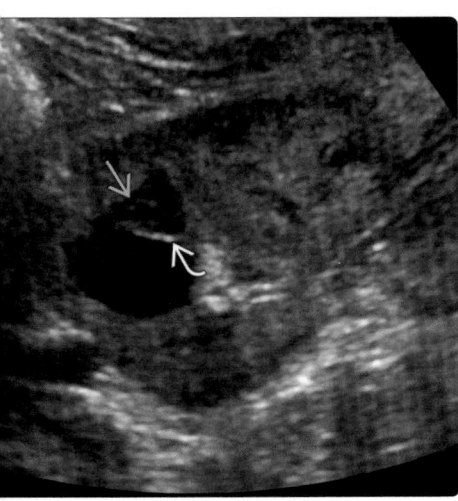

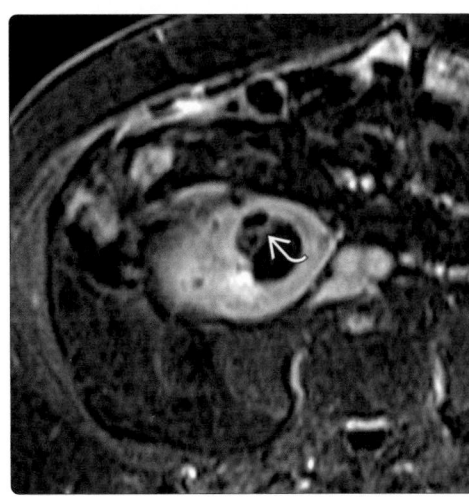

(Left) Longitudinal US in a transplant kidney shows a complex upper pole cystic lesion with a septation ⬈ and nodule ➡, which is suspicious for potential malignancy. (Right) Transverse T1 C+ MR subtraction image in the same patient shows the presence of enhancement within the septations ⬈, consistent with a Bosniak III lesion.

KEY FACTS

TERMINOLOGY

- Presence of 3 or more renal cysts per kidney in patients with chronic kidney disease (CKD) who do not have hereditary cystic disease
- Occurs predominantly in patients on long-term dialysis (peritoneal or hemodialysis)
- Can be seen in up to 13% of patients with CKD prior to dialysis

IMAGING

- Ultrasound as initial investigation for establishing diagnosis in patients on dialysis
- Multiple bilateral small cysts in normal-sized or atrophic, echogenic kidneys
  - Simple cysts: Well-defined round lesions with posterior acoustic enhancement, distinct echogenic posterior wall, lack of internal echoes
  - Hemorrhagic cysts: May contain visible internal echoes or debris

- Malignant transformation of cysts typically manifests as papillary growth within the cyst
- Cysts scattered in both renal cortex and medulla
- Renal size may be enlarged due to increase in size and number of cysts
- Contrast enhanced ultrasound (CEUS), CECT, or CEMR are required to evaluate complex cysts and distinguish from renal cell carcinoma (RCC)

TOP DIFFERENTIAL DIAGNOSES

- Multiple simple cysts
- Adult polycystic kidneys disease (ADPKD)
- von Hippel-Lindau disease
- Tuberous sclerosis (TS)
- Medullary cystic disease

CLINICAL ISSUES

- Renal cell carcinoma occurs in up to 7% of patients with acquired cystic kidney disease (ACKD)

(Left) US shows a markedly echogenic kidney ➡ with multiple small cortical and medullary cysts ➡. Many of these contain peripheral calcifications ➡, more common in ACKD than in age-related simple renal cysts. One of these is entirely calcified ➡. (Right) Longitudinal US shows the lateral aspect of the left kidney ➡ in a patient with ACKD. A large exophytic complex cyst ➡ with internal echoes is suspicious for malignancy, despite the lack of color flow. Surgical pathology confirmed a papillary renal cell carcinoma.

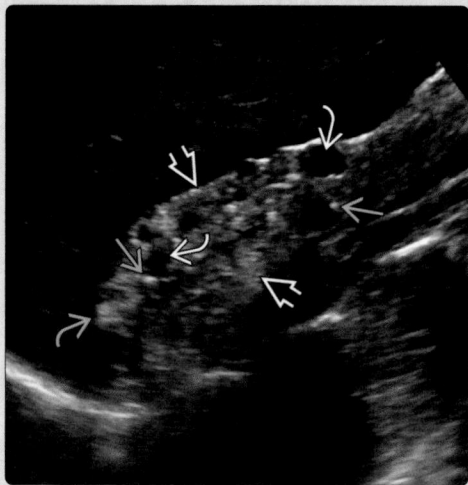
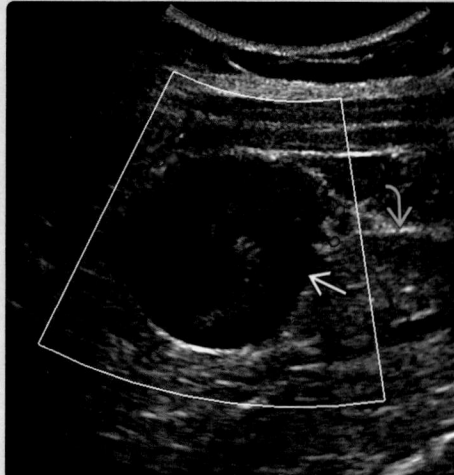

(Left) Longitudinal color Doppler image shows multiple cysts ➡ within an echogenic kidney ➡. The inferior cyst has internal echoes ➡ and lack of color flow, consistent with a hemorrhagic cyst, common in patients with ACKD. (Right) Coronal CT image in the same patient shows the corresponding hyperdense ➡ cyst in the mid to lower pole. There was no evidence of enhancement on this multiphase CT scan, which is consistent with a hemorrhagic cyst.

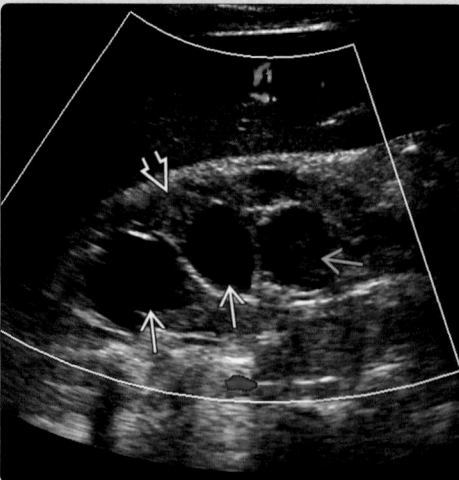
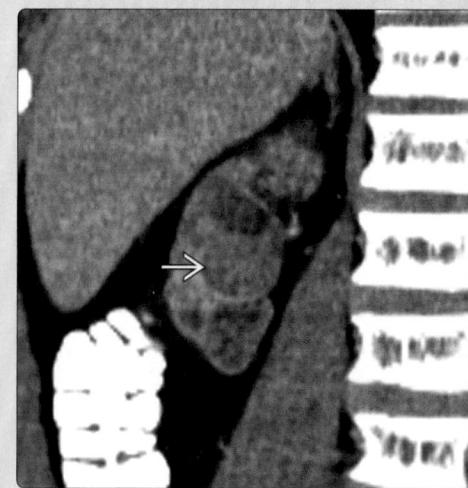

TERMINOLOGY

Abbreviations

- Acquired cystic kidney disease (ACKD)

Synonyms

- Acquired cystic disease of uremia

Definitions

- Presence of 3 or more renal cysts per kidney in patients with chronic kidney disease (CKD) who do not have hereditary cystic disease
- Occurs predominantly in patients on long-term dialysis (peritoneal or hemodialysis)

IMAGING

General Features

- Best diagnostic clue
  - Small kidneys with multiple small cysts bilaterally
  - Advanced stage: Large kidneys as cysts increase in size and number
- Location
  - Bilateral; in areas of scarring throughout cortex and medulla
- Size
  - Usually < 1 cm, up to 3 cm
- Morphology
  - Simple cyst: Round, fluid-filled lesion with imperceptible walls
  - Complex cyst: Internal debris, septations, calcifications, wall thickening

Ultrasonographic Findings

- Grayscale ultrasound
  - Multiple bilateral small cysts in normal size or atrophic, echogenic kidneys
  - Cysts scattered in both renal cortex and medulla
  - Renal size may be enlarged due to increase in size and number of cysts
    - In advanced stage, appearance may resemble adult polycystic kidney disease (ADPKD)
  - Simple cysts: Well-defined round lesions with posterior acoustic enhancement, distinct echogenic posterior wall, lack of internal echoes
  - Hemorrhagic cysts: May contain internal echoes or nodular debris
    - Distinction from neoplasm not always possible
  - Cyst rupture: May bleed into renal pelvis or retroperitoneum resulting in hematuria or retroperitoneal hematoma, respectively
  - Malignant transformation of cysts typically manifests as papillary growth within the cyst
- Color Doppler
  - Presence of internal flow signal distinguishes tumor from hemorrhagic cyst
  - Power Doppler more sensitive than color Doppler to detect slow flow
- Contrast enhanced ultrasound (CEUS)
  - Increased sensitivity for detecting malignancy compared to unenhanced US and CECT
  - Not nephrotoxic, can be used in end-stage renal disease

  - No internal enhancement in simple and complex cysts (other than thin smooth septa)
  - Contrast uptake within cystic lesion is suspicious for malignancy

CT Findings

- Well-defined, thin-walled, nonenhancing lesions, < 20 HU
- ± cyst wall calcifications, ± luminal high density from crystal deposition
- Superior to ultrasound for detection of small tumors
  - Neoplasms enhance with contrast, typically more heterogeneous
  - Hyperdense cysts may be difficult to distinguish from solid lesions unless contrast is administered

MR Findings

- Best imaging test to evaluate for enhancing lesions, but contrast use may be limited secondary to risk of nephrogenic systemic fibrosis (NSF)
- Simple cyst: T1 hypointense, T2 hyperintense, homogeneous
- Hemorrhagic cyst: Variable T1 and T2 signal dependent upon age of hemorrhage
- CEMR: No enhancement

Imaging Recommendations

- Best imaging tool
  - Ultrasound as initial investigation for establishing diagnosis in patients on dialysis
  - CEUS, CECT, or CEMR to evaluate complex cysts and distinguish from renal cell carcinoma (RCC)
- Protocol advice
  - No widely accepted guidelines for screening of dialysis patients for ACKD or RCC

DIFFERENTIAL DIAGNOSIS

Multiple Simple Cysts

- Rarely as numerous as in ACKD
- Normal size kidneys with normal echogenicity
- Renal function not impaired
- Incidence increases with increasing age

Adult Polycystic Kidney Disease (ADPKD)

- Hereditary disorder characterized by multiple renal cysts and various systemic manifestations
- Cysts and kidneys are larger in size than in ACKD
- Differential features favoring ADPKD
  - Family history; presence of renal failure
  - Cysts in other organs: Liver (75%), pancreas (10%), spleen, ovaries
  - Intracranial aneurysms

von Hippel-Lindau Disease

- Autosomal dominant multisystemic disorder
- Multiple renal cysts, cysts in other organs
- Kidneys are normal in size and functional
- Hemangioblastomas: Cerebellar, spinal, and retinal
- Multifocal renal cell carcinomas, pheochromocytomas

Tuberous Sclerosis (TS)

- Multiple bilateral renal cysts
- Multiple small fat-containing renal angiomyolipomas

- Cerebral paraventricular calcifications

Medullary Cystic Disease

- Rare disease associated with progressive salt wasting nephropathy, renal insufficiency
- Cysts may be too small to be seen; visible cysts occur only in medulla
- Kidneys are almost invariably small in size
- Clinically, progressive renal failure in young patients

PATHOLOGY

General Features

- Etiology
  - Destruction of functional renal tissue, with compensatory hypertrophy of normal nephrons
  - Proliferation of epithelial cells from proximal renal tubules
    - Increased circulating growth factors and proto-oncogene activation
  - Fluid accumulation and expansion of renal tubule leads to cyst formation
    - Obstruction of tubules by oxalate crystals, interstitial fibrosis, or hyperplasia
    - Altered compliance of tubular basement membrane
    - Eventually loses connection with parent tubule to become isolated sac

Gross Pathologic & Surgical Features

- Atrophic kidneys with multiple small cysts, renal cortex > medulla, containing clear fluid or hemorrhage

Microscopic Features

- Cysts lined by single layer of flattened or cuboidal epithelium
- Papillary projections from cyst wall are common
- Calcium oxalate deposition in cyst walls

CLINICAL ISSUES

Presentation

- Most common signs/symptoms
  - Most patients with ACKD are asymptomatic
  - History of chronic renal failure and long-term dialysis
- Other signs/symptoms
  - Hematuria, flank pain, fever if complications occur

Demographics

- Gender
  - M > F ~ 3:1
- Epidemiology
  - Prevalence of ACKD in dialysis patients
    - 10-20% after 3 years
    - 40-60% after 5 years
    - > 90% after 10 years
  - Can be seen in up to 13% of patients with CKD prior to dialysis
  - Equal incidence in hemodialysis and peritoneal dialysis

Natural History & Prognosis

- Size and number of cysts correlate with duration of dialysis but not with renal disease
- Complications

- Intracystic hemorrhage in up to 50% of patients
- Cyst infection
- Rupture with retroperitoneal hemorrhage (13% of patients)
- Renal stones
- Malignant transformation to RCC
  - Develops in up to 7% of patients with ACKD over period of 7-10 years
  - Less aggressive than classical RCC, more commonly papillary RCC with infrequent metastasis (5-7%)
    - Acquired cystic disease associated RCC: New subtype exclusive to ACKD and long term dialysis
  - Risk of is higher in patients with cysts enlarging the renal volume
- Prognosis: In absence of RCC, dependent upon course of underlying renal disease

Treatment

- Asymptomatic simple and complex cysts require no treatment
- Bleeding and rupture usually treated conservatively
- Painful cysts may require drainage
- Infected cysts may require antibiotics and drainage
- Persistent and severe hemorrhage necessitates nephrectomy or renal artery embolization
- Bosniak category III and IV cysts require surgical exploration and nephrectomy
  - ~ 50% of category III cysts are malignant (RCC)
- Renal transplantation prevents formation of new cysts but does not decrease malignant potential of existing cysts
  - Prevents formation of new cysts; existing cysts may regress
  - Malignant potential may increase as result of immunosuppression

DIAGNOSTIC CHECKLIST

Consider

- Correlate with history to exclude hereditary cystic disease
- CT or US screening of asymptomatic patients for RCC and ACKD

Image Interpretation Pearls

- Bilateral, multiple small cysts in small to normal-sized echogenic kidneys
- Differentiate hemorrhagic cysts from small RCC

SELECTED REFERENCES

1. Wood CG 3rd et al: CT and MR Imaging for Evaluation of Cystic Renal Lesions and Diseases. Radiographics. 35(1):125-41, 2015
2. Cokkinos DD et al: Contrast enhanced ultrasound of the kidneys: what is it capable of? Biomed Res Int. 2013:595873, 2013
3. Singanamala S et al: Should screening for acquired cystic disease and renal malignancy be undertaken in dialysis patients? Semin Dial. 24(4):365-6, 2011
4. Katabathina VS et al: Adult renal cystic disease: a genetic, biological, and developmental primer. Radiographics. 30(6):1509-23, 2010
5. Ishikawa I et al: Twenty-year follow-up of acquired renal cystic disease. Clin Nephrol. 59(3):153-9, 2003
6. Nascimento AB et al: Rapid MR imaging detection of renal cysts: age-based standards. Radiology. 221(3):628-32, 2001
7. Choyke PL: Acquired cystic kidney disease. Eur Radiol. 10:1716-1721, 2000.

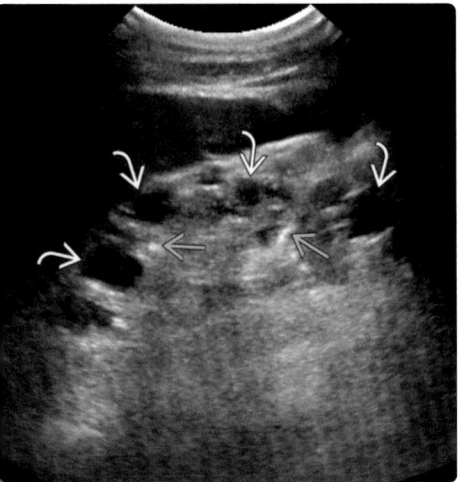

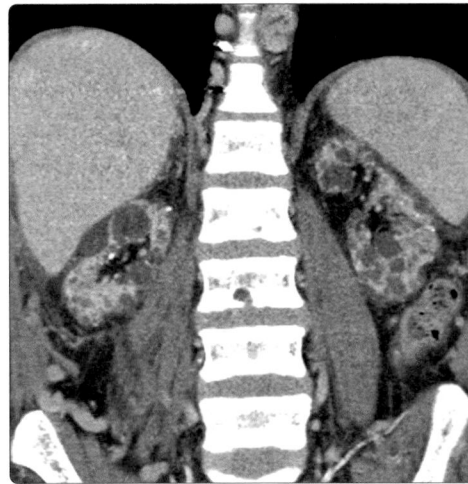

(Left) *Longitudinal ultrasound shows multiple cortical cysts* ⇲ *within an echogenic kidney in a patient with ESRD. Scattered parenchymal calcifications* ⇥ *are visible. Although the kidney is atrophic, the apparent renal size is increased secondary to the numerous cysts.* (Right) *Coronal CECT scan in the same patient demonstrates the bilateral nature of ACKD, with typical numerous small cysts throughout both kidneys.*

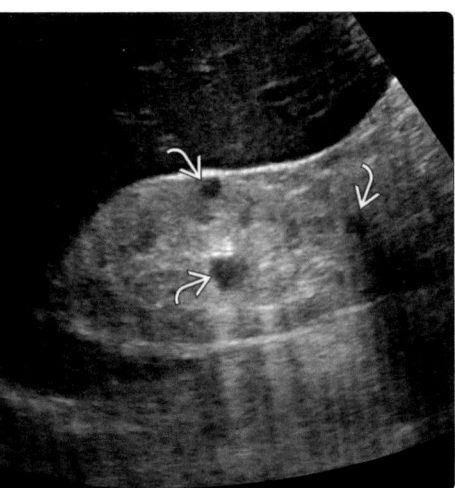

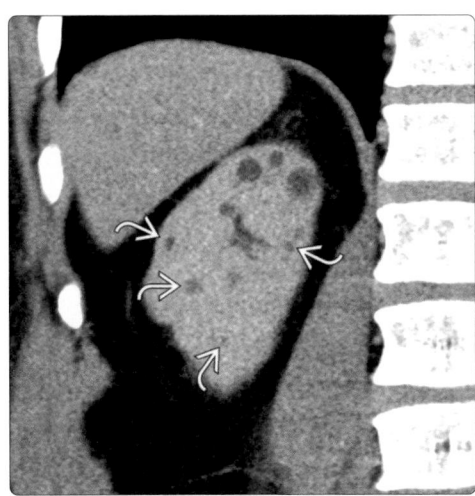

(Left) *Longitudinal ultrasound shows a markedly echogenic kidney consistent with ESRD. While 3 cysts are identified* ⇲*, many subcentimeter cysts are not clearly visible with ultrasound.* (Right) *Coronal delayed-phase CT image in the same patient better depicts the numerous tiny cysts* ⇲*, which were not clearly visible with ultrasound.*

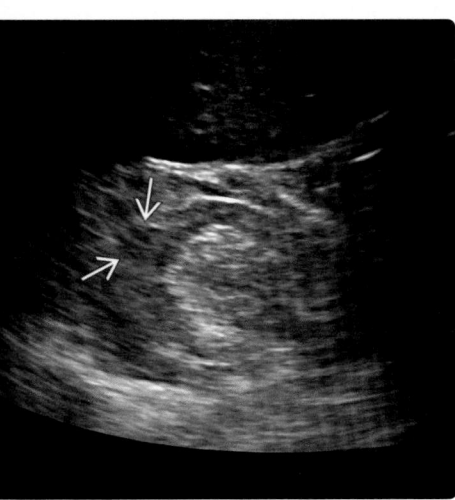

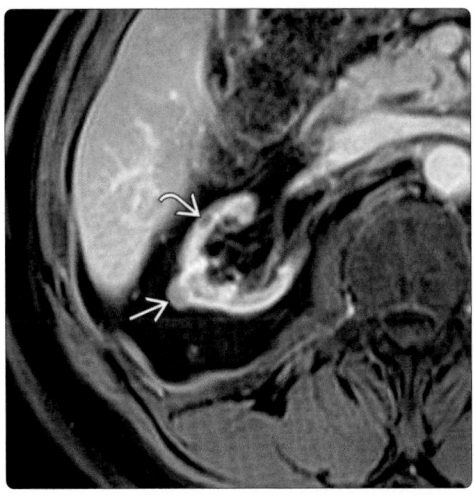

(Left) *Ultrasound can be limited in evaluating small lesions. Multiple small cysts are present in this patient with ESRD, but not clearly identified with ultrasound. In particular, there is a small peripheral solid lesion that even in retrospect is not well identified* ⇲*.* (Right) *Axial T1W contrast-enhanced MR image in the same patient more clearly shows the enhancing mass* ⇲ *consistent with RCC. An additional smaller cortical cyst* ⇲ *was not clearly visible on the ultrasound.*

Multilocular Cystic Nephroma

TERMINOLOGY

- Rare nonhereditary benign cystic renal neoplasm containing epithelial and stromal components

IMAGING

- Encapsulated multilocular cystic renal mass herniating into renal hilum
- Grayscale ultrasound
  - Numerous anechoic cysts with hyperechoic septa
  - Occasionally more solid-appearing due to numerous tiny cysts causing acoustic interfaces
- Fine vessels may be seen within septa on color Doppler
- Contrast uptake within septa and wall on CEUS
- CT: Large, well-defined multiloculated cystic mass, ± calcification, ± capsular enhancement
- T1WI: Multiloculated hypointense mass (clear fluid) with variable signal intensity (blood or protein)

TOP DIFFERENTIAL DIAGNOSES

- Cystic renal cell carcinoma (RCC)
- Mixed epithelial and stromal tumor (MEST)
- Cystic Wilms tumor

CLINICAL ISSUES

- Present with hematuria, abdominal/flank pain, palpable mass
- Complications
  - Obstructive uropathy, infection, hemorrhage
- Cured with complete surgical excisionblane
- Bimodal age and sex distribution: 2-4 years old, M>F; 40-60 years old, F>>M

DIAGNOSTIC CHECKLIST

- Appears as Bosniak class 3 or 4 cystic mass
- May be indistinguishable from cystic renal carcinoma
- Presence of enclosing capsule distinguishes MLCN from almost all other cystic renal masses

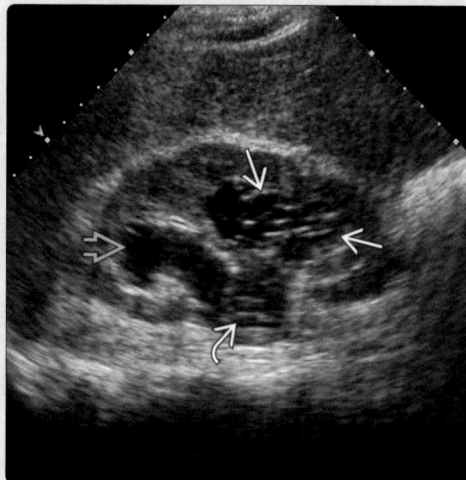
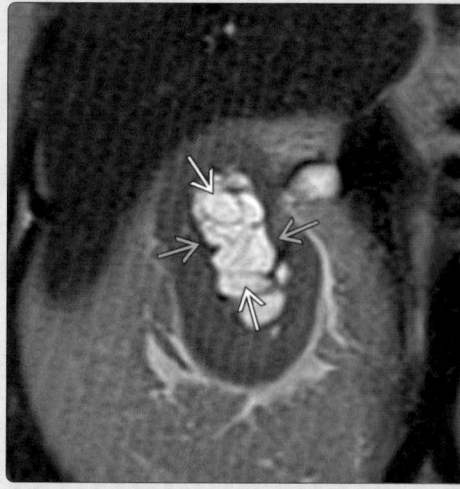

(Left) Longitudinal view of the right kidney reveals numerous small anechoic cystic locules ➡ in the lower pole, separated by echogenic septa, comprising a MLCN. This herniates into the renal hilum ➡, with associated obstruction of the renal pelvis leading to upper pole calyectasis ➡. (Right) Coronal T2-weighted MR in the same patient demonstrates multiple hyperintense cystic locules ➡ surrounded by a well-defined hypointense fibrous capsule ➡.

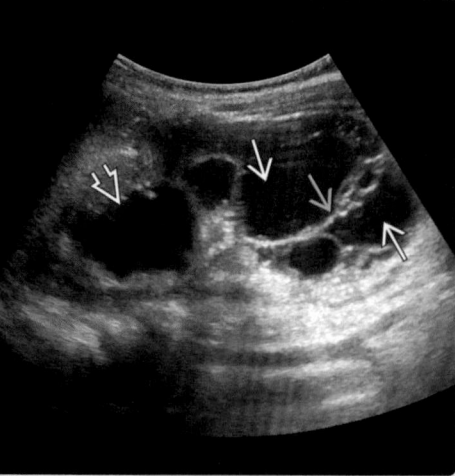
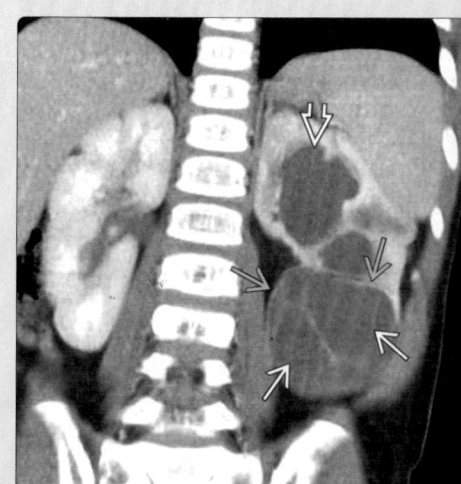

(Left) Longitudinal ultrasound view of the left kidney reveals multiple large anechoic cysts in the lower pole ➡ separated by thick septae ➡, consistent with MLCN. The upper pole cystic structure ➡ represents calyceal dilatation secondary to mass effect from the MLCN. (Right) Coronal contrast-enhanced CT image in the same patient showing multiple large cystic locules ➡ in the lower pole, surrounded by a thick fibrous capsule ➡. Mass effect leads to calyceal dilatation in the upper pole ➡.

TERMINOLOGY

Abbreviations

- Multilocular cystic nephroma (MLCN)

Synonyms

- Cystic nephroma, multilocular cystic renal tumor, cystic hamartoma

Definitions

- Rare, nonhereditary, benign, cystic renal neoplasm containing epithelial and stromal components

IMAGING

General Features

- Best diagnostic clue
  - Encapsulated multilocular cystic renal mass herniating into renal hilum (renal vein or ureter)
- Size
  - Entire lesion: Few cm to > 30 cm (average: 10 cm)
  - Individual locules: Few millimeters to 2.5 cm
- Morphology
  - Unilateral solitary cystic mass with thick fibrous capsule ± herniation into renal pelvis

Ultrasonographic Findings

- Grayscale ultrasound
  - Large, well-defined, multiloculated cystic mass
  - Numerous anechoic cysts with hyperechoic septa
  - Hyperechoic thick fibrous capsule
  - Occasionally more solid-appearing due to numerous tiny cysts causing acoustic interfaces
- Color Doppler
  - Fine vessels may be seen within septa
- Contrast enhanced ultrasound (CEUS)
  - Contrast uptake within septa and wall

CT Findings

- Large, well-defined, multiloculated cystic mass, rare calcification, ± capsular enhancement
- Distortion of collecting system, ± obstruction
- Small locules/proteinaceous material within cysts → may appear as solid mass, nonenhancing

MR Findings

- T1WI: Multiloculated hypointense mass (clear fluid) with variable signal intensity (blood or protein)
- T2WI: Hyperintense (clear fluid) or variable (blood or protein) with hypointense capsule and septa (fibrous tissue)
- T1WI C+: Enhancement of thin or thick septa

DIFFERENTIAL DIAGNOSIS

Cystic Renal Cell Carcinoma (RCC)

- Cysts in RCC usually not enclosed by capsule
- Enhancing nodules favor RCC over MLCN

Mixed Epithelial and Stromal Tumor (MEST)

- More solid components, mimicking cystic RCC

Cystic Wilms Tumor

- Numerous thick septa; thinner in MLCN

Localized Cystic Renal Disease

- Conglomerate of simple cysts simulating multilocular cystic mass, usually unilateral
- Lacks well-defined pseudocapsule around cysts
- Renal parenchyma is present between cysts

Multicystic Dysplastic Kidney (MCDK)

- Nonfunctional kidney replaced by multiple cysts and dysplastic tissue
- Sonographically, appears as small kidney consisting of multiple cysts or echogenic kidney if cysts are too tiny to be visualized

Simple Renal Cysts

- No surrounding capsule

PATHOLOGY

General Features

- Etiology
  - Steroid hormonal influence: Estrogens

Staging, Grading, & Classification

- WHO classification: Grouped with MEST (mixed epithelial stromal tumors)

Gross Pathologic & Surgical Features

- Thick fibrous capsule
- "Honeycombed" noncommunicating cysts of varying size with intervening septa < 5 mm
- No solid component or necrosis

CLINICAL ISSUES

Presentation

- Most common signs/symptoms
  - Hematuria, abdominal/flank pain, palpable mass
  - May be asymptomatic

Demographics

- Bimodal age and sex distribution
  - Children M:F = 3:1, age 2-4 years old
  - Adults F:M = 8:1, peak age 40-60 years old

Natural History & Prognosis

- Complications
  - Obstructive uropathy, infection
  - Hemorrhage
- Good prognosis following excision
  - Local recurrence usually due to incomplete excision

Treatment

- Cured with complete surgical excision

SELECTED REFERENCES

1. Wood CG 3rd et al: CT and MR Imaging for Evaluation of Cystic Renal Lesions and Diseases. Radiographics. 35(1):125-41, 2015
2. Wilkinson C et al: Adult multilocular cystic nephroma: Report of six cases with clinical, radio-pathologic correlation and review of literature. Urol Ann. 5(1):13-7, 2013
3. Lane BR et al: Adult cystic nephroma and mixed epithelial and stromal tumor of the kidney: clinical, radiographic, and pathologic characteristics. Urology. 71(6):1142-8, 2008
4. Hopkins JK et al: Best cases from the AFIP: cystic nephroma. Radiographics. 24(2):589-93, 2004

Acute Pyelonephritis

IMAGING

- Findings of acute pyelonephritis (AP) are almost always asymmetric
- Renal enlargement with loss of corticomedullary (CM) differentiation on US and CT
- Geographic areas of altered echogenicity on US
- Urothelial thickening on US and CT
- In general, ultrasound is much more sensitive for causes (obstruction) and complications (abscess) of AP than for AP itself, which is a clinical diagnosis
- Many kidneys with pyelonephritis will be sonographically normal
- Foci of gas in parenchyma (rare) could indicate emphysematous pyelonephritis; treat as urologic emergency
- Altered nephrogram on CT, classically striated, best seen in excretory phase
- Microabscesses or areas of necrosis can emerge after 1-2 weeks of infection

PATHOLOGY

- Most common organism: *Escherichia coli*
- Route of spread of infection: Ascending (85%) > hematogenous (15%)
- Risk factors include obstruction, ureteric reflux, diabetes, pregnancy, lower UTI

CLINICAL ISSUES

- Positive urine culture for bacilli is typical
- Remember, especially in children, absence of lower UTI does not exclude pyelonephritis

DIAGNOSTIC CHECKLIST

- Pyelonephritis usually asymmetric; sonographic changes may be subtle in acute setting
- Focused US evaluation for ureteral stones if AP is suspected, including transvaginal images for distal ureter stones, because presence of stones would alter management

(Left) Transverse US of the kidney exhibits a geographic area of increased echogenicity in the anterior interpolar region ⟹ in an area of focal pyelonephritis. (Right) Longitudinal US of the kidney illustrates diffuse loss of corticomedullary differentiation, crescentic perinephric fluid ⟹, and urothelial thickening ⟹ in a patient with acute pyelonephritis.

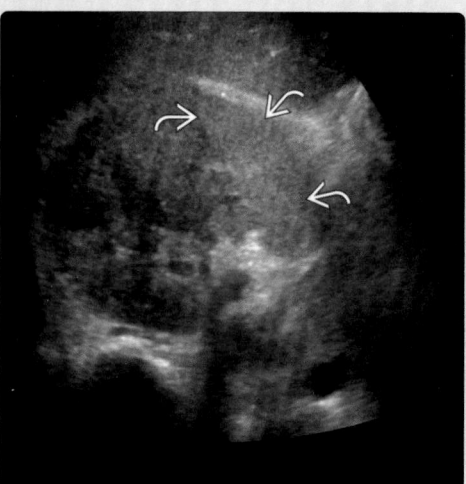
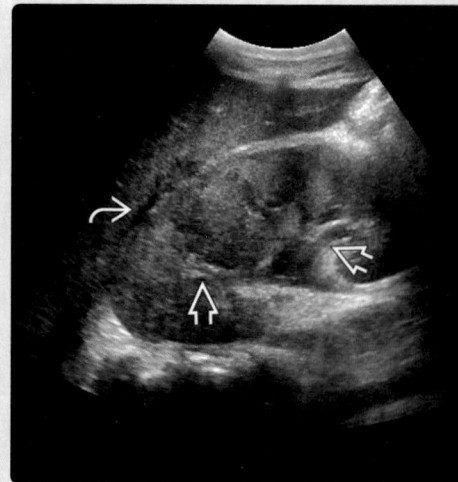

(Left) Longitudinal US of the kidney illustrates a focal, wedge-shaped area of increased echogenicity ⟹ in a patient with pyelonephritis, (Right) Longitudinal color Doppler US of the same kidney shows a focal area of diminished color flow ⟹ corresponding to the hyperechoic wedge in an area of infection.

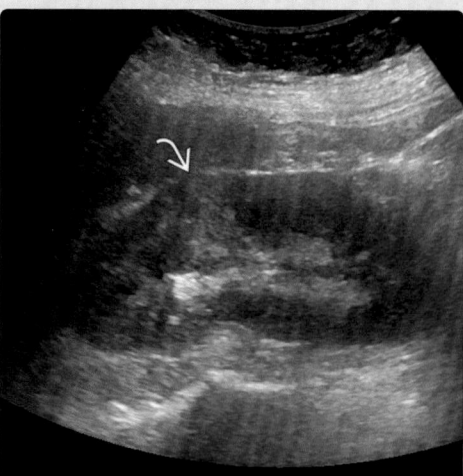
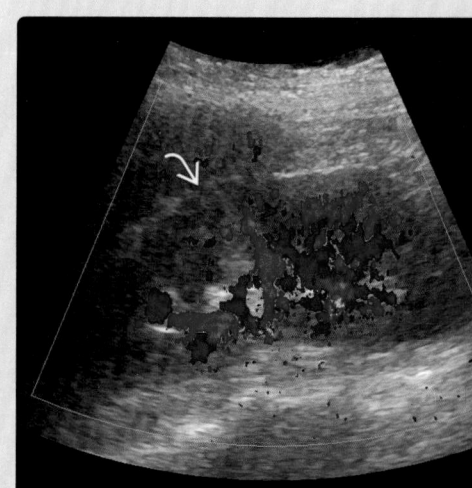

TERMINOLOGY

Abbreviations

Acute pyelonephritis (AP)

Definitions

Renal parenchymal infection

Different from pyelitis (inflammation of renal pelvis) or pyonephrosis (infection plus collecting system obstruction)

IMAGING

General Features

Best diagnostic clue
- Findings of AP are almost always asymmetric
  - Renal enlargement with loss of corticomedullary (CM) differentiation
  - Geographic areas of altered echogenicity, attenuation, or signal depending on modality
  - Urothelial thickening
- Perinephric inflammatory changes may be subtle but are almost always present

Location
- Usually unilateral
- No side or polar predominance
- Infection affects entire cortex, from sinus to capsule
  - Pelvis and ureter may or may not be involved

Ultrasonographic Findings

Grayscale ultrasound
- In general, ultrasound is much more sensitive for causes (obstruction) and complications (abscess) of pyelonephritis than for pyelonephritis itself, which is a clinical diagnosis
- Many kidneys with pyelonephritis will be sonographically normal
- Asymmetric global or focal swelling
- Altered echogenicity and diminished corticomedullary differentiation
- Microabscesses or areas of necrosis can emerge after 1-2 weeks of infection
- Perinephric fat may be unusually echogenic due to edema and inflammatory cell infiltrate
- Thin, anechoic rim of perinephric fluid sometimes seen
- Foci of gas in parenchyma (rare) could indicate emphysematous pyelonephritis
  - Treat as urologic emergency
- Pyelonephritis plus collecting system dilatation indicate pyonephrosis (pus under pressure), a surgical emergency

Color Doppler
- Although kidney is inflamed, parenchyma is usually hypovascular
- Slight elevation in arcuate artery resistive index can be seen but is not as specific or sensitive as diagnostic criterion
- Renal vein thrombosis is an occasional complication

CT Findings

NECT
- May see perinephric stranding or renal enlargement
- May be occult
- Important to check for stones
  - Stone may cause outflow obstruction
  - Tiny fragment can be nidus of infection after lithotripsy
- CECT
  - Global or focal renal enlargement, sometimes with sinus obliteration
  - Altered nephrogram, classically striated, best seen in excretory phase
    - Wedge-shaped areas of low attenuation may mimic infarcts
    - Striated nephrogram arises from partial obstruction of tubules by white blood cells and debris
  - Urothelial thickening in pelvis or ureter
  - Perinephric or periureteric fat stranding or edema
  - Look for asymmetric thickening of renal fascia

Nuclear Medicine Findings

- No utility in acute setting
  - DMSA cortical scans can be used to assess scarring; usually seen in kids with chronic reflux
  - Technetium-99 DTPA or MAG-3 scans provide functional information in kidney damaged by chronic infection

Imaging Recommendations

- Best imaging tool
  - CT is most sensitive for subtle parenchymal changes in acute pyelonephritis, but with increased radiation and expense; usually not necessary
  - Ultrasound is useful to rule out obstruction or abscess, particularly in children or other radiation-sensitive contexts
- Protocol advice
  - Initial investigation by ultrasound followed by CT if needed (for delineation of complications)
  - Watch for asymmetry between kidneys over phases of enhancement and excretion on multiphasic CT or MR

DIFFERENTIAL DIAGNOSIS

Acute Tubular Necrosis (ATN)

- Due to ischemia or nephrotoxicity
- AP usually not associated with decline in renal function, but ATN is

Lymphoma

- Diffuse: Enlarged kidney and ↓ echogenicity
- Multifocal: Enlarged kidney and hypoechoic masses
- Look for adjacent retroperitoneal adenopathy

Acute Renal Infarction

- Global or segmental vascular defect on color Doppler imaging in normal/enlarged kidney

PATHOLOGY

General Features

- Etiology
  - Most common organism: *Escherichia coli*
  - Route of spread of infection: Ascending (85%) > hematogenous (15%)
  - Risk factors include obstruction, ureteric reflux, diabetes, pregnancy, lower UTI

Gross Pathologic & Surgical Features

- Polar abscesses: Microabscesses on renal surface
- Narrowed calyces and enlarged kidney

Microscopic Features

- Mononuclear cell infiltrate and fibrosis
  - Accumulated neutrophils in tubules can coalesce and be passed in urine as casts
- Interstitial or tubular necrosis

CLINICAL ISSUES

Presentation

- Most common signs/symptoms
  - Fever, malaise, dysuria, flank pain, and tenderness are typical
    - Young children may have nonspecific symptoms: Fussiness and poor feeding
    - Elderly patients may present with mental status changes or failure to thrive
- Lab data
  - Serum: ↑ ESR, ↑ WBC, ↑ proteinuria
  - Urine: ↑ WBC, WBC casts, proteinuria, positive urine culture for bacilli
    - Remember: Especially in children, absence of lower UTI does not exclude AP

Demographics

- Age
  - Common in adults (also seen in children)
- Gender
  - F > M
- Epidemiology
  - ↑ incidence: M > 65 years, F < 40 years
  - Pregnant women are at increased risk for upper UTI due to hormonal changes affecting ureteral peristalsis and gravid uterus causing ureteral compression
  - Diabetic patients are at increased risk for upper and lower UTI

Natural History & Prognosis

- Good
  - Potential complications
    - Abscess formation
    - Renal vein thrombosis
    - Pyonephrosis
    - Cortical scarring
  - Rare complications, more common in patients with diabetes mellitus
    - Papillary necrosis
    - Emphysematous pyelonephritis

Treatment

- Acute: Antibiotic therapy

DIAGNOSTIC CHECKLIST

Consider

- Focused US evaluation for ureteral stones if pyelonephritis is suspected, including transvaginal images for distal ureter stones
  - Presence of stones alters management

Image Interpretation Pearls

- Pyelonephritis usually asymmetric
- Sonographic changes may be subtle in acute setting

SELECTED REFERENCES

1. Lee YJ et al: Unilateral and bilateral acute pyelonephritis: differences in clinical presentation, progress and outcome. Postgrad Med J. 90(1060):80-5 2014
2. Faletti R et al: Diffusion-weighted imaging and apparent diffusion coefficient values versus contrast-enhanced MR imaging in the identification and characterisation of acute pyelonephritis. Eur Radiol. 23(12):3501-8, 2013
3. Fontanilla T et al: Acute complicated pyelonephritis: contrast-enhanced ultrasound. Abdom Imaging. 37(4):639-46, 2012
4. Ifergan J et al: Imaging in upper urinary tract infections. Diagn Interv Imaging. 93(6):509-19, 2012
5. Chen KC et al: The role of emergency ultrasound for evaluating acute pyelonephritis in the ED. Am J Emerg Med. 29(7):721-4, 2011
6. Cavorsi K et al: Acute pyelonephritis. Ultrasound Q. 26(2):103-5, 2010
7. Dell'Atti L et al: Clinical use of ultrasonography associated with color Doppler in the diagnosis and follow-up of acute pyelonephritis. Arch Ital Urol Androl 82(4):217-20, 2010
8. Craig WD et al: Pyelonephritis: radiologic-pathologic review. Radiographics. 28(1):255-77; quiz 327-8, 2008
9. Demertzis J et al: State of the art: imaging of renal infections. Emerg Radiol 14(1):13-22, 2007
10. Browne RF et al: Imaging of urinary tract infection in the adult. Eur Radiol. 1 Suppl 3:E168-83, 2004
11. Dacher JN et al: Power Doppler sonographic pattern of acute pyelonephritis in children: comparison with CT. AJR Am J Roentgenol. 166(6):1451-5, 1996
12. Talner LB et al: Acute pyelonephritis: can we agree on terminology? Radiology. 192(2):297-305, 1994

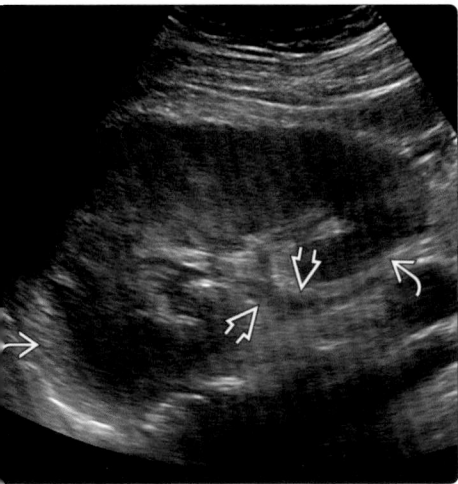

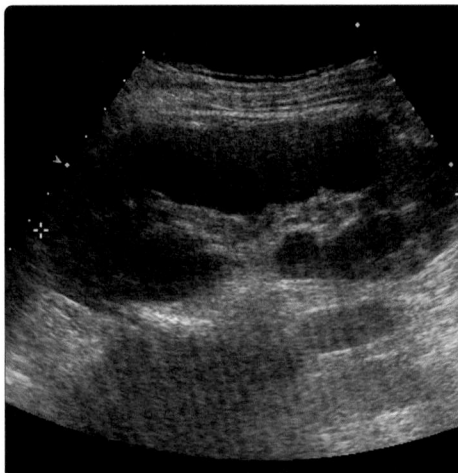

(Left) Longitudinal US shows there is almost no corticomedullary differentiation in this infected and edematous kidney. Urothelial thickening ⮕ is seen in the renal pelvis and proximal ureter. The inflamed perinephric fat is quite echogenic ⬈. (Right) Longitudinal US shows this kidney is diffusely hypoechoic and edematous due to pyelonephritis.

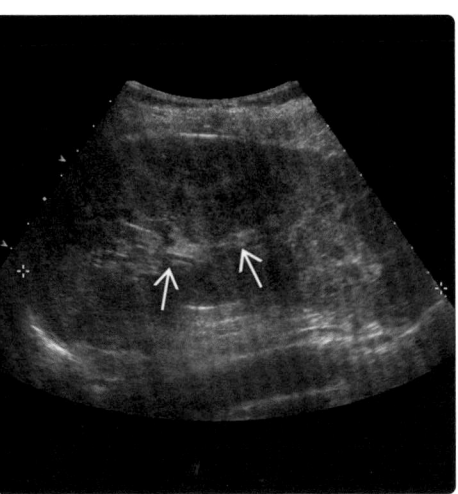

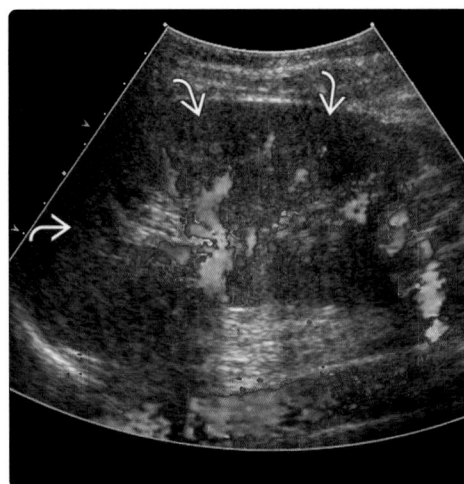

(Left) Longitudinal US shows this patient with acute pyelonephritis has an enlarged, hypoechoic kidney with decreased corticomedullary differentiation. The renal sinus is flattened ⮕ due to diffuse renal edema. (Right) Longitudinal color Doppler US shows there is little peripheral Doppler flow ⮕ in the same patient with an edematous kidney and acute pyelonephritis.

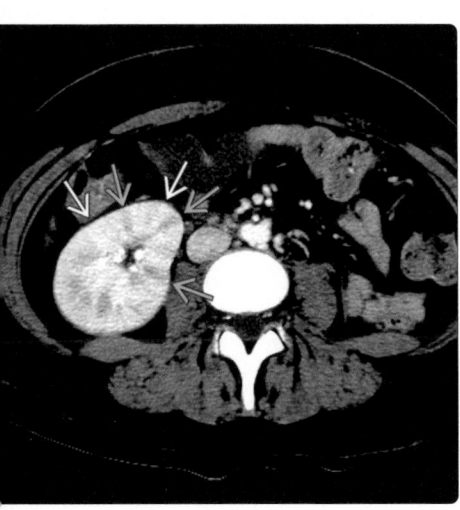

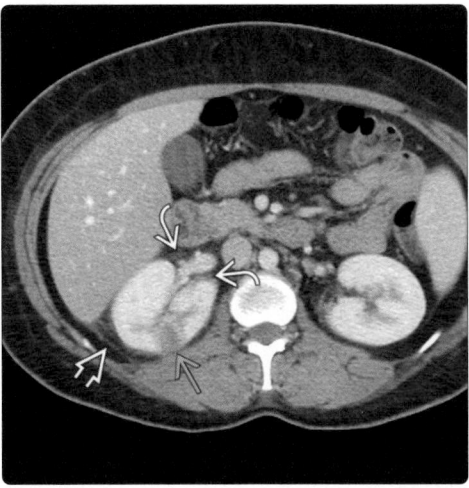

(Left) Axial CECT shows a classic diffuse "striated nephrogram" in a patient with acute pyelonephritis. Note the alternating bands of hypo- ⮕ and hyperenhancing ⮕ parenchyma. (Right) Focal, wedge-shaped enhancement defect in the right kidney ⮕ is accompanied by subtle perinephric stranding ⬈ and thickening of posterior renal fascia ⮕ in this patient with acute pyelonephritis. These findings help to distinguish acute pyelonephritis from renal infarcts.

TERMINOLOGY

- Purulent &/or necrotic intraparenchymal or perinephric collection arising from unresolved pyelonephritis

IMAGING

- Complex cystic mass, may be sharply marginated or more permeative
- Rim may be hypervascular or vessels may course to edge of lesion and stop
- Findings of pyelonephritis (renal enlargement, lack of corticomedullary differentiation, and urothelial thickening) may be present
- Internal echogenic foci with "comet tail" may represent gas-forming organisms within abscess

PATHOLOGY

- Ascending urinary tract infections (80%)
  - Corticomedullary abscess by *Escherichia coli* or *Proteus* species

- Hematogenous spread (20%)
  - Cortical abscess by *Staphylococcus aureus*

CLINICAL ISSUES

- Abscess emerges after 10-14 days of untreated or undertreated urinary tract infection, not on 1st day of symptoms
- Antibiotic therapy, usually IV ± percutaneous drainage
- Surgical drainage or nephrectomy are rarely needed

DIAGNOSTIC CHECKLIST

- Many abscesses appear mass-like and may mimic neoplasms but are usually associated with > 1-week history of infection, minimal internal vascularity, and associated inflammatory changes

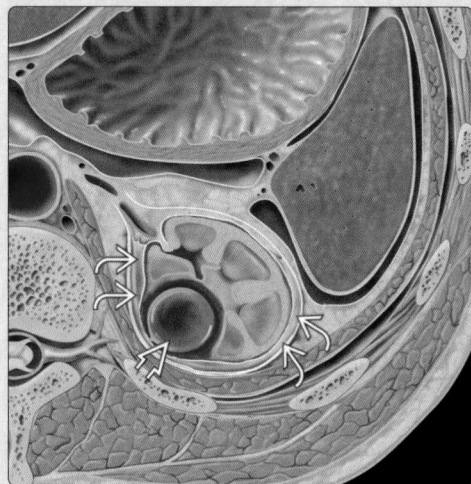 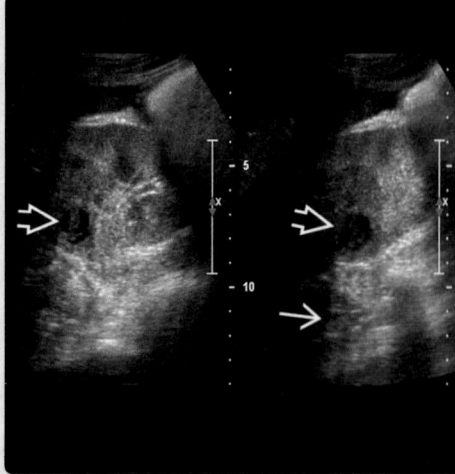

(Left) *Graphic shows a pus-filled cavity within the renal parenchyma* ➡ *and purulent material in the perinephric space* ➡. (Right) *Transverse and longitudinal images of the kidney show a well-circumscribed, hypoechoic mass in the posterior kidney* ➡. *Note the posterior acoustic enhancement* ➡.

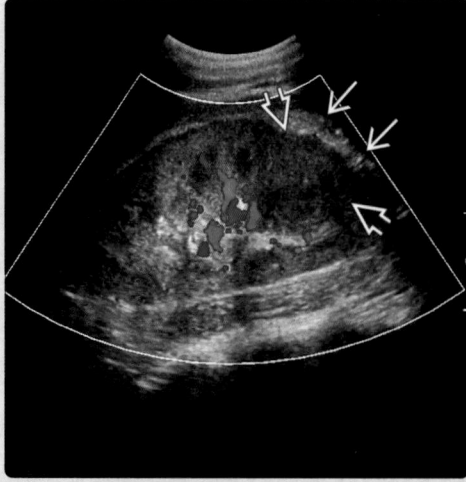 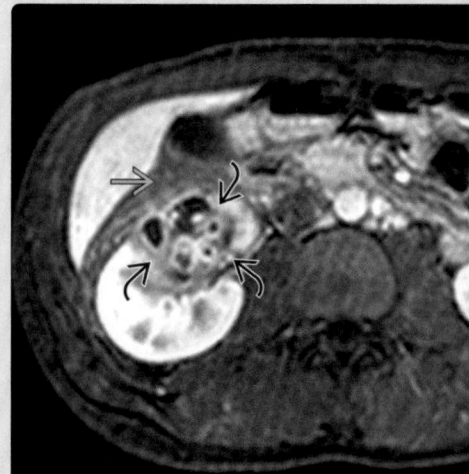

(Left) *Color Doppler US shows lack of vascularity within a lower pole hypoechoic mass (abscess collection)* ➡. *Note the echogenic surrounding fat, indicative of perinephric inflammation* ➡. (Right) *T1 C+ FS MR in the same patient shows an irregular lower pole mass containing multiple rim-enhancing locules* ➡. *Because of the resemblance to cystic renal neoplasm, biopsy was performed and abscess was confirmed. However, note the inflammatory change in the anterior pararenal space* ➡, *favoring infection.*

TERMINOLOGY

Definitions

Purulent &/or necrotic intraparenchymal or perinephric collection arising from unresolved pyelonephritis

IMAGING

General Features

Best diagnostic clue
o Well-defined, centrally avascular hypoechoic area with irregular wall and internal debris
Location
o Single > multiple; unilateral > bilateral

Ultrasonographic Findings

Grayscale ultrasound
o Complex cystic mass, may be sharply marginated or more permeative
o Anechoic/hypoechoic ± weak acoustic enhancement
o May contain echogenic internal debris, septations, or loculations
o Internal echogenic foci with "comet tail" may represent gas-forming organisms within abscess
o Findings of pyelonephritis (renal enlargement, lack of corticomedullary differentiation, and urothelial thickening) may be present
o Perinephric fat may appear hyperechoic and fascial planes thickened due to inflammation
Color Doppler
o Rim may be hypervascular or vessels may course to edge of lesion and stop
o Little to no internal vascularity

CT Findings

NECT
o Round, well-defined, low-attenuation masses ± gas within collection
o Perinephric inflammatory change
CECT
o Focal hypodense area ± wall enhancement
o Perinephric reaction or extension
– Edema or obliteration of perinephric fat
– Thickened Gerota fascia and perinephric septa

Imaging Recommendations

Best imaging tool
o CT for perinephric extension; ultrasound for guided aspiration
Protocol advice
o Initial examination is ultrasound; CT for further investigation

DIFFERENTIAL DIAGNOSIS

Renal Cell Carcinoma (RCC)

Hypervascular mass; usually asymptomatic
Lack of inflammatory change favors this diagnosis over abscess

Metastases and Lymphoma

Hypovascular with variable echogenicity
Often multiple, whereas most abscesses are solitary

Hemorrhagic Cyst or Proteinaceous Cyst

- Appearance of lesion itself indistinguishable from abscess
- Should not have associated inflammatory changes or history of fever, flank pain, etc.

PATHOLOGY

General Features

- Etiology
  o Ascending urinary tract infections (80%)
    – Corticomedullary abscess by *Escherichia coli* or *Proteus* species
  o Hematogenous spread (20%)
    – Cortical abscess by *Staphylococcus aureus*
- Associated abnormalities
  o Urolithiasis (20-60%)

Microscopic Features

- Necrotic glomeruli & polymorphonuclear infiltration

CLINICAL ISSUES

Presentation

- Most common signs/symptoms
  o Fever, flank/abdominal pain, chills, and dysuria

Demographics

- Age
  o All; M = F

Natural History & Prognosis

- Complications: Abscess rupture into pelvis, perinephric space, retroperitoneum, or peritoneal space
- Prognosis is good if therapy is prompt
  o Good (early therapy); poor (delayed or insufficient therapy)

Treatment

- Antibiotic therapy, usually IV ± percutaneous drainage
- Surgical drainage or nephrectomy are rarely needed

DIAGNOSTIC CHECKLIST

Consider

- Clinical history & urinalysis for work-up of diagnosis
- Imaging-guided aspiration

Image Interpretation Pearls

- Many abscesses appear mass-like and may mimic neoplasms but are usually associated with > 1-week history of infection, minimal internal vascularity, and associated inflammatory changes

SELECTED REFERENCES

1. Fontanilla T et al: Acute complicated pyelonephritis: contrast-enhanced ultrasound. Abdom Imaging. 37(4):639-46, 2012
2. Heller MT et al: Acute conditions affecting the perinephric space: imaging anatomy, pathways of disease spread, and differential diagnosis. Emerg Radiol. 19(3):245-54, 2012
3. Demertzis J et al: State of the art: imaging of renal infections. Emerg Radiol. 14(1):13-22, 2007

Emphysematous Pyelonephritis

TERMINOLOGY

- Gas-forming upper UTI involving renal parenchyma &/or perinephric space

IMAGING

- Highly echogenic areas within renal sinus and parenchyma with "dirty" shadowing
- Ring-down artifacts: Air bubbles trapped in fluid
- Perinephric fluid collections may be seen
- Type I (33%): Parenchymal replacement by gas, ± crescent of subcapsular or perinephric gas
- Type II (66%): Renal or perirenal fluid abscesses with bubbly gas pattern ± gas within renal pelvis
- CT is ideal to determine location and extent of renal and perirenal gas
- Evaluation for psoas abscess and spinal osteomyelitis is essential

TOP DIFFERENTIAL DIAGNOSES

- Emphysematous pyelitis
  - Gas is limited to renal collecting system and pelvis, not parenchyma
  - Less clinically serious than emphysematous pyelonephritis, unless obstructed

PATHOLOGY

- Single or mixed organism(s) infection
- *Escherichia coli* (68%), *Klebsiella pneumoniae* (9%)
- *Proteus mirabilis, Pseudomonas, Enterobacter, Candida, Ilostridia* species

CLINICAL ISSUES

- Extremely ill at presentation: Fever, flank pain, hyperglycemia, acidosis, dehydration and electrolyte imbalance

(Left) *Ill-defined hyperechoic material in the posterior renal cortex ➡ causes posterior acoustic shadowing ⬈. However, the shadowing is much less dense, or obscuring, than would be expected for something like a calcification of this size.* (Right) *As on the transverse image, gas in the central left kidney ➡ is highly echogenic with posterior "dirty" shadowing ⬈. The renal sinus is obscured and it is hard to differentiate emphysematous pyelonephritis from emphysematous pyelitis on this image.*

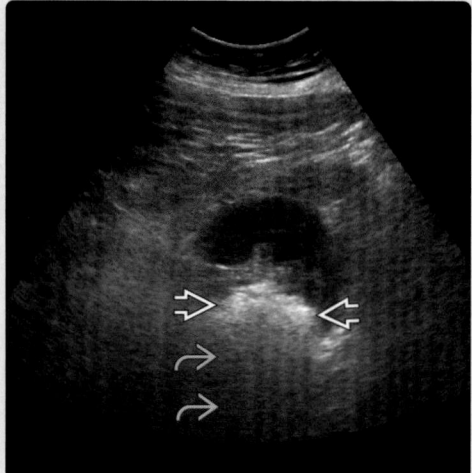
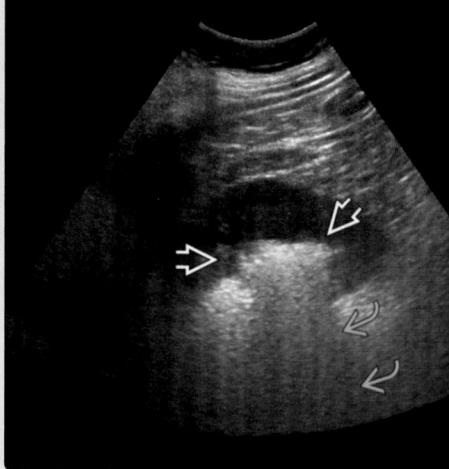

(Left) *NECT in the same patient shows gas in the renal parenchyma ➡ and pelvis ⬈. The adjacent posterior renal fascia is thickened by edema and inflammation, but there is no perinephric collection ⬈.* (Right) *Sagittal reconstruction CT shows a lobulated area of intraparenchymal gas ➡ with sparing of the renal sinus fat ⬈.*

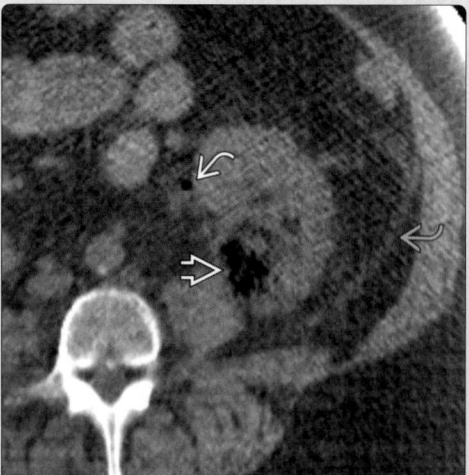
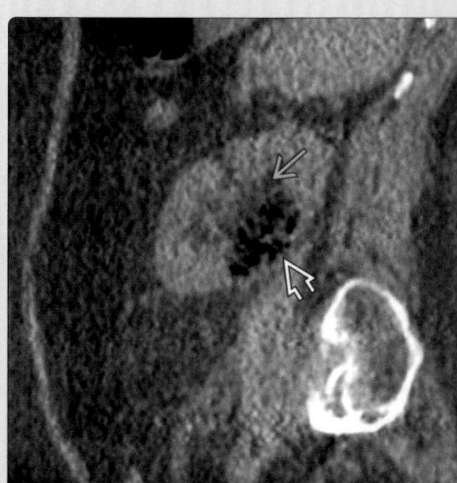

TERMINOLOGY

Abbreviations

Emphysematous pyelonephritis (EPN)

Definitions

Gas-forming upper urinary tract infection involving renal parenchyma &/or perinephric space

IMAGING

General Features

Location
○ Unilateral > bilateral (5-7% of cases)

Ultrasonographic Findings

Grayscale ultrasound
○ Highly echogenic areas within renal sinus and parenchyma with "dirty" shadowing
○ Ring-down artifacts: Air bubbles trapped in fluid
○ Gas in perinephric space or perinephric collections may obscure kidney

Color Doppler
○ Twinkling artifact: May mimic stones

Radiographic Findings

Radiography
○ Gas in parenchyma ± perinephric space

CT Findings

2 types of emphysematous pyelonephritis
○ Type I (33%): Parenchymal replacement by gas, ± subcapsular or perinephric gas
○ Type II (66%): Renal or perirenal abscesses with gas, ± gas within renal pelvis

Intraparenchymal, intracaliceal, and intrapelvic gas

Gas may extend into subcapsular, perinephric, pararenal, contralateral retroperitoneal spaces

MR Findings

T1WI, T2WI: Foci of gas are signal voids on all sequences
T2WI: Perinephric edema ± fluid collections

Imaging Recommendations

Best imaging tool
○ CT is ideal to determine location and extent of renal and perirenal gas
○ Evaluation for psoas abscess and spinal osteomyelitis is essential

DIFFERENTIAL DIAGNOSIS

Renal Calculus

Discrete echogenic focus with sharp distal acoustic shadowing

Nephrocalcinosis

Generalized increased echogenicity of renal pyramid ± shadowing

Papillary Necrosis

Single or multiple cystic cavities in medullary pyramids continuous with calyces
Sloughed papillae: Echogenic, nonshadowing

Emphysematous Pyelitis

- Gas limited to renal collecting system and pelvis, not parenchyma
- Usually less clinically serious than EPN

Benign Gas in Renal Pelvis

- May arise from recent interventions

PATHOLOGY

General Features

- Etiology
  ○ Single or mixed organism(s) infection
    – *Escherichia coli* (68%), *Klebsiella pneumoniae* (9%)
    – *Proteus mirabilis, Pseudomonas, Enterobacter, Candida, Ilostridia* species
  ○ Risk factors
    – Recurrent or chronic UTIs
    – Immunocompromised: Diabetes mellitus (87-97%)
    – Ureteral obstruction (20-40%): Calculi, stenosis
  ○ Pathogenesis
    – Pyelonephritis → ischemia and low oxygen tension → anaerobe proliferation in anaerobic environment → CO_2 production

Gross Pathologic & Surgical Features

- Suppurative necrotizing infection of renal parenchyma and perirenal tissue with multiple cortical abscesses

CLINICAL ISSUES

Presentation

- Most common signs/symptoms
  ○ Extremely ill at presentation: Fever, flank pain, hyperglycemia, acidosis, dehydration, and electrolyte imbalance
  ○ Hypoalbuminemia and need for emergent hemodialysis are independent predictors of mortality

Natural History & Prognosis

- Complications: Generalized sepsis
- Prognosis: Poor
  ○ Mortality: 66% with type I, 18% with type II

Treatment

- Antibiotic therapy; nephrectomy for type I
  ○ Conservative management fails in at least 1/3 of cases
- CT-guided drainage procedures for type II

SELECTED REFERENCES

1. Lu YC et al: Predictors of failure of conservative treatment among patients with emphysematous pyelonephritis. BMC Infect Dis. 14:418, 2014
2. Lin YC et al: Risk factors of renal failure and severe complications in patients with emphysematous pyelonephritis-a single-center 15-year experience. Am J Med Sci. 343(3):186-91, 2012
3. Chen KC et al: The role of emergency ultrasound for evaluating acute pyelonephritis in the ED. Am J Emerg Med. 29(7):721-4, 2011
4. Ubee SS et al: Emphysematous pyelonephritis. BJU Int. 107(9):1474-8, 2011
5. Grayson DE et al: Emphysematous infections of the abdomen and pelvis: a pictorial review. Radiographics. 22(3):543-61, 2002

(Left) *Abdominal radiograph shows a mottled gas pattern ➡ projecting over the expected location of the left renal fossa in a patient with emphysematous pyelonephritis.* (Right) *On grayscale US imagining, multiple punctate and highly echogenic foci of gas ➡ are seen in a subcapsular collection compressing the lower pole of the right kidney ➡ in a different patient. These echogenic foci are nondependent (floating in fluid) and were seen to move with real-time imaging.*

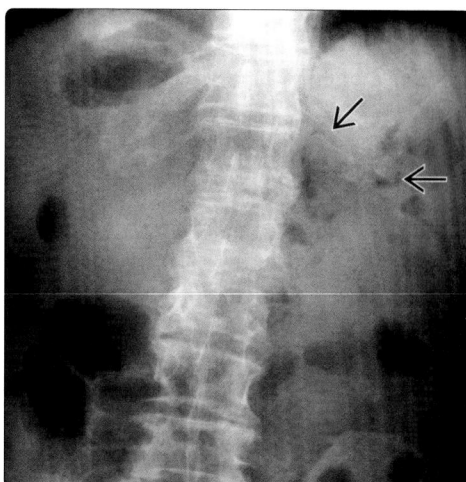
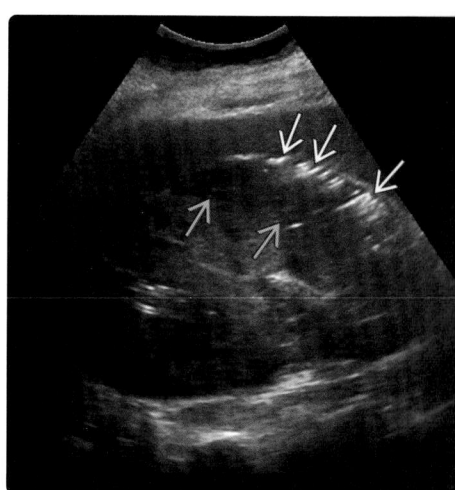

(Left) *Doppler US in the same patient shows color signal related to twinkling artifact associated with the gas bubbles ➡. To prevent confusion with true vascular flow, spectral tracings should be obtained. In this case, the waveform demonstrated noise (not shown), which verified that this area of color was artifactual and not true vascular flow.* (Right) *Axial NECT in the same patient confirms multiple foci of gas ➡ in the subcapsular collection, which compresses the renal contour ➡.*

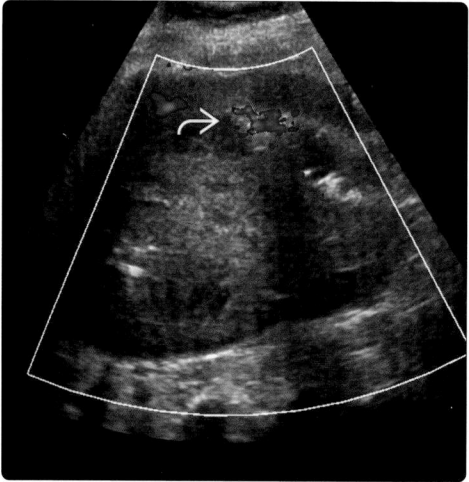
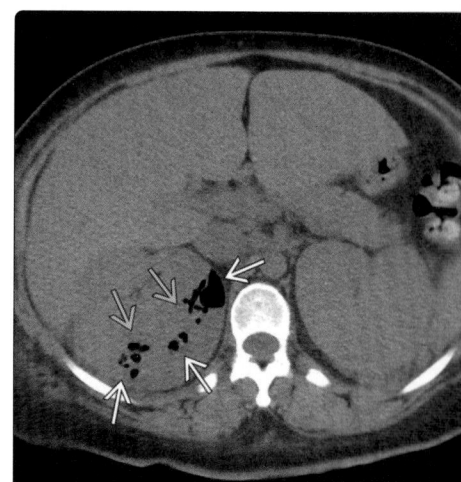

(Left) *CECT shows a markedly enlarged right kidney ➡ with a delayed and faint nephrogram compared to the contralateral side. Multiple foci of gas in the upper pole parenchyma ➡ confirm the diagnosis of emphysematous pyelonephritis.* (Right) *Dynamic renal scan images in the same patient show near absence of activity in the infected right kidney ➡ (patient is prone) with normal uptake and excretion on the left ➡. This study was performed as part of surgical planning for right nephrectomy.*

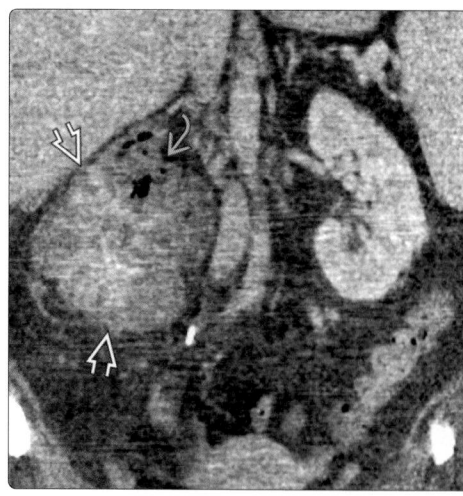
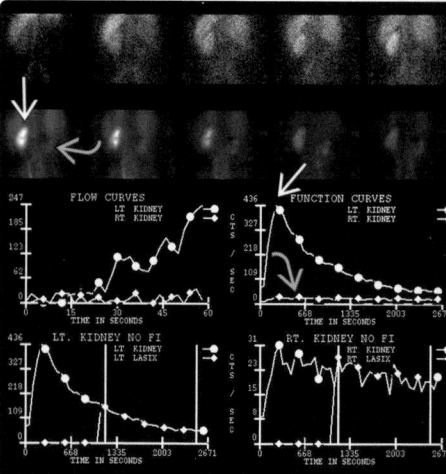

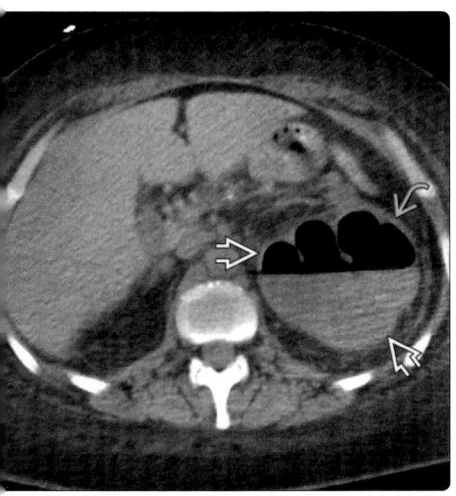

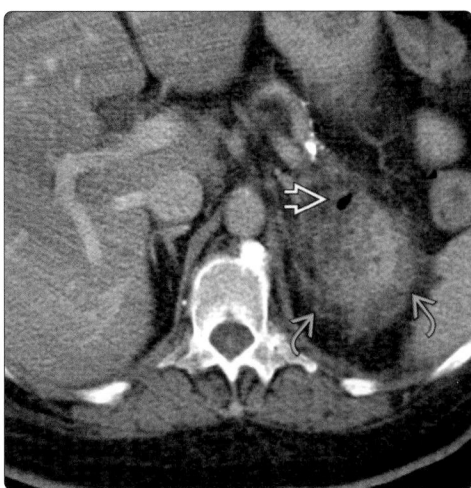

(Left) *On noncontrast CT, chronic obstruction and infection in this patient's left kidney have caused marked cortical thinning ➘, with replacement of pelvis and parenchyma by a contained gas and fluid collection ➭.* (Right) *Axial CT in another patient with emphysematous pyelonephritis shows focal intraparenchymal gas ➭ in the upper pole of the left kidney. Note surrounding inflammatory changes ➘, which suggests this infection is chronic.*

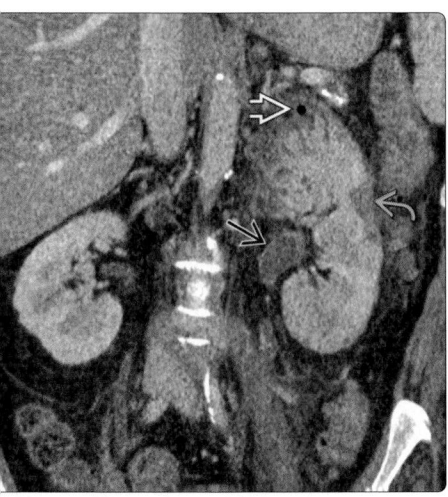

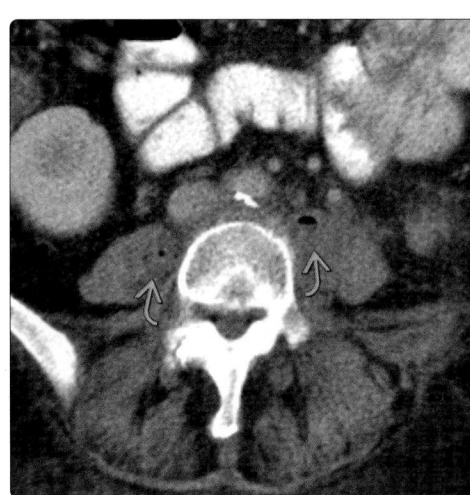

(Left) *Coronal CT from the same patient again illustrates minimal intraparenchymal gas ➭. Also note other signs of infection including marked enlargement of the left kidney, delayed nephrogram, cortical abscess ➘, and urothelial thickening of the renal pelvis ➭.* (Right) *Axial CT more inferiorly in the same patient shows foci of gas within thick-walled collections in both psoas muscles ➘ associated with the patient's emphysematous pyelonephritis.*

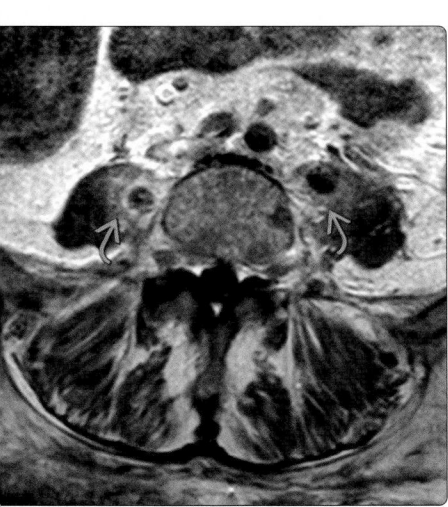

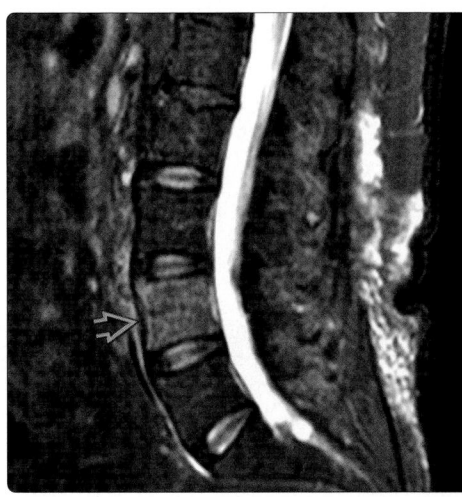

(Left) *Axial post-contrast T1 weighted MR in the same patient at a similar level confirms bilateral psoas abscesses ➘.* (Right) *Sagittal T2-weighted MR in the same patient reveals abnormal hyperintense signal in the adjacent L4 vertebral body ➘, indicating developing osteomyelitis. This diabetic patient with emphysematous pyelonephritis, psoas abscesses, and vertebral body osteomyelitis presented with sepsis and severe back pain.*

TERMINOLOGY

- Obstructed renal collecting system containing pus or infected urine

IMAGING

- Presence of mobile debris and layering of low-amplitude echoes within dilated collecting system on US
- Dilated collecting system containing intermediate- or high-density material on CT
- Enlarged kidney with perinephric inflammatory changes on CT

TOP DIFFERENTIAL DIAGNOSES

- Sterile hydronephrosis
- Complex renal cyst
- Urothelial carcinoma

PATHOLOGY

- Stagnant urine becomes infected, filled with white blood cells, bacteria, debris, and pus

- Chronic > acute ureteral obstruction
- Etiology
  - Young adult: Calculus or ureteropelvic junction obstruction or duplicated collecting system more common
  - Elderly: Malignant ureteral stricture other mechanical obstruction

CLINICAL ISSUES

- Delay in diagnosis and treatment leads to irreversible renal parenchymal damage and renal failure
  - Progress to bacteremia or septic shock and can lead to 25-50% mortality
- Symptoms include fever, chills, flank pain
- Most common organism: *E. Coli*
- Treatment: Percutaneous nephrostomy
- Diabetes is a risk factor for worse clinical outcomes
- Early diagnosis and drainage are crucial to prevent bacteremia and septic shock

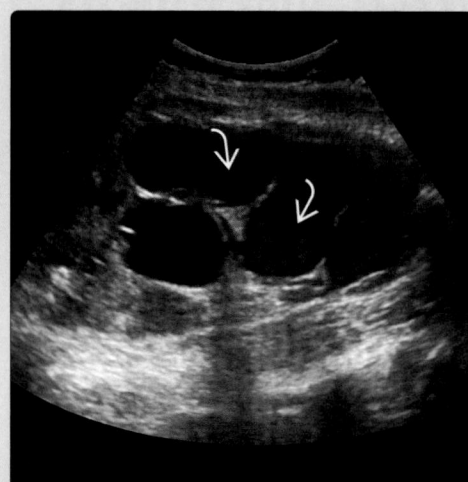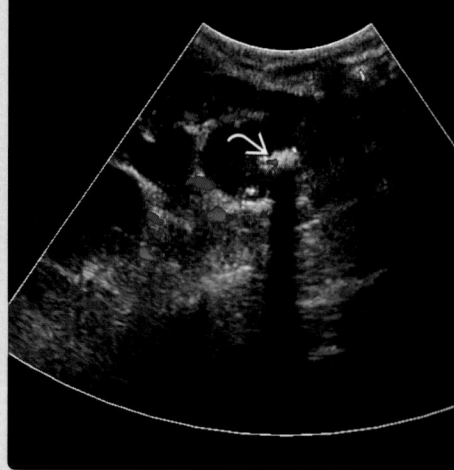

(Left) *Debris layers dependently in a mass-like fashion ⊅ in this case of pyonephrosis in an adult patient with multiple sclerosis on grayscale US imaging.* (Right) *Note the twinkling artifact on the surface of stone ⊅ in this high-PRF Doppler ultrasound.*

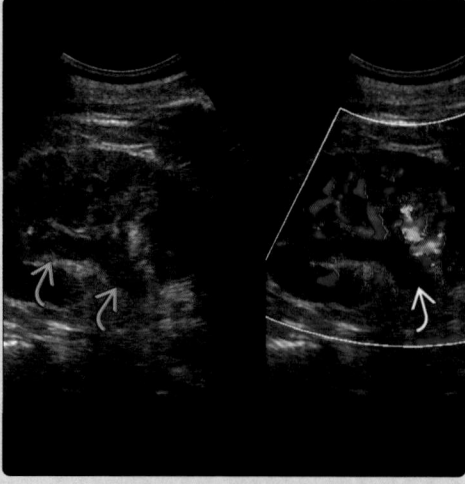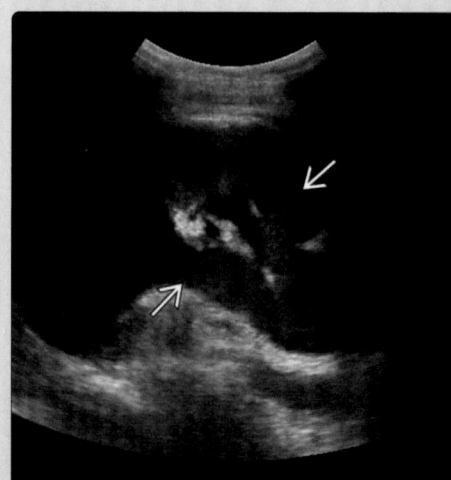

(Left) *Longitudinal grayscale and color Doppler US show abnormal echogenic material within a mildly dilated collecting system ⊅. Note absence of internal vascularity ⊅, helping to distinguish this from tumor in the renal pelvis.* (Right) *Transverse ultrasound of the kidney with the patient in the left lateral decubitus position shows a distinct pus-urine level ⊅ in the dilated system in this patient with prostate cancer and pyonephrosis.*

TERMINOLOGY

Definitions

Obstructed renal collecting system containing pus or infected urine

IMAGING

General Features

Best diagnostic clue
- o Presence of mobile debris and layering of low-amplitude echoes within dilated collecting system

Ultrasonographic Findings

Grayscale ultrasound
- o Hydronephrosis, ± hydroureter, with internal debris
- o Most consistent finding: Low-level mobile echoes
- o Echogenic pus layering in dependent portion of collecting system
- o Associated stone or gas sometimes seen
- o Urothelial thickening of renal pelvis or ureter

Color Doppler
- o Resistive indices may be elevated

CT Findings

Dilated collecting system containing intermediate- or high-density material

Enlarged kidney with perinephric inflammatory changes

Delayed nephrogram on affected side

Gas or perinephric abscess may also be seen

DIFFERENTIAL DIAGNOSIS

Sterile Hydronephrosis

Anechoic dilated collecting system, no dependent internal echoes

Urothelial Carcinoma

Solid tumor with vascularity within dilated collecting system

Note that mucinous tumors may precisely mimic appearance of pyonephrosis

Longstanding hydronephrosis or pyonephrosis also predisposes to squamous tumors

Complex Renal Cyst

Echoes/solid component/septum within cyst

No communication with renal pelvis or adjacent calyces

PATHOLOGY

General Features

Etiology
- o Chronic > acute ureteral obstruction
  - – Calculus, congenital ureteropelvic junction obstruction, or duplicated collecting system in young adult
  - – Malignant ureteral stricture or other mechanical obstruction in elderly
- o Stagnant urine becomes infected, filled with white blood cells, bacteria, debris, and pus
  - – Ascending urinary tract infection
  - – Blood-borne bacterial pathogen

Associated abnormalities

- o Complications: Renal abscess, perinephric abscess, xanthogranulomatous pyelonephritis, fistula to duodenum, colon, or pleura

Microscopic Features

- Purulent exudate composed of sloughed urothelium and inflammatory cells from early formation of microabscesses and necrotizing papillitis

CLINICAL ISSUES

Presentation

- Most common signs/symptoms
  - o Fever, chills, flank pain
- Other signs/symptoms
  - o Pyuria, leukocytosis, bacteriuria

Demographics

- Epidemiology
  - o Most common organism: *E. Coli*

Natural History & Prognosis

- Progress to bacteremia or septic shock leads to 25-50% mortality
- Delay in diagnosis and treatment leads to irreversible renal parenchymal damage and renal failure
- Diabetes is a risk factor for worse clinical outcomes
- Nuclear medicine scans can be used to assess residual function after acute illness is treated

Treatment

- Early diagnosis and drainage are crucial to prevent bacteremia and septic shock
- Percutaneous nephrostomy is typical therapy

DIAGNOSTIC CHECKLIST

Image Interpretation Pearls

- May be indistinguishable from noninfected hydronephrosis
  - o Proceed to percutaneous nephrostomy for urine microscopy and culture if patient is clinically septic

SELECTED REFERENCES

1. Das CJ et al: Multimodality imaging of renal inflammatory lesions. World J Radiol. 6(11):865-73, 2014
2. Kim SH et al: Serious acute pyelonephritis: a predictive score for evaluation of deterioration of treatment based on clinical and radiologic findings using CT. Acta Radiol. 53(2):233-8, 2012
3. Li AC et al: Emergent percutaneous nephrostomy for the diagnosis and management of pyonephrosis. Semin Intervent Radiol. 29(3):218-25, 2012
4. Browne RF et al: Imaging of urinary tract infection in the adult. Eur Radiol. 14 Suppl 3:E168-83, 2004
5. Paterson A: Urinary tract infection: an update on imaging strategies. Eur Radiol. 14 Suppl 4:L89-100, 2004
6. Wang IK et al: The use of ultrasonography in evaluating adults with febrile urinary tract infection. Ren Fail. 25(6):981-7, 2003

Xanthogranulomatous Pyelonephritis

TERMINOLOGY

- Chronic renal inflammation usually associated with longstanding urinary calculus obstruction (75%)
- Renal parenchyma is gradually replaced by lipid-laden macrophages
- Diffuse (> 80%) and focal (< 20%) forms
- 3 stages of XGP: Intrarenal → perirenal → perinephric ± retroperitoneal involvement

IMAGING

- Staghorn calculus with renal enlargement and perirenal fibrofatty proliferation on CT
- Multiple focal low-attenuating renal masses with rim enhancement on CT
- Renal sinus fat obliterated with large central "staghorn" calculus on any modality
- Perinephric extension ± adjacent organs or structures may include sinus tracts or abscesses

- Diffusely enlarged kidney with hypoechoic round masses replacing normal parenchyma on US
- Ultrasound ideal at initial investigation; CT good for assessing excretory function and retroperitoneal involvement

PATHOLOGY

- Lipid-laden "foamy" macrophages, diffuse infiltration of plasma cells and histiocytes

CLINICAL ISSUES

- Flank pain, fever, palpable mass & weight loss
- Rare complications: Hepatic dysfunction, extrarenal extension, fistulas
- Long-term chronic process with good prognosis if treated, and rare mortality
- Antibiotic treatment is sometimes effective
- Severe disease or perinephric extension usually requires nephrectomy

(Left) Graphic shows lower pole XGP with a longstanding ureteropelvic obstruction by a large staghorn stone ➡, causing replacement of parenchyma by collections of foamy macrophages ➡. (Right) Transverse color Doppler US shows a dilated collecting system ➡ with internal debris and an obstructing stone ➡ at the ureterovesical junction. The parenchyma is replaced by cystic spaces containing debris ➡. Note the lack of vascularity in the expected region of renal parenchyma.

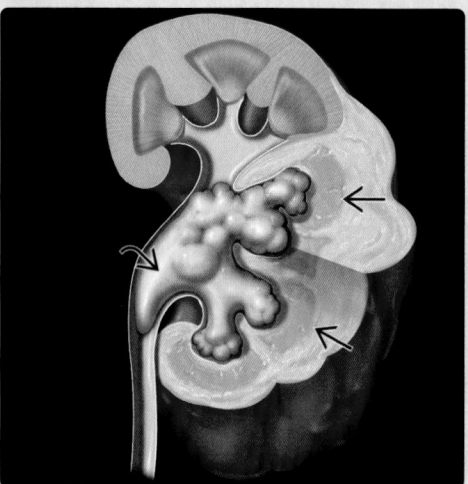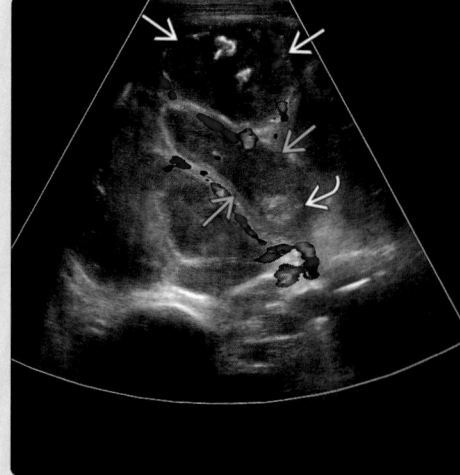

(Left) Two ultrasounds in another patient show cystic intraparenchymal spaces ➡ peripheral to calculi (calipers) in central renal pelvis. Color Doppler US shows twinkling artifact ➡ with stones. (Right) Axial CECT shows a large central calculus ➡, near-complete replacement of parenchyma by cystic collections ➡, and formation of an abscess and sinus tract ➡ necessitating into adjacent abdominal wall. Proliferation of perinephric fat ➡ in this otherwise cachectic patient is a response to chronic inflammation.

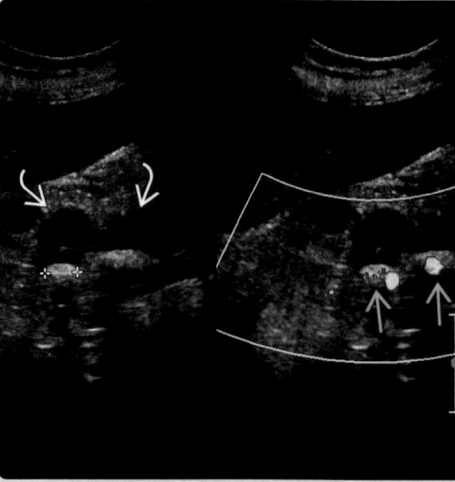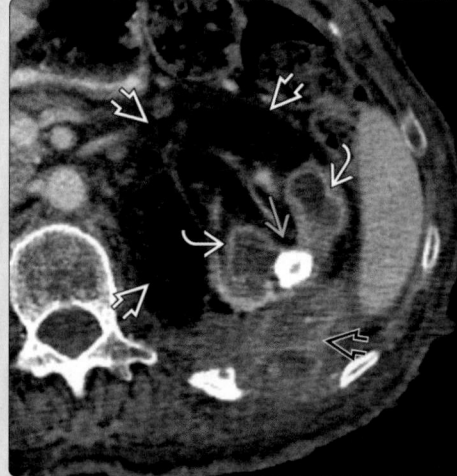

TERMINOLOGY

Abbreviations

Xanthogranulomatous pyelonephritis (XGP/XGPN)

Definitions

Chronic renal inflammation usually associated with longstanding urinary calculus obstruction (75%)

Renal parenchyma is gradually replaced by lipid-laden macrophages

o Greek prefix "xantho-" refers to yellow color of fat

Diffuse (> 80%) and focal (< 20%) forms

o Diffuse: Due to obstruction at ureteropelvic junction

o Focal or segmental: Due to obstruction of single infundibulum or 1 moiety of duplex system

3 stages of XGP: Intrarenal → perirenal → perinephric ± retroperitoneal involvement

IMAGING

General Features

Best diagnostic clue

o Staghorn calculus with renal enlargement and perirenal fibrofatty proliferation

Location

o Unilateral (most cases) > bilateral

Ultrasonographic Findings

Grayscale ultrasound

o Appearance varies depending on pattern of XGP

o Diffusely enlarged kidney; highly reflective central calculus

o Anechoic or hypoechoic round masses replacing normal parenchyma

o Parenchymal thinning ± hydrocalyces or pyonephrosis

o Segmental XGP: Anechoic or hypoechoic masses surrounding calculus-obstructing calyx

o Perinephric inflammatory tissue ± fluid collection

CT Findings

Multiple focal low-attenuating renal masses with rim enhancement

o Pockets of lipid-laden macrophages appear cystic on CT and may mimic hydronephrosis

Impaired contrast excretion into collecting system

Renal sinus fat obliterated with large central "staghorn" calculus

Perinephric extension ± adjacent organs or structures may include sinus tracts or abscesses

Imaging Recommendations

Best imaging tool

o Ultrasound ideal at initial investigation; CT good for assessing excretory function and retroperitoneal involvement

DIFFERENTIAL DIAGNOSIS

Renal Neoplasm

XGP may simulate cystic renal cell carcinoma

Urothelial cancer obstructing pelvis or secondarily invading parenchyma may look similar

- Renal lymphoma may appear very similar to XGP due to its low density on CT

Pyonephrosis or Renal Abscess

- Pyonephrosis: Purulent material within collecting system, usually no staghorn
- Renal abscess: Ill-defined hypoechoic masses, acute rather than chronic presentation

Papillary Necrosis

- Due to analgesic abuse, diabetes mellitus, chronic pyelonephritis, and sickle cell anemia

PATHOLOGY

General Features

- Etiology
  o Chronic obstruction of ureteropelvic junction by longstanding calculus
    – Complication by secondary infection
  o Pyonephrosis leads to mucosal destruction, extension into adjacent cortex & medulla, and papillary necrosis

Microscopic Features

- Lipid-laden "foamy" macrophages, diffuse infiltration of plasma cells and histiocytes

CLINICAL ISSUES

Presentation

- Most common signs/symptoms
  o Flank pain, fever, palpable mass, & weight loss

Demographics

- Epidemiology
  o Peak age: 40-50 years; F > M

Natural History & Prognosis

- Rare complications: Hepatic dysfunction, extrarenal extension, fistulas
- Long-term chronic process with good prognosis if treated, and rare mortality

Treatment

- Antibiotic treatment is sometimes effective
- Severe disease or perinephric extension usually requires nephrectomy

DIAGNOSTIC CHECKLIST

Consider

- Histologic diagnosis in equivocal XGP

SELECTED REFERENCES

1. Ifergan J et al: Imaging in upper urinary tract infections. Diagn Interv Imaging. 93(6):509-19, 2012
2. Arvind NK et al: Laparoscopic nephrectomy in xanthogranulomatous pyelonephritis: 7-year single-surgeon outcome. Urology. 78(4):797-801, 2011
3. Li L et al: Xanthogranulomatous pyelonephritis. Arch Pathol Lab Med. 135(5):671-4, 2011
4. Kim JC: US and CT findings of xanthogranulomatous pyelonephritis. Clin Imaging. 25(2):118-21, 2001

TERMINOLOGY

- Urinary tract infection (UTI) by mycobacterium tuberculosis via hematogenous spread from primary focus, usually lungs

IMAGING

- Depends on stage of disease; may range from caliectasis, abscess, cavities, calcifications, and strictures in urinary tract
- Early stage: Normal kidney or small focal cortical lesions with poorly defined border ± calcification
- Progressive stage: Papillary destruction with echogenic masses near calyces
- Mural thickening ± ureteric and bladder involvement, associated stricture → hydronephrosis
- Small, fibrotic, thick-walled bladder
- Small, shrunken kidney, "paper-thin" cortex and dystrophic calcification in collecting system
- CECT with CT urogram (CTU) is useful in diagnosing and assessing severity

- Heavily calcified caseous mass surrounded by thin parenchymal shell → "putty kidney"
- Hydrocalyces or "phantom calyx" (nonopacification of caly: due to infiltration and obliteration) proximal to infundibul: stricture
- Late stages: Small, poor-functioning, scarred kidneys with dystrophic calcification
- CT (CTU) has replaced IVP for diagnosis and to rule out complications (strictures, abscess) and extrarenal manifestation
- Ultrasound useful in assessing complications (renal absces: hydronephrosis)

TOP DIFFERENTIAL DIAGNOSES

- Papillary necrosis
- Pyonephrosis
- Xanthogranulomatous pyelonephritis (XGP)
- Cystitis

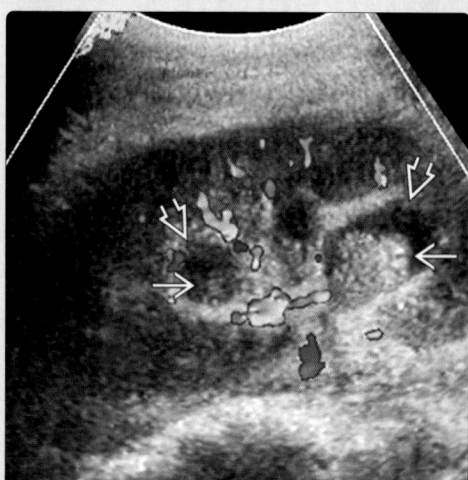
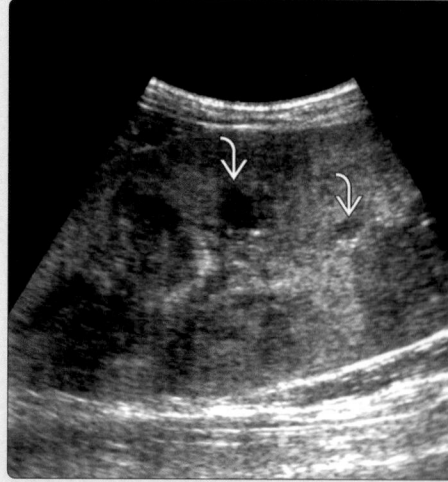

(Left) Longitudinal transabdominal Color Doppler ultrasound shows renal TB with mild hydronephrosis ➡ and avascular internal echogenic debris ➡. (Courtesy A. Pandya, MD.) (Right) Longitudinal transabdominal ultrasound shows renal TB with distorted renal parenchyma. There are small, irregular, hypoechoic lesions ➡, which represent cavities connecting to the collecting system.

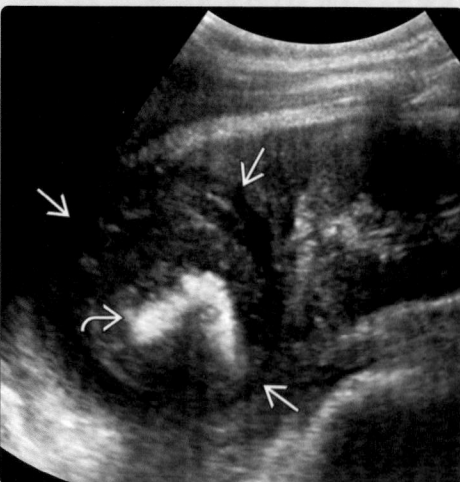
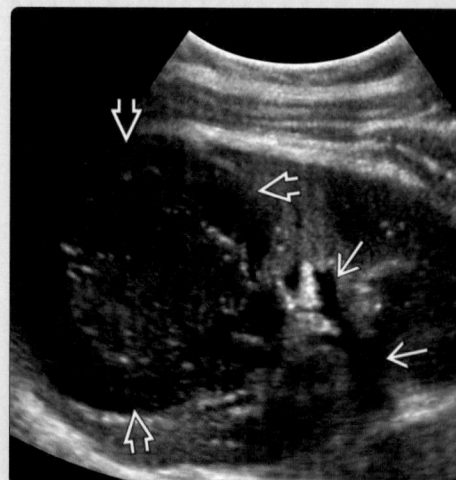

(Left) Longitudinal transabdominal ultrasound shows renal TB with a large cavity in the upper renal pole ➡ containing gas ➡ consistent with abscess. (Courtesy A. Pandya, MD.) (Right) Longitudinal transabdominal ultrasound shows a large cavity with internal debris ➡ in the upper renal pole. Note the mild hydronephrosis ➡. (Courtesy A. Pandya, MD.)

TERMINOLOGY

Abbreviations
- Urinary tract tuberculosis (TB)

Synonyms
- Renal TB, urinary bladder tuberculosis

Definitions
- Urinary tract infection (UTI) by mycobacterium tuberculosis via hematogenous spread from primary focus, usually lungs
- Ureteral and bladder disease are secondary to renal involvement
- Earliest form of bladder TB starts around ureteral orifice

IMAGING

General Features
- Best diagnostic clue
  - Depends on stage of disease; may range from caliectasis, abscess, cavities, calcifications, and strictures in urinary tract
- Location
  - Kidney, ureter, and bladder (~ 14-41% of extrapulmonary TB)
  - Usually bilateral involvement but can also be unilateral

Ultrasonographic Findings
- Grayscale ultrasound
  - Appearance is nonspecific and variable based on stage
  - **Early**: Normal kidney or small focal cortical lesions with poorly defined border ± calcification
  - **Progressive**
    - Papillary destruction with echogenic masses near calyces
    - Distorted renal parenchyma, manifest as pyelonephritis with edematous kidney
    - Irregular hypoechoic masses connecting to collecting system (pseudotumor)
    - Mural thickening ± ureteric and bladder involvement, associated stricture → hydronephrosis
    - Small, fibrotic, thick-walled bladder
    - Echogenic foci or calcification (granulomas) in bladder wall near ureteric orifice
  - **Late**
    - Small, shrunken kidney, "paper-thin" cortex and dystrophic calcification in collecting system
    - May resemble chronic renal disease
  - US less sensitive than CT in detection of isoechoic parenchymal masses, small cavities, calyceal/ureteral abnormalities
  - US unable to evaluate renal function
  - Useful to evaluate pelvic inflammation, especially in women

Radiographic Findings
- IVP
  - Early: Irregular calyceal contour due to erosion moth-eaten appearance
  - Progressive
    - Irregular tract formation from calyx to papilla
    - Large irregular cavities with extensive destruction due to papillary necrosis
    - Hydrocalyces or "phantom calyx" (nonopacification of calyx due to infiltration and obliteration) proximal to infundibular stricture
    - Sharp kink at pelviureteric junction due to scarring ("Kerr kink")
    - Delayed contrast excretion
    - Fibrosis and stricture of renal pelvis or ureter → beaded ureter, focal calcification, or hydronephrosis
    - Small volume bladder
  - Late
    - Heavily calcified caseous mass surrounded by thin parenchymal shell → "putty kidney"
    - Small, shrunken, scarred, nonfunctioning kidney with dystrophic calcification (autonephrectomy)

CT Findings
- CECT
  - CECT with CT urogram (CTU) is useful in diagnosing and assessing severity
  - Moth-eaten calyces, cavities, and renal parenchymal masses better appreciated
  - Amputated infundibulum due to stricture
  - Assessment of renal function (delayed nephrogram and contrast excretion)
  - Multifocal ureteral stricture causing hydronephrosis
  - Better assessment of wall thickening and calcification along urinary tract
  - Late stages: Small, poor-functioning, scarred kidneys with dystrophic calcification
  - Better assessment of extrarenal manifestation in retroperitoneum and pelvis

Imaging Recommendations
- Best imaging tool
  - IVP described to have high sensitivity (88%) in detecting TB manifestation; in fact, majority of imaging features have been described on IVP
  - CECT with CTU has been shown to be more useful in assessing the severity and extrarenal complications
    - CTU may evolve as preferred imaging modality in evaluation of GU TB
  - Ultrasound: Often used for monitoring disease progression and complication (like hydronephrosis)
- Protocol advice
  - IVP described as primary investigation; however, CT (CTU) may evolve as a preferred imaging modality in diagnosis and evaluation of complications and extrarenal manifestation; US useful in assessing complications (renal abscess, hydronephrosis)

DIFFERENTIAL DIAGNOSIS

Papillary Necrosis
- Sonographically, necrotic papilla depicted as echogenic nonshadowing lesion surrounded by fluid in medulla

Pyonephrosis
- Dependent echoes and fluid debris level within dilated collecting system
- Gas within collecting system

Xanthogranulomatous Pyelonephritis (XGP)

- Enlarged kidney with highly reflective central echo complex containing calculus
- Both XGP and renal TB show thickening of perirenal fasciae and spread of inflammation into adjacent organs

Chronic Cystitis

- US: Irregularly thickened bladder wall and reduced bladder volume
- Emphysematous cystitis: Highly reflective intramural gas in bladder wall

PATHOLOGY

General Features

- Etiology
  - Infection by mycobacterium tuberculosis by hematogenous spread from pulmonary TB
  - Occasionally, *Mycobacterium bovis* and *Mycobacterium avium-intracellulare* (MAIC)
  - Reactivation of prior blood-borne dormant tubercle bacilli
- Associated abnormalities
  - Males: Prostatitis, epididymitis, or orchitis
  - Females: Salpingitis, endometritis, or oophoritis (pelvic inflammatory disease)
- Reactivation of dormant mycobacterium TB, which spread into medulla causing papillitis
- Necrotizing papillae sloughed into calyces can both infect and obstruct calyces, ureters, and bladder
- Ulceration of calyx gives typical ulcerocavernous lesion
- Fibrosis causes obstructive strictures leading to hydronephrosis or pyonephrosis
- Infundibular stricture may result in chronic renal abscesses
- Healing results in fibrous tissue and calcium salts being deposited, producing calcified masses
- Diffuse renal involvement with parenchymal destruction and calcification

Gross Pathologic & Surgical Features

- Late stage: Small, irregular, fibrocalcific kidney

Microscopic Features

- Cortical granulomas consist of Langerhans giant cells surrounded by lymphocytes and fibroblasts
- Papillary destruction extending into collecting system with extensive fibrosis
- Multifocal infundibular, pelvic and ureteric fibrotic strictures
- Diffuse parenchymal destruction and calcification

CLINICAL ISSUES

Presentation

- Most common signs/symptoms
  - Asymptomatic common
  - Earliest symptom: Frequency
  - Recurrent UTI: Flank pain, dysuria, fever
  - Sterile pyuria; gross painless hematuria
- Other signs/symptoms
  - Malaise, anorexia, weight loss, night sweats, hypertension

- Prostatic enlargement ± tenderness (male)
- Infertility, pelvic pain, or abnormal menstrual bleeding (female)

Demographics

- Age
  - Usually 2nd-4th decades, due to longer latency betwee pulmonary disease and renal manifestation
- Epidemiology
  - < 2% in developed countries
  - > 20% in developing countries
  - M:F = 2:1

Natural History & Prognosis

- Renal infection → obstructive uropathy → renal failure
- Complications: Hydronephrosis, abscess formation, hypertension, extrarenal spread
- Low mortality but high morbidity
- High relapse rate in patients with poor nutritional status and social condition
- Extrarenal manifestation like pelvic inflammatory diseases in women

Treatment

- Antituberculosis chemotherapy usually followed by surgic intervention
- Surgical intervention
  - Percutaneous balloon stenting for strictures
  - Partial or total nephrectomy to remove large foci of infection in renal calcifications or for extensive renal damage
  - Cystectomy and substitution cystoplasty for extensive bladder damage

DIAGNOSTIC CHECKLIST

Consider

- TB if concurrent multiple abnormalities exist in urinary trac or in patient with known tubercular disease
- Chest radiography to look for primary TB focus
- Biopsy of lesions, urinalysis, and culture

Image Interpretation Pearls

- Abnormalities in multiple sites: Renal parenchymal mass/cavitation ± hydrocalyces/hydronephrosis ± UT calcifications ± small and thick-walled bladder

SELECTED REFERENCES

1. Merchant S et al: Tuberculosis of the genitourinary system-Urinary tract tuberculosis: Renal tuberculosis-Part I. Indian J Radiol Imaging. 23(1):46-63, 2013
2. Merchant S et al: Tuberculosis of the genitourinary system-Urinary tract tuberculosis: Renal tuberculosis-Part II. Indian J Radiol Imaging. 23(1):64-77, 2013
3. Vijayaraghavan SB et al: Spectrum of high-resolution sonographic features of urinary tuberculosis. J Ultrasound Med. 23(5):585-94, 2004
4. Wang LJ et al: Imaging findings of urinary tuberculosis on excretory urography and computerized tomography. J Urol. 169(2):524-8, 2003
5. Wise GJ et al: Genitourinary manifestations of tuberculosis. Urol Clin North Am. 30(1):111-21, 2003
6. Goel A et al: Autocystectomy following extensive genitourinary tuberculos presentation and management. Int Urol Nephrol. 34(3):325-7, 2002
7. Izbudak-Oznur I et al: Renal tuberculosis mimicking xanthogranulomatous pyelonephritis: ultrasonography, computed tomography and magnetic resonance imaging findings. Turk J Pediatr. 44(2):168-71, 2002
8. Premkumar A et al: CT and sonography of advanced urinary tract tuberculosis. AJR Am J Roentgenol. 148(1):65-9, 1987

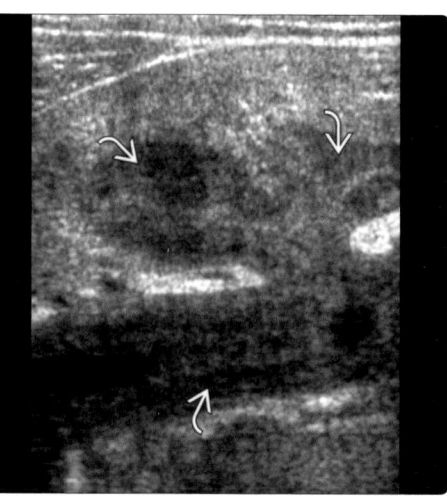

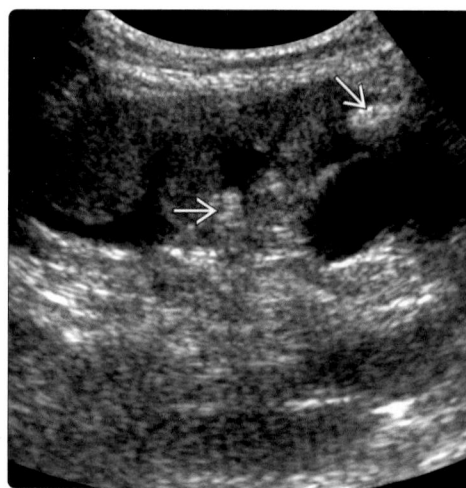

(Left) Longitudinal high-resolution ultrasound shows gross mucosal thickening ➡ in the collecting system of a patient with fulminant renal TB. The appearance may mimic pyonephrosis or neoplasm. (Right) Longitudinal transabdominal ultrasound shows renal TB with papillary involvement. Echogenic nonshadowing lesions ➡ surrounded by fluid in renal medulla suggest papillary necrosis.

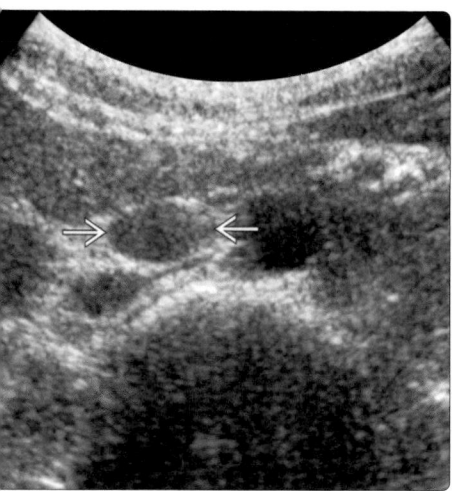

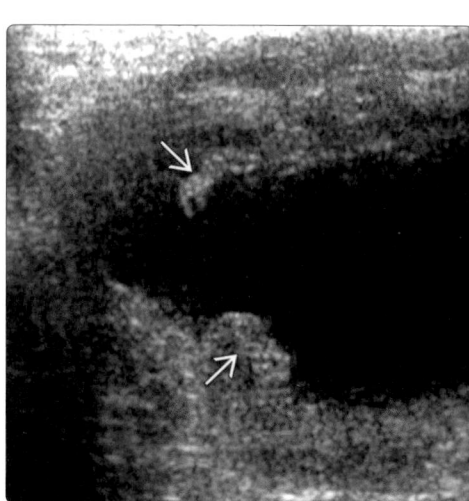

(Left) Transverse transabdominal ultrasound shows an enlarged, paraaortic lymph node ➡ in a patient with renal TB. Associated lymphadenopathy is common and may be either reactive or infective. (Right) Transverse transabdominal ultrasound shows TB of the bladder with an irregularly thickened bladder wall ➡. Its appearance may be indistinguishable from other forms of bacterial cystitis.

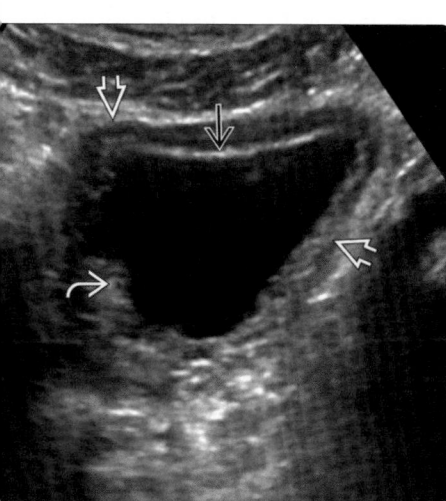

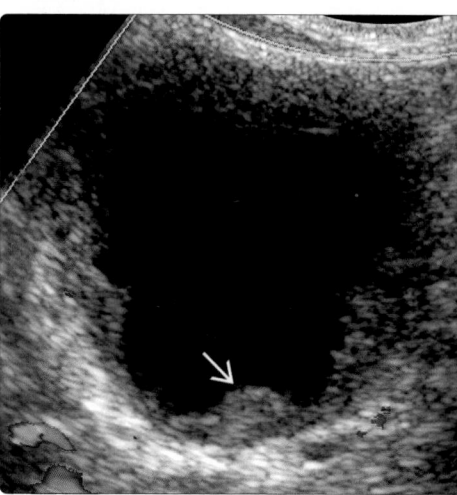

(Left) Transverse oblique transabdominal ultrasound of the bladder in this patient with known GU tuberculosis shows diffuse wall thickening ➡ with mucosal irregularity ➡ and echogenicity, likely calcification ➡. (Right) Longitudinal transabdominal ultrasound shows a urinary bladder infected by TB. There is irregular mucosal thickening near the ureteric orifice ➡, which is the earliest site for onset of disease.

KEY FACTS

TERMINOLOGY

- Malignant tumor arising from proximal tubular epithelium
- Most common primary renal malignancy

IMAGING

- Clear cell adenocarcinoma (60-70%)
- Papillary (5-15%)
- Chromophobe (5%)
- Variable appearance: Solid, cystic, or complex
- Macroscopic fat practically excludes renal cell carcinoma (RCC)
- Clear cell RCC: Hypervascular, heterogeneous, mixed enhancement pattern with both enhancing soft tissue components and areas of necrosis
- Papillary RCC: Hypovascular, typically homogeneous; may be partly cystic
- Increasing role of percutaneous biopsy in selecting patients for treatment or surveillance based on subtype

- RCC may be initially detected by US but CECT and MR are primary tools for characterization and staging
- In select patients, US may be used for screening and follow-up depending on body habitus
- MR/US preferred over CT for long-term surveillance based on radiation concerns
- Ultrasound may be useful in characterizing complex cystic lesions, which are indeterminate or equivocal on CECT or MR
- Use Doppler (color/power/pulsed) for detection of internal vascularity

TOP DIFFERENTIAL DIAGNOSES

- Renal angiomyolipoma
- Transitional cell carcinoma (TCC)
- Renal oncocytoma
- Renal metastases and lymphoma
- Column of Bertin

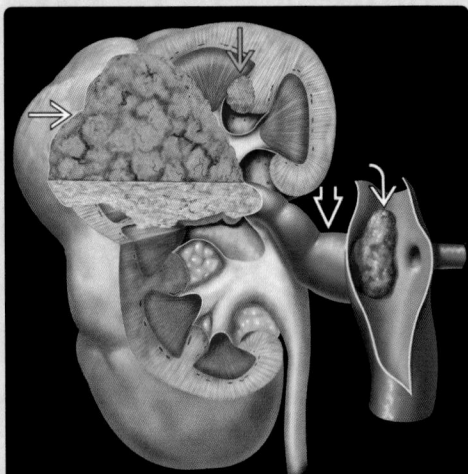
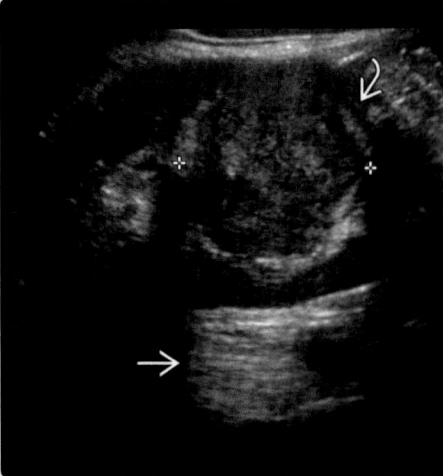

(Left) *Graphic shows a lobulated, solid, upper pole renal carcinoma ➡. The renal vein ➡ is expanded with tumor thrombus, which extends into the inferior vena cava ➡. A 2nd tumor nodule is seen ➡.* **(Right)** *Longitudinal ultrasound in a patient with clear cell renal carcinoma shows a solid, slightly hyperechoic mass within the calipers. There is an incomplete hypoechoic rim ➡. Note posterior acoustic enhancement ➡.*

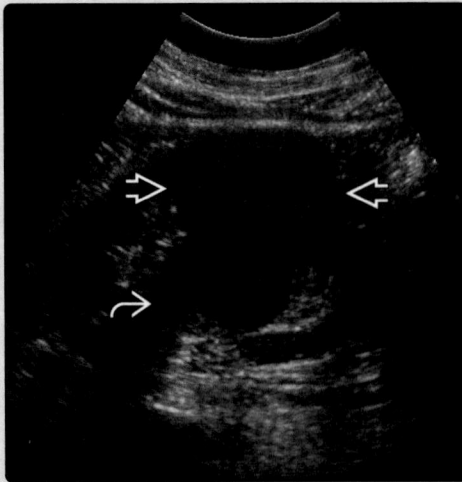
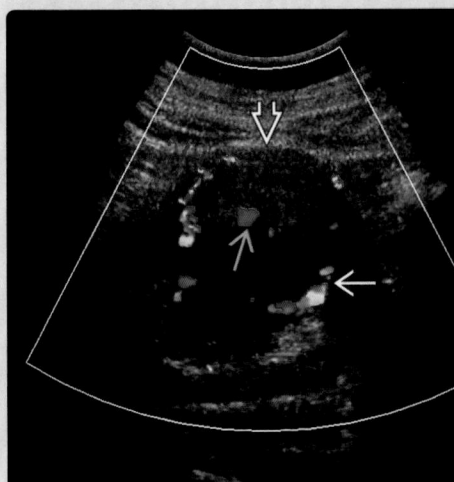

(Left) *Longitudinal ultrasound shows an exophytic, homogeneous, hypoechoic chromophobe renal cell carcinoma (RCC) ➡ with infiltration and distortion of the renal sinus fat ➡.* **(Right)** *Transverse ultrasound of the same patient shows a solid, hypoechoic, exophytic chromophobe RCC ➡ with peripheral ➡ and internal color flow ➡.*

TERMINOLOGY

Abbreviations

- Renal cell carcinoma (RCC)

Synonyms

- Renal cell adenocarcinoma, hypernephroma

Definitions

- Malignant tumor arising from proximal tubular epithelium

IMAGING

General Features

- Best diagnostic clue
  - Hypervascular solid renal mass
  - Macroscopic fat practically excludes RCC
  - Extension into veins
- Location
  - Renal cortex
  - Tumors usually solitary but may be multifocal (6-25%) or bilateral (~ 4%)
- Morphology
  - Usually solid mass; variants are cystic (< 5%)
- Subtypes include
  - Clear cell adenocarcinoma (60-70%)
  - Papillary (5-15%)
  - Chromophobe (5%)
  - Collecting duct (< 1%), unclassified (4%)

Ultrasonographic Findings

- Grayscale ultrasound
  - Variable appearance: Solid, cystic or complex
  - Hyperechoic (48%), isoechoic (42%), or hypoechoic (10%)
  - Small tumors are usually hyperechoic; simulate angiomyolipoma (AML)
  - Large tumors tend to be hypoechoic, exophytic with anechoic necrotic areas
  - Hypoechoic rim resembling "pseudocapsule"
  - Cystic variant: Unilocular or multilocular, fluid-debris levels (hemorrhage and necrosis), thick and irregular wall or septations, nodules
- Color Doppler
  - Discernible tumor vascularity; most prominent around tumor periphery, < renal parenchyma
    - Contrast-enhanced ultrasound can improve detection of neovascularity

CT Findings

- NECT
  - Solid or complicated cystic mass, hyperdense, isodense, or hypodense compared to renal tissue
  - Heterogeneous mass (hemorrhage and necrosis)
  - Calcifications have high positive predictive value for malignancy when amorphous and in solid components
  - Intratumoral fat is extremely rare and associated with osseous metaplasia
- CECT
  - Degree of enhancement most valuable in differentiating RCC subtypes
  - Clear cell RCC: Hypervascular, heterogeneous, mixed enhancement pattern with both enhancing soft tissue components and areas of necrosis
    - Enhances more than other subtypes
  - Papillary RCC: Hypovascular, typically homogeneous; may be partly cystic
  - Cystic RCC variants: Uni-/multilocular cystic mass with thick wall and nodular component, enhancing smooth or nodular septa
  - RCC occasionally diffusely infiltrative or infiltrates collecting system
  - Lucent rim (pseudocapsule)
  - Direct extension to renal vein (RV) (20-35%), inferior vena cava (IVC) (4-10%), adjacent muscles, and viscera

MR Findings

- Isointense (60%) on T1WI and T2WI or hyperintense (40%) on T2WI
- Hypointense band/rim on T1WI (25%) and T2WI (60%)
- T1WI C+: Enhances, usually less than renal tissue

Image-Guided Biopsy

- Increasing role in selecting patients for treatment or surveillance based on subtype
- Performed in setting of widely metastatic disease or when there is another malignancy
- Used to confirm diagnosis prior to ablative therapy, as up to 30% of small solid renal masses are benign

Imaging Recommendations

- Best imaging tool
  - RCC may be initially detected by US but CECT and MR are primary tools for characterization and staging
  - In select patients, US may be used for screening and follow-up depending on body habitus
  - MR/US preferred over CT for long-term surveillance based on radiation concerns
- Protocol advice
  - Ultrasound may be useful in characterizing complex cystic lesions, which are indeterminate or equivocal on CECT or MR
    - Use Doppler (color/power/pulsed) for detection of internal vascularity
    - Contrast-enhanced ultrasound sensitivity of 96% for classifying complex cystic renal masses

DIFFERENTIAL DIAGNOSIS

Renal Angiomyolipoma

- Homogeneous, well-defined, noncalcified, echogenic cortical mass with occasional posterior acoustic shadowing
- Characteristic macroscopic fat confirmed with CT or MR
- Both AML with minimal fat and RCC can contain microscopic fat on chemical shift imaging; AML with minimal fat usually hypointense on T2WI MR

Transitional Cell Carcinoma (TCC)

- Infiltrative tumor involving renal parenchyma may be indistinct from infiltrative RCC
- Renal pelvic filling defect, irregular narrowing of collecting system, hypovascular

Renal Oncocytoma

- No imaging criteria to accurately differentiate from RCC

Renal Metastases and Lymphoma

- Metastases: Usually hypovascular; infiltrative or multiple
- Lymphoma: Usually multiple or bilateral; hypovascular solid masses, typically associated with lymphadenopathy

Column of Bertin

- Isoechoic; located in mid 1/3 of kidney

Multilocular Cystic Nephroma

- Morphologically indistinguishable from cystic RCC but different demographics

Complex Renal Cyst

- Septated cyst ± calcification ± internal hemorrhage or high density ± thick wall

Renal Abscess

- Renal enlargement with complex cystic mass
- Differentiated by clinical history and urinalysis

PATHOLOGY

General Features

- Etiology
  - Risk factors: Most sporadic but can be hereditary (~ 4%)
    - Genetics: von Hippel-Lindau (VHL) disease, hereditary papillary RCC, Birt-Hogg-Dubé syndrome, tuberous sclerosis, sickle cell trait
    - Advanced age
    - Long-term dialysis/acquired cystic renal disease, kidney transplantation
    - Environmental/chemical: Smoking, obesity, diethylstilbestrol, lead, cadmium, diuretic use, HIV infection

Staging, Grading, & Classification

- TNM classification system of RCC (American Joint Committee on Cancer, 2002)
- Fuhrman (nuclear) grade: Most common system for grading RCC, based on appearance of nuclei (uniform to bizarre) and presence of nucleoli

Gross Pathologic & Surgical Features

- Completely solid to cystic mass with irregular, lobulated margins
- Heterogeneous appearance with hemorrhage and necrosis

Microscopic Features

- Clear cell RCC: Cells with clear cytoplasm from high glycogen and lipid content
- Papillary RCC: Small cells with scant cytoplasm arranged in papillae

CLINICAL ISSUES

Presentation

- Most common signs/symptoms
  - Gross hematuria (60%), flank pain (40%), palpable flank mass (30-40%); classical triad (< 10%)
  - Fever, anorexia, weight loss, malaise, nausea, vomiting
  - Most tumors now detected incidentally and are smaller

- Other signs/symptoms
  - Varicocele formation (tumor thrombus in left renal vein or IVC)
  - Hypertension, hepatopathy (Stauffer syndrome), paraneoplastic syndromes (hypercalcemia or polycythemia)
  - 30% present with symptomatic metastases

Demographics

- Age
  - 50-70 years of age
- Gender
  - M:F = 2:1, slightly higher in African Americans
- Epidemiology
  - 8th most common malignancy affecting adults, most common primary renal malignancy
  - 3-4% of all cancers
  - 24-45% of VHL patients develop RCC, which are multifocal and bilateral

Natural History & Prognosis

- Prognosis: 5-year survival rate (SR): Stage I: 96%; stage II: 82%; stage III: 64%; stage IV: 23%
- Larger tumors, bilateral or multiple RCCs have poorer SR
- Clear cell RCCs have greatest metastatic potential and chromophobe tumors have best overall prognosis
- Metastases: Lungs most common; lymph nodes, bones, liver, brain, adrenal glands, or pancreas
- Tumor may recur locally or in contralateral kidney

Treatment

- Radical or partial nephrectomy (equally as efficacious)
  - Indications for partial nephrectomy include ≤ 4 cm size, peripheral location, exophytic extension, no invasion of vessels or lymph nodes
- Radiofrequency ablation and cryoablation

DIAGNOSTIC CHECKLIST

Consider

- Suspect RCC in solid renal lesions with internal vascularity calcifications

Image Interpretation Pearls

- Evaluate complex cystic lesions for solid nodules and internal color flow
  - CECT and enhanced MR for lesion characterization and staging

SELECTED REFERENCES

1. Allen BC et al: Characterizing solid renal neoplasms with MRI in adults. Abdom Imaging. 39(2):358-87, 2014
2. Kang SK et al: Solid renal masses: what the numbers tell us. AJR Am J Roentgenol. 202(6):1196-206, 2014
3. Klatte T et al: The contemporary role of ablative treatment approaches in the management of renal cell carcinoma (RCC): focus on radiofrequency ablation (RFA), high-intensity focused ultrasound (HIFU), and cryoablation. World J Urol. 32(3):597-605, 2014
4. Patel U et al: Imaging in the follow-up of renal cell carcinoma. AJR Am J Roentgenol. 198(6):1266-76, 2012
5. Ng CS et al: Renal cell carcinoma: diagnosis, staging, and surveillance. AJR Am J Roentgenol. 191(4):1220-32, 2008

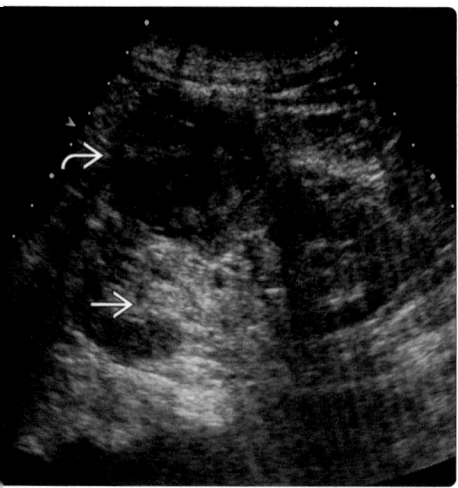
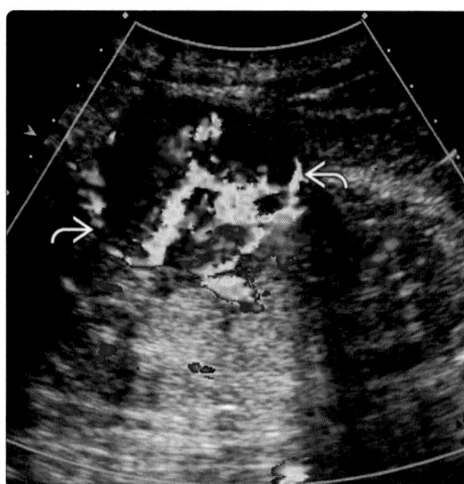

(Left) Longitudinal US shows exophytic, heterogeneous clear cell renal carcinoma ➡. There is some posterior acoustic enhancement from internal cystic/necrotic components ➡. (Right) Color Doppler US in the same patient with exophytic heterogeneous renal carcinoma ➡ shows prominent internal and peripheral color flow.

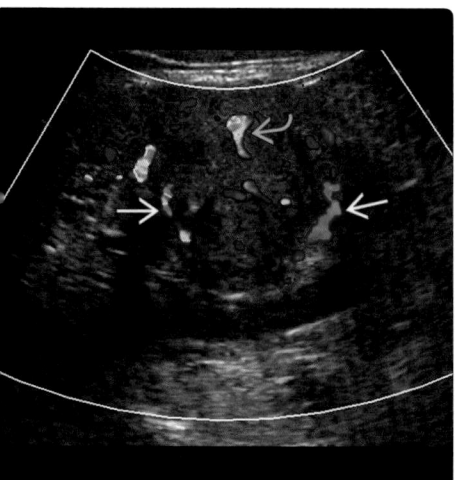
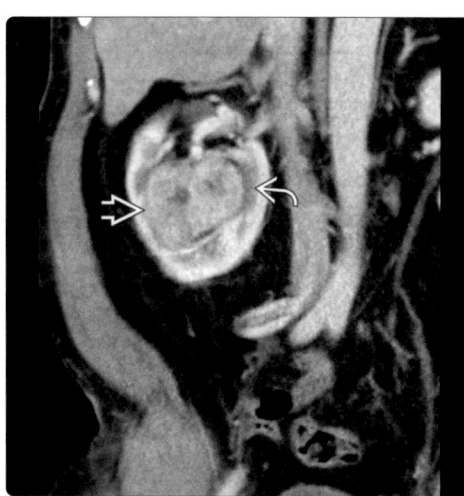

(Left) Longitudinal color Doppler ultrasound in a patient with clear cell RCC shows prominent peripheral ➡ and internal ➡ vascularity within a solid mass. (Right) Coronal CECT of the same patient shows a lobulated, well-defined, enhancing intrarenal RCC ➡. Note the hypodense rim ➡.

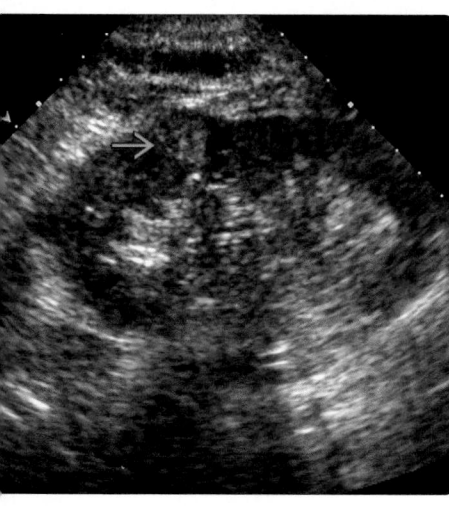
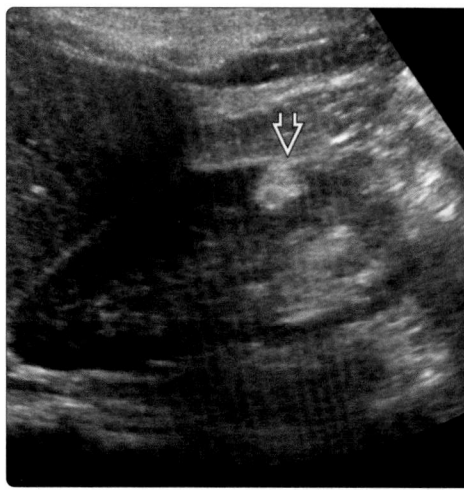

(Left) Longitudinal ultrasound shows a small, hyperechoic, partly exophytic clear cell RCC ➡, which may be mistaken for an angiomyolipoma. These can be distinguished by confirming the presence of macroscopic fat with CT or MR. (Right) Longitudinal ultrasound in a patient with angiomyolipoma shows a small, cortical, hyperechoic lesion ➡. Echogenicity was higher than the preceding RCC. No color flow was detected. CT or MR can confirm the diagnosis.

IMAGING

- Typically multiple and small, bilateral, hypoenhancing renal masses
- More likely to be endophytic, compared to renal cell carcinoma (RCC), which is more likely exophytic
- Large exophytic metastases may be encountered
- Mostly avascular or hypovascular
- Increased uptake in F-18-2-fluoro-2-deoxy-glucose (FDG) scan
- Melanoma metastasis: Hypervascular; may stimulate RCC
- Perinephric infiltration from tumor extension or hemorrhage may be seen (melanoma)

TOP DIFFERENTIAL DIAGNOSES

- Primary renal malignancy
- Renal angiomyolipoma
- Renal cyst
- Renal lymphoma or leukemia
- Renal infection
- Renal infarction

CLINICAL ISSUES

- Usually asymptomatic; may have hematuria or microhematuria (12-31%)
- Most are clinically occult and found on imaging or at autopsy
- Most common malignant renal tumor at autopsy (7-13% of autopsies), 20% of patients dying of disseminated malignancy
- Lung cancer most common primary site followed by breast, gastric cancer, melanoma, and lymphoma
- Prognosis very poor

DIAGNOSTIC CHECKLIST

- Multiple renal masses likely to be metastases in presence of nonrenal primary cancer and widespread systemic metastases

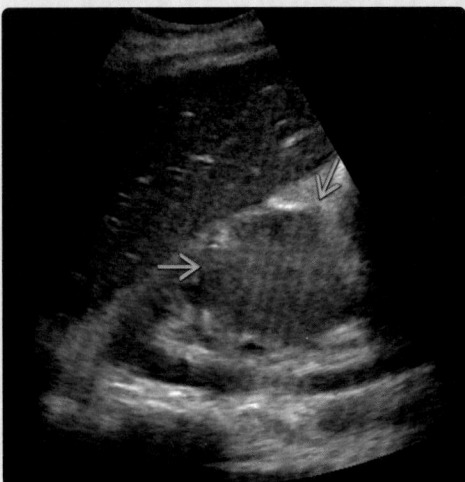
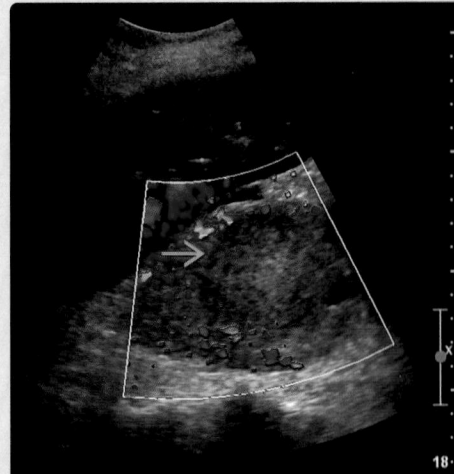

(Left) *Longitudinal US of the right kidney shows a mid pole solid, homogeneous, slightly hyperechoic mass ➡ representing metastatic melanoma. This cannot be distinguished from renal cell carcinoma (RCC).* **(Right)** *Corresponding color Doppler US shows no significant color flow within the mass ➡. While the grayscale features are indistinguishable from RCC, metastases are typically hypovascular compared to RCC.*

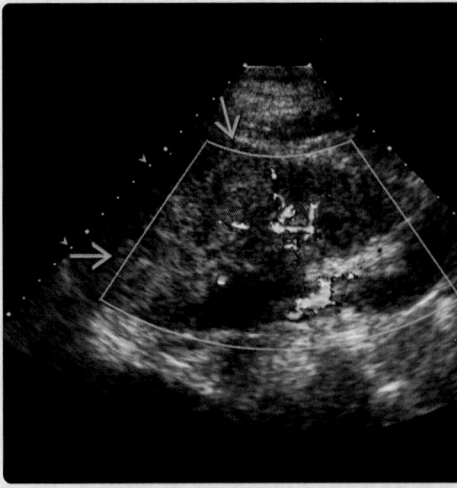
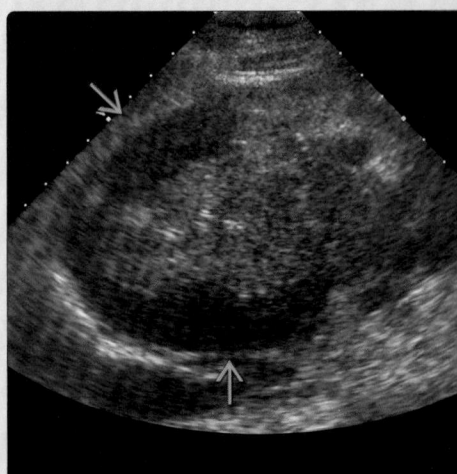

(Left) *Color Doppler ultrasound shows a large, echogenic renal metastasis ➡, which is hypovascular. There is preservation of the renal contour. Renal metastases are usually smaller and less echogenic and may be difficult to detect with ultrasound.* **(Right)** *Longitudinal US shows an enlarged, globular kidney with hypoechoic infiltration of the cortex ➡ by multiple myeloma. Note relative preservation of the sinus fat.*

IMAGING

General Features

Best diagnostic clue
- Imaging findings are nonspecific
- Typically multiple and small, bilateral, hypoenhancing renal masses
- More likely to be endophytic, compared to renal cell carcinoma (RCC), which is more likely exophytic
- Large exophytic metastases may be encountered
- Perinephric infiltration from tumor extension or hemorrhage may be seen (more common in melanoma)
- Most patients have metastatic tumor at other locations

Ultrasonographic Findings

Grayscale ultrasound
- Usually small and round, may be wedge-shaped
- Usually cortical; rarely disrupting renal contour or capsule
- May be hypoechoic, hyperechoic, or sonographically occult
- Occasionally infiltrative

Color Doppler
- Mostly avascular or hypovascular, using low flow Doppler settings
- Melanoma metastasis can be hypervascular; may simulate RCC

CT Findings

Usually small, bilateral, and multifocal

Iso- to hypodense on NECT, poorly enhancing

Cystic/necrotic or hypervascular variants depending on primary malignancy

Widespread extrarenal metastases usually present

Nuclear Medicine Findings

PET
- Increased uptake in F-18-2-fluoro-2-deoxy-glucose (FDG) scan, extrarenal lesions in majority

DIFFERENTIAL DIAGNOSIS

Primary Renal Neoplasms

RCC: Solitary renal cortical mass, hypervascular, usually exophytic, may be necrotic

Transitional cell carcinoma: Infiltrative mass + obstruction of collecting system

Renal Angiomyolipoma

Majority are echogenic due to intratumoral fat content

May also be multiple or bilateral

Renal Cyst

Anechoic, lacking color flow, can be multiple

Renal Lymphoma or Leukemia

Multifocal or infiltrative masses, ± perirenal masses or lymphadenopathy

Renal Infection

Focal pyelonephritis may mimic metastasis

Clinical picture of infection is key for diagnosis

Renal Infarction

Avascular, wedge-shaped renal lesion

PATHOLOGY

General Features

- Etiology
  - Dissemination of advanced primary malignancy; hematogenous > direct spread

Microscopic Features

- Varies based on primary cancer
- Metastases are distinctly different from primary renal cell cancers on cytological smears

CLINICAL ISSUES

Presentation

- Most common signs/symptoms
  - Usually asymptomatic; may have hematuria or microhematuria (12-31%)
- Other signs/symptoms
  - Most found on imaging or at autopsy
  - Acute pain or hypotension from perinephric hemorrhage

Demographics

- Epidemiology
  - Most common malignant renal tumor at autopsy (7-13% of autopsies), 20% of patients dying of disseminated malignancy
  - Lung cancer most common primary site followed by breast, gastric, and melanoma

Natural History & Prognosis

- Prognosis very poor
- More common in patients with higher stage of nonrenal malignancy

Treatment

- Chemotherapy or palliative treatment
- Nephrectomy if metastasis is small and isolated

DIAGNOSTIC CHECKLIST

Consider

- Multiple renal masses likely to be metastases in presence of nonrenal primary cancer and widespread systemic metastases
- Single renal mass in patient with nonrenal malignancy could be metastasis or synchronous primary renal malignancy
  - Differentiation between the above can be made with CT or US-guided percutaneous biopsy if this directly influences treatment

SELECTED REFERENCES

1. Roy A et al: Common and uncommon bilateral adult renal masses. Cancer Imaging. 12:205-11, 2012
2. Patel U et al: Synchronous renal masses in patients with a nonrenal malignancy: incidence of metastasis to the kidney versus primary renal neoplasia and differentiating features on CT. AJR Am J Roentgenol. 197(4):W680-6, 2011

Renal Angiomyolipoma

IMAGING

- Discrete intrarenal mass containing macroscopic fat
- Few mm to very large
- Triphasic angiomyolipoma (AML) histopathology: Varying amounts of dysmorphic blood vessels, smooth muscle, and mature adipose tissue; can be classified radiologically into "classic" and "fat-poor" subtypes
- Classic AML: Contains fat measuring < -10 HU on NECT
- Fat-poor subtype ("AML with minimal fat"): Insufficient amount of fat to be detected by conventional CT or MR imaging

TOP DIFFERENTIAL DIAGNOSES

- Renal cell carcinoma
- After acute hemorrhage, RCC or AML may be indistinguishable if no fat is detected
- Wilms tumor
- Renal oncocytoma
- Deep cortical scar

- Cortical milk of calcium cyst (MCC)

CLINICAL ISSUES

- Most common benign solid renal neoplasm
- Majority detected as incidental finding on imaging or during screening of tuberous sclerosis
- 80% sporadic, prevalence 0.2%, 4th-6th decades; usually unilateral and solitary
- Sporadic form more common in females than males (F:M = 3:1)
- 20% associated with tuberous sclerosis complex (TSC); mean age younger; 55-75% of patients with TSC will have AML by 3rd decade; any subtype of AML, multiple and bilateral
- Tend to grow faster when > 4 cm
- Size > 4 cm or aneurysm size > 5 mm found to predict bleeding
- AML associated with TSC more likely to need some form of treatment

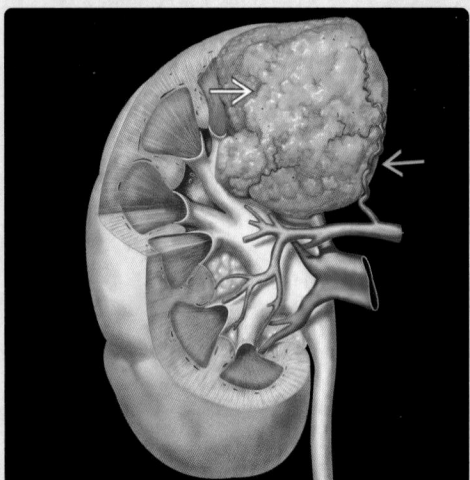
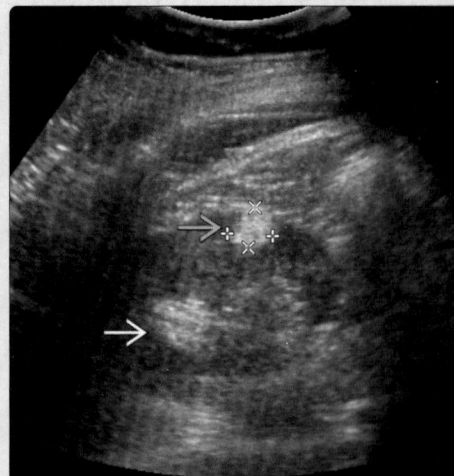

(Left) Graphic shows a vascular renal mass containing predominantly adipose ➡ components. Note the tortuous feeding artery ➡ arising from the main renal artery. (Right) Transverse US shows a small, well-marginated, hyperechoic mass ➡ characteristic of angiomyolipoma (AML). Note the similar appearance to the renal sinus fat ➡.

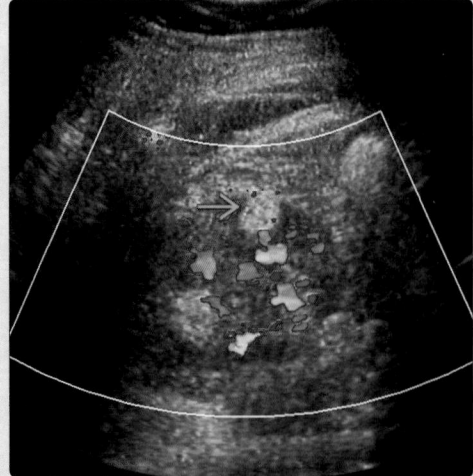
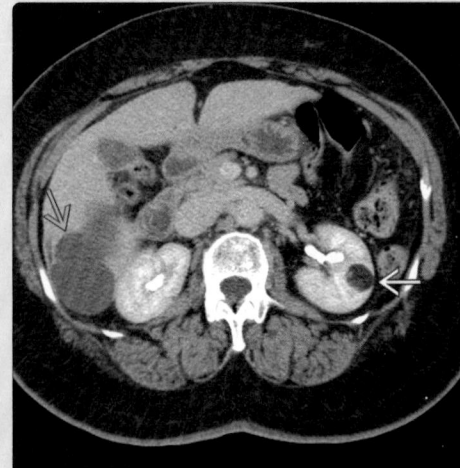

(Left) Corresponding transverse color Doppler US shows no significant color flow in the small AML ➡. (Right) Axial CECT in delayed phase shows an asymptomatic classic fat-containing AML ➡ in the mid left kidney. Liver cysts ➡ are noted incidentally.

TERMINOLOGY

Abbreviations

- Angiomyolipoma (AML)

IMAGING

General Features

- Best diagnostic clue
  - Discrete intrarenal mass containing macroscopic fat
- Location
  - Renal cortex
- Size
  - Few mm to very large
- Heterogeneous group of benign neoplasms with varying pathologic, radiologic, and clinical characteristics
- Triphasic AML: Composed of varying amounts of dysmorphic blood vessels, smooth muscle, and mature adipose tissue; can be classified radiologically into "classic" and "fat-poor" subtypes
  - Classic AML: Contains fat detectable by imaging
  - Fat-poor AML ("AML with minimal fat"): Insufficient amount of fat to be detected by conventional CT or MR imaging; divided into 3 categories
    - Hyperattenuating AML: Abundant smooth muscle component; average size 3 cm
    - Isoattenuating AML: Interspersed fat within smooth muscle; shows chemical shift suppression mimicking clear cell renal cell carcinoma (RCC)
    - AML with epithelial cysts: Extremely rare; cystic components and few, if any, fat cells
- Epithelioid AML: Extremely rare subtype

Ultrasonographic Findings

- Grayscale ultrasound
  - Echogenicity depends on amount of fat
  - Classic AML: Renal lesion of similar echogenicity to renal sinus fat
    - Small < 3 cm: Round, well-marginated, hyperechoic renal cortical lesion
    - Larger: More lobulated and exophytic
    - Acoustic shadowing in 21-33% of AML (not in RCC)
    - Hypoechoic rim and intratumoral cysts suggest RCC
  - Hemorrhage in perinephric space and retroperitoneum from tumor rupture
- Color Doppler
  - Tortuous dilated vessels, aneurysms

CT Findings

- NECT
  - Classic AML: Contains fat measuring < -10 HU
    - Appearance depends on proportion of fat, blood vessel, and smooth muscle components
    - Region of interest measurements of thin sections or histogram analysis may be needed to detect fat
      □ Hemorrhage may obscure fat
  - Fat-poor AML
    - Hyperattenuating AML: High attenuation on CT
    - Isoattenuating AML: Isoattenuation to renal tissue
  - Calcification very rare in AML, suggests RCC
- CECT
  - Varied enhancement pattern based on amount of fat and vascular components
  - Extension of tumor into inferior vena cava (IVC) is rare
- CTA
  - Aneurysmal renal vessels may be seen

MR Findings

- T1WI
  - Classic AML: Hyperintense with signal loss on fat suppression
- T2WI
  - Classic AML: Isointense to fat, suppress with fat suppression
  - Fat-poor AML: Hypointense, do not suppress with fat suppression
- T1WI C+
  - Variable enhancement
- Chemical shift
  - India ink artifact at border of mass indicates AML; however, signal loss throughout mass (that does not suppress with fat suppression) could represent clear cell RCC or AML

Angiographic Findings

- Vascular tumor with long tortuous arteries and aneurysms, active bleeding rarely seen
- Current role is for embolization of bleeding AML or for prophylaxis in larger AML at risk of bleeding

Imaging Recommendations

- Best imaging tool
  - CT/MR more specific than US
  - Ultrasound may be used for screening and monitoring of AML, depending on body habitus
- Protocol advice
  - Echogenic masses detected by ultrasound should be further evaluated with CT or MR to confirm presence of fat
  - Consider fat-poor AML if solid, enhancing mass is hypointense on T2WI

DIFFERENTIAL DIAGNOSIS

Renal Cell Carcinoma

- May be echogenic on US but rarely contains fat
  - Fat typically associated with coarse calcification while AML are very rarely calcified
- RCC may engulf renal sinus fat
- Ablated RCC may be replaced by fat, history and prior imaging are essential
- After acute hemorrhage, RCC or AML may be indistinguishable if no fat is detected

Perirenal Liposarcoma

- Large exophytic AML may resemble retroperitoneal liposarcoma
- Smooth compression of kidney & extension beyond perirenal space favor liposarcoma
- Identification of enlarged/bridging renal vessels and aneurysms favor AML
- Beak of renal tissue around fatty mass or small cortical defect at interface of mass with kidney favor AML

Wilms Tumor

- Pediatric renal tumor that rarely contains fat

Renal Oncocytoma

- Solid renal tumor that rarely contains fat
- Well-defined, homogeneous, hypoechoic to isoechoic masses
- Central scar cannot be confidently identified on ultrasound

Deep Cortical Scar

- Echogenic cortical defect ± underlying dilated calyx

Cortical Milk of Calcium Cyst (MCC)

- Round, echogenic, avascular lesion with ring-down artifact, debris level, or acoustic enhancement

PATHOLOGY

General Features

- Etiology
  - Family of perivascular epithelioid cell tumors (PEComa)
- Genetics
  - Associated with tuberous sclerosis complex (TSC)

Gross Pathologic & Surgical Features

- Round, lobulated, yellow-to-gray color secondary to fat content

Microscopic Features

- Classic triphasic AML: Varying proportions of angioid, myoid, and lipoid components
- Fat-poor AML: May be composed almost entirely of smooth muscle
- Epithelioid angiomyolipoma: Composed of numerous atypical epithelioid muscle cells and few or no fat cells

CLINICAL ISSUES

Presentation

- Most common signs/symptoms
  - Majority detected as incidental finding on imaging or during screening of tuberous sclerosis
  - May present with acute abdomen, flank pain, or flank mass from spontaneous bleeding
  - Hematuria
- Other signs/symptoms
  - Hypertension & chronic renal failure

Demographics

- Age
  - Mean: 5th decade
- Gender
  - Sporadic form more common in females than males (F:M = 3:1)
  - In TSC, M:F = 1:1
- Epidemiology
  - Most common benign solid renal neoplasm
  - 80% sporadic, prevalence 0.2%, 4th-6th decades; usually unilateral and solitary
  - 20% associated with TSC; mean age younger; 55-75% of patients with TSC will have AML by 3rd decade; any subtype of AML, multiple and bilateral, also associated with lymphangioleiomyomatosis

Natural History & Prognosis

- Slow-growing tumors
- Tend to grow faster when > 4 cm
  - Rapid tumor growth associated with increased angiogenesis leading to vessel dilation, formation, and aneurysms
  - Size > 4 cm or aneurysm > 5 mm found to predict bleeding
- AML associated with TSC more likely to need some form of treatment
  - Tend to grow more rapidly (1.25 cm/yr) compared to sporadic AML (0.19 cm/yr)
  - Recurrent bleed more likely with TSC 43%, whereas sporadic AMLs typically do not rebleed
- Complications: Hemorrhage and rupture
- Prognosis
  - Usually good after partial or complete nephrectomy
  - Poor with hemorrhage, rupture, no treatment

Treatment

- If asymptomatic, conservative treatment unless there are complications
  - No consensus on which asymptomatic AML need follow-up
  - Follow-up not needed in tumors < 2 cm, except in young patients with TSC
- Tumor size > 4 cm or symptomatic: Selective arterial embolization or partial nephrectomy
- Spontaneous bleeding treated with transarterial embolization

DIAGNOSTIC CHECKLIST

Image Interpretation Pearls

- Well-circumscribed, discrete fatty renal mass
- Current practice is to confirm presence of fat with CT or MR, as RCC can also be echogenic on US
- Presence of posterior shadowing from renal lesion on US is more suggestive of AML than RCC
- Intratumoral hemorrhage may mask small amount of fat leading to misdiagnosis of RCC

SELECTED REFERENCES

1. Fittschen A et al: Prevalence of sporadic renal angiomyolipoma: a retrospective analysis of 61,389 in- and out-patients. Abdom Imaging. 39(5):1009-13, 2014
2. Hocquelet A et al: Long-term results of preventive embolization of renal angiomyolipomas: evaluation of predictive factors of volume decrease. Eur Radiol. 24(8):1785-93, 2014
3. Jinzaki M et al: Renal angiomyolipoma: a radiological classification and update on recent developments in diagnosis and management. Abdom Imaging. 39(3):588-604, 2014
4. Kaler KS et al: Angiomyolipoma with caval extension and regional nodal involvement: Aggressive behaviour or just rare natural history? Case report and review of literature. Can Urol Assoc J. 8(3-4):E276-8, 2014
5. Maclean DF et al: Is the follow-up of small renal angiomyolipomas a necessary precaution? Clin Radiol. 69(8):822-6, 2014
6. Ouzaid I et al: Active surveillance for renal angiomyolipoma: outcomes and factors predictive of delayed intervention. BJU Int. 114(3):412-7, 2014

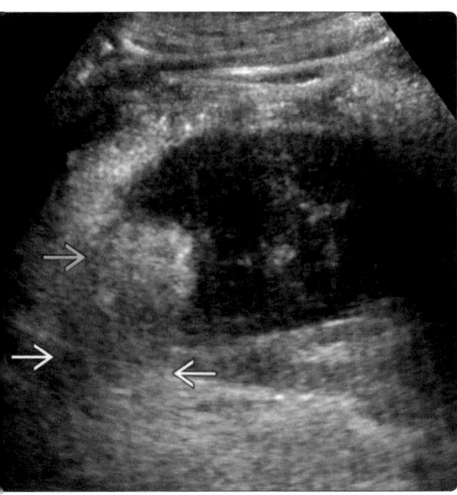

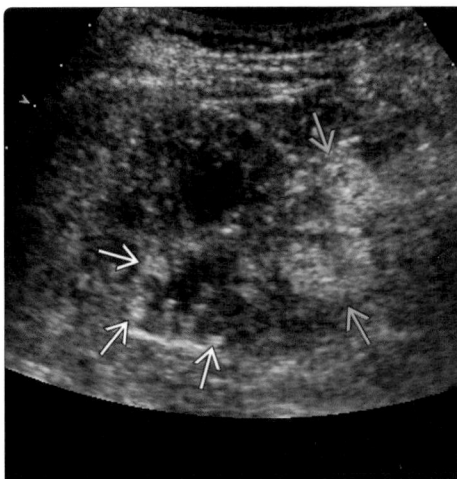

(Left) *Longitudinal ultrasound shows an echogenic AML ➡ in the upper pole of the kidney. Note the subtle posterior acoustic shadowing ➡.* **(Right)** *Longitudinal ultrasound of the kidney in a patient with tuberous sclerosis shows an exophytic echogenic AML ➡. The renal cortex is increased in echogenicity with multiple small, echogenic foci ➡ representing smaller AML.*

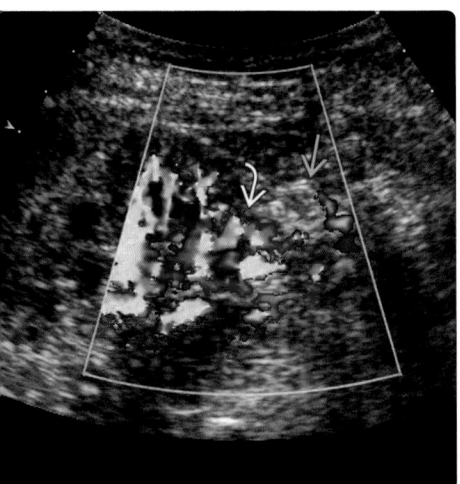

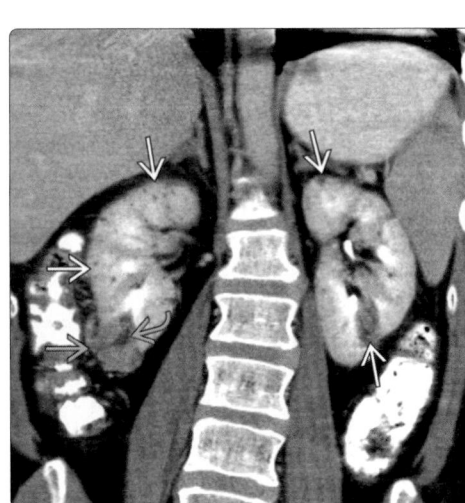

(Left) *Longitudinal color Doppler ultrasound of the same patient with tuberous sclerosis shows an exophytic echogenic AML ➡. Bridging renal vessels ➡ supply the AML.* **(Right)** *Coronal-delayed phase CECT in a patient with tuberous sclerosis shows an exophytic AML ➡, which is mostly solid with a few areas containing fat ➡. Multiple other AML are present ➡, largest in the left lower pole.*

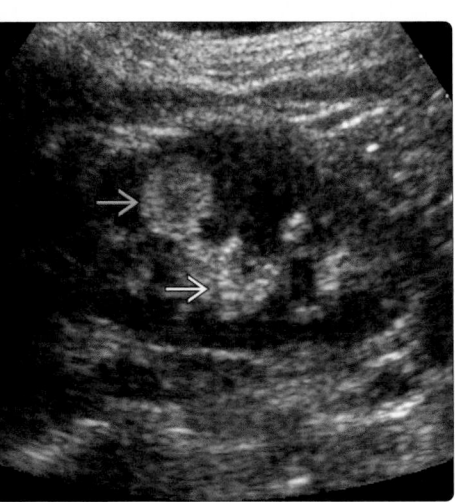

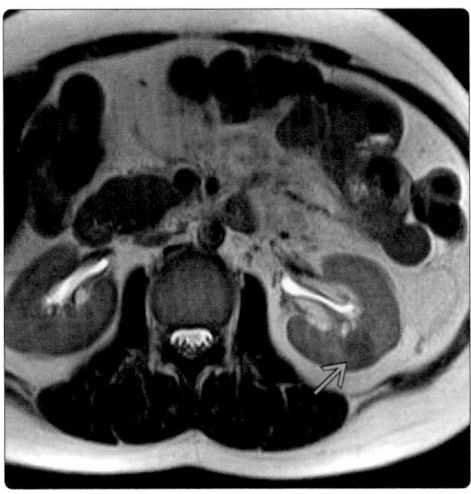

(Left) *Longitudinal US shows a hyperechoic nonshadowing mass ➡ in the left kidney. The mass is less echogenic than renal sinus fat ➡. This is a nonspecific appearance, but the most likely causes would be AML or RCC. Further imaging with CT or MR is needed.* **(Right)** *Axial non fat-suppressed T2 HASTE MR in the same patient shows that the lesion ➡ has low T2 signal. This was a fat-poor AML at partial nephrectomy.*

Upper Tract Urothelial Carcinoma

TERMINOLOGY

- Malignant tumor of transitional epithelium extending from calyces to ureteral orifices

IMAGING

- Hypovascular infiltrative tumor with minimal enhancement; lack of vascularity does not exclude TCC
- Typically causes hydronephrosis and calyceal dilatation
- Diffusely infiltrating renal mass with preservation of the renal contour
- CT/CTU superior to excretory urography or ultrasound
- MRU: Alternative to CTU in patients with iodinated contrast allergy

TOP DIFFERENTIAL DIAGNOSES

- Renal cell carcinoma (RCC)
- Blood clot or hemonephrosis
- Urothelial thickening

PATHOLOGY

- Renal pelvis: 8%, ureter: 2%
- Hallmark of TCC is multifocality and highest recurrence rate of any cancer

CLINICAL ISSUES

- Gross or microscopic hematuria (70-80%), flank pain (20-40%), lumbar mass (10-20%)
- Most common sites of recurrence for upper tract urothelial carcinoma (UTUC) include bladder (22-47%) and contralateral collecting system (2-6%)

DIAGNOSTIC CHECKLIST

- Important to define location of tumor (renal pelvis, mid ureter, distal ureter), extent of tumor (intraluminal vs. extraluminal), ± hydroureteronephrosis, ± invasion into contiguous organs
- Screen entire excretory system for synchronous tumors

(Left) Graphic shows a multifocal TCC involving the upper pole calyces and the proximal ureter. Hydronephrosis ± hydrocalyces are commonly associated with upper tract TCC. (Right) Longitudinal ultrasound of the left kidney shows dilated calyces ⇗ and cortical loss ⇥ secondary to a poorly defined hyperechoic mass in the renal pelvis ⇥. The patient had liver metastases from this upper tract urothelial cancer.

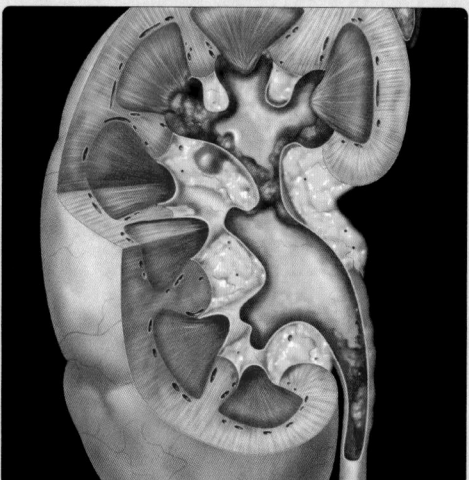
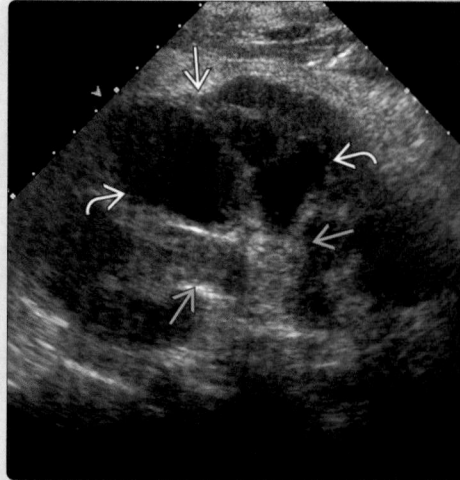

(Left) Longitudinal ultrasound shows the left kidney in a 45-year-old woman with liver failure from metastatic urothelial cancer. Lung and bone metastases were also present. The kidney is enlarged and hydronephrotic. A lobulated/papillary hyperechoic mass ⇥ extends from the renal pelvis into calyces. (Right) Longitudinal ultrasound of the right kidney shows lower pole hydronephrosis ⇥. The sinus fat in the upper 1/2 of the kidney is infiltrated by indistinct urothelial cancer ⇥.

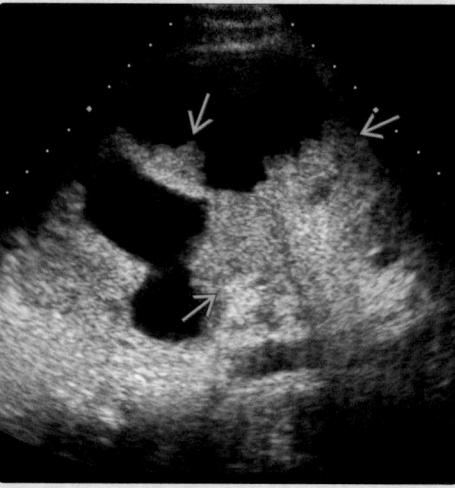
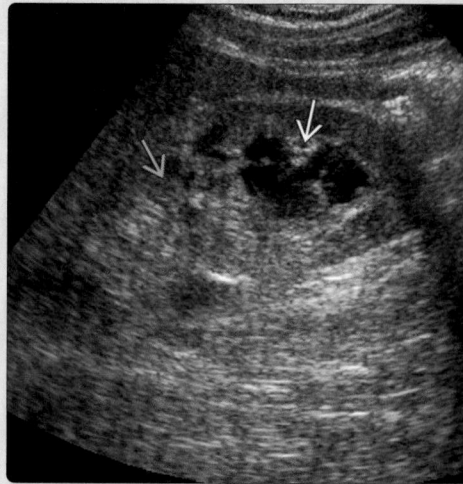

TERMINOLOGY

Abbreviations
Upper tract urothelial carcinoma (UTUC)

Synonyms
Upper tract transitional cell carcinoma (TCC)

Definitions
Malignant tumor of transitional epithelium extending from calyces to ureteral orifices

IMAGING

General Features
Best diagnostic clue
- Intraluminal mass or focal urothelial thickening in any part of collecting system
- Multicentric with synchronous tumors in upper urinary tract and bladder
- Diffusely infiltrating renal mass with preservation of renal contour

Location
- Renal pelvis 8%, ureter 2%, (90-95% of UC occurs in bladder)
- 2-4% of patients with bladder cancer develop UTUC; 40% of patients with UTUC develop bladder cancer

Ultrasonographic Findings
Grayscale ultrasound
- Less sensitive than CT for identifying or characterizing renal masses
- Soft tissue mass in echogenic renal sinus, which may be hyper-, iso- or hypoechoic to renal parenchyma
  - Markedly hyperechoic due to squamous metaplasia with formation of keratin pearls, non-shadowing
- Typically causes hydronephrosis and calyceal dilatation
  - Difficult to visualize if small and nonobstructing
- More aggressive tumors may infiltrate diffusely but preserve renal contour
  - May be indistinguishable from renal cell carcinoma (RCC), lymphoma, or metastases
- Focal hypoechogenicity of adjacent renal cortex reflects local invasion
- Contrast-enhanced US: Slow wash-in, fast wash-out and low enhancement degree typical
- Upper ureter
  - Focal urothelial thickening with secondary hydronephrosis

Color Doppler
- Most hypo- or avascular; lack of vascularity does not exclude TCC
- Detection of internal color flow excludes blood clot, fungus ball, pus, calculi

Pyelography
Intravenous pyelography superseded by CT urography (CTU)
Retrograde pyelography performed during cystoscopy and ureteroscopy
Renal pelvis
- Single or multiple discrete filling defects; surface is usually irregular, stippled, serrated or frond like
- Stipple sign: Contrast within interstices of tumor
- Oncocalyx: Ballooned tumor-filled calyx
- Phantom calyx: Unopacified calyx from obstruction of calyceal infundibulum
- Ureter
  - Smooth or irregular, eccentric or circumferential stricture, non-tapering margins, filling defects
  - Champagne glass/goblet sign: Dilatation distal to luminal tumor caused by slow growing tumor expanding ureteral lumen

CT Findings
- CECT
  - Hypovascular infiltrative tumor with minimal enhancement; preserved renal shape
  - Sessile, flat, or polypoid solid mass ± hydronephrosis ± calcification
  - Invasion of renal sinus fat and parenchyma
  - Fine encrusted calcifications that may be mistaken for renal calculi
- CT urography
  - Superior to excretory urography or ultrasound
  - Eccentric or circumferential wall thickening or mass of renal pelvis or ureter
  - Focal filling defects ± hydronephrosis
  - Crust-like rims: Contrast in curvilinear calyceal spaces around periphery of tumor

MR Findings
- Alternative to CTU in patients with iodinated contrast allergy
- Combination of T2-weighted and contrast-enhanced sequences for optimum sensitivity
- Isointense to the renal parenchyma on T1- and T2WI
- Enhancing lesion with similar morphology as described for CT
- Diffusion-weighted sequences may add value when contrast cannot be used

Imaging Recommendations
- Best imaging tool
  - Upper tract tumors detected primarily using CTU
  - CT preferred for staging or follow up, although MR/U is viable alternative
  - Chest imaging important for staging and follow up as lung most common site of visceral metastases
- Protocol advice
  - Vigilant monitoring for metachronous lesions and local recurrence for UTUC

DIFFERENTIAL DIAGNOSIS

Renal Cell Carcinoma (RCC)
- Usually hypervascular and more heterogeneous (solid/cystic/calcified); vascular invasion more typical
- Difficult to distinguish infiltrative RCC from TCC
- However, RCC is more exophytic and has mass effect with contour distortion

Blood Clot or Hemonephrosis
- Same echogenicity as tumor but mobile, avascular, and resolves over time

Urothelial Thickening

- Occurs in renal transplant rejection, urinary tract infection, reflux, chronic obstruction, other malignancies

Pyonephrosis

- Echogenic debris within dilated calyces, signs of infection

Fungus Ball

- Echogenic, avascular, poorly shadowing masses

Sloughed Papilla

- Filling defects in calyces
- Destruction of apex of pyramid → irregular cavitation and sinus formation between papilla and calyx

Lymphoma

- May also invade renal sinus; usually disseminated disease

Calculus

- Echogenic with posterior shadowing

Other Benign Lesions of Urinary Tract

- Endometriosis, malakoplakia, tuberculosis, fibroepithelial polyp, xanthogranulomatous pyelonephritis

PATHOLOGY

General Features

- Etiology
  o Risk factors: Tobacco use, aromatic amines, arsenic ingestion, Balkan nephropathy, phenacetin abuse, Chinese herbs, cyclophosphamide treatment, recurrent infections, and stones
- Genetics
  o Linked to hereditary nonpolyposis colorectal carcinoma (Lynch syndrome) and some genetic polymorphisms

Staging, Grading, & Classification

- Ta: Noninvasive papillary carcinoma, tis: Carcinoma in situ
- T1: Tumor invades lamina propria
- T2: Tumor invades muscularis
- T3: Renal pelvis: Tumor invades beyond the muscularis into peripelvic fat or renal parenchyma
  o Ureter: Tumor invades beyond muscularis into periureteric fat
- T4: Tumor invades adjacent organs, pelvic or abdominal wall, or through the kidney into perinephric fat
- N0: None; N1: Single node < 2 cm; N2: Single node 2-5 cm or to multiple nodes > 5 cm; N3: Node > 5 cm
- M0: No distant metastasis; M1: Distant metastases

Gross Pathologic & Surgical Features

- Hallmark of TCC is multifocality and highest recurrence rate of any cancer
- Spectrum ranging from noninvasive papillary tumors (papillary urothelial tumors of low-malignant potential, low-grade papillary UC, high-grade papillary UC) through flat lesions (carcinoma in situ [CIS]) to invasive carcinomas
- 60% of UTUC are invasive at diagnosis compared with only 15-25% of bladder tumors
- Spread by direct invasion and lymphatic route

Microscopic Features

- 3 grades: Papillary urothelial neoplasm of low malignant potential, low grade, and high grade; most are high grade

Urine Cytology

- Less sensitive than for bladder UC

CLINICAL ISSUES

Presentation

- Most common signs/symptoms
  o Gross or microscopic hematuria (70-80%), flank pain (20-40%), lumbar mass (10-20%)

Demographics

- Age
  o Peak incidence: 70-80 years (M:F = 3:1)
- Epidemiology
  o TCC accounts for 90% of all urothelial tumors but only 10% of all renal tumors

Natural History & Prognosis

- Most common sites of recurrence for UTUC include bladder (22-47%) and contralateral collecting system (2-6%)
- 5-year survival depends on tumor location: Renal pelvis: 83%, ureter: 72%

Treatment

- Radical nephroureterectomy with bladder cuff excision ± intravesical chemotherapy
- Metastases: chemotherapy ± radiation
- Endoscopic ablation in highly selected low-grade cases

DIAGNOSTIC CHECKLIST

Consider

- Multifocality of UC in upper and lower urinary tract

Image Interpretation Pearls

- Important to define location of tumor (renal pelvis, mid ureter, distal ureter), extent of the tumor (intraluminal vs. extraluminal), ± hydroureteronephrosis, ± invasion into contiguous organs
- Screen entire excretory system for synchronous tumors
- Imaging follow-up for metachronous tumors

SELECTED REFERENCES

1. Gayer G et al: The renal sinus–transitional cell carcinoma and its mimickers on computed tomography. Semin Ultrasound CT MR. 35(3):308-19, 2014
2. Rouprêt M et al: European guidelines on upper tract urothelial carcinomas: 2013 update. Eur Urol. 63(6):1059-71, 2013
3. Xue LY et al: Evaluation of renal urothelial carcinoma by contrast-enhanced ultrasonography. Eur J Radiol. 82(4):e151-7, 2013
4. Lee EK et al: Imaging of urothelial cancers: what the urologist needs to know. AJR Am J Roentgenol. 196(6):1249-54, 2011
5. Vikram R et al: Imaging and staging of transitional cell carcinoma: part 2, upper urinary tract. AJR Am J Roentgenol. 192(6):1488-93, 2009
6. Park S et al: The impact of tumor location on prognosis of transitional cell carcinoma of the upper urinary tract. J Urol. 171(2 Pt 1):621-5, 2004

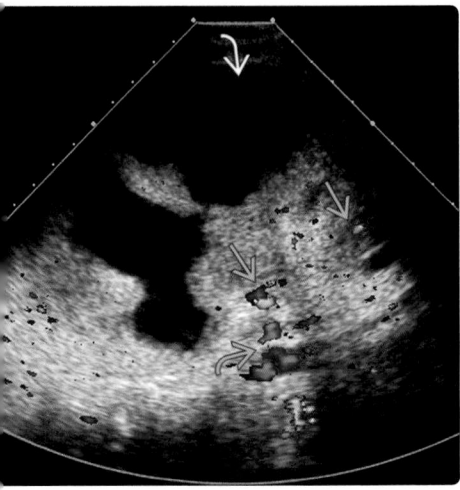

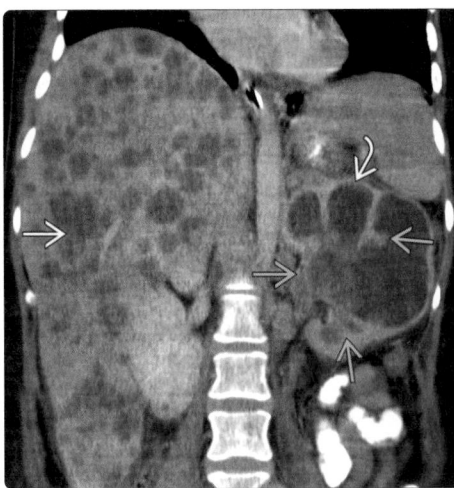

(Left) *Color Doppler ultrasound of metastatic urothelial cancer shows vascular flow in the mass ➡, confirming that this is a tumor. Note the severe hydronephrosis ⇗ and renal vascular pedicle ➡.* (Right) *Coronal delayed phase CECT shows metastatic urothelial cancer of the left renal pelvis. The pelvic mass extends into the calyces ➡. There is severe hydronephrosis and cortical thinning ⇗ as well as hepatomegaly and liver metastases ➡.*

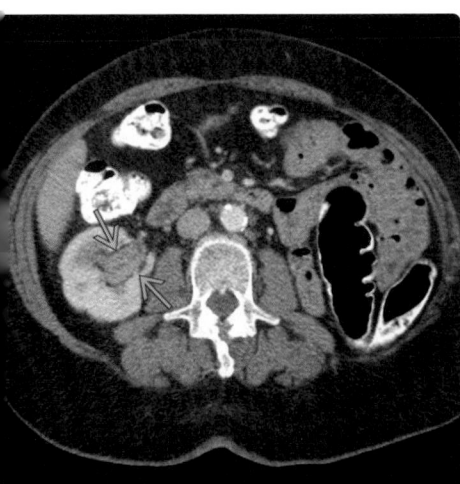

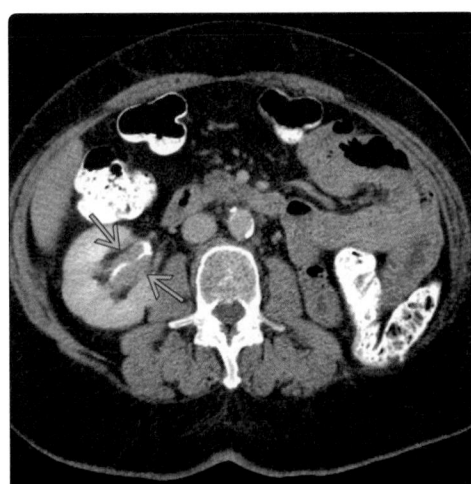

(Left) *Axial CECT in the portal venous phase shows circumferential wall thickening of the right renal pelvis ➡, representing urothelial carcinoma. Note the left nephrectomy for urothelial carcinoma.* (Right) *Axial CT urogram in the same patient differentiates the contrast-filled lumen from the tumor in the wall of the renal pelvis ➡. There was no invasion of renal parenchyma.*

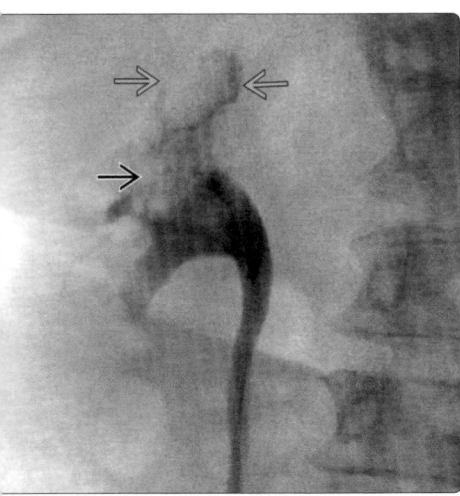

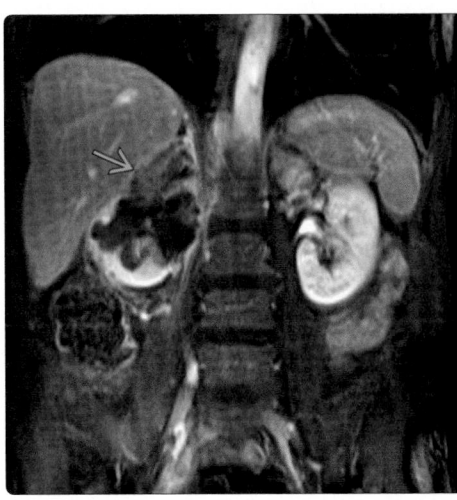

(Left) *Retrograde pyelogram of UTUC shows a dilated upper pole calyx with a filling defect from the tumor oncocalyx ➡. There is a tumor extending into the renal pelvis, with stippling of contrast in the interstices ➡.* (Right) *Coronal delayed phase T1 C+ MR shows infiltrating urothelial carcinoma. The renal shape and contour are preserved. The tumor ➡ is hypoenhancing.*

TERMINOLOGY

- Primary: Involvement of kidneys without evidence of other organ or nodal involvement; extremely rare: <1%
- Secondary: Dissemination of extrarenal lymphoma; more common

IMAGING

- Multiple hypoenhancing/hypoechoic masses, may see posterior acoustic enhancement
- Direct extension from retroperitoneal adenopathy, associated hydronephrosis
- Solitary hypoenhancing/hypoechoic mass
- Bilateral renal enlargement
- Perinephric disease
- Vascular invasion rare
- Image-guided biopsy important to differentiate from other solid renal masses and determine medical or surgical management

TOP DIFFERENTIAL DIAGNOSES

- Renal cell carcinoma
- Transitional cell carcinoma
- Metastases

PATHOLOGY

- Usually non-Hodgkin lymphoma, typically B-cell or Burkitt type; involvement by Hodgkin disease very rare

CLINICAL ISSUES

- Majority are asymptomatic and renal function unaffected
- Identification of extrarenal nodal and extranodal disease is key to diagnosis

DIAGNOSTIC CHECKLIST

- Consider clinical history, presence of another malignancy, extent of disease

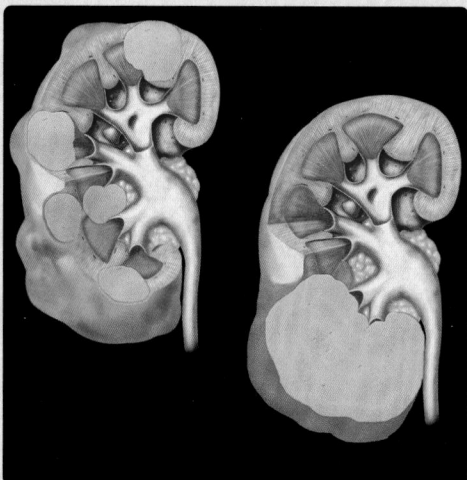

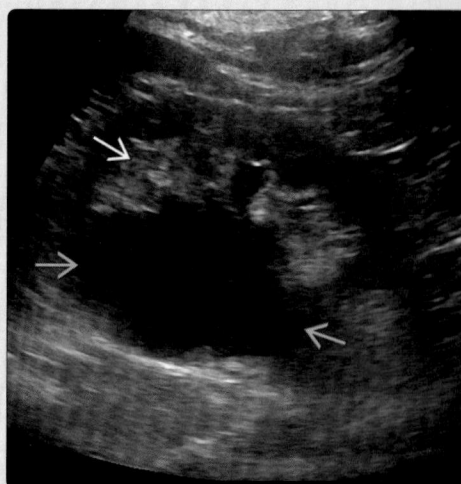

(Left) Graphic shows different manifestations of renal lymphoma. Multiple masses are depicted in variable locations in renal parenchyma (left), whereas a solitary mass replaces a lobar segment (right). (Right) US shows a markedly hypoechoic mass ⇨ medial to the left kidney. The mass infiltrates the sinus fat ⇨. It could be misinterpreted as being cystic, but there are internal echoes. Color Doppler should be used to find internal vascularity.

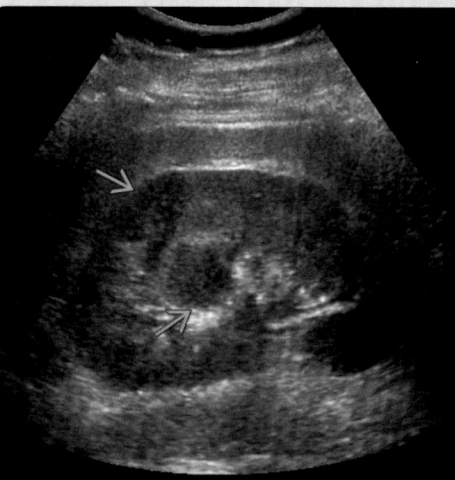

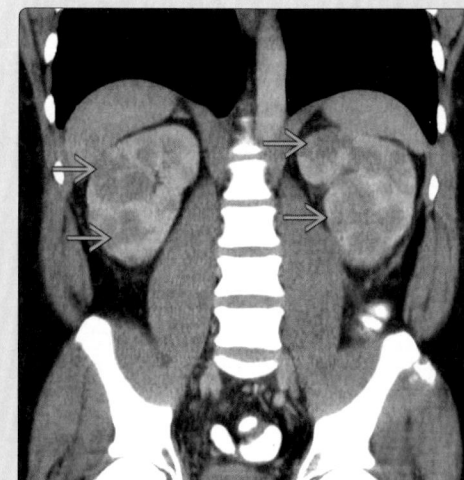

(Left) Longitudinal US shows an enlarged right kidney with loss of normal morphology. There are multiple ill-defined solid hypoechoic masses ⇨ secondary to Burkitt lymphoma. (Right) Portal phase CECT in the coronal plane of the same patient with Burkitt lymphoma shows multiple hypodense deposits of lymphoma in both kidneys ⇨. The masses are distributed in the cortex and medulla.

TERMINOLOGY

Abbreviations

Primary renal lymphoma (PRL); secondary renal lymphoma (SRL)

Definitions

Lymphoma: Malignant tumor of lymphocytes
Primary: Involvement of kidneys without evidence of other organ or nodal involvement
o Extremely rare; < 1% of extranodal lymphoma
Secondary: Dissemination of extrarenal lymphoma by hematogenous spread (90%) or direct extension via retroperitoneal lymphatic channels
o Non-Hodgkin lymphoma >> Hodgkin disease

IMAGING

General Features

Morphology
o Multiple hypoenhancing/hypoechoic masses (50-60%)
o Direct extension from retroperitoneal adenopathy (25-30%), associated hydronephrosis
o Solitary hypoenhancing/hypoechoic mass (10-25%)
o Bilateral renal enlargement (nephromegaly) (20%)
  – More common in Burkitt lymphoma
o Perinephric disease (< 10%); rind of homogeneous perinephric soft tissue
  – May be limited to thickening of Gerota fascia or plaques and nodules in perirenal space
o Renal sinus predominant: Uncommon, no vascular invasion, milder hydronephrosis

Ultrasonographic Findings

Grayscale ultrasound
o Typically hypoechoic and homogeneous mass
o Homogeneity of lymphoma results in few tissue interfaces to insonating beam; there may even be posterior acoustic enhancement
o Solitary or multiple masses
  – Small lesions may be confused with medullary pyramids, renal cysts, or abscesses
o Direct invasion: Hypoechoic mass extending from retroperitoneum or perirenal space into renal parenchyma or sinus
o Nephromegaly: Globular enlargement with heterogeneous echotexture and loss of normal echogenic appearance of renal sinus fat
  – Diffuse uniform increase in echogenicity may simulate renal parenchymal disease
o Perirenal lymphoma: Hypoechoic soft tissue of variable thickness surrounding kidney
Color Doppler
o Displacement of normal renal cortical vessels with little vascularity within lesions
o Soft tissue surrounding renal hilar vessels or vena cava without significant compromise

CT Findings

Mildly hyperdense to normal kidney on unenhanced CT
Hypovascular mass, unlike clear cell renal cell carcinoma (RCC)

o Note hypovascular subtypes of RCC, such as papillary and chromophobe
• Despite large infiltrative retroperitoneal and perinephric space masses, vena cava and renal vein are rarely invaded, unlike RCC
• Nephromegaly with diffuse infiltration and heterogeneous enhancement
• Difficult to differentiate from transitional cell carcinoma (TCC) when epicenter of disease is in renal sinus
• Splenomegaly or lymphadenopathy at other sites in SRL
• Extranodal involvement of gastrointestinal tract, brain, liver, and bone marrow
• Calcification and cystic change are rare

MR Findings

• Low to intermediate signal on both T1 and T2
• Heterogeneous high signal may be seen on T2WI
• May show restricted diffusion
• T1 C+: Heterogenous enhancement, less than that of cortex
• Ideal for detecting synchronous osseous disease

Image-Guided Biopsy

• Important role to differentiate from other solid renal masses and determine medical or surgical management
• US is ideal for guidance, but CT may be needed for deeper lesions or lesions not visible on US
• Fine-needle aspiration supplemented by core biopsies: High sensitivity and specificity
  o Immunochemistry, flow cytometry, and histopathology drive specific therapies
• Renal mass biopsy not necessary in widespread lymphoma unless renal mass is atypical or patient has 2nd malignancy

Nuclear Medicine Findings

• PET/CT
  o Important role in evaluation of both nodal and extranodal lymphoma
  o Used for initial staging, evaluation of treatment response, and detection of recurrence in some subtypes of lymphoma
  o More sensitive than conventional anatomic imaging
  o 18F-FDG uptake much higher on average in renal lymphoma (SUV mean 6.37) compared to RCC (SUV mean 2.58)

Imaging Recommendations

• Best imaging tool
  o CECT is modality of choice for initial diagnosis and staging of renal lymphoma
    – Combined with 18F-FDG PET for initial staging, assessment of response and detection of recurrence
  o MR is alternative in patients with impaired renal function; avoids radiation exposure

DIFFERENTIAL DIAGNOSIS

Renal Cell Carcinoma

• Round or oval cortical solid or cystic mass ± central necrosis
• Typically hypervascular, however, some subtypes are hypovascular
• Propensity to vascular invasion

Transitional Cell Carcinoma

- Centered in collecting system; may be infiltrative and extend into renal cortex; more likely to cause collecting system obstruction

Metastases

- Lung, breast, gastric cancer, and melanoma

Other Malignant Lymphoproliferative Diseases

- Myeloma: Diffuse infiltration, solitary or multiple masses
- Leukemia: Enlarged kidney from diffuse infiltration

Renal Infection

- Pyelonephritis, renal abscess, septic emboli
- May present as single or multiple lesions; differentiated by clinical history and urinalysis

Perirenal Hematoma, Extramedullary Hematopoiesis, Retroperitoneal Sarcoma

- May simulate perirenal lymphoma

PATHOLOGY

General Features

- GU system commonly affected by extranodal spread of lymphoma; kidney is most commonly involved
- Usually non-Hodgkin lymphoma, typically B-cell or Burkitt type; involvement by Hodgkin disease very rare
- Renal tissue is devoid of lymphoid tissue; lymphatics within renal capsule, perinephric fat, or lymphocytes in areas of chronic inflammation may account for renal involvement
- Modes of renal spread include hematogenous and direct contiguous extension

Gross Pathologic & Surgical Features

- Enlarged kidney ± distortion of renal contour
- Expansion of fat caused by homogeneous yellowish tumor infiltration

CLINICAL ISSUES

Presentation

- Most common signs/symptoms
  - Majority are asymptomatic and renal function unaffected
  - Rarely present with acute renal failure; rapid improvement in renal function post treatment
  - Hematuria, flank pain, palpable mass, or renal insufficiency
- Other signs/symptoms
  - Fever, weight loss, ↑ serum lactate dehydrogenase, lymphopenia

Demographics

- Age
  - Any (middle-aged to elderly more common)
- Gender
  - Prevalence equal in both sexes
- Epidemiology
  - SRL: 30-60% silent renal disease in case of widespread lymphoma based on autopsy series; imaging manifestation occurs only in 1-8%

- PRL: More common in middle-aged men; may present with renal failure in absence of other causes of renal impairment
- Predisposing factors
  - Immunocompromised (post organ transplantation, HIV), prior treatment for malignancy, autoimmune disorders, viruses such as Epstein-Barr virus

Natural History & Prognosis

- Complications
  - Renal or perinephric hemorrhage, renal obstruction, renovascular hypertension, acute renal failure
- Prognosis
  - Good prognosis with early diagnosis and chemotherapy
  - Tumor size > 10 cm, involvement of renal hilum and diffuse infiltration associated with poorer prognosis
  - Involvement of kidneys at time of initial presentation of B-cell lymphoma may be associated with high incidence of CNS relapse; diagnosis may alter treatment regimen

Treatment

- Chemotherapy ± radiation therapy

DIAGNOSTIC CHECKLIST

Consider

- Clinical history, any other malignancy, extent of disease
- Overlapping features of renal metastases, renal lymphoma and primary renal carcinoma
- Ultrasound-guided renal biopsy for definitive diagnosis

Image Interpretation Pearls

- Always look for evidence of multisystem involvement in liver, lung, CNS, bone marrow and gastrointestinal tract

SELECTED REFERENCES

1. Ganeshan D et al: Imaging of primary and secondary renal lymphoma. AJR Am J Roentgenol. 201(5):W712-9, 2013
2. Kostakoglu L et al: State-of-the-Art Research on "Lymphomas: Role of Molecular Imaging for Staging, Prognostic Evaluation, and Treatment Response". Front Oncol. 3:212, 2013
3. Bach AG et al: Prevalence and patterns of renal involvement in imaging of malignant lymphoproliferative diseases. Acta Radiol. 53(3):343-8, 2012
4. Ye XH et al: 18F-FDG PET/CT evaluation of lymphoma with renal involvement: comparison with renal carcinoma. South Med J. 103(7):642-9, 2010
5. El-Sharkawy MS et al: Renal involvement in lymphoma: prevalence and various patterns of involvement on abdominal CT. Int Urol Nephrol. 39(3):929-33, 2007
6. Sheth S et al: Imaging of renal lymphoma: patterns of disease with pathologic correlation. Radiographics. 26(4):1151-68, 2006

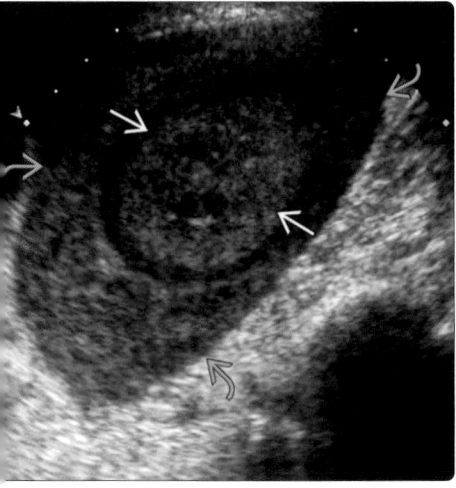
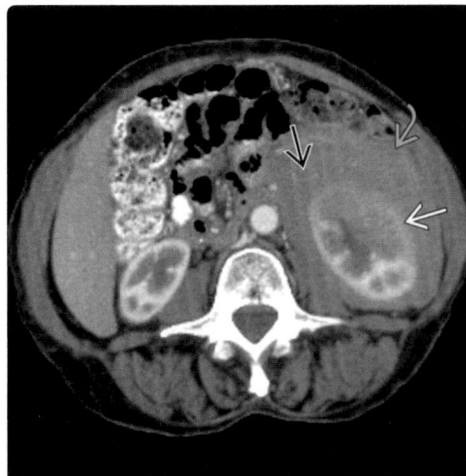

(Left) *Longitudinal ultrasound shows the left kidney* ➡ *surrounded by a thick perirenal rind of tumor* ⬈. *Percutaneous biopsy showed B-cell lymphoma.* (Right) *CECT of the same patient with B-cell lymphoma shows the perirenal lymphoma* ⬈ *infiltrating the kidney* ➡. *There are patent arteries* ➡ *within the perirenal mass, which helps distinguish solid tumor from perirenal hemorrhage.*

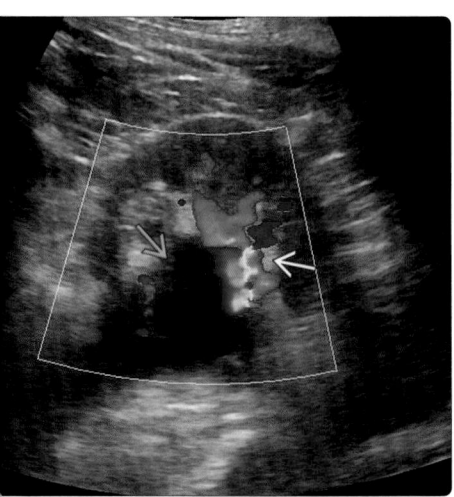
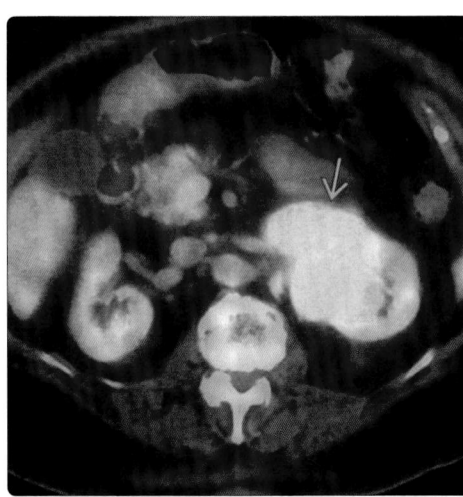

(Left) *Transverse color Doppler US shows renal hilar follicular lymphoma* ⬈. *The mass is hypovascular and displaces hilar vessels* ➡. (Right) *Axial fused FDG PET/CT shows follicular lymphoma. There is avid FDG uptake (SUV = 22) in the mass at the left renal hilum* ⬈. *Pathologic nodes were also present in the pelvis and mesentery (not shown).*

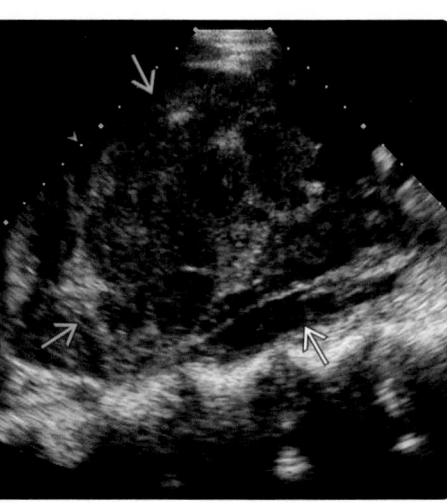
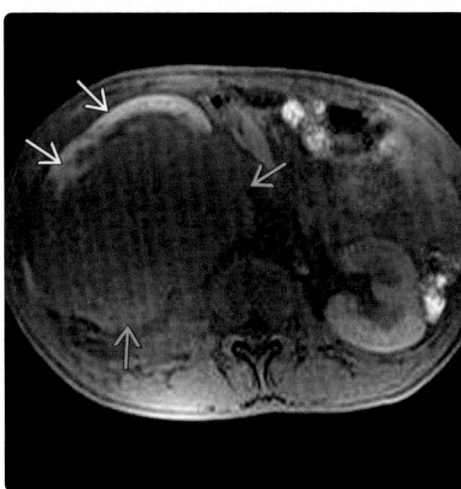

(Left) *Longitudinal US of the right renal fossa in patient with HIV infection shows a heterogenous solid mass* ⬈, *which was large B-cell lymphoma on biopsy. No normal kidney is seen. The psoas muscle is preserved* ➡. (Right) *Axial T1 FS MR of the same patient with large B-cell lymphoma shows a rim of preserved renal tissue* ➡ *anterior to the large mass* ⬈. *The patient could not receive intravenous contrast because of poor renal function.*

Renal Artery Stenosis

TERMINOLOGY

- Hemodynamically significant narrowing of renal arterial lumen

IMAGING

- Poststenotic "jet" and turbulent flow on color Doppler US
  - Abnormally high peak systolic velocity with angle-corrected spectral Doppler in main renal artery immediately distal to stenosis
  - Peak systolic velocity in and immediately distal to stenosis ≥ 180-200 cm/sec
  - Accurate Doppler angle ≤ 60° essential for velocity measurements
- Diminished downstream systolic peaks
  - Abnormally low peak systolic velocity in arcuate arteries with diminished resistive indices (RI)
  - Tardus et parvus waveform shape, late and small systolic peaks

  - Low resistive index < 0.5 (compare with other kidney) due to dampened systolic peaks and normal diastolic flow
  - Prolonged acceleration time (time to peak systole) > 0.07 seconds
  - Acceleration index (AI) < 3 m/s²

PATHOLOGY

- Atherosclerosis
  - Ostium or proximal 2 cm of renal artery
- Fibromuscular dysplasia
  - Most common mid or distal main renal artery
- Aortic dissection
- Aortic aneurysm (renal artery compression)
- Thromboembolism
- Other vasculitides
- Retroperitoneal fibrosis
- Trauma with renal artery dissection

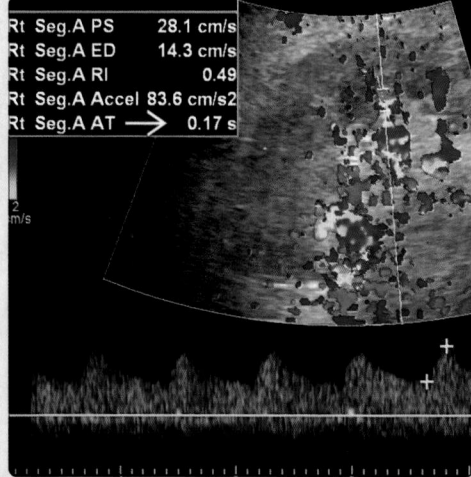
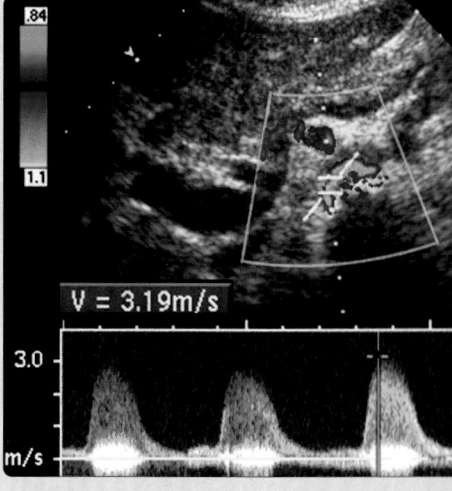

(Left) *Renal artery stenosis and parvus tardus due to aortic dissection are shown. Note the prolonged acceleration time* ➡. (Right) *Spectral Doppler ultrasound in another patient shows a peak systolic velocity of 319 cm/sec at location of aliasing, consistent with high grade stenosis. The renal:aortic ratio was 4.0.*

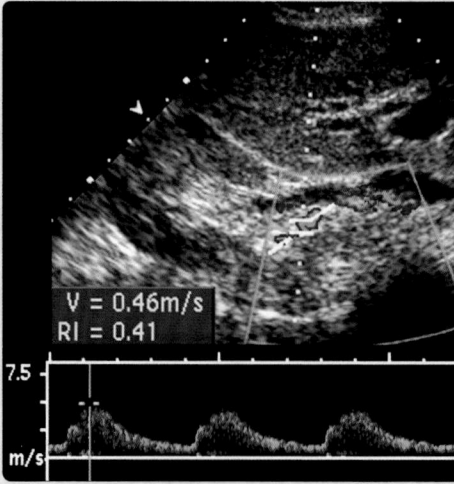
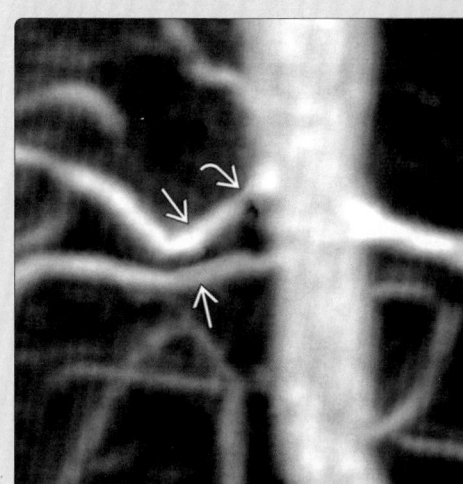

(Left) *Transverse spectral Doppler ultrasound in the same patient illustrates diminished systolic peaks and resistive indices (RI) < 0.5 distal to the right renal artery stenosis.* (Right) *Oblique maximum intensity projection from MRA shows duplicated right renal arteries* ➡, *with the more superior exhibiting a significant stenosis* ➡. *It is easy to envision why renal artery duplication is often missed with US and complicates assessment of intrarenal flow dynamics.*

TERMINOLOGY

Abbreviations
- Renal artery stenosis (RAS)

Definitions
- Hemodynamically significant narrowing of renal arterial lumen

IMAGING

General Features
- Best diagnostic clue
  - Poststenotic "jet" and turbulent flow on color Doppler US
    - Abnormally high peak systolic velocity with angle-corrected spectral Doppler in main renal artery immediately distal to stenosis
  - Diminished downstream systolic peaks
    - Abnormally low peak systolic velocity in distal main and arcuate arteries with diminished resistive indices (RI)
- Location
  - Ostium/intramural: Primary aortic disease
  - Atherosclerosis: Within 2 cm of ostium
  - Fibromuscular dysplasia (FMD): Distal renal artery (RA), hilar branches

Ultrasonographic Findings
- Grayscale ultrasound
  - Asymmetric kidneys (unilateral length < 8 cm or difference > 2 cm)
  - Diffusely increased parenchymal echogenicity (limited to chronic, severe ischemia)
  - Occasional string of beads appearance of arterial wall in FMD (requires excellent visualization)
- Pulsed Doppler
  - Normal renal artery peak systolic velocity 75-125 cm/sec
  - Doppler criteria ≥ 50-60% diameter stenosis
    - Peak systolic velocity in and immediately distal to stenosis ≥ 180-200 cm/sec
    - Renal/aortic ratio > 3.5 (peak systole in RAS/peak systole in aorta at level of renal arteries)
    - Poststenotic Doppler spectral broadening
  - Intrarenal Doppler waveform signs of significant RAS
    - These downstream effects are very different from the poststenotic high velocity jet
    - Tardus et parvus waveform shape, late and small systolic peaks
      - Prolonged acceleration time (time to peak systole) > 0.07 seconds
      - Low resistive index < 0.5 (compare with other kidney) due to dampened systolic peaks and normal diastolic flow
      - Acceleration index (AI) < 3 m/s²
    - Cannot accurately diagnose RAS **solely** by intrarenal arterial waveform analysis
  - Doppler angle ≤ 60° essential to measure velocity
- Color Doppler
  - Color shift/color aliasing in renal artery at site of stenosis: High velocity flow

  - Poststenotic turbulence, possibly with soft tissue reverberation

Angiographic Findings
- Contrast enhanced MRA, CTA, or DSA
  - Atherosclerotic lesions: Focal eccentric/concentric stenosis
  - Fibromuscular dysplasia: Most commonly serial ridges or string of beads pattern, may have associated aneurysms
  - Focal dephasing on phase contrast MR analogous to aliasing in poststenotic jet

Imaging Recommendations
- Best imaging tool
  - Imaging goal: Accurately diagnose ≥ 50-60% diameter renal artery stenosis
  - Ultrasound may be used for screening, followed by contrast-enhanced MRA or CTA
  - DSA may be needed for accurate FMD diagnosis in distal RA, hilar branches due to higher spatial resolution
  - Duplex ultrasound problems
    - Technically difficult/high exam failure rate
    - Failure to recognize duplicate RAs and collaterals, which will alter arcuate artery waveforms
    - Inadequate visualization for distal/hilar RAS
    - Wide reported accuracy range; best results for proximal (atherosclerosis-related) RAS
- Protocol advice
  - **Imaging for RAS (regardless of modality) is indicated only after appropriate clinical screening**

DIFFERENTIAL DIAGNOSIS

Primary Hypertension
- Renal arteries normal

Chronic Parenchymal Renal Disease Unrelated to Renal Artery Stenosis
- Parenchymal hyperechogenicity and atrophy from interstitial fibrosis
- Elevated resistive index (> 0.7) interlobar/arcuate arteries
- Usually bilateral unless there is a local insult such as infection, trauma, radiation, etc.

Aortic Dissection
- Possible ostial/intramural obstruction, may be dynamic
- Dissection flap may extend into RA
- US findings: Dissection plane/2 lumens seen on color Doppler US

Renal Artery Occlusion
- Etiology
  - Subsequent to RAS
  - Embolic
  - Primary aortic disease
- US findings
  - Absent RA on color Doppler US
  - Absent or very diminished arterial signals in kidney if acute
  - Intrarenal Doppler signals may be normal if chronic (collateralized)
  - Renal atrophy if chronic

PATHOLOGY

General Features

- Etiology
  - Atherosclerosis
    - Ostium (aortic plaque) or proximal 2 cm of renal artery
    - RAS bilateral in 30-40% of atherosclerosis cases
  - FMD
    - Medial fibroplasia 70-80% FMD; intimal hyperplasia: 10-15%; subadventitial fibroplasia 10-15%
    - Most common mid or distal main renal artery ± hilar branches
    - Right RA > left; bilateral 2/3 of cases
  - Aortic dissection
  - Aortic aneurysm (renal artery compression)
  - Thromboembolism (more likely leads to occlusion than renal artery stenosis)
  - Other vasculitides (e.g., Takayasu, polyarteritis nodosa, congenital intimal fibroplasia)
  - Retroperitoneal fibrosis
  - Trauma with renal artery dissection

Staging, Grading, & Classification

- Hemodynamically significant arterial stenosis: Pressure/flow reducing lesion
- Hemodynamically significant RAS: ≥ 50-60% diameter reduction

Gross Pathologic & Surgical Features

- Atherosclerosis
  - Eccentric or circumferential plaque in proximal RA
  - Possible turbulence-related poststenotic dilatation
- Medial fibroplasia FMD
  - String of beads appearance
- Renal parenchymal atrophy (renal length ≤ 8 cm) moderate/severe RAS

Microscopic Features

- Atherosclerotic plaque: Subintimal fibrofatty plaque, possibly calcified
- Medial fibroplasia FMD: Fibrous ridges with intervening media thinning/aneurysmal dilatation

CLINICAL ISSUES

Presentation

- Most common signs/symptoms
  - No signs or symptoms specific for RA hypertension
  - Clinical scenarios suggesting RA hypertension and **justifying RA imaging**
    - Hypertension in child or young adult
    - Hypertension uncontrolled with 3 or more drugs
    - Previously controlled hypertension newly uncontrollable
    - Rapidly worsening (malignant) hypertension
    - Hypertension with deteriorating renal function
- Other signs/symptoms
  - Unilateral small kidney

Demographics

- Age
  - Atherosclerosis: > age 50 years
  - FMD: Usually young adulthood
- Gender
  - Atherosclerosis: Male predominance
  - FMD: Female predominance
- Epidemiology
  - RAS most common cause of secondary hypertension (1-4% of all HTN)
    - Called "renovascular hypertension"
  - Atherosclerosis
    - Most common cause of RAS (60-90% of cases)
  - FMD
    - 2nd most common cause of RAS overall (10-30% cases)
    - Most common cause of renovascular hypertension in children and young adults

Natural History & Prognosis

- Atherosclerosis: Poor prognosis after RAS angioplasty/surgery
  - Mixed results for hypertension control, poor results for arresting decline in renal function
    - Debate continues about role of stents vs. angioplasty
  - Impossible to predict who is likely to respond, visually successful treatment not always associated with clinical improvement
- FMD: Good prognosis after RAS angioplasty
  - Hypertension improved or medically controllable
  - Recurrent stenosis possible

Treatment

- Angiotensin converting enzyme (ACE) inhibitors
- Transluminal angioplasty: 80% RAS correction rate for nonostial lesions; 25-30% ostial
- Surgical revascularization: 80-90% success rate (bypass stenosis)

DIAGNOSTIC CHECKLIST

Consider

- RAS/RA occlusion with unilateral small kidney

Image Interpretation Pearls

- Atherosclerotic RAS: Proximal 2 cm of RA
- FMD-RAS: Mid or distal RA ± intrarenal branches and string of beads appearance

SELECTED REFERENCES

1. Albert TS et al: An international multicenter comparison of time-SLIP unenhanced MR angiography and contrast-enhanced CT angiography for assessing renal artery stenosis: the renal artery contrast-free trial. AJR Am J Roentgenol. 204(1):182-8, 2015
2. Chrysant GS et al: Proper patient selection yields significant and sustained reduction in systolic blood pressure following renal artery stenting in patients with uncontrolled hypertension: long-term results from the HERCULES trial. J Clin Hypertens (Greenwich). 16(7):497-503, 2014
3. Voiculescu A et al: Duplex ultrasound findings before and after surgery in children and adolescents with renovascular hypertension. Ultrasound Med Biol. 40(12):2786-93, 2014
4. Granata A et al: Doppler ultrasound and renal artery stenosis: An overview. Ultrasound. 12(4):133-43, 2009

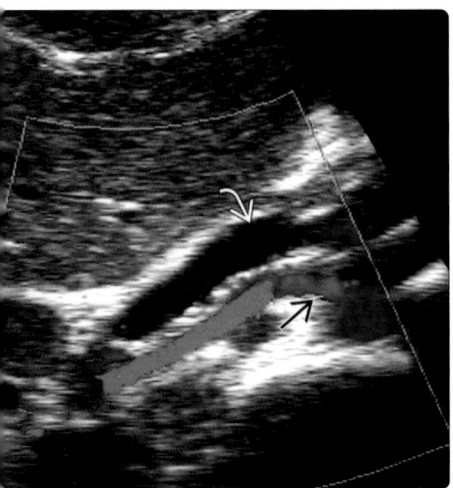

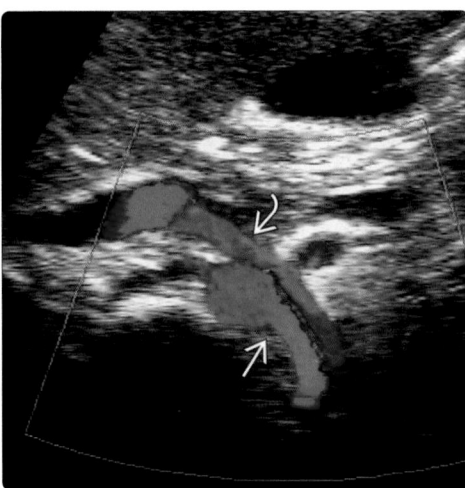

(Left) *Oblique color Doppler ultrasound shows a normal right renal artery, which consistently arises from the anterolateral aspect of the aorta ➡ and travels posterior to the IVC and left renal vein ⬈.* (Right) *Oblique color Doppler ultrasound shows the origin of the left renal artery ➡, which varies from anterolateral to posterolateral, but always lies posterior to the left renal vein ⬈.*

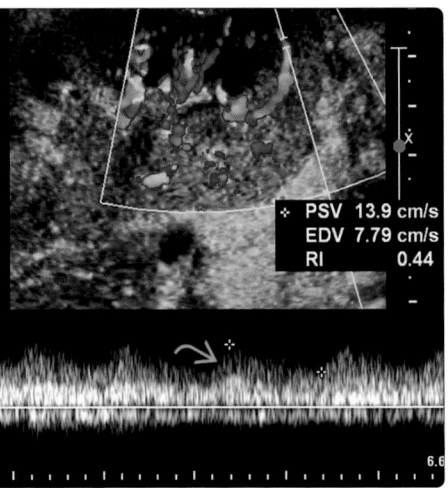

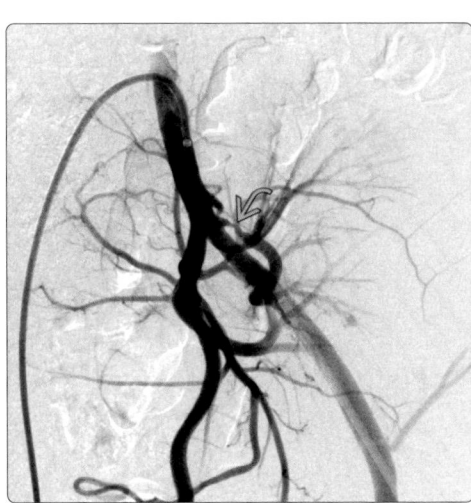

(Left) *Spectral Doppler ultrasound of a downstream (arcuate) artery demonstrates a slow upstroke ➡ and RI < 0.5 in a transplant kidney with renal artery stenosis.* (Right) *Left common iliac artery injection shows a high-grade stenosis of the transplant renal artery ➡, which arises from the external iliac. This was angioplastied, with some improvement in transplant function.*

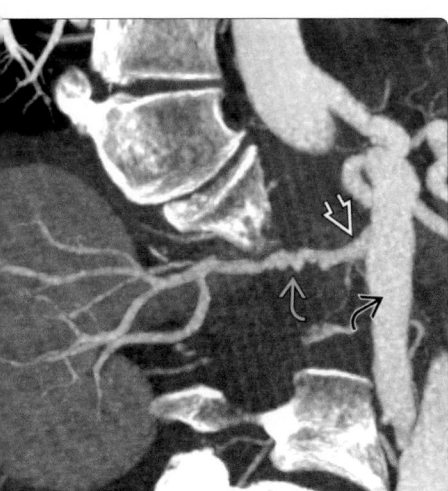

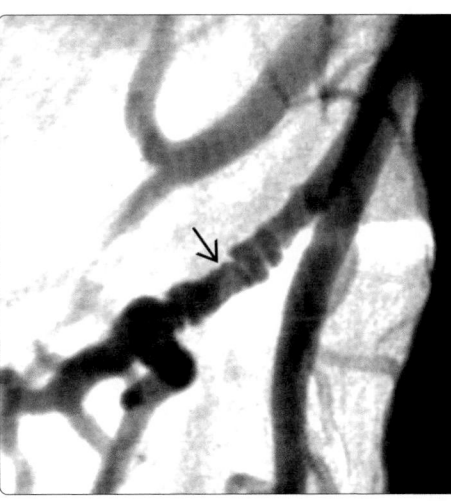

(Left) *Coronal MIP in a 30-year-old woman with fibromuscular dysplasia shows an irregular corrugated or beaded appearance of the mid right renal artery ➡, with relative sparing of the ostium and proximal portion of artery ⬈. This patient's aneurysmal SMA is also seen in the image ➡.* (Right) *In another patient with FMD, oblique DSA shows a series of ridges in the distal right renal artery ➡. This is a middle-aged woman with poorly controlled hypertension. FMD is more common on the right, but is often bilateral.*

TERMINOLOGY

- Clot formation in renal vein

IMAGING

- Unilateral > bilateral
- Kidney enlarged acutely in 75% cases
- Renal vein dilated acutely
- Possible inferior vena cava (IVC) thrombus extension
- **Altered renal artery spectral waveforms**
  - ↑ systolic pulsatility (narrow, sharp systolic peaks)
  - Persistent retrograde diastolic flow
- Do not mistake splenic vein for left renal vein
  - Splenic vein **anterior** to superior mesenteric artery
  - Left renal vein **posterior** to superior mesenteric artery

PATHOLOGY

- Nephrotic syndrome: Most common cause of renal vein thrombosis in adults

- Hypovolemia/renal hypoperfusion: Most common cause of renal vein thrombosis in children
- Risk in neonates is associated with fetal distress, perinatal asphyxia, diabetic mothers, and volume contraction

CLINICAL ISSUES

- Outcome depends on cause, time to diagnosis, duration of occlusion, recanalization, collateralization
- Prognosis overall good; frequent spontaneous recovery
- Anticoagulation: Heparin then Coumadin or low molecular weight heparin for maintenance
- Thrombolysis/surgical thrombectomy: Heroic measure for life-threatening situations
- Suprarenal caval filter (IVC thrombus)

DIAGNOSTIC CHECKLIST

- Persistent diastolic flow reversal in renal artery suggests renal vein thrombosis

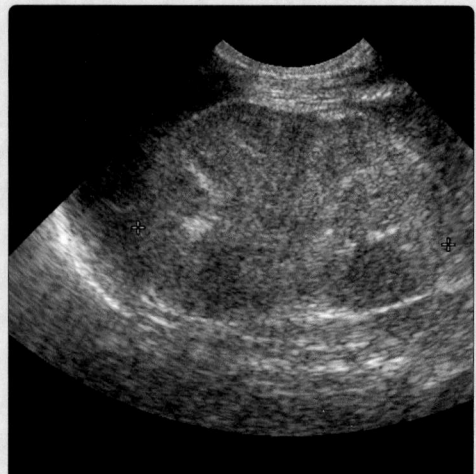
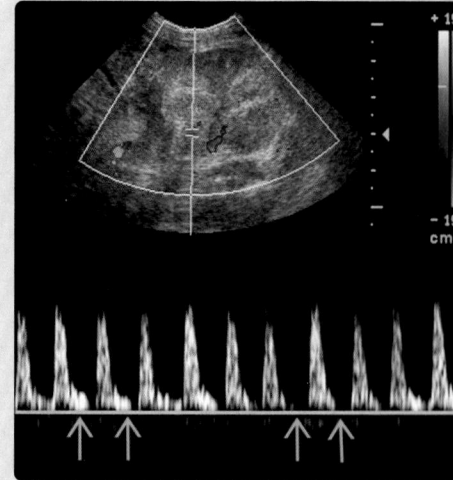

(Left) *Longitudinal ultrasound of the left kidney in a premature infant shows an edematous and nearly featureless kidney caused by acute renal vein thrombosis.* (Right) *Spectral Doppler at the renal hilum in the same patient shows absent end diastolic flow ➡, which corresponds to an elevated resistive index of 1.0. In contrast, the contralateral kidney (not shown) had a spectral tracing with substantial diastolic flow above baseline with a normal resistive index (RI) of 0.65.*

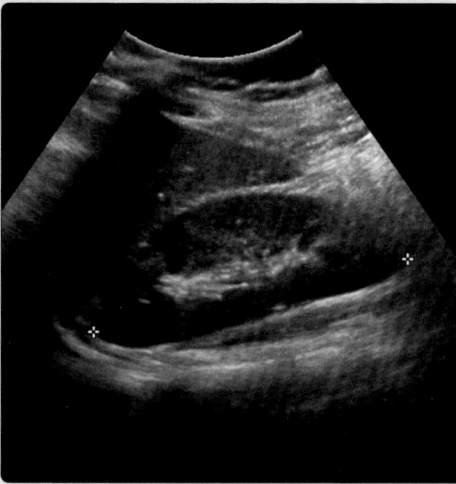
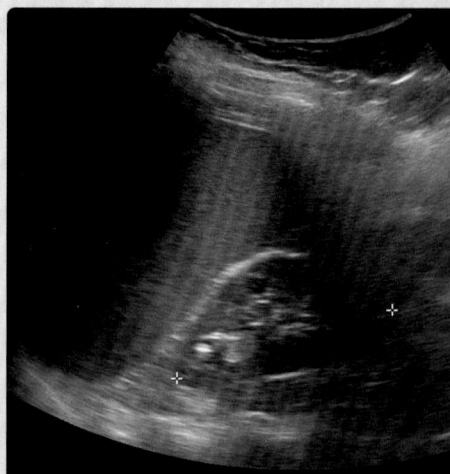

(Left) *Ten years later, longitudinal grayscale ultrasound in the same patient shows a mildly hypertrophied contralateral (right) kidney at 10.5 cm long (calipers). Note that in adults, this type of subsequent compensatory hypertrophy would not be expected.* (Right) *The left kidney (calipers) in the same patient who had venous thrombosis during the neonatal period has grown very little, now quite small in size for the patient's age, measuring 5.1 cm in length.*

TERMINOLOGY

Abbreviations
- Renal vein thrombosis (RVT)

Definitions
- Clot formation in renal vein (RV)

IMAGING

General Features
- Best diagnostic clue
  - o Echogenic material in RV with absence of flow on color Doppler US
  - o Reversal of diastolic flow on spectral Doppler tracing of renal artery is indirect sonographic finding of RVT
- Location
  - o Unilateral > bilateral
  - o Left renal vein > right renal vein, probably because it is longer
  - o Possible inferior vena cava (IVC) thrombus extension
- Size
  - o Kidney enlarged acutely in 75% cases
  - o RV dilated acutely
  - o May see shrunken, scarred kidney chronically

Ultrasonographic Findings
- Grayscale ultrasound
  - o **Acute thrombosis**
    - – Renal enlargement
      - □ Venous congestion → edema → renal enlargement
      - □ Enlargement varies & depends on degree of RV obstruction
    - – Altered parenchymal echogenicity (3 patterns)
      - □ Diffusely hypoechoic, no corticomedullary differentiation
      - □ Diffusely heterogeneous (if extensive hemorrhage and necrosis)
      - □ Linear echogenic "streaks" radiating from hilum (thrombosed parenchymal veins)
    - – Renal vein distended (faintly echogenic material)
    - – IVC thrombus extension (uncommon)
  - o **Subacute thrombosis**
    - – ↑ cortical echogenicity, ↑ corticomedullary contrast (after 10-14 days)
    - – Reduced RV size, increased thrombus echogenicity
  - o **Chronic thrombosis**
    - – Appearance depends on amount of renal damage, degree of RV flow restoration
      - □ Normal grayscale appearance
      - □ ↑ parenchymal echogenicity
      - □ ↓ kidney size (scar)
- Pulsed Doppler
  - o **Altered renal artery spectral waveforms**
    - – ↑ systolic pulsatility (narrow, sharp systolic peaks)
    - – Persistent retrograde diastolic flow
  - o Focal ↑ flow velocity around thrombus if nonocclusive
- Color Doppler
  - o **Acute occlusive thrombus**
    - – Absent RV blood flow
    - – May see "tram-track" (small flow channels around thrombus)
  - o **Acute nonocclusive thrombus**
    - – Thrombus "filling defect" in RV flow column
    - – May see aliasing from ↑ flow velocity around thrombus
  - o **Subacute/chronic**
    - – Variable restoration of flow, depending on degree of lysis
    - – Possible collateral veins (hilar, capsular-retroperitoneal, renal-splenic)

Other Modality Findings
- CT
  - o Noncontrast CT may show enlargement and high attenuation of thrombosed vessel
  - o Perinephric &/or perivascular edema
  - o Delayed nephrogram compared to contralateral side
  - o Filling defect at portal venous phase may be hard to distinguish from flow artifacts
  - o Delayed phase imaging (2-5 minutes) most sensitive for venous thrombosis
- MR
  - o Absence of flow voids in thrombosed vessel
  - o Perivascular edema on T2WI
  - o Direct visualization of clot on delayed post-contrast images

Imaging Recommendations
- Best imaging tool
  - o Color Doppler and spectral Doppler US for initial diagnosis
  - o CT/MR for comprehensive assessment, follow-up
- Protocol advice
  - o Do not mistake splenic vein for left renal vein (LRV)
    - – Splenic vein **anterior** to superior mesenteric artery
    - – LRV **posterior** to superior mesenteric artery
  - o Doppler angle (60° or less), pulse repetition frequency, and gain must be appropriate for low velocity flow

DIFFERENTIAL DIAGNOSIS

Renal Vein Tumor Invasion
- Renal cell carcinoma is most common cause of renal vein tumor invasion; Wilms and urothelial tumors less common
- RV distended by faintly echogenic tumor (looks like thrombus)
- May see tumor vessels in RV with color Doppler
- Kidney may be infiltrated, enlarged

Renal Parenchymal Infiltration
- Diffusely enlarged, hypoechoic kidney, loss of corticomedullary differentiation
- Parenchymal appearance identical to RVT but vein is patent
- Infiltrative processes involving kidney that can mimic RVT include: Lymphoma, renal cell carcinoma, urothelial carcinoma, and amyloid

Pyelonephritis
- Enlarged, hypoechoic kidney, loss of corticomedullary differentiation
- Appearance identical to RVT, but RV patent

o Note, however, that RVT can be a complication of infection

Urinary Tract Obstruction

- Possible kidney enlargement
- Normal echogenicity maintained acutely
- Dilated pelvis/calyces almost always seen

PATHOLOGY

General Features

- Etiology
  - o Nephrotic syndrome: Most common cause of RVT in adults
    - – Especially membranous glomerulonephritis
  - o Hypovolemia/renal hypoperfusion: Most common cause of RVT in children
    - – Dehydration, sepsis, hemorrhage, pericarditis, CHF
  - o Risk in neonates is associated with fetal distress, perinatal asphyxia, diabetic mothers, and volume contraction
  - o Abdominal/renal trauma
  - o Mechanical RV compression
  - o Postoperative renal transplantation
  - o Spontaneous or iatrogenic hypercoagulable states (malignancy-related, pregnancy, genetic, systemic diseases, drugs)

Gross Pathologic & Surgical Features

- Congested, enlarged kidney acutely → scarred, small kidney chronically

Microscopic Features

- Acute: Vascular congestion, edema → tissue necrosis, hemorrhage
- Chronic: Fibrosis, dystrophic calcification

CLINICAL ISSUES

Presentation

- Most common signs/symptoms
  - o Acute
    - – Flank/abdominal pain, nausea, vomiting
    - – Mass (enlarged kidney)
    - – Proteinuria, hematuria, acute renal failure
  - o Chronic
    - – Asymptomatic (if RVT unilateral or with complete recovery)
    - – Renal failure/hypertension
- Other signs/symptoms
  - o Related to acute pulmonary embolization (most common RVT complication)

Demographics

- Age
  - o Adults (most common) or children < 2 years of age
- Epidemiology
  - o Nephrotic syndrome is underlying cause of 16-42% of RVT
  - o Dehydration/sepsis most common cause of RVT in children < 2 years of age

Natural History & Prognosis

- Sparse data, small anecdotal clinical series
- Outcome depends on cause, time to diagnosis, duration of occlusion, recanalization, collateralization
- Prognosis overall good; frequent spontaneous recovery

Treatment

- Anticoagulation: Heparin then Coumadin or low molecular weight heparin for maintenance
- Thrombolysis/surgical thrombectomy: Heroic measure for life-threatening situations
- Suprarenal caval filter (IVC thrombus)

DIAGNOSTIC CHECKLIST

Consider

- RVT with diffusely enlarged, hypoechoic/heterogeneous kidney

Image Interpretation Pearls

- Persistent diastolic flow reversal in renal artery suggests RVT

SELECTED REFERENCES

1. Jones JA et al: Late onset of renal vein thrombosis after renal transplantation. Ultrasound Q. 30(3):228-9, 2014
2. Moudgil A: Renal venous thrombosis in neonates. Curr Pediatr Rev. 10(2):101-6, 2014
3. Sciascia S et al: Renal involvement in antiphospholipid syndrome. Nat Rev Nephrol. 10(5):279-89, 2014
4. Horrow MM et al: Immediate postoperative sonography of renal transplant vascular findings and outcomes. AJR Am J Roentgenol. 201(3):W479-86, 2013
5. Leschied JR et al: 99mTc MAG3 renography demonstrating return to normal renal function following resolution of renal vein thrombosis. Clin Nucl Med. 37(4):382-4, 2012
6. Yang GF et al: Thromboembolic complications in nephrotic syndrome: imaging spectrum. Acta Radiol. 53(10):1186-94, 2012
7. Sidhu R et al: Imaging of renovascular disease. Semin Ultrasound CT MR. 30(4):271-88, 2009
8. Urban BA et al: Three-dimensional volume-rendered CT angiography of the renal arteries and veins: normal anatomy, variants, and clinical applications. Radiographics. 21(2):373-86; questionnaire 549-55, 2001
9. Heiss SG et al: Contrast-enhanced three-dimensional fast spoiled gradient-echo renal MR imaging: evaluation of vascular and nonvascular disease. Radiographics. 20(5):1341-52; discussion 1353-4, 2000
10. Kawashima A et al: CT evaluation of renovascular disease. Radiographics. 20(5):1321-40, 2000
11. Zigman A et al: Renal vein thrombosis: a 10-year review. J Pediatr Surg. 35(11):1540-2, 2000
12. Chait A et al: Renal vein thrombosis. Radiology. 90(5):886-96, 1968

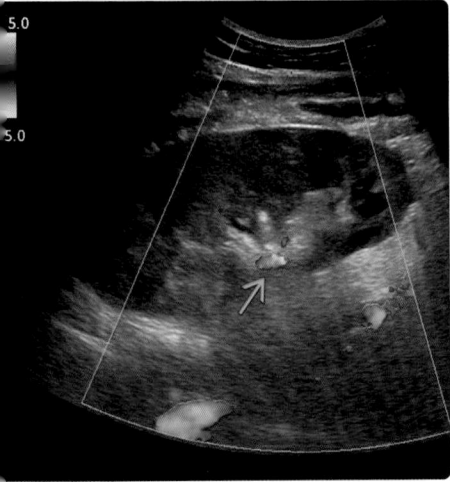

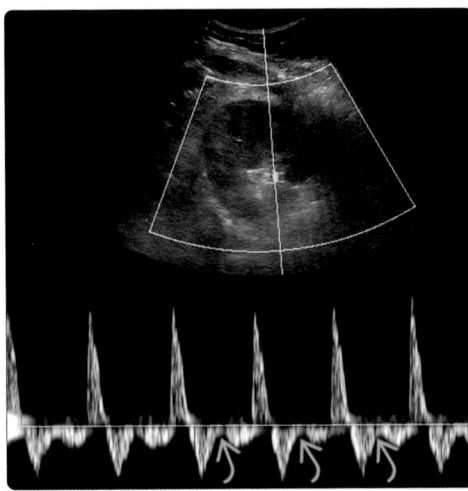

(Left) *Longitudinal color Doppler ultrasound of a renal transplant on postoperative day 1 reveals no detectable parenchymal vascularity. The only area of detectable vascularity is an arterial signal at the hilum* ➡. **(Right)** *Spectral Doppler in the same patient reveals pandiastolic reversal of flow* ➡ *in the main renal artery which occurred secondary to acute renal vein thrombosis. Renal vein patency could not be restored in this patient and the patient required explantation on day 3.*

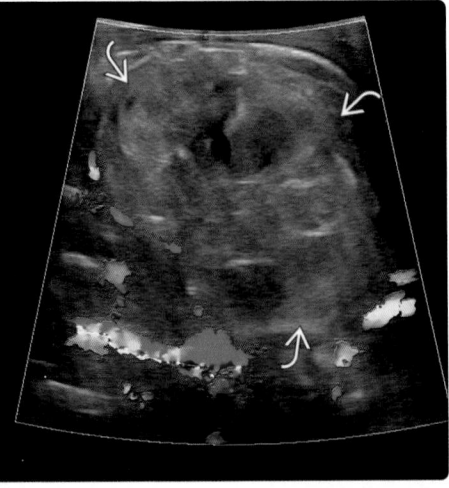

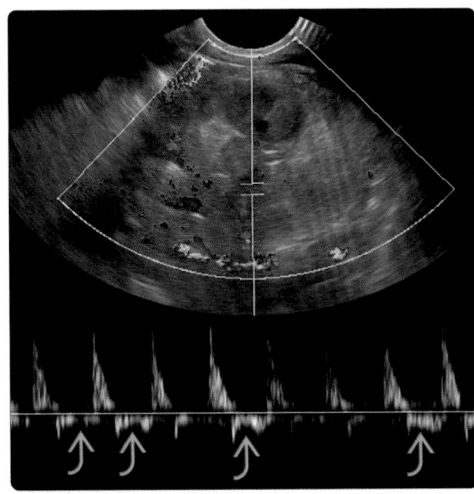

(Left) *Color Doppler ultrasound of the left upper quadrant in a 33-week premature infant shows an irregular and hypovascular mass* ➡. *The mass was only minimally reniform and was described as a tumor on an outside hospital imaging report.* **(Right)** *Spectral Doppler in the same patient shows pandiastolic reversal of flow* ➡ *in the renal artery secondary to acute renal vein thrombosis. This unfortunate infant also suffered an ipsilateral adrenal hemorrhage (not shown).*

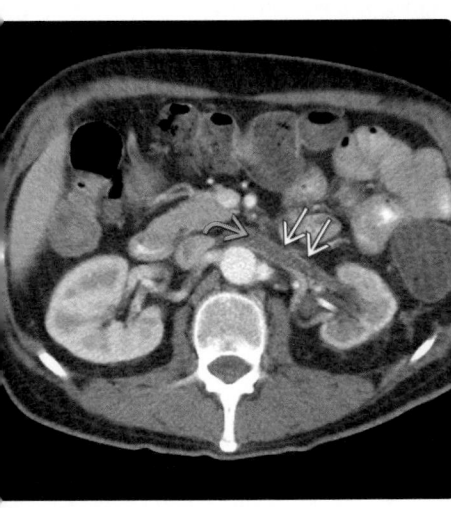

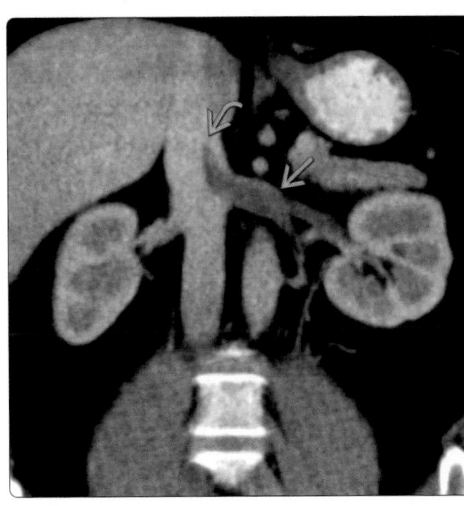

(Left) *This patient had chronic renal obstruction (now stented) and infections due to a bladder tumor. Axial contrast-enhanced CT shows a tubular, low-density filling defect in the left renal vein* ➡, *with at most minimal flow around the periphery of the clot* ➡. **(Right)** *Coronal reformatted CT in a different patient with nephrotic syndrome shows diffuse left renal vein thrombosis* ➡, *with extension into the IVC* ➡. *This patient later suffered a small pulmonary embolism.*

TERMINOLOGY

- Global or focal renal hypoperfusion → tissue ischemia and eventually, parenchymal loss

IMAGING

- Sonographic diagnosis is difficult; evaluation by CT/MR more common
- ± alteration in grey scale appearance with ↓ corticomedullary differentiation
- Focally diminished or absent Doppler flow
- May involve all or part of 1 kidney
- Insults to accessory renal arteries tend to cause polar infarcts
- Wedge shaped, corresponding to vascular territory in kidney
- May be hypoechoic or hyperechoic, depending on timing
- When focal, tends to be wedge shaped and extend all the way from hilum to capsule
- Focal or global loss of parenchymal flow

- Optimize settings to detect slow flow

PATHOLOGY

- Arterial disease: Trauma, atherosclerosis, vasculitis, dissection
- Embolism: Endocarditis, arrhythmias with clot
- Thrombosis: Trauma or hypercoagulability
- Iatrogenic: Small polar arteries may be sacrificed in AAA repair or transplant harvest

DIAGNOSTIC CHECKLIST

- Clinical context will usually help to exclude the other items in differential diagnosis
- Look for ancillary signs of infection or trauma on CT exams to narrow the differential
- Small polar infarcts are common after endovascular repair of AAA

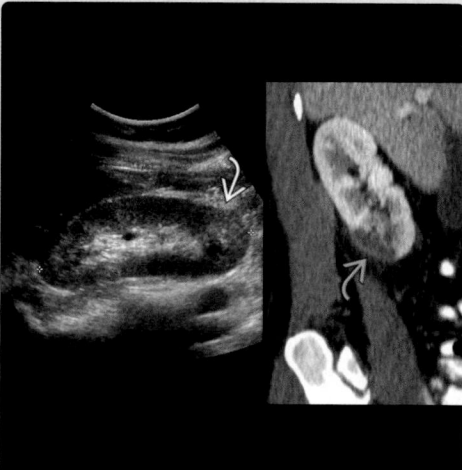
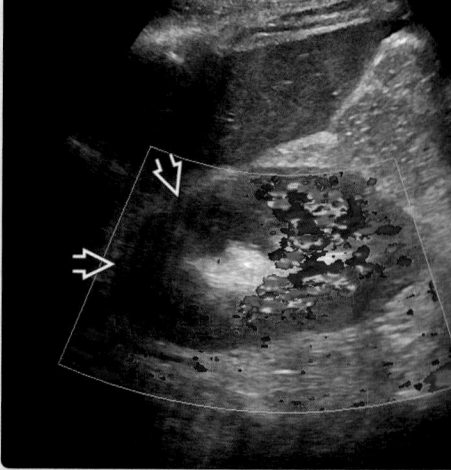

(Left) US shows a subtle, wedge-shaped, hyperechoic infarct ➡ in the lower pole of the right kidney in a patient with dilated cardiomyopathy. Correlative CECT demonstrates the corresponding enhancement defect ➡. Note the preserved capsular enhancement, a.k.a. the cortical rim sign, due to patent capsular arteries that perfuse the capsule. (Right) Absent color Doppler flow ➡ is shown in the upper pole of a patient with segmental renal infarct.

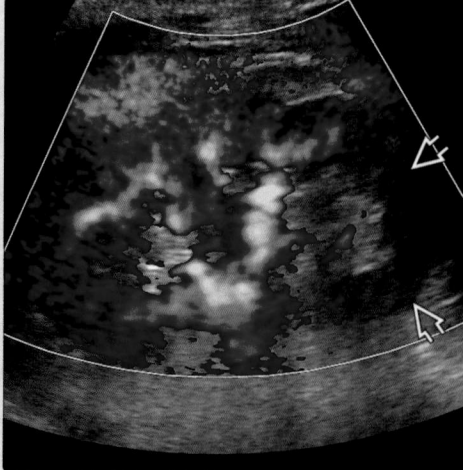
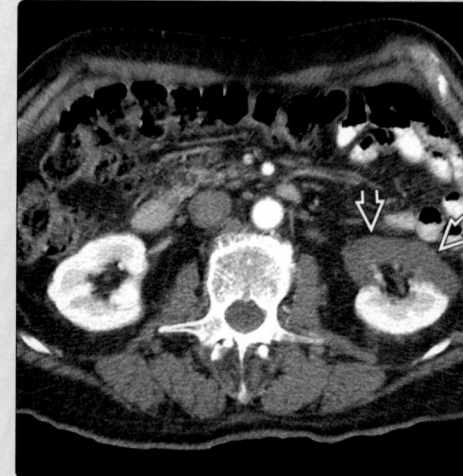

(Left) Absent power Doppler flow ➡ is shown in the lower pole of a patient with renal infarct from atrial fibrillation. Power Doppler is most sensitive for slow flow and should be used as a confirmatory test when infarct is suspected. (Right) Contrast-enhanced CT in the same patient shows absent perfusion ➡ in the anterior cortex of the kidney.

TERMINOLOGY

Definitions

- Global or focal renal hypoperfusion → tissue ischemia and eventually, parenchymal loss

IMAGING

General Features

Best diagnostic clue
- Sonographic diagnosis is difficult; evaluation by CT/MR more common
- ± alteration in gray scale appearance with ↓ corticomedullary differentiation
- Focally diminished or absent Doppler flow

Location
- May involve all or part of 1 kidney
- Insults to accessory renal arteries tend to → polar infarcts

Size
- Variable

Morphology
- Wedge shaped, corresponding to vascular territory in kidney

Ultrasonographic Findings

Grayscale ultrasound
- Diminished corticomedullary differentiation
- May be hypoechoic or hyperechoic, depending on timing
- When focal, tends to be wedge shaped and extend all the way from hilum to capsule

Color Doppler
- Focal or global loss of parenchymal flow
- Optimize settings to detect slow flow
  - Use power Doppler for increased sensitivity
- CEUS used to assess perfusion where available

CT Findings

CECT
- Decreased attenuation, delayed or absent nephrogram
- Delayed or absent excretion if global infarct
- CTA may demonstrate a vascular lesion

Imaging Recommendations

Best imaging tool
- Color and power Doppler helps distinguish ischemia from other renal pathologies
- CECT has best sensitivity to evaluate infarction and causes

Protocol advice
- Doppler parameters must be optimized to detect slow flow

DIFFERENTIAL DIAGNOSIS

Pyelonephritis

- Clinical context is key; often has urothelial thickening
- Focal nephritis may appear similar, wedge-shaped, echogenic

Radiation Effects

- Tend to be nonanatomic in distribution, rather than segmental

Renal Neoplasm

- More commonly round or ovoid + color flow within lesion

Renal Laceration

- Antecedent trauma history, perinephric fluid is common

PATHOLOGY

General Features

- Etiology
  - Arterial disease: Trauma, atherosclerosis, vasculitis, dissection
  - Embolism: Endocarditis, arrhythmias with clot
  - Thrombosis: Trauma or hypercoagulability
  - Iatrogenic: Small polar arteries may be sacrificed in AAA repair or transplant harvest

Staging, Grading, & Classification

- Clinical significance depends on volume of renal parenchyma lost

Gross Pathologic & Surgical Features

- Ischemic tissue is pale or white grossly
- Long term, renal scarring, and cortical lobulation results

CLINICAL ISSUES

Presentation

- Most common signs/symptoms
  - Often asymptomatic, depends on etiology
- Other signs/symptoms
  - Flank pain, hypertension; hematuria

Demographics

- Age
  - Given variety of causes, can occur at all ages

Natural History & Prognosis

- Segmental infarcts are well tolerated and rarely have long term sequelae
- Global infarct can result in "auto nephrectomy"

Treatment

- May include medical management, angioplasty &/or endovascular stenting

DIAGNOSTIC CHECKLIST

Consider

- Clinical context will usually help to exclude the other items in differential diagnosis

Image Interpretation Pearls

- Look for ancillary signs of infection or trauma on CT exams to narrow the differential
- Small polar infarcts are common after endovascular repair of AAA

SELECTED REFERENCES

1. Piccoli GB et al: Renal infarction versus pyelonephritis in a woman presenting with fever and flank pain. Am J Kidney Dis. 64(2):311-4, 2014
2. Stenberg B et al: Post-operative 3-dimensional contrast-enhanced ultrasound (CEUS) versus Tc99m-DTPA in the detection of post-surgical perfusion defects in kidney transplants - preliminary findings. Ultraschall Med. 35(3):273-8, 2014

TERMINOLOGY

- Hemorrhagic collection in perinephric spaces: Subcapsular, perirenal, anterior and posterior pararenal

IMAGING

- Avascular solid or cystic masses in 1 or more perinephric spaces
- Echogenicity of blood changes over time
- Sonographic features vary over time
  - Acute: Highly echogenic perinephric mass
  - Subacute: Partial liquefaction, echogenic debris, retractile clot with thick septa
  - Chronic: May be almost anechoic
- Useful to assess perfusion in compressed kidney
- Sometimes reveals etiologies such as pseudoaneurysm

TOP DIFFERENTIAL DIAGNOSES

- Lymphoma infiltration
- Cystic lymphangioma

- Perinephric abscess

PATHOLOGY

- Causes include trauma, renal biopsy, renal cyst or tumor rupture, anticoagulation, aneurysm rupture

CLINICAL ISSUES

- Treatment varies with etiology
- Hematoma without underlying significant pathology usually resolves spontaneously
- Flank pain, often severe, palpable mass, shock
- Diminished hematocrit may prompt evaluation
- Subcapsular hematoma may cause hypertension

DIAGNOSTIC CHECKLIST

- Must identify underlying etiology in spontaneous perinephric hematoma to exclude malignancy

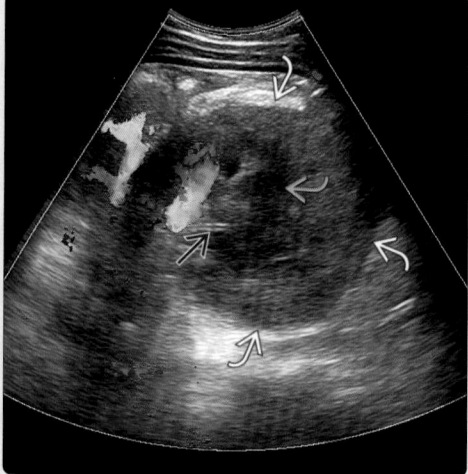
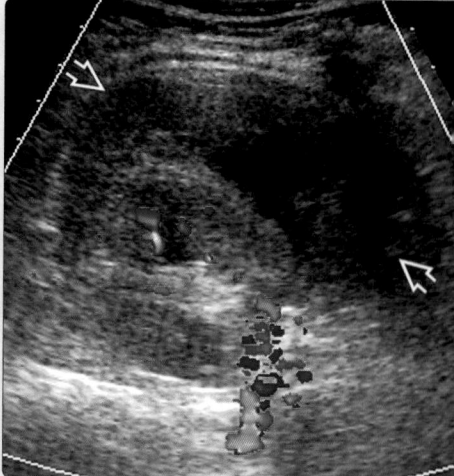

(Left) *Transverse color Doppler US of a 6 year old after stent placement ➡ shows a grossly enlarged renal contour ➡ due to large echogenic perinephric hematoma. The relatively hypoechoic kidney is seen in the center of the mass ➡, demonstrating how hyperechoic acute blood can obscure normal structures.* (Right) *Transverse color Doppler US shows a large, spontaneous perinephric hematoma with mixed echogenicity ➡. Note occult RCC must be considered in spontaneous hemorrhage.*

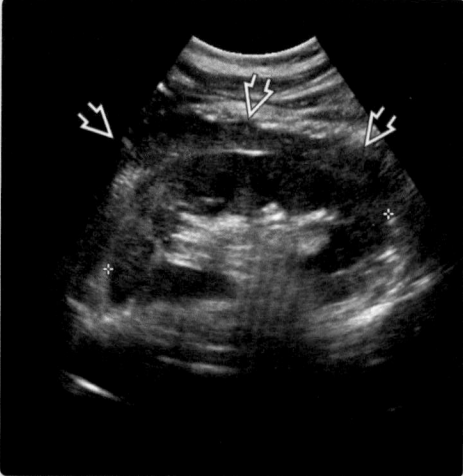
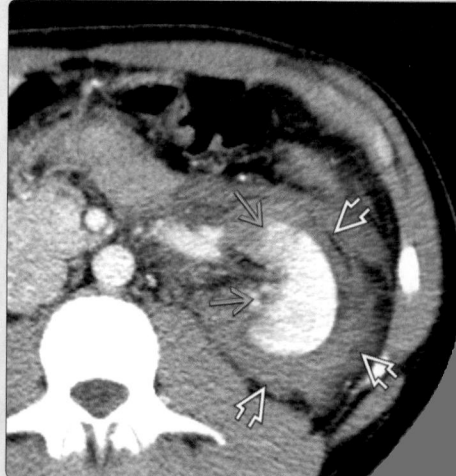

(Left) *Longitudinal US in a young man with left flank pain after collision during a soccer game illustrates a thick, irregular soft tissue rind ➡ of blood surrounding the left kidney.* (Right) *CT confirms an extensive perinephric hematoma ➡ in the same patient, with associated renal lacerations ➡.*

Perinephric Hematoma

TERMINOLOGY

Definitions

Hemorrhagic collection in perinephric spaces: Subcapsular, perirenal, anterior and posterior pararenal

IMAGING

General Features

Best diagnostic clue
- Avascular solid or cystic masses in 1 or more perinephric spaces
  - Echogenicity of blood changes over time

Ultrasonographic Findings

Grayscale ultrasound
- Sonographic features vary over time
  - Acute: Highly echogenic perinephric mass
  - Subacute: Partial liquefaction, echogenic debris, retractile clot with thick septa
  - Chronic: May be almost anechoic

Color Doppler
- Useful to assess perfusion in compressed kidney
- Subcapsular collection will indent and compress renal contour, causing Page kidney
- Sometimes reveals etiologies such as pseudoaneurysm
- No vascular flow within hematoma

CT Findings

CECT
- Highly sensitive for detection of perinephric fluid collection, its extent, and underlying causes
- In trauma or suspected active bleeding: Delayed images to evaluate for pooling of extravasated vascular or excreted urinary contrast
- Hematoma: High attenuation (> 28 HU) may show hematocrit level

Imaging Recommendations

Best imaging tool
- CT is diagnostic method of choice
- US is ideal adjunct to CT and can guide aspiration to determine nature of fluid collection

Protocol advice
- US is initial investigation for perinephric fluid collection and guided aspiration
- CT is required to identify cause of perinephric hematoma or characterize fluid collections
- Angiography is offered for superselective embolization of bleeding tumor
- For suspected occult renal cell carcinoma (RCC) as cause of hematoma, consider follow-up ± biopsy by US or CT

DIFFERENTIAL DIAGNOSIS

Lymphoma Infiltration

Lymphoma may completely encircle kidney, producing hypoechoic collar

Cystic Lymphangioma

Multilocular cystic lesion, occurs anywhere in retroperitoneum

Perinephric Abscess

- Subacute complication of pyelonephritis; difficult or impossible to differentiate from hematoma by US

PATHOLOGY

General Features

- Etiology
  - Causes include trauma, renal biopsy, renal tumor rupture, renal cyst rupture, anticoagulant therapy, aortic aneurysm rupture

CLINICAL ISSUES

Presentation

- Most common signs/symptoms
  - Flank pain, often severe, palpable mass, shock
- Other signs/symptoms
  - Diminished hematocrit may prompt evaluation
  - Subcapsular hematoma may cause hypertension

Natural History & Prognosis

- Hematoma without underlying significant pathology usually resolves spontaneously with good prognosis

Treatment

- Subcapsular or perinephric hematoma: Treatment varies with etiology
  - Extrafascial nephrectomy for malignant tumors or extensive hemorrhage
  - Superselective embolization or covered stent for active bleeding with clinical instability
  - Managed conservatively in benign entities

DIAGNOSTIC CHECKLIST

Consider

- Must identify underlying etiology in spontaneous perinephric hematoma to exclude malignancy

Image Interpretation Pearls

- US provides noninvasive means of assessing fluid collection resolution over time

SELECTED REFERENCES

1. Kozminski MA et al: Symptomatic Subcapsular and Perinephric Hematoma Following Ureteroscopic Lithotripsy for Renal Calculi. J Endourol. ePub, 2014
2. Lee SW et al: Experience of ultrasonography-guided percutaneous core biopsy for renal masses. Korean J Urol. 54(10):660-5, 2013
3. Sunga KL et al: Spontaneous retroperitoneal hematoma: etiology, characteristics, management, and outcome. J Emerg Med. 43(2):e157-61, 2012
4. Chan YC et al: Management of spontaneous and iatrogenic retroperitoneal haemorrhage: conservative management, endovascular intervention or open surgery? Int J Clin Pract. 62(10):1604-13, 2008
5. Shih WJ et al: Spontaneous subcapsular and intrarenal hematoma demonstrated by various diagnostic modalities and monitored by ultrasonography until complete resolution. J Natl Med Assoc. 92(4):200-5, 2000

TERMINOLOGY

- Benign prostatic hyperplasia (BPH)
  - Term reserved for histopathological pattern of smooth muscle and epithelial cell proliferation
  - Hyperplasia is correct term since BPH is characterized by increased number of epithelial stromal cells in periurethral area of prostate (not hypertrophy, which means increase in size)

IMAGING

- Sonographic appearance of BPH is variable, depending on histopathologic changes
- Ultrasound cannot reliably differentiate BPH from prostate cancer
- Ultrasound may be used to measure prostate size and PVR as well as evaluate for upper tract obstruction in men with BPH and renal insufficiency
- Estimated prostate volume: Prolate ellipsoid formula: Width x height x length x ∏/6 = W x H x L x 0.52

TOP DIFFERENTIAL DIAGNOSES

- Prostate carcinoma
- Bladder carcinoma
- Prostatitis

PATHOLOGY

- Bladder outlet obstruction from BPH may occur from urethral constriction from increased smooth muscle tone and resistance (dynamic component) &/or urethral compression from gland enlargement (static component)
- Possible bladder sequelae: Trabeculation, diverticula, calculi, detrusor muscle failure
- Possible upper tract changes: Ureterectasis, hydronephro
  - Can be from secondary vesicoureteral reflux, obstructic from muscular hypertrophy or angulation at ureterovesical junction, sustained high pressure bladder storage

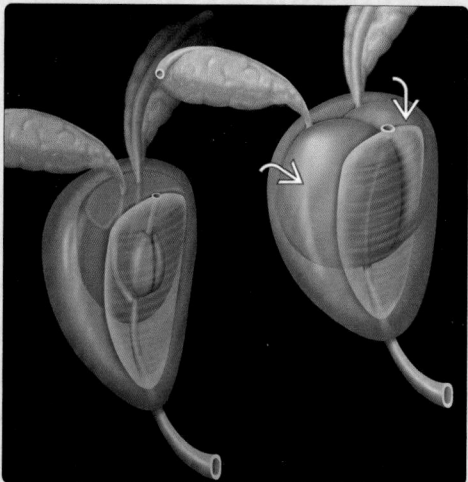
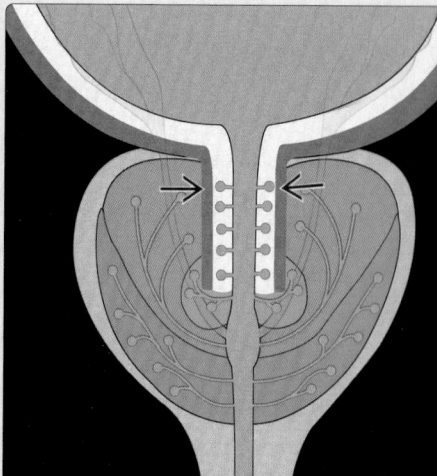

(Left) *Graphic shows a normal (left) and hyperplastic (right) prostate gland with enlargement of the transition zone (blue ➜) surrounding the urethra. Central zone is in orange, peripheral zone is in green, and anterior fibromuscular stroma is in yellow.* (Right) *Graphic shows zonal anatomy in coronal plane. The urethra from the bladder neck to verumontanum is surrounded by the preprostatic sphincter ➡, which contains periurethral glands. The TZ and periurethral glands are the sites of origin of BPH.*

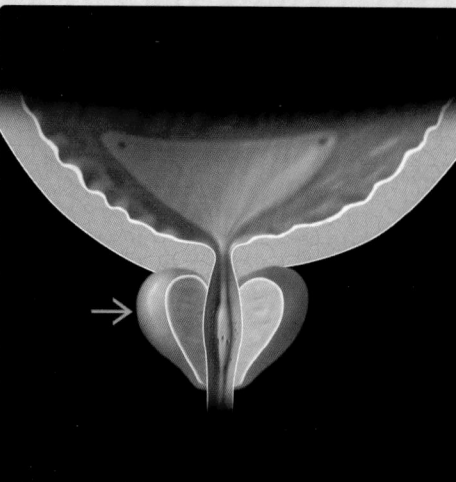
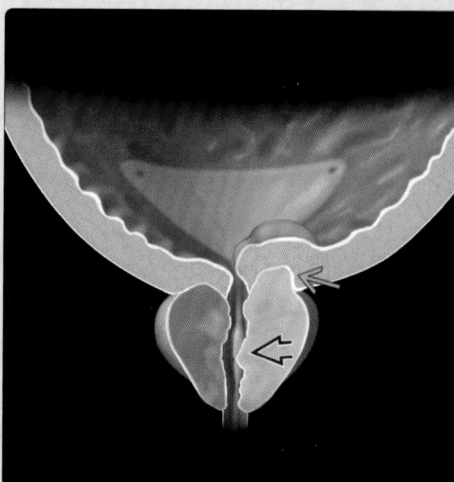

(Left) *Coronal graphic shows the normal prostate ➡ with smooth contours and widely patent prostatic urethra.* (Right) *Nodular enlargement of the periurethral glands and TZ cause external compression of the prostatic urethra ➡ and elevation of the bladder base ➡. Nodular protrusion into the bladder (a.k.a. enlarged "median lobe") → can ball-valve into the urethra and cause severe obstructive symptoms.*

TERMINOLOGY

Abbreviations

Benign prostatic hyperplasia (BPH)

Synonyms

Prostatism; glandular and stromal hyperplasia

Hyperplasia is correct term since BPH is characterized by increased number of stromal and glandular cells (not hypertrophy, which means increase in size)

Definitions

BPH reserved for histopathological pattern of smooth muscle and epithelial cell proliferation in TZ and periurethral glands

Prostatism historically applied to almost all symptoms of micturition disorder in older men

○ Term implies prostate as cause of problem, which may not be the case (e.g., neurologic abnormalities)

Lower urinary tract symptoms (LUTS) applies to any patient with urinary symptoms, regardless of age or sex; does not specify underlying etiology

○ Storage LUTS: Frequency, urgency, nocturia

○ Voiding LUTS: Hesitancy, straining, slow stream, intermittent or interrupted flow, terminal dribbling, sensation of incomplete emptying

BPE: Benign prostate enlargement: Usually presumptive diagnosis based on prostate size

BPO: Benign prostate obstruction: Enlarged gland with obstruction that has been proven by urodynamics

BOO: Bladder outlet obstruction: Generic term for any cause of subvesical obstruction, including BPO

IMAGING

General Features

Best diagnostic clue

○ Enlarged prostate with nodular enlargement in transition zone &/or periurethral region

Size

○ Normally the size of walnut or golf ball, ~ 20-30 g

○ May be as large as 500 g

Morphology

○ Inverted conical shape with base at urethrovesical junction and apex at urogenital diaphragm

○ Lobular configuration was previously used but distinct lobes do not exist

  – Currently used only in context of BPH → lateral &/or median lobe enlargement

  – Replaced by zonal anatomy with morphologic, functional, and pathologic significance

○ Prostate is divided into glandular zones and single stromal zone (anterior fibromuscular stroma)

  – Peripheral zone (PZ): ~ 70% normal glandular prostate

    □ Extends from base to apex along posterolateral aspect and surrounds distal urethra

  – Central zone (CZ): ~ 25% normal glandular prostate

    □ Cone-shaped with widest portion making majority of prostatic base, surrounds ejaculatory ducts

  – Transition zone (TZ): ~ 5% normal glandular prostate

    □ 2 separate glands immediately external to preprostatic urethra (from bladder neck to verumontanum)

  – Periurethral glands: < 1% normal glandular prostate

    □ Glands entirely contained within smooth muscle of preprostatic sphincter

  – Historically, "inner gland" refers to periurethral glands and TZ, and "outer gland" refers to CZ and PZ

    □ In radiology, "central gland" refers to periurethral glands, TZ, and CZ; correlates to imaging findings

  – Origin of BPH is confined to periurethral glands & TZ

    □ Volumetric contribution of TZ and CZ changes with age → enlarged TZ compresses CZ

  – Pseudocapsule ("surgical capsule"): Visible boundary between central gland and PZ

  – "Median lobe" seen as an intraluminal bladder component of BPH; may originate from TZ or periurethral glands

Radiographic Findings

- IVP
  ○ Elevated bladder floor with medially lifted distal ureters yield J-shaped or fishhook ureters

CT Findings

- NECT
  ○ Enlarged prostate ± calcification
    – Enlarged "median lobe" may protrude into bladder lumen.
- CECT
  ○ Enlarged prostate with mass effect on bladder base

MR Findings

- T1WI
  ○ Enlarged prostate
- T2WI
  ○ Heterogeneous T2 signal within TZ: Varied appearance correlates to variable histologic composition
    – BPH nodules show different signal behaviors depending on epithelial and stromal components
    – BPH characterized by septation of individual nodules, which can be seen as T2 dark rim
    – Classic BPH nodule = round or oval-shaped lesion with well-defined T2 dark rim
  ○ Difficult to distinguish BPH from central gland cancer
    – Look for "erased charcoal" sign suggestive of carcinoma
- DWI
  ○ BPH nodules may show restricted diffusion
- T1WI C+
  ○ Does not reliably differentiate BPH nodule from cancer

Ultrasonographic Findings

- Grayscale ultrasound
  ○ Prostate ultrasound most commonly used for transrectal ultrasound (TRUS)-guided biopsies and volume estimation
  ○ Estimate prostate volume using prolate ellipsoid formula: Width x height x length x 0.52
    – 1 cc of prostate tissue ~ 1 gram
  ○ On TRUS, normal prostate is homogeneous with relatively more hyperechoic peripheral zone

- o Sonographic appearance of BPH is variable, depending on histopathologic changes
  - – Diffusely enlarged TZ; heterogeneous, nodular
  - – ± calcification of corpora amylacea → prostatic calculi
  - – ± cystic degeneration of BPH nodules
- o Potential secondary changes of bladder and upper urinary tracts are best seen transabdominally
  - – Possible bladder findings: Wall thickening/trabeculation, diverticula, stones, abnormal postvoid residual (PVR)
  - – Possible upper tract changes: Ureteral dilation, hydronephrosis
- Color Doppler
  - o Normal prostate is moderately vascular
  - o Vascularity is usually higher in malignancy and prostatitis than in BPH
- Power Doppler
  - o Cannot reliably differentiate BPH from prostatic cancer

Imaging Recommendations

- Best imaging tool
  - o Ultrasound is typically not needed in BPH management but may be obtained to investigate BPH as cause of renal insufficiency → measure prostate size and PVR, evaluate for upper tract obstruction

DIFFERENTIAL DIAGNOSIS

Prostate Carcinoma

- Commonly originates in PZ (70%)
- Classically described as hypervascular hypoechoic PZ nodule but is difficult to differentiate cancer from BPH, prostatitis and other nonmalignant entities

Prostatitis

- Variable, may be normal
  - o Main role of US is to exclude prostatic abscess
- Acute: Enlarged gland; diffuse or focal hypoechogenicity with focal or global hypervascularity; may mimic carcinoma
- Chronic: Abnormalities may be diffuse or only in the periurethral or peripheral areas
  - o Scattered hypoechoic areas in PZ; hyperechoic regions with hypoechoic halos; focal or diffuse hypervascularity; ejaculatory duct calcifications; thick/irregular capsule

Bladder Carcinoma

- Enlarged median lobe in BPH simulates bladder mass

PATHOLOGY

General Features

- Etiology
  - o Nodular periurethral stromal and epithelial hyperplasia
  - o BOO from BPH may occur from urethral constriction from increased smooth muscle tone and resistance (dynamic) &/or urethral compression from gland enlargement (static)
  - o All BPH nodules develop in TZ or periurethral region

Gross Pathologic & Surgical Features

- Enlarged, rubbery gland at prostatectomy

Microscopic Features

- Hyperplastic nodules due to glandular &/or fibrous or muscular stromal proliferation

CLINICAL ISSUES

Presentation

- Most common signs/symptoms
  - o Asymptomatic or LUTS
  - o Size of prostate does not correlate with severity of symptoms or urodynamic changes
- Other signs/symptoms
  - o Urinary incontinence: Overflow or urge
  - o Hematuria
  - o UTI
  - o Acute urinary retention
- Clinical profile
  - o Enlarged prostate on rectal exam
  - o May have elevated prostate-specific antigen (PSA)
  - o Possible bladder sequelae: Trabeculation, diverticula, calculi, detrusor muscle failure
  - o Possible upper tract changes: Ureterectasis, hydronephrosis
    - – Can be from secondary vesicoureteral reflux, obstruction from muscular hypertrophy or angulatio at ureterovesical junction, sustained high pressure bladder storage

Demographics

- Epidemiology
  - o Affects 70% of men by age 60-69 years; 80% of those aged 70-80 years; 90% men aged 80-90 years

Natural History & Prognosis

- May lead to detrusor muscle failure, renal insufficiency

Treatment

- Options, risks, complications
  - o Noninvasive: No therapy if asymptomatic or no bothersome symptoms
    - – If bothersome symptoms, then drug therapy is first line
  - o Minimal invasive & surgical options if drug therapy fails
    - – Transurethral: Resection of the prostate (TURP), incision of the prostate (TUIP), microwave thermotherapy (TUMT), needle ablation (TUNA), lase
    - – Embolization
    - – Simple prostatectomy, open or robot-assisted

DIAGNOSTIC CHECKLIST

Consider

- Prostate carcinoma or prostatitis

Image Interpretation Pearls

- Median lobe hyperplasia may simulate bladder mass

SELECTED REFERENCES

1. Trabulsi E, Halpern E, Gomella L. (2012). Ultrasonography and Biopsy of the Prostate. In Campbell-Walsh Urology (10th ed., pp. 2735-2747). Philadelph Saunders.
2. Roehrborn, C. (2012). Benign Prostatic Hyperplasia. In Wein AJ, et al (Ed), Campbell-Walsh Urology (10th edition, pp 2570-2610). Philadelphia: Saunders.

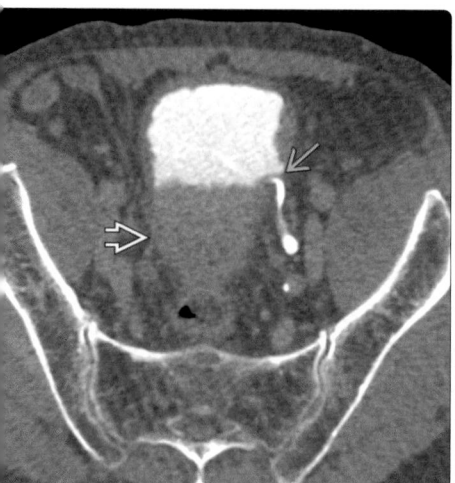

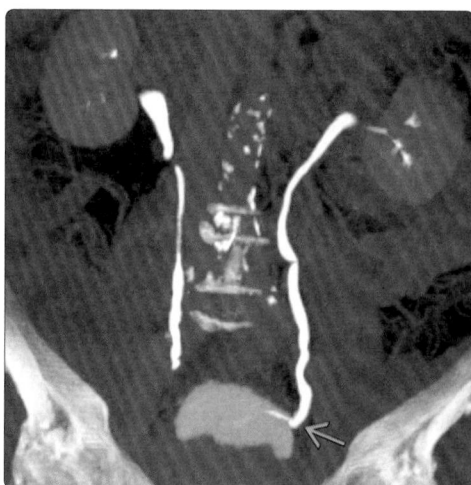

(Left) *Axial CT shows the base of an enlarged prostate ➡. Prostatomegaly causes anterior displacement of the distal left ureter ➡ at the ureterovesical junction.* (Right) *Coronal MIP of the same patient demonstrates the "fishhook" or J-shaped appearance of the distal left ureter ➡ due to elevation of the bladder base and ureterovesical junction from an enlarged prostate.*

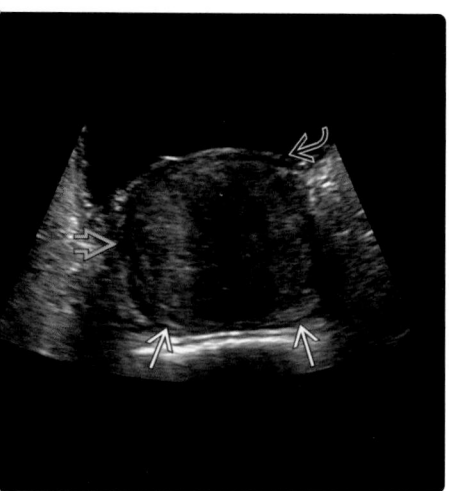

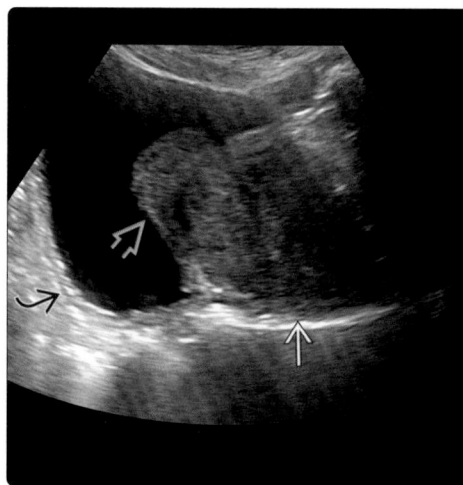

(Left) *Transabdominal ultrasound shows nodular enlargement of central gland ➡ with compression of the slightly more hyperechoic PZ ➡. Note elevation of bladder base ➡ due to mass effect.* (Right) *Sagittal US in the same patient shows nodular enlargement of the TZ and periurethral glands with "median lobe" protrusion into the bladder base ➡. This can ball-valve into the urethra, causing severe obstructive symptoms. The compressed PZ is seen posteriorly ➡. Note bladder wall thickening ➡.*

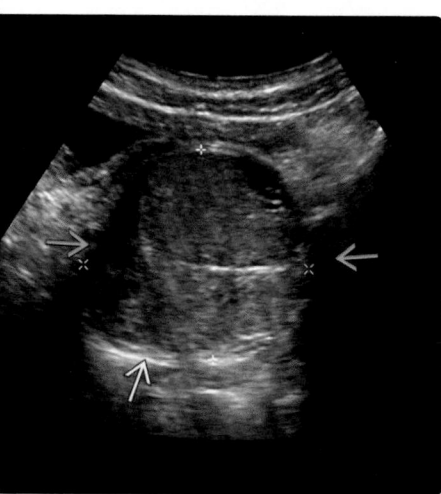

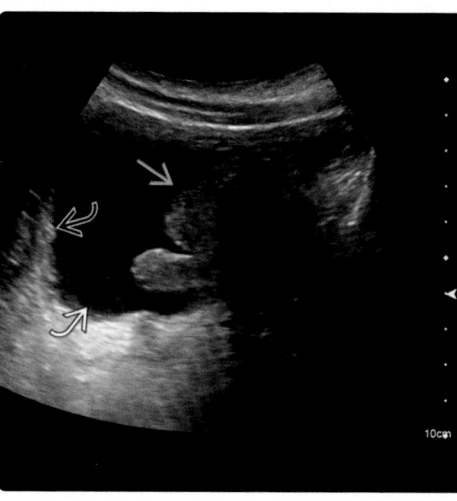

(Left) *Transverse transabdominal ultrasound shows enlargement of the well-defined TZ ➡. The severely compressed more hyperechoic PZ ➡ is seen posteriorly.* (Right) *Sagittal US in the same patient shows the "median lobe" of BPH protruding into the bladder base lumen ➡, which may simulate a polypoid bladder mass. There is thickening of the bladder wall ➡. Low-level intraluminal echoes ➡ correspond to patient's known urinary tract infection.*

Prostatic Carcinoma

IMAGING

- Location of prostate cancer: Peripheral zone (PZ) 70-80%, transition zone (TZ) 20%, central zone (CZ) 1-5%
- Transrectal ultrasound (TRUS) is imaging of choice to guide biopsy in evaluation for PCa but performs poorly in cancer detection and staging
- Calculate prostate volume using largest cross-sectional image in transverse and mid sagittal planes: Transverse x AP x long x 0.52
- MR is most sensitive imaging technique for PCa diagnosis and staging
  - PZ: T2 dark lesion with restricted diffusion; TZ: "Erased charcoal" sign on T2WI
- Targeted MR-guided and MR/ultrasound fusion-guided biopsy is promising for increasing detection of high-risk prostate cancer while reducing detection of low-risk cancer compared with standard biopsy

PATHOLOGY

- Most common noncutaneous malignancy in western world; 2nd most common cause of cancer deaths among men
- 95% of tumors are acinar adenocarcinoma
- Staging based on TNM, PSA at time of diagnosis, and Gleason score

CLINICAL ISSUES

- Management is complex due to difficulty in accurate staging and in predicting speed of disease progression
- Despite having higher volumes and PSA values at diagnosis, TZ cancers are less likely to be associated with seminal vesicle, extraprostatic and lymphovascular invasion

DIAGNOSTIC CHECKLIST

- Classic description of hypoechoic prostate lesion for PCa is less valuable in PSA era when cancer is diagnosed earlier; greater than 30-40% PCa are invisible on TRUS

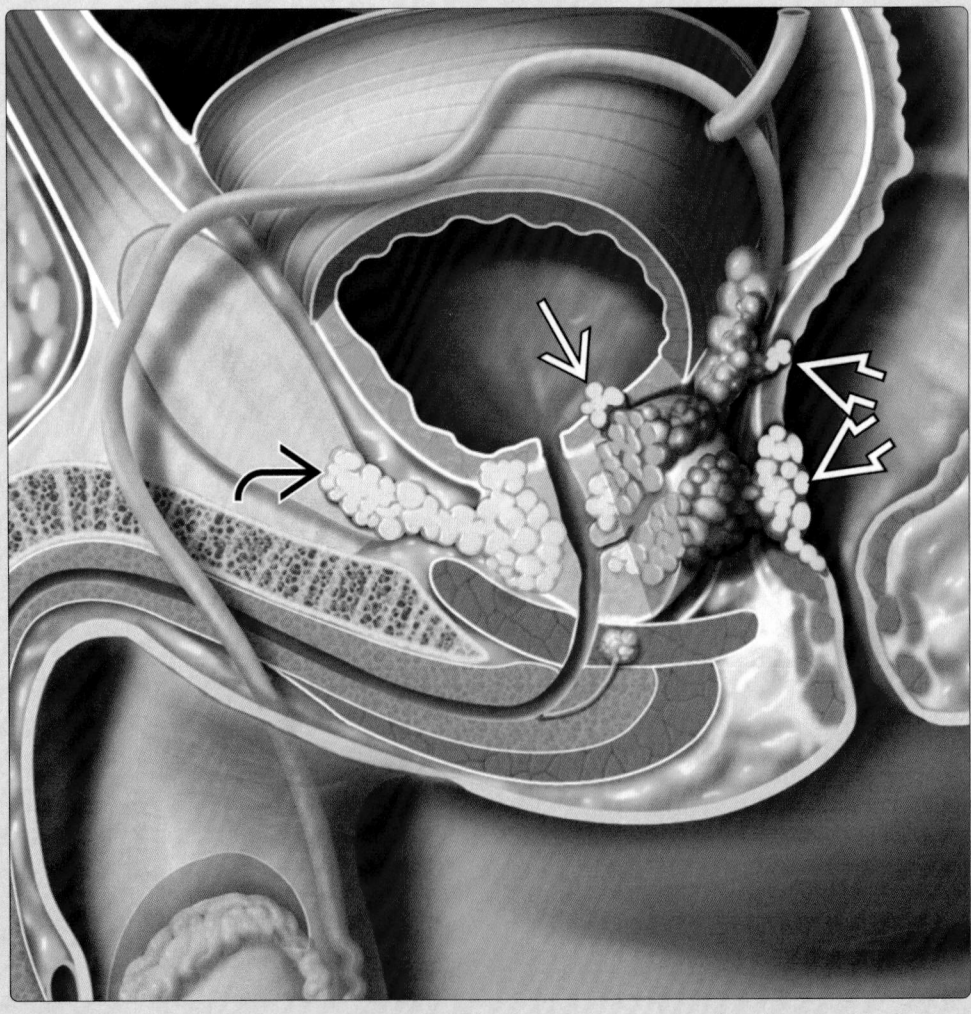

Longitudinal graphic shows advanced prostatic carcinoma (PCa) with extracapsular spread to the adjacent pelvic structures such as the bladder ➡, rectal wall ➡, and symphysis pubis ➡.

TERMINOLOGY

Abbreviations

Prostate carcinoma (PCa)

Synonyms

Prostate adenocarcinoma

IMAGING

General Features

Best diagnostic clue
- MR: Peripheral zone (PZ): T2 dark lesion with restricted diffusion; central gland: "Erased charcoal" sign on T2WI

Location
- PZ 70-80%, transition zone (TZ) 20-25%, central zone (CZ) 1-5%

Targeted MR-guided and MR/ultrasound fusion-guided biopsy is promising for increasing detection of high-risk prostate cancer while reducing detection of low-risk cancer compared with standard biopsy

Ultrasonographic Findings

Grayscale ultrasound
- Transrectal ultrasound (TRUS) is imaging modality of choice to guide biopsy but performs poorly in cancer detection and staging; also used to guide focal therapies
  - TRUS-guided biopsy considered "blind" or "random" since it is usually not targeted to specific abnormality
- Traditional description of PCa is hypoechoic PZ lesion; difficult to identify central gland tumors due to heterogeneity from benign prostatic hyperplasia (BPH)
  - Now with earlier cancer detection with PSA, studies have shown that hypoechoic lesions are not pathognomonic for cancer, as was once thought
  - PCa can appear as hypoechoic (60-70%), isoechoic/invisible (30-40%), rarely hyperechoic ± asymmetric capsular bulging or irregularity
  - Probability of hypoechoic lesion being PCa is 17-57%

Color Doppler
- PCa may be hypervascular; however, absence does not exclude Ca, and other benign entities (e.g., prostatitis) may also be hypervascular

Power Doppler
- No advantages over color Doppler

CT Findings

Not accurate in detection of cancer within prostate

Glazer et al showed mass-like PZ enhancement is predictive of higher-grade (≥ Gleason 4 + 3) cancer

Evaluate local/distant staging only among patients with intermediate- or high-risk disease
- Clinical stage ≥ T2b vs. 3 (differing guidelines), Gleason ≥ 8, PSA > 10 vs. 20, or chance of lymph node involvement > 20% (based on nomograms)

MR Findings

MR is most sensitive imaging technique for prostate cancer diagnosis and staging: Prostate Imaging and Reporting and Data System (PI-RADS) 1-5

Prostatic cancer is best seen on T2WI and DWI
- Abnormal low T2 signal in normally high signal PZ with corresponding reduced diffusion
  - Differential for T2 dark lesion in PZ: Biopsy-related hemorrhage, changes from hormone therapy, prostatitis, atrophy, fibrosis
- "Erased charcoal" sign in TZ: Focal, homogeneous low T2 signal lesion with ill-defined margins

- T1WI: Precontrast: Evaluate for post-biopsy hemorrhage; dynamic postcontrast: Hypervascular lesion corresponding to T2/DWI abnormality

- MR useful for staging
  - T stage: Organ confined (≤ T2 disease) vs. extending beyond gland (≥ T3 disease); signs of extraprostatic extension: Bulging prostatic contour, irregular or spiculated margin, obliteration of rectoprostatic angle, asymmetry or invasion of neurovascular bundle, seminal vesicle or bladder wall invasion
  - Pelvic and retroperitoneal lymph nodes
  - Osteoblastic bone metastases: Low signal intensity on both T1WI and T2WI

- Post-biopsy changes (e.g., hemorrhage, inflammation) may complicate interpretation of prostate MR for staging; at least 6 weeks interval between biopsy and MR should be considered for staging

Nuclear Medicine Findings

- Bone scan
  - Tc-99m MDP planar bone scan is standard imaging modality for diagnosis of bone metastases: Sensitivity 62-89%, specificity 57%; reflects osteoblastic response in cortex, misses early marrow disease
  - Should only be performed in patients with high-risk disease or symptoms of bony involvement: Clinical stage ≥ T2c vs. 3 (differing guidelines), Gleason ≥ 8, PSA > 10 vs. 20, or bony symptoms
  - Tc-99m MDP SPECT (single-photon emission CT) improves sensitivity (92%) and specificity (82%)

- PET/CT
  - Main role of PET/CT is in primary staging and evaluation for biochemically recurrent disease; not helpful in diagnosis or T staging
  - 18F-FDG PET/CT: Limited utility due to relatively low glucose metabolism of most PCa
  - 18F-NaF PET/CT: For bone metastases; higher diagnostic accuracy, but arguably more expensive than bone scan + SPECT
  - 11C-choline PET/CT: Limited accessibility, requires on site cyclotron; may detect disease in nonenlarged nodes and early marrow involvement; evaluation for suspected recurrent disease

Imaging Recommendations

- Best imaging tool
  - MR is most sensitive imaging technique for prostate cancer diagnosis and staging
  - TRUS is imaging modality of choice for prostate biopsy

DIFFERENTIAL DIAGNOSIS

Benign Prostatic Hyperplasia

- Hyperplasia of TZ and periurethral glands; heterogeneous, nodular enlargement ± cystic degeneration, calcification

Prostatitis

- Acute and chronic prostatitis can mimic prostate cancer

- PZ: Can cause ↓ signal on both T2WI and ADC map, may also be hypervascular

Atrophy

- From normal aging or chronic inflammation
- Typically wedge-shaped areas of ↓ T2 signal and mildly ↓ ADC map signal from loss of glandular tissue (but typically not as low as in cancer) ± contour retraction

Fibrosis

- Can occur after inflammation, may appear as wedge- or band-shaped low signal on T2WI

Prostatic Intraepithelial Neoplasia (PIN)

- Dysplasia of epithelial lining of prostate glands
- Management of high-grade PIN is controversial; PCa diagnosis on rebiopsy is similar to that in men whose initial biopsies were normal

Atypia (a.k.a. Atypical Small Acinar Proliferation [ASAP])

- Descriptive term: When needle biopsy shows findings highly suspicious for, but not diagnostic of, PCa
- If other cores are negative, then short interval follow-up rebiopsy, since ~ 40% of men with atypia will have PCa diagnosed on rebiopsy

PATHOLOGY

General Features

- Etiology
  - Unknown: Advancing age, hormonal influence, environmental and genetic factors play role
- Most common noncutaneous malignancy in western world, 2nd most common cause of cancer deaths among men

Staging, Grading, & Classification

- Staging based on TNM, PSA at time of diagnosis, and Gleason score
- Grading by Gleason score: 2 values given; 1st is predominant histologic pattern, 2nd is next most prevalent histologic pattern; each value ranging from 1-5 (least to most abnormal)
- T stage
  - T1: Clinically localized (tumor not palpable on DRE)
  - T2: Tumor confined to prostate
  - T3: Locally invasive beyond prostatic capsule
  - T4: Tumor is fixed or invades adjacent structures other than seminal vesicles, such as external sphincter, rectum, bladder, levator muscles, &/or pelvic wall
- N stage: N0: No nodal metastases, N1: Metastasis in regional nodes
- M stage: M0: No distant metastasis, M1: Metastasis to nonregional lymph nodes, bones, or other sites

Microscopic Features

- 95% of tumors are acinar adenocarcinoma

CLINICAL ISSUES

Presentation

- Most common signs/symptoms
  - Early: Asymptomatic, elevated PSA on screening

  - Advanced: Problems urinating, hematospermia, hematuria, pelvic pain/discomfort, urinary incontinence, erectile dysfunction, bone pain, rarely rectal obstruction
  - In general, most agree TRUS-guided prostate biopsy should be performed when abnormal DRE or elevated PSA (> 4.0 ng/ml)
    - Complications of TRUS-guided prostate needle biopsy: Sepsis (1-4%), hematuria (most common), rectal bleeding, vasovagal episode, hematospermia
- Diagnosis: Pathology
- Current methods of prostate cancer detection: DRE, serum PSA level, TRUS-guided biopsy ± MR

Demographics

- Age
  - Average age at diagnosis is 66, rare before age 40
- Ethnicity
  - African Americans > non-Hispanic whites > Asian American and Hispanic/Latino
- Epidemiology
  - Heterogeneous disease, and most men with disease will ultimately die of other causes

Natural History & Prognosis

- 5-year relative survival rates
  - Localized to prostate (AJCC stages I and II): Nearly 100%
  - Regional stage (AJCC stage III and stage IV cancers without distant disease): Nearly 100%
  - Distant stage (rest of AJCC stage IV cancers = distant disease): 28%
- Despite having higher volumes and PSA values at diagnosis, TZ cancers are less likely to be associated with seminal vesicle, extraprostatic and lymphovascular invasion

Treatment

- Management is complex due to difficulty in accurate staging and in predicting speed of disease progression
- Options: Watchful waiting, targeted local therapies, radical prostatectomy, various forms of radiation, hormonal treatment, chemotherapy, combined approach

DIAGNOSTIC CHECKLIST

Image Interpretation Pearls

- Classic description of hypoechoic prostate lesion for PCa is less valuable in PSA era when cancer is diagnosed earlier; greater than 30-40% PCa are invisible on TRUS

SELECTED REFERENCES

1. Trabulsi EJ et al: Enhanced transrectal ultrasound modalities in the diagnosis of prostate cancer. Urology. 76(5):1025-33, 2010
2. Trabulsi E, Halpern E, Gomella L. Ultrasonography and Biopsy of the Prostate. In Campbell-Walsh Urology (10th ed., pp. 2735-2747). Philadelphia:Saunders.
3. Harvey CJ et al: Applications of transrectal ultrasound in prostate cancer. Br J Radiol. 85 Spec No 1:S3-17, 2012
4. Onur R et al: Contemporary impact of transrectal ultrasound lesions for prostate cancer detection. J Urol. 172(2):512-4, 2004
5. Wollin DA et al: Guideline of Guidelines: Prostate Cancer Imaging. BJU Int. ePub, 2015
6. Bouchelouche K et al: Advances in imaging modalities in prostate cancer. Curr Opin Oncol. ePub, 2015

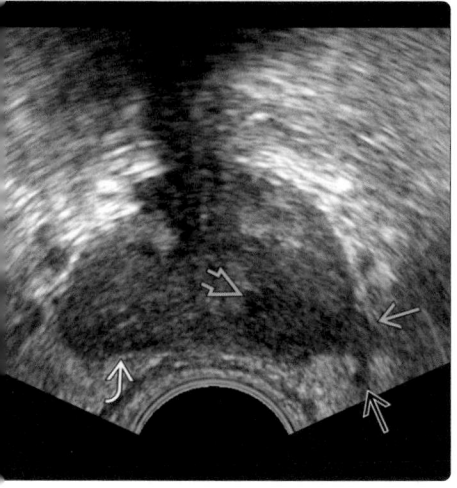
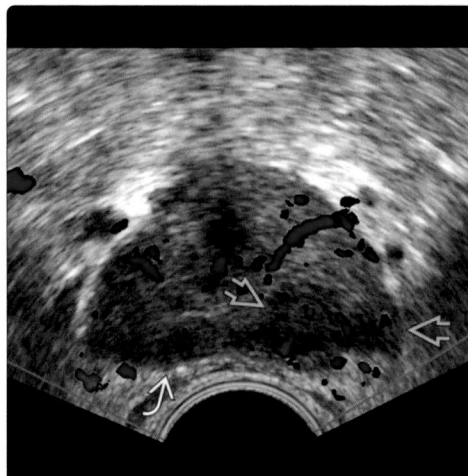

(Left) *Transverse TRUS shows a hypoechoic left PZ lesion* ⇨ *with capsular bulging and nodularity extending into the adjacent fat* ⇨ *and left neurovascular bundle (NVB)* ⇨. *A smaller hypoechoic lesion is seen in the right PZ* ⇨. (Right) *Corresponding Doppler ultrasound shows focal hypervascularity* ⇨ *in the left PZ lesion. The right PZ lesion is mildly hypervascular* ⇨. *Prostatectomy revealed multifocal PCa, including Gleason 5 + 5 adenocarcinoma with left extraprostatic extension and lymphovascular and perineural invasion.*

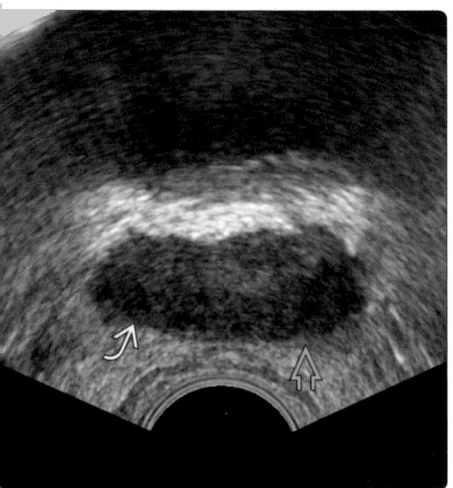
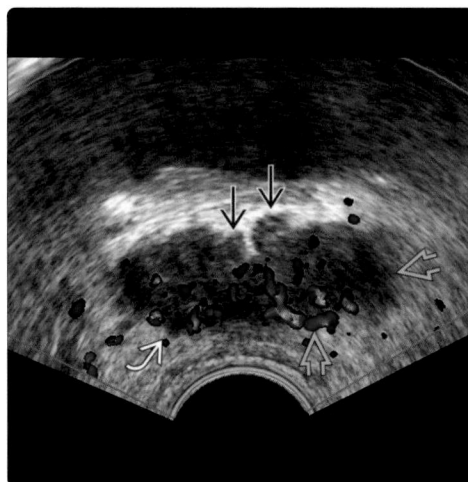

(Left) *Transverse TRUS shows cranial extension of the hypoechoic right* ⇨ *and left* ⇨ *PZ lesions into the base and seminal vesicles (SV) with left focal bulging and contour irregularity.* (Right) *Transverse TRUS, slightly higher at the level of the base and seminal vesicles, shows corresponding hypervascularity in abnormal hypoechoic regions in the right* ⇨ *and left* ⇨ *PZ lesions & SV* ⇨. *Bilateral SV invasion was confirmed at prostatectomy. SV invasion (stage T3B) increases probability of recurrence after treatment.*

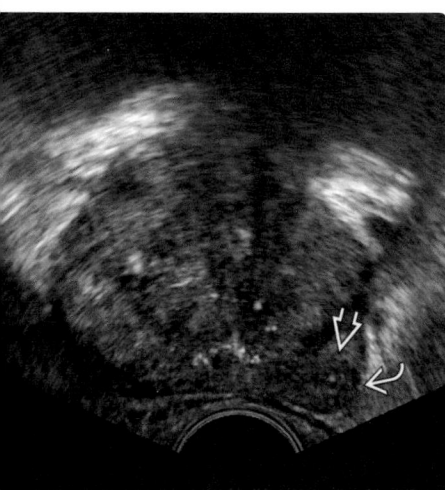
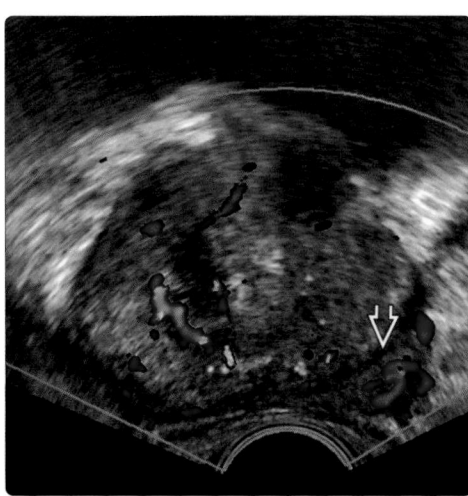

(Left) *Transverse TRUS shows focal hypoechogenicity in the left PZ* ⇨ *with mild bulging of the contour* ⇨. (Right) *Corresponding color Doppler ultrasound shows focal hypervascularity in this region* ⇨. *Pathology from targeted biopsies of this region showed focal prostatitis.*

(Left) *Heterogeneous T2 signal intensity is seen within the transition zone (TZ) with findings of glandular and stromal hyperplasia. The ill-defined homogeneous T2 hypointense region on anterior TZ, consistent with "erased charcoal" sign, is seen. Note BPH nodule with a smoothly marginated T2 dark rim ➡️ uniformly T2-hyperintense PZ ➡️ and neurovascular bundles ➡️.* (Right) *Focal, ill-defined region of homogeneous T2 hypointensity in the anterior TZ corresponds to focal hypervascularity on the color map ➡️.*

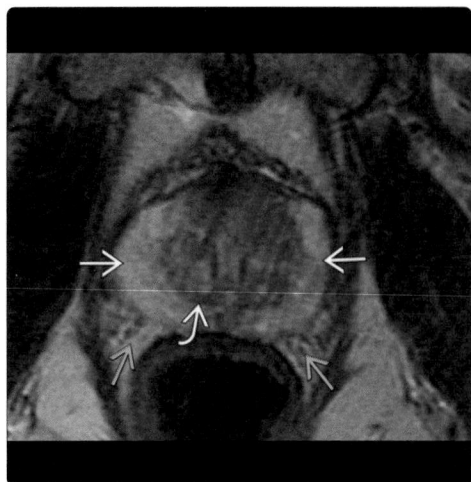
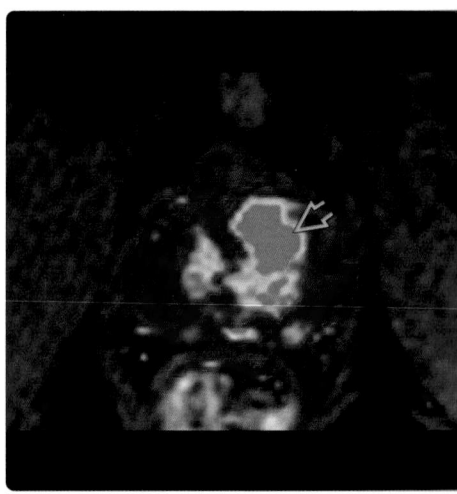

(Left) *Focal, ill-defined region of homogeneous T2 hypointensity and hypervascularity in the anterior TZ shows restricted diffusion ➡️.* (Right) *Corresponding low signal is shown on ADC map ➡️. Targeted MR-US fusion biopsy of this lesion showed Gleason 4 + 4 adenocarcinoma.*

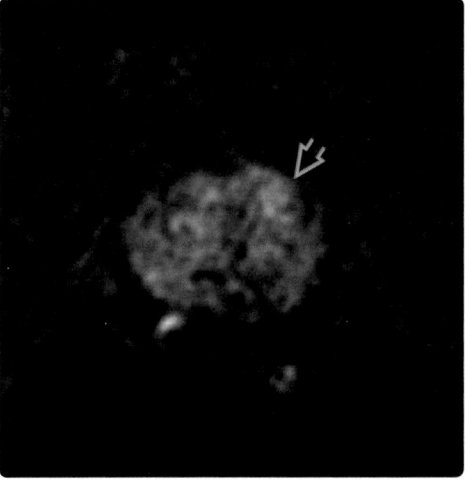
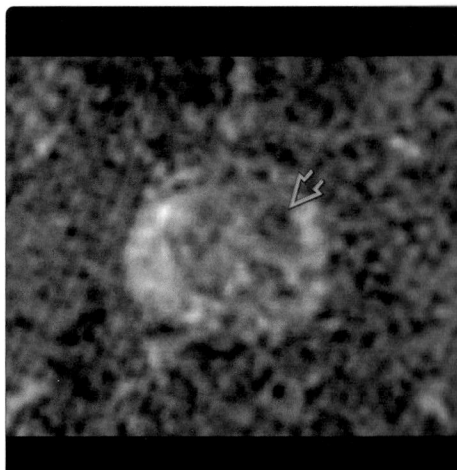

(Left) *Transverse TRUS shows a small, rounded, hypoechoic lesion in the left TZ ➡️. Targeted MR/US fusion biopsy of this lesion revealed benign tissue. Extensive PZ calcifications ➡️ are present.* (Right) *Transverse TRUS in a different patient shows a larger hypoechoic lesion (outlined in red) within the left TZ. Pathology from a targeted MR/US fusion biopsy showed Gleason 4 + 5 adenocarcinoma.*

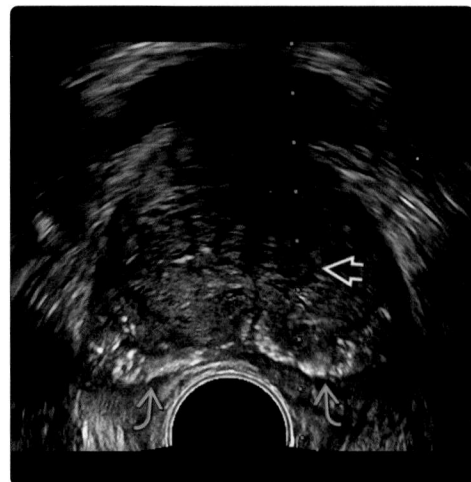
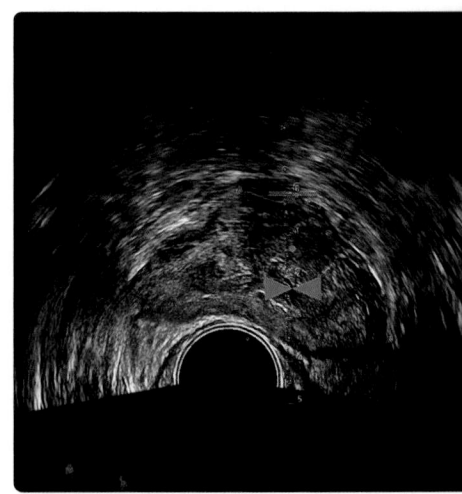

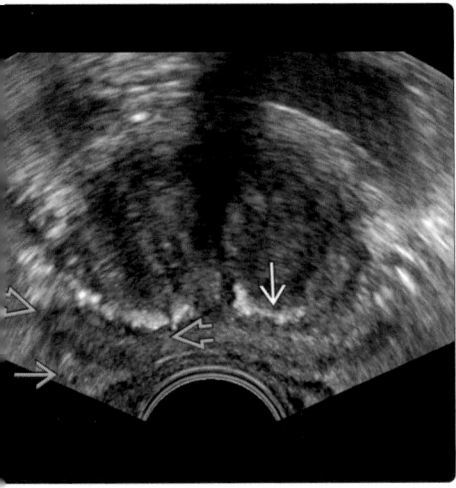

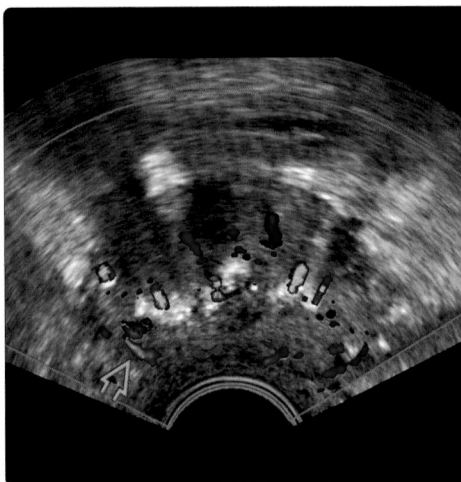

(Left) *Transverse transrectal ultrasound of the mid prostate shows a subtle focal region of hypoechogenicity in the right PZ ⇒. Shadowing calcified corpora amylacea along the surgical capsule ➡ demarcates the boundary between the central gland and PZ. The right neurovascular bundle ⇒ is not involved.* (Right) *Corresponding color Doppler ultrasound shows focal hypervascularity in the right PZ hypoechoic lesion ⇒. Targeted biopsy to this region showed Gleason 3 + 3 adenocarcinoma.*

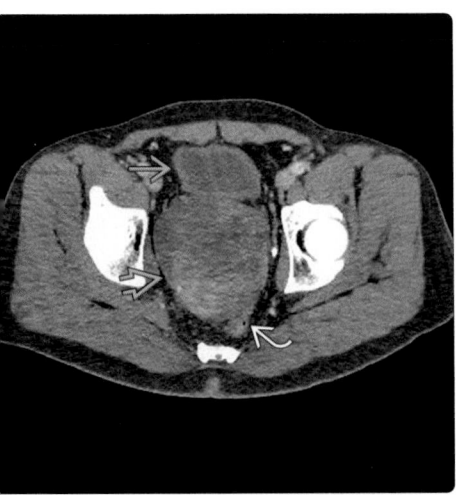

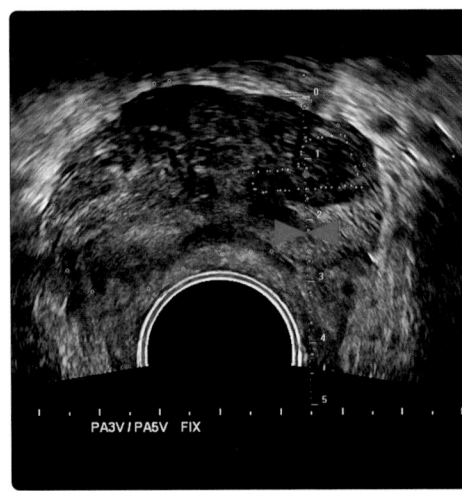

(Left) *Axial CECT shows a large heterogeneously enhancing prostate mass with regions of necrosis ⇒. The urinary bladder ⇒ is separate, and the rectosigmoid colon ➡ is laterally displaced by the mass. Pathology showed spindle cell synovial sarcoma.* (Right) *Transverse transrectal ultrasound shows a focal hypoechoic lesion in the left TZ (partly outlined by dotted yellow line). The ruler corresponds to the biopsy needle path. Pathology from a targeted MR/US fusion biopsy showed Gleason 4 + 4 adenocarcinoma.*

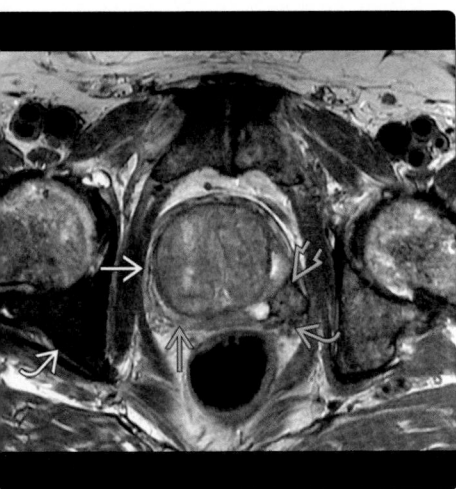

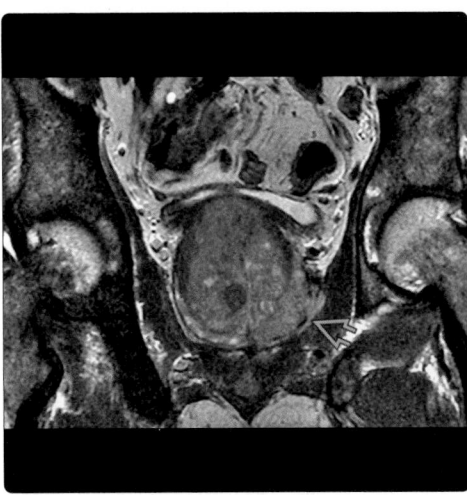

(Left) *Axial T3 MR shows an enlarged prostate with an irregular left PZ mass with extraprostatic extension ⇒ and left NVB invasion ➡. Note: TZ hyperplasia ➡ compressing the PZ ⇒ and heterogeneous bone marrow signal intensity, with markedly hypointense right acetabulum ➡, in keeping with widespread osseous metastases (later shown with bone scan).* (Right) *Coronal T2 MR in same patient shows the left PZ mass with extraprostatic tumor ⇒ indenting the left levator ani, stage 3 prostate cancer.*

Bladder Carcinoma

TERMINOLOGY

- Malignant tumor of bladder (95% transitional cell carcinoma)

IMAGING

- Focal bladder wall thickening with intraluminal extension as a mass on US, CT, or MR
- Grayscale US: Immobile polypoidal or broad-based mass along bladder wall, may present as focal wall thickening
- Color Doppler US shows increased vascularity in large tumors, power Doppler more sensitive in detection of vascularity in small tumors
  - Useful for bladder tumor screening in patients with schistosomiasis, tumor within diverticulum
- CTU: better delineation as intraluminal filling defect, screening upper urinary tract
- MR: T1WI isointense to muscle/bladder wall, T2WI slightly hyperintense to muscle, early post-gadolinium enhancement

- High accuracy for locoregional spread, accuracy of approximately 85% in differentiating nonmuscle invasive from muscle invasive tumor
- ± enlarged (> 10 mm) metastatic lymph nodes

TOP DIFFERENTIAL DIAGNOSES

- Benign prostatic hypertrophy (BPH)
- Bladder debris &/or blood clot
- Extrinsic tumor/mass
- Bladder inflammation

PATHOLOGY

- Superficial (70-80%) and are usually papillary (70%)

CLINICAL ISSUES

- Painless hematuria, may have hydronephrosis

DIAGNOSTIC CHECKLIST

- Check kidneys, ureters for synchronous and metachronous tumors

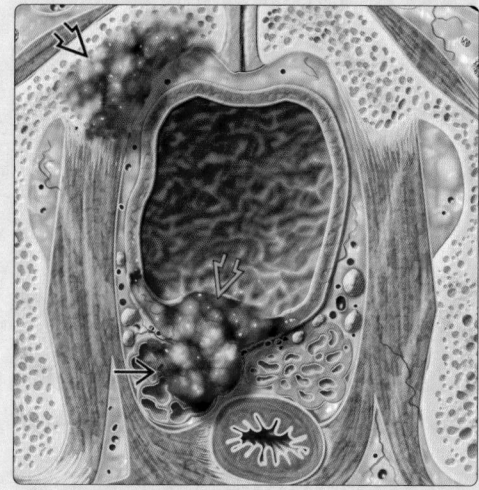 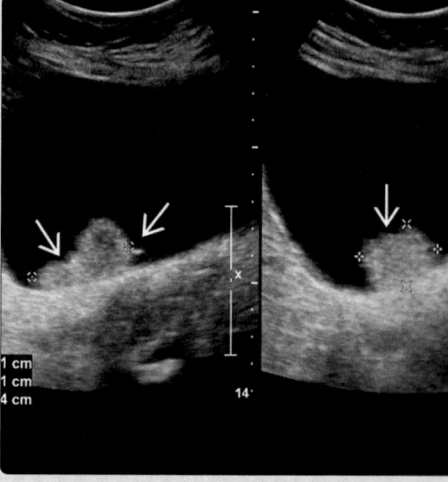

(Left) Graphic shows an irregular bladder tumor ⊘ infiltrating beyond the muscular layer of the bladder wall and invading the right seminal vesicle ⊘. There is a hematogenous metastasis to the right pubic symphysis ⊘. (Right) Transverse and longitudinal transabdominal ultrasound of the bladder shows a broad-based, immobile, polypoidal mass (bladder transitional cell cancer) ⊘.

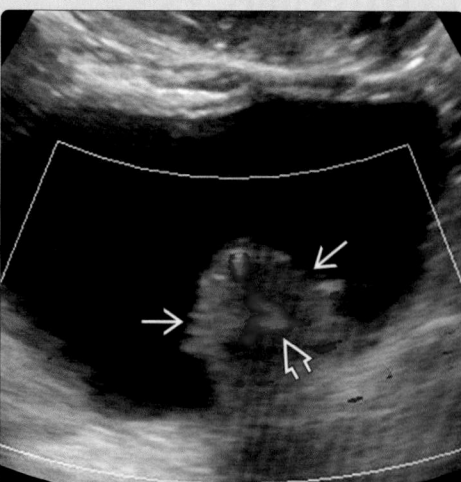 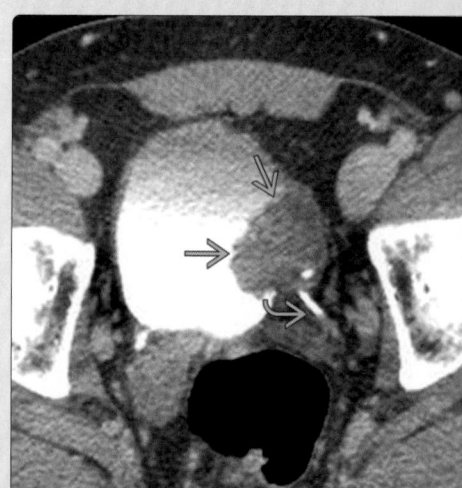

(Left) Transverse transabdominal color Doppler ultrasound of the bladder shows a solid intraluminal mass ⊘ with internal vascularity ⊘ consistent with bladder carcinoma. (Right) Axial CT urography of the pelvis in the same patient confirms the lobulated mass ⊘ arises from the left posterolateral bladder wall. Margins are well-delineated as a filling defect in the contrast-opacified bladder. The left ureter ⊘ is noted.

TERMINOLOGY

Definitions

Malignant tumor of bladder

IMAGING

General Features

Best diagnostic clue
- Focal bladder wall thickening with intraluminal extension as mass on US, CT, or MR

Ultrasonographic Findings

Grayscale ultrasound
- Focal, immobile, polypoid or broad-based mass along bladder wall; may present as focal wall thickening
- Mass may be heterogeneous with mixed echogenicity

Color Doppler
- Color Doppler shows increased vascularity in large tumors, power Doppler may be useful to detect vascularity in small tumors

Reported sensitivities range from 50-90%, with higher sensitivity for tumor > 5 mm

US may be useful in detection of tumor arising from bladder diverticulum, provided diverticulum is optimally fluid filled
- Diverticular tumor may be inaccessible by cystoscopy due to narrow neck of diverticulum

Poor sensitivity in detecting tumors near bladder base in males with prostatic enlargement
- Transrectal ultrasound differentiates bladder tumors from prostatic lesion, although MR has higher sensitivity
- Bladder tumors and prostatic enlargement may coexist and bladder tumors may invade prostate

Transvaginal or transrectal US: To assess bladder wall mass if suprapubic visualization is poor
- Poor transabdominal visualization may be due to obesity, scars on wall, and poor bladder distension

Recent advances: 3D US rendering may help to discriminate between superficial and muscle invasive carcinoma
- Contrast-enhanced ultrasound has shown higher accuracy than baseline ultrasound

Negative ultrasound in patient with hematuria and no identified renal/bladder stone does not exclude bladder cancer

Radiographic Findings

IVP
- Currently less commonly used
- Scout radiograph may show punctate or speckled calcification on fronds of villous, papillary tumors, and linear calcification in sessile tumor
- Nonspecific filling defects within bladder
- May be used to detect upper tract disease

Cystography
- ± bladder diverticulum (2-10% contain neoplasm)

CT Findings

Sessile or pedunculated soft tissue mass projecting into lumen with post-contrast enhancement
- CTU better delineation as intraluminal filling defect

- ± enlarged (> 10 mm) metastatic lymph nodes; extravesical tumor extension
- Fine punctate calcification in tumor; may suggest mucinous adenocarcinoma
- Ring pattern of calcification; may suggest pheochromocytoma
- Poor accuracy for locoregional spread
- Sensitivity of 85% and specificity of 94% for detecting bladder tumor
- False-negatives with flat lesion, < 1 cm, local inflammation, fibrosis, scar tissue
- Urachal adenocarcinoma-lobulated mass arising from midline ventral dome of bladder with exophytic component

MR Findings

- T1WI
  - Tumor has intermediate signal intensity (isointense to bladder wall)
  - Bone marrow metastases; similar signal intensity as primary tumor
- T2WI
  - Tumor has slightly higher signal than bladder wall or muscle, lower than urine
  - Invasion of prostate, seminal vesicle, rectum, uterus, vagina: ↑ signal intensity
  - T2 images helpful in determination of tumor infiltration of perivesical fat
  - Confirm bone marrow metastases
- DWI
  - More accurate than T2WI for organ-confined and higher-stage tumors
  - Low ADC value suggests high-grade tumor; may be used to assess early treatment response with increased ADC value
- T1WI C+
  - Early enhancement relative to bladder wall
  - Hyperenhancement of perivesical infiltration, including nodal and bone invasion
- ± enlarged (> 10 mm) metastatic lymph nodes
- Unable to differentiate stage T1 from stage T2, acute edema or hyperemia from 1st week post biopsy
- High accuracy for locoregional spread; accuracy ~ 85% in differentiating nonmuscle-invasive from muscle-invasive tumor

Imaging Recommendations

- Best imaging tool
  - US: Useful for bladder tumor screening in patients with schistosomiasis, tumor within diverticulum
  - CTU: Screening upper urinary tract
  - MR: Preferred modality for local staging

DIFFERENTIAL DIAGNOSIS

Benign Prostatic Hypertrophy (BPH)

- Enlarged median lobe of prostate may appear as irregular mass lying free within bladder in some planes
- On angling transducer caudad, enlarged prostatic median lobe can be shown to be part of prostate gland

Bladder Sludge/Blood Clot

- Mobile avascular nonshadowing intraluminal mass

Extrinsic Tumor/Mass

- Rectal, ovarian, vaginal tumor or fibroids overlying bladder; may simulate bladder carcinoma (CT/MR helpful)

Bladder Inflammation

- Cystitis may cause diffuse wall thickening and internal debris
  - Asymmetric bladder wall should be viewed with suspicion for tumor

PATHOLOGY

General Features

- Etiology
  - Risk factors
    - Environment: Smoking (most common association)
    - Infection: Schistosomiasis, chronic cystitis
    - Iatrogenic: Cyclophosphamide, radiation therapy
    - Occupation: Chemical, dye (e.g., aniline dye), rubber and textile industries
- 95% of bladder neoplasms are malignant
- Types of bladder carcinoma
  - Transitional cell carcinoma (90-95%), a.k.a. urothelial cancer
  - Squamous cell carcinoma (5%)
  - Adenocarcinoma (2%): Urachal origin, secondary to cystitis glandularis, or secondary to extrophy
  - Carcinosarcoma
  - Other rare tumors: Carcinoid, rhabdoid, small cell, metastases (GI tract, melanoma)
- Types of nonepithelial bladder carcinoma
  - Pheochromocytoma
  - Leiomyosarcoma
  - Embryonal rhabdomyosarcoma (most common bladder neoplasm in children)
  - Lymphoma

Staging, Grading, & Classification

- TNM classification of bladder carcinoma
  - T0: No tumor
  - Tis: Carcinoma in situ
  - Ta: Papillary tumor confined to mucosa (epithelium)
  - T1: Invasion of lamina propria (subepithelial connective tissue)
  - T2: Invasion of inner half of muscle (detrusor)
  - T2b: Invasion of outer half of muscle
  - T3a: Microscopic invasion of perivesical fat
  - T3b: Macroscopic invasion of perivesical fat
  - T4a: Invasion of surrounding organs
  - T4b: Invasion of pelvic or abdominal wall
  - N1-3: Pelvic lymph node metastases
  - N4: Lymph node metastases above bifurcation
  - M1: Distant metastases

Gross Pathologic & Surgical Features

- Superficial (70-80%) and are usually papillary (70%)
- Invasive (20-30%), infiltrating in/beyond muscular layer of wall

CLINICAL ISSUES

Presentation

- Most common signs/symptoms
  - Painless microscopic or macroscopic hematuria
  - Tumor involving ureterovesical junction → hydronephrosis (flank pain); urethral orifice → urinary retention

Demographics

- Age
  - 50-60 years of age
  - Increasing incidence in patients < 30 years of age
- Gender
  - M:F = 4:1
- Ethnicity
  - Caucasian to African American ratio = 1.5:1

Natural History & Prognosis

- Complications
  - Hydronephrosis, incontinence, and urethral stricture
- Prognosis
  - 5-year survival rate: 82% in all stages combined
    - 94% in localized stages
    - 48% in regional stages
    - 6% in distant stages

Treatment

- < T2: Local endoscopic resection ± intravesical instillation of bacille Calmette-Guérin (BCG) therapy
- T2 to T4a: Radical cystectomy or radiotherapy (cure)
- > T4b: Chemotherapy or radiotherapy ± adjuvant surgery (palliative)

DIAGNOSTIC CHECKLIST

Consider

- Immobile soft tissue mass in bladder ± vascularity
- Distinction of benign from malignant tumor by cystoscopy ± biopsy
- CT/MR used for staging for treatment and prognosis
- Check kidneys, ureters for synchronous and metachronous tumors

Image Interpretation Pearls

- MR is superior in locoregional staging and used in patients with high-grade stage T1 or > stage T2

SELECTED REFERENCES

1. Hafeez S et al: Advances in bladder cancer imaging. BMC Med. 11:104, 2013
2. Verma S et al: Urinary bladder cancer: role of MR imaging. Radiographics. 32(2):371-87, 2012
3. Nicolau C et al: Accuracy of contrast-enhanced ultrasound in the detection of bladder cancer. Br J Radiol. 84(1008):1091-9, 2011
4. Tekes A et al: Dynamic MRI of bladder cancer: evaluation of staging accuracy. AJR Am J Roentgenol. 184(1):121-7, 2005
5. Wagner B et al: Staging bladder carcinoma by three-dimensional ultrasound rendering. Ultrasound Med Biol. 31(3):301-5, 2005
6. Koraitim M et al: Transurethral ultrasonographic assessment of bladder carcinoma: its value and limitation. J Urol. 154(2 Pt 1):375-8, 1995
7. Kim B et al: Bladder tumor staging: comparison of contrast-enhanced CT, T1 and T2-weighted MR imaging, dynamic gadolinium-enhanced imaging, and late gadolinium-enhanced imaging. Radiology. 193(1):239-45, 1994

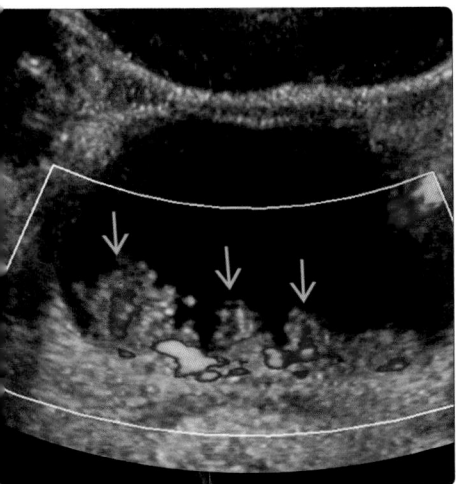
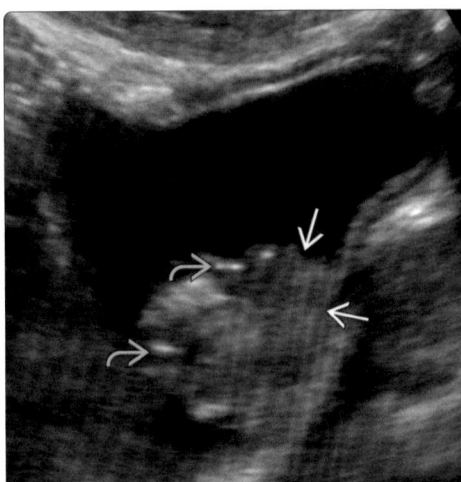

(Left) *Transverse transabdominal power Doppler ultrasound shows multiple immobile, vascular, polypoid masses* ➡ *arising from the urinary bladder consistent with bladder carcinoma.* **(Right)** *Longitudinal transabdominal ultrasound of the bladder shows a polypoid, intraluminal bladder carcinoma* ➡ *with punctate calcifications* ➡.

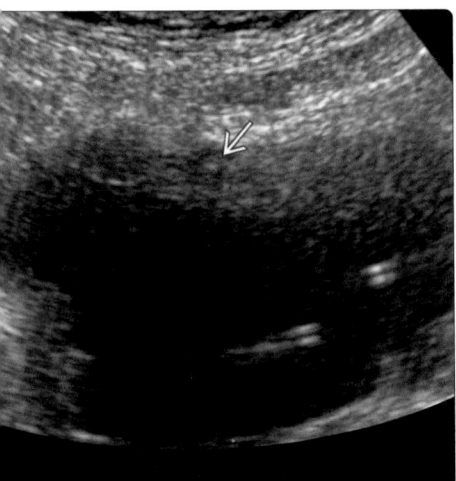
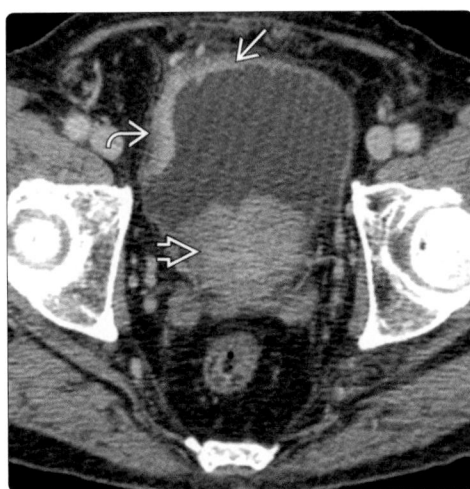

(Left) *Transverse transabdominal ultrasound shows biopsy-proven bladder cancer seen as focal areas of wall thickening over the lateral and anterior wall* ➡ *of the urinary bladder.* **(Right)** *Transverse CECT in the same patient shows the lateral* ➡ *and anterior bladder wall* ➡ *thickening proven to represent bladder cancer. Note benign hypertrophy of the prostate* ➡ *at the base of the urinary bladder.*

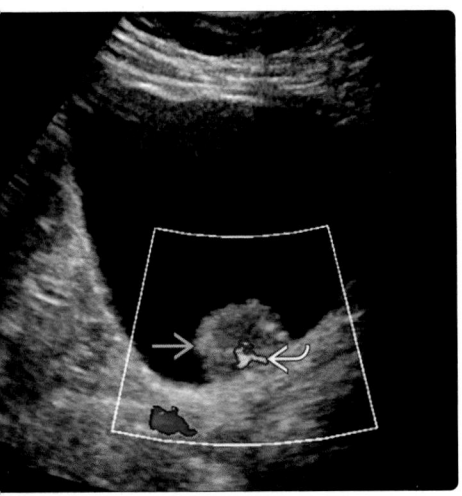
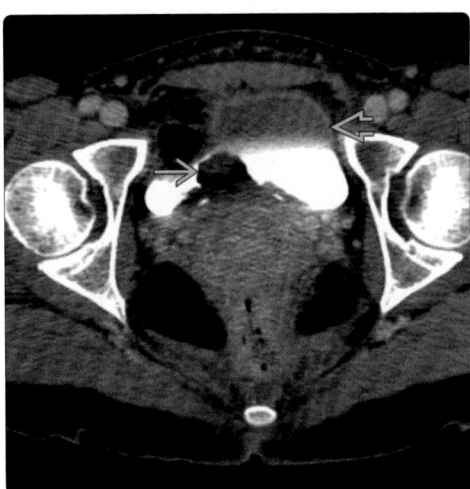

(Left) *Longitudinal color Doppler transabdominal ultrasound of the bladder shows a intraluminal bladder cancer* ➡ *with internal vascularity* ➡. **(Right)** *Axial CT urography through pelvis in the same patient confirms the bladder cancer as a large filling defect* ➡ *in a contrast-opacified bladder* ➡.

Ureterocele

KEY FACTS

TERMINOLOGY

- Cystic balloon-like dilatation of intramural portion of distal ureter bulging into bladder
- **Orthotopic ureterocele (less common)**: Normal insertion at trigone and otherwise normal ureter
- **Ectopic ureterocele (more common)**: Inserts below trigone
- Duplicated collecting system in 80%

IMAGING

- Ectopic: 50% in bladder and 50% in posterior urethra; 10% bilateral
- US/CT: Thin-walled, cystic intravesical mass continuous with distal ureter
- Changes in size with degree of ureteral dilation
- Dilated ureter in ectopic lower moiety, changes in size with degree of ureteral dilation
- IVP/cystogram: Orthotopic ureterocele: Cobra-head deformity

- ○ Drooping lily sign: Displacement of reflux opacified lower pole moiety by dilated upper pole moiety
- T2W MR: Superior to demonstrate ectopic ureter extending from poorly functioning moiety invisible on other imaging
- US: Obtain images when bladder is reasonably full
- Cystogram: Images during early bladder filling; overfilling may collapse, obscure, or invert low-pressure ureterocele

PATHOLOGY

- Single system ectopic ureteroceles: Associated with cardiac and genital anomalies
- Complete duplicated system: Commonly upper moiety ureter associated with ureterocele

DIAGNOSTIC CHECKLIST

- Look for ureterocele in reasonably full bladder if duplex renal system detected

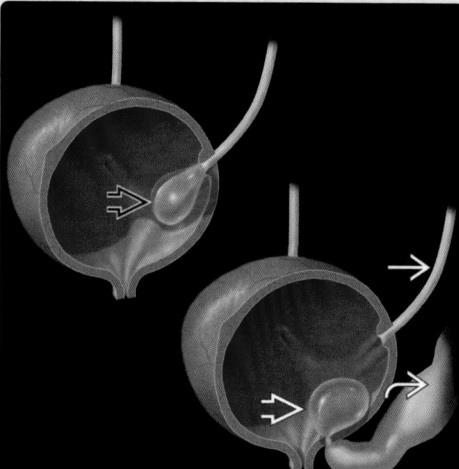
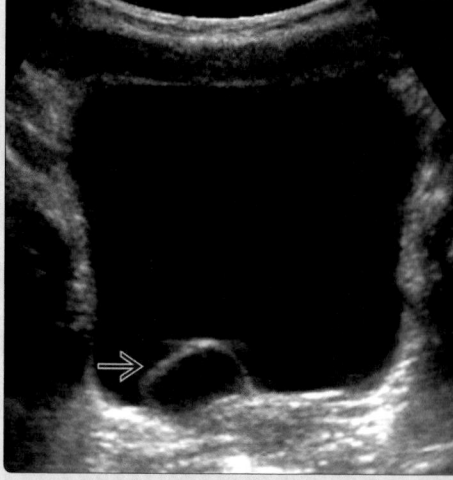

(Left) Upper graphic shows orthotopic ureterocele ⇨ at trigone in single system. Lower graphic shows ectopic ureterocele ⇥ with hydroureter ⇥ of the upper moiety, inserting inferior and medial to the lower moiety ureter ⇥ in duplex system. (Right) Transabdominal transverse ultrasound of the pelvis shows typical ureterocele ⇨ as a balloon-like cyst within the urinary bladder.

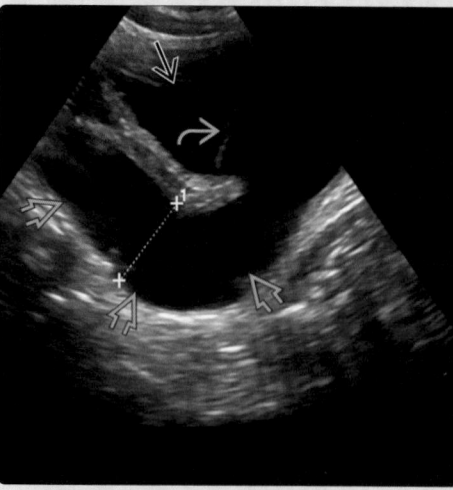
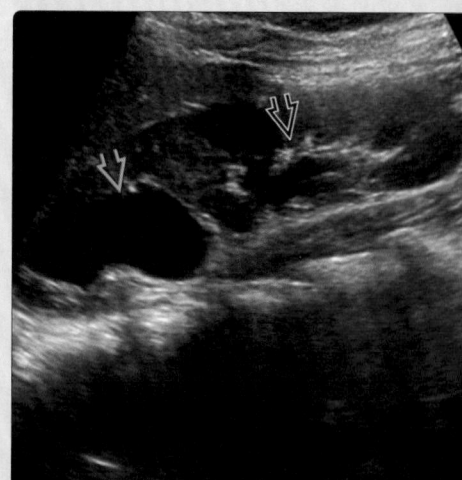

(Left) Transabdominal longitudinal oblique ultrasound shows a typical ureteric duplex system associated with a ureterocele ⇨ within the bladder ⇥ at the distal end of the upper pole moiety ureter. The ureter is dilated ⇥. (Right) Transabdominal longitudinal ultrasound through the right kidney in the same patient shows duplex collecting system with dilated upper moiety ⇥ and nondilated lower moiety ⇥.

TERMINOLOGY

Definitions

Cystic balloon-like dilatation of intramural portion of distal ureter bulging into bladder

Orthotopic ureterocele (less common): Normal insertion at trigone and otherwise normal ureter
- Single ureter system
- Bilateral in ~ 30% cases

Ectopic ureterocele (more common): Inserts below trigone
- Duplicated collecting system in 80%
  - Upper moiety ureter often inserts medial and distal to superior moiety ureter
  - Male: Insertion at bladder neck, prostatic urethra, vas deferens, or seminal vesicle
    - No wetting in males as insertion always above external sphincter
  - Female: Insertion in distal urethra, vaginal vestibule, vagina, cervix, uterus, or fallopian tube
    - Wetting in females only if insertion below external sphincter
- Single nonduplicated system in 20%
  - Small/poorly functioning kidney, may be invisible on imaging
- Cecoureterocele: Ectopic submucosal ureterocele extending to urethra, with intravesical opening

IMAGING

General Features

Best diagnostic clue
- Orthotopic: Thin-walled sac-like cystic structure continuous with distal ureter
- Ectopic: Continuous with hydronephrotic obstructive (usually upper) moiety and hydroureter in duplex system

Location
- Ectopic: 50% in bladder and 50% in posterior urethra; 10% bilateral
  - Males: Insertion always above external sphincter

Size
- 1 to a few cm in diameter

Morphology
- Smooth, round, or ovoid

Ultrasonographic Findings

Grayscale ultrasound
- Thin-walled, cystic intravesical mass continuous with distal ureter
- Dilated ureter in ectopic lower moiety, changes in size with degree of ureteral dilation
- Midline intravesical tubular structure may be seen, leading to outlet obstruction (cecoureterocele)
- Occasionally, in full bladder, ureteroceles may invert, giving an appearance similar to diverticulum
  - Inverted ureterocele reverts to its usual appearance upon partial emptying of bladder
- Wall thickening secondary to edema from impacted stone/infection
- Ectopic ureteroceles inserting outside bladder mimic pelvic cyst

- Color Doppler
  - Demonstrates ureteric jet from tip of ureterocele

Radiographic Findings

- Intravenous pyelogram (IVP)/cystography
  - Orthotopic ureterocele: Cobra-head deformity
    - Ballooned distal ureter projecting into lumen of bladder with surrounding radiolucent halo
  - Ectopic ureterocele: Smooth, radiolucent intravesicular mass mostly near bladder base
    - May evert during voiding and mimic diverticulum
    - Lumen opacification depends on function of upper pole moiety
    - Drooping lily sign: Displacement of reflux opacified lower pole moiety by dilated upper pole moiety
    - Voiding cystourethrogram may also show reflux in lower pole moiety in duplex system

CT Findings

- CECT
  - Thin-walled intravesicular cystic mass at ureterovesical junction (UVJ)

MR Findings

- T2WI
  - Intravesicular cystic mass at UVJ
    - Ectopic: May see ectopic insertion into bladder neck, urethra, vagina, etc.
  - Maximum-intensity projection (MIP) image demonstrates relative positions of upper and lower moiety ureters in duplex system
    - Superior to demonstrate ectopic ureter extending from poorly functioning moiety invisible on other imaging
    - Ureterocele may be masked by fluid within urinary bladder
- Contrast-enhanced MR urography
  - Best for detection of ureterocele in duplex system
  - Intravesicular cyst filled by contrast with surrounding halo within bladder during early filling phase
  - Continuous with hydronephrotic upper moiety and hydroureter if function of upper pole moiety preserved
  - Poor or no excretion by upper pole of duplex kidney if dysplastic

Imaging Recommendations

- Best imaging tool
  - US and CT/MR Urography
- Protocol advice
  - US: Obtain images when bladder is reasonably full
  - Cystogram: Image during early bladder filling; overfilling may collapse, obscure, or invert low-pressure ureterocele

DIFFERENTIAL DIAGNOSIS

Foley Catheter

- Characteristic shape of Foley catheter with round distal balloon in bladder

Pseudoureterocele

- From distal ureteral obstruction (stone or tumor), thicker poorly defined halo/lucency around distal ureter

Prolapsing Ureterocele: Vaginal Mass in Females

- Bladder diverticulum: Indistinguishable from everted ureterocele
  - Sac formed by herniation of bladder mucosa, connects to bladder cavity via neck
  - Does not return to intravesical position after micturition
- Gartner duct cyst: Cyst in vaginal wall
  - Transvaginal US defines origin

PATHOLOGY

General Features

- Etiology
  - Congenital anomaly
  - Simple type: Secondary to obstruction or stricture (adults) at terminal ureter
- Associated abnormalities
  - Single system ectopic ureteroceles: Cardiac and genital anomalies
  - Complete duplicated system: Commonly upper moiety ureter associated with ureterocele
    - Obstruction leading to hydronephrosis and hydroureter
    - Occasional dysplastic small upper pole moiety with hydroureter
    - Lower pole moiety ureter has orthotopic insertion associated with hydronephrosis due to reflux (Weigert-Meyer rule)

Staging, Grading, & Classification

- Orifice type: Stenotic, sphincteric, sphincterostenotic, cecoureterocele
  - Sphincteric: Orifice distal to bladder neck
  - Cecoureterocele: Intravesical orifice; submucosal extension to urethra

Gross Pathologic & Surgical Features

- Simple ureteroceles: Pinpoint orifices but no significant obstruction
- Ectopic ureteroceles: Often obstructed, with dysplasia of upper pole kidney
- Ureteric orifice, which is narrowed, usually opens at tip, occasionally at base
- Sometimes portion of ureter extends distal to ureterocele to open in ectopic position in bladder or urethra

Microscopic Features

- Thin wall: Covered by bladder mucosa and lined by ureteral mucosa
- Less common: Mucosal layer only or mucosal and thin muscularis layer

CLINICAL ISSUES

Presentation

- Most common signs/symptoms
  - Orthotopic: Usually asymptomatic; incidental finding
  - Ectopic ureteroceles: UTI, incontinence, vaginal mass
- Other signs/symptoms
  - Rarely, prolapse into bladder neck/urethra, causing obstruction
- Clinical profile
  - Ectopic: Infant or child with UTI or sepsis

Demographics

- Age
  - Ectopic: Median age 3 months at diagnosis
    - Often diagnosed with prenatal ultrasound
- Gender
  - Ectopic ureterocele with duplicated system M:F = 1:4
- Epidemiology
  - US: 1:12,000-1:5,000

Natural History & Prognosis

- Severe obstruction: Primarily ectopic ureteroceles
  - Dysplasia of obstructed upper pole moiety in complete duplex system

Treatment

- Options, risks, complications
  - Obstructed ureteroceles may cause stasis and stone formation

DIAGNOSTIC CHECKLIST

Consider

- Look for ureterocele in reasonably full bladder if duplex renal system detected
- Big ureterocele may occupy the entire bladder mimicking bladder itself, especially if bladder is empty

Image Interpretation Pearls

- Long axis of ectopic ureterocele points to side of origin

SELECTED REFERENCES

1. Adeb M et al: Magnetic resonance urography in evaluation of duplicated renal collecting systems. Magn Reson Imaging Clin N Am. 21(4):717-30, 201
2. Shebel HM et al: Cysts of the lower male genitourinary tract: embryologic and anatomic considerations and differential diagnosis. Radiographics. 33(4):1125-43, 2013
3. Esfahani SA et al: Precise delineation of ureterocele anatomy: virtual magnetic resonance cystoscopy. Abdom Imaging. 36(6):765-70, 2011
4. Taori K et al: Prolapsed simple ureterocele: evaluation by transvaginal voiding sono-urethrography. J Clin Ultrasound. 39(9):544-7, 2011
5. Zougkas K et al: Assessment of obstruction in adult ureterocele by means of color Doppler duplex sonography. Urol Int. 75(3):239-46, 2005
6. Bolduc S et al: The predictive value of diagnostic imaging for histological lesions of the upper poles in duplex systems with ureteroceles. BJU Int. 91(7):678-82, 2003
7. do Nascimento H et al: Magnetic resonance in diagnosis of ureterocele. Int Braz J Urol. 29(3):248-50, 2003
8. Shimoya K et al: Diagnosis of ureterocele with transvaginal sonography. Gynecol Obstet Invest. 54(1):58-60, 2002
9. Madeb R et al: Evaluation of ureterocele with Doppler sonography. J Clin Ultrasound. 28(8):425-9, 2000
10. Zerin JM et al: Single-system ureteroceles in infants and children: imaging features. Pediatr Radiol. 30(3):139-46, 2000
11. Davidson AJ et al: Radiology of the kidney and genitourinary tract. 3rd ed. Philadelphia, W.B. Saunders. 213-6, 1999
12. Abrahamsson K et al: Bladder dysfunction: an integral part of the ectopic ureterocele complex. J Urol. 160(4):1468-70, 1998

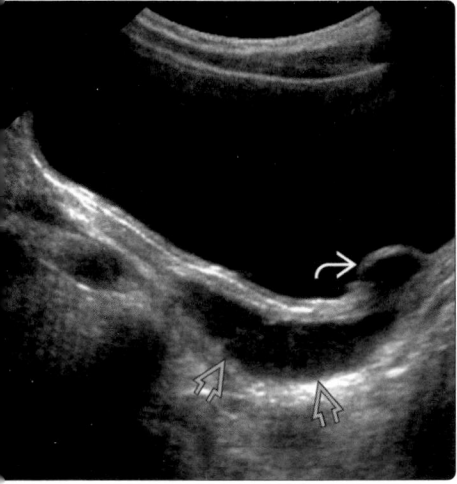

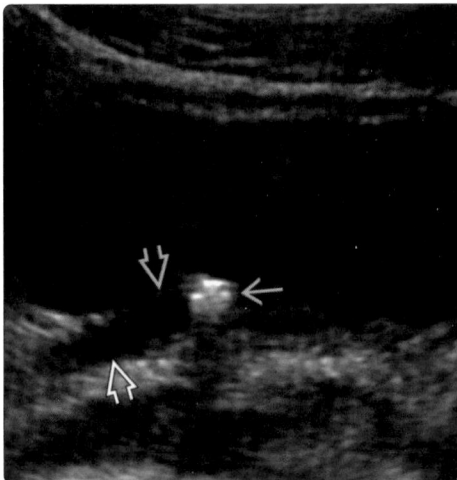

(Left) *Transabdominal longitudinal ultrasound shows a small ureterocele* ⇒ *with upstream ureteral dilation* ⇒. (**Right**) *Transverse oblique transabdominal ultrasound shows an echogenic stone impacted at the right ureterovesical junction* ⇒ *with upstream ureteral dilation* ⇒. *Focal bulge at the intramural segment of the ureter is compatible with pseudoureterocele* ⇒.

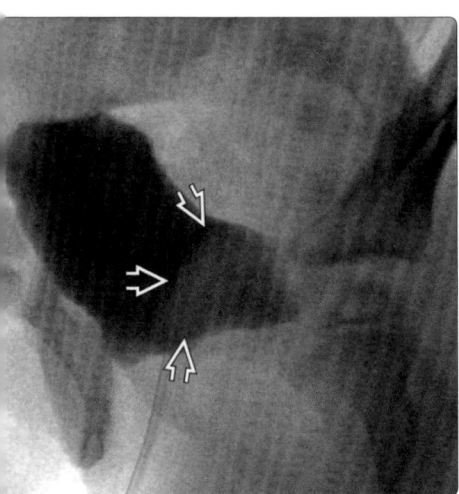

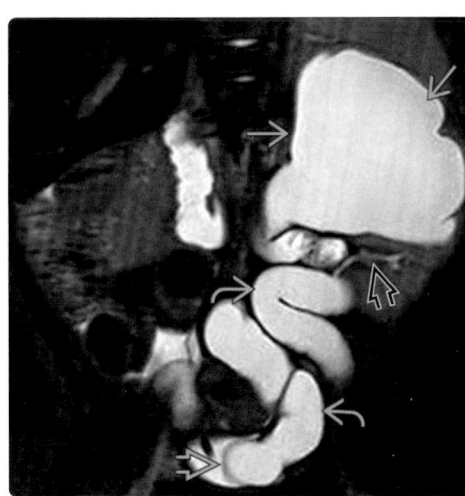

(Left) *Voiding cystourethrogram shows a round filling defect* ⇒ *within the urinary bladder compatible with a ureterocele.* (**Right**) *Coronal heavily T2-weighted MR shows left renal duplex collecting system with dilated upper moiety* ⇒ *and decompressed lower moiety* ⇒. *The upper moiety is seen continuous with significantly dilated and tortuous ureter* ⇒ *seen terminating in an intravesical ureterocele* ⇒.

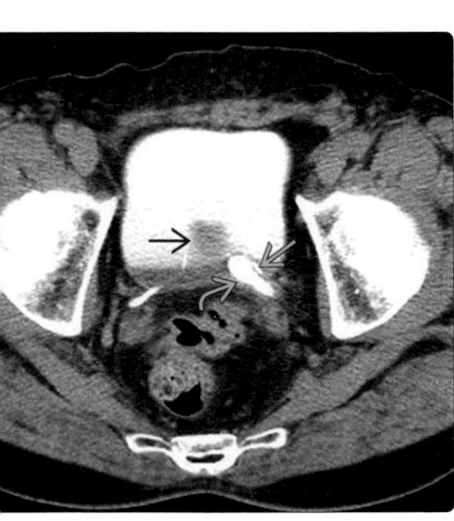

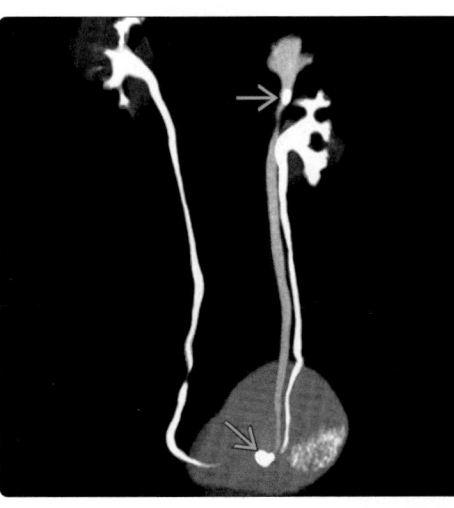

(Left) *Axial CT urogram through the pelvis shows left duplex system with the upper moiety terminating in a ureterocele* ⇒ *that contained calculi. The lower moiety ureter is nondilated and seen terminating adjacent to the ureterocele* ⇒. *Note the prostatic impression at the bladder base* ⇒. (**Right**) *3D reformatted MIP image of the CT Urogram (posterior view) shows the duplicated left collecting system with calculi in the ureteropelvic junction* ⇒ *and in the ureterocele of upper moiety.*

Bladder Diverticulum

TERMINOLOGY

- Saccular outpouching from herniation of bladder mucosa and submucosa through muscular wall of bladder

IMAGING

- Most commonly near ureterovesical junction (UVJ)
- US: Anechoic outpouching from bladder with narrow or wide neck, may empty with micturition
- May contain calculi, hematoma, or tumor
- Color Doppler shows ureteral jet to and from diverticulum to bladder
- CT/MR: Fluid attenuation outpouching from bladder
- Usually fills with contrast on excretory post-contrast phase

TOP DIFFERENTIAL DIAGNOSES

- Urachus
- Everted ureterocele
- Paraovarian cysts in female
- Pelvic cysts in male

PATHOLOGY

- Acquired: Most common secondary to chronic bladder outlet obstruction (60%)
- Congenital: Hutch diverticulum (40%)
- Vesicoureteral reflux (VUR)

CLINICAL ISSUES

- Narrow-neck diverticula: Urinary stasis → complications such as infection, stone, and ureteral obstruction
- Secondary inflammation predisposes to development of carcinoma within diverticulum
- Complications
  - Carcinoma
  - Vesicoureteral reflux
  - Ureteral obstruction

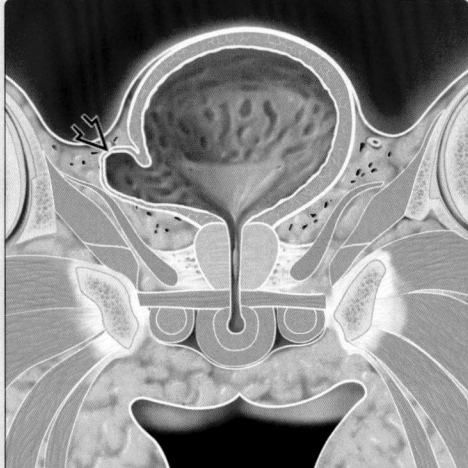
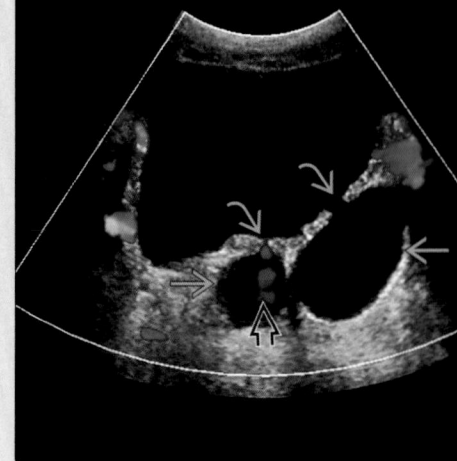

(Left) Graphic shows a diverticulum ⇨ arising from the lateral bladder wall, due to herniation of the mucosa and submucosa through the muscular wall. (Right) Transabdominal transverse oblique ultrasound of the urinary bladder shows 2 left posterolateral diverticula ⇨ with narrow necks ⇨. One of the diverticula shows a urinary jet as Doppler signal into the diverticulum ⇨.

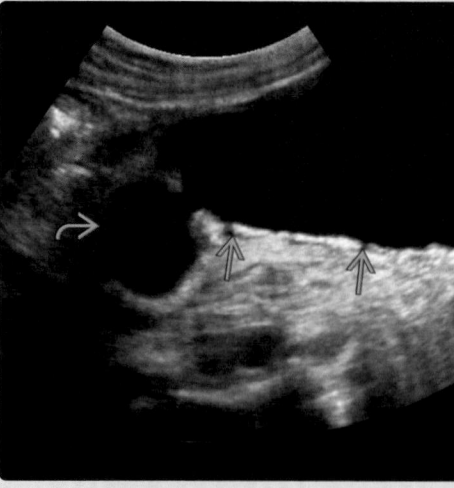
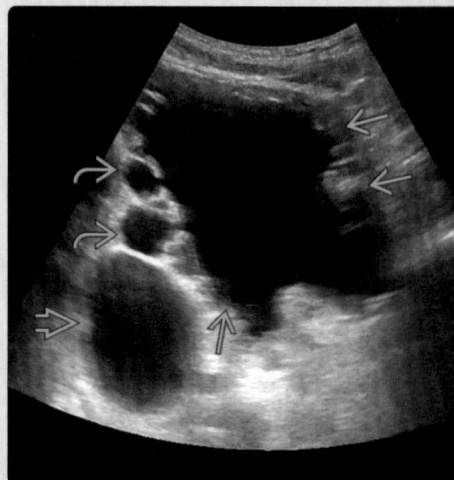

(Left) Transabdominal longitudinal oblique ultrasound of the urinary bladder shows a posterior wall diverticulum ⇨. Note mild wall trabeculation of the bladder ⇨ in this patient with prostatomegaly resulting in chronic bladder outlet obstruction. (Right) Transabdominal transverse oblique ultrasound in a patient with neurogenic urinary bladder shows a trabeculated bladder wall ⇨ with multiple small ⇨ and 1 large diverticula ⇨.

Bladder Diverticulum

TERMINOLOGY

Abbreviations
Bladder diverticula/outpouching

Definitions
Saccular outpouching from herniation of bladder mucosa and submucosa through muscular wall of bladder
Communicates with bladder lumen via wide or narrow neck

IMAGING

General Features
Best diagnostic clue
o Perivesical cystic mass with communication to bladder lumen
Location
o Most commonly near ureterovesical junction (UVJ)
Size
o Variable size; can exceed size of bladder
Morphology
o Single or multiple
o Smooth wall

Ultrasonographic Findings
Grayscale ultrasound
o Anechoic outpouching from bladder with narrow or wide neck
o May empty with micturition
o Internal echogenicity of diverticulum varies depending on its contents
o May contain calculi, hematoma, or tumor
Color Doppler
o Urine may be seen flowing into and out of diverticulum
  − Color Doppler jet connecting bladder to diverticulum very useful to distinguish diverticulum from other paravesical masses
  − Power Doppler may show vascularity within tumors that can mimic bladder diverticulum

Radiographic Findings
IVP
o Opacifies with excreted contrast unless obstructed
o Medial deviation of ipsilateral ureter
o Intraluminal stones, debris, or tumor appear as filling defects
Cystogram
o Oblique films may show configuration of diverticulum neck

Fluoroscopic Findings
Voiding cystourethrogram
o Rarely used, evaluates diverticulum if ultrasound cannot differentiate it from pelvic/adnexal cyst

CT Findings
CECT
o Fluid attenuation outpouching from bladder
o Usually fills with contrast on excretory phase (CT urogram)

MR Findings
T1WI
o Exophytic low-intensity mass isointense to urine
T2WI
o High signal mass contiguous with bladder
o May see dephasing with motion of urine flowing between it and bladder lumen

Imaging Recommendations
• Best imaging tool
  o Ultrasound, CT urogram
• Protocol advice
  o Check emptying of diverticulum on post-void studies

DIFFERENTIAL DIAGNOSIS

Urachus
• Cord-like embryonic remnant that connects anterior bladder dome with umbilicus
• Characteristic midline position
• Depending on patency can be seen as diverticulum, cyst, or fistula

Everted Ureterocele
• Continuous with ureter
• Assumes its more usual appearance of bulging into bladder upon partial bladder emptying

Paraovarian Cysts in Female
• Vestigial remnant of Wolffian duct in mesosalpinx
• No communication with bladder
• No change with micturition

Pelvic Cysts in Male
• Transrectal US defines origins and shows no communication with bladder
• Prostatic utricle cyst
  o Dilatation of prostatic utricle
  o Midline
  o Associated with urogenital anomalies
• Müllerian cyst
  o Arise from remnants of müllerian duct
  o May extend lateral to midline
• Seminal vesicle cyst
  o Wolffian duct anomaly
  o Usually large and solitary

PATHOLOGY

General Features
• Etiology
  o Acquired: Most common secondary to chronic bladder outlet obstruction (60%)
    − Associated with weakening of muscle layers from long-standing bladder outlet obstruction
    − **Children**
      □ Posterior urethral valves
      □ Large ureterocele
      □ Neurogenic bladder
      □ Bladder neck stenosis
    − **Adults**
      □ Secondary to prostatic enlargement
      □ Post-traumatic urethral stricture
      □ Neurogenic bladder

– May occur anywhere
  □ Most common near ureteric orifices
– Associated with syndromes
  □ Prune-belly syndrome
  □ Ehlers-Danlos
  □ Menkes kinky-hair syndrome
  □ Diamond-Blackfan syndrome
○ Congenital: Hutch diverticulum (40%)
  – Weakness in detrusor muscle in paraureteric region
  – Associated ± vesicoureteric reflux
● Associated abnormalities
  ○ Vesicoureteral reflux (VUR)

Gross Pathologic & Surgical Features

● Bladder mucosa and submucosa herniates through weak areas in wall
● Typically located at areas of congenital weakness of muscular wall at ureteral meatus or periureteral (posterolateral) bladder wall

Microscopic Features

● Uroepithelial lining

CLINICAL ISSUES

Presentation

● Most common signs/symptoms
  ○ Usually asymptomatic
● Other signs/symptoms
  ○ Hematuria due to complications
    – Calculi
    – Tumor due to chronic inflammation (in older patients)
  ○ Large fluid-filled diverticulum may present with pelvic mass and may cause bladder outlet obstruction
● Clinical profile
  ○ Older male with benign prostatic hyperplasia (BPH)
  ○ Spinal cord injury patient (neurogenic bladder)

Demographics

● Age
  ○ 6th and 7th decade
● Gender
  ○ M:F = 9:1
● Epidemiology
  ○ Prevalence 1.7% in children
  ○ Multiple diverticula in children
    – Neurogenic dysfunction
    – Posterior urethral valves
    – Prune belly syndrome

Natural History & Prognosis

● Wide neck diverticula
  ○ Empty readily with bladder
● Narrow neck diverticula
  ○ Urinary stasis → complications such as infection, stone and ureteral obstruction
● Secondary inflammation predisposes to development of carcinoma within diverticulum
● Tumors in diverticula have worse prognosis
  ○ Poorly formed wall and absence of muscle layer leads to more rapid local invasion into surrounding perivesical fat

Treatment

● Options, risks, complications
  ○ Complications
    – Carcinoma
    – Vesicoureteral reflux
    – Ureteral obstruction
  ○ Indications for surgery
    – Persistent infection
    – Stone formation
    – Ureteral obstruction

DIAGNOSTIC CHECKLIST

Consider

● Look for internal debris or filling defects, which may be calculi, hematoma, or tumor

Image Interpretation Pearls

● Differentiated from pelvic cysts by demonstration of diverticulum neck connecting to bladder in appropriate plane
  ○ CTU or cystogram can help in differentiation

SELECTED REFERENCES

1. Shebel HM et al: Cysts of the lower male genitourinary tract: embryologic and anatomic considerations and differential diagnosis. Radiographics. 33(4):1125-43, 2013
2. Alexander RE et al: Bladder diverticulum: clinicopathologic spectrum in pediatric patients. Pediatr Dev Pathol. 15(4):281-5, 2012
3. Debenedectis CM et al: Incidental genitourinary findings on obstetrics/gynecology ultrasound. Ultrasound Q. 28(4):293-8, 2012
4. Aslam F et al: Acute urinary retention as a result of a bladder diverticulum. Int J Urol. 13(5):628-30, 2006
5. Pace AM et al: Congenital vesical diverticulum in a 38-year-old female. Int Urol Nephrol. 37(3):473-5, 2005
6. Yang JM et al: Transvaginal sonography in the diagnosis, management and follow-up of complex paraurethral abnormalities. Ultrasound Obstet Gynecol. 25(3):302-6, 2005
7. Shukla AR et al: Giant bladder diverticula causing bladder outlet obstruction in children. J Urol. 172(5 Pt 1):1977-9, 2004
8. Wang CW et al: Pitfalls in the differential diagnosis of a pelvic cyst: lessons from a post-menopausal woman with bladder diverticulum. Int J Clin Pract. 58(9):894-6, 2004
9. Cappele O et al: A study of the anatomic features of the duct of the urachus. Surg Radiol Anat. 23(4):229-35, 2001
10. Yu JS et al: Urachal remnant diseases: spectrum of CT and US findings. Radiographics. 21(2):451-61, 2001
11. Maynor CH et al: Urinary bladder diverticula: sonographic diagnosis and interpretive pitfalls. J Ultrasound Med. 15(3):189-94, 1996
12. Bellah RD et al: Ureterocele eversion with vesicoureteral reflux in duplex kidneys: findings at voiding cystourethrography. AJR Am J Roentgenol. 165(2):409-13, 1995
13. Itoh N et al: Spontaneous rupture of a bladder diverticulum: ultrasonographic diagnosis. J Urol. 152(4):1206-7, 1994
14. Levine D et al: Using color Doppler jets to differentiate a pelvic cyst from a bladder diverticulum. J Ultrasound Med. 13(7):575-7, 1994
15. Dondalski M et al: Carcinoma arising in urinary bladder diverticula: imaging findings in six patients. AJR Am J Roentgenol. 161(4):817-20, 1993
16. Farhi J et al: Giant diverticulum of the bladder simulating ovarian cyst. Int J Gynaecol Obstet. 36(1):55-7, 1991
17. Dragsted J et al: Urothelial carcinoma in a bladder diverticulum evaluated by transurethral ultrasonography. Scand J Urol Nephrol. 19(2):153-4, 1985

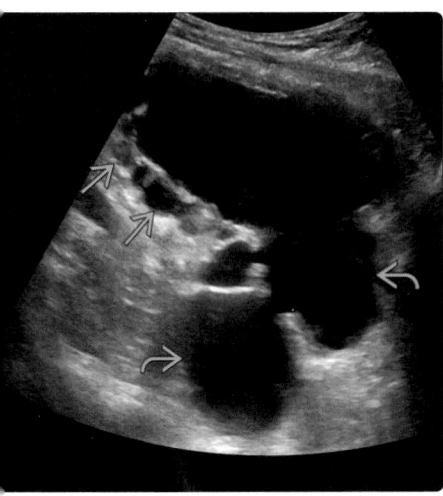
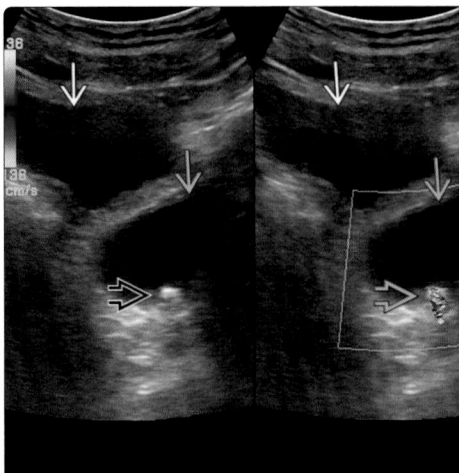

(Left) *Transabdominal longitudinal oblique ultrasound of the urinary bladder shows multiple small diverticula ⊟ and 2 large right posterolateral diverticula ⊟.* (Right) *Transabdominal transverse oblique ultrasound of the urinary bladder ⊟ shows a left posterolateral bladder diverticulum ⊟ containing layering stones seen as echogenic foci on grayscale ⊟ and with twinkling artifact on color Doppler imaging ⊟.*

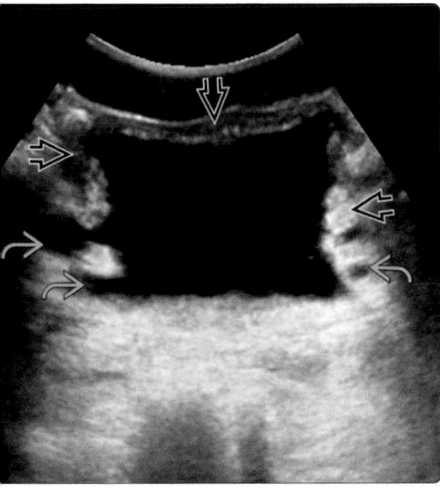
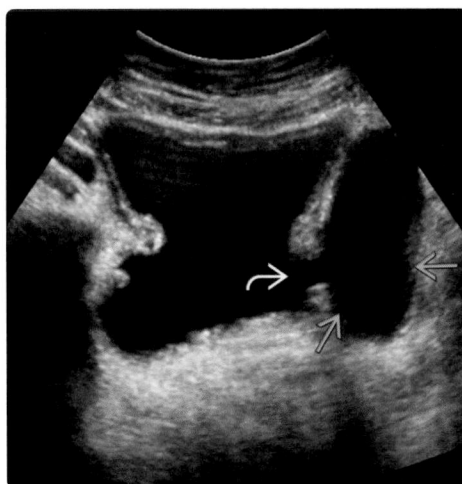

(Left) *Transabdominal transverse ultrasound in a patient with a neurogenic bladder shows thick-walled trabeculations ⊟ and multiple diverticula ⊟.* (Right) *Transabdominal transverse ultrasound of the urinary bladder shows a large left lateral diverticulum ⊟ with narrow neck communication ⊟ with the urinary bladder.*

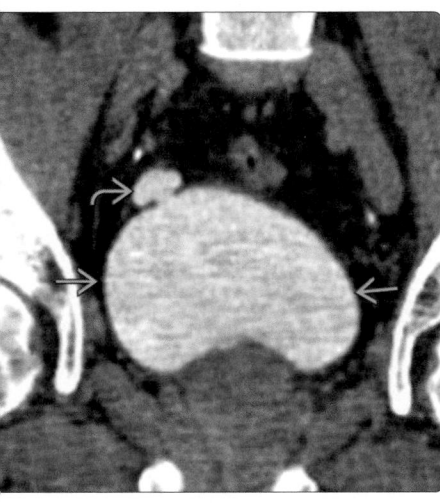
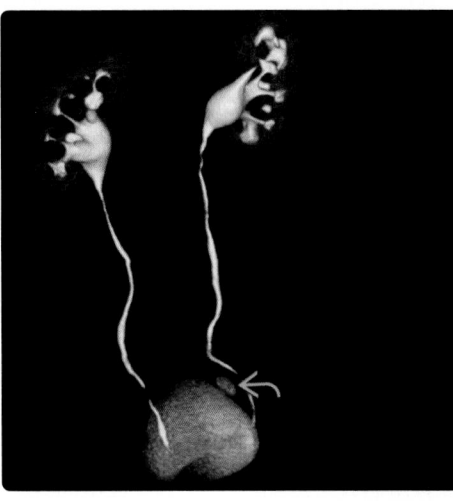

(Left) *Coronal reformatted CT urogram image through the pelvis shows excreted contrast opacified urinary bladder ⊟ with a small right posterior bladder diverticulum ⊟ that also fills with contrast.* (Right) *Volume-rendered 3D reformatted image in the same patient depicts the right posterior bladder diverticulum ⊟ arising near the bladder dome.*

KEY FACTS

TERMINOLOGY

- Concretions of mineral salts/crystal within bladder lumen

IMAGING

- Mobile avascular echogenic focus/foci in bladder with acoustic shadowing on US
- Smooth round or ovoid laminated calcification in bladder region on plain radiograph
- Associated bladder wall thickening and internal echoes or debris may be seen
- Calcific density in bladder, of varying size and shape, often lamellated on NECT or CECT
- Low signal intensity on all MR sequences

TOP DIFFERENTIAL DIAGNOSES

- Bladder neoplasm
- Blood clot
- Fungal ball
- Prostatomegaly

PATHOLOGY

- Stasis: Bladder outlet obstruction, neurogenic bladder, bladder diverticula
- Infection, especially proteus mirabilis

CLINICAL ISSUES

- Most asymptomatic
- May present with hematuria, suprapubic pain, and repeated UTI
- Complication: Malignant bladder tumors in patients with stones from indwelling Foley catheters

DIAGNOSTIC CHECKLIST

- Carcinoma resulting from chronic bladder irritation may coexist with bladder stone

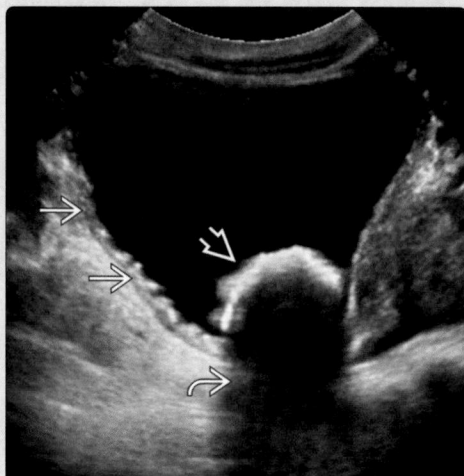
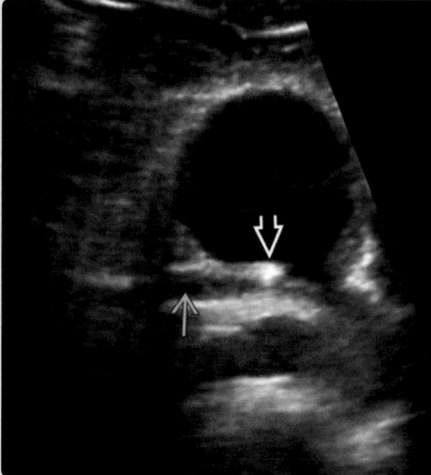

(Left) Longitudinal transabdominal ultrasound shows a large, echogenic stone ➡ within the urinary bladder. The stone is lobulated in contour and associated with posterior acoustic shadowing ➡. Note the diffuse bladder wall thickening ➡ related to chronic bladder outlet obstruction, a known risk factor for development of bladder calculi. (Right) Transverse oblique transabdominal US of the bladder shows a partly obstructing stone ➡ at the right UVJ and mildly dilated upstream ureter ➡.

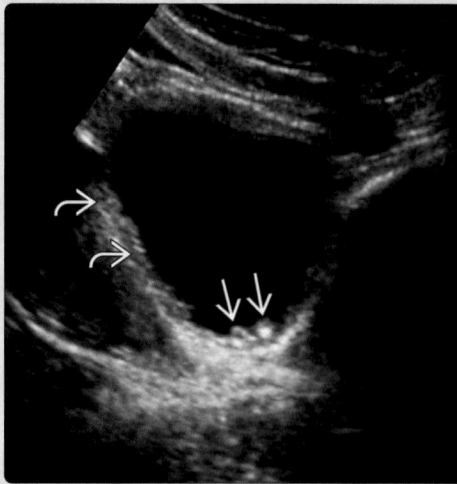
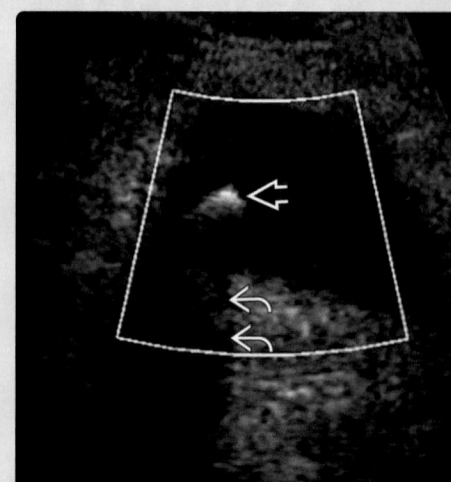

(Left) Longitudinal transabdominal ultrasound shows multiple tiny layering echogenic stones ➡ within the urinary bladder. Note the mild bladder wall thickening ➡. (Right) Longitudinal oblique transabdominal ultrasound shows a small, echogenic stone ➡ with posterior acoustic shadowing ➡ seen adherent to the bladder wall.

TERMINOLOGY

Synonyms

Bladder stones, vesical calculi, cystolithiasis

Definitions

Concretions of mineral salts/crystal within bladder lumen

IMAGING

General Features

Best diagnostic clue
- Mobile avascular echogenic focus/foci in bladder with acoustic shadowing on US
- Smooth, round or ovoid, lamellated calcification in bladder region on plain radiograph

Location
- Bladder lumen: Usually midline with patient supine
  - Eccentric location in patients with bladder augmentation or diverticulum

Size
- Variable (tiny migrated renal stones to large inherent bladder stones)

Morphology
- Round, oval, spiculated, lamellated, faceted

Ultrasonographic Findings

Grayscale ultrasound
- Mobile, avascular, crescentic echogenic focus with sharp acoustic shadowing
- Occasionally stone adheres to bladder wall due to inflammation
- Associated bladder wall thickening and internal echoes or debris in bladder lumen may be seen
- Edema of ureterovesical junction may be seen with recent passage of ureteral stone into bladder

Radiographic Findings

Radiography
- Solitary or multiple calcifications overlying bladder region
- Mostly radiopaque but opacity can be variable; radiolucent stone = cystine or uric acid stone

CT Findings

Calcific density in bladder, of varying size and shape, often lamellated on NECT or CECT
- Filling defect on CT urogram

MR Findings

All pulse sequences: Signal void(s) in bladder, typical filling defect on T2WI

DIFFERENTIAL DIAGNOSIS

Bladder Neoplasm

Focal immobile mass in bladder, with internal vascular flow

Blood Clot

Avascular hypo-/hyperechoic foci without posterior acoustic shadowing, ± internal echoes
History of hematuria can be helpful clue

Fungal Ball

- Rare entities occurring in diabetics or immunocompromised patients
- Medium echogenicity, nonshadowing, rounded mobile lesions within bladder

Prostatomegaly

- Median lobe hypertrophy may indent bladder base, mimicking stone

PATHOLOGY

General Features

- Etiology
  - Stasis: Bladder outlet obstruction, neurogenic bladder, bladder diverticula
    - Concentrated, stagnant urine crystallizes in bladder
  - Migrated renal calculi
  - Infection, especially proteus mirabilis
  - Foreign bodies: Act as nidus for crystal growth
  - Bladder augmentation: Local metabolic derangement
- Most are mixture of calcium oxalate and calcium phosphate
- Infection stones: Magnesium ammonium phosphate ("struvite")

CLINICAL ISSUES

Presentation

- Most common signs/symptoms
  - Most asymptomatic
  - May present with hematuria, suprapubic pain, and repeated UTI

Demographics

- Gender
  - M > F

Natural History & Prognosis

- Complication: Malignant bladder tumors in patients with stones from indwelling Foley catheters

DIAGNOSTIC CHECKLIST

Image Interpretation Pearls

- Carcinoma resulting from chronic bladder irritation may coexist with bladder stone

SELECTED REFERENCES

1. Celik S et al: Association between ureteral jet dynamics and nonobstructive kidney stones: a prospective-controlled study. Urology. 84(5):1016-20, 2014
2. Shih CJ et al: Urinary calculi and risk of cancer: a nationwide population-based study. Medicine (Baltimore). 93(29):e342, 2014
3. Hammad FT et al: Bladder calculi: did the clinical picture change? Urology. 67(6):1154-8, 2006
4. Schwartz BF et al: The vesical calculus. Urol Clin North Am. 27(2):333-46, 2000

TERMINOLOGY

- Bilharziasis, parasitic infection
- Infection of urinary system by parasite *Schistosoma hematobium*

IMAGING

- Imaging findings mirror pathologic course
  - Acute phase: Nodular bladder wall thickening
  - Chronic phase: Contracted, fibrotic, thick-walled bladder with calcifications
- Calcifications of bladder wall (4-56%)
  - ± calcification of ureter (34%), seminal vesicle (late)
  - Calcification best seen on NECT
- Mucosal irregularity, inflammatory pseudopolyps of bladder
- Ureteritis cystica, distal ureteric stricture
- Noncompliant, small-capacity bladder with significant postvoid residual

TOP DIFFERENTIAL DIAGNOSES

- Bladder calculi
- Bladder carcinoma
- Cystitis
  - Emphysematous cystitis

PATHOLOGY

- Cercariae pass from snail (intermediate host) to water and penetrate human skin
- Pass into lymphatics, lungs, and liver and migrate to pelvic venous plexus → bladder wall vessels

CLINICAL ISSUES

- Endemic in Middle East, India, Africa, Central America, and South America
- Diagnosis is confirmed by identifying ova of parasite in urine
- Squamous cell carcinoma of bladder is late complication

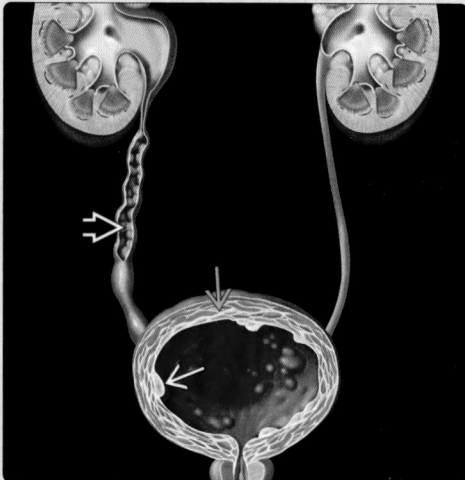
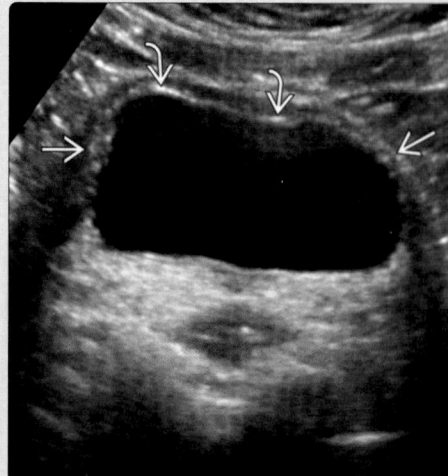

(Left) Graphic shows a markedly thickened urinary bladder wall with inflammatory polyps ➡ and mural calcifications ➡. Ureteritis cystica changes ➡ are present in the dilated right ureter. (Right) Transverse transabdominal ultrasound of the bladder shows mild diffuse wall thickening ➡ with linear echogenicity in the wall ➡ from subtle wall calcification in a patient with schistosomiasis.

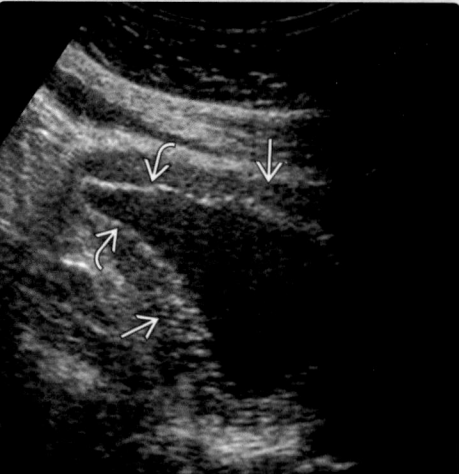
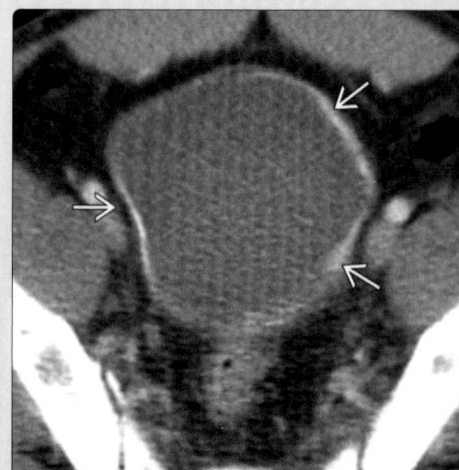

(Left) Longitudinal transabdominal ultrasound of the bladder shows diffuse wall thickening ➡ with linear mucosal echogenicity ➡ from calcification in a patient with schistosomiasis.(Courtesy E. Wassal, MD, and A Abdelaziz, MD.) (Right) Axial CECT shows diffuse bladder wall calcification ➡, consistent with chronic phase of schistosomiasis infection.

Schistosomiasis, Bladder

TERMINOLOGY

Synonyms

Bilharziasis, parasitic infection

Definitions

Infection of urinary system by parasite *Schistosoma hematobium*

IMAGING

General Features

Best diagnostic clue
- Curvilinear bladder wall calcification in patient from endemic area

Imaging findings correspond to pathologic course
- Acute phase: Nodular bladder wall thickening
- Chronic phase: Contracted, thick-walled bladder with calcifications

Ultrasonographic Findings

Noncompliant, thick-walled, small-capacity bladder with significant postvoid residual

Echogenic calcification within bladder wall

Hydronephrosis and hydroureter due to distal ureteric stricture

Radiographic Findings

Calcifications of bladder wall (4-56%)

± calcification of ureter (34%), seminal vesicle (late)

Fluoroscopic Findings

Mucosal irregularity, inflammatory pseudopolyps of bladder

Ureteritis cystica, distal ureteric stricture

Vesicoureteric reflux

CT Findings

NECT
- Best delineation of extent of bladder calcification, mural pathology, ureteral involvement

DIFFERENTIAL DIAGNOSIS

Bladder Calculi

Mobile echogenic focus within bladder lumen

Bladder Carcinoma

Irregular wall thickening ± focal mass with vascularity

Associated lymphadenopathy ± multiple sites of involvement

Urachal Carcinoma

Intramural exophytic mass arising from dome of bladder extending toward umbilicus

May have focal calcification

Cystitis

Diffuse or focal hypoechoic thickening of bladder wall; no wall calcification

Clinical, not imaging distinction

Emphysematous Cystitis

Infection by gas-forming organism

- Echogenic foci within area of bladder, wall thickening with ring-down shadowing
- Gas in bladder wall or lumen easily detected on CT

PATHOLOGY

General Features

- Etiology
  - Female parasite discharges eggs into urine and feces
  - Ova hatch into miracidia, infecting fresh water snails (intermediate host)
  - Cercariae pass from snail to water and penetrate human skin
  - Pass into lymphatics, lungs, and liver and migrate to pelvic venous plexus
  - Ultimately eggs are deposited and erode into bladder wall

Microscopic Features

- Encapsulated eggs in bladder wall/vessels cause inflammatory granulomatous reaction
- Fibrosis traps ova in tunica propria of bladder wall where ova die and calcify

CLINICAL ISSUES

Presentation

- Most common signs/symptoms
  - Frequency, urgency, dysuria, hematuria

Demographics

- Epidemiology
  - Endemic in Middle East, India, Africa, Central America, and South America

Natural History & Prognosis

- Squamous cell carcinoma of bladder is late complication

Treatment

- Drugs: Praziquantel, metrifonate

DIAGNOSTIC CHECKLIST

Image Interpretation Pearls

- Degree of hydronephrosis and irregularity of bladder wall correlates strongly with prevalence and intensity of *S. hematobium* infection, microhematuria, and proteinuria

SELECTED REFERENCES

1. Rinaldi G et al: New Research Tools for Urogenital Schistosomiasis. J Infect Dis. 211(6):861-869, 2015
2. Sabe I et al: New concept of schistosomiasis lesions of urinary bladder versus development of bladder cancer. J Egypt Soc Parasitol. 38(1):85-102, 2008
3. Gouda I et al: Bilharziasis and bladder cancer: a time trend analysis of 9843 patients. J Egypt Natl Canc Inst. 19(2):158-62, 2007
4. Mungadi IA et al: Urinary bladder cancer and schistosomiasis in North-Western Nigeria. West Afr J Med. 26(3):226-9, 2007
5. Wong-You-Cheong JJ et al: From the archives of the AFIP: Inflammatory and nonneoplastic bladder masses: radiologic-pathologic correlation. Radiographics. 26(6):1847-68, 2006
6. Degremont A et al: Value of ultrasonography in investigating morbidity due to Schistosoma haematobium infection. Lancet. 1(8430):662-5, 1985

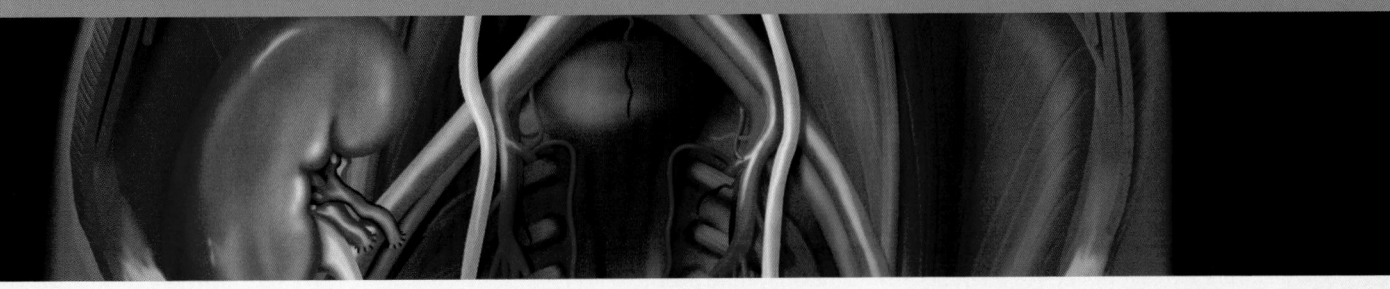

PART II
SECTION 6
Kidney Transplant

Imaging Anatomy

Renal transplants are placed in the pelvis where they are readily accessible for ultrasound imaging. The transplant renal artery is typically anastomosed end to side to the external iliac artery and the renal vein to the external iliac vein. The transplant ureter anastomosis is at the dome of the bladder. The ureter is not usually visible unless it is dilated or contains a stent. Stents may be placed if the surgeon is concerned about the integrity of the ureteral anastomosis.

The first renal transplant or solitary renal transplants are preferentially placed in the right pelvis, where the iliac vessels are more superficial, in an extraperitoneal location. Second transplants or those accompanied by a pancreas transplant are typically placed in the left pelvis. Patients may have dual simultaneous bilateral transplants or sequential transplants, in both iliac fossae. Pediatric donor kidneys are harvested en bloc with the intervening aorta and vena cava, leaving the renal vascular pedicle intact. They appear as two small, closely opposed kidneys in one iliac fossa with intervening aorta and vena cava anastomosed to iliac artery and vein. These kidneys are intraperitoneal. When patients have had multiple failed renal transplants, the newest transplant may be placed intraperitoneally with anastomoses to aorta and vena cava.

The renal transplant appears like a normal kidney but is oriented obliquely. The position of the hilum is variable; it can be facing medially or laterally, depending on size match between the donor and recipient. Renal pyramids are well seen and are hypoechoic to renal cortex and sinus fat. Color perfusion should be seen up to the arcuate arteries. Doppler shows a low-resistance arterial waveform with continuous flow throughout the cardiac cycle. The resistive index is normally < 0.7 and tends to be higher in the main renal artery than in the intrarenal arteries. The renal vein and intrarenal venous waveforms are monophasic or slightly undulating with the respiratory and cardiac cycle.

Gas may be seen in the renal pelvis or calyces secondary to reflux from the bladder in the setting of bladder catheterization.

Anatomy-Based Imaging Issues

At baseline, it is crucial to determine if there are any variations to the standard surgery. These include accessory renal arteries separately anastomosed to the iliac artery or arterial reconstruction onto a patch of aortic graft or interposed vein graft. Accessory veins are much less common.

Mild dilatation of the collecting system is not uncommon early after transplantation and is more commonly seen in the renal pelvis. Calyceal dilatation is a more concerning sign. Dilated calyces should be distinguished from cortical cysts or sinus cysts, by demonstrating communication with the renal pelvis. Hypoechoic pyramids should not be mistaken for calyces. Color Doppler should be used to rule out a vascular lesion mimicking a cyst. If the bladder is distended and there is dilatation of renal pelvis or ureter, the patient should be rescanned after emptying the bladder.

Pathologic Issues

Pathologic evaluation of renal transplant biopsy is the gold standard for the diagnosis of nonsurgical noninfectious causes of renal transplant dysfunction. Evaluation includes histology, immunofluorescence, immunohistochemistry, and electron microscopy.

In the first few days after transplantation, acute tubular necrosis is the most common cause of delayed function. Hyperacute rejection is not common with current screening. After the first three-five days, acute cell mediated rejection and acute antibody mediated rejection occur. Pathological evaluation is key to making an accurate diagnosis of rejection so that the antirejection therapy can be tailored to the patient. The Banff classification for rejection is in wide use. Toxic effects from calcineurin inhibitors (used to counter rejection) may be manifest as tubulopathy or thrombotic microangiopathy on biopsy.

In the first year after transplantation, recurrent glomerular disease (such as focal segmental glomerulosclerosis) can significantly impact graft survival and can be diagnosed by biopsy. Polyomavirus nephropathy is an important cause of chronic graft failure, secondary to viruses such BK and JC viruses. Later allograft dysfunction can result from a combination of all the above with the addition of hypertension, pyelonephritis, and post-transplant lymphoproliferative disorder.

Pathology-Based Imaging Issues

Imaging is not sensitive or specific for differentiating parenchymal causes of dysfunction; biopsy is required.

Imaging Protocols

Curved transducers are ideal for evaluation, using as high a frequency as allowed by body habitus and depth of the kidney, typically between 2-5 MHz but up to 8 MHz if feasible. A linear transducer may be used for focused assessment of a lesion. Use of compound and harmonic imaging can improve image quality and decrease artifacts.

Patients are typically imaged supine but the decubitus position is very helpful to mitigate the presence of intervening gas or pannus. Additionally, in the immediate postoperative period, wound staples and dressings may prevent optimal access. Grayscale evaluation of the renal transplant should include assessment of renal size, cortical echogenicity, presence of hydronephrosis or hydroureter, and perinephric collections. The bladder should also be evaluated for degree of distension, wall thickness, and intraluminal content such as stent, clot, or debris.

Color Doppler is essential for identification of vessels and to determine patency and luminal narrowing. The iliac artery and vein are assessed in color Doppler and Doppler waveforms are obtained. More detailed devaluation of the iliac artery waveforms may be obtained if there is a suspicion for iliac artery dissection or atherosclerosis.

The main renal artery or arteries are evaluated with color and spectral Doppler for patency and the presence of stenosis. Stenosis most commonly occurs at the renal artery to iliac artery anastomosis and causes aliasing in color Doppler with elevation of peak systolic velocity on spectral Doppler. This is compared to the peak systolic velocity in the iliac artery. Downstream effects can be observed, notably the tardus parvus waveform in the intrarenal arteries, which is quantified using the acceleration index and the resistive index.

Starting at the renal hilum and progressing toward the cortex the intrarenal arteries are the segmental, interlobar, arcuate, and interlobular arteries. Doppler waveforms are obtained of these arteries with measurements of the resistive index. Such measurements may be obtained in the upper, mid, and lower

le when there are multiple supplying arteries. Intrarenal
ins are also documented but are less important.

Clinical Implications

trasound is the method of choice for imaging renal
ansplants. The most common indication is poor renal
nction such as elevated creatinine and drop in urine output.
her indications include fever, urinary tract infection, pain,
evated white cell count, and dropping hemoglobin and
matocrit. Occasionally, patients will present with swelling
er the graft or leakage from the wound. Hypertension and
uit are later indications for ultrasound.

s not possible to accurately diagnose rejection with
trasound. The main purpose of ultrasound is to exclude
her causes of renal dysfunction and facilitate ultrasound-
ided biopsy for the definitive diagnosis.

trasound can accurately and promptly detect vascular
mplications. It is the first-line imaging modality for
rombosis, renal artery stenosis, and arteriovenous fistula
ut may be limited by body habitus. Evaluation of arterial
ortoiliac inflow is best obtained with enhanced CT and MR if
nal function permits. Fluid collections and hydronephrosis
e readily detected but ultrasound is limited for infection and
mor detection.

omplications of renal transplantation can be classified based
timing since transplantation. **Immediate** complications
cur from the time of surgery to the first postoperative
eek. The most frequent immediate complications are:
- Hemorrhage
- Graft thrombosis (arterial or venous)
- Delayed graft function/acute tubular necrosis/primary
  graft non-function
- Hyperacute rejection

arly complications occur between 1 week and 1 month after
ansplantation. These include:
- Acute rejection
- Drug toxicity (calcineurin inhibitors)
- Vascular complications: Graft thrombosis, post-biopsy
  arteriovenous fistula or pseudoaneurysm
- Surgical complications: Ureteral leak or stricture;
  perinephric hematoma, seroma, lymphocele; urinary
  tract or systemic infection (can occur at any time)

ate complications are defined as occurring after 1 month.
he most common complications are:
- Complications of biopsy: Arteriovenous fistula and
  pseudoaneurysm
- Ureteral stricture
- Renal artery stenosis
- Polyoma virus nephropathy
- Chronic rejection
- Malignancy: Post-transplant lymphoproliferative
  disorder, renal and bladder cancer

Differential Diagnosis

. is uncommon for a specific diagnosis to be made from a
ingle ultrasound examination with exceptions such as renal
rtery or vein thrombosis. In most patients, knowledge of the
linical presentation and laboratory tests is essential for
arrowing the differential diagnosis and suggesting further
ests to the clinician.

Urothelial Thickening
- Infection

- Rejection
- Post relief of obstruction
- Secondary to stent
- Urothelial malignancy

Dilated Renal Pelvis
- Stricture
- Stone
- Extrinsic compression

Abnormal Blood Flow
- Arterial or venous thrombosis
- Arterial or venous stenosis
- Arteriovenous fistula
- Pseudoaneurysm
- Acute and chronic rejection
- Acute tubular necrosis

Fluid Collections
- Seroma
- Urinoma
- Lymphocele
- Hematoma

Poor Renal Function With Normal Ultrasound
- Acute tubular necrosis
- Acute and chronic rejection
- Drug toxicity
- Virus nephropathy
- Infection

Renal Transplant Mass
- Renal carcinoma
- Sloughed papilla
- Fungus ball
- Urothelial carcinoma
- Lymphoma
- Post-transplant lymphoproliferative disorder
- Infection: Non-liquefied abscess, granulomatous
  infection

Selected References

1. Naesens M et al: Intrarenal resistive index after renal transplantation. N Engl J Med. 370(7):677-8, 2014
2. Rodgers SK et al: Ultrasonographic evaluation of the renal transplant. Radiol Clin North Am. 52(6):1307-24, 2014
3. Williams WW et al: Clinical role of the renal transplant biopsy. Nat Rev Nephrol. 8(2):110-21, 2012
4. Cosgrove DO et al: Renal transplants: what ultrasound can and cannot do. Ultrasound Q. 24(2):77-87; quiz 141-2, 2008
5. Irshad A et al: A review of sonographic evaluation of renal transplant complications. Curr Probl Diagn Radiol. 37(2):67-79, 2008
6. Gao J et al: Intrarenal color duplex ultrasonography: a window to vascular complications of renal transplants. J Ultrasound Med. 26(10):1403-18, 2007

(Left) *Longitudinal ultrasound shows hypoechoic pyramids* ➡️ *arranged around the echogenic renal sinus* ➡️ *of a normal renal transplant. The cortex* ➡️ *is intermediate in echogenicity between the pyramids and the sinus fat. The iliacus muscle is noted* ➡️ *in this child.* **(Right)** *Longitudinal ultrasound shows an adult renal transplant. Pyramids* ➡️ *are evident and should not be mistaken for calyces. The renal sinus* ➡️ *is more echogenic than the renal cortex* ➡️.

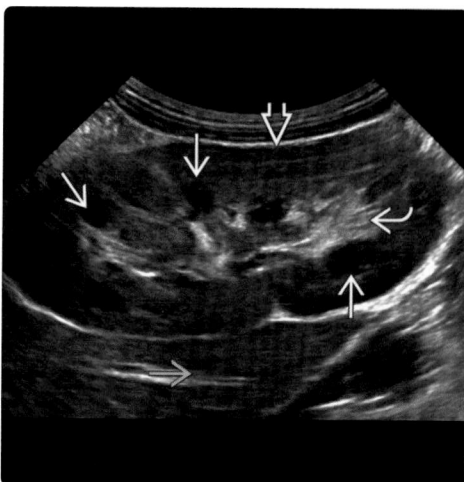
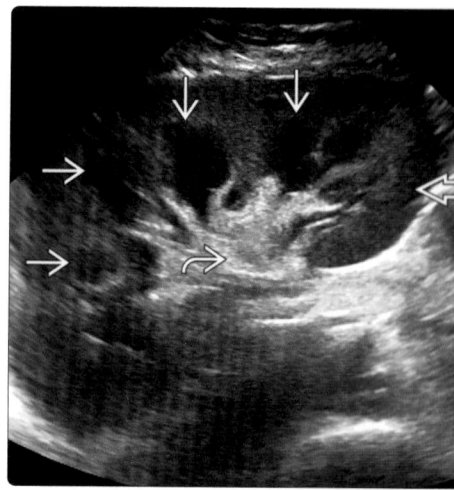

(Left) *Longitudinal color Doppler ultrasound shows color flow extending from the renal sinus to the cortex representing the normal arborization of intrarenal vessels from segmental* ➡️ *to arcuate arteries* ➡️. *The renal vein* ➡️ *and venous tributaries are also well seen.* **(Right)** *Power Doppler ultrasound is more sensitive to vascular flow, showing more detail of the interlobular arteries* ➡️. *The iliac artery* ➡️ *and renal artery anastomosis* ➡️, *segmental* ➡️ *and interlobar* ➡️ *arteries are demonstrated.*

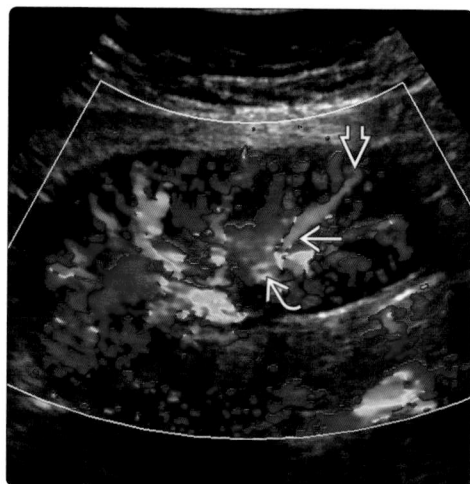
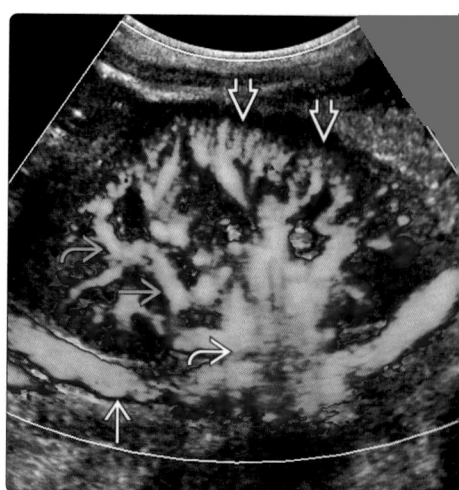

(Left) *Longitudinal color Doppler ultrasound of the vascular pedicle shows the iliac artery* ➡️ *and renal artery* ➡️, *and the iliac vein* ➡️ *and main renal vein* ➡️. **(Right)** *Transverse oblique color Doppler ultrasound shows the course of the main renal artery* ➡️. *Angulation and tortuosity can make Doppler interrogation challenging. The renal transplant* ➡️ *is echogenic.*

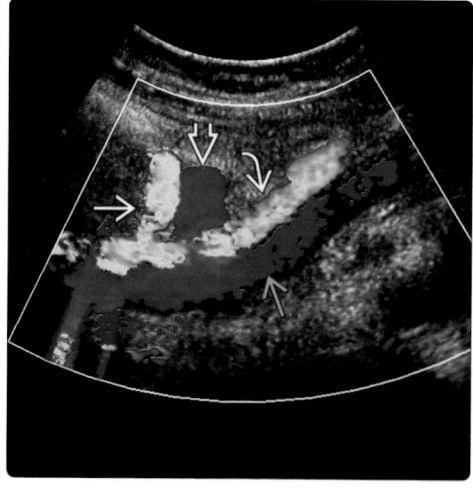
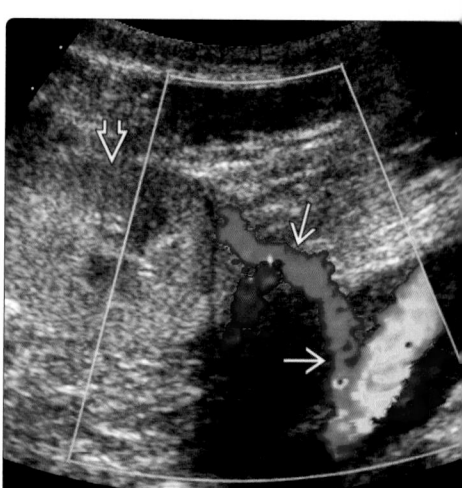

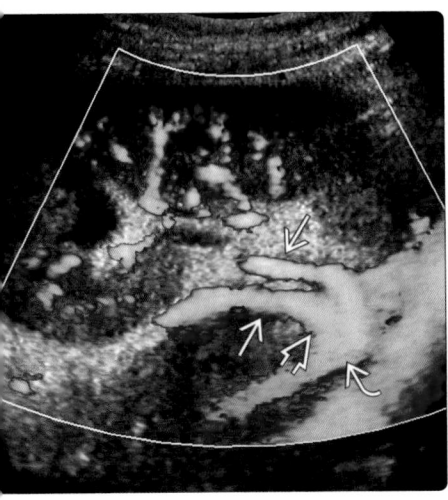

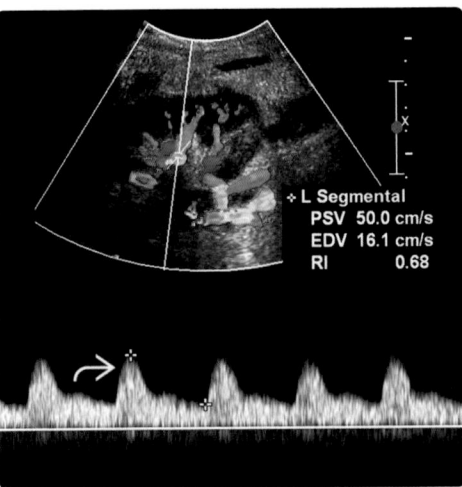

(Left) Longitudinal oblique power Doppler ultrasound through the arterial anastomosis shows two renal arteries ➡ arising from a common patch ➡ sewn to the iliac artery ➡. (Right) Doppler ultrasound shows a segmental renal artery with measurement of the resistive index (RI). Normal RI is < 0.7. The waveform ➡ should be antegrade throughout the cardiac cycle.

L Segmental
PSV 50.0 cm/s
EDV 16.1 cm/s
RI 0.68

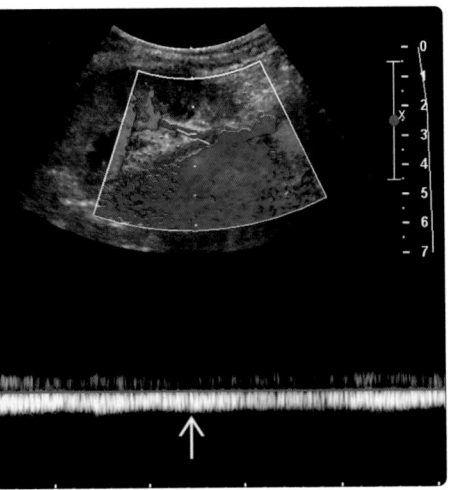

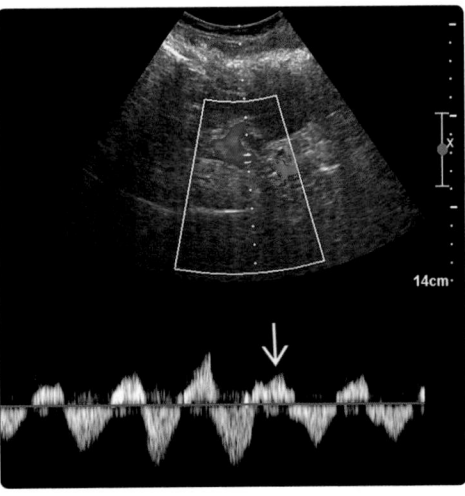

(Left) Spectral Doppler ultrasound shows a normal monophasic renal vein waveform ➡. (Right) Spectral Doppler ultrasound shows a pulsatile biphasic renal vein waveform ➡. This should not be mistaken for an arterial waveform.

14cm

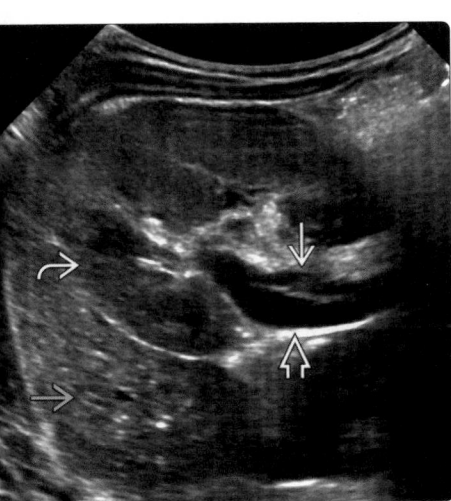

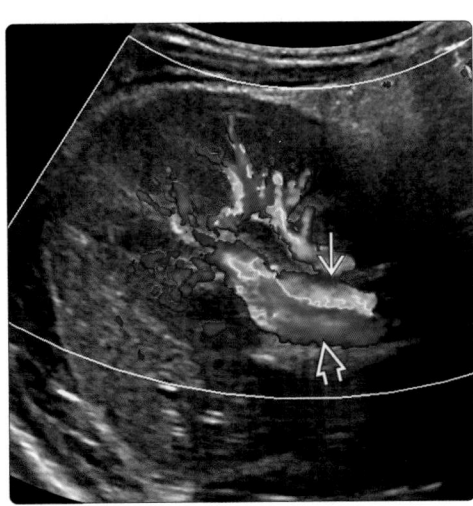

(Left) Transverse ultrasound through the hilum of the renal transplant shows the anechoic lumen of the segmental renal artery ➡ and vein ➡. The cortex ➡ is isoechoic to the iliacus muscle ➡ in this child. (Right) Transverse color Doppler ultrasound through the mid renal transplant shows normal color flow in the segmental renal artery ➡ and vein ➡.

(Left) Longitudinal ultrasound of the renal pelvis shows a stent ➡ within the pelvis and ureter. Stents are more difficult to detect when the ureter does not contain fluid. (Right) Longitudinal ultrasound of a renal transplant shows urothelial thickening ➡ and gas within a calyx. Ring down artifact ➡ allows detection of small amounts of gas, which has refluxed from the bladder. Urothelial thickening is most commonly secondary to infection and rejection.

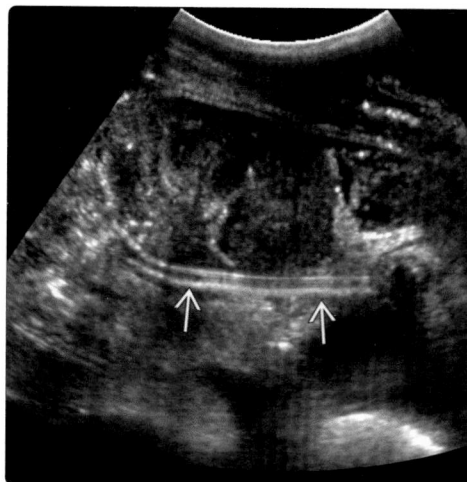
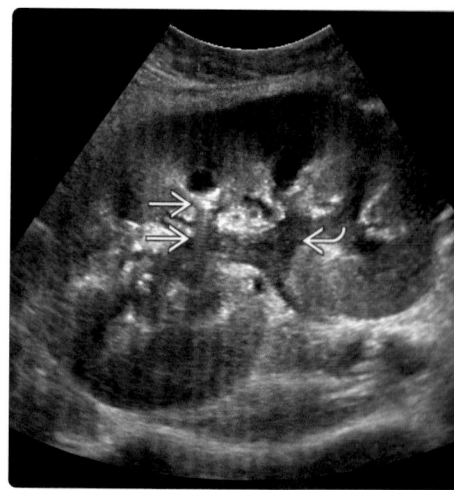

(Left) Longitudinal ultrasound of a renal transplant shows urothelial thickening in the dilated renal pelvis ➡. Consider infection, rejection, and obstruction, and evaluate the entire ureter. (Right) Longitudinal ultrasound of a patient with simultaneous renal and pancreatic transplant shows diffuse circumferential urothelial thickening ➡ after removal of a ureteral stent. There is increased echogenicity of the transplant kidney ➡ and perinephric fluid ➡.

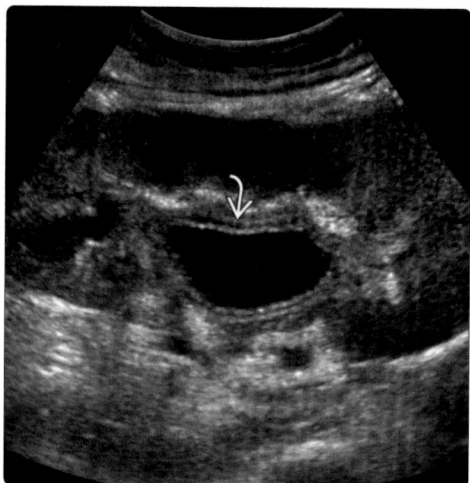
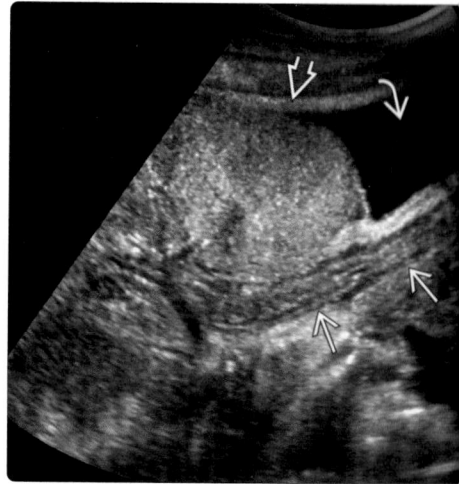

(Left) Longitudinal color Doppler ultrasound shows a renal transplant with hydronephrosis ➡. Color Doppler can distinguish dilated vessels from fluid-filled collecting system. (Right) Transverse color Doppler ultrasound shows a dilated proximal ureter ➡. This should be traced to the bladder to determine the level of obstruction. The lower pole calyx is dilated ➡.

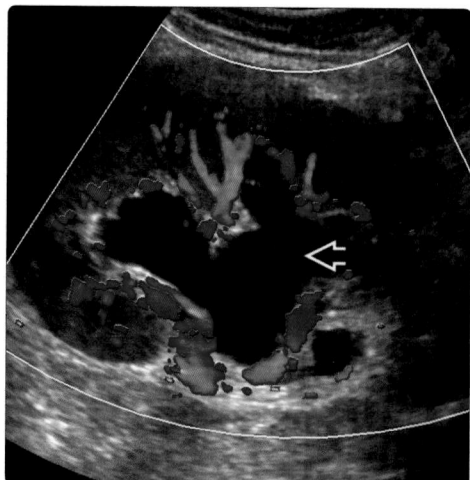
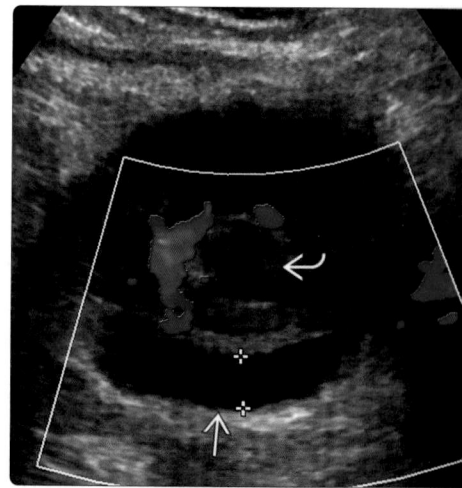

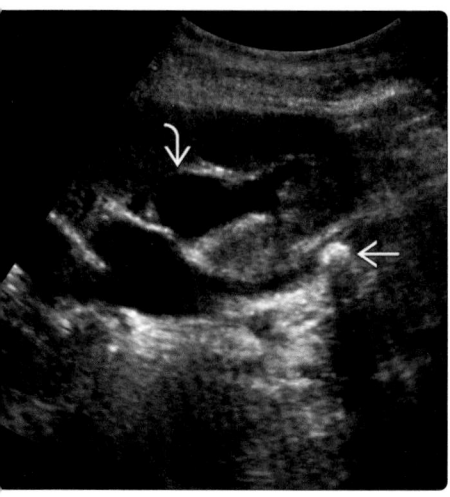

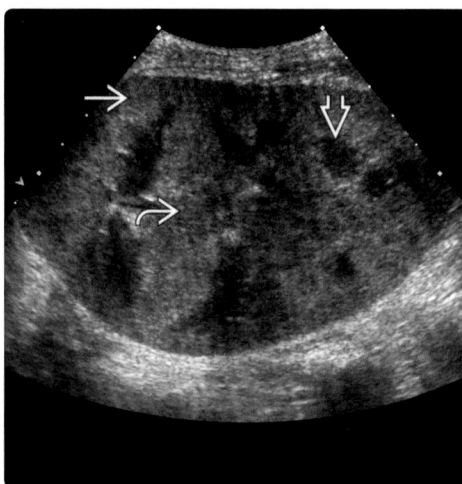

(Left) Longitudinal ultrasound shows a calculus ➡ obstructing the transplant ureter. There is moderate hydronephrosis ➡. (Right) Longitudinal ultrasound of a poorly functioning renal transplant shows increased cortical echogenicity ➡ and decreased echogenicity of the sinus fat ➡ with prominent pyramids ➡. Biopsy showed acute rejection.

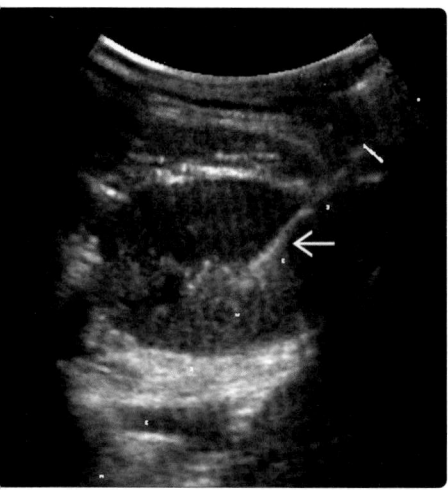

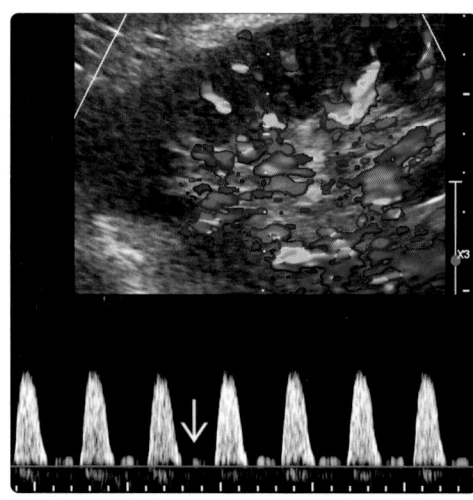

(Left) Transverse ultrasound with a needle guide shows a biopsy needle ➡ in the lower pole cortex. An adequate biopsy should include at least 10 glomeruli and 2 arteries with 2 separate cores through the cortex. (Right) Doppler ultrasound shows a renal transplant with poor function in the early postoperative phase. Absence of diastolic flow ➡ was secondary to acute tubular necrosis causing delayed graft function.

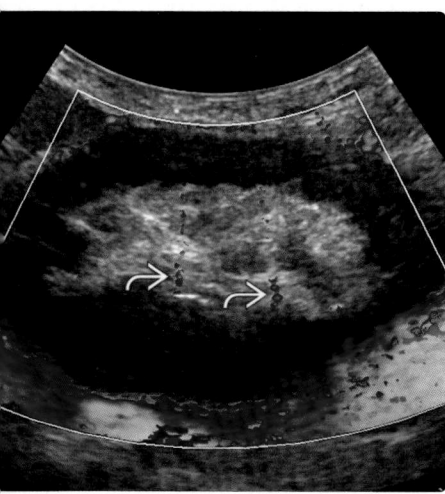

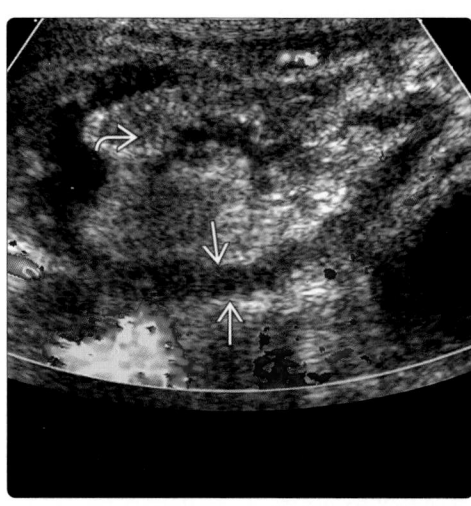

(Left) Power Doppler ultrasound performed for poor transplant function shows a normal-sized kidney with no internal flow consistent with acute vascular thrombosis. Artifacts ➡ should be interrogated with Doppler to confirm that they do not represent true flow. (Right) Longitudinal color Doppler ultrasound of a failed renal transplant demonstrates marked cortical thinning ➡, sinus lipomatosis ➡, and absence of color flow. This was not acute thrombosis.

TERMINOLOGY

- Dilated renal pelvis and calyces, usually secondary to obstruction

IMAGING

- Over 90% at ureterovesical anastomosis and distal 1/3 of ureter
- Low-level echoes within lumen suggest pus (pyonephrosis) or blood (hemonephrosis)
- Highly echogenic shadowing intraluminal structures represent stones
- Highly echogenic, weakly shadowing masses, suggest fungal balls
- Ultrasound is sensitive and specific for hydronephrosis
- Ultrasound may be limited for site of obstruction and cannot provide functional information
- Antegrade nephrostogram is gold standard in differentiating fixed from transient obstruction and for localizing site obstruction

- o Usually combined with ultrasound guidance to access collecting system
- MR/MRU comprehensive high-resolution evaluation of entire urinary tract, including distal to obstruction

TOP DIFFERENTIAL DIAGNOSES

- Nonobstructive dilatation
- Pyo- or hemonephrosis
- Ureteral calculi
- Urothelial thickening
- Transitional cell carcinoma (TCC)
- Renal sinus cysts
- Prominent hilar vessels

DIAGNOSTIC CHECKLIST

- Ultrasound is first-line imaging modality for renal transplant dysfunction in immediate postoperative period or for follow-up

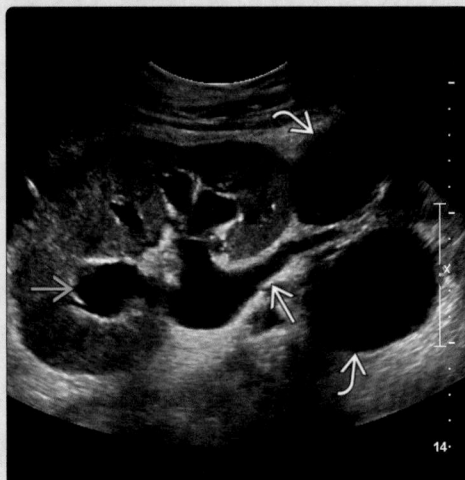
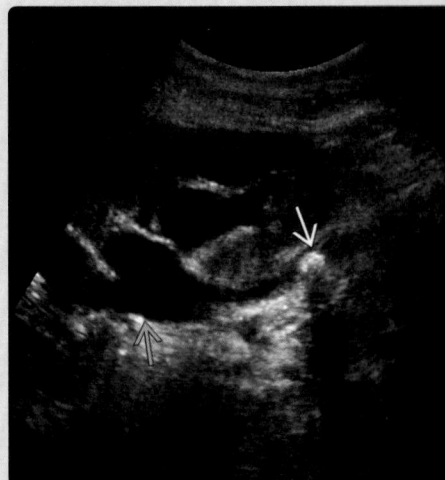

(Left) Longitudinal ultrasound shows mild to moderate hydronephrosis ➡ in a renal transplant. The ureter ➡ is dilated secondary to obstruction by a fluid collection ➡, which wrapped around the ureter. (Right) Longitudinal ultrasound shows mild to moderate hydronephrosis ➡ secondary to a shadowing calculus ➡ in the transplant ureter.

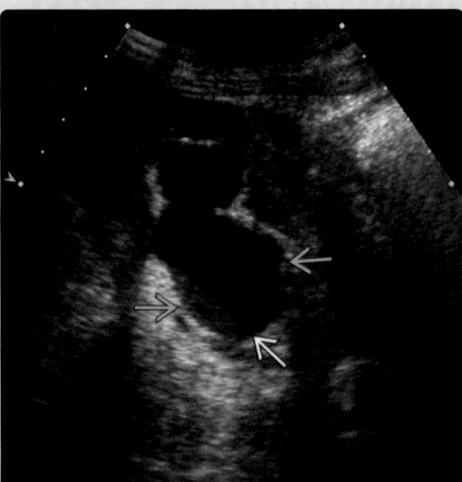
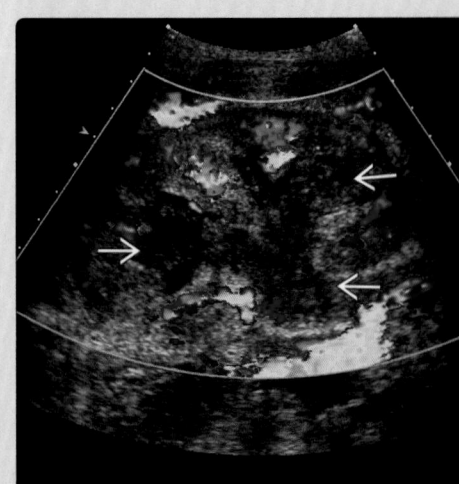

(Left) Transverse ultrasound shows a debris level ➡ within a dilated renal pelvis ➡. This was secondary to infection in a chronically dilated collecting system. (Right) Longitudinal ultrasound shows a dilated renal pelvis and calyces, which are filled with avascular hypoechoic clot ➡. The hemonephrosis was secondary to a renal transplant biopsy.

TERMINOLOGY

Definitions

Dilated renal pelvis and calyces, usually secondary to obstruction
- ± hydroureter

IMAGING

General Features

Best diagnostic clue
- Dilated fluid-filled renal pelvis and calyces, persisting when bladder is empty

Location
- Over 90% at ureterovesical anastomosis and distal 1/3 of ureter

Ultrasonographic Findings

Grayscale ultrasound
- Fluid-filled dilatation of renal pelvis branching into dilated calyces
- Hydroureter may be present, producing avascular tubular structure arising from renal hilum and extending toward bladder
- Note that distended bladder may cause functional obstruction or reflux resulting in hydronephrosis
  - Repeat scan with bladder empty
- Low-level echoes within lumen suggest pus (pyonephrosis) or blood (hemonephrosis)
  - Clot may also be present in ureter and bladder
  - Debris from infection may layer dependently
- Highly echogenic shadowing intraluminal structures represent stones
  - However, small stones may be very difficult to detect
- Highly echogenic, weakly shadowing masses suggest fungal balls
- Ultrasound is sensitive and specific for hydronephrosis
- Ultrasound may be limited for site of obstruction and cannot provide functional information

Color Doppler
- Useful to distinguish hilar vessels from dilated renal pelvis
- Use Color Doppler to distinguish clot or debris from solid tumor
  - Useful to demonstrate tiny vessels within urothelial tumors
- Elevated resistive index (RI) > 0.7 may occur in obstructive uropathy, but RI is nonspecific and rarely diagnostic
- "Twinkling" artifact allows confident diagnosis of calculus

Nonvascular Interventions

Antegrade nephrostogram is gold standard in differentiating fixed from transient obstruction and for localizing site of obstruction

Invasive test requiring direct puncture of lateral calyx and injection of iodinated contrast medium into collecting system

Usually combined with ultrasound guidance to access collecting system

- Insertion of percutaneous nephrostomy catheter allows decompression of urine until definitive therapy, which can be performed through same access
- Antegrade pyelography not performed in acute infection

CT Findings

- Use of iodinated contrast limited by poor renal function
- More sensitive for fluid collections and calculi
- CT nephrostography useful for delineation of stricture length and surrounding pathology

MR Findings

- T2WI
  - High signal in fluid-filled pelvis and calyces
  - Highly sensitive for fluid collection and allows differentiation between hydronephrosis and renal cysts
  - Comprehensive high-resolution evaluation of entire urinary tract, including distal to obstruction
    - Localization of obstruction is superior to ultrasound
  - Fast sequences allow diagnostic study in poorly cooperative patients
- MR urogram (MRU) can be performed without contrast (T2WI) or with contrast (T1WI C+ FS)
  - Avoids potential side effects of iodinated contrast medium administration but with risk for nephrogenic systemic fibrosis in poor renal function
- Functional MR techniques not yet in wide clinical use

Nuclear Medicine Findings

- Tc-99m MAG3 renogram
- Can differentiate true obstruction from nonobstructive dilatation
- Provides functional information

Imaging Recommendations

- Best imaging tool
  - Ultrasound is first-line imaging modality for allograft dysfunction both in early postoperative period and later
  - Sensitive and specific for hydronephrosis but may be limited for location and cause of obstruction
- Protocol advice
  - If bladder is distended, re-evaluate for hydronephrosis when empty
  - Look for transition zone and cause for obstruction, such as fluid collection, stone, or clot
  - Consider antegrade pyelography or MAG3 renogram to differentiate obstruction from dilatation
  - MR or CT for level of obstruction (MR preferred [no ionizing radiation] but CT in wide use)

DIFFERENTIAL DIAGNOSIS

Nonobstructive Dilatation

- May be seen early due to atony and denervation
- Associated with distended bladder
  - Resolves on bladder emptying

Pyo- or Hemonephrosis

- Dilated calyceal system filled with low-level echoes
- Clinical picture important for diagnosis

Ureteral Calculi

- Typical echogenic shadowing stone

- More common from deceased donor transplants

Urothelial Thickening

- Secondary to acute rejection or infection
- Regular laminated wall thickening in renal pelvis or ureter
- If grossly thickened, can mimic hydronephrosis

Transitional Cell Carcinoma (TCC)

- Patients usually present with painless hematuria
- Hypoechoic urothelial tumor is solid with internal color Doppler flow
- Typically causes hydronephrosis

Renal Sinus Cysts

- Peripelvic or renal sinus cysts may mimic hydronephrosis
- Differentiate by showing lack of communication between cystic lesions and collecting system

Prominent Hilar Vessels

- Mimicking dilated ureter
- Easily differentiated from dilated ureter with aid of color Doppler imaging

PATHOLOGY

General Features

- Etiology
  - Postoperative ureteral anastomotic edema and denervation may cause transient early hydronephrosis
  - Fixed strictures of distal ureter and ureterovesical anastomosis most commonly from ischemia, scarring, surgical technique or rejection
    - Distal ureter has tenuous vascular supply
  - Luminal causes of obstruction include blood clot, calculus, sloughed papilla, or fungus ball
  - Extrinsic obstruction may be secondary to perigraft fluid collections, fibrosis, or ureteral kinking
  - Reflux, infection, and decreased ureteral tone may cause nonobstructive dilatation
- Associated abnormalities
  - Acute or chronic rejection
  - Infection
  - Hemorrhage
  - Nephrolithiasis (1-2%)
  - Urothelial tumors

Gross Pathologic & Surgical Features

- Early strictures typically secondary to ureteral ischemia or surgical technical complication
- Later stenosis from rejection, drugs, or infection such as BK infection
- Ureteral edema or intraluminal blood clot
- Cortical thinning if hydronephrosis is longstanding and severe

CLINICAL ISSUES

Presentation

- Most common signs/symptoms
  - Rising creatinine level may prompt ultrasound
  - Diagnosis often incidental
- Other signs/symptoms
  - Rarely painful as allograft is denervated

- Occasional tenderness, particularly if infected
- Signs of infection

Demographics

- Epidemiology
  - Ureteral obstruction occurs in 3-6% of renal allografts
    - Most common in first 6 months after transplantation

Natural History & Prognosis

- Ureteral strictures rarely lead to allograft loss if diagnosed and treated promptly

Treatment

- Initial percutaneous nephrostomy to relieve obstruction and until infection resolves
  - Antegrade nephrostogram to confirm diagnosis and delineate location and length of stricture
  - Antegrade stent followed by balloon dilatation of stricture
  - Retrograde stent and balloon dilatation more technically challenging
- Surgical reconstruction required for long or recurrent strictures
- Drainage of collections causing obstruction
- Removal of intrinsic obstruction such as clot, calculus
- Ureteral stent or Foley catheterization with bladder irrigation for hemonephrosis

DIAGNOSTIC CHECKLIST

Consider

- Ultrasound is first-line imaging modality for renal transplant dysfunction in immediate postoperative period or for follow-up
- MR/MRU is complementary to ultrasound to evaluate causes of obstruction
- Ultrasound-guided antegrade nephrostogram for initial drainage and access for later interventional procedures

Image Interpretation Pearls

- Look for full bladder, stones, clot, or collections as potential causes of hydronephrosis

SELECTED REFERENCES

1. Aktaş A: Transplanted kidney function evaluation. Semin Nucl Med. 44(2):129-45, 2014
2. Duty BD et al: The current role of endourologic management of renal transplantation complications. Adv Urol. 2013:246520, 2013
3. Ferreira Cassini M et al: Lithiasis in 1,313 kidney transplants: incidence, diagnosis, and management. Transplant Proc. 44(8):2373-5, 2012
4. Eufrásio P et al: Surgical complications in 2000 renal transplants. Transplant Proc. 43(1):142-4, 2011
5. Cosgrove DO et al: Renal transplants: what ultrasound can and cannot do. Ultrasound Q. 24(2):77-87; quiz 141-2, 2008
6. Kobayashi K et al: Interventional radiologic management of renal transplant dysfunction: indications, limitations, and technical considerations. Radiographics. 27(4):1109-30, 2007
7. Kamath S et al: Papillary necrosis causing hydronephrosis in renal allograft treated by percutaneous retrieval of sloughed papilla. Br J Radiol. 78(928):346-8, 2005

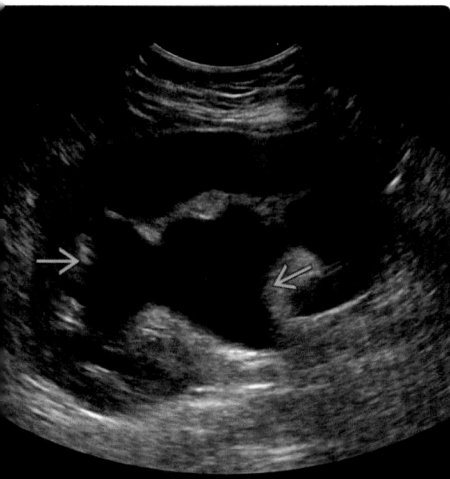

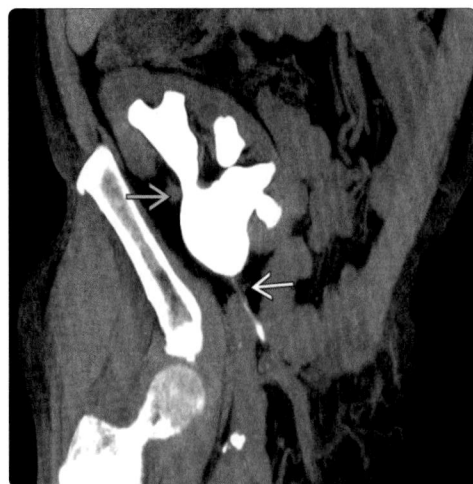

(Left) *Longitudinal ultrasound of a renal transplant shows dilatation of the renal pelvis and calyces* ⇒ *secondary to a long ureteral stricture.* (Right) *MIP of a CT antegrade nephrostogram in the same patient shows severe hydronephrosis* ⇒ *in a renal transplant. There is a long fibrous stricture of the transplant ureter* ⇒. *Surgical reconstruction was required.*

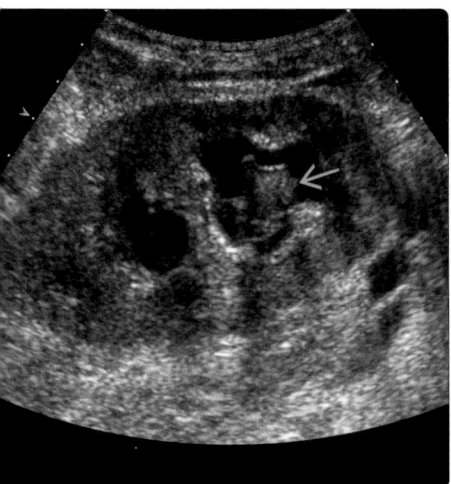

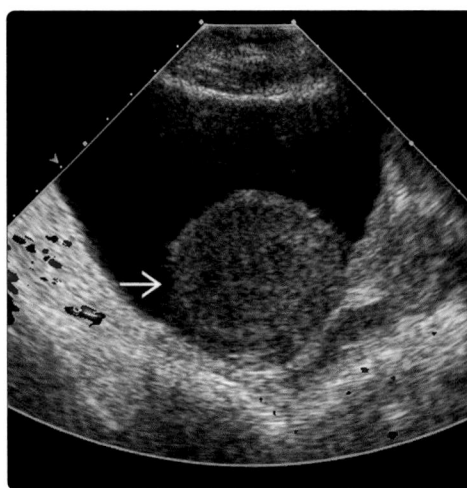

(Left) *Longitudinal ultrasound of a renal transplant shows debris* ⇒ *within a dilated renal pelvis. The patient had gross hematuria after a percutaneous biopsy. It is important to look for an arteriovenous fistula in this context.* (Right) *Transverse color Doppler ultrasound of the bladder in the same patient with hematuria after a renal transplant biopsy shows a large, avascular clot* ⇒ *in the bladder.*

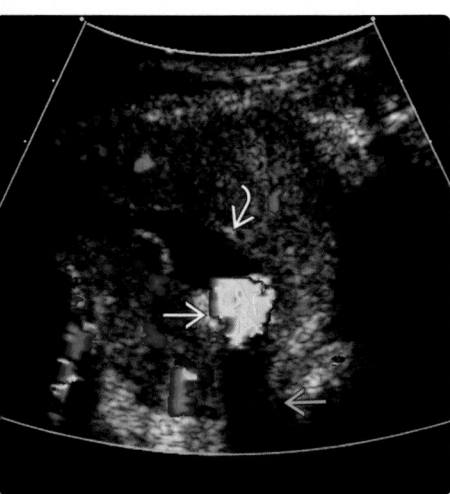

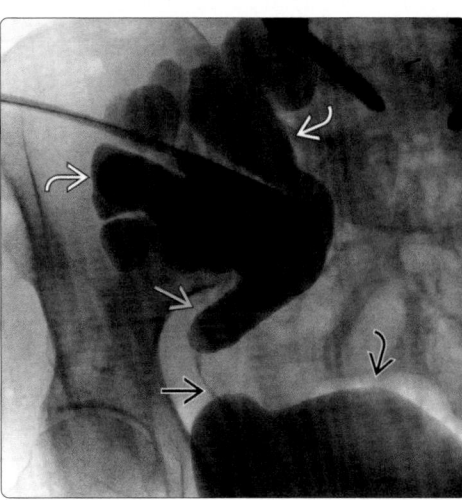

(Left) *Transverse color Doppler ultrasound shows a calculus causing mild hydronephrosis* ⇒ *in a renal transplant. The calculus exhibits twinkling artifact* ⇒ *and posterior acoustic shadowing* ⇒. (Right) *Percutaneous nephrostogram shows a dilated renal pelvis and blunted calyces* ⇒. *There was an obstructing calculus visible as a round filling defect* ⇒. *Contrast is seen in the nondilated ureter* ⇒ *below the calculus and in the bladder* ⇒.

Perigraft Fluid Collections

TERMINOLOGY

- Perigraft fluid collections (PFC) include hematomas, seromas, urinomas, lymphoceles, and abscesses
- Depending on size and location, PFC may cause mass effect on allograft resulting in hydronephrosis or graft dysfunction
- Lymphoceles, most common PFC, occur in 5-15% patients, usually after 4 weeks
- Urinomas occur in 2-5% of patients secondary to anastomotic leak or ureteric ischemia within first 2 weeks

IMAGING

- US is first-line modality for evaluating graft dysfunction, excellent for PFC
- Collection of simple or complex fluid around renal allograft, typically walled off
- CT superior for larger collections, local consequences, as well as other abdominopelvic complications

- Multidetector CT urography (CTU) superior to intravenous pyelogram in detecting urine leaks and ureteral obstruction
- Contrast cystography can demonstrate ureterovesical anastomotic leak
- Definitive diagnosis established by US-guided needle aspiration
- Aspiration of PFC to drain the collection and rule out infection
- Aspirate should be tested for creatinine, markedly elevated in urine leak

TOP DIFFERENTIAL DIAGNOSES

- Ovarian cysts
- Renal cyst
- Peritoneal inclusion cyst
- Penile prosthesis reservoir
- Pseudomyxoma peritonei

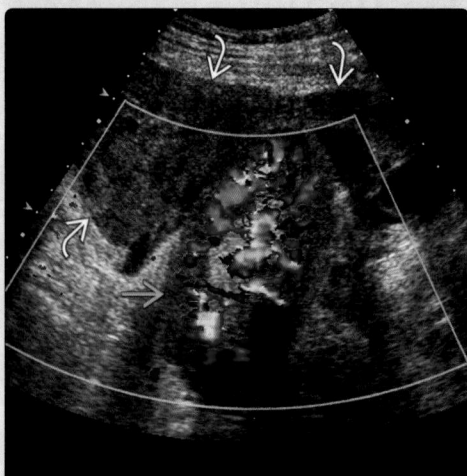

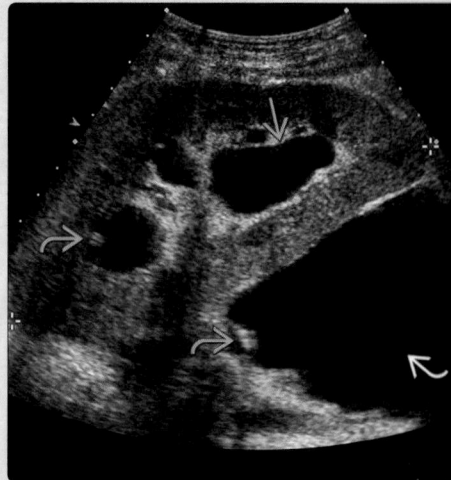

(Left) *Longitudinal color Doppler US shows a right lower quadrant renal allograft ➡️. The allograft is well perfused despite a large, acute, echogenic perinephric hematoma ➡️. (Right) Longitudinal US shows a renal allograft with moderate hydronephrosis ➡️. The transplant ureter was compressed by a large lymphocele ➡️, and a ureteral stent is present ➡️.*

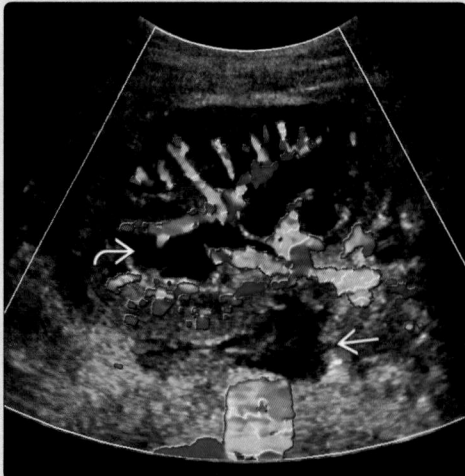

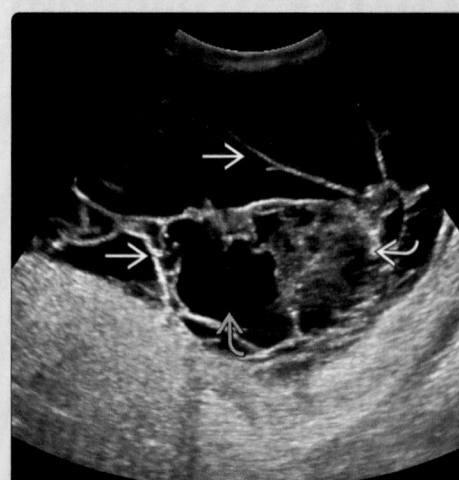

(Left) *Longitudinal color Doppler US shows a renal transplant with mild hydronephrosis ➡️. Although there was a small hematoma ➡️ posterior to the transplant, this was not the cause of the hydronephrosis. (Right) Longitudinal US shows a chronic hematoma in the right pelvis. There are multiple thick and irregular septations ➡️ with more solid, avascular areas ➡️. Some loculi contain echogenic fluid ➡️.*

TERMINOLOGY

Abbreviations

- Perigraft fluid collections (PFC)

Definitions

- Not uncommon in early postoperative period and usually asymptomatic
- PFC include hematomas, seromas, urinomas, lymphoceles, and abscesses
- Depending on size and location, PFC may cause mass effect on allograft resulting in hydronephrosis or graft dysfunction
- Hematomas/seromas: Normal sequela of surgery often small, seen immediately after transplantation
- Lymphoceles, most common PFC, occur in 5-15% patients, usually after 4 weeks
  - Frequently cause hydronephrosis due to extrinsic ureteral compression
- Urinomas occur in 2-5% of patients secondary to anastomotic leak or ureteric ischemia within first 2 weeks
- Abscesses occur later in postoperative period with clinical evidence of infection
  - Bacterial or fungal infection not uncommon in renal transplant patients due to immunosuppression

IMAGING

General Features

- Best diagnostic clue
  - Collection of simple or complex fluid around renal allograft, typically walled off
  - Appearance and complications of PFC depend on composition and location
  - Definitive diagnosis established by ultrasound-guided needle aspiration
- Location
  - Variable
- Size
  - Variable
- Morphology
  - Depends on composition of PFC

Ultrasonographic Findings

- Grayscale ultrasound
  - Fluid characteristics when simple: Anechoic or hypoechoic with posterior enhancement
  - Internal echoes when complex
  - Seromas: Typically anechoic and small
    - May contain low-level echoes if infected
  - Hematomas: Echogenicity depends on age of collections
    - Acute hematomas appear as echogenic heterogeneous collection
    - Crescentic perigraft fluid collection or ovoid collection
    - Upon maturation, hematomas become cystic containing low-level internal echoes and thin or thick fibrin strands with retracting clot
  - Lymphoceles: Well defined and anechoic but may be septated
    - Located near renal vascular pedicle
  - Urinomas: Usually localized anechoic collection

- Undetectable when small, may produce urinary ascites as they enlarge
- Typically adjacent to ureter and separate from bladder
- Rarely septated unless infected
  - Abscesses: Typically complex thick-walled cystic structures with irregular outline and echogenic internal debris
    - Can form adjacent to, or remote from, graft
- Color Doppler
  - Useful to differentiate complex PFC from complex cystic masses by demonstrating vascularity within masses

Ultrasound-Guided Aspiration

- Aspiration to drain collection and exclude infection
- Aspirate should be tested for creatinine, markedly elevated in urine leak
- Aspirate from hematoma or lymphocele has creatinine level comparable to serum

Nonvascular Interventions

- Percutaneous sclerosis
  - Therapeutic option for recurrent lymphoceles

Fluoroscopic Findings

- Contrast cystography can demonstrate ureterovesical anastomotic leak
- After percutaneous access, antegrade pyelography (AP) can be used to detect more proximal leaks

CT Findings

- Collection with CT attenuation between 10-24 HU suggestive of lymphoceles or seromas
- Collection with high CT attenuation (> 28 HU) most likely hematoma
- Abscesses or chronic hematomas have variable HU values
- CT superior for larger collections, local consequences, as well as other abdominopelvic complications
  - Wider FOV, less limited by body habitus and acoustic window
- Multidetector CT urography (CTU) superior to intravenous pyelogram in detecting urine leaks and ureteral obstruction
- CT cystography or CT nephrostography have high sensitivity for ureteral leaks

Nuclear Medicine Findings

- Technetium-99m mercaptoacetyltriglycine (Tc-99m MAG) study
  - Progressive radiotracer activity in abnormal collection is diagnostic of urinoma
  - Large photopenic defect compressing graft kidney is suggestive of PFC

Imaging Recommendations

- Best imaging tool
  - US is first-line modality for evaluating graft dysfunction, excellent for PFC
  - US guidance for aspiration (CT guided if US is not feasible)
- Protocol advice
  - CT may be performed as general survey for abscess or complications

DIFFERENTIAL DIAGNOSIS

Ovarian Cysts

- Coexisting ovarian cysts may produce features simulating lymphoceles or hematomas, including
  - Functional cysts ± hemorrhage
  - Cystadenomas
  - Endometriomas

Renal Cyst

- Exophytic large renal cortical cyst may mimic PFC

Peritoneal Inclusion Cyst

- Also called peritoneal pseudocysts or inflammatory pelvic cysts
- Variable appearance that can simulate hydro- or pyosalpinx, paraovarian cysts, and malignant ovarian neoplasm
- Variable size; may be large, filling entire pelvis and extending into abdomen

Penile Prosthesis Reservoir

- Diagnosis based on history and presence of tubing

Pseudomyxoma Peritonei

- Rare intraabdominal disease characterized by dissecting gelatinous ascites and multifocal peritoneal deposits that secrete mucin
- Originates from perforated appendiceal epithelial tumor, which may be benign, borderline, or malignant
- Patients present with abdominal pain and distension
- Sonographically manifests as complex echogenic ascites

Tuberculous Peritonitis

- Associated with ascites that may be free or loculated, anechoic, or contains fine fibrin strands

PATHOLOGY

General Features

- Etiology
  - Lymphoceles form when normal lymphatics are disrupted during perivascular dissection or after incomplete ligation of pelvic lymphatics
  - Urinomas result from urine leaks at ureterovesical junction (UVJ) secondary to ischemia and necrosis of distal ureter
  - Abscesses can be due to fungal or bacterial infection
  - Hematomas may develop from venous or arterial bleeders, from surgical complications or bleeding diathesis
- Associated abnormalities
  - Ureteral compression and hydronephrosis
  - Vascular compression with graft or leg edema or ischemia
  - Compartment syndrome with graft dysfunction

CLINICAL ISSUES

Presentation

- Most common signs/symptoms
  - Lymphoceles: Majority asymptomatic
  - Urinomas: Pain, swelling, discharge from wound
  - Abscesses: Fever, abdominal pain, raised white cell count
  - Hematomas or seromas: Usually asymptomatic
- Other signs/symptoms
  - Lymphoceles: Palpable mass, leg pain, edema, impaired renal function

Natural History & Prognosis

- Lymphoceles are usually slow growing, occurring within 1 year of transplantation
  - May recur after catheter drainage
  - Sclerotherapy after percutaneous aspiration and drainage may reduce recurrence rate
- Urinomas require intervention
- Small hematomas and seromas resolve spontaneously
- Abscesses usually resolve following treatment

Treatment

- Most PFC are small and asymptomatic, require careful observation only, and will resolve with single aspiration
- Aggressive treatment reserved for symptomatic PFC that may result in allograft dysfunction
- Lymphoceles usually require no therapy unless symptomatic
  - Noninfected: Open surgical drainage, percutaneous aspiration ± sclerotherapy, and laparoscopic marsupialization
  - Infected: Percutaneous drainage
- Urinomas: Short-term urinary diversion with nephrostomy or ureteral stenting if small
  - Large, or those associated with complete disruption of ureteroneocystostomy: Surgical reimplantation
  - Surgically not feasible: Long-term urinary diversion with nephrostomy or ureteral stenting
- Abscesses: Percutaneous drainage followed by antibiotic therapy
- Small hematomas and seromas usually require no therapy
  - Active bleeding requires surgery

DIAGNOSTIC CHECKLIST

Consider

- Definitive diagnosis established by needle aspiration
- Important to exclude obstructive uropathy

Image Interpretation Pearls

- Appearance, location, and occurrence of PFC after transplantation are useful clues to diagnosis

SELECTED REFERENCES

1. Eufrásio P et al: Surgical complications in 2000 renal transplants. Transplant Proc. 43(1):142-4, 2011
2. Irshad A et al: An overview of renal transplantation: current practice and use of ultrasound. Semin Ultrasound CT MR. 30(4):298-314, 2009
3. Cosgrove DO et al: Renal transplants: what ultrasound can and cannot do. Ultrasound Q. 24(2):77-87; quiz 141-2, 2008
4. Akbar SA et al: Complications of renal transplantation. Radiographics. 25(5):1335-56, 2005

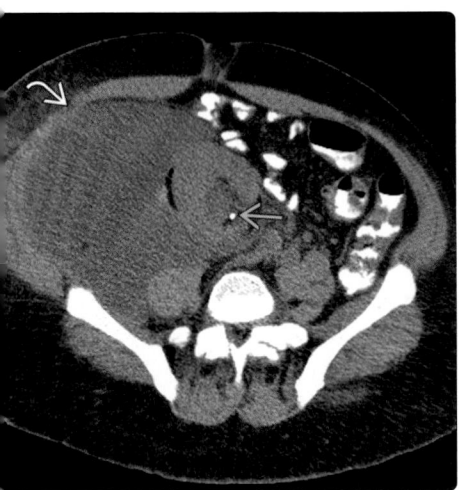

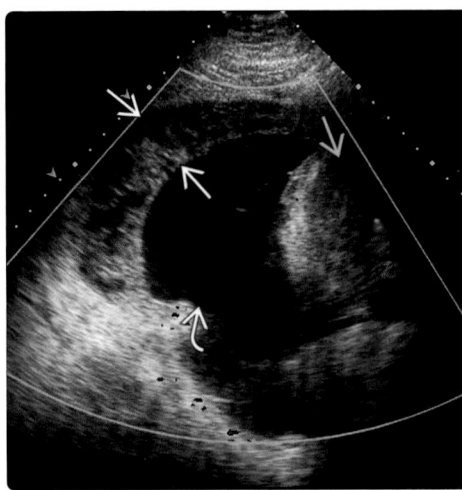

(Left) *Axial NECT shows a large fluid collection representing a lymphocele ➡ in the right pelvis. The renal allograft is displaced medially. Hydronephrosis is present despite the ureteral stent ➡.* (Right) *Transverse color Doppler US shows the same patient after drainage of the lymphocele ➡. Although the lymphocele is smaller, the wall is much thicker ➡. The renal transplant is perfused ➡.*

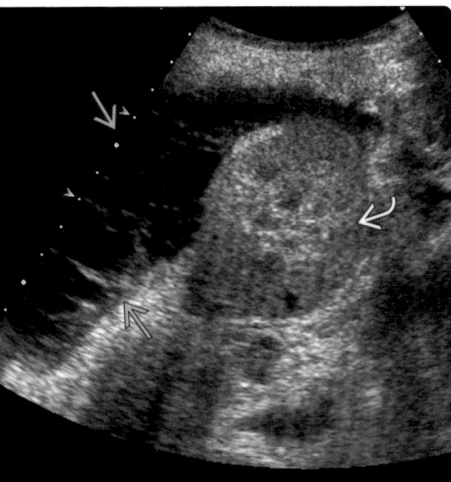

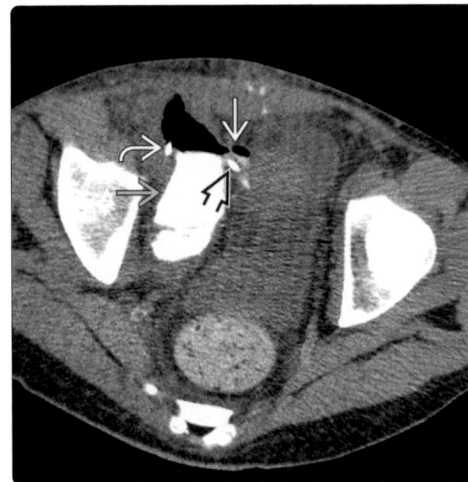

(Left) *Longitudinal oblique US shows a large, septated urinoma ➡ anterior to an unremarkable renal transplant ➡. Fluid aspirated from the collection had a high creatinine level.* (Right) *Axial CT cystogram shows contrast leaking ➡ from the bladder at the ureterovesical anastomosis. The collection of air and contrast ➡ lateral to the bladder is a urinoma. A drain ➡ is present in the collection and there is a ureteral stent ➡.*

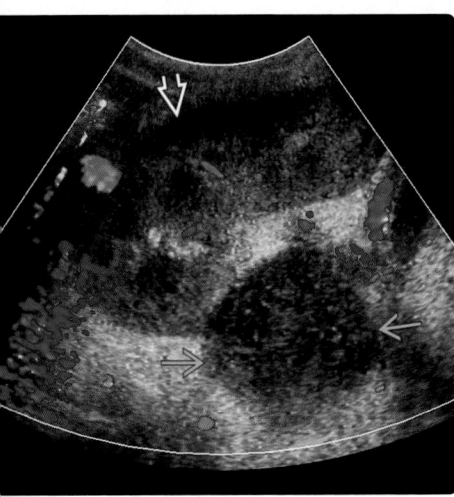

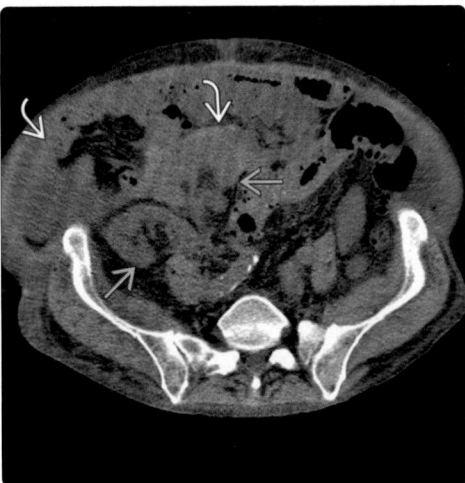

(Left) *Longitudinal color Doppler US shows a small hematoma ➡ deep to the renal transplant ➡ in a patient on anticoagulants. The hematoma was asymptomatic.* (Right) *Axial NECT shows a patient with pediatric en bloc renal transplants ➡ who developed intraperitoneal hemorrhage ➡ after percutaneous biopsy. Hemorrhagic ascites tracked into the lower pelvis (not shown).*

KEY FACTS

IMAGING

- Most commonly at arterial anastomosis
- Focal elevation of peak systolic velocity (PSV) with post-stenotic turbulence
- Color aliasing and soft tissue vibration at area of stenosis
- Elevated PSV in stenotic area > 250-300 cm/sec
- Secondary sign: Tardus parvus intrarenal waveforms = slow systolic upstroke and decreased peak velocity
  - Low resistive index (RI) < 0.5
- Color, power, spectral Doppler US is screening modality for transplant renal artery stenosis (TRAS)
- Careful attention to Doppler angle to ensure accurate PSV measurements
- Supplemented by CTA and MRA
  - More comprehensive vascular evaluation including iliac arteries and aorta
- Catheter angiography is gold standard but is invasive with potential complications

TOP DIFFERENTIAL DIAGNOSES

- Abrupt renal artery curves and kinks
- Pseudo renal artery stenosis

PATHOLOGY

- Surgical injury during harvesting or transplantation
- Immune mediated vascular damage from rejection
- Older renal donors
- Predisposing recipient factors: Atherosclerosis, diabetes, obesity, increasing age

CLINICAL ISSUES

- 2-10% of transplants
- Present with hypertension, acute renal failure or progressive decline in renal function
- May have bruit in vicinity of transplant/iliac artery
- Increased patient morbidity and mortality if untreated

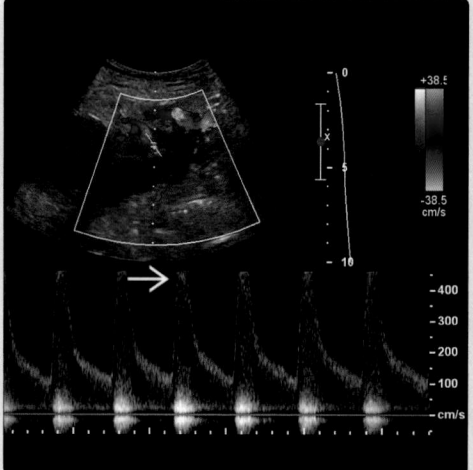
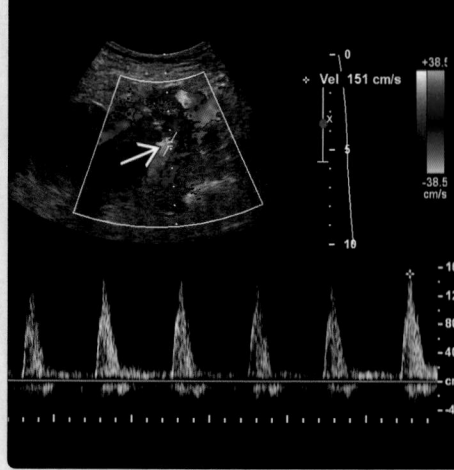

(Left) Longitudinal spectral Doppler ultrasound shows the main renal artery 3 weeks after cadaveric renal transplant in an 82-year-old man. The peak systolic velocity ➡ in the main renal artery exceeds 400 cm/s with aliasing of the Doppler spectrum indicating a significant artery stenosis. Renal function was poor. (Right) Longitudinal spectral Doppler ultrasound of the same patient with renal artery stenosis shows the peak systolic velocity of the external iliac artery ➡ was 151 cm/s with a renal artery to iliac artery ratio > 2.6.

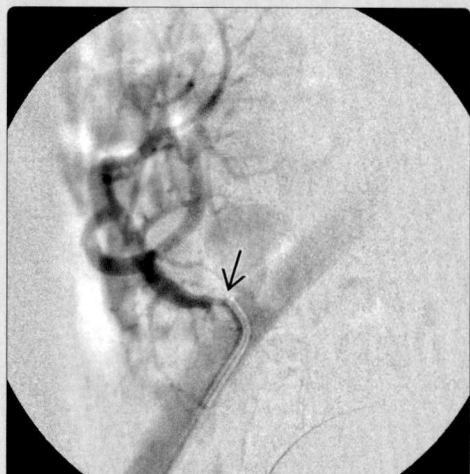
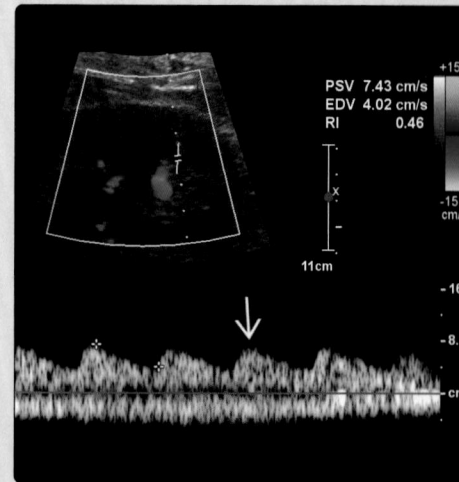

(Left) Digital subtraction angiography of the same patient confirms stenosis at the renal artery anastomosis ➡ estimated to be > 80%. This was successfully angioplastied. (Right) Doppler ultrasound of an interlobar artery in a renal transplant with renal artery stenosis shows tardus parvus ➡ with a low resistive index of 0.46.

TERMINOLOGY

Abbreviations

- Transplant renal artery stenosis (TRAS)

Definitions

- Narrowing of the transplant renal artery (TRA)

IMAGING

General Features

- Best diagnostic clue
  o Focal elevation of peak systolic velocity (PSV) with post-stenotic turbulence
- Location
  o Most commonly at arterial anastomosis
  o Can occur anywhere along transplant artery or there may be diffuse involvement
  o In iliac artery proximal to renal artery graft (pseudo TRAS)
- Surgical anatomy
  o End of graft artery-to-side of external iliac artery most common
    – Performed in living donor and cadaveric grafts
  o Patch of donor aorta along with single or multiple renal arteries anastomosed with recipient external iliac artery
    – Cadaveric graft only
  o End of graft artery-to-end of internal iliac artery or branch uncommon
    – Living donor or cadaveric graft

Ultrasonographic Findings

- Grayscale ultrasound
  o Appearance usually normal
- Color Doppler
  o Color aliasing at area of stenosis
  o Soft tissue vibration adjacent to stenosis
- Spectral Doppler
  o Direct criteria: Elevated PSV in stenotic area > 250-300 cm/sec
    – Wide range of PSV in normal graft arteries: 60-200 cm/sec
  o Renal artery to iliac PSV ratio > 1.8-3.5
  o Sensitivity 87-94%, specificity 86-100 for > 50% stenosis
  o Moderate to severe post-stenotic turbulence
  o Indirect criteria: tardus parvus intrarenal waveforms = slow systolic upstroke and decreased peak velocity
    – Quantified by acceleration index, acceleration time, and resistive index (RI)
      □ Prolonged systolic acceleration time > 0.1 s and decreased acceleration index < 3 m/s²
      □ Low RI < 0.5
    – Acceleration index and acceleration time less specific than PSV of main renal artery and should not be used as signs of TRAS in isolation
    – Note that sensitivity and specificity depend on specific Doppler criteria
  o More proximal stenosis such as common iliac or external iliac stenosis may cause tardus parvus in main renal artery and intrarenal arteries
- Ideal screening modality

- Contrast-enhanced US
  o Fast and noninvasive evaluation of graft perfusion
  o Time for contrast arrival and rate of inflow correlate with degree of stenosis
  o Use is not limited by renal function

Nuclear Medicine Findings

- Isotope renography: Lower sensitivity (75%(and specificity (67%) for TRAS
- Prolonged tracer transit using MAG3

CT Findings

- CTA
  o Comprehensive vascular evaluation including iliac arteries and aorta
  o 3-dimensional images with high spatial resolution, can be rotated for optimal angle
  o Accurate, noninvasive
  o Limited by nephrotoxicity, streak artifact from metal

MR Findings

- MRA
  o Comprehensive vascular evaluation
  o 3-dimensional images which can be manipulated for optimal angle
  o High sensitivity (67-100%) and high specificity (75-100%)
  o No radiation or nephrotoxic iodinated contrast agents
    – However, limited by risk of nephrogenic systemic fibrosis when renal function is abnormal
  o Artifacts from surgical clips and metal prostheses may lead to overestimate of stenosis or nondiagnostic study
- Nonenhaned MRA techniques increasing in diagnostic value and accuracy
  o For patients with abnormal glomerular filtration rate in whom gadolinium based contrast agents are best avoided

Angiographic Findings

- Catheter angiography is gold standard but is invasive with potential complications
- Confirms stenosis (> 50% stenosis on angiography considered significant)
- Pull back pressure gradient across stenosis > 10-20 mmHg suggests significant stenosis
- Carbon dioxide angiography useful to limit amount of iodinated contrast
- Endovascular intervention can be performed

Imaging Recommendations

- Best imaging tool
  o Color, power, spectral Doppler US is screening modality for TRAS
- Protocol advice
  o Careful attention to Doppler angle to ensure accurate PSV measurements
  o Optimization of pulse repetition frequency and gain is essential

DIFFERENTIAL DIAGNOSIS

Abrupt Renal Artery Curves and Kinks

- Curves and kinks can elevate peak velocity without stenosis

- Renal torsion or graft malposition may result in functional arterial stenosis
- May be initially evaluated with CTA or MRA
- However, may need confirmatory angiography to determine functional significance
- Be wary of diagnosing flow-limiting stenosis in absence of post-stenotic flow disturbance

Pseudo Renal Artery Stenosis

- Stenosis proximal to renal artery causing diminished flow
- Diffuse atherosclerosis in aorta, common or external iliac artery

Transplant Arteriovenous Fistula

- Typically intrarenal area of color aliasing and tissue vibration
- High-velocity low-resistance waveform
- Post biopsy

PATHOLOGY

General Features

- Etiology
  - Surgical injury during harvesting or transplantation
    - Anastomotic technical problems, reaction to suture, clamp injury
    - Angulation, kink or twist
    - Mechanical compression resulting in turbulent flow
  - Immune-mediated vascular damage from rejection
  - Neointimal hyperplasia
  - Older renal donors are more likely to have renal artery stenosis
  - More common in living renal donor transplants: No patch of donor aorta
  - Predisposing recipient factors include atherosclerosis, diabetes, obesity, increasing age

Gross Pathologic & Surgical Features

- Arterial wall fibrosis → luminal narrowing
- Diffuse arterial disease from cell mediated immune injury

Microscopic Features

- Surgical injury, inflammation, arterial wall fibrosis, thrombus

CLINICAL ISSUES

Presentation

- Most common signs/symptoms
  - Any time after transplantation but peaks at 6 months and usually within 3 years
    - Hypertension is the principal symptom; newly developed, progressive, or resistant to therapy
    - Acute renal failure
    - Progressive decline in renal function
      □ Renal failure after ACE inhibitor
    - Bruit in vicinity of transplant/iliac artery
    - Heart failure
    - Volume overload
    - Flash pulmonary edema

Demographics

- Epidemiology
  - Most common graft vascular complication

- 2-10% of transplants

Natural History & Prognosis

- Main cause of graft loss given current success of antirejection therapy
- Increased patient morbidity and mortality if untreated
- Excellent prognosis with successful treatment of stenosis/surgical revision

Treatment

- Percutaneous transluminal angioplasty
  - ± stent
    - 5-10% complication rate
- Surgical repair second line
- Iliac stenosis may also be treated with angioplasty and stent

DIAGNOSTIC CHECKLIST

Consider

- Curves and kinks mimicking transplant renal artery stenosis

Image Interpretation Pearls

- Look for focal elevation in peak renal artery velocity compared to iliac artery velocity **and** post stenotic turbulence

SELECTED REFERENCES

1. Chen W et al: Transplant renal artery stenosis: clinical manifestations, diagnosis and therapy. Clin Kidney J. 8(1):71-8, 2015
2. Gaddikeri S et al: Comparing the diagnostic accuracy of contrast-enhanced computed tomographic angiography and gadolinium-enhanced magnetic resonance angiography for the assessment of hemodynamically significant transplant renal artery stenosis. Curr Probl Diagn Radiol. 43(4):162-8, 2014
3. Rodgers SK et al: Ultrasonographic evaluation of the renal transplant. Radiol Clin North Am. 52(6):1307-24, 2014
4. Glebova NO et al: Endovascular interventions for managing vascular complication of renal transplantation. Semin Vasc Surg. 26(4):205-12, 2013
5. Kobayashi K et al: Interventional radiologic management of renal transplant dysfunction: indications, limitations, and technical considerations. Radiographics. 27(4):1109-30, 2007
6. Li JC et al: Evaluation of severe transplant renal artery stenosis with Doppler sonography. J Clin Ultrasound. 33(6):261-9, 2005
7. de Morais RH et al: Duplex Doppler sonography of transplant renal artery stenosis. J Clin Ultrasound. 31(3):135-41, 2003
8. Patel U et al: Doppler ultrasound for detection of renal transplant artery stenosis-threshold peak systolic velocity needs to be higher in a low-risk or surveillance population. Clin Radiol. 58(10):772-7, 2003
9. Loubeyre P et al: Transplanted renal artery: detection of stenosis with color Doppler US. Radiology. 203(3):661-5, 1997
10. Baxter GM et al: Colour Doppler ultrasound in renal transplant artery stenosis: which Doppler index? Clin Radiol. 50(9):618-22, 1995
11. Gottlieb RH et al: Diagnosis of renal artery stenosis in transplanted kidneys: value of Doppler waveform analysis of the intrarenal arteries. AJR Am J Roentgenol. 165(6):1441-6, 1995

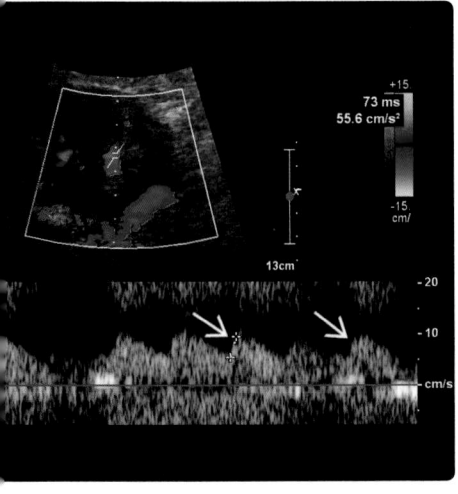

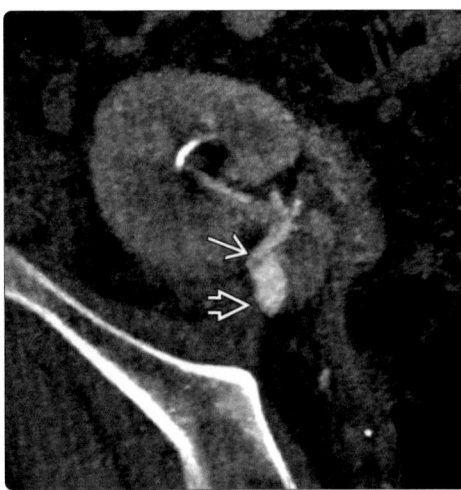

(Left) *Doppler ultrasound of a segmental lower pole artery in a renal transplant with renal artery stenosis shows tardus parvus* ➜ *with a decreased acceleration index of 55.6 cm/s².* **(Right)** *CT arteriogram performed after Doppler ultrasound tardus parvus after living unrelated renal transplant. There is a twist in the proximal renal artery* ➡. *The iliac artery* ➡ *was normal. The kidney was abnormally rotated at surgery.*

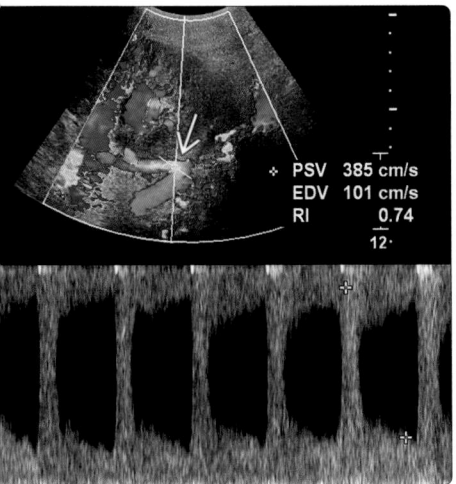

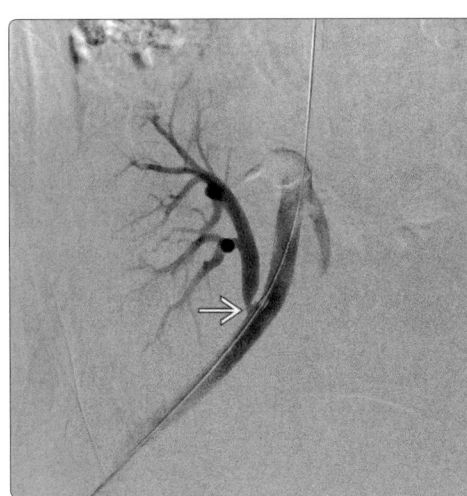

(Left) *Doppler ultrasound of the renal artery anastomosis in a patient with acute kidney injury 1 year after cadaver transplantation is shown. Color and Doppler aliasing are noted at the anastomosis* ➡ *with peak velocities exceeding 385 cm/s.* **(Right)** *Digital subtraction angiography of the same patient confirms a high-grade (90%) stenosis at the anastomosis* ➡. *This was treated with angioplasty.*

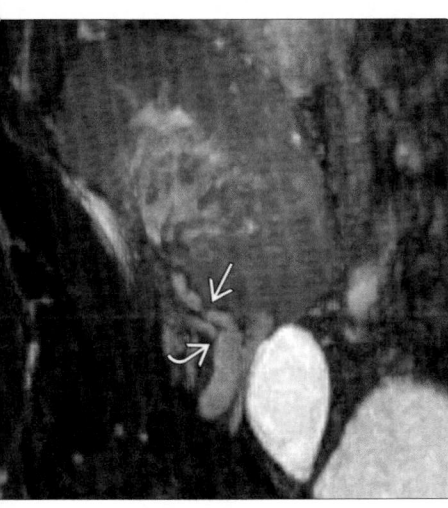

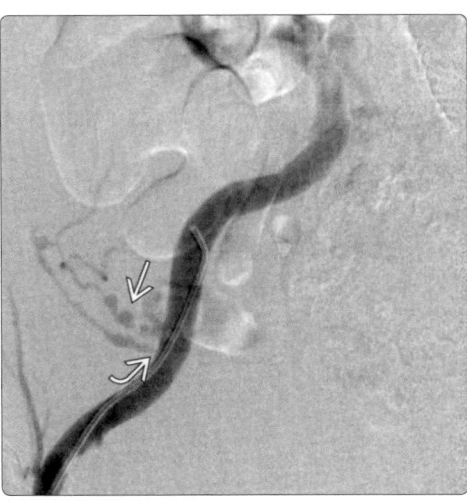

(Left) *Coronal unenhanced MRA performed after suspected renal artery stenosis on Doppler ultrasound shows delayed graft function and hypertension 3 months after cadaveric renal transplant. There are 2 renal arteries with a significant stenosis of the inferior origin* ➡ *and diffuse irregularity of the superior artery* ➡. **(Right)** *Digital subtraction angiography of the same patient confirms the diffusely abnormal superior artery* ➡ *with alternating stenoses/dilatation as well as the more focal stenosis* ➡ *of the inferior artery.*

Transplant Renal Artery Thrombosis

TERMINOLOGY

- Occlusion of transplant renal artery secondary to thrombus

IMAGING

- Absence of blood flow in main renal artery
- Diffuse absence of parenchymal perfusion on color or power Doppler
- If involving accessory renal artery
  o Segmental wedge-shaped peripheral area of decreased color flow
- US is first-line imaging modality for complications of renal transplantation
- Optimize color and spectral Doppler settings for slow flow

TOP DIFFERENTIAL DIAGNOSES

- Transplant renal vein thrombosis
- Acute rejection/acute tubular necrosis
- Hyperacute rejection

CLINICAL ISSUES

- Rare < 1%
- Abrupt onset of oliguria, decreased function, pain and swelling of allograft
- Poor prognosis, graft loss is usual when single main artery thrombosed
  o Transplant nephrectomy
  o Thrombectomy or thrombolysis rarely successful unless diagnosis made early
- Accessory or segmental arterial thrombosis: Ischemia and subsequent atrophy

DIAGNOSTIC CHECKLIST

- Severe acute rejection or tubular necrosis may cause propagating small vessel thrombosis resulting in infarction and mimic transplant renal artery thrombosis (TRAT)
- Urgent finding requiring prompt communication

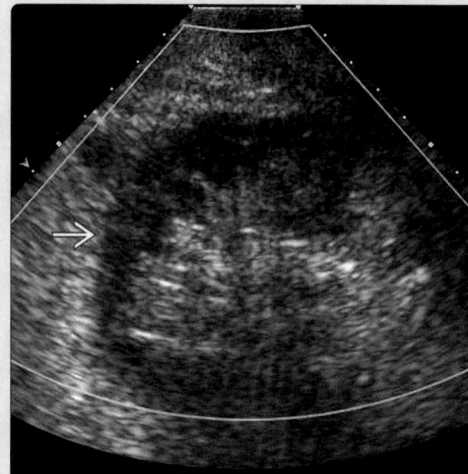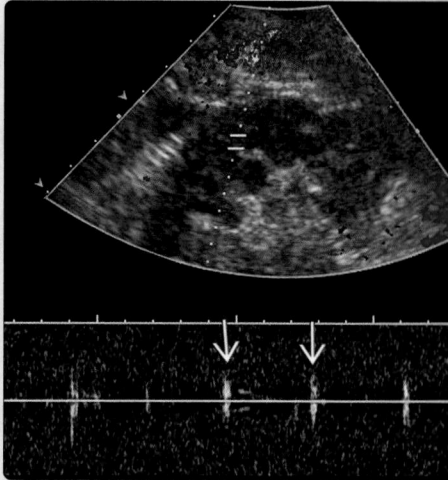

(Left) Longitudinal color Doppler US in the 1st day after renal transplantation shows no color flow in the allograft ➔ secondary to early thrombosis in a hypercoagulable patient. (Right) Longitudinal pulsed Doppler ultrasound of the same patient shows no intrarenal arterial flow. Noise ➔ was transmitted to the kidney.

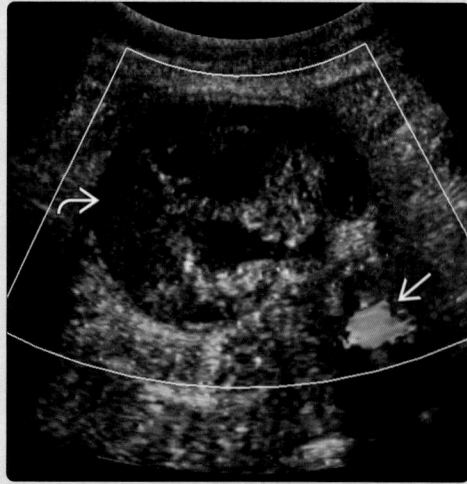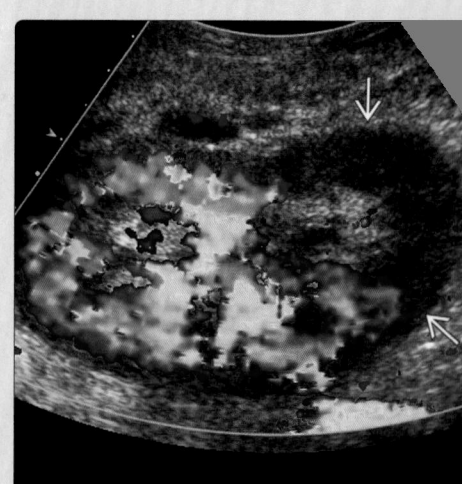

(Left) Transverse color Doppler ultrasound of a thrombosed recent renal transplant shows an edematous allograft ➔ with no internal color flow. The iliac artery ➔ is patent. (Right) Longitudinal color Doppler ultrasound shows a renal allograft with segmental ischemia of the lower pole ➔ secondary to thrombosis of an accessory renal artery. Absence of color flow is noted in the lower 1/2 of the allograft.

TERMINOLOGY

Abbreviations

Transplant renal artery thrombosis (TRAT)

Definitions

Occlusion of transplant renal artery secondary to thrombus

IMAGING

General Features

Best diagnostic clue
- Absence of blood flow in renal artery
- Absence of color flow in transplant kidney

Location
- Main artery or distal branch
- May involve accessory renal artery causing segmental ischemia
- Important to know surgical vascular anatomy
  - Single or multiple renal arteries
  - End of graft artery-to-side of external iliac artery anastomosis most common
  - Patch of donor aorta (with single or multiple renal arteries attached)-to-side of external iliac artery
  - Venous interposition graft
  - End of graft artery-to-end of internal iliac artery, common iliac artery or aorta less common

Ultrasonographic Findings

Grayscale ultrasound
- Enlarged hypoechoic allograft
- Hypoechoic peripheral wedge-shaped areas

Color Doppler
- Nonvisualization of entire renal transplant artery and vein
  - Diffuse absence of parenchymal perfusion on color or power Doppler
  - Segmental wedge-shaped peripheral areas of decreased color flow when accessory or distal arteries are occluded
- Thrombosis of distal artery with patent flow proximally (will progress to complete thrombosis)

Spectral Doppler
- Absence of Doppler signal in complete thrombosis
- Blunted low-resistance waveforms in ischemic areas (collateral flow)
- Absence of venous flow

Imaging Recommendations

Best imaging tool
- US is first-line imaging modality for complications of renal transplantation

Protocol advice
- Optimize color and spectral Doppler settings for slow flow

DIFFERENTIAL DIAGNOSIS

Transplant Renal Vein Thrombosis

Many features in common but arterial reversed diastolic flow is present early in renal vein thrombosis

Acute Rejection/Acute Tubular Necrosis

- Markedly diminished flow in renal parenchyma with high resistive index or reversed diastolic flow

Hyperacute Rejection

- Typically occurs during surgery or soon after resulting in graft thrombosis

PATHOLOGY

General Features

- Etiology
  - Early postoperative period
    - Surgical technique: Kinking, twisting, or dissection of renal artery, trauma to iliac artery, thromboembolism
    - Hypercoagulable state, hypotension
    - Intentional or inadvertent ligation of small accessory arteries
    - Transplant torsion
  - Later: Severe rejection

Gross Pathologic & Surgical Features

- Infarcted kidney

CLINICAL ISSUES

Presentation

- Most common signs/symptoms
  - Abrupt onset of oliguria, decreased function, pain and swelling of allograft

Demographics

- Epidemiology
  - Rare < 1%

Natural History & Prognosis

- Poor prognosis, graft loss is usual when single main artery is thrombosed
- Accessory or segmental arterial thrombosis: Ischemia and subsequent atrophy

Treatment

- Transplant nephrectomy
- Thrombectomy or thrombolysis rarely successful unless diagnosis made early

DIAGNOSTIC CHECKLIST

Consider

- Severe acute rejection or tubular necrosis may cause propagating small vessel thrombosis resulting in infarction and mimic TRAT

Image Interpretation Pearls

- Urgent finding requiring prompt communication

SELECTED REFERENCES

1. Rodgers SK et al: Ultrasonographic evaluation of the renal transplant. Radiol Clin North Am. 52(6):1307-24, 2014
2. Low G et al: Imaging of vascular complications and their consequences following transplantation in the abdomen. Radiographics. 33(3):633-52, 2013
3. Eufrásio P et al: Surgical complications in 2000 renal transplants. Transplant Proc. 43(1):142-4, 2011

Transplant Renal Vein Thrombosis

IMAGING

- Enlarged, edematous, hypoechoic kidney due to outflow obstruction
- Absence or decreased color flow in renal vein at hilum
- Patent renal artery early, later the renal artery will thrombose also
- High systolic arterial peaks with flow reversal in diastole
- Color, power, spectral Doppler US is first-line imaging modality for complications of renal transplantation

TOP DIFFERENTIAL DIAGNOSES

- Acute, severe rejection or delayed graft function
- Iliac vein thrombosis or renal vein compression

PATHOLOGY

- Surgical injury or technical problem
- Compression by fluid collection
- Hypovolemia, hypercoagulable state

- Thrombus propagation from common femoral/external iliac vein

CLINICAL ISSUES

- Abrupt onset of graft tenderness and swelling, decreased function
- Usually within 1st week, most commonly within 48 hours of transplantation
- ≤ 4% of transplants
- Poor prognosis even with prompt diagnosis and thrombectomy/surgical revision
- May progress to rupture with hemorrhage and hypovolemia

DIAGNOSTIC CHECKLIST

- Consider renal vein thrombosis when there is a sudden drop in urine output in early postoperative period
- Reversal of arterial diastolic flow and absence of venous flow confirms this diagnosis

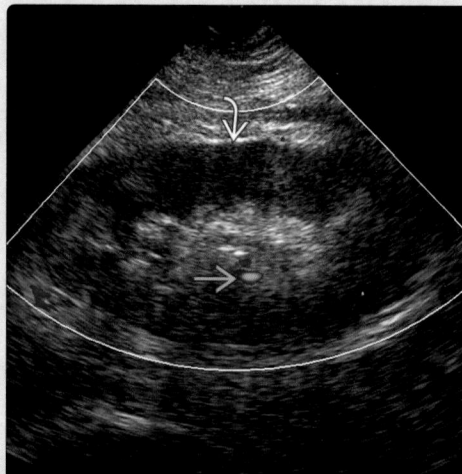
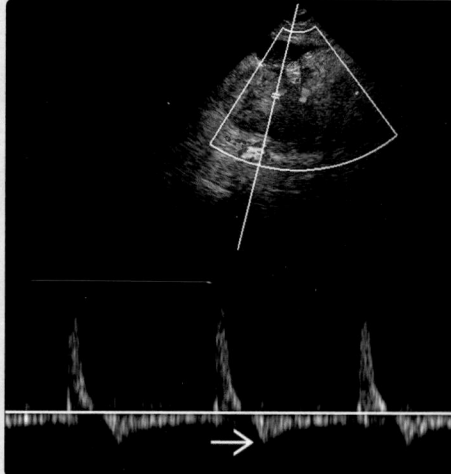

(Left) Longitudinal power Doppler ultrasound of the renal allograft in a patient who developed pain and anuria is shown. Minimal color flow ⇨ is seen in the allograft ➚, which is edematous. (Right) Longitudinal Doppler of the same patient shows abnormal segmental arterial waveform with narrow systolic peaks and reversal of flow ➦ in diastole. The renal vein was thrombosed.

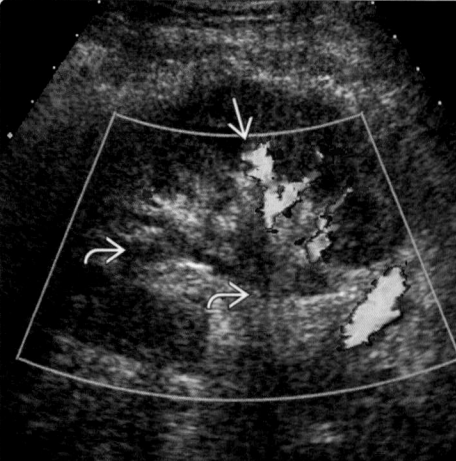
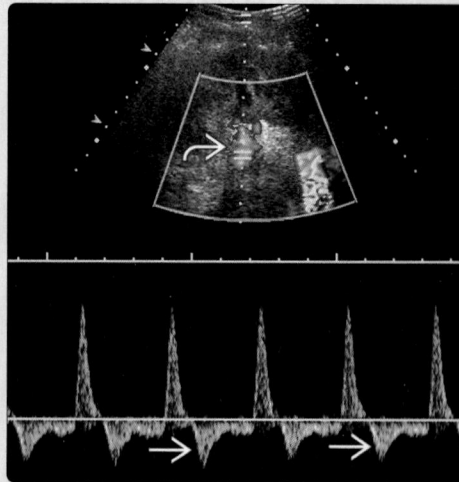

(Left) Longitudinal color Doppler ultrasound shows renal vein thrombosis in a renal allograft. Thrombus can be seen in the main renal vein ➦ extending into segmental veins. Arterial flow ➦ was still detected in the lower pole. (Right) Longitudinal color Doppler ultrasound of the same patient is shown. The main renal artery ➦ was patent but the waveform is abnormal with reversal of diastolic flow ➦.

Transplant Renal Vein Thrombosis

TERMINOLOGY

Abbreviations

- Transplant renal vein thrombosis (TRVT)

Definitions

- Occlusion of transplant renal vein due to thrombus formation

IMAGING

General Features

- Best diagnostic clue
  - Absence of blood flow in renal vein
  - Abnormal renal artery waveform with reversal of diastolic flow
- Location
  - Entire vessel
  - Segmental thrombus (rarely caught early)

Ultrasonographic Findings

- Grayscale ultrasound
  - Enlarged, edematous, hypoechoic kidney due to outflow obstruction
  - Renal vein distended by low echogenicity thrombus
  - Renal rupture with hemorrhage if late
- Color Doppler
  - Absence or decreased color flow in renal vein at hilum
    - Patent renal artery early, later the renal artery will thrombose also
    - Absent to severely diminished parenchymal color flow
- Spectral Doppler
  - Absent venous waveforms at renal hilum and in parenchyma
  - High systolic arterial peaks with flow reversal in diastole

Imaging Recommendations

- Best imaging tool
  - Color, power, spectral Doppler US is first-line imaging modality for complications of renal transplantation
- Protocol advice
  - Optimize color and spectral Doppler settings for slow flow

DIFFERENTIAL DIAGNOSIS

Acute, Severe Rejection or Delayed Graft Function

- Vascular resistance in renal parenchyma markedly increased
  - Diminished, absent, or reversed arterial flow in kidney hilum/intrarenal arteries
  - Renal vein is patent

Iliac Vein Thrombosis or Venous Compression

- Thrombus in ipsilateral iliac or femoral vein
- Extrinsic compression by fluid collection or hematoma

PATHOLOGY

General Features

- Etiology
  - Surgical injury or technical problem
    - Kinking, angulation, or trauma to vein

- Compression by fluid collection (e.g., hematoma, lymphocele): Less common
    - May result in compartment syndrome
  - Hypovolemia, hypercoagulable state
  - Thrombus propagation from common femoral/external iliac vein
  - Rejection
- Associated abnormalities
  - Marked graft congestion/edema
  - Adjacent fluid collections

Gross Pathologic & Surgical Features

- Large vein thrombus extending into smaller veins

Microscopic Features

- Hemorrhagic necrosis

CLINICAL ISSUES

Presentation

- Most common signs/symptoms
  - Abrupt onset of graft tenderness and swelling, decreased function
    - Hematuria, oliguria, proteinuria
  - Usually within 1st week, most commonly within 48 hours of transplantation

Demographics

- Epidemiology
  - ≤ 4% of transplants

Natural History & Prognosis

- Poor prognosis even with prompt diagnosis and thrombectomy/surgical revision
- May progress to rupture with hemorrhage and hypovolemia

Treatment

- Thrombectomy, surgical revision

DIAGNOSTIC CHECKLIST

Consider

- Renal vein thrombosis when there is a sudden drop in urine output in early postoperative period

Image Interpretation Pearls

- Reversal of arterial diastolic flow and absence of venous flow confirms this diagnosis
- Additional imaging causes needless delay

SELECTED REFERENCES

1. Rodgers SK et al: Ultrasonographic evaluation of the renal transplant. Radiol Clin North Am. 52(6):1307-24, 2014
2. Low G et al: Imaging of vascular complications and their consequences following transplantation in the abdomen. Radiographics. 33(3):633-52, 2013
3. Eufrásio P et al: Surgical complications in 2000 renal transplants. Transplant Proc. 43(1):142-4, 2011
4. Kobayashi K et al: Interventional radiologic management of renal transplant dysfunction: indications, limitations, and technical considerations. Radiographics. 27(4):1109-30, 2007

TERMINOLOGY

- Abnormal direct communication between artery and vein

IMAGING

- Usually in renal parenchyma; may be extrarenal
- Not usually visible when small
- Large arteriovenous fistulas (AVF) are serpiginous vessels
- Feeding artery shows high-velocity, low-resistance waveform with spectral broadening
- Pulsatile arterialized flow in draining vein when large
- Best detected when background normal color flow is suppressed by using higher Doppler scale
- Perivascular tissue vibration producing color in adjacent tissues
- Catheter angiography is gold standard for diagnosis, allows endovascular treatment

TOP DIFFERENTIAL DIAGNOSES

- Pseudoaneurysm

- Renal artery stenosis

PATHOLOGY

- Complication of percutaneous transplant biopsy or insertion of nephrostomy

CLINICAL ISSUES

- Post-biopsy incidence: 1-18%
- Most asymptomatic or present with hematuria
- 50% disappear within 48 hours; 70% resolve spontaneous within 1-2 years
- Observation with serial ultrasound for majority
- 30% symptomatic and persistent
- Treated with superselective embolization of feeding arter

(Left) Longitudinal ultrasound of the lower pole of a renal allograft shows a large, serpiginous, anechoic structure ➡ extending from the sinus to the cortex. (Right) Longitudinal color Doppler ultrasound of the same patient shows that the serpiginous structure ➡ fills in with color, representing an intrarenal arteriovenous fistula. This was confirmed with spectral Doppler.

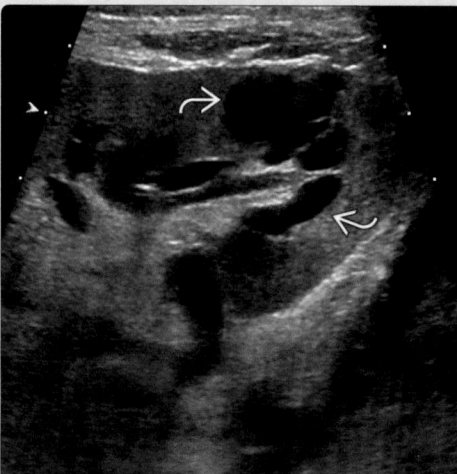
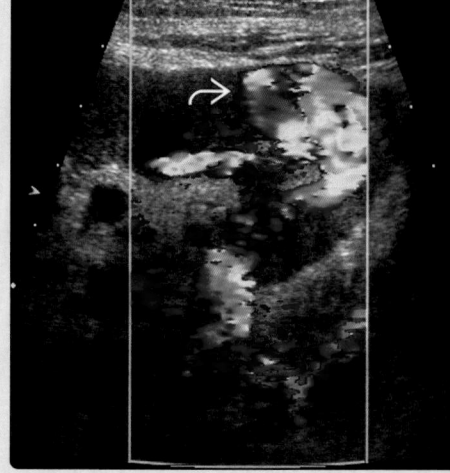

(Left) Longitudinal power Doppler ultrasound of a renal allograft with a lower pole arteriovenous fistula ➡ obscured by perivascular color bleeding shows that there is surrounding tissue vibration ➡. (Right) Longitudinal spectral Doppler of an arteriovenous fistula ➡ presenting as a small area of increased color flow relative to background shows a characteristic high-velocity, low-resistance turbulent waveform.

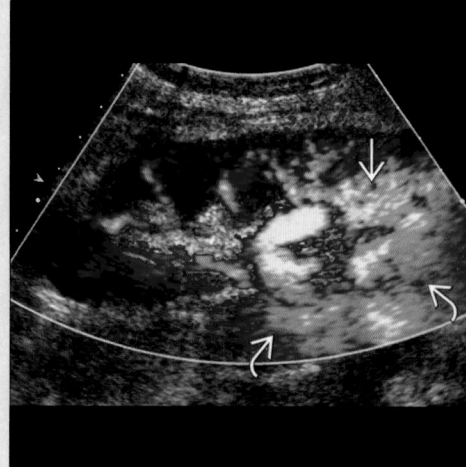
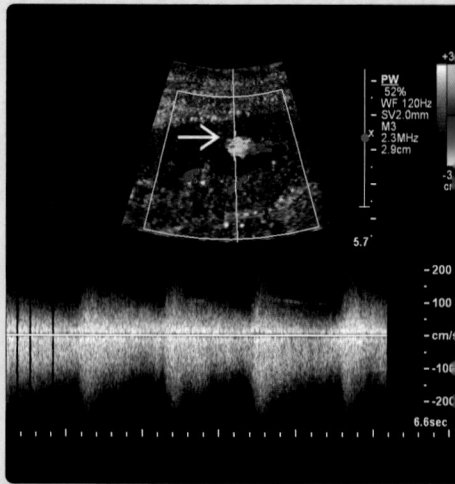

Renal Transplant Arteriovenous (AV) Fistula

TERMINOLOGY

Abbreviations
- Arteriovenous fistula (AVF)

Definitions
- Abnormal direct communication between artery and vein

IMAGING

General Features
- Best diagnostic clue
  - Focal area of increased color Doppler
- Location
  - Usually in renal parenchyma, may be extrarenal
- Size
  - Variable
- Morphology
  - Round when small, tubular when large

Ultrasonographic Findings
- Grayscale ultrasound
  - Not usually visible when small
  - Large AVFs are tubular serpiginous fluid filled structures
- Pulsed Doppler
  - Feeding artery shows high-velocity, low-resistance waveform with spectral broadening
  - Pulsatile arterialized flow in draining vein when large
- Color Doppler
  - Focal aliasing at site of AVF
    - Best detected when background normal color flow is suppressed by using higher Doppler scale
  - Perivascular tissue vibration producing color in adjacent tissues

Angiographic Findings
- Gold standard for diagnosis and first-line for treatment
- Abnormal communication between artery and vein with early venous opacification
- More sensitive than ultrasound for complex AVF

Imaging Recommendations
- Best imaging tool
  - Color Doppler sonography for detection
  - Confirmed by characteristic Doppler waveform
- Protocol advice
  - Optimize detection by suppressing background normal color flow

CTA and MRA
- Require injection of contrast media
- Arterial phase phase blush with early venous filling

DIFFERENTIAL DIAGNOSIS

Pseudoaneurysm
- Spherical intra- or extraparenchymal vascular lesion with yin-yang flow on color Doppler
- Feeding artery shows to and fro waveform

Renal Artery Stenosis
- Narrowing of the renal anastomosis with increased peak systolic velocity
- Poststenotic spectral broadening ± tardus parvus

PATHOLOGY

General Features
- Etiology
  - Complication of percutaneous transplant biopsy or insertion of nephrostomy
  - Increased risk with number of biopsies, hypertension, central renal biopsies, and renal medullary disease
  - Rarely surgical complication, usually anastomotic
- Associated abnormalities
  - AVF may coexist with intrarenal pseudoaneurysm

CLINICAL ISSUES

Presentation
- Most common signs/symptoms
  - Most asymptomatic
- Other signs/symptoms
  - Hematuria
  - Clot colic causing urinary tract obstruction
  - Hypertension/renal dysfunction/heart failure from steal phenomenon in large AVF
  - Rupture

Demographics
- Epidemiology
  - Post-biopsy incidence: 1-18%

Natural History & Prognosis
- 50% disappear within 48 hours, 70% resolve spontaneously within 1-2 years
- 30% symptomatic and persistent
- Extrarenal/sinus AVF larger, unlikely to resolve spontaneously

Treatment
- Observation with serial ultrasound for majority
- Superselective embolization of the feeding artery (coils, cyanoacrylate, glue)
- Surgery: Higher complication rate

DIAGNOSTIC CHECKLIST

Consider
- AVF when patients develop hematuria after renal transplant biopsy

Image Interpretation Pearls
- High-velocity, low-resistance waveform with perivascular color Doppler tissue vibration

SELECTED REFERENCES
1. Rodgers SK et al: Ultrasonographic evaluation of the renal transplant. Radiol Clin North Am. 52(6):1307-24, 2014
2. Glebova NO et al: Endovascular interventions for managing vascular complication of renal transplantation. Semin Vasc Surg. 26(4):205-12, 2013
3. Dimitroulis D et al: Vascular complications in renal transplantation: a single-center experience in 1367 renal transplantations and review of the literature. Transplant Proc. 41(5):1609-14, 2009
4. Kobayashi K et al: Interventional radiologic management of renal transplant dysfunction: indications, limitations, and technical considerations. Radiographics. 27(4):1109-30, 2007

Renal Transplant Pseudoaneurysm

TERMINOLOGY

- Contained rupture secondary to defect in artery wall

IMAGING

- Usually in renal parenchyma, rarely extrarenal
- Usually ≤ 1 cm
- Extrarenal pseudoaneurysm (PA) may be larger
- Mimics simple or complex renal cyst
- High velocity jet into sac with internal turbulent flow
- To-and-fro waveform in neck
- Swirling yin-yang internal flow
- Saccular, round or ovoid
- Pulsations or swirling internal echoes
- Internal clot when large
- CTA/MRA
  - Outpouching from arterial lumen enhancing during arterial phase
  - Provide more information about state of arterial tree as well as size and morphology of pseudoaneurysm

TOP DIFFERENTIAL DIAGNOSES

- Cyst
- Arteriovenous fistula
- Perinephric collection

PATHOLOGY

- Intrarenal: Iatrogenic injury during biopsy or percutaneous procedure

CLINICAL ISSUES

- Most asymptomatic
- Hematuria, abnormal renal function
- Pain, bleeding/hypotension from rupture

DIAGNOSTIC CHECKLIST

- Increased risk of rupture when extrarenal and > 2 cm
- Always turn on color Doppler when evaluating renal cystic lesions

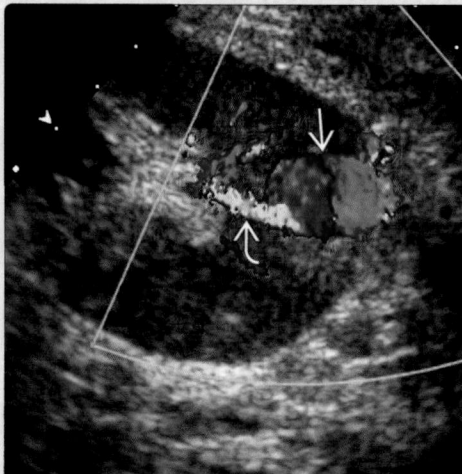
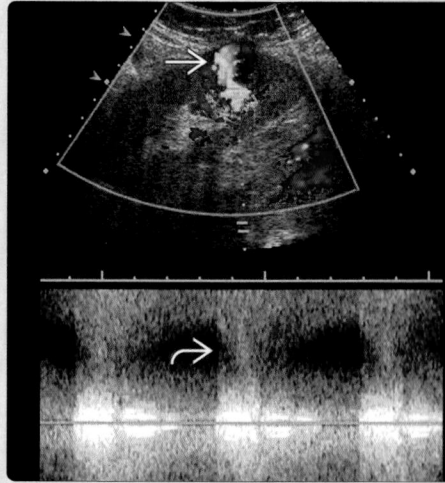

(Left) *Longitudinal color Doppler ultrasound shows a pseudoaneurysm ➡ in the lower pole of a renal transplant. Yin-yang internal swirling flow is present. Color aliasing is noted in the feeding artery ⤴.* (Right) *Longitudinal spectral Doppler ultrasound of a pseudoaneurysm ➡ shows disorganized turbulent flow ⤴ at the base of the pseudoaneurysm.*

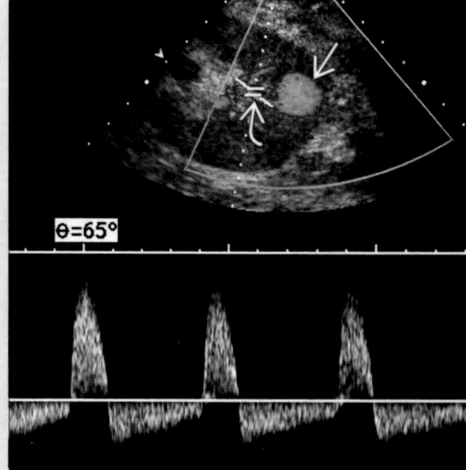
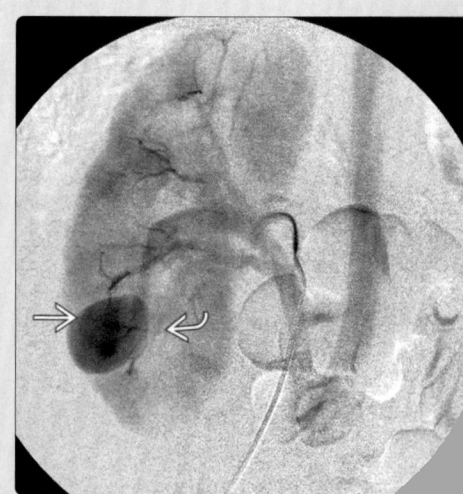

(Left) *Longitudinal Doppler ultrasound shows a pseudoaneurysm ➡ in the lower pole of a renal transplant. To-and-fro flow ⤴ in the neck is characteristic.* (Right) *Digital subtracted selective renal arteriogram shows a pseudoaneurysm ➡ filling from a lower pole artery ⤴. This was embolized.*

TERMINOLOGY

Abbreviations

- Pseudoaneurysm (PA)

Definitions

- Contained rupture secondary to defect in artery wall

IMAGING

General Features

- Best diagnostic clue
  - Focal outpouching from artery
- Location
  - Usually in renal parenchyma, rarely extrarenal
- Size
  - Usually ≤ 1 cm
  - Extrarenal PA may be larger
- Morphology
  - Saccular or fusiform
  - Narrow or wide neck

Ultrasonographic Findings

- Grayscale ultrasound
  - Mimics simple or complex renal cyst
  - Pulsations or swirling internal echoes
  - Internal clot when large
- Pulsed Doppler
  - High velocity jet into sac
  - Internal turbulent flow
  - To-and-fro waveform in neck
- Color Doppler
  - Swirling yin-yang internal flow
  - Aliasing in neck

Angiographic Findings

- Ovoid or spherical outpouching from artery
- May contain intraluminal thrombus

Imaging Recommendations

- Best imaging tool
  - Color Doppler sonography for screening
  - Angiography for confirmation and endovascular intervention
- Protocol advice
  - Always turn on color Doppler when evaluating renal cystic lesions

CTA and MRA

- Outpouching from arterial lumen enhancing during arterial phase
- Provide more information about state of arterial tree as well as size and morphology of pseudoaneurysm
- Noninvasive but require intravenous contrast

DIFFERENTIAL DIAGNOSIS

Cyst

- Anechoic, thin walled with posterior enhancement
- No flow on color Doppler

Arteriovenous Fistula

- May coexist with PA

- Low-resistance, high-velocity waveform
- Pulsatile draining vein

Perinephric Collection

- Cystic ± internal echoes
- Avascular

PATHOLOGY

General Features

- Etiology
  - Intrarenal: Iatrogenic injury during biopsy or percutaneous procedure
  - Extrarenal: Surgical complication at anastomosis or infection (mycotic)
  - Rarely secondary to trauma, inflammation, or neoplasm in renal transplants
- Associated abnormalities
  - Arteriovenous fistula (AVF) or multiple PA

Microscopic Features

- Confined by organized thrombus or fibrous tissue

CLINICAL ISSUES

Presentation

- Most common signs/symptoms
  - Most asymptomatic
- Other signs/symptoms
  - Hematuria, abnormal renal function
  - Pain, bleeding/hypotension from rupture
  - Bruit or pulsatile mass if large

Demographics

- Epidemiology
  - Less frequent than AVF
  - Extrarenal < 1%

Natural History & Prognosis

- Smaller PA: Self-limiting with spontaneous thrombosis
- Larger or enlarging PA: More prone to rupture

Treatment

- Selective embolization
- Thrombin injection

DIAGNOSTIC CHECKLIST

Consider

- Increased risk of rupture when extrarenal and > 2 cm

Image Interpretation Pearls

- To-and-fro flow in neck is diagnostic of PA

SELECTED REFERENCES

1. Rodgers SK et al: Ultrasonographic evaluation of the renal transplant. Radiol Clin North Am. 52(6):1307-24, 2014
2. Glebova NO et al: Endovascular interventions for managing vascular complication of renal transplantation. Semin Vasc Surg. 26(4):205-12, 2013
3. Aktas S et al: Analysis of vascular complications after renal transplantation. Transplant Proc. 43(2):557-61, 2011
4. Rivera M et al: Asymptomatic large extracapsular renal pseudoaneurysm following kidney transplant biopsy. Am J Kidney Dis. 57(1):175-8, 2011
5. Jin KB et al: Delayed presentation of arteriovenous fistula and pseudoaneurysms in a renal transplant patient 10 years after percutaneous allograft biopsy. Transplant Proc. 40(7):2444-5, 2008

IMAGING

- No specific imaging characteristics
- Ultrasound-guided renal biopsy is gold standard
- Acute rejection (AR): Nonspecific allograft edema, urothelial thickening; elevated resistive index may be present but is not specific
- Chronic rejection (CR): Cortical atrophy, increased echogenicity, calcification
- Color perfusion may be decreased in AR or CR
- Tc-99m MAG3 renogram may show decreased perfusion and uptake but is nonspecific

TOP DIFFERENTIAL DIAGNOSES

- Acute tubular necrosis/delayed graft function
- Infection
- Calcineurin inhibitor toxicity

PATHOLOGY

- Adequate biopsy sample requires at least 10 glomeruli and 2 arteries with 2 separate cores through cortex
- Acute cellular rejection: T lymphocyte interstitial infiltratio tubulitis, and arteritis
- Acute humoral antibody-mediated rejection: transmural arteritis and fibrinoid necrosis
- CR: Vascular sclerosis, fibrosis, and tubular atrophy

CLINICAL ISSUES

- Elevation of creatinine
- Oliguria or anuria
- Fever, graft tenderness, or swelling
- 14% in first 3-6 months
- Acute cellular rejection most common, after 1st postoperative week

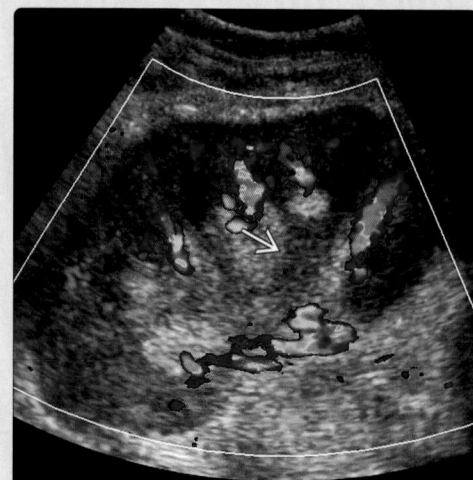
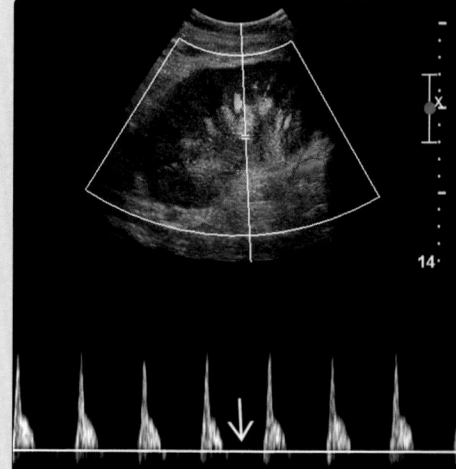

(Left) *Longitudinal color Doppler ultrasound of a renal transplant with oliguria secondary to acute rejection shows global decrease in color flow. The renal pelvic urothelium is thick ➡. (Right) Longitudinal pulsed Doppler ultrasound of the same renal transplant shows a high-resistance arterial waveform with absence of flow in diastole ➡.*

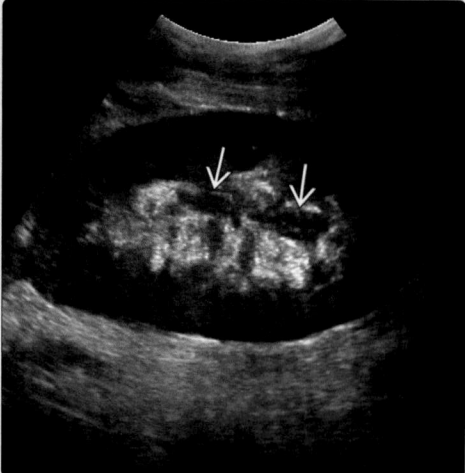
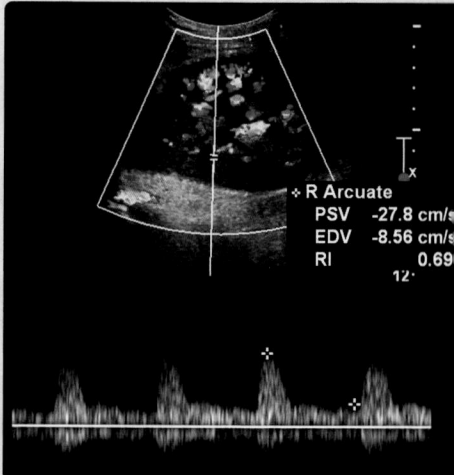

(Left) *Longitudinal ultrasound of a living related renal transplant with biopsy-proven moderate acute cell-mediated rejection is shown. Other than urothelial thickening ➡, the kidney appears normal. (Right) Longitudinal pulsed Doppler ultrasound of the same patient shows normal diastolic flow and a resistive index within normal limits at 0.69.*

IMAGING

General Features

Best diagnostic clue
- No specific imaging characteristics

Ultrasonographic Findings

Grayscale ultrasound
- Acute rejection (AR): Nonspecific allograft edema, urothelial thickening
- Chronic rejection (CR): Cortical atrophy, increased echogenicity, calcification

Pulsed Doppler
- Resistive index (RI) measured in segmental, interlobar and arcuate arteries
- AR: Elevated RI may be present but is not specific
- Elevated RI > 0.80 associated with increased risk of failure or death with functioning graft chronic allograft nephropathy (CAN), may be related to recipient factors

Color Doppler
- May be decreased in AR or CR

Nuclear Medicine Findings

Tc-99m MAG3 renogram may show decreased perfusion and uptake but is nonspecific

Imaging Recommendations

Best imaging tool
- Ultrasound-guided renal biopsy is gold standard

DIFFERENTIAL DIAGNOSIS

Acute Tubular Necrosis/Delayed Graft Function

Clinical diagnosis
May have decreased diastolic flow

Infection

Clinical diagnosis, positive urine cultures
Thickened urothelium, mild dilatation of ureter and pelvis

Calcineurin Inhibitor Toxicity

Clinical diagnosis

PATHOLOGY

General Features

Acute cellular rejection: T-cell-mediated reaction

Staging, Grading, & Classification

Acute cellular rejection: T-cell-mediated reaction
Acute antibody-mediated rejection: Immediate "hyperacute" or delayed "accelerated acute" due to preformed antibodies
- Caused by donor-specific antibody to graft microvascular antigens complement activation

Chronic allograft nephropathy: Final common pathway of different insults to transplant resulting in progressive failure, including chronic rejection

Gross Pathologic & Surgical Features

Adequate biopsy sample requires at least 10 glomeruli and 2 arteries with 2 separate cores through cortex
Acute cellular rejection: T lymphocyte interstitial infiltration, tubulitis, and arteritis

- Acute humoral antibody-mediated rejection: transmural arteritis and fibrinoid necrosis
- Chronic rejection: Vascular sclerosis, fibrosis, and tubular atrophy

CLINICAL ISSUES

Presentation

- Most common signs/symptoms
  - Elevation of creatinine
  - Oliguria or anuria
  - Fever, graft tenderness or swelling

Demographics

- Epidemiology
  - Reduced problem with modern therapy
  - 14% in first 3-6 months
  - Acute cellular rejection most common, after 1st postoperative week

Natural History & Prognosis

- Varying severity
- Acute rejection

Treatment

- Depends on type of rejection

Risk Factors

- Immune sensitization, ABO incompatible transplants, prior transplantation

DIAGNOSTIC CHECKLIST

Consider

- Failed renal transplant as cause of a solid pelvic mass (± calcifications)

SELECTED REFERENCES

1. Naesens M et al: Intrarenal resistive index after renal transplantation. N Engl J Med. 370(7):677-8, 2014
2. Rodgers SK et al: Ultrasonographic evaluation of the renal transplant. Radiol Clin North Am. 52(6):1307-24, 2014
3. McArthur C et al: Early measurement of pulsatility and resistive indexes: correlation with long-term renal transplant function. Radiology. 259(1):278-85, 2011
4. Radermacher J et al: The renal arterial resistance index and renal allograft survival. N Engl J Med. 349(2):115-24, 2003

Delayed Renal Graft Function

TERMINOLOGY

- Oliguria, poor clearance, and need for dialysis in 1st week after transplantation

IMAGING

- Clinical diagnosis with no specific imaging findings
- May have elevated resistive indices or absence of diastolic flow
- Renal transplant may be edematous
- Ultrasound with Doppler serves to exclude other causes of renal transplant dysfunction
- Look for hemorrhage, vascular thrombosis, or hydronephrosis
- Tc-99m mertiatide scintigraphy: Normal perfusion with accumulation of activity in renal parenchyma
  - Minimal if any excretion

PATHOLOGY

- 21% incidence in deceased donor transplantation, 2-5% after living donor transplantation
- Most common cause is acute tubular necrosis: 70-90%
- Risk factors
  - Donor age, harvest injury, preservation
  - Injury at procurement, organ preservation methods, warm and cold ischemia time

CLINICAL ISSUES

- Present with oliguria, lack of renal function
- DGF has significant impact on long-term graft and patient survival
- May be complicated by vascular thrombosis
- Treatment is supportive with dialysis as indicated

DIAGNOSTIC CHECKLIST

- Early biopsy (3-5 days in high-risk patients) to detect coexisting early rejection

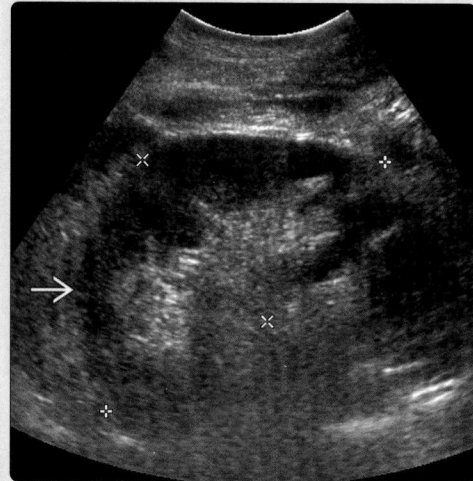 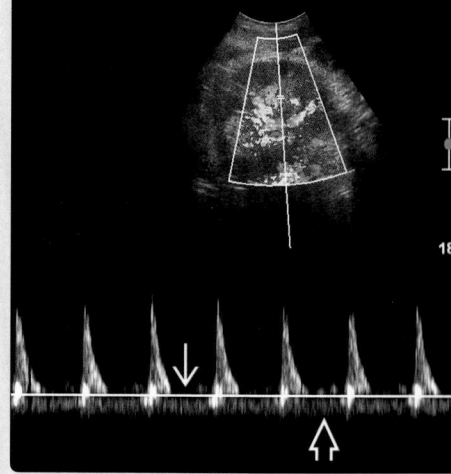

(Left) Longitudinal ultrasound shows a nonfunctioning renal transplant ➡ on the 1st postoperative day. The transplant appears normal. (Right) Pulsed Doppler ultrasound in the same patient with delayed graft function shows absence of diastolic flow ➡ and narrow systolic peaks. Venous flow ➡ is present.

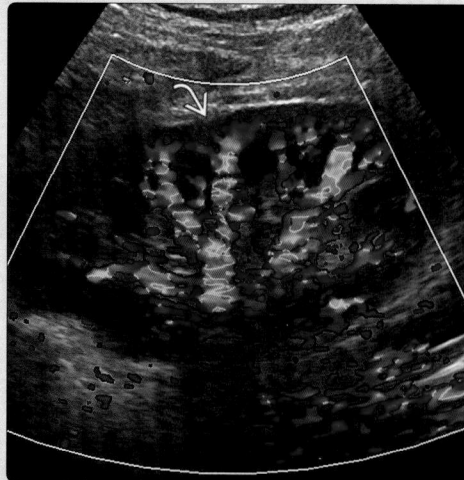 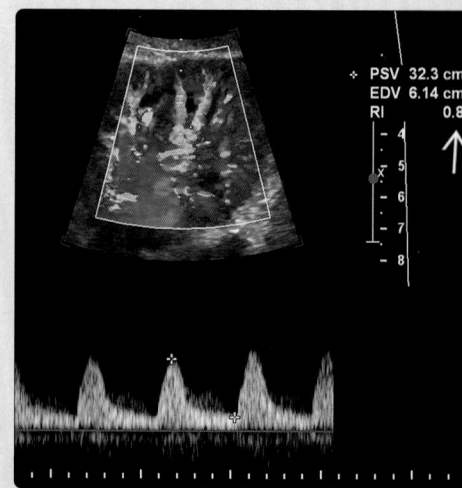

(Left) Longitudinal color Doppler ultrasound shows a nonfunctioning renal transplant ➡ with delayed graft function. The transplant is perfused, excluding vascular thrombosis as a cause of dysfunction. There was also no hydronephrosis or collection. (Right) Pulsed Doppler ultrasound shows an elevated resistive index of 0.81 ➡ in delayed graft function. Perfusion is normal. Resistive index is the ratio of peak systolic velocity minus end diastolic velocity to peak systolic velocity.

TERMINOLOGY

Abbreviations

- Delayed graft function (DGF)

Definitions

- Oliguria, poor clearance, and need for dialysis in 1st week after transplantation

IMAGING

General Features

- Best diagnostic clue
  - Clinical diagnosis with no specific imaging findings

Ultrasonographic Findings

- Renal transplant may be edematous
- May have elevated resistive indices or absence of diastolic flow
- Look for hemorrhage, vascular thrombosis, or hydronephrosis

Nuclear Medicine Findings

- Normal perfusion with accumulation of activity in renal parenchyma using Tc-99m mertiatide
- Minimal if any excretion

Imaging Recommendations

- Best imaging tool
  - Doppler ultrasound to exclude other causes of renal transplant dysfunction

PATHOLOGY

General Features

- Etiology
  - Ischemia/reperfusion injury resulting in tubular damage

Risk Factors

- Donor: Age, cause of death, comorbidities
- Injury at procurement, organ preservation methods, warm and cold ischemia time

CLINICAL ISSUES

Presentation

- Most common signs/symptoms
  - Oliguria, lack of renal function

Demographics

- Epidemiology
  - 21% incidence in deceased donor transplantation, 2-5% after living donor transplantation
  - < 5% of kidneys never function: Primary nonfunction
- Most common cause is acute tubular necrosis: 70-90%

Natural History & Prognosis

- Significant impact on long-term graft and patient survival
- Increased incidence of acute rejection
- May be complicated by vascular thrombosis

Treatment

- Supportive with dialysis as needed

DIAGNOSTIC CHECKLIST

Consider

- Early biopsy (3-5 days in high-risk patients) to detect coexisting early rejection

SELECTED REFERENCES

1. Granata A et al: Renal transplant vascular complications: the role of Doppler ultrasound. J Ultrasound. 18(2):101-7, 2015
2. Granata A et al: Renal transplantation parenchymal complications: what Doppler ultrasound can and cannot do. J Ultrasound. 18(2):109-16, 2015
3. Ninet S et al: Doppler-based renal resistive index for prediction of renal dysfunction reversibility: A systematic review and meta-analysis. J Crit Care. 30(3):629-35, 2015
4. Shakeri Bavil A et al: The inability of an early post-transplantation intrarenal resistive index to predict renal allograft function at 12 weeks after engraftment in young adults. Acta Radiol. ePub, 2015
5. Cano H et al: Resistance index measured by Doppler ultrasound as a predictor of graft function after kidney transplantation. Transplant Proc. 46(9):2972-4, 2014
6. Rodgers SK et al: Ultrasonographic evaluation of the renal transplant. Radiol Clin North Am. 52(6):1307-24, 2014
7. Schwenger V et al: Contrast-enhanced ultrasonography in the early period after kidney transplantation predicts long-term allograft function. Transplant Proc. 46(10):3352-7, 2014
8. Uliel L et al: Nuclear medicine in the acute clinical setting: indications, imaging findings, and potential pitfalls. Radiographics. 33(2):375-96, 2013
9. Cosgrove DO et al: Renal transplants: what ultrasound can and cannot do. Ultrasound Q. 24(2):77-87; quiz 141-2, 2008

PART II
SECTION 7
Adrenal Gland

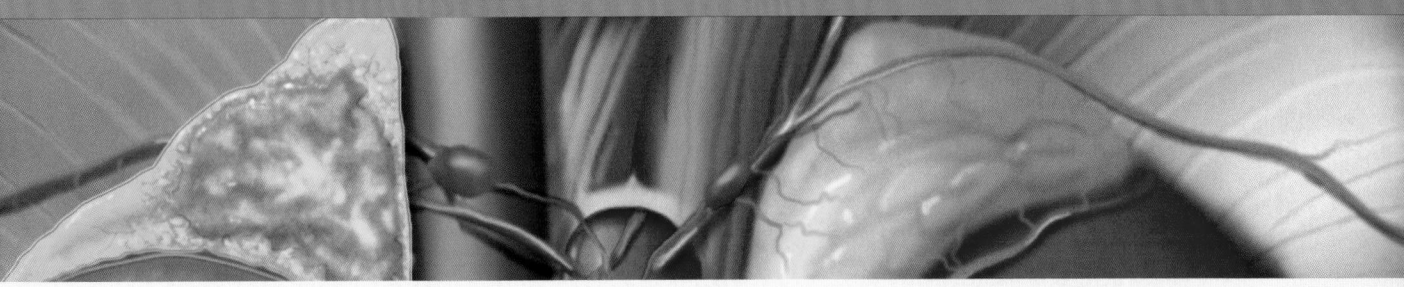

Adrenal Hemorrhage

IMAGING

- May be unilateral or bilateral
- Variable appearance depending on age of hemorrhage
- US: Nonspecific, avascular hypoechoic, hyperechoic or heterogeneous lesion
- CT/MR: Can better characterize hemorrhagic contents of lesion, increasing specificity

TOP DIFFERENTIAL DIAGNOSES

- Adrenal adenoma
- Pheochromocytoma
- Myelolipoma
- Primary adrenal or metastatic tumors
- Adjacent neoplasm
- Adrenal lymphoma

PATHOLOGY

- Nontraumatic pathogenesis: Vascular dam of abundant arterial supply and limited venous drainage

CLINICAL ISSUES

- Relatively uncommon condition but potentially catastrophic event
  - Bilateral in 15% of individuals who die of shock
  - Can result in adrenal insufficiency
- More common in neonates than children & adults
  - Most common cause of adrenal mass in infancy
- Occurs secondary to traumatic (more common) & nontraumatic causes
  - Traumatic hemorrhage: Blunt abdominal trauma
    - 25% of patients with blunt abdominal trauma have adrenal hemorrhage
    - Unilateral in 80% of cases: Right (85%), left (15%)
  - Nontraumatic hemorrhage (often bilateral)
    - Stress, bleeding disorders, adrenal tumors
    - Neonatal stress (birth asphyxia), idiopathic
    - Meningococcal septicemia (Waterhouse-Friderichsen syndrome)

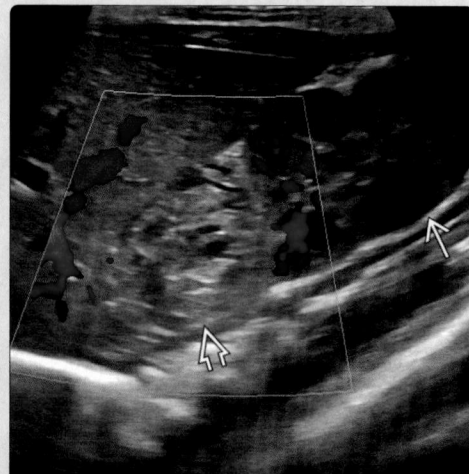
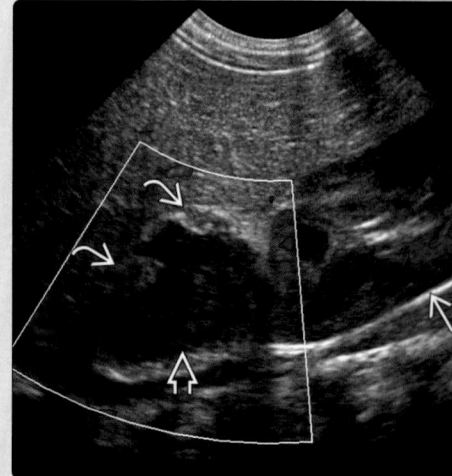

(Left) Longitudinal color Doppler ultrasound shows an avascular, heterogeneously hyperechoic, right suprarenal lesion ⬅. Note right kidney ➡. *(Right)* Longitudinal color Doppler ultrasound shows a heterogeneous, avascular right suprarenal lesion with a hypoechoic center ➡ and irregular echogenic components along the periphery ➡. Note right kidney ➡.

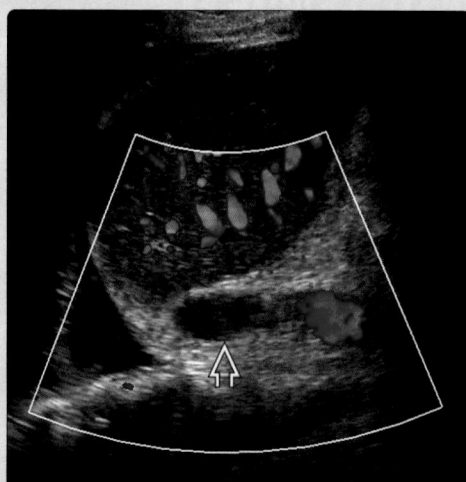
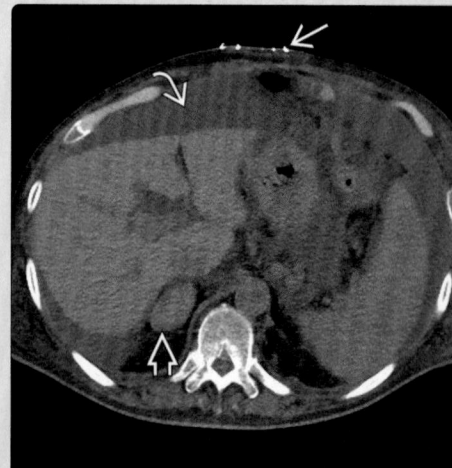

(Left) Longitudinal color Doppler ultrasound shows a well-defined hypoechoic lesion in the right adrenal gland with no vascular flow ➡. *(Right)* Axial NECT in the same patient demonstrates a well-defined, hyperdense, right adrenal hematoma ➡. Note skin staples ➡ in the abdominal wall from recent liver transplantation as well as ascites ➡.

TERMINOLOGY

Abbreviations

- Adrenal hemorrhage (AH), adrenal hematoma

Definitions

- Hemorrhage within adrenal gland or adrenal tumor

IMAGING

General Features

- Best diagnostic clue
  - Well-defined, avascular homogeneous or heterogeneous adrenal mass in proper clinical context

Ultrasonographic Findings

- Grayscale ultrasound
  - Unilateral or bilateral
  - Round or oval, well-defined adrenal mass with variable echogenicity depending on stage of hemorrhage
    - Acute hematoma: Hyperechoic
    - Subacute hematoma: Mixed echogenicity ± central hypoechoic area
    - Chronic hematoma: Hypo- or anechoic cyst-like lesion
      - ± curvilinear/eggshell calcification &/or internal echoes or layering debris
  - Asymmetric adeniform enlargement of adrenal gland
  - May see adjacent area(s) of ill-defined hypoechoic fluid or fluid collections related to adjacent organs (e.g., liver or kidney)
  - Displacement & mass effect on kidney & IVC
- Color Doppler
  - Avascular on color Doppler
  - Secondary adrenal hemorrhage shows variable vascularity of underlying adrenal tumor
    - Adrenal carcinoma/pheochromocytoma; usually hypervascular
    - Myelolipoma/adrenal cyst; hypo- to avascular
  - ± extension of thrombus into IVC

CT Findings

- Acute or subacute hematoma
  - Round or oval mass of high attenuation (50-90 HU)
  - May show heterogeneous density with evolving/layering hyperdensity
  - No enhancement with contrast
  - Periadrenal fat infiltration
  - Thickening of adjacent diaphragmatic crura
  - ± associated upper abdominal trauma findings
    - Pneumothorax, hydropneumothorax, rib fracture
    - Contusion of lung, liver, spleen, or pancreas
- Chronic hematoma
  - Decreases in size and attenuation over time, leading to
    - Adrenal atrophy
    - Hemorrhagic pseudocyst = thin-rimmed collection with central hypoattenuation close to simple fluid
  - Lack of enhancement
  - Calcification: Usually seen after 1 year in adults
    - Neonates: Seen within 1-2 weeks after trauma
- ± underlying adrenal mass (pheochromocytoma, adrenal carcinoma, myelolipoma, or cyst)
  - Intralesional calcification and enhancing components suggest underlying tumor

MR Findings

- T1 & T2WI: Varied signal based on age of hematoma
- Acute hematoma (< 7 days after onset)
  - T1WI: Isointense or slightly hypointense
  - T2WI: Markedly hypointense
- Subacute hematoma (7 days to 7 weeks after onset)
  - T1WI: Hyperintense; due to free methemoglobin
  - T2WI: Markedly hyperintense; due to serum & clot
  - Large hematoma: Irregular clot lysis; multilocular, fluid-fluid levels
- Chronic hematoma (beyond 7 weeks after onset)
  - T1 & T2WI: Hyperintense hematoma; due to persistence of free methemoglobin
  - T1 & T2WI: Hypointense rim; due to hemosiderin deposition in fibrous capsule
- Gradient-echo imaging
  - Demonstrates "blooming" effect (magnetic susceptibility) due to hemosiderin deposition
- T1WI C+ FS: Can be helpful in detecting intralesional enhancement

Nuclear Medicine Findings

- PET/CT: May show increased activity due to inflammatory reaction from fat necrosis
  - Look for lack of associated enhancing mass to exclude underlying tumor
  - Can see calcification with underlying tumor or chronic adrenal hematoma

Imaging Recommendations

- Best imaging tool
  - US for initial screening & detection followed by CT/MR for further characterization
    - Left adrenal gland can be difficult to see on US, & small lesions may be obscured
- Protocol advice
  - CT: Thin sections < 3 mm
  - MR: Include gradient-echo imaging to look for susceptibility artifact

DIFFERENTIAL DIAGNOSIS

Adrenal Adenoma

- Hypoechoic mass on US and homogeneously hypodense on CT ± calcification
- However, lacks associated findings of adjacent fluid collection or periadrenal fat stranding
- Shows avid enhancement with contrast

Pheochromocytoma

- Variable appearance; purely solid (68%), complex (16%), & cystic tumor (16%)
- Large tumors may appear purely solid with homogeneous (46%) or heterogeneous (54%) echo pattern
- Predominantly cystic lesions are due to chronic hemorrhage & necrotic debris (± fluid-fluid levels)

Myelolipoma

- Well-defined homogeneous echogenic mass (when fat cells predominate)

- Heterogeneous mass (when myeloid cells predominate)

Adrenal Metastases

- Most frequently occurring hemorrhagic adrenal neoplasm
- Lung cancer most common hemorrhagic metastasis; RCC, breast, colon, and melanoma also possibilities
- Melanoma: Intrinsic T1 hyperintense may mimic hemorrhage; appears hypervascular with contrast

Adjacent Neoplasm

- Renal cell carcinoma, angiomyolipoma, hepatocellular carcinoma, atypical hepatic hemangioma

Adrenal Lymphoma

- Nonspecific US appearance with increased density on CT
- Typically bilateral and in setting of systemic disease

PATHOLOGY

General Features

- Etiology
  - Nontraumatic pathogenesis: Vascular dam of abundant supply (3 arteries) and limited drainage (1 vein)
    - Stress or adrenal tumor → ↑ adrenocorticotrophic hormone → ↑ arterial blood flow + limited venous drainage → hemorrhage
    - Stress or tumor → ↑ catecholamines → adrenal vein spasm → stasis → thrombosis → hemorrhage
    - Coagulopathies → ↑ venous stasis → thrombosis → hemorrhage
  - Causes
    - Blunt abdominal trauma (right gland > left gland)
    - Anticoagulation therapy
    - Antiphospholipid antibody syndrome & disseminated intravascular coagulopathy
    - Stress: Recent surgery, sepsis, burns, hypotension, steroids, pregnancy
    - After liver transplantation (commonly seen in right gland due to ligation of right adrenal vein)
    - Primary adrenal or metastatic tumors: Pheochromocytoma, metastases, adenoma, myelolipoma, adrenal carcinoma
    - Adrenal hyperplasia
    - Complication of venous sampling or biopsy
    - Neonates (most common adrenal mass in infancy)
      □ Difficult labor or delivery; asphyxia or hypoxia
      □ Renal vein thrombosis
      □ Hemorrhagic disorders; meningococcal septicemia (Waterhouse-Friderichsen syndrome)

Gross Pathologic & Surgical Features

- Hematoma, enlarged gland, peri-adrenal stranding

Microscopic Features

- Necrosis of all 3 cortical layers + medullary cells

CLINICAL ISSUES

Presentation

- Most common signs/symptoms
  - Nonspecific: Abdominal, flank, or back pain, nausea, and vomiting
  - Fever, tachycardia, hypotension
  - Acute abdomen
    - Guarding, rigidity, rebound tenderness
  - Confusion, disorientation, shock in late phase
  - Acute adrenal insufficiency
    - Fatigue, anorexia, nausea, & vomiting
  - Waterhouse-Friderichsen syndrome: Rapidly developing adrenal failure that can lead to death
    - Petechial and purpuric rash, disseminated intravascular coagulation, fever, septic shock
  - Rarely, asymptomatic; incidental finding (imaging)

Demographics

- Age
  - Occurs in any age group but more common in neonates
    - Incidence: 1.7-3% per 1,000 births
  - Nontraumatic (40-80 years); traumatic (20-30 years)
- Gender
  - M:F = 2:1
- Epidemiology
  - Autopsy studies: 0.3-1.8% of unselected cases
  - 15% of individuals who die of shock
  - 2% of orthotopic liver transplantations

Natural History & Prognosis

- Complications
  - Adults: Adrenal crisis; neonate: death (> blood loss)
  - Prerenal azotemia, adrenal abscess, shock
- Prognosis
  - Depends on etiology rather than extent of hemorrhage
  - Often self-limiting, resolving over time
  - 16-50% of patients with bilateral hemorrhage develop life-threatening adrenal insufficiency
  - Overall mortality rate: 15%
    - Waterhouse-Friderichsen syndrome: 55-60%

Treatment

- Medical: Correct fluid, electrolytes, & treat underlying cause
- Surgical: Adrenalectomy (open or laparoscopic)
  - Surgery not typically required, except in adrenal tumors

DIAGNOSTIC CHECKLIST

Consider

- Check for history of trauma, anticoagulant therapy, coagulopathies, malignancies, stress, recent surgery, adrenal tumor
- Change over time is suggestive of acute adrenal hemorrhage; check prior examinations or follow-up studies for evolution

Image Interpretation Pearls

- US: Avascular adrenal lesion of variable echogenicity with relevant clinical features
- CT/MR: CT density and MR signal intensity vary with age of hematoma

SELECTED REFERENCES

1. Hammond NA et al: Imaging of adrenal and renal hemorrhage. Abdom Imaging. ePub, 2015
2. Jordan E et al: Imaging of nontraumatic adrenal hemorrhage. AJR Am J Roentgenol. 199(1):W91-8, 2012
3. To'o KJ et al: Imaging of traumatic adrenal injury. Emerg Radiol. 19(6):499-503, 2012

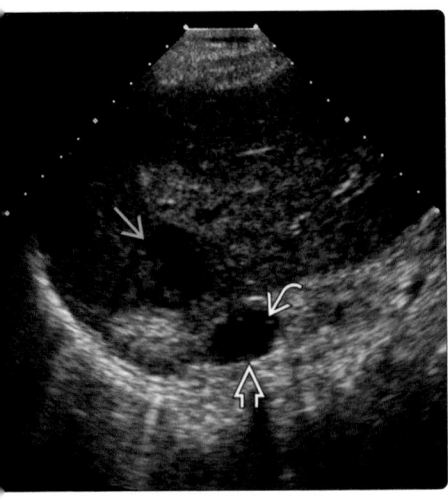
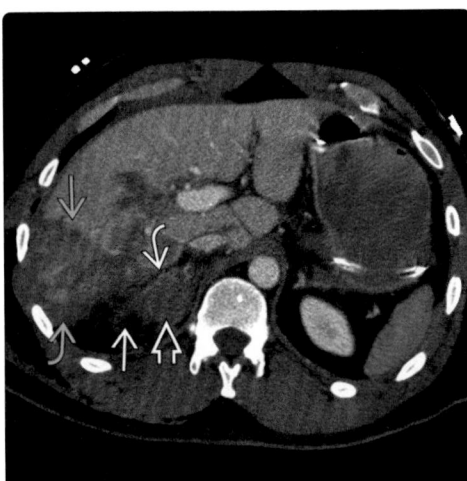

(Left) *Longitudinal transabdominal ultrasound shows a very hypoechoic right suprarenal lesion ⇒ with low-level internal echoes ⇗, compatible with evolving hematoma. Note the complex intrahepatic collection ⇥.* (Right) *Axial CECT in the same patient shows a nonenhancing, hypodense right adrenal lesion ⇒ with irregular enhancement of the lateral limb of the gland ⇗. Note the surrounding periadrenal fat infiltration ⇗, hepatic contusion ⇥, and perihepatic fluid ⇨ in this patient post trauma.*

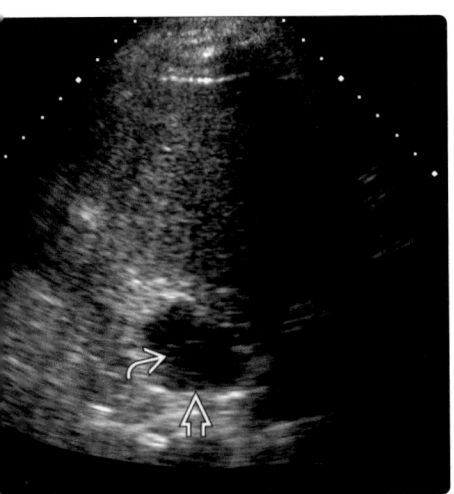
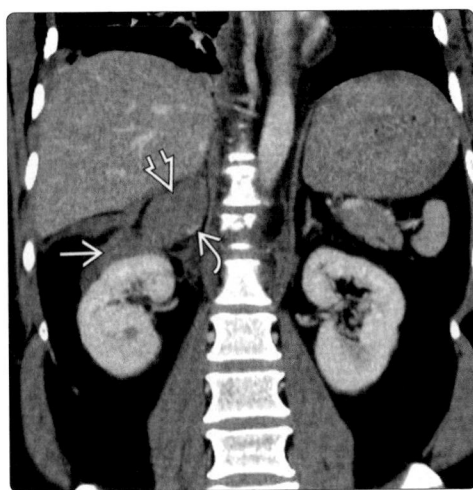

(Left) *Transverse transabdominal ultrasound in a patient after a motor vehicle collision shows a well-demarcated hypoechoic right adrenal lesion ⇒ with low-level internal echoes ⇗.* (Right) *Coronal CECT in the same patient shows a nonenhancing oval hypodense lesion ⇒ in the right adrenal gland. Note focal preservation of normal adrenal enhancement ⇗ along the medial peripheral margin. Ill-defined periadrenal fluid tracks to the perirenal space ⇗.*

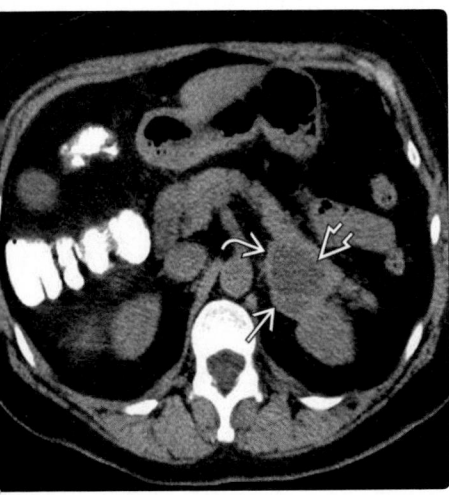
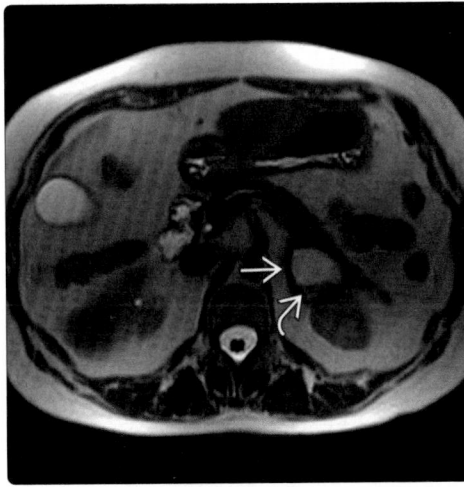

(Left) *Axial NECT shows a well-circumscribed, oval left adrenal lesion ⇒ with heterogeneous density. Note the well-defined peripheral rim ⇗ with central low attenuation and layering hyperdense debris level ⇗.* (Right) *Axial T2 HASTE MR shows a well-defined left adrenal lesion with a T2-dark rim ⇒ characteristic of chronic hemorrhage. Note the T2-hyperintense internal contents with layering T2-dark debris ⇗.*

Myelolipoma

TERMINOLOGY

- Definition: Rare benign tumor consisting of macroscopic fat interspersed with hematopoietic elements

IMAGING

- Appearance varies depending on admixture of fatty and soft tissue components
- US typically shows homogeneously hyperechoic mass, but it may be heterogeneous iso- or hypoechoic
- CT typically shows well-defined, heterogeneous mass with macroscopic fat that is diagnostic
- MR characterizes intratumoral fat best on fat-suppressed sequences

TOP DIFFERENTIAL DIAGNOSES

- Adrenal hemorrhage
- Pheochromocytoma
- Liposarcoma
- Renal angiomyolipoma

- Adrenal adenoma
- Adrenal metastases

PATHOLOGY

- Contains mature fat cells with variable mixture of myeloid cells, erythroid cells, and megakaryocytes

CLINICAL ISSUES

- Usually found incidentally
- Clinical signs are usually absent except in rare cases of hemorrhage and rupture

DIAGNOSTIC CHECKLIST

- Confirm that fat-containing lesion arises from adrenal gland and not adjacent organs or retroperitoneum
- Adrenal mass with discrete focus of macroscopic fat is virtually diagnostic of myelolipoma

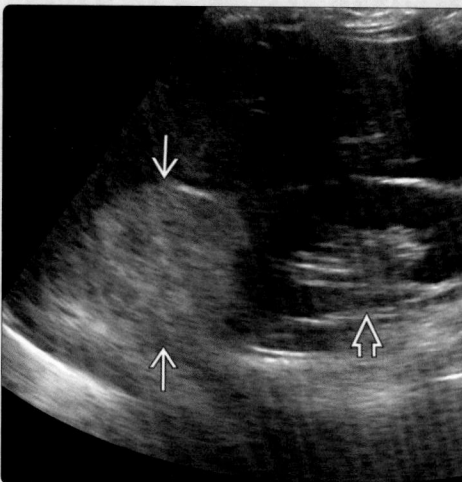
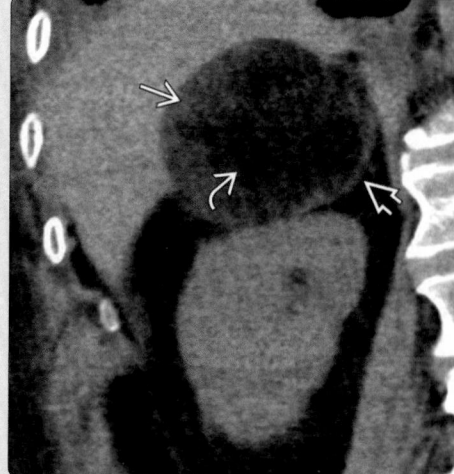

(Left) Longitudinal ultrasound of a myelolipoma shows a lobulated, well-defined, heterogeneously hyperechoic mass ⮞ above the right kidney ⮞. (Right) Coronal CT demonstrates a heterogeneous, encapsulated, suprarenal mass ⮞ containing ill-defined, "smoky" soft tissue elements ⮞ and macroscopic fat ⮞.

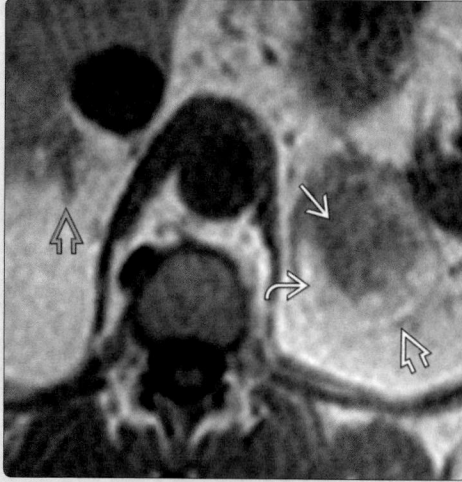
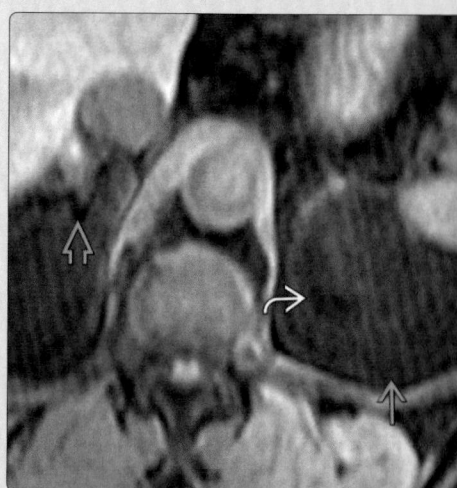

(Left) Axial T1 MR shows an encapsulated, unilateral, left adrenal mass ⮞ containing heterogeneous components. Central soft tissue shows central T1 hypointensity ⮞, while peripheral intratumoral fat shows T1 hyperintensity ⮞. Note the normal-appearing right adrenal gland ⮞. (Right) Axial T1 MR with fat saturation shows signal drop of the retroperitoneal fat ⮞ and in the peripheral components of the mass ⮞, confirming the presence of intratumoral fat. Note the normal-appearing right adrenal gland ⮞.

TERMINOLOGY

Definitions

Rare benign tumor composed of mature fat tissue and hematopoietic elements (myeloid and erythroid cells)

IMAGING

General Features

- Best diagnostic clue
  o Heterogeneous fat-containing adrenal mass
- Location
  o Adrenal gland (85%): Thought to arise in zona fasciculata of adrenal cortex
  o Typically unilateral, only very rarely bilateral: 10:1
  o Extraadrenal (15%): Retroperitoneal (12%) and intrathoracic (3%)
  o Possible right-sided predilection
- Size
  o Usually 2-10 cm, rarely 10-20 cm

Ultrasonographic Findings

- Grayscale ultrasound
  o Well-defined, homogeneous, hyperechoic suprarenal mass (when predominantly composed of fatty tissue)
  o When small, difficult to distinguish from echogenic retroperitoneal fat
  o Apparent diaphragm disruption: Propagation speed artifact; decreased sound velocity through fatty mass leads to this appearance, usually seen when tumor > 4 cm
  o Heterogeneous mass (when myeloid cells predominate), may be isoechoic or hypoechoic
  o Heterogeneous echo pattern may also be due to internal hemorrhage (common), ± calcification
- Color Doppler
  o Avascular to hypovascular adrenal mass

Radiographic Findings

- Radiography
  o Lucent mass with rim of residual normal adrenal cortex
  o May see calcification due to previous hemorrhage

CT Findings

- CT appearance usually characteristic
  o Typically appears as heterogeneous fat-containing adrenal mass
    – Macroscopic fat within tumor is diagnostic
    – Low attenuation of fat density (-30 to -90 HU)
    – Amount of fat is widely variable: Completely fat, to > 1/2 fat (50%), to only a few tiny foci of fat in soft tissue mass (10%)
- Usually well-defined mass with recognizable capsule
- Interspersed "smoky" areas of higher CT values than those of retroperitoneal fat because of presence of hematopoietic tissue in myelolipoma
- Mass may have attenuation values between fat and water due to diffusely mixed fat and myeloid elements
- Higher density areas may be seen with hemorrhage
- Punctate calcification in 25-30% of cases
- Occasionally the mass may appear to extend into retroperitoneum

- Thin sections are recommended (to avoid volume averaging) if fatty tissue is not predominant
  o Or consider pixel mapping

MR Findings

- Varied MR appearance depending on mixture of elements
  o Fat within mass is hyperintense on T1- and T2WI
  o Hematopoietic elements are T1 hypointense and moderately hyperintense on T2WI
- Fat-suppressed sequences best demonstrate intratumoral fat
- Opposed-phase sequences can be helpful for characterizing presence of both fat and water
  o India ink artifact at boundary of fat and water confirms diagnosis
  o If mass is predominantly composed of mature fat cells with little intracellular water from soft tissue, little to no loss of signal seen on opposed phase sequence
- Soft tissue elements enhance avidly after intravenous administration of gadolinium-based contrast

Angiographic Findings

- Conventional
  o Differentiate myelolipoma from retroperitoneal liposarcoma by determining origin of blood supply and vascularity of tumors

Imaging Recommendations

- Best imaging tool
  o Optimally imaged with NECT or MR with fat-suppression sequence
- Protocol advice
  o Ultrasonography may be useful in diagnosis of large tumors; however, CT or MR are better in detecting smaller masses

DIFFERENTIAL DIAGNOSIS

Adrenal Hemorrhage

- Usually well defined and round in shape
- Acute: Hyperechoic or heterogeneous in echogenicity
- Chronic: Well defined, hypoechoic, cystic, or calcified
- Often in setting of blunt abdominal trauma, bleeding disorder, stress, or underlying tumor
- Best characterized with CT or MR

Pheochromocytoma

- Variable appearance: Purely solid (68%), complex (16%), and cystic tumor (16%)
- Small tumor: Round, solid, well-circumscribed mass with uniform echogenicity
- Large tumor may appear as purely solid mass of homogeneous (46%) or heterogeneous (54%) echo pattern
- Highly vascular; prone to hemorrhage and necrosis

Adjacent Neoplasm

- Renal angiomyolipoma
  o Well-defined, fat-containing, hyperechoic lesion arising exophytically from upper pole of kidney
  o Multiplanar CT or MR best demonstrates claw of renal parenchyma around part of lesion
- Renal cell carcinoma (RCC)
  o Well-defined mass of variable echogenicity

- o When large may appear heterogeneous due to areas of necrosis and hemorrhage
- o Multiplanar CT or MR best characterizes origin from adjacent kidney
- Liposarcoma
  - o Retroperitoneal primary sarcoma in perirenal space
  - o Displaces or invades adrenal gland as opposed to arising from it
- Retroperitoneal teratoma
  - o Uncommon neoplasm composed of mixed dermal elements derived from 3 germ cell layers
  - o Fat-fluid (sebum) level and chemical shift between fat and fluid are pathognomonic

Adrenal Adenoma

- Well-defined, small, solid, round, hypoechoic adrenal mass
- Lipid-rich adenoma shows greater signal loss on chemical shift MR, while myelolipoma shows greater signal loss with fat saturated sequences

Adrenal Metastases/Lymphoma

- Metastases: Usually < 5 cm, variable appearance, may be hypervascular on color Doppler
  - o Usually known to have primary malignancy elsewhere
- Lymphoma: Discrete or diffuse mass, adrenal shape maintained
  - o Often bilateral with retroperitoneal masses or retroperitoneal tumor engulfing adrenal

Adrenal Carcinoma

- Rare, unilateral, solid mass with heterogeneous echogenicity
- Exceedingly rare cases may contain macroscopic fat
- Areas of necrosis and hemorrhage ± calcification (> 30%)

PATHOLOGY

General Features

- Etiology
  - o Best hypothesis: Metaplasia of adrenal cortical cells resulting from chronic stress or degeneration
  - o Secondary hypothesis: Myelolipoma represents site of extramedullary hematopoiesis
- Associated abnormalities
  - o Adrenal collision tumors: Independently coexisting neoplasms without significant tissue admixture (e.g., adrenal adenoma and myelolipoma)
  - o Endocrine disorders in 7%; Cushing syndrome, congenital adrenal hyperplasia (21-hydroxylase deficiency), and Conn syndrome
  - o Nonhyperfunctioning adenoma 15%

Gross Pathologic & Surgical Features

- Mass with pseudocapsule; contains fat and soft tissue components

Microscopic Features

- Mature fat cells with variable mixture of myeloid cells, erythroid cells, megakaryocytes, and occasional lymphocytes; no malignant cells

CLINICAL ISSUES

Presentation

- Most common signs/symptoms
  - o Usually asymptomatic and incidental finding on CT, MR, or US (9% of adrenal incidentalomas)
  - o Acute abdomen: Rupture with hemorrhage (rare)
- Other signs/symptoms
  - o Pain from necrosis, hemorrhage, or compression of structures

Demographics

- Age
  - o Usually in older age group: 50-70 years
  - o Uncommon in patients younger than 30 years
- Gender
  - o Occur with equal frequency in men and women
- Epidemiology
  - o Autopsy incidence: 0.2-0.4%

Natural History & Prognosis

- Complication: Rupture with hemorrhage usually when > 4 cm
- Prognosis: Excellent
- No malignant transformation

Treatment

- When diagnosis is certain and patient is asymptomatic, surgery is not necessary
- If symptomatic, enlarging, or > 7 cm, surgery indicated due to increased risk of bleeding and rupture

DIAGNOSTIC CHECKLIST

Consider

- Differentiate from other fat-containing tumors, most importantly retroperitoneal liposarcoma

Image Interpretation Pearls

- Well-marginated fat-containing adrenal mass is virtually diagnostic
- Diagnosis: CT or MR; biopsy prone to sampling error
- Presence of tumoral fat confirms diagnosis of this benign lesion, obviating need for further work-up

SELECTED REFERENCES

1. Katabathina VS et al: Adrenal collision tumors and their mimics: multimodality imaging findings. Cancer Imaging. 13(4):602-10, 2013
2. Aron D et al: Adrenal incidentalomas. Best Pract Res Clin Endocrinol Metab. 26(1):69-82, 2012
3. Song JH et al: The incidental adrenal mass on CT: Prevalence of adrenal disease in 1049 consecutive adrenal masses in patients with no known malignancy. AJR 190: 1163-1168; 2008
4. Daneshmand S et al: Adrenal myelolipoma: diagnosis and management. Ur J. 3(2):71-4, 2006

Myelolipoma

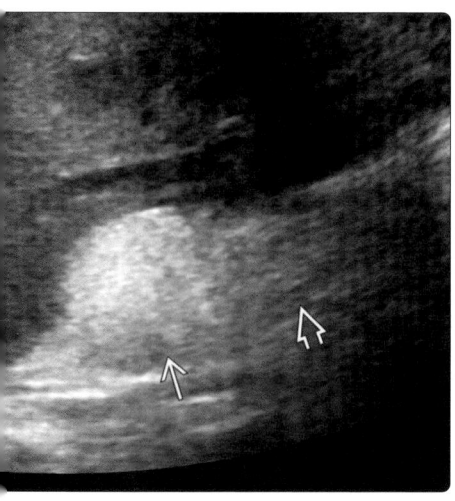
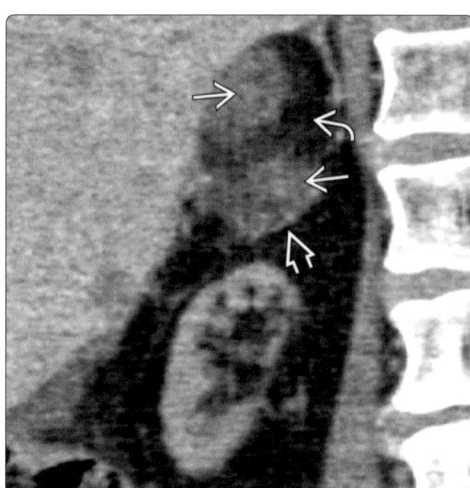

(Left) *Longitudinal US shows a lobulated hyperechoic right adrenal myelolipoma* ➡. *Note the adjacent liver echogenicity and atrophic right kidney* ➡. (Right) *Coronal CT shows an encapsulated, heterogeneous myelolipoma* ➡ *with fat* ➡ *and soft tissue components* ➡.

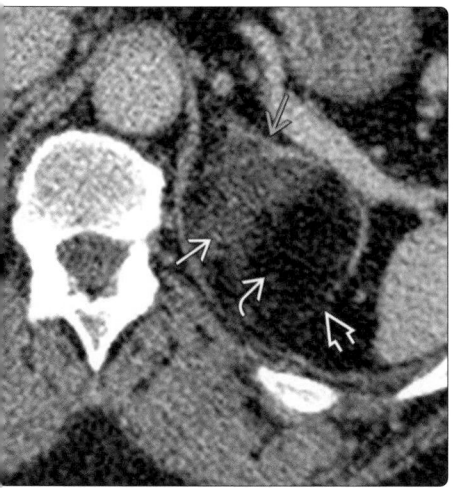
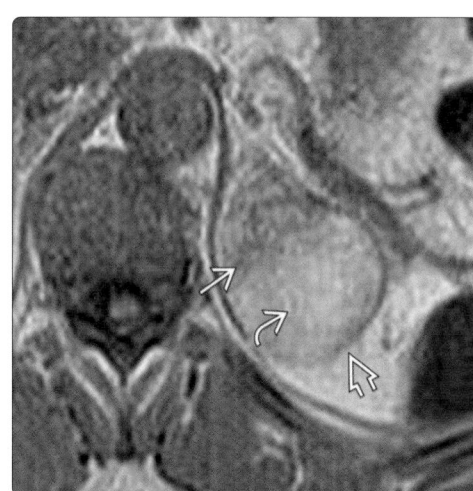

(Left) *Axial CT shows fat* ➡ *within a myelolipoma* ➡ *arising from the lateral limb of the left adrenal gland* ➡. *Note the ill-defined soft tissue component* ➡. (Right) *Axial T1 in-phase MR shows hyperintensity* ➡ *of fat within the mass* ➡ *seen on CT. Wispy soft tissue components show T1 isointensity* ➡.

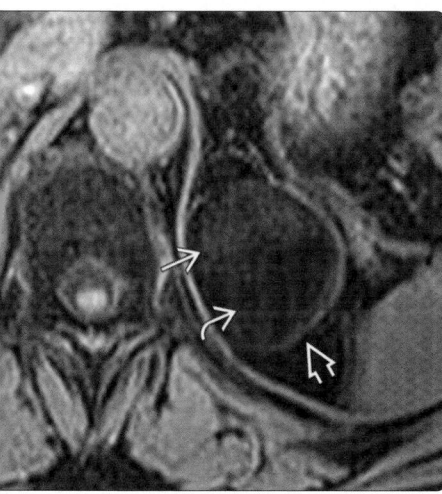
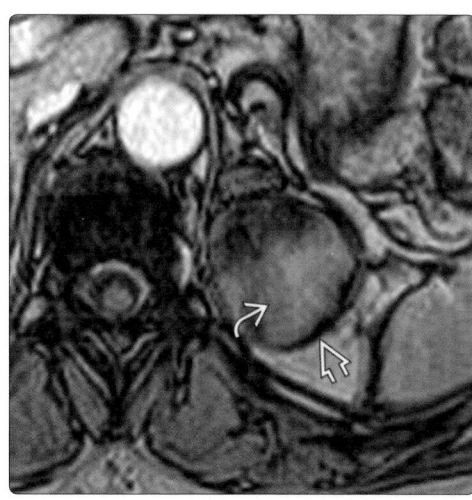

(Left) *Axial T1 MR with fat saturation shows signal drop* ➡ *of the fat-containing components of the myelolipoma* ➡. *Wispy soft tissue components show T1 isointensity* ➡. (Right) *Axial opposed-phase T1 MR shows no drop in signal of the macroscopic fat elements* ➡. *Note the India ink etching artifact at the interface between the fat and soft tissue elements of the myelolipoma* ➡.

Adrenal Adenoma

TERMINOLOGY

- Synonym: Adrenocortical adenoma

IMAGING

- May suggest diagnosis based on US; however, no specific sonographic features distinguish adenomas from other adrenal lesions
- US: Typically small, smoothly marginated, homogeneous, and hypoechoic
  - Size is particularly important: Smaller adrenal lesions tend to be benign; > 4 cm more likely malignant
  - Size stability over 12 months supports benignity
- CT and MR: Best imaging tool
  - Lipid-rich adenomas are best characterized with NECT or chemical shift MR
  - Lipid-poor adenomas can be characterized with CECT with 10-min delayed-phase imaging

CLINICAL ISSUES

- Adrenal adenoma may be detected due to hyperfunctioning activity
  - Cushing syndrome, Conn syndrome, or virilization syndromes
- More commonly detected as incidental finding
  - Increased detection in recent years due to greater imaging utilization

DIAGNOSTIC CHECKLIST

- Benign vs. malignant: Consider size and stability
  - Comparison with any available prior imaging may help to establish stability over 12 month period and avoid unnecessary additional testing
- Attenuation < 10 HU on NECT → lipid-rich adenoma
- Signal drop on T1 out-of-phase MR → lipid-rich adenoma
- > 60% absolute washout on 10-min delayed-phase CECT → lipid-rich and lipid-poor adenomas

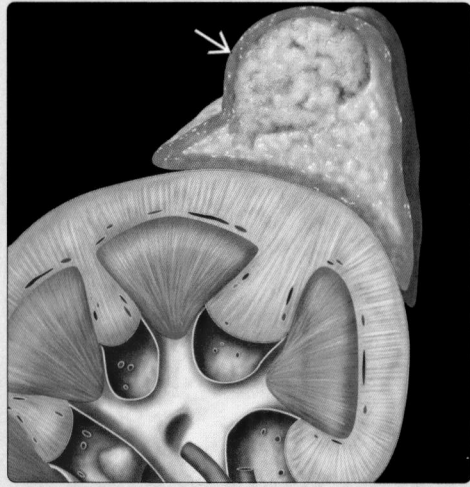
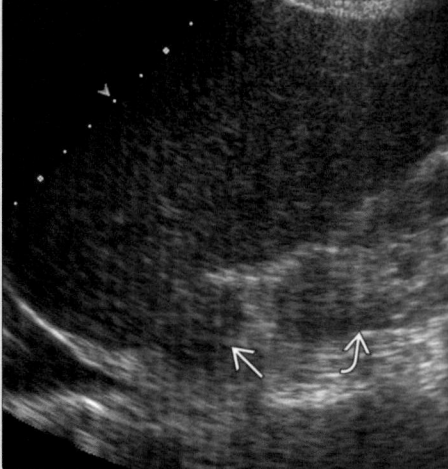

(Left) *Graphic shows a small, homogeneous, solid nodule* ➡ *arising from the peripheral adrenal gland. Note the oval shape and smooth margin typical of an adrenal adenoma.* (Right) *Longitudinal transabdominal US shows a well-circumscribed, homogeneous solid mass* ➡ *above the right kidney* ➡.

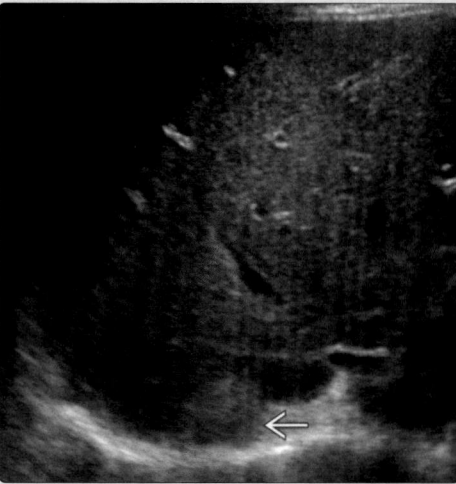
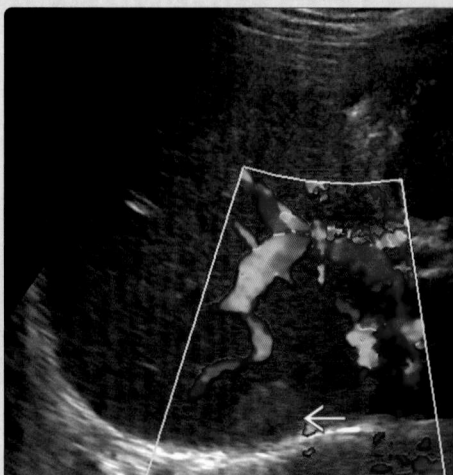

(Left) *Transverse transabdominal US shows a well-demarcated, homogeneous right adrenal mass* ➡*, which is mildly hyperechoic relative to the liver.* (Right) *Transverse color Doppler US in the same patient shows that the lesion* ➡ *is relatively hypovascular.*

TERMINOLOGY

Synonyms

- Adrenocortical adenoma

Definitions

- Extremely common, benign tumor of adrenal cortex

IMAGING

General Features

- Best diagnostic clue
  - Small, well-circumscribed, homogeneous adrenal mass
- Location
  - Can be bilateral (10%)
- Size
  - Varies from 2-5 cm
  - Smaller lesions are seen with Conn syndrome, usually < 2 cm (20% < 1 cm)
- Morphology
  - Typically small, round, or oval, smoothly marginated, and homogeneous
  - Size is particularly important: Smaller adrenal lesions tend to be benign; > 4 cm more likely malignant
    - Size stability over 12 months supports benignity

Ultrasonographic Findings

- Nonspecific sonographic appearance
- Well-circumscribed, solid, oval-shaped mass, typically < 3 cm
- Usually homogeneous and hypoechoic
  - Or slightly heterogeneous with mixed echogenicity
- Atypically can appear more heterogeneous
  - Possibly with hemorrhage/necrosis or calcification (rare)
  - Necrosis is seldom seen in small adenoma

CT Findings

- Usually small (< 3 cm) and homogeneous
- Smoothly marginated and well defined
- Atypical features: Large size (> 3 cm), hemorrhage, cystic degeneration, calcification
- **NECT**: CT characteristics depend on lipid content
  - Lipid-rich adenomas (70-90%): Attenuation < 10 HU is characteristic and diagnostic
  - Lipid-poor adenoma (10-30%): Variable attenuation from 10-30 HU or higher, more nonspecific appearance
  - May see glandular atrophy bilaterally in setting of Cushing syndrome
- **CECT**: Avid enhancement with rapid de-enhancement
  - Characteristic pattern of lesion washout when comparing enhancement on portal venous phase to attenuation at 10 min post injection: > 60% absolute percent washout
    - (Lesion attenuation on enhanced CT - lesion attenuation on delayed CT) / (lesion attenuation on enhanced CT - lesion attenuation on unenhanced CT) x 100%
    - Diagnostic for adenoma
    - Independent of lipid content

MR Findings

- T1WI: Chemical shift MR can confirm presence of intracellular lipid
  - Shows signal dropout on out-of-phase imaging
    - Compare lesion to spleen or muscle (SI of liver may be affected by lipid deposition)
  - Diagnostic for adrenal adenomas containing lipid
- T1WI C+: No established dynamic enhancement characteristics for MR

Nuclear Medicine Findings

- PET/CT
  - No increased uptake of FDG
  - Useful in differentiating from malignant lesions (↑ uptake)

Angiographic Findings

- Adrenal venography: Adrenal vein sampling in setting of Conn syndrome
  - Can distinguish unilateral vs. bilateral aldosterone secretion
  - Higher aldosterone:cortisol ratio than peripheral sample = abnormal

Imaging Recommendations

- Best imaging tool
  - NECT and CECT or MR
- Protocol advice
  - Full adrenal mass CT protocol should include NECT and CECT (with 10 min delayed phase)
    - Check attenuation on NECT before contrast administration to eliminate unnecessary imaging
    - Use thin sections (3 mm) to better assess small lesions
  - Chemical shift MR can also be used to characterize indeterminate adrenal nodules with attenuation of 10-30 HU
  - CECT with 10 min delayed-phase imaging should be used to characterize indeterminate adrenal nodules with CT attenuation > 30 HU
- Recommendations for evaluating nonspecific incidental adrenal nodules (ACR)
  - ≤ 1 cm can be ignored
  - 1-4 cm needs further evaluation or follow-up to establish stability
  - ≥ 4 cm should undergo biopsy or PET

DIFFERENTIAL DIAGNOSIS

Adrenal Metastases

- Unilateral or bilateral; more often hypoechoic than echogenic
- ± necrosis or hemorrhage
- Usually known to have malignancy elsewhere, although adenoma is still more common even in setting of known cancer
- NECT: Metastases can mimic lipid-poor adenoma
- CECT: Shows prolonged washout pattern, < 60% on 10 min delayed phase

Adrenal Lymphoma

- Unilateral or bilateral masses
- Usually secondary spread to adrenal with evidence of lymphoma elsewhere
- Unilateral primary lymphoma (non-Hodgkin) rare

Adrenal Hemorrhage

- Chronic hematoma may mimic adenoma: Well defined, oval, and hypoechoic on US
- No enhancement on CECT or CEMR

Adrenal Myelolipoma

- Can be small or large; asymptomatic
- Often homogeneous but typically more hyperechoic
- CT shows macroscopic fat, which is diagnostic
- Lipid-rich adenoma shows greater signal loss on chemical shift MR, whereas myelolipoma shows greater signal loss on fat-saturated sequences

Pheochromocytoma

- Typically large, > 3 cm in most cases
- Small tumors may be homogeneous isoechoic/hypoechoic
- Characteristically very hyperintense on T2WI
- Prone to hemorrhage and necrosis
- Characteristic clinical syndrome and endocrine dysfunction

Adrenal Carcinoma

- Rare; most commonly large and heterogeneous
- When small, can appear homogeneously hypoechoic

PATHOLOGY

General Features

- Classified as nonfunctioning vs. functioning
  - Most are nonfunctioning (normal hormone levels)
  - 15% are functional and produce hormones
    - Glucocorticoids result in Cushing syndrome
    - Mineralocorticoids result in Conn syndrome
    - Androgens result in virilization of women or feminization of men
  - Cushing syndrome
    - 15-25% are due to adrenal adenoma; usually > 2 cm
    - More commonly due to adrenal hyperplasia
  - Conn syndrome (primary hyperaldosteronism)
    - 80% are due to adrenal adenoma; often < 2 cm
    - 20% are due to adrenal hyperplasia

Gross Pathologic & Surgical Features

- Encapsulated, well-circumscribed, tan-yellow, ovoid mass
- Necrosis and hemorrhage are rare

Microscopic Features

- 70% show high intracytoplasmic lipid content
- 30% are atypical with lipid-poor features

CLINICAL ISSUES

Presentation

- Most common signs/symptoms
  - Most commonly: Asymptomatic, incidental finding
    - Accounts for > 90% of all incidentalomas
  - Hypertension and weakness with Conn syndrome
  - Moon facies, truncal obesity, purple striae, and buffalo hump with Cushing syndrome
- Other signs/symptoms
  - Lab data: ↑ aldosterone, cortisol, &/or androgens

Demographics

- Age
  - Prevalence of adenoma increases with age
  - Peak at 60-69 years, decreasing thereafter
- Gender
  - M = F
- Epidemiology
  - Most common adrenal tumor
  - Detected with increasing frequency in recent years due to increased use of CT and MR
  - Occurs in up to 9% of population (autopsy studies)
  - ↑ incidence in patients with diabetes or HTN

Natural History & Prognosis

- Excellent prognosis when incidental and nonhyperfunctioning

Treatment

- No treatment when asymptomatic incidental finding
- Laparoscopic removal of gland if hyperfunctioning
  - Unilateral aldosterone secretion on adrenal vein sampling may be treated surgically

DIAGNOSTIC CHECKLIST

Consider

- Small, asymptomatic adrenal nodule most likely to represent adrenal adenoma
- Consider comparison with any available prior imaging to establish stability over 12 month period and avoid unnecessary additional testing

Image Interpretation Pearls

- No specific sonographic features distinguish adenomas from other adrenal lesions
  - May suggest diagnosis for small, well-circumscribed, homogeneous lesion on US
- CT and MR show specific patterns that can confirm
  - Lipid-rich adenomas
    - NECT: < 10 HU
    - Chemical shift MR: Signal drop on out-of-phase T1
  - Lipid-rich and lipid-poor adenomas
    - 10 min delayed-phase CECT: > 60% washout on 10 min delay

SELECTED REFERENCES

1. Lattin GE Jr et al: From the radiologic pathology archives: Adrenal tumors and tumor-like conditions in the adult: radiologic-pathologic correlation. Radiographics. 34(3):805-29, 2014
2. Berland LL et al: Managing incidental findings on abdominal CT: white paper of the ACR incidental findings committee. J Am Coll Radiol. 7(10):754-73, 2010
3. Johnson PT et al: Adrenal mass imaging with multidetector CT: pathologic conditions, pearls, and pitfalls. Radiographics. 29(5):1333-51, 2009
4. Caoili EM, et al. Adrenal masses: characterization with combined unenhanced and delayed enhanced CT. Radiology 2002; 222:629-33.

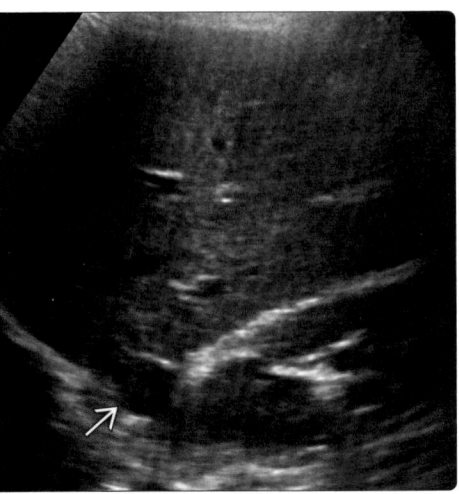
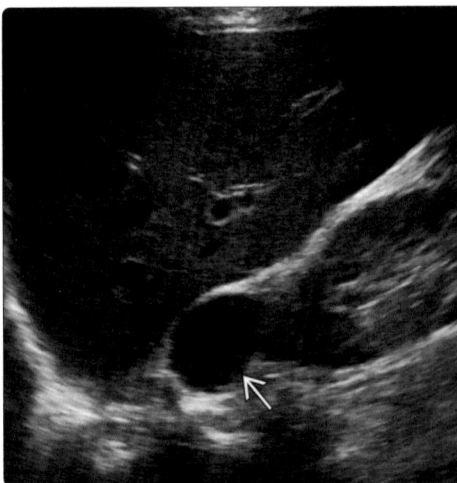

(Left) *Longitudinal transabdominal US shows an incidentally found, small, round, homogeneous hypoechoic mass in the right adrenal gland ➡, which was proven to be an adenoma on NECT.* (Right) *Longitudinal transabdominal US shows a well-circumscribed, homogeneously hypoechoic right adrenal mass ➡. Adenoma was considered. However, the appearance is nonspecific and indistinguishable from other small adrenal lesions. Biopsy revealed adrenal lymphoma.*

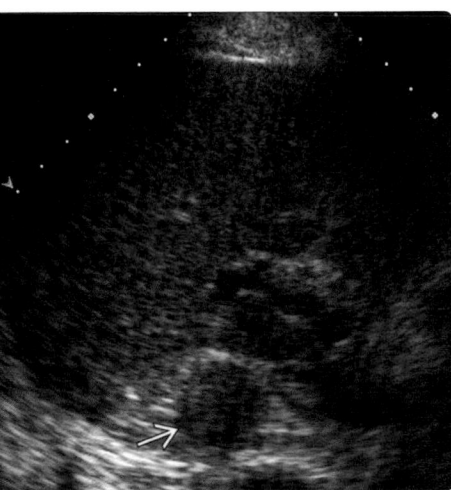
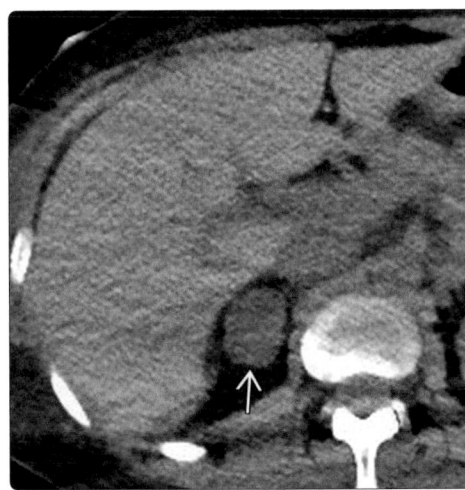

(Left) *Transverse transabdominal US shows a round, smoothly marginated, hypoechoic mass ➡. The size of the lesion and its nonspecific appearance prompted further evaluation.* (Right) *Corresponding axial noncontrast CT shows a smoothly marginated, homogeneous, low-density right adrenal mass ➡, which did not have an attenuation < 10 HU.*

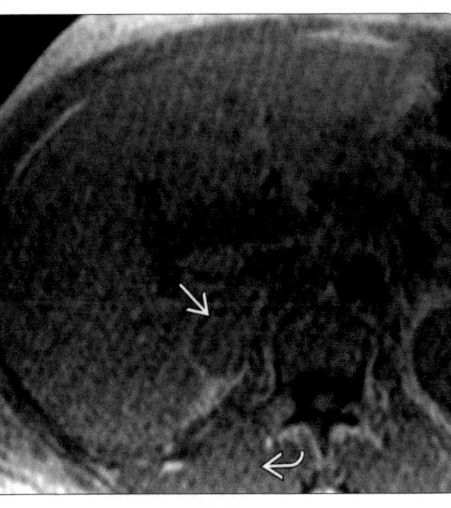
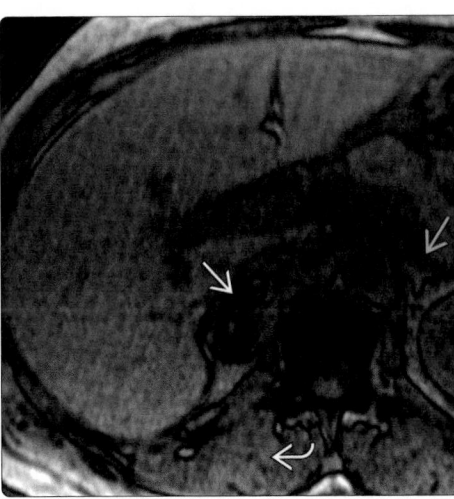

(Left) *Axial T1 in-phase MR in the same patient shows homogeneous T1 signal in the lesion ➡, which is isointense to muscle ➡.* (Right) *Corresponding opposed-phase T1 MR shows marked signal drop within the lesion ➡ compared with muscle ➡, diagnostic of intracellular lipid within an adrenal adenoma. Note normal left adrenal gland ➡.*

Adrenal Cyst

TERMINOLOGY

- Descriptive term for simple or complex cystic lesion in adrenal gland

IMAGING

- General features: Well-defined, round, uni-/multilocular, thin-walled, suprarenal cyst
- US: Avascular, anechoic or hypoechoic lesion with thin wall and posterior acoustic enhancement
  - Low-level internal echoes, calcification, fluid-fluid levels, and septations suggest recent hemorrhage
- CT: Nonenhancing, thin-walled, homogeneous, low-density lesion with attenuation values < 20 HU
  - Higher or mixed attenuation cyst contents → hemorrhage, intracystic debris, crystals; ± calcification
- MR: Nonenhancing with uniform low T1, high T2 SI
  - Hemorrhage shows variable T1 signal
- Concerning features: Complicated cyst, ≥ 5 cm size, internal echogenicity, or thick wall (≥ 3 mm) → suspect malignancy

- Imaging recommendation
  - US for initial screening and follow-up
  - CT and MR for further characterization

TOP DIFFERENTIAL DIAGNOSES

- Necrotic adrenal tumor
- Adjacent cystic lesions
- Adrenal adenoma

CLINICAL ISSUES

- Typically clinically silent
- Often increases in size over time; not indicative of malignancy
- Usually conservative management: No standard follow-up imaging recommendations
- Treatment reserved for cysts with malignant features, > 5 cm, or in symptomatic patients with endocrine abnormalities or complications

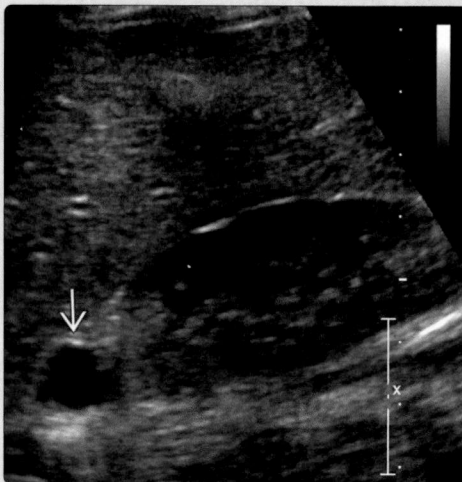
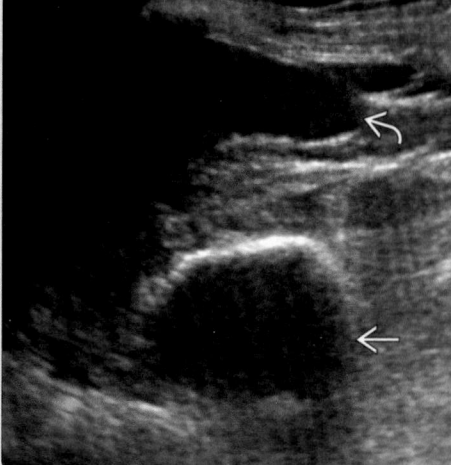

(Left) Sagittal transabdominal ultrasound shows a well-circumscribed anechoic lesion with a thin wall and posterior acoustic enhancement ➡ immediately superior to the right kidney, compatible with an adrenal cyst. (Right) Longitudinal transabdominal ultrasound shows a well-defined left adrenal cyst ➡. Note adjacent spleen ➡.

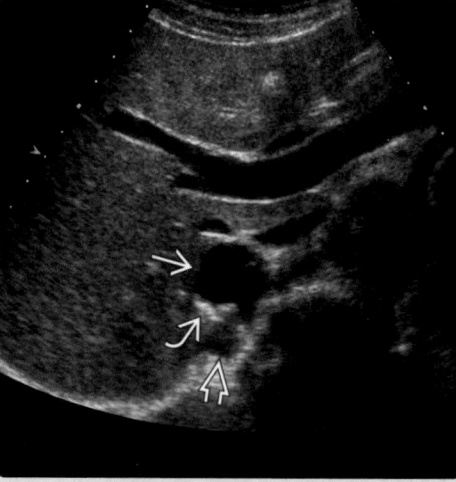
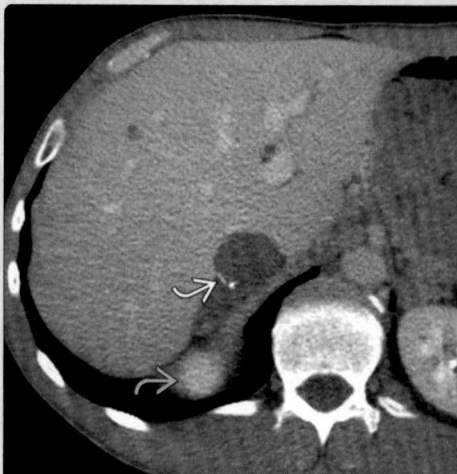

(Left) Transverse oblique transabdominal ultrasound shows a complex, septated cystic lesion ➡ above the right kidney (not included in the field of view). Note the hyperechoic foci ➡ associated with the septum and low-level echoes in the smaller cystic component ➡. (Right) Corresponding axial CT confirms the cystic nature of the complex lesion arising from the right adrenal gland. Note calcification associated with the septum ➡. Upper pole of the right kidney ➡.

Adrenal Cyst

TERMINOLOGY

Definitions

Descriptive term for simple or complex cystic lesion in adrenal gland

IMAGING

General Features

- Best diagnostic clue
  - Rounded, uni-/multilocular, thin-walled, suprarenal cyst
- Location
  - Unilateral > bilateral (8-10%)
- Size
  - Majority ≤ 5 cm (50%), up to 20 cm

Ultrasonographic Findings

- Grayscale ultrasound
  - Well-defined, anechoic or hypoechoic, uni-/multilocular; with thin wall and posterior acoustic enhancement
  - Low-level internal echoes, hyperechoic foci (calcification), fluid-fluid levels, and septations suggest recent hemorrhage
  - Complicated cyst, ≥ 5 cm size, internal echogenicity or thick wall (≥ 3 mm): ↑ concern for malignancy
- Color Doppler shows no internal flow

CT Findings

- NECT
  - Well circumscribed with thin wall, homogeneous low density (water or near-water density < 20 HU)
  - Higher or mixed attenuation cyst contents → hemorrhage, intracystic debris, crystals
  - Calcification seen in 15-30%
    - Rim-like or nodular (51-69%), centrally along septations (19%), punctate within intracystic hemorrhage (5%)
- CECT: No central enhancement ± wall enhancement

MR Findings

- Uncomplicated: Uniformly T1 hypointense, T2 hyperintense
- Hemorrhage: Variable T1 hyperintensity
- Centrally nonenhancing on T1WI C+

Imaging Recommendations

- Best imaging tool
  - US for initial screening and follow-up
  - CT and MR for further characterization

DIFFERENTIAL DIAGNOSIS

Necrotic Adrenal Tumor

- Primary: Pheochromocytoma or adrenal carcinoma
- Metastatic tumor (e.g., melanoma metastases)
- Cystic neuroblastoma in appropriate age group (rare)
- Complex wall with heterogeneous contents and enhancing components

Adjacent Cystic Lesions

- Hepatic or renal cyst; pancreatic tail pseudocyst, splenic artery pseudoaneurysm, splenic varices, GI duplication cyst; gastric diverticulum
- Multiplanar CT or MR can help better characterize origin

Adrenal Adenoma

- Well defined and homogeneous with density < 30 HU on CT
- Shows avid enhancement without wall

PATHOLOGY

General Features

- Etiology
  - Endothelial lining (~ 45%): Lymphangioma (majority) and hemangioma
  - Epithelial lining (~ 9%): True simple cyst; types include congenital glandular or retention cyst, embryonal cyst, cystic adenoma, or mesothelial inclusion cyst
  - Pseudocyst (~ 39%): Prior hemorrhage or infarction
  - Parasitic cyst (~ 7%): Usually due to disseminated *Echinococcus granulosus* infection

CLINICAL ISSUES

Presentation

- Most common signs/symptoms
  - Usually clinically silent
  - Abdominal or flank pain due to mass effect
- Other signs/symptoms
  - Retroperitoneal hemorrhage
  - Hypertension associated with adrenal cyst

Demographics

- Age
  - 3rd to 6th decade of life
- Epidemiology
  - Uncommon with autopsy incidence of 0.073%
  - Imaging prevalence of about 1%

Natural History & Prognosis

- Complications: Hypertension, infection, rupture with retroperitoneal hemorrhage, intracystic hemorrhage
- Prognosis: Excellent
- Increase in size over time frequently seen with benign cysts and is not indicative of malignancy

Treatment

- Usually conservative management: No standard follow-up imaging recommendations
  - Hormonal work-up to assess activity of lesion
- Treatment reserved for cysts with malignant features, > 5 cm, or in symptomatic patients with endocrine abnormalities or complications
  - Ultrasound-guided percutaneous cyst aspiration; ± injection of sclerosing agent
    - Cyst-fluid analysis may yield adrenal steroids or cholesterol: Diagnostic of adrenal cyst
    - Therapeutic for cyst without malignant features
  - Surgical resection; laparoscopic approach

SELECTED REFERENCES

1. Lattin GE Jr et al: From the radiologic pathology archives: adrenal tumors and tumor-like conditions in the adult: radiologic-pathologic correlation. Radiographics. 34(3):805-29, 2014
2. Ricci Z et al: Adrenal cysts: natural history by long-term imaging follow-up. AJR Am J Roentgenol. 201(5):1009-16, 2013

Pheochromocytoma

TERMINOLOGY

- Definition: Rare catecholamine-secreting tumor arising from chromaffin cells of adrenal medulla
- Termed **paraganglioma** if extraadrenal

IMAGING

- Best diagnostic clue
  - Adrenal mass in setting of clinical symptoms or biochemical abnormality
    - Paroxysmal headache, palpitations, sweating
    - ↑ levels of 24-hr urine-fractionated metanephrines
- **"Imaging chameleon"**: Variable US/CT/MR appearance; mimics other lesions
  - Commonly solid and hypervascular ± cystic change, necrosis, and calcification
  - Can be purely cystic
- **First-line**: CT or MR
- **US**: Comparable to CT in detecting adrenal tumors; limited for extraadrenal disease

- **I-123 MIBG**: For extraadrenal, metastatic, or recurrent disease

TOP DIFFERENTIAL DIAGNOSES

- Adrenal adenoma
- Adrenal metastases or lymphoma
- Adrenocortical carcinoma
- Adrenal neuroblastoma
- Adrenal granulomatous infection

DIAGNOSTIC CHECKLIST

- Remembered as **"rule of 10s"**
  - 10% extraadrenal (paraganglioma)
  - 10% bilateral (suggesting hereditary disease)
  - 10% pediatric (also suggests hereditary disease)
  - 10% contain calcification
  - 10% malignant (higher for extraadrenal cases)
  - 25% familial (previously thought to be 10%)

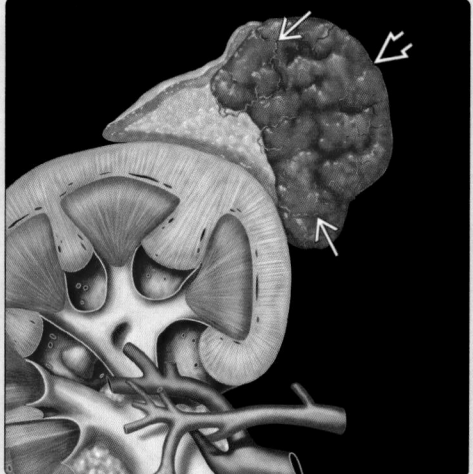
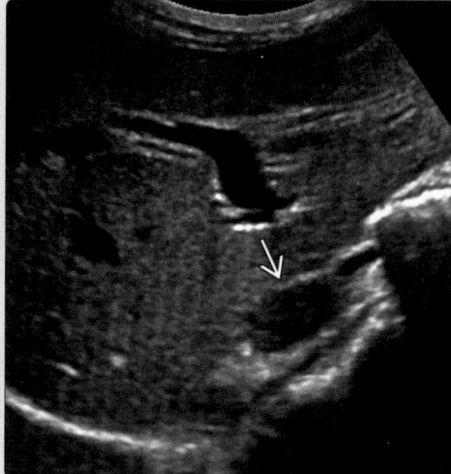

(Left) Graphic shows a typical pheochromocytoma ➡, moderate in size, with a well-circumscribed margin and solid appearance. Note hypervascularity ➡ of the mass, which commonly results in necrosis and cystic change. (Right) Transverse transabdominal ultrasound demonstrates a well-circumscribed, homogeneous hypoechoic adrenal mass ➡. The appearance is nonspecific, but the patient presented with elevated catecholamines and hypertensive urgency, suggesting a diagnosis of pheochromocytoma.

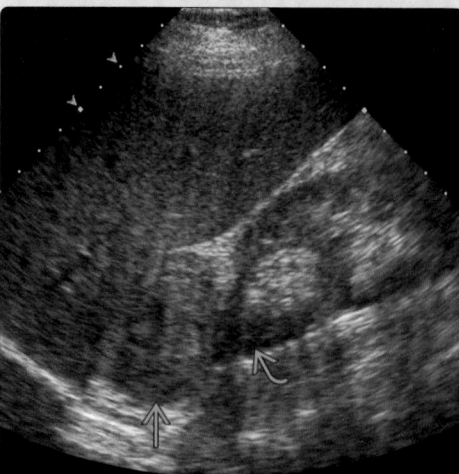
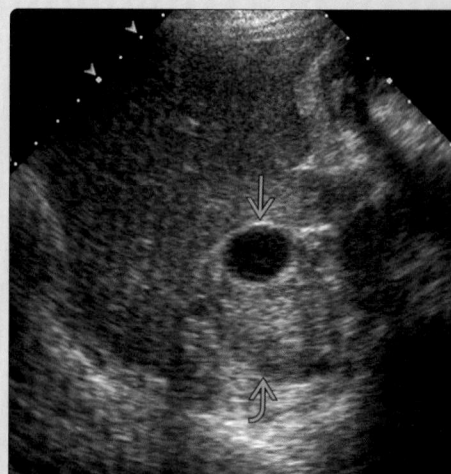

(Left) Longitudinal transabdominal ultrasound shows a well-demarcated, solid right adrenal mass ➡, which was proven to be a pheochromocytoma. It is hyperechoic to the renal cortex ➡. (Right) Transverse transabdominal ultrasound of a right adrenal pheochromocytoma shows a large, well-defined echogenic mass ➡ with an anechoic cystic area representing necrosis ➡.

TERMINOLOGY

Definitions

Paraganglioma: Neuroendocrine tumor arising from paraganglia anywhere in sympathetic chain

Pheochromocytoma: Adrenal medullary paraganglioma

- Arises from catecholamine-secreting chromaffin cells of adrenal medulla

IMAGING

General Features

Best diagnostic clue
- Adrenal mass in setting of clinical symptoms or biochemical abnormality

Location
- Paragangliomas occur along **sympathetic chain**: Neck to urinary bladder
- Majority are **subdiaphragmatic** (98%)
  - Adrenal (90%); extraadrenal (10%)
    □ Aortic bifurcation: Organ of Zuckerkandl, 2.5%
- Typically unilateral
- Bilateral: Commonly with hereditary conditions; 10% of sporadic cases

Size
- Variable: Up to 15 cm (typically 3-5 cm)

Morphology
- Well-circumscribed, encapsulated tumor
- Variable size & appearance, "chameleon tumors"
  - Commonly solid and hypervascular ± cystic change, necrosis, and calcification
  - Can be purely cystic
- Pheochromocytomas and paragangliomas demonstrate similar imaging features but vary in location

Ultrasonographic Findings

Grayscale ultrasound
- Variable appearance: Solid (75%) > solid/cystic or cystic
  - Iso-/hypoechoic (77%) or hyperechoic (23%) to kidney
- Small tumors: Solid, well-circumscribed; uniform echoes
- Large tumors: Solid; homogeneous (46%) or heterogeneous (54%) echo pattern
  - Complex echo pattern: Necrosis (hypoechoic) &/or hemorrhage (hyperechoic)
- Can be predominantly cystic lesions due to chronic hemorrhage and necrotic debris (fluid-fluid level)
- Overlying bowel gas can obscure extraadrenal masses
- Always evaluate bladder wall, renal hilum, and organ of Zuckerkandl at origin of inferior mesenteric artery

Color Doppler
- Hypervascular
- Compression/invasion of IVC/renal vein
  - Seen with both benign & malignant tumors

CT Findings

NECT: Well-defined mass with low soft tissue attenuation
- Generally attenuation > 10 HU; however, rarely intracellular fat may result in lower attenuation
- ±: ↑ density (hemorrhage), ↓ density (cystic degeneration; necrosis), calcification (rare; 10%)

- **CECT**: Marked enhancement; may be heterogeneous due to hemorrhage/necrosis
  - Variable washout characteristics: Can show rapid washout that mimics adenoma
  - No convincing evidence that IV injection of iodinated contrast precipitates hypertensive crisis (previous belief)

MR Findings

- **T1WI**: **Isointense** to muscle & hypointense to liver
  - Variable signal intensity if necrosis/hemorrhage present
  - If microscopic fat present (rare), chemical shift signal loss may mimic adenoma
- **T2WI**: T2 hyperintense due to ↑ water content (cystic/liquefactive necrosis)
  - Classic "**light-bulb**" appearance of marked T2-bright SI, variably seen (11-65%)
  - 35% have low T2 SI (isointense to spleen)
  - **Most common**: heterogeneously enhancing lesion with multiple high-SI pockets
- **T1WI C+**: Characteristic "**salt and pepper**" pattern
  - **Salt** (enhancing parenchyma); **pepper** (↑ vascular flow voids due to hypervascular tumor)

Nuclear Medicine Findings

- **First-line**: I-123 metaiodobenzylguanidine (**MIBG**)
  - Norepinephrine analog
  - After 24-72 hours: ↑ uptake of I-123 MIBG in tumor
  - Useful for extraadrenal, metastatic, recurrent disease
  - Sensitivity (79-88%); specificity (~ 100%)
- 2nd line: In-111 Pentetreotide, FDG PET, DOPA analogs

Imaging Recommendations

- Best imaging tool
  - **US**: Comparable sensitivity to CT for detection of adrenal disease; poor detection of extraadrenal tumors
  - **NE + CECT**: Overall 93-100% sensitive; however, up to 40% extraadrenal lesions may be missed on CT
  - **I-123 MIBG**: Superior detection of extraadrenal, metastatic, &/or recurrent disease
- Protocol advice
  - Include aortic bifurcation in CT/MR field of view to evaluate for paragangliomas

DIFFERENTIAL DIAGNOSIS

Adrenal Adenoma

- Most common adrenal lesion; benign
- Pheochromocytomas tend to be larger than adenomas
- Cystic and rare microscopic fat-containing pheochromocytomas **may also be** hypodense on NECT
- Adenoma: Characteristic CT washout & MR signal dropout

Adrenal Metastases

- Most common malignant adrenal neoplasm (27% of all cancer)
- Typically bilateral; delayed contrast washout

Adrenal Lymphoma

- Large infiltrative, bilateral masses; adrenals maintain shape
- 25% secondary to non-Hodgkin lymphoma; primary is rare

Adrenocortical Carcinoma

- Rare; aggressive; large, unilateral, heterogeneous solid with necrosis; hemorrhage ± calcification
- ↑ T1 and ↓ T2 signal (as with "classic" pheochromocytomas)
- Aggressive, often with IVC extension

Adrenal Neuroblastoma

- Large pediatric adrenal mass; calcification (80-90%)

Adrenal Granulomatous Infection

- TB, histoplasmosis, other fungal diseases; usually bilateral
  - Acute (hypoechoic masses) or chronic (small & calcified)

PATHOLOGY

General Features

- Associated abnormalities
  - Majority are sporadic
  - 25% have autosomal dominant gene mutation
    - **Multiple endocrine neoplasia, type II (MEN2)**
      - □ *MEN2* mutation; 50% have pheochromocytoma
      - □ Medullary thyroid carcinoma; hyperparathyroidism; neuromas and marfanoid habitus
    - **von Hippel-Lindau (VHL) disease**
      - □ *VHL* tumor suppressor gene, 10-20% risk
      - □ Multiple benign and malignant tumors
    - **Neurofibromatosis, type I**
      - □ Rare cause of pheochromocytomas (1% risk)
      - □ Cutaneous/plexiform neurofibromas, optic nerve gliomas, peripheral nerve sheath tumors, gastrointestinal stromal tumor
    - **Pheochromocytoma-paraganglioma syndromes**
      - □ Mutations of succinate dehydrogenase gene family (*SDHB* and *SDHD*)
      - □ ↑ incidence of extraadrenal tumors and head/neck paragangliomas
      - □ 50% risk of malignant pheochromocytomas
- Most are benign; 10% are malignant
  - Diagnosis of malignancy is based solely on presence of direct local tumor invasion or metastatic disease
  - Extraadrenal paragangliomas are more likely to be malignant

Gross Pathologic & Surgical Features

- Range of appearances: Small, well-circumscribed, yellow-tan lesion confined to adrenals; large, hemorrhagic, cystic-necrotic masses

Microscopic Features

- Predominantly chromaffin cells; occasionally spindle cells are dominant feature
  - Term pheochromocytoma refers to dusky color of cells stained with chromium salts
- No single histologic feature of pheochromocytoma consistently predicts malignancy

CLINICAL ISSUES

Presentation

- Most common signs/symptoms
  - Majority are asymptomatic; symptoms may be episodic or paroxysmal
  - Classic triad (arises from adrenergic excess)
    - Paroxysmal headache, palpitations, sweating
    - 90% specific but uncommon (only present in 10.0-36.5% of patients)
- Other signs/symptoms
  - Hypertensive crisis: Palpitations, tremors, arrhythmias, pain, myocardial infarction
- Lab data
  - Tumors typically secrete norepinephrine > epinephrine
  - **↑ levels of 24-hour urine-fractionated metanephrine**
    - 90-97% sensitivity; 69-98% specificity

Demographics

- Age
  - Sporadic cases, 3rd and 4th decades (mean age: 44 year
  - Hereditary cases (mean age: 25 years)
  - 10% are found in children
- Gender
  - Slight female predilection (M:F = 1:1.4)
- Epidemiology
  - Incidence (exact unknown): Estimated at 2-8 cases/1 million people/year
    - 0.1-0.6% of hypertensive adults
  - Majority of pheochromocytomas are likely asymptomati (incidentalomas)
    - Autopsy occurrence rates 10-17%

Natural History & Prognosis

- Hypertensive crises and cardiovascular complications ↑ morbidity/mortality
- Prognosis
  - Noninvasive and nonmetastatic: Typically favorable
    - Postoperatively: 50% have persistent hypertension; 16% recur within 10 years of resection
  - Malignant tumors: 54% 5-year survival rate

Treatment

- Symptomatic therapy: α-adrenergic blockade and calcium channel antagonists
- Laparoscopic resection/debulking for both benign and malignant tumors
- Adjuvant therapy (malignant tumors): I-131 MIBG therapy chemotherapy (cyclophosphamide, vincristine, dacarbazine

DIAGNOSTIC CHECKLIST

Consider

- Imaging characteristics can **mimic** other diagnoses; labs essential for diagnosis

Image Interpretation Pearls

- Extraadrenal tumors arise anywhere along sympathetic ganglia (neck to bladder); include in search pattern

SELECTED REFERENCES

1. Lattin GE Jr et al: From the radiologic pathology archives: adrenal tumors and tumor-like conditions in the adult: radiologic-pathologic correlation. Radiographics. 34(3):805-29, 2014
2. Leung K et al: Pheochromocytoma: the range of appearances on ultrasound CT, MRI, and functional imaging. AJR Am J Roentgenol. 200(2):370-8, 2013
3. Raja A et al: Multimodality imaging findings of pheochromocytoma with associated clinical and biochemical features in 53 patients with histologically confirmed tumors. AJR Am J Roentgenol. 201(4):825-33, 2013

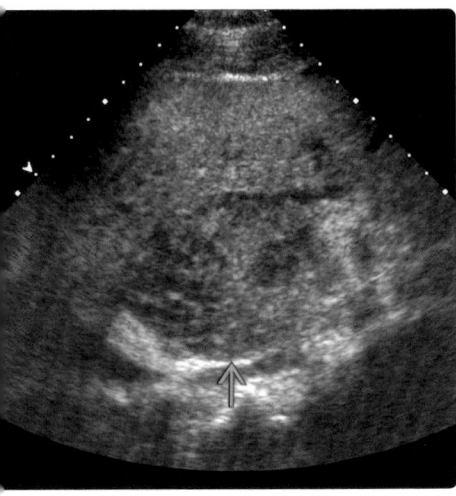

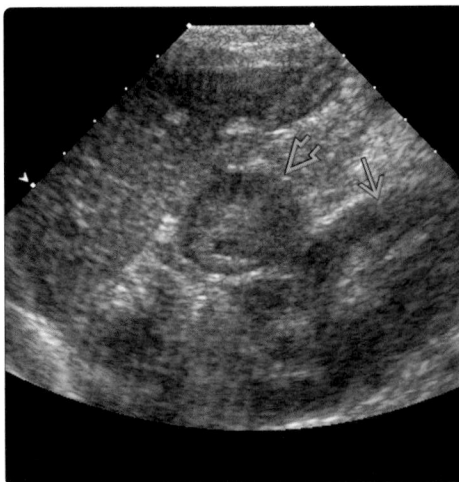

(Left) *Longitudinal transabdominal ultrasound demonstrates a heterogeneous adrenal mass* ➡️ *with mixed echogenicity due to necrosis and hemorrhage in the large pheochromocytoma.* (Right) *Longitudinal transabdominal ultrasound demonstrates an oval, well-circumscribed heterogeneous mass* ➡️, *which is anterior to the left kidney* ➡️, *proven to be a paraganglioma.*

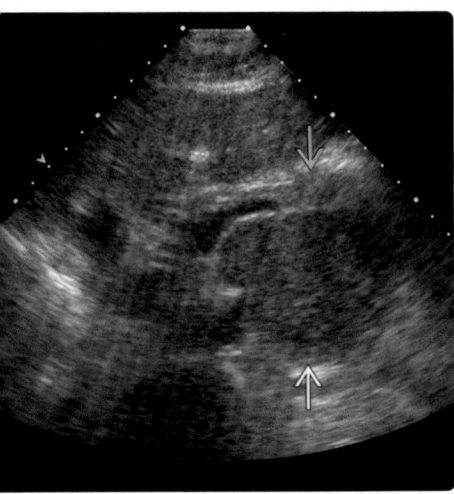

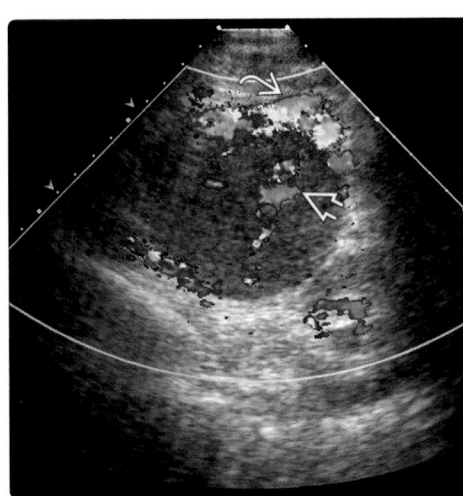

(Left) *Transverse transabdominal ultrasound shows a large, well-circumscribed, solid hypoechoic mass* ➡️ *in the left retroperitoneum displacing the pancreas anteriorly* ➡️. (Right) *Transverse transabdominal color Doppler ultrasound in the same patient shows hypervascularity of the mass* ➡️, *which is anteromedial to the left kidney and was a paraganglioma. Note mass effect on the splenic vein, which courses over the mass* ➡️.

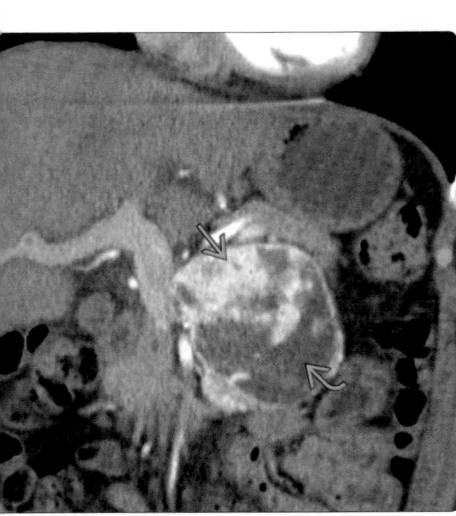

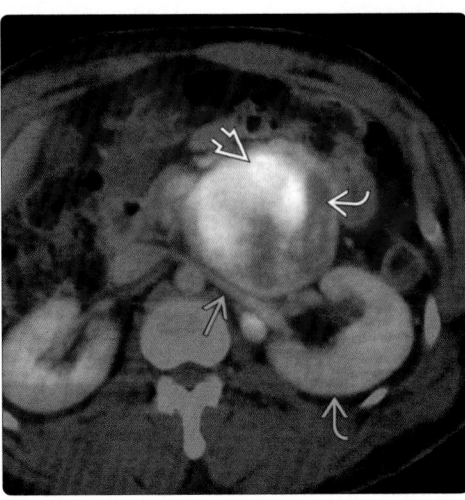

(Left) *Corresponding coronal CECT shows the large, well-defined mass, with avidly enhancing solid portions* ➡️ *and large hypodense areas of necrosis* ➡️, *resulting in a very heterogeneous appearance.* (Right) *Corresponding axial fused PET/CT demonstrates ↑ radiotracer uptake* ➡️ *within the solid portions of the tumor, whereas the necrotic areas appear photopenic* ➡️. *The mass is distinct from the left kidney* ➡️, *but notice abutment/narrowing of the main left renal vein* ➡️.

Adrenal Carcinoma

TERMINOLOGY

- Adrenal carcinoma
- **Synonyms**: Adrenocortical carcinoma; adrenal cancer
- **Definition**: Rare, aggressive tumor arising from adrenal cortex, often with local invasion and distant metastases

IMAGING

- US may be used for initial screening in patients with abdominal pain but offers limited ability to characterize or differentiate from other adrenal masses
- Best imaging tool: **CECT** or **CEMR**
- Large heterogeneous necrotic adrenal mass ± calcification venous invasion and metastases
  - Metastases to regional lymph nodes, liver, lung, bone

TOP DIFFERENTIAL DIAGNOSES

- Pheochromocytoma
- Adrenal metastases
- Adrenal adenoma
- Adrenal lymphoma
- Ganglioneuroma
- Neuroblastoma (in children)
- Myelolipoma
- Adrenal hemorrhage

CLINICAL ISSUES

- **Rare**: < 0.2% of all cancers
- **Bimodal** distribution: < 5 years old (1st peak) and 30-50 years old (2nd peak); slightly more common in women
- **Associated syndromes**: Cushing, female virilization, Conn, male feminization
- Definitive treatment (all stages): En bloc resection

DIAGNOSTIC CHECKLIST

- Rule out other more common diagnoses, e.g., adenoma, hemorrhage, neuroblastoma in child
- **Inferior vena cava (IVC) invasion** (best depicted on MR) is **crucial** for surgical planning

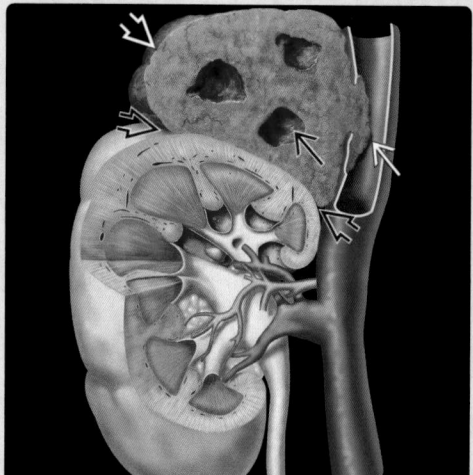
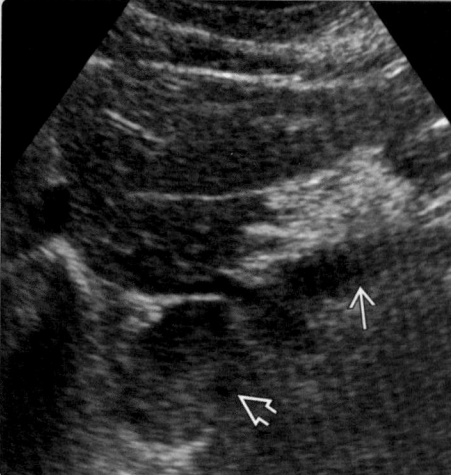

(Left) *Longitudinal graphic shows a large right adrenal carcinoma (AC)* ➡ *with areas of necrosis* ➡, *tumor invasion into the IVC* ➡, *and compression of the right renal upper pole* ➡. **(Right)** *Longitudinal transabdominal US demonstrates a large, well-demarcated solid echogenic mass* ➡. *Its large size makes adenoma less likely, but the US appearance is otherwise nonspecific and could represent a variety of adrenal masses. CT showed features specific for AC, which was confirmed at surgical resection. IVC is shown* ➡.

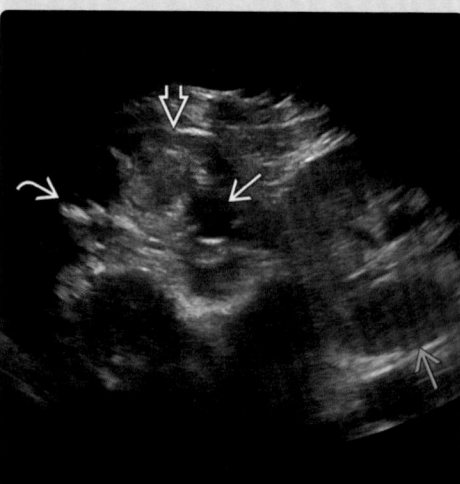
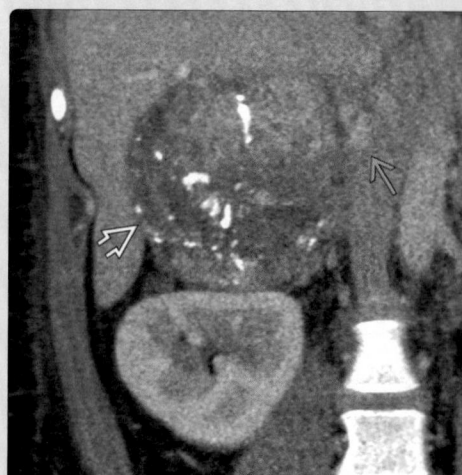

(Left) *Longitudinal transabdominal ultrasound demonstrates a large, heterogenous right adrenal mass* ➡ *with hypoechoic areas of necrosis* ➡. *Note the radiating stellate echogenicity and calcification* ➡. *Right kidney is shown* ➡. **(Right)** *Corresponding coronal CECT shows a large heterogenous right adrenal mass* ➡ *with internal necrosis and intratumoral calcification. Note invasion of the IVC* ➡.

Adrenal Carcinoma

TERMINOLOGY

Synonyms

- Adrenocortical carcinoma (ACC); adrenal cancer

Definitions

- Malignant neoplasm arising from adrenal cortex

IMAGING

General Features

- Best diagnostic clue
  - Large, heterogeneous, unilateral solid mass with local invasion (inferior vena cava [IVC] invasion) and metastases
- Location
  - Suprarenal, 90-98% unilateral (left slightly > right gland)
  - Metastases: Liver, lung, regional lymph nodes, bone
- Size
  - Large (average size: 9 cm; 70% > 6 cm)
    - Functioning tumors usually smaller (≤ 5 cm) than nonfunctioning tumors (≥ 10 cm) at presentation
- Morphology
  - Typically well defined with aggressive-appearing features
    - Size > 4 cm, irregular margins, intratumoral necrosis/hemorrhage, calcification, heterogeneous enhancement, regional/venous invasion → IVC invasion (9-19% cases at presentation)
  - Displaces adjacent structures: Compresses kidney

Ultrasonographic Findings

- Grayscale ultrasound
  - Small tumors: Homogeneous, hypoechoic, similar to renal cortex
  - Large tumors: Heterogeneous, hypoechoic/anechoic areas (necrosis &/or hemorrhage), and echogenic
  - Scar sign: Predominantly echogenic pattern with radiating linear echoes; suggests carcinoma
- Color Doppler
  - Invasion/occlusion of adrenal vein, renal vein, and IVC; ± intraluminal tumor thrombus

CT Findings

- **NECT**: Rarely attenuate < 10 HU (98% specificity for identifying benign adenomas)
- **CECT**: Retain IV contrast material with absolute and relative washout of < 60% and < 40%, respectively, at 15 min
  - Heterogeneous, primarily peripheral enhancement due to central necrosis and hemorrhage
    - Necrosis invariably present in tumors ≥ 6 cm
  - Mass effect ± regional invasion, IVC thrombus, metastatic disease
    - Nodes, liver, lungs, bone
- Calcifications (30%); coarse or micro, usually central

MR Findings

- **T1WI**: Predominately isointense/hypointense to liver parenchyma; often heterogeneous (necrosis)
  - High T1 signal indicates hemorrhage
- **T2WI**: Hyperintense to liver parenchyma; heterogeneous
- **T1WI C+**: Avid enhancement with delayed washout

- Chemical shift imaging
  - Functioning tumors may contain small regions of intracytoplasmic lipid → small, nonuniform areas of signal loss (< 30% of lesion)
    - Similar pattern seen in lipid-poor adenomas
    - **Not seen**: Uniform signal loss (i.e., lipid-rich adenomas)
- **MR spectroscopy**: Potential for distinguishing adenomas, pheochromocytomas, ACCs, and metastases

Nuclear Medicine Findings

- **FDG PET combined with CECT**
  - Sensitivity of 100% and specificity of 87-97% for identifying malignant adrenal masses
  - Detection of distant metastases (present in 1/3 of patients at presentation)
- Novel PET tracer 11C metomidate for adrenocortical tissue
  - Uptake seen in adenomas and ACCs but **not** in pheochromocytomas and metastases

Imaging Recommendations

- Best imaging tool
  - CT or MR for complete characterization
    - US (initial screening)
  - MR is superior to CT in delineating invasion of IVC, renal vein, and interface with adjacent kidney/liver
- Study of choice to **exclude** adenoma: NE + CECT

DIFFERENTIAL DIAGNOSIS

Pheochromocytoma

- Can be large and heterogeneous, similar to adrenal carcinoma (AC)
  - Less commonly shows calcification, seen in 10%
- 91% are functional → recognized biochemically
- Bilateral in multiple endocrine neoplasia (MEN) 2A and 2B (not MEN1)

Adrenal Metastases

- Most common adrenal malignancy
- Consider if **bilateral** involvement and known 1° present
  - Lung is most common primary

Adrenal Adenoma

- Small ACs can appear well defined and homogeneously hypoechoic
- Adenoma rarely shows calcification
- May be distinguished by CT washout and chemical shift imaging (sensitivity 75-98%; specificity 92-100%)

Adrenal Lymphoma

- Most commonly: Non-Hodgkin diffuse large B cell
- Large, bilateral masses maintain adeniform shape

Ganglioneuroma

- In children and young adults (60% before 20 years)
- CECT: Large solid lesion with homogeneous enhancement
- MR: T2 heterogeneous hyperintensity, T1 C+ shows late gradual enhancement
- Punctate or discrete calcification; no vessel involvement

Neuroblastoma

- Pediatric population; calcification is hallmark

ion

soft tissue masses with cystic changes ±

histoblastomas usually bilateral but can be

wever, can be

ements predominate and

due to macroscopic fat,

...al Hemorrhage

- Heterogeneous on US depending on age of hemorrhage
- AC can contain hemorrhagic elements due to necrosis
- CT and MR show lack of enhancement

PATHOLOGY

General Features

- Etiology
  ○ Most ACs are sporadic
- Genetics
  ○ More likely to be aneuploid or tetraploid
  ○ Genetic syndromes can ↑ incidence of AC
    - Beckwith-Wiedemann, Li-Fraumeni, Carney, familial adenomatous polyposis, MEN1

Staging, Grading, & Classification

- Surgical staging system may offer better prognostic accuracy than TMN staging
  ○ **Stage I**: Diameter ≤ 5 cm, no local invasion
  ○ **Stage II**: Diameter > 5 cm, no local invasion
  ○ **Stage III**: Any size + local invasion or nodes
  ○ **Stage IV**: Any size + local invasion & nodes or metastases

Gross Pathologic & Surgical Features

- Tumor weight > 500 g, grossly lobulated cut surface, necrosis, calcification, and hemorrhage **favor** malignancy

Microscopic Features

- Architectural disarray, ↑ mitotic rate, nuclear pleomorphism/atypia, hyperchromasia, capsular invasion, and venous or sinusoidal invasion **favor** malignancy
- May contain intracytoplasmic lipid or macroscopic fat
  ○ Due to cortisol/related fatty precursors in hormonally active tumors or coexisting myelolipomatous tissue

CLINICAL ISSUES

Presentation

- Most common signs/symptoms
  ○ 65-85% are nonfunctioning at presentation (adults)
    - Large, palpable mass (40-50%)
      □ Mass effect symptoms: Pain, fullness
    - Incidental mass on imaging exam (0-25%)
    - Late detection: 30% with metastases at presentation
- Other signs/symptoms
  ○ Functional tumors (85% of children; 15-30% of adults)
    - **Cushing syndrome** (30-40%): ↑ cortisol
      □ Moon facies, truncal obesity, striae, and buffalo hump

- **Virilization in females** (20-30%): ↑ androgens
  □ 95% of girls with functioning AC present with virilization
- 10-20% present with Cushing syndrome & virilization
  □ Cortisol & androgen cosecretion **favors** malignancy
- **Conn syndrome** (2%): 1° hyperaldosteronism
- **Feminization in males** (2%): ↑ androgens
- Other clinical syndromes: Hypoglycemia, polycythemia, and nonglucocorticoid-related insulin resistance

Demographics

- Age
  ○ Bimodal distribution
    - < 5 years old (1st peak) and 30-50 years old (2nd peak)
- Gender
  ○ Slightly more common in women (M:F = 1:1.5)
  ○ Functioning: F > M; nonfunctioning: M > F
- Epidemiology
  ○ Rare: 0.05-0.20% of all cancers
  ○ 1 per 1,500 adrenal tumors is malignant

Natural History & Prognosis

- Rapid growth with local invasion and distant metastases
- Tumor thrombus: IVC and renal vein (best seen on MR)
- **5-year post-resection survival**
  ○ **Stage I and II**: 65%; **stage III**: 40%; **stage IV**: 10%
- 5-year survival for pediatric ACs > adults (54% vs. 38%)
  ○ Pediatric ACs tend to be **less** aggressive

Treatment

- **Definitive treatment for all stages**: En bloc resection ± adjacent invaded organs
  ○ **Open adrenalectomy** favored over laparoscopic
    - High rate of recurrence/peritoneal carcinomatosis associated with laparoscopic procedures
- Chemotherapy: Primary and adjuvant therapy
  ○ Mitotane = adrenolytic
- Radiotherapy: Local recurrence, incomplete/indeterminate resection, bone metastases

DIAGNOSTIC CHECKLIST

Consider

- AC is rare; rule out common diagnoses
  ○ For example, adenoma, hemorrhage, neuroblastoma
- Differentiation may be difficult on US

Image Interpretation Pearls

- Large masses: More likely to be malignant (> 4 cm → 70%)
  ○ Excluding myelolipoma and pheochromocytoma, which are usually recognizable
- Vascular invasion and IVC extension may be seen at presentation

Reporting Tips

- **IVC invasion** (best depicted on MR; seen in 9-19% of cases) is **crucial** for surgical planning

SELECTED REFERENCES

1. Ganeshan D et al: Current update on cytogenetics, taxonomy, diagnosis, and management of adrenocortical carcinoma: what radiologists should know. AJR Am J Roentgenol. 199(6):1283-93, 2012

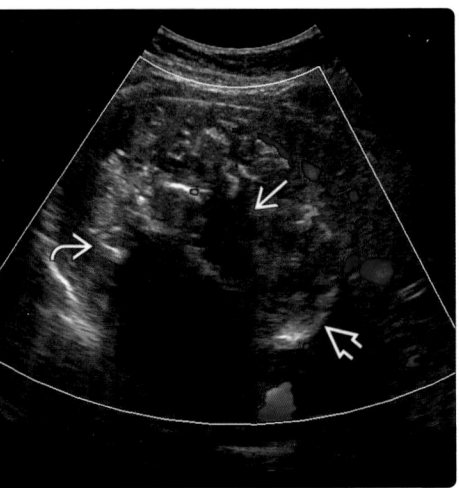

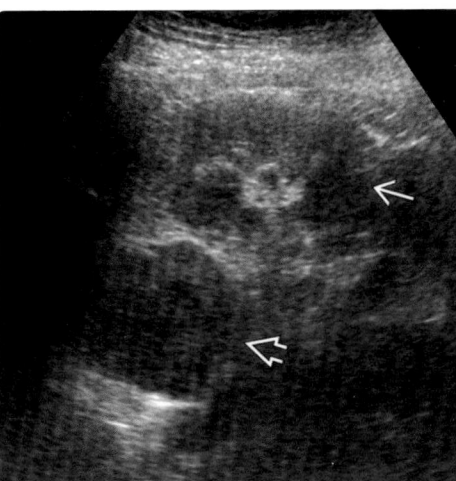

(Left) Transverse transabdominal color Doppler ultrasound shows a large, heterogeneous adrenal mass ⮕ with minimal peripheral flow, central hypoechoic areas of necrosis ⮕, and scattered calcification ⮕. (Right) Longitudinal decubitus transabdominal ultrasound demonstrates a large nonspecific hypoechoic adrenal mass ⮕. The upper pole of the right kidney is shown ⮕.

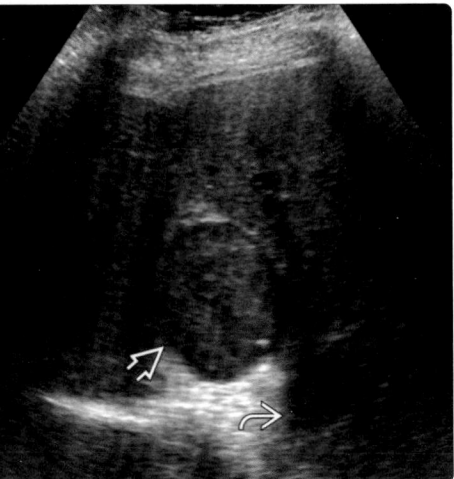

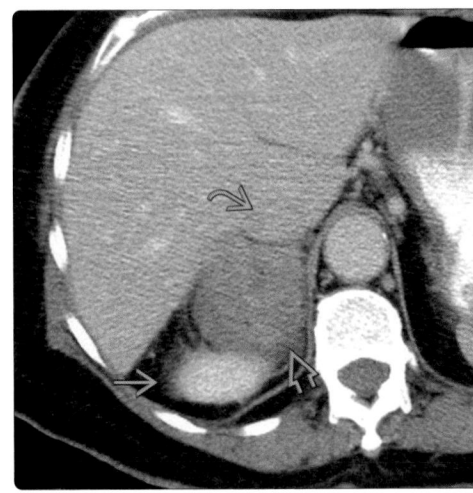

(Left) Transverse transabdominal ultrasound shows a well-circumscribed, solid isoechoic to liver adrenal mass ⮕, which was proven to be AC. The IVC ⮕ appeared spared at this level. (Right) Corresponding axial CECT shows a large, hypodense right adrenal mass ⮕ with infiltration of the surrounding fat. Tumor extension into the IVC ⮕ is difficult to see on the CT. The upper pole of the right kidney is shown ⮕.

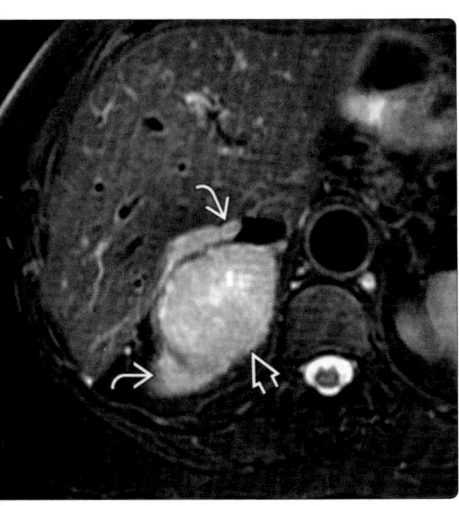

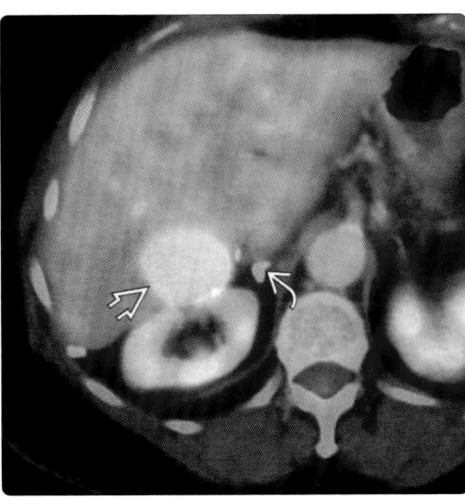

(Left) Corresponding axial T2 FS MR better demonstrates T2-hyperintense tumor thrombus in an accessory hepatic vein extending to the IVC ⮕. The mass ⮕ shows homogeneous T2 bright signal as well. Surgery confirmed invasion of segment VI of the liver with tumor thrombus reaching the IVC. (Right) Postoperative, follow-up axial PET/CT performed 5 months later shows a new metabolically active mass ⮕ in the surgical bed compatible with recurrent disease. Note the surgical clips ⮕.

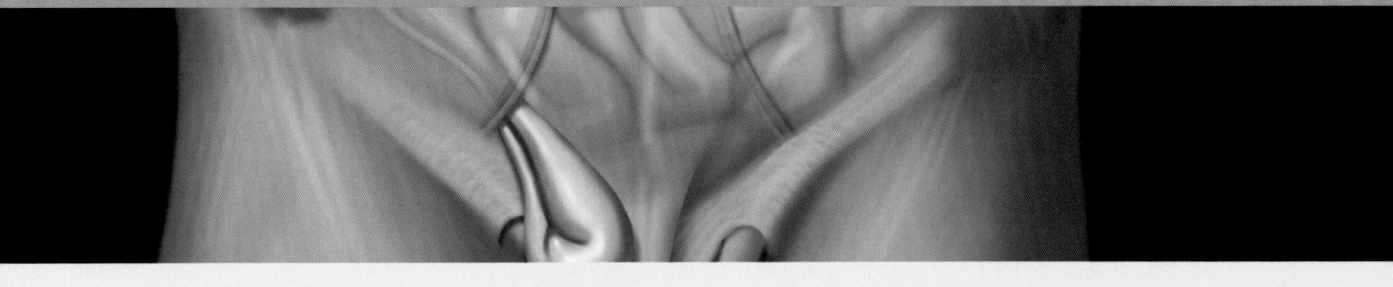

PART II
SECTION 8

Abdominal Wall/Peritoneal Cavity

Anatomy-Based Imaging Issues

Abdominal Wall

The anterolateral muscles of the abdominal wall are the external oblique, internal oblique and the transversus abdominis muscles. The aponeuroses of the internal oblique and transversus abdominis join medially to form the rectus sheath which contains the paired rectus abdominis muscles. These muscle groups protect the abdominal organs and assist in trunk flexion, twisting, walking and sitting as well as increasing intraabdominal pressure.

The linea alba is a midline raphe between the two rectus muscles. The linea semilunaris/spigelian fascia is a vertical fibrous band at the lateral edge of rectus sheath. These are sites of weakness and locations of abdominal wall hernias. Midline hernias through the linea alba include epigastric, umbilical and hypogastric hernias. Lateral hernias through the spigelian fascia are spigelian hernias. Deep to muscle layer is the transversalis fascia, followed by the extraperitoneal fascia and fat and the parietal peritoneum.

The inguinal ligament is the inferior edge of the external oblique aponeurosis, running from the anterior superior iliac spine to the pubic tubercle. The inguinal canal runs between the external oblique and the transversalis fascia, above the inguinal ligament. The inguinal canal begins at the deep inguinal ring and opens medially and inferiorly at the superficial inguinal ring. The deep inguinal ring is a defect in the transversalis fascia half way between the anterior superior iliac spine and the pubic tubercle. It is lateral to the inferior epigastric artery which is a key landmark for hernia evaluation. The Hesselbach triangle lies medial to the inferior epigastric artery, lateral to the rectus sheath and above the inguinal ligament. Indirect inguinal hernias pass through the deep inguinal ring to emerge at the superficial inguinal ring with a neck lateral to the inferior epigastric artery. Direct inguinal hernias emerge through Hesselbach triangle, medial to the inferior epigastric artery. Femoral hernias pass through the femoral canal, inferior to the inguinal ligament and medial to the femoral vein.

The posterior abdominal wall muscles are the psoas major and minor, iliacus and quadratus lumborum. They assist in hip flexion, maintenance of posture and lateral trunk flexion. Paraspinal muscles are the three columns of the erector spinae: Iliocostalis, longissimus and spinalis which extend the vertebral column. The latissimus dorsi arises from the thoracolumbar fascia lateral to the erector spinae. Lumbar hernias arise in two lumbar triangles: Superior (Grynfeltt) below the 12th rib, lateral to erector spinae and medial to the internal oblique muscle; inferior (Petit) above iliac crest between latissimus dorsi medially and external oblique laterally.

Peritoneal Cavity

The peritoneal cavity is a potential space between abdominal visceral and parietal peritoneum. It is divided into greater and lesser sacs which communicate at the foramen of Winslow. Compartments include right and left supramesocolic and inframesocolic spaces, paracolic gutters and pelvic cavity. The peritoneal cavity normally contains a small amount of lubricating fluid. Fluid collects in dependent pouches of the peritoneal cavity such as the pouch of Douglas (rectouterine pouch) and Morison pouch (hepatorenal pouch). This is where fluid should be sought initially. With increasing volumes of intraperitoneal fluid, fluid will spill over into all recesses and spaces.

The greater omentum and lesser omentum are folds of peritoneum that drape from the stomach. The greater omentum extends to cover the transverse colon and the small bowel and serves to contain inflammation or tumor. The lesser omentum extends from the lesser curve to the liver and proximal duodenum. The mesentery is a layer of peritoneum that encloses mobile bowel, connecting it to the posterior abdominal wall. The ascending and descending colon are not mobile and are retroperitoneal. Ligaments connect viscera to each other or to the abdominal wall, folds are peritoneal reflections. In the absence of ascites, sonographic evaluation of these normal structures is limited.

Pathologic Issues

Ultrasound has many advantages for imaging of the anterior abdominal wall and peritoneal cavity. For the abdominal wall real-time, high-resolution ultrasound and the dynamic ability to provoke hernias makes it an ideal imaging test. For fluid detection, ultrasound is highly sensitive within limitations of body habitus.

One of the most common indications for imaging the abdominal wall and groin is for the evaluation of hernias. The most common hernias are acquired inguinal and incisional hernias. Risk factors include abdominal wall laxity and increased intraabdominal pressure, prior surgery and trauma. Femoral and umbilical hernias are not uncommon. Congenital hernias are typically umbilical and indirect inguinal hernias. Other than confirming the clinically suspected diagnosis, ultrasound can determine the type of hernia and contents as well as complications such as strangulation.

Ultrasound is often used for the evaluation of lumps and swelling. Masses include lipomas and other soft tissue tumor, fat necrosis, epidermal inclusion cysts, endometriosis, desmoid tumors, and metastases. Careful search for tumor blood flow and comparison to the other asymptomatic side are recommended. Some lesions have characteristic findings, others require further imaging or biopsy.

Other indications for ultrasound of the abdominal wall include suspected fluid collections or abscesses. Ultrasound can be an ideal modality for localized fluid collections, able to detect internal contents and vascularity. Hematomas and abscesses are more complex than seromas.

Ultrasound of the peritoneal cavity usually consists of a search for ascites or acute hemorrhage (as in the FAST scan after abdominal trauma). Complexity of ascites, peritoneal nodularity or discrete soft tissue masses may suggest causes for the ascites, such as carcinomatosis or bacterial peritonitis.

Imaging Protocols

Prior to imaging, a good clinical history is obtained. Specific details regarding location and onset of symptoms and exacerbating factors are very important. The study can then be tailored to the patient.

Abdominal Wall

A high-frequency (8-15 MHz) linear transducer is required. The trapezoid format and extended field of view/panoramic format are very useful techniques for imaging larger structures. Curvilinear lower frequency transducers may also be required for larger lesions. More penetration and deeper field of view are needed for deeper lesions. For complex and ore extensive masses and collections CT or MR are indicated ven their wider field and depth of view. Furthermore, CT and R are less limited by body size and not limited by gas which ay be present in a hernia or abdominal wall abscess.

tients should be examined supine initially with images in ansverse and longitudinal planes. Hernias should be stinguished from soft tissue masses by position, sonographic ppearance and dynamic maneuvers. Evaluation for groin or odominal wall hernia is not complete without provocative aneuvers such as Valsalva, coughing or standing positions. ompression with the transducer is used to determine ducibility of hernias; however, too much probe pressure ay reduce a hernia and prevent detection unless provocative aneuvers are utilized. Stored cine clips are very useful for view. For the posterior abdominal wall, patients are initially aged prone. Comparison to the other side is very helpful for hernias and subtle masses.

roin hernias: Initially, the transducer is oriented transversely d over the lateral rectus muscle half way between the mbilicus and pubis. The inferior epigastric artery and vein are entified posterior to the rectus muscle and followed eriorly as they course laterally. Spigelian hernias are located ong the lateral edge of the rectus muscle, typically where e inferior epigastric artery is lateral to the muscle. Where e inferior epigastric artery arises from the external iliac tery localizes the deep inguinal ring. The transducer is then tated to be parallel and perpendicular to the inguinal canal. direct inguinal hernias arise between the external iliac artery d the proximal inferior epigastric artery. Moving the ansducer inferomedially identifies the superficial inguinal ng. Direct inguinal hernias protrude through here, inferior d medial to the inferior epigastric artery. Next the ansducer is placed below and parallel to the the inguinal nal and evaluation is made for femoral hernias. The phenofemoral junction identifies the femoral canal. Most moral hernias are medial to the common femoral vein. At all ese locations, systematic evaluation is made at rest and uring Valsalva. Hernia size and contents such as fat, fluid or eristalsing bowel are assessed. Tenderness and reducibility e evaluated. Evaluation of the asymptomatic contralateral otential hernia sites are recommended.

cisional or ventral hernias: A similar protocol with dynamic aneuvers is used at the site of symptoms. Incisional hernias cur at surgical sites and penetrate through muscle. They ay be quite large and may require a curvilinear transducer or T when complex or complicated by strangulation. In the idline a true hernia should be distinguished from rectus astasis which stretches the linea alba along its entire length. oigastric or ventral hernias are more focal.

asses: Targeted ultrasound for masses includes high solution gray scale imaging supplemented by color and ower Doppler. Panoramic techniques can be very helpful to ow the relationship of the mass to surrounding structures.

uid collections/hematomas: In addition to above, look for wirling or mobile internal echoes with compression of the ollection, which is a sign of an abscess or acute bleeding. ematomas in the rectus sheath may be associated with tive bleeding, which may be detected with color Doppler if ofuse.

eritoneal Cavity
2-5 MHz curvilinear transducer is typically required to assess e deeper recesses of the peritoneal cavity unless the patient

is small. The anterior peritoneum or superficial intraperitoneal lesions can be evaluated with a linear higher frequency 8-15 MHz transducer.

Ascites: The most common indication for ultrasound of the peritoneal cavity is a search for ascites. Right and left upper and lower quadrants and the midline pelvis are assessed for free fluid. Fluid initially collects in the hepatorenal recess and rectovesical pouch spilling over into the rest of the peritoneal cavity as the volume increases. Causes of ascites such a hepatic cirrhosis or hepatic congestion may be detected during the search for fluid. In the setting of abdominal trauma, ultrasound is used to screen for intraperitoneal bleeding.

Ascites is complex when it contains internal echoes and septations. This may be secondary to infection (bacterial or fungal peritonitis), hemorrhage or malignancy. Ultrasound guidance is useful to target the paracentesis for most diagnostic value.

Tumor: Malignant ascites is complex and associated with omental or peritoneal masses and nodules. A careful search for these ancillary signs and a primary tumor such as ovarian carcinoma is recommended. A more specific tissue diagnosis may be derived from biopsy of the solid masses.

Selected References

1. Arend CF: Static and dynamic sonography for diagnosis of abdominal wall hernias. J Ultrasound Med. 32(7):1251-9, 2013
2. Robinson A et al: Meta-analysis of sonography in the diagnosis of inguinal hernias. J Ultrasound Med. 32(2):339-46, 2013
3. Wagner JM et al: Accuracy of sonographic diagnosis of superficial masses. J Ultrasound Med. 32(8):1443-50, 2013

(Left) *Transverse ultrasound shows the right inguinal area over an intermittent lump. During the Valsalva maneuver, fat and peristalsing bowel* ➡ *were seen to bulge inferomedially from the origin of the inferior epigastric artery* ➡ *on the external iliac artery* ➡*, compatible with an indirect inguinal hernia.* **(Right)** *Transverse panoramic ultrasound shows the abdominal wall of a lump developing after umbilical hernia repair. The lump corresponds to a small fluid collection* ➡*. The abdominal fascia* ➡ *was intact.*

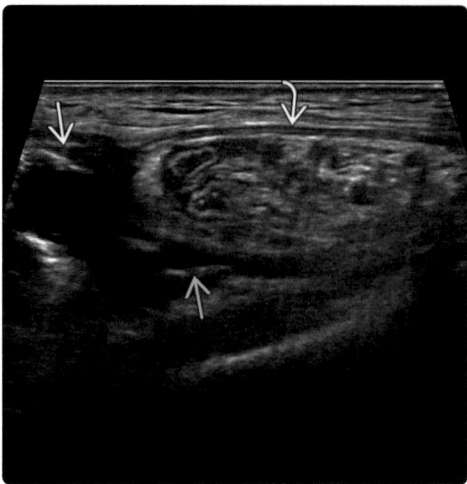
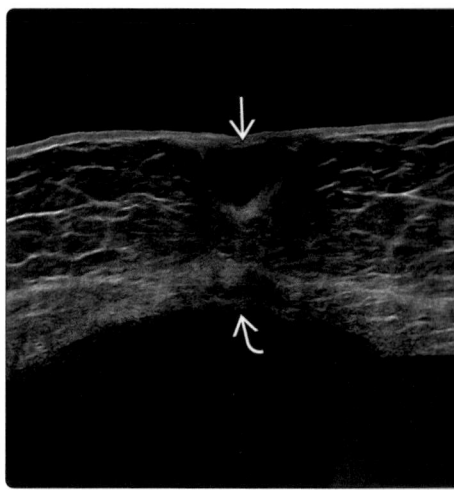

(Left) *Transverse ultrasound of the right upper quadrant performed for painful mass shows an ovoid collection with internal echoes* ➡*. No flow was seen on color Doppler. The liver* ➡ *and gallbladder* ➡ *were normal.* **(Right)** *NECT in the same patient on anticoagulants confirms a hematoma* ➡ *in the right rectus sheath. There is surrounding fat stranding* ➡*.*

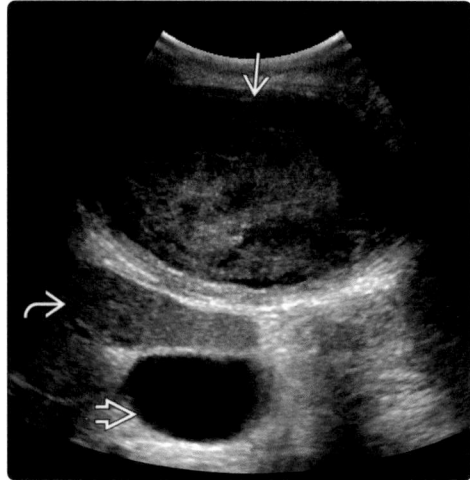
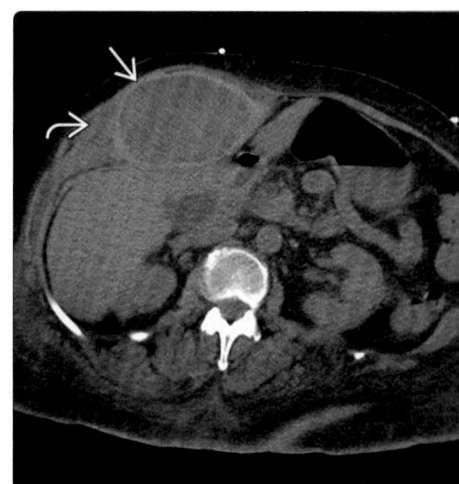

(Left) *Transverse high-resolution color Doppler ultrasound of an umbilical mass shows a lobulated soft tissue mass* ➡*, which was firm and had internal vascularity. Biopsy showed an epithelioid sarcoma.* **(Right)** *NECT in the same patient shows the umbilical metastasis* ➡*; however, CT also showed diffuse omental tumor* ➡ *but no ascites, which would have enhanced detection of the omental mass.*

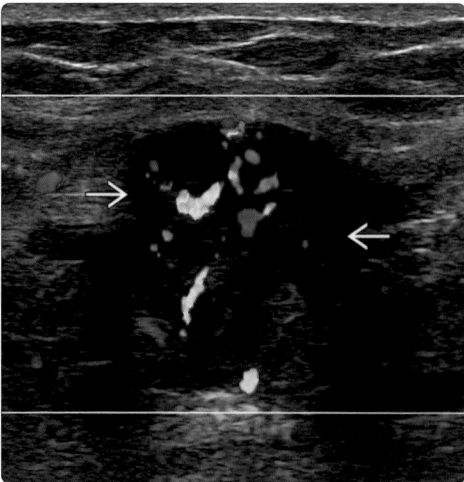
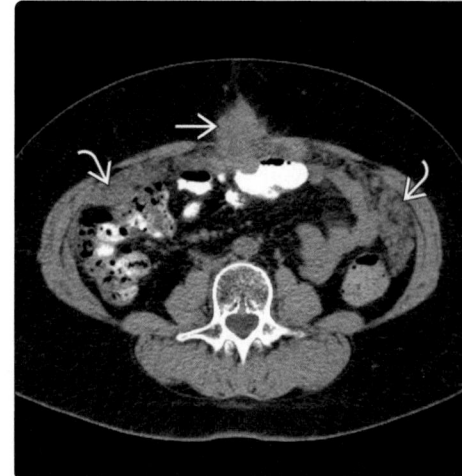

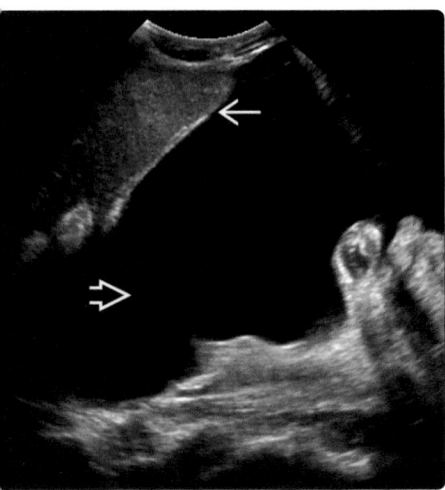

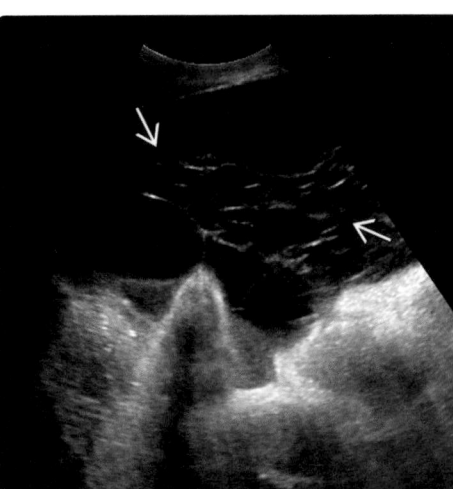

(Left) *Longitudinal ultrasound of the right upper quadrant shows a large amount of simple ascites in Morison pouch ➡. The liver transplant surface ➡ was smooth.*
(Right) *Transverse ultrasound of the right lower quadrant shows septated ➡ ascites secondary to prior hemorrhage from a ruptured spleen. Septa may preclude therapeutic drainage.*

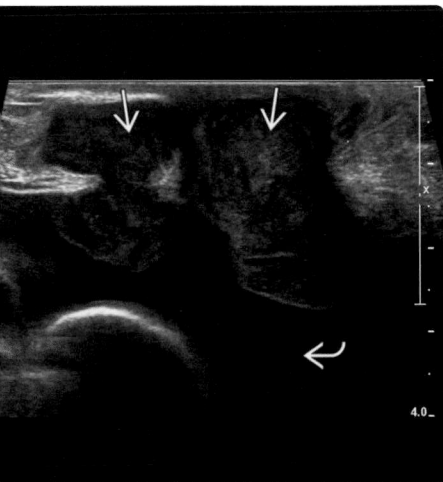

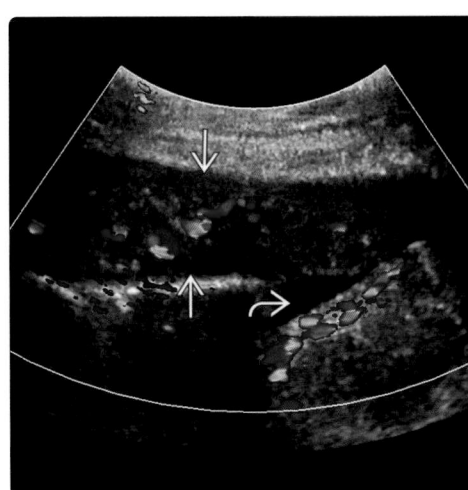

(Left) *Longitudinal high-resolution ultrasound of the anterior abdominal wall shows 2 peritoneal metastases ➡ growing through the abdominal wall. There was also ascites ➡ from metastatic pancreatic carcinoma.* (Right) *Transverse color Doppler ultrasound of the right upper quadrant shows a plaque of soft tissue ➡ against the peritoneum. Color flow was present in this omental cake from mucinous carcinoma. Ascites ➡ increases sensitivity for detection of peritoneal metastases.*

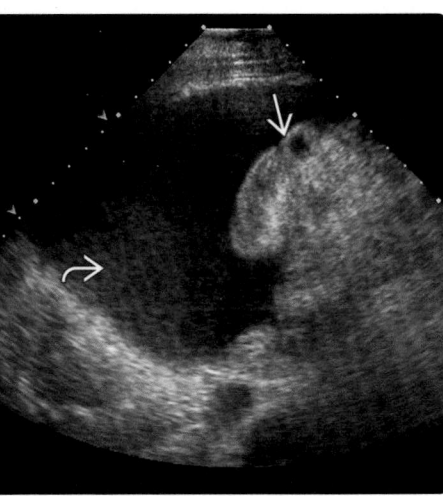

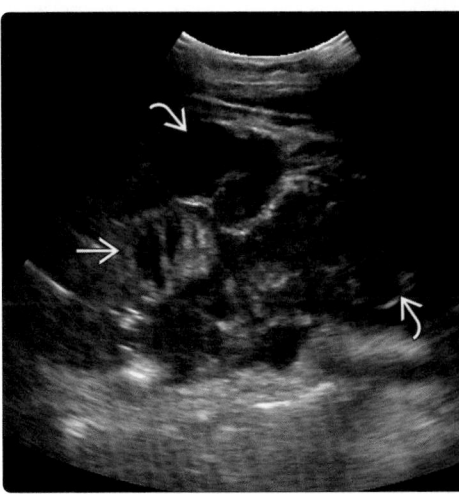

(Left) *Transverse ultrasound of the right lateral mid abdomen shows echogenic ascites ➡ from acute hemorrhage. There were multiple hepatocellular carcinomas in this cirrhotic patient. Normal bowel ➡ is noted.* (Right) *Transverse ultrasound of the left lower quadrant shows complex ascites ➡ from carcinomatosis. There are thick, irregular septa with adherent bowel ➡.*

KEY FACTS

TERMINOLOGY

- Hernia: Weakness or defect in fibromuscular wall with protrusion of an organ or part of an organ through the defect

IMAGING

- Midline hernias
  - Epigastric: Between xiphisternum and umbilicus
  - Umbilical: Umbilical or immediate paraumbilical region
  - Hypogastric: Between umbilicus and pubic symphysis
- Lateral hernias
  - Spigelian
  - Lumbar: Occur in 2 potentially weak areas of flank
- Incisional hernia: Located at surgical incisional site
- Complications: Incarceration, strangulation, bowel obstruction
- Ultrasound first-line imaging for smaller hernias or children
  - Uniquely dynamic, real-time examination; repeatable, widely available, inexpensive

- Use of maneuvers such as Valsalva or standing position to improve detection of hernias
- CT for larger deep-seated hernias and complications and obese patients
- MR similar to CT but can use dynamic sequences during Valsalva

TOP DIFFERENTIAL DIAGNOSES

- Abdominal wall tumor
- Abdominal wall abscess or seroma
- Abdominal wall or rectus sheath hematoma
- Divarication (diastasis) of rectus abdominis muscles

DIAGNOSTIC CHECKLIST

- Determine nature of herniated content (omentum, bowel site/size of abdominal wall defect

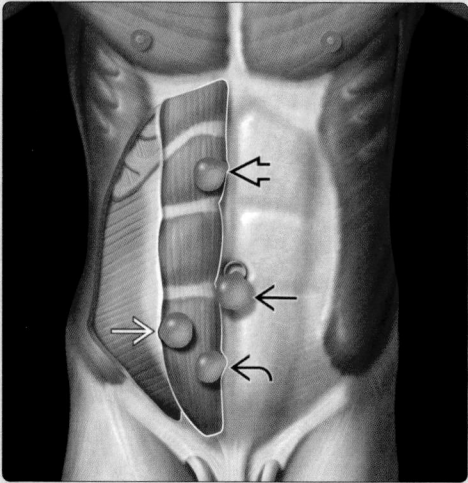
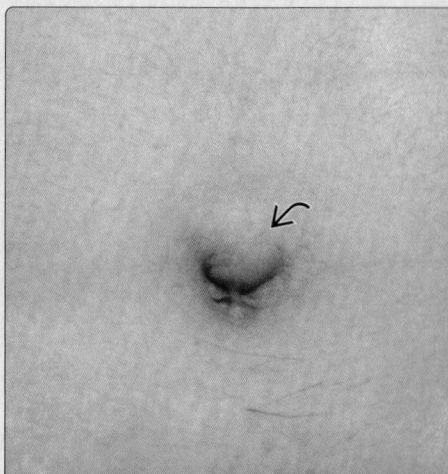

(Left) Graphic shows a paraumbilical hernia ⊇ arising from the umbilicus area. The locations of epigastric ⊇, spigelian ➡, and hypogastric ⊇ hernias are also shown for reference. (Right) Clinical photograph shows a typical appearance of a small paraumbilical hernia in an adult with swelling ⊇ at the superior aspect of the umbilicus.

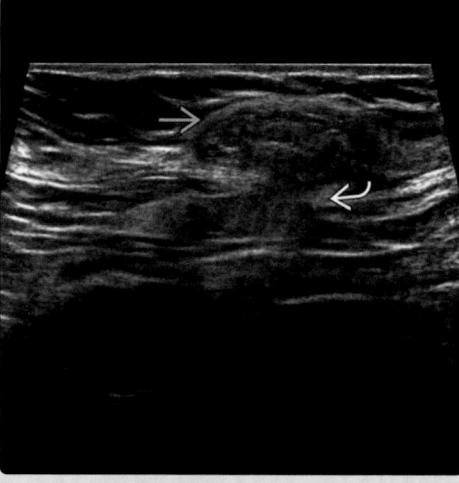
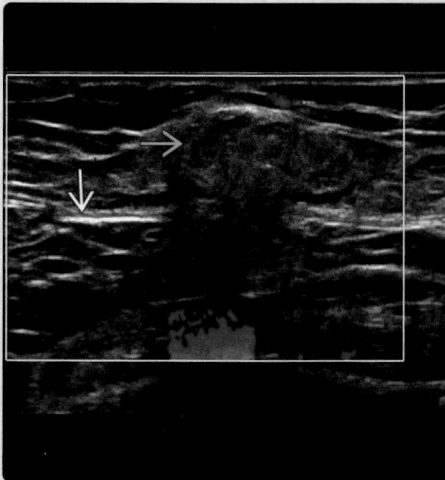

(Left) Longitudinal ultrasound of a recurrent periumbilical hernia in a young woman following 2 pregnancies. Omental fat ⊇ protrudes through a narrow defect ➡ in the linea alba accentuated by the Valsalva maneuver. (Right) Longitudinal color Doppler ultrasound of the same recurrent periumbilical hernia. The linea alba is better seen as a thin echogenic line ➡ with a small defect. No color flow is seen in the herniated omentum ⊇, not necessarily indicative of strangulation as fat is usually hypovascular.

TERMINOLOGY

Definitions

Hernia: Weakness or defect in fibromuscular wall with protrusion of an organ/part of an organ through defect
- Reducible: Recedes spontaneously or with external pressure (manual or transducer)
- Incarcerated: Nonreducible
- Strangulated: Compromised vascular supply of hernia contents

Classification: Midline versus lateral hernias

IMAGING

General Features

Best diagnostic clue
- Abdominal wall lump due to tissue protruding though a defect in abdominal wall

Location
- Midline hernias
  - Epigastric: Between xiphisternum and umbilicus
  - Umbilical: Umbilical or immediate paraumbilical region
  - Hypogastric: Between umbilicus and pubic symphysis
- Lateral hernias
  - Spigelian
    - Defect in transversus abdominis aponeurosis just lateral to rectus sheath (linea semilunaris)
    - Most commonly located near arcuate line
  - Lumbar: Occur in 2 potentially weak areas of flank
    - Superior lumbar triangle (Grynfeltt hernia) bounded by erector spinae medially, 12th rib superiorly, and internal oblique muscle laterally
    - Inferior lumbar triangle (Petit hernia) bounded by latissimus dorsi muscle medially, iliac crest inferiorly, and external oblique muscle laterally
- Incisional hernia: Located at surgical incisional site

Morphology
- Epigastric hernia
  - Usually small and contains extraperitoneal fat that protrudes through linea alba (fatty hernia of linea alba)
  - May occasionally be large and contain bowel
- Umbilical hernia
  - Umbilical in children
    - Peritoneal content protrudes through patent umbilical ring
  - Paraumbilical or periumbilical in adults
    - Extraperitoneal fat ± peritoneal contents protrude through 1 side of umbilical ring
- Hypogastric hernia
  - Very uncommon
- Spigelian hernia
  - Usually extends into subcutaneous layer, though may pass between transversus abdominis and internal oblique muscles, or may extend into rectus sheath
    - Can present as flank lump if extends laterally
  - Sometimes secondary to trauma
  - More prone to strangulation
- Lumbar hernia
  - Usually painless due to wide hernial neck
  - Secondary to trauma or surgery

- Incisional hernia
  - Occurs in 10-30% of postoperative patients
  - May occur years after surgery, though usually within 1st year
  - May go unnoticed by patient and be incidentally detected on imaging
    - Can be very large

Ultrasonographic Findings

- Grayscale ultrasound
  - High resolution linear transducer; reserve curvilinear lower frequency for large hernias/overview
    - Extended field of view (panoramic) for larger hernias, diastasis recti
  - Identify relevant muscles and fascial planes
  - Show content of hernia (omentum, bowel, properitoneal fat, fluid), site/size of abdominal wall defect and complications
    - Omental fat: Echogenic/hypoechoic tissue without peristalsis
    - Bowel: "Target" echo pattern with central echoes due to air in lumen and visible peristalsis
      - May see valvulae conniventes (small bowel) or feculent content (large bowel)
      - Variable appearances due to air-fluid content
  - Use of maneuvers such as Valsalva or standing position to improve detection of hernias
    - Document with cine clips
  - Check for reducibility by applying pressure
  - Complications: Irreducible hernia may become obstructed or strangulated
    - Uncommon in noninguinal abdominal wall hernias
    - Obstructed hernia: Absence of bowel peristalsis, narrow neck, dilated bowel, fluid
    - Strangulated hernia: Absence of color Doppler flow within bowel wall or mesentery, swollen bowel wall, aperistalsis, fluid, echogenic fat
      - Note that absence of color flow is a late sign and nonstrangulated fat containing hernias do not show flow
    - Other signs are also unreliable, making it difficult to assess strangulation on ultrasound

CT Findings

- Accurate at assessing presence of hernia and identifying sac contents as well as site and size of abdominal wall defect
  - Useful for assessing larger deep-seated hernias and complications
- Hernias may be less evident in supine position but CT can be performed during Valsalva

MR Findings

- Similar to CT but can use dynamic sequences during Valsalva

Imaging Recommendations

- Best imaging tool
  - Ultrasound first-line imaging for smaller hernias or children
    - Uniquely dynamic, real-time examination; repeatable, widely available, inexpensive

- o CT most useful for large or complex hernias or in larger patients: Better for bowel complications
- o MR similar anatomic information to CT but dynamic
- Protocol advice
  - o Identify anatomical layers, localize focal abdominal wall defect, compare with opposite side (if possible), and identify hernial contents
    - Use light transducer pressure to minimize reduction of hernia
    - Routine use of Valsalva maneuver to accentuate hernia and examine contents
    - Examine in standing position if this clinically accentuates hernia or if no hernia detected while supine
    - Measure size of hernial sac and fascial defect
    - If bowel content, check for complications (irreducibility/obstruction/strangulation)

DIFFERENTIAL DIAGNOSIS

Abdominal Wall Tumor

- Primary (lipoma, desmoid tumor, endometriosis) or secondary tumor (scar metastasis, melanoma metastases, Sister Mary Joseph nodule)
- Differentiate by location, lack of fascial defect or change with Valsalva
- Thin capsule encircling lipoma distinguishes it from fat herniating through an abdominal wall defect (also has a neck)

Abdominal Wall Abscess or Seroma

- No fascial defect present

Abdominal Wall or Rectus Sheath Hematoma

- Post-traumatic or spontaneous: Bleeding of epigastric vessels or muscle tear
- No fascial defect present, no change with Valsalva

Divarication (Diastasis) of Rectus Abdominis Muscles

- Bulging of abdominal cavity due to stretching and thinning of linea alba
  - o Particularly in elderly multiparous women

Dilated Abdominal Wall Vessels

- Compressible, tubular, vascular flow

Suture Granuloma

- Incisional, lack of fascial defect or change with Valsalva
- Echogenic internal suture may be detected

PATHOLOGY

General Features

- Etiology
  - o Primary: Congenital defect; epigastric and umbilical
  - o Secondary
    - Weak abdominal wall musculature
      - □ Chronic increased intraabdominal pressure, abdominal distension (cirrhosis, ascites), muscle laxity (obesity, old age, pregnancy)
      - □ Physical exertion, chronic cough, prostatism, or constipation
    - Trauma: Blunt force or hyperextension strain

- □ Sudden ↑ in intraabdominal pressure
- □ Insufficient to penetrate skin but strong enough t disrupt muscle and fascia
- Postoperative abdominal wall weakness, surgical sca suture dehiscence, wound infection

CLINICAL ISSUES

Presentation

- Most common signs/symptoms
  - o Abdominal bulge increasing in size with ↑ in intraabdominal pressure
  - o Reducible swelling, positive cough impulse
  - o Discomfort, pain, intermittent intestinal obstruction

Demographics

- Age
  - o Umbilical hernia: Young children
  - o Paraumbilical hernia: Adults
  - o Epigastric hernia: 20-50 years
  - o Incisional hernia: More frequent in elderly
- Gender
  - o Epigastric hernia is 2x more common in males
- Epidemiology
  - o Most common abdominal wall lesion seen in ultrasound practice

Natural History & Prognosis

- ~ 1/3 of umbilical hernias close within 1 month of birth an rarely persist beyond 3-4 years
- All other hernias persist and frequently enlarge with time
- 20% need emergency repair for incarceration and strangulation
  - o Less common with very small (< 1 cm) or very large hernia necks

Treatment

- Repair of muscle/fascial defect: Open or laparoscopic technique, meshplasty
- Intestinal obstruction/strangulated hernia; urgent exploratory laparotomy

DIAGNOSTIC CHECKLIST

Consider

- Abdominal wall hernia if posterior margin of any abdomin wall mass cannot be seen on ultrasound

Image Interpretation Pearls

- Check for abdominal wall defect, hernial sac contents, peristaltic movement, and vascularity (if bowel)

SELECTED REFERENCES

1. Murphy KP et al: Adult abdominal hernias. AJR Am J Roentgenol. 202(6):W506-11, 2014
2. Yeh DD et al: Hernia emergencies. Surg Clin North Am. 94(1):97-130, 2014
3. Arend CF: Static and dynamic sonography for diagnosis of abdominal wall hernias. J Ultrasound Med. 32(7):1251-9, 2013
4. Lee RK et al: Ultrasound of the abdominal wall and groin. Can Assoc Radiol 64(4):295-305, 2013
5. Stavros AT et al: Dynamic ultrasound of hernias of the groin and anterior abdominal wall. Ultrasound Q. 26(3):135-69, 2010
6. Muysoms FE et al: Classification of primary and incisional abdominal wall hernias. Hernia. 13(4):407-14, 2009

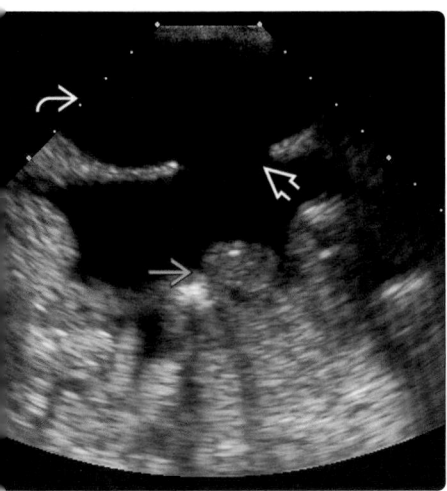

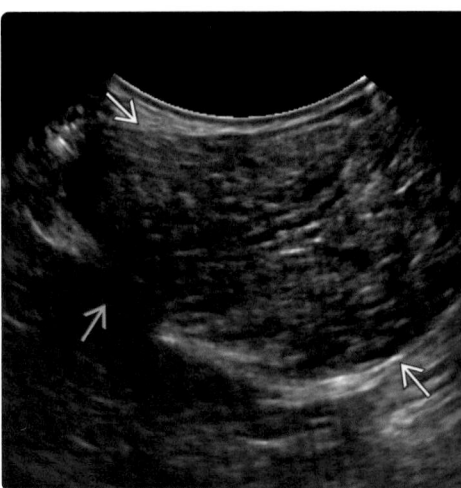

(Left) *Transverse ultrasound of a patient with cirrhosis and ascites. There is a large umbilical hernia containing ascites ⊇ protruding through a defect in the linea alba at the umbilicus ⊇. There is no bowel in the hernia. The intraabdominal bowel ⊇ is not dilated.* (Right) *Longitudinal ultrasound of a large midline hernia containing fat ⊇. Due to its size, the hernia was imaged with a curvilinear transducer. The defect in the abdominal wall is still visualized ⊇.*

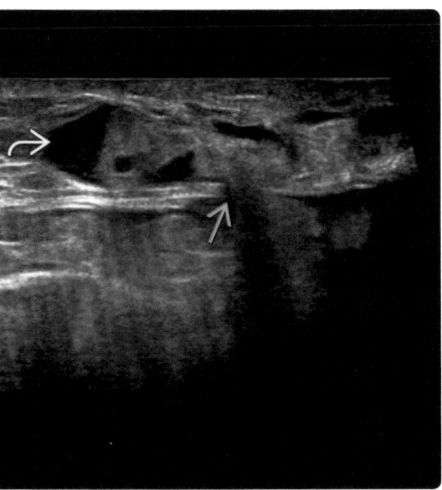

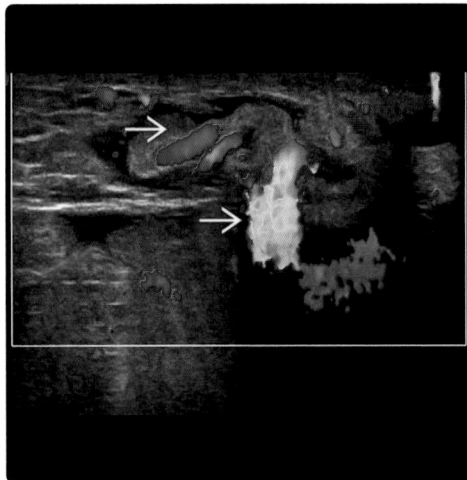

(Left) *Longitudinal ultrasound of a painful umbilical hernia ⊇ containing fluid and soft tissue in a patient with cirrhosis and portal hypertension. The defect in the linea alba is small ⊇. No peristalsis was seen.* (Right) *Longitudinal color Doppler ultrasound of the same patient with portal hypertension. Umbilical hernias are a site of weakness through which collateral veins ⊇ may herniate. Although tender, the veins were not thrombosed.*

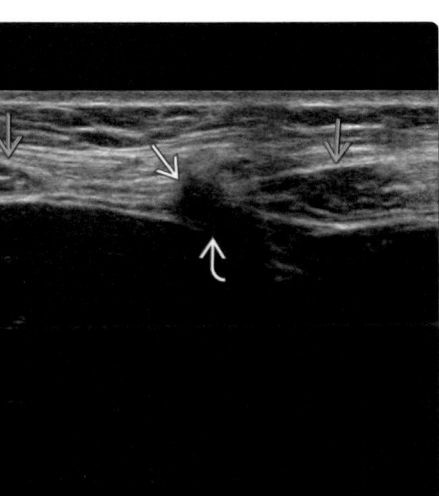

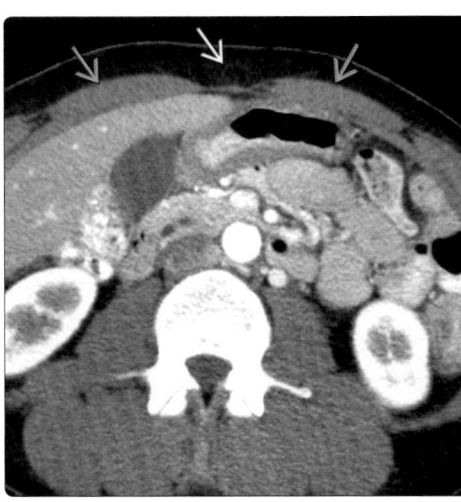

(Left) *Transverse focused ultrasound shows a small epigastric hernia ⊇ extending though a defect ⊇ in the linea alba. Rectus muscles ⊇ are shown.* (Right) *Axial CECT of the same patient confirms the small fat-containing epigastric hernia ⊇ within the midline. The defect in the linea alba is not seen. Rectus muscles ⊇ are intact.*

(Left) *Transverse ultrasound of the umbilical region shows a fat-containing symptomatic periumbilical hernia. Note the narrow neck ⊸.* **(Right)** *Transverse panoramic ultrasound shows a midline incisional hernia ➡ containing bowel. The hernia developed after laparotomy complicated by wound infection. The rectus muscles ➡ are widely separated.*

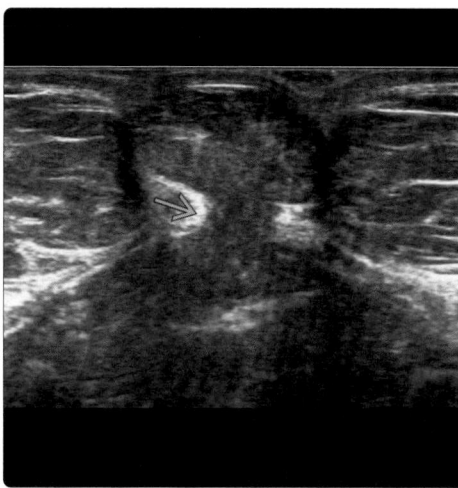
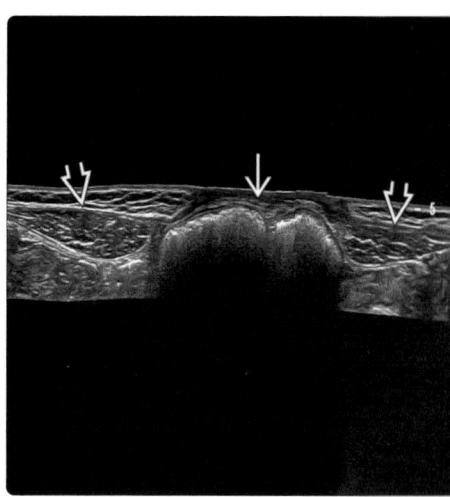

(Left) *Transverse ultrasound shows a wide neck to a midline hernia containing bowel ➡. This was an incisional hernia. The right rectus muscle is shown ⊸.* **(Right)** *Axial CECT of the same patient shows the broad incisional hernia ➡ containing undilated small bowel. The rectus muscles are atrophied ⊸.*

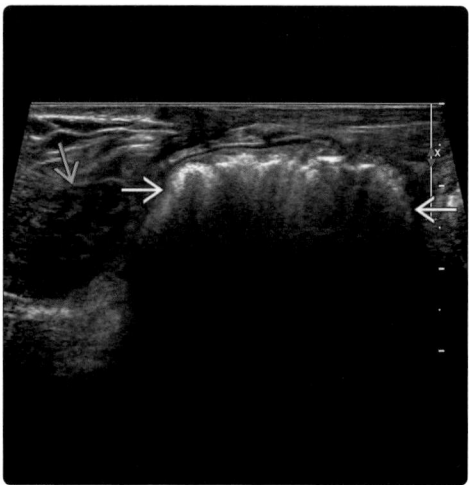
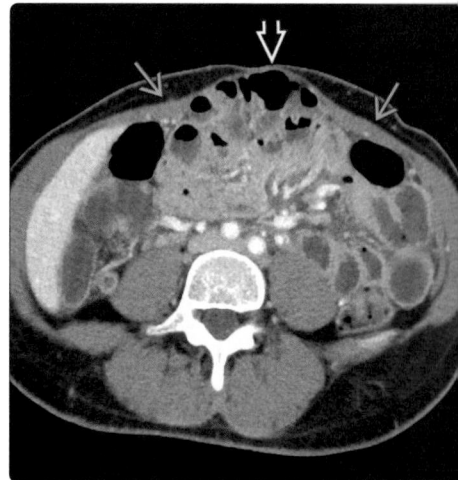

(Left) *Axial CECT showing an incarcerated periumbilical hernia ⊸ with dilated small bowel ➡ proximal to the hernia and in the hernia ➡. The herniated bowel wall shows enhancement and there was no strangulation at surgery.* **(Right)** *Coronal CECT following aortic aneurysm surgery shows a very large incisional hernia ➡ containing undilated small bowel. Sigmoid thickening ⊸ from C. Difficile colitis is noted.*

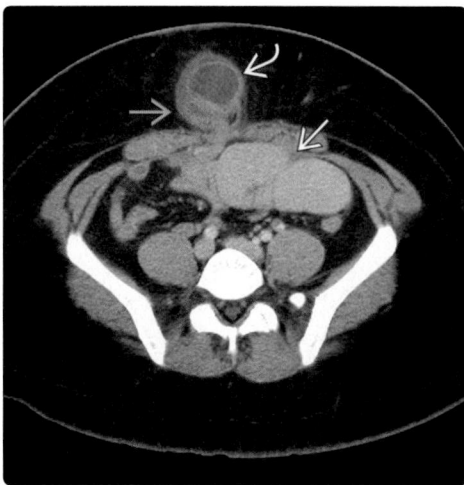
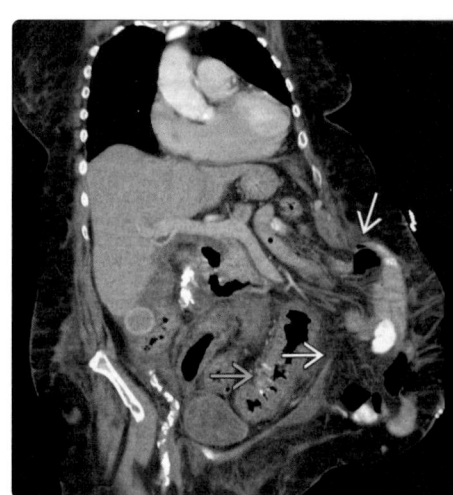

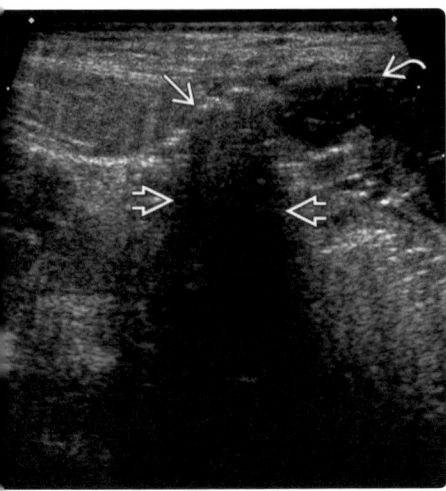
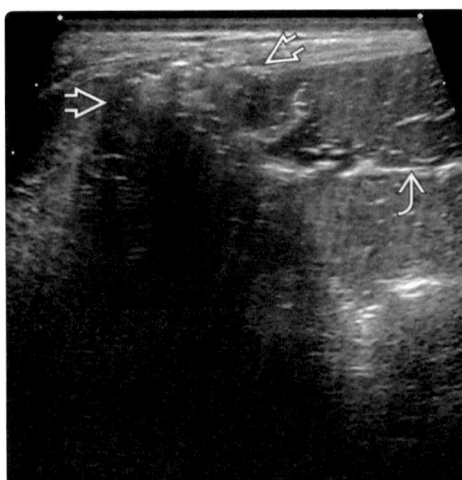

(Left) *Transverse ultrasound at rest shows a medium-sized traumatic right spigelian hernia* ⟶ *bulging through the linea semilunaris/transversus abdominis aponeurosis* ⟶. *The rectus abdominis muscle* ⟶ *is shown.* **(Right)** *Transverse ultrasound during Valsalva shows the same post-traumatic right spigelian hernia* ⟶, *which has enlarged. The intact rectus abdominis muscle* ⟶ *is shown. The change with Valsalva is more evident on real-time imaging.*

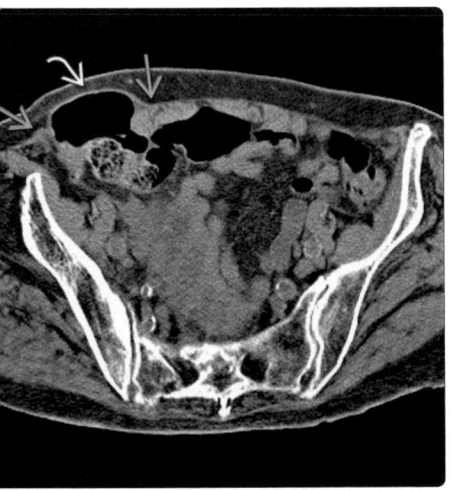
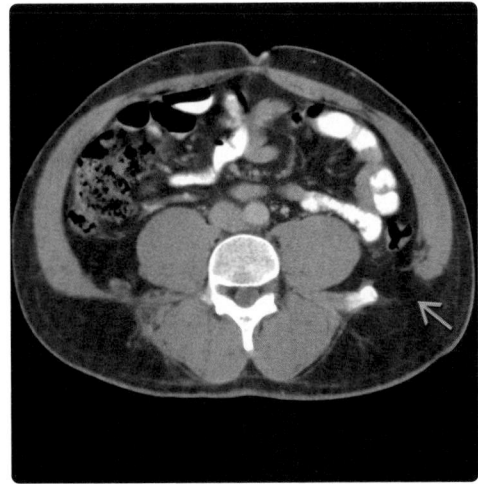

(Left) *Axial CT obtained after a traumatic right hip fracture shows a spigelian hernia* ⟶ *containing colon. The hernia defect lies between the rectus and oblique muscles* ⟶. **(Right)** *Axial NECT shows a fat-containing superior lumbar hernia* ⟶ *(Grynfeltt hernia).*

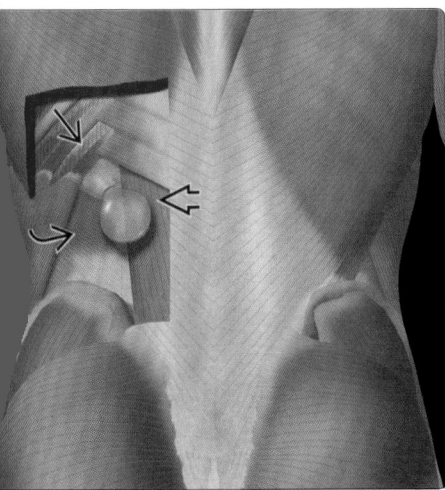
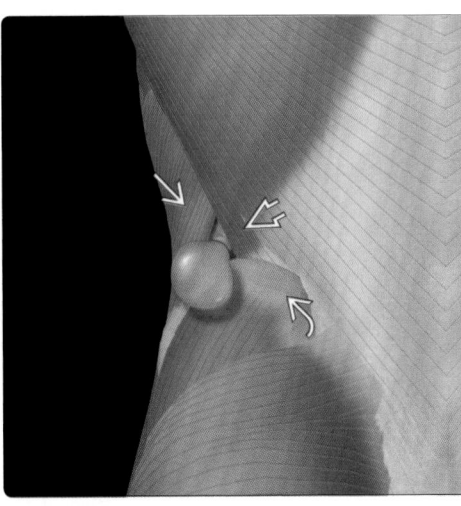

(Left) *Graphic shows a superior lumbar hernia (Grynfeltt hernia) arising from the superior lumbar triangle bounded by the erector spinae muscle medially* ⟶, *the 12th rib superiorly* ⟶, *and the internal oblique muscle laterally* ⟶. **(Right)** *Graphic shows an inferior lumbar hernia (Petit hernia) arising from the inferior lumbar triangle bounded by the latissimus dorsi muscle medially* ⟶, *the iliac crest inferiorly* ⟶, *and the external oblique muscle laterally* ⟶.

KEY FACTS

TERMINOLOGY

- Hernia: Weakness or defect in fibromuscular wall with protrusion of organ or part of organ through defect
- Reducible hernia: Decrease in hernia size with decreased intraabdominal pressure or application of external pressure
- Incarcerated: Nonreducible
- Strangulated: Compromised vascular supply of hernia contents

IMAGING

- Indirect inguinal hernia passes through deep inguinal ring, extends along inguinal canal, and emerges at superficial inguinal ring
- Direct inguinal hernia passes through transversalis fascial defect in Hesselbach triangle
- Femoral hernia passes through femoral canal into superomedial thigh
- Ultrasound accurate at detecting hernia sac and contents as well as fascial defect at rest or with provocative maneuvers

- ○ Increase in hernia size during cough, Valsalva maneuver or standing
- Color Doppler helps identify inferior epigastric artery and its relationship to hernia neck for inguinal hernias
- CT or MR: Useful if ultrasound is equivocal, better for detecting alternative causes of symptoms

TOP DIFFERENTIAL DIAGNOSES

- Lipoma of spermatic cord
- Encysted hydrocele canal of Nück
- Inguinal canal lesions

CLINICAL ISSUES

- Obstruction or strangulation more common with femoral hernias due to narrow neck

(Left) Graphic shows 3 types of groin hernia: Direct ➡ and indirect ➡ inguinal hernias arise above the inguinal ligament ➡, medial and lateral to the inferior epigastric vessels ➡ respectively; femoral hernias ➡ arise below the inguinal ligament medial to femoral vessels ➡. (Right) Transverse ultrasound of the right groin shows a direct inguinal hernia containing small bowel ➡. The hernia neck was medial to the inferior epigastric vessels ➡. The small bowel was only seen during Valsalva or while standing.

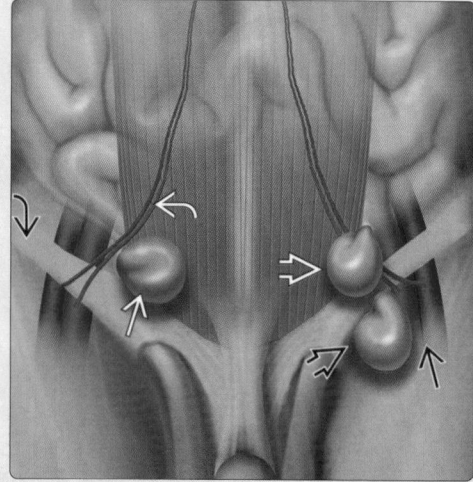
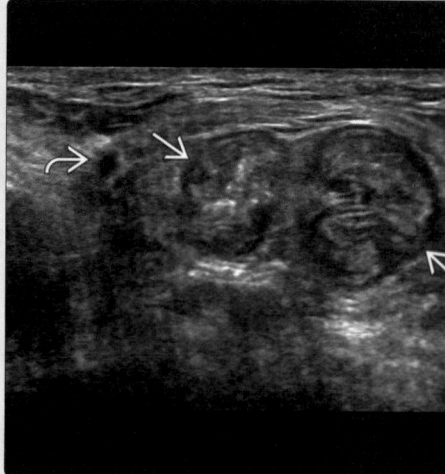

(Left) Transverse ultrasound shows a left direct-type inguinal hernia ➡ containing bowel. The neck ➡ of the hernia lies medial to the inferior epigastric vessels ➡. (Right) Transverse color Doppler ultrasound of the same left direct inguinal hernia ➡ during Valsalva maneuver is shown. The hernia sac is larger. The hernia neck ➡ is medial to the inferior epigastric vessels ➡. Direct inguinal hernias rarely obstruct.

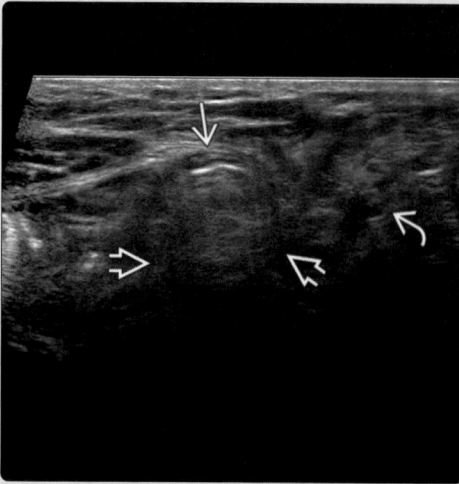
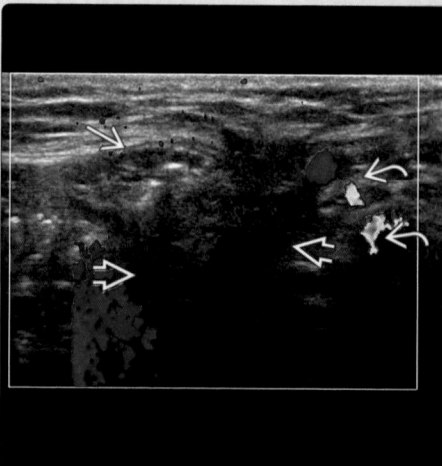

TERMINOLOGY

Definitions

Hernia: Weakness or defect in fibromuscular wall with protrusion of organ or part of organ through defect
o Groin hernias include indirect and direct inguinal hernias and femoral hernia

Reducible: Hernia recedes spontaneously or with external pressure (manual or transducer)

Incarcerated: Nonreducible

Strangulated: Compromised vascular supply of hernia contents

IMAGING

General Features

Location
o **Inguinal canal**
  – ~ 4 cm long, ~ 1.2 cm above inguinal ligament, runs from anterior superior iliac spine to pubic tubercle
    □ Contains spermatic cord and ilioinguinal nerve in males, round ligament of uterus and ilioinguinal nerve in females
o **Femoral canal**
  – ~ 2 cm long, just medial to femoral vein, deep and distal to inguinal ligament
o **Indirect inguinal hernia**
  – Passes through deep inguinal ring, extends along inguinal canal, and emerges at superficial inguinal ring
  – Neck is lateral to inferior epigastric artery and above inguinal ligament
  – In males, usually extends along spermatic cord to scrotum
  – In females, may extend along round ligament to labia majora
o **Direct inguinal hernia**
  – Passes through transversalis fascial defect in Hesselbach triangle
  – Protrudes anteriorly through abdominal wall
  – Wide neck medial to inferior epigastric artery and above inguinal ligament
  – Does not pass into spermatic cord and generally does not extend to scrotum
o **Femoral hernia**
  – Passes through femoral canal into superomedial thigh
  – Narrow neck medial to femoral vein and below inguinal ligament
o **Double hernia**
  – Simultaneous occurrence of direct and indirect inguinal hernia in same groin saddlebag hernia

Ultrasonographic Findings

Grayscale ultrasound
o Accurate at detecting hernia sac and contents, as well as fascial defect at rest or with provocative maneuvers
  – Increase in hernia size during cough, Valsalva maneuver, or standing
o Contents
  – Omental fat: Echogenic without peristalsis

  – Bowel loops: Layers; "target" echo pattern with strong central echoes representing air or fluid in lumen
    □ Bowel peristalsis best assessed in real time
  – Fluid
o Reducible hernia: Decrease in hernia size with decrease in intraabdominal pressure or application of external pressure to hernial sac with transducer
o Nonobstructed hernia: Active peristalsis ± movement of intestinal contents
o Strangulated hernia: Thickened sac, fluid, thickened bowel, echogenic fat
o Obstructed hernia: Absence of peristalsis or hyperperistaltic loops in hernia, dilated/thick bowel loops in hernia sac or abdomen
• Color Doppler
o Helps identify inferior epigastric artery and its relationship to hernia sac
  – Differentiates direct and indirect inguinal hernias
o Strangulated hernia: Absence of vascularity within bowel wall and mesentery is late sign

CT and MR

• Equivalent performance for most hernias but CT uses ionizing radiation
• Obtained after nondiagnostic ultrasound; better for detecting alternative causes of symptoms or complicated hernias
• Dynamic ultrasound more sensitive for smaller reducible hernias

Radiographic Findings

• Radiography
o Gas-filled intestinal loops projecting over groin
o ± small or large bowel obstruction
• Herniography/peritoneography
o Injection of soluble low-osmolar contrast medium into peritoneal cavity
o Invasive but superior modality for occult inguinal hernias

Imaging Recommendations

• Best imaging tool
o Ultrasound should be initial tool, accurate provided that strict systematic approach is used
  – Dynamic but operator dependent
  – 97% sensitivity, 85% specificity, and 93% positive predictive value for diagnosis of groin hernia
  – Lower accuracy for determining type of hernia (indirect inguinal, direct inguinal, femoral)
  – Pure fat hernia most difficult to diagnose
o CT or MR if ultrasound is equivocal
• Protocol advice
o High-resolution linear transducer
o Start lateral to rectus muscle and identify inferior epigastric artery (IEA)
  – Follow IEA down to origin on external iliac artery; this is deep inguinal ring
o Orient transducer parallel to inguinal ligament
o Scan caudad over femoral vessels, look for femoral hernia medially at saphenofemoral junction
o Scan cephalad, find origin of inferior epigastric artery off medial femoral artery, look for indirect inguinal hernia

- o Scan medially for superficial ring and look for direct inguinal hernia
- o At each area, examine at rest and during Valsalva maneuver for presence of hernia or laxity
- o Examine other side if hernia found, examine sites of tenderness
- o Cine clips strongly advised
- o Repeat with patient standing, more sensitive for fluid in hernia

DIFFERENTIAL DIAGNOSIS

Lipoma of Spermatic Cord

- No change with Valsalva maneuver, not reducible
- Usually no deep extension into peritoneal cavity

Encysted Hydrocele Canal of Nück

- Processus vaginalis extends from peritoneal cavity to scrotum in embryo
  - o Normally obliterates in cord while scrotal component persists as tunica vaginalis
  - o Failure of obliteration leads to fluid distension within cord, known as encysted hydrocele canal of Nück
    - – Filled with anechoic fluid, no change with Valsalva maneuver, not reducible
    - – No deep extension into peritoneal cavity

Inguinal Canal Lesions

- Benign and malignant tumors: Neurofibroma, desmoid, metastases, lymphadenopathy, lymphoma, sarcomas
- Undescended testis
- Miscellaneous: Varicocele, abscess, hematoma, granuloma, scar

PATHOLOGY

General Features

- Etiology
  - o Multifactorial
    - – Chronic: Increased intraabdominal pressure from abdominal distension (ascites)
      - □ Weak abdominal musculature: Chronic cough, prostatism, constipation, manual labor, pregnancy, steroids, collagen abnormality, smoking
    - – Acute: Sudden severe increase in intraabdominal pressure
  - o Indirect inguinal hernia: Congenital due to persistence of processus vaginalis in infants and children

Gross Pathologic & Surgical Features

- Sac contents: Commonly omentum, ascites, small bowel, or mobile colon segments (sigmoid, cecum, appendix), rarely bladder, ovary
  - o Littre hernia: Meckel diverticulum in sac
  - o Richter hernia: Only portion of bowel circumference (antimesenteric portion) in sac

CLINICAL ISSUES

Presentation

- Most common signs/symptoms
  - o Groin lump or discomfort with positive cough impulse (allows clinical diagnosis)

- – Continuous or intermittent
- Other signs/symptoms
  - o Features of intestinal obstruction

Demographics

- Age
  - o Indirect inguinal hernia tend to occur in young to middle aged individuals
  - o Prevalence of direct inguinal hernia increases with increasing age
  - o Femoral hernia is more common in middle-aged to elderly individuals
- Gender
  - o Indirect inguinal hernia is 5-10x more common in males
  - o Direct inguinal hernia nearly always occurs in males
  - o Femoral hernia is more common in females
    - – However, indirect inguinal hernia is most common hernia in females
- Epidemiology
  - o Hernia repair is most common surgical procedure in US
  - o 5% of males develop groin hernia
  - o 75% of all hernias inguinal, indirect to direct 5:1
  - o 10-15% femoral
  - o Inguinal hernia in children is always result of patent processus vaginalis and is thus indirect hernia extending to scrotal sac

Natural History & Prognosis

- Recurrence rate after repair: 1-15%
  - o Direct inguinal hernia may develop after repair of indirect inguinal hernia
- Complications: Obstruction, strangulation
  - o Indirect inguinal hernias account for 15% of intestinal obstruction cases
  - o Obstruction or strangulation more common with femoral hernias due to narrow neck

Treatment

- Laparoscopic or open hernia repair

DIAGNOSTIC CHECKLIST

Consider

- Relation of hernia neck to inferior epigastric artery for inguinal hernias
- Femoral hernia: Below inguinal ligament

SELECTED REFERENCES

1. Arend CF: Static and dynamic sonography for diagnosis of abdominal wall hernias. J Ultrasound Med. 32(7):1251-9, 2013
2. Jain N et al: Ultrasound of the abdominal wall: what lies beneath? Clin Rad 68(1):85-93, 2013
3. Robinson A et al: Meta-analysis of sonography in the diagnosis of inguinal hernias. J Ultrasound Med. 32(2):339-46, 2013
4. Stavros AT et al: Dynamic ultrasound of hernias of the groin and anterior abdominal wall. Ultrasound Q. 26(3):135-69, 2010
5. Bhosale PR et al: The inguinal canal: anatomy and imaging features of common and uncommon masses. Radiographics. 28(3):819-35; quiz 913, 2008

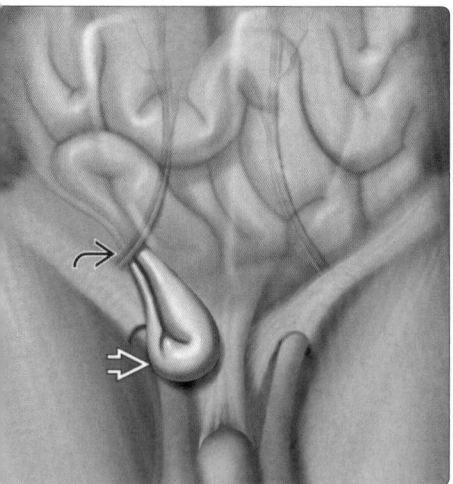

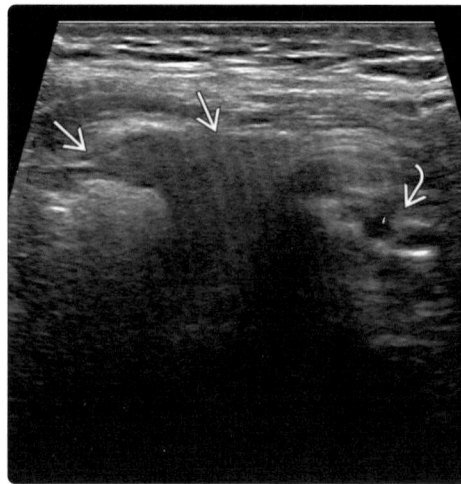

(Left) *Graphic shows a direct inguinal hernia* ➦. *Note that the neck of a direct inguinal hernia is medial to the inferior epigastric vessels* ➡. *A direct inguinal hernia passes through the transversalis fascial defect in the Hesselbach triangle.* (Right) *Transverse ultrasound of the left groin obtained during Valsalva maneuver shows there is fat containing a direct inguinal hernia* ➡ *medial to the inferior epigastric vessels* ➡.

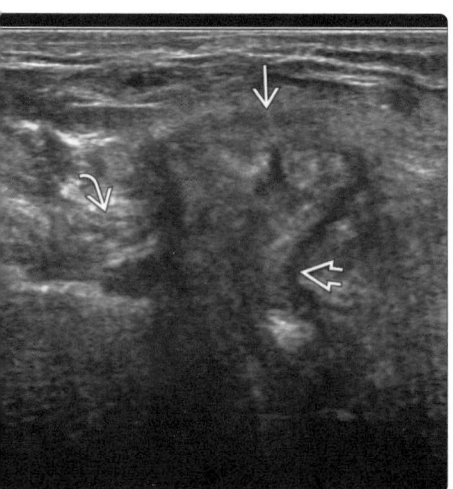

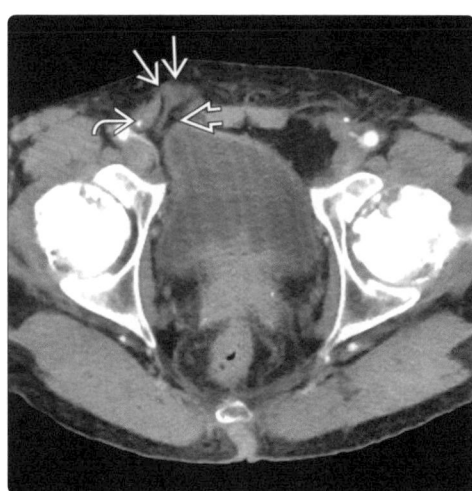

(Left) *Transverse ultrasound shows a right direct inguinal hernia* ➡ *containing bowel . The neck* ➡ *of the hernia lies medial to the epigastric vessels* ➡. (Right) *Axial CECT of the same patient obtained for another reason shows a right direct inguinal hernia* ➡ *containing fat and fluid. Bowel was not seen. The neck* ➡ *of the hernia lies medial to the epigastric artery* ➡. *Lack of dynamic maneuvers limits CT.*

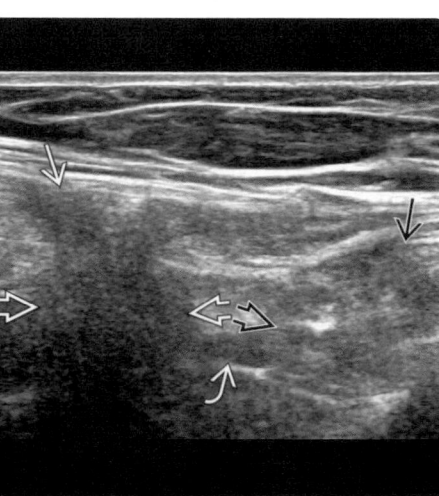

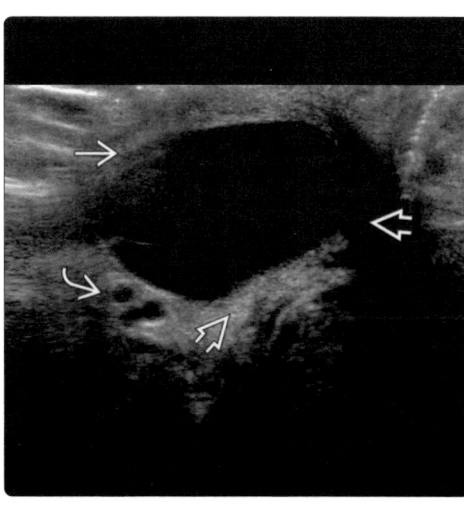

(Left) *Transverse ultrasound shows concurrent left direct* ➡ *and indirect* ➡ *inguinal hernias, both containing mesenteric fat. The necks of the indirect* ➡ *and direct* ➡ *hernias lie lateral and medial to the epigastric vessels* ➡, *respectively. This is known as a saddlebag hernia.* (Right) *Transverse ultrasound shows a left indirect-type inguinal hernia* ➡ *containing fluid and fat (not shown). The neck* ➡ *of the hernia lies lateral to the epigastric veins and artery* ➡.

(Left) *Graphic shows an indirect inguinal hernia entering the right scrotal sac. Note that the neck* ➡ *of an indirect inguinal hernia lies lateral to the inferior epigastric vessels* ⬈. **(Right)** *Longitudinal ultrasound of the right groin performed during Valsalva shows an indirect inguinal hernia containing bowel* ➡ *with fluid inferiorly* ➡. *There was normal peristalsis.*

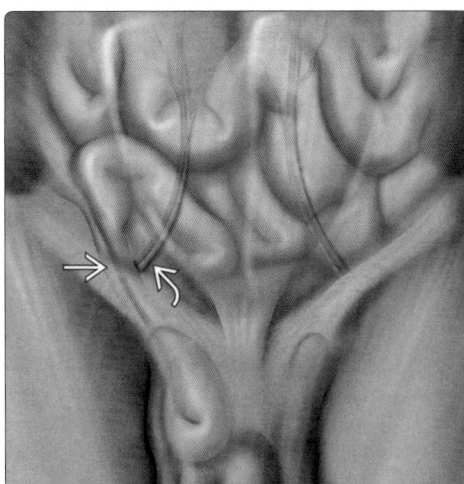
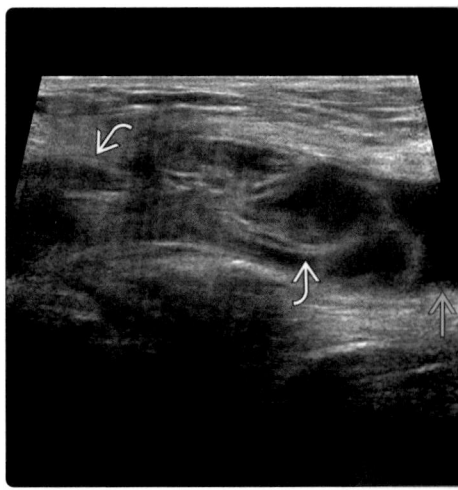

(Left) *Longitudinal ultrasound shows a large indirect-type inguinal hernia* ➡ *extending into the upper scrotal region. There is gas within bowel* ➡ *in the hernia sac. Shadowing from gas* ➡ *may obscure hernia contents.* **(Right)** *Coronal CECT in the same patient confirms the presence of cecum* ➡ *but also terminal ileum* ➡ *in the right indirect inguinoscrotal hernia* ➡.

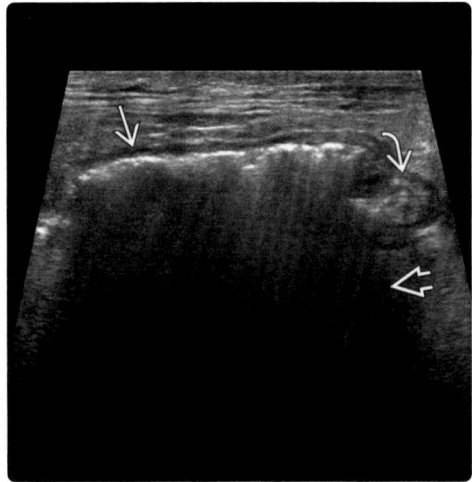
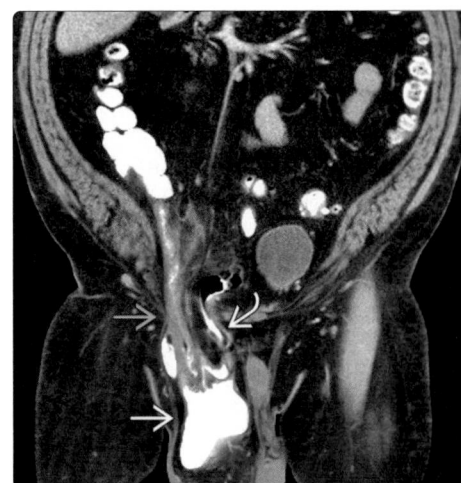

(Left) *Transverse ultrasound of the scrotum in a patient with an incarcerated right indirect inguinal hernia. There are thick dilated edematous bowel loops* ➡ *with surrounding fluid in the scrotum. Left hydrocele was also noted* ➡. *The testis was ischemic.* **(Right)** *Longitudinal panoramic ultrasound of the left groin in a boy shows a patent processus vaginalis resulting in a left indirect inguinal hernia containing fat* ➡ *and fluid* ➡. *The testis is displaced inferiorly* ➡.

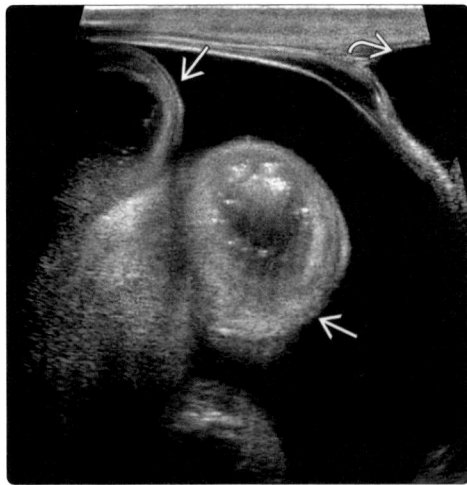
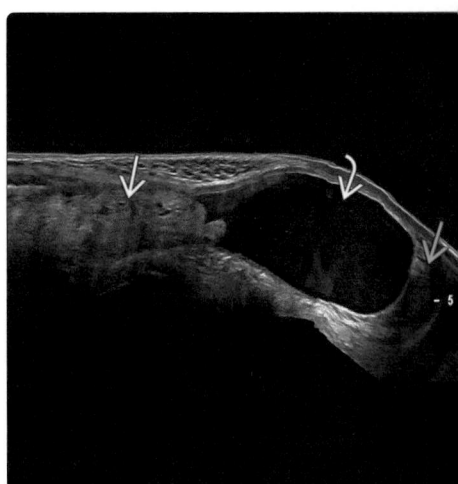

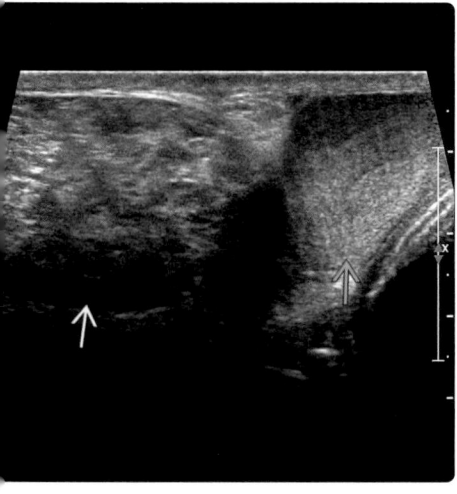
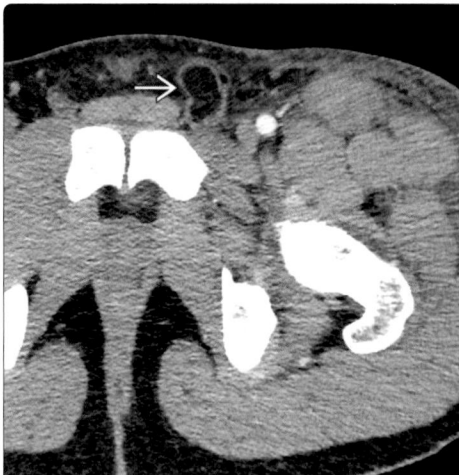

(Left) Longitudinal ultrasound shows a left indirect inguinal hernia extending into the scrotum in an adult male. The herniated fat ⇒ abuts the testis ➡. (Right) Axial CECT of the same patient performed for trauma to the leg shows an indirect inguinal hernia containing fat ⇒. The hernia was asymptomatic.

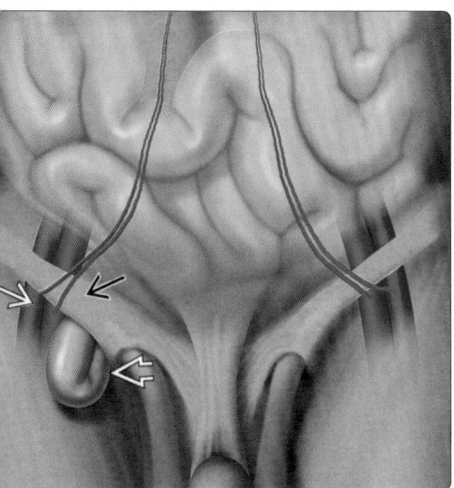
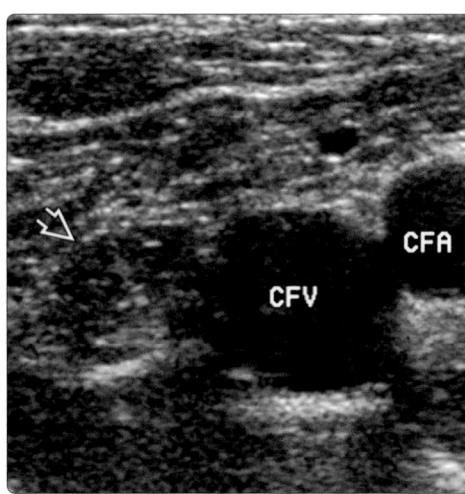

(Left) Graphic shows a femoral hernia ⇒. Note that the neck of the femoral hernia is medial to the common femoral vein ⇒ and inferior to the inguinal ligament ➡. (Right) Transverse oblique ultrasound of the femoral canal with the patient standing shows a femoral hernia ⇒ containing mesenteric fat. The hernia is medial to the common femoral vein (CFV) and artery (CFA). (Courtesy C. Rapp, RDMS, FAIUM, FSDMS.)

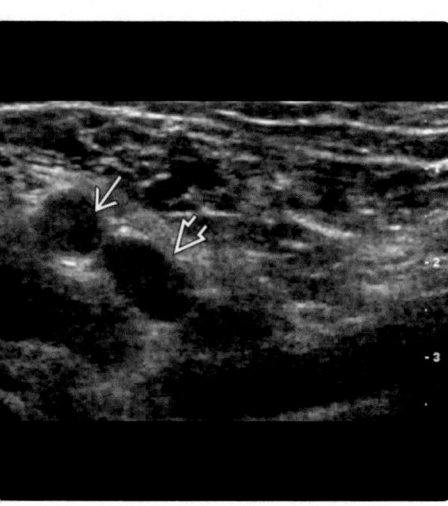
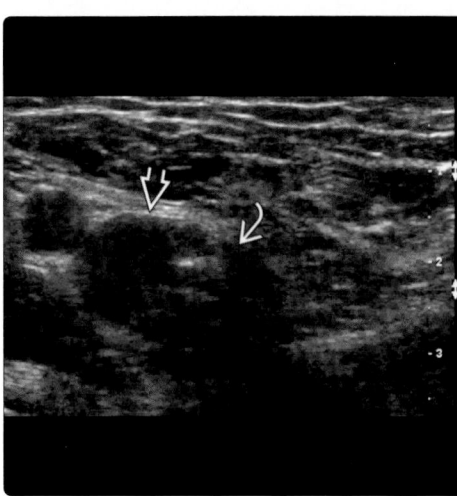

(Left) Transverse oblique ultrasound of the right femoral canal at rest shows a normal, common femoral vein ⇒ and artery ➡ with no hernia. (Courtesy of C. Rapp, RDMS, FAIUM, FSDMS.) (Right) Transverse oblique ultrasound of the right femoral canal during Valsalva shows a small femoral hernia ⇒ medial to the common femoral vein ⇒. (Courtesy C. Rapp, RDMS, FAIUM, FSDMS.)

TERMINOLOGY

- Abnormal accumulation of fluid within peritoneal cavity

IMAGING

- Fluid collects in most dependent locations unless there are loculations
- Pelvis: In pouch of Douglas
- Free-flowing: Fluid insinuates itself between organs and is shaped by surrounding structures
- US accurate at detecting, localizing, and characterizing ascites; quantification more subjective
- Simple: Anechoic; homogeneous, freely mobile, deep acoustic enhancement
- Complicated: Echogenic fluid with coarse or fine internal echoes, layering debris or particulate material, septa
- Small free fluid in cul-de-sac; physiologic in women
- Look for associated hepatic disease, peritoneal masses, or adherent bowel

TOP DIFFERENTIAL DIAGNOSES

- Hemoperitoneum
- Infectious ascites
- Malignant ascites
- Pseudomyxoma peritonei

PATHOLOGY

- Traditionally classified as transudative or exudative ascites based on protein content
- Serum Albumin Ascites Gradient (SAAG) is difference between serum and ascites albumin, now widely used to differentiate causes of ascites

DIAGNOSTIC CHECKLIST

- Imaging alone cannot characterize nature or cause of peritoneal fluid collections; sampling is required

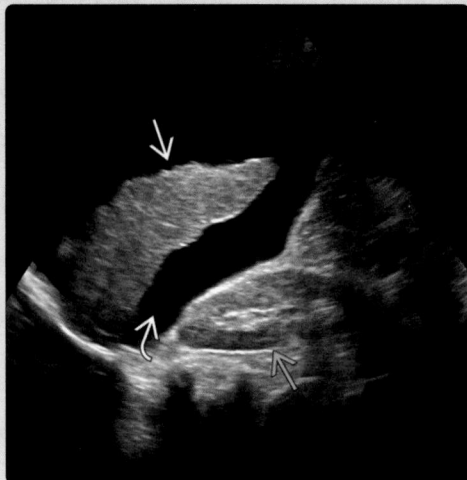
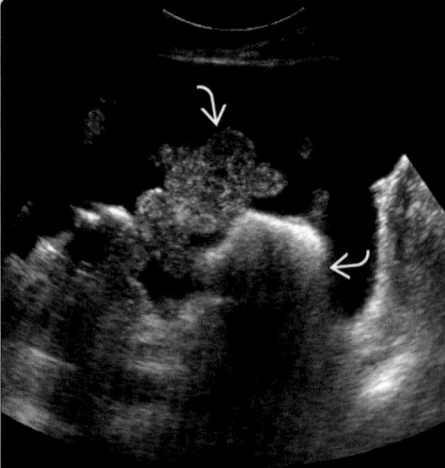

(Left) Longitudinal ultrasound shows the right upper quadrant in a patient with cirrhosis and ascites. The liver contour is nodular ➡. Ascites surrounds the liver and fills Morison pouch ➡. The right kidney ➡ appears echogenic secondary to acoustic enhancement. (Right) Transverse ultrasound shows the left lower quadrant in a patient with end-stage liver disease. There is free fluid surrounding the bowel ➡ with no mass effect.

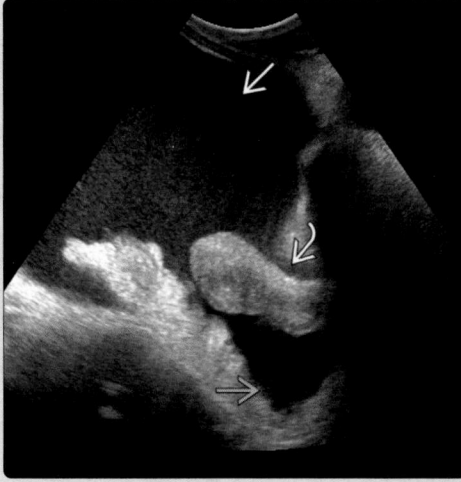
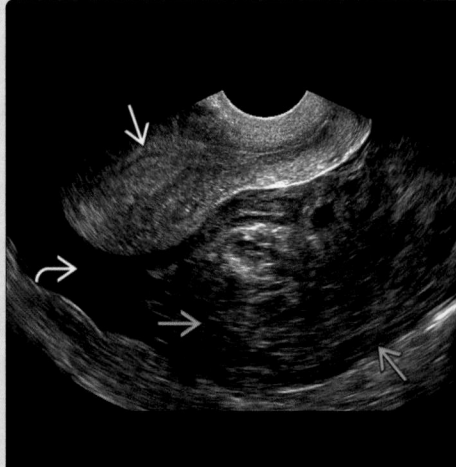

(Left) Longitudinal ultrasound of the pelvis in a patient with cirrhosis shows a large volume of complex ascites ➡ containing low-level echoes. Paracentesis showed hemorrhage. Ascites extends into the cul-de-sac ➡. The uterus ➡ is normal. (Right) Longitudinal transvaginal ultrasound shows the pelvis in a ruptured ectopic pregnancy. There is free anechoic fluid in the upper pelvis ➡ with clotted blood ➡ in the dependent pouch of Douglas. Endometrial thickening is noted in the uterus with no intrauterine sac ➡.

Ascites

TERMINOLOGY

Definitions

Abnormal accumulation of fluid within peritoneal cavity

IMAGING

General Features

- Best diagnostic clue
  - Free fluid in peritoneal cavity
- Location
  - Fluid collects in most dependent locations unless there are loculations
  - Dependent spaces: Pouch of Douglas in pelvis; Morison pouch (hepatorenal fossa) in upper abdomen, paracolic gutters
  - Subphrenic spaces: Not dependent, but fill due to suction effect of diaphragmatic motion
  - Lesser sac usually does not fill with ascites unless tense ascites, local source (gastric ulcer or pancreatitis)
    - Otherwise due to carcinomatosis or infected ascites
- Morphology
  - Free-flowing: Fluid insinuates itself between organs and is shaped by surrounding structures
    - No mass effect
  - Loculated: Rounded, bulging contour, encapsulated
    - Does not conform to organ margins
    - Mass effect on adjacent organs
  - Fluid can also be chylous, hemorrhagic, bilious, pancreatic, urine, or cerebrospinal fluid
  - Malignant ascites and pseudomyxoma peritonei more complex with solid components

Ultrasonographic Findings

- Grayscale ultrasound
  - US accurate at detecting, localizing, and characterizing ascites; quantification more subjective
    - Fluid in dependent recesses, shifts with patient movement, compresses with increased transducer pressure
  - Characterization of ascites: Simple or complicated
    - Simple: Anechoic; homogeneous, freely mobile, deep acoustic enhancement
      - Usually transudate
    - Complicated: Echogenic fluid with coarse or fine internal echoes, layering debris or particulate material, septa
      - Usually exudate
      - Appearance of hemorrhagic ascites varies with time of onset and transducer frequency
      - Can be anechoic or hyperechoic initially, ± clots, anechoic later
    - Loculated ascites: Encapsulated, internal thick or thin septa
      - Secondary to adhesions, chronic ascites, malignancy, infection
      - Rounded margins with mass effect, frequently displacing adjacent structures, less compressible
      - Malignant ascites: Tethered matted bowel, peritoneal masses; concordant fluid in greater and lesser sac

- Small free fluid in cul-de-sac; physiologic in women
- Massive ascites: Small bowel loops arrayed on either side of vertically floating mesentery
- Transverse & sigmoid colon usually float on top of fluid
- Cerebrospinal fluid ascites: Small amounts of free fluid normal with ventriculoperitoneal shunt
  - Localized/loculated collection around tip of shunt tube is pathologic, implies adhesions
- Pancreatic ascites: Peripancreatic, lesser sac, anterior pararenal space
  - Disruption of pancreatic duct or severe pancreatitis

Radiographic Findings

- Plain abdominal films insensitive for small amounts of ascites
  - Direct signs
    - Obliteration of hepatic angle
    - Hellmer sign: Displacement of lateral edge of liver medially, away from thoracoabdominal wall
  - Indirect signs: Diffuse abdominal haziness; bulging of flanks; poor visualization of psoas & renal outline
    - Centralization of floating gas-containing small bowel or separation of small bowel loops

CT Findings

- Simple ascites: Low-density free fluid 0-30 Hounsfield units
  - Centralization of bowel loops; triangular configuration within leaves of mesentery
  - Massive ascites; distends peritoneal spaces
- Complex ascites
  - Exudates: Density of ascitic fluid increases with increasing protein content
  - Hemorrhagic ascites: High density with layering ± active bleeding
  - Chylous ascites: Less than 0 HU
  - Bilious ascites: Less than 20 HU; typically in right or left supramesocolic spaces
  - Urine ascites: Nonspecific appearance but delayed CECT can confirm diagnosis

Nonvascular Interventions

- US-guided therapeutic & diagnostic paracentesis

Imaging Recommendations

- Best imaging tool
  - US for detection & characterization of peritoneal fluid collections
  - US guidance for paracentesis
- Protocol advice
  - Look for associated hepatic disease, peritoneal masses, or adherent bowel

DIFFERENTIAL DIAGNOSIS

Hemoperitoneum

- Trauma, ruptured aneurysm, ruptured ectopic pregnancy, ruptured liver mass, postsurgical bleeding, anticoagulant therapy
- Fluid debris level may develop if patient in supine position for a long time
- Massive hemorrhage: Large echogenic mass (clots), later heterogeneous (lysis)

Infected Ascites

- Postoperative, bacterial peritonitis, tuberculosis, acquired immunodeficiency syndrome, fungal infections
- Fluid with internal echoes, debris, loculations, multiple septa
- Peritoneal thickening, matted bowel loops, abscess

Malignant Ascites

- Known malignancy, accounts for ~ 10% of refractory ascites
- Lesions in other organs and lymph nodes; primary mass such as ovary, gut, pancreas
- Loculated collections; fluid in greater & lesser sac
- Bowel loops tethered along abdominal wall
- Thickening of peritoneum; peritoneal seeding or masses

Pseudomyxoma Peritonei

- Gelatinous mucinous accumulation in peritoneal cavity secondary to benign or malignant mucin-producing neoplasm
- Echogenic fluid (nonmobile echoes), masses with cystic spaces or calcification, echogenic septa, liver scalloping, and bowel displacement

Peritoneal Inclusion Cyst

- Loculated fluid collections in pelvis

PATHOLOGY

General Features

- Etiology
  - Traditionally classified as transudative or exudative ascites based on protein content
  - Transudate: Clear or straw colored (protein < 25 g/L)
  - Causes: Cirrhosis, heart failure, nephrotic syndrome
    - Cirrhosis and portal hypertension is most common cause (81%)
      - Budd-Chiari syndrome, portal vein thrombosis, alcoholic hepatitis, fulminant hepatic failure
    - Cardiac: Congestive heart failure, constrictive pericarditis, cardiac tamponade
    - Renal: Nephrotic syndrome, chronic renal failure
    - Hypoalbuminemia; protein-losing enteropathy
  - Exudate: Yellowish/hemorrhagic (protein > 25 g/L)
  - Causes: Exudate from inflamed or neoplastic peritoneum
    - Neoplasm: Colon, gastric, pancreatic, hepatic, ovarian; metastatic disease (breast/lung, etc.)
    - Infections: Bacterial, fungal, parasitic, tuberculosis
    - Trauma: Blunt, penetrating, or iatrogenic
      - Diagnostic/therapeutic peritoneal lavage
      - Bile ascites: Trauma, cholecystectomy, biliary or hepatic surgery, biopsy, percutaneous drainage
      - Urine ascites: Trauma to bladder or collecting system, instrumentation
      - Cerebrospinal fluid: Ventriculoperitoneal shunts
      - Chylous: Trauma (blunt, penetrating, surgical), inflammatory, idiopathic
    - Bowel pathology: Ischemia, inflammation, obstruction

Gross Pathologic & Surgical Features

- Serum Albumin Ascites Gradient (SAAG) is difference between serum and ascites albumin; more useful for diagnosis of portal hypertension

- SAAG < 11g/L = normal portal portal pressure; SAAG >11g/L = portal hypertension
- Hemorrhagic: Serosanguineous, erythrocytes > 10,000/mm³
- Spontaneous bacterial peritonitis: Cloudy, neutrophils ≥ 250 /mm³ (500/mm³ threshold more specific); cultures negative in 40%
- Chylous: Yellowish white or milky, triglycerides > 2.25 mmol/L
- Pancreatitis: Dark brown-black, amylase > 2000 U/L
- Pseudomyxoma peritonei: Gelatinous, mucinous

CLINICAL ISSUES

Presentation

- Most common signs/symptoms
  - Asymptomatic, abdominal discomfort & distension, weight gain
- Physical examination: Bulging flanks, flank dullness, fluid thrill, umbilical hernia, penile or scrotal edema
- Diagnosis: Paracentesis (US guidance or blind tap)
  - All patients with new onset ascites should have a paracentesis
  - In chronic ascites, fever, abdominal pain, leucocytosis, renal insufficiency, or encephalopathy are indications for paracentesis
  - Fluid analysis: Protein, albumin, lactate dehydrogenase, glucose, amylase, cytology, pH, triglycerides, cell count, culture

Natural History & Prognosis

- Ascites is associated with increased mortality and morbidity in chronic liver disease
- Complication: Spontaneous bacterial peritonitis, respiratory compromise, anorexia, hepatorenal syndrome

Treatment

- Sodium restriction & diuretics
- Refractory cases: Large volume paracentesis
  - Peritoneovenous shunting; LeVeen, Denver
  - Transjugular intrahepatic portosystemic shunting (TIPS)
  - IVC or hepatic vein stenting (Budd-Chiari syndrome)

DIAGNOSTIC CHECKLIST

Consider

- Imaging alone cannot characterize nature or cause of peritoneal fluid collections; sampling is required

SELECTED REFERENCES

1. Runyon BA et al: Introduction to the revised American Association for the Study of Liver Diseases Practice Guideline management of adult patients with ascites due to cirrhosis 2012. Hepatology. 57(4):1651-3, 2013
2. Tirkes T et al: Peritoneal and retroperitoneal anatomy and its relevance for cross-sectional imaging. Radiographics. 32(2):437-51, 2012
3. Levy AD et al: Secondary tumors and tumorlike lesions of the peritoneal cavity: imaging features with pathologic correlation. Radiographics. 29(2):347-73, 2009
4. Runyon BA et al: Management of adult patients with ascites due to cirrhosis: an update. Hepatology. 49(6):2087-107, 2009
5. Hanbidge AE et al: US of the peritoneum. Radiographics. 23(3):663-84; discussion 684-5, 2003
6. Practice Guidelines from American Association for the Study of Liver Diseases

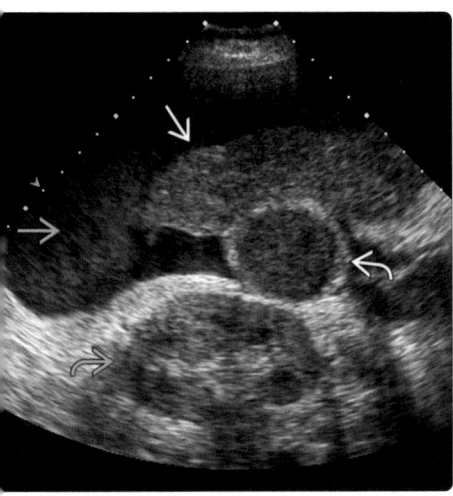
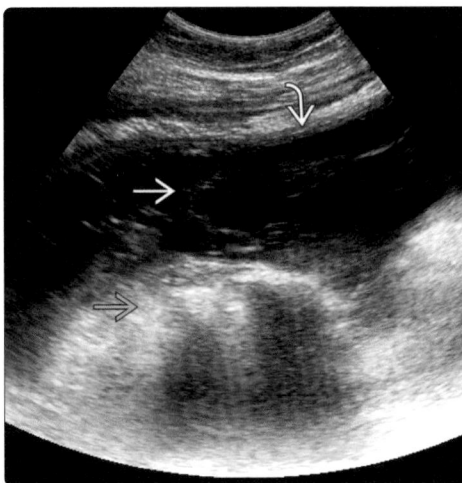

(Left) Transverse ultrasound of the right upper quadrant shows a small cirrhotic liver ➡. There is hemorrhagic ascites ➡, which should raise suspicion for a bleeding hepatocellular carcinoma. The gallbladder ➡ is sludge filled and thick walled. Also note the echogenic right kidney ➡. (Right) Transverse ultrasound shows the right mid abdomen in a patient with sepsis and abdominal pain. Ascites ➡ is loculated and septated ➡ with bowel displacement ➡. Paracentesis revealed Pseudomonas peritonitis from bowel perforation.

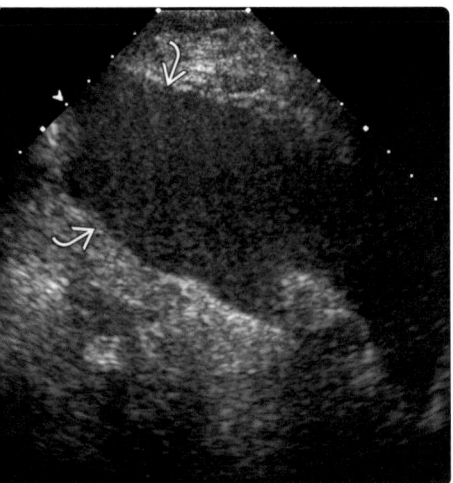
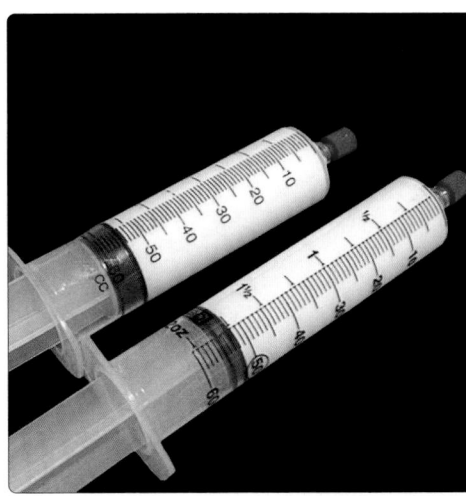

(Left) Transverse ultrasound shows the left lateral abdomen in a patient with abdominal distension after a 2nd renal transplant. Ascites with low-level echoes ➡ was nonloculated and mobile. (Right) Diagnostic paracentesis of the same patient shows milky fluid compatible with chylous ascites. This can be confirmed by measuring the triglyceride level in the fluid.

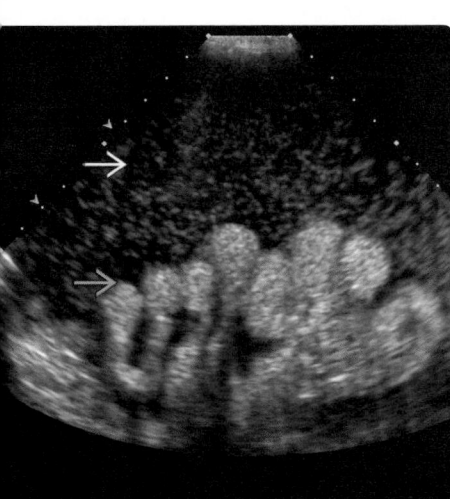
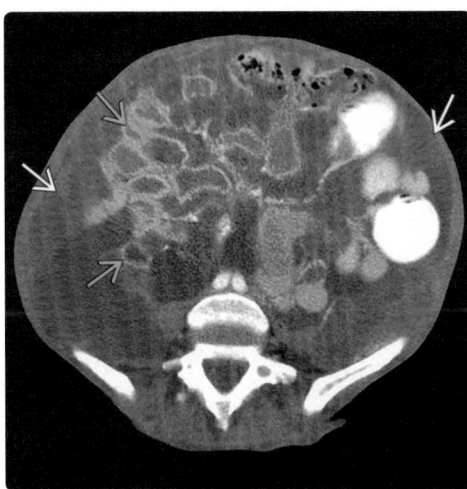

(Left) Transverse ultrasound shows the right mid abdomen in a patient with pseudomyxoma peritonei from mucinous appendiceal carcinoma. The peritoneal fluid contains multiple low-level echoes ➡, which were not mobile. Adjacent bowel ➡ is displaced posteriorly. (Right) Axial CECT of the same patient shows loculated low-density mucinous fluid ➡ with mass effect on bowel ➡.

KEY FACTS

TERMINOLOGY

- Peritoneal spread of tumor from epithelial malignancy resulting in peritoneal thickening, omental infiltration, serosal implants, and ascites

IMAGING

- Implants develop where peritoneal fluid collects: Dome of liver, omentum, paracolic gutters, and pelvic recesses
- Omental involvement may be nodular or diffuse, producing an omental cake
- Peritoneal masses may be solid, cystic, or mixed, depending on primary neoplasm
- Hypoechoic rind-like thickening of peritoneum
- Ascites: Complex with septations or internal echoes (jiggle with transducer pressure)
- Dissemination of tumor also occurs via hematogenous, contiguous, or lymphatic spread

- Diagnosis may be obtained by US-guided aspiration of peritoneal fluid or fine-needle/core biopsy of omental cake/peritoneal masses
- Color Doppler confirms that omental/peritoneal deposits are solid; improves biopsy yield when viable tumor is targeted

TOP DIFFERENTIAL DIAGNOSES

- Pseudomyxoma peritonei
- Peritoneal mesothelioma
- Peritoneal tuberculosis
- Peritoneal sarcomatosis
- Peritoneal lymphomatosis

CLINICAL ISSUES

- Present with abdominal distension and pain, weight loss, malaise, fever
- May have elevated tumor markers such as CA125 or CEA
- Prognosis variable depending on primary tumor, but generally poor prognosis

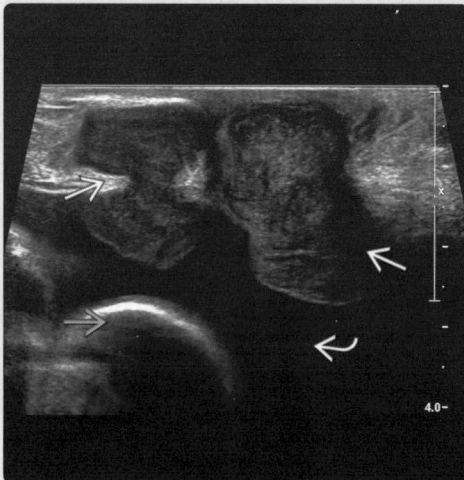
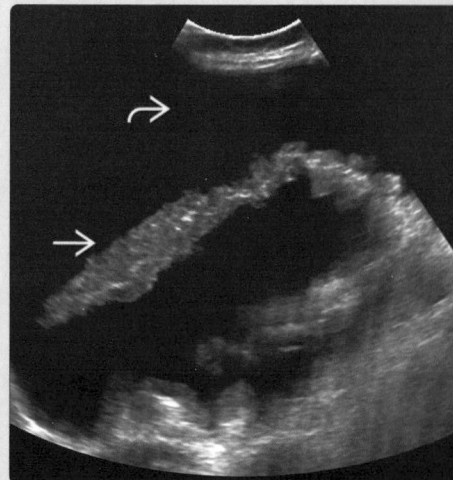

(Left) Longitudinal ultrasound of the midline anterior abdominal wall in a patient with metastatic pancreatic neuroendocrine carcinoma shows there are 2 peritoneal soft tissue implants growing through the anterior abdominal wall ➡ with adjacent ascites ➡ and bowel ➡. (Right) Longitudinal ultrasound of the right upper quadrant inferior to the liver shows ascites ➡ and a thick lobular omental cake ➡ from pancreatic carcinomatosis.

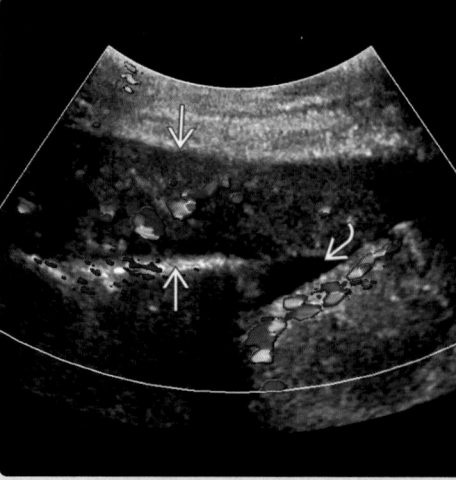
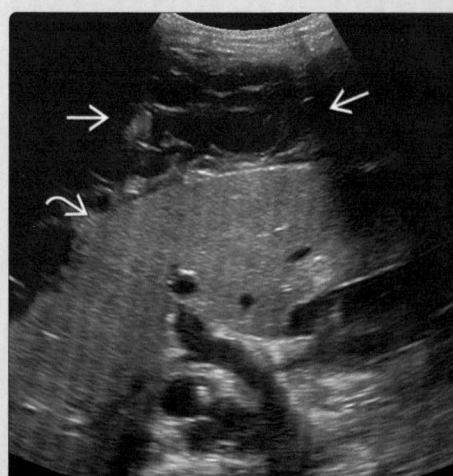

(Left) Transverse color Doppler ultrasound of the midline anterior abdominal wall in a patient with ovarian carcinomatosis and an omental cake ➡. Color flow is present within the omentum. A small amount of ascites ➡ is noted. (Right) Transverse ultrasound of the right upper quadrant shows complex septated ascites ➡ anterior to the liver ➡, representing mucinous carcinomatosis from appendiceal carcinoma.

TERMINOLOGY

Definitions

- Peritoneal spread of tumor from epithelial malignancy resulting in peritoneal thickening, omental infiltration, serosal implants, and ascites
- Krukenberg tumor: Bilateral ovarian metastases from hematogenous or lymphatic spread from signet ring gastric carcinoma (less commonly breast)

IMAGING

General Features

- Best diagnostic clue
  - Omental cake
  - Cystic or solid peritoneal masses or peritoneal thickening
  - Ascites, mesenteric infiltration
- Location
  - Implants develop where peritoneal fluid collects: Dome of liver, omentum, paracolic gutters, and pelvic recesses
  - Dissemination of tumor also occurs via hematogenous, contiguous, or lymphatic spread
    - To peritoneum, adjacent organs, and mesentery
- Size
  - Variable: Tiny nodules to large confluent omental or peritoneal masses
- Morphology
  - Omental involvement may be nodular or diffuse, producing an omental cake
  - Peritoneal masses may be solid, cystic, or mixed, depending on primary neoplasm

Ultrasonographic Findings

- Grayscale ultrasound
  - Omentum: Thickened and hypoechoic or heterogeneous with preserved islands of echogenic fat
  - Peritoneum
    - Hypoechoic rind-like thickening of peritoneum
    - Discrete implants: Irregular nodular masses along parietal and visceral peritoneum
      □ Usually grow inward towards peritoneal cavity; may grow outwards and invade abdominal wall
      □ Pouch of Douglas, Morison pouch, and right subphrenic space commonly involved
    - Psammomatous calcification in peritoneal implants seen in ovarian serous carcinoma (up to 40% with stage III/IV disease)
  - Ascites: Complex with septations or internal echoes (jiggle with transducer pressure)
    - May be only finding early on
    - Improves conspicuity of peritoneal implants, which may not be detectable when small
  - Thickening of mesenteric leaves due to desmoplastic reaction; typically mesenteric side of terminal ileum
    - May give "sunburst" appearance
  - ± enlarged hypoechoic retroperitoneal and mesenteric lymph nodes (more common in lymphomatosis)
  - Primary neoplasm may be evident, e.g., ovarian, appendiceal, pancreatic, or GI malignancies
- Color Doppler

  - Confirms that omental/peritoneal deposits are solid; improves biopsy yield when viable tumor is targeted

Nuclear Medicine Findings

- FDG PET/CT: Increased metabolic activity in masses or along neoplastic peritoneum, most useful in lymphoma

CT Findings

- Ascites, stranding of peritoneal fat, nodular or diffuse thickening of peritoneum with enhancement
- Omental cake or omental nodules, streaky increased density of omentum
- Infiltrated or spiculated mesentery or mass
- Thick, fixed bowel wall ± bowel obstruction

MR Findings

- T1WI
  - Low signal ascites; medium signal omental cake, nodules, and masses
- T2WI
  - Intermediate signal peritoneal mass, nodule, or omental cake with high signal ascites
- DWI
  - Tumors may variably restrict diffusion depending on primary neoplasm and presence of necrosis
- T1WI C+
  - Abnormal linear or nodular hyperenhancement of peritoneum
  - Variable enhancement of nodules and masses

Nonvascular Interventions

- US-guided diagnostic and therapeutic aspiration of peritoneal fluid
- US-guided fine-needle or core biopsy of omental cake or peritoneal masses

Imaging Recommendations

- Best imaging tool
  - CECT: Superior for cancer staging
- Protocol advice
  - Optimum CECT requires oral and intravenous contrast, CEMR is alternative
  - US ideal for guiding diagnostic and therapeutic aspiration or tissue biopsy
  - US may follow CT/MR for detailed search of primary tumor involving ovaries, gallbladder, and bile ducts

DIFFERENTIAL DIAGNOSIS

Pseudomyxoma Peritonei

- Secondary to neoplasm, secreting mucin most commonly appendiceal, or ovarian primary neoplasm
- Low-density loculated complex ascites exerting mass effect reflecting gelatinous peritoneal fluid
  - Curvilinear surface calcification highly suggestive
- Scalloping of lateral contour of liver and spleen
- Peritoneal nodules, omental invasion

Peritoneal Mesothelioma

- 25% of mesotheliomas are peritoneal; most common in middle-aged males; associated with asbestos exposure

- Similar to carcinomatosis: Thick nodular masses involving anterior parietal peritoneum, becoming confluent and cake-like
- Large solid omental and mesenteric masses often infiltrating bowel and mesentery
- Smaller volume of ascites
- Look for associated pleural calcification (sign of asbestos exposure)

Peritoneal Tuberculosis

- Ileocecal mural thickening, matted, hypoperistaltic small bowel loops, necrotic lymph nodes, splenomegaly, or splenic calcifications favor tuberculosis
- Wet type (90%): Ascites with increased density ± mesenteric nodes
- Fixed fibrotic type (7%): Smooth thickening of peritoneum, nodular mesenteric masses, loculated ascites ± calcification
- Dry type (3%): Peritoneal fibrosis

Peritoneal Sarcomatosis

- Peritoneal spread of sarcoma most commonly from gastrointestinal stromal tumors, liposarcoma, and leiomyosarcoma
- Discrete well-defined masses with more smooth outlines, typically > 2 cm
- Less ascites, peritoneal thickening, omental cake, serosal implants, and lymphadenopathy than carcinomatosis

Peritoneal Lymphomatosis

- Rare peritoneal spread of lymphoma, typically aggressive non-Hodgkin (diffuse large B cell most common)
- Bulky omental thickening or smooth peritoneal nodules (typically > 5 cm), less ascites
- Lymphadenopathy, mesenteric masses ("sandwiching" vessels), and splenomegaly help distinguish from carcinomatosis and sarcomatosis
- Intense FDG uptake, nodular or diffuse

PATHOLOGY

General Features

- Etiology
  - Metastatic disease to peritoneal surfaces, omentum, and mesentery
  - Most commonly from ovarian, colorectal, gastric, breast and pancreatic cancer
    - Less common: Lung and renal carcinoma
  - Sarcomas and lymphomas may also spread intraperitoneally
- Genetics
  - Colorectal, endometrial, and ovarian cancers related to Lynch syndrome

Staging, Grading, & Classification

- Peritoneal metastases indicate stage IV disease (excluding ovarian carcinoma)

Gross Pathologic & Surgical Features

- Infiltrating masses of peritoneal surfaces, omentum, and mesentery
- Omental cake: Replacement of omental fat by tumor and fibrosis
- Ascites: Clear or turbid and thick (viscous/gelatinous)

Microscopic Features

- Varies according to primary tumor
  - Most commonly adenocarcinoma

CLINICAL ISSUES

Presentation

- Most common signs/symptoms
  - Abdominal distension and pain, weight loss, malaise, fever
- Other signs/symptoms
  - Progression of known malignancy
- Clinical profile
  - New presentation: Diagnosis may be made by paracentesis or tissue sampling of mass
  - May have elevated tumor markers such as CA125 or CEA

Demographics

- Age
  - Adults generally > 40 years
  - Younger patients with hereditary syndromes
- Gender
  - More common in females than males, due to ovarian carcinoma

Natural History & Prognosis

- Variable, depending on primary tumor; poor prognosis in general
- Progressive if untreated
- Complication: Bowel obstruction

Treatment

- Depends on pathology
- Cytoreductive surgery ± hyperthermic intraperitoneal chemotherapy
- Combination of systemic and intraperitoneal chemotherapy

DIAGNOSTIC CHECKLIST

Consider

- Peritoneal sarcomatosis if there are large, well-defined smooth, intraperitoneal masses with no omental involvement and minimal ascites
- Peritoneal lymphomatosis if there are also large mesenteric and retroperitoneal nodal masses and splenomegaly
- TB peritonitis if there is ileocecal involvement, necrotic, or calcified lymph nodes

SELECTED REFERENCES

1. Wasnik AP et al: Primary and secondary disease of the peritoneum and mesentery: review of anatomy and imaging features. Abdom Imaging. 40(3):626-42, 2015
2. Diop AD et al: CT imaging of peritoneal carcinomatosis and its mimics. Diagn Interv Imaging. ePub, 2014
3. O'Neill AC et al: Differences in CT features of peritoneal carcinomatosis, sarcomatosis, and lymphomatosis: retrospective analysis of 122 cases at a tertiary cancer institution. Clin Radiol. 69(12):1219-27, 2014
4. Vicens RA et al: Multimodality imaging of common and uncommon peritoneal diseases: a review for radiologists. Abdom Imaging. ePub, 2014
5. Cabral FC et al: Peritoneal lymphomatosis: CT and PET/CT findings and how to differentiate between carcinomatosis and sarcomatosis. Cancer Imaging. 13:162-70, 2013
6. Oei TN et al: Peritoneal sarcomatosis versus peritoneal carcinomatosis: imaging findings at MDCT. AJR Am J Roentgenol. 195(3):W229-35, 2010

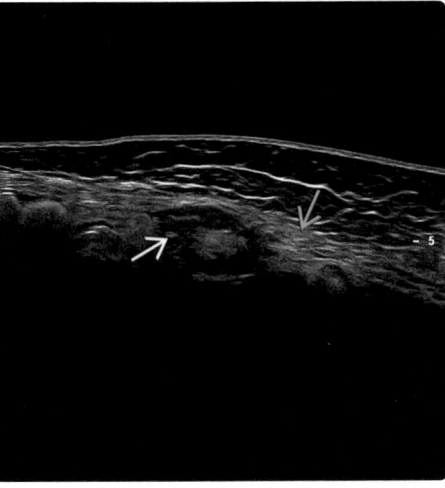

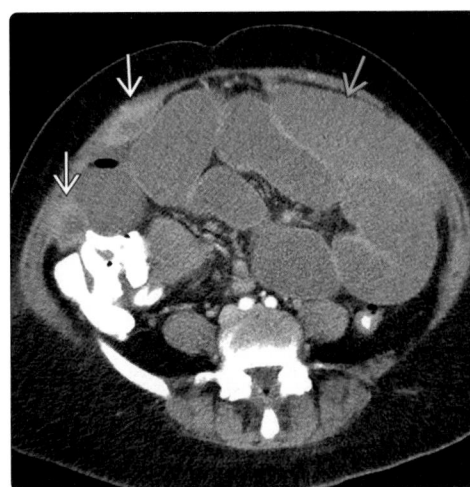

(Left) *Longitudinal panoramic ultrasound of the right abdominal abdominal wall in a patient with metastatic squamous cervical carcinoma. There is a peritoneal metastasis ➜ invading the abdominal wall fascia ⇥.* **(Right)** *CECT of the same patient shows multiple peritoneal metastases ➜ and small bowel obstruction ⇥. The metastasis causing the obstruction is not shown.*

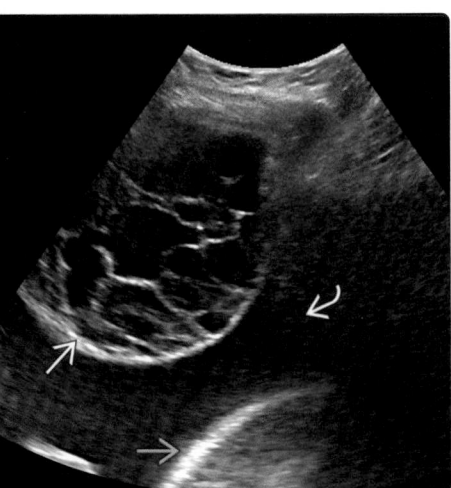

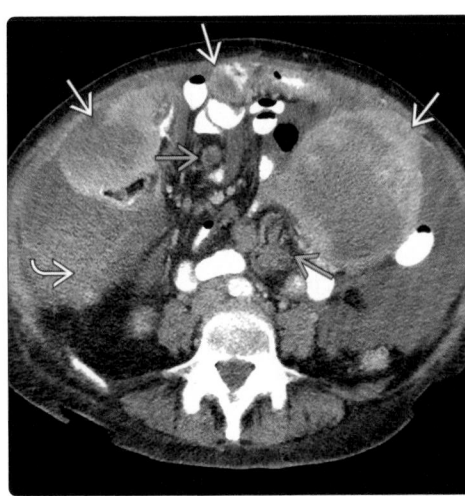

(Left) *Longitudinal ultrasound of the pelvis in a patient with recurrent endometrial carcinoma in the peritoneal cavity shows a septated cystic peritoneal mass ➜ and ascites ➛. A more solid mass ⇥ is deeper.* **(Right)** *Axial CECT of the same patient shows ascites ➛ and multiple peritoneal masses ➜ with central cystic change. There is minimal adenopathy ⇥.*

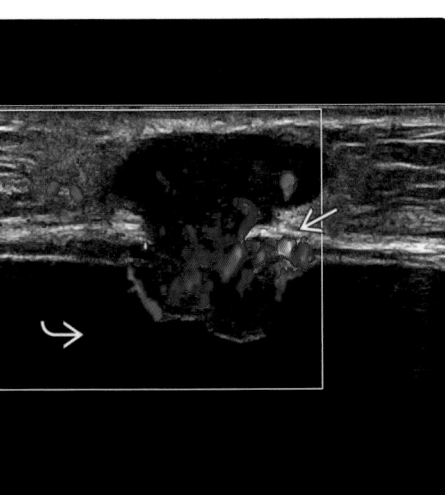

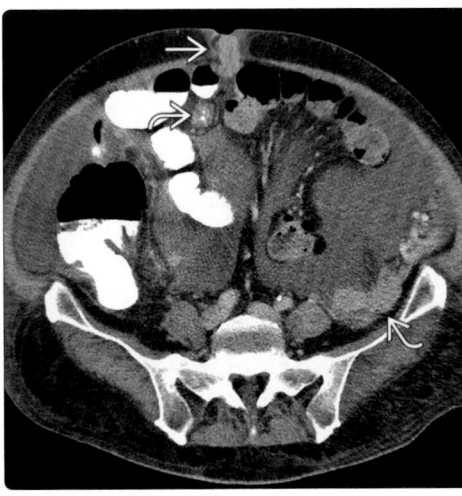

(Left) *Transverse color Doppler ultrasound of a peritoneal metastasis invading the abdominal wall ➛ in a patient with pancreatic neuroendocrine carcinoma shows the mass is well perfused. The presence of ascites ➛ improves detection of peritoneal masses.* **(Right)** *Axial CECT of the same patient shows the superficial metastasis extending through the umbilicus ➜, but also multiple other intraperitoneal metastases ➛, one of which is calcified.*

(Left) *Transverse ultrasound of the upper abdomen shows a thickened heterogeneous omentum* ➡ *with underlying bowel* ➡. *Core biopsies showed mucinous adenocarcinoma.* **(Right)** *Axial CECT of the same patient shows the extent of the omental cake* ➡. *The omentum contains soft tissue and fat densities. A large amount of ascites* ➡ *is present.*

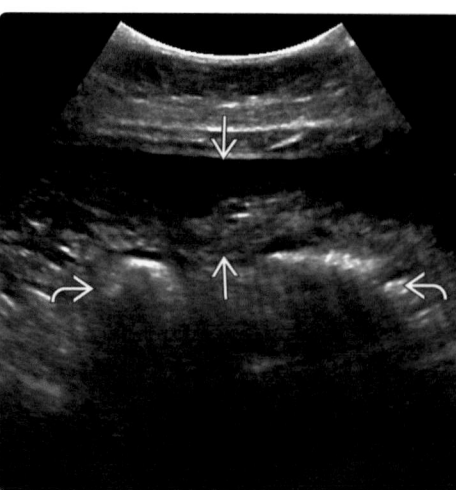
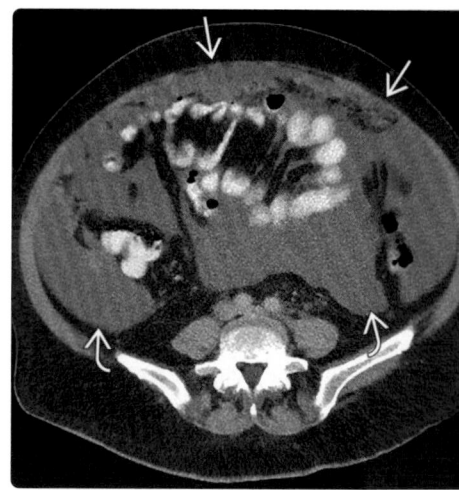

(Left) *Panoramic transverse ultrasound (same patient) of the upper abdomen shows the extent of the hypoechoic omental cake* ➡ *displacing bowel* ➡ *posteriorly.* **(Right)** *Axial NECT of a patient with a renal transplant and abdominal distension* ➡ *shows an extensive omental cake displacing bowel* ➡. *Ascites* ➡ *is mild. Omental biopsy confirmed ovarian carcinoma.*

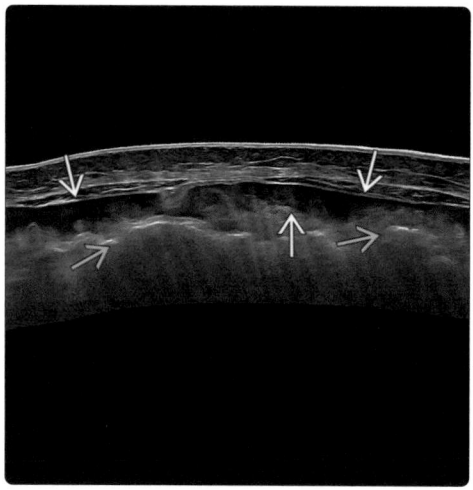
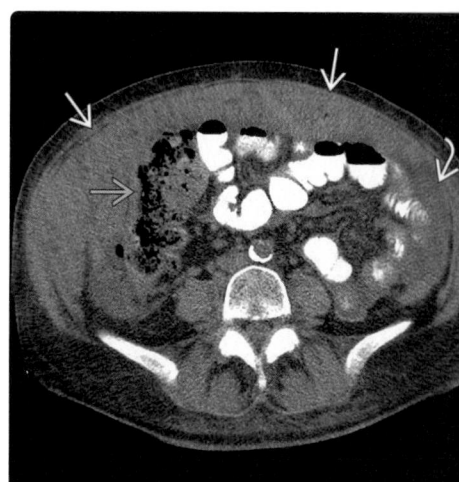

(Left) *Axial NECT of the same patient confirms thickening of the peritoneum* ➡ *and a large pelvic mass* ➡. *The lower pole of a renal transplant* ➡ *is noted.* **(Right)** *Transvaginal ultrasound of a patient with ovarian carcinomatosis shows that in the left adnexa there is a soft tissue plaque* ➡ *along the peritoneum as well as a solid mass* ➡. *Surrounding ascites contains low-level echoes* ➡.

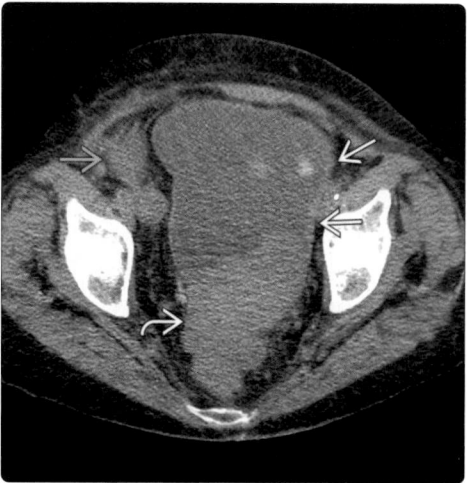
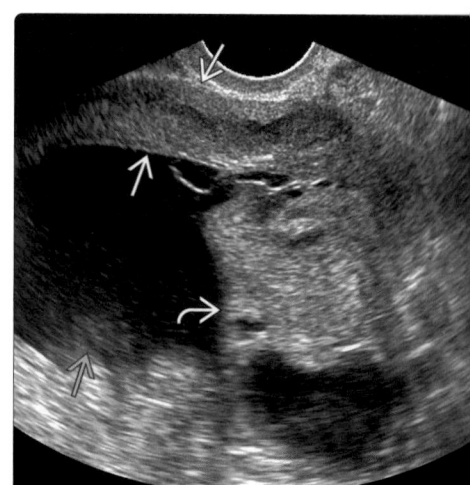

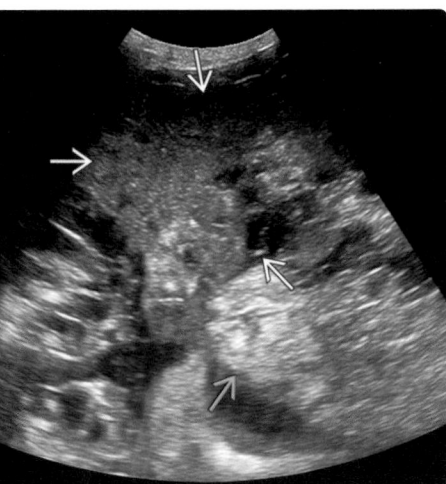

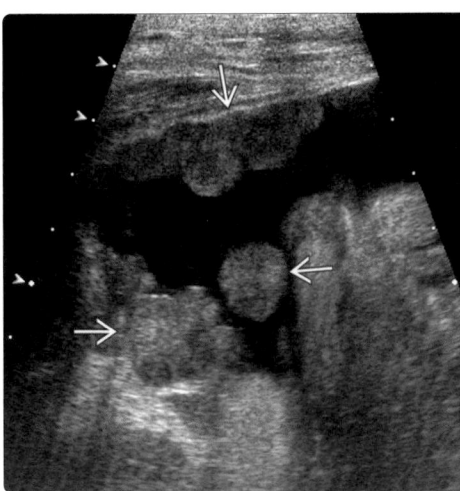

(Left) *Transverse ultrasound shows gelatinous ascites* ➡️ *in pseudomyxoma peritonei. Mobile echoes were seen in real-time, confirming the liquid content. Bowel is displaced* ➡️. **(Right)** *Transverse ultrasound of the right lower quadrant shows ascites and multiple peritoneal nodules* ➡️ *from recurrent native kidney renal cell carcinoma in a renal transplant recipient.*

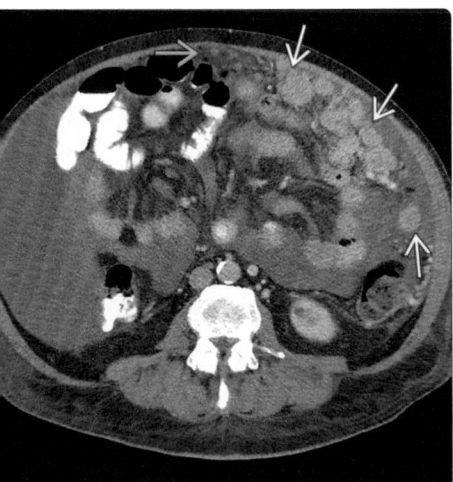

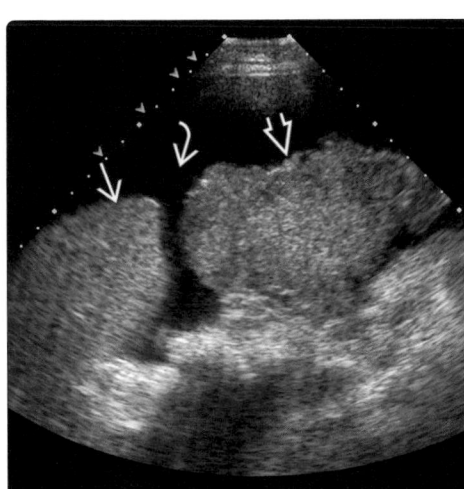

(Left) *Axial CECT in a patient with metastatic pancreatic neuroendocrine tumor shows multiple peritoneal nodules* ➡️ *of varying sizes with ascites. There is infiltration of the omentum* ➡️. **(Right)** *Longitudinal ultrasound of the right abdomen shows ascites* ➡️ *around the liver* ➡️ *and outlining a solid intraperitoneal metastasis* ➡️ *from recurrent renal cell carcinoma.*

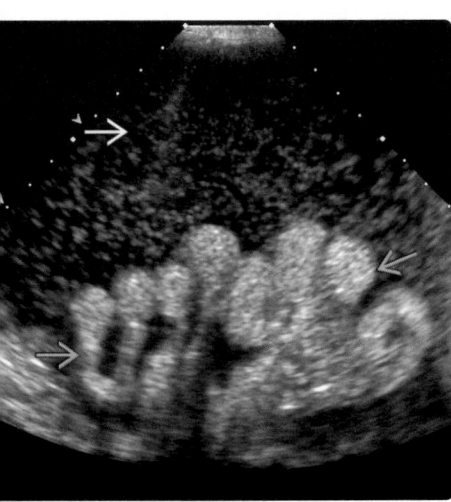

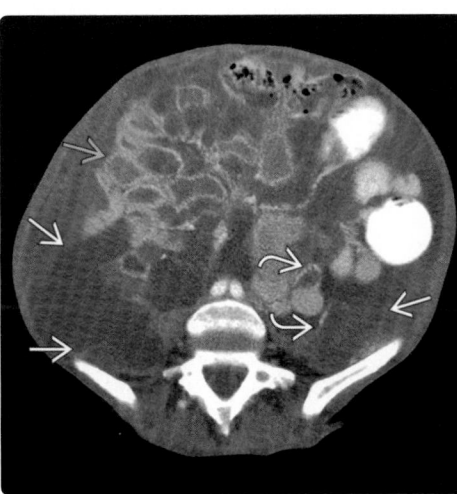

(Left) *Transverse ultrasound of the pelvis in a patient with pseudomyxoma peritonei from appendiceal adenocarcinoma shows ascites contains multiple low-level echoes* ➡️ *and exerts mass effect on the small bowel* ➡️. *Pushing and releasing the transducer will induce jiggling of the ascites.* **(Right)** *Axial CECT of the same patient shows septations in the low-density gelatinous ascites* ➡️ *with subtle calcifications* ➡️. *The small bowel is clumped* ➡️.

Peritoneal Space Abscess

TERMINOLOGY

- Localized abdominal collection of pus

IMAGING

- Typical intraperitoneal spaces are cul-de-sac, Morison pouch, and subphrenic spaces
- Complex fluid collection with internal low-level echoes, membranes, or septations
- Bright linear echoes with reverberation artifacts representing gas bubbles; highly suggestive of infection
- Dependent echoes representing debris may produce a fluid-fluid level or gas may produce an air-fluid level
- Inflamed fat adjacent to abscess presents as echogenic mass
- Hypervascular periphery, avascular center of abscess; adjacent inflamed fat may be hyperemic
- Bedside US: For critically ill or postoperative patients, can be effective screening tool to localize intraperitoneal abscess or collections

- CECT: More sensitive for deeper, larger, or gas-containing collections and as screening test
- CECT: Oral and IV contrast for best accuracy

TOP DIFFERENTIAL DIAGNOSES

- Loculated ascites
- Lymphocele
- Biloma
- Other fluid collections
- Necrotic tumor/peritoneal carcinomatosis
- Gossypiboma
- Oxidized cellulose packing or other hemostatic agents

CLINICAL ISSUES

- Most common in postoperative setting
- Increases with age, diabetes, and immunocompromised patients

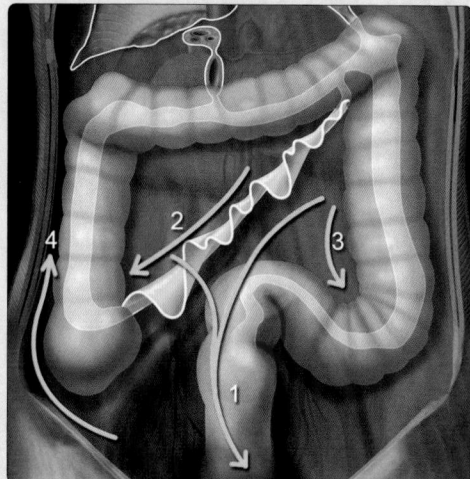
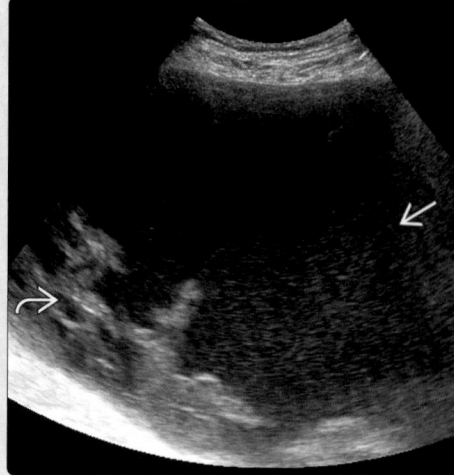

(Left) *Graphic shows preferential sites of peritoneal collections in the abdomen and pelvis. 1) Rectovesical or rectouterine pouch; 2) Right inframesocolic space; 3) Left inframesocolic space; 4) Right paracolic gutter.* (Right) *Transverse ultrasound of the midabdomen shows a large complex fluid collection with low-level echoes ➡ and irregular avascular mural debris ⊅. This was a chronic abscess.*

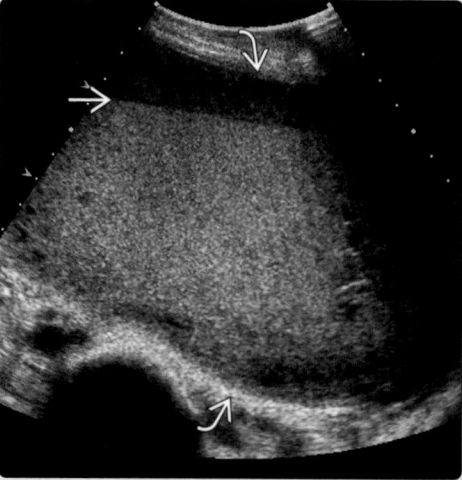
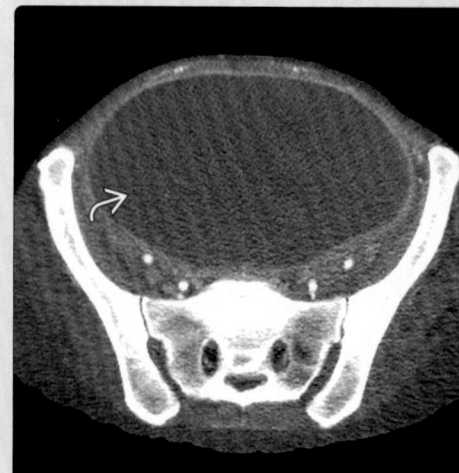

(Left) *Transverse ultrasound of the pelvis in a woman with fever and pain after gastrectomy for carcinoma is shown. There is a huge abscess ⊅ with a fluid-fluid level ➡. This was successfully drained percutaneously.* (Right) *CECT of the same patient confirms the extent of the abscess ⊅, but it does not show the fluid-fluid level.*

TERMINOLOGY

Definitions

Localized abdominal collection of pus

IMAGING

General Features

Best diagnostic clue
- Fluid collection with mass effect ± gas bubbles or air-fluid level

Location
- Anywhere within abdominal cavity
- Typical intraperitoneal spaces are cul-de-sac, Morison pouch, and subphrenic spaces

Size
- Highly variable; 2-15 cm in diameter or diffuse peritoneal collection

Morphology
- Hypoechoic or anechoic fluid collection ± septations and debris

Ultrasonographic Findings

- Grayscale ultrasound
  - Complex fluid collection with internal low-level echoes, membranes, or septations
  - Dependent echoes representing debris may produce fluid-fluid level
  - Bright linear echoes with reverberation artifacts representing gas bubbles; highly suggestive of infection
  - Inflamed fat adjacent to abscess presents as echogenic mass
    - Usually seen with abscesses due to appendicitis, diverticulitis, complicated acute cholecystitis, inflammatory bowel disease, and pancreatitis
  - Bacterial peritonitis: Primary or secondary to other intraabdominal infection or perforated viscus
    - Ascites with internal echoes from particulate debris or pus, loculations, internal septations, gas
    - Diffuse thickening of peritoneum (parietal and visceral), mesentery, and omentum
  - Postoperative peritoneal abscess
    - Close to site of surgery, around the tip of drainage catheter (if blocked), dependent parts of peritoneal cavity (supine patients)
  - Tuberculous peritonitis: Matted bowel loops with heterogeneous interbowel exudate
    - ± necrotic lymphadenopathy (mesenteric and retroperitoneal), may progress to liquefaction and abscess formation
  - Sclerosing peritonitis: Major complication of continuous ambulatory peritoneal dialysis (CAPD) with secondary infection
    - Hyperperistaltic bowel loops with both free and loculated ascites (earlier sign)
    - Later: Matted, clumped bowel loops tethered to posterior abdominal wall by uniformly echogenic enveloping membrane (1-4 mm thick)
- Color Doppler
  - Hypervascular periphery, avascular center of abscess; adjacent inflamed fat may be hyperemic

Radiographic Findings

- Radiography
  - Insensitive
  - Abnormal gas collection with air-fluid level
  - Soft tissue "mass" or focal ileus
  - Subphrenic abscess: Pleural effusion and lower lobe atelectasis

Fluoroscopic Findings

- Abscess sinogram
  - Useful after percutaneous drainage, defines residual cavity
  - Detection of fistulas to bowel, pancreas, or biliary duct

CT Findings

- Low-attenuation fluid collection with peripheral rim enhancement
- ± gas/mass effect/fat stranding

MR Findings

- T2-bright fluid collection with enhancing rim post contrast
- High T1 signal suggests hemorrhagic, proteinaceous, or mucinous content

Nonvascular Interventions

- US-guided: Diagnostic or therapeutic aspiration and percutaneous abscess drainage (PAD)

Nuclear Medicine Findings

- In-111 WBC scan preferred
  - Persistent nonphysiologic activity, focal or diffuse
- Tc-99m-labeled HMPAO WBC: Alternative for pediatric patients or patients with inflammatory bowel disease

Imaging Recommendations

- Best imaging tool
  - CECT: More sensitive for deeper, larger, or gas-containing collections and as screening test
  - Bedside US: For critically ill or postoperative patients, can be effective screening tool to localize intraperitoneal abscess or collections
    - US may be suboptimal due to limited patient mobility, open wounds, dressings, drainage tubes, paralytic ileus
  - MR: Alternative to CT for patients with contrast allergy or impaired renal function
- Protocol advice
  - CECT: Oral and IV contrast for best accuracy
  - US: Evaluation of dependent portion of peritoneal cavity or area surrounding operative site with transabdominal and transvaginal probes
  - Scanning over sites of tenderness improves detection, abscesses tender with transducer pressure

DIFFERENTIAL DIAGNOSIS

Loculated Ascites

- Evidence for cirrhosis or chronic liver disease
- Passively conforms to peritoneal space
- May contain septations and thinner, smoother wall

Lymphocele

- History of lymph node dissection or vascular surgery, adjacent to transplant kidneys
- Fluid collections along lymphatic drainage that may occur lateral to bladder
- Usually anechoic but may be multilocular

Biloma

- History of biliary or hepatic surgery
- Perihepatic fluid collection commonly in gallbladder fossa or Morison pouch
- Hypoechoic rounded collections or complex cystic collections

Other Fluid Collections

- Pseudocyst: History and signs of pancreatitis, may be complex with debris or hemorrhage, may be infected
- Hematoma: May be indistinguishable from abscess, aspiration required to exclude infection

Necrotic Tumor/Peritoneal Carcinomatosis

- Known primary malignancy, not febrile; associated with ascites, peritoneal nodularity, omental cake

Gossypiboma

- Gas- and fluid-containing collection around retained surgical gauze or cotton with history of abdominal surgery
- May be asymptomatic or present with acute or subacute infection
- Ultrasound: Heterogeneous; cystic with internal linear echogenicity or solid with hypoechoic and bright echoes; acoustic shadowing from gas, calcification, or fibrosis
- Characteristic radiopaque marker on radiography or CT, variable surrounding "mass" with fluid or gas

Oxidized Cellulose Packing or Other Hemostatic Agents

- History of surgery with use of such agents in preceding month
- Highly reflective mass lesion with posterior reverberation
- May have associated hypoechoic rim of fluid
- Gas density on CT or radiography

PATHOLOGY

General Features

- Etiology
  - Postoperative (most common) or post traumatic
    - Bowel anastomotic leak or bowel ischemia
    - Dropped gall stones; late presentation with abscess or fistula
  - Bowel perforation
    - Appendicitis, diverticulitis, Crohn disease, peptic ulcer
  - Complication of pancreatitis
  - Extension from visceral abscess: Liver, spleen, gallbladder, kidney, tubo-ovarian
  - Spontaneous bacterial peritonitis becoming loculated
  - CAPD with secondary infection

Staging, Grading, & Classification

- Organism: Bacterial, fungal, amebic
- Related to organ of origin (i.e., liver abscess)
- Intraperitoneal or extraperitoneal

- Communicating
  - Fistula to GI tract or biliary/pancreatic ducts

Gross Pathologic & Surgical Features

- Pus collection; often polymicrobial from enteric organisms
- Often confined by adherent omentum or bowel loops
- May or may not have peripheral fibrocapillary capsule

Microscopic Features

- Polymorphonuclear leukocytes (PMN) and white cell debris
- Bacteria, fungi, or parasites

CLINICAL ISSUES

Presentation

- Most common signs/symptoms
  - Fever, chills, abdominal pain, tachycardia, ↓ blood pressure if septic
- Clinical profile
  - Leukocytosis, with blood/peritoneal cultures and ↑ ESR

Demographics

- Epidemiology
  - Most common in postoperative setting
  - Increases with age, diabetes, and immunocompromise

Natural History & Prognosis

- Variable depending on extent of abscess, patient immune system status, and comorbidities, good prognosis when small and confined
- May progress to sepsis, septic shock, septic inflammatory response syndrome, and multiorgan failure

Treatment

- Dependent upon etiology, size of abscess, and patient factors
- Broad spectrum antibiotics
- Percutaneous ultrasound or CT-guided drainage
- Surgical drainage and washout

DIAGNOSTIC CHECKLIST

Consider

- Iatrogenic hemostatic agents or dilated hypoperistaltic bowel as mimic of gas-containing collection
- Other loculated fluid collections, such as pseudocyst, biloma, hematoma

Image Interpretation Pearls

- Appropriate clinical context and aspiration of collection required for diagnosis

SELECTED REFERENCES

1. Weledji EP et al: The challenge of intra-abdominal sepsis. Int J Surg. 11(4):290-5, 2013
2. Tirkes T et al: Peritoneal and retroperitoneal anatomy and its relevance for cross-sectional imaging. Radiographics. 32(2):437-51, 2012
3. Manzella A et al: Imaging of gossypibomas: pictorial review. AJR Am J Roentgenol. 193(6 Suppl):S94-101, 2009
4. Arnold AC et al: Postoperative Surgicel mimicking abscesses following cholecystectomy and liver biopsy. Emerg Radiol. 15(3):183-5, 2008

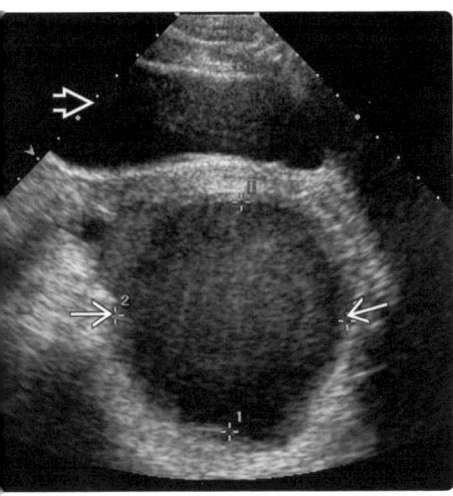
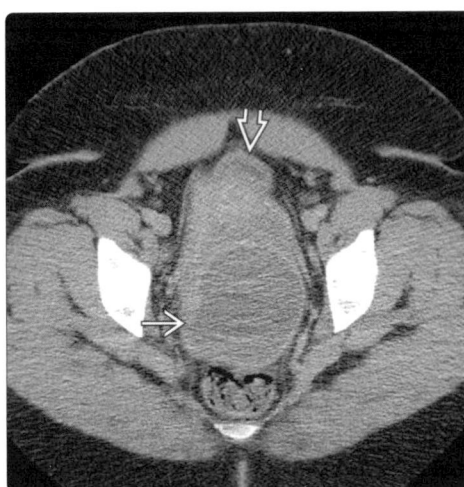

(Left) Transverse ultrasound of the pelvis in a diabetic woman postdilatation and curettage is shown. A thick-walled abscess is present in the cul-de-sac ➡, posterior to the bladder ➡. (Right) CECT of the same patient confirms the thick-walled abscess ➡. The bladder ➡ is empty.

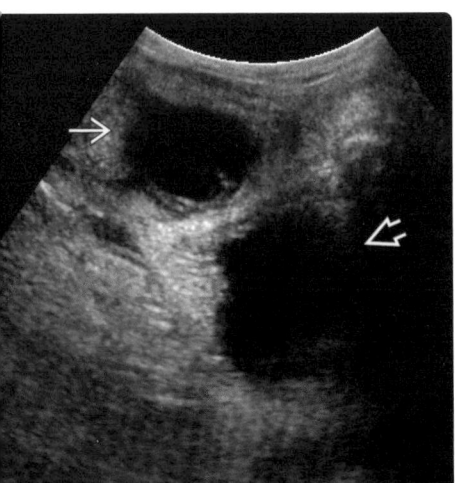
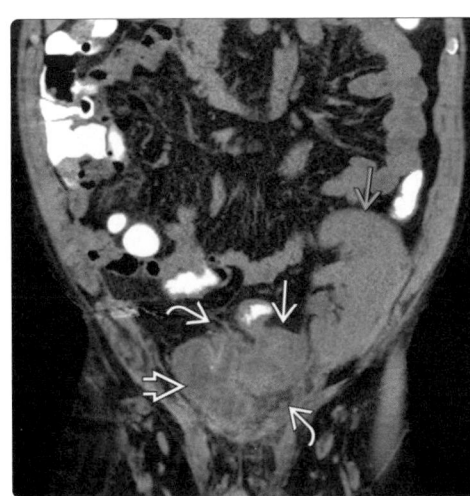

(Left) Longitudinal ultrasound of the midline pelvis in a patient with a renal transplant and a diverticular abscess ➡ is shown. The fat between the abscess and the bladder ➡ is inflamed. (Right) Coronal NECT of the same patient shows the abscess ➡ between the renal transplant ➡ and the bladder ➡. Inflammatory fat stranding ➡ is easier to recognize on NECT.

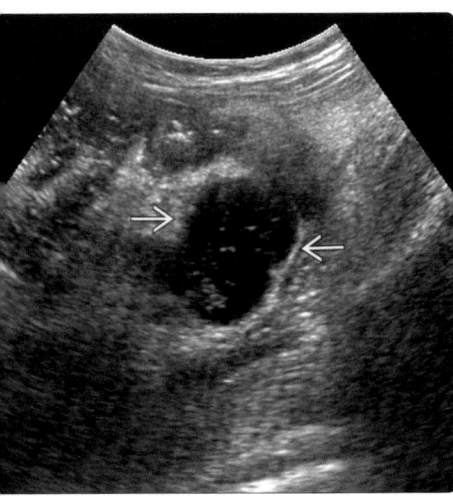
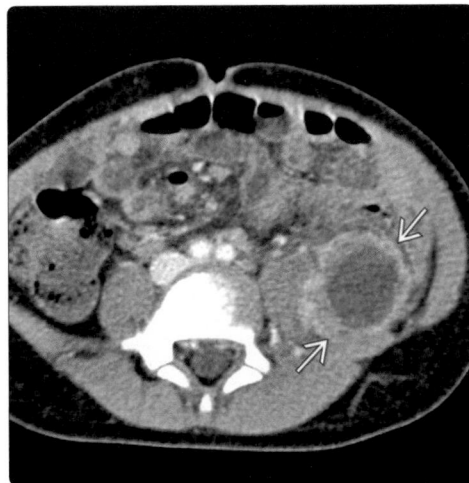

(Left) Transverse ultrasound of the left pelvis in a child post recent surgery for complicated appendicitis shows a unilocular fluid collection ➡ with internal echoes. (Right) CECT of the same patient confirms the collection but is superior at depicting the thick enhancing wall ➡ and adjacent structures.

KEY FACTS

TERMINOLOGY

- Vascular compromise of greater omentum (may be primary or secondary)

IMAGING

- Noncompressible focal echogenic fat at site of maximal tenderness
- CECT demonstrates focal fat haziness or, more commonly, a large (> 5 cm) nonenhancing heterogeneous omental mass with fat stranding
- Central dot sign may be present (central echogenic/hyperattenuating focus representing central engorged or thrombosed vessel/hemorrhage)

TOP DIFFERENTIAL DIAGNOSES

- Acute appendicitis
- Acute cholecystitis
- Right-sided diverticulitis
- Epiploic appendagitis

PATHOLOGY

- Primary OI may result from venous channel kinking or omental torsion (resulting in vascular compromise)
- Secondary OI may result from torsion due to: (a) attachment to an acquired lesion (e.g., surgical scar and neoplasm), (b) trauma, or (c) hernial incarceration

CLINICAL ISSUES

- Typical radiological appearances are diagnostic and management is conservative

DIAGNOSTIC CHECKLIST

- Typical cross-sectional appearances with normal appearances to adjacent structures
- Absence of symptoms and signs of sepsis
- Differentiate from more common causes of acute abdominal pain (especially acute appendicitis and acute cholecystitis)
- Most common in right side of abdomen

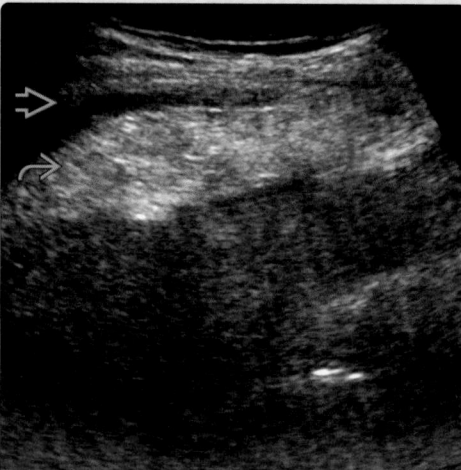
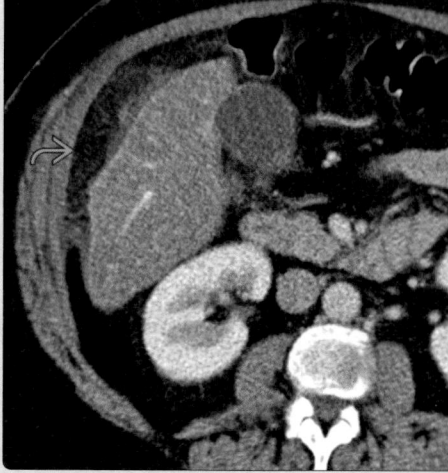

(Left) Transabdominal ultrasound of the right upper quadrant in a patient presenting with acute right-sided upper abdominal pain shows an echogenic elliptical mass ⊞ deep to the anterior abdominal wall ⊟. The adjacent gallbladder appeared normal (not shown). (Right) Axial CECT of the same patient shows haziness to the omental fat ➡ in the right upper quadrant corresponding to the ultrasound abnormality. Note the adjacent thin-walled, normal-appearing gallbladder.

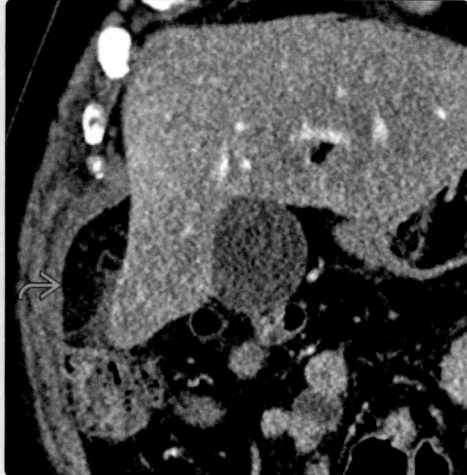
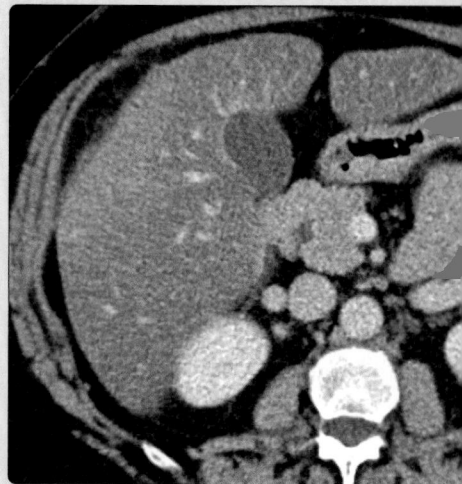

(Left) Coronal MPR from the same patient shows omental fat with haziness giving a mass-like ➡ appearance. Note the normal thin-walled gallbladder. (Right) Follow-up study after 3 months shows interval improvement with slow resolution of the radiological changes.

TERMINOLOGY

Abbreviations

- Omental infarction (OI)

Definitions

- Primary (idiopathic) OI refers to vascular compromise of omentum, ± torsion
- Secondary OI may result from torsion due to: (a) attachment to acquired lesion (e.g., surgical scar and neoplasm), (b) trauma, or (c) hernial incarceration

IMAGING

General Features

- Best diagnostic clue
  - Ovoid/cake-like predominantly fat attenuation/density omental mass
- Location
  - Located between abdominal wall and colon, usually on right side
    - 82% lower and 15% upper quadrant
- Size
  - Usually > 5 cm (3.5-10 cm)

Imaging Recommendations

- Best imaging tool
  - CECT is often diagnostic, non-operator dependent, and allows better depiction/interrogation
  - Focused high-resolution ultrasound at point of maximal tenderness with typical ultrasound appearances can be diagnostic
  - Often clinically unsuspected and ultrasound may be initially performed to exclude alternative diagnosis (e.g., appendicitis or cholecystitis)

CT Findings

- CECT
  - Abnormal omental fat located between rectus abdominis and colon
    - Appearances may be of focal fat haziness or, more commonly, a large (> 5 cm) nonenhancing heterogeneous omental mass with fat stranding
  - Central dot sign may be present (central hyperattenuating focus representing central engorged or thrombosed vessel/hemorrhage)
  - Normal appearances to adjacent colon, gallbladder, and appendix
  - Less commonly there may be free fluid and minimal colonic reactive thickening

Ultrasonographic Findings

- Grayscale ultrasound
  - Noncompressible focal echogenic fat with mass-like appearances, located directly beneath abdominal wall, at site of maximal tenderness
  - Color flow mapping shows mass to be avascular
    - Peripheral hyperemia may be present
  - Poorly defined nodular or linear hypoechoic avascular areas within hyperechoic mass

DIFFERENTIAL DIAGNOSIS

Acute Appendicitis

- Dilated noncompressible appendix (> 6 mm) ± appendicolith
- Ancillary findings: Periappendiceal fat stranding, reactive cecal/terminal ileal thickening, free fluid, ± appendicular abscess

Acute Cholecystitis

- Thick-walled gallbladder with pericholecystic edema/free fluid

Right-Sided Diverticulitis

- Presence of right-sided diverticula with associated colonic thickening

Epiploic Appendagitis

- Focal lesion (< 5 cm) located adjacent to sigmoid colon in majority of cases
- Presence of hyperattenuating ring sign representing inflamed visceral peritoneum, absent in OI

CLINICAL ISSUES

Presentation

- Most common signs/symptoms
  - Constant nonradiating right flank/lower abdominal pain gradually increasing in intensity over a few days
  - Local peritonism ± palpable mass
  - Radiological features lag clinical improvement
- Other signs/symptoms
  - Commonly afebrile, mild leukocytosis

Demographics

- Age
  - Adult predominance; 15% of cases occur in pediatric population
- Gender
  - Male predominance (2:1)
- Precipitating factors
  - Primary OI
    - Obesity (irregular accumulations of omental fat), anatomical omental variations (including accessory and bifid omentum and narrowed omentum pedicle)
  - Secondary OI
    - Hernia, neoplasm, adhesions, trauma, or postsurgical

Treatment

- Conservative management with nonsteroidal therapy

SELECTED REFERENCES

1. Yoo E et al: Greater and lesser omenta: normal anatomy and pathologic processes. Radiographics. 27(3):707-20, 2007
2. Baldisserotto M et al: Omental infarction in children: color Doppler sonography correlated with surgery and pathology findings. AJR Am J Roentgenol. 184(1):156-62, 2005
3. Singh AK et al. Acute Epiploic Appendagitis and Its Mimics. Radiographics. 25(6): 1521-34, 2005
4. Grattan-Smith JD et al: Omental infarction in pediatric patients: sonographic and CT findings. AJR Am J Roentgenol. 178(6):1537-9, 2002

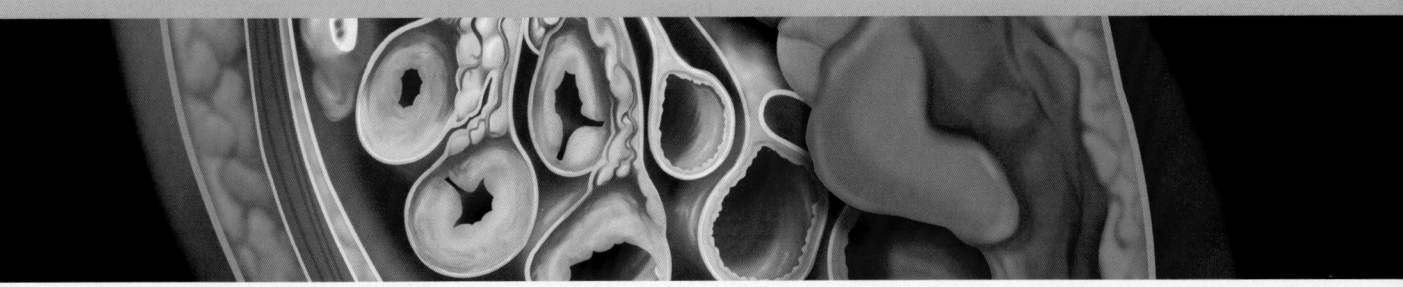

PART II
SECTION 9
Bowel

Introduction

Assessment of the bowel with ultrasound has been undervalued due to the commonly held perception that artifact (notably from gas in the lumen of the bowel) will limit visibility. The lack of awareness of normal and diseased bowel, limited technical expertise, and prolonged time of study are some compounding factors that have lead to a significant inconsistency in radiology departments for the application of ultrasound in the assessment of the bowel. US is safe, noninvasive, inexpensive, and does not use ionizing radiation. Real-time images can be obtained to provide a dynamic assessment. With the appropriate skills and knowledge, ultrasound has a valuable role in the assessment of patients with suspected and known bowel diseases. US remains the first-line imaging modality in acute abdominal conditions, particularly in Europe, hence a systematic approach and familiarity of the sonographic appearances of the spectrum of diseases affecting the bowel is crucial.

Anatomy-Based Imaging Issues

The gut is a long, tortuous, confluent hollow viscus that has a reproducible stratified layered pattern on ultrasound referred to as the gut signature. This alternating layered pattern corresponds to distinct histological layers of the normal bowel wall.

Five sonographic layers are identified as alternating hyperechoic and hypoechoic layers. These consecutive layers from innermost (layer 1) to outermost (layer 5) are listed below.

- Layer 1: Interface of lumen and mucosa
- Layer 2: Muscularis mucosa
- Layer 3: Submucosa
- Layer 4: Muscularis propria
- Layer 5: Serosa

There are typically three hyperechoic layers (layer 1, 3, and 5). These three hyperechoic layers are the interface of the lumen and mucosa, submucosa and serosa. The hypoechoic layers (layers 2 and 4) represent the two respective muscular layers; the muscularis mucosa (inner) and muscularis propria (outer), respectively.

The number of visible layers depends on:

- Frequency of transducer
- Proximity of transducer to gut wall

The trade off between the improved resolution with a high-frequency probe is the depth of penetration of the sound beam. It is ideal to maximize the frequency to obtain the best permissible resolution; however, this is reliant on the body habitus of the patient.

On a routine 5 MHz curvilinear probe, the transverse section of the bowel demonstrates a stratified target-like appearance with an inner hyperechoic layer representing the submucosa and a hypoechoic outer rim of the muscularis propria.

Using high-resolution linear transducer (12-18 MHz), the five distinct layers can be readily appreciated. On axial imaging, a pattern of concentric rings of alternating bands of hyper and hypoechoic rings can be seen.

The technological advances in transducers, combined with endoscopy, have lead to the evolution of endoscopic ultrasound technique. This represents the combined endoscopic and ultrasound assessment of the gut wall. The direct contact of the ultrasound transducer with the gut wall and high-frequency transducer allows for a focused assessment of a lesion, depiction of the depth of penetration in relation to the gut wall layers and lumen. In addition, histological assessment with needle biopsy is now also possible using this minimally invasive technique.

Normal bowel has an average maximal single wall thickness of 3-5 mm dependent on the degree of distension.

Fixed points of the bowel are easier to assess with transabdominal ultrasound: C loop of the duodenum, ileocecal junction, rectum, and recto sigmoid.

Features of small bowel loops are the central location, presence of valvulae conniventes, and active bowel peristalsis. In contrast, the colon has a heterogenous haustral pattern associated with a prominent linear arc of gas and posterior reverberation artefact.

Clinical Implications

US of the bowel:

- Can be part of routine abdominal scan for nonspecific broad range of abdominal symptoms
- Has an established focused role in suspected acute GI conditions, such as acute appendicitis, pyloric stenosis, and intussusception, especially in children and young adults
- Can be used for dedicated assessment of chronic gut-related disorders

In patients with Crohn disease, ultrasound has a role in:

- Detection of disease
- Evaluation of disease extent
- Detection of complication such as formation of abscess fistula, or obstruction
- Assessment of activity and follow-up of disease

Given the increasing use of ultrasound as the first-line modality, in addition to the standard assessment of the solid abdominal viscera, it is crucial for the operator to have an understanding of the principles of bowel ultrasound to avoid overlooking a GI tract-related diagnosis. The value is significantly felt in the younger population where ultrasound is much better tolerated and can significantly reduce the radiation burden of unjustified CT scans.

One of the inherent strengths of performing ultrasound is the instant clinical history and specific detail that is directly available from the patient. Ultrasound becomes an extension of the clinical examination and facilitates the diagnostic process. With accurate history and clinical signs, the operator can formulate a tailored approach to the ultrasound examination. Note that sonographic findings often overlap, hence the clinical history is crucial to determine the accurate diagnosis.

Imaging Technique

Routine transabdominal assessment of the bowel is typically performed after assessment of the solid abdominal viscera. The assessment of the bowel starts by using a standard 5 MHz curvilinear transducer. While scanning, it is important to optimize the settings, in particular the focal point and dynamic contrast, to enhance image quality. Recognizing useful landmarks such as the interface of the peritoneum with the abdominal wall and the psoas muscle provides an indicator of the depth of assessment and is helpful to avoid any confusion at the outset.

Given the relatively fixed position of the colon, the examination begins with identifying the cecum in the right lower quadrant. The characteristic blind ending arc of large bowel gas can be identified, which leads into the terminal ileum. The colon is first assessed systematically by performing a sweep along the entire path of the colon down to the sigmoid colon and rectum in the pelvis. The rectum can be visualized with a full bladder, which serves as an acoustic window. In certain circumstances, the transvaginal probe can be used to assess the rectum and pelvic loops of bowel that are obscured by bowel gas or adipose tissue on transabdominal scan. This process is repeated in a retrograde manner. When indicated, a focused assessment is performed of the appendix and terminal ileum. Then the small bowel is visualized with a generalized sweep over the four quadrants of the abdominal cavity.

Low-graded sonographic compression is applied when scanning the bowel. Normal bowel is readily compressible, shows peristaltic activity, and dispels intraluminal gas. This is a crucial observation in contrast to abnormal bowel, which is usually thick walled, rigid, demonstrates reduced peristalsis, and remains in a relatively fixed position. This technique also allows for the demonstration of localized peritonism, which increases the index of suspicion for underlying focal pathology.

Careful attention is required for the detection of thickened segments looking for alterations in the gut signature or focal mass lesions, in particular at sites of tenderness. Bowel presets that offer higher contrast images or adjustment of gain allow for the clearer demonstration of the gut signature and changes related to pathology. Any thickened segment should be assessed in two orthogonal planes. The effect on the gut wall layers should be scrutinized and the length of involved bowel documented.

The adjacent fat planes in thickened segments should be assessed for useful secondary signs, such as presence of extramural spread of disease, tracts, collection, enlarged lymph nodes, and inflamed hyperechoic fat. The inflamed hyperechoic fat is a useful clue and draws attention to the underlying thickened loop of bowel. These regions of interest should be reassessed more thoroughly using a high-frequency 5-12 MHz linear probe. While there is increased resolution, note that there is limited depth of penetration as a trade off determined by the body habitus.

Doppler assessment provides additional information regarding the vascularity of the bowel wall and adjacent fat; however, this technique has a limited sensitivity due to artifact. Increased vascularity is typically seen in infectious or inflammatory thickening and absence of flow can potentially indicate bowel ischemia. These findings require correlation with the underlying clinical context and baseline ultrasound images.

Contrast-enhanced ultrasound (CEUS) is now is being used to provide a more detailed and dynamic assessment of vascularity of thickened segments of bowel. CEUS is the application of intravenous contrast agent to conventional grayscale ultrasound imaging. The agent used is highly reflective, gas-filled microbubbles. The microbubbles enhance intravascular contrast by increasing ultrasound backscatter. The contrast agent can demonstrate intravascular blood flow as well as different phases of organ and bowel enhancement similar to CT and MR, hence disease activity and perfusion can

be assessed. This is a quick and safe technique, which can be performed at the bedside with no risk of nephrotoxicity.

The motility of bowel loops should be assessed. Ultrasound is a dynamic study and offers real-time imaging. US has a significant advantage over CT and MR, which can be hampered by artifact from spasm that may mimic a stricture.

The examination is completed with assessment of the stomach. The stomach and small bowel may be reassessed after providing the patient with oral fluid intake. Dedicated bowel ultrasound following luminal distension with water (US enterography) provides contrast, which allows for characterization of the gut wall and lumen. Routine use of this technique may not be feasible due to time constraints.

Limitations

Limited visualization when large amount of subcutaneous adipose tissue is present
- Hinders penetration of ultrasound waves, resulting in poor image quality
- Graded compression challenging

Overlying intraluminal bowel gas:
- May mask deep-seated pathology, such as retro-cecal appendicitis

Pathology-Based Imaging Issues

Meticulous assessment of the bowel wall thickness, effect on the gut signature and motility, in conjunction with the clinical history, forms the basis of ultrasound evaluation of the gut.

Benign disease: Inflammatory conditions
- Long segment involvement
- Uniform thickening
- Preservation and exaggeration of gut signature

Neoplastic disease; bowel carcinoma
- Short segment involvement
- Eccentric, asymmetric, and irregular mural thickening

These are general guidelines. Some conditions may overlap; for instance, in chronic sigmoid diverticulitis, the findings may mimic a cancer. With ischemia, there may be disruption of the layers due to bowel infarction.

Motility is typically reduced in both inflammatory and neoplastic conditions.

Ultrasound is useful in identifying fluid-filled, dilated loops of bowel in underlying bowel obstruction. The dilated loops can be traced downstream to identify the site and cause of obstruction at the transition point. Motility of the dilated loops is useful to distinguish ileus from a mechanical obstruction.
- Pitfall: Dilated loops can be adynamic in prolonged obstruction

Using these fundamental principles to approach bowel assessment, together with the clinical picture, an accurate diagnosis can be made.

Selected References

1. Muradali D et al: US of gastrointestinal tract disease. Radiographics. 35(1):50-68, 2015
2. O'Malley ME et al: US of gastrointestinal tract abnormalities with CT correlation. Radiographics. 23(1):59-72, 2003
3. Puylaert JB: Acute appendicitis: US evaluation using graded compression. Radiology. 158(2):355-60, 1986

(Left) *US depicts suboptimal resolution of bowel ⇨. This is due to a careless wide field of view and poor depth control, hence there is loss of detail of the bowel near the abdominal wall ⇨ and poor orientation. Image optimization is a key step in bowel ultrasound.* **(Right)** *US in the same patient following adjustment of the depth and field of view denotes normal cecum ⇨ and characteristic bowel gas pattern ⇨. There is normal compression of the terminal ileum between the abdominal wall and psoas muscle.*

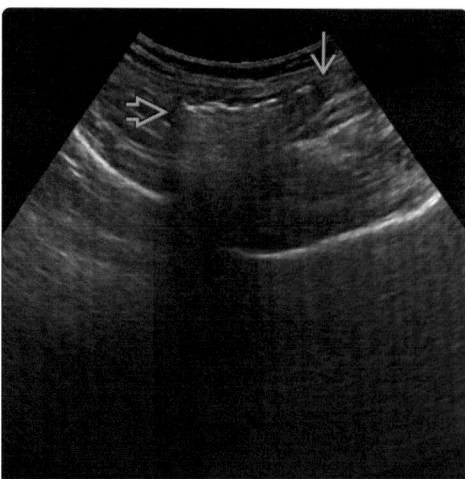
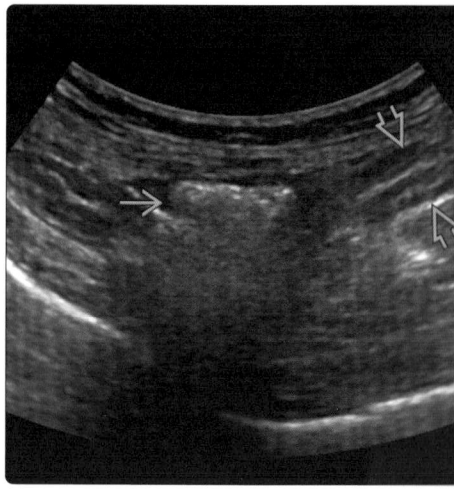

(Left) *Axial US in the right lower quadrant denotes useful landmarks of the peritoneal cavity. Note abdominal wall interface with the peritoneum ⇨ and the margin ⇨ with the psoas muscle ➡. Terminal ileum (TI) ⇨ is also shown. It is important to identify landmarks for correct anatomic orientation.* **(Right)** *Ileocecal junction ➡ is shown in the same patient using a 12 MHz linear transducer. TI ➡ and cecum ⇨ are noted. High-resolution transducer allows demonstration of the gut signature.*

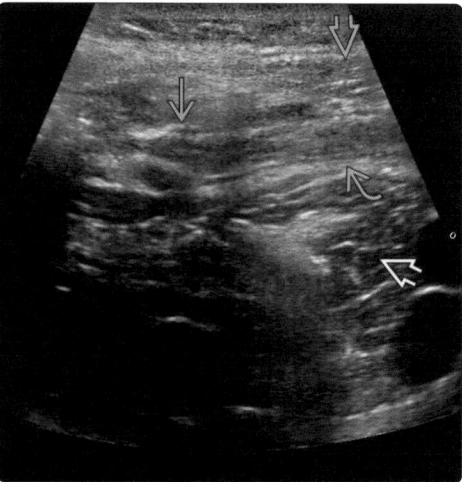
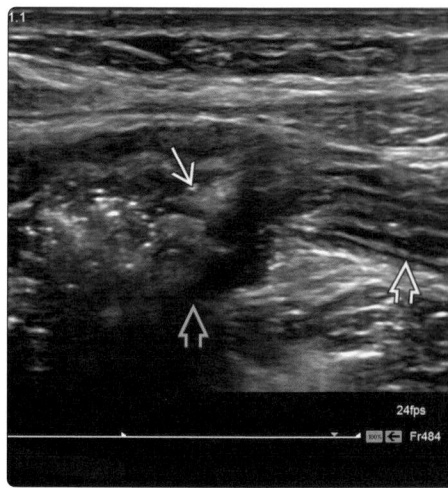

(Left) *Short axis US using linear high-resolution 12 MHz shows Crohn colitis. Calipers denote the single wall thickness of the colon. Note the exaggerated stratified layers of the colonic wall, a hallmark of benign inflammatory disease.* **(Right)** *Corresponding long axis US in same patient outlines the full thickness of the colon ⇨. This demonstrates preservation of the gut signature, a feature of benign inflammatory thickening. It is important to assess thickened segments in 2 orthogonal planes.*

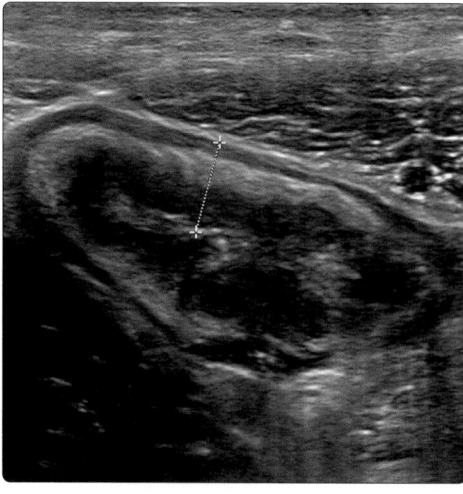
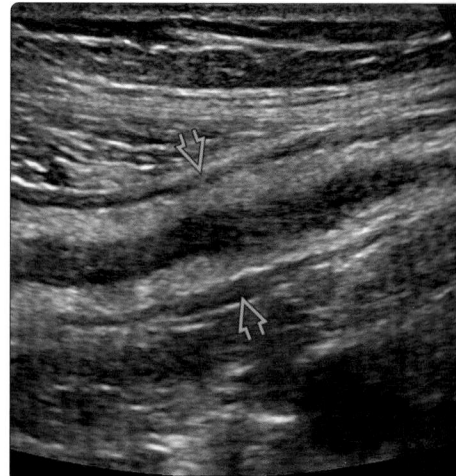

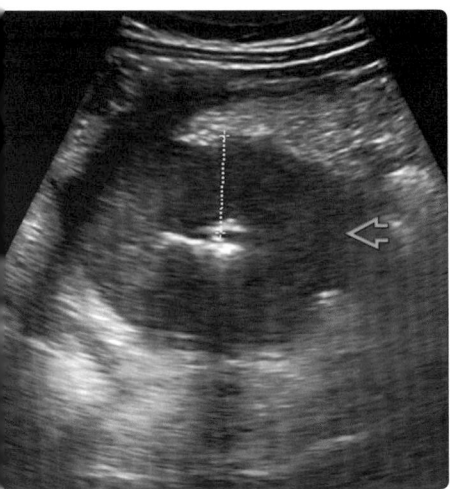

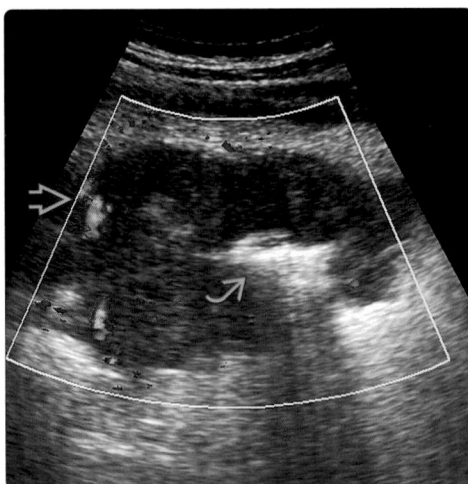

(Left) Abnormal circumferential thickening of the right colon ⇒ is shown. Calipers indicate the single wall thickness. Note the loss of the stratified layers of the bowel and lobular outline. These are hallmarks of neoplastic disease. (Right) Corresponding color Doppler US shows the relatively hypovascular nature of the colonic mass ⇒. Note linear arc of gas with reverberation artifact ⇒ denoting the stenosed ulcerated lumen.

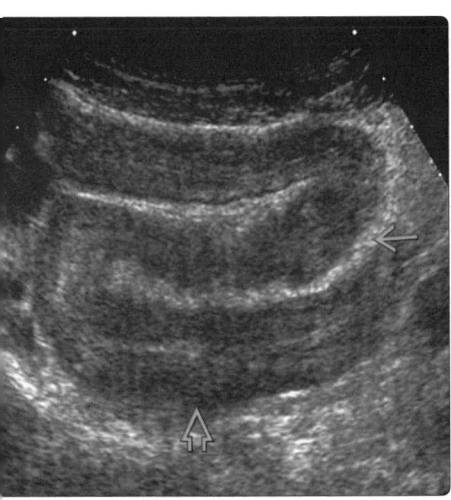

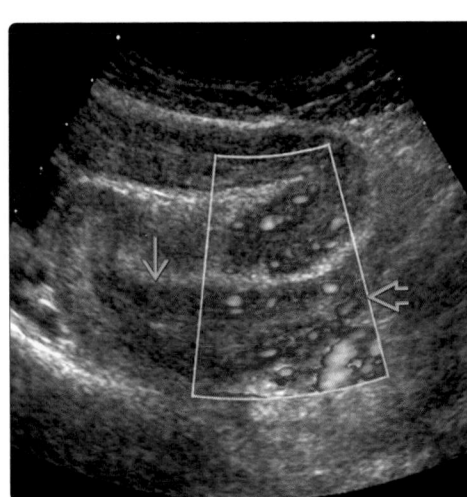

(Left) Axial US demonstrates long segment confluent thickening of centrally placed small bowel in a patient with known Crohn disease. Thickened segment ⇒ is angulated and rigid with surrounding hyperemic fat ⇒. This makes the thickened bowel more conspicuous. (Right) Corresponding US in the same patient shows increased vascularity ⇒ in keeping with a significant active inflammatory component. Note that with the presence of significant inflammation, there maybe loss of the gut wall layers ⇒.

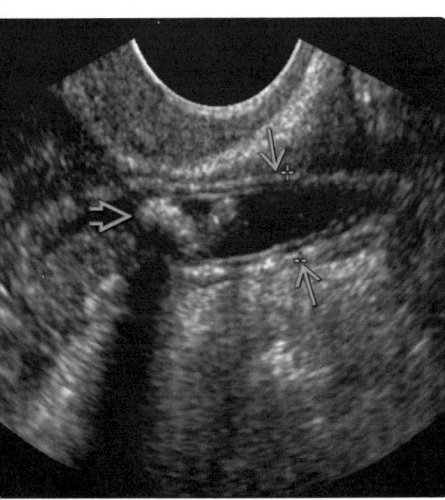

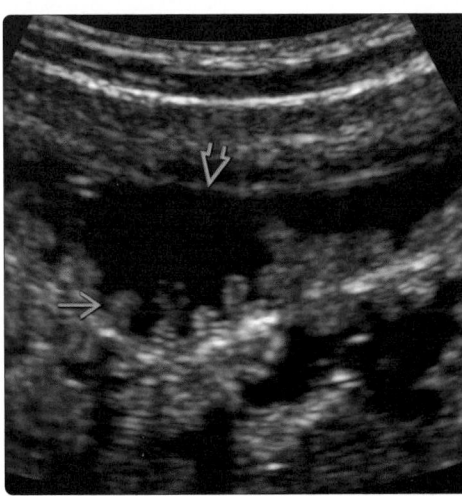

(Left) Transvaginal US (TVUS) shows a distended pelvic appendix ⇒ with calcified appendicoliths ⇒ in the base, in keeping with an acute pelvic appendicitis. This was not visible on abdominal US, hence the value of TVUS. (Right) Thickening of the valvulae conniventes ⇒ in the distal ileum and dilatation of the distal ileum with fluid ⇒ are shown in a patient with known celiac disease. This reversal of the small bowel folds and dilatation with fluid from impaired motility is clearly seen and well recognized in celiac disease.

Appendicitis

TERMINOLOGY

- Acute inflammation of appendix, which may be precipitated by obstruction of lumen

IMAGING

- US: Thick-walled noncompressible appendix (outer diameter ≥ 7 mm)
  - Periappendiceal edema seen as echogenic fat
  - Increased vascularity on power Doppler
- CT: Distension &/or wall thickening; single wall thickness > 3 mm
  - Hyperenhancement of wall
  - Periappendiceal inflammation seen as fat stranding
- Additional findings: Appendicolith, periappendiceal fluid
- US technique: Abdominal scan with graded compression
- US method 1st choice in children, thin young adults, and pregnant patients
- CT performed for patients with inconclusive US, if complications suspected, or in obese patients

- MR: Useful in pregnancy

TOP DIFFERENTIAL DIAGNOSES

- Mesenteric adenitis
- Cecal diverticulitis/ileocolitis
- Appendicular mucocele
- Normal appendix with mucosal lymphoid hyperplasia
- Appendiceal/cecal carcinoma
- Pelvic inflammatory disease
- Segmental omental infarction/epiploic appendagitis
- Meckel diverticulitis

PATHOLOGY

- Could be obstructive or nonobstructive

CLINICAL ISSUES

- Periumbilical pain migrating to RLQ; peritoneal irritation a McBurney point; atypical signs in 1/3 of patients
- Prognosis
  - Excellent with early surgery

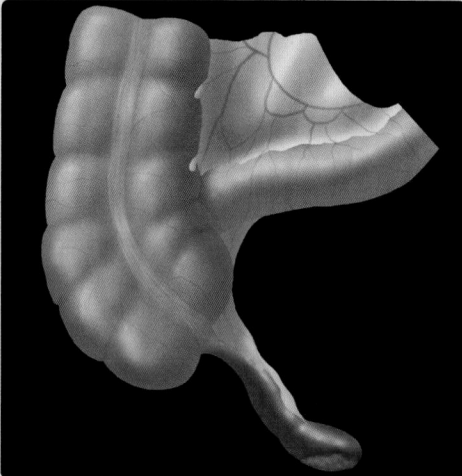
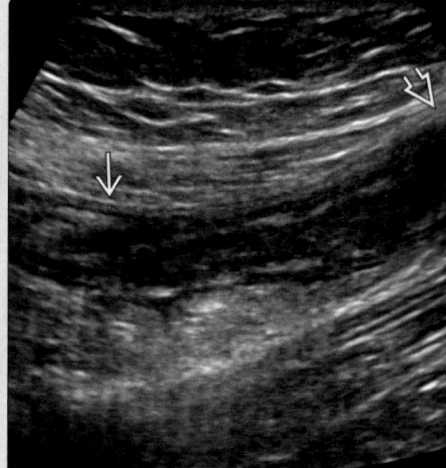

(Left) *Graphic shows the typical location and morphology of an inflamed appendix. The direction of the tip of the appendix and length can vary.* (Right) *Axial ultrasound through the right iliac fossa shows a thick-walled blind-ending ➡ tubular structure representing an inflamed appendix. Note the mural stratification ➡ and the base invaginating into the medial cecal wall.*

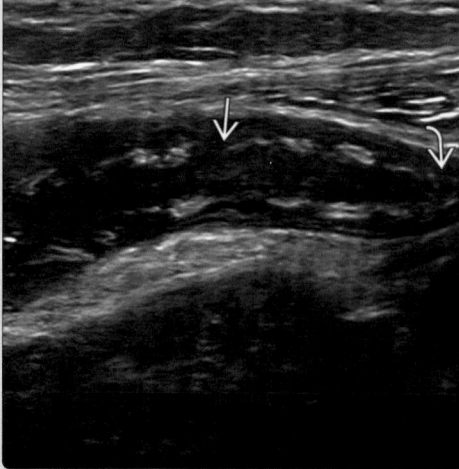
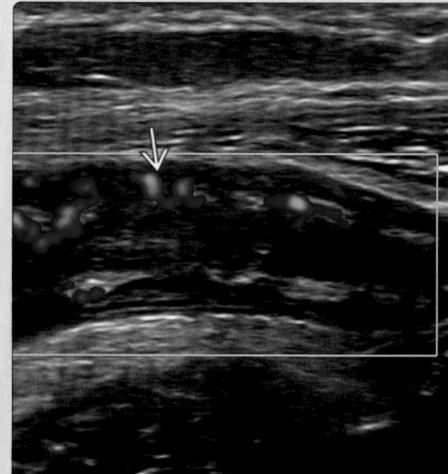

(Left) *In this axial oblique US of the same patient, note the blind-ending tip ➡ and mural stratification ➡.* (Right) *Power Doppler ultrasound of the inflamed appendix shows increased flow ➡.*

TERMINOLOGY

Definitions

- Acute inflammation of appendix, which may be precipitated by obstruction of lumen

IMAGING

General Features

- Best diagnostic clue
  - US
    - Thick-walled noncompressible appendix (outer diameter ≥ 7 mm)
      □ Lumen may or may not be distended
    - Periappendiceal edema seen as echogenic fat
    - Increased vascularity on power Doppler
  - CT
    - Distension &/or wall thickening; single wall thickness > 3 mm
      □ Wall thickening more reliable than maximum outer diameter
    - Hyperenhancement of wall
    - Periappendiceal inflammation seen as fat stranding
  - Additional findings include appendicolith, periappendiceal fluid
  - Increased caliber alone is not reliable indicator: Must be considered alongside history and other imaging findings
- Location
  - Base between ileocecal valve and cecal apex
    - Position of tip variable, depending upon length and direction
- Size
  - Length ranges between 2-20 cm
  - Wall thickening when inflamed
- Morphology
  - Blind-ending, worm-like extension of cecum

Ultrasonographic Findings

- Grayscale ultrasound
  - Thickened noncompressible appendix
    - Outer diameter > 7 mm, single wall thickness > 3 mm
    - May or may not be distended
    - Echogenic periappendiceal fat
    - Mural stratification seen in early stages
  - Sonographic McBurney sign over inflamed appendix
  - Gangrenous appendicitis: Loss of mural stratification
  - "Tip appendicitis": Changes involving only tip
  - Appendicolith may be present: Echogenic focus, with distal acoustic shadowing
    - Seen in obstructive type
    - When present, increased risk of perforation
  - Perforated appendicitis
    - Identifying appendix can be difficult
    - Marked periappendiceal inflammatory change
    - Fluid collection/abscess (thick echogenic fluid ± gas)
    - Loose appendicolith may be seen in collection
  - Additional findings: Dilated adynamic small bowel loops in right lower quadrant (RLQ), associated thickening of adjacent bowel

- False-negative US: Aberrant location of appendix, appendiceal perforation, early inflammation limited to appendix tip
- False-positive US: Distended noninflamed appendix from gas, fluid, and feces; thickened appendix from lymphoid hyperplasia
- Doppler
  - Increased flow on power Doppler within wall of appendix and periappendiceal inflamed fat
- Transvaginal US: For visualization of pelvic appendix

Radiographic Findings

- Radiography
  - Infrequently diagnostic
  - Appendicolith may be visible in 5-10% of patients

CT Findings

- CECT
  - Wall thickening
    - May or may not be distended
  - Hyperenhancement of appendiceal wall
    - Mural stratification seen in early stages
  - Periappendiceal fat stranding and fluid
  - Appendicolith
    - Can be seen as incidental finding
      □ In isolation not diagnostic of appendicitis
  - Arrowhead sign
    - Focal symmetric thickening of medial cecal wall at base of appendix
- Entire appendix should be scrutinized
  - "Tip appendicitis" may be early manifestation
- Excellent for identifying complications

MR Findings

- Overlap with CT findings

Imaging Recommendations

- Best imaging tool
  - US method 1st choice in children, thin young adults, and pregnant patients
  - CT performed for patients with inconclusive US, if complications suspected, or in obese patients
  - MR helpful during pregnancy; alternative to CT in children/young adults
- Protocol advice
  - US: Transabdominal scan with graded compression
  - CT: Optimal CT technique controversial
  - MR: Adding DWI improves reader sensitivity

DIFFERENTIAL DIAGNOSIS

Mesenteric Adenitis

- Enlarged and clustered lymph nodes in mesentery and RLQ
- Normal appendix
- May have ileal/cecal wall thickening due to GI involvement
- Diagnosis of exclusion, as other inflammatory conditions may show enlarged reactive mesenteric nodes

Cecal Diverticulitis

- Focal pericecal inflammatory changes
- Mild cecal wall thickening
- Visualization of thickened cecal diverticulum

Ileocolitis

- Mural thickening of cecum and terminal ileum; increased mural flow on color Doppler
  - Crohn disease
  - Infectious (e.g., *Campylobacter*, *Yersinia*, tuberculosis)

Appendicular Mucocele

- Well-encapsulated cystic mass, ± wall calcification
- No periappendiceal inflammation
- Onion skin appearance of mucus in lumen

Normal Appendix With Mucosal Lymphoid Hyperplasia

- Associated with infectious/inflammatory GI tract conditions
- Appendix may be thick walled; thick, smooth, inner hypoechoic band; no luminal distension
- Absent periappendiceal inflammatory changes/no hyperenhancement in wall

Appendiceal/Cecal Carcinoma

- Soft tissue density mass infiltrating &/or occluding appendicular lumen
- Usually little surrounding inflammatory infiltration
- Local and regional enlarged lymph nodes

Pelvic Inflammatory Disease

- Complex adnexal/tubo-ovarian mass
- Dilated fallopian tube with fluid-fluid level (pyosalpinx)

Ruptured Right Adnexal Ectopic Pregnancy

- Echogenic tubal ring and increased tubal mural vascularity, ± fetal pole (± cardiac activity)

Segmental Omental Infarction (SOI)/Epiploic Appendagitis (EA)

- Mass-like echogenic omentum in SOI, smaller echogenic mass in EA with focal tenderness
- Absent or minimal adjacent bowel wall changes

Meckel Diverticulitis

- Imaging findings may overlap with acute appendicitis
- No association with cecum

PATHOLOGY

General Features

- Etiology
  - Multifactorial
    - Ischemic mucosal damage, bacterial overgrowth, luminal obstruction (appendicolith or Peyer patches)
  - Secondary/reactive appendicitis
    - Crohn disease, reactive to adjacent inflammation

Staging, Grading, & Classification

- Could be obstructive or nonobstructive
- Gangrenous when there is necrosis

Gross Pathologic & Surgical Features

- Thickened appendix, which may or may not be distended
  - Appendicolith may be present

Microscopic Features

- Leukocyte infiltration of appendiceal wall
- Mucosal ulceration, necrosis if gangrenous

CLINICAL ISSUES

Presentation

- Most common signs/symptoms
  - Periumbilical pain migrating to RLQ; peritoneal irritatio at McBurney point; atypical signs in 1/3 patients
  - Anorexia, nausea, vomiting, diarrhea, fever
- Clinical profile
  - White blood cells may or may not be elevated

Demographics

- Age
  - All ages affected
- Gender
  - M = F
- Epidemiology
  - 7% of all individuals in Western world develop appendicitis during their lifetime

Natural History & Prognosis

- Treatment
  - Surgery if nonperforated or if minimal perforation
  - Antibiotic therapy alternative to surgery in nonobstructive appendicitis in some centers
  - Percutaneous drainage if well-localized abscess > 3 cm
  - Antibiotic therapy if periappendiceal soft tissue inflammation and no abscess
- Complications
  - Gangrene and perforation; abscess formation
  - Peritonitis; septicemia; liver abscess, pyelophlebitis
  - Bowel obstruction; hydronephrosis
- Prognosis
  - Excellent with early surgery

DIAGNOSTIC CHECKLIST

Consider

- Appendicitis in right clinical context when inflamed fat is seen in RLQ
  - Use graded compression to identify inflamed appendix
  - Nonvisualization of inflamed appendix does not rule ou appendicitis
- Other possible causes when no features to suggest appendicitis
- Perforated appendicitis when there is inflamed echogenic fat with fluid collection in right iliac fossa

Image Interpretation Pearls

- Blind-ended, aperistaltic, thick-walled tubular structure wi gut signature
  - May or may not be distended
- Sonographic McBurney sign with focal pain over appendix
- Presence of appendicolith associated with periappendicea inflammation is diagnostic of appendicitis

SELECTED REFERENCES

1. Park NH et al: Ultrasonography of normal and abnormal appendix in children. World J Radiol. 3(4):85-91, 2011
2. Pinto Leite N et al: CT evaluation of appendicitis and its complications: imaging techniques and key diagnostic findings. AJR Am J Roentgenol. 185(2):406-17, 2005
3. Andersson RE: Meta-analysis of the clinical and laboratory diagnosis of appendicitis. Br J Surg. 91(1):28-37, 2004

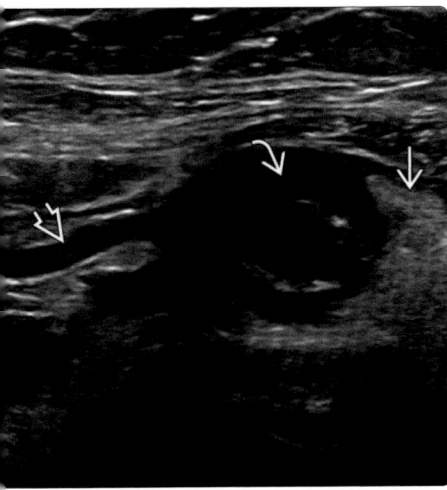
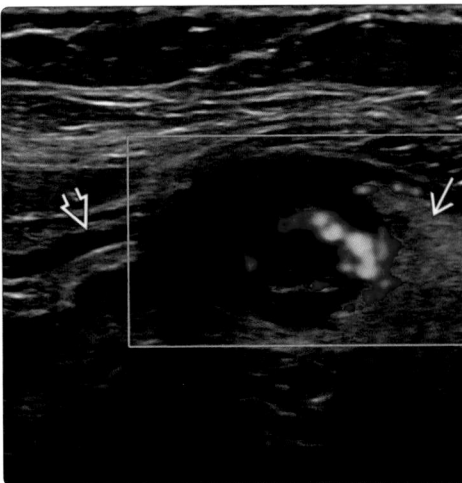

(Left) *Axial ultrasound through an inflamed appendix demonstrates a target-like ➡ appearance due to the preservation of mural stratification. Note the surrounding echogenic inflamed fat ➡ and a thickened inflamed parietal layer ➡ of the peritoneum, which is in contact with the inflamed appendix.* (Right) *Axial ultrasound of an inflamed appendix demonstrates increased mural flow on power Doppler. Note the surrounding echogenic inflamed fat ➡ and thickened parietal peritoneum ➡.*

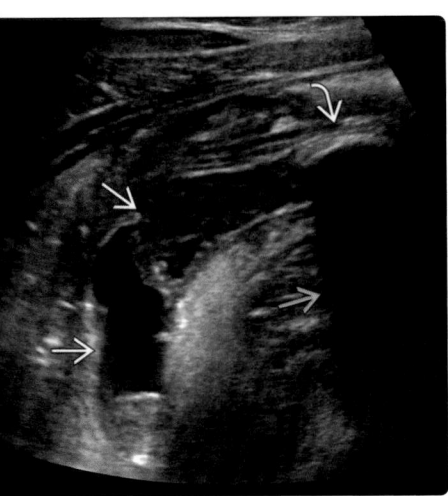
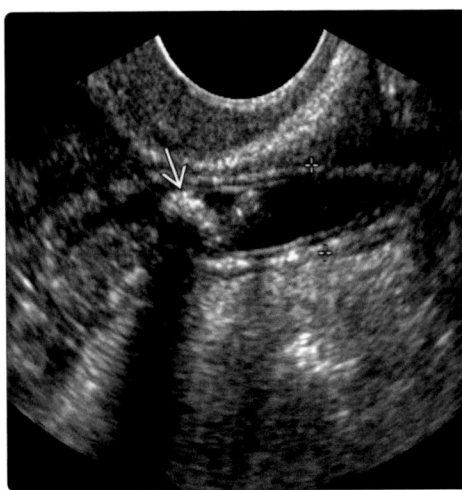

(Left) *In this ultrasound of obstructive appendicitis, note the distended appendix with an appendicolith ➡ at the base, curvilinear echogenicity with posterior acoustic shadowing ➡, and lumen distended with purulent exudate and debris ➡.* (Right) *Transvaginal ultrasound depicts a distended inflamed pelvic appendix with an appendicolith ➡ within the lumen, representing acute pelvic appendicitis. Note the stratified mural appearance to the appendicular wall.*

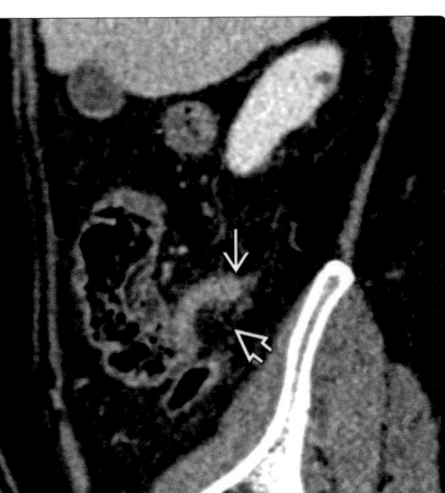
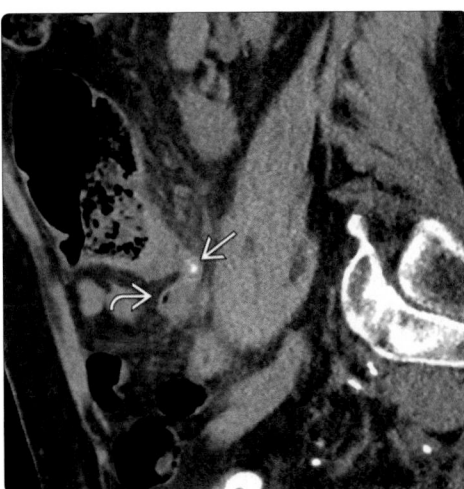

(Left) *Sagittal CECT reconstruction shows a thickened appendix ➡ with periappendicular fat stranding ➡ representing retrocecal acute appendicitis; ultrasound has a limited role in identifying these.* (Right) *Sagittal NECT reconstruction in a different patient shows a distended appendix with an appendicolith ➡ at the base and surrounding fat stranding representing acute appendicitis. Note the focus of gas within the lumen ➡.*

(Left) *Axial NECT through the right iliac fossa in the same patient demonstrates the inflamed, distended appendix* ➡️. *Note the poor definition of the wall and gas within the lumen.* (Right) *Coronal MPR NECT in the same patient shows the increased density and stranding in the surrounding fat* ➡️ *and a tiny focus of extra luminal gas* ➡️, *appearances representing gangrenous appendicitis on CT.*

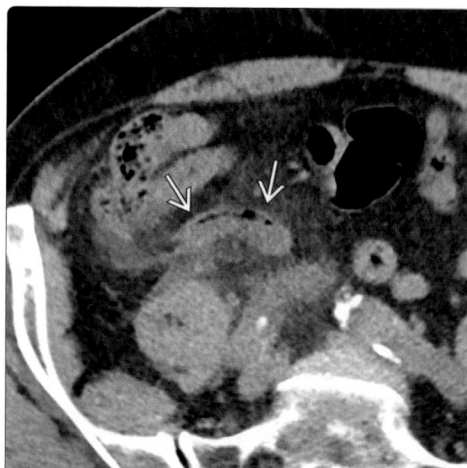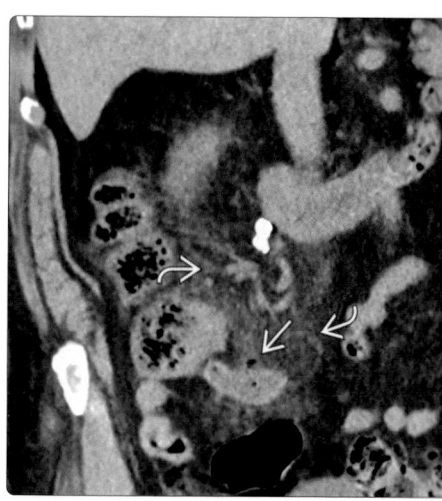

(Left) *Ultrasound through the right iliac fossa in a patient with previous appendectomy shows an inflamed, distended appendicular stump* ➡️ *containing luminal purulent exudate* ➡️. *Note the reactive thickening of the cecal pole* ➡️ *surrounding echogenic fat. (Courtesy A. Law, MD).* (Right) *Coronal CECT shows an inflamed appendicular stump* ➡️ *with an appendicolith* ➡️ *at the base. Note the surrounding inflammatory fat stranding and reactive thickening of the cecum* ➡️. *The ileocecal valve* ➡️ *is seen.*

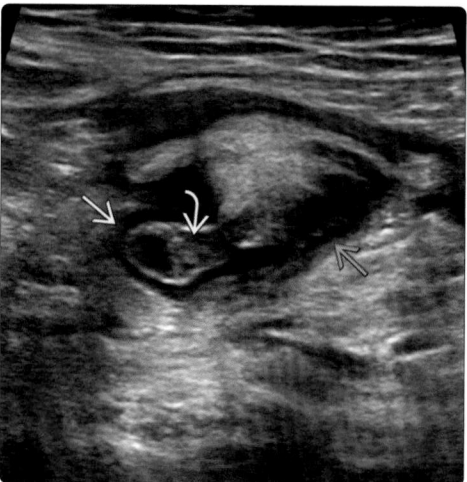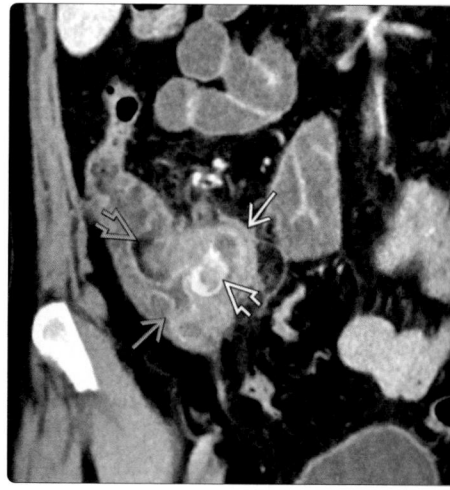

(Left) *Axial ultrasound through the right iliac fossa depicts phlegmonous appendicitis with a central collection* ➡️ *containing a loose appendicolith* ➡️ *secondary to appendicular perforation. (Courtesy V. Rudralingam, MD.)* (Right) *Axial CECT from the same patient shows the phlegmon* ➡️ *with a central loose calcific appendicolith* ➡️.

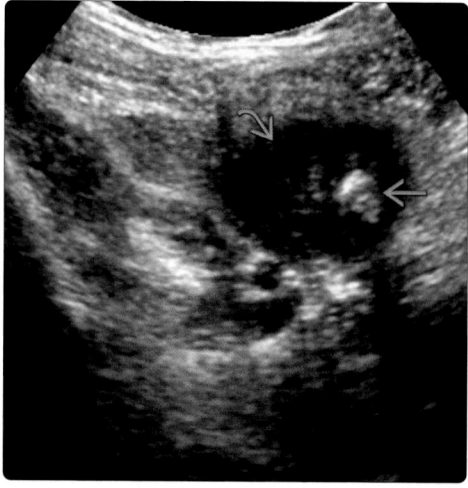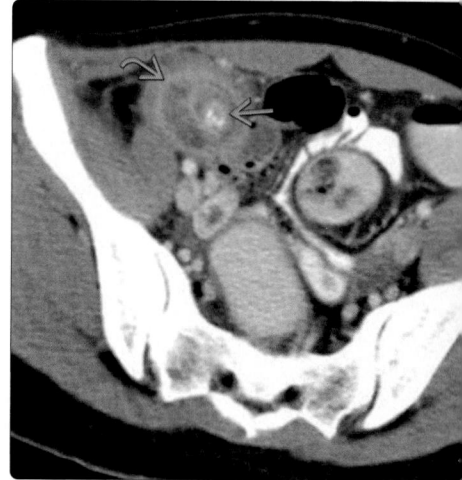

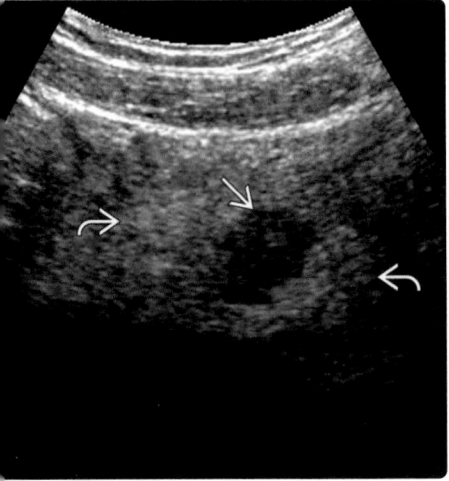
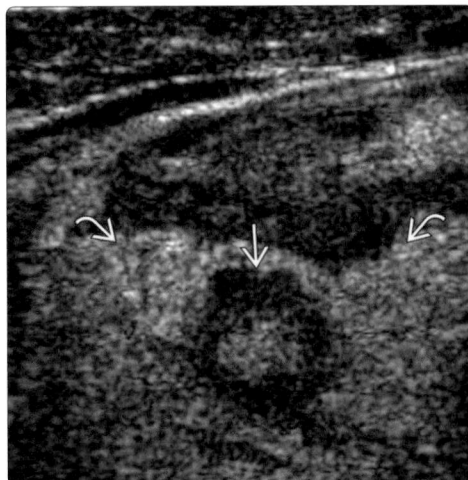

(Left) *Axial ultrasound shows an appendicular tip* ➡ *with loss of the stratified mural appearance representing gangrenous "tip appendicitis." Note the surrounding echogenic inflamed fat* ➡. (Right) *Oblique axial ultrasound in the same patient shows a more proximal part of the appendix with an inflamed thickened wall* ➡ *and surrounding inflamed echogenic fat* ➡. *(Courtesy V. Rudralingam, MD.)*

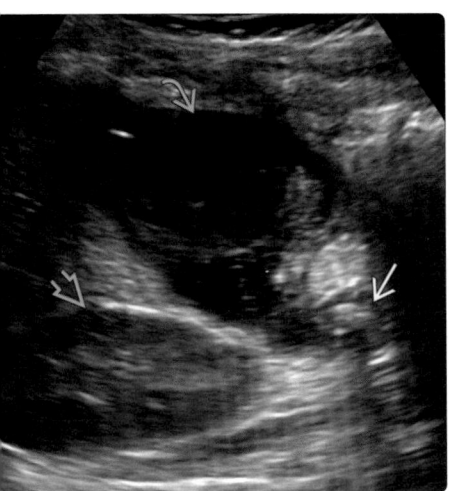
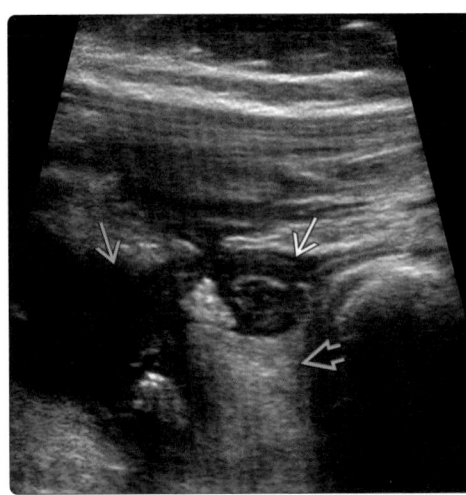

(Left) *Sagittal oblique ultrasound through the right flank shows an abscess* ➡ *with debris and an appendicolith* ➡ *at the dependent part from perforated appendicitis. Note the abscess extending cranially anterior to the right kidney* ➡. *(Courtesy A. Law, MD.)* (Right) *Sagittal oblique ultrasound in the same patient (at a lower level) shows the proximal part of the inflamed appendix* ➡, *the adjacent collection* ➡ *from tip perforation, and the surrounding inflamed fat* ➡. *(Courtesy A. Law, MD.)*

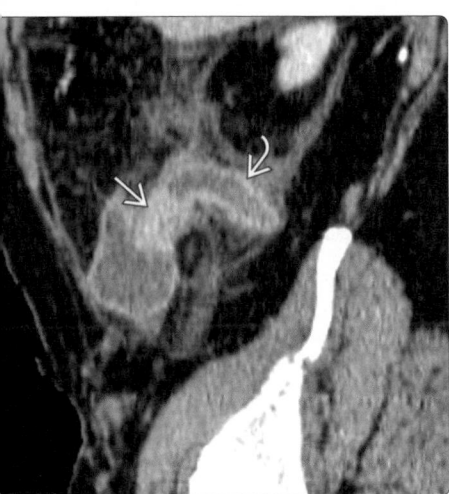
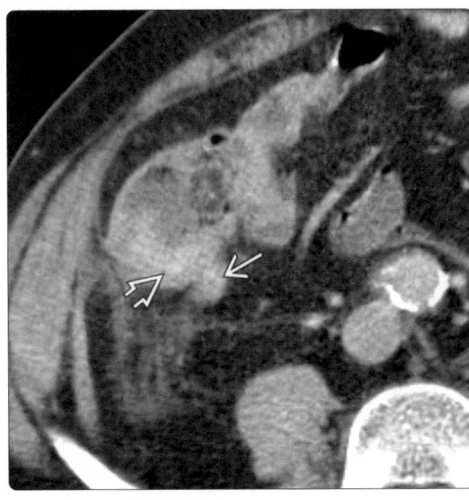

(Left) *Sagittal CECT shows an inflamed, distended appendix* ➡ *with surrounding periappendicular inflammatory changes. Note soft tissue* ➡ *at the base of the appendix that is causing the obstruction.* (Right) *Axial CECT through the appendicular base from the same patient shows the soft tissue* ➡ *at the appendicular base in continuity with eccentric soft tissue thickening* ➡ *involving the posterior wall of the cecum. At surgery, there was an infiltrative cecal carcinoma, causing obstruction and infection.*

TERMINOLOGY

- Distension of appendiceal lumen as result of mucin accumulation

IMAGING

- Distended tubular or pear-shaped cystic intraperitoneal structure in right lower quadrant, traced from medial wall of cecal pole
- Presence of calcification in wall strongly supports diagnosis of appendicular mucocele
- Concentric layering of dense mucoid material gives onion skin appearance on ultrasound
- Contrast-enhanced CT scan is best imaging tool

TOP DIFFERENTIAL DIAGNOSES

- Cystic ovarian neoplasm
- Hydrosalpinx
- Tubo-ovarian abscess
- Duplication cyst

- Appendiceal obstruction from appendiceal carcinoma
- Obstructive acute appendicitis
- Mesenteric cyst

PATHOLOGY

- Commonly caused by epithelial proliferation, which could be benign or malignant
- Less commonly secondary to obstructive causes

CLINICAL ISSUES

- Most common presentation is right lower quadrant pain o palpable mass
- Frequently discovered incidentally
- Pseudomyxoma peritonei (PMP): Serious complication of spontaneous or iatrogenic rupture of appendicular mucocele (benign or malignant)
- Preoperative differentiation of benign and malignant mucoceles challenging

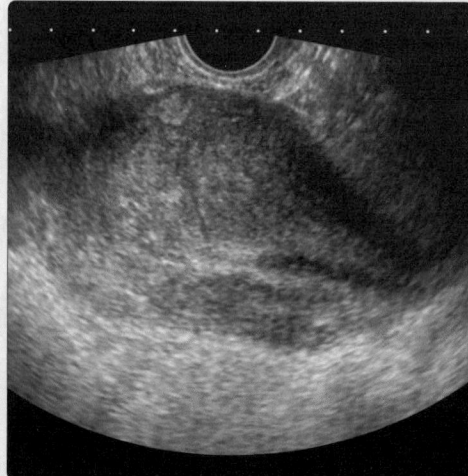 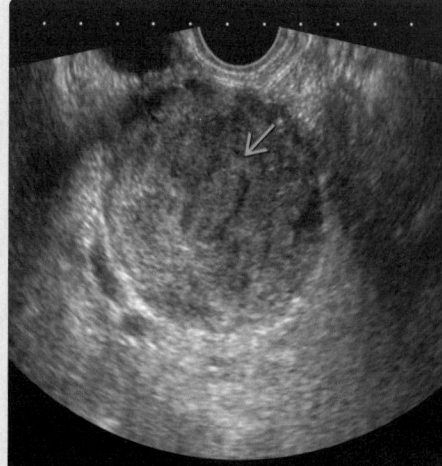

(Left) Longitudinal transvaginal ultrasound shows well-marginated, complex, cystic mass containing dense mucoid material giving onion skin appearance. (Right) Transvaginal axial ultrasound image shows the central echogenic inspissated mucoid material ➡.

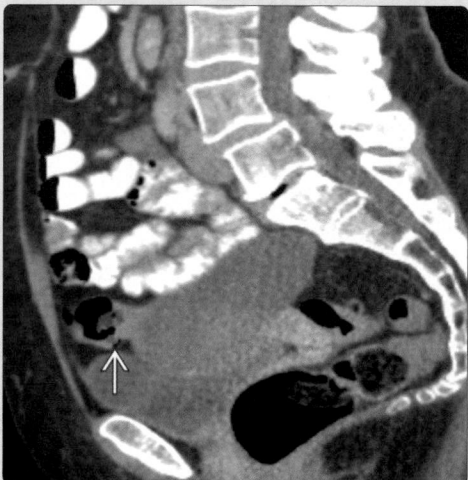 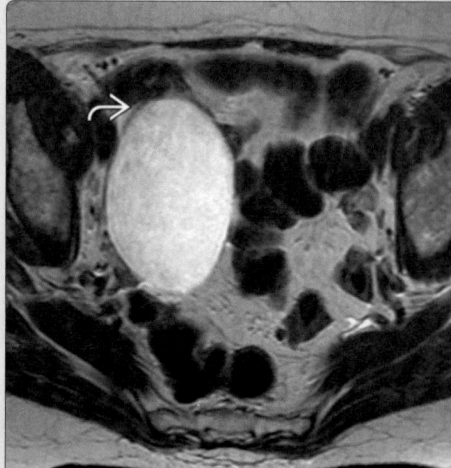

(Left) Sagittal MPR image from a CECT of the same patient shows a tubular cystic structure with the base ➡ attached to the cecal pole. Note the central homogeneous low attenuation. (Right) T2 axial image in the same patient shows the cystic mass with contents of uniform high signal intensity. The base ➡ traced to the cecal pole.

TERMINOLOGY

Definitions

Distension of appendiceal lumen as result of mucin accumulation
- Macroscopic description and not pathologic diagnosis

IMAGING

General Features

Best diagnostic clue
- Distended tubular, round or pear-shaped cystic intraperitoneal structure in right lower quadrant traced from cecal pole
- Presence of calcification in wall strongly supports diagnosis

Location
- Right lower quadrant of abdomen

Size
- Transverse diameter: 1.5-7.0 cm
  - Giant mucoceles can grow up to 25 cm in size

Morphology
- Tubular, round or pear-shaped cystic structure

Ultrasonographic Findings

Grayscale ultrasound
- Cystic tubular or pear-shaped structure
  - ± acoustic shadowing from mural calcification
- Intraluminal contents can have a variable appearance
  - Typically low-level echoes
  - Sometimes concentric layering of dense mucoid material producing onion skin appearance
- Transvaginal pelvic ultrasound improves image quality and helps to differentiate from ovarian cystic masses in women with pelvic appendiceal mucoceles
- Soft tissue thickening and irregularity of mucocele wall suggest malignancy
- Fecalith or appendicolith may be visible in obstructive type (simple mucocele)
- Echogenic surrounding inflamed fat seen in acute obstructive type and in inflamed or perforated appendicular mucoceles

CT Findings

CECT
- Cystic tubular, round or pear-shaped, well-encapsulated mass with base indistinguishable from appendicular base
- Central homogeneous low attenuation (15-25 HU) with peripheral enhancing wall
- Wall calcification seen in < 50% of cases
  - Calcification can be punctate or curvilinear
- Atypical features reflect secondary complication, such as infection/perforation, malignancy, or unusual underlying pathology
  - Soft tissue thickening and irregularity of wall
  - Soft tissue stranding in surrounding fat
- Intraluminal gas bubbles or air-fluid level within mucocele are indicative of super added infection
- Myxoglobulosis is rare mucocele variant where there are multiple intraluminal, small, pearly filling defects, which may be visible on CT if calcified

- Intussusception into colon is rare complication of appendiceal mucocele
  - Cystic leading point may be visible
- Dense calcific appendicolith or fecalith may be visible in simple obstructive form of appendiceal mucocele
- **CTC**
  - On 3D endoluminal view mucoceles cause smooth impression in medial aspect of cecal pole, suggesting extramucosal or extrinsic compression
    - Similar appearance also noted at endoscopy

MR Findings

- T1WI
  - Cystic structure with base indistinguishable from appendix
  - Contents homogeneous and hypo- or isointense
  - Wall calcification less apparent
- T2WI
  - Contents homogeneous and hyperintense
- T1WI C+
  - Enhancing wall
  - Centrally homogeneous and hypo- or isointense

Imaging Recommendations

- Best imaging tool
  - Contrast-enhanced CT scan
    - Relationship of cystic mass and cecum is easily identified, especially with multiplanar reformations
    - More sensitive in detecting wall calcification
- Protocol advice
  - Contrast-enhanced CT of abdomen and pelvis
    - Oral contrast optional

DIFFERENTIAL DIAGNOSIS

Cystic Ovarian Neoplasm

- Appendicular mucoceles are intraperitoneal and can mimic cystic ovarian and tubal masses in females
  - Appendix identified separately
  - Right gonadal vessels traced to cystic mass

Hydrosalpinx

- Tubular structure traced to uterine cornu with narrow medial and wide distal ends
- Hydrosalpinx has partial folds and small mural nodules producing characteristic 'cogwheel' appearance
- Appendix identified separately

Tubo-Ovarian Abscess

- Usually bilateral
- Multilocular thick-walled collections with internal debris and peripheral hyperemia
- Clinical signs and symptoms of infection

Duplication Cyst

- Thin walled with all 3 layers of the bowel wall (gut signature), sometimes visible on trans abdominal ultrasound
- May or may not be adjacent to bowel

Appendiceal Obstruction From Appendiceal Carcinoma/Cecal Carcinoma

- Distended appendix

- Infiltrative mass ± enlarged nodes

Obstructive Acute Appendicitis

- Peri appendiceal echogenic fat
- Focal tenderness and clinical findings

Mesenteric Cyst

- Usually lymphangioma
- Closely associated with bowel wall
- Septations seen on ultrasound and MR

Distended Meckel Diverticulum

- Appendix identified separately
- Fluid-filled tubular structure with base in antimesenteric border of distal ileum

PATHOLOGY

General Features

- Etiology
  - Commonly caused by epithelial proliferation, which could be benign or malignant
  - Less commonly secondary to obstructive causes
    - Fecalith or appendicolith
    - Inflammatory or fibrotic narrowing
    - Rarely from deep infiltrative endometriosis

Staging, Grading, & Classification

- Simple mucocele secondary to inflammation and nonneoplastic obstruction (simple retention cysts)
  - Rarely exceed 2.0 cm in diameter
- Mucocele secondary to
  - Focal or diffuse mucosal hyperplasia
  - Low-grade mucinous cystadenoma (low-grade appendiceal mucinous neoplasm [LAMN])
  - Mucinous cystadenocarcinoma
- Classification of appendiceal mucinous neoplasms is controversial and terminology inconsistent
- Simple mucocele and mucocele secondary to mucosal hyperplasia are referred to as nonneoplastic mucocele
- Mucocele secondary to LAMN is referred to as benign neoplastic mucocele
- Mucocele secondary to mucinous cystadenocarcinoma is referred to as malignant mucocele

Gross Pathologic & Surgical Features

- Round or oval cystic mass with thick fibrous capsule
- Lumen filled with translucent yellowish mucoid fluid

CLINICAL ISSUES

Presentation

- Most common signs/symptoms
  - Frequently discovered incidentally
    - Asymptomatic in 25% patients
  - Most common presentation is right lower quadrant pain or palpable mass
    - Found in up to 50% patients
- Other signs/symptoms
  - Superinfection of tumoral mucocele may clinically resemble nontumoral acute appendicitis
  - Simple mucoceles secondary to obstruction and inflammation can clinically present as acute appendicitis
  - Rarely presents as intussusception

Demographics

- Age
  - Middle aged or older
- Gender
  - More frequent in females
- Epidemiology
  - Reported prevalence in appendectomy specimens is 0.2 0.3%

Natural History & Prognosis

- Pseudomyxoma peritonei (PMP): Serious complication of spontaneous or iatrogenic rupture of appendicular mucocele, which could be benign or malignant
  - Incidence of perforation and PMP is ~ 20% in benign mucinous cystadenomas and 6% in malignant cystadenocarcinoma
- Appendiceal mucocele is associated with increased incidence of colon adenocarcinoma

Treatment

- Options, risks, complications
  - Treatment of choice for simple mucocele is appendectomy
  - Cecectomy is performed for benign mucoceles
  - Right hemicolectomy is performed for mucinous cystadenocarcinoma
    - Open laparotomy is preferred to avoid perforation, which has risk of pseudomyxoma peritonei
  - Preoperative differentiation of benign and malignant mucoceles challenging
    - Irregular wall and internal soft tissue nodularity of mucoceles suggestive of malignant mucoceles
    - Frozen section useful

DIAGNOSTIC CHECKLIST

Consider

- Appendicular mucocele in differential diagnosis of cystic right lower quadrant mass

Image Interpretation Pearls

- Cystic tubular or pear-shaped cystic structure in right lower quadrant
- Base indistinguishable from appendix
- Calcification in wall suggestive of appendicular mucocele
- Echogenic contents with onion skin sign on ultrasound specific for appendicular mucocele
- Appendicolith seen at base in simple appendicular mucocele of obstructive type
- Irregular wall and internal soft tissue nodularity of mucoceles suggestive of malignant mucocele

SELECTED REFERENCES

1. Attarde V et al: Sonographic appearance of a giant appendicular mucocele. Clin Ultrasound. 39(5):290-2, 2011
2. Caspi B et al: The onion skin sign: a specific sonographic marker of appendiceal mucocele. J Ultrasound Med. 23(1):117-21; quiz 122-3, 2004
3. Wang H et al: Appendiceal mucocele: A diagnostic dilemma in differentiat malignant from benign lesions with CT. AJR Am J Roentgenol. 201(4):W59 5, 2013
4. Pickhardt PJ et al: Primary neoplasms of the appendix: radiologic spectrum of disease with pathologic correlation. Radiographics. 23(3):645-62, 2003

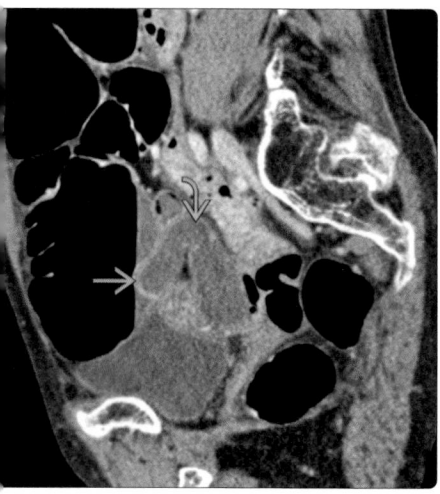

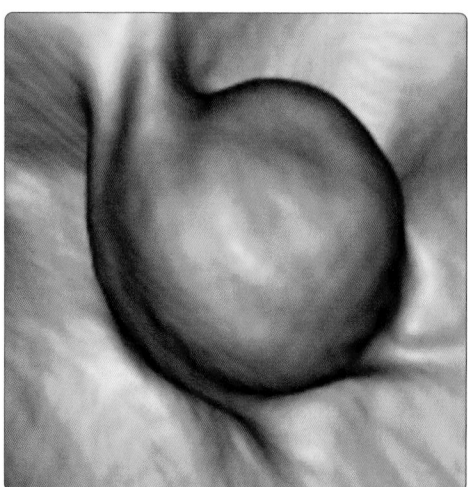

(Left) *Sagittal MPR image from a CT colonography study performed for anemia shows an incidental appendicular mucocele. The base ➡ of the distended appendix ⊡ projects into the cecal lumen.* (Right) *Endoluminal view from the prone series of the same study demonstrates smooth extrinsic compression into the cecal lumen.*

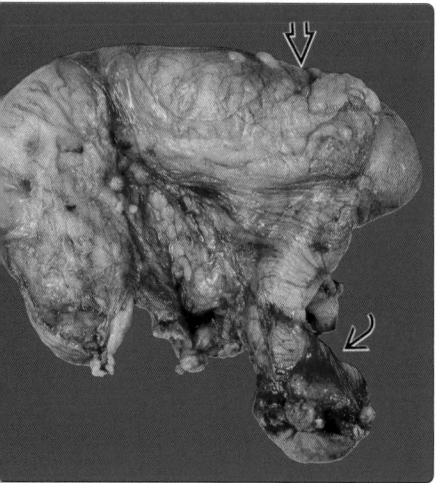

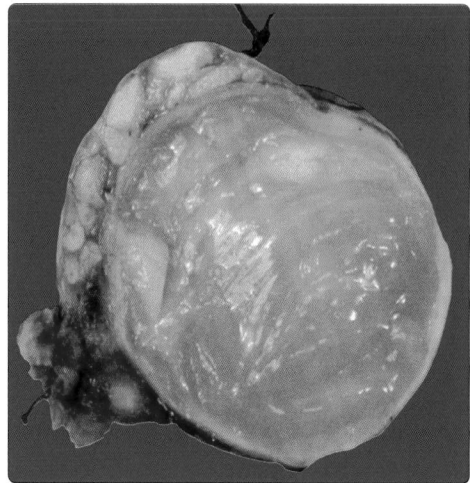

(Left) *Photograph of gross specimen shows resected appendicular mucocele ➡ attached to the cecum ⊡.* (Right) *Macroscopic cross section of the resected specimen shows the typical appearance of the yellowish, jelly-like mucinous content. Histology confirmed low-grade mucinous tumor of the appendix.*

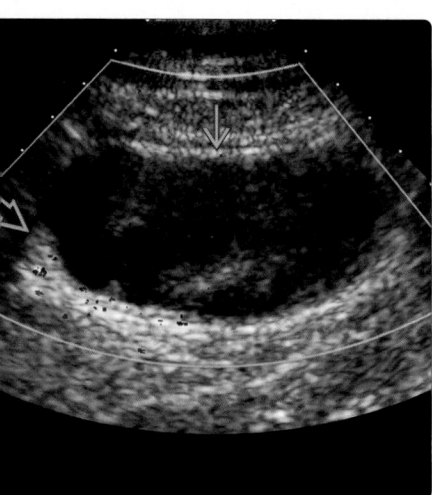

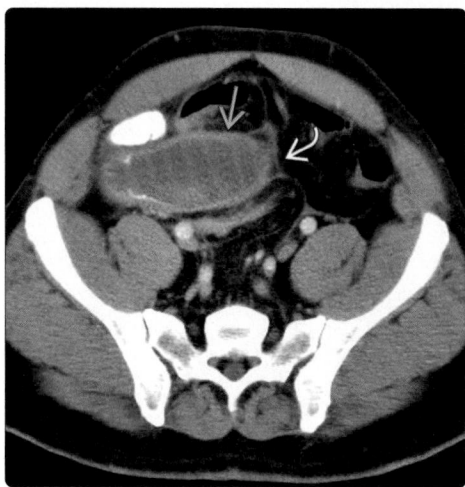

(Left) *Longitudinal color Doppler ultrasound of the right lower quadrant in a patient who presented with fullness shows mucocele ➡ containing mixed echogenicity contents with no internal color flow. Note the posterior acoustic enhancement ⊡.* (Right) *Axial CECT in the portal venous phase of a mucocele ➡ with fine mural calcification shows mild surrounding fat infiltration ➡.*

Intussusception

TERMINOLOGY

- Invagination or telescoping of 1 segment of gastrointestinal tract and its mesentery (intussusceptum) into lumen of adjacent distal segment (intussuscipiens)

IMAGING

- "Bowel within bowel" appearance
- Occurs anywhere from stomach to rectum
- Ultrasound: High sensitivity (98-100%) and specificity (88-100%); first-line in children
- Concentric parallel rings of bowel wall (target, doughnut, or bull's-eye sign)
- Layering of fluid trapped between compressed bowel segments
- Signs of vascular compromise with reduced or absent mural vascularity of intussusceptum; indicates risk of ischemia/infarction and perforation

TOP DIFFERENTIAL DIAGNOSES

- Tumor, inflammation, infection

PATHOLOGY

- Children: Idiopathic in 95%
- Adults: Identifiable etiology in 90%, lead point, or underlying condition such as celiac or Whipple disease
- Transient intussusception: Nonobstructing, spontaneous resolution

CLINICAL ISSUES

- Children: Acute pain, palpable mass, "red currant jelly" stools
- Adults: Insidious, vague abdominal symptoms, vomiting, red blood in stool
- Complications: Obstruction, bowel ischemia, or infarction
- Surgery indicated where lead point identified or complications evident on CT

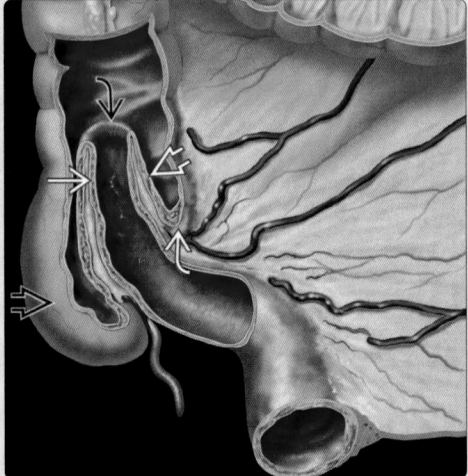
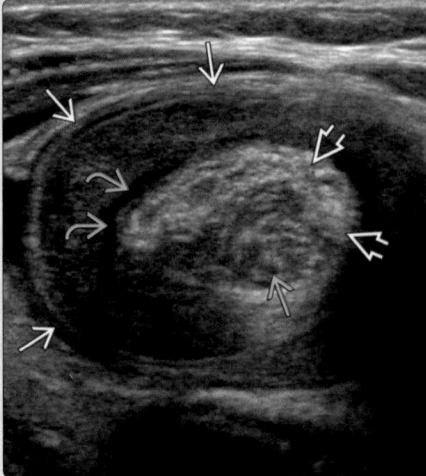

(Left) Graphic shows ileo-colic intussusception. Note entering layer ➡, returning layer ➡, and apex ➡ of intussusceptum (terminal ileum). Intussuscipiens (cecum) ➡ and neck of intussusception ➡ are noted. (Right) Transverse transabdominal US shows classic "bowel within bowel" appearance of ileocolic intussusception. Note the inner intussusceptum (ileum ➡ and mesentery ➡) and outer intussuscipiens (hypoechoic layer of edematous bowel ➡) and intervening fluid ➡.

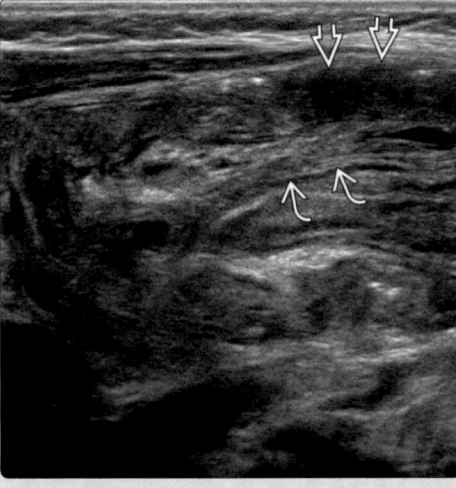
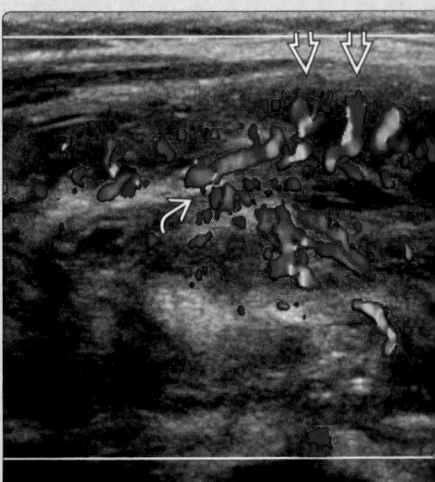

(Left) Longitudinal transabdominal US shows the layers of bowel wall involved in the intussusception. Outer layer of edematous bowel wall ➡ (intussuscipiens) and compressed inner layers ➡ (intussusceptum) are noted. (Right) Longitudinal color Doppler US shows intussusception. Hyperemia of edematous outer intussuscipiens ➡ and inner layers of intussusceptum ➡ is noted. Presence of vascularity is favorable for bowel viability and potential reducibility. (Courtesy V. Godhamgaonkar, MD.)

TERMINOLOGY

Definitions

Invagination or telescoping of 1 segment of gastrointestinal tract and its mesentery (intussusceptum) into lumen of adjacent distal segment (intussuscipiens)

IMAGING

General Features

Best diagnostic clue
- Sausage-shaped mass (longitudinal) and target or doughnut appearance (transverse) on cross section

Location
- Occurs anywhere from stomach to rectum
- Tends to occur at junctions between free-moving and fixed segments (retroperitoneum or adhesional)
- Categories: Enteric, ileocolic, ileocecal, colonic
- Adults: Most commonly enteroenteric and ileocolic
- Children: Most commonly ileocolic (75%)

Morphology
- "Bowel within bowel" appearance
- Adults: 90% have pathological trigger (lead point or predisposing condition)
- Children: 95% idiopathic (lymphoid hyperplasia in mesenteric adenitis)
- Transient intussusception: Nonobstructing, self-limiting

Ultrasonographic Findings

Grayscale ultrasound
- High sensitivity (98-100%) & specificity (88-100%)
- Particularly useful in pediatric population (gold standard)
  - Diagnostic and therapeutic, avoiding radiation
  - Usually subhepatic complex structure, > 5 cm, displacing bowel loops
- Transverse
  - Concentric parallel rings of bowel wall (target, doughnut, or bull's-eye sign)
  - Hypoechoic outer layer of edematous bowel
  - Layering of hypoechoic fluid trapped between compressed bowel segments
  - Echogenic crescent of intussuscepted mesenteric fat (crescent within doughnut sign)
- Longitudinal
  - Multiple parallel, hypoechoic, and echogenic stripes (sandwich sign)
  - Curved with eccentric fat or imaged obliquely, giving rise to pseudokidney sign
  - Enlarged hypoechoic mesenteric lymph nodes give appearance of renal medullary pyramids
- Additional features
  - Central lead point lesion or lymph nodes
  - Small volume of free fluid (common)
  - Perforation: Large-volume ascites, debris, and free gas
- US-guided hydrostatic nonsurgical reduction (NSR)
  - Increasing use of saline solution under ultrasound guidance; avoids ionizing radiation
  - Limited by presence of excessive bowel gas, depending on site of intussusception

  - Outer wall thickness < 1 cm, lymph nodes < 1 cm within intussusception & minimal internal trapped fluid associated with higher success rate of NSR
- Transient intussusception
  - No significant bowel edema, fat, or lymph nodes; segment involved often shorter and smaller diameter
  - Spontaneous resolution may be observed on US, particularly in pediatric population in small bowel intussusception (SBI), so-called benign SBIs
- Color Doppler
  - Mesenteric vessels trapped between entering and returning limbs of intussusceptum
  - Reduced or absent mural vascularity of intussusceptum indicative of vascular compromise, ischemia with risk of infarction and perforation
  - Absence of vascularity in intussusceptum is good predictor of irreducibility

Radiographic Findings

- Radiography
  - Elongated soft tissue mass
  - Intraluminal air between walls of intussusceptum and intussuscipiens, air crescent sign

Fluoroscopic Findings

- Fluoroscopic contrast enema
  - No longer gold standard investigation in children; therapeutic use only
  - Edematous mucosal folds of returning limb outlined by contrast in lumen, giving rise to coiled spring appearance
  - Contraindicated in perforation
- Fluoroscopic-guided hydrostatic/contrast/pneumatic NSR
  - Water-soluble contrast, barium, or air enema

CT Findings

- Multiplanar viewing essential and confirms presence or absence of lead point
  - Soft tissue sausage-shaped mass (longitudinal)
  - "Bowel within bowel" configuration with concentric rings axial to plane of intussusception, ultrasound equivalent of target sign
  - Complications: Signs of ischemia/infarct (variable wall enhancement, edema), perforation (free gas, fluid)
  - Transient intussusception may be incidental finding

Imaging Recommendations

- Best imaging tool
  - Ultrasound: 1st modality in pediatrics but operator dependent and limited by distended bowel
  - CT: Often 1st investigation in adults presenting acutely; high sensitivity and specificity and accessible

DIFFERENTIAL DIAGNOSIS

Tumor

- Bowel-related masses
  - Malignant: Adenocarcinoma, carcinoid tumor, lymphoma, GIST
  - Benign: Lipoma & adenoma
  - Metastases to bowel
    - Antimesenteric border of small bowel
    - From malignant melanoma, lung, and breast cancer

Inflammatory

- Appendicular mass
  - Right iliac fossa mass ± inflamed appendix/appendicolith, inflamed periappendiceal fat ± fluid
- Inflammatory bowel disease
  - Thickened bowel wall with preservation of gut signature and creeping fat

Infection

- Enteritis/colitis
  - Long segment involvement
  - *Clostridium difficile* colitis particularly, because of degree of thickening and submucosal edema

PATHOLOGY

General Features

- Etiology
  - Children
    - Idiopathic (95%)
      - Enlarged lymphoid tissue post infection; rare before 3 months of age (passive immunity)
      - Other causes: Abnormal motility, early weaning, prematurity, hyperperistalsis, hypertrophied Peyer patches
    - Lead point (5%)
      - Meckel diverticulum, polyp, enteric duplication cyst, appendicitis, Henoch-Schönlein purpura, inspissated meconium, gastrojejunal feeding tubes
  - Adults: Identifiable etiology in 90%
    - Lead point
      - Malignant: Primary polypoid adenocarcinoma (more commonly colon), metastases (melanoma, breast, lung), and lymphoma (more commonly small bowel)
      - Benign: GIST, polyp, lipoma, leiomyoma, adenoma of appendix, appendiceal stump granuloma
      - Higher incidence of malignant lesions in large bowel and benign lesions in small bowel
      - Congenital: Meckel diverticulum, duplication cyst, ectopic pancreas
      - Inflammatory: Colitis, chronic ulcers, epiploic appendagitis, cystic fibrosis
      - Trauma: Mural hematoma
      - Postoperative: Suture lines, ostomy closure sites, submucosal edema
      - Long intestinal tubes
    - Nonlead point intussusception
      - Abnormal bowel motility, electrolyte imbalance, fasting, chronic dilated loop
      - Miscellaneous: Scleroderma, celiac and Whipple disease
    - Transient intussusception
      - Often incidental finding in asymptomatic patient
      - No lead point identified, dysrhythmic peristalsis
      - Usually short segment, no proximal dilatation or obstruction
      - Spontaneous resolution, rarely requiring surgical treatment

Gross Pathologic & Surgical Features

- Invaginated bowel ± lead point

CLINICAL ISSUES

Presentation

- Most common signs/symptoms
  - Adults (5%): Accounts for < 2% adult obstructions
    - Insidious, vague abdominal symptoms to intermitten pain, vomiting, red blood in stool
  - Children (95%): Accounts for 80% cases of infantile obstruction, most common pediatric abdominal surgica emergency
    - Triad: Acute pain, palpable mass, "red currant jelly" stools

Natural History & Prognosis

- Complications: Obstruction, bowel ischemia/infarction, perforation, & peritonitis
- Option to rescan after few hours if pain subsiding
- Prompt treatment (reduction or surgery) associated with good prognosis and low recurrence rate
- Poor prognosis if vascular compromise (ischemia & perforation)

Treatment

- Surgery indicated where lead point identified or complications evident on CT
- Children
  - Hydrostatic or pneumatic reduction (US/fluoroscopy)
  - If nonreducible, consider open surgical reduction or resection
- Adults
  - Surgery usually indicated as high incidence of underlyinç lesion
  - Intraoperative reduction may minimize extent of bowel resection, reducing risk of short bowel syndrome
  - No treatment for transient intussusception as spontaneous resolution

DIAGNOSTIC CHECKLIST

Consider

- Intussusception: When classical target or doughnut sign is seen on US or CT in appropriate clinical setting
- Exclude lead point lesion, vascular compromise, and complications of ischemia

SELECTED REFERENCES

1. Aref H et al: Transient small bowel intussusception in an adult: case report with intraoperative video and literature review. BMC Surg. 15(1):36, 2015
2. Kim JS et al: [Conservative management of adult small bowel intussusception detected at abdominal computed tomography.] Korean J Gastroenterol. 65(5):291-6, 2015
3. Hannon E et al: UK intussusception audit: a national survey of practice and audit of reduction rates. Clin Radiol. 69(4):344-9, 2014
4. Potts J et al: Small bowel intussusception in adults. Ann R Coll Surg Engl. 96(1):11-4, 2014
5. Park NH et al: Ultrasonographic findings of small bowel intussusception, focusing on differentiation from ileocolic intussusception. Br J Radiol. 80(958):798-802, 2007
6. Choi SH et al: Intussusception in adults: from stomach to rectum. AJR Am J Roentgenol. 183(3):691-8, 2004

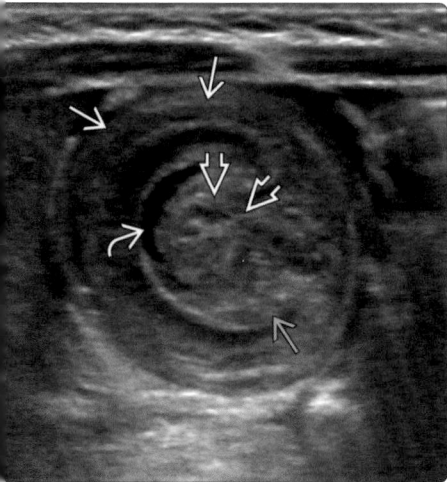

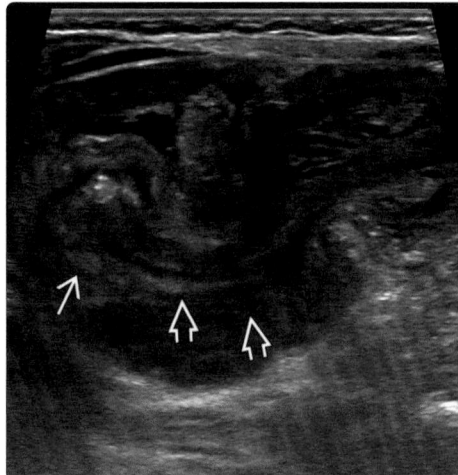

(Left) *Transverse transabdominal US shows classic "bowel within bowel" appearance of ileocolic intussusception. Note the compressed inner loop ⇒ and outer edematous layer with ⇒ intervening crescent of fluid ⇒ and mesenteric fat ⇒.* (Right) *Longitudinal transabdominal US shows layering appearance of the bowel walls involved in the intussusception ⇒. Lymph nodes seen close to the apex of the intussusceptum ⇒.*

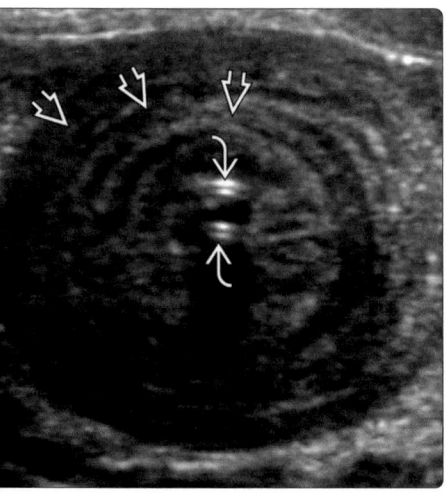

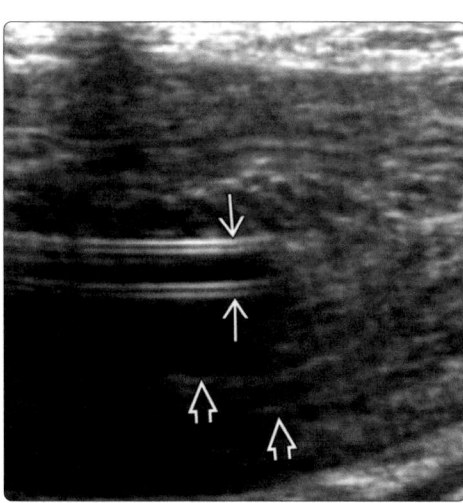

(Left) *Transverse transabdominal US shows classic target appearance of ileoileal intussusception. Note concentric rings axial to the plane of intussusception ⇒ and central naso-jejunal tube tip ⇒, the trigger for intussusception.* (Right) *Longitudinal transabdominal US in the same patient shows layering appearance of the bowel walls involved in the intussusception ⇒ and central naso-jejunal tube tip, trigger for intussusception ⇒.*

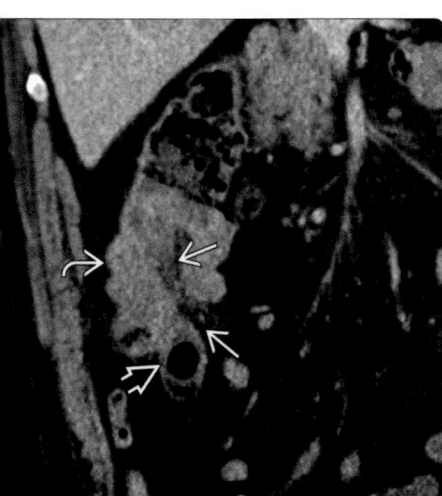

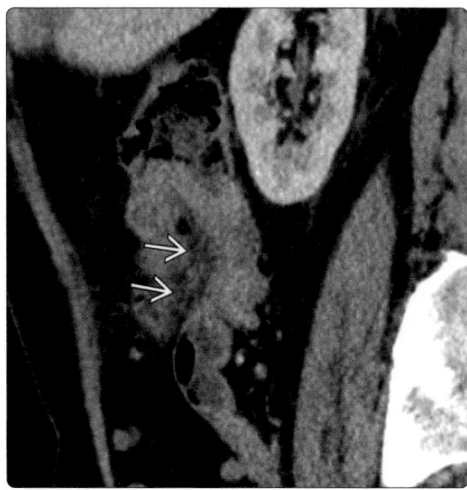

(Left) *Coronal MPR CT demonstrates ileocecal intussusception, the terminal ileum ⇒ invaginating into the thickened cecum/proximal ascending colon ⇒. The intussusceptum drags the mesenteric fat with it ⇒. Underlying ileocecal junction adenocarcinoma was found at surgery.* (Right) *Sagittal MPR CT in the same patient shows ileocecal intussusception with mesenteric fat pulled into intussuscipiens with mesenteric vessels ⇒. Resultant vascular compromise predisposes to ischemia.*

Epiploic Appendagitis

TERMINOLOGY

- Ischemic infarction of epiploic appendage (may be primary or secondary)

IMAGING

- Noncompressible avascular hyperechoic oval mass, adjacent to colon, deep to region of maximal tenderness
- Normal or mild localized asymmetric thickening of adjacent colonic wall
- Peripheral 2-3 mm hypoechoic/hyperattenuating rim of inflamed visceral peritoneum: Hyperattenuating ring sign
- Central focus of hypoechogenicity/hyperattenuation (central engorged or thrombosed vessel &/or central areas of hemorrhage): Central dot sign

TOP DIFFERENTIAL DIAGNOSES

- Segmental omental infarction
- Diverticulitis
- Appendicitis

- Sclerosing mesenteritis
- Primary tumors and mesocolon metastases
- Pelvic inflammatory disease

PATHOLOGY

- Torsion of epiploic appendage along its long axis with impairment of its vascular supply and subsequent venous thrombosis or spontaneous central vein thrombosis resulting in necrosis

DIAGNOSTIC CHECKLIST

- Differentiate from more common causes of acute abdominal pain (especially acute appendicitis and diverticulitis)
- Pericolonic avascular ovoid fatty lesion with visceral peritoneal thickening at site of maximal tenderness
- Most common in sigmoid but not limited to left colon

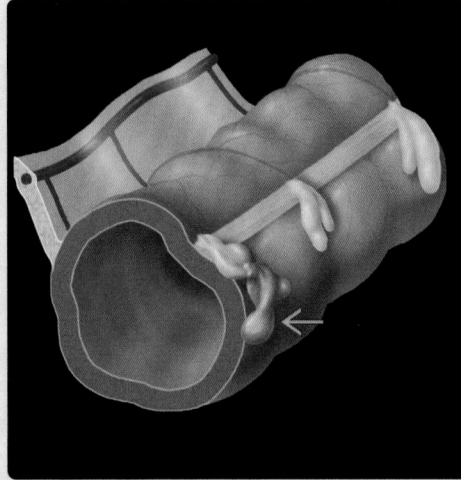
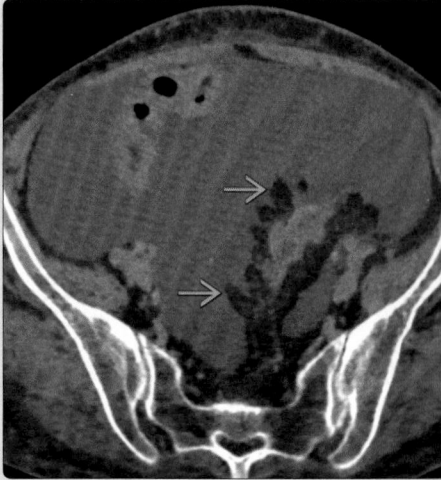

(Left) Graphic shows a torsed and infarcted epiploic appendage ➡ and 2 adjacent normal appendages. (Right) Axial NECT shows normal sigmoid colon epiploic appendages ➡ of fat density outlined by ascites.

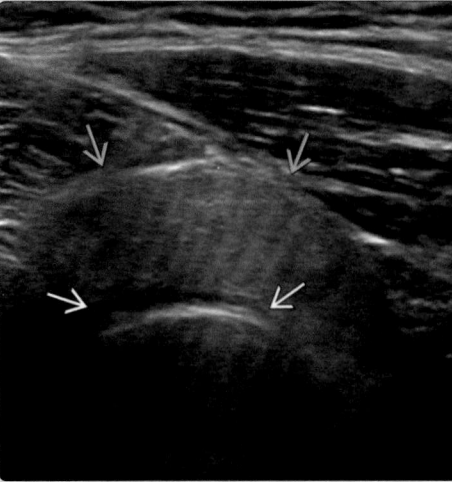
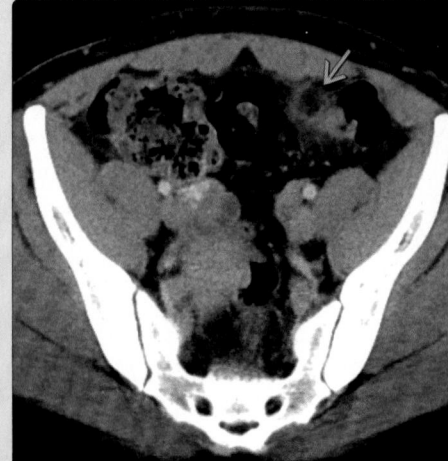

(Left) Grayscale transabdominal ultrasound at the point of maximal tenderness in a patient with clinically suspected ovarian torsion shows an ovoid hyperechoic mass ➡ adherent to the colonic wall ➡. (Right) Axial CECT of the same patient demonstrates an ovoid fat-density lesion with a hyperattenuating rim and surrounding inflammation ➡ abutting the sigmoid colon consistent with epiploic appendagitis.

TERMINOLOGY

Abbreviations

- Epiploic appendagitis (EA)

Synonyms

- Appendicitis epiploicae

Definitions

- Primary EA refers to ischemic infarction of epiploic appendage secondary to either torsion or spontaneous central draining vein thrombosis
- Secondary EA is caused by inflammation of adjacent structure

IMAGING

General Features

- Best diagnostic clue
  - Fat-containing ovoid structure with surrounding mesenteric fat stranding adjacent to colonic wall
- Location
  - Rectosigmoid junction (57%)
  - Ileocecal region (26%)
  - Ascending colon (9%)
  - Transverse colon (6%)
  - Descending colon (2%)
- Morphology
  - Epiploic appendages are small (0.5-5 cm long and 1-2 cm thick), fat-containing, peritoneal outpouchings arising from antimesenteric serosal colonic surface
  - In acute EA, appendage becomes swollen with mean diameter of 1.5-3.5 cm

Ultrasonographic Findings

- Grayscale ultrasound
  - Noncompressible hyperechoic oval mass adjacent to colon
  - Hypoechoic rim of inflamed visceral peritoneum (93%) deep to region of maximal tenderness
  - May contain central hypoechoic areas of hemorrhagic change
  - Adjacent absent or minimal bowel wall thickening with local mass effect
- Color Doppler
  - Absence of central blood flow (useful differentiating feature from secondary epiploic appendagitis)
- Contrast-enhanced ultrasound
  - Rim of peripheral arterial hyperenhancement
  - Central nonenhancing hypoechoic regions

CT Findings

- CECT
  - Ovoid pericolonic fat-density lesion measuring < 5 cm abutting antimesenteric colonic wall
  - Localized mass effect on adjacent bowel wall
  - Central dot sign: Central hyperattenuating focus representing central engorged or thrombosed vessel &/or central areas of hemorrhage
  - Hyperattenuating ring sign: 2-3 mm hyperdense rim surrounding ovoid lesion representing inflamed visceral peritoneum
  - Surrounding inflammatory changes: Fat stranding, parietal peritoneal thickening, and mild localized asymmetric adjacent colonic wall thickening

Imaging Recommendations

- Best imaging tool
  - When clinically suspected, focused high-resolution ultrasound is preferred, especially in younger age group
    - Often CT is performed in acute setting, if diagnosis is clinically unsuspected
  - CT is performed for patients with inconclusive US findings
  - CT aids differentiation from alternative pathology and aids identification of secondary complications
- Protocol advice
  - Focused high-resolution ultrasound examination at point of maximum tenderness: Searching for noncompressible avascular hyperechoic oval mass with hypoechoic rim
  - Standard portal venous phase CECT

DIFFERENTIAL DIAGNOSIS

Segmental Omental Infarction

- Localized greater omental infarction secondary to torsion, trauma, or central venous occlusion
- Lesion is centered within omentum and predominantly occurs in right upper quadrant
- Focal lesion is larger (mean diameter: 7 cm)
- Absence of hyperattenuating ring sign
- Central dot sign may be present
- Can occur in pediatric population (15%)

Appendicitis

- Identification of abnormally noncompressible, inflamed appendix with thickened enhancing wall
- ± calcified appendicolith
- Pericecal inflammation
- Increased color Doppler flow

Diverticulitis

- Secondary inflammation of epiploic appendages may be seen
- Longer segment of colonic wall thickening
- Abscess formation more common
- May lead to colonic obstruction
- Tends to affect older patients (> 50 years)
- More likely to have elevated WBC count

Sclerosing Mesenteritis

- Distortion and thickening of small bowel mesenteric root
- Does not abut colonic wall
- Fat ring sign: Traversing mesenteric vessels have surrounding spared fat halo
- Punctate calcification (rare) and small volume (usually < 5 mm) adjacent lymph nodes

Primary Tumors and Mesocolon Metastases

- Multiplicity and ill-defined margins
  - Lesions tend to be hypoechoic
- Centered on omentum and may be adherent to ventral surface of colon
- History of primary neoplasm and absence of acute abdominal pain at presentation

Pelvic Inflammatory Disease

- Usually occurs in women of childbearing age
- Bilateral tubo-ovarian masses
- May have reactive inflammation to perienteric and pericolonic fat
- Usually presents with systemic symptoms
- Associated with presence of intrauterine contraceptive device

PATHOLOGY

General Features

- Etiology
  - Torsion of epiploic appendage along its long axis with impairment of its vascular supply and subsequent venous thrombosis
  - Spontaneous central vein thrombosis resulting in necrosis (also possible)

Gross Pathologic & Surgical Features

- Acute infarction with inflammation, fat necrosis, vessel thrombosis, and hemorrhagic suffusion
- Torsion is seldom seen intraoperatively

CLINICAL ISSUES

Presentation

- Most common signs/symptoms
  - Abrupt onset of very localized abdominal pain, most frequently left lower quadrant, gradually resolving over 3-10 days
  - Palpable mass (10-30%)
  - Obesity and strenuous exercise are recognized risk factors
- Other signs/symptoms
  - Mild or absent systemic symptoms and signs
- Clinical profile
  - White cell count may be normal or mildly elevated

Demographics

- Age
  - 4th-5th decades of life
- Gender
  - Male predominance (M:F = 4:1)
- Epidemiology
  - True incidence is unknown but is less than < 1%

Natural History & Prognosis

- Prognosis
  - Usually self-limiting condition with clinical recovery within 10 days
  - CT findings may persist beyond 6 months
    - Calcified mobile "stone" in dependent peritoneal recesses may persist long-term
- Complications are rare but may include
  - Abscess formation
  - Adhesions
  - Bowel obstruction
  - Intussusception
  - Peritonitis

Treatment

- Conservative management with oral anti-inflammatory medication
- Antibiotics are not routinely indicated

DIAGNOSTIC CHECKLIST

Image Interpretation Pearls

- Noncompressible avascular hyperechoic oval mass, adjacent to colon, deep to region of maximal tenderness
- Normal or mild localized asymmetric thickening of adjacent colonic wall
- Peripheral 2-3 mm hypoechoic/hyperattenuating rim of inflamed visceral peritoneum
- Central focus of hypoechogenicity/hyperattenuation (central engorged or thrombosed vessel &/or central areas of hemorrhage)

SELECTED REFERENCES

1. Menozzi G et al: Contrast-enhanced ultrasound appearance of primary epiploic appendagitis. J Ultrasound. 17(1):75-6, 2014
2. Oztunali C et al: Radiologic findings of epiploic appendagitis. Med Ultrason. 15(1):71-2, 2013
3. Kamaya A et al: Imaging manifestations of abdominal fat necrosis and its mimics. Radiographics. 31(7):2021-34, 2011
4. Sand M et al: Epiploic appendagitis–clinical characteristics of an uncommon surgical diagnosis. BMC Surg. 7:11, 2007
5. Singh AK et al: CT appearance of acute appendicitis. AJR Am J Roentgenol. 183(5):1303-7, 2004
6. Boardman J et al: Radiologic-pathologic conference of Keller Army Community Hospital at West Point, the United States Military Academy: torsion of the epiploic appendage. AJR Am J Roentgenol. 180(3):748, 2003
7. Rioux M et al: Primary epiploic appendagitis: clinical, US, and CT findings in 1 cases. Radiology. 191(2):523-6, 1994
8. Carmichael DH et al: Epiploic disorders. Conditions of the epiploic appendages. Arch Surg. 120(10):1167-72, 1985
9. Thomas JH et al: Epiploic appendagitis. Surg Gynecol Obstet. 138(1):23-5, 1974
10. Fieber SS et al: Appendices epiploicae: clinical and pathological considerations; report of three cases and statistical analysis on one hundred five cases. AMA Arch Surg. 66(3):329-38, 1953

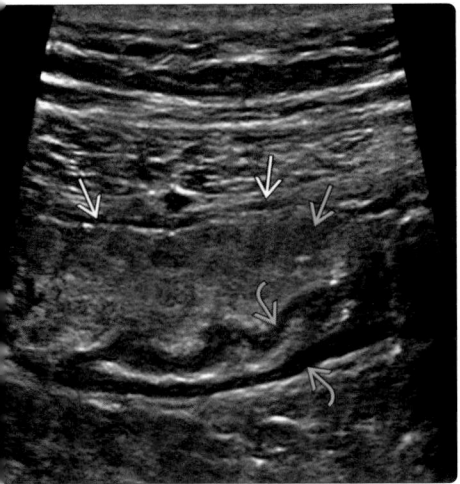

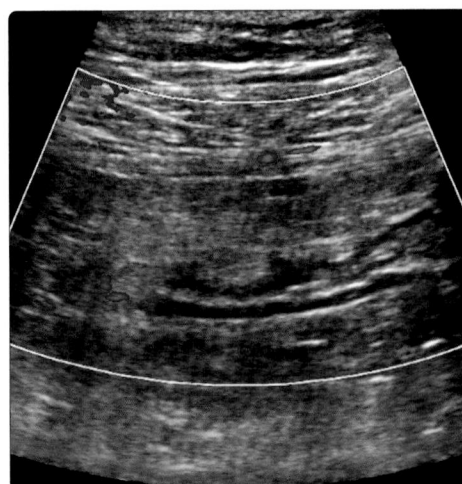

(Left) *Grayscale ultrasound shows a well-defined echogenic mass* ➡ *with a hypoechoic rim of visceral peritoneal thickening* ➡ *and central ill-defined hypoechoic foci. Note the normal hypoechoic layers representing the muscularis propria of the sigmoid colon* ➡. **(Right)** *Color Doppler ultrasound shows the mass to be avascular.*

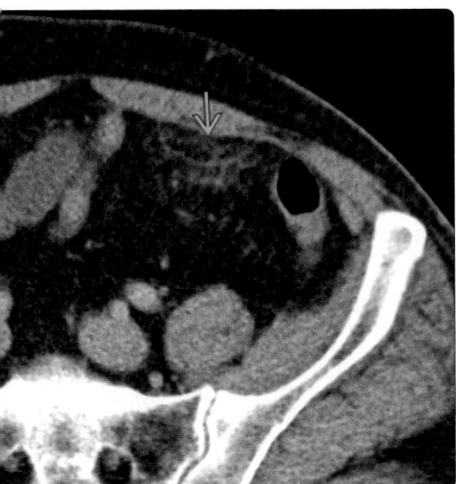

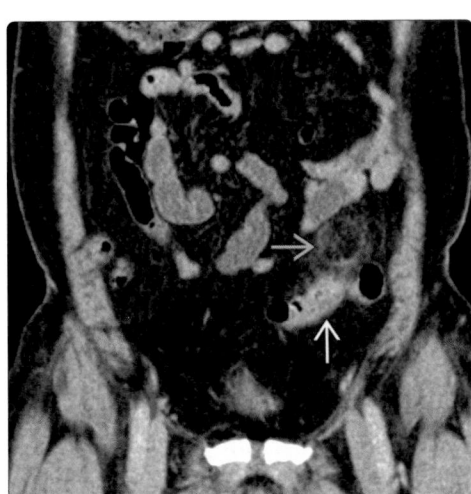

(Left) *Axial CECT in the same patient demonstrates the typical radiological appearances of epiploic appendagitis (EA) with surrounding fat stranding* ➡. *Note the normal adjacent sigmoid colon.* **(Right)** *Corresponding coronal MPR showing the EA* ➡ *and its intimate relationship to the normal adjacent sigmoid colon* ➡.

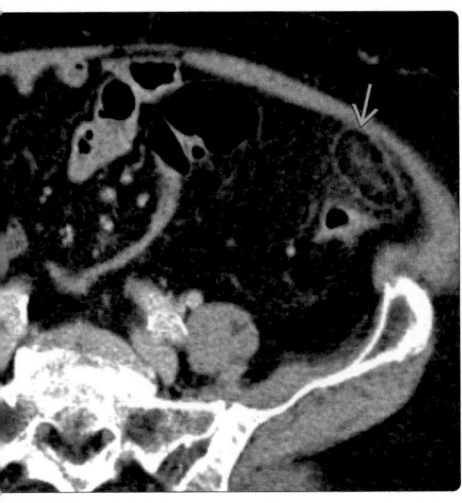

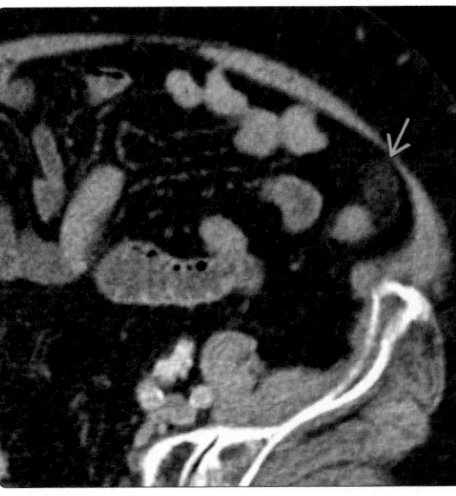

(Left) *Axial CECT in a patient with suspected diverticulitis shows a focal fat-containing lesion* ➡ *with peripheral hyperattenuation (hyperattenuating ring sign) and central linear hyperdensity (equivalent to the central dot sign when seen en face). Note the adjacent fat stranding.* **(Right)** *Follow-up axial CECT in the same patient performed at 8-month interval demonstrates improvement but persistent radiological features* ➡. *This case illustrates the slow resolution of EA radiological signs.*

Diverticulitis

TERMINOLOGY

- Evidence of inflammation in thick-walled colonic segment centered around colonic diverticulosis

IMAGING

- Hypertrophy of muscularis propria with sac-like outpouchings represents underlying colonic diverticulosis
- Diverticulitis
  - US: Colonic diverticulosis with adjacent inflamed echogenic pericolic fat
  - CECT: Significant fat stranding centered around diverticula with background mural hypertrophy

TOP DIFFERENTIAL DIAGNOSES

- Colon cancer
- Colitis
- Acute appendicitis
- Epiploic appendagitis and segmental omental infarction

PATHOLOGY

- Due to localized microperforation of inflamed colonic diverticulum secondary to impacted fecalith

CLINICAL ISSUES

- Clinical presentation
  - Acute lower abdominal pain, localization dependent on site of inflammation
  - Fever, diarrhea, and rectal bleeding
- Majority settle with conservative management
- Complications: Abscess, fistula, stricture, obstruction, perforation with purulent or fecal peritonitis

DIAGNOSTIC CHECKLIST

- Consider diverticulitis in differential diagnosis of acute abdomen presenting with lower abdominal pain
- Typical US and CECT diagnostic of diverticulitis
- Look for complications, and beware of mimics, e.g., colon carcinoma

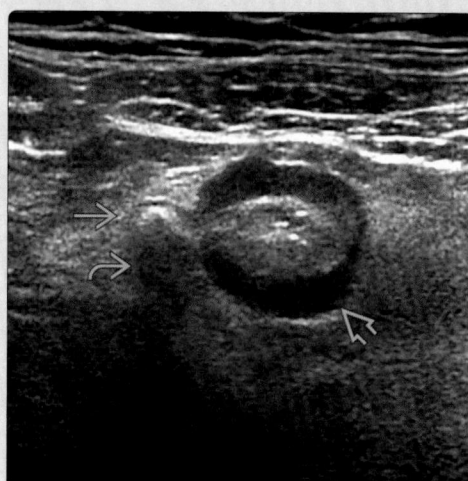
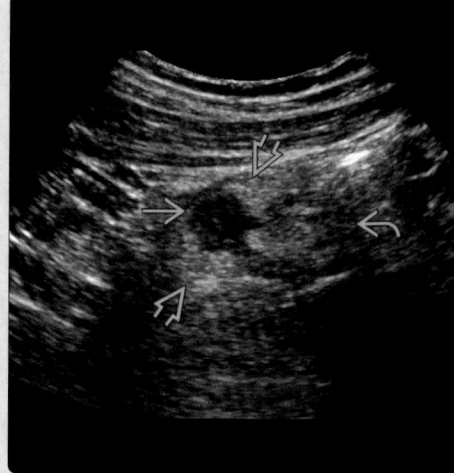

(Left) Diverticulosis can be identified by thickened colon with a pronounced hypoechoic muscularis propria layer ➡ containing diverticulum; note focal outpouching containing gas ➡. Note the linear echogenic foci with posterior reverberation artifact ➡. No surrounding acute inflammation can be seen. (Right) Acute diverticulitis can be identified by hypoechoic outpouching ➡ arising from the adjacent colon ➡ with surrounding inflamed echogenic fat ➡. Patient had localized peritonism.

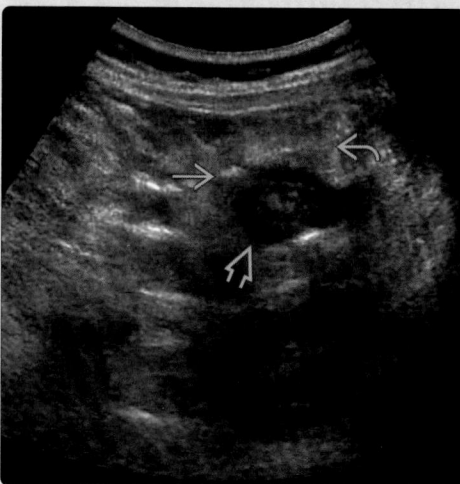
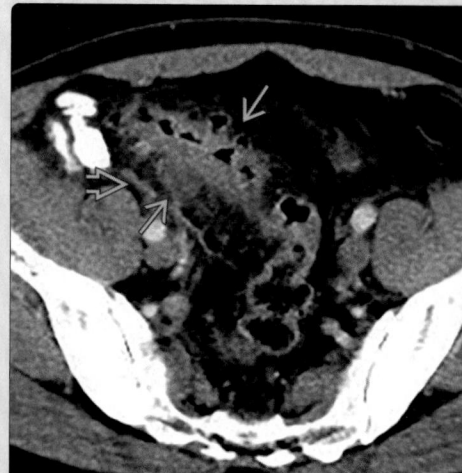

(Left) Hypertrophied muscularis propria ➡ of colonic wall shows acute sigmoid diverticulitis. Linear arc-like echo ➡ projects beyond colonic wall, showing gas. Note surrounding echogenic fat ➡. (Right) Acute sigmoid diverticulitis is shown by thick-walled sigmoid colon containing multiple diverticula with surrounding fat stranding and hyperemia ➡. Note the adjacent reactive thickening of the parietal peritoneum ➡. The mobile position of sigmoid colon mimics clinical presentation of acute appendicitis.

TERMINOLOGY

Definitions

- Diverticulum: Focal sac-like outpouching
- Diverticulosis: Presence of colonic diverticula in absence of acute signs or symptoms
- Diverticulitis: Inflammation of colonic diverticulum resulting in clinical signs

IMAGING

General Features

- Best diagnostic clue
  - Evidence of inflammation in thick-walled colonic segment centered around diverticula
- Location
  - Diverticula
    - Can occur anywhere in colon
      □ Most common in sigmoid and left colon
- Size
  - Usually 3-5 mm
  - > 4 cm referred to as giant diverticulum
- Morphology
  - Can be solitary or multiple
  - Diverticula
    - Herniation of mucosa and submucosa bounded by thin layer of serosa
      □ Referred to as pulsion type or false diverticula
      □ Typically at point of weakness where perforating vessels enter teniae coli
  - Right-sided diverticulum
    - Multiple: Pulsion type (false diverticula)
    - Solitary: Congenital and true diverticulum; containing all layers of bowel wall
  - Giant colonic diverticulum
    - Congenital (true)
    - Acquired (pulsion type with ball valve-type effect)

Ultrasonographic Findings

- Diverticulosis
  - Thickened colon
    - Pronounced hypoechoic muscularis propria layer representing muscular hypertrophy
    - Early feature and can precede development of diverticula; prediverticulosis
  - Diverticula
    - Often inconspicuous, masked by gas from overlapping bowel loops
    - Linear echogenic foci with reverberation artifact protruding out from colonic wall represent gas
    - Hypoechoic colonic outpouching with heterogeneous echogenic foci representing gas and fecalith
- Acute diverticulitis
  - Features of diverticulosis with adjacent inflamed echogenic pericolic fat
  - Hyperemia on color Doppler assessment
  - Inflamed pericolic fat
    - Striking echogenic appearance with localized tenderness draws operator to underlying abnormality
    - Results in localized tenderness and draws operator to underlying abnormality

- Accentuates hypoechoic muscularis propria and inflamed diverticula
  - Complications
    - Abscess: Loculated fluid collection that may contain gas and debris
    - Fistula: Linear tract outlined by gas or fluid between thickened colon and adjacent structure

Radiographic Findings

- Giant diverticulum (thin-walled, air-filled structure) may be incidental finding

CT Findings

- CECT
  - Diverticulosis
    - Segmental mural thickening reflecting muscular hypertrophy and shortening of colon
      □ May be seen without diverticula
    - Diverticula
      □ Focal outpouchings may contain gas, fecalith, or mixture of both
  - Acute diverticulitis
    - Significant pericolonic fat stranding and edema centered around preexisting colonic diverticulosis
- CTA
  - Performed in cases of acute lower GI bleeding
- CT colonography
  - Diverticulosis/diverticulitis
    - 2D: Features overlap with conventional CT
    - Impacted fecalith in diverticulum or inverted diverticulum may mimic polyp

Imaging Recommendations

- Best imaging tool
  - CT is best imaging tool in assessment of acute diverticulitis, severity, and complications
  - US is valuable in initial assessment of patients with acute abdominal pain, which includes diverticulitis
  - Typical features on ultrasound are diagnostic of acute, uncomplicated diverticulitis
  - If US is inconclusive or coexistent complications are suspected, recommend further imaging with CT
- Protocol advice
  - CT
    - Portal-phase CECT with multiplanar assessment
  - US
    - Initial overview of abdominal viscera and bowel with curvilinear probe followed by focused assessment of bowel using high-resolution linear probe, typically where maximally tender
    - Transvaginal scan can demonstrate features of acute diverticulitis in pelvic colon

DIFFERENTIAL DIAGNOSIS

Colonic Tumor

- Short-segment colonic mural thickening with destruction of gut wall layers (gut signature) on ultrasound
- Can be difficult to distinguish from diverticulitis because of overlapping findings
- Presence of localized mass with pericolonic lymph nodes favors tumor

Colitis

- Presence of inflammatory colonic thickening typically in absence of diverticula
- Etiology infectious, inflammatory, or ischemic
- Thickened long segment of colon with exaggeration of gut signature surrounded by echogenic inflamed fat

Acute Appendicitis

- In clinical context, findings of thickened and distended appendix ± calcified appendicolith are diagnostic
- Blind-ending, noncompressible tubular structure (> 7 mm in caliber) arising from cecum with surrounding echogenic fat seen on ultrasound
- CT: Dilated, thick-walled appendix with periappendiceal fat stranding

Acute Epiploic Appendagitis (AEA) and Segmental Omental Infarction (SOI)

- Localized infarction of appendices epiploicae (AEA) or greater omentum (SOI) secondary to torsion, trauma, or venous occlusion
- AEA typically in antimesenteric border of colon and SOI in greater omentum
- Typically between 1-4 cm in AEA and larger (> 7 cm) in SOI with significant focal tenderness
- Ultrasound: Echogenic mass without any adjacent bowel wall thickening
- CECT: Ovoid fat density lesion with marked surrounding fat stranding and relative sparing of colonic wall
- Recognizing AEA and SOI on imaging is crucial because these are self-limiting and management is conservative

PATHOLOGY

General Features

- Acute diverticulitis
  - Impacted fecalith in diverticulum triggers localized inflammation and microperforation
  - Progressive pericolic inflammation and infection result in abscess formation
  - Perforation can also lead to generalized peritonitis

CLINICAL ISSUES

Presentation

- Most common signs/symptoms
  - Acute lower abdominal pain
    - Localization of pain dependent on site of inflammation
      □ Typically left iliac fossa pain in classic acute sigmoid diverticulitis
  - Fever, diarrhea, rectal bleeding (due to proximity of inflamed diverticula to perforating vessels)
- Other signs/symptoms
  - Diverticulosis typically asymptomatic

Demographics

- Ethnicity
  - Prevalent in Western society associated with low dietary fiber intake and has multifactorial etiology
  - Right-sided diverticulum; more common in young adults and in Asian population

- Epidemiology
  - Diverticulosis; increases with age; < 5% before 40 years to > 65% by 80 years of age
  - ~ 25% with diverticulosis will become symptomatic
  - Diverticulosis of right colon occurs at rate of 6-14%

Natural History & Prognosis

- Acute diverticulitis
  - Majority settle with conservative management
- Complications
  - Abscess, fistula, stricture, obstruction, perforation with purulent or fecal peritonitis

Treatment

- Acute, uncomplicated diverticulitis
  - Conservative: Intravenous antibiotics and analgesia
- Radiological intervention; US or CT guided
  - To drain abscess and control localized sepsis
- Surgery
  - Decision based on clinical status and findings on CT
    - Perforation with generalized peritonitis usually Hinchey stage 3 and 4 disease
  - Considered in mechanical large bowel obstruction or fistula

DIAGNOSTIC CHECKLIST

Consider

- Acute diverticulitis
  - Differential diagnosis of acute abdomen presenting with lower abdominal pain
  - Cause of generalized peritonitis or pneumoperitoneum
  - Cause of pelvic abscess ± evidence of fistula in pelvic viscera
  - Source of liver abscess secondary to ascending portal pyemia

Image Interpretation Pearls

- Ultrasound
  - Pronounced hypoechoic muscular layer of colonic wall containing diverticula with surrounding inflamed echogenic fat accompanied with localized tenderness
- CT: Thick-walled colon containing diverticula with surrounding fat stranding

Reporting Tips

- Look for complications
- Beware of carcinoma in background of diverticulosis

SELECTED REFERENCES

1. Klarenbeek BR et al: Review of current classifications for diverticular disease and a translation into clinical practice. Int J Colorectal Dis. 27(2):207-14, 201.
2. Puylaert JB: Ultrasound of colon diverticulitis. Dig Dis. 30(1):56-9, 2012
3. Goh V et al: Differentiation between diverticulitis and colorectal cancer: quantitative CT perfusion measurements versus morphologic criteria–initial experience. Radiology. 242(2):456-62, 2007
4. West AB et al: The pathology of diverticulosis coli. J Clin Gastroenterol. 38(5 Suppl):S11-6, 2004
5. Pereira JM et al: Disproportionate fat stranding: a helpful CT sign in patients with acute abdominal pain. Radiographics. 24(3):703-15, 2004
6. O'Malley M et al: Ultrasound of gastrointestinal tract abnormalities with CT correlation. RadioGraphics. 23(1):59-72, 2003
7. Horton KM et al: CT evaluation of the colon: inflammatory disease. RadioGraphics. 20(2):399-418, 2000

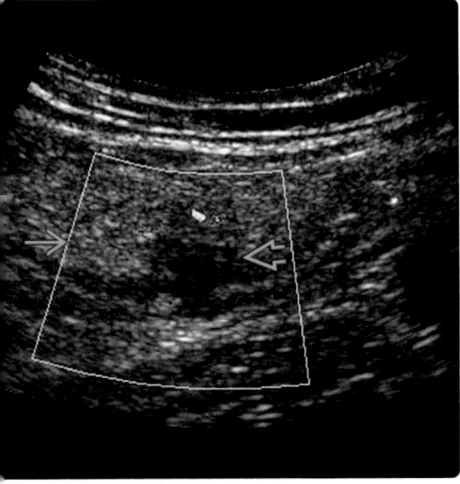

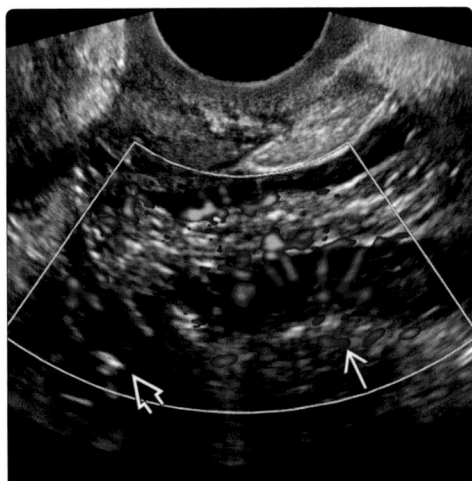

(Left) *Acute diverticulitis is shown by hyperemia on color Doppler US surrounding hypoechoic diverticulum ⇨. Hyperechoic fat ⇨ surrounding diverticulum reflects acute inflammation.* (Right) *Transvaginal ultrasound shows hypertrophied muscularis propria in sigmoid colon containing diverticula ⇨. Power Doppler demonstrates significant mural and pericolonic hyperemia ⇨. Features are consistent with acute diverticulitis.*

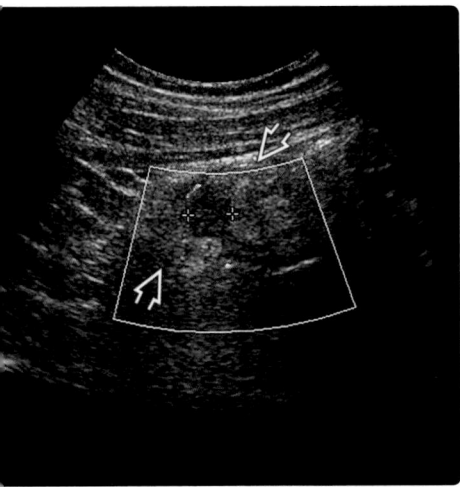

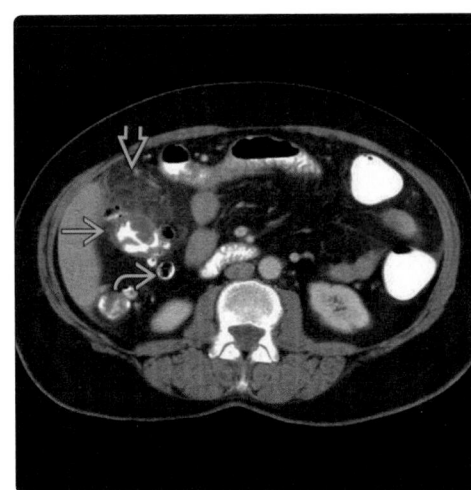

(Left) *Right-sided diverticulitis is shown by calipers outlining hypoechoic diverticulum arising from the right colon. There is surrounding hyperemia on the color Doppler assessment. Echogenic fat ⇨ accentuates the diverticulum.* (Right) *Axial CECT of the same patient demonstrates right-sided colonic diverticulitis. The thick-walled ascending colon ⇨ contains multiple diverticula ⇨ with surrounding pericolic fat stranding ⇨.*

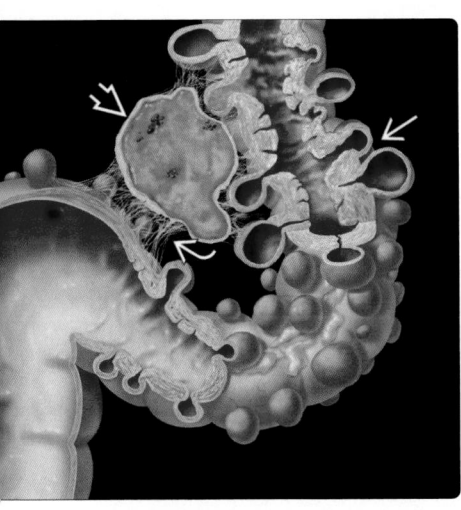

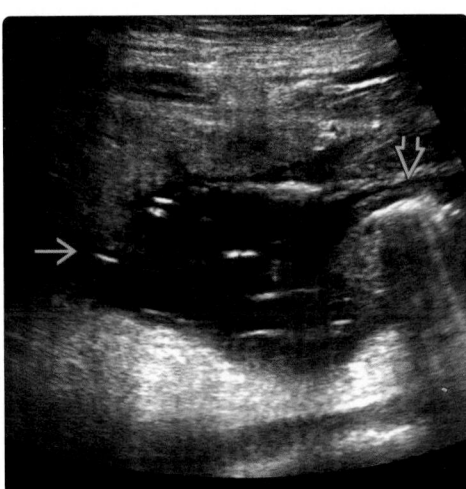

(Left) *Acute sigmoid diverticulitis with pericolonic abscess is shown by the thick-walled sigmoid colon ⇨ containing multiple diverticula. Localized fat stranding ⇨ and pericolic abscess ⇨ can also be seen.* (Right) *Pericolic abscess is shown by fluid collection adjacent to the colon ⇨ containing highly reflective echoes, consistent with gas within a pericolic abscess ⇨.*

Crohn Disease

TERMINOLOGY

- Chronic, relapsing granulomatous inflammatory disease with predominant involvement of gastrointestinal tract

IMAGING

- Ultrasound
  - Bowel wall thickening
    - Adults: > 3 mm
    - Children: Small bowel thickness > 2.5 mm and large bowel wall thickness > 2 mm
  - Loss of normal bowel wall stratification
  - Hyperemia of bowel wall correlates with disease activity
  - Thickening/increased echogenicity of mesentery
- Can occur anywhere from mouth to anus
- Involvement: Terminal ileum (95%), colon (22-55%), rectum (14-50%)
- Look for skip lesions: Normal bowel between areas of involved bowel

- Fistulas (enteroenteric, enteromesenteric, enterocutaneous, enterovesical, enterovaginal)
- Phlegmon/abscess
- Undiagnosed or suspected patients stratified into high or low risk based on symptoms, laboratory values, physical exam, and family history
  - Low risk: Ultrasound or MRE recommended
  - High risk: MRE or CTE
- Newly diagnosed patients
  - MRE or CTE

DIAGNOSTIC CHECKLIST

- Penetrating &/or stricturing disease alters clinical management
- Evaluate for associated abnormalities in other organs (primary sclerosing cholangitis, arthritis, gallstones, and urolithiasis)

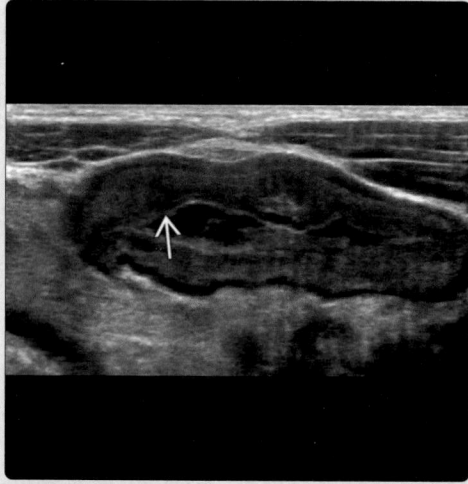
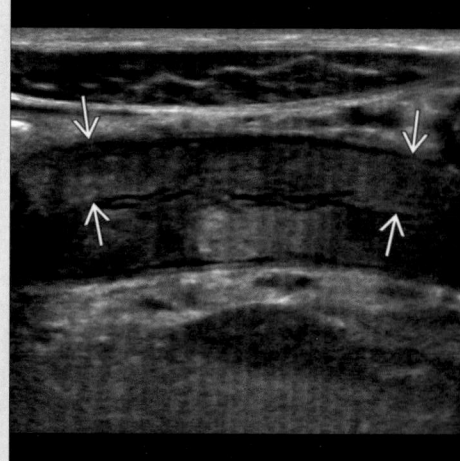

(Left) Short-axis ultrasound of the sigmoid colon shows marked thickening ➡ of the wall and loss of normal stratification. (Right) Long-axis ultrasound shows marked thickening ➡, loss of bowel wall stratification, and luminal narrowing in this 17 year old with Crohn disease.

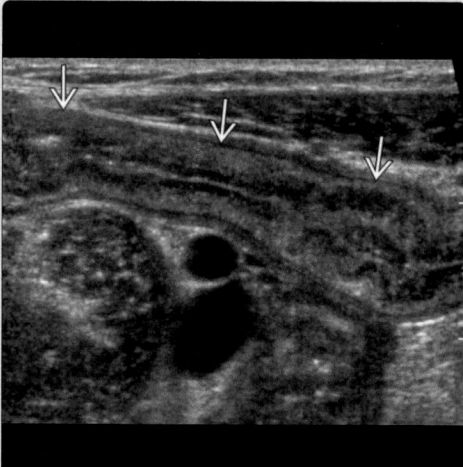
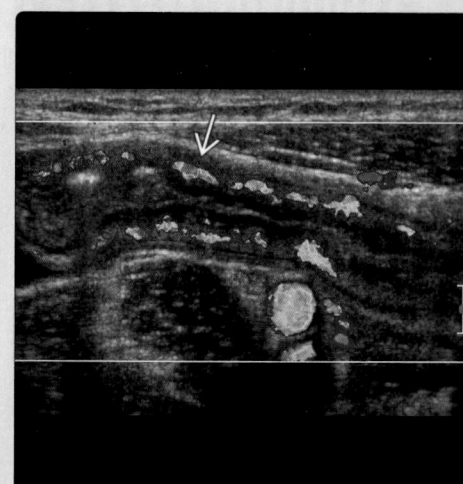

(Left) Grayscale long-axis oblique ultrasound shows a thickened terminal ileum ➡. (Right) Color Doppler ultrasound in the same patient shows hyperemia ➡ in the terminal ileum compatible with active inflammation.

Crohn Disease

TERMINOLOGY

Synonyms

- Terminal ileitis, regional enteritis, ileocolitis

Definitions

- Chronic, relapsing granulomatous inflammatory disease with predominant involvement of gastrointestinal tract

IMAGING

General Features

- Best diagnostic clue
  - Bowel wall thickening
    - Adults: > 3 mm
    - Children: Small bowel thickness > 2.5 mm and large bowel wall thickness > 2 mm
- Location
  - From mouth to anus
    - Involvement: Terminal ileum (95%), colon (22-55%), rectum (14-50%)
      - Small bowel alone (30-35%), small bowel and colon (50-60%), colon alone (20%)
    - Increased small bowel involvement in younger patients (80% vs. 60%)
  - Look for skip lesions: Normal bowel between areas of involved bowel

Ultrasonographic Findings

- Grayscale ultrasound
  - Mural
    - Bowel wall thickening
    - Increased or decreased echogenicity of bowel wall
    - Loss of normal bowel wall stratification
    - Ulceration
    - Fistula/sinus tract
    - Intramural abscess
    - Luminal narrowing
    - Postinflammatory polyps can form during healing of extensive ulcerative disease
  - Extramural
    - Thickening/increased echogenicity of mesentery
    - Separation of bowel loops
    - Fistulas (enteroenteric, enteromesenteric, enterocutaneous, enterovesical, enterovaginal)
    - Lymphadenopathy
    - Phlegmon/abscess
  - Decreased/absent peristalsis of involved bowel
- Color Doppler
  - Hyperemia of bowel wall and mesentery
    - Correlates with disease activity as angiogenesis and inflammation are directly correlated
- Contrast material-enhanced ultrasonography
  - Improves sensitivity for detecting inflammation
  - Objective quantification for assessing degree of inflammation and for follow-up
- Elastography
  - Able to detect changes of fibrosis in affected bowel wall segments

Fluoroscopic Findings

- Upper GI/small bowel series

- Aphthous ulcers: Earliest macroscopic change, central punctate barium with surrounding edema (target/bull's eye)
- Cobblestone appearance: Linear and transverse ulcers with spared surrounding mucosa (pseudopolyps)
- Luminal narrowing, ulceration; penetrating disease: Fistula or sinus tract

CT Findings

- CECT or CT enterography (CTE)
  - Wall thickening
  - Engorgement of vasa recta ("comb" sign)
  - Inflammation in mesentery
  - Reactive lymphadenopathy
  - Penetrating disease: Fistulae, sinus tracks, phlegmon/abscess
  - Luminal narrowing ± obstruction
  - Perianal disease
  - Enhancement of bowel wall; "target" or "double halo" sign

MR Findings

- MR enterography (MRE)
  - Similar findings to CT but without using ionizing radiation
  - Can assess peristalsis on free-breathing coronal sequences
  - Useful in evaluating perianal involvement

Imaging Recommendations

- Best imaging tool
  - Undiagnosed or suspected patients stratified into high or low risk based on symptoms, laboratory values, physical exam, and family history
    - Low risk: Ultrasound or MRE recommended
    - High risk: MRE or CTE
  - Newly diagnosed patients
    - MRE or CTE
  - Patients with established diagnosis of Crohn disease
    - Acute/emergent assessment: CT
    - Monitoring/longstanding complications: MRE
- Protocol advice
  - Ultrasound
    - High-resolution, high-frequency linear transducer (> 10 MHz)
      - Convex transducer for better penetration as needed (3-8 MHz)
    - Encourage clear, noncarbonated beverages prior to exam to help distend bowel
    - Graded compression
    - Harmonic imaging: Wide band preferred
    - Clips for assessment of bowel motility

DIFFERENTIAL DIAGNOSIS

Infectious Colitis

- *Shigella, Salmonella, Campylobacter, Escherichia coli* O157:H, *Yersinia*, parasites, amebiasis
- *Clostridium difficile* if recent antibiotic use
- Cytomegalovirus in immunocompromised patients
- Tuberculosis: Narrowed terminal ileum and cecum

Ulcerative Colitis

- Pancolitis without stricture, fistula, or sinus tract
- "Backwash" ileitis
- Continuous (no skip areas)

Lymphoma

- Non-Hodgkin lymphoma more common

Mesenteric Adenitis

- Common cause of right lower quadrant pain
- Enlarged lymph nodes ± ileal wall thickening

Appendicitis

- Dilated appendix ± appendicolith, periappendiceal inflammation ± abscess

PATHOLOGY

General Features

- Etiology
  - Exact etiology unknown but likely multifactorial
  - Possible causes
    - Environmental: Nutrition, smoking (4x increase), lifestyle
    - Immunobiologic: Altered bowel flora, abnormal response to unknown antigen
- Genetics
  - Familial disposition
  - Many susceptibility loci for Crohn disease found on numerous chromosomes
  - High rate of concordance in monozygotic twins
- Associated abnormalities
  - Extraintestinal disorders: Pyoderma gangrenosum, erythema nodosum, anemia, iritis/uveitis, primary sclerosing cholangitis, polyarticular and axial arthropathy, vitamin deficiency, nephrolithiasis
  - Associated autoimmune disorders: Asthma, autoimmune thyroiditis, vasculitis, multiple sclerosis, type 1 diabetes, psoriasis

Staging, Grading, & Classification

- Radiologic
  - Active inflammatory
  - Perforating and fistulizing
  - Fibrostenotic
  - Reparative and regenerative
- Disease severity scored clinically using Crohn Disease Activity Index and Pediatric Crohn Disease Activity Index
- Fecal markers (calprotectin and lactoferrin) helpful in diagnosis and monitoring disease

Gross Pathologic & Surgical Features

- Clearly defined normal segments of bowel between diseased segments ("skip lesions")
- Early: Aphthous ulcers, lymphoid hyperplasia and edema, fissures, and transmural inflammation
- Later: Transmural bowel wall inflammation, deep ulcers/fistulas, mesenteric inflammation
- Chronic: Fibrotic change, stricture formation
- Microscopic features
  - Edema, inflammation, and noncaseating granulomas

CLINICAL ISSUES

Presentation

- Most common signs/symptoms
  - Recurrent abdominal pain and diarrhea
- Other signs/symptoms
  - Malabsorption: Interrupted enterohepatic circuit with diminished absorption of bile salts in terminal ileum
    - Weight loss, fatigue, poor growth/weight gain in children, anemia, anorexia, nutritional deficiencies
  - Erythema nodosum and pyoderma gangrenosum
  - Obstruction

Demographics

- Age
  - 18-25 years, 20-30% of patients present under age of 20, smaller peak 50-80 years
- Gender
  - M = F
- Ethnicity
  - More common in Caucasian, Jewish populations
- Epidemiology
  - Incidence: ~ 5 cases/100,000 population
  - Smoking: More aggressive disease phenotype

Natural History & Prognosis

- Increased risk of small bowel and colorectal cancer

Treatment

- Medical treatment: Mesalamine, steroids, antibiotics, probiotics
  - Bowel rest
  - Immunomodulators and biologic therapies for severe/refractory disease
- Surgical treatment reserved for abscesses, complex perianal/internal fistulas unresponsive to medical therapy, fibrostenotic strictures with obstructive symptoms
- Surveillance colonoscopy

DIAGNOSTIC CHECKLIST

Consider

- Associated abnormalities in other organs (primary sclerosing cholangitis, arthritis, renal/biliary stones)

Image Interpretation Pearls

- Penetrating &/or stricturing disease alters clinical management

SELECTED REFERENCES

1. Baumgart DC et al: US-based Real-time Elastography for the Detection of Fibrotic Gut Tissue in Patients with Stricturing Crohn Disease. Radiology. 141929, 2015
2. Anupindi SA et al: Imaging in the evaluation of the young patient with inflammatory bowel disease: what the gastroenterologist needs to know. J Pediatr Gastroenterol Nutr. 59(4):429-39, 2014
3. Anupindi SA et al: Common and uncommon applications of bowel ultrasound with pathologic correlation in children. AJR Am J Roentgenol. 202(5):946-59, 2014
4. Novak KL et al: The role of ultrasound in the evaluation of inflammatory bowel disease. Semin Roentgenol. 48(3):224-33, 2013
5. Rodgers PM et al: Transabdominal ultrasound for bowel evaluation. Radiol Clin North Am. 51(1):133-48, 2013
6. Baumgart DC et al: Crohn's disease. Lancet. 380(9853):1590-605, 2012

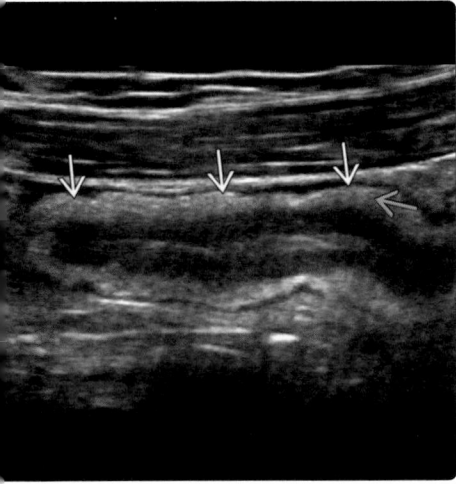

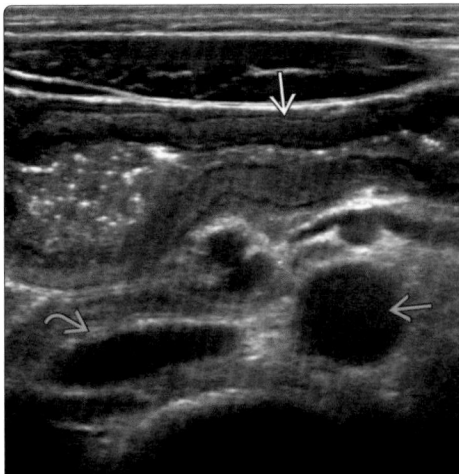

(Left) *Long-axis ultrasound shows a markedly thickened terminal ileum ➡. Note that even though thickened, there is preservation of some of the mural stratification seen in normal bowel. Echogenic submucosa ⮕ is present and thought to be related to lymphedema.* (Right) *Long-axis ultrasound of the transverse colon shows mild thickening of the wall with some loss of the normal stratified appearance of the bowel wall ➡. The aorta ⮕ and vena cava ⮕ are noted.*

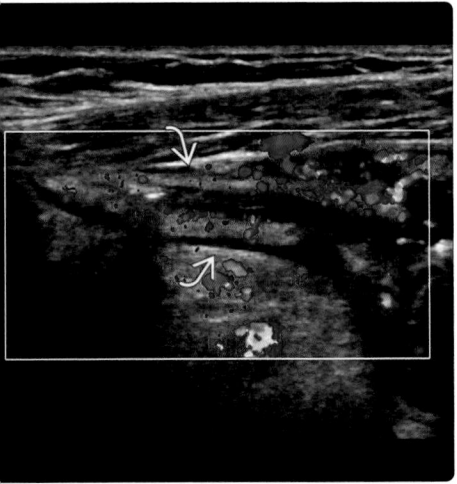

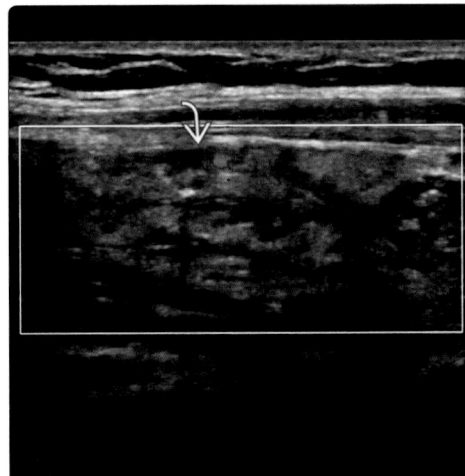

(Left) *Color Doppler US of the terminal ileum shows bowel wall thickening ➡ and hyperemia, which is compatible with acute inflammation.* (Right) *Color Doppler US from the same patient after treatment shows continued wall thickening ➡ but markedly reduced color Doppler blood flow consistent with interval decrease in active inflammation.*

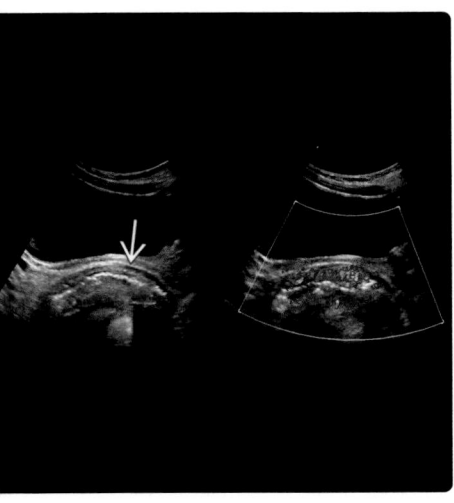

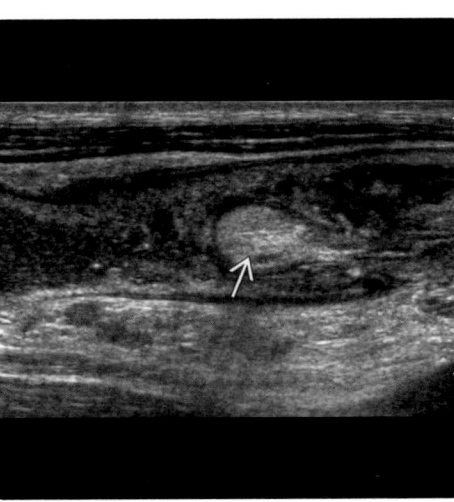

(Left) *Long-axis ultrasound of the rectum using the bladder as a window shows thickening of the rectum ➡. Color Doppler ultrasound at the same location shows hyperemia of the thickened wall.* (Right) *Long-axis ultrasound shows thickening and loss of bowel wall stratification in the terminal ileum. Additionally, there is an inflammatory polyp ➡ protruding into the lumen. These polyps can form in the healing phase of extensive ulcerative disease.*

(Left) *Grayscale ultrasound shows inflamed terminal ileum* ⮕ *with a fistula* ➡ *to another loop of small bowel.* (Right) *Transabdominal ultrasound shows a small fluid collection* ⮕ *in the mesentery with multiple connections* ➡ *to the adjacent bowel*

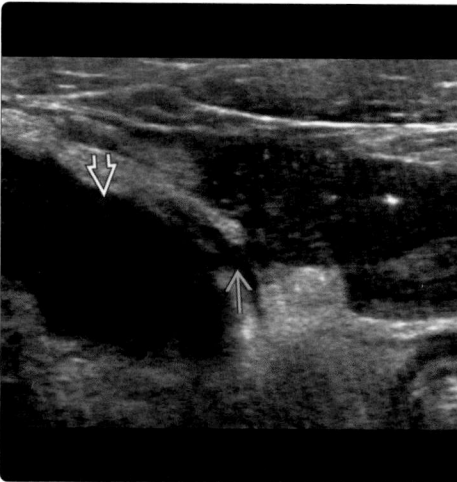
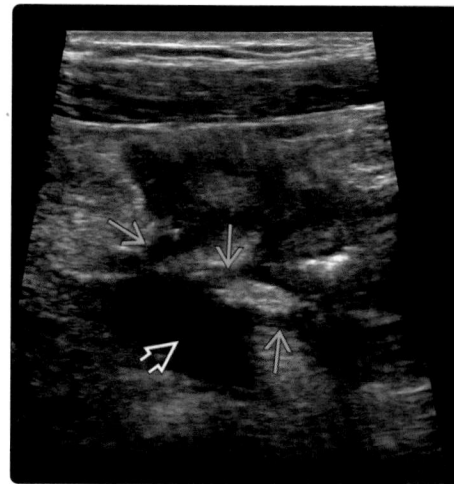

(Left) *A heterogeneous fluid collection* ⮕ *is seen in inflamed mesentery next to a thick-walled loop of ileum* ➡. *Note the echogenic gas bubbles in the wall of the bowel representing a site of deep ulceration/fistula* ➡. (Right) *Grayscale ultrasound shows a hypoechoic line* ⮕ *connecting 2 adjacent loops of bowel* ➡ *compatible with an enteroenteric fistula*

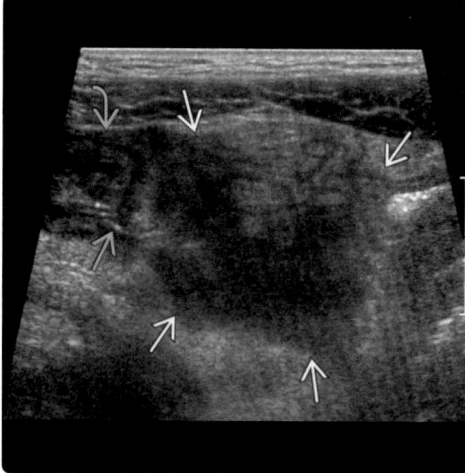
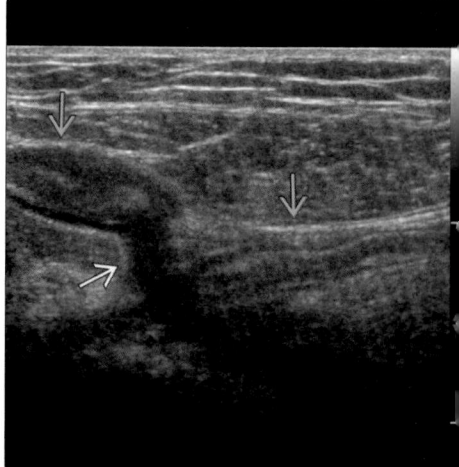

(Left) *Long-axis ultrasound shows marked thickening of the sigmoid colon* ➡. *Numerous round hypoechoic mural lesions are seen* ➡. (Right) *Color Doppler ultrasound in the same patient is shown. The round hypoechoic mural lesions are avascular* ➡ *along with marked hyperemia of the bowel wall raising concern that these were intramural abscesses.*

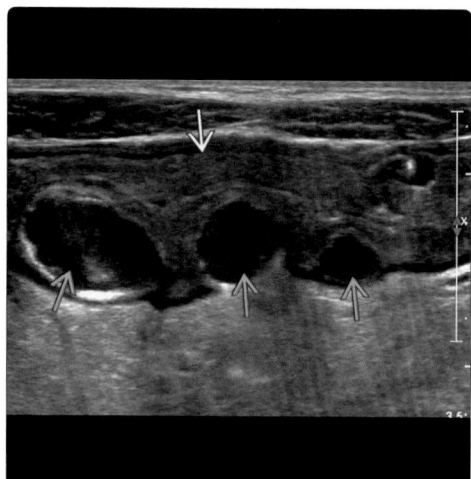
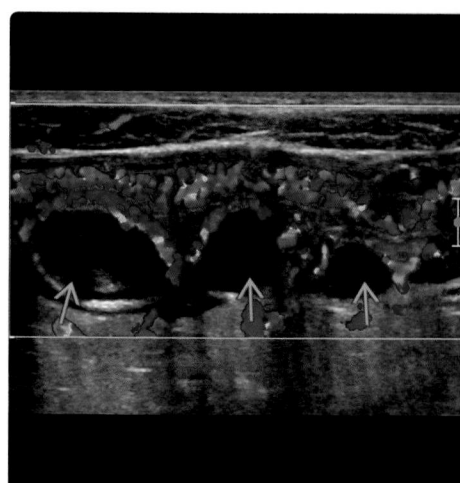

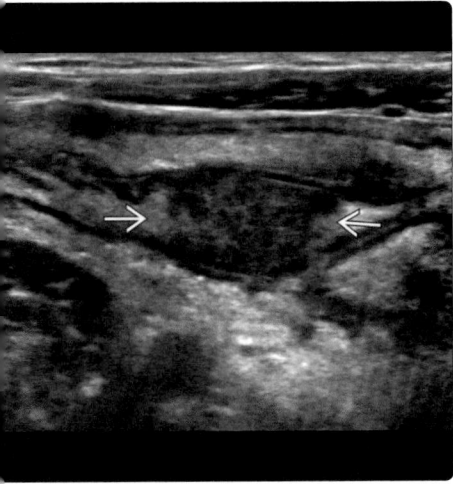
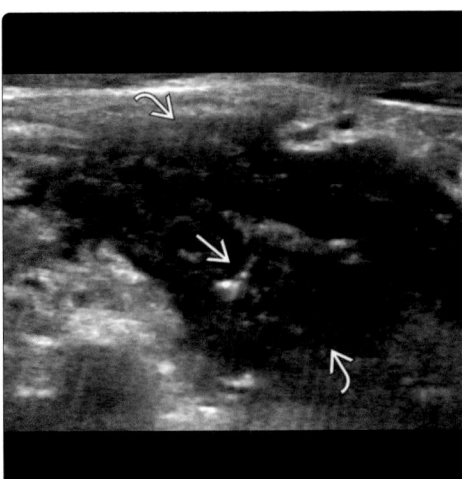

(Left) *Long-axis ultrasound of the terminal ileum shows thickening of the bowel wall. Although a long segment of bowel was thickened, note the focal area of decreased echogenicity and loss of bowel wall stratification indicative of severe subacute inflammation* ➡. **(Right)** *Grayscale ultrasound shows a markedly thickened and diffusely hypoechoic terminal ileum* ➡ *with loss of the normal bowel wall stratification. Small bubbles of gas are also seen within the bowel wall consistent with an area of ulceration* ➡.

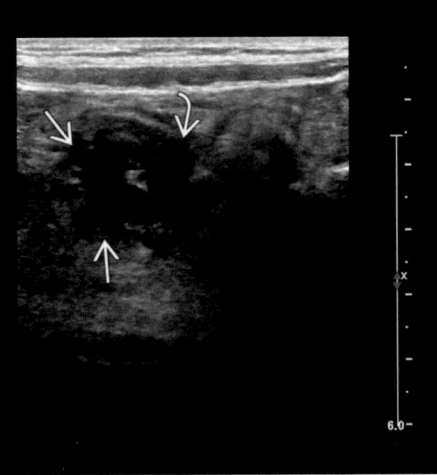
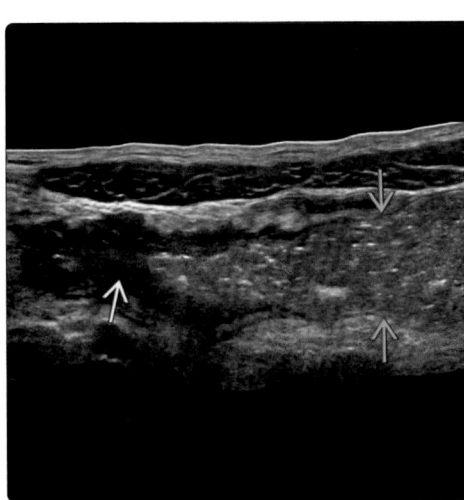

(Left) *Short-axis ultrasound of the terminal ileum in the same patient shows the marked thickening of the bowel wall and loss of normal stratification* ➡. *The irregular and spiculated serosal border* ➡ *of the wall is indicative of severe transmural inflammation.* **(Right)** *A panoramic view of the terminal ileum in the same patient shows the markedly thickened terminal ileum with resultant narrowing of the lumen* ➡. *There is dilation of the more proximal, upstream, ileum reflecting some degree of obstruction* ➡.

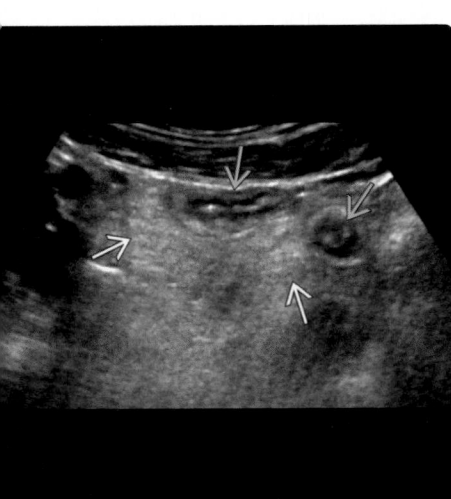
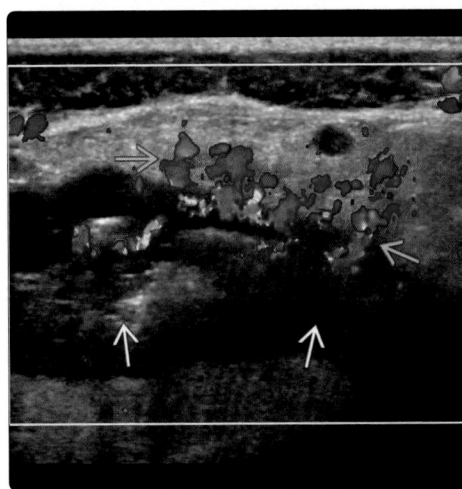

(Left) *Grayscale ultrasound shows thickened bowel loops* ➡. *There is thickening and increased echogenicity of the surrounding mesentery* ➡. **(Right)** *Long-axis US shows a thickened loop of sigmoid colon* ➡. *There is increased echogenicity of the adjacent mesentery with hyperemia of the vasa recta* ➡ *correlating to the "comb" sign on CTE or MRE.*

TERMINOLOGY

- Malignant lesion of colon or rectum

IMAGING

- Best diagnostic clue: Focal segmental thickening or mass lesion of colon or rectum
- US image interpretation pearls
  - Irregular hypoechoic lesion causing abrupt, segmental loss of normal wall stratification
  - Extramural extension of tumor
  - Locoregional lymph node involvement
- Staging: CECT
- Metastases: Most commonly to regional lymph nodes, liver, and lung

TOP DIFFERENTIAL DIAGNOSES

- Diverticulitis
- Inflammatory bowel disease
- Colonic lymphoma

- Gastrointestinal stromal tumors
- Intussusception
- Infectious colitis
- Ischemic colitis

CLINICAL ISSUES

- Most common signs and symptoms
  - Hematochezia
  - Altered bowel habit; abdominal pain
  - Weight loss
- Staged using AJCC TNM, Modified Astler Collier (MAC), or Dukes staging systems
- 5-year survival: 50-60% depending on stage

DIAGNOSTIC CHECKLIST

- If colon cancer is detected sonographically, evaluate liver for metastases at time of initial US scan
- Recommend CECT for complete staging
- Recommend colonoscopy for histologic confirmation

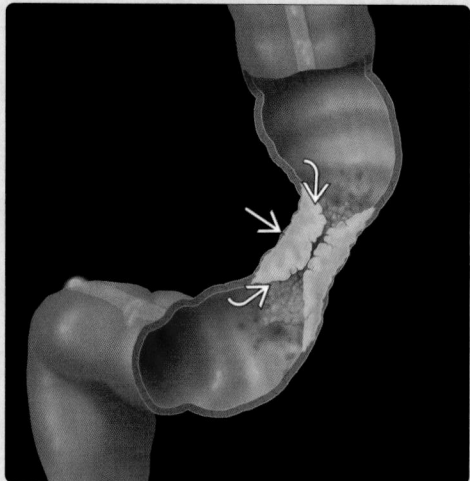
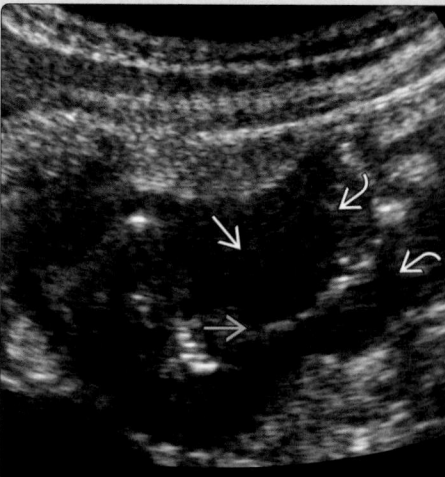

(Left) *Graphic illustrates a circumferential tumor ➡ of the colon with luminal narrowing. Note "shouldering" at both ends ➡.* (Right) *Longitudinal ultrasound in a patient with ascending colon tumor shows asymmetrical annular hypoechoic thickening to a short segment of colon. There is loss of colonic mural stratification ➡, and effacement of echogenic lumen ➡. Note "shouldering" at the ends of the lesion ➡.*

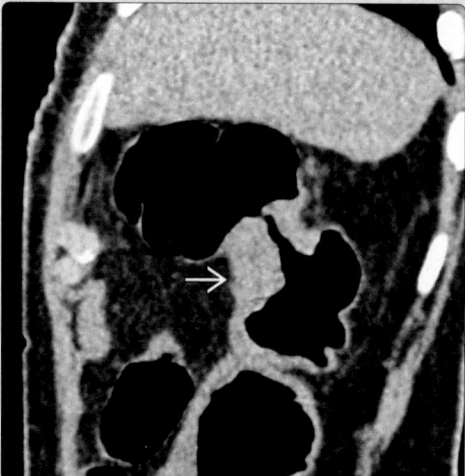
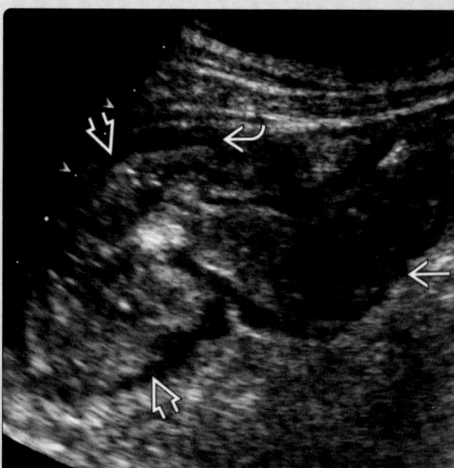

(Left) *Sagittal CT reformat from the same patient depicts the ascending colon "apple core" tumor ➡. Note "shouldering" at both ends and the luminal narrowing.* (Right) *The terminal ileum ➡ and cecum ➡ from the same patient proximal to the tumor demonstrates mural edema secondary to obstruction, but note the preserved mural stratification ➡.*

TERMINOLOGY

Synonyms

Colorectal, colon(ic), or rectal cancer, neoplasia, malignancy

Definitions

Malignant lesion of colon or rectum

IMAGING

General Features

Best diagnostic clue
o Focal segmental thickening or mass lesion of colon/rectum

Location
o Ascending colon: 30%
o Sigmoid colon: 25%
o Rectum: 20%
o Descending colon: 15%
o Transverse colon: 10%

Morphology
o Circumferential, annular, "apple core," semiannular, eccentric, sessile, pedunculated, exophytic, desmoplastic

Ultrasonographic Findings

Normal colonic wall seen on US as 5 distinct alternating hyperechoic and hypoechoic layers: Gut signature

Colon cancer is seen on US as
o Irregular hypoechoic lesion causing abrupt, segmental loss of normal wall stratification
o Irregular wall thickening that may be eccentric or circumferential affecting short segment
o Hyperechoic foci representing intraluminal gas or feces may be seen within hypoechoic mass (pseudokidney appearance)
o Dilatation of prestenotic segment
o Disappearance of colonic haustra
o Increased vascularity may be seen with Color Doppler

Staging of colon cancer with US
o Tis: Focal hypoechoic lesion in contact with mucosa or deep mucosa
o T1: Focal hypoechoic lesion infiltrating submucosa, but without involvement of muscularis propria (MP)
o T2: Focal hypoechoic lesion infiltrating MP
o T3: Focal hypoechoic lesion penetrating MP but not involving adjacent organs
o T4: Focal hypoechoic lesion penetrating serosal surface

Perifocal or regional hypoechoic lymph nodes with loss of normal nodal architecture

Radiographic Findings

Double-contrast barium enema
o Annular: Focal circumferential luminal narrowing with irregular margins and acute shouldering (apple core)
o Semiannular: Eccentric luminal narrowing with irregular margins
o Intraluminal: Flat lesion with broad base (sessile) or lesion with stalk (pedunculated) protruding into lumen
o Exophytic: Focal defect or "puckering" indicating base of lesion
o Desmoplastic: Luminal distortion, tethering, and angulated margins of lumen

CT Findings

- CECT
  o Intraluminal: Early cancers or cancerous polyps seen as intraluminal lesions
  o Mural: Focal asymmetric, irregular, or circumferential thickening of colonic wall
  o Extramural
    – Perilesional fat stranding
    – Nodular or broad-based extramural tissue extension into pericolonic fat
    – Expansion of draining veins by tumor indicative of extramural venous invasion
    – Infiltration of adjacent organs
  o Metastatic deposits: Typically to liver, lung, and bone
  o Nodal deposits
- CT colonography
  o Small polyps or lesions appear as intraluminal filling defects
  o Mural and extramural changes overlap with CECT findings

MR Findings

- Typically used for local staging of rectal cancer
  o Useful for T staging and relationship to circumferential resection margin (CRM)
    – Relationship to CRM dictates management and need for adjuvant chemoradiotherapy
- Mesorectal and pelvic side wall nodal metastases
  o Loss of round morphology
  o Loss of homogenous signal
  o Demonstrate restricted diffusion
- Extramural venous invasion
  o Intermediate signal tumor extends into and expands adjacent veins

Imaging Recommendations

- Best imaging tool
  o MR for local staging of rectal cancer
  o CT for local staging of colon cancer
  o CT and PET/CT for evaluation of metastatic disease
  o US not routinely used for diagnosis or staging; cancer may be detected incidentally on routine US examination for evaluation of abdominal pain
    – Endoanal US has role in T staging of rectal cancer

DIFFERENTIAL DIAGNOSIS

Diverticulitis

- Background diverticulosis
- Wall thickening, adjacent inflammatory changes, and reactive lymph nodes can mimic colonic cancer
- Longer segment of thickening (> 10 cm)

Inflammatory Bowel Disease (IBD)

- Bowel wall thickening is more symmetrical and may affect longer segment
- Involvement of terminal ileum favors Crohn disease
- Increase in fatty submucosal layer with preservation of gut signature
- Penetrating ulcers seen in IBD may breach serosa, but is more focal, less broad based, and not seen in association with hypoechoic mass

- Multisegmental involvement in Crohn disease

Colonic Lymphoma

- Hypoechoic/anechoic; single or multifocal
- Typically circumferential with destruction of gut signature
- Transition from tumor to normal bowel is gradual
- Dilatation of lumen
- Bulky mesenteric/retroperitoneal nodes

Gastrointestinal Stromal Tumors

- Rare in large bowel
- Rounded mural mass; exophytic or project into lumen
- Large central necrotic cavity may communicate with lumen
- No lymph node enlargement

Intussusception

- "Bowel-within-bowel" appearance
- Eccentrically placed crescentic echogenicity representing intussuscepted mesentery

Infectious Colitis

- Longer segment of involvement
- Accordion sign in *Clostridium difficile* colitis may be seen on CT or US

Colonic Ischemia

- Can demonstrate hypoechoic segmental bowel thickening, mimicking colon cancer
- Location: Watershed regions, splenic flexure; rectal sparing
- Color Doppler may demonstrate absence of arterial flow
- Pneumatosis or portal venous gas

PATHOLOGY

General Features

- Etiology
  - Adenoma-carcinoma sequence: Benign adenoma progressing to malignant transformation
  - Risk factors
    - Colonic polyps
    - Family history of colorectal cancer (CRC)
    - Inflammatory bowel disease
    - Diet: High fat, low roughage, high alcohol
    - Inherited conditions: Familial adenomatous polyposis (FAP) and hereditary nonpolyposis colon cancer (HNPCC) account for 5% of CRCs

Staging, Grading, & Classification

- AJCC TNM stage
- Modified Astler Collier staging (MAC)
  - Original MAC was based on the modified Dukes classification
- Original Dukes classification
  - A: Tumor limited to bowel wall
  - B: Tumor extending through bowel wall
  - C: Nodal metastasis

CLINICAL ISSUES

Presentation

- Most common signs/symptoms
  - Hematochezia, altered bowel habit, weight loss, tenesmus, abdominal pain (from bowel obstruction or perforation)
- Other signs/symptoms
  - Asymptomatic and detected through screening programs.

Demographics

- Epidemiology
  - 2nd and 3rd most common cancers in Europe and United States, respectively (Europe: 183,000; USA: 79,000 new cases per year)

Natural History & Prognosis

- 5-year survival: 50-60%.
- 30-50% of patients either present with or develop distant metastases in liver &/or lungs

Treatment

- Surgery
  - 85% of patients undergo resection with curative intent
- Chemotherapy
- Radiotherapy

DIAGNOSTIC CHECKLIST

Consider

- Colonic carcinoma in differential of short segment bowel wall thickening

Image Interpretation Pearls

- Short segment thickening
- Asymmetric thickening
- Loss of gut signature
- Extramural tumor extension
- Local lymph nodes

Reporting Tips

- Recommend colonoscopy for histologic confirmation
- Recommend CECT for confirmation and complete staging when US suspicious for colonic cancer
- EUS &/or MR for locoregional staging of rectal cancer

SELECTED REFERENCES

1. Shibasaki S et al: Use of transabdominal ultrasonography to preoperatively determine T-stage of proven colon cancers. Abdom Imaging. ePub, 2014
2. Martínez-Ares D et al: Ultrasonography is an accurate technique for the diagnosis of gastrointestinal tumors in patients without localizing symptoms. Rev Esp Enferm Dig. 101(11):773-86, 2009
3. Smith NJ et al: Preoperative computed tomography staging of nonmetastatic colon cancer predicts outcome: implications for clinical trials. Br J Cancer. 96(7):1030-6, 2007
4. O'Malley ME et al: US of gastrointestinal tract abnormalities with CT correlation. Radiographics. 23(1):59-72, 2003

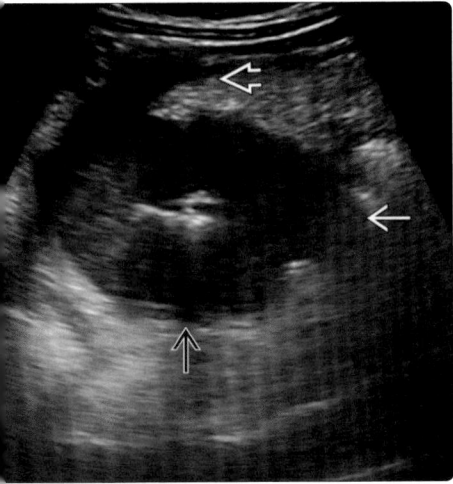
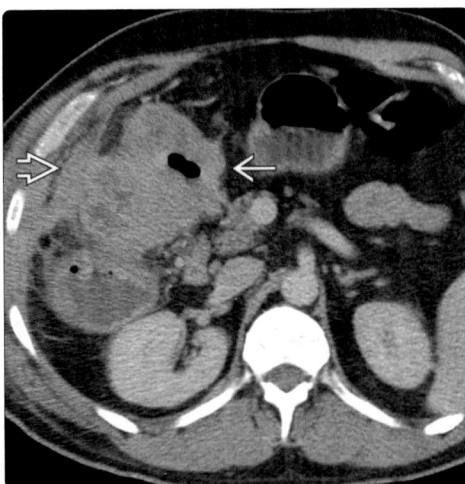

(Left) *Hepatic flexure tumor is shown. There is circumferential hypoechoic thickening and loss of the normal mural stratification ➡. There are extramural nodular tongues of tumor extending into the pericolonic fat medially ➡, and also extending to involve the peritoneum laterally ➡, indicating T4 disease.* (Right) *Hepatic flexure tumor on CECT from the same patient shows circumferential thickening to the colon ➡, with involvement and thickening to the right parietal peritoneum ➡, in keeping with T4 disease.*

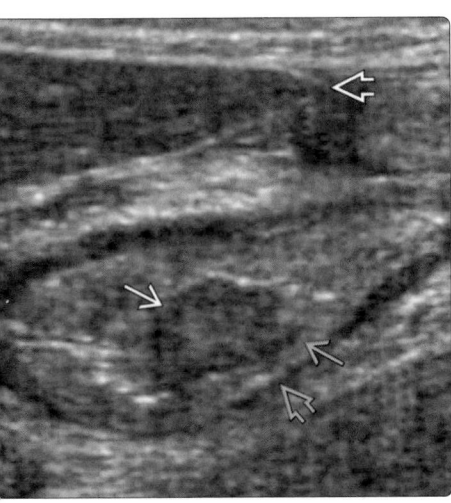
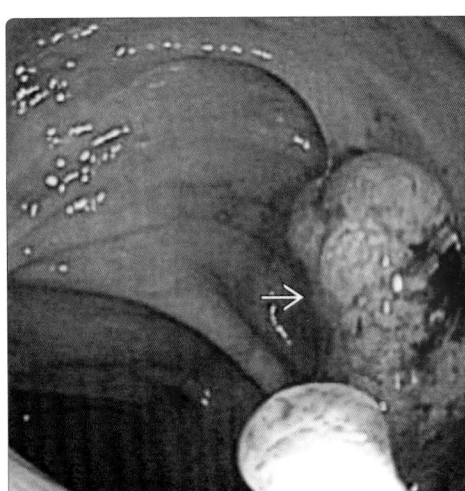

(Left) *US in a patient with polypoidal carcinoma shows a hypoechoic lesion within the lumen of the transverse colon ➡. The echogenic submucosa ➡ and the hypoechoic muscularis propria ➡ are intact, indicating T1 disease. Note the inferior edge of the liver ➡.* (Right) *Endoluminal colonoscopic image depicting the polypoidal lesion ➡ in the same patient represents a polypoidal carcinoma. (Courtesy V. Rudralingam, MD).*

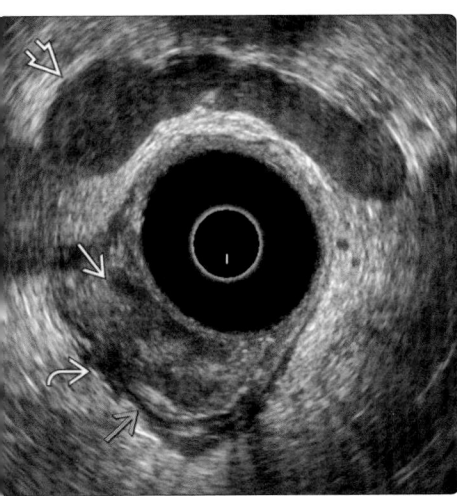
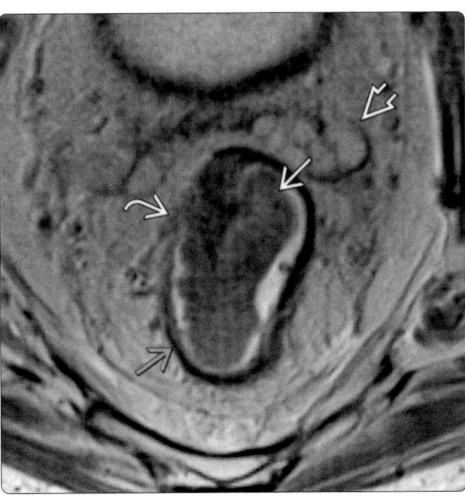

(Left) *Transrectal ultrasound shows a large polypoidal tumor ➡ with extramural tumor ➡ breaching the outer hypoechoic muscularis propria layer ➡, indicating a T3 tumor. Note the seminal vesicles ➡.* (Right) *T2-weighted MR from the same patient shows the intermediate intensity polypoidal tumor ➡ with extramural tongue of tissue ➡ extending beyond the low-signal muscularis propria ➡ into the mesorectal fat, representing T3 tumor. Note the seminal vesicles ➡.*

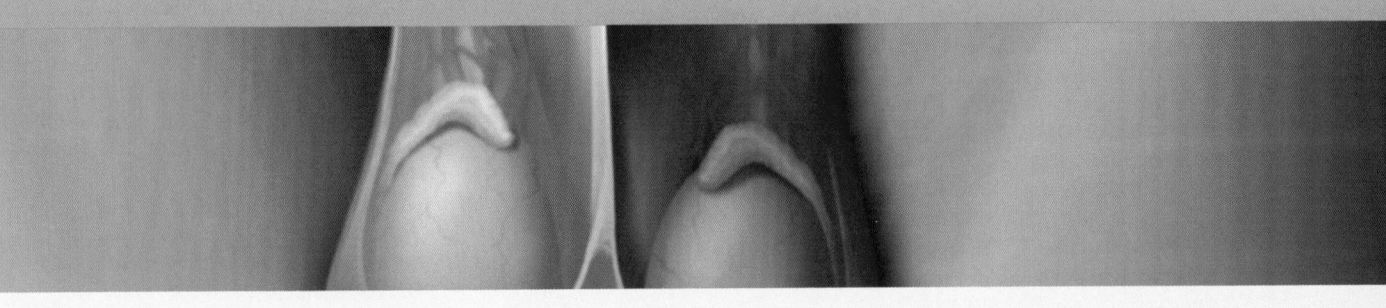

Introduction

High-frequency transducer sonography, using grayscale along with pulsed and color Doppler, is the imaging modality of choice for evaluating patients who present with scrotal pathology. Scrotal ultrasound (US) is often requested in an emergency setting in cases of acute scrotal pain. The leading differential diagnoses in such a scenario include testicular torsion, acute epididymoorchitis, and traumatic injury (in the setting of preceding trauma). In the nonacute setting, scrotal ultrasound is often requested for evaluation of chronic testicular pain or a palpable scrotal mass. The differential diagnoses of a palpable mass includes testicular neoplasm, benign or malignant, and extratesticular masses including paratesticular lesions and inguinal hernia.

Clinical correlation with history and symptoms is an extremely important aspect of scrotal sonography.

Ultrasound Technique for Scrotal Evaluation

Scrotal US is performed with the patient in the supine position and the scrotum supported by a towel placed between the thighs. Optimal results are obtained with a 9-15 MHz high-frequency linear-array transducer. Scanning is performed with the transducer in direct contact with the skin with copious amounts of gel; if necessary, a stand-off pad can be used for evaluation of superficial lesions. A curvilinear lower frequency transducer may be used for supplementary evaluation when the scrotum is too large to be evaluated with a linear high resolution transducer.

The testes are examined in at least two planes, i.e., the longitudinal and transverse axes. The size and echogenicity of each testis and epididymis are compared with those on the opposite side. Scrotal skin thickness is evaluated for symmetricity as well as focal or diffuse edema. Color Doppler and pulsed Doppler parameters are optimized to display low-flow velocities and demonstrate blood flow in the testes and surrounding scrotal structures. Color Doppler ultrasound should include comparison of bilateral testicular spectral Doppler tracings. Power Doppler US may also be used to demonstrate intratesticular blood flow in patients with an acute scrotum, particularly in evaluation for torsion or infarct.

When evaluating patients who present with an acute scrotum, the asymptomatic side should be scanned first in order to set the grayscale and color Doppler gain settings to allow comparison with the affected side, remembering that testicular torsion can be a bilateral process in 2% of patients. Transverse images with portions of each testis on the same image should be acquired in grayscale and color Doppler modes. Additional techniques, such as use of the Valsalva maneuver or upright positioning, can be used as needed for venous evaluation. Power Doppler sonography uses the amplitude of the Doppler signal independent of flow directionality. Therefore, power Doppler sonography has greater sensitivity than standard color Doppler for detecting low-flow states and provides essential information in diagnosis of complete testicular torsion.

Clinical Perspective

Acute Scrotal Pain

In an emergency setting, acute scrotal pain should prompt one to assess the scrotum for epididymoorchitis, testicular torsion, and traumatic injury. History and physical examination are critical in making the correct diagnosis along with the sonographic appearance of the scrotum. Although acute epididymoorchitis and acute testicular torsion present similarly with acute onset of unilateral testicular pain, epididymoorchitis may be accompanied with fever &/or a Prehn sign (relief of pain with elevation of scrotum above the level of pubic symphysis). Moreover, the sonographic appearances for both diagnoses are very distinct: Edema with increased vascularity in epididymoorchitis, and edema with absent or reduced flow in torsion. A potential pitfall for testicular torsion is torsion-detorsion syndrome wherein the testis may detorse spontaneously, resulting in reactive hyperemia, which can appear sonographically similar to epididymoorchitis. An appropriate history preceding the clinical presentation may lead to the correct diagnosis. Torsion-detorsion syndrome will typically present with intermittent symptoms of pain and discomfort. epididymoorchitis will present with constant or worsening pain. Associated findings of inflammation in the ipsilateral scrotum, such as scrotal skin thickening and pyocele, also favors epididymoorchitis.

Diagnosis of a traumatic scrotal injury is usually not difficult with a prior history of trauma (blunt or penetrating). The purpose of performing an ultrasound after trauma is to determine whether surgical exploration is required. Most cases with testicular rupture (tunica albuginea disruption) will need to be surgically repaired. In addition, large hematoceles or large hematomas resulting in nonviable testis may require surgical evacuation &/or debridement. Presence of color Doppler flow in the testis helps determine viability. It is extremely important to follow all such cases to resolution, as some hematomas may become infected and form an abscess.

Chronic/Nonacute Scrotal Pathology

In a nonacute setting, patients often present with an enlarged scrotum, palpable mass, or mild scrotal pain. An enlarged scrotum may be related to a hydrocele, spermatocele, scrotal wall edema, or inguinal hernia. In the setting of a palpable mass, ultrasound is extremely sensitive in detecting the presence of an intratesticular neoplasm, which is a malignancy until proven otherwise. Mild scrotal pain is often related to a varicocele, which can easily be diagnosed with color Doppler and Valsalva maneuvers.

Summary

The ability of ultrasound to diagnose the pathogenesis of the acute scrotum is unsurpassed by any other imaging modality. Ultrasound is the first-line imaging study performed in patients with acute scrotum. Knowledge of the normal and pathologic sonographic appearance of the scrotum and an understanding of the proper technique are essential for accurate diagnosis of an acute scrotum. High-frequency transducer sonography combined with color and power Doppler sonography provides information essential to reach a specific diagnosis in patients with testicular torsion, epididymoorchitis, and scrotal trauma.

Selected References

1. Appelbaum L et al: Scrotal ultrasound in adults. Semin Ultrasound CT MR. 34(3):257-73, 2013
2. American Institute of Ultrasound in Medicine et al: AIUM practice guideline for the performance of scrotal ultrasound examinations. J Ultrasound Med. 30(1):151-5, 2011
3. Bhatt S et al: Role of US in testicular and scrotal trauma. Radiographics. 28(6):1617-29, 2008
4. Dogra V et al: Acute painful scrotum. Radiol Clin North Am. 42 (2): 349-63, 2004
5. Dogra VS et al: Sonography of the scrotum. Radiology. 227(1):18-36, 2003

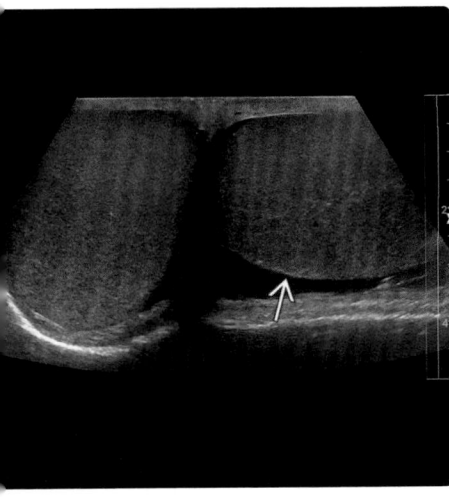

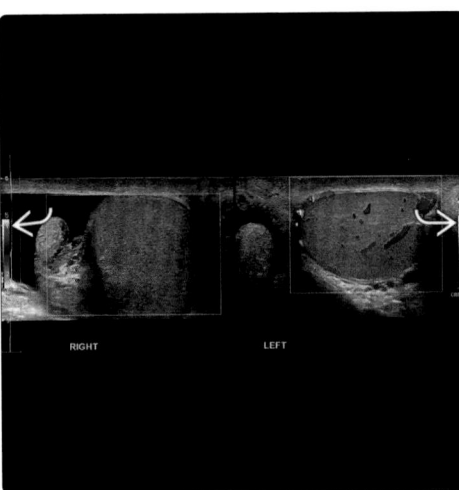

(Left) *Transverse grayscale ultrasound of the scrotum shows an abnormal axis of the left testis* ➡ *compared to the right. Patient was confirmed to have acute left testicular torsion. Torsed testis may change its axis and be located more horizontally.* (Right) *Transverse color Doppler ultrasound of bilateral testes shows a complete absence of flow in the right testis, suggestive of acute testicular torsion. It is important to examine both testes using the same color scale* ➡ *and same color Doppler gain settings.*

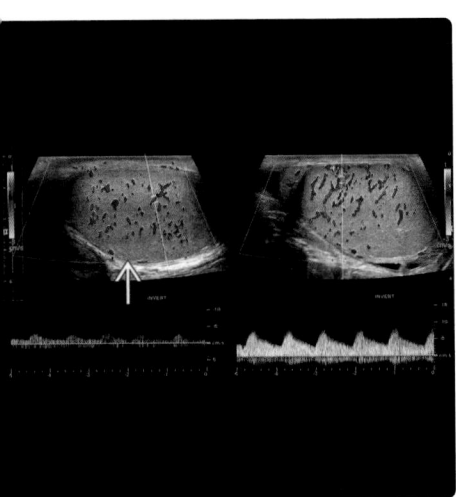

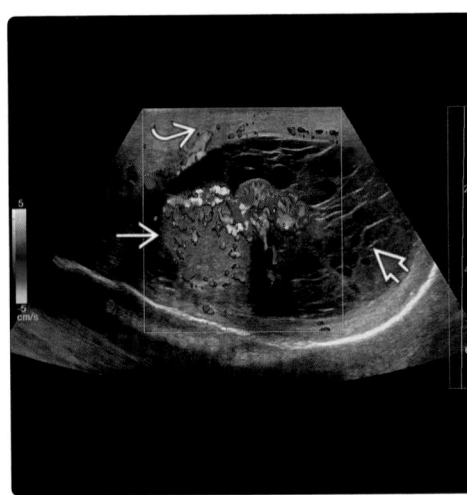

(Left) *Evaluation of both testes side by side using the same scale is essential to detect slight asymmetry in blood flow. This patient shows decreased flow on the right side* ➡*, surgically confirmed to be right-sided partial testicular torsion.* (Right) *Color Doppler ultrasound of the left testis demonstrates hyperemia* ➡ *of the testis and epididymis, along with associated complex hydrocele* ➡ *and skin thickening* ➡*. Findings suggest acute epididymoorchitis in the setting of acute left-sided pain.*

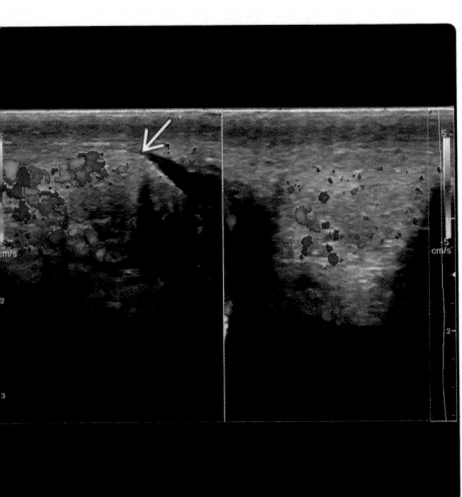

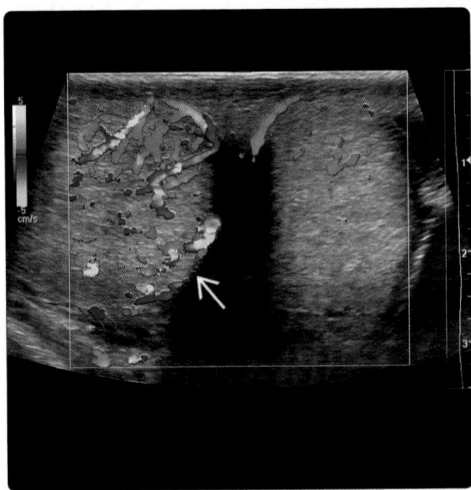

(Left) *Color Doppler ultrasound of bilateral epididymal tails shows enlarged right epididymis with increased blood flow* ➡*. Comparison of both sides using the same scale is essential to detect asymmetry in size and vascularity.* (Right) *Color Doppler ultrasound of testes in the same patient shows increased blood flow on the right side* ➡*. In a patient with acute right-sided pain, findings suggest acute epididymoorchitis.*

IMAGING

- Most common neoplasm in males between ages 15-34 years
- Mostly unilateral; contralateral tumor develops eventually in 8%
- Seminoma is most common pure germ cell tumor of testis
- On ultrasound, seminomas are usually well-defined, hypoechoic, solid without calcification or tunica invasion
- Tumor < 1.5 cm is commonly hypovascular, and tumors > 1.6 cm are more often hypervascular
- Embryonal cell carcinoma are aggressive tumors, may invade tunica albuginea and distort testicular contour
- US is used to identify and characterize scrotal mass; CT or MR for metastatic staging; PET to evaluate post-treatment residual masses
- Lymph nodes < 1 cm are suspicious if located in typical drainage areas; left renal hilus and right retrocaval in location

PATHOLOGY

- Associated with cryptorchidism, previous contralateral cancer; possible association with mumps orchitis, microlithiasis, and family history of tumor

CLINICAL ISSUES

- Beta hCG is elevated in pure or mixed embryonal carcinoma or choriocarcinoma; also in 15-20% of those with advanced seminoma
- Elevated α-fetoprotein (AFP) levels above 10,000 microg/L are found almost exclusively in patients with NSGCTs (not seen with pure seminomas) and hepatocellular carcinoma
- Lactate dehydrogenase (LDH) has independent prognostic significance: Increased levels reflect tumor burden, growth rate, and cellular proliferation

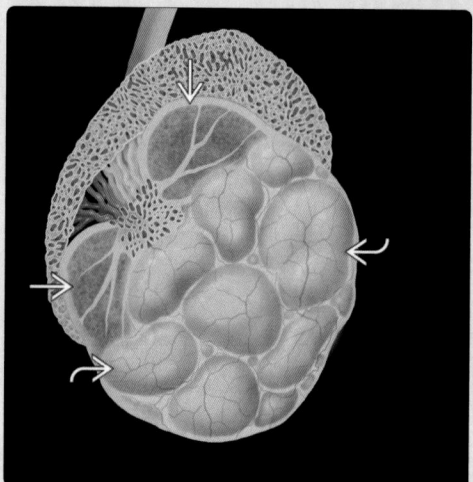
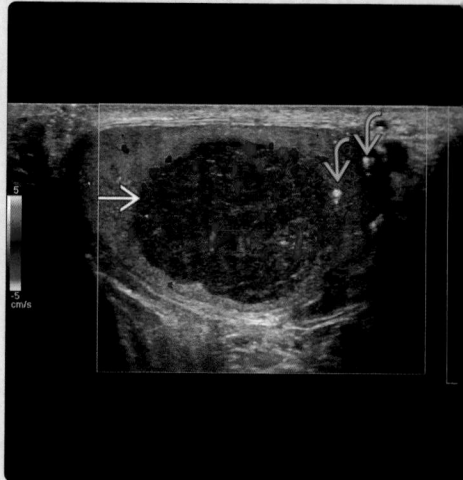

(Left) *Graphic shows a multilobulated testicular mass ➡. Note the compressed and near-complete replacement of normal testicular parenchyma ➡. (Right) Longitudinal color Doppler ultrasound of the right testis demonstrates a well-defined hypoechoic solid mass ➡ with mild internal vascularity. Imaging features are classic for a seminoma. A few scattered microliths ➡ are also seen in the noninvolved portion of the testicle.*

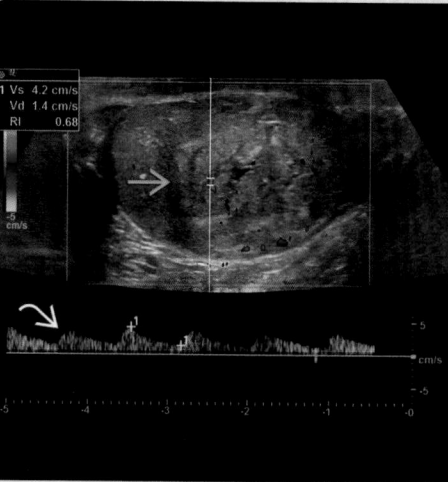
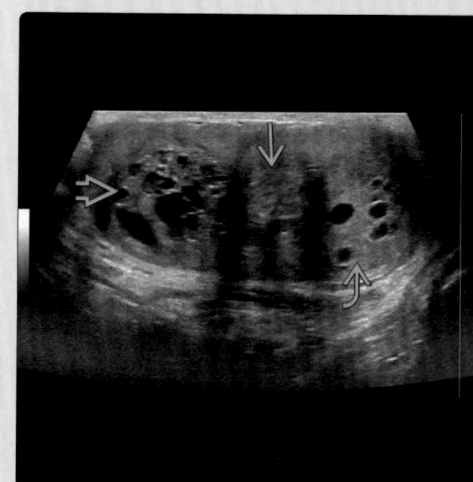

(Left) *Sagittal color Doppler ultrasound of the right testicle demonstrates a predominantly solid, heterogeneous mass ➡ with internal arterial vascularity ➡. Pathology revealed a mixed germ cell tumor with 95% embryonal component and 5% teratoma. (Right) Sagittal grayscale US of the left testicle demonstrates multifocal masses with 3 different sonographic patterns including solid ➡, multiple cystic foci ➡, and solid and cystic foci ➡. Pathology revealed MGCT with 55% embryonal, 35% teratoma, and 10% yolk sac.*

TERMINOLOGY

Abbreviations

- Germ cell tumor (GCT)
- Mixed germ cell tumor (MGCT)

Definitions

- Malignant germ cell tumor of testis

IMAGING

General Features

- Best diagnostic clue
  o Discrete hypoechoic or mixed echogenic testicular mass, ± vascularity
- Morphology
  o Most common neoplasm in males between ages 15-34 years
  o Mostly unilateral; contralateral tumor develops eventually in 8%
  o Seminoma is most common pure germ cell tumor of testis
    – Bilateral in 1-3%, almost always asynchronous

Ultrasonographic Findings

- Grayscale ultrasound
  o Seminoma
    – Typically well-defined, homogeneously hypoechoic, solid mass without calcification or tunica invasion
      □ With high-resolution US some lesions show a heterogeneous echo pattern, ± lobulation
    – May be solitary or multifocal masses
    – May very rarely undergo necrosis and appear partly cystic
  o Teratoma/teratocarcinoma
    – Well-defined, anechoic/complex heterogeneous cystic mass
    – Cystic areas, calcification (cartilage, immature bone) ± fibrosis characterize teratoma/teratocarcinoma
  o Embryonal cell carcinoma
    – Heterogeneous, predominantly solid mass, of mixed echogenicity
    – Poorly marginated, 1/3 have cystic necrosis
    – Coarse calcification infrequently seen
    – Embryonal cell carcinoma are aggressive tumors, may invade tunica albuginea and distort testicular contour
  o Yolk sac tumor
    – Most common testicular neoplasm in pediatric population
    – Seen in pure form in children, while almost always admixed with other germ cell elements in adults
  o Choriocarcinoma
    – Mixed echogenicity, heterogeneous mass
    – Cystic areas with calcification common
    – Hemorrhage with focal necrosis is typical feature of choriocarcinoma
    – Usually rare in pure form; occurs with mixed GCT in 8%
    – Highly malignant
- Color Doppler
  o Tumor < 1.5 cm is commonly hypovascular, and tumors > 1.6 cm are more often hypervascular
  o Disorganized flow is typical
  o Cystic areas are avascular

CT Findings

- CECT
  o Useful for staging retroperitoneal, nodal, and pulmonary metastases
  o Low-attenuation nodes
  o Even nodes < 1 cm suspicious if located in typical drainage areas; left renal hilus and right retrocaval in location
  o Helpful to identify retroperitoneal recurrence &/or "growing teratoma" syndrome

MR Findings

- T2WI
  o Useful for identifying nodal metastases
  o Moderate high signal intensity lymphadenopathy in retroperitoneum
  o Seminoma is multinodular, hypointense
  o Intratumoral low signal band-like structures representing fibrovascular septa

Nuclear Medicine Findings

- PET
  o Helpful to reduce false-negative CT study
    – May aid in differentiating residual tumor from scar in treated patients

Imaging Recommendations

- Best imaging tool
  o US to identify and characterize scrotal mass; CT or MR for metastatic staging; PET to evaluate post-treatment residual masses
- Protocol advice
  o High-frequency (9-15 MHz) linear array transducer

DIFFERENTIAL DIAGNOSIS

Epidermoid Cyst

- Cystic cavity lined by stratified squamous epithelium
- "Onion skin" appearance due to alternating layers of keratin and desquamated squamous cells
- May have calcified rim, no enhancement on MR

Lymphoma

- Older age group, most common tumor of testes in men > 60 years
- 50% of cases bilateral, often multiple lesions, associated with lymphadenopathy masses elsewhere
- Hypoechoic and hypervascular on color Doppler

Subacute Hematoma

- History of trauma, associated hematocele
- Hypoechoic on US

Segmental Infarct

- Acute pain, no palpable mass
- Infarct is typically hypoechoic, focal avascular area on color Doppler

Focal Orchitis

- Irregular hypoechoic area within testis, enlarged epididymis

- Increased vascularity on color Doppler without displacement of vessels
- Reactive hydrocele with low-level echoes, scrotal wall thickening

PATHOLOGY

General Features

- Etiology
  - Associated with cryptorchidism, previous contralateral cancer; possible association with mumps orchitis, microlithiasis, and family history of tumor
- Genetics
  - Family history increases risk
- Associated abnormalities
  - Gynecomastia, prepubescent virilization
- 95% of testicular tumors are malignant germ cell tumors
- Single histologic subtype in 65% of tumors (seminoma most common)
- Multiple subtypes in 35%

Staging, Grading, & Classification

- Stage I (A): Tumor confined to testis
- Stage II (B): Tumor metastatic to nodes below diaphragm
- Stage IIA (B1): Retroperitoneal node enlargement < 2 cm (5 cm³)
- Stage IIB (B2): Retroperitoneal node enlargement > 2 cm x < 5 cm (10 cm³)
- Stage IIC (B3): Retroperitoneal node enlargement > 5 cm
- Stage III (C): Tumor metastatic to lymph nodes above diaphragm
- Stage IIIA (C1): Metastases confined to lymphatic system
- Stage IIIB or IV: Extranodal metastases

Gross Pathologic & Surgical Features

- Solid or solid/cystic intratesticular mass
- 10-15% have epididymis or spermatic cord involvement
- Bilateral in 2-3% of cases

CLINICAL ISSUES

Presentation

- Most common signs/symptoms
  - Palpable mass in testis, painless enlarging mass
  - Dull pain (27%)
  - Acute pain (10%)
- Other signs/symptoms
  - Gynecomastia, virilization
- Clinical profile
  - Young male with palpable testicular mass, elevated serum tumor markers
    - 3 serum tumor markers have established roles in management of men with testicular GCTs
    - Beta subunit of human chorionic gonadotropin (beta-hCG)
      - Elevated in pure or mixed embryonal carcinoma or choriocarcinoma; also in 15-20% of those with advanced seminoma
    - Alpha fetoprotein (AFP)
      - Elevated levels above 10,000 microg/L are found almost exclusively in patients with NSGCTs (not seen with pure seminomas)
      - Elevated AFP is most often seen with yolk sac tumor and less often embryonal tumors
    - Lactate dehydrogenase (LDH)
      - Elevated in 40-60% of men with testicular GCTs

Demographics

- Age
  - Seminomatous tumor: Average age 40.5 years
  - Nonseminomatous tumor: 20-30 years
  - Endodermal sinus tumor/teratoma: 1st decade
- Ethnicity
  - Increased incidence in Caucasian and Jewish males
- Epidemiology
  - Most common cancer in men aged 15-34
  - 1% of all cancers in men, 4-6% of all male genitourinary tumors, 4th most common cause of death from malignancy between 15-34 years
  - Seminomas most common in men 35-39 years, most common tumor in undescended testis
  - Seminomas rare before 10 years and after 60 years

Natural History & Prognosis

- 95% 5-year survival rate overall
- Metastases at presentation is seen in 4-14% of individuals
  - Distant spread occurs along testicular lymphatics
  - Hematogenous dissemination (usually late) to lung, bone, brain
  - Choriocarcinoma has proclivity for early hematogenous spread especially to brain, death usually within 1 year of diagnosis
- Growing teratoma syndrome: Evolution of mixed germ cell tumor into mature teratoma after chemotherapy (in 40%) followed by interval growth despite maintaining benign histologic type

Treatment

- Seminoma very sensitive to radiotherapy ± chemotherapy
- Radical orchiectomy; retroperitoneal node dissection for nonseminomatous tumor
- Radiotherapy or chemotherapy for metastatic disease

SELECTED REFERENCES

1. Kreydin EI et al: Testicular cancer: what the radiologist needs to know. AJR Am J Roentgenol. 200(6):1215-25, 2013
2. McDonald MW et al: Testicular tumor ultrasound characteristics and association with histopathology. Urol Int. 89(2):196-202, 2012
3. Sohaib SA et al: Imaging studies for germ cell tumors. Hematol Oncol Clin North Am. 25(3):487-502, vii, 2011
4. Sohaib SA et al: The role of imaging in the diagnosis, staging, and management of testicular cancer. AJR Am J Roentgenol. 191(2):387-95, 2008
5. Dalal PU et al: Imaging of testicular germ cell tumours. Cancer Imaging. 6:124-34, 2006
6. Jones RH et al: Part I: testicular cancer–management of early disease. Lancet Oncol. 4(12):730-7, 2003
7. Woodward PJ et al: From the archives of the AFIP: tumors and tumorlike lesions of the testis: radiologic-pathologic correlation. Radiographics. 22(1):189-216, 2002

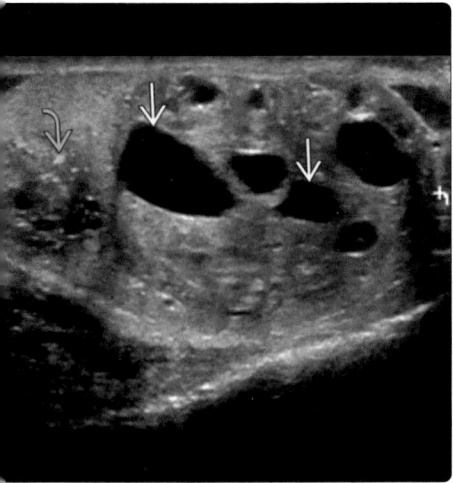

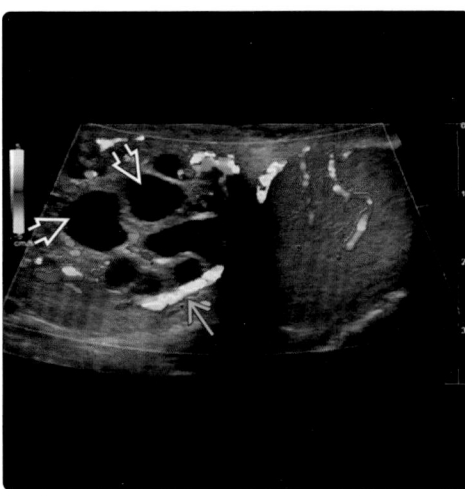

(Left) *Longitudinal grayscale ultrasound of the testis in a patient with a cystic teratoma shows a complex heterogeneous mass with cystic areas* ⮕ *of varying sizes and small echogenic foci* ⇗. (Right) *Transverse color Doppler ultrasound of both testes in a side-by-side configuration shows a right-sided teratoma with cystic spaces* ⮕ *and associated increased vascularity* ⇗.

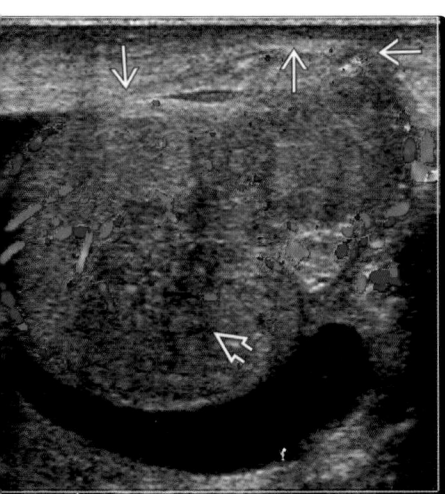

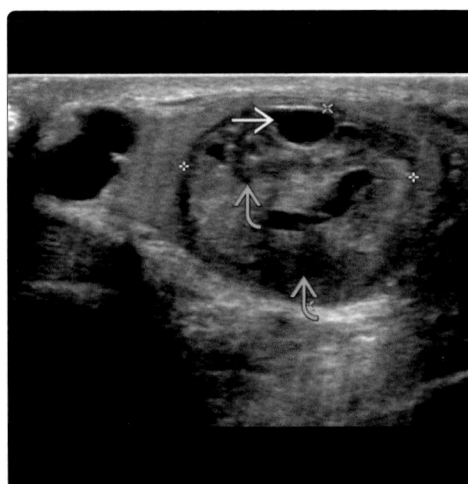

(Left) *Transverse color Doppler ultrasound of the testis demonstrates a poorly defined hypoechoic mass* ⮕ *with internal vascularity. The mass invades the tunica albuginea* ⮕ *and involves the scrotal wall.* (Right) *Longitudinal grayscale ultrasound of the testis shows a heterogeneous well-defined mass with cystic* ⮕ *as well as hypoechoic areas* ⇗. *Pathology revealed a mixed germ cell tumor with choriocarcinoma and mature teratoma.*

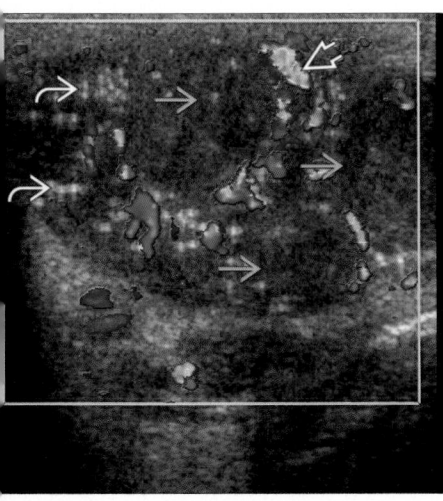

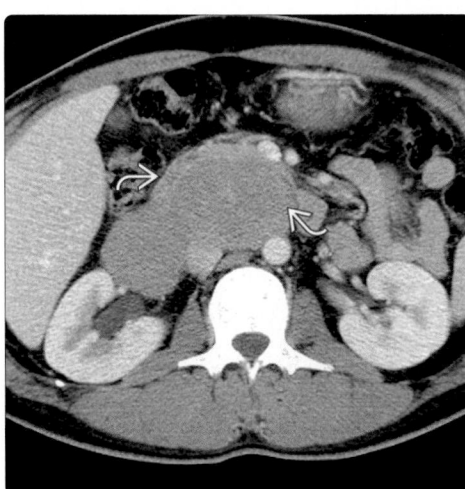

(Left) *Longitudinal color Doppler ultrasound of the right testis with multifocal seminoma shows multiple hypoechoic masses* ⮕ *with background microlithiasis* ⮕, *predominantly peripheral vascularity* ⮕, *and minimal internal vascularity within the hypoechoic masses.* (Right) *Axial CECT of the mid abdomen shows a conglomerate of metastatic paraaortic and retroperitoneal low-density lymph nodes* ⮕ *in a patient with testicular cancer.*

Gonadal Stromal Tumors, Testis

TERMINOLOGY

- Gonadal stromal tumors arise from nongerm cell elements

IMAGING

- May be indistinguishable from germ cell tumors on grayscale ultrasound
  o Leydig cell tumors
    - Small, solid, hypoechoic intratesticular mass
  o Sertoli cell tumors
    - Small, hypoechoic mass with occasional hemorrhage, which may lead to heterogeneity and cystic components
  o Gonadoblastoma
    - Stromal tumor in conjunction with germ cell tumor, usually mixed sonographic features
- High-resolution US (≥ 7.5 MHz) is best imaging tool for detection of gonadal stromal neoplasms

CLINICAL ISSUES

- 30% of patients with gonadal stromal tumors have endocrinopathy secondary to testosterone or estrogen production by tumor presenting with
  o Precocious virilization in children
  o Gynecomastia, impotence, ↓ libido in adults
- Majority of these tumors are benign
- Orchidectomy is preferred treatment

DIAGNOSTIC CHECKLIST

- Consider stromal tumor in any patient with endocrinopath and testicular mass

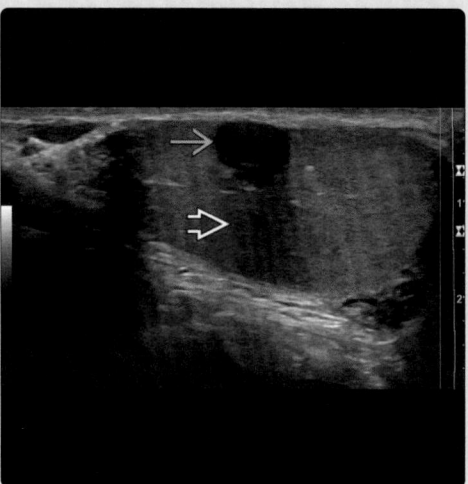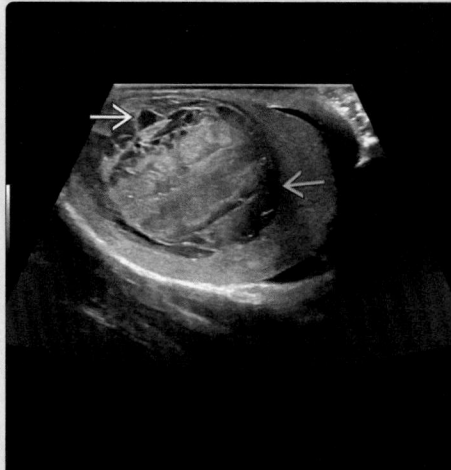

(Left) Sagittal grayscale ultrasound of the right testis in a 16-year-old male demonstrates a well-defined, hypoechoic mass ➡ with some posterior acoustic shadowing ➡. Pathology after orchiectomy confirmed it to be a benign sex cord stromal tumor (unclassified type). (Right) Sagittal grayscale ultrasound in a 16-year-old male demonstrates a well-defined, predominantly solid mass ➡ with some interspersed cystic areas ➡. Pathology confirmed it to be a granulosa cell tumor (adult type).

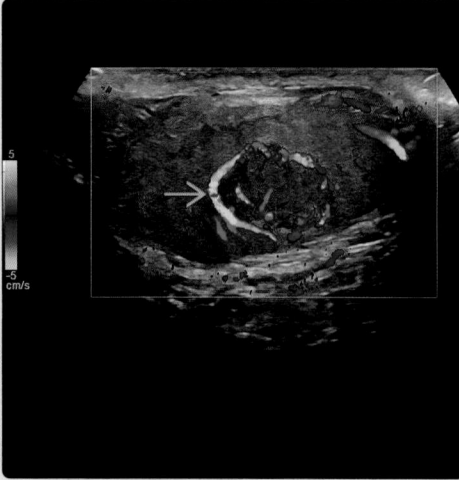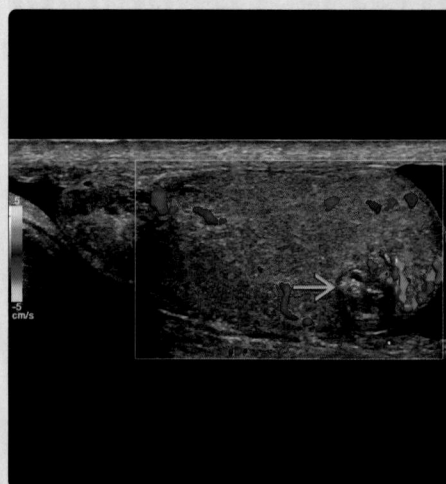

(Left) Sagittal color Doppler ultrasound of the right testis in a 33-year-old man demonstrates a well-defined, hypoechoic, solid mass with marked internal vascularity ➡. Pathology confirmed it to be a Leydig cell tumor. (Right) Sagittal color Doppler ultrasound shows the right testis with a partially calcified mass ➡ and minimal to no internal vascularity. Pathology confirmed a Sertoli cell tumor.

TERMINOLOGY

Abbreviations

Gonadal stromal tumors (GST)

Synonyms

Also called nongerm cell tumors, interstitial cell tumors, or sex cord tumors

Definitions

Leydig cell tumor (LCT): Arises from interstitial cells

Sertoli cell tumor (SCT): Arises from sustentacular cells lining seminiferous tubules

Granulosa cell tumor (GCT): Rare sex cord tumor

Gonadoblastoma: Contains both stromal and germ cell elements

IMAGING

General Features

Location
- o Bilateral in 3%

Size
- o Benign tumors: Usually < 3 cm
- o Malignant tumors: Usually > 5 cm

Morphology
- o Well circumscribed, round/lobulated

Ultrasonographic Findings

Grayscale ultrasound
- o May be indistinguishable from germ cell tumors
- o LCT: Small, solid, hypoechoic intratesticular mass
  - Larger tumors: Hemorrhage or necrosis leads to heterogeneous echo pattern
  - May occasionally show cystic change
- o SCT: Small, hypoechoic mass, hemorrhage may lead to heterogeneity
  - Solid and cystic components
  - ± punctate calcification; large, calcified mass in large-cell calcifying Sertoli cell tumor
- o GCT: Well-defined hypoechoic mass with solid and cystic components
- o Adult testicular GCTs are rare sex cord-stromal tumors

MR Findings

T2WI: Low signal intratesticular mass ± high signal fibrous capsule rim and high signal intensity foci internally secondary to central scars

Imaging Recommendations

Best imaging tool
- o High-resolution US (9-15 MHz)

DIFFERENTIAL DIAGNOSIS

Testicular Germ Cell Tumors

May be indistinguishable from stromal tumors on US

Testicular Metastases, Lymphoma, Leukemia

Often multiple; otherwise indistinguishable

Intratesticular Hematoma

Scrotal trauma, no internal color flow in hematoma

PATHOLOGY

General Features

- Associated abnormalities
  - o LCT: Klinefelter syndrome
  - o SCT: Peutz-Jeghers syndrome and Carney syndrome
- Leydig cell tumors: 3% of all testicular tumors
  - o 90% benign, 3% bilateral
  - o Most common, may produce testosterone
- Sertoli cell tumors: 1% of all testis tumors
  - o 85-90% benign
  - o May produce estrogen/müllerian inhibiting factor
- Granulosa cell tumor: Rare
  - o Juvenile GCTs are typically benign; 20% of testicular adult GCTs have been reported to present malignant behavior

CLINICAL ISSUES

Presentation

- Most common signs/symptoms
  - o Painless testicular enlargement
  - o 30% of patients have endocrinopathy secondary to testosterone or estrogen production by tumor
    - Gynecomastia, impotence, ↓ libido in adults

Demographics

- Age
  - o LCT: 30-60 years; 25% occur before puberty
  - o SCT: All age groups; 1/3 < 12 years
  - o GCT: Juvenile type in infants; adult type in patients aged 16-77 years

Natural History & Prognosis

- Malignant tumors metastasize in same pattern as testicular germ cell tumors

Treatment

- Orchidectomy or testis-sparing surgery

DIAGNOSTIC CHECKLIST

Image Interpretation Pearls

- Consider stromal tumor in any patient with endocrinopathy and testicular mass

SELECTED REFERENCES

1. Miliaras D et al: Adult type granulosa cell tumor: a very rare case of sex-cord tumor of the testis with review of the literature. Case Rep Pathol. 2013:932086, 2013
2. Leonhartsberger N et al: Increased incidence of Leydig cell tumours of the testis in the era of improved imaging techniques. BJU Int. 108(10):1603-7, 2011
3. Tallen G et al: High reliability of scrotal ultrasonography in the management of childhood primary testicular neoplasms. Klin Padiatr. 223(3):131-7, 2011
4. Maizlin ZV et al: Leydig cell tumors of the testis: gray scale and color Doppler sonographic appearance. J Ultrasound Med. 23(7):959-64, 2004
5. Carmignani L et al: High incidence of benign testicular neoplasms diagnosed by ultrasound. J Urol. 170(5):1783-6, 2003
6. Woodward PJ et al: From the archives of the AFIP: tumors and tumorlike lesions of the testis: radiologic-pathologic correlation. Radiographics. 22(1):189-216, 2002
7. Ulbright TM et al. Tumors of the testis, adnexa, spermatic cord, and scrotum. In: Atlas of Tumor Pathology. Washington, DC: Armed Forces Institute of Pathology. 1–290, 1999

(Left) *Sagittal grayscale ultrasound of the right testis in a 33-year-old man demonstrates a well-defined, hypoechoic, solid mass ➡. Pathology confirmed it to be a Leydig cell tumor.* **(Right)** *Sagittal grayscale ultrasound of the right testis in a young male demonstrates a solid cystic mass ➡ with some echogenic areas with calcification ➡. Pathology confirmed it to be a Sertoli cell tumor.*

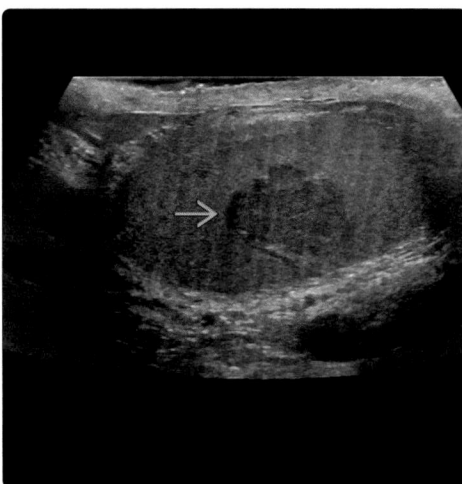 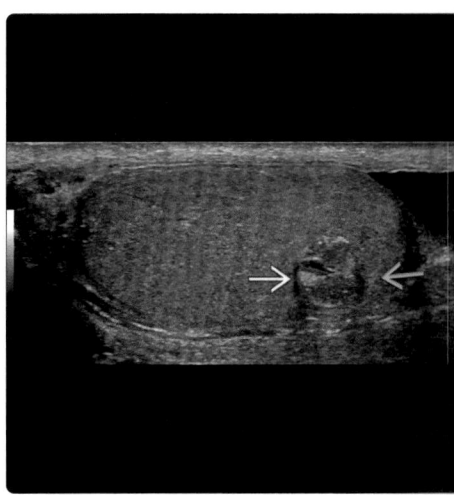

(Left) *Transverse color Doppler ultrasound of the right testis in a 16-year-old male demonstrates a well-defined, hypoechoic, solid mass ➡ with minimal internal vascularity. Pathology confirmed it to be a benign sex cord stromal tumor (unclassified type).* **(Right)** *Sagittal color Doppler ultrasound of the testicular mass shows no internal vascularity. Pathology confirmed it to be an adult granulosa cell tumor.*

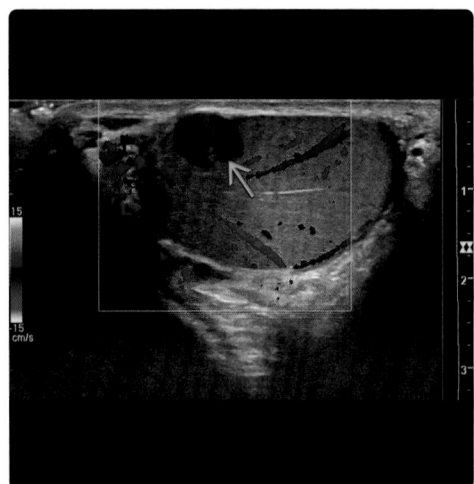 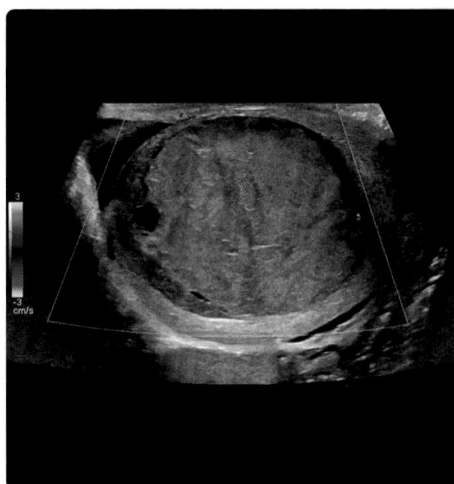

(Left) *Transverse grayscale ultrasound of the testis in a 12-year-old boy demonstrates a well-defined, heterogeneous, hypoechoic, solid mass ➡.* **(Right)** *Corresponding transverse color Doppler ultrasound of the testis demonstrates internal vascularity in this well-defined, heterogeneous, hypoechoic, solid mass ➡. Pathology confirmed a Leydig cell tumor.*

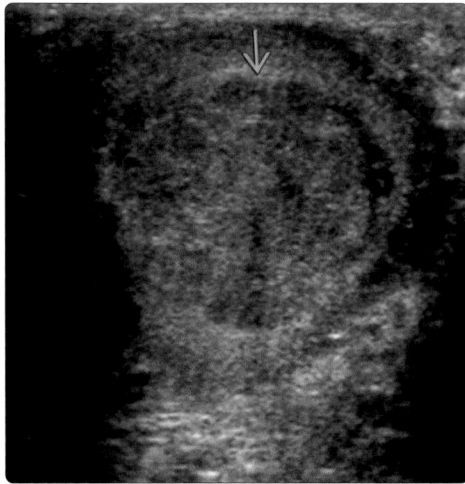 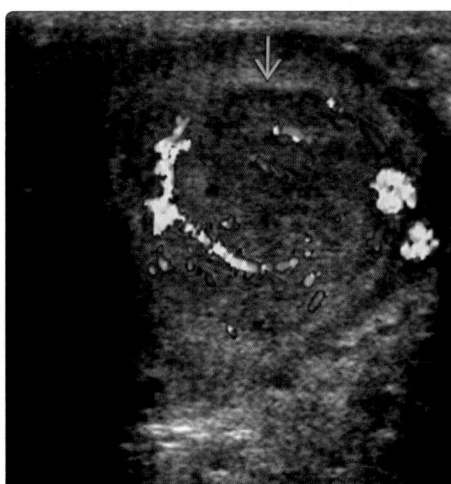

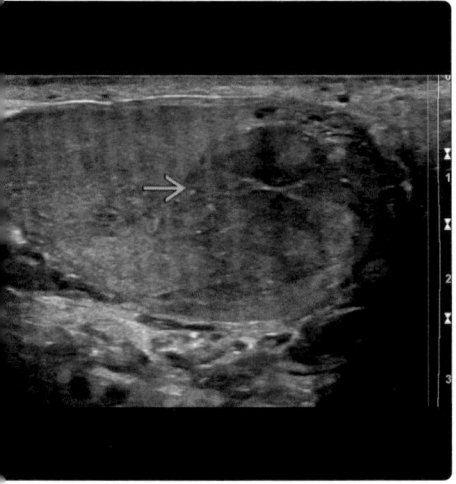 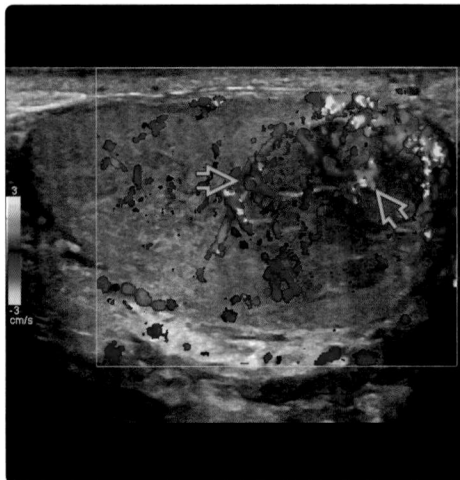

(Left) *Sagittal grayscale ultrasound of the left testis in this 18-year-old man demonstrates a hypoechoic, solid mass ➡. (Right) Corresponding color Doppler ultrasound of the left testis in the same patient shows presence of marked internal vascularity ➡. Pathology confirmed a Leydig cell tumor.*

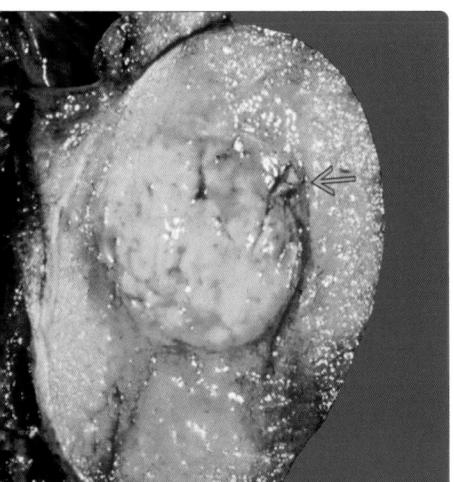 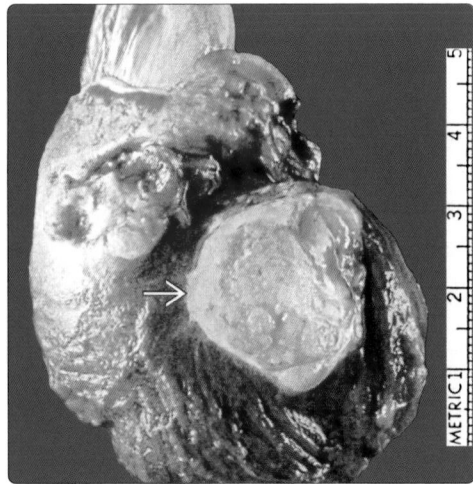

(Left) *Leydig cell tumor (LCT) is often a well-circumscribed mass with a homogeneous yellow-tan cut surface. Focal cystic change is present ➡. Hemorrhage or necrosis is lacking. LCT often do not replace the entire testis.* (Right) *A well-circumscribed Sertoli cell tumor with a tan-white firm cut surface ➡ is shown. The gross finding is different from Leydig cell tumor, which usually is tan-brown to yellow due to high lipid content.*

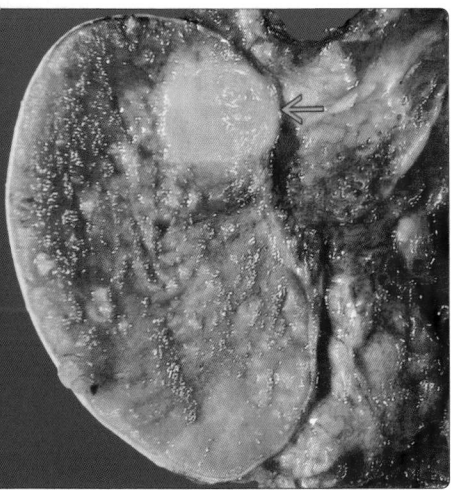 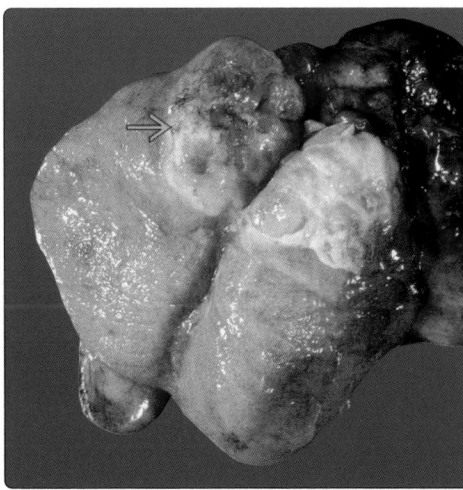

(Left) *Granulosa cell tumor shows a well-circumscribed, homogeneous, tan-white nodule ➡. The tumor is small and, like many sex cord stromal tumors, does not extensively involve the testis. Hemorrhage and necrosis are lacking.* (Right) *Gross photo shows a well-circumscribed, unclassified sex cord stromal tumor (SCST) ➡. It has heterogeneous, soft, tan nodular areas with dense white fibrotic septa. SCSTs frequently do not replace the entire testis.*

Testicular Lymphoma/Leukemia

TERMINOLOGY

- Infiltrative neoplasm of testis in which tumor cells surround and compress seminiferous tubules and normal testicular vessels

IMAGING

- Bilateral, solid, hypoechoic, hypervascular nodules/masses
- Diffuse hypoechoic testis with hypervascularity
- Striated pattern
- Testicular shape not altered
- Normal testicular vessels with straight course crossing through lesions
- Comparison of both testes to look for asymmetry in sizes and echogenicity

PATHOLOGY

- Most commonly secondary lymphomatous involvement of testis; rarely primary

- Lymphoma behaves similar to leukemia with abnormal cell diffusely infiltrating interstitium with compression of seminiferous tubules without causing their destruction
- Testis is "sanctuary organ": Blood gonad barrier limits accumulation of chemotherapeutic agents

CLINICAL ISSUES

- Stages IE and IIE: Orchidectomy
- Stage IIIE and IVE: Systemic chemotherapy using cyclophosphamide, doxorubicin, vincristine, and prednisolone
- Radiation in symptomatic and bulky deposits
- Lymphoma accounts for approximately 5% of all testicular tumors
- Most common bilateral testicular tumor

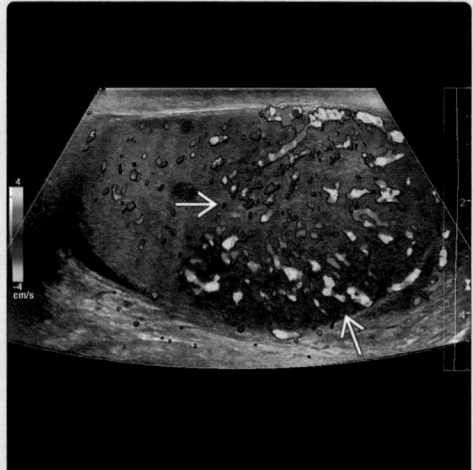
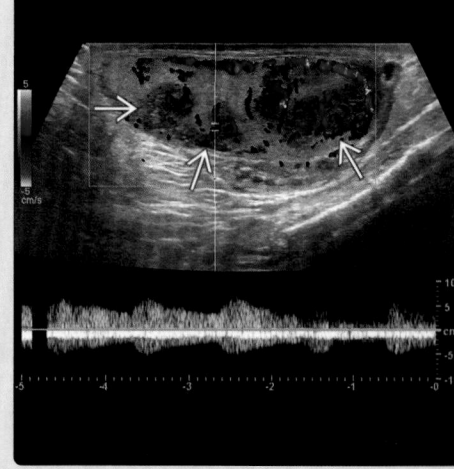

(Left) Sagittal color Doppler ultrasound of the right testis in a 56-year-old man with non-Hodgkin lymphoma shows a hypervascular focal mass ➡ in the inferior pole with focal enlargement of testis. Note that the shape of the testis is maintained. Pathology confirmed lymphoma. (Right) Sagittal color Doppler ultrasound of the left testis in a 65-year-old man shows multiple hypervascular hypoechoic masses ➡ in the testis. Pathology confirmed lymphoma.

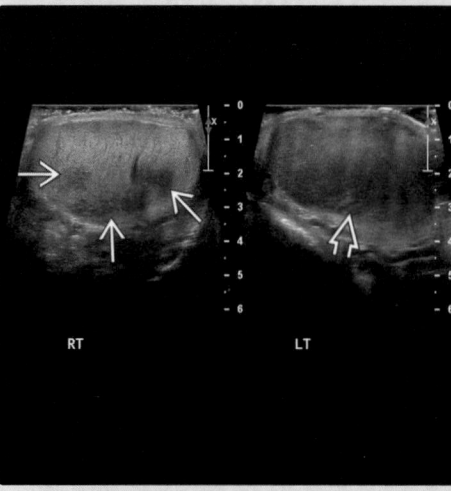
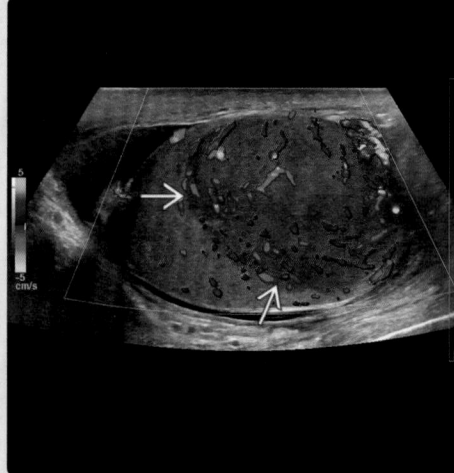

(Left) Sagittal grayscale ultrasound of the testes in a 60-year-old man with non-Hodgkin lymphoma shows bilateral hypoechoic masses, multifocal on the right ➡ and diffuse infiltrative on the left ➡. (Right) Sagittal color Doppler ultrasound of the right testis in a 51-year-old man with known history of acute myeloid leukemia shows a hypervascular focal hypoechoic mass ➡ in the inferior pole. Pathology confirmed acute myeloid leukemia.

TERMINOLOGY

Synonyms

- B-cell lymphoma of testis

Definitions

- Infiltrative neoplasm of testis in which tumor cells surround and compress seminiferous tubules and normal testicular vessels

IMAGING

General Features

- Best diagnostic clue
  - Bilateral, solid, hypoechoic, hypervascular nodules/masses
  - Diffuse hypoechoic testis with hypervascularity

Ultrasonographic Findings

- Grayscale ultrasound
  - Unifocal or multifocal hypoechoic lesions
  - Diffuse enlarged testis with diffuse decreased echogenicity
  - Striated pattern
  - Testicular shape not altered
- Color Doppler
  - Hypervascular lesions
  - Normal testicular vessels with straight course crossing through lesions

Imaging Recommendations

- Best imaging tool
  - Ultrasound
- Protocol advice
  - Comparison of both testes to look for asymmetry in sizes and echogenicity

Nuclear Medicine Findings

- Increased FDG uptake on PET

DIFFERENTIAL DIAGNOSIS

Epididymoorchitis

- Enlarged and heterogeneous testis and epididymis
- Hypervascular
- Associated findings: Complex hydrocele, skin thickening
- Clinical findings of acute scrotum at time of presentation

Primary Testicular Neoplasm

- Solid or mixed solid-cystic discrete mass; ± calcifications
- May have increased vascularity

Granulomatous Orchitis (Tuberculosis)

- Multiple hypoechoic nodules
- Testis and epididymis involved

PATHOLOGY

General Features

- Etiology
  - Most commonly secondary lymphomatous involvement of testis; rarely primary
  - Testis is "sanctuary organ": Blood gonad barrier limits accumulation of chemotherapeutic agents

  - Most commonly described in children with acute lymphoblastic leukemia
- Associated abnormalities
  - May have enlarged lymph nodes in other parts of body

Gross Pathologic & Surgical Features

- Solid, tannish-white mass
- Lymphoma behaves similar to leukemia with abnormal cells diffusely infiltrating interstitium with compression of seminiferous tubules without causing their destruction

CLINICAL ISSUES

Presentation

- Most common signs/symptoms
  - Painless testicular mass/enlargement
- Other signs/symptoms
  - Weight loss, night sweats, fever, anorexia

Demographics

- Age
  - Lymphoma: 20-80 years
    - Most common malignant tumor of testis in elderly
  - Leukemia: Seen in childhood
- Epidemiology
  - Lymphoma accounts for approximately 5% of all testicular tumors
  - Most common bilateral testicular tumor

Natural History & Prognosis

- Primary lymphoma: 5-year survival rate of 12%

Treatment

- Stages IE and IIE: Orchidectomy
- Stage IIIE and IVE: Systemic chemotherapy using cyclophosphamide, doxorubicin, vincristine, and prednisolone
- Radiation in symptomatic and bulky deposits
- CNS prophylaxis should be considered

DIAGNOSTIC CHECKLIST

Consider

- Primary testicular neoplasm
- Orchitis if pain and fever present

Image Interpretation Pearls

- Bilateral, uni- or multifocal, or infiltrative hypoechoic mass(es) with increased vascularity
- Maintained testicular contour

SELECTED REFERENCES

1. Bertolotto M et al: Grayscale and color Doppler features of testicular lymphoma. J Ultrasound Med. 34(6):1139-45, 2015
2. Liu KL et al: Imaging diagnosis of testicular lymphoma. Abdom Imaging. 31(5):610-2, 2006
3. Mazzu D et al: Lymphoma and leukemia involving the testicles: findings on gray-scale and color Doppler sonography. AJR Am J Roentgenol. 164(3):645-7, 1995

Epidermoid Cyst

TERMINOLOGY

- Rare, benign, keratin-containing lesion of controversial origin

IMAGING

- High-resolution US (≥ 10 MHz) is imaging modality of choice
- **Grayscale US**
  - Characteristic onion skin or target/bull's eye appearance of avascular testicular mass
  - Unilocular cyst containing keratin; fibrous wall
  - Sharply circumscribed, encapsulated round "mass"
- **Color Doppler US**
  - Avascular, no blood flow demonstrable
- Most commonly intratesticular, but rarely may be extratesticular

TOP DIFFERENTIAL DIAGNOSES

- Tunica albuginea cyst
  - Located within tunica, solitary, unilocular, and anechoic

- Germ cell tumor
  - Heterogeneous mass with vascularity seen on Doppler
- Testicular granuloma
  - Most probably due to TB, usually multiple

CLINICAL ISSUES

- May occur at any age; 2nd-4th decade most common
- 1-2% of all testicular tumors
- No malignant potential
- Enucleate 1st if lesions < 3 cm with characteristic US appearance and no color flow; testis can be spared if
  - Frozen sections of lesion are consistent with epidermoid cyst
  - No evidence of malignancy within or surrounding lesion
  - Negative tumor markers (AFP, β-HCG)

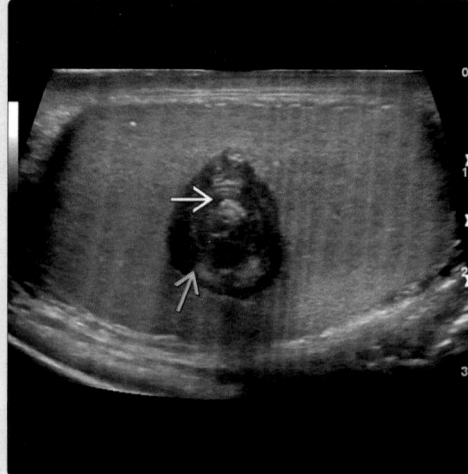
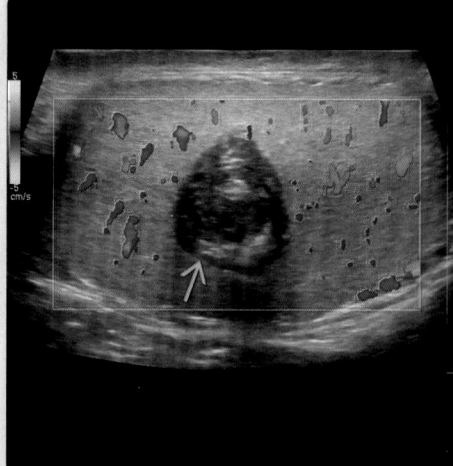

(Left) *Sagittal grayscale ultrasound of the testis demonstrates a unilocular, well-demarcated intratesticular epidermoid cyst ➡. The central hyperechoic focus ➡ corresponds to keratin. The surrounding testicular parenchyma is normal in echogenicity.* (Right) *Color Doppler ultrasound of the same lesion ➡ demonstrates no internal vascularity, which further supports the diagnosis of epidermoid cyst.*

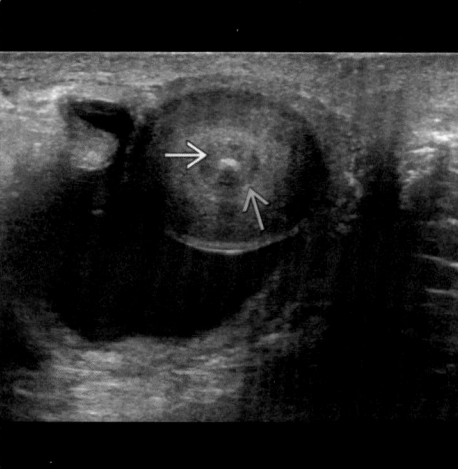
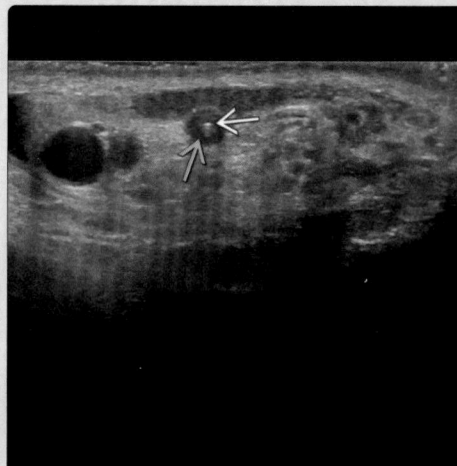

(Left) *Sagittal ultrasound of a patient with a painless scrotal lump demonstrates a circumscribed, oval, extratesticular epidermoid cyst with a classic "onion-skin" appearance ➡ and central echogenic focus ➡. (Right) Sagittal grayscale ultrasound of the right epididymis in a different patient demonstrates a circumscribed, oval lesion ➡ with characteristic bull's eye appearance of an epidermoid cyst. The central hyperechoic focus ➡ is consistent with keratin.*

TERMINOLOGY

Synonyms

- Monodermal dermoid, keratin/cyst of testis

Definitions

- Rare, benign, keratin-containing lesion of controversial origin

IMAGING

General Features

- Best diagnostic clue
  - Characteristic onion skin or target/bull's eye appearance of avascular testicular mass
- Location
  - Most commonly intratesticular, but rarely may be extratesticular
- Size
  - 0.5-10.5 cm in diameter
- Morphology
  - Unilocular cyst containing keratin; fibrous wall

Ultrasonographic Findings

- Grayscale ultrasound
  - Sharply circumscribed, encapsulated round "mass"
  - 4 ultrasound appearances varying with maturation, compactness, and amount of keratin present
    - Type 1: Classic onion- skin appearance (concentric hypoechoic and hyperechoic rings)
    - Type 2: Densely calcified echogenic mass with posterior acoustic shadowing
    - Type 3: Target/bull's-eye appearance (cystic appearing lesion with echogenic center; secondary to compact keratin/calcification)
    - Type 4: Mixed pattern
- Color Doppler
  - Avascular, no blood flow demonstrable

MR Findings

- Can have a bull's-eye or onion skin appearance similar to what is seen on ultrasound; however
  - What appears bright on ultrasound (central keratin and fibrous capsule) has low signal on both T1WI and T2WI
  - What appears dark on ultrasound (desquamated cellular debris with ↑ water and fat content) has high signal on T1WI and T2WI
- Does not enhance → differentiates cyst from neoplasms

Imaging Recommendations

- Best imaging tool
  - High-resolution US (≥ 10 MHz)

DIFFERENTIAL DIAGNOSIS

Tunica Albuginea Cyst

- Located within tunica, solitary, unilocular, and anechoic

Germ Cell Tumor

- Heterogeneous mass with vascularity seen on Doppler
- Testicular teratoma may have overlapping appearance with epidermoid but typically much larger

Testicular Granuloma

- Most probably due to TB, usually multiple

PATHOLOGY

General Features

- Etiology
  - Controversial etiology
  - Prevailing theory: Monodermal teratoma composed entirely of ectoderm
  - Alternate theories
    - Metaplasia of seminiferous tubules or rete testis
    - Due to abnormal closure of neural groove

Microscopic Features

- Unilocular cyst surrounded by fibrous wall composed at least partially of squamous epithelium
- Contains keratin and desquamated material

CLINICAL ISSUES

Presentation

- Most common signs/symptoms
  - Painless tumor, incidentally noted, may cause diffuse testicular enlargement, negative tumor markers

Demographics

- Age
  - May present at any age; 2nd-4th decade most common
- Epidemiology
  - 1-2% of all testicular tumors
  - 3% of all pediatric tumors

Natural History & Prognosis

- No malignant potential

Treatment

- Enucleate 1st if lesions < 3 cm with characteristic US appearance and no color flow
- Testis can be spared if
  - Frozen sections of lesion are consistent with epidermoid cyst
  - No evidence of malignancy within or surrounding lesion
  - Negative tumor markers (AFP, β-HCG)

DIAGNOSTIC CHECKLIST

Image Interpretation Pearls

- Onion skin appearance in well-circumscribed testicular mass on US
- Avascular benign mass on color Doppler

SELECTED REFERENCES

1. Bhatt S et al: Imaging of non-neoplastic intratesticular masses. Diagn Interv Radiol. 2011 Mar;17(1):52-63. Epub 2010 Jun 30. Review. Erratum in: Diagn Interv Radiol. 17(4):388, 2011
2. Loberant N et al: Bilateral testicular epidermoid cysts. J Clin Imaging Sci. 1:4, 2011
3. Manning MA et al: Testicular epidermoid cysts: sonographic features with clinicopathologic correlation. J Ultrasound Med. 29(5):831-7, 2010
4. Loya AG et al: Epidermoid cyst of the testis: radiologic-pathologic correlation. Radiographics. 24 Suppl 1:S243-6, 2004

Tubular Ectasia of Rete Testis

TERMINOLOGY

- Dilated rete testis
- Cystic transformation of rete testis

IMAGING

- Frequently bilateral
  - Usually asymmetric involvement
- Branching tubules converging at mediastinum testis
  - Dilated tubules create lace-like or "fishnet" appearance
- Adjacent parenchyma is normal
- Associated ipsilateral spermatoceles are common
- Tubules are avascular and fluid filled
  - No flow on color Doppler imaging
- MR performed for confirmation if cystic malignant neoplasm cannot be ruled out

TOP DIFFERENTIAL DIAGNOSES

- Testicular carcinoma

- Mixed germ cell tumors with teratomatous component will often have cystic areas
  - Does not form network of tubules
- Intratesticular varicocele
  - Characteristic color flow on Doppler
- Testicular infarct
  - Avascular wedge-shaped area with sharp borders

CLINICAL ISSUES

- Generally nonpalpable and asymptomatic
- May be found when doing ultrasound for related issue, such as epididymal cyst

DIAGNOSTIC CHECKLIST

- Important to distinguish tubular ectasia from malignancy to prevent unnecessary orchiectomy

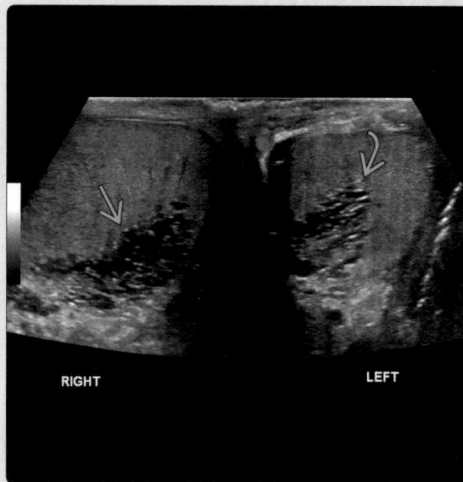
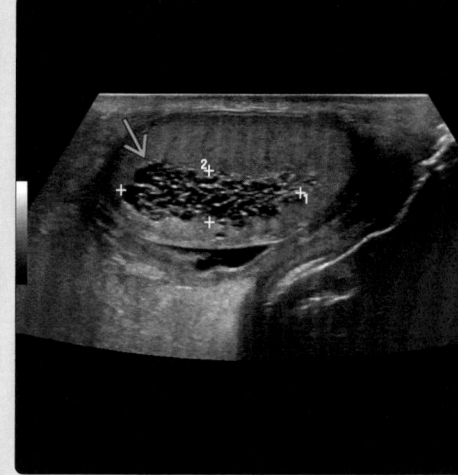

(Left) *Transverse grayscale ultrasound of the testes demonstrates bilateral tubular ectasia of the rete testis, which is slightly asymmetric, right ➡ greater than left ➡.* (Right) *Sagittal grayscale ultrasound of the left testis demonstrates cystic areas ➡ within the mediastinum testis, consistent with tubular ectasia of the rete testis.*

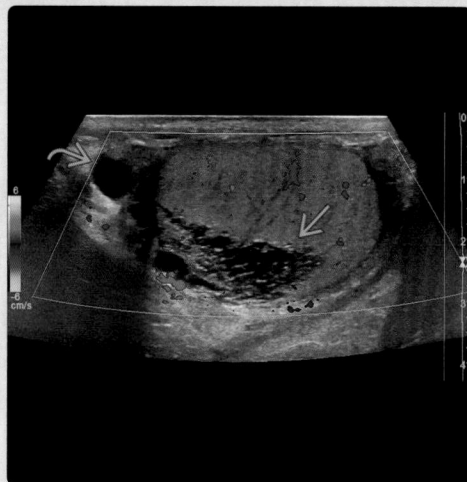
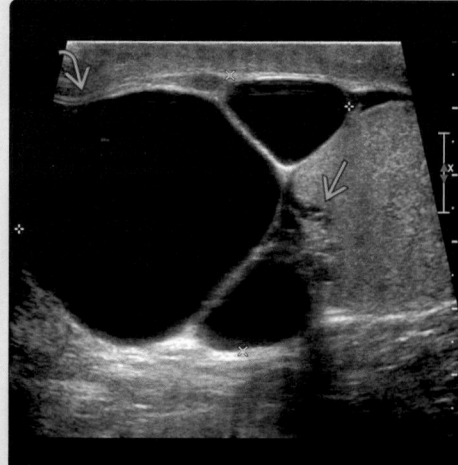

(Left) *Transverse color Doppler ultrasound of the right testicle demonstrates avascular cystic areas within the testis ➡ with a cystic area within the epididymal head ➗. These findings are consistent with tubular ectasia of the rete testis with associated spermatocele.* (Right) *Sagittal grayscale ultrasound of the epididymal head demonstrates large spermatoceles ➡ with partially visualized tubular ectasia ➡.*

TERMINOLOGY

Synonyms

- Dilated rete testis
- Cystic transformation of rete testis

IMAGING

General Features

- Best diagnostic clue
  - Variably sized network of dilated tubules near mediastinum testis with no flow on color Doppler
- Location
  - Posterior near mediastinum testis
  - Frequently bilateral
- Size
  - Can replace large portion of normal parenchyma
  - Variably sized cystic spaces
- Morphology
  - Branching tubules converging at mediastinum testis
  - Characteristic appearance and location make it possible to distinguish this benign condition from malignancy

Ultrasonographic Findings

- Grayscale ultrasound
  - Longitudinal plane shows branching tubular structures along mediastinum
    - Dilated tubules create lace-like or "fishnet" appearance
  - Adjacent parenchyma is normal
    - Differentiates it from cystic malignant masses, which have abnormal rind of parenchyma
  - Associated ipsilateral spermatoceles are common
    - May also see intratesticular cysts
- Color Doppler
  - Tubules are avascular and fluid filled, hence no color flow
  - Normal flow in adjacent testicular parenchyma

MR Findings

- MR performed for confirmation if cystic malignant neoplasm cannot be ruled out
- T1 and proton density-weighted Images: Hypointense to testis
- T2WI: Iso- to hyperintense to testis → nearly invisible
  - Malignant testicular neoplasms → solid portions hypointense on T2WI; have dark fibrous capsule

Imaging Recommendations

- Best imaging tool
  - High-resolution US (≥ 7.5 MHz) is imaging modality of choice
- Protocol advice
  - Longitudinal plane shows morphology of tubules far better than transverse plane
    - Appears more mass-like and has greater likelihood of causing confusion when viewed in transverse plane
  - Always use color Doppler to look for areas of abnormal parenchymal flow

DIFFERENTIAL DIAGNOSIS

Testicular Carcinoma

- Mixed germ cell tumors with teratomatous components will often have cystic areas
- Does not form network of tubules
- Surrounding parenchyma is abnormal
  - Will have abnormal flow on color Doppler

Intratesticular Varicocele

- Multiple intratesticular anechoic serpiginous tubules with characteristic color flow on Doppler, particularly during Valsalva maneuver
- Will have associated extratesticular varicocele

Testicular Infarct

- Avascular hypoechoic mass, as sequelae of any previous vascular insult
- Sharp, linear borders demarcate area

PATHOLOGY

General Features

- Etiology
  - Partial or complete efferent ductule obstruction → ectasia → eventually cystic transformation
  - May be associated with epididymal obstruction due to inflammation or trauma
- Associated abnormalities
  - Spermatocele
  - Epididymal cyst
  - Intratesticular cyst

CLINICAL ISSUES

Presentation

- Most common signs/symptoms
  - Generally nonpalpable and asymptomatic
  - May be found when doing ultrasound for related issue, such as epididymal cyst or spermatocele

Demographics

- Age
  - Middle-aged to elderly men most commonly affected

DIAGNOSTIC CHECKLIST

Image Interpretation Pearls

- Important to distinguish tubular ectasia from malignancy to prevent unnecessary orchiectomy

SELECTED REFERENCES

1. Bhatt S et al: Imaging of non-neoplastic intratesticular masses. Diagn Interv Radiol. 2011 Mar;17(1):52-63. Epub 2010 Jun 30. Review. Erratum in: Diagn Interv Radiol. 17(4):388, 2011
2. Bhatt S et al: Sonography of benign intrascrotal lesions. Ultrasound Q. 22(2):121-36, 2006
3. Woodward PJ et al: From the archives of the AFIP: tumors and tumorlike lesions of the testis: radiologic-pathologic correlation. Radiographics. 22(1):189-216, 2002
4. Dogra VS et al: Benign intratesticular cystic lesions: US features. Radiographics. 21 Spec No:S273-81, 2001
5. Tartar VM et al: Tubular ectasia of the testicle: sonographic and MR imaging appearance. AJR Am J Roentgenol. 160(3):539-42, 1993

Testicular Microlithiasis

TERMINOLOGY

- Microcalcifications composed of hydroxyapatite, located within the spermatic tubules

IMAGING

- On ultrasound, seen as discrete, punctate, nonshadowing echogenic foci scattered within testicular parenchyma
- Majority are idiopathic; previous infection or trauma may also be responsible
- Clusters of microliths may represent testicular tumors even when no soft tissue mass can be identified
- Adjacent hypoechoic foci, if seen, could represent neoplasia
- High resolution US (≥ 7.5 MHz) is modality of choice

TOP DIFFERENTIAL DIAGNOSES

- Scrotal pearls (scrotoliths)
- Large-cell calcifying Sertoli cell tumor
- Testicular granuloma

PATHOLOGY

- Testicular neoplasia in 18-75%, intratubular germ cell neoplasia (IGCN), germ cell version of carcinoma in situ

CLINICAL ISSUES

- Presence of microlithiasis alone in absence of other risk factors is not indication for regular scrotal ultrasound, further sonographic screening or biopsy
- US is recommended in follow-up of patients with risk factors, which includes personal/family history of GCT, maldescent or undescended testes, orchidopexy, testicular atrophy

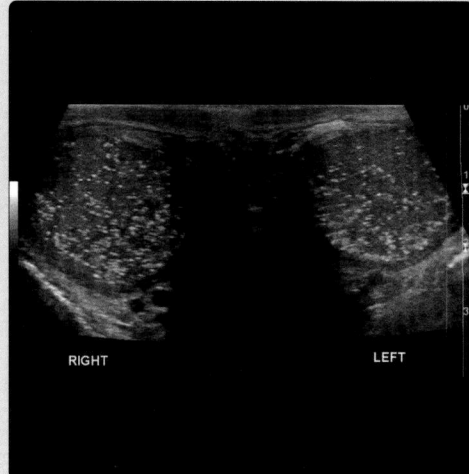
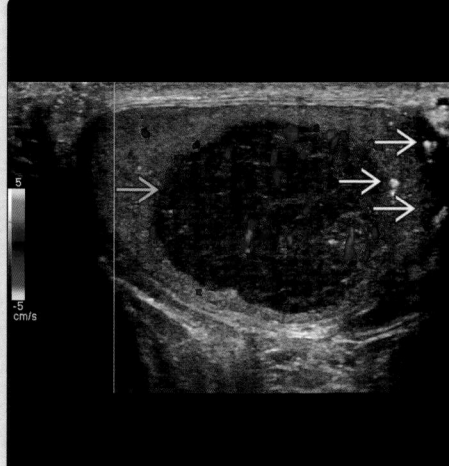

(Left) *Transverse grayscale ultrasound of bilateral testes demonstrates extensive microlithiasis.* (Right) *Sagittal color Doppler ultrasound of the right testis demonstrates a large hypoechoic mass ➡ in a background of microlithiasis ➡. Pathology confirmed a classic seminoma.*

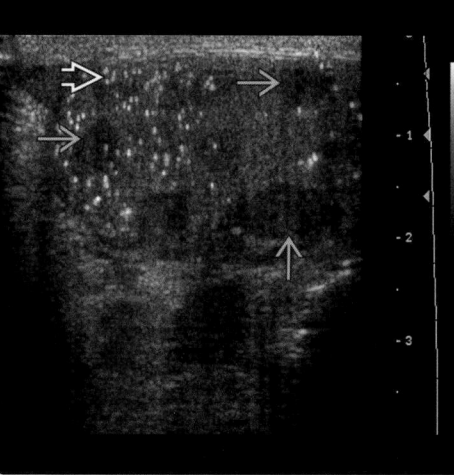
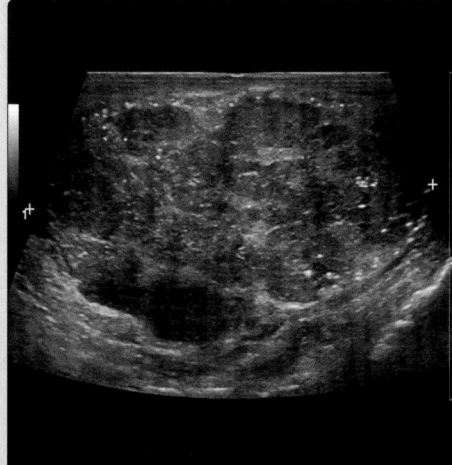

(Left) *Sagittal grayscale ultrasound of the right testis demonstrates multifocal hypoechoic masses ➡ in a background of microlithiasis with clustering at the superior pole ➡. Pathology after orchiectomy confirmed multifocal seminoma.* (Right) *Sagittal grayscale ultrasound of the right testis demonstrates an enlarged testis infiltrated with a hypoechoic mass in a background of microlithiasis. Pathology after orchiectomy confirmed a seminoma*

TERMINOLOGY

Definitions

- Testicular microlithiasis (TML): Presence of 5 or more microliths or microcalcifications in whole testis or 5 or more microliths per FOV

IMAGING

General Features

- Best diagnostic clue
  - Discrete, punctate, nonshadowing echogenic foci scattered within testicular parenchyma
- Location
  - Either unilateral or bilateral
- Size
  - 1-3 mm
- Morphology
  - Asymmetrically distributed, peripheral predominance, impalpable
  - Microcalcifications, composed of hydroxyapatite, formed within spermatic tubule lumina
  - Multilayered envelope, composed of stratified collagen fibers, is considered to be responsible for absence of acoustic shadowing
  - Majority are idiopathic; previous infection or trauma may also be responsible

Ultrasonographic Findings

- Grayscale ultrasound
  - Small hyperechoic foci diffusely scattered throughout testicular parenchyma
    - 1-3 mm echogenic foci, no shadowing
    - May occasionally see "comet-tail" artifact
    - May be peripheral or segmental in distribution
    - Clusters of microliths may represent testicular tumor (carcinoma in situ) without soft tissue mass
      □ Clusters of microliths adjacent to solid mass suggests germ cell tumor (GCT)

Imaging Recommendations

- Best imaging tool
  - High resolution US (≥ 7.5 MHz) is modality of choice
  - Microliths are not visible on MR

DIFFERENTIAL DIAGNOSIS

Scrotal Pearls (Scrotoliths)

- Extratesticular calcified bodies within scrotum with no clinical significance; result from inflammation of tunica vaginalis or torsion of appendix testis

Large Cell Calcifying Sertoli Cell Tumor

- Gonadal stromal tumor, often bilateral and multifocal
- Most common cause of intratesticular macrolithiasis, mass may be almost completely calcified

Testicular Granuloma

- TB epididymoorchitis may produce intrascrotal calcifications and scrotal sinus tract

PATHOLOGY

General Features

- Etiology
  - Exact cause is unknown
    - Defect in phagocytic activity of Sertoli cells leads to degenerated intratubular debris, genetic mutation, or sequela of testicular tubular degeneration
  - Debris accumulates as glycoprotein and calcium layers
- Genetics
  - Associated with Klinefelter syndrome, Down syndrome, male pseudohermaphroditism, cryptorchidism, McCune-Albright syndrome, Peutz Jeghers syndrome
- Associated abnormalities
  - Testicular neoplasia in 18-75%, intratubular germ cell neoplasia (IGCN)
  - Testicular microlithiasis rarely associated with extratesticular tumors, such as epididymal or abdominal neoplasms in absence of testicular tumor

CLINICAL ISSUES

Presentation

- Most common signs/symptoms
  - Asymptomatic, incidentally seen on US for other scrotal abnormalities

Demographics

- Age
  - Usually seen in older boys and adolescents
  - Rare in boys younger than 2 years
- Epidemiology
  - 0.6%, increased detection due to frequent use of high-frequency ultrasonography

Natural History & Prognosis

- Concurrent germ cell tumor in up to 40%
- Follow-up US recommended in patients with risk factors
  - Personal/ family history of GCT, maldescent or undescended testes, orchidopexy, testicular atrophy

Treatment

- No treatment or follow-up or biopsy in absence of risk factors of testicular malignancy
- If associated with hypoechoic mass, surgical biopsy, or orchiectomy

SELECTED REFERENCES

1. Richenberg J et al: Testicular microlithiasis imaging and follow-up: guidelines of the ESUR scrotal imaging subcommittee. Eur Radiol. 25(2):323-30, 2015
2. Cooper ML et al: Testicular microlithiasis in children and associated testicular cancer. Radiology. 270(3):857-63, 2014
3. Chiang LW et al: Implications of incidental finding of testicular microlithiasis in paediatric patients. J Pediatr Urol. 8(2):162-5, 2012
4. Richenberg J et al: Testicular microlithiasis: is there a need for surveillance in the absence of other risk factors? Eur Radiol. 22(11):2540-6, 2012
5. Silveri M et al: Management and follow-up of pediatric asymptomatic testicular microlithiasis: are we doing it well? Urol J. 8(4):287-90, 2011
6. Tan IB et al: Testicular microlithiasis predicts concurrent testicular germ cell tumors and intratubular germ cell neoplasia of unclassified type in adults: a meta-analysis and systematic review. Cancer. 116(19):4520-32, 2010
7. Dagash H et al: Testicular microlithiasis: what does it mean clinically? BJU Int. 99(1):157-60, 2007

(Left) *Transverse grayscale ultrasound of the bilateral testes demonstrates an atrophic left testis* ➡️ *with bilateral microlithiasis* ➡️. *Annual screening ultrasound is indicated due to increased risk for cancer in an atrophic testicle with microlithiasis.* **(Right)** *Transverse grayscale ultrasound demonstrates the left undescended testis* ➡️ *in the left inguinal canal with microlithiasis* ➡️. *This needs to be annually screened by ultrasound due to increased risk for cancer.*

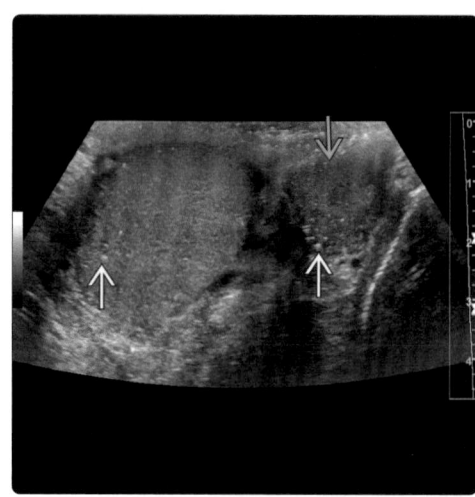 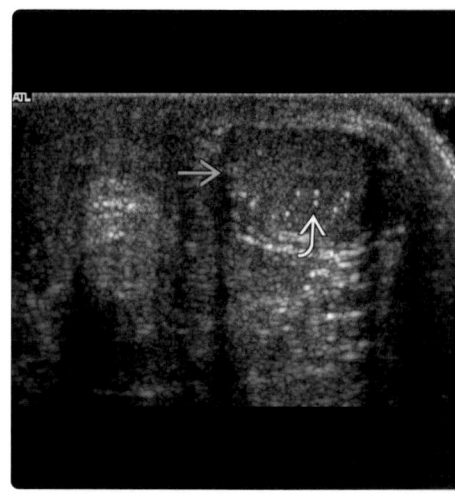

(Left) *Transverse grayscale ultrasound of the scrotum demonstrates a single left-sided testis* ➡️ *with microlithiasis* ➡️. *The patient had a history of right orchiectomy for germ cell tumor and was being screened annually for increased risk of cancer.* **(Right)** *Sagittal grayscale ultrasound shows the left testis with macrocalcifications* ➡️ *and a large, hypoechoic mass* ➡️ *confirmed to be a seminoma.*

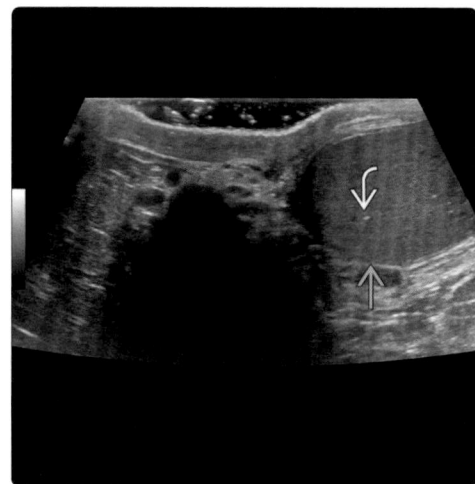 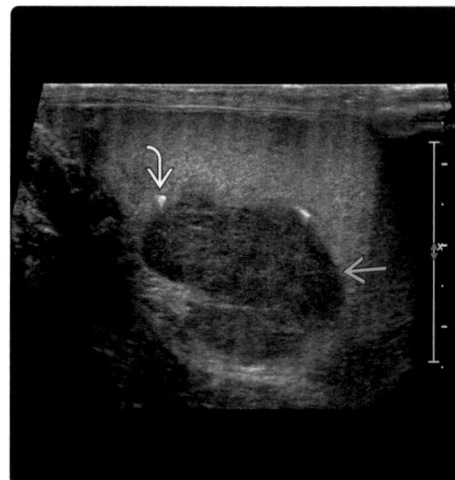

(Left) *Sagittal grayscale ultrasound of the right testis demonstrates scattered micro-* ➡️ *and macrocalcifications* ➡️. *The left testis was normal without microlithiasis. The patient was followed up with an annual ultrasound.* **(Right)** *Sagittal grayscale ultrasound follow-up in the same patient after 3 years demonstrated development of a large heterogeneous mass* ➡️. *Pathology confirmed a mixed germ cell tumor (95% embryonal, 5% teratoma).*

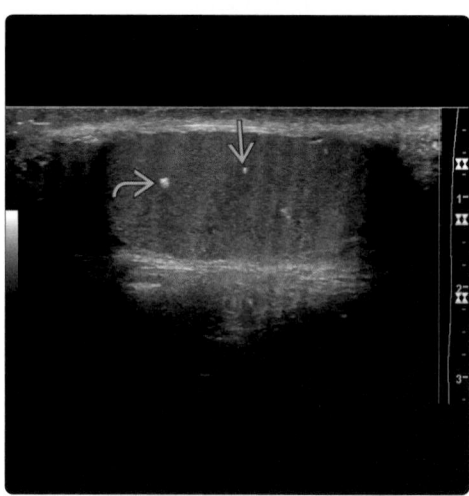 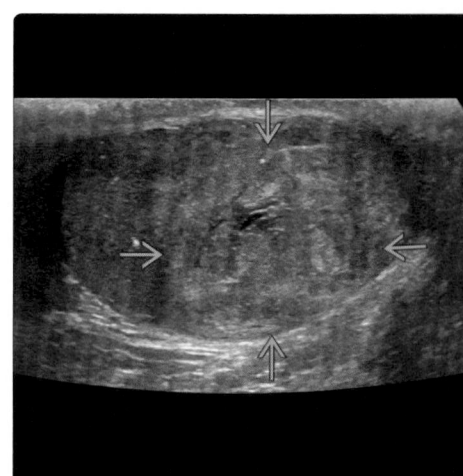

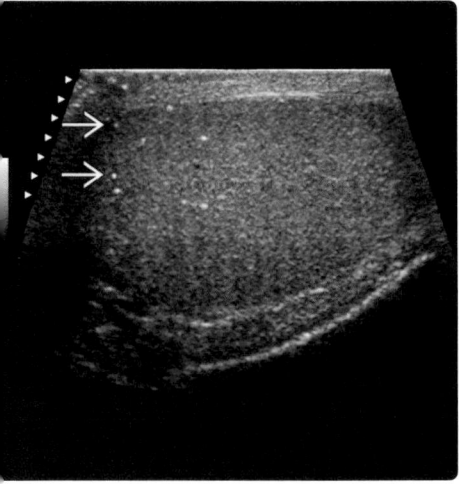

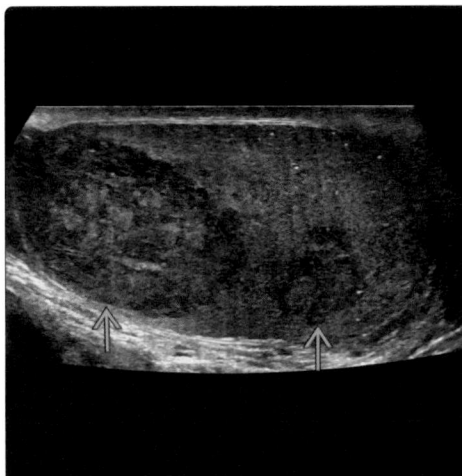

(Left) *Transverse grayscale ultrasound of the left testis demonstrates clustered microlithiasis* ➡. *The patient had a history of right orchiectomy for germ cell tumor and was being followed-up by ultrasound on an annual basis.* (Right) *Sagittal grayscale ultrasound follow-up on the same patient after 11 years demonstrates development of multiple hypoechoic masses* ➡. *Pathology confirmed multifocal seminoma.*

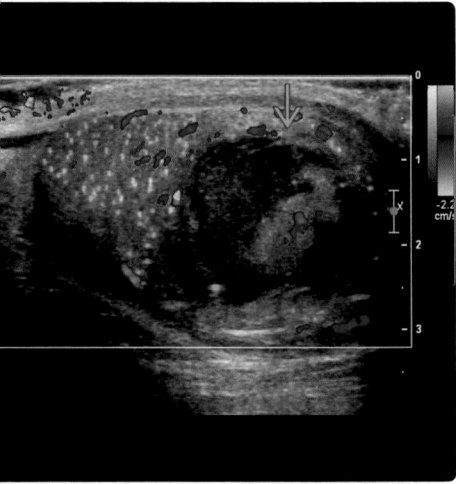

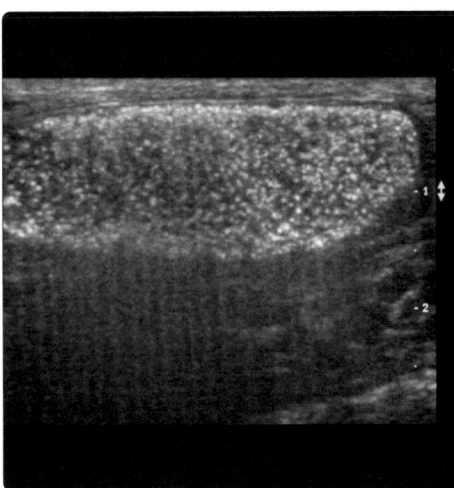

(Left) *Sagittal color Doppler ultrasound of the right testis demonstrates a large hypoechoic mass* ➡ *in the background of extensive microlithiasis. Pathology confirmed a classic seminoma.* (Right) *Sagittal grayscale ultrasound of the right testis demonstrates diffuse extensive microlithiasis. This limits adequate assessment of the testicular parenchyma for tumor, hence these must be referred to specialist centers for alternate methods of future screening.*

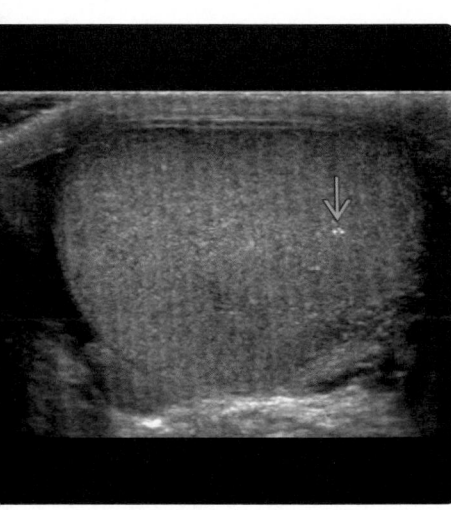

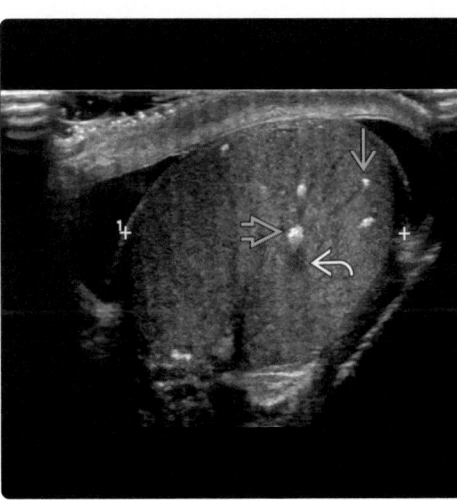

(Left) *Transverse grayscale ultrasound of the left testis demonstrates an isolated microlith* ➡ *in the parenchyma. This does not meet the definition of testicular microlithiasis and is likely a sequela of prior infection or trauma.* (Right) *Transverse grayscale ultrasound of the left testis demonstrates presence of microcalcifications* ➡ *and macrocalcifications* ➡ *(with shadowing* ➡*). Patients with any intratesticular calcification should be considered to be at higher risk of a testicular malignancy.*

Testicular Torsion/Infarction

TERMINOLOGY

- Spontaneous or traumatic twisting of testis & spermatic cord within scrotum, resulting in vascular occlusion/infarction

IMAGING

- Absent or decreased abnormal testicular blood flow on color Doppler US
- Findings vary with duration and degree of rotation of cord
- Unilateral in 95% of patients
- Role of spectral Doppler is limited; may be helpful to detect partial torsion; in partial torsion of 360° or less, spectral Doppler may show diminished diastolic arterial flow
- Spiral twist of spermatic cord cranial to testis and epididymis causing torsion knot or whirlpool pattern of concentric layers

PATHOLOGY

- Varying degrees of ischemic necrosis & fibrosis depending on duration of symptoms
- Undescended testes have an increased risk of torsion
- Intravaginal torsion: Common type, most frequently occurs at puberty

CLINICAL ISSUES

- Acute scrotal/inguinal pain; swollen, erythematous hemiscrotum without recognized trauma
- Reducing time lag between onset of symptoms and time of surgical or manual detorsion is of utmost importance in preserving viable testis
- Nonviable testicle usually removed; higher risk of subsequent torsion on contralateral side
- Venous obstruction occurs 1st, followed by obstruction of arterial flow, which leads to testicular ischemia

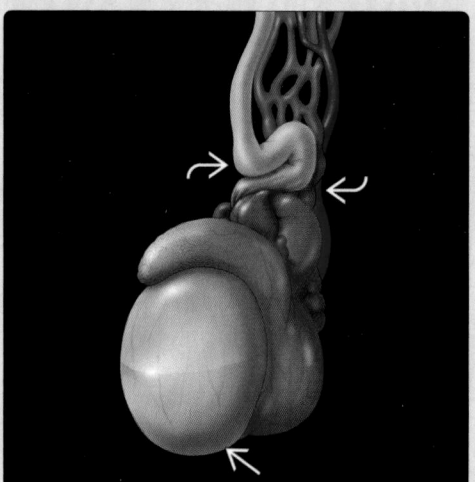
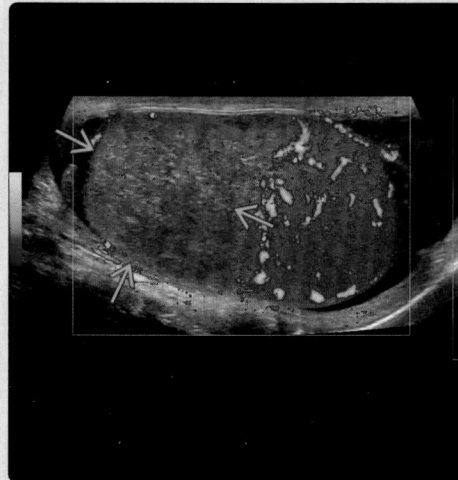

(Left) Graphic shows spiral twist ⟹ of the spermatic cord with torsion, leading to venous congestion and compromised blood supply to the testis ➡. (Right) Sagittal power Doppler ultrasound of the left testis in a young male with intermittent symptoms of left testicular pain demonstrates a large focal avascular heterogeneous area ⟹ consistent with infarct that is likely secondary to intermittent torsion.

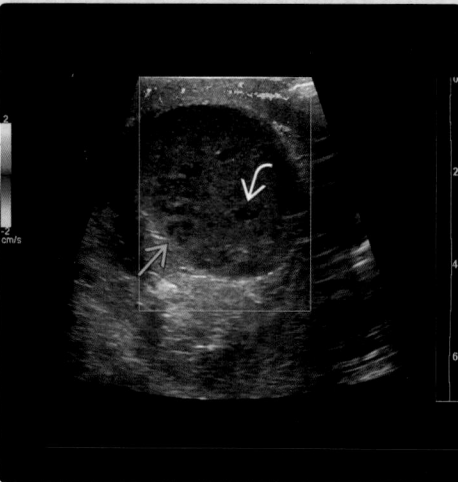
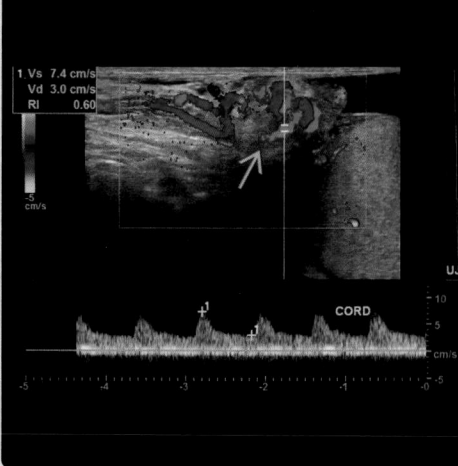

(Left) Transverse color Doppler ultrasound of the testis in a young male with an acute painful scrotum for 48 hours shows a heterogeneous avascular testis ⟹ with cystic areas ⟹, consistent with an infarcted testis with necrosis secondary to torsion. (Right) Sagittal color Doppler ultrasound superior to the left testis in a young male with acute painful scrotum shows a whirlpool sign ⟹ secondary to a twisted spermatic cord. Patient was manually detorsed followed by bilateral orchidopexy.

TERMINOLOGY

Definitions

Spontaneous or traumatic twisting of testis & spermatic cord within scrotum, resulting in vascular occlusion/infarction

IMAGING

General Features

Best diagnostic clue
- Absent or decreased abnormal testicular blood flow on color Doppler US

Location
- Unilateral in 95% of patients

Morphology
- Complete/incomplete torsion
- Types according to location of torsion knot
  - Intravaginal torsion: Torsion knot within tunica vaginalis
  - Extravaginal torsion: Torsion knot outside tunica vaginalis

Ultrasonographic Findings

- Grayscale ultrasound
  - Testicular torsion
    - Findings vary with duration and degree of rotation of cord
    - Grayscale appearance during acute phase (critical phase) may be normal
    - Spiral twist of spermatic cord cranial to testis and epididymis causing torsion knot or whirlpool pattern of concentric layers
    - Enlarged testis and epididymis (heterogeneous echotexture, most often decreased echogenicity)
    - Edema of scrotal wall, secondary hydrocele
    - Intratesticular necrosis, hemorrhage or fragmentation if delayed diagnosis missed torsion
    - At 24 hours after onset changes like congestion, hemorrhage, and infarction are seen
    - Hypoechoic areas associated with testicular infarction may have striated appearance (due to accentuation of septa within the testis)
    - Normal testicular echogenicity is strong predictor of testicular viability; decreased and heterogeneous testicular echogenicity correlates with worse prognosis and may indicate nonviability
    - Subacute phase (1-10 days): Testis echogenicity decreases in initial 4-5 days, then may show focal or diffuse infarction; epididymis may remain echogenic
    - Chronic phase: Small atrophied homogeneously hypoechoic testis; enlarged echogenic epididymis
  - Testicular infarction
    - Diffusely hypoechoic small testis or focal wedge-shaped hypoechoic area in infarcted testis
    - Hyperechoic regions (hemorrhage/fibrosis), focal infarctions may have striated appearance
- Color Doppler
  - Color Doppler is very useful to establish diagnosis of testicular torsion
  - In acute torsion sensitivity, 80-90%; 10% of patients with early or partial torsion have normal exam

- Setup optimized for detection of slow flow (low pulse repetition frequency, low wall filter, high Doppler gain)
  - Absent or decreased or abnormal flow
  - Comparison with contralateral spermatic cord and testis is mandatory
  - In subacute or chronic torsion: No flow in testis and increased flow in paratesticular tissues, including epididymis-cord complex and dartos fascia
  - Role of spectral Doppler is limited; may be helpful to detect partial torsion; in partial torsion of 360° or less, spectral Doppler may show diminished diastolic arterial flow
  - Use of intravascular ultrasound contrast agents may improve sensitivity for detecting blood flow in testes
  - Increased flow may be seen in the affected testis in a case of torsion-detorsion syndrome: Correlation with clinical history of preceding intermittent ipsilateral pain is helpful clue

Nuclear Medicine Findings

- Tc-99m pertechnetate: Dynamic flow imaging at 2-5 second intervals for 1 minute (vascular phase); 5-minute intervals for tissue phase; sensitivity 80-90%
  - Can detect reduced or absent testicular flow in 94-99%
  - In testicular torsion, rounded cold area and halo of dartos perfusion is seen

Imaging Recommendations

- Best imaging tool
  - US with high-frequency linear transducer & color/power Doppler
- Protocol advice
  - Compare grayscale, color Doppler appearances to contralateral normal testis

DIFFERENTIAL DIAGNOSIS

Testicular Trauma

- Hematocele, irregular contours, heterogeneous parenchymal echogenicity
- Avascular fracture plane

Testicular Abscess (Epididymoorchitis)

- Thick-walled, hypoechoic focus with low-level internal echoes, thickened tunica albuginea
- Enlarged hypoechoic epididymis with increased flow on color Doppler

Testicular Tumor

- Focal hypoechoic mass with heterogeneous areas
- Abnormal vascularity within mass

Torsion of Appendix Testis or Appendix Epididymis

- Presents with acute scrotum
- Small firm nodule that is palpable on superior aspect of testis that exhibits bluish discoloration through overlying skin, called the blue dot sign
- Hyperechoic mass with central hypoechoic area adjacent to testis or epididymis, reactive hydrocele, skin thickening, and peripheral hyperemia

PATHOLOGY

General Features

- Etiology
  - Most occur spontaneously; rarely occurs due to traumatic etiology
- Varying degrees of ischemic necrosis & fibrosis depending on duration of symptoms
- Undescended testes have increased risk of torsion
- Exocrine and endocrine function is substandard in men with history of unilateral torsion; the following 3 theories explain the contralateral disease noted in torsion
  - Unrecognized or unreported repeated injury to both testes
  - Preexisting pathologic condition predisposing both testes to abnormal spermatogenesis and torsion of spermatic cord
  - Induction of pathologic changes in contralateral testis by retention of injured testis

Staging, Grading, & Classification

- Intravaginal torsion: Common type, most frequently occurs at puberty
  - Torsion occurs within tunica vaginalis
  - 2 predisposing conditions
    - Long stalk of mesentery or spermatic cord leading to anomalous suspension of testis
    - Bell clapper deformity where tunica vaginalis completely encircles epididymis, distal spermatic cord, and testis rather than attaching to posterolateral aspect of testis
  - Anomalous testicular suspension is bilateral in 50-80%
  - 10-fold increased incidence of torsion in undescended testis after orchiopexy
- Extravaginal torsion: Exclusively in newborns
  - No bell clapper deformity
  - Torsion occurs outside tunica vaginalis when testes and gubernacula are not fixed and are free to rotate
  - Infarcted and necrotic testis at birth

Gross Pathologic & Surgical Features

- Purple, edematous, ischemic testicle, may rapidly reperfuse when manually detorsed

Microscopic Features

- Hemorrhagic, interstitial edema; necrosis

CLINICAL ISSUES

Presentation

- Most common signs/symptoms
  - Acute scrotal/inguinal pain; swollen, erythematous hemiscrotum without recognized trauma
  - Pain not relieved by elevation of scrotum
  - Absent cremasteric reflex
- Clinical profile
  - Young male with acute scrotal pain

Demographics

- Epidemiology
  - Infant & adolescent boys most often affected

Natural History & Prognosis

- Testis usually turns medially up to 1,080°, 3 full revolutions
  - Venous obstruction occurs 1st, followed by obstruction of arterial flow, which leads to testicular ischemia
  - Diminished blood flow in testis with twist of 180° or less
  - Testicular viability depends on degree of torsion and duration of symptoms
- Surgical emergency: Testicular infarction if not treated promptly

Treatment

- Surgical exploration; detorsion; bilateral orchidopexy if viable testicle
  - Nonviable testicle usually removed; higher risk of subsequent torsion on contralateral side
- Delaying surgical intervention worsens intraoperative testicular salvage rate and extent of subsequent testicular atrophy
- Reducing time lag between onset of symptoms and time of surgical or manual detorsion is of utmost importance in preserving viable testis
- Salvage rate of testis vs. time interval between onset of pain and surgery
  - 80-100% → < 6 hours
  - 76% → 6-12 hours
  - 20% → 12-24 hours
  - 0% → > 24 hours

DIAGNOSTIC CHECKLIST

Consider

- Normal US (grayscale & Doppler) does not exclude early or partial torsion
  - Repeat examination at 1-4 hour intervals if conservatively managed

Image Interpretation Pearls

- Decreased or absent flow on Doppler ultrasound

SELECTED REFERENCES

1. Esposito F et al: The "whirlpool sign", a US finding in partial torsion of the spermatic cord: 4 cases. J Ultrasound. 17(4):313-5, 2014
2. Yusuf GT et al: A review of ultrasound imaging in scrotal emergencies. J Ultrasound. 16(4):171-8, 2013
3. Yagil Y et al: Role of Doppler ultrasonography in the triage of acute scrotum in the emergency department. J Ultrasound Med. 29(1):11-21, 2010
4. Schalamon J et al: Management of acute scrotum in children–the impact of Doppler ultrasound. J Pediatr Surg. 41(8):1377-80, 2006
5. Vijayaraghavan SB: Sonographic differential diagnosis of acute scrotum: real-time whirlpool sign, a key sign of torsion. J Ultrasound Med. 25(5):563-74, 2006
6. Dogra V et al: Acute painful scrotum. Radiol Clin North Am. 42(2):349-63, 2004
7. Dogra VS et al: Torsion and beyond: new twists in spectral Doppler evaluation of the scrotum. J Ultrasound Med. 23(8):1077-85, 2004
8. Dogra VS et al: Sonography of the scrotum. Radiology. 227(1):18-36, 2003
9. Arce JD et al: Sonographic diagnosis of acute spermatic cord torsion. Rotation of the cord: a key to the diagnosis. Pediatr Radiol. 32(7):485-91, 2002

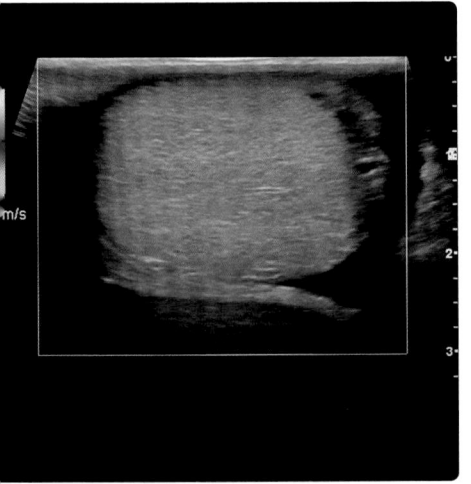

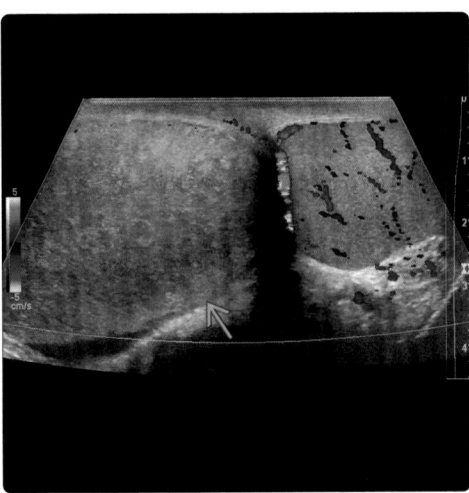

(Left) *Transverse color Doppler ultrasound of the left testis in a male with an acute painful scrotum for 2 hours shows complete absence of internal blood flow. Note the normal grayscale homogeneous appearance of the parenchyma that is suggestive of a potentially viable testis.* (Right) *Transverse color Doppler ultrasound of both testes shows an enlarged heterogeneous avascular right testis ⬡ with an abnormal line. Patient was symptomatic for 24 hours; testis could not be salvaged after detorsion.*

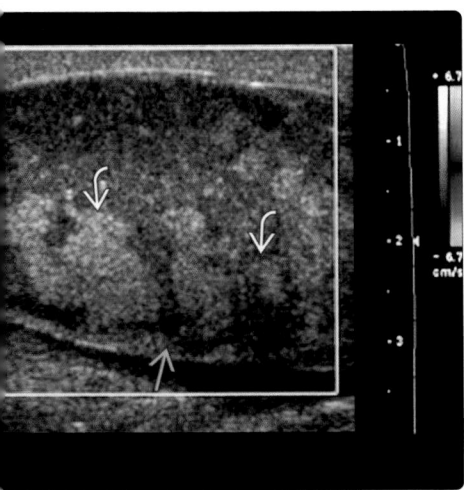

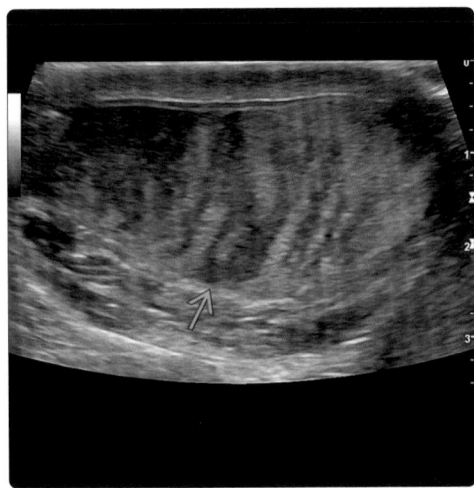

(Left) *Sagittal color Doppler ultrasound of the left testis shows an enlarged heterogeneous avascular testis ⬡ with multiple hyperechoic areas ⬡. Pathology confirmed it to be a hemorrhagic infarction of the testis with torsion > 360° degrees.* (Right) *Sagittal grayscale ultrasound of the right testis shows an enlarged heterogeneous right testis ⬡ with a striated appearance suggestive of partial infarcts. The patient had a history of partial testicular torsion.*

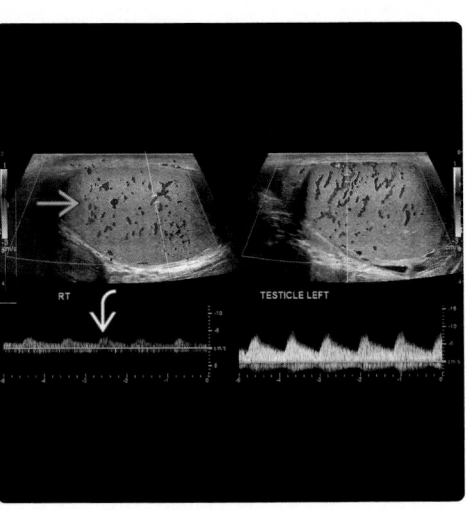

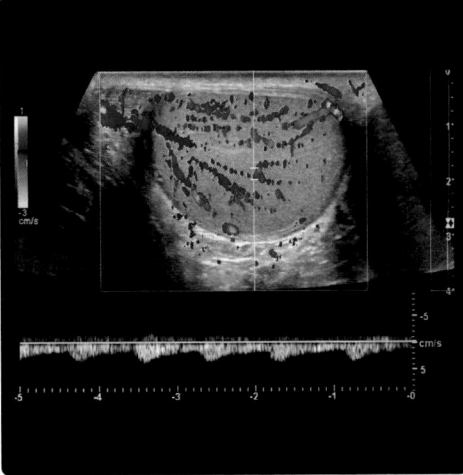

(Left) *Sagittal color Doppler ultrasound of both testes in a young male with right testicular pain shows an asymmetric blood flow with reduced flow to the right testis ⬡, as seen on color flow and spectral waveform ⬡. This was surgically confirmed to be partial right testicular torsion of 180°.* (Right) *Transverse color Doppler ultrasound of the right testis after detorsion shows reactive hyperemia.*

TERMINOLOGY

- Cryptorchidism, cryptorchism
- Definition: Incomplete descent of testis into base of scrotum

IMAGING

- Unilateral or bilateral absence of testis in scrotum
- Located anywhere from kidney to inguinal canal, inguinal canal most common (80%)
  o Bilateral in 10%
- Ultrasound features: Ovoid homogeneous, hypoechoic, well-circumscribed structure smaller than normal descended testis
- MR: Useful for detecting intraabdominal testis, if not seen by ultrasound

TOP DIFFERENTIAL DIAGNOSES

- Inguinal lymphadenopathy
- Inguinal hernia

- Anorchia: Absent testis

PATHOLOGY

- Undescended testis: Arrest of testis along its normal path of descent
- Ectopic testis: Testis located outside its normal path of descent

CLINICAL ISSUES

- Complications
  o Incidence of testicular cancer: 1:1,000-1:2,500
  o Torsion
  o Atrophy/infertility
  o Trauma
- Treatment
  o Orchiopexy before age 2 to preserve fertility
  o Orchiectomy: Consider in patients aged 12-50 years

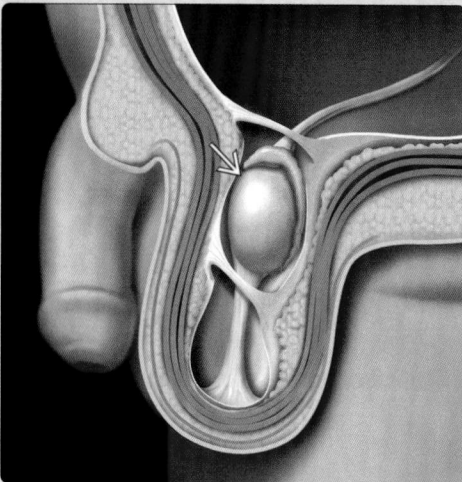
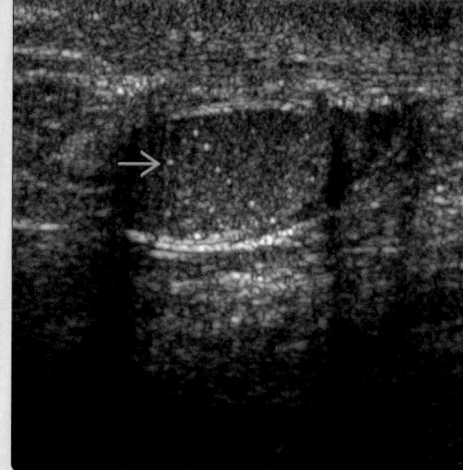

(Left) Graphic shows a testis ➡ at a high scrotal location due to incomplete descent. An undescended testis may be located anywhere from the kidney to the inguinal canal. (Right) Grayscale ultrasound demonstrates an undescended testis with numerous (> 5 per field) punctate, nonshadowing hyperechoic foci ➡, consistent with microlithiasis. Testicular microlithiasis in a cryptorchid testis is associated with increased risk of development of testicular carcinoma. This testis will need routine follow-up.

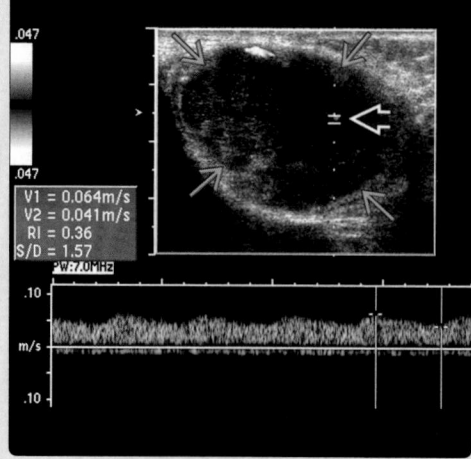
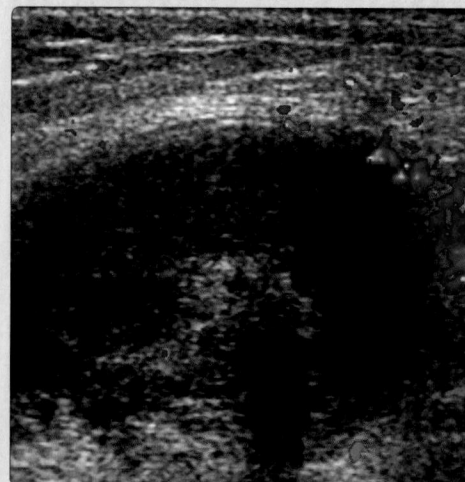

(Left) Spectral Doppler of a cryptorchid testis demonstrates a hypoechoic intratesticular mass ➡ with internal blood flow ➡ pathologically confirmed to be a seminoma. (Right) Color Doppler shows a cryptorchid testis. The heterogenous echogenicity and lack of color flow within this testis is consistent with testicular torsion.

TERMINOLOGY

Synonyms

Cryptorchidism, cryptorchism

Definitions

Incomplete descent of testis into base of scrotum

IMAGING

General Features

Best diagnostic clue
- Unilateral or bilateral absence of testis in scrotum

Location
- Anywhere from kidney to inguinal canal, inguinal canal most common (80%)
- Bilateral in 10%
- Unilateral more common on right (70%)

Ultrasonographic Findings

- Grayscale ultrasound
  - Absence of testicle/spermatic cord within scrotal sac
  - Ovoid homogeneous, less echogenic, well-circumscribed structure smaller than normal descended testis
    - Identify echogenic line of the mediastinum testis to distinguish cryptorchid testis from other inguinal masses on US
    - Lack of surrounding fluid and compression by adjacent structures make the testicular margins less defined than normally located testes
    - Testes < 1 cm cannot be detected
  - Undescended testis in adults exhibit different degrees of atrophy with altered parenchymal echogenicity
  - Associated with microlithiasis; neoplastic foci, if present may be detected

MR Findings

- MR imaging should be used in US-negative cases
- T1WI: Low signal intensity ovoid mass; T2WI: High signal intensity ovoid mass

DIFFERENTIAL DIAGNOSIS

Inguinal Lymphadenopathy

- Most common groin "mass" seen in multiple pathologies

Inguinal Hernia

- Direct/indirect inguinal hernia, bowel/omentum as hernia content

Anorchia: Absent Testis

- Congenital or prior resection

PATHOLOGY

General Features

- Etiology
  - Interruption of embryologic testicular descent from abdomen into scrotal sac
- Associated abnormalities
  - Renal agenesis/ectopia, prune belly syndrome, hypospadias

Staging, Grading, & Classification

- Undescended testis: Arrest of testis along its normal path of descent
  - Abdomen, inguinal canal, external inguinal ring, prescrotal, upper scrotal
  - 80% palpable, 20% unpalpable
- Ectopic testis: Testis located outside its normal path of descent
  - Superficial inguinal pouch, perineal, perirenal, thigh

CLINICAL ISSUES

Demographics

- Epidemiology
  - Testis may be absent from scrotum in 4% of newborns (spontaneous descent in 1st few months)
  - More common in preterm infants

Natural History & Prognosis

- Complications
  - Cancer: Incidence is 1:1,000-1:2,500
    - 5-7x ↑ risk of malignant neoplasm in cryptorchid testis; ~ 20% of tumors occur in the contralateral descended testis (also at an increased risk)
    - Untreated UDT → seminoma is most common tumor
    - UDT treated with orchiopexy → nonseminomatous tumors more common (such as embryonal)
  - Torsion
  - Atrophy/infertility: Infertility more common with bilateral UDT
  - Trauma

Treatment

- Orchiopexy before age 2 to preserve fertility
  - Prepubertal males (≤ 12 years) who undergo orchiopexy have 2-6x decreased relative risk of developing testicular cancer compared to patients who undergo orchiopexy after age 12
- Orchiectomy
  - Consider in patients aged 12-50 years
  - Biopsy can be performed in patients ≥ 10 years to determine if orchiectomy is indicated

SELECTED REFERENCES

1. Abacı A et al: Epidemiology, classification and management of undescended testes: does medication have value in its treatment? J Clin Res Pediatr Endocrinol. 5(2):65-72, 2013
2. Ekenze SO et al: The utility of ultrasonography in the management of undescended testis in a developing country. World J Surg. 37(5):1121-4, 2013
3. Singal AK et al: Undescended testis and torsion: is the risk understated? Arch Dis Child. 98(1):77-9, 2013
4. Abbas TO et al: Role of ultrasonography in the preoperative assessment of impalpable testes: a single center experience. ISRN Urol. 2012:560216, 2012
5. Canning DA: Re: Diagnostic performance of ultrasound in nonpalpable cryptorchidism: a systematic review and meta-analysis. J Urol. 187(4):1434, 2012
6. Mansour SM et al: Does MRI add to ultrasound in the assessment of disorders of sex development? Eur J Radiol. 81(9):2403-10, 2012
7. Tasian GE et al: Diagnostic imaging in cryptorchidism: utility, indications, and effectiveness. J Pediatr Surg. 46(12):2406-13, 2011
8. Tasian GE et al: Imaging use and cryptorchidism: determinants of practice patterns. J Urol. 185(5):1882-7, 2011
9. Nguyen HT et al: Cryptorchidism: strategies in detection. Eur Radiol. 9(2):336-43, 1999

Epididymitis/Orchitis

TERMINOLOGY

- Inflammation of epididymis &/or testis

IMAGING

- Test of choice: Color Doppler US; high frequency transducers (9-15 MHz)
- Diffuse or focal hyperemia in body and tail of epididymis ± increased vascularity of testis (compare with contralateral testis if subtle)
- Starts within tail of epididymis → body → testis
- Orchitis is usually secondary, occurring in 20-40% of epididymitis due to contiguous spread of infection
  - Can cause vascular compromise → ischemia → testicular infarction → sonographic features indistinguishable from testicular torsion
  - Reversal of arterial diastolic flow of testis is ominous finding associated with testicular infarction

TOP DIFFERENTIAL DIAGNOSES

- Testicular torsion
- Testicular lymphoma
- Testicular trauma

CLINICAL ISSUES

- Commonest cause of acute scrotal pain in adolescent boys and adults (15-35 years)
- Males 14 to 35 years of age: Most commonly caused by *Neisseria gonorrhoeae* and *Chlamydia trachomatis*
- Scrotal swelling, erythema; fever; dysuria
  - Scrotal pain due to epididymitis is usually relieved after elevation of testes (scrotum) over symphysis pubis (Prehn sign)
  - Associated lower urinary tract infection and its symptoms, urethral discharge
- Prognosis excellent if treated early with antibiotics; follow-up scans to exclude abscess if no improvement

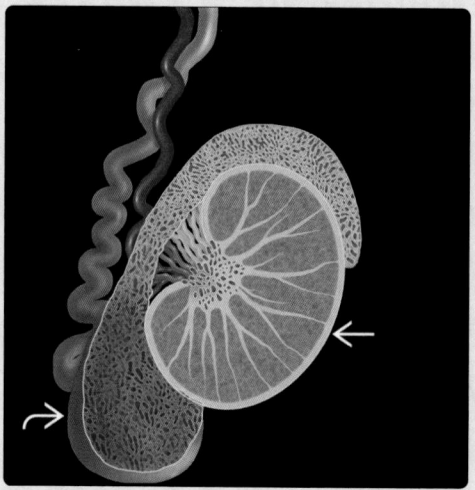 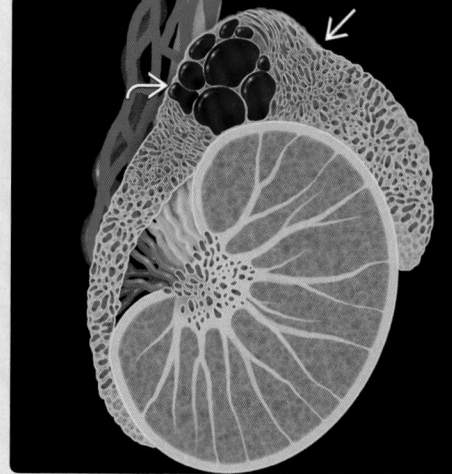

(Left) *Graphic shows an enlarged and inflamed epididymis* ⇗ *enveloping the testis posteriorly. Note that the testis* ⇒ *appears normal in size and configuration.* (Right) *Graphic shows an irregularly enlarged epididymis* ⇒ *with focal cystic areas* ⇒ *indicating early liquefaction and necrosis.*

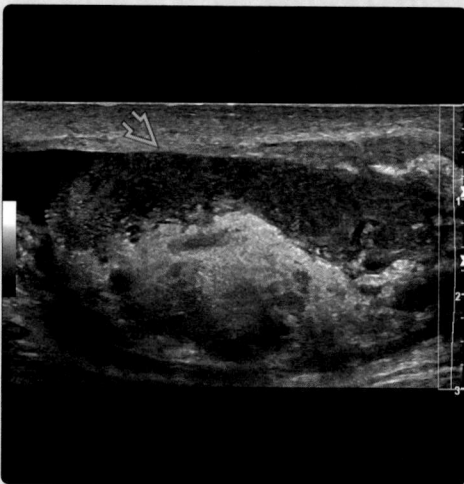 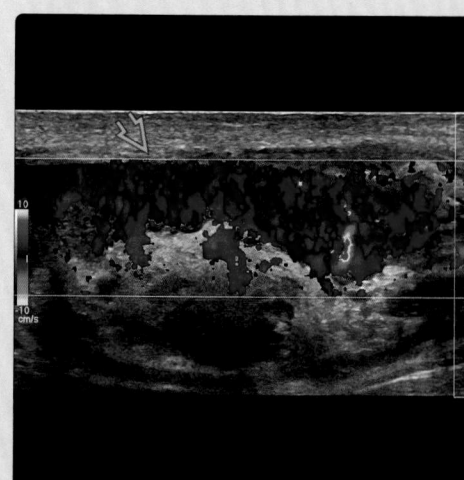

(Left) *Sagittal grayscale ultrasound of the right scrotum demonstrates a thickened heterogeneous and hypoechoic epididymis* ⇨. (Right) *Color Doppler of the epididymis in the same patient reveals marked hyperemia* ⇨ *of the epididymis consistent with acute epididymitis.*

TERMINOLOGY

Synonyms

Acute scrotum, orchitis, epididymo-orchitis

Definitions

Infectious inflammation of epididymis &/or testis

IMAGING

General Features

Best diagnostic clue
o Enlarged, hyperemic epididymis &/or testis on color Doppler US

Location
o Early epididymitis often involves tail of epididymis
o Orchitis is usually secondary, occurring in 20-40% of epididymitis due to contiguous spread of infection
  – Primary orchitis is caused by mumps and is usually bilateral

Size
o Epididymis typically 2-3x larger than normal

Morphology
o Focal enlargement of tail or diffuse enlargement of entire epididymis

Ultrasonographic Findings

Grayscale ultrasound
o Epididymitis: Primarily involved in epididymo-orchitis
  – Acute: Enlarged epididymis, ↓ echogenicity, coarse heterogeneous echotexture due to edema & hemorrhage
  – Chronic epididymitis: Enlarged hyperechoic epididymis
o Orchitis: Follows in 20-40% of epididymitis due to contiguous spread of infection
  – Focal or diffuse
    □ Focal: Hypoechoic area adjacent to enlarged portion of epididymis
    □ Diffuse: Testis is diffusely enlarged with heterogenous echotexture, thickening of tunica albuginea (in severe infection)
  – Edematous, congested testes contained within rigid tunica albuginea → ↑ intratesticular pressure
    □ Heterogeneous parenchymal echogenicity (predominantly hyperechoic initially and hypoechoic later) and septal accentuation visible as hypoechoic bands
    □ May lead to venous occlusion
    □ Can cause vascular compromise → ischemia → testicular infarction → sonographic features indistinguishable from testicular torsion (flow preserved in epididymis compared to torsion where flow is absent in both testis and epididymis)
o Spermatic cord may be inflamed and may appear hypoechoic with associated hyperechoic fat within
o Reactive hydrocele containing low-level internal echoes, septae, thickening of tunical layers ± skin edema; all represent changes of periorchitis

Color Doppler
o Diffuse or focal hyperemia in body and tail of epididymis ± increased vascularity of testis → highly sensitive and specific for epididymo-orchitis
o Inflammation of epididymis and testis is associated with ↓ vascular resistance compared with healthy individuals
  – Resistive index (RI) < 0.5 (normal RI in testis ≥ 0.5)
o Signs of infarction in cases with severe epididymo-orchitis
  – Relatively avascular areas within hyperemic testis or epididymis suggests focal infarction, which may be round or wedge shaped
  – Reversal of arterial diastolic flow of testis (seen with obstruction of venous outflow/venous infarction) is ominous finding associated with testicular infarction

Nuclear Medicine Findings

- Tc-99m: 90% accurate in differentiating torsion from epididymitis
  o Increased flow within testicular vessels and vas deferens on flow study
  o Markedly increased perfusion through spermatic cord vessels (testicular + deferential arteries)
  o Curvilinear increased activity laterally in hemiscrotum on static images (also centrally if testis is involved)

Imaging Recommendations

- Best imaging tool
  o Color Doppler US; high frequency transducers (9-15 MHz)
- Protocol advice
  o Comparison with contralateral testis is useful when increase in vascularity is subtle

DIFFERENTIAL DIAGNOSIS

Testicular Torsion

- Absent or diminished color Doppler flow, "twist" of spermatic cord in inguinal region
- Epididymis may be enlarged with no vascularity on color Doppler US

Testicular Lymphoma

- Often large in size at time of diagnosis, commonly occurs in association with disseminated disease
- Heterogeneous echo pattern; often bilateral; involvement of epididymis and spermatic cord is common; hemorrhage and necrosis is rare

Testicular Trauma

- History of trauma; acute pain
- Focal hypoechoic avascular area on color Doppler; rupture of tunica albuginea associated hematocele

PATHOLOGY

General Features

- Etiology
  o Ascending genitourinary tract infection
    – In males 14 to 35 years of age, disease is most frequently caused by *Neisseria gonorrhoeae* and *Chlamydia trachomatis*
    – In prepubertal boys, men over 35 years of age, and men who practice anal intercourse, disease is most frequently caused by *Escherichia coli*

- Other causes: *Pseudomonas, Klebsiella, Proteus mirabilis, Staphylococcus aureus, Mycobacterium tuberculosis*, Mumps virus
  o Bacterial seeding occurs directly in cases with genitourinary (GU) anomaly and presumably hematogenously in cases without demonstrable anomaly
  o Primary orchitis is rare and caused by mumps (usually bilateral)
  o Traumatic epididymitis: Similar findings as infectious epididymitis
    - However, patient will have preceding history of scrotal trauma ± additional traumatic features such as hematocele &/or testicular injury
    - Conservative management: Antibiotics not needed
    - Should not be confused with infectious epididymitis
  o Drugs such as amiodarone hydrochloride may cause chemical epididymitis
  o Strenuous physical activity
  o Pelvic/inguinal surgery

Staging, Grading, & Classification

- Epididymitis: Isolated epididymitis, focal or diffuse
  o Acute/chronic epididymitis
- Orchitis or combined epididymitis & orchitis
  o Primary: Isolated orchitis (may be seen in boys with mumps)
  o Secondary: Infection spread from adjacent epididymis
  o Acute/chronic orchitis or epididymo-orchitis

Gross Pathologic & Surgical Features

- Treated surgically only if abscess forms despite antibiotic treatment

Microscopic Features

- Inflammatory infiltrate of testis and epididymis

CLINICAL ISSUES

Presentation

- Most common signs/symptoms
  o Commonest cause of acute scrotal pain in adolescent boys and adults
  o Scrotal swelling, erythema; fever; dysuria
    - Prehn sign: Scrotal pain due to epididymo-orchitis is usually relieved after elevation of scrotum over symphysis pubis → may help clinically to differentiate from torsion
  o Associated lower urinary tract infection and its symptoms, urethral discharge
- Other signs/symptoms
  o Pyuria (95%), prostatic tenderness (infrequent)
  o ↑ CRP can help distinguish epididymo-orchitis from testicular torsion (sensitivity 96%, specificity 94%)
  o Positive urinalysis for WBC and bacteria; may have elevated WBC

Demographics

- Age
  o Most commonly 15-35 years
- Epidemiology
  o Most frequently seen in sexually active young men; also seen in infants and boys

Natural History & Prognosis

- Prognosis excellent if treated early with antibiotics
- Complications
  o Abscess formation (epididymal abscess: 6%, testicular abscess: 6%), microabscesses are usually seen in low-grade infection such as tuberculosis and in immunocompromised host
  o Testicular infarction
    - Venous infarction: Due to venous outflow obstructio
    - Thrombosis of main testicular artery or its branches secondary to chronic inflammation
    - Gangrene is rare but a known complication
  o Gonadal vein thrombosis
  o Pyocele
  o Late testicular atrophy (21%)
  o Recurrent infection may lead to infertility

Treatment

- Antibiotic therapy; follow-up scans to exclude abscess if no improvement
- Work-up for GU anomalies in younger children and recurrent cases
- Bed rest, scrotal elevation, analgesics

DIAGNOSTIC CHECKLIST

Consider

- Torsion if low or absent flow within testis

Image Interpretation Pearls

- Hyperemic and enlarged epididymis &/or testis

SELECTED REFERENCES

1. Avery LL et al: Imaging of penile and scrotal emergencies. Radiographics. 33(3):721-40, 2013
2. Boettcher M et al: Differentiation of epididymitis and appendix testis torsio by clinical and ultrasound signs in children. Urology. 82(4):899-904, 2013
3. D'Andrea A et al: US in the assessment of acute scrotum. Crit Ultrasound J. Suppl 1:S8, 2013
4. Yusuf G et al: Global testicular infarction in the presence of epididymitis: clinical features, appearances on grayscale, color Doppler, and contrast-enhanced sonography, and histologic correlation. J Ultrasound Med. 32(1):175-80, 2013
5. Aganovic L et al: Imaging of the scrotum. Radiol Clin North Am. 50(6):1145-65, 2012
6. Yagil Y et al: Role of Doppler ultrasonography in the triage of acute scrotum in the emergency department. J Ultrasound Med. 29(1):11-21, 2010
7. Thinyu S et al: Role of ultrasonography in diagnosis of scrotal disorders: a review of 110 cases. Biomed Imaging Interv J. 5(1):e2, 2009
8. Trojian TH et al: Epididymitis and orchitis: an overview. Am Fam Physician. 79(7):583-7, 2009
9. Aso C et al: Gray-scale and color Doppler sonography of scrotal disorders in children: an update. Radiographics. 25(5):1197-214, 2005
10. Dogra V et al: Acute painful scrotum. Radiol Clin North Am. 42(2):349-63, 2004
11. Dogra VS et al: Sonography of the scrotum. Radiology. 227(1):18-36, 2003
12. Chung JJ et al: Sonographic findings in tuberculous epididymitis and epididymo-orchitis. J Clin Ultrasound. 25(7):390-4, 1997
13. Gordon LM et al: Traumatic epididymitis: evaluation with color Doppler sonography. AJR Am J Roentgenol. 166(6):1323-5, 1996
14. Bukowski TP et al: Epididymitis in older boys: dysfunctional voiding as an etiology. J Urol. 154(2 Pt 2):762-5, 1995

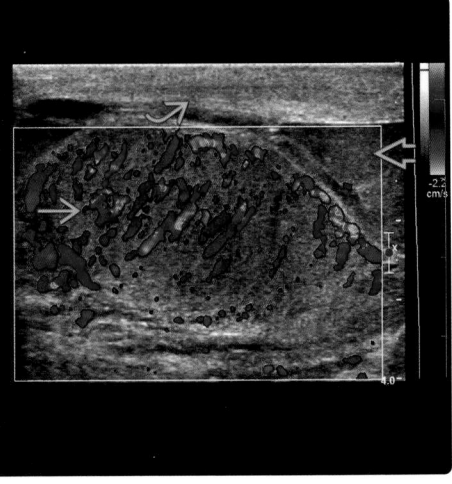

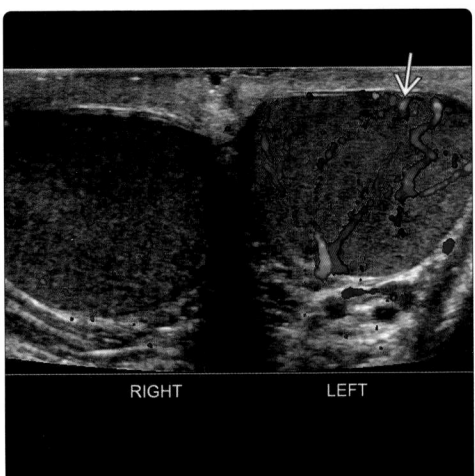

(Left) *Sagittal color Doppler US image of the right testis in a young man with acute scrotal pain shows an enlarged testis with diffuse hyperemia ➡, which is a typical appearance for acute orchitis. In addition, this patient has a complex hydrocele ➡ and overlying skin thickening ➡.* (Right) *Side-by-side color Doppler image of the testicles bilaterally shows the left testicle is markedly hyperemic ➡ in comparison to the right, consistent with left-sided orchitis.*

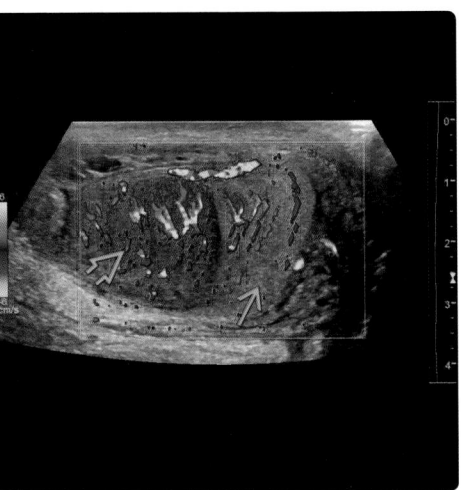

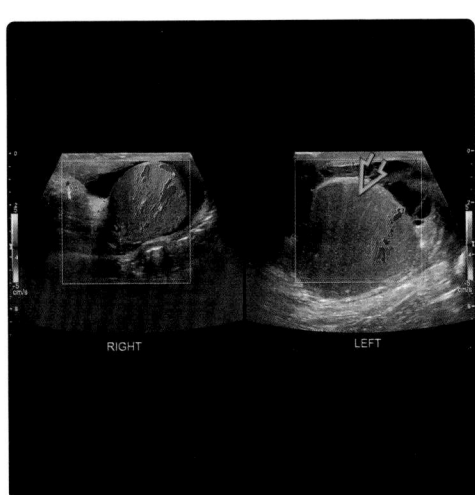

(Left) *Color Doppler reveals a round focal hypoechoic region within the right testicle with increased vascularity ➡. Normal testicular parenchyma can be seen adjacent to this area ➡. This was a case of focal orchitis.* (Right) *Color Doppler of bilateral testes demonstrates heterogenous echogenicity and decreased vascularity within the left testicle ➡ consistent with testicular infarction. This was the sequela of venous thrombosis secondary to orchitis.*

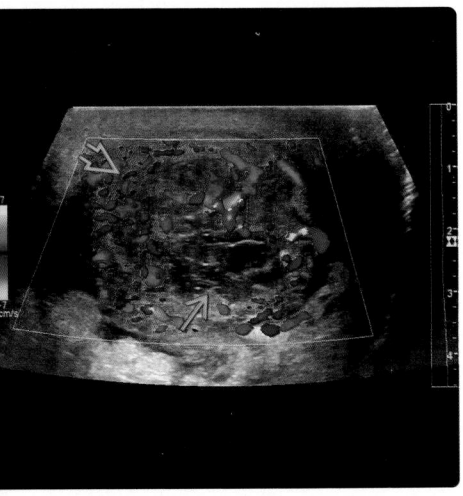

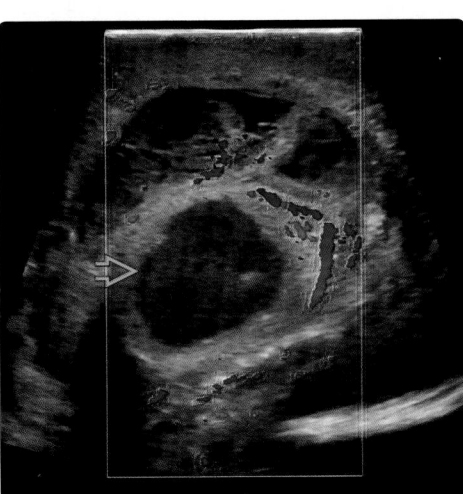

(Left) *Color Doppler of the left epididymis reveals a markedly hyperemic tail ➡ with a heterogenous hypoechoic lesion centrally ➡. The findings are consistent with epididymitis complicated by an epididymal abscess.* (Right) *Color Doppler of the left testis in a patient who presented with acute epididymo-orchitis reveals a hypoechoic, thick-walled lesion within the testicle ➡ consistent with a testicular abscess.*

IMAGING

- Heterogeneous testicular parenchyma or contour abnormality of testis in setting of scrotal trauma
  - Disruption of tunica albuginea is very specific for testicular rupture
- Extratesticular hematocele: Most common finding in scrotum after blunt injury
- US appearance of hematoma depends on time elapsed since trauma
- Intra- or extratesticular air in scrotum, missile track &/or foreign bodies (bullet/pellet) is indicative of penetrating injury
- Spermatic cord hematoma appears as heterogeneous avascular mass superior to testis
- Color Doppler is useful to determine viable portions of testis

PATHOLOGY

- Sports injuries (> 50%), vehicular and ballistic trauma, and iatrogenic

CLINICAL ISSUES

- Unless repaired within 72 hours, salvage rate only 45%
- Follow-up of conservatively treated testicular hematomas essential due to increased risk of infection, which may resu in orchiectomy
- Orchiectomy (total or partial) is performed for nonviable testis in testicular rupture
- Surgical exploration and drainage must be performed for large intratesticular hematomas
- Tumors may be discovered after trauma, consider tumor if there is internal color flow in an intratesticular lesion

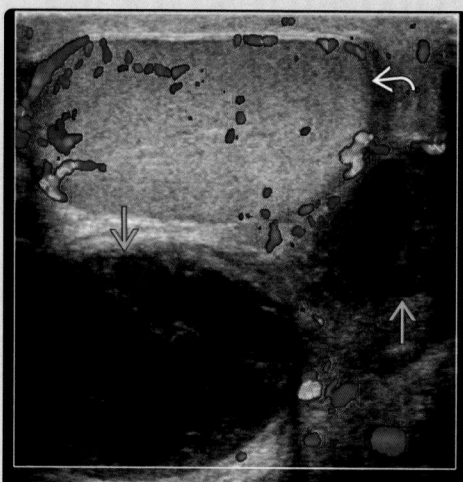
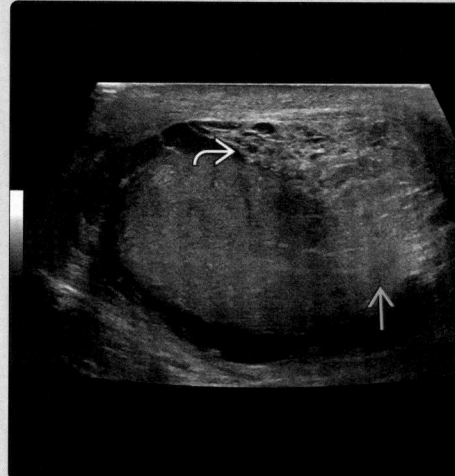

(Left) *Transverse color Doppler ultrasound of the scrotum demonstrates 2 large, extratesticular avascular fluid collections (hematomas)* ⮕ *in the scrotal cavity. The patient was status post recent vasectomy with new onset scrotal swelling. Testis* ⮕ *is normal.* (Right) *Sagittal ultrasound of the right testis after a MVC demonstrates heterogeneous testicular parenchyma* ⮕ *with indistinct tunica albuginea and adjacent hematocele* ⮕. *Surgery confirmed a testicular rupture.*

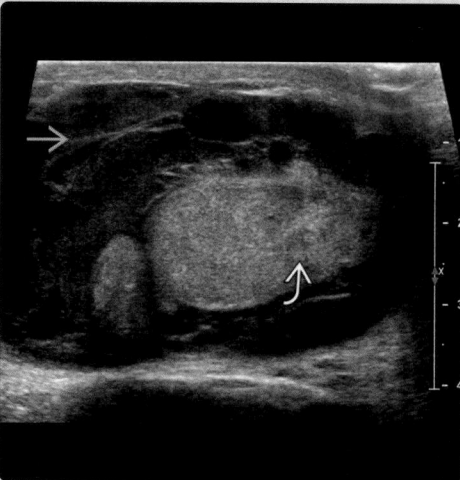
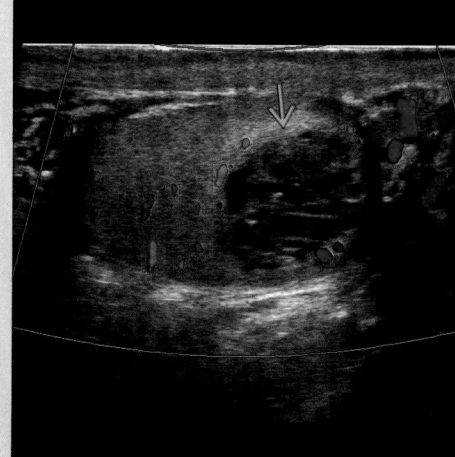

(Left) *Sagittal grayscale ultrasound of the right scrotal cavity shows a large, complex extratesticular fluid collection* ⮕, *consistent with hematocele. Mildly heterogeneous testis* ⮕ *is suggestive of contusion/hematoma.* (Right) *Color Doppler ultrasound of the right testis shows an avascular complex fluid collection* ⮕ *consistent with an intratesticular hematoma. The patient was continually followed until resolution of this hematoma.*

Scrotal Trauma

TERMINOLOGY

Definitions

Rupture of tunica albuginea, extrusion of testicular tissue into scrotal sac, collection of blood in tunica vaginalis or scrotal wall

IMAGING

General Features

Best diagnostic clue
- Heterogeneous parenchymal echogenicity of testis or contour abnormality of testis in presence of history of scrotal trauma

Morphology
- Irregularity of testicular contour and focal or diffuse heterogeneity in testis &/or epididymis
- Extratesticular hematocele: Most common finding in scrotum after blunt injury

Ultrasonographic Findings

Grayscale ultrasound
- Hematocele: Hemorrhage contained within layers of tunica vaginalis
- Testicular rupture
  - Disruption of tunica albuginea
  - Contour abnormality of testis due to testicular extrusion
  - Heterogeneous testicular echotexture and echogenicity
- Testicular fracture
  - Discrete linear or irregular fracture plane within testis (17%)
- Testicular dislocation
  - Unilateral > > bilateral
  - Most commonly from high-impact injury against fuel tank in motorcycle accidents
- Testicular torsion
  - Trauma-induced torsion in 5-8% cases
- Testicular hematoma
  - US appearance depends on time elapsed since trauma
- Penetrating trauma
  - Intra- or extratesticular air in scrotum, missile track &/or foreign bodies (bullet/pellet)
- Epididymal injury: Focal epididymal enlargement with reduced echogenicity & abnormal position in relation to testis
- Scrotal wall hematoma: Focal wall thickening or loculated collection within wall
- Spermatic cord hematoma: Heterogeneous avascular mass superior to testis

Color Doppler
- Distorted intratesticular vascularity with interruption of vessels in area of injury due to injury to tunica vasculosa
  - Useful to determine viable portions of testis

Imaging Recommendations

Best imaging tool
- High-resolution US (9-15 MHz)

DIFFERENTIAL DIAGNOSIS

Testicular Torsion
- ↓ overall vascularity compared to normal testis

Epididymoorchitis
- Acute or chronic pain without history of trauma, enlarged hypoechoic epididymis with increased vascularity in epididymis and testis on color Doppler

Testicular Abscess
- Focal ill-defined, thick-walled mass and necrotic center

PATHOLOGY

General Features
- Etiology
  - Sports injuries (> 50%), vehicular and ballistic trauma, and iatrogenic
  - Blunt trauma impales scrotal contents to symphysis pubis or pubic rami, pelvic fracture
  - Penetrating trauma includes sharp objects such as knives, bullets, animal bites, self mutilation; gunshot injuries most common
  - Iatrogenic injuries from inguinal herniorrhaphy and orchiectomy

CLINICAL ISSUES

Presentation
- Most common signs/symptoms
  - Acute scrotal hematoma following blunt trauma

Natural History & Prognosis
- Unless repaired within 72 hours, salvage rate only 45%
- Follow-up of conservatively treated testicular hematomas is essential due to increased risk of infection, which may result in orchiectomy

Treatment
- Drainage: Large hematocele
- Orchiectomy (total or partial): Nonviable testis in testicular rupture
- Surgical exploration and drainage: Large intratesticular hematomas

DIAGNOSTIC CHECKLIST

Image Interpretation Pearls
- Irregularity of testicular contour, heterogeneous parenchyma and echogenic collection in tunica vaginalis

SELECTED REFERENCES

1. Avery LL et al: Imaging of penile and scrotal emergencies. Radiographics. 33(3):721-40, 2013
2. D'Andrea A et al: US in the assessment of acute scrotum. Crit Ultrasound J. 5 Suppl 1:S8, 2013
3. Bhatt S et al: Role of US in testicular and scrotal trauma. Radiographics. 28(6):1617-29, 2008
4. Deurdulian C et al: US of acute scrotal trauma: optimal technique, imaging findings, and management. Radiographics. 27(2):357-69, 2007
5. Buckley JC et al: Use of ultrasonography for the diagnosis of testicular injuries in blunt scrotal trauma. J Urol. 175(1):175-8, 2006
6. Pepe P et al: Does color Doppler sonography improve the clinical assessment of patients with acute scrotum? Eur J Radiol. 60(1):120-4, 2006

(Left) *Grayscale ultrasound of the testis after a Lacrosse ball injury demonstrates a disrupted tunica albuginea ⇨, heterogeneous testicular parenchyma ⮎, and a contour abnormality ⬈, consistent with testicular rupture.* **(Right)** *Corresponding color Doppler ultrasound in the same patient shows the extruded testicular parenchyma ⇨ to be avascular, suggestive of nonviable portions.*

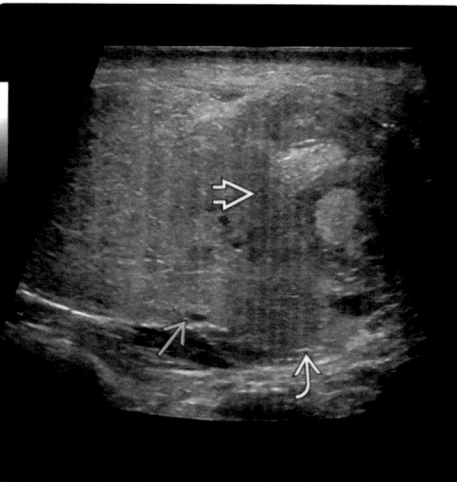
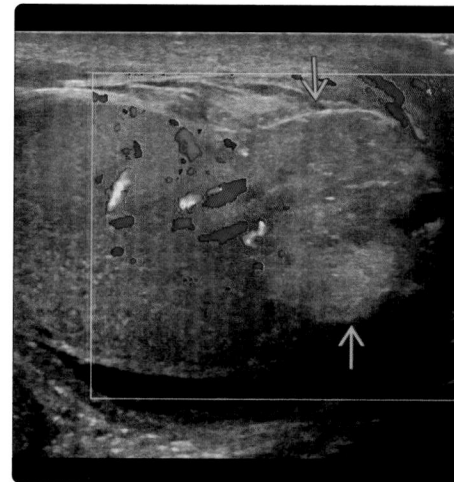

(Left) *Transverse grayscale ultrasound of bilateral testes shows a normal right testis ⇨ and a heterogeneous left testis ⮎ with disrupted tunica albuginea ⬈ consistent with testicular rupture.* **(Right)** *Color Doppler ultrasound of the scrotal cavity in the same patient with testicular rupture demonstrates a complex extratesticular fluid collection, consistent with an associated hematocele.*

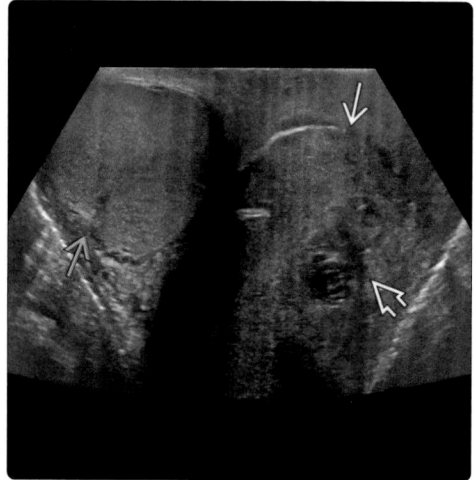
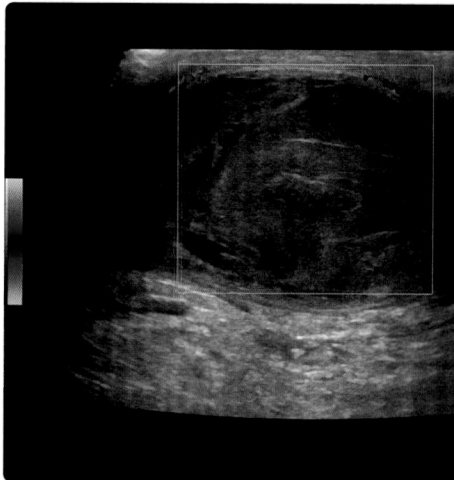

(Left) *Transverse grayscale ultrasound of the testis after blunt trauma shows a well-defined echogenic lesion ⮎ in the parenchyma.* **(Right)** *Corresponding color Doppler ultrasound in the same patient confirms that the lesion is avascular ⮎, suggestive of an acute intratesticular hematoma. The patient was sequentially followed until resolution. In cases of focal intratesticular hematomas, follow-up to resolution is recommended to exclude underlying neoplasm.*

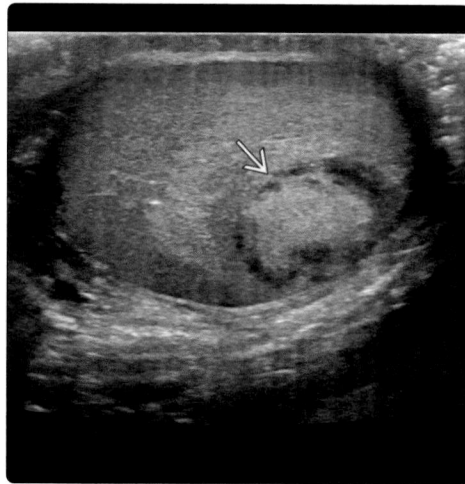
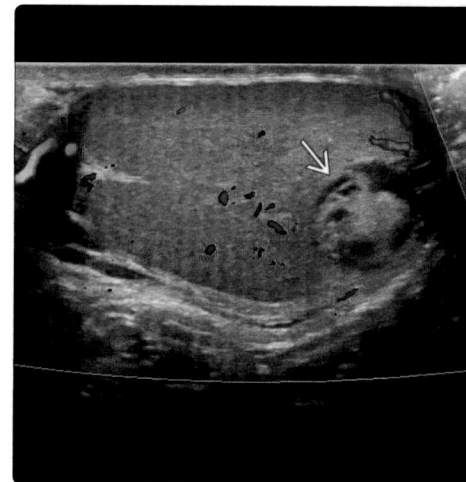

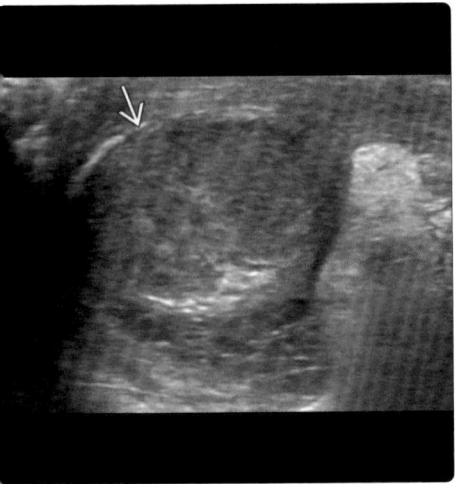

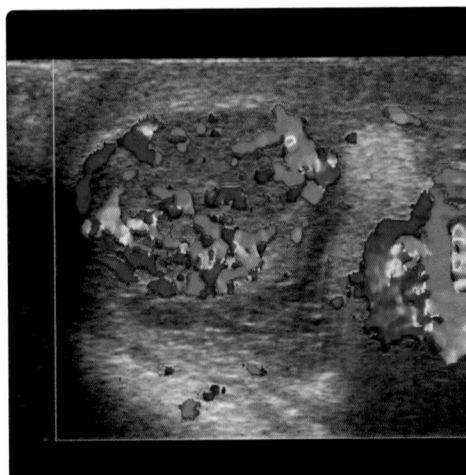

(Left) *Transverse grayscale ultrasound of the epididymis in a patient with blunt trauma to the scrotum demonstrates an enlarged and heterogeneous epididymis ➡. (Right) Corresponding color Doppler ultrasound demonstrates marked hyperemia of the epididymis, suggestive of traumatic epididymitis.*

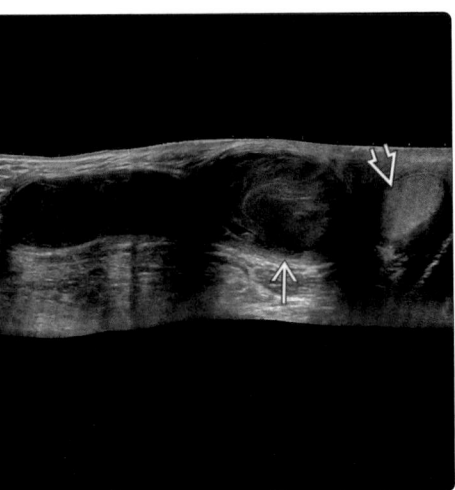

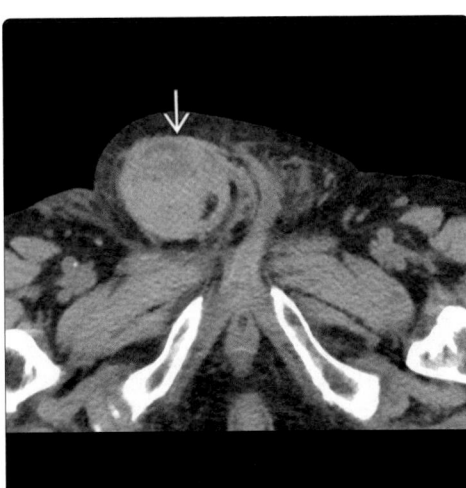

(Left) *Sagittal grayscale panoramic ultrasound of the right scrotum after inguinal herniorrhaphy demonstrates a large, complex fluid collection ➡ extending from the superior pole of the testis ➡ into the groin. Surgery confirmed a spermatic cord hematoma. (Right) Corresponding axial NECT at the level of the groin shows a large, high-attenuation mass ➡ involving the right spermatic cord, consistent with a spermatic cord hematoma*

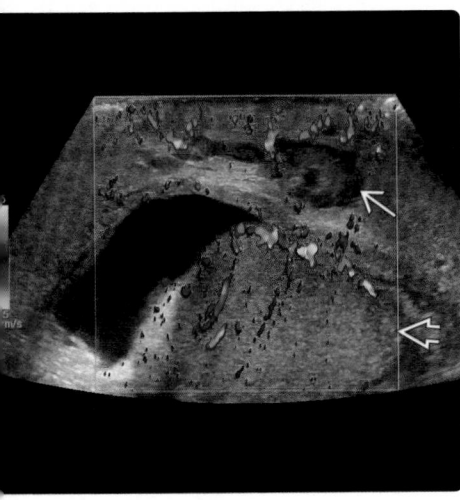

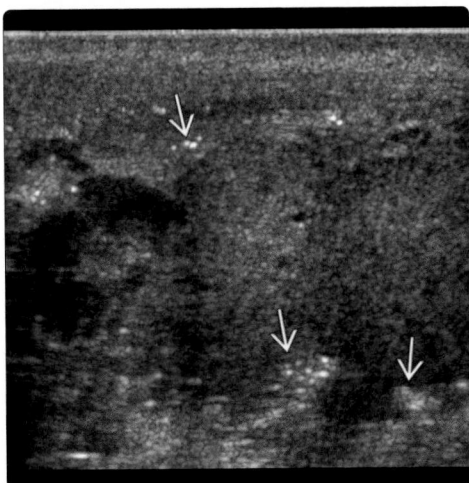

(Left) *Color Doppler ultrasound of the right scrotum after blunt trauma shows a complex avascular collection ➡ in the scrotal wall, suggestive of a scrotal wall hematoma. Testis ➡ was normal. (Right) Transverse grayscale ultrasound of the testis in a patient with gun shot injury to the thigh shows multiple echogenic foci ➡ in the scrotum suggestive of gas. Surgery confirmed presence of an associated testicular rupture.*

Hydrocele

TERMINOLOGY

- Congenital or acquired serous fluid contained within layers of scrotal tunica vaginalis

IMAGING

- Scrotal fluid surrounding testis, except for "bare area" where tunica vaginalis does not cover testis and is attached to epididymis
- Intrascrotal, external to testis and epididymis
- Not within scrotal wall
- Specific anatomic location: Tunica vaginalis
- Simple or complex avascular fluid
- High-resolution US (9-15 MHz) is modality of choice

PATHOLOGY

- Congenital or communicating hydrocele is due to failure of processus vaginalis to close
- Secondary occurrence in adults due to epididymitis, trauma, surgery, or tumor

- Simple fluid collection within tunica vaginalis
- Chronic cases show thickened tunica with septation
- Complex fluid may be seen in acute infection or afterward
- Scrotal hematoma may be slow to resolve and manifest as complex collection

CLINICAL ISSUES

- Congenital hydroceles usually resolve by 18 months of age
- 25-50% of acquired hydroceles are associated with trauma
- 10% of testicular tumors have associated hydrocele
- Surgical hydrocelectomy: Open drainage of fluid and oversewing of hydrocele sac edges
- Aspiration and sclerotherapy: Less invasive approach with slightly higher risk of recurrence

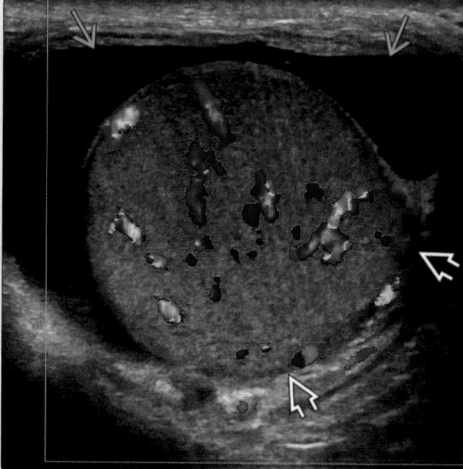
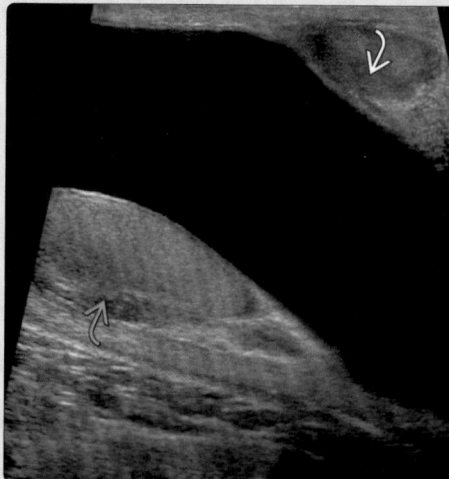

(Left) *Transverse color Doppler ultrasound shows simple-appearing fluid ➡ in a small hydrocele. Note that the fluid does not surround the testicle along the bare area ⧨ where the tunica vaginalis does not cover the testicle and is attached to the epididymis.* (Right) *Massive simple hydrocele in a 90-year-old man compresses the right testis ➡ along the scrotal wall. The left testis ⧨ is also visible in this image.*

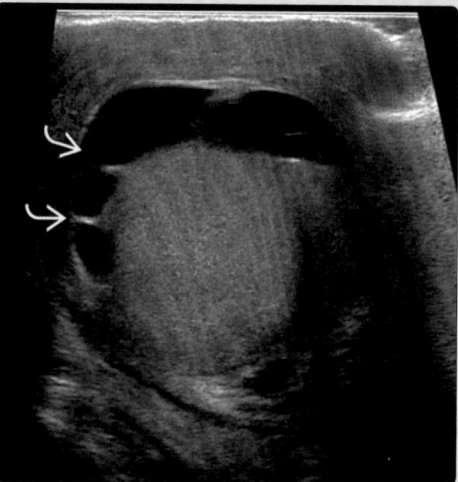
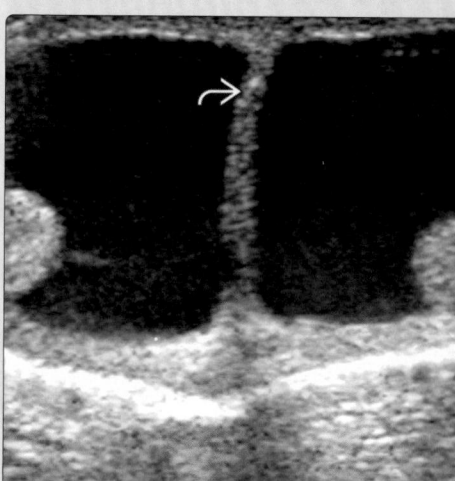

(Left) *Thin septations ⧨ are shown within a minimally complex hydrocele in a patient with epidydimo-orchitis.* (Right) *Transverse ultrasound in a newborn boy shows symmetrical hydrocele in both hemiscrotums with clear separation ⧨ between right and left scrotal sac, characteristic of neonatal hydrocele.*

TERMINOLOGY

Definitions

Congenital or acquired serous fluid contained within layers of scrotal tunica vaginalis

IMAGING

General Features

Best diagnostic clue
- Scrotal fluid surrounding testis, except for "bare area" where tunica vaginalis does not cover testis and is attached to epididymis

Location
- Intrascrotal, external to testis and epididymis
- Not within scrotal wall
- Specific anatomic location: Tunica vaginalis

Morphology
- Simple or complex avascular fluid

Ultrasonographic Findings

Grayscale ultrasound
- Acute hydrocele (AH): Crescentic anechoic fluid collection surrounding anterolateral aspect of testis
  - Usually testis displaced posteromedially
- Chronic hydrocele (CH): Low-level, mobile echoes
  - Cholesterol crystals presumed to cause these low-level mobile echoes and cannot be distinguished from inflammatory debris; beware of artifacts on color Doppler
  - Diffuse scrotal wall thickening, parietal calcifications and scrotoliths
  - Septations may be present, should be avascular

Power Doppler
- May demonstrate movement of internal debris in chronic hydrocele

MR Findings

T1WI
- Low signal intrascrotal collection with no enhancement

T2WI
- Homogeneous high signal collection when fluid is simple, may be intermediate when chronic or complex

Imaging Recommendations

High-resolution US (9-15 MHz) is modality of choice

DIFFERENTIAL DIAGNOSIS

Pyocele

Septated fluid with low-level internal echoes
Associated with epididymitis, intrascrotal abscess, and clinical signs of inflammation

Hematocele

Complex echogenic fluid in tunica vaginalis on US
Associated with trauma, torsion, and infarct

Scrotal Hernia

Peristalsing bowel or echogenic omentum within scrotum

PATHOLOGY

General Features

- Etiology
  - Embryology-anatomy
    - Congenital or communicating hydrocele is due to failure of processus vaginalis to close
    - Secondary occurrence in adults due to epididymitis, trauma, surgery, or tumor
- Simple fluid collection within tunica vaginalis
- Chronic cases show thickened tunica with septation
  - Complex fluid may be seen in acute infection or afterwards
  - Scrotal hematoma may be slow to resolve and manifest as complex collection

CLINICAL ISSUES

Presentation

- Most common signs/symptoms
  - Asymptomatic (painless) scrotal mass/enlargement

Demographics

- Epidemiology
  - Congenital hydroceles usually resolve by 18 months of age
  - 25-50% of acquired hydroceles are associated with trauma
  - 10% of testicular tumors have associated hydrocele

Treatment

- Surgical hydrocelectomy: Open drainage of fluid and oversewing of hydrocele sac edges
- Aspiration and sclerotherapy: Less invasive approach with slightly higher risk of recurrence

DIAGNOSTIC CHECKLIST

Image Interpretation Pearls

- Anechoic fluid collection in tunica vaginalis along anterolateral aspect of testis

SELECTED REFERENCES

1. Rafailidis V et al: Sonography of the scrotum: from appendages to scrotolithiasis. J Ultrasound Med. 34(3):507-18, 2015
2. Koutsoumis G et al: Primary new-onset hydroceles presenting in late childhood and pre-adolescent patients resemble the adult type hydrocele pathology. J Pediatr Surg. 49(11):1656-8, 2014
3. Shakiba B et al: Aspiration and sclerotherapy versus hydrocoelectomy for treating hydrocoeles. Cochrane Database Syst Rev. 11:CD009735, 2014
4. Naji H et al: Decision making in the management of hydroceles in infants and children. Eur J Pediatr. 171(5):807-10, 2012
5. Rizvi SA et al: Role of color Doppler ultrasonography in evaluation of scrotal swellings: pattern of disease in 120 patients with review of literature. Urol J. 8(1):60-5, 2011
6. Garriga V et al: US of the tunica vaginalis testis: anatomic relationships and pathologic conditions. Radiographics. 29(7):2017-32, 2009
7. Woodward PJ et al: From the archives of the AFIP: extratesticular scrotal masses: radiologic-pathologic correlation. Radiographics. 23(1):215-40, 2003

Spermatocele/Epididymal Cyst

KEY FACTS

TERMINOLOGY

- Spermatocele: Retention cyst of rete testis or epididymis containing spermatozoa
- Epididymal head cyst: Collection of simple fluid

IMAGING

- Protocol advice: Grayscale US with color Doppler imaging
- US findings
  - Simple or complex cystic mass: May be multiseptated; may contain diffuse, low-level echoes due to spermatozoa
  - "Falling snow" sign: Mechanically moving particulate material within cyst due to acoustic radiation force from color Doppler

PATHOLOGY

- Etiology: Unknown, may reflect scarring secondary to either epididymitis, trauma, or vasectomy

- Associated abnormalities: Dilation of rete testis within mediastinum of testis

CLINICAL ISSUES

- Most common signs/symptoms: Painless scrotal mass
  - Rare hypofertility or torsion
- Treatment: Most can be observed if asymptomatic
  - Surgery (spermatocelectomy) only if sufficiently large to cause discomfort

DIAGNOSTIC CHECKLIST

- Image interpretation pearls: Cystic mass in head of epididymis, either simple or with "falling snow" sign on color Doppler US
- Cystic extratesticular lesions almost always benign; if no vascularized soft tissue elements, not neoplasm

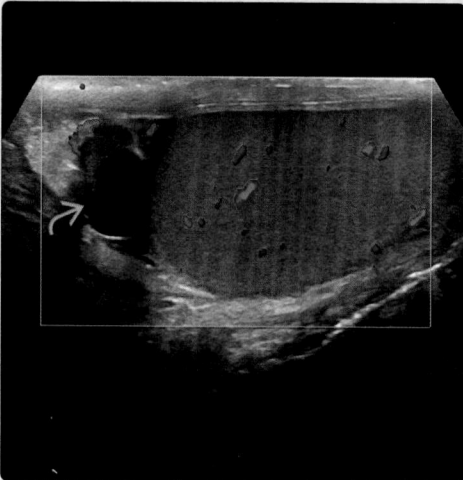
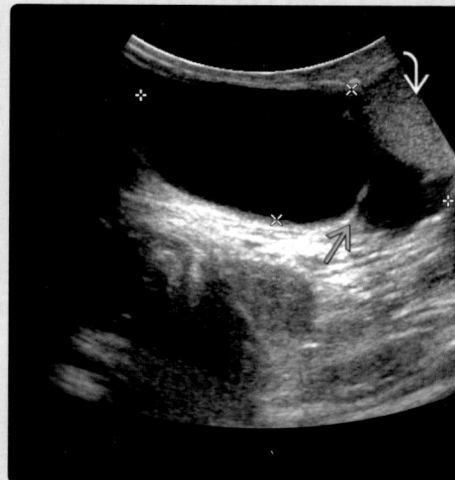

(Left) *Typical appearance of an incidentally discovered and clinically unimportant epididymal cyst is shown. Note the well-circumscribed, anechoic, avascular lesion* ⟶ *in the epididymal head.* (Right) *Large epididymal cyst (calipers) is shown with a single thin septation* ⟶ *in the right hemiscrotum, displacing the testis* ⟶ *inferiorly. Note that the abdominal probe rather than the high-frequency linear probe was needed to capture this large lesion.*

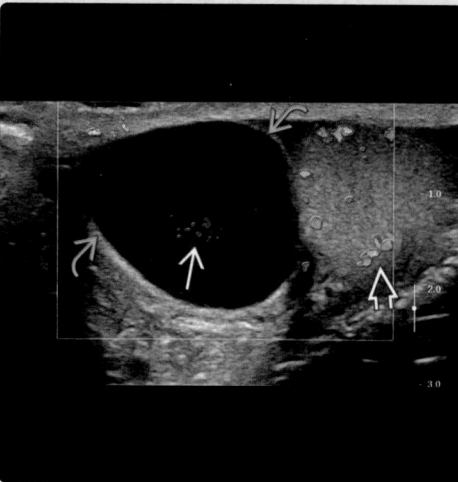
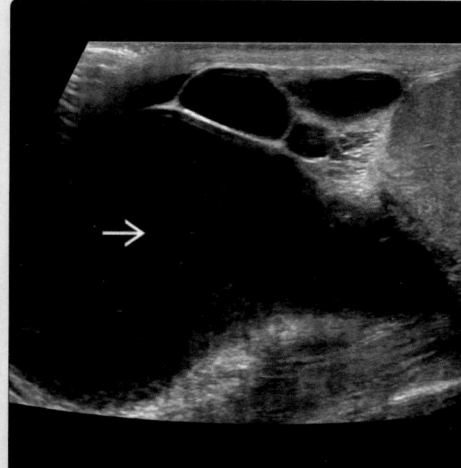

(Left) *Large spermatocele* ⟶ *superior to right testis* ⟶ *contains punctate low-level echoes with corresponding Doppler artifact* ⟶. *These punctate foci were mobile in real time.* (Right) *Longitudinal grayscale ultrasound demonstrates a complex, multiseptate cystic mass with numerous locules containing debris* ⟶, *characteristic findings for a spermatocele.*

TERMINOLOGY

Definitions

- Spermatocele: Retention cyst of rete testis or epididymis containing spermatozoa
- Epididymal head cyst: Collection of simple fluid

IMAGING

General Features

- Best diagnostic clue
  - Simple or minimally complex cystic mass within head of epididymis
- Location
  - Head of epididymis
- Size
  - 3 mm to 10 cm
- Morphology
  - Epididymal head cysts are anechoic, thin walled, and avascular
  - Spermatoceles may contain linear septations and internal debris

Imaging Recommendations

- Best imaging tool
  - US
- Protocol advice
  - Grayscale US with color Doppler imaging

Ultrasonographic Findings

- Simple or complex cystic mass: May be multiseptated; may contain diffuse; low-level echoes due to spermatozoa
- "Falling snow" sign: Mechanically moving particulate material within cyst due to acoustic radiation force from color Doppler

DIFFERENTIAL DIAGNOSIS

Hematocele

- History of trauma
- Complex fluid collection within tunica vaginalis
- Contains echogenic clot and fibrin strands

Pyocele

- Associated with epididymoorchitis with hyperemia and enlargement of epididymis &/or testis
- Complex fluid collection located within tunica vaginalis
- Contains white-cell debris and fibrinous strands producing linear septations and low-level echoes

Hydrocele

- Simple or complex intrascrotal fluid collection within tunica vaginalis

Cyst of Tunica Albuginea

- Usually small (2-5 mm) simple cyst between layers of tunica albuginea

PATHOLOGY

General Features

- Etiology
  - Scarring secondary to either epididymitis, trauma, or vasectomy

- Associated abnormalities
  - Dilation of rete testis within mediastinum of testis

Gross Pathologic & Surgical Features

- Complex cystic mass containing simple fluid or milky fluid and spermatozoa, depending on type

CLINICAL ISSUES

Presentation

- Most common signs/symptoms
  - Painless scrotal mass
    - Rare hypofertility or torsion
  - Cystic masses can be transilluminated like hydroceles at physical exam

Demographics

- Age
  - Any age can be affected
- Epidemiology
  - Very common; present in 20-40% of men

Treatment

- Most can be observed if asymptomatic
- Surgery (spermatocelectomy) only if sufficiently large to cause discomfort

DIAGNOSTIC CHECKLIST

Consider

- Abscess: Correlate with recent epididymitis and ongoing hyperemia
- Inguinal hernia: Should vary with Valsalva maneuver and exhibit expected gut signature or echogenic fat

Image Interpretation Pearls

- Cystic mass in head of epididymis with "falling snow" sign on color Doppler US
- Cystic extratesticular lesions almost always benign; if no vascularized soft tissue elements, not neoplasm

SELECTED REFERENCES

1. Yang JR et al: Comparison between Open Epididymal Cystectomy and Minimal Resection of Epididymal Cysts Using a Scrotoscope: A Clinical Trial for the Evaluation of a New Surgical Technique. Urology. ePub, 2015
2. Erikci V et al: Management of epididymal cysts in childhood. J Pediatr Surg. 48(10):2153-6, 2013
3. Rioja J et al: Adult hydrocele and spermatocele. BJU Int. 107(11):1852-64, 2011
4. Valentino M et al: Cystic lesions and scrotal fluid collections in adults: Ultrasound findings. J Ultrasound. 14(4):208-15, 2011
5. Posey ZQ et al: Rate and associations of epididymal cysts on pediatric scrotal ultrasound. J Urol. 184(4 Suppl):1739-42, 2010
6. Sista AK et al: Color Doppler sonography in evaluation of spermatoceles: the "falling snow" sign. J Ultrasound Med. 27(1):141-3, 2008
7. Smart JM et al: Ultrasound findings of masses of the paratesticular space. Clin Radiol. 63(8):929-38, 2008

Adenomatoid Tumor

TERMINOLOGY

- Benign solid paratesticular tumor of mesenchymal origin

IMAGING

- Solid intrascrotal mass, usually extratesticular
- Location
  - Epididymis: Most common location overall
  - May arise in tunica albuginea
  - Rarely intratesticular or other locations such as spermatic cord and prostate
- Imaging appearance
  - Rounded or ovoid
  - Well circumscribed
  - Varying echogenicity
  - Gentle transducer pressure may show mass can move independently of testis
  - Refractive edge shadows on grayscale US
  - Hypovascular or avascular on color Doppler US
  - Size: 5 mm to 5 cm

TOP DIFFERENTIAL DIAGNOSES

- Leiomyoma
- Lipoma
- Cystadenoma

CLINICAL ISSUES

- Most common solid mass in epididymis
  - 36% of all paratesticular tumors
- Slowly enlarges over years
- Most surgically excised to confirm diagnosis
- Some urologists and patients elect surveillance
- Age: 20 years and older
  - Mean age 36
  - Rarely seen in boys

DIAGNOSTIC CHECKLIST

- Consider leiomyoma

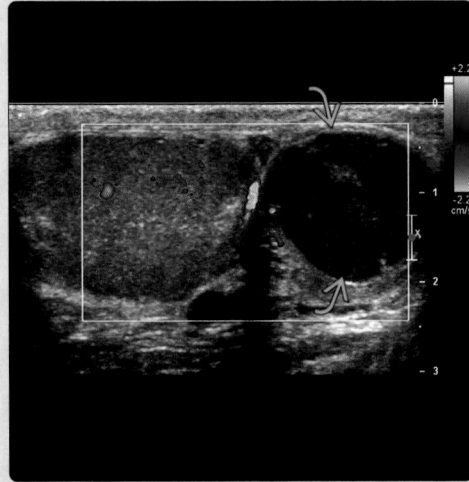
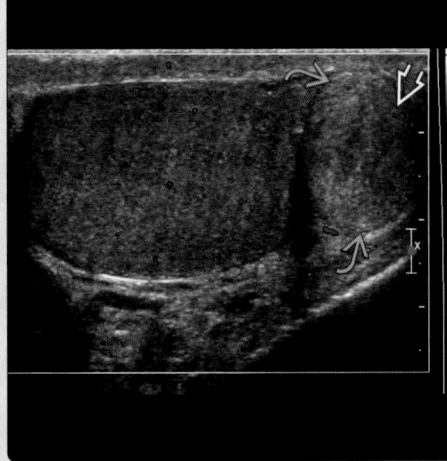

(Left) This palpable hypoechoic adenomatoid tumor ⧉ located in the in tail of the epididymis in a 41-year-old man has no demonstrable internal vascularity. (Right) This 50-year-old man had 5 years of ultrasound surveillance for a presumed adenomatoid tumor. This ovoid, well-circumscribed mass ⧉ in the tail of the epididymis is isoechoic to testis and shows minimal internal vascularity ⧉. Note the very different echogenicity compared to the otherwise similar patient shown previously.

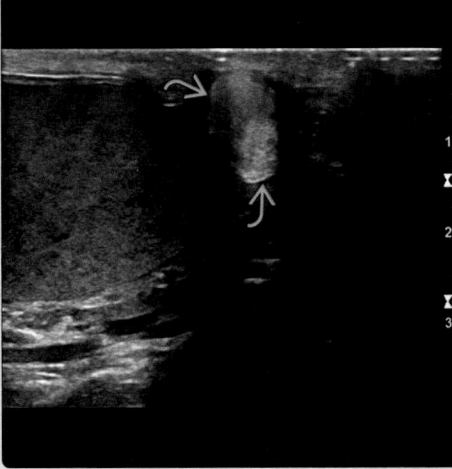
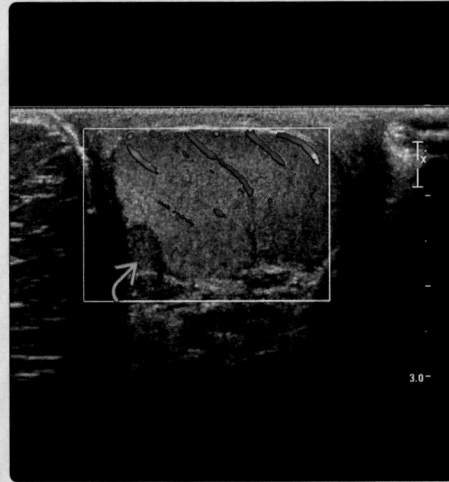

(Left) This hyperechoic ovoid adenomatoid tumor ⧉ in the tail of the epididymis was an incidental finding in a 37-year-old man. (Right) This adenomatoid tumor of the tunica albuginea ⧉ was incidentally noted on a pelvic MR in a 12-year-old boy. The lesion is equally endophytic and exophytic to the testis as it is centered in the tunica. Note minimal internal vascularity.

TERMINOLOGY

Definitions

Benign solid paratesticular tumor of mesenchymal origin

IMAGING

General Features

Best diagnostic clue
- Solid intrascrotal mass, usually extratesticular

Location
- Epididymis: Most common location overall
  - Most commonly in tail
- Tunica albuginea
- Rarely intratesticular or other locations such as spermatic cord and prostate

Size
- 5 mm to 5 cm

Morphology
- Rounded or ovoid
- Well circumscribed

Imaging Recommendations

Best imaging tool
- US

Protocol advice
- Grayscale US with color Doppler imaging

Ultrasonographic Findings

Solid mass within epididymis or tunica, varying echogenicity
- Gentle transducer pressure may show mass can move independently of testis

Hypovascular or avascular on color Doppler US

Refractive edge shadows on grayscale US

DIFFERENTIAL DIAGNOSIS

Leiomyoma

Solid or cystic, may contain calcifications

Most often located in epididymal head

Lipoma

45% of all paratesticular masses

Composed of mature fat cells
- Homogeneous and hyperechoic on US
- High signal on T1-weighted MR

Cystadenoma

Reported in 60% of men with von Hippel-Lindau disease

May occur sporadically, typically in middle age

May be primarily cystic, or mixed solid and cystic on US

PATHOLOGY

General Features

Etiology
- Unknown
- Believed to be mesothelial in origin

Gross Pathologic & Surgical Features

Solid, homogeneous, yellowish nodule with smooth surface
- Most common location is tail of epididymis

Rarely may occur in tunica, testis, or spermatic cord

- Generally not encapsulated

Microscopic Features

- Lesion composed of irregular tubules lined with flattened and cuboid epithelial or endothelial cells
- Keratin positive on immunoperoxidase stains
- Cells are positive for mesothelial related markers (calretinin, HMBE1)
- Increasing recognition that FNA can provide accurate diagnosis

CLINICAL ISSUES

Presentation

- Most common signs/symptoms
  - Many patients are asymptomatic
  - Slowly growing palpable mass
- Other signs/symptoms
  - 5% of patients present with pain

Demographics

- Age
  - 20 years and older: Mean age 36
  - Rarely seen in boys
- Gender
  - Masses of similar histology may arise in female genital tract as well
- Epidemiology
  - Most common solid mass in epididymis
  - 36% of all paratesticular tumors

Natural History & Prognosis

- Slowly enlarges over years

Treatment

- Most are surgically excised to confirm diagnosis, usually testis-sparing
- Some urologists and patients elect surveillance
- Emerging role for FNA

DIAGNOSTIC CHECKLIST

Consider

- Leiomyoma

Image Interpretation Pearls

- Solid paratesticular mass
- Hypovascular or avascular on color Doppler US

SELECTED REFERENCES

1. Makkar M et al: Adenomatoid tumor of testis: A rare cytological diagnosis. J Cytol. 30(1):65-7, 2013
2. Gupta S et al: Aspiration cytology of adenomatoid tumor of epididymis: An important diagnostic tool. J Surg Case Rep. 2012(4):11, 2012
3. Wasnik AP et al: Scrotal pearls and pitfalls: ultrasound findings of benign scrotal lesions. Ultrasound Q. 28(4):281-91, 2012
4. Park SB et al: Imaging features of benign solid testicular and paratesticular lesions. Eur Radiol. 21(10):2226-34, 2011
5. Evans K: Rapidly growing adenomatoid tumor extending into testicular parenchyma mimics testicular carcinoma. Urology. 64(3):589, 2004
6. Williams SB et al: Adenomatoid tumor of the testes. Urology. 63(4):779-81, 2004

Varicocele

TERMINOLOGY

- Dilatation of pampiniform plexus > 2-3 mm due to congestion and retrograde flow in internal spermatic vein

IMAGING

- Dilated serpiginous veins at superior pole testis
- "Flash" of color Doppler with Valsalva
- Left (78%), right (6%), bilateral (16%)
- Varicose veins are > 2-3 mm diameter, increase in size with Valsalva

PATHOLOGY

- Primary: Incompetent venous valve near junction of left renal vein (LRV) and IVC
- Secondary: Obstruction of LRV by renal or adrenal tumor, nodes or rarely SMA compression

CLINICAL ISSUES

- Most frequent cause of male infertility

- Vague scrotal discomfort or pressure, primarily when standing
- 10-15% of men in USA have varicoceles
- Subclinical varicocele in 40-75% of infertile men
- Catheter embolization, surgical treatment, or sclerotherap if symptomatic
- Emerging research suggests even subclinical varicoceles should be treated

DIAGNOSTIC CHECKLIST

- Consider left renal vein occlusion by tumor in elderly male patient presenting with recent onset varicocele
- Valsalva essential for diagnosis of small varicoceles
- Varicocele diagnosed when vessel > 2 mm during quiet respiration in supine position

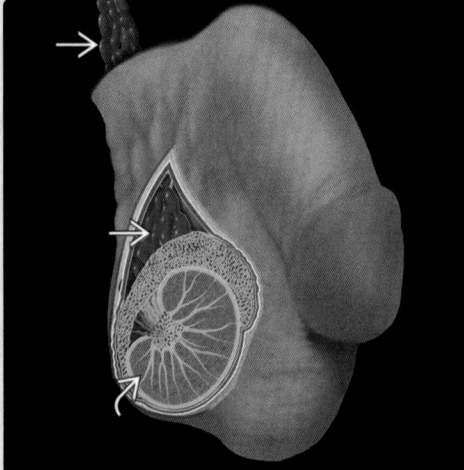
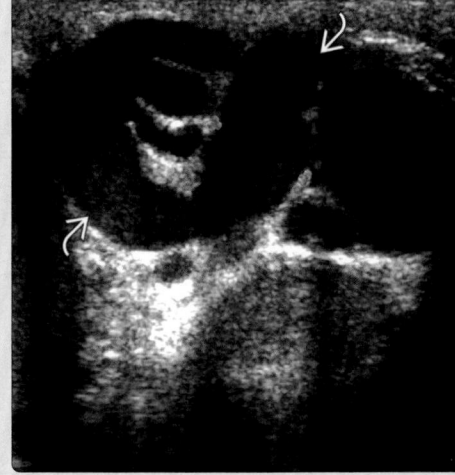

(Left) Graphic shows dilated, tortuous varicose veins of the pampiniform plexus ➡ in the spermatic cord and along the posterosuperior aspect of the testis ➡. (Right) Oblique grayscale ultrasound through cord, in supine position with normal respiration, shows a dilated, tortuous principal vein ➡ in pampiniform plexus measuring 7.5 mm in caliber.

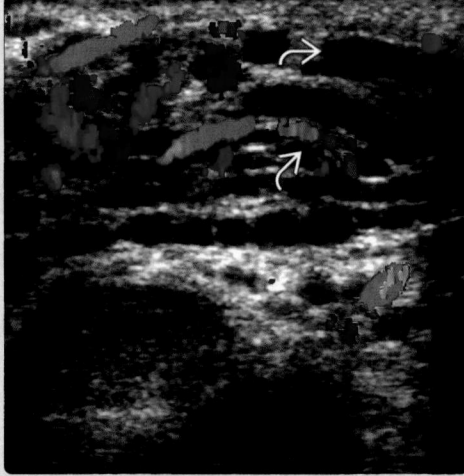
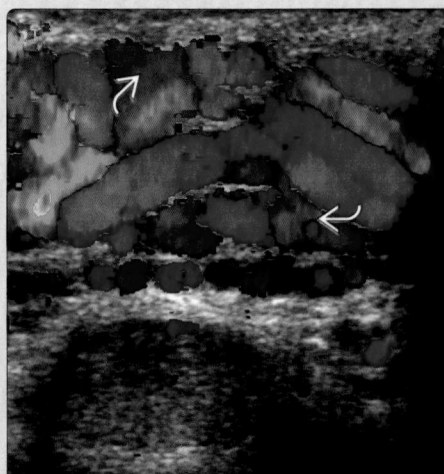

(Left) Longitudinal color Doppler ultrasound shows multiple serpiginous, dilated veins ➡ in the pampiniform plexus of the cord, along the posterosuperior aspect of testis in supine position during normal respiration. (Right) Longitudinal color Doppler ultrasound in the same patient shows flow ➡ in these dilated veins during Valsalva, indicative of moderate varicocele. Blood flow in the varicocele is slow and may be detected only with low Doppler settings.

TERMINOLOGY

Definitions

- Dilatation and tortuosity of pampiniform plexus > 2-3 mm due to congestion and retrograde flow in internal spermatic vein

IMAGING

General Features

- Best diagnostic clue
  - Dilated serpiginous veins adjacent to superior pole testis
  - "Flash" of color Doppler with Valsalva
- Location
  - Left (78%), right (6%), bilateral (16%)
  - Can extend along spermatic cord to inferior scrotal sac or rarely may have intratesticular varicocele
- Size
  - Varicose veins are > 2-3 mm diameter, increase in size with Valsalva

Ultrasonographic Findings

- Grayscale ultrasound
  - US should be performed in supine and standing positions
    - Hypoechoic, tubular structures superior and lateral to testis
  - ± low-level internal echoes due to slow flow and formation of red cell rouleaux
  - Scan retroperitoneum for mass
- Color Doppler
  - Detection approaches 100% with color Doppler US
  - Slow flow may be visible only with Valsalva

Other Modality Findings

- Catheter venography demonstrates dilated venous channels
- Enhancing tubular structures may be seen on CECT or MR

Imaging Recommendations

- Best imaging tool
  - US with color Doppler
- Protocol advice
  - Resting and Valsalva color Doppler

DIFFERENTIAL DIAGNOSIS

Tubular Ectasia/Rete Testis

- Normal variant: Dilated tubules of mediastinum &/or testis
- No flow on color Doppler

Testicular Torsion

- Absent or decreased flow to testis on color Doppler
- Enlarged, hypoechoic testis

Epididymitis

- Enlarged epididymis with increased flow on color Doppler
- Flow does not show change with Valsalva

PATHOLOGY

General Features

- Etiology

  - Primary: Incompetent venous valve near junction of left renal vein (LRV) and IVC
    - Left testicular vein is longer than right, enters LRV at right angle, sometimes arches over LRV
  - Secondary: Obstruction of LRV by renal or adrenal tumor, nodes, or rarely SMA compression
- Pathophysiology: Engorged veins have 3 distinct mechanisms of potential testicular damage
  - Increased heat: Warms blood heats testes
  - Oxidative stress: Reactive oxygen species (ROS)
  - Hemodynamics: ↑ venous pressure ↓ arterial inflow

Staging, Grading, & Classification

- Grading of varicoceles
  - Small varicocele: Palpable only with Valsalva maneuver
  - Moderate varicocele: Palpable with patient standing
  - Large varicocele: Visible through scrotal skin, and palpable with patient standing

CLINICAL ISSUES

Presentation

- Most common signs/symptoms
  - Most frequent cause of male infertility
  - Vague scrotal discomfort or pressure, primarily when standing

Demographics

- Age
  - Primary: Idiopathic > 15 years
  - Secondary: < 40 years or elderly
- Epidemiology
  - 10-15% of men in USA have varicoceles
  - Subclinical varicocele in 40-75% of infertile men

Natural History & Prognosis

- Excellent prognosis in treated cases

Treatment

- Catheter embolization, surgical treatment, or sclerotherapy if symptomatic
- Emerging research suggests even subclinical varicoceles should be treated

DIAGNOSTIC CHECKLIST

Consider

- Left renal vein occlusion by tumor in elderly male patient presenting with recent onset varicocele

Image Interpretation Pearls

- Valsalva essential for diagnosis of small varicoceles
- Varicocele diagnosed when vessel > 2 mm during quiet respiration in supine position

SELECTED REFERENCES

1. Cantoro U et al: Reassessing the role of subclinical varicocele in infertile men with impaired semen quality: a prospective study. Urology. 85(4):826-30, 2015
2. Kim YS et al: Efficacy of scrotal Doppler ultrasonography with the Valsalva maneuver, standing position, and resting-Valsalva ratio for varicocele diagnosis. Korean J Urol. 56(2):144-9, 2015
3. Karami M et al: Determination of the best position and site for color Doppler ultrasonographic evaluation of the testicular vein to define the clinical grades of varicocele ultrasonographically. Adv Biomed Res. 3:17, 2014

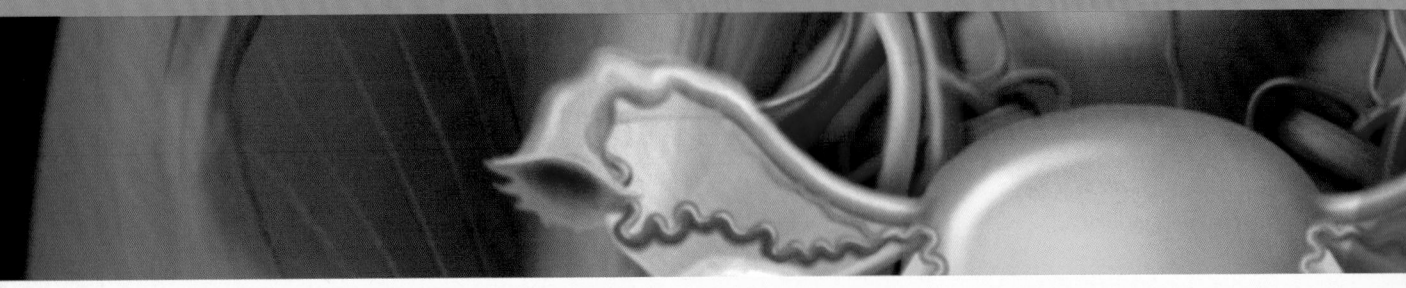

PART II
SECTION 11
Female Pelvis

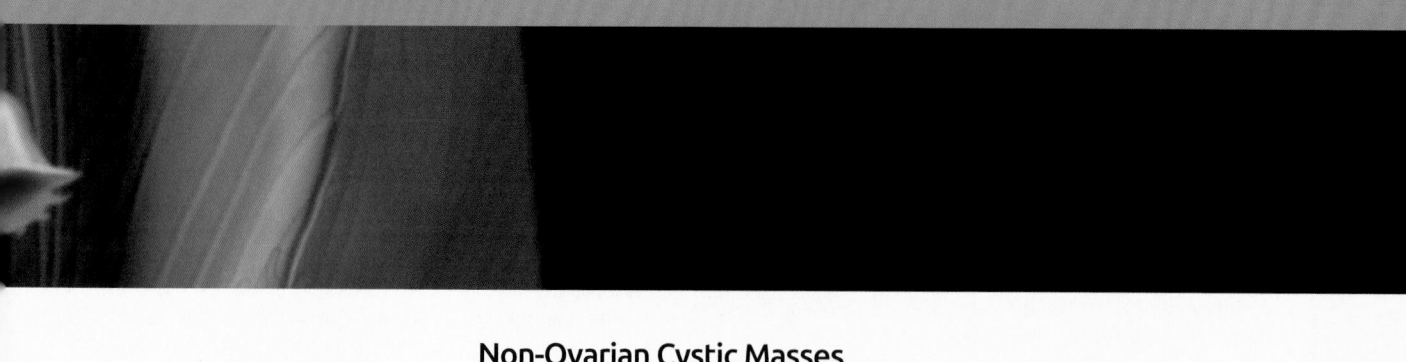

Imaging Anatomy

Uterus

The position of the uterus is variable and affected by the bladder filling, parity, fibroids, and bowel. Most commonly, the uterus lies in the midline with the fundus pointing towards the anterior abdominal wall and the external os pointing towards the rectum (anteversion and anteflexion). The opposite configuration (retroversion and retroflexion) is also commonly encountered and sometimes the uterus moves during the ultrasound exam. Both variants of uterine position are well imaged at endovaginal sonography because the transducer can be placed in the anterior or posterior vaginal fornices and close to the uterine serosa, allowing for high-frequency and high-resolution imaging. The uterus may also be in a neutral position, which is often the most difficult to image because the fundus points superiorly, away from the transducer. In this position, the fundus is at quite some depth from the vaginal fornix, making it difficult to penetrate with the higher frequencies of endovaginal transducers. In this situation, the patient or sonographer can apply pressure to the anterior abdominal wall to try and move the uterus to a favorable position.

Ovaries

The position of the ovaries is also variable and can be affected by the bladder filling, parity, uterine position, and pathology. The ovaries are generally found along the pelvic sidewall, adjacent to the external iliac vessels. The broad ligament, fallopian tube, and mesosalpinx are found between the ovary and uterus. These structures are often not seen as discrete anatomy when normal and are generally a heterogenous hyperechoic area containing variable-sized traversing vascularity. The ovaries are often found by scanning in the transverse plane and following the broad ligament laterally. During pregnancy, the ovaries move superiorly, out of the pelvis. In some women, they do not return to the ovarian fossa. Occasionally, an ovary will not be seen by transvaginal ultrasound, but will be well seen by transabdominal scanning because of a high position in the pelvis. In postmenopausal women, the ovaries may be difficult to identify because of a combination of atrophy, high position, &/or intervening bowel gas. In general, when the ovary is not identified, additional cross-sectional imaging can be avoided because it can be safely assumed that no significant mass exists since ovarian cancer does not present as a small ovarian mass.

Imaging Protocols

The pelvic ultrasound begins with a transabdominal exam typically using a curved low-frequency transducer. The patient is asked to fill her bladder prior to the exam such that the bladder displaces the small bowel and creates a sonographic window through which the uterus and adnexa are better seen. It should be noted that an overdistended bladder can push the uterus and ovaries far posteriorly and hinder evaluation. The patient is then asked to void in preparation for the endovaginal ultrasound. An endovaginal ultrasound routinely should be performed for all indications, though occasionally the anatomy is seen sufficiently by transabdominal imaging and an ultrasound can be avoided. In general, there are no absolute contraindications to endovaginal scanning, but it is generally not used in virginal women.

Images are always acquired in the sagittal (longitudinal) and transverse planes. It is important to remember that

depending on the angulation of the endovaginal transducer and lie of the uterus, the transverse view may be more in the coronal or coronal oblique plane with respect to the patient, rather than a true axial plane. The uterus should be measured and then evaluated for myometrial lesions such as fibroids (leiomyomas). The endometrium should be measured in the longitudinal plane perpendicular to the endometrial stripe, so as not to falsely elongate the true thickness. If fluid or blood is present in the endometrial cavity, it should be excluded from the measurement. The endometrium should also be evaluated for masses, cysts, or abnormal vascularity. The cervix should be imaged in two planes. Imaging of the vagina is not a routine part of pelvic ultrasonography, but can be performed transabdominally, endovaginally with minimal insertion of the transducer, or translabially. The ovaries should be scanned in two orthogonal planes and measured in three dimensions. Finally, the cul-de-sac should be imaged to evaluate for free fluid, hemorrhage, or masses.

Anatomy-Based Imaging Issues

Endometrium

The endometrium varies significantly in thickness and echogenicity depending on the phase of the menstrual cycle. Immediately after menstruation, the endometrium is seen as a thin echogenic line (1-2 mm) representing the 2 coapted layers of endometrium. In the proliferative phase, under the influence of estrogen, the endometrium starts to thicken. In the late proliferative phase, just prior to ovulation (day 14), the endometrium has a distinctive trilaminar or striated appearance with alternating hyper- and hypoechoic lines. After ovulation, when progesterone is produced, the endometrium becomes thicker and hyperechoic, losing definition of the layers. During menstruation, the endometrium sloughs and fluid and mobile debris may be seen in the cavity.

Ovaries

The ovaries are also under the influence of the menstrual cycle and normal physiologic changes are commonly encountered at ultrasound and should not be mistaken for pathology. In the follicular phase (day 0-14), one or more dominant follicles develop. Ovulation occurs on day 14. The follicle then becomes a corpus luteum which either supports an early pregnancy or regresses. A developing follicle is typically a simple cyst less than three cm (although can occasionally be larger) and should not be mistaken for a pathologic cyst or cancer.

Indications for Pelvic Ultrasound

Clinical indications for pelvic ultrasound include the following:

- Acute or chronic pelvic pain
- Pelvic masses
- Abnormal bleeding (dysmenorrhea, menorrhagia, amenorrhea)
- Pregnancy (infertility, normal, complicated, postpartum)
- Intrauterine device evaluation
- Pelvic inflammatory disease
- Difficult clinical exam of the pelvis
- Congenital uterine anomalies
- Endocrine abnormality (polycystic ovaries)
- Screening for malignancy in high-risk patients

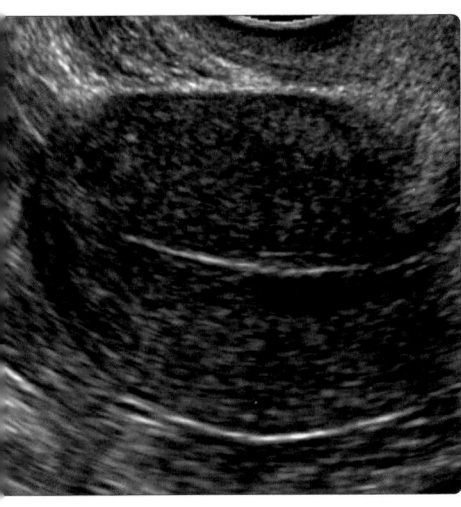
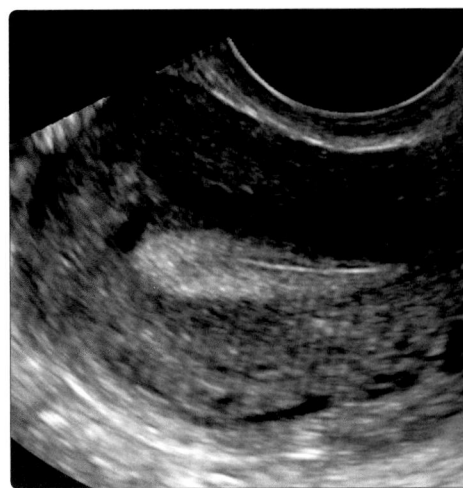

(Left) *Day 4: Longitudinal endovaginal grayscale ultrasound of the uterus shows a uniformly thin 1 mm endometrium at the end of menstruation when the endometrium is at its thinnest.* (Right) *Day 11: Longitudinal endovaginal ultrasound shows the typical appearance of the mildly thickened endometrium in the proliferative phase.*

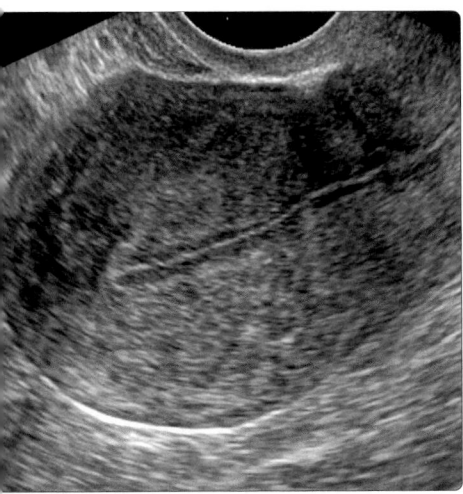
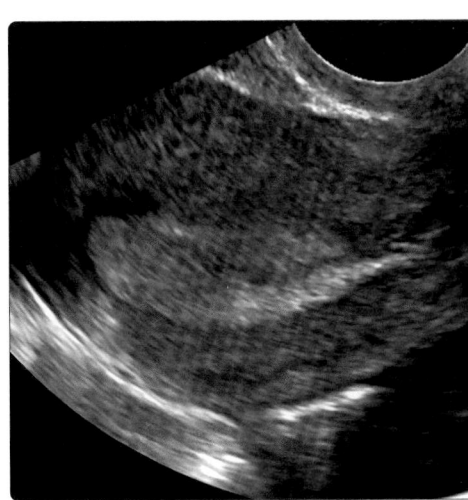

(Left) *Day 15: Longitudinal endovaginal ultrasound shows the trilaminar appearance of the endometrium in the periovulatory phase of the menstrual cycle. Of note, this is the best phase to detect endometrial polyps because they stand out as a hyperechoic lesion against a background hypoechoic endometrium.* (Right) *Day 28: Longitudinal endovaginal ultrasound shows a thickened and uniformly hyperechoic endometrium that is typical of the secretory phase just prior to menstruation.*

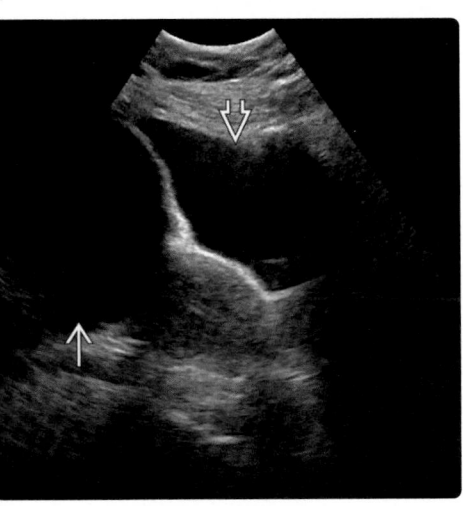
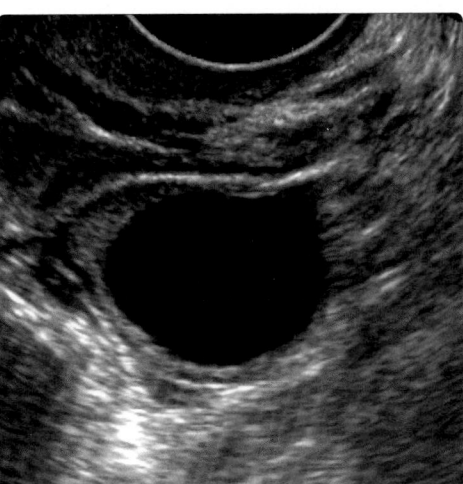

(Left) *Longitudinal transabdominal ultrasound shows the importance of starting the scan with transabdominal imaging prior to endovaginal scanning. This large cystic right ovarian mass ➡ (borderline ovarian tumor) above the bladder ➡ was only seen transabdominally and not seen by endovaginal imaging.* (Right) *Transverse endovaginal US shows 2.5 cm anechoic simple ovarian cyst representing a developing dominant follicle just prior to ovulation. This should not be confused with a pathologic cyst.*

KEY FACTS

TERMINOLOGY

- Most common pathologic process of cervix
- Mucus-filled cystic dilatation of endocervical gland
- Tunnel cluster: Type of nabothian cyst characterized by complex multicystic dilatation of endocervical glands

IMAGING

- Best imaging clue: Circumscribed superficial unilocular cyst in wall of cervix
  - Often multiple
  - Average size: 10-15 mm
- Important to identify relationship between nabothian cyst and endocervical canal
- Debris within cysts is common
- Use color Doppler if cyst appears potentially solid

TOP DIFFERENTIAL DIAGNOSES

- Adenoma malignum (minimal deviation adenocarcinoma)
- Endocervical hyperplasia

- Uterine cervicitis
- Cystic endometrial polyp
- Cervical cancer
- Cervical ectopic pregnancy
- Abortion in progress

CLINICAL ISSUES

- Nabothian cysts are rarely symptomatic
- More common in women who have had children
- Treatment is rarely necessary

DIAGNOSTIC CHECKLIST

- Requires further evaluation with MR if
  - Solid components
  - Copious vaginal discharge
  - Deep cervical invasion

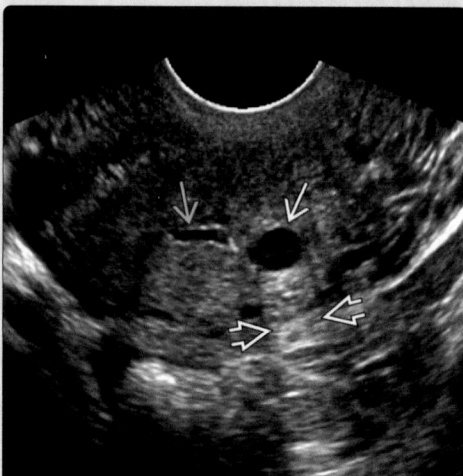
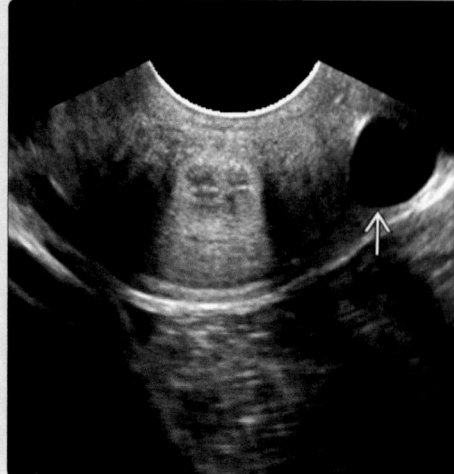

(Left) *Transverse transvaginal ultrasound through the cervix shows a well-circumscribed simple nabothian cyst* ➡ *with posterior acoustic enhancement* ➡, *separate from the fluid-filled endocervical canal* ➡. **(Right)** *Transverse transvaginal US shows a simple nabothian cyst* ➡ *at the lateral margin of the cervix. Real-time imaging helped confirm the location within the cervical stroma; however, this image demonstrates the potential for misdiagnosis as an ovarian follicle.*

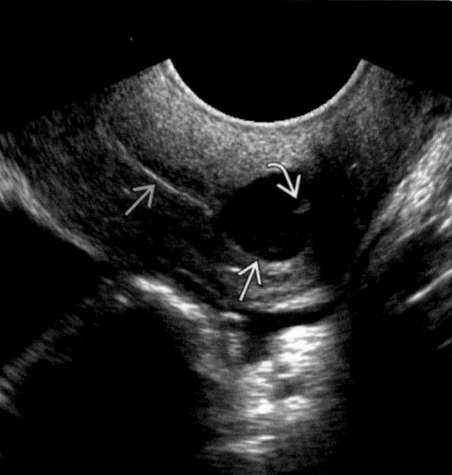
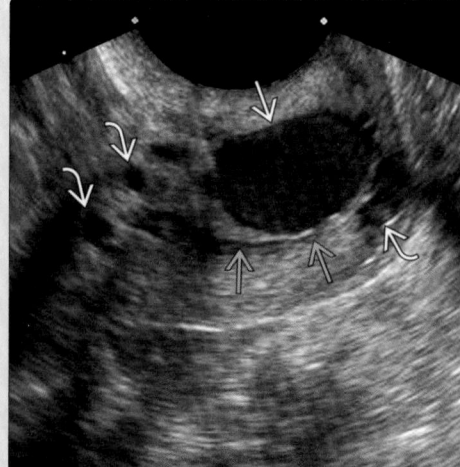

(Left) *Transverse transvaginal US shows a complex nabothian cyst* ➡ *with internal echoes and peripheral debris* ➡, *consistent with inspissated mucus. The cyst is adjacent to the cervical canal* ➡. **(Right)** *Longitudinal transvaginal US shows a large complex nabothian cyst* ➡ *with homogeneous internal echoes, in addition to multiple smaller nabothian cysts* ➡. *The cervical canal is minimally displaced but remains visible* ➡.

TERMINOLOGY

Synonyms

- Retention cyst
- Cervical cyst
- Ovula nabothi
- Nabothian follicle

Definitions

- Mucus-filled cystic dilatation of endocervical gland
- Tunnel cluster: Type of nabothian cyst characterized by complex multicystic dilatation of endocervical glands

IMAGING

General Features

- Best diagnostic clue
  - Circumscribed superficial unilocular cyst in wall of cervix
- Location
  - Usually superficial, along endocervical canal or ectocervix
    - Superficial cysts visible on speculum exam
  - Anterior, posterior or lateral cervical lip
    - Not in cervical canal
  - Deep cysts only visible with imaging
- Size
  - Usually 10-15 mm in diameter
  - Rarely > 4 cm
  - Often multiple
- Morphology
  - May distort endocervical canal
  - Can mimic multicystic mass
  - Can enlarge cervix if large or multiple

Ultrasonographic Findings

- Grayscale ultrasound
  - Simple superficial cervical cystic lesion
    - Imperceptible thin wall
    - Posterior acoustic enhancement (increased through transmission)
    - Anechoic fluid most common
    - Can have proteinaceous debris
      - Diffusely echogenic
    - Rare septations
      - More likely multiple cysts than true septations
  - Large nabothian cysts
    - Can occupy most of cervix
    - Displaces endocervical canal
      - Rare cause of cervical stenosis
    - Can mimic cervical os dilatation
      - Confusing in pregnancy
  - Multiple cysts common
    - Can obscure endocervical canal
    - May mimic adnexal or cervical cystic mass
      - Multiple lateral cysts
      - Identification of separate ovary necessary
- Color Doppler
  - Absence of internal or peripheral flow

MR Findings

- T1WI: Variable, often mildly increased signal intensity
- T2WI: High signal intensity secondary to mucous

- T1WI C+: No enhancement

CT Findings

- NECT: Usually isodense or hypodense to cervix
- CECT: Nonenhancing hypodense cervical lesion

Imaging Recommendations

- Best imaging tool
  - TV ultrasound
  - MR helpful for complicated cases
    - Intravenous contrast required to differentiate from neoplasm
    - Identify separate ovary
- Protocol advice
  - Identify relationship between nabothian cyst and endocervical canal
    - If fluid in canal, consider alternate diagnosis
  - Debris within cysts is common
    - Not associated with malignancy
  - Use color Doppler if cyst appears potentially solid

DIFFERENTIAL DIAGNOSIS

Adenoma Malignum (Minimal Deviation Adenocarcinoma)

- Low-grade mucinous carcinoma affecting deep endocervical glands
- Multilocular cystic mass in cervix
- Deeply penetrating into cervical stroma; distinguish from more superficial nabothian cysts
- Typical clinical presentation of copious watery vaginal discharge
- Associated with Peutz-Jeghers syndrome

Endocervical Hyperplasia

- Thickening of endocervical mucosa ± cystic change
- Associated with oral progestational agents, pregnancy, and postpartum
- Appearance can overlap with adenoma malignum

Uterine Cervicitis

- Clinical: Tenacious, yellow or turbid, jelly-like discharge
- Associated with pelvic pressure or discomfort
- Can appear as retention cysts in cervix

Cystic Endometrial Polyp

- May contain cysts and arise from, or prolapse into, cervix
- Endocavitary mass; not within cervical stroma
- Doppler shows flow in stalk

Cervical Cancer

- Bulky large cervix, difficult to identify cervical canal
  - Cervical width > 4 cm
- Solid mass much more common than cystic
- Endometrial fluid from cervical stenosis
- Mucin producing carcinoma can mimic nabothian cyst
  - Both are high signal on T2WI MR
  - Carcinoma enhances irregularly

Cervical Ectopic Pregnancy

- Implantation of conceptus within cervical stroma
- Thick-walled cystic mass
  - Echogenic rim

- o Doppler shows trophoblastic flow
- Internal sac structures often visible
  - o Yolk sac
  - o Embryo, ± cardiac activity

Abortion in Progress

- Detached gestational sac in cervical canal
  - o Teardrop shape
- Internal sac structures sometimes visible
  - o Yolk sac
  - o Embryo
    - Cardiac activity almost always absent
    - If living embryo, must rule out cervical ectopic
- No trophoblastic flow around sac
  - o If blood flow seen, must rule out cervical ectopic

PATHOLOGY

General Features

- Etiology
  - o Healing process of chronic cervicitis
    - Endocervical glands become covered by squamous epithelium
    - Columnar epithelial cells continue to secrete mucus
    - Trapped mucus becomes cyst
  - o Tunnel cluster
    - Most commonly, result of stimulatory effects during pregnancy
    - Type A: Small, nondilated tunnels
    - Type B: Obstruction of type A tunnels leads to larger cysts
  - o Progestogenic therapy
    - Due to failure of cyclic flow of cervical mucus

Gross Pathologic & Surgical Features

- Yellow or white cysts on surface of cervix
- Round cysts with clear fluid

Microscopic Features

- Lined by columnar epithelium
- Retained mucus
- Tunnel cluster
  - o Type A: Small-caliber tunnels lined by tall columnar epithelium
  - o Type B: Cystic tunnels lined by cuboidal or flattened cells

CLINICAL ISSUES

Presentation

- Most common signs/symptoms
  - o Rarely symptomatic
  - o Incidental finding
    - Superficial cysts observed by gynecologist during speculum exam
    - Deep cysts seen incidentally during transvaginal ultrasound
  - o Large cysts may be palpable
- Other signs/symptoms
  - o Enlarged cervix
    - Patient discomfort
    - Cervical stenosis
  - o Rarely infected

Demographics

- Age
  - o Women of reproductive age
  - o More common in women who have had children
  - o Tunnel clusters almost always in multigravid women > 3 years old
- Epidemiology
  - o Most common pathologic process of cervix

Natural History & Prognosis

- Slow growing, do not resolve spontaneously

Treatment

- Rarely necessary
- Symptomatic nabothian cysts
  - o Electrocautery
  - o Cryotherapy
  - o Drainage

DIAGNOSTIC CHECKLIST

Consider

- Nabothian cysts are common
- Requires further evaluation with MR if
  - o Solid components
  - o Copious vaginal discharge
  - o Deep cervical invasion

Image Interpretation Pearls

- Well-defined, small, unilocular simple cysts in cervix
- Superficial location along cervical canal
- Large cysts can mimic endocervical fluid
  - o Identify cervical canal separate from cyst
- Pregnant patients may have other significant cervical problems

SELECTED REFERENCES

1. Bin Park S et al: Multilocular cystic lesions in the uterine cervix: broad spectrum of imaging features and pathologic correlation. AJR Am J Roentgenol. 195(2):517-23, 2010
2. Dujardin M et al: Cystic lesions of the female reproductive system: a review. JBR-BTR. 93(2):56-61, 2010
3. Rezvani M et al: Imaging of cervical pathology. Top Magn Reson Imaging. 21(4):261-71, 2010
4. Sosnovski V et al: Complex Nabothian cysts: a diagnostic dilemma. Arch Gynecol Obstet. 279(5):759-61, 2009
5. Oguri H et al: MRI of endocervical glandular disorders: three cases of a deep nabothian cyst and three cases of a minimal-deviation adenocarcinoma. Magn Reson Imaging. 22(9):1333-7, 2004
6. Li H et al: Markedly high signal intensity lesions in the uterine cervix on T2-weighted imaging: differentiation between mucin-producing carcinomas and nabothian cysts. Radiat Med. 17(2):137-43, 1999
7. Janus C et al: Nabothian cysts stimulating an adnexal mass. Clin Imaging. 13(2):157-8, 1989
8. Fogel SR et al: Sonography of Nabothian cysts. AJR Am J Roentgenol. 138(5):927-30, 1982

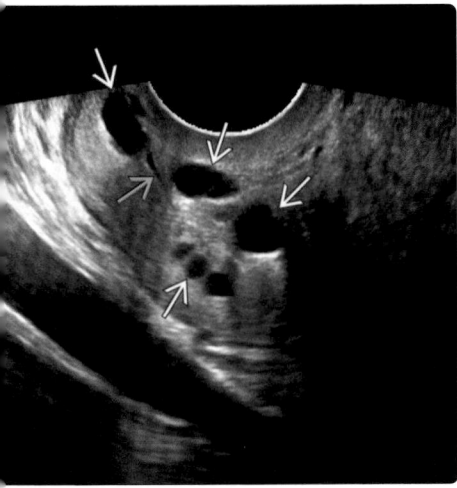

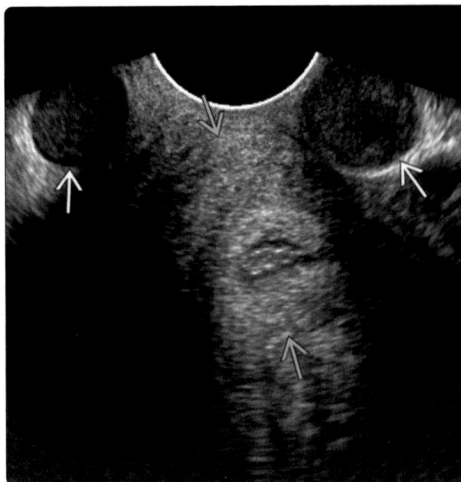

(Left) *Longitudinal US of a retroverted uterus shows multiple simple nabothian cysts ➡. As in this case, multiple cysts can make visualization of the cervical canal ⊡ difficult.* (Right) *Transverse transvaginal US shows 2 complex cysts ➡ at the periphery of the cervix ⊡. These were initially confused for ovarian follicles, until the ovaries were definitively identified later during the scan.*

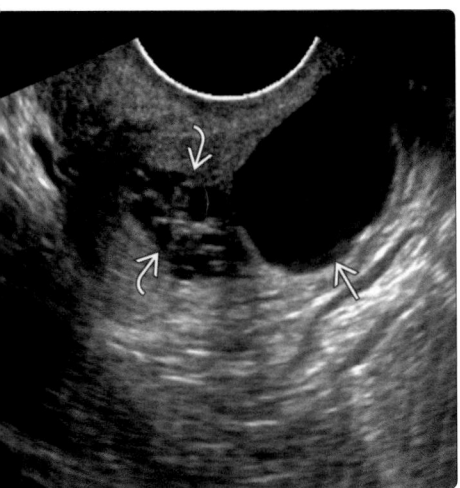

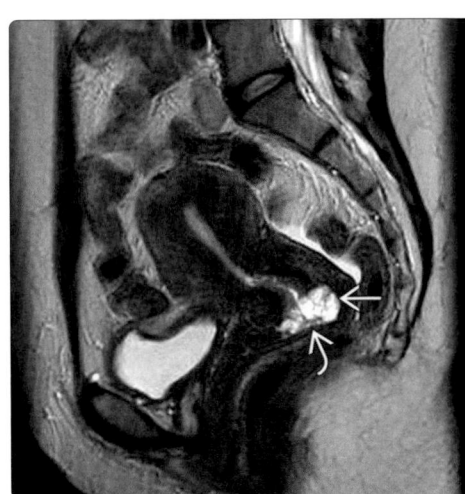

(Left) *Transverse transvaginal US shows a single large nabothian cyst ➡ with multiple more central small cysts ➡, which mimic a multilocular cystic mass and obscure the cervical canal.* (Right) *Sagittal T2 HASTE MR shows multiple small T2-bright nabothian cysts ➡ at the ectocervix ➡. These were an incidental finding.*

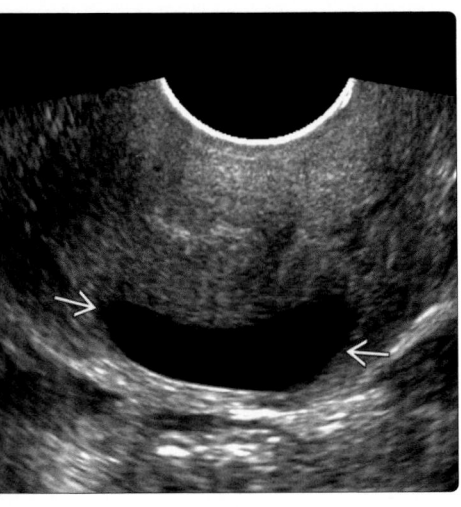

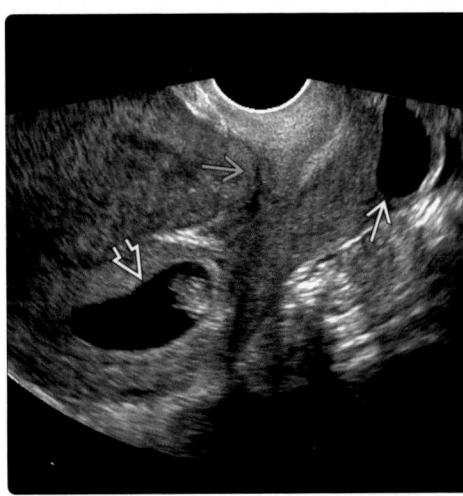

(Left) *Transverse transvaginal US through the cervix in a pregnant patient shows an ovoid cyst ➡, potentially mimicking a cervical ectopic. The thin wall, lack of internal components, and lack of flow confirm that this is a nabothian cyst.* (Right) *Longitudinal US in the same patient shows the nabothian cyst ➡ as well as the intrauterine gestational sac ➡. Note the distortion and shadowing related to a cesarean section scar ⊡.*

IMAGING

- Soft tissue mass: Hypoechoic or isoechoic ± necrosis
- Hydro- or hematometra from cervical obstruction
- MR is best modality for local staging and planning of radiation therapy
  - Tumor: Intermediate to high signal mass replacing dark cervical stroma on T2-weighted sequences
  - Accuracy superior to FIGO staging for size, parametrial extension, lymph nodes
- In experienced hands, ultrasound may be superior to MR for local staging and is more widely available than MR
- PET/CT best modality for overall staging: Nodal disease, liver, bone, and lung metastases
- Revised FIGO staging uses information from CT or MR; cystoscopy and sigmoidoscopy not mandatory

TOP DIFFERENTIAL DIAGNOSES

- Cervical fibroid
- Cervical polyp
- Endometrial cancer
- Primary cervical lymphoma
- Adenoma malignum/minimal deviation adenocarcinoma
- Neuroendocrine/small cell carcinoma

PATHOLOGY

- Approximately 80-90% are squamous carcinoma
- Arise at squamocolumnar junction
- Precursor lesions
  - Cervical intraepithelial neoplasia (CIN) grades I-III

CLINICAL ISSUES

- Abnormal bleeding, pain, or discharge
- Detected by screening cytology from Pap smear
  - ± testing for high-risk HPV

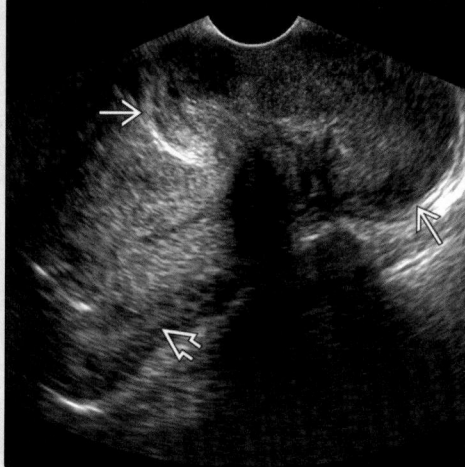
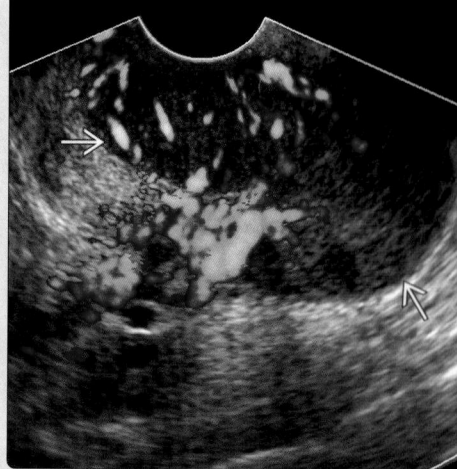

(Left) Sagittal transvaginal ultrasound shows a bulky soft tissue mass in the cervix ➡, proven to be squamous cell carcinoma. The body of the uterus ⮕ was unremarkable. (Right) Parasagittal transvaginal power Doppler ultrasound shows abundant vascularity within the anterior portion of the cervical carcinoma ➡.

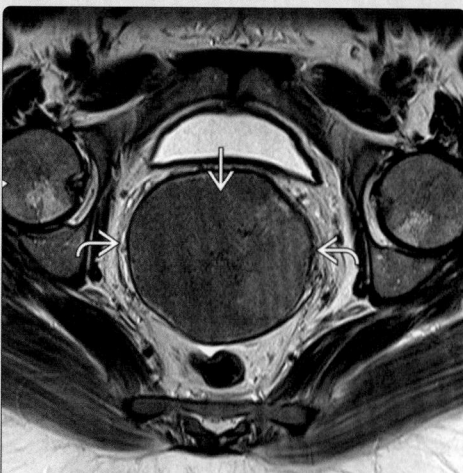
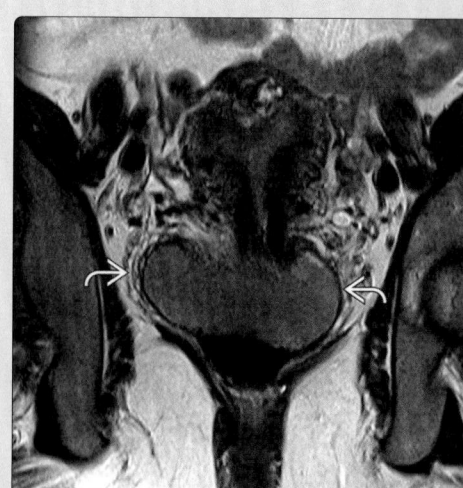

(Left) Axial oblique T2 TSE MR of the same patient shows a large (7 cm) tumor with intermediate signal intensity ➡. The low signal intensity cervical stroma ➡ is thinned but preserved. No parametrial invasion was found at surgery. (Right) Coronal T2 TSE parallel to the endometrium in the same patient confirms the lack of parametrial invasion ⮕ despite the large size of the tumor.

Cervical Carcinoma

IMAGING

General Features

Best diagnostic clue
- Mass involving cervical stroma

Ultrasonographic Findings

Grayscale ultrasound
- Soft tissue mass, hypoechoic or isoechoic ± necrosis, less commonly hyperechoic
- Mass extending into upper vagina
- Invasion of posterior bladder wall
- Invasion of anterior rectal wall
- Enlarged lymph nodes
- Hydro- or hematometra from cervical obstruction
- Hydronephrosis implies stage IIIB disease

3D
- May be used to assess tumor volume before/after therapy

Color/power Doppler
- Abundant internal color flow
- Vascularity may predict response to therapy
- Useful for detection of isoechoic tumors

Ultrasound to guide treatment
- Placement of interstitial radiation therapy devices
- Guidance for dilatation of postradiation cervical/vaginal stenosis

CT Findings

CECT
- For whole body staging: Nodal disease, liver, bone, and lung metastases
- Less sensitive for local staging
  - Soft tissue mass ± necrosis

MR Findings

- T2WI
  - Tumor: Intermediate to high signal mass replacing dark cervical stroma
    - Look for disruption of dark stromal "ring" on true axial images of cervix
- DWI
  - Tumor and lymphadenopathy: High signal on DWI with low ADC
- T1WI C+
  - Variable, smaller tumors enhance more than larger tumors
- Study of choice for identification of disease beyond cervix
- Accuracy for tumor size: 93%
- Parametrial invasion: Accuracy: 88-97%, specificity: 93%, negative predictive value (NPV): 94-100%
- High negative predictive value for bladder and rectal invasion: 100%
- Essential for patients being considered for trachelectomy
- Ideal for radiation planning

Nuclear Medicine Findings

- PET/CT
  - Study of choice for whole body staging, especially lymph nodes
  - May reduce unnecessary surgical interventions/change therapeutic approach
  - For restaging after therapy and follow-up

Imaging Recommendations

- Best imaging tool
  - MR is best modality for local staging and planning of radiation therapy
  - Accuracy superior to FIGO staging for size, parametrial extension, lymph nodes
  - PET/CT best modality for overall staging
  - In experienced hands, ultrasound may be superior to MR for local staging and is more widely available than MR
- Protocol advice
  - Optimize MR study by
    - Obtaining images perpendicular to cervix
    - Distending vagina with water soluble gel

DIFFERENTIAL DIAGNOSIS

Cervical Fibroid

- Similar appearance to myometrium
- Prolapsed endocavitary fibroid may mimic cervical mass
- Fibroid may arise from cervical stroma, producing subserosal or submucosal mass

Cervical Polyp

- May originate in cervical canal or prolapse from endometrial cavity
- Similar echogenicity to endometrium and cervical mucosa
- Feeding vessel and internal cysts may be visible

Endometrial Cancer

- Direct extension to cervix
- Epicenter of mass will be in uterus

Primary Cervical Lymphoma

- Solid mass with relative preservation of cervical canal
- Aggressive surgery not required
- Responds to chemotherapy/radiation therapy

Adenoma Malignum/Minimal Deviation Adenocarcinoma

- Rare well-differentiated adenocarcinoma of cervix
- Early dissemination/poor prognosis
- Arises from columnar epithelium
- Barrel-shaped multicystic lesion deep in cervical stroma with solid components
  - May be mistaken for nabothian cysts (more superficial)

Neuroendocrine/Small Cell Carcinoma

- More aggressive
- Lymphadenopathy and metastases more extensive
- Related to smoking

Cervical Metastasis

- Fallopian tube, ovary, primary peritoneal carcinoma
- Differentiate by histology and presence of other tumor

PATHOLOGY

General Features

- Precursor lesions

- o Low- and high-grade intraepithelial lesions
- o Cervical intraepithelial neoplasia (CIN) grades I-III

Staging, Grading, & Classification

- Traditional FIGO staging: Clinical examination, examination under anesthesia ± cystoscopy, sigmoidoscopy
- Revised FIGO staging uses information from CT or MR; cystoscopy and sigmoidoscopy not mandatory
  - o Stage I: Confined to cervix
    - – IA: Invasive but only diagnosed at microscopy
    - – IB: Clinically visible lesion; IB1 < 4 cm, IB2 > 4 cm
  - o Stage II: Beyond uterus but not to pelvic sidewall or lower 1/3 of vagina
    - – IIA: No parametrial invasion
      - □ IIA1 tumor < 4 cm, IIA2 > 4 cm
    - – IIB: Parametrial invasion
  - o Stage III
    - – IIIA: Lower 1/3 of vagina
    - – IIIB: Pelvic side wall (within 3 mm of obturator internus, levator ani or pyriformis muscles, or iliac vessels) **or** hydronephrosis/nonfunctioning kidney
  - o Stage IV: Bladder/rectal involvement or distant metastases (lung, liver, bones)
- Presence of pelvic or paraaortic lymphadenopathy alters prognosis but not FIGO stage

Gross Pathologic & Surgical Features

- Arises at squamocolumnar junction
  - o Endocervical in older women with supravaginal and lateral tumor growth
  - o Ectocervical in younger patients with exophytic growth inferiorly into vagina

Microscopic Features

- Approximately 80-90% are squamous carcinoma
- Approximately 10-20% are adenocarcinoma (~ 1-3% adenoma malignum)

Prognostic factors

- Tumor size
- Parametrial and pelvic side wall invasion
- Bladder or rectal invasion
- Lymph node metastases

CLINICAL ISSUES

Presentation

- Most common signs/symptoms
  - o Abnormal bleeding, pain, or discharge
- Other signs/symptoms
  - o Often asymptomatic
  - o Detected by screening cytology from Pap smear
  - o Following primary screening for high risk human papilloma virus (HPV) infections

Demographics

- Epidemiology
  - o 3rd most common gynecologic malignancy in USA and most common gynecologic malignancy worldwide, detected at more advanced stages
  - o Screening and prevention has decreased mortality and morbidity significantly in developed countries
  - o Average age at diagnosis is 50

- o Risk factors
  - – HPV infection most important risk factor
  - – Early onset sexual activity, multiple partners
  - – Smoking, immunosuppression, HIV infection

Natural History & Prognosis

- 10-20% of CIN 3 progress to invasive cancer if untreated
- Papanicolaou test screening alone or cotesting with high risk HPV tests are mainstay of detection
- Treatment is successful if cancer is detected early
- 5-year survival rate: Early stage: 91%; locally advanced: 57% and metastatic disease: 16%
- Pathways of spread
  - o Lymphatic: Parametrial/obturator/internal-external iliac
  - o Direct invasion: Vagina/bladder/uterosacral ligaments to rectum

Treatment

- Prevention: Vaccine for oncogenic HPV strains 16 and 18
- Loop electrosurgical excision procedure (LEEP) procedure or cone biopsy
  - o To further evaluate abnormal Pap smear or abnormal findings at colposcopy
  - o To excise transformation zone
- Microinvasive disease IA1: Cone biopsy or trachelectomy (for fertility sparing) or simple hysterectomy
  - o MR essential for patient selection prior to trachelectomy
- Lower than stage IIA: Radical hysterectomy and bilateral pelvic lymphadenectomy
  - o Variations of chemotherapy and radiotherapy
- Bulky stage IB2 and IIA2 > 4 cm: Chemoradiation
- Stage IIB or higher: Radiation therapy ± concomitant or neoadjuvant chemotherapy

DIAGNOSTIC CHECKLIST

Consider

- Traditional FIGO staging: Error rates up to 65% for stage III
- Detection of tumor beyond cervix is key for imaging, as this determines surgical vs. nonsurgical treatment

Image Interpretation Pearls

- Do not mistake transposed ovaries for peritoneal masses or adenopathy
  - o Patient with history of cervical cancer and radiation therapy

SELECTED REFERENCES

1. Dutta S et al: Image-guided radiotherapy and -brachytherapy for cervical cancer. Front Oncol. 5:64, 2015
2. Koh WJ et al: Cervical Cancer, Version 2. J Natl Compr Canc Netw. 13(4):395-404, 2015
3. Kusmirek J et al: PET/CT and MRI in the imaging assessment of cervical cancer. Abdom Imaging. ePub, 2015
4. Epstein E et al: Early-stage cervical cancer: tumor delineation by magnetic resonance imaging and ultrasound - a European multicenter trial. Gynecol Oncol. 128(3):449-53, 2013
5. Thomeer MG et al: Clinical examination versus magnetic resonance imaging in the pretreatment staging of cervical carcinoma: systematic review and meta-analysis. Eur Radiol. 23(7):2005-18, 2013
6. Freeman SJ et al: The revised FIGO staging system for uterine malignancies: implications for MR imaging. Radiographics. 32(6):1805-27, 2012
7. Park SB et al: Sonographic findings of uterine cervical lymphoma manifesting as multinodular lesions. Clin Imaging. 36(5):636-8, 2012

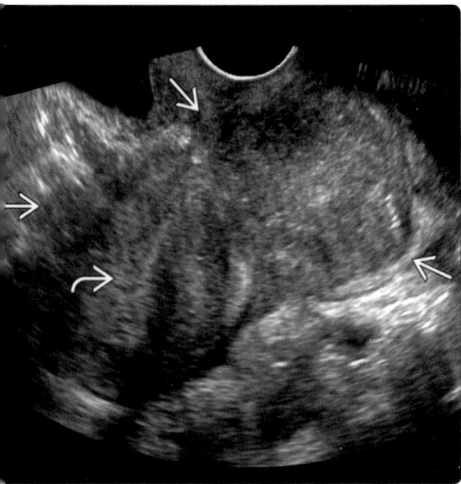

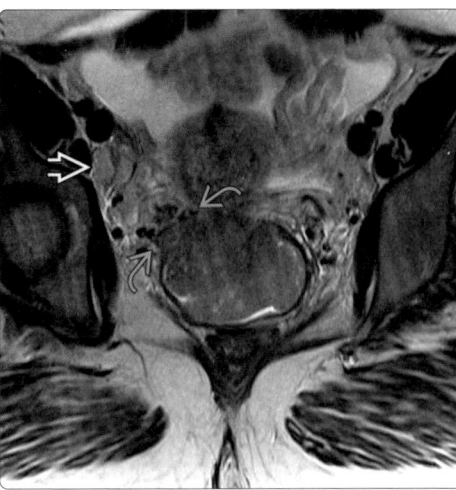

(Left) *Longitudinal transvaginal ultrasound demonstrates a large cervical carcinoma ➡. Local staging cannot be determined. There is no hematometra ➡.* (Right) *Coronal oblique T2 TSE MR through the cervix shows frank parametrial extension ➡ on the right where the tumor transgresses the low signal cervical stroma. There were pathologic external iliac nodes ➡.*

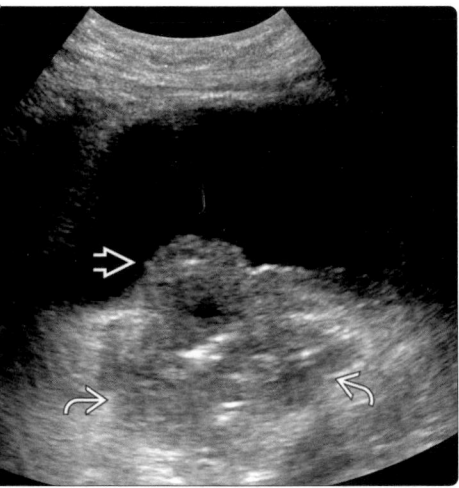

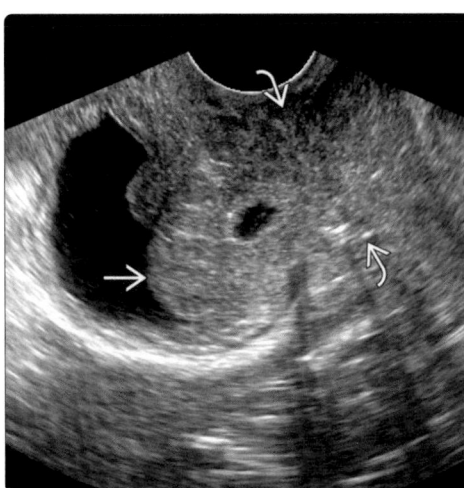

(Left) *Transverse transabdominal ultrasound of the bladder in a patient with hematuria and vaginal bleeding shows a lobulated mass in the posterior bladder ➡ and a mass containing gas ➡ posterior to the bladder.* (Right) *Longitudinal transvaginal ultrasound of the same patient confirms that the bladder mass ➡ is contiguous with a cervical mass ➡, which was biopsy-proven to be squamous cell carcinoma.*

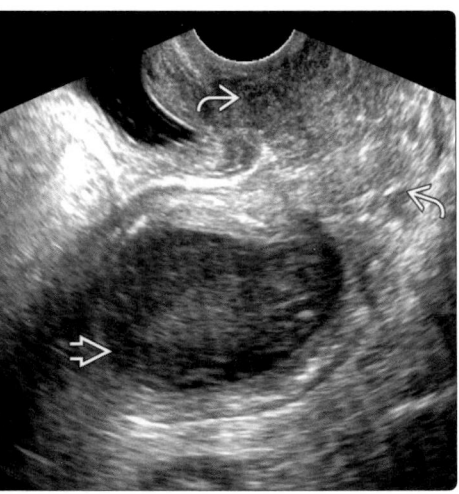

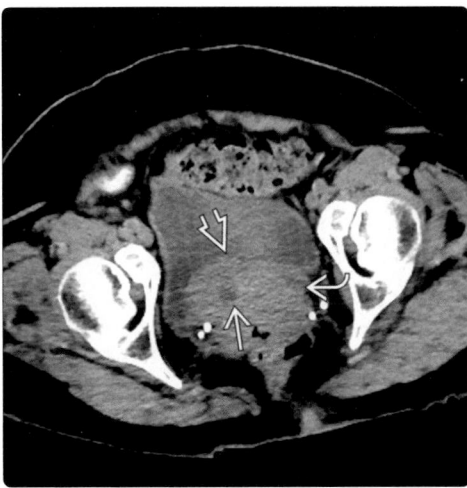

(Left) *Longitudinal transvaginal ultrasound of the uterus in the same patient shows hematometra ➡ secondary to the cervical carcinoma ➡.* (Right) *Axial NECT the same patient shows the cervical mass ➡ with a cystic component ➡, but it is difficult to determine if there is frank bladder invasion ➡.*

(Left) *Longitudinal transabdominal ultrasound shows an enlarged cervix ➡ relative to the uterus ➡ in a patient with profuse vaginal bleeding.* **(Right)** *Sagittal transvaginal ultrasound of the same patient shows the cervix ➡ to be enlarged and hyperechoic to the myometrium ➡. The endometrium ➡ is thin.*

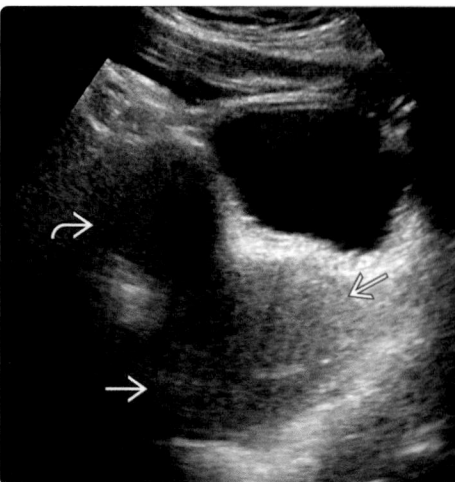
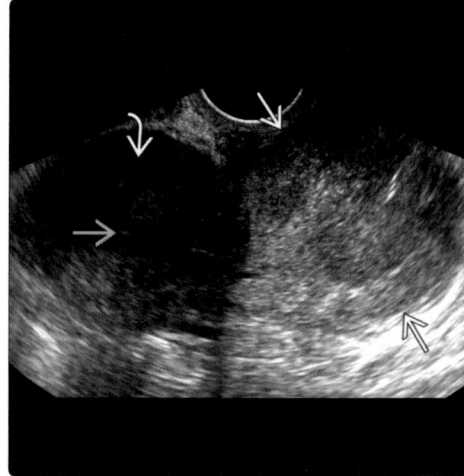

(Left) *Coronal oblique transvaginal ultrasound of the same patient shows that the mass ➡ infiltrates the entire cervix. Small cystic foci are present ➡.* **(Right)** *Coronal T2 FSE MR parallel to the endometrium in a patient with HIV and CIN 3 shows the normal cervical high signal mucosa ➡ and intact low signal intensity stroma ➡.*

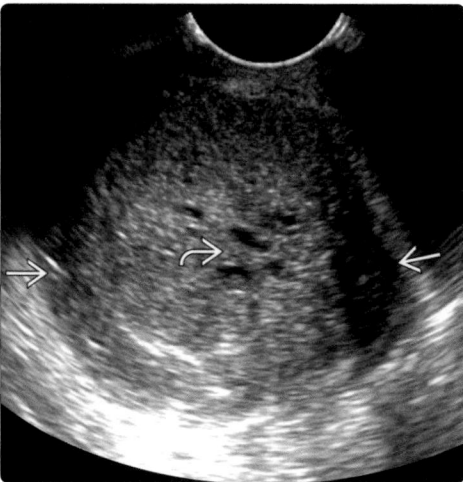
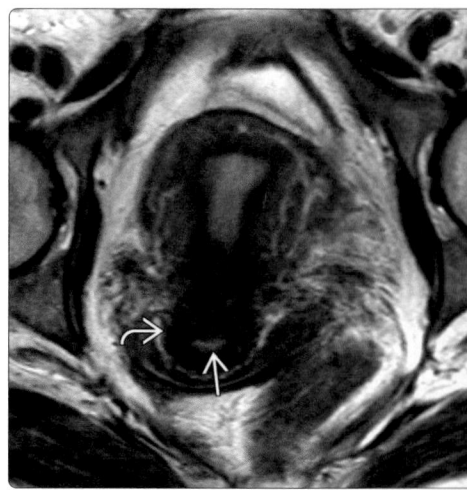

(Left) *Coronal oblique TSE perpendicular to the cervix ("doughnut" view) shows a mass with intermediate T2 signal intensity ➡ that extends through the cervical stroma ➡ on the right and into the parametrium.* **(Right)** *Axial FDG PET/CT of the same patient shows increased metabolic activity in the primary tumor ➡ (SUV 15.6) posterior to the bladder ➡.*

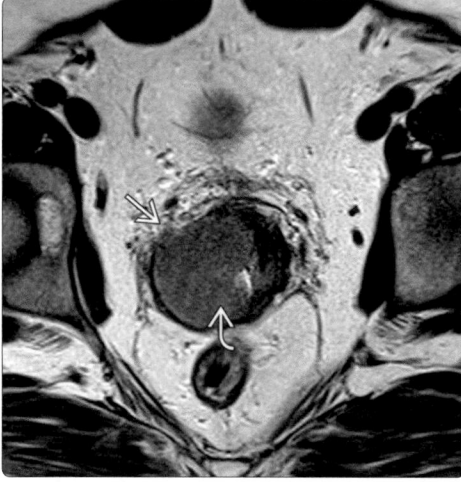
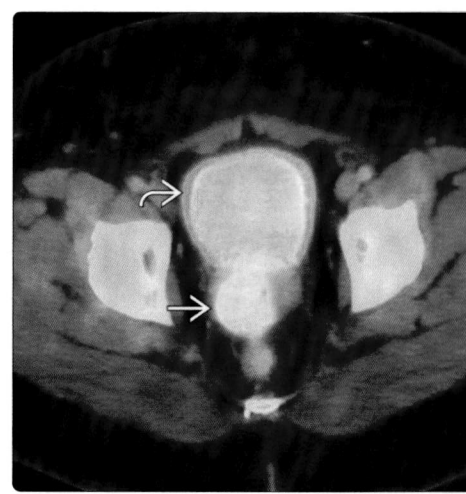

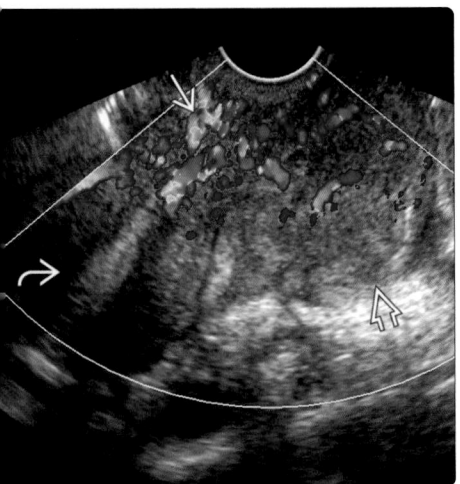

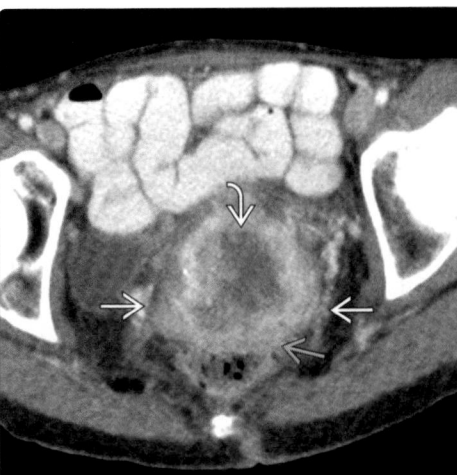

(Left) *Longitudinal transvaginal ultrasound demonstrates a large hypervascular cervical carcinoma ➡. Posteriorly, there was less color flow ➡. The endometrium was normal ➡.* (Right) *Axial CECT of the same patient better shows necrosis ➡ in the tumor. There is infiltration of the parametrium ➡ bilaterally, not reaching the pelvic side wall. No fat plane is seen between the tumor and the rectum ➡; however, the rectal mucosa was not involved.*

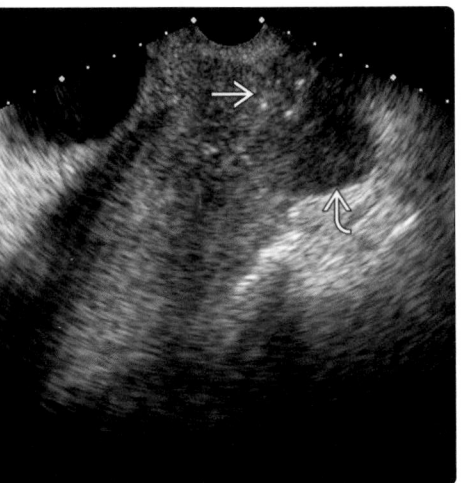

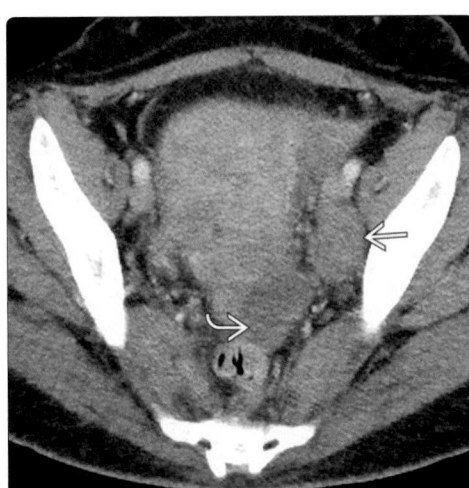

(Left) *Sagittal transvaginal ultrasound shows a lobulated hypoechoic carcinoma protruding from the posterior cervix ➡. Gas was noted within the tumor ➡ secondary to tumor necrosis.* (Right) *Axial CECT of the same patient shows the posterior extent of the cervical carcinoma ➡ and pathologic left pelvic adenopathy ➡.*

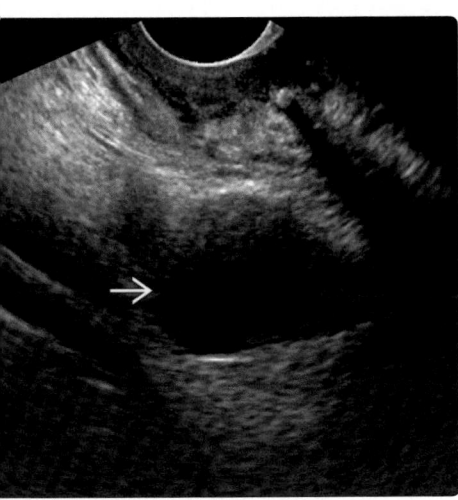

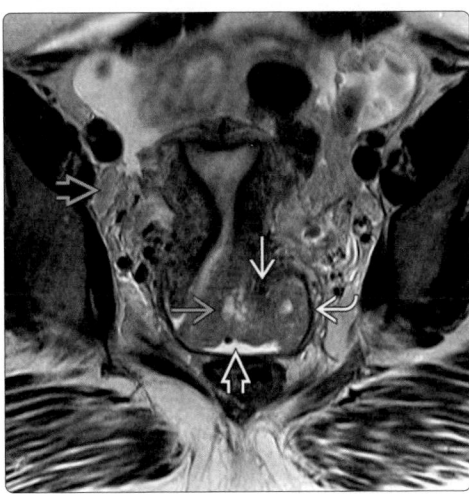

(Left) *Sagittal transvaginal ultrasound shows that the left pelvic node ➡ is cystic secondary to necrosis, not uncommon in squamous carcinoma. Be careful not to misinterpret a node as an ovary.* (Right) *Coronal oblique T2 TSE MR parallel to the endometrium shows an eccentric cervical carcinoma ➡ extending into the vaginal fornix ➡ that contained gel ➡. Cystic foci are noted in the tumor ➡. Right external iliac nodes ➡ were malignant.*

TERMINOLOGY

- Ectopic endometrial tissue within myometrium with adjacent smooth muscle hyperplasia
- May have diffuse involvement or focal mass (adenomyoma)

IMAGING

- Best diagnostic clue: Uterine enlargement with poor definition of endometrial-myometrial interface
- Ultrasound
  - Globular uterine enlargement
  - Heterogeneous myometrial echotexture
  - Loss of endomyometrial interface due to thickening of junctional zone
  - May be asymmetric; if mass-like, often emanates from endomyometrial junction
    - May be difficult to differentiate from leiomyoma
- T2WI MR: Thickened junctional zone > 12 mm ± T2-bright foci

TOP DIFFERENTIAL DIAGNOSES

- Leiomyoma
- Diffuse myometrial hypertrophy due to parity
- Endometrial cancer
- Metastasis to uterine corpus
- Endometrial hyperplasia

CLINICAL ISSUES

- Commonly associated with endometriosis
- Uterine artery embolization may be effective
- Hysterectomy definitive treatment

DIAGNOSTIC CHECKLIST

- Abnormal myometrial echogenicity, most commonly hypoechoic, due to smooth muscle hyperplasia
- Loss of endomyometrial interface due to thickening of junctional zone
- If findings are equivocal, obtain MR to evaluate for thickened junctional zone

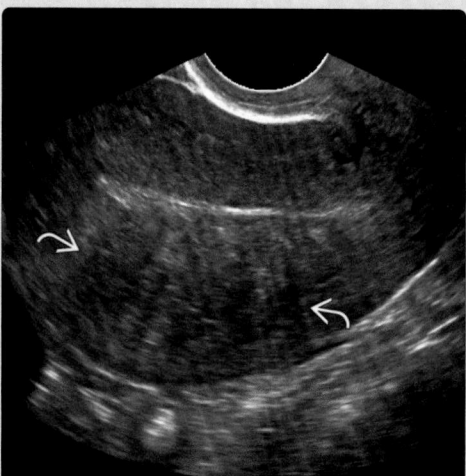
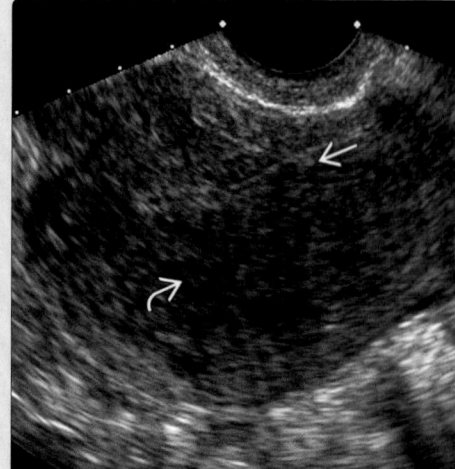

(Left) Longitudinal transvaginal US demonstrates asymmetric posterior greater than anterior linear bands of echogenicity and shadowing ➜ without a focal mass, consistent with adenomyosis. (Right) Longitudinal transvaginal US demonstrates asymmetric posterior myometrial thickening with subtle shadowing ➜ without a defined mass. The endomyometrial border is partially obscured ➡.

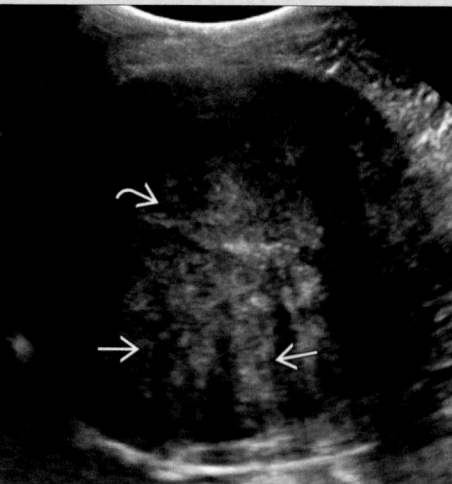
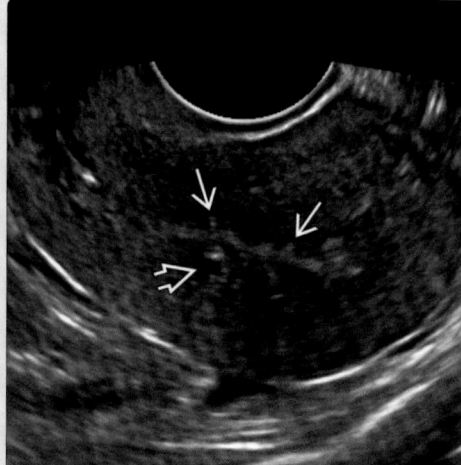

(Left) Transverse transabdominal US demonstrates poor delineation of the endomyometrial border ➜, and diffuse myometrial thickening with areas of band-like shadowing ➡. (Right) Longitudinal transvaginal US demonstrates subtle invaginations of the endometrium into the myometrium ➡, diagnostic of adenomyosis. Presence of a subendometrial cyst ➤ is also highly specific.

TERMINOLOGY

Synonyms

Uterine endometriosis

Endometriosis interna

Definitions

Heterotopic endometrial tissue within myometrium with adjacent smooth muscle hyperplasia

IMAGING

General Features

Best diagnostic clue
- Uterine enlargement with poor definition of endometrial-myometrial interface
- Myometrial cysts in up to 50%
  - Usually subendometrial

Location
- Diffuse or asymmetric myometrial involvement
  - Superficial type: Involving < 1/3 of myometrial thickness
  - Deep type: Invasion > 1/3 of myometrial thickness
  - When asymmetric, posterior > anterior myometrium
- May be more focal and mass-like, resulting in adenomyoma
  - Often near endomyometrial junction

Size
- Variable

Morphology
- If confluent/diffuse, globular enlarged uterus with smooth external contour
- If focal, commonly elliptical myometrial mass

Ultrasonographic Findings

Globular uterine enlargement

Heterogeneous myometrial echotexture
- Hypoechoic smooth muscle hyperplasia
- Echogenic linear striations due to endometrial extension into myometrium

Loss of endomyometrial interface due to thickening of junctional zone

Cysts within myometrium
- Anechoic, usually subendometrial
- Highly specific for diagnosis
- Distinguish from uterine veins, which are peripheral, have color flow

Disordered or uncircumscribed myometrial vascular pattern on color Doppler

If mass-like, difficult to differentiate from leiomyoma but less distinct
- Often emanates from endomyometrial junction
- Penetrating vessels without mass effect on color Doppler
- Not calcified

Tender with probe pressure

MR Findings

Thickened junctional zone (> 12 mm) on T2WI, diffuse or focal

Focal areas of T2 increased signal due to dilated endometrial glands

- May have focal areas of T1 increased signal due to hemorrhage
- If mass-like, difficult to differentiate from leiomyoma
  - Often near junctional zone
  - T2 hypointense due to smooth muscle hyperplasia
  - Similar enhancement patterns as leiomyoma

Fluoroscopic Findings

- Hysterosalpingography (HSG)
  - Small diverticula extending from endometrial cavity

Saline-Infused Hysterosonography

- Saline and bubbles may fill linear tracks in myometrium, producing "myometrial cracks"

Imaging Recommendations

- Best imaging tool
  - US best initial study for patients with pelvic symptoms
    - Transvaginal ultrasound best to evaluate endomyometrial interface
  - MR for equivocal, difficult, or nondiagnostic cases
    - T2WI best to evaluate junctional zone
    - Less limited by size of uterus and patient
    - More comprehensive evaluation of fibroid burden
    - Not limited by shadowing
- Protocol advice
  - Cine clips with slow sweep are helpful for subtle findings such as streaky shadowing and small myometrial cysts
  - Evaluate for uterine tenderness

DIFFERENTIAL DIAGNOSIS

Leiomyoma

- US: Well-defined mass in submucosal, subserosal, or mural location
  - May be difficult to distinguish from adenomyoma
- Often multiple, with lobular external uterine contour
- Can be calcified with peripheral vascularity
- MR: Low T1/T2 signal with nonthickened junctional zone

Diffuse Myometrial Hypertrophy

- Endometrial-myometrial borders maintained
- Junctional zone remains well defined
- Heterogeneous myometrium without other findings

Endometrial Cancer

- Irregularly thickened heterogeneous endometrium
- Possible invasion into myometrium with loss of endomyometrial interface

Metastasis to Uterine Corpus

- Rare, most commonly breast, gastric cancers and lymphoma
- Lymphoma rarely primary
  - Hypoechoic infiltration, preserves contour with less mass effect on endomyometrial interface

Endometrial Hyperplasia

- Thickened endometrium, may have cystic appearance
- Typically preserved endomyometrial interface

PATHOLOGY

General Features

- Etiology
  - Ectopic endometrial tissue within myometrium
  - Reactive hypertrophy and hyperplasia of surrounding smooth muscle
  - Etiology poorly understood, but may involve invagination of endometrium directly into myometrium vs. de novo development from müllerian rests
- Associated abnormalities
  - Endometriosis

Gross Pathologic & Surgical Features

- Enlarged and boggy uterus
  - With thickened myometrial wall and islands of endometrial bleeding
- Adenomyoma may resemble leiomyoma, but cannot be easily excised

Microscopic Features

- Ectopic endometrial tissue within myometrium at least 1 low-power field from endomyometrial interface
- Adjacent smooth muscle hypertrophy and hyperplasia

CLINICAL ISSUES

Presentation

- Most common signs/symptoms
  - Diffusely enlarged uterus, may be tender
  - Often associated with menorrhagia
    - Less commonly dysmenorrhea or metrorrhagia
  - Commonly associated with endometriosis
  - Controversial association with infertility
- Other signs/symptoms
  - Often mistaken for fibroids given similar symptoms and ultrasound findings

Demographics

- Age
  - Pre- or perimenopausal
- Epidemiology
  - Often have coexistent leiomyomas
  - Most commonly multiparous
  - Association with cesarean sections

Treatment

- Medical treatment with oral contraceptives or gonadotropin releasing hormone agonists to control symptoms
- Adenomyosis cannot be resected
- Hysterectomy is definitive treatment
- Uterine artery embolization is effective alternative treatment
  - Results not as reproducible as for leiomyoma

DIAGNOSTIC CHECKLIST

Consider

- Enlarged, tender uterus in patient with menorrhagia

Image Interpretation Pearls

- Loss of endomyometrial interface due to thickening of junctional zone
- Abnormal myometrial echogenicity, most commonly hypoechoic, due to smooth muscle hyperplasia
- Echogenic linear striations due to endometrial extension into myometrium
- If findings are equivocal, obtain MR to evaluate for thickened junctional zone (> 12 mm is diagnostic)
  - However, diagnosis can be made at lower threshold if T1/T2-bright foci or linear high T2 signal striations are present

SELECTED REFERENCES

1. Van den Bosch T et al: Terms and definitions for describing myometrial pathology using ultrasonography. Ultrasound Obstet Gynecol. ePub, 2015
2. Boeer B et al: Differences in the clinical phenotype of adenomyosis and leiomyomas: a retrospective, questionnaire-based study. Arch Gynecol Obstet. 289(6):1235-9, 2014
3. Genc M et al: Adenomyosis and accompanying gynecological pathologies. Arch Gynecol Obstet. ePub, 2014
4. Pistofidis G et al: Distinct types of uterine adenomyosis based on laparoscopic and histopathologic criteria. Clin Exp Obstet Gynecol. 41(2):113-8, 2014
5. Riggs JC et al: Cesarean section as a risk factor for the development of adenomyosis uteri. J Reprod Med. 59(1-2):20-4, 2014
6. Levy G et al: An update on adenomyosis. Diagn Interv Imaging. 94(1):3-25, 2013
7. Taran FA et al: Adenomyosis: Epidemiology, Risk Factors, Clinical Phenotype and Surgical and Interventional Alternatives to Hysterectomy. Geburtshilfe Frauenheilkd. 73(9):924-931, 2013
8. Naftalin J et al: How common is adenomyosis? A prospective study of prevalence using transvaginal ultrasound in a gynaecology clinic. Hum Reprod. 27(12):3432-9, 2012
9. Smeets AJ et al: Long-term follow-up of uterine artery embolization for symptomatic adenomyosis. Cardiovasc Intervent Radiol. 35(4):815-9, 2012
10. Stamatopoulos CP et al: Value of magnetic resonance imaging in diagnosis of adenomyosis and myomas of the uterus. J Minim Invasive Gynecol. 19(5):620-6, 2012
11. Manyonda IT et al: Uterine Artery Embolization versus Myomectomy: Impact on Quality of Life-Results of the FUME (Fibroids of the Uterus: Myomectomy versus Embolization) Trial. Cardiovasc Intervent Radiol. Epub ahead of print 2011

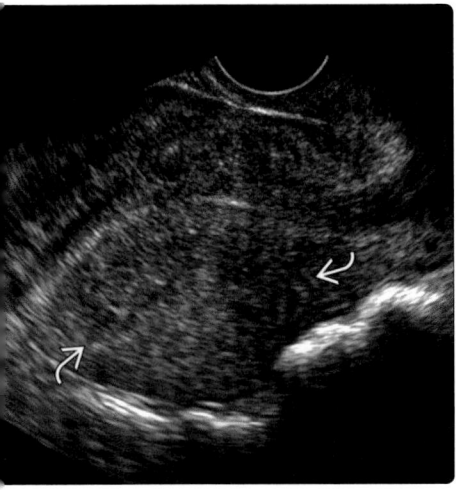
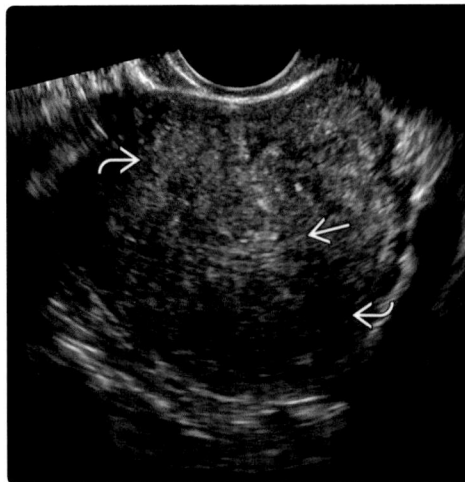

(Left) Longitudinal transvaginal US demonstrates asymmetric posterior enlargement of the uterus body/fundus ⮣ without a defined mass. (Right) Transverse transvaginal US shows diffuse heterogeneity and thickening of the myometrium ⮣ without a focal mass. The endomyometrial border is obscured ➔.

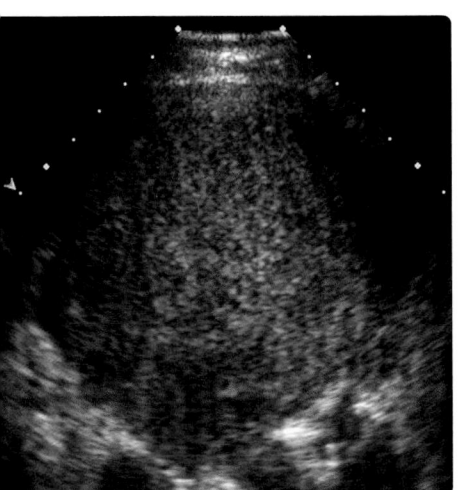
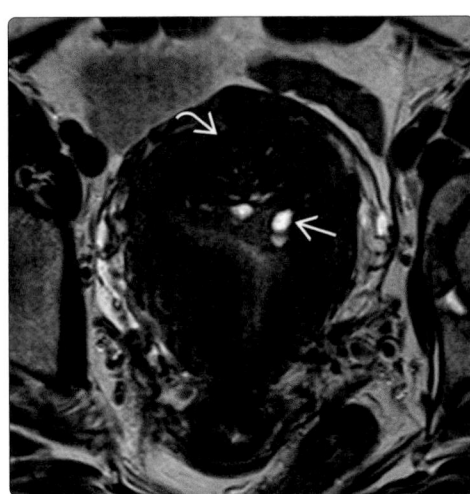

(Left) Transabdominal US shows uterine enlargement and diffuse heterogeneity of the uterine parenchyma with nonvisualization of the endometrium. (Right) Axial T2WI MR in the same patient demonstrates diffuse but asymmetric thickening of the fundal junctional zone ⮣ with subendometrial cysts ➔, diagnostic of adenomyosis.

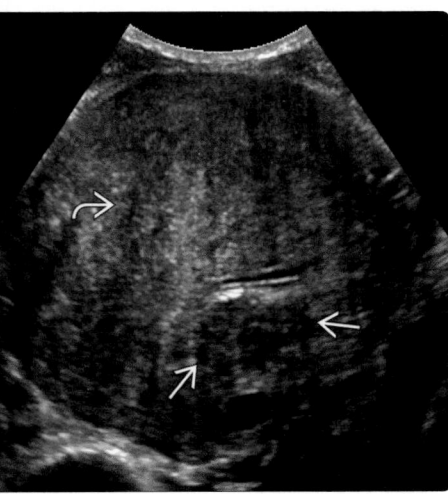
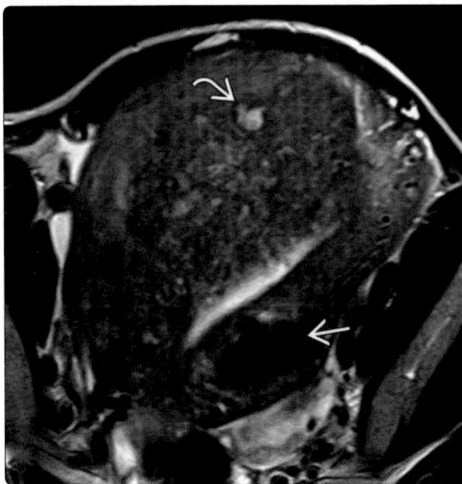

(Left) Transabdominal US shows diffuse heterogeneity of the uterus with asymmetric anterior myometrial thickening with linear refractive shadows ⮣, consistent with adenomyosis. A well-defined hypoechoic mass with posterior shadowing in the posterior fundus ➔ is consistent with an intramural fibroid. (Right) Axial T2WI MR in the same patient better demonstrates heterogeneity of the anterior uterine myometrium with thickening and cysts ⮣ as well as the posterior intramural fibroid ➔.

Leiomyoma

TERMINOLOGY

- Benign smooth muscle neoplasm of uterus

IMAGING

- Ultrasound (transabdominal and transvaginal) initial study of choice
  - Circumscribed mass, hypoechoic to myometrium with posterior acoustic shadowing
  - Variable location: Submucosal, intramural, subserosal, intracavitary, pedunculated, cervical, or broad ligament
- MR
  - Low T2 signal from smooth muscle proliferation
  - Variable enhancement on post-contrast imaging
  - High signal on T1WI if hemorrhage; high signal on T2WI if cystic degeneration

TOP DIFFERENTIAL DIAGNOSES

- Adenomyosis
- Focal myometrial contraction
- Leiomyosarcoma
- Uterine duplication

CLINICAL ISSUES

- Symptoms primarily related to leiomyoma location, size, &/or growth
- Can undergo rapid growth during pregnancy
- For bulk symptoms or bleeding, management includes uterine artery embolization, myomectomy, or hysterectomy
- If greater than 50% of submucosal leiomyoma is within endometrial cavity, will require hysteroscopy for removal

DIAGNOSTIC CHECKLIST

- If borders are not well delineated, consider adenomyosis
- SIS to evaluate submucosal leiomyomas
- MR prior to uterine artery embolization, and to evaluate multiple or complex leiomyomas
- Consider malignant form if rapidly growing uterine mass in postmenopausal woman

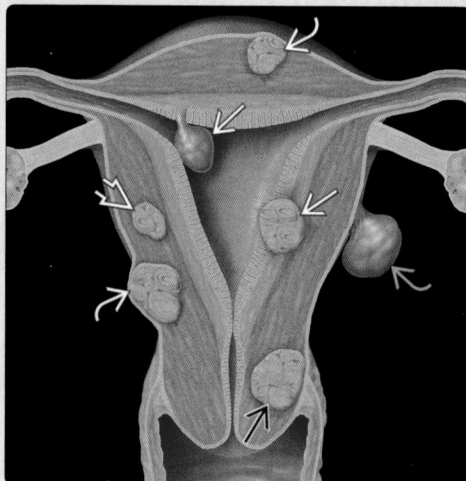
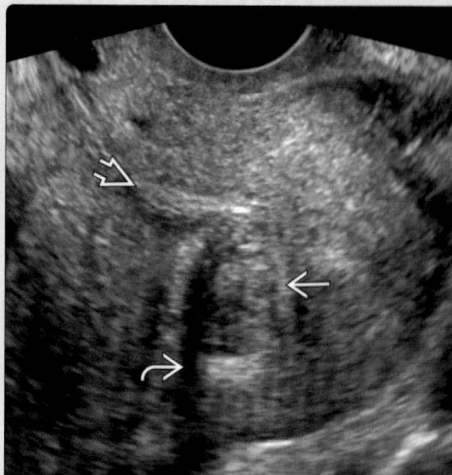

(Left) *Coronal graphic shows various leiomyoma locations including submucosal and endocavitary ➡, subserosal ➡ and pedunculated ➡, and mural ➡ and cervical ➡. Note the whorled consistency.* (Right) *Transvaginal ultrasound demonstrates a hypoechoic, slightly heterogeneous mass ➡ without significant distortion of the endometrium ➡, consistent with an intramural leiomyoma. Note the posterior acoustic shadowing ➡.*

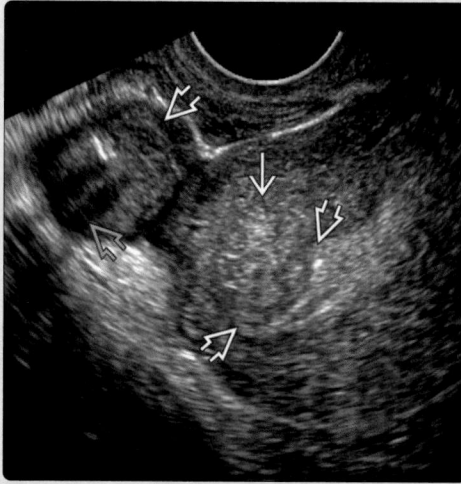
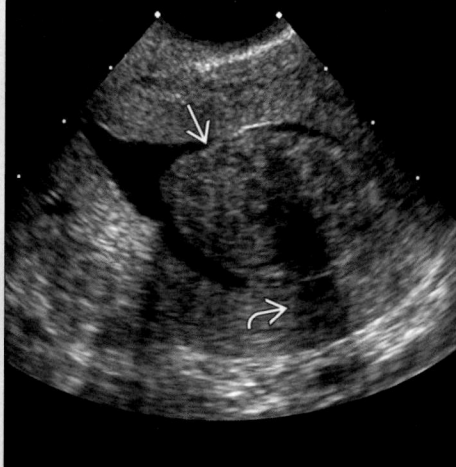

(Left) *Transvaginal ultrasound demonstrates a hypoechoic subserosal pedunculated leiomyoma ➡ with posterior acoustic shadowing ➡. An isoechoic submucosal leiomyoma ➡ causes distortion of the endometrium.* (Right) *Saline-infused sonohysterography (SIS) clearly demonstrates the intracavitary location of a hypoechoic submucosal leiomyoma ➡. Posterior shadowing ➡ is the result of fibrous tissue, not calcifications.*

TERMINOLOGY

Abbreviations
- Myoma

Synonyms
- Fibroid
- Myoma
- Uterine fibroma

Definitions
- Benign smooth muscle neoplasm of uterus

IMAGING

General Features
- Best diagnostic clue
  - Circumscribed uterine wall mass
- Location
  - Can develop anywhere within uterine smooth muscle
    - Submucosal: In close contact with endometrium
    - Intramural: Most common, entirely within myometrium
    - Subserosal: Bulges externally from uterine surface
  - Can also be exophytic/pedunculated, intracavitary, cervical, or within broad ligament
- Size
  - Extremely variable, subcentimeter to > 10 cm
- Morphology
  - Distortion of uterine contour and enlargement of uterus (subserosal or intramural)
  - Narrowing and distortion of endometrium (submucosal or intramural)
  - Mimics solid adnexal mass (pedunculated or broad ligament leiomyoma)

Ultrasonographic Findings
- Circumscribed mass, hypoechoic to myometrium
  - Poor posterior acoustic transmission
  - May demonstrate shadowing even without associated calcifications
  - Shadowing can limit utility of transvaginal ultrasound
- Bulky uterine enlargement from large or multiple leiomyomas
- Variable location: Submucosal, intramural, subserosal, intracavitary, pedunculated, cervical, or broad ligament
  - Submucosal: Mass effect on endometrium, may obstruct endometrial canal if intracavitary
  - Subserosal: Distorts uterine contour, especially if large
  - Pedunculated: At risk for torsion with vascular connection visible on color Doppler
  - Cervical: Unlike nabothian cyst, will have internal blood flow
  - Broad ligament: May be confused for solid ovarian mass, unless ovary identified separately
- May appear heterogeneous if cystic degeneration or hemorrhage
- Lipoleiomyoma: Variant of leiomyoma with variable amount of fat
  - May be hyperechoic due to significant fat component
  - May be confused for dermoid if exophytic/pedunculated
- Peripheral vascularity on color Doppler
  - Submucosal fibroid tends to have multiple feeding vessels compared to single feeding vessel for endometrial polyp
  - Vascular stalk helps characterize pedunculated leiomyoma
  - Ischemia/degeneration: Decreased or absent color flow

Saline Infusion Sonohysterography (SIS)
- Helpful in characterizing submucosal fibroids
  - Leiomyomas more hypoechoic than endometrial polyps and associated with shadowing
  - Echogenic endometrial lining covers surface of leiomyoma
  - Multiple feeding vessels rather than linear stalk-like vascularity
- Hysteroscopic resection if > 50% of myoma is intracavitary

Angiographic Findings
- Peripherally vascular masses, may have dual supply from both uterine arteries
- May have additional vascular supply from ovarian arteries

CT Findings
- Enlarged uterus, may be lobular
- Fibroid attenuation
  - Often similar attenuation to uterus on unenhanced scan
  - Variable enhancement after contrast
  - Heterogeneous if cystic degeneration, hemorrhage
  - May contain coarse, dense calcifications, especially in older women or after degeneration

MR Findings
- Low T1/T2 signal from smooth muscle proliferation
- Variable enhancement on post-contrast imaging
  - Usually less than surrounding myometrium
- High signal on T1WI if hemorrhage; high signal on T2WI if cystic degeneration
- Expected appearance after uterine artery embolization: Decreased volume and enhancement

Imaging Recommendations
- Best imaging tool
  - Ultrasound initial study of choice
    - Transabdominal to evaluate for pedunculated or subserosal leiomyomas, which may be missed on transvaginal imaging alone
    - Transvaginal best to evaluate submucosal leiomyomas
      - May be limited by extensive shadowing
  - Sonohysterography to evaluate submucosal leiomyomas
  - MR as supplement
    - Prior to uterine artery embolization: Evaluate for enhancement and map fibroids
    - Multiple or complex features, limited ultrasound
- Protocol advice
  - Use both transabdominal and transvaginal ultrasound (TVUS)
  - Determine size, location, and effect of myomas on endometrium
    - At least largest 3 myomas should be measured as index lesions
    - Report size of submucosal interface; size of stalk if pedunculated

o Consider renal ultrasound to exclude hydronephrosis when uterus is large

DIFFERENTIAL DIAGNOSIS

Adenomyosis

- Ectopic endometrial tissue; is similar in appearance to leiomyoma when mass-like
- Often elliptical in shape; arises near endomyometrial junction if focal
- More commonly associated with tender/painful uterus

Focal Myometrial Contraction

- Focal bulge of myometrium during pregnancy, resolves over time
- Isoechoic to surrounding myometrium
- Affects internal myometrial appearance more than external contour

Leiomyosarcoma

- Rapidly growing uterine mass, older or postmenopausal woman
- Typically heterogeneous, with necrosis and hemorrhage, can be similar to leiomyoma
- Rare tumor, not thought to arise from preexisting leiomyoma
- Look for signs of tumor spread

Uterine Duplication

- Bicornuate uterus: 1 horn can mimic leiomyoma
- Empty horn during pregnancy can also appear similar to leiomyoma
- Can differentiate by central endometrial line, but noncavitary horns will lack endometrium

PATHOLOGY

Gross Pathologic & Surgical Features

- Well-circumscribed, grayish-white mass with whorled cut surface
- Red degeneration: Infarction and hemorrhage

Microscopic Features

- Whorled appearance of smooth muscle bundles with interspersed vascular connective tissue
- May demonstrate areas of degeneration or calcification

CLINICAL ISSUES

Presentation

- Most common signs/symptoms
  o Symptoms primarily related to leiomyoma location, size, &/or growth
    - Submucosal: Dysfunctional uterine bleeding
    - Subserosal: Bulk symptoms, including urinary urgency &/or constipation
    - Pedunculated: Can have severe pain from torsion
    - Degeneration of leiomyoma can also cause pelvic pain
    - Cornual leiomyoma may cause tubal obstruction
  o Parasitic leiomyoma: Separate from uterine stalk and obtain vascular supply from adjacent pelvic structure (e.g., omentum)
  o Can undergo rapid growth during pregnancy

- Low-lying leiomyomas can block birth canal (myoma previa), requiring cesarean section
- May result in failure of implantation, loss of pregnancy, placental abruption

Demographics

- Age
  o Increase in size and frequency with age
- Epidemiology
  o 25-30% incidence in United States
  o Higher incidence in African American women
  o 77% incidence in hysterectomy specimens

Natural History & Prognosis

- May grow during pregnancy
- Involute after menopause and calcify

Treatment

- Hormonal therapy can be used for symptomatic relief
- For bulk symptoms or bleeding, management includes uterine artery embolization, myomectomy, and hysterectomy
  o Similar rate of success and less morbidity associated with uterine artery embolization
- If greater than 50% of submucosal leiomyoma is within endometrial cavity, will require hysteroscopy for removal

DIAGNOSTIC CHECKLIST

Consider

- If borders are not well delineated, consider adenomyosis

Image Interpretation Pearls

- Circumscribed mass, hypoechoic to myometrium, with posterior acoustic shadowing
- SIS to better characterize submucosal leiomyomas
- MR prior to uterine artery embolization, and to evaluate multiple or complex leiomyomas
- Consider malignant form if rapidly growing uterine mass in postmenopausal woman

Reporting Tips

- If multiple, report at least 3 largest index leiomyomas
- Report size of submucosal component and size of stalk if pedunculated

SELECTED REFERENCES

1. Van den Bosch T et al: Terms and definitions for describing myometrial pathology using ultrasonography. Ultrasound Obstet Gynecol. ePub, 2015
2. Akbulut M et al: Clinical and pathological features of lipoleiomyoma of the uterine corpus: a review of 76 cases. Balkan Med J. 31(3):224-9, 2014
3. Choi HJ et al: Is uterine artery embolization for patients with large myomas safe and effective? A retrospective comparative study in 323 patients. J Vasc Interv Radiol. 24(6):772-8, 2013
4. Islam MS et al: Uterine leiomyoma: available medical treatments and new possible therapeutic options. J Clin Endocrinol Metab. 98(3):921-34, 2013
5. Ly A et al: Atypical leiomyomas of the uterus: a clinicopathologic study of 51 cases. Am J Surg Pathol. 37(5):643-9, 2013
6. Deshmukh SP et al: Role of MR imaging of uterine leiomyomas before and after embolization. Radiographics. 32(6):E251-81, 2012
7. Manyonda IT et al: Uterine Artery Embolization versus Myomectomy: Impact on Quality of Life-Results of the FUME (Fibroids of the Uterus: Myomectomy versus Embolization) Trial. Cardiovasc Intervent Radiol. Epub ahead of print, 2011
8. Stamatopoulos CP et al: Value of magnetic resonance imaging in diagnosis of adenomyosis and myomas of the uterus. J Minim Invasive Gynecol. 19(5):620-6, 2012

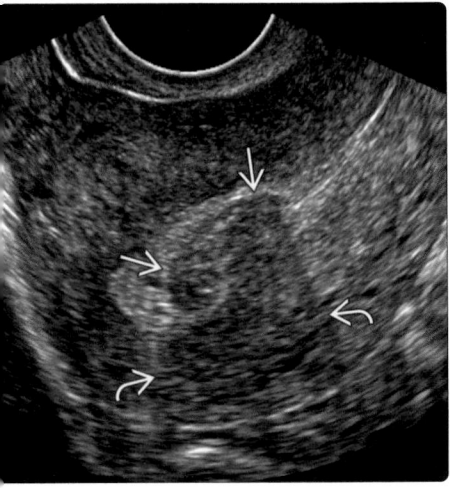
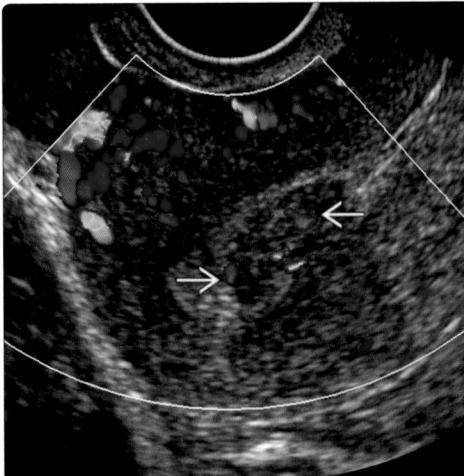

(Left) *Transvaginal ultrasound shows a hypoechoic mass within the endometrial cavity* ➡ *with posterior shadowing* ➡ *, consistent with a submucosal/intracavitary leiomyoma.* (Right) *Color Doppler ultrasound of the same patient demonstrates multiple vessels within the leiomyoma* ➡ *.*

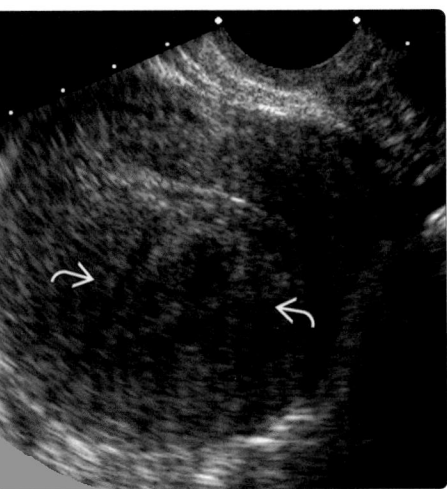
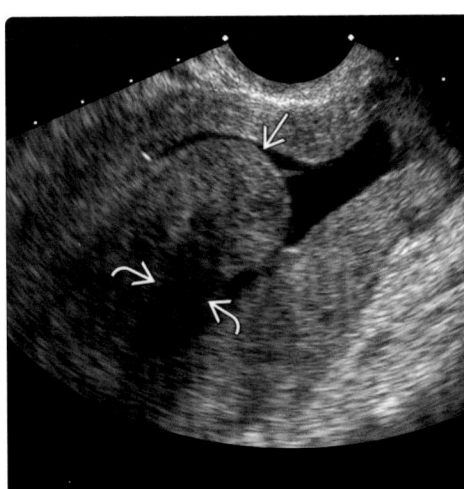

(Left) *Endovaginal ultrasound demonstrates a poorly defined, heterogeneous mass in the posterior uterine fundus with streaky shadowing* ➡ *. The appearance overlaps with adenomyosis.* (Right) *Saline-infused sonohysterography in the same patient confirms an intracavitary mass* ➡ *with posterior shadowing* ➡ *, consistent with submucosal leiomyoma.*

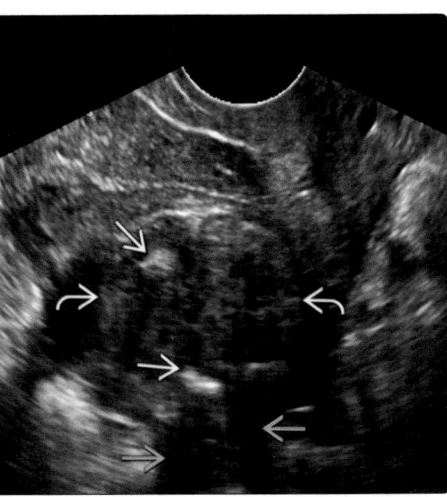
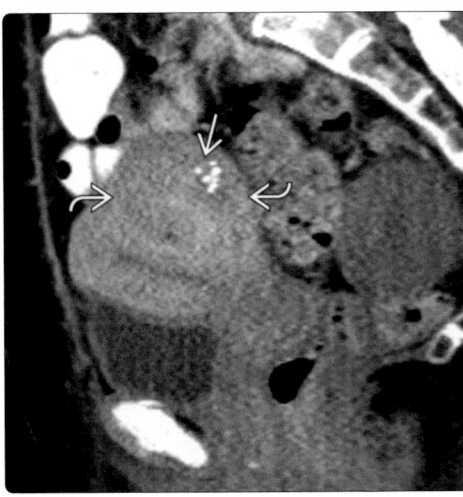

(Left) *Transvaginal ultrasound demonstrates a circumscribed, heterogeneous mass* ➡ *with areas of increased echogenicity consistent with calcifications* ➡ *and shadowing* ➡ *consistent with an intramural leiomyoma.* (Right) *Sagittal CT reconstruction of the pelvis in the same patient better demonstrates calcifications* ➡ *within the posterior intramural leiomyoma* ➡ *. Note the mass effect on the uterus and surrounding structures.*

(Left) *Transvaginal ultrasound demonstrates a hypoechoic pedunculated mass* ➡ *with a broad-based attachment* ⮕ *to the uterine fundus, consistent with a subserosal fibroid.* **(Right)** *Color Doppler ultrasound in the same patient demonstrates the vascular pedicle from the uterus supplying the leiomyoma* ➡*.*

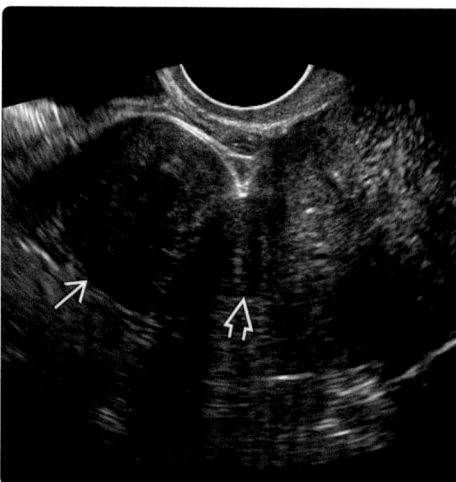
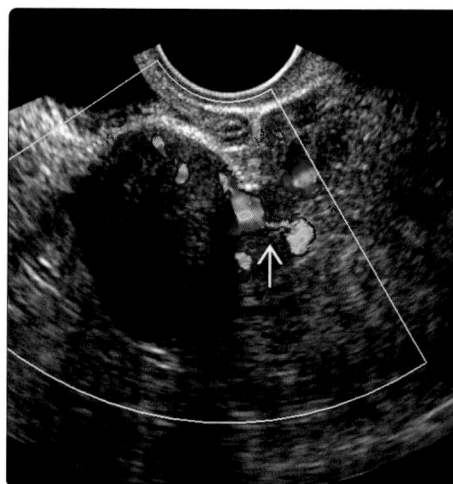

(Left) *Transverse transabdominal ultrasound in a patient with acute pain shows a heterogeneous hypoechoic mass* ➡ *with posterior shadowing* ➡ *in the left pelvis superior to the uterus, corresponding to the area of pain. The medial hypoechoic structure is the dome of the distended bladder* ⮕*.* **(Right)** *Sagittal CT reconstruction in the same patient better demonstrates a thin stalk from the uterus* ⮕ *to a pedunculated, nonenhancing mass* ➡*, consistent with fibroid torsion and possible necrosis.*

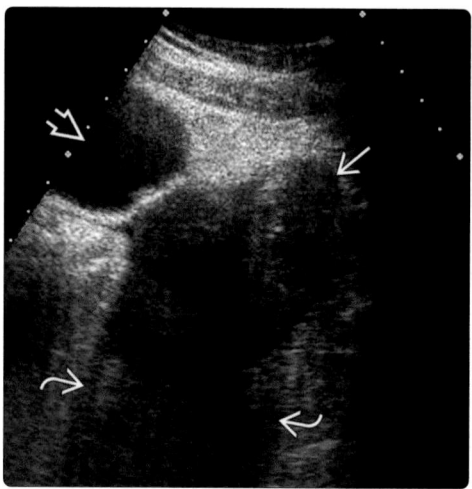
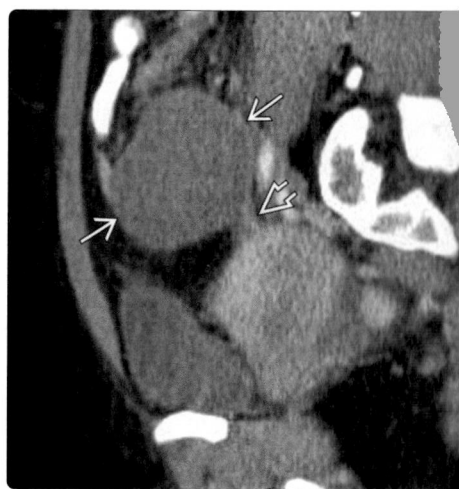

(Left) *Transabdominal longitudinal ultrasound in a patient with pelvic pain demonstrates a large, hypoechoic mass with posterior shadowing* ➡ *arising superiorly from the uterus* ⮕*. The mass is not entirely included in the FOV.* **(Right)** *Coronal NECT reconstruction in the same patient better demonstrates a large subserosal fibroid* ➡*, exceeding the size of the uterus* ⮕*.*

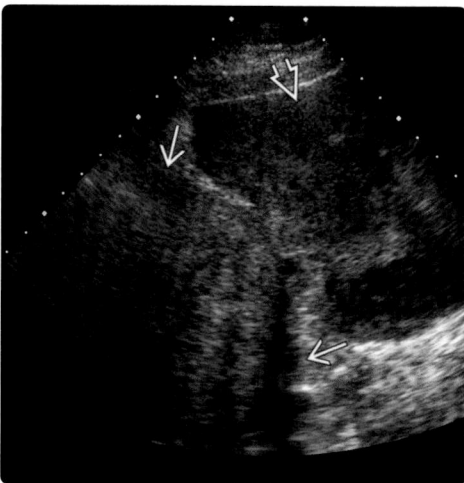
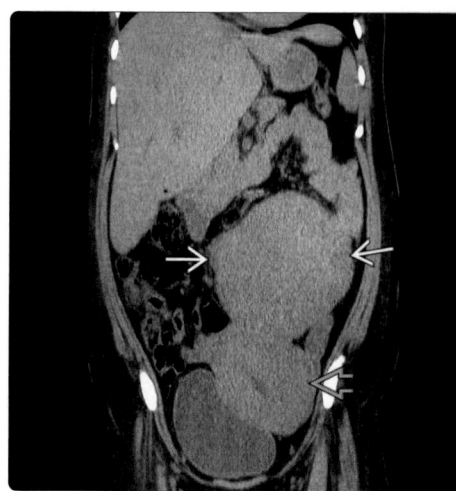

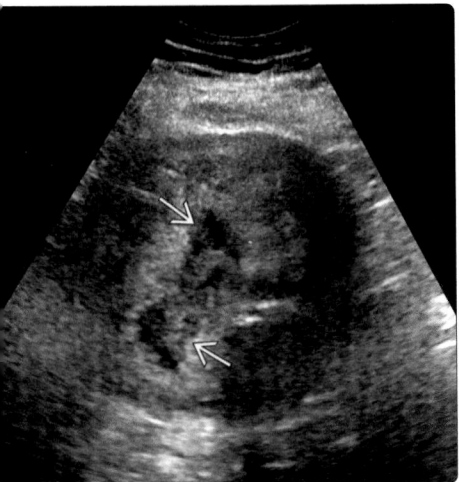

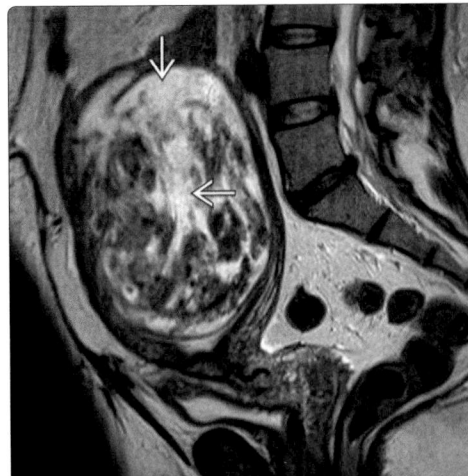

(Left) *Transverse transabdominal ultrasound demonstrates a mixed echogenicity mass with areas of internal cystic change ➡, suggestive of a degenerating leiomyoma.* (Right) *Sagittal T2WI in the same patient demonstrates a heterogenous appearance of the large intramural leiomyoma, with large areas of increased T2 signal ➡ consistent with cystic degeneration.*

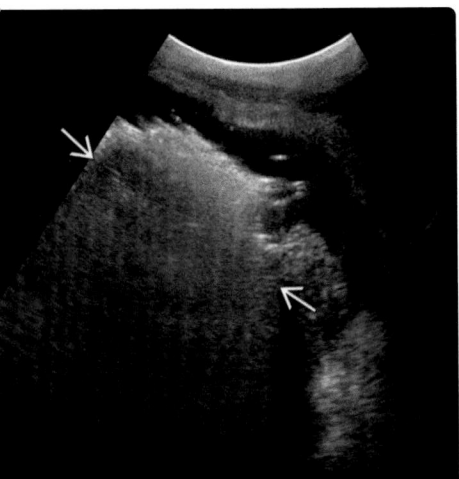

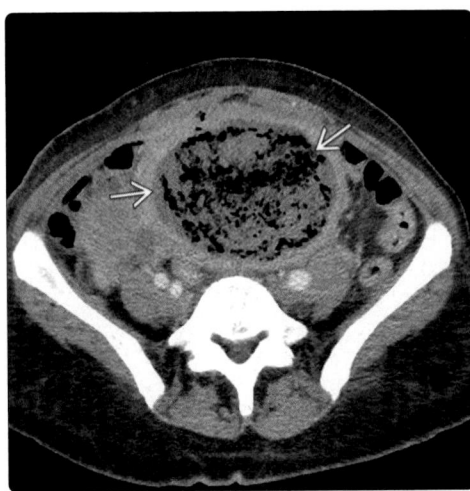

(Left) *Transabdominal ultrasound after uterine artery embolization (UAE) demonstrates a large region of increased echogenicity with poor acoustic penetration and incomplete "dirty shadowing" ➡ consistent with gas.* (Right) *Axial CECT on the same patient demonstrates extensive gas ➡ throughout the nonenhancing leiomyoma, consistent with postembolization necrosis and infection, as the patient had fever and leucocytosis.*

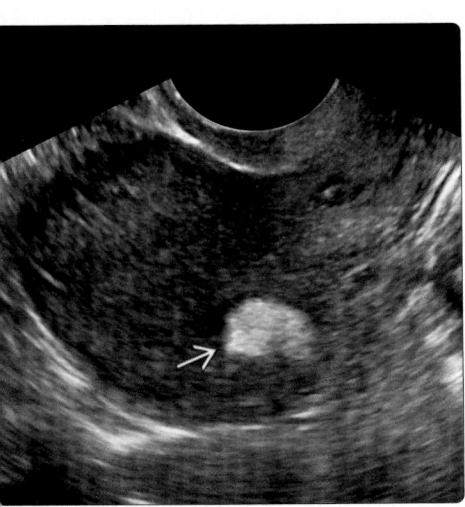

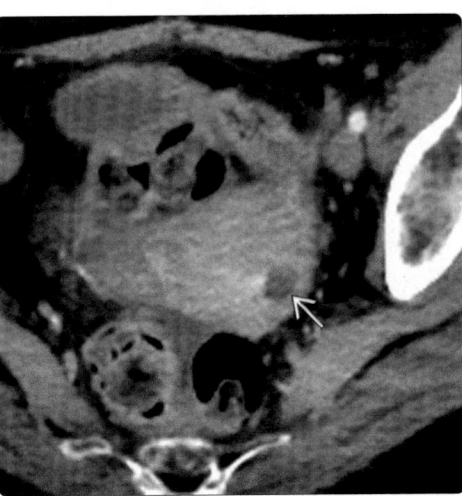

(Left) *Longitudinal transvaginal ultrasound demonstrates an echogenic circumscribed mass in the posterior uterus ➡ without shadowing, suggestive of a fat-containing lesion. Close attention should be made to the location of the mass to avoid confusion with an ovarian dermoid.* (Right) *Axial CECT of the same patient confirms a low-attenuation, fat-containing mass in the posterior aspect of the uterus ➡, consistent with a lipoleiomyoma.*

TERMINOLOGY

- Müllerian duct anomalies (MDA)
  - Series of uterine malformations resulting from abnormal development, fusion, or resorption of müllerian ducts
- MDA types
  - Müllerian agenesis or hypoplasia
  - Unicornuate uterus
  - Uterus didelphys
  - Bicornuate uterus
  - Septate uterus
  - Arcuate uterus

IMAGING

- Best diagnostic clue: Abnormal configuration of endometrial cavity ± abnormal external contour of uterus
- 3D ultrasound is vital for correct diagnosis
- MR to clarify anatomy, relationship of pelvic organs

TOP DIFFERENTIAL DIAGNOSES

- Imperforate hymen
- Cervical stenosis
- Pyometra

PATHOLOGY

- MDAs occur during 1 of 3 phases of development
  - Organogenesis phase: Uterine agenesis, hypoplasia, unicornuate
  - Fusion phase: Didelphys, bicornuate
  - Septal resorption phase: Septate, arcuate
- Renal anomalies in ~ 30%

DIAGNOSTIC CHECKLIST

- Determining outer uterine contour is essential to distinguish septate vs. bicornuate uterus
- Image renal fossae to assess for unilateral agenesis

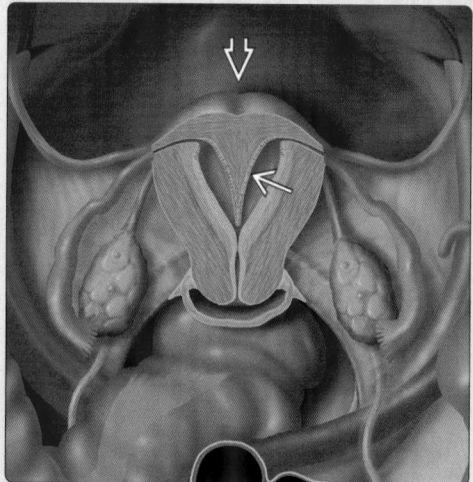
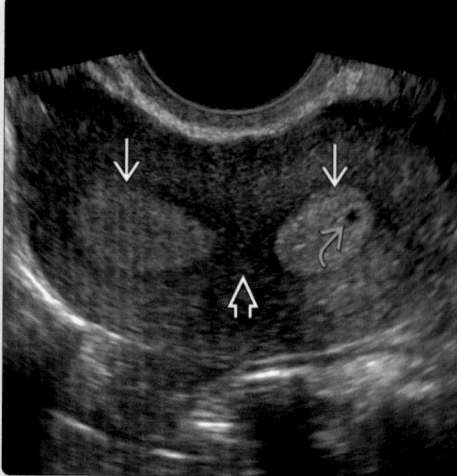

(Left) *Graphic of a septate uterus shows minimal indentation on the uterine fundus* ➡. *There is myometrium in the superior aspect of the septum, although normal zonal anatomy is not present in this portion* ➡. **(Right)** *Transverse ultrasound shows 2 endometrial cavities* ➡ *separated by myometrial tissue* ➡. *An early gestational sac* ➡ *is present on the left side. Evaluation of the external uterine contour was necessary to confirm this as a septate uterus.*

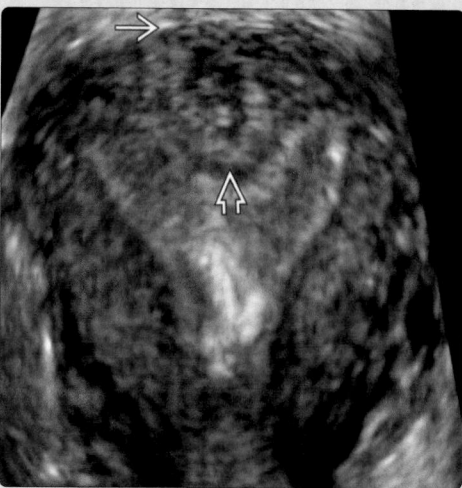
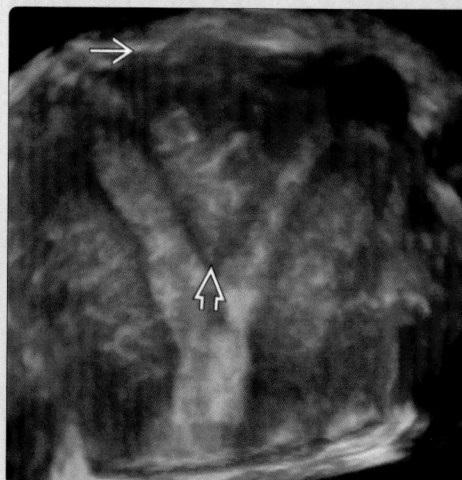

(Left) *3D ultrasound with coronal MIP rendering shows a muscular septum* ➡ *indenting the fundal endometrium. The coronal reconstruction readily depicts the normal convex outer uterine contour* ➡ *of this septate uterus.* **(Right)** *3D ultrasound with cut-surface volume rendering shows a deep muscular septum* ➡ *extending into the fundal endometrium, with a normal convex outer uterine contour* ➡, *consistent with septate uterus.*

TERMINOLOGY

Abbreviations

Müllerian duct anomalies (MDA)

Synonyms

Uterine fusion anomalies

Definitions

MDA: Series of uterine malformations resulting from abnormal development, fusion, or resorption of müllerian ducts

o Unicornuate, bicornuate, didelphys uterus ± cervical/vaginal malformation

IMAGING

General Features

Best diagnostic clue

o Abnormal configuration of endometrial cavity ± abnormal external contour of uterus

Ultrasonographic Findings

Grayscale ultrasound

o Arcuate uterus
  – Most common MDA
  – Minimal indentation of fundal endometrium
  – Normal external uterine contour
o Septate uterus
  – 2nd most common MDA
  – 2 endometrial cavities, septum of variable length and thickness
    □ Thin fibrous septum variably present
  – May be difficult to discern outer uterine contour: Imaging overlap with bicornuate uterus
    □ Convex outer uterine contour or cleft < 1 cm
    □ Intercornual angle < 75° suggests septate uterus
o Bicornuate uterus
  – 3rd most common MDA
  – 2 symmetric uterine horns, fused inferiorly
  – May be difficult to discern outer uterine contour: Imaging overlap with septate uterus
    □ Deep fundal cleft > 1 cm
    □ Intercornual angle > 105° suggests bicornuate uterus
    □ Intercornual distance > 4 cm favors bicornuate uterus
  – May have single cervix (unicollis) or duplication (bicollis)
o Unicornuate uterus
  – Curved and elongated banana-shaped single uterine horn and endometrium
  – Hypoplastic contralateral horn often present
    □ Hematometros (HM) when obstructed
    □ May or may not communicate with unicornuate horn
o Uterus didelphys
  – 2 separate noncommunicating divergent uterine horns
  – Deep fundal cleft
  – 2 cervices
  – Vaginal septum in 75%
    □ Hematometrocolpos (HC) if obstructed
o Müllerian agenesis or hypoplasia
  – Absent or small rudimentary uterus
  – ± hematometros
o DES uterus (T shaped)
  – Nonspecific appearance on 2D US
• 3D
  o Vital for correct diagnosis of MDA
    – True coronal plane allows for better sonographic evaluation of uterine fundal contour

MR Findings

• Appearance dependent upon MDA type
• T2WI: Best for visualizing outer uterine contour, zonal anatomy
• T1WI: High signal endometrium indicates hematometros when obstructed

CT Findings

• MPR images can demonstrate outer uterine contour and endometrial cavity but not study of choice

Fluoroscopic Findings

• Hysterosalpingography: Variable appearance of uterine cavity/cavities depending upon MDA type
  o Limited as outer uterine contour not visible

Imaging Recommendations

• Best imaging tool
  o Ultrasound as initial imaging test
  o MR to clarify anatomy, relationship of pelvic organs
    – Better than ultrasound in defining uterine contour, identifying rudimentary uterine horns
• Protocol advice
  o Ultrasound
    – 3D essential to evaluate uterine fundal contour
    – Limited until puberty, secondary to small uterine size
  o MR
    – T1 and T2WI to evaluate anatomy, blood products
      □ True coronal images of uterus to evaluate fundal contour
    – Include renal fossae on coronal views

DIFFERENTIAL DIAGNOSIS

Imperforate Hymen

• Uterus/vagina distended with mucous secretions or blood
• Not associated with MDA
• Need to differentiate from low transverse vaginal septum

Cervical Stenosis

• Can cause obstruction and distortion of endometrial cavity, mimicking MDA

Pyometra

• Associated with fever, elevated white cell count
• Clinical diagnosis as complex fluid on imaging, may be pus or blood

PATHOLOGY

General Features

• Etiology

American Fertility Society Classification System of Müllerian Duct Anomalies

Category	Type	Definition
Class I	Agenesis or hypoplasia	Complete or segmental agenesis, or variable uterovaginal hypoplasia
Class II	Unicornuate uterus	Partial or complete unilateral hypoplasia
Class III	Uterus didelphys	Duplication of uterus
Class IV	Bicornuate uterus	Incomplete fusion of superior uterovaginal canal
Class V	Septate uterus	Incomplete resorption of uterine septum
Class VI	Arcuate uterus	Near complete resorption of uterine septum/normal variant
Class VII	T-shaped uterus	In utero Diethylstilbestrol (DES) exposure

(The American Fertility Society classification system is the most widely utilized and accepted.

The American Fertility Society classifications of adnexal adhesions, distal tubal occlusion, tubal occlusion secondary to tubal ligation, tubal pregnancies, müllerian anomalies and intrauterine adhesions. Fertil Steril. 49(6):944-55, 1988)

- o Müllerian duct structures
  - – Fallopian tubes, uterus, cervix, upper 2/3 of vagina
- o MDAs occur during 1 of 3 phases of development
  - – Organogenesis phase: Uterine agenesis, hypoplasia, unicornuate
  - – Fusion phase: Didelphys, bicornuate
  - – Septal resorption phase: Septate, arcuate
- Associated abnormalities
  - o Renal anomalies in 30-50%
    - – Renal agenesis most common
    - – Ectopic kidney, horseshoe kidney, duplicated collecting system, renal dysplasia also possible
  - o Endometriosis if obstruction present
  - o Mayer-Rokitansky-Kuster-Hauser syndrome
    - – Most common etiology of class I MDA
    - – Complete vaginal agenesis
    - – 90% have uterine agenesis; 10% with rudimentary horn
  - o Obstructed hemivagina-ipsilateral renal agenesis (OHVIRA)
    - – Associated with class III MDA
    - – Unilateral obstructing transverse vaginal septum → hematometrocolpos
    - – Ipsilateral renal agenesis

CLINICAL ISSUES

Presentation

- Most common signs/symptoms
  - o Asymptomatic
  - o Presents at menarche
    - – Primary amenorrhea or dysmenorrhea
    - – Uterus didelphys → duplicated vagina → normal menses through unobstructed side with progressive distension of obstructed side
  - o Obstetric-/fertility-related
    - – Recurrent spontaneous abortions/infertility
    - – Malpresentation, premature labor, intrauterine growth restriction
    - – Ectopic pregnancy
- Other signs/symptoms
  - o Cyclical pelvic pain and pressure
  - o Distended uterus/vagina → mass effect → acute urinary retention

Demographics

- Epidemiology
  - o 1-5% prevalence in general population
    - – Up to 25% in women with recurrent pregnancy loss and infertility
    - – Prevalence of subtypes depends on method of diagnosis and patient population
  - o Vaginal agenesis = 1:5,000

Natural History & Prognosis

- Depends on underlying malformation
- Associated with endometriosis if obstruction
  - o Increased incidence of infertility/ectopic pregnancy
  - o Chronic pelvic pain

Treatment

- MR to verify diagnosis and assess extent of associated malformation
- MDA repair varies with malformation
  - o Simple septal resection to more complex vaginal reconstruction
  - o Creation of perineal opening/vaginoplasty
  - o Uterine surgery may be required to improve chances of successful pregnancy

DIAGNOSTIC CHECKLIST

Consider

- MDA in patients with recurrent miscarriage or infertility
- HM/HC should be evaluated for in any young female with cyclical pelvic pain
- Image renal fossae to assess for unilateral agenesis

Image Interpretation Pearls

- Determining outer uterine contour is essential to distinguish septate vs. bicornuate uterus
- Determine presence of communication between endometrial cavities
- Determine if 1 or 2 cervices

SELECTED REFERENCES

1. Sakhel K et al: Begin with the basics: role of 3-dimensional sonography as a first-line imaging technique in the cost-effective evaluation of gynecologic pelvic disease. J Ultrasound Med. 32(3):381-8, 2013
2. Behr SC et al: Imaging of müllerian duct anomalies. Radiographics. 32(6):E233-50, 2012

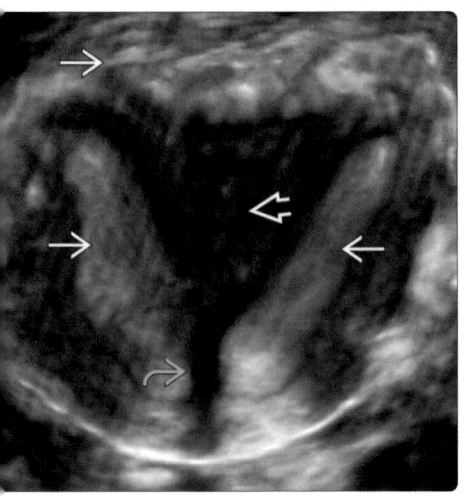

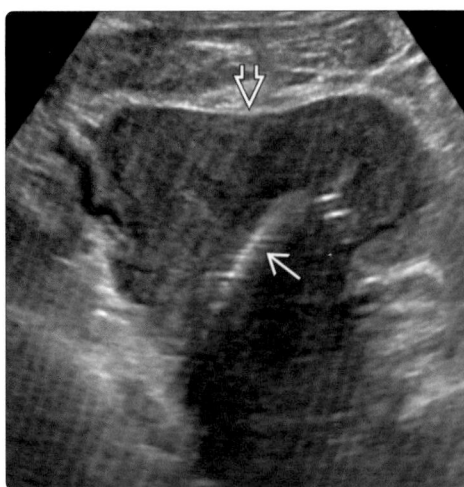

(Left) *3D ultrasound with coronal MIP rendering showing a large wedge of myometrium ⇲ separating the 2 endometrial cavities. Inferiorly is a thin hypoechoic fibrous continuation of the septum ⇲. The convex outer uterine contour ⇲ is maintained in this septate uterus.* (Right) *Transverse oblique ultrasound obtained coronal to the uterus shows the stem of an IUD ⇲ projecting into the left endometrium. The outer contour is only minimally indented ⇲ in this septate uterus.*

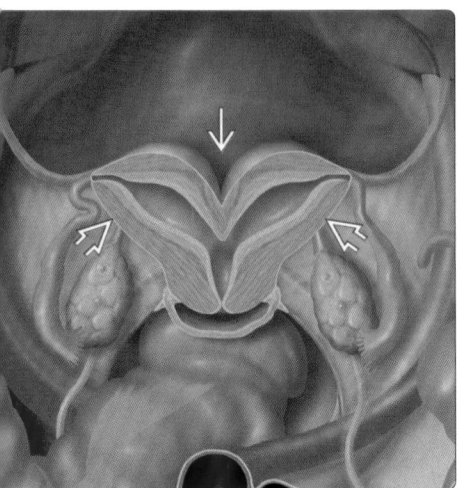

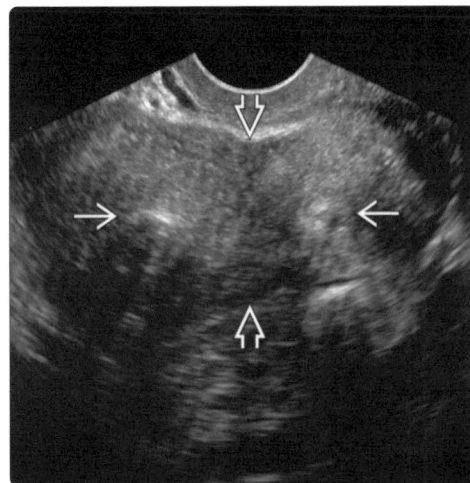

(Left) *Graphic of a bicornuate uterus demonstrates a deep external fundal cleft ⇲ and 2 symmetric cornua ⇲ that are fused inferiorly.* (Right) *Transverse transvaginal ultrasound shows 2 widely separated endometrial cavities ⇲. The outer contour of the uterus appears indented anteriorly and posteriorly ⇲, suggesting a bicornuate uterus; however, the fundus could not be adequately evaluated.*

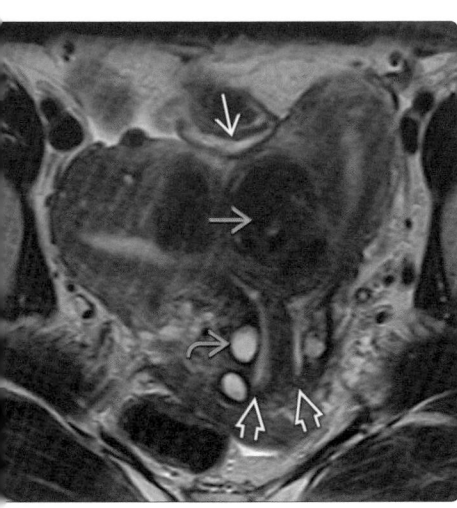

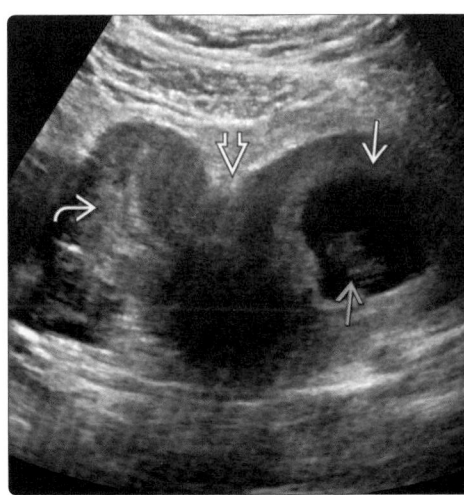

(Left) *Coronal T2 MR image in the same patient confirms a fundal indentation ⇲ and wide separation of the endometrial cavities > 110° as well as 2 cervices ⇲ in this patient with bicornuate bicollis uterus. Fibroids ⇲ and nabothian cysts ⇲ are also present.* (Right) *Transverse transabdominal ultrasound shows wide separation ⇲ of the uterine horns with a 9-week pregnancy ⇲ in the left horn ⇲ and endometrial thickening in the right horn ⇲. There was a single cervix (not shown) confirming a bicornuate unicollis uterus.*

(Left) *Slightly oblique transverse transvaginal ultrasound showing separation of the endometrium as well as indentation of the external uterine contour* ➡, *consistent with bicornuate uterus. An early gestational sac is present in the left horn* ➡. **(Right)** *Transvaginal ultrasound obtained coronal to a slightly deviated uterus shows a gestational sac within 1 uterine horn* ➡ *and fluid and debris within the other* ➡. *The fundal indentation of this bicornuate uterus is visible superiorly* ➡.

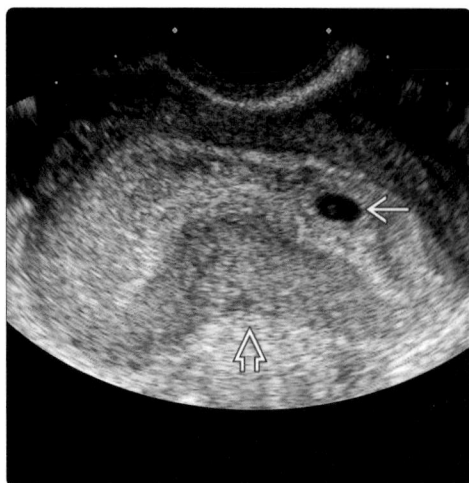
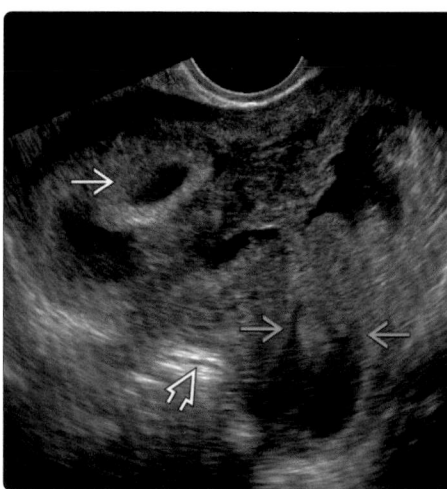

(Left) *Coronal transvaginal ultrasound in a complex case shows a normal endometrium* ➡ *on the left side with thick muscle* ➡ *connecting to another horn, which lacked the normal endometrial line* ➡. *The precise anatomy was not able to be defined sonographically. The left ovary was normal* ➡. **(Right)** *Right sagittal ultrasound of the right adnexa in the same patient shows a complex cystic right ovarian mass* ➡, *consistent with an endometrioma.*

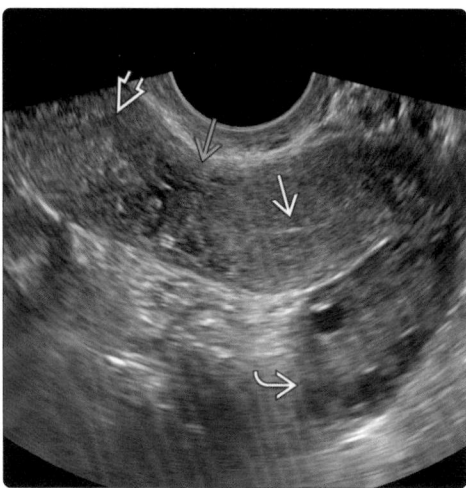
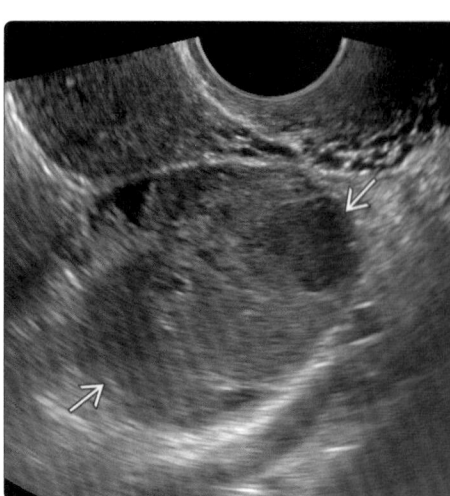

(Left) *T2 MR in the same patient better depicts the anatomy, showing a normal left horn* ➡ *and an obstructed right horn with distended endometrium* ➡ *and associated right endometrioma with T2 shading* ➡. *This was a unicornuate uterus with a noncommunicating cavitary right horn.* **(Right)** *Hysterosalpingogram shows only the endometrial cavities* ➡; *however, the degree of separation > 110° is consistent with a bicornuate uterus. There is normal free spillage of contrast bilaterally* ➡.

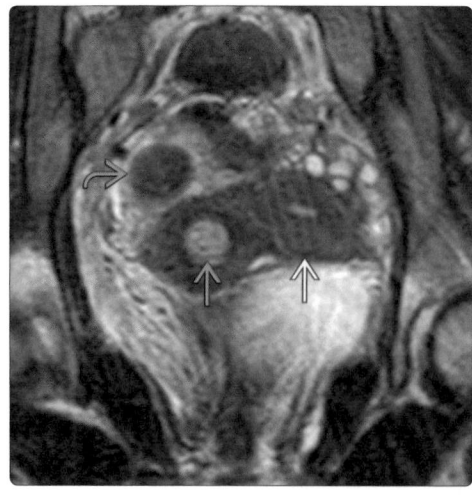
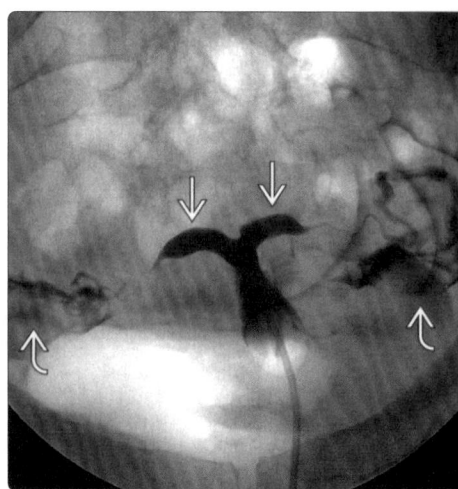

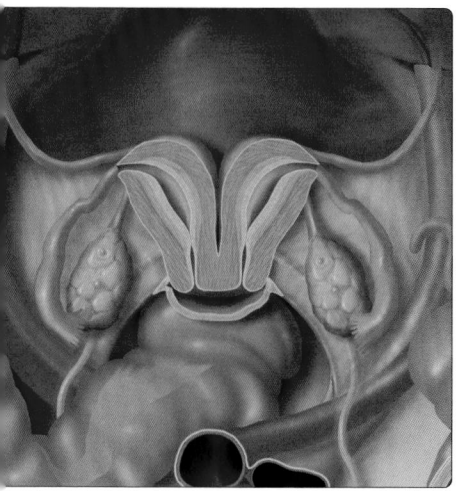
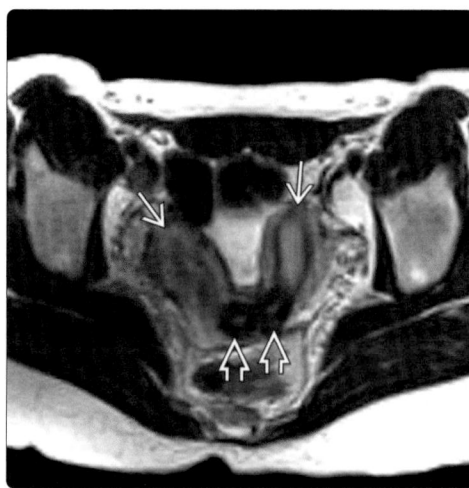

(Left) Graphic of a uterus didelphys shows complete duplication of uterine horns and cervices with no communication of the endometrial cavities. (Right) Axial MR image shows 2 completely separated uterine horns ➡ with 2 cervices ➡, consistent with uterus didelphys.

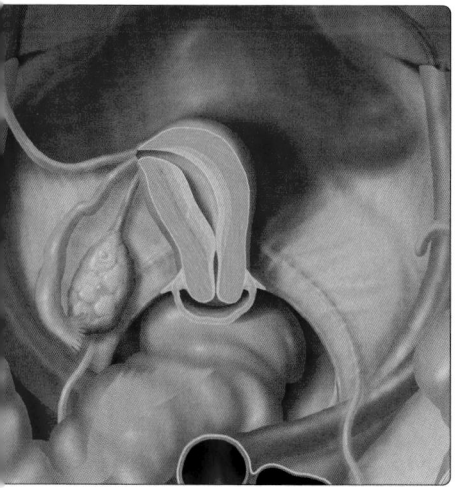
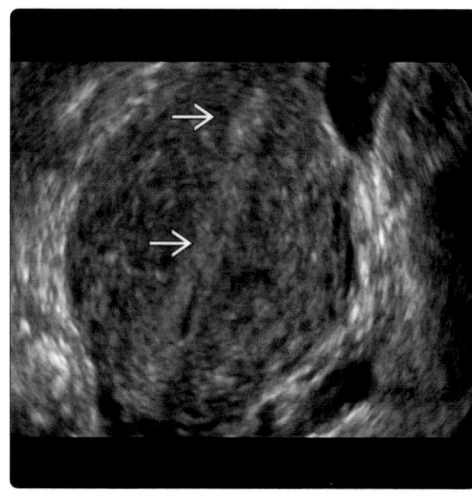

(Left) Graphic of a unicornuate uterus shows a small uterus shifted off midline with smooth tapering of fundal myometrium. The endometrial canal communicates with a solitary fallopian tube. (Right) 3D ultrasound acquisition with coronal reconstruction shows a thin, straight endometrium ➡ communicating with only 1 identifiable cornua, consistent with unicornuate uterus.

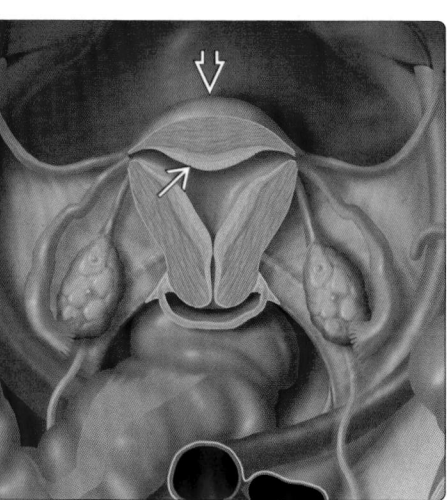
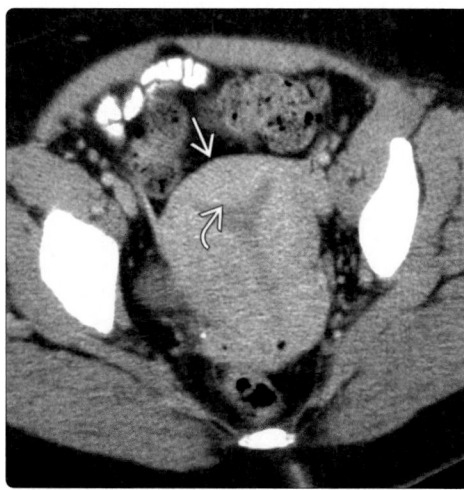

(Left) Graphic of an arcuate uterus shows normal convex contour of the uterine fundus ➡. There is indentation of the fundal endometrium < 1 cm without a true septum ➡. (Right) Axial CECT shows minimal indentation ➡ of the fundal endometrium, of < 1 cm, with a normal external uterine contour ➡.

KEY FACTS

TERMINOLOGY

- Hematometrocolpos: Distension of uterus and vagina by accumulated blood

IMAGING

- US best for initial evaluation or to confirm CT findings
  - HM appears thick-walled due to surrounding myometrium
  - HC is lower in pelvis and appears thin-walled compared to HM
  - Mixed echogenicity material within uterine &/or vaginal cavities
  - No flow: Presence of flow should raise concern for mass
- MR best to confirm blood products, absence of solid mass
- MR best to clarify anatomy, relationship of pelvic organs

TOP DIFFERENTIAL DIAGNOSES

- Pyometra
- Endometritis
- Muco/hydrometrocolpos
- Gestational trophoblastic disease
- Retained products of conception
- Complex adnexal mass

PATHOLOGY

- Imperforate hymen
- Müllerian duct anomaly
- Cloacal malformation
- Cervical/vaginal stenosis

CLINICAL ISSUES

- Presents at puberty if associated with MDA
- Presents later if associated with cervical cancer

DIAGNOSTIC CHECKLIST

- Distended uterine &/or vaginal cavities with heterogeneou avascular material
- HM/HC should be considered in young female patients wit lower abdominal symptoms or back pain

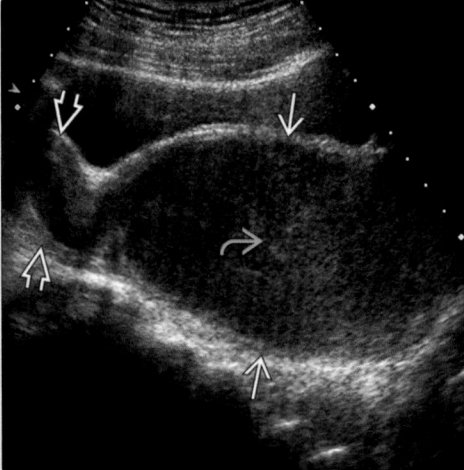
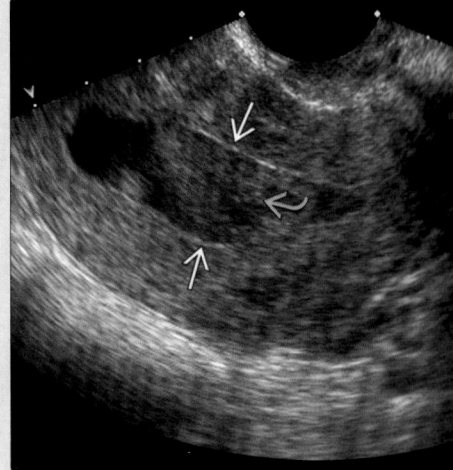

(Left) *Longitudinal transabdominal US in a patient with vaginal atresia shows a distended vagina with thin walls ⇥ containing hypoechoic heterogeneous fluid ⇗ consistent with hematocolpos. Note the thicker walls of the distended uterine cavity ⇥. (Right) Longitudinal transvaginal ultrasound in a patient with uterine fibroids and irregular bleeding shows a distended endometrial cavity ⇥ containing hypoechoic fluid and echogenic material ⇗ consistent with hematometros.*

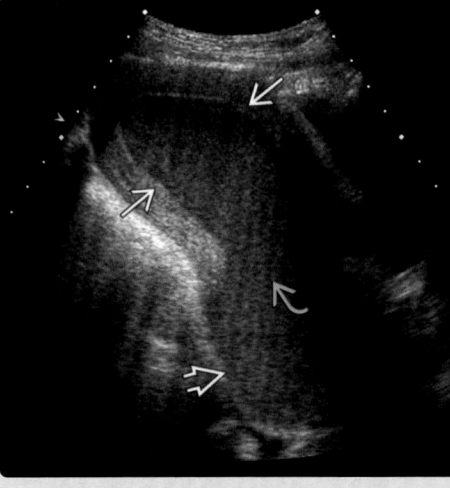
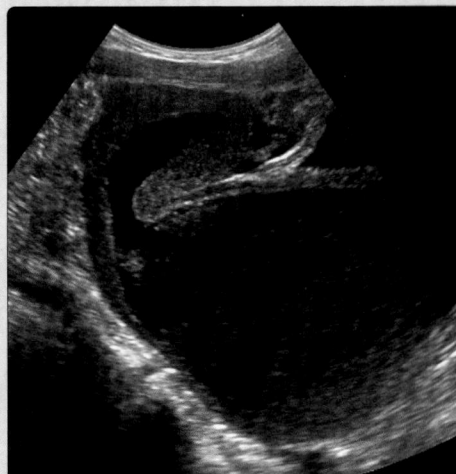

(Left) *Longitudinal transabdominal ultrasound of the uterus shows distention of the uterine ⇥ and cervical ⇥ cavities with homogeneous echogenic material ⇗, consistent with hematometros in this patient with cervical stenosis. (Right) Longitudinal transabdominal in a patient with imperforate hymen shows a markedly distended cervical canal containing hypoechoic, heterogeneous fluid, consistent with hematocolpos. There is less severe distention of the uterine cavity.*

Hematometrocolpos

TERMINOLOGY

Abbreviations

- Hematometra (HM)
- Hematocolpos (HC)
- Müllerian duct anomaly (MDA)
- Cloacal malformation (CM)

Definitions

- HM: Distension of uterine cavity by blood products
- HC: Distension of vagina by blood products
- Hematometrocolpos: Distension of uterus and vagina by accumulated blood

IMAGING

General Features

- Best diagnostic clue
  - Echogenic fluid within distended uterus ± vagina

Ultrasonographic Findings

- Grayscale ultrasound
  - Distended uterine &/or vaginal cavities
    - HM appears thick-walled due to surrounding myometrium
    - HC is lower in pelvis and appears thin-walled compared to HM
  - Mixed echogenicity material within uterine &/or vaginal cavities
    - Blood products of varying age
  - Fetal diagnosis reported
    - Thin bulging membrane separating labia
    - Distended vagina
    - May be associated with ascites attributed to uterine reflux via fallopian tubes versus associated distal urinary obstruction
- Color Doppler
  - No flow: Presence of flow should raise concern for mass
- 3D allows better sonographic evaluation of uterine fundal contour
  - Vital for diagnosis of MDA

MR Findings

- Distended uterus &/or vaginal cavities
  - T1WI: Isointense to hyperintense material
  - T2WI: Hyperintense, but less than simple fluid
- T1 C+: No enhancement of endometrial/vaginal contents

CT Findings

- Nonspecific: Requires further work-up with US or MR
- Enlarged distended uterus
  - May mimic a fluid collection, distended rectum, or mass

Imaging Recommendations

- Best imaging tool
  - US for initial evaluation or to confirm CT findings
  - MR best to confirm blood products, absence of solid mass
  - MR best to clarify anatomy, relationship of pelvic organs
- Protocol advice
  - Ultrasound
    - Consider use of translabial scans
    - Some reports of transrectal sonography
  - MR
    - Include renal images on coronal scout views
    - True coronal images of uterus to evaluate fundal contour for MDA
    - Distend vagina with Surgilube if possible, helpful to inject even if tiny perineal orifice
    - Contrast necessary if there is concern for an underlying mass

DIFFERENTIAL DIAGNOSIS

Pyometra

- Associated with fever, elevated white cell count
- Clinical diagnosis, imaging cannot distinguish pus vs. blood
- Does not involve vagina

Endometritis

- Seen after childbirth, uterine instrumentation
- Look for gas bubbles within endometrial cavity
- Not associated with amenorrhea
- Does not involve vagina

Muco/Hydrometrocolpos

- Uterus/vagina distended with mucous secretions, not blood
- Most commonly associated with imperforate hymen
- Hymenal membrane appears white
  - HC/HM hymenal membrane appears bluish due to accumulated blood products

Gestational Trophoblastic Disease

- Uterus distended by complete mole, has typical snowstorm appearance, not echogenic fluid
- Invasive mole typically hypervascular mass invading myometrium
  - Myometrium may be thinned in HM but is intact
- Does not involve vagina

Retained Products of Conception

- History of recent delivery
- Solid perfused tissue
- Retained clot is hypoechoic, nonvascular, smaller in volume than that seen with HM
- Does not involve vagina

Complex Adnexal Mass

- Always identify organ of origin of adnexal mass
  - Most are ovarian: Normal uterus can be identified separately
  - Pedunculated fibroids with cystic degeneration can be confusing
    - Not associated with amenorrhea
    - Look for vessels from myometrium to mass
    - Often other fibroids in uterine corpus in addition to pedunculated
  - If normal uterus is not identified could "mass" be abnormal uterus?
- May require MR to visualize normal ovaries
  - If large complex pelvic mass
  - If vaginal sonography not possible

PATHOLOGY

General Features

- Etiology
  - Imperforate hymen
    - Most frequent cause of vaginal outflow obstruction
  - Müllerian duct anomaly
    - Vaginal septum: Transverse or vertical
    - Vaginal agenesis
    - Cervical agenesis
    - Uterus didelphys with obstructed hemivagina is most confusing as normal menstruation occurs through nonobstructed side
  - Cloacal malformation
    - Confluence of rectum, vagina, and urethra into single common channel
    - Often septated or bilobed due to müllerian duplication
    - Up to 50% present with hydrocolpos at birth
    - Obstruction due to vaginal stenosis after reconstruction, stenosis of persistent urogenital sinus (no previous reconstruction), or cervical stenosis
  - Cervical/vaginal stenosis
    - Post radiation therapy for gynecologic/colorectal malignancies
    - Post reconstructive surgery
    - Vaginal stenosis described in chronic graft-vs.-host disease
- Associated abnormalities
  - Renal anomalies
  - Endometriosis

CLINICAL ISSUES

Presentation

- Most common signs/symptoms
  - Primary amenorrhea
  - Cyclical pelvic pain/pressure
  - Low back pain
- Other signs/symptoms
  - Urinary retention secondary to pressure on bladder/ureters
  - Constipation secondary to pressure on rectum
  - Presents at puberty if associated with MDA
    - Uterus didelphys → duplicated vagina → normal menses through unobstructed side with progressive distension of obstructed side
  - Presents later if associated with cervical cancer
    - Average age at diagnosis of CxCA is 50 years
    - Radiation therapy induced cervical/vaginal stenosis develops within a year of therapy

Demographics

- Epidemiology
  - Imperforate hymen 1:1,000
  - Vaginal agenesis 1:5,000
  - CM occurs exclusively in females, 1:20,000 live births
  - Vaginal stenosis occurs in up to 88% of cervical cancer patients treated with radiation therapy

Natural History & Prognosis

- Depends on underlying etiology
  - Imperforate hymen easily corrected
  - CM requires complex repair with multiple surgeries
  - MDA repair varies with malformation: Simple septal resection to more complex vaginal reconstruction
- Associated with endometriosis
  - Increased incidence of infertility/ectopic pregnancy
  - Chronic pelvic pain

Treatment

- Avoid aspiration as risk of infection → pyocolpos/pyometra
- Imperforate hymen
  - Cruciate incision with marsupialization of edges to vaginal wall
  - Simple incision inadequate → does not guarantee complete drainage → risk of infection
- MDA
  - Incision/removal of vaginal septum
  - Creation of perineal opening/vaginoplasty
  - Uterine surgery may also be required to improve chances of successful pregnancy
- Radiation therapy related
  - Topical estrogen, anti-inflammatory ointment
  - Serial vaginal dilators
- CM
  - Surgical challenge is to create 3 perineal openings with functional vagina, bladder/bowel control
  - Individual anatomy will direct reconstructive approach

DIAGNOSTIC CHECKLIST

Consider

- HM/HC should be considered in young female patients with lower abdominal symptoms or back pain

Image Interpretation Pearls

- Distended uterine &/or vaginal cavities with heterogeneous avascular material

SELECTED REFERENCES

1. Sakhel K et al: Begin with the basics: role of 3-dimensional sonography as a first-line imaging technique in the cost-effective evaluation of gynecologic pelvic disease. J Ultrasound Med. 32(3):381-8, 2013
2. Behr SC et al: Imaging of müllerian duct anomalies. Radiographics. 32(6):E233-50, 2012
3. Marcal L et al: Mullerian duct anomalies: MR imaging. Abdom Imaging. 36(6):756-64, 2011
4. Drakonaki EE et al: Hematocolpometra due to an imperforate hymen presenting with back pain: sonographic diagnosis. J Ultrasound Med. 29(2):321-2, 2010
5. Junqueira BL et al: Müllerian duct anomalies and mimics in children and adolescents: correlative intraoperative assessment with clinical imaging. Radiographics. 29(4):1085-103, 2009
6. Dane C et al: Imperforate hymen-a rare cause of abdominal pain: two cases and review of the literature. J Pediatr Adolesc Gynecol. 20(4):245-7, 2007
7. Sherer DM et al: Acquired hematometra and hematotrachelos in an adolescent with dysfunctional uterine bleeding. J Ultrasound Med. 25(12):1599-602, 2006
8. Prada Arias M et al: Uterus didelphys with obstructed hemivagina and multicystic dysplastic kidney. Eur J Pediatr Surg. 15(6):441-5, 2005
9. Warne SA et al: Long-term gynecological outcome of patients with persistent cloaca. J Urol. 170(4 Pt 2):1493-6, 2003

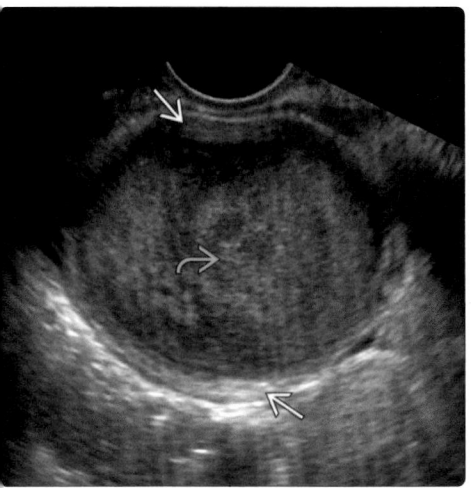

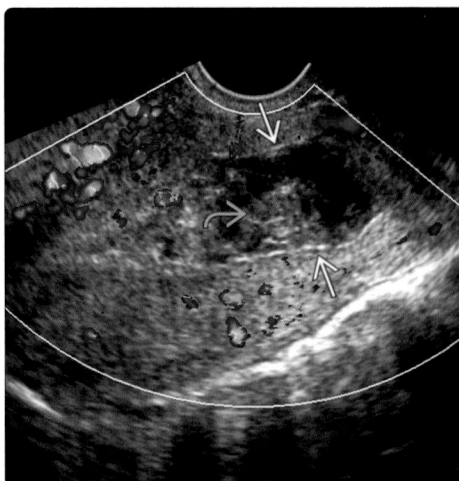

(Left) *Transverse transvaginal ultrasound shows distention of the cervix ➡️ with homogeneous echogenic material ➡️ consistent with hematometros in this patient with cervical stenosis.* (Right) *Longitudinal transvaginal US of the uterus shows mixed echogenicity material ➡️ distending the lower uterine segment ➡️, consistent with hematometros. The patient had recently undergone a D&C procedure.*

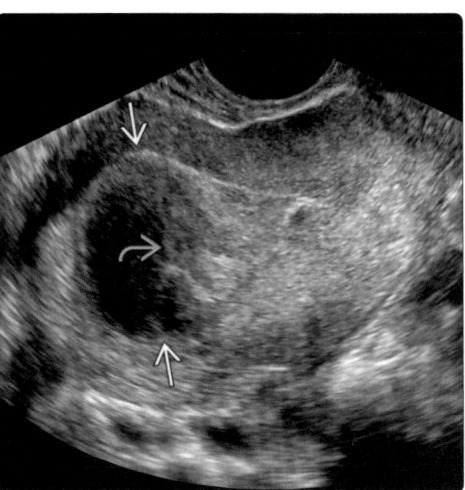

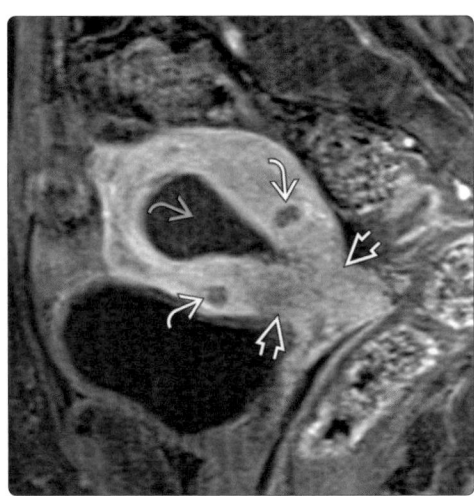

(Left) *Longitudinal transvaginal ultrasound shows heterogeneous mixed echogenicity material ➡️ distending the uterine cavity ➡️. The lack of blood flow on color Doppler (not shown) confirms hematometros.* (Right) *Sagittal T1-weighted MR following contrast administration confirms the lack of enhancement within the endometrial cavity ➡️. Two small fibroids are incidentally noted ➡️. The cause of hematometros was a cervical carcinoma, visible as subtle hypoenhancement with ill-defined borders ➡️.*

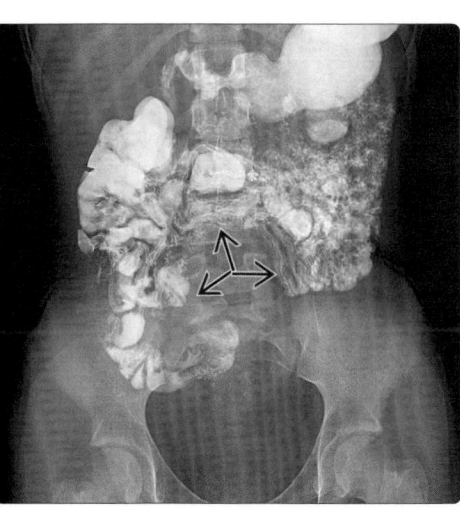

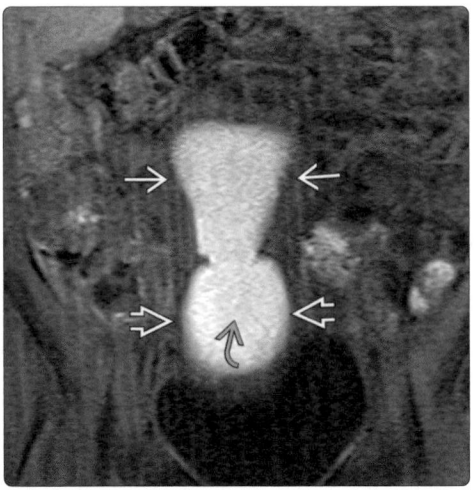

(Left) *Radiograph obtained as part of a small-bowel series in a young female with abdominal pain and suspected inflammatory bowel disease shows displacement of bowel from the lower abdomen ➡️, suggesting an underlying mass.* (Right) *Coronal T1-weighted MR in the same patient reveals a dilated uterus ➡️ and vagina ➡️ filled with high signal intensity material ➡️, consistent with hematometrocolpos. The patient was diagnosed with imperforate hymen.*

KEY FACTS

TERMINOLOGY

- Focal hyperplastic overgrowth of endometrial tissue
- Saline infusion sonohysterography: SHG, SIS

IMAGING

- Focal echogenic endometrial thickening or mass with feeding vessel
- Schedule US/SHG within first 10 days of menstrual cycle in menstruating females
- Ultrasound features
  - Echogenic area in endometrium during proliferative phase of menstrual cycle
  - Hyperechoic line sign: Full/partial echogenic rim around area of endometrial thickening highly specific for endocavitary mass
  - Color Doppler: Single feeding vessel in stalk
- Saline infusion sonohysterography
  - Best technique to differentiate focal from diffuse endometrial thickening

TOP DIFFERENTIAL DIAGNOSES

- Endometrial carcinoma
- Endometrial hyperplasia
- Submucosal fibroid
- Gestational trophoblastic disease
- Retained products of conception

CLINICAL ISSUES

- Etiology of up to 30% of cases of postmenopausal bleeding

DIAGNOSTIC CHECKLIST

- SHG for endometrial thickening, particularly if no cysts or feeding vessel on US
- MR/TVS/color Doppler may help to distinguish polyp from carcinoma
- Cancer may coexist with benign disease
  - Biopsy required: Benign polyps cannot be differentiated from polyps with atypical hyperplasia

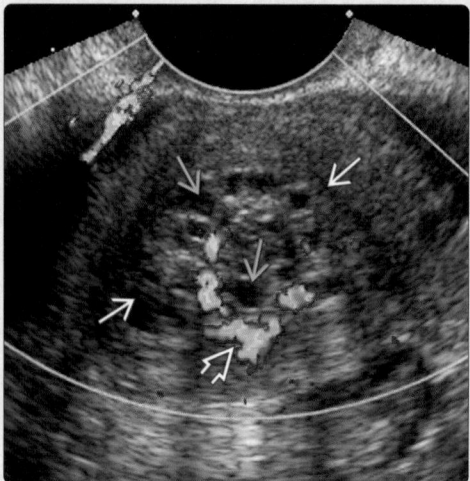
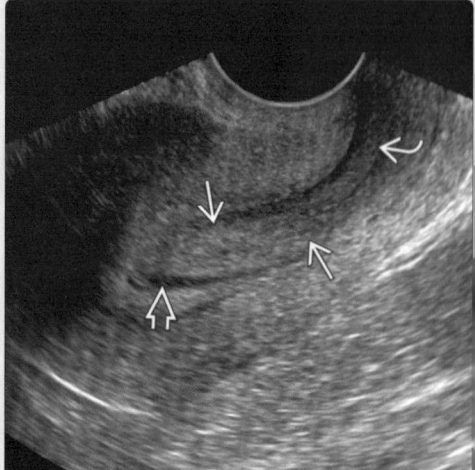

(Left) *Transverse transvaginal color Doppler US shows an endometrial polyp ➡ with a vascular pedicle ➡ denoting the location of attachment to the endometrial wall. Internal cystic spaces ➡, as in this case, are typically associated with a benign etiology.* (Right) *Longitudinal transvaginal ultrasound shows an elongated polyp ➡, partially surrounded by fluid ➡, filling the endometrial cavity and prolapsing through the cervical canal ➡.*

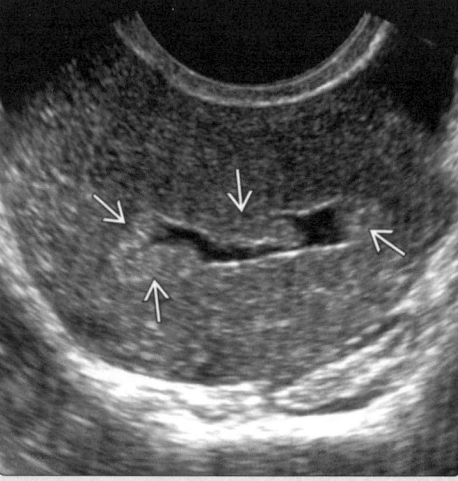
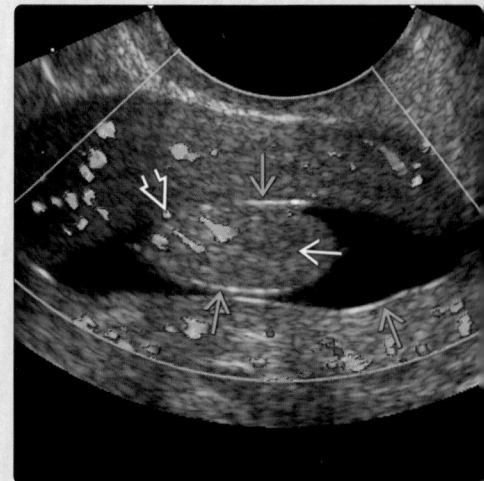

(Left) *Transverse transvaginal ultrasound during saline infusion sonohysterography demonstrates multiple sessile polyps ➡ within the endometrial cavity. Four are visible on this single image.* (Right) *Sagittal transvaginal ultrasound during saline infusion sonohysterography demonstrates a single pedunculated polyp within the cavity ➡. Color Doppler shows the vascular pedicle ➡, denoting the site of attachment. The echogenic line sign is seen at multiple interfaces lying perpendicular to the ultrasound beam ➡.*

TERMINOLOGY

Abbreviations

- Endometrial polyp (EP)

Definitions

- Focal hyperplastic overgrowth of endometrial tissue
- Saline infusion sonohysterography (SHG, SIS): Ultrasound of uterus after distension of cavity with sterile saline

IMAGING

General Features

- Best diagnostic clue
  - Focal echogenic endometrial thickening or mass with feeding vessel
- Size
  - Variable: May be tiny or large enough to fill entire uterine cavity
- Morphology
  - Pedunculated or sessile
    - May prolapse into cervical canal
  - Oval or fusiform rather than round
    - Round mass more likely to be submucosal fibroid
  - Multiple in 20% of patients

Ultrasonographic Findings

- Grayscale ultrasound
  - Echogenic area in endometrium during proliferative phase of menstrual cycle
    - Proliferative endometrium is normally hypoechoic
    - Secretory endometrium is echogenic, may obscure small polyp
  - Pedunculated or sessile, solitary or multiple
  - Small "cystic" areas within polyp due to dilated endometrial glands
    - Strong correlation with benignity
  - Hyperechoic line sign
    - Full/partial echogenic rim around area of endometrial thickening highly specific for endocavitary mass
    - Thought to be compressed endometrium vs. interface of mass with cavity
    - Does not differentiate between masses (polyp vs. fibroid)
- Color Doppler
  - Single feeding vessel in stalk may be evident
    - Divides into smaller vessels within polyp
- 3D
  - Useful for "global view"
  - 3D shows multiple polyps better than 2D
  - Useful during SHG especially if multiple lesions
- Sonohysterography
  - Best technique to differentiate focal from diffuse endometrial thickening
  - Focal
    - Polypoid with thin stalk
    - Sessile: If broad-based resection is more complex than simple snare
  - Diffuse
    - Symmetric thickening: "Blind" office biopsy with Pipelle or similar implement

    - Asymmetric: Requires visually directed biopsy of thickest area
  - Uterine contraction is a response to cavitary distention → endometrial "wrinkles"
    - May be mistaken for sessile polyps

MR Findings

- T2WI
  - Hyperintense, with polyp lower signal intensity than normal endometrium
    - Central fibrous core (low signal intensity) within endometrial cavity
    - Intratumoral cysts (high signal intensity) seen more frequently in polyps than carcinomas

Imaging Recommendations

- Best imaging tool
  - Transvaginal sonography (TVS), SHG
- Protocol advice
  - TVS
    - Schedule scans early in menstrual cycle if possible
      - □ Endometrium is thin and hypoechoic
    - If postmenopausal on hormone replacement therapy (HRT) schedule immediately after withdrawal bleed
    - If postmenopausal not on HRT schedule at any time
  - SHG
    - Schedule within first 10 days of menstrual cycle in menstruating females
      - □ Avoids risk of displacing an early pregnancy
    - Suggest patient take analgesic (nonsteroidal anti-inflammatory) 1 hour prior to procedure to minimize discomfort
  - MR with T2 FS if SHG cannot be performed
- Thick echogenic endometrium in premenopausal female
  - > 15 mm → abnormal → SHG to determine type of biopsy
  - 11-15 mm is indeterminate → follow-up after menstrual period
  - Normal endometrium will slough post menstrually
  - Persistent thickening of increased echogenicity → SHG

DIFFERENTIAL DIAGNOSIS

Thickened Endometrium

- Endometrial carcinoma
  - Irregular endometrial thickening
  - Often mixed hyper/hypoechoic areas, lack of tumoral cysts
  - Invasion into myometrium is highly suggestive of carcinoma
- Endometrial hyperplasia
  - More likely diffuse than focal process
  - Often asymptomatic

Intracavitary Mass

- Submucosal fibroid
  - Hypoechoic mass with shadowing; less echogenic than endometrial stripe
  - Spherical rather than oval/fusiform
  - Layer of endometrium covers surface of fibroid
  - Disrupts endometrial-myometrial interface
  - Multiple feeding vessels arise from inner myometrium
- Gestational trophoblastic disease

- o Positive pregnancy test
- o Often associated with hyperemesis
- o Beta human chorionic gonadotrophin levels may be extremely high
- o 25% association with theca lutein cysts
- Retained products of conception
  - o Associated with history of recent gestation
  - o Often prominent feeding vessels from myometrium to "mass"
  - o May have positive pregnancy test

PATHOLOGY

General Features

- Etiology
  - o Associated with Tamoxifen treatment in postmenopausal women
    - – Premenopausal women taking Tamoxifen for breast cancer are not at increased risk for endometrial cancer
  - o Lynch syndrome (hereditary nonpolyposis colon cancer) case report of EP containing cancer

Gross Pathologic & Surgical Features

- Circumscribed overgrowth of endometrial mucosa ± stromal tissue
- Protrudes into cavity on fibrovascular stalk

Microscopic Features

- Foci of atypical hyperplasia may be seen within polyps

CLINICAL ISSUES

Presentation

- Most common signs/symptoms
  - o Abnormal bleeding
    - – Intermenstrual
    - – Postcoital
    - – Postmenopausal
- Other signs/symptoms
  - o Atypical glandular cells of endometrial origin on Papanicolaou smear
    - – Indication for endometrial biopsy as 40% incidence of significant pathology

Demographics

- Epidemiology
  - o EP → 30% of postmenopausal bleeding

Natural History & Prognosis

- Polyp site/number/diameter do not correlate with symptomatology
- Often asymptomatic
  - o 36.1% of postmenopausal women
  - o 44.4% of reproductive-aged women
- Frequent finding in infertile patients
  - o Controversial if etiologic factor or if resection improves outcome
  - o Endometrial polyps < 1.5 cm diameter discovered during ovarian stimulation do not negatively affect pregnancy/implantation outcomes in intracytoplasmic sperm injection (ICSI) cycles

Treatment

- Progestin therapy
- Polypectomy
  - o Outpatient procedure is safe and better tolerated than operating room hysteroscopic resection
- Hysterectomy if atypical pathology/carcinoma
- Observation, particularly in older asymptomatic patients

DIAGNOSTIC CHECKLIST

Consider

- SHG for endometrial thickening, particularly if no cysts or feeding vessel
- MR/TVS/color Doppler may help to distinguish polyp from carcinoma
  - o Cancer may coexist with benign disease

Image Interpretation Pearls

- Focal or diffuse echogenic endometrial thickening with "hyperechoic line" sign
- Single feeding vessel
- Intratumoral cysts suggestive of polyp, rare in carcinoma
- Benign polyps cannot be differentiated from polyps with atypical hyperplasia; biopsy required
- Beware of endometrial "wrinkles," which can be mistaken for sessile polyps
  - o Uterine contraction is a response to cavitary distention → "wrinkles"

SELECTED REFERENCES

1. Fang L et al: Value of 3-dimensional and power Doppler sonography for diagnosis of endometrial polyps. J Ultrasound Med. 32(2):247-55, 2013
2. Van den Bosch T et al: Pre-sampling ultrasound evaluation and assessment of the tissue yield during sampling improves the diagnostic reliability of office endometrial biopsy. J Obstet Gynaecol. 32(2):173-6, 2012
3. Costa-Paiva L et al: Risk of malignancy in endometrial polyps in premenopausal and postmenopausal women according to clinicopathologic characteristics. Menopause. 18(12):1278-82, 2011
4. La Sala GB et al: Diagnostic accuracy of sonohysterography and transvaginal sonography as compared with hysteroscopy and endometrial biopsy: a prospective study. Minerva Ginecol. 63(5):421-7, 2011
5. Cil AP et al: Power Doppler properties of endometrial polyps and submucosal fibroids: a preliminary observational study in women with known intracavitary lesions. Ultrasound Obstet Gynecol. 35(2):233-7, 2010
6. Grimbizis GF et al: A prospective comparison of transvaginal ultrasound, saline infusion sonohysterography, and diagnostic hysteroscopy in the evaluation of endometrial pathology. Fertil Steril. 94(7):2720-5, 2010
7. Lee SC et al: The oncogenic potential of endometrial polyps: a systematic review and meta-analysis. Obstet Gynecol. 116(5):1197-205, 2010
8. Tamura-Sadamori R et al: The sonohysterographic difference in submucosal uterine fibroids and endometrial polyps treated by hysteroscopic surgery. J Ultrasound Med. 26(7):941-6; quiz 947-8, 2007
9. American College of Obstetricians and Gynecologists Committee on Gynecologic Practice: ACOG committee opinion. No. 336: Tamoxifen and uterine cancer. Obstet Gynecol. 107(6):1475-8, 2006
10. Hassa H et al: Are the site, diameter, and number of endometrial polyps related with symptomatology? Am J Obstet Gynecol. 194(3):718-21, 2006
11. Fong K et al: Transvaginal US and hysterosonography in postmenopausal women with breast cancer receiving tamoxifen: correlation with hysteroscopy and pathologic study. Radiographics. 23(1):137-50; discussion 151-5, 2003

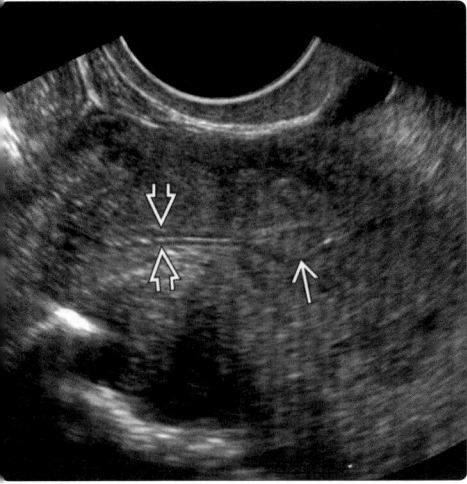

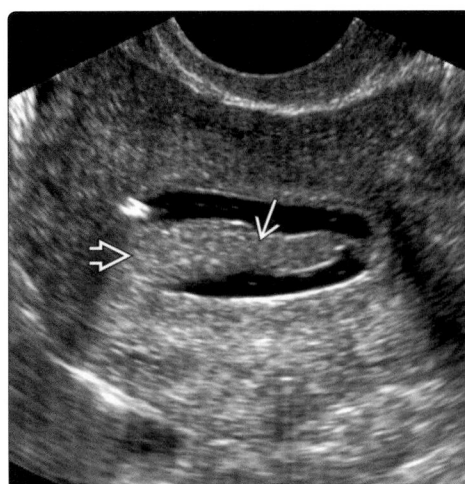

(Left) *Longitudinal transvaginal ultrasound shows focal nonspecific thickening of the endometrium ➡ in a patient with dysfunctional uterine bleeding. The majority of the endometrium is atrophic, with a thin trilaminar appearance ➡.* (Right) *Longitudinal transvaginal ultrasound during saline infusion in the same patient reveals an elongated pedunculated polyp ➡ with a small stalk ➡ corresponding to the focal area of endometrial thickening.*

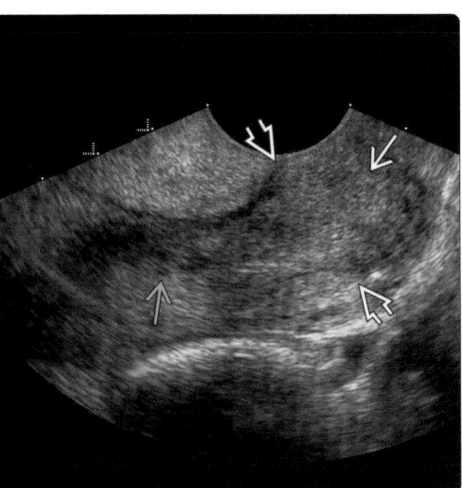

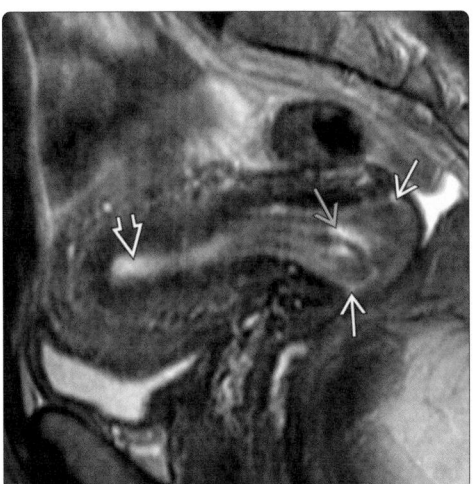

(Left) *Longitudinal transvaginal ultrasound of the cervix shows a large polyp ➡ prolapsing through the external os ➡. Small internal cystic spaces ➡ are visible near the internal os.* (Right) *Sagittal T2-weighted MR in the same patient shows the polyp protruding through the cervical canal ➡. The polyp is hypointense relative to the normal endometrium ➡, with the exception of internal cystic spaces ➡.*

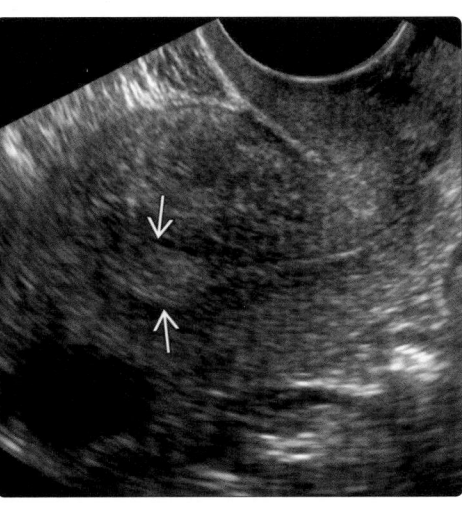

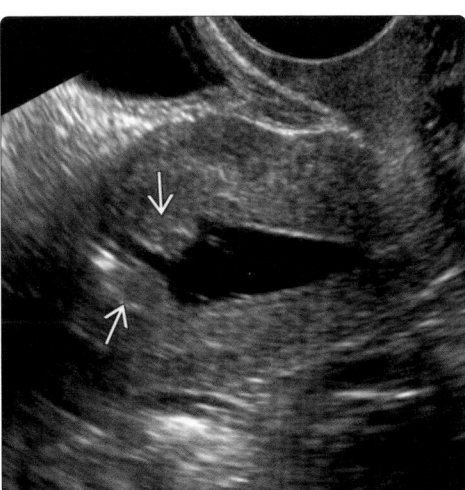

(Left) *Longitudinal transvaginal ultrasound shows nonspecific focal thickening ➡ in the upper endometrium, which could be secondary to hyperplasia, a polyp, or carcinoma.* (Right) *Longitudinal transvaginal ultrasound in the same patient following saline infusion ➡ reveals 2 sessile polyps ➡ corresponding to the region of focal endometrial thickening.*

(Left) *Longitudinal transvaginal ultrasound of the endometrium in a patient with menorrhagia shows a hyperechoic endometrial polyp with a hyperechoic line sign* ⮩. *The endometrium is proliferative* ⮕. **(Right)** *Longitudinal transvaginal color Doppler ultrasound of the same polyp shows the vascular pedicle* ⮕ *with early branching.*

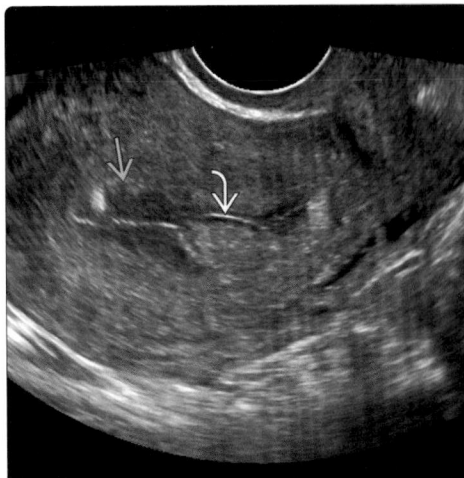
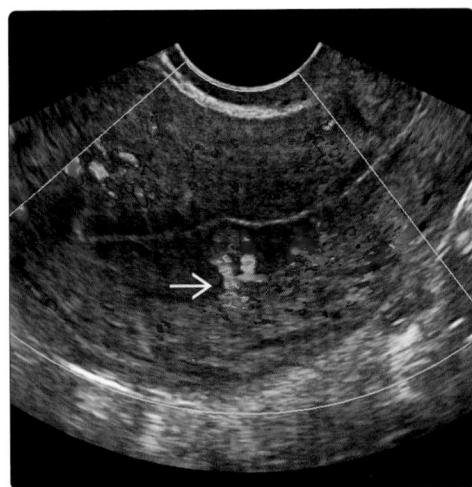

(Left) *Longitudinal transvaginal ultrasound shows a cystic endometrial polyp* ⮕ *with a hyperechoic line sign* ⮩. **(Right)** *Longitudinal transvaginal ultrasound of a patient with postmenopausal bleeding shows that the uterus is retroverted and contains a partially cystic endometrial polyp* ⮕. *This was treated by D&C.*

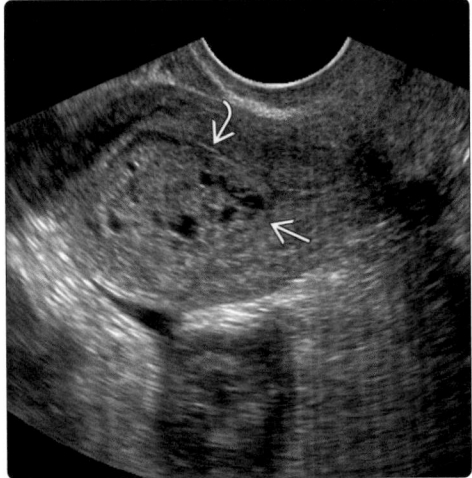
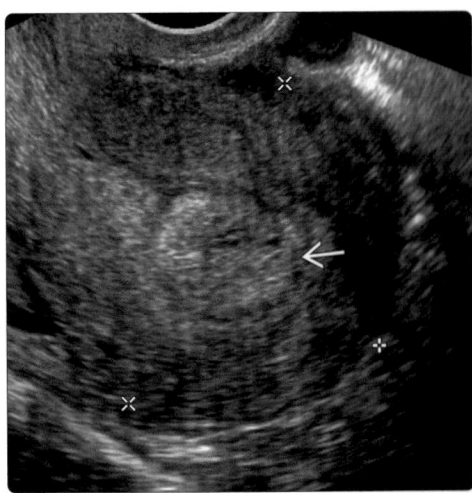

(Left) *Sagittal T2 HASTE MR demonstrates a thickened heterogenous endometrium with lower signal intensity from a polyp* ⮕. *A small cyst in noted in the junctional zone* ⮩ *that is compatible with adenomyosis.* **(Right)** *Post-contrast fat-suppressed sagittal MR confirms the enhancing polyp* ⮕, *which has internal cystic change* ⮩.

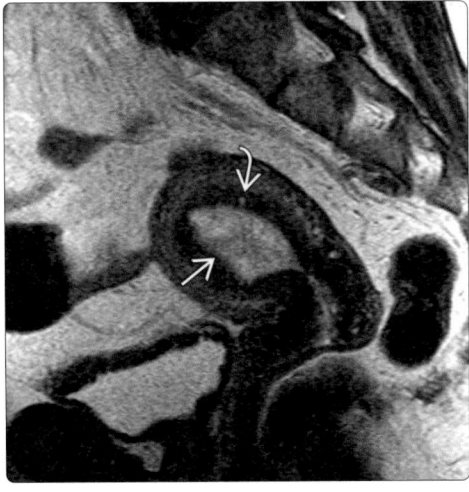
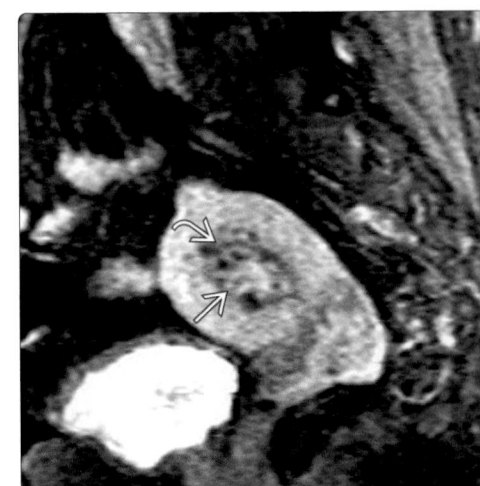

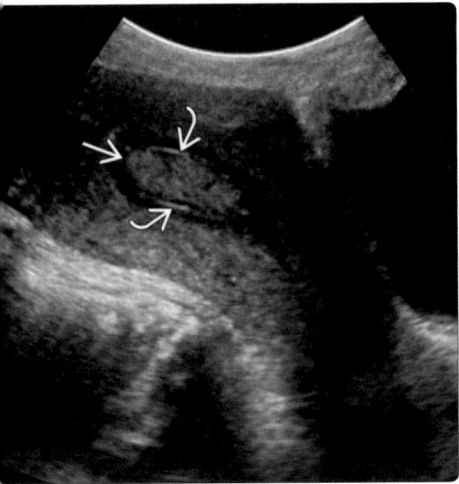

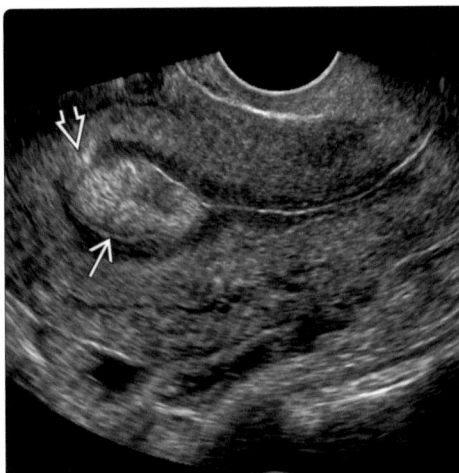

(Left) *Transabdominal pelvic ultrasound in a patient with menorrhagia shows an echogenic endometrial mass ➡ with the echogenic line sign ↗. (Right) Transvaginal pelvic ultrasound in the same patient confirms a large endometrial polyp ➡ attached to the fundus ⇒.*

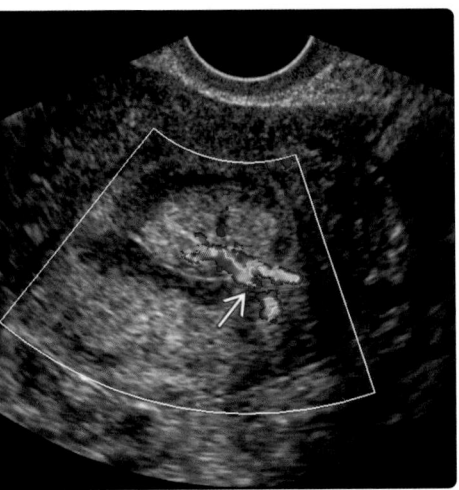

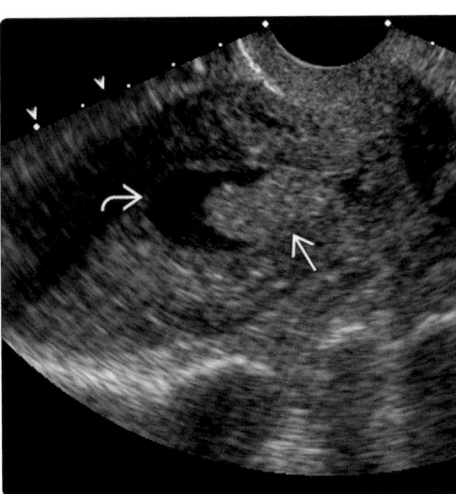

(Left) *Coronal color Doppler ultrasound of the same patient shows the vessels ➡ in the pedicle of the polyp. (Right) Longitudinal ultrasound of a postmenopausal woman with vaginal spotting. There is fluid/blood ➡ within the endometrial cavity outlining a polyp ➡.*

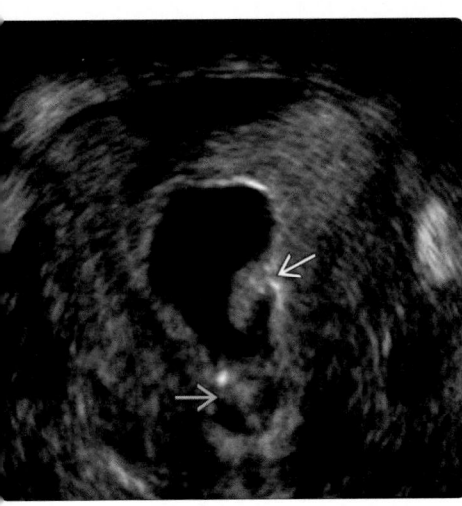

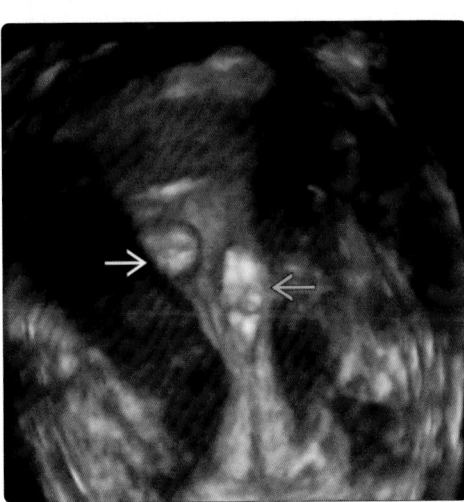

(Left) *Coronal oblique reconstruction of saline infusion sonohysterography (SHG) shows a pedunculated polyp ➡. The endometrium is otherwise normal. A catheter balloon is noted in the lower segment ⊡. (Right) Volume-rendered coronal reconstruction obtained during sonohysterography shows a sessile polyp ➡ and the catheter balloon ⊡.*

Endometrial Carcinoma

TERMINOLOGY

- Malignant proliferation of abnormal endometrial glands

IMAGING

- Mass in endometrial cavity with internal color flow
- Endometrial thickening: Mixed echogenicity more suspicious than homogeneous
- Smooth margins in early stage disease (stage 1A)
- Disruption of subendometrial halo suggests myometrial invasion (stage 1B)
- Multiple feeding vessels

TOP DIFFERENTIAL DIAGNOSES

- Endometrial hyperplasia
- Endometrial polyp
- Submucosal fibroid
- Uterine sarcoma
- Adenomyosis

PATHOLOGY

- Majority are adenocarcinoma, 75% endometrioid type (associated with estrogen stimulation)
- Serous (papillary serous), clear cell types also occur (not associated with estrogen stimulation)

CLINICAL ISSUES

- Postmenopausal women with abnormal vaginal bleeding
- Most common gynecologic malignancy

DIAGNOSTIC CHECKLIST

- Irregularly thickened endometrial echo complex in postmenopausal patient with vaginal bleeding
- Imaging alone cannot differentiate hyperplasia from carcinoma
- > 5 mm bilayer thickness in postmenopausal patient with vaginal bleeding → biopsy
- Transvaginal ultrasound (TVUS) for initial detection
- MR for local staging; CECT for lymphadenopathy, mets

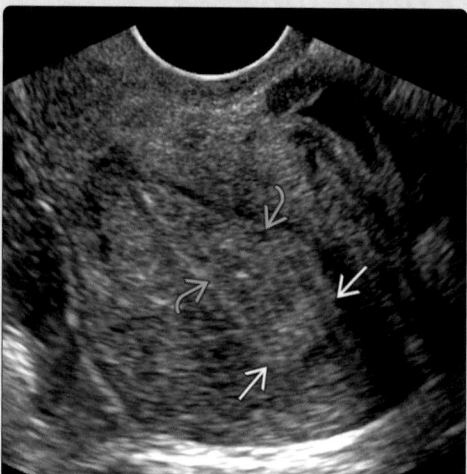
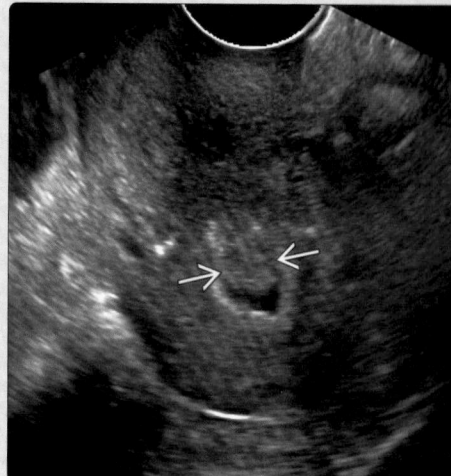

(Left) Longitudinal transvaginal ultrasound in a woman with irregular vaginal bleeding shows a thickened endometrium. The fundal endometrium is echogenic ➡ but with subtle heterogeneity and hypoechogenicity inferiorly ⬈. Biopsy confirmed endometrioid carcinoma. (Right) Longitudinal transvaginal US of a retroverted uterus in a patient with postmenopausal bleeding shows a polypoid mass ➡ distending the uterine cavity. Endocervical curettage confirmed endometrioid carcinoma.

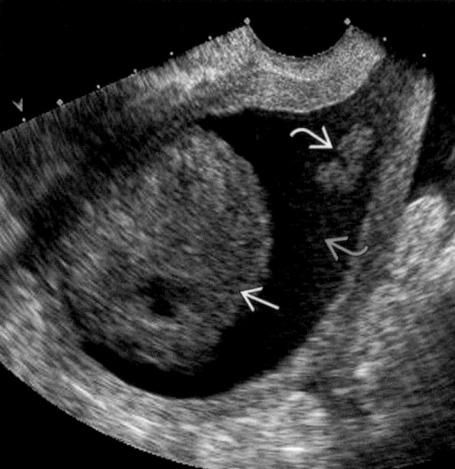
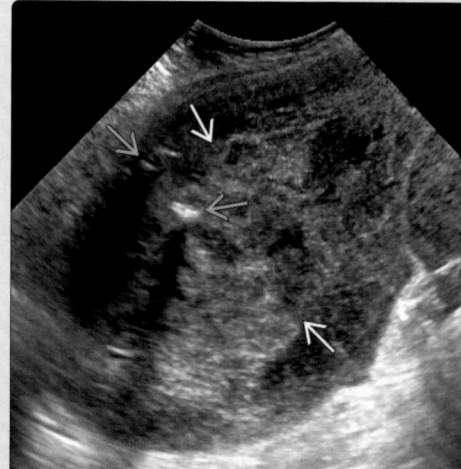

(Left) Longitudinal transvaginal US shows a large polypoid mass ➡ within the endometrial cavity, with an additional smaller inferior mass ⬈, the latter leading to obstructive hematometros ⬈. Pathology revealed carcinosarcoma. (Right) Transabdominal ultrasound shows an internally heterogeneous mixed echogenicity mass ➡ expanding the uterine cavity, with poorly defined margins and internal calcifications ⬈. Pathology confirmed endometrial sarcoma.

Endometrial Carcinoma

TERMINOLOGY

Abbreviations

Endometrial carcinoma (EC)

Definitions

Malignant proliferation of abnormal endometrial glands

IMAGING

General Features

- Best diagnostic clue
  - Mass in endometrial cavity with internal color flow
  - Irregularly thickened endometrial echo complex in postmenopausal patient with vaginal bleeding
- Location
  - Can invade myometrium, cervix, parametrial structures
- Morphology
  - Polypoid masses or diffuse endometrial thickening

Ultrasonographic Findings

Grayscale ultrasound
- Thickened endometrium
  - Focal thickening more concerning than diffuse
  - Areas of mixed echogenicity more suspicious than homogeneous hyperechogenicity
- Endometrial-myometrial interface
  - Smooth margins in early stage disease (stage 1A)
  - Disruption of subendometrial halo suggests myometrial invasion (stage 1B)
- Hematometros if obstruction of uterine cavity or cervix
Pulsed Doppler
- Not specific: Significant overlap with benign etiologies
- Color Doppler
  - Multiple feeding vessels

CT Findings

- Focal or diffuse endometrial thickening
- Centrally located uterine mass hypoenhancing to myometrium
- Useful for assessment of lymphadenopathy and metastases
  - Limited in early disease detection and in local staging

MR Findings

- T1WI
  - Hypo- or isointense to normal endometrium/myometrium
  - Hematometros is hyperintense
- T2WI
  - Hypo- or isointense to normal endometrium
  - Intact junctional zone excludes deep myometrial invasion
- DWI
  - Restricted diffusion in tumor and lymphadenopathy
- T1WI C+
  - Hypoenhancing relative to myometrium in early and equilibrium phase
  - Myometrial invasion: Hypoenhancing tissue extending through junctional zone
  - Distinguish enhancing tumor from nonenhancing endometrial blood
- Loss of zonal anatomy is potential pitfall in postmenopausal women, those on tamoxifen therapy

Nuclear Medicine Findings

- F-18 FDG PET is useful for detecting metastases, surveillance for recurrence

Imaging Recommendations

- Best imaging tool
  - Transvaginal sonography (TVS) for initial detection
  - High resolution T2WI and C+ MR for local staging
  - CECT or MR (contrast enhanced and diffusion weighted) to evaluate for lymphadenopathy, metastatic disease
- Protocol advice
  - Must see entire endometrium
    - Measure on sagittal section of uterus at widest point
    - Exclude hypoechoic inner myometrium in measurement
    - Exclude endometrial cavity fluid from measurement
  - If inadequate TVS (5-10%) → additional evaluation with sonohysterography (SHG) or MR
  - In postmenopausal women bilayer thickness > 5 mm merits biopsy
  - Saline-infusion sonohysterography (SHG) useful in triage
    - Diffuse thickening: Blind endometrial biopsy
    - Focal thickening: Hysteroscopic biopsy necessary to ensure sampling of abnormal area

DIFFERENTIAL DIAGNOSIS

Endometrial Hyperplasia

- Imaging cannot differentiate hyperplasia from carcinoma, particularly stage 1A
- More likely homogeneous thickening

Endometrial Polyp

- More likely to be focal oval or fusiform mass than diffuse thickening
- Look for single feeding vessel in fibrovascular stalk
- Internal cystic components more likely than in carcinoma

Submucosal Fibroid

- Hypoechoic mass/masses in cavity
- Mass arises from myometrium, displaces but does not expand endometrium
- SHG: "Rind" of endometrium covers fibroid surface

Uterine Sarcoma

- Usually larger, heterogeneous, more aggressive
- Much less common than uterine carcinoma

Adenomyosis

- Based in myometrium, can mimic stage 1B carcinoma with extension into myometrium
- Myometrial/subendometrial cysts
- Bulky uterus with areas of acoustic shadowing

PATHOLOGY

General Features

- Etiology
  - Risk factors
    - Obesity, diabetes, hypertension, chronic anovulation
    - Polycystic ovarian syndrome: Controversial causative association vs. 2 diseases with similar risk factors
    - Prior pelvic radiation

- o Atypical hyperplasia
  - – Confers 25% risk of developing endometrial cancer
  - – Hyperplasia without atypia → 2% risk
- o Endometrioid subtypes: Unopposed estrogen stimulation
  - – Hormone replacement therapy without progestins
  - – Early menarche and late menopause
  - – Tamoxifen
  - – Estrogen-secreting tumors
- Genetics
  - o *P53* suppressor gene: Nonendometrioid subtypes
    - – More common in African American women, associated with poorer outcomes
  - o Hereditary nonpolyposis colorectal cancer syndrome (HNPCC) (Lynch syndrome)
  - o PTEN-hamartoma tumor syndrome (Cowden syndrome)
    - – More common in Caucasian women, associated with better outcomes
  - o Peutz-Jeghers syndrome (PJS)

Staging, Grading, & Classification

- Stage I: Confined to uterus
- Stage II: Spread to involve cervix but not beyond uterus
- Stage III: Spread beyond uterus confined to true pelvis
- Stage IV: Disseminated metastases or bladder/bowel involvement

Microscopic Features

- Majority are adenocarcinoma, 75% endometrioid type (associated with estrogen stimulation)
- Serous (papillary serous), clear cell types also occur (not associated with estrogen stimulation)
  - o Older patients, more aggressive behavior
  - o Serous type invades lymphovascular spaces → metastasizes without invasion of deep myometrium

CLINICAL ISSUES

Presentation

- Most common signs/symptoms
  - o Abnormal bleeding in 90%
- Other signs/symptoms
  - o Endometrial cells on Papanicolaou smear
  - o Symptoms related to metastases in advanced disease
- Clinical profile
  - o Postmenopausal women with abnormal vaginal bleeding

Demographics

- Age
  - o Most common in 50-65-year-old age group
    - – 75% postmenopausal, 25% premenopausal
- Epidemiology
  - o Most common gynecologic malignancy
  - o 4th most common cancer in women
  - o Western affluent societies, least common in India/Southeast Asia

Natural History & Prognosis

- Depends on stage at diagnosis
  - o Stage I or II: 5-year survival 96%
  - o Stage III: 5-year survival 63%
  - o Stage IV: 5-year survival 8%

- African American woman tend to have worse outcome than Caucasian women
  - o Mortality rates 1.8x greater
  - o Higher stage at diagnosis
  - o More aggressive types (papillary serous, clear cell)

Treatment

- Stage dependent
  - o Stage I or II: Surgical ± radiation therapy (XRT)
  - o Stage III: Combined surgery, XRT
  - o Stage IV: Combined surgery, chemotherapy, XRT
- Surgery
  - o Hysterectomy, bilateral salpingo-oophorectomy, lymphadenectomy
  - o Surgical staging vital as imaging misses microscopic disease

DIAGNOSTIC CHECKLIST

Consider

- Endometrial cancer is most serious cause of PMB
  - o 10% of women with PMB will have endometrial cancer
  - o Other etiologies include hyperplasia, polyps, atrophy, or fibroids
- TV US is good test to detect EC
  - o Use of 5 mm bilayer thickness as threshold for intervention will detect 96% of EC
  - o Safe to use TV US as initial diagnostic test
    - – Better tolerated than endometrial biopsy
  - o Normal endometrium with bilayer thickness < 5 mm
    - – Negative test for endometrial cancer
    - – Obviates need for additional testing in patient with PMB and nondiagnostic office biopsy

Image Interpretation Pearls

- Imaging alone cannot differentiate hyperplasia from carcinoma
- Cancer may arise within endometrial polyp

SELECTED REFERENCES

1. Kabil Kucur S et al: Role of endometrial power Doppler ultrasound using the international endometrial tumor analysis group classification in predicting intrauterine pathology. Arch Gynecol Obstet. 288(3):649-54, 2013
2. Breijer MC et al: Capacity of endometrial thickness measurement to diagnose endometrial carcinoma in asymptomatic postmenopausal women: a systematic review and meta-analysis. Ultrasound Obstet Gynecol. 40(6):621-9, 2012
3. Van den Bosch T et al: Pre-sampling ultrasound evaluation and assessment of the tissue yield during sampling improves the diagnostic reliability of office endometrial biopsy. J Obstet Gynaecol. 32(2):173-6, 2012
4. Jacobs I et al: Sensitivity of transvaginal ultrasound screening for endometrial cancer in postmenopausal women: a case-control study within the UKCTOCS cohort. Lancet Oncol. 12(1):38-48, 2011
5. Menzies R et al: Significance of abnormal sonographic findings in postmenopausal women with and without bleeding. J Obstet Gynaecol Can. 33(9):944-51, 2011
6. Odeh M et al: Three-dimensional endometrial volume and 3-dimensional power Doppler analysis in predicting endometrial carcinoma and hyperplasia. Gynecol Oncol. 106(2):348-53, 2007
7. Barwick TD et al: Imaging of endometrial adenocarcinoma. Clin Radiol. 61(7):545-55, 2006
8. Messiou C et al: MR staging of endometrial carcinoma. Clin Radiol. 61(10):822-32, 2006

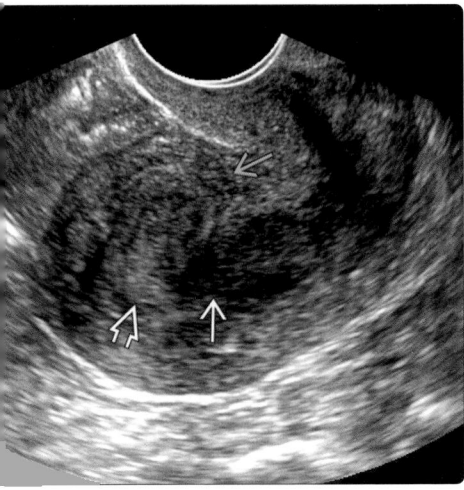
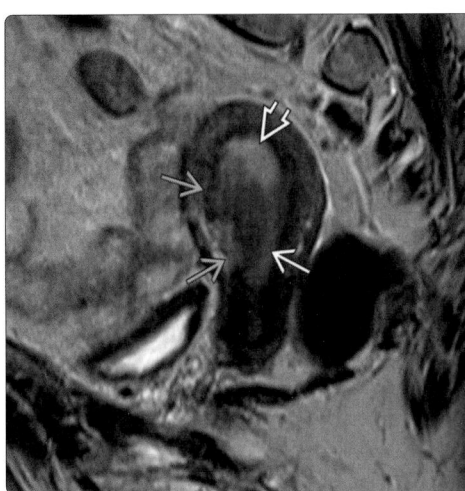

(Left) *Longitudinal transvaginal ultrasound shows a heterogeneous hypoechoic mass ➡ distending the uterine cavity. The anterior myometrial border ➡ is indistinct, suggesting invasion. A small amount of echogenic endometrium is visible ➡.* (Right) *Sagittal T2-weighted MR in the same patient shows hypointense tumor ➡, hyperintense endometrium ➡, and disruption of the anterior junctional zone ➡ consistent with myometrial invasion. Pathology revealed endometrioid and papillary features.*

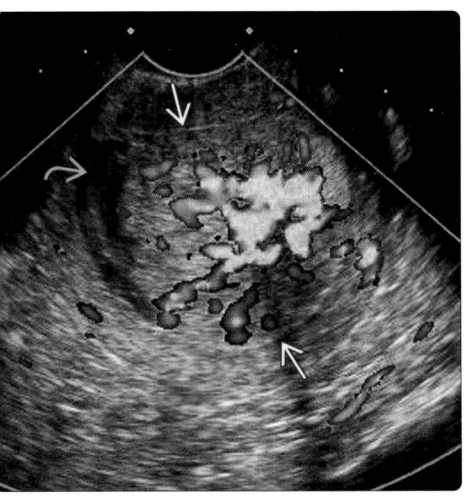
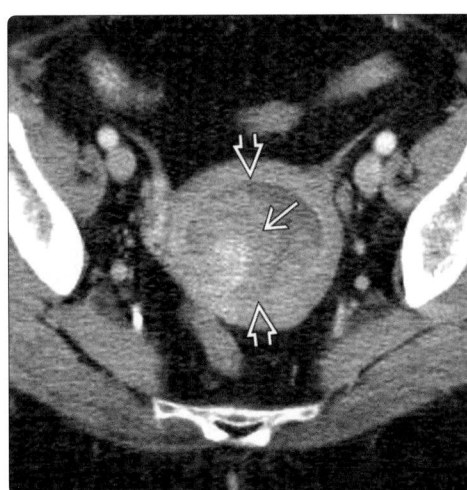

(Left) *Transverse transvaginal color Doppler US shows a highly vascular echogenic mass distending the endometrial cavity ➡, which pathology revealed endometrioid-type carcinoma. Myometrial invasion was not identified on the ultrasound. There is minimal hematometros ➡.* (Right) *Transverse CT in the same patient shows the enhancing endometrial mass ➡ within the expanded endometrial cavity ➡. No lymphadenopathy was identified.*

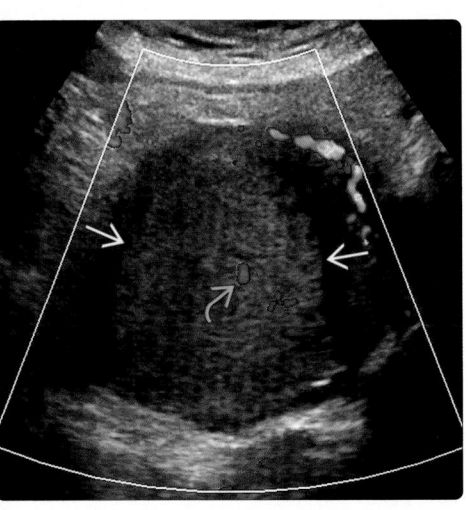
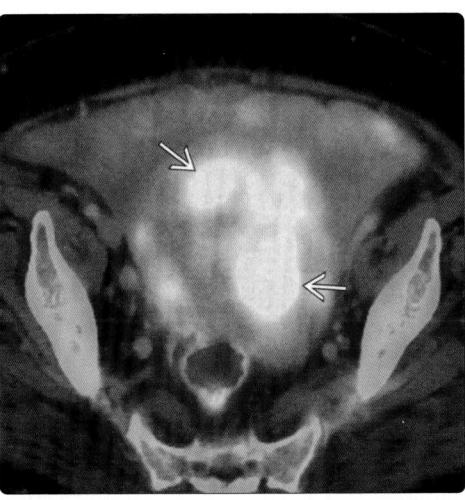

(Left) *Transverse transabdominal color Doppler US in a postmenopausal patient who presented with abdominal distention shows a large echogenic mass ➡ distending the uterine cavity, with minimal internal flow ➡. Pap smear and biopsy were consistent with clear cell carcinoma.* (Right) *Fused axial FDG PET/CT in the same patient reveals significant metabolic activity within the uterine mass ➡. Peritoneal metastases were also discovered (not shown).*

Endometritis

TERMINOLOGY

- Polymicrobial infection resulting from ascending spread of organisms from cervix into uterus

IMAGING

- Findings often normal or nonspecific
  - Endometrial gas and fluid in a patient with postpartum fever and pelvic pain
  - Thickened, heterogeneous endometrium
- Imaging usually ordered to look for complications: Pyometrium, abscess, retained products of conception (RPOC)

TOP DIFFERENTIAL DIAGNOSES

- RPOC
- Intrauterine blood/clot
- Asymptomatic postpartum endometrial gas
- Endometrial calcifications
- Other causes of postpartum fever

PATHOLOGY

- Generally caused by ascending spread of organisms through cervix or incision site into uterus

CLINICAL ISSUES

- Fever and pain in postpartum period (most common)
  - More common following cesarean section than vaginal delivery
- Occasionally associated with pelvic inflammatory disease (PID) in nonobstetric patient
- Rarely leads to development of pelvic septic thrombophlebitis

DIAGNOSTIC CHECKLIST

- Endometritis is predominantly a clinical diagnosis
- In appropriate clinical setting (postpartum fever and pain) the presence of endometrial fluid and bubbles is highly suggestive of endometritis

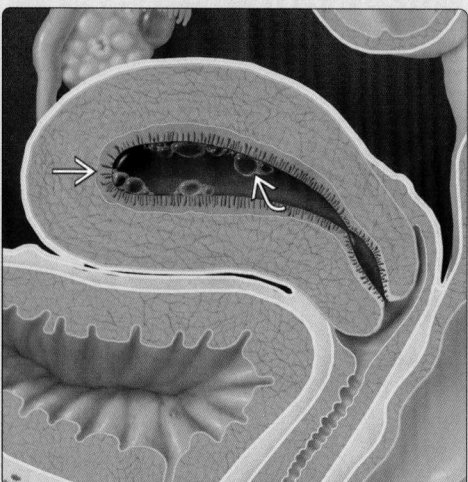
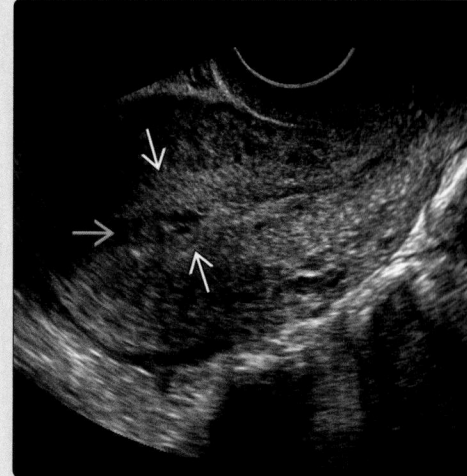

(Left) Graphic shows findings in endometritis including hyperemia of the endometrium ➡, with associated fluid and gas bubbles ➡ in the endometrial cavity. (Right) Longitudinal transvaginal ultrasound shows nonspecific endometrial thickening ➡ and fluid ➡ in this patient with clinical endometritis, evidenced by vaginal discharge and pelvic pain.

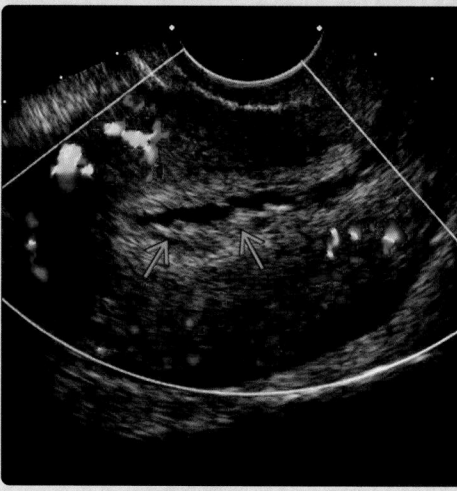
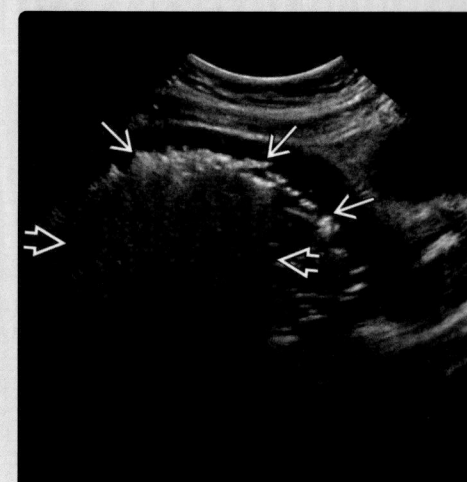

(Left) Longitudinal transvaginal ultrasound with color Doppler shows fluid and debris ➡ within the endometrial cavity in a patient with clinical endometritis following D&C. (Right) Transabdominal longitudinal ultrasound shows extensive gas within the uterus, visible as echogenic foci ➡ with heterogeneous posterior shadowing ➡ "dirty shadowing." The patient presented with pelvic pain and vaginal discharge following recent fibroid embolization.

TERMINOLOGY

Synonyms

Endometrial infection

Definitions

Polymicrobial infection resulting from ascending spread of organisms from cervix into uterus

IMAGING

General Features

Best diagnostic clue
o Endometrial gas and fluid in patient with postpartum fever and pelvic pain

Primarily clinical diagnosis
o Often no imaging findings in uncomplicated endometritis
o Primary role of imaging is to evaluate for complications

Ultrasonographic Findings

Pain may limit ability to perform transvaginal examination

Endometrium may appear normal

Findings often nonspecific
o Thickened, heterogeneous endometrium
o Endometrial fluid
o Fluid in cul-de-sac

Hyperechoic foci within endometrial cavity ± shadowing
o Intracavitary gas, inflammatory debris
 – Gas bubbles alone are not diagnostic
 – Endometrial gas is a normal finding for up to 3 weeks postpartum and is present in up to 21% of healthy patients
o Large amount of echogenic fluid suspicious for pyometra

Color Doppler
o May see increased flow, but not always present
o Lack of ↑ flow does not rule out endometritis

Findings overlap with retained products of conception (RPOC)
o RPOC is a risk factor for developing endometritis
o Patients may have both RPOC and endometritis

If associated with pelvic inflammatory disease (PID), may see tubo-ovarian abscess

CT Findings

Nonspecific, most useful for complications (abscess) or alternative diagnosis

Uterine enlargement, heterogeneous density

Distended endometrial cavity
o May see air-fluid or fluid-fluid level (pus, hematoma)

Inflammatory changes around uterus better seen than with ultrasound

MR Findings

T1WI: Low signal uterus and endometrial fluid

T2WI: Myometrium increased in signal intensity with loss of junctional zone

Intense enhancement with gadolinium

Imaging Recommendations

Best imaging tool
o Transvaginal ultrasound

Protocol advice
o Always use color Doppler to evaluate for possible RPOC
o Thorough scan of adnexa to look for parametrial or tubo-ovarian abscess

DIFFERENTIAL DIAGNOSIS

Retained Products of Conception

- Echogenic endometrial mass
- Significant overlap in findings with endometritis
- High-velocity, low-resistance flow
  o Not always present
- Presents with postpartum bleeding
  o Simple RPOC should not have fever, ↑ white count
- May have RPOC with superimposed infection

Intrauterine Blood/Clot

- Seen in up to 24% of asymptomatic postpartum patients
- May also be seen with endometritis
- Should not have fever, ↑ white count
- Changes rapidly with resolution on follow-up scans

Asymptomatic Postpartum Endometrial Gas

- Seen in up to 21% of healthy patients in postpartum period
- May be present up to 3 weeks postpartum
- Should not have fever, ↑ white count

Endometrial Calcifications

- Incidental finding in asymptomatic patient
- Curvilinear calcifications along endometrium
- Often history of prior instrumentation (D&C)

Other Causes of Postpartum Fever

- Ovarian vein thrombosis
- Atelectasis
- Pneumonia
- Pyelonephritis
- Appendicitis

PATHOLOGY

General Features

- Etiology
  o Generally caused by ascending spread of organisms through cervix or incision site into uterus
   – May extend to involve myometrium and parametrium
  o More common following cesarean section than vaginal delivery
  o May progress from chorioamnionitis
  o Monomicrobial infection may occur in first 24-36 hours
   – Group B Streptococcus
  o Most infections are polymicrobial
   – Both aerobic and anaerobic
   – Occurs in first 48 hr
  o Common causative agents
   – Vaginal flora, including those associated with bacterial vaginosis
   – Neisseria gonorrhoeae
   – Enterococcus
   – Chlamydia and tuberculosis often seen in chronic endometritis
   – Etiologic agent(s) often never identified

CLINICAL ISSUES

Presentation

- Most common signs/symptoms
  - Fever (> 100.4° F) within 36 hours following delivery
  - Pelvic/abdominal pain
  - Uterine tenderness on physical exam and during ultrasound
  - ↑ white blood cell count
- Other signs/symptoms
  - Malodorous lochia
  - Vaginal bleeding
  - Vaginal discharge
  - Tachycardia
- Clinical profile
  - Endometritis occurs in 2 clinical settings
    - Fever and pain in postpartum period (most common)
    - Associated with PID in nonobstetric patient

Demographics

- Epidemiology
  - Most common cause of postpartum fever
  - Occurs in 1-3% of vaginal deliveries
  - Much more common following cesarean section (15-20%)
    - Prophylactic antibiotics highly effective in reducing risk of endometritis after cesarean section
    - 50-60% of women undergoing cesarean section without antibiotics will develop endometritis
  - Risk factors in obstetric patients
    - Cesarean section
    - Preexisting lower genital tract infection
    - Prolonged labor
    - Prolonged rupture of membranes
    - RPOC
    - Retained clots
  - Risk factors in nonobstetric patients
    - 70-90% of patients with PID have coexistent endometritis
    - May also occur after invasive gynecologic procedure
    - Intrauterine device
  - Uterine artery embolization
    - Both infectious and noninfectious endometritis reported in 0.5% of cases after uterine artery embolization
  - Chronic endometritis may occur
    - Associated with RPOC in obstetric population
    - In nonobstetric population associated with intrauterine device

Natural History & Prognosis

- Cure rates approach 95% with appropriate therapy
- May extend to myometrium/parametrium if untreated or if caused by drug-resistant organisms
  - Potential complications include pyometrium and pelvic abscess
- Rarely leads to development of pelvic septic thrombophlebitis
  - 1-2% of cases of endometritis
  - Associated with parametrial spread of infection

Treatment

- Parenteral broad spectrum antibiotics
  - 90-95% defervesce with 48-72 hr
  - Therapy continued until patient is afebrile for 24-48 hr and white blood cell count returns to normal
- Persistent fever
  - Resistant organism → triple antibiotic therapy
  - Abscess → surgical or percutaneous drainage
- RPOC, uterine hematoma → evacuation
- Septic thrombophlebitis → anticoagulation in addition to antibiotics

DIAGNOSTIC CHECKLIST

Consider

- Endometritis is predominantly a clinical diagnosis
  - Imaging findings frequently normal in uncomplicated endometritis
- Imaging usually ordered to look for complications
  - Pyometrium
  - Abscess
  - RPOC

Image Interpretation Pearls

- In appropriate clinical setting (postpartum fever and pain) the presence of endometrial fluid and bubbles is highly suggestive of endometritis
- Conversely, endometrial gas in asymptomatic postpartum patient is likely normal

SELECTED REFERENCES

1. Plunk M et al: Imaging of postpartum complications: a multimodality review AJR Am J Roentgenol. 200(2):W143-54, 2013
2. Cicchiello LA et al: Ultrasound evaluation of gynecologic causes of pelvic pain. Obstet Gynecol Clin North Am. 38(1):85-114, viii, 2011
3. Müngen E et al: Postabortion Doppler evaluation of the uterus: incidence and causes of myometrial hypervascularity. J Ultrasound Med. 28(8):1053-60, 2009
4. Vandermeer FQ et al: Imaging of acute pelvic pain. Clin Obstet Gynecol. 52(1):2-20, 2009
5. Rufener SL et al: Sonography of uterine abnormalities in postpartum and postabortion patients: a potential pitfall of interpretation. J Ultrasound Med. 27(3):343-8, 2008
6. Faro S: Postpartum endometritis. Clin Perinatol. 32(3):803-14, 2005
7. Ledger WJ: Post-partum endomyometritis diagnosis and treatment: a review. J Obstet Gynaecol Res. 29(6):364-73, 2003
8. Savelli L et al: Transvaginal sonographic appearance of anaerobic endometritis. Ultrasound Obstet Gynecol. 21(6):624-5, 2003
9. Eckert LO et al: Endometritis: the clinical-pathologic syndrome. Am J Obstet Gynecol. 186(4):690-5, 2002

Endometritis

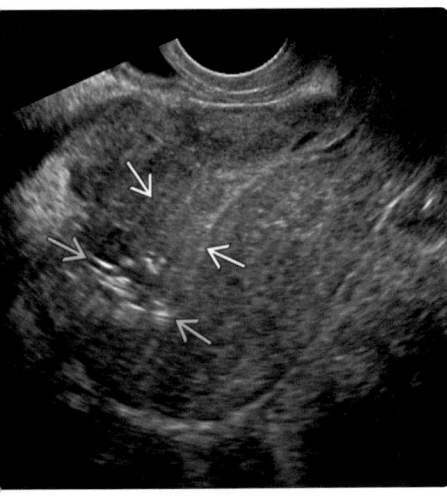
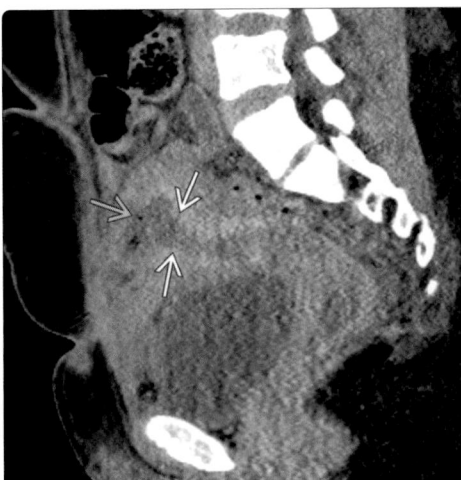

(Left) Longitudinal transvaginal ultrasound shows endometrial thickening ➡ and scattered foci of gas ⇨ in a patient following recent cesarean section 3 weeks earlier. (Right) Sagittal unenhanced CT in the same patient demonstrates the low-density thickened endometrium ➡ with a scattered foci of gas ⇨.

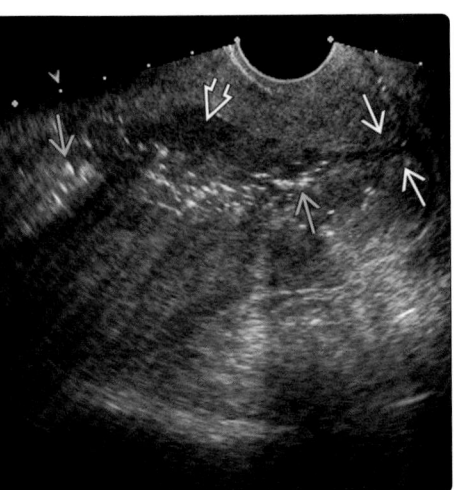
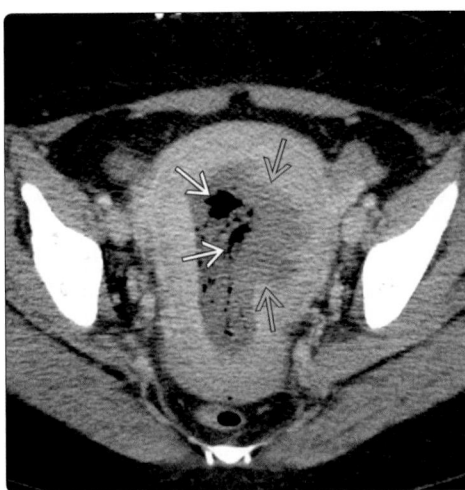

(Left) Longitudinal transvaginal ultrasound shows extensive gas ⇨ and heterogeneous material ➡ in the endometrial cavity; consistent with pyometrium, extending to the cervical os ➡. The patient presented with foul-smelling vaginal discharge and pelvic pain, with no history of recent pregnancy or instrumentation. (Right) Axial unenhanced CT in the same patient shows the endometrial gas ➡ as well as extension into the myometrium ⇨.

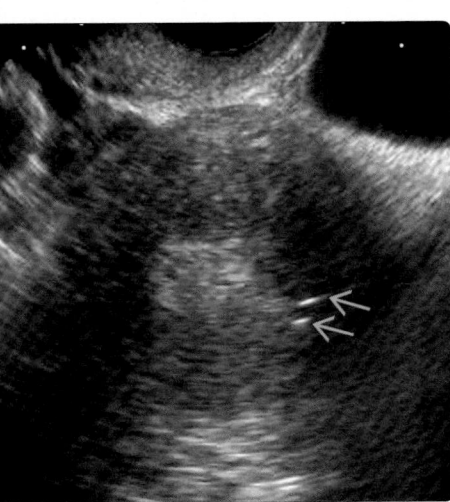
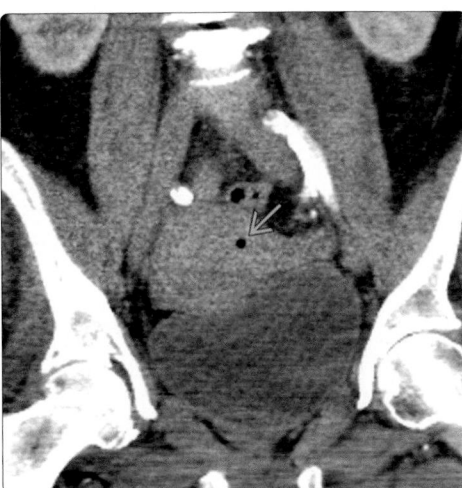

(Left) Transverse endovaginal ultrasound shows only subtle gas ⇨ in the left cornua region in this patient with pelvic pain and vaginal discharge, which is consistent with clinical endometritis. (Right) Coronal unenhanced CT in the same patient more clearly demonstrates the focus of gas ⇨ in the left fundal region.

KEY FACTS

TERMINOLOGY

- 2 types of IUDs in United States
  - Copper-containing
  - Levonorgestrel-releasing
- Device inserted into endometrial cavity to prevent pregnancy
- T-shaped polyethylene frame with polyethylene monofilament string

IMAGING

- US
  - IUD stem is linear bright echo aligned with endometrial cavity
  - If difficult to visualize, look for shadowing
  - ≤ 3 mm between top of IUD and fundal endometrium
  - Arms/cross bars extend laterally at fundus
- Radiography
  - KUB helps to differentiate IUD expulsion from perforation

- Image from diaphragm to pelvis
- Differentiates expulsion from perforation when IUD is not seen in uterus on US
- CT: May be helpful in select cases to evaluate for complications related to perforation and intraabdominal IUD
- Perforation
  - IUD above pelvic brim, far lateral, or anterior/posterior

CLINICAL ISSUES

- Complications
  - Displacement (25%)
  - Embedment (18%)
  - Uterine expulsion (10%)
  - Complete perforation (0.1%)

DIAGNOSTIC CHECKLIST

- Entire IUD should be visualized within endometrial cavity with arms in appropriate orientation

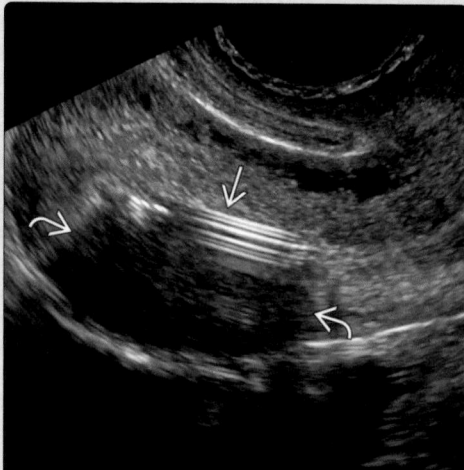
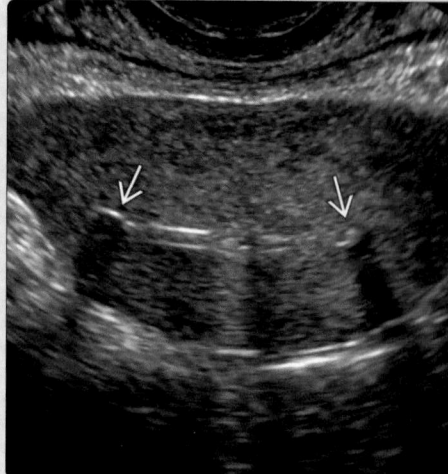

(Left) *Longitudinal endovaginal US shows the typical appearance of well positioned IUD stem* ➡ *as an area of reverberation and posterior acoustic shadowing* ➡. (Right) *Transverse US in the same patient shows normal position of arms/cross bars* ➡ *extending laterally along the endometrial cavity at the fundus pointing towards the cornua. Note shadowing at the ends that are typical of the levonorgestrel-releasing IUD.*

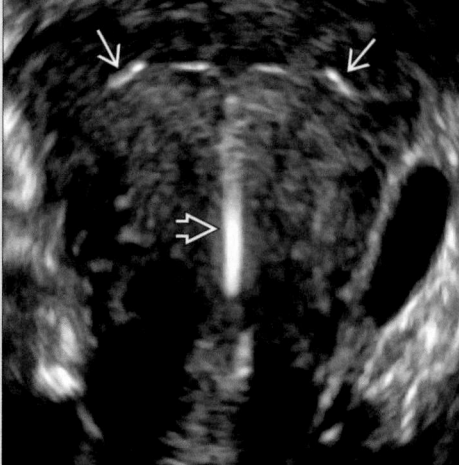
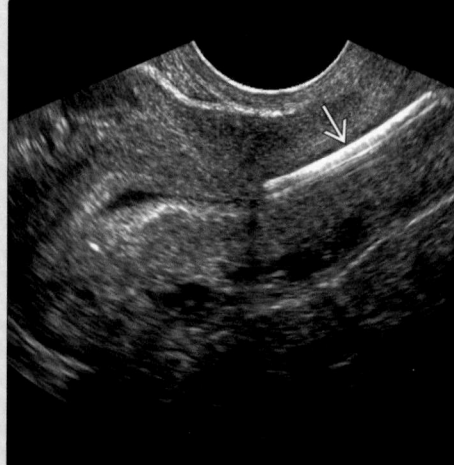

(Left) *3D MPR US shows an IUD in its entirety in the appropriate position, with the stem* ➡ *positioned longitudinally along the canal, the arms* ➡ *pointing towards the cornua, and the proximal end ≤ 3mm from the fundal endometrium.* (Right) *Longitudinal endovaginal US shows an abnormally low IUD* ➡ *in the lower uterine segment extending into the cervix. Note the echogenic signature that is typical of a copper IUD.*

TERMINOLOGY

Abbreviations

Intrauterine device (IUD)
Levonorgestrel-releasing intrauterine system (LNG-IUS)

Definitions

IUD
- Device inserted into endometrial cavity to prevent pregnancy
- T-shaped polyethylene frame with polyethylene monofilament string
- 2 types of IUDs in United States
  - Copper-containing (Paragard, Ortho-McNeil Pharmaceutical, Inc., Raritan, NJ)
    - Copper wire wrapped around stem
  - Levonorgestrel-releasing (Mirena, Shering, AG Pharmaceutical, Germany)
    - Levonorgestrel-containing collar around stem
- Other IUDs
  - Plastic IUDs and Lippes loop IUD (older)
  - Round IUD of stainless steel ring in fundus with straight shaft in lower endometrium (commonly used in China)
- Mechanism of action: Primarily prevents fertilization
  - Also has spermicidal effects and implantation inhibiting effects
  - Partially inhibit ovulation (Mirena only)
  - Copper devices ↑ copper levels → change in cervical mucus, affecting sperm motility and irritating endometrium

IMAGING

General Features

US
- Longitudinal image
  - IUD stem is straight and aligned with endometrial cavity
  - ≤ 3 mm between top of IUD and fundal endometrium
  - Copper IUD is echogenic and easily seen as linear bright echo
  - Levonorgestrel-containing IUD is harder to see, often seen as shadowing between echogenic proximal and distal ends
- Transverse image
  - IUD arms/cross bars extend laterally at fundus towards cornua
- String may be seen as linear bright echo or reverberation in cervix

Radiography
- Radiopaque: Image from diaphragm to pelvis
- Differentiates expulsion from perforation when IUD is not seen in uterus on US
- Perforation
  - IUD above pelvic brim, far lateral, or anterior/posterior
  - 90° or 180° rotation of IUD is less specific

CT: May be helpful in select cases to evaluate for complications related to perforation and intraabdominal IUD

- MR: IUD can be seen as signal void but should not be used primarily to evaluate position

Imaging Recommendations

- Best imaging tool
  - Transvaginal ultrasound for IUD position
  - KUB for IUD expulsion/perforation
- Protocol advice
  - Ultrasound for IUD
    - If IUD is difficult to visualize sonographically, look for shadowing
    - Posterior shadowing best visualized when scanning perpendicular to long axis of IUD
    - 3D sonography helpful for diagnosis of embedment and displacement
    - 3D is helpful for reconstructing true coronal imaging of uterus

CLINICAL ISSUES

Presentation

- IUD
  - Pain and abnormal bleeding is common within 1st few months of placement
  - Indications for imaging
    - String not visualized on exam
    - Prolonged pain/dyspareunia
      - Malpositioned or perforated
    - Irregular menses/dysmenorrhea
    - Infection
- IUD complications
  - Displacement (25%)
    - Low IUDs may spontaneously migrate into more appropriate position
  - Uterine expulsion (10%)
    - Confirm expulsion with KUB
  - Embedment (18%)
    - IUD penetrates endometrium into myometrium without extension through uterine serosa
  - Complete perforation (0.1%)
    - IUD penetrates through uterine serosa and is partially or completely in peritoneal cavity

Demographics

- Epidemiology
  - IUDs are most common method of reversible contraception worldwide
    - Used by 23%
  - Less common in US
    - Used by 7.7%
  - Synchronous pregnancy
    - 2/100 women per year of IUD use

SELECTED REFERENCES

1. Boortz HE et al: Migration of intrauterine devices: radiologic findings and implications for patient care. Radiographics. 32(2):335-52, 2012
2. Benacerraf BR et al: Three-dimensional ultrasound detection of abnormally located intrauterine contraceptive devices which are a source of pelvic pain and abnormal bleeding. Ultrasound Obstet Gynecol. 34(1):110-5, 2009

(Left) *Longitudinal endovaginal US of the cervix shows a linear echogenic line ➡ in the cervical canal with reverberation. This is the normally positioned string of the IUD, which may be seen and should not be confused with abnormal position of the device.* (Right) *Coronal 3D US shows a malpositioned copper IUD in the lower uterine segment and cervix with arms extending into the myometrium ➡.*

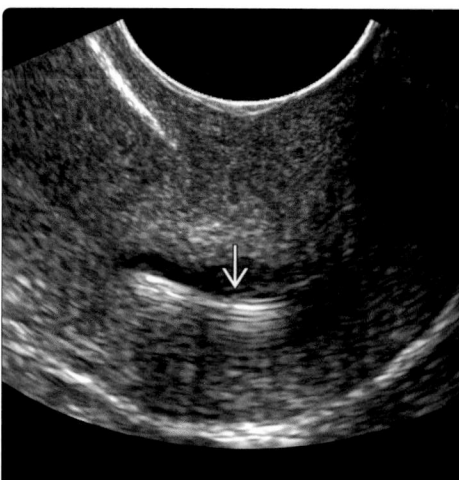
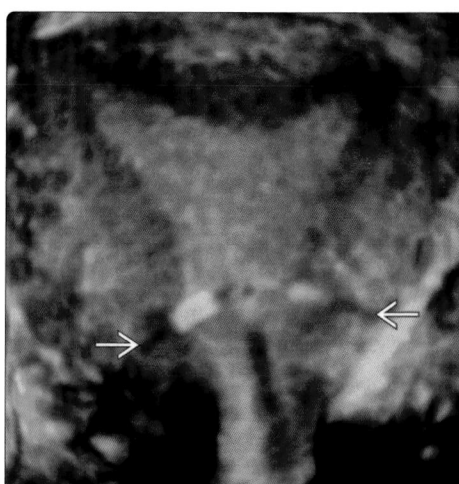

(Left) *Longitudinal endovaginal US in a 28-year-old patient with a missing IUD string and pelvic pain shows an empty endometrial cavity with no IUD.* (Right) *Longitudinal endovaginal US of the left adnexa in the same patient shows echogenic linear structure representing the IUD stem ➡ adjacent to the left ovary ➡.*

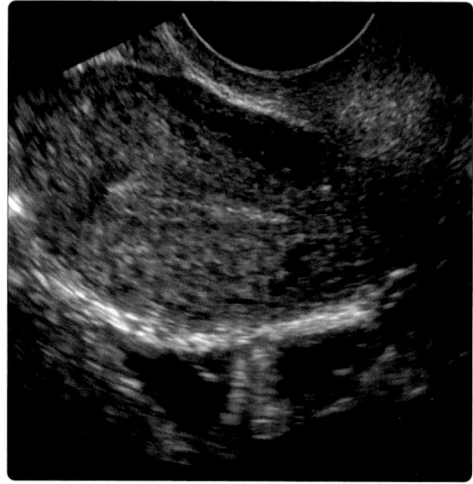
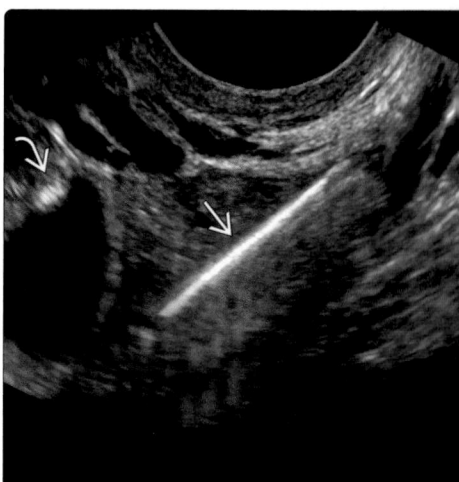

(Left) *Abdominal radiograph in the same patient confirms a perforated IUD ➡ in the left adnexa. Note the position of the IUD is too far lateral and too high above the pelvic brim.* (Right) *Intraoperative photograph looking caudal obtained during laparoscopy in the same patient shows forceps grasping the copper IUD in the left adnexa. Note healed perforation site on posterior uterine body ➡ and inflamed broad ligament ➡.*

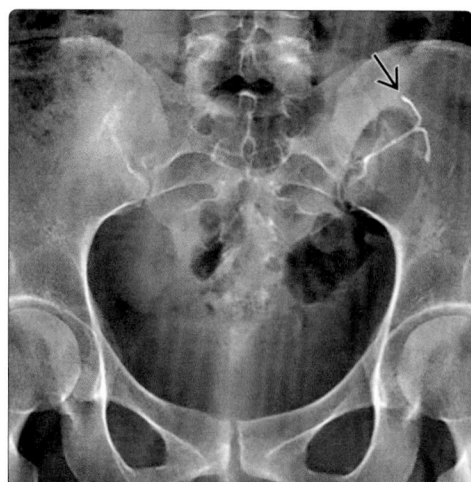
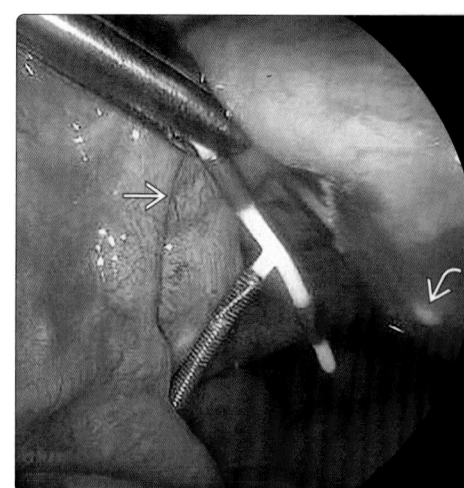

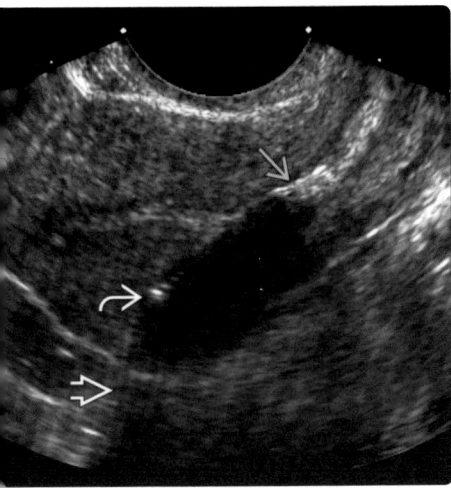

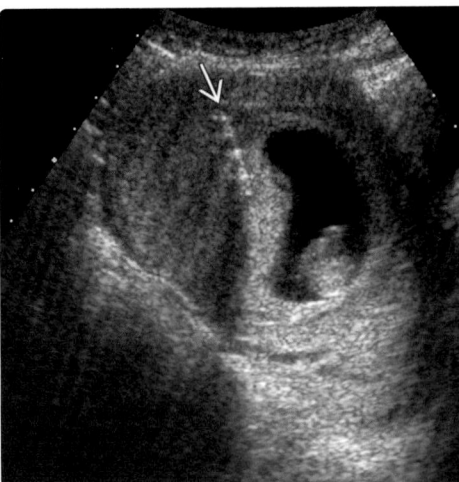

(Left) *Longitudinal endovaginal US shows an IUD* ➡ *penetrating the posterior uterine body myometrium with only the distal stem* ➡ *remaining intracavitary. Shadowing* ➡ *from the IUD may help to identify its location when the stem is not well visualized.* (Right) *Transabdominal US shows an IUD* ➡ *present in the endometrial canal with synchronous early intrauterine pregnancy. The IUD can be left in place or removed; it is controversial which is the best practice at this time.*

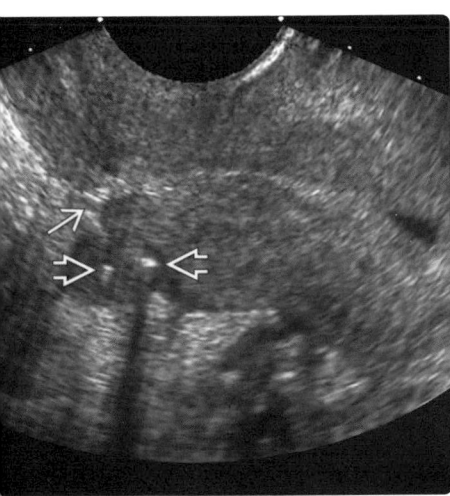

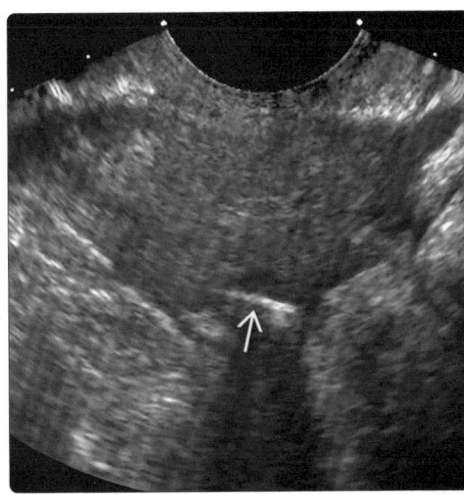

(Left) *Longitudinal endovaginal US shows a retroverted uterus with a cesarean section scar* ➡. *The IUD is not seen in the endometrial cavity. Two subtle echogenic shadowing foci are seen near the scar and uterine serosa* ➡. (Right) *Transverse US of the lower uterine segment in the same patient shows the IUD stem* ➡ *to better advantage, perforating through the cesarean section scar. Prior cesarean section is said to not increase the risk of perforation, but these likely happen at the time of placement.*

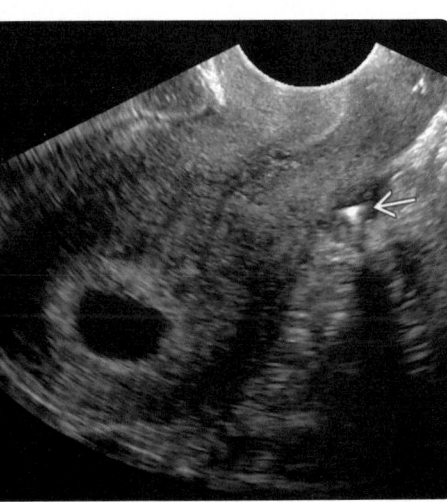

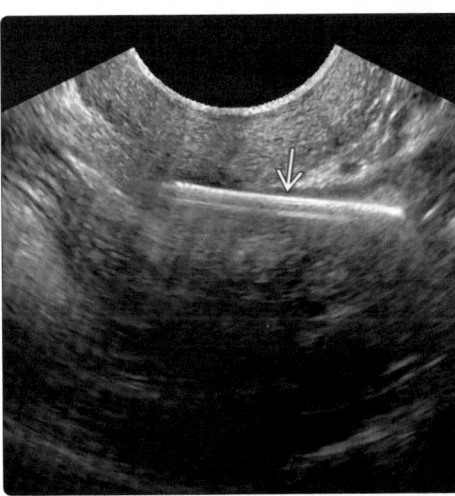

(Left) *Longitudinal endovaginal US shows early intrauterine pregnancy in a patient who has an IUD. The strings were not seen on clinical exam. An echogenic focus in the cul-de-sac* ➡ *with reverberation is seen.* (Right) *Transverse endovaginal US of the cul-de-sac in the same patient shows the perforated IUD* ➡. *When there is a missing IUD, careful scanning should be done to locate it. If not found, a KUB should be performed as the IUD may be beyond the FOV of the transducer.*

Tubal Ectopic Pregnancy

TERMINOLOGY

- Synonyms: Ectopic pregnancy (EP); tubal pregnancy

IMAGING

- Adnexal findings seen in majority of cases
  o Commonly heterogeneous adnexal mass
  o Tubal ring sign: Less common but more specific, especially if clearly distinct from ovary
- May see pseudosac in uterus (only 10-20% of cases)
  o Intrauterine fluid collection more likely represents intrauterine pregnancy (IUP)
- Pregnancy not definitively identified in 5-10% of cases

TOP DIFFERENTIAL DIAGNOSES

- Exophytic corpus luteum of pregnancy
- Incidental adnexal mass
- Bowel
- Intrauterine pregnancy

CLINICAL ISSUES

- Must correlate US findings with human chorionic gonadotropin (hCG) levels
  o hCG > 3,000 mIU/mL and no IUP
    − EP vs. failing IUP vs. early multiple gestation
  o Lower hCG level and no IUP
    − EP vs. early or failing IUP
  o Single hCG measurement in unreliable in distinguishing IUP (nonviable or viable) from EP
  o Follow serial hCG levels in indeterminate cases, with repeat US if rising

DIAGNOSTIC CHECKLIST

- Confirm extraovarian origin of adnexal ring-like mass
- Reserve treatment for visualized abnormality
- Be cautious in considering nonspecific intrauterine collection to be pseudosac of EP
- Consider favoring more likely diagnosis of IUP in medically stable patient and follow with US

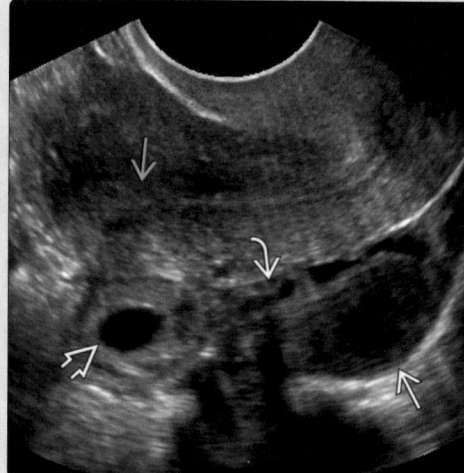
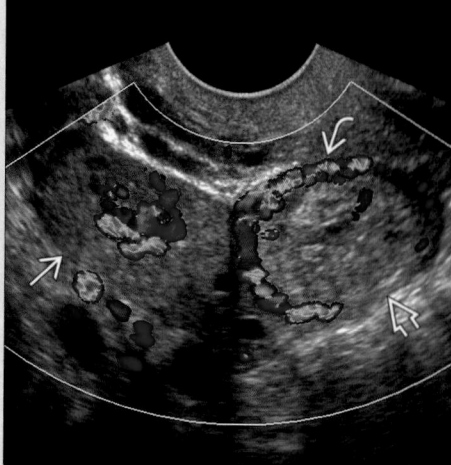

(Left) Sagittal transvaginal ultrasound shows an empty uterus ⮕ and an echogenic ring-like mass ⮕ adjacent to the ovary with a hemorrhagic corpus luteum ⮕. Note the small amount of echogenic fluid in the pelvis ⮕. (Right) Transverse transvaginal color Doppler ultrasound shows an echogenic round mass ⮕ adjacent to, and separate from, the right ovary ⮕ with a ring of blood flow, described as the "ring of fire" ⮕ of an ectopic pregnancy (EP).

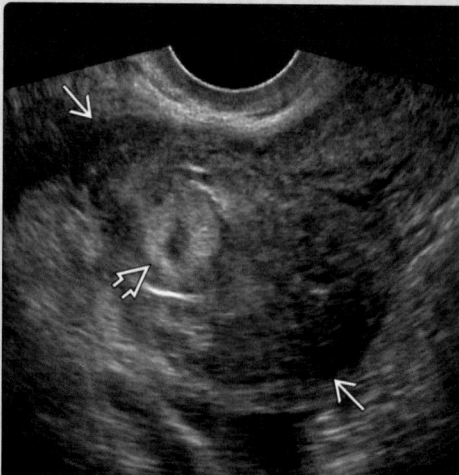
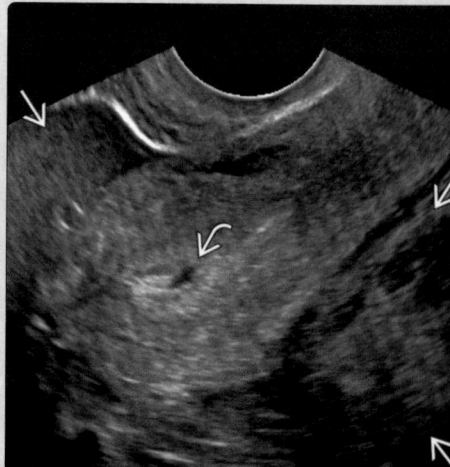

(Left) Tranverse transvaginal ultrasound shows a heterogeneous mass in the right adnexa consistent with a blood clot ⮕ encasing an echogenic tubal ring ⮕. (Right) Sagittal transvaginal ultrasound shows a large amount of echogenic fluid ⮕ surrounding the uterus, compatible with clot in a patient with ruptured EP. Note the small pseudosac ⮕ in the uterus.

TERMINOLOGY

Synonyms

Ectopic pregnancy (EP); tubal pregnancy

Definitions

Implantation of embryo within fallopian tube

IMAGING

General Features

Best diagnostic clue
- No intrauterine pregnancy (IUP)
- Heterogeneous adnexal mass separate from ovary
- Echogenic fluid in cul-de-sac (blood)

Location
- 95% of EPs occur within fallopian tube
- 75-80% ampullary, 10-15% isthmic, 5% fimbrial, 2-4% interstitial

Ultrasonographic Findings

Uterine findings with EP
- Thick echogenic endometrium
  - Decidual reaction
  - Endometrial or decidual cysts: Can mimic intrauterine gestational sac (GS)
- Pseudogestational sac sign (10-20% of tubal EP)
  - Teardrop-shaped fluid collection, centrally located in endometrial cavity; surrounding echogenic decidua
  - No intra- or double decidual sac sign of IUP
    - However, these signs are often absent with IUP and not necessary for diagnosis
  - Debris or clot may mimic yolk sac or embryo
- IUP and coexistent EP extremely rare
  - Greater risk (1-3%) occur with assisted reproduction

Adnexal findings in 80-95% of tubal EP
- Heterogeneous extraovarian mass: Most common but least specific finding of EP
  - Represents hematoma in or around EP
  - Elongated, tubular configuration if in fallopian tube
  - Color Doppler may show vascular ring of EP within adnexal hematoma
- Tubal ring sign: Echogenic ring separate from ovary (2nd most common finding)
  - With yolk sac ± embryo, increases specificity to 100%
  - Usually more echogenic than ovarian stroma or corpus luteum (CL)
  - Color Doppler: "Ring of fire" = circumferential vascularity
    - Usually incomplete ring, with focal or minimal vascular flow
    - May help identify mass obscured by bowel or hematoma
  - Pulsed Doppler: High-velocity, low-resistance flow

Ovary findings with tubal EP
- CL when exophytic can mimic EP
  - Thick-walled cystic structure in ovary
  - Variable appearance: Anechoic → complex hemorrhagic cyst
  - Wall thicker and more hypoechoic than with EP
  - Color and spectral Doppler findings overlap with EP
    - "Ring of fire" with relatively high peak systolic and high end diastolic velocities
  - Approximately 2/3 of EP on same side as CL
- Echogenic fluid in cul-de-sac: Hemoperitoneum
  - Small amount may be seen with normal IUP
  - Larger hemoperitoneum: EP vs. ruptured CL
    - Does not necessarily indicate rupture of EP
      - Retrograde bleeding/leaking from tube vs. rupture
      - Moderate or large amount hemoperitoneum, suspect rupture
  - Clotted blood often mass-like
    - Color flow may help locate hidden EP
  - May be isolated positive finding in 15% of patients
- Pregnancy of unknown location (PUL) in 5-10% of cases
  - No IUP, normal adnexa, no cul-de-sac fluid

Imaging Recommendations

- Best imaging tool
  - Transvaginal ultrasound + color Doppler
    - 91% of EP accurately diagnosed
- Protocol advice
  - Correlate findings with human chorionic gonadotropin (hCG) levels
    - Usually see IUP > 2000 mIU/mL; but with no IUP, single measurement does not reliably distinguish EP from IUP (viable or nonviable)
    - < 3000 mIU/mL presumptive treatment should not be undertaken; risk of disrupting normal IUP
    - > 3000 mIU/mL and no IUP unlikely; most likely diagnosis is nonviable IUP → follow-up hCG and US
  - Obtain sagittal cul-de-sac view in every case to look for echogenic blood
    - May need ↑ gain settings to see echoes
    - Scan abdomen when hemoperitoneum present to assess degree
  - Color Doppler
    - Can help identify small EP or EP engulfed by clot
  - Use endovaginal probe as palpation tool: "Slide test"
    - EP moves independent of ovary; CL moves with ovary
  - Optimize transvaginal ultrasound (TVUS) search for yolk sac (YS) in tubal ring; increases specificity to 100%
    - Magnify image, adjust focal zone and gain, apply pressure to anterior abdominal wall to move mass closer to transducer, and eliminate bowel artifact

DIFFERENTIAL DIAGNOSIS

Corpus Luteum of Pregnancy

- Wall usually more hypoechoic than with EP
- Peripheral flow in wall only and tends to be more continuous ring
- Intraovarian origin as opposed to extraovarian mass
  - "Claw" sign of ovarian parenchyma partially surrounds exophytic CL
  - Intraovarian CL moves with ovary vs. EP, which moves separately

Incidental Adnexal Mass

- Dermoid: Complex mass with fat, fluid, and calcification
- Neoplasm: Complex mass with nodularity, thick septations, and vascular flow
- Paraovarian cyst

- Interligamentous fibroid

Bowel

- Watch for peristalsis

Intrauterine Pregnancy

- Intradecidual sac sign, double decidual sac sign
  - May help identify an IUP, but not necessary for diagnosis
  - Nonspecific intrauterine fluid collection has greater odds of being gestational sac (GS) than pseudosac
  - Look for eccentricity and curved edges to increase likelihood further
- Perigestational hemorrhage is common
  - Resembles pseudosac
- Anechoic cul-de-sac fluid: Considered physiologic

PATHOLOGY

General Features

- Etiology
  - Abnormal blastocyst implantation within fallopian tube due to delay or obstruction to transit

CLINICAL ISSUES

Presentation

- Most common signs/symptoms
  - Classic triad: Pelvic pain (most common presentation), vaginal bleeding, palpable mass; nonspecific
  - Cardiovascular shock: Highly specific sign of rupture
- Other signs/symptoms
  - When hCG > 3,000 mIU/mL IRP and no IUP
    - Differential: EP vs. failing IUP vs. multiple gestation
  - Lower hCG level and negative US
    - Differential: EP vs. viable or nonviable IUP
  - Obtain follow-up hCG and US in indeterminate cases
    - Levels double every 2-3 days with normal IUP; slower rise with EP
    - Dropping levels suggest failing pregnancy
  - No lower limit below which rupture is not seen; do not delay US due to low hCG level
  - Maternal serum progesterone levels
    - Helps predict normal IUP vs. EP/failing IUP
    - Cannot differentiate EP from failed IUP
    - < 5 ng/mL = nonviable pregnancy in 100%
    - Office curettage can rule out failed IUP
    - > 25 ng/mL excludes ectopic with 97.5% sensitivity

Demographics

- Epidemiology
  - 1.4% of all pregnancies are ectopic
  - 5-20% incidence if patient presents with pain/bleeding
  - 10-40% risk in fertility patients
  - Abnormal tube is risk factor for tubal ectopic
    - Chronic salpingitis, salpingitis isthmica nodosa, tubal surgery, prior EP

Natural History & Prognosis

- Delayed diagnosis → ↑ morbidity and death
  - Fatality rate has ↓ from 3.5 to 1:1,000
- Prognosis for future pregnancies
  - 80% will have future IUP; 15-20% will have future EP

- 24% of all EP may spontaneously resolve
  - More likely if hCG levels < 1,000 mIU/mL IRP
  - Must follow dropping hCG levels very carefully

Treatment

- Medical treatment with methotrexate (MTX)
  - Patient must be hemodynamically stable
  - No evidence for tube rupture: Little or no free fluid
  - 90% success rate for early, unruptured, small ectopic
    - EP < 4 cm
    - hCG levels < 5,000 mIU/mL
    - ≤ 8 weeks gestation
  - 30% failure rate if living embryo
  - Ultrasound after treatment is often confusing: Mass possible up to 3 months after treatment
    - ↑ hemorrhage around EP; ↑ size of EP due to hemorrhage and edema
    - US only if suspected tubal rupture
  - Multiple doses may be necessary
- Surgical therapy
  - Salpingectomy: Segment of tube removed and reconnected if possible → only choice for ruptured EP
  - Salpingotomy: Small lengthwise incision in tube for removal of EP
- Ultrasound-guided local injection
  - MTX or potassium chloride (KCl)
    - Injected directly into gestational sac
  - Live ectopic + unruptured tube
    - Combined with systemic MTX increases success rate over systemic MTX alone

DIAGNOSTIC CHECKLIST

Consider

- In setting of PUL, single hCG measurement is unreliable in distinguishing IUP (nonviable or viable) from EP; reserve treatment for visualized abnormality
- Follow serial hCG levels in indeterminate cases
  - Repeat US if hCG levels are rising
  - Dropping levels suggest failing pregnancy
- No lower limit hCG level for EP, often found with hCG level < 1,000 mIU/mL → do not delay US

Image Interpretation Pearls

- Presence of IUP is best negative predictor of EP in general population
- Any extraovarian mass with empty uterus and hCG level > 2000 mIU/mL should be viewed with suspicion
- Be aware of (and beware of) CL mimic; can be cause of pain
- Be cautious in categorizing nonspecific intrauterine collection as pseudosac of EP
  - Consider favoring more likely diagnosis of IUP in medically stable patient

SELECTED REFERENCES

1. Ko JK et al: Time to revisit the human chorionic gonadotropin discriminator level in the management of pregnancy of unknown location. J Ultrasound Med. 33(3):465-71, 2014
2. Doubilet PM et al: Diagnostic criteria for nonviable pregnancy early in the first trimester. N Engl J Med. 369(15):1443-51, 2013
3. Rana P et al: Ectopic pregnancy: a review. Arch Gynecol Obstet. 288(4):747-57, 2013

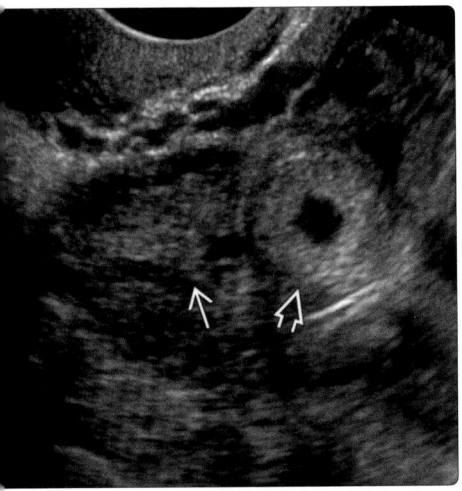

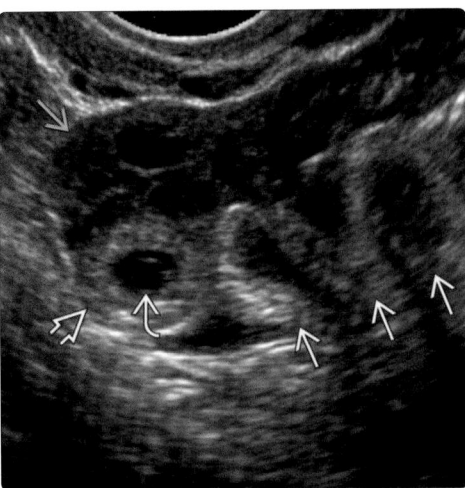

(Left) *Transverse transvaginal ultrasound shows a tubal ring* ⟹ *adjacent to the right ovary* ⟹. *Applying pressure with the transducer while scanning in this region confirmed that the ring-like mass moved separate from the ovary. Note its hyperechoic appearance relative to the ovary and the corpus luteum below.* (Right) *Transverse oblique transvaginal ultrasound shows echogenic bowel loops* ⟹ *obscuring the tubal ring* ⟹ *of an ectopic pregnancy adjacent to the right ovary* →. *Note the yolk sac (YS) in the gestational sac* ⤴.

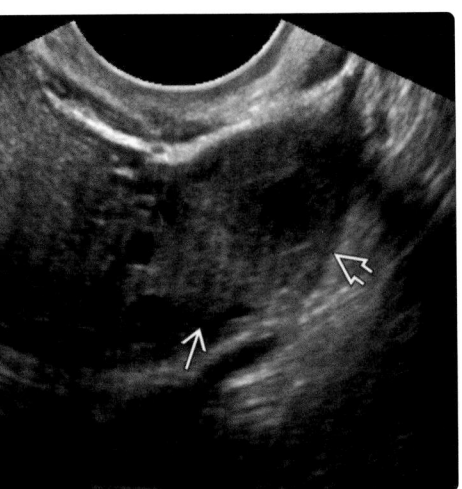

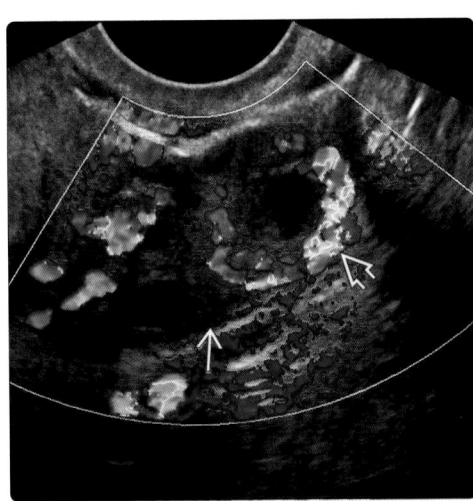

(Left) *Transverse transvaginal ultrasound shows a thick-walled cystic structure* ⟹ *within the left ovary* ⟹, *compatible with a corpus luteum. Applying pressure with the transducer while scanning in this region confirmed that this structure moved with the ovary. Note its hypoechoic appearance relative to the tubal ring above.* (Right) *Transverse color Doppler transvaginal ultrasound shows the "ring of fire"* ⟹ *associated with the corpus luteum in the left ovary* →.

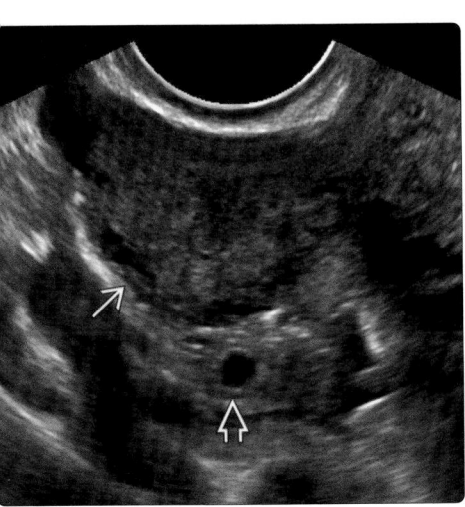

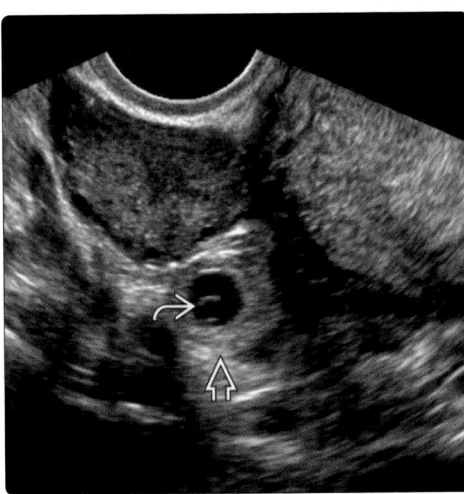

(Left) *Transverse oblique transvaginal ultrasound shows a small, subtle echogenic ring* ⟹ *posterior to the right ovary* →. *The absence of pelvic fluid and lack of associated mass suggest the tube is intact. Methotrexate (MTX) was used for treatment.* (Right) *Follow-up transvaginal ultrasound in the same patient shows interval growth of the gestational sac* ⟹ *in the right adnexa, which now contains a YS* ⤴ *and is compatible with MTX treatment failure.*

(Left) *Transverse transvaginal ultrasound shows a gestational sac ⇒ outside of the adjacent empty uterus →. Note the embryo in the gestational sac ⇒.* **(Right)** *Transverse oblique M-mode ultrasound in the same patient shows cardiac activity in the live ectopic.*

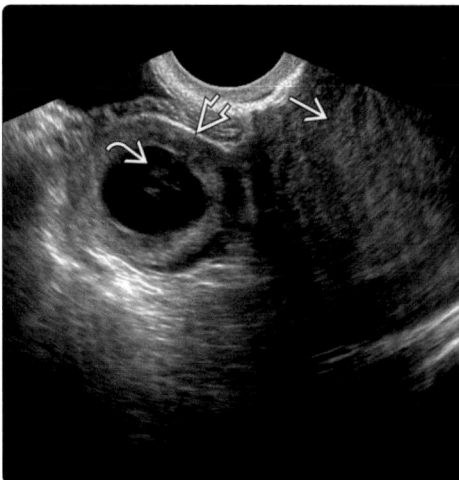
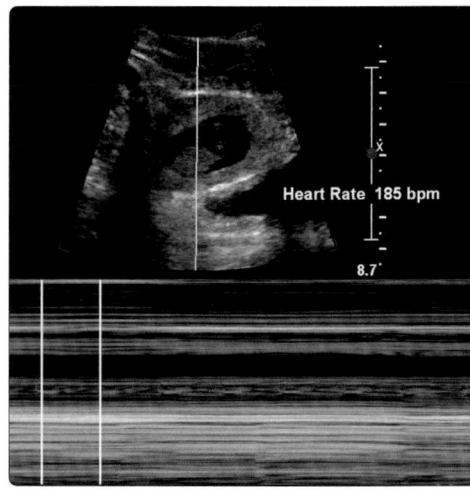

(Left) *Sagittal oblique transvaginal ultrasound shows a heterogeneous mass in the right adnexa ⇒.* **(Right)** *Transverse color Doppler ultrasound in the same patient shows a ring of vascular flow ⇒, which aides in localization of the tubal ring → that is obscured by the surrounding clot ⇒.*

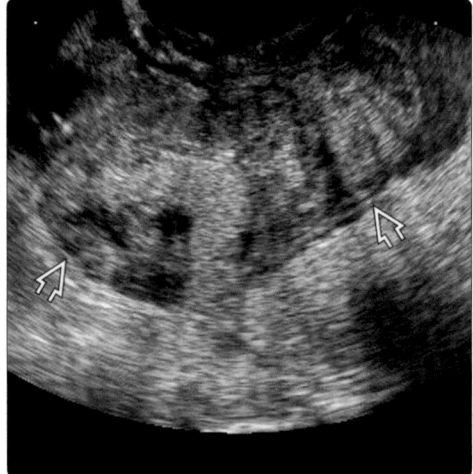
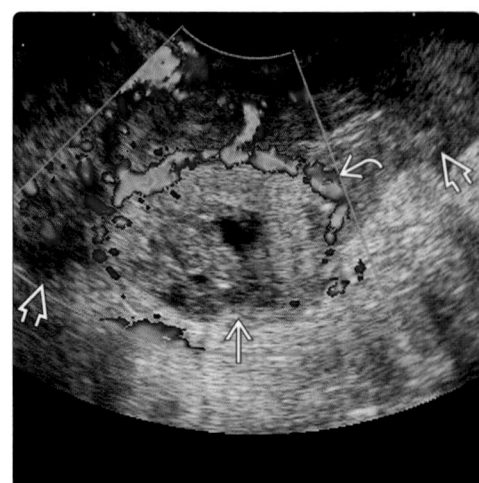

(Left) *Magnified transverse ultrasound of the tubal ring in the same patient demonstrates an embryo (calipers) in the ruptured ectopic.* **(Right)** *Sagittal transvaginal ultrasound shows the empty uterus ⇒ with a large amount of echogenic free fluid ⇒ in the cul-de-sac.*

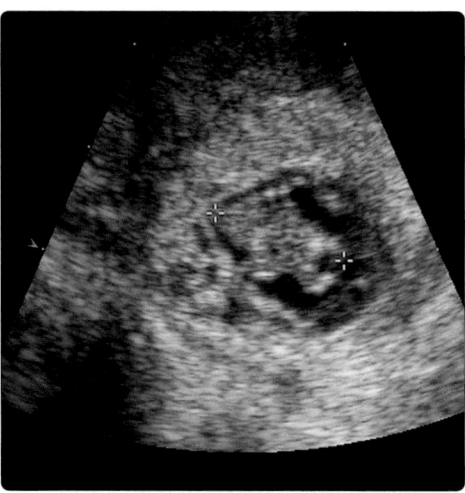
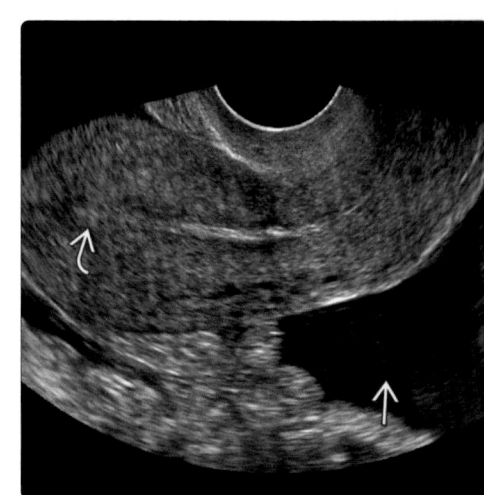

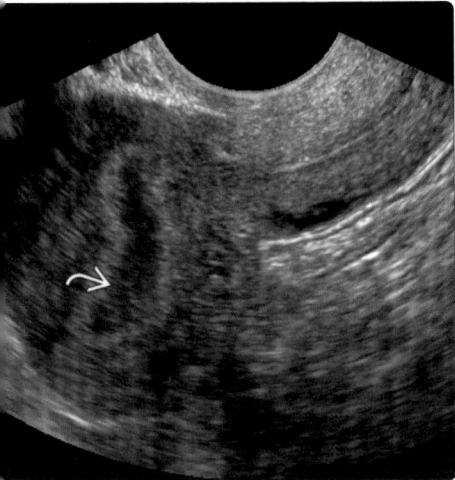

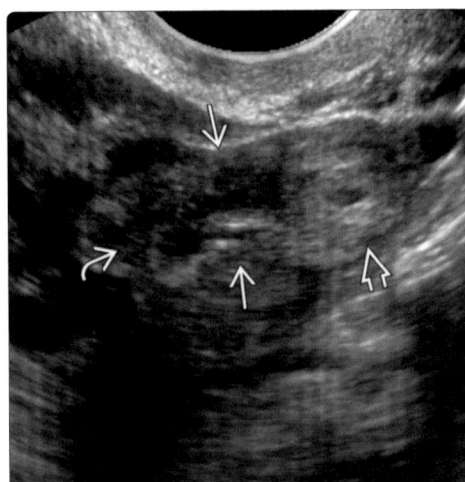

(Left) *Sagittal transvaginal ultrasound of the uterus shows fluid in the endometrial cavity with low-level echoes ⇗, compatible with a pseudosac.* (Right) *Sagittal oblique transvaginal ultrasound of the left adnexa shows an echogenic ring-like mass ⇒ within a thickened tube ⇒ containing echogenic fluid ⇒.*

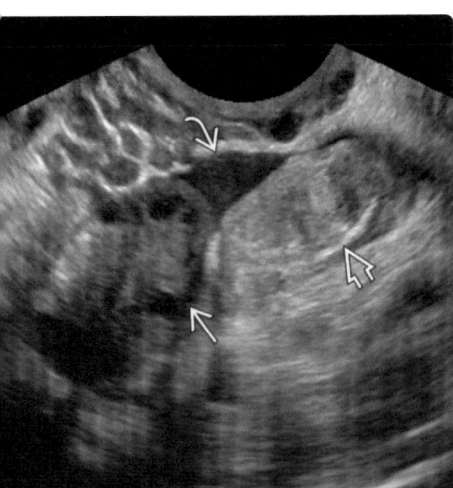

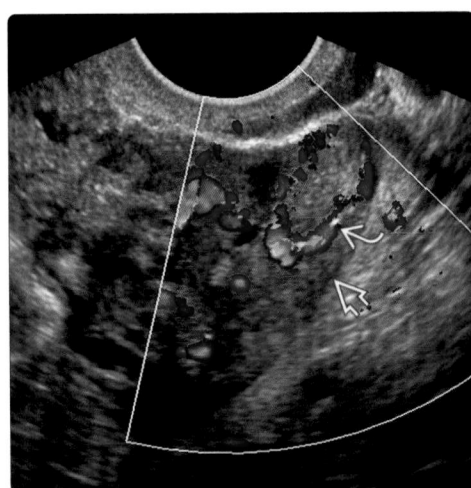

(Left) *Transverse transvaginal ultrasound of the right adnexa shows a hyperechoic tubular mass ⇒ adjacent to the right ovary ⇒. Note the small amount of adjacent echogenic free fluid ⇒.* (Right) *Transverse color Doppler ultrasound in the same patient shows a ring of vascular flow ⇒ in the tubal mass ⇒.*

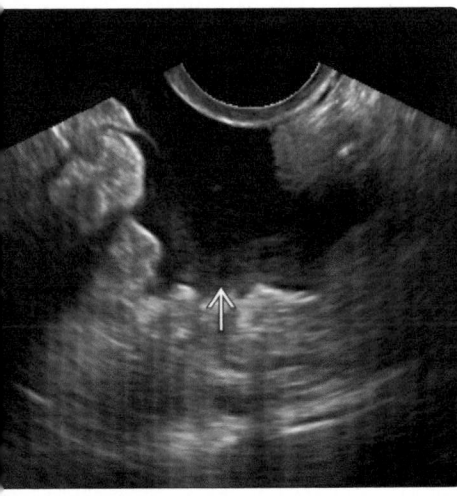

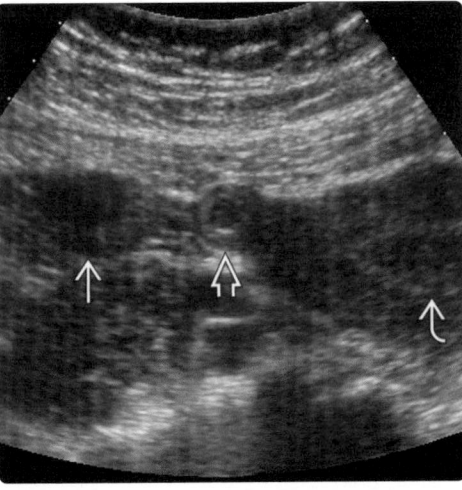

(Left) *Sagittal transvaginal ultrasound shows pelvic free fluid with low-level echoes ⇒ that are compatible with moderate hemoperitoneum, which could be due to bleeding from the tube or rupture.* (Right) *Longitudinal oblique transabdominal ultrasound of the pelvis was repeated after transvaginal imaging showed no evidence of IUP ⇗ in a patient with hCG > 2000mIU/mL. A small echogenic ring ⇒ could only be seen with transabdominal imaging above the uterus and separate from the left ovary ⇒.*

TERMINOLOGY

- **Interstitial ectopic pregnancy (EP)**: Pregnancy occurring in intramural portion of fallopian tube
- **Cornual EP**: Pregnancy in cornua of an anomalous uterus
- **Uterine scar EP**: Implantation of pregnancy at site of previous uterine surgery
- **Cervical EP**: Gestational sac (GS) in wall of the cervix
- **Ovarian EP**: GS implanted on ovary
- **Abdominal EP**: Implantation in peritoneal cavity
- **Heterotopic pregnancy**: Concurrent intrauterine and ectopic pregnancies

IMAGING

- Best diagnostic clues on ultrasound (US)
  - Interstitial: Interstitial line sign = echogenic line from endometrium to ectopic sac
  - Cornual: Occurs with uterine mullerian duct anomaly
  - Scar EP: Eccentrically located GS at site of C-section scar
  - Cervical EP: GS eccentric to the endocervical canal

- 3D ultrasound: Improves visualization of gestational sac in relation to the intrauterine cavity
- MR: Reserved for problem solving when US findings are equivocal or preoperative planning for large ectopics

TOP DIFFERENTIAL DIAGNOSES

- Intrauterine pregnancy vs. interstitial or scar EP
- Tubal ectopic vs. interstitial EP
- Septate uterus vs. interstitial EP
- Abortion in progress vs. cervical EP
- Corpus luteum vs. ovarian EP

CLINICAL ISSUES

- Overall, increased morbidity and mortality compared to usual tubal EP
  - Improved blood supply in setting of unusual EP often allows GS to grow larger and present later
- Diagnosis of unusual ectopic pregnancy can be difficult; must have a high degree of suspicion, especially in a high-risk patient

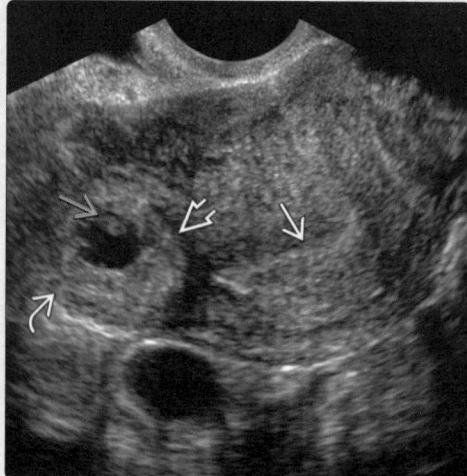
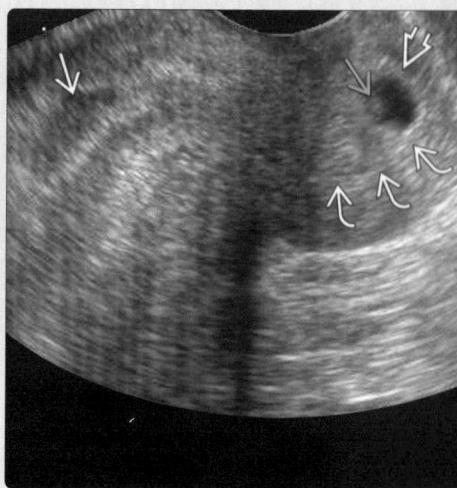

(Left) Transverse transvaginal US of an interstitial EP shows an eccentrically located GS ➡ with a fetal pole ➡ protruding from the lateral aspect of the uterus, separate from the empty endometrial cavity ➡. Note thinned overlying myometrium ➡. (Right) Longitudinal transvaginal ultrasound of a cervical EP shows an empty uterus ➡ with a round, eccentrically located gestational sac ➡ in the anterior wall of the cervix. Note thin central curved line of the endocervical canal ➡ and fetal pole ➡.

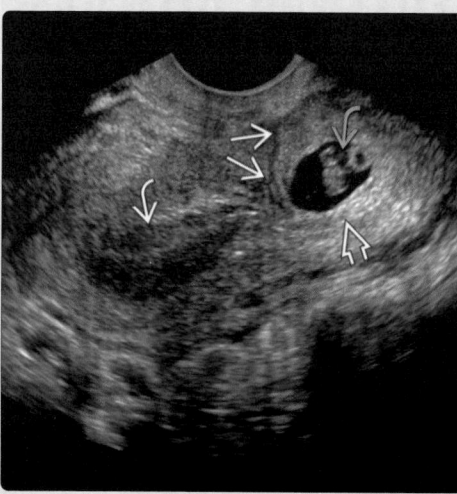
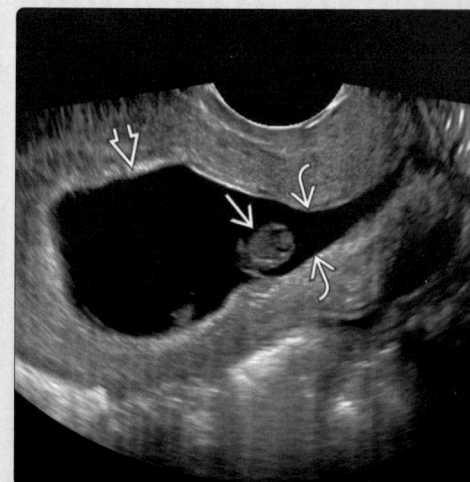

(Left) Longitudinal transvaginal US of a cesarean section scar ectopic, shows an eccentrically located gestation sac ➡ within the lower anterior uterine myometrium at the site of a cesarean section scar ➡. Note the yolk sac and fetal pole ➡ and empty endometrial cavity ➡. (Right) Longitudinal transvaginal US shows an abortion in progress with a centrally located, tear-drop shaped gestational sac ➡ spanning the lower uterine cavity and endocervical canal. Note wide open internal os ➡ and fetal pole ➡.

TERMINOLOGY

Definitions

- **Interstitial ectopic pregnancy (EP)**: Preferred term for pregnancy occurring in interstitial (intramural) portion of fallopian tube
  - Synonym: Intramural ectopic pregnancy
- **Cornual EP**: Often used interchangeably with interstitial ectopic; more appropriately applied to pregnancy in the cornua of an abnormal uterus (horn of uni- or bicornuate uterus or lateral half of septate uterus)
- **Angular pregnancy**: Pregnancy implanted at lateral angle of uterine cavity by ostium, medial to interstitial tube
- **Uterine scar EP**: Implantation of pregnancy at the site of previous uterine surgery, e.g., myomectomy or cesarean section (C-section)
  - Synonyms: Scar EP, C-section scar EP
- **Cervical EP**: Gestational sac (GS) implanted in the wall of the cervix below the level of the internal cervical os
- **Ovarian EP**: Intraovarian implantation of a GS
- **Abdominal EP**: Implantation in the peritoneal cavity
  - Primary: Direct peritoneal implantation; secondary: Re-implantation of ruptured extrauterine pregnancy in peritoneal cavity (more common than primary form)
- **Heterotopic pregnancy**: Concurrent intrauterine and ectopic pregnancies

IMAGING

General Features

- Best diagnostic clues
  - Interstitial: Interstitial line sign = echogenic line from endometrium to ectopic sac
  - Cornual: Occurs with uterine mullerian duct anomaly
  - Scar EP: Eccentrically located GS at site of C-section scar
  - Cervical EP: GS eccentric to the endocervical canal
- Size
  - Generally larger than tubal EP
- Location
  - Vast majority of EP occurs in the fallopian tube (95-99%): Ampullary, isthmic, or fimbriated portions
  - Unusual locations: Interstitial/intramural portion of tube, myometrial scar, wall of cervix, ovary, abdominal cavity

Ultrasonographic Findings

- Interstitial EP: GS eccentrically located in myometrium of uterine fundus separate from endometrium
  - Interstitial line sign: Thin echogenic line representing interstitial portion of the tube extending from the ectopic GS to cornua of empty endometrial cavity
  - More commonly, see separation between echogenic border of endometrium and outer echogenic edge of GS
  - GS with thinned overlying myometrium (< 5 mm)
    - Bulge of outer contour or serosa of myometrium
    - GS: Can be large ± YS or embryo; or may appear as an echogenic mass (trophoblastic tissue and hematoma)
  - 3D ultrasound (US): Improves ability to localize GS and visualize intramural portion of the fallopian tube
  - Doppler findings: Highly vascular trophoblastic tissue
    - May see prominent arcuate vessels in outer third of myometrium

- Pulsed Doppler: High-velocity, low-resistance waveform
- Cornual EP: Eccentrically located with similar appearance to interstitial pregnancy but in anomalous uterus
  - Visualization of uterine anomaly necessary for diagnosis
  - 3D US: Improves visualization of uterine cavity and fundus in order to diagnose congenital uterine anomalies and location of GS
- Angular pregnancy: GS located in the uterine cavity deviated towards the lateral angle with thin overlying myometrium
  - 3D US: Improves visualization of the gestational sac in relation to the intrauterine cavity
  - GS may descend into the endometrial cavity on subsequent studies
- Scar EP: GS located in the anterior myometrium of the lower uterine segment eccentric to the endometrium, in patient status-post C-section
  - Myometrium between bladder and GS: Thinned or absent
  - Triangular configuration of C-section scar at implantation site; possibly with fluid along edge
  - Sac may extend into endometrial cavity or beyond serosal surface of the uterus
- Cervical EP: GS in the wall of the cervix, adjacent to endocervical canal; closed internal os
  - Later presentation → hourglass-shaped uterus: Uterine body = top of hourglass, bulging cervical EP = bottom, waist = level of internal os
  - Color Doppler: Peritrophoblastic perfusion ± feeding vessel from the cervical wall
- Ovarian EP: GS (± YS &/or embryo) surrounded by ovarian parenchyma
  - Moves with the ovary when gentle pressure applied during TV examination
  - Very difficult to diagnose by ultrasound; most cases diagnosed intraoperatively
- Abdominal EP: EP at site of pain outside adnexa
  - May be best seen transabdominally
- Heterotopic pregnancy: Consider in patient undergoing assisted reproduction
  - Can be tubal, interstitial, scar, cervical, or less commonly ovarian or abdominal

MR Findings

- GS: Eccentric, thick-walled cystic structure with T2 hyperintense wall
  - Separated from endometrium by junctional zone in interstitial pregnancy and scar EP
- Corpus luteum: Wall shows low T2 signal intensity
- Associated hematoma: Intermediate to high signal on T1 and low T2 signal

Imaging Recommendations

- Always document location of sac with respect to endometrium in both transverse and longitudinal planes
- Measure surrounding myometrium if it appears thin
- Use 3D ultrasound if available
  - High concordance between 3D US and MR; and more rapid access and lower cost
- If diagnosis is unclear: MR or short term follow-up
- Target transabdominal US to area of pain if outside adnexa

- o Look for hemoperitoneum around the liver
- MR: Generally not necessary and avoided in first trimester unless clinical situation warrants
  - o Consider when ultrasound findings are equivocal or preoperative planning for large ectopics
    - – Can delineate anatomy, location of placenta, and vascular supply before intervention
  - o Useful in evaluating for congenital uterine anomalies

DIFFERENTIAL DIAGNOSIS

Intrauterine Pregnancy vs. Interstitial

- High or eccentric implantation can be confusing
- Should always have normal myometrial coverage
- Angular pregnancy: May descend or grow into cavity

Tubal Ectopic vs. Interstitial EP

- Can be confusing if adjacent to uterine cornua
- Use ultrasound probe to gently separate structures

Septate Uterus vs. Interstitial EP

- Implantation in one horn gives eccentric appearance
- Myometrium completely surrounds GS
- 3D US helpful in showing 2 uterine cavities

Scar EP vs. IUP or Abortion in Progress

- Thin overlying myometrium or uterine serosa
- May bulge uterine contour at C-section scar if large enough
- If not diagnosed, reports of becoming placenta accreta

Abortion in Progress vs. Cervical EP

- Centrally located products of conception, ± open internal os; may move during the examination
  - o May be displaced with gentle pressure
- Cardiac activity and trophoblastic flow are more suggestive of cervical EP with vascularity from adjacent cervical tissue
  - o Cardiac activity occasionally seen with Ab in progress

Corpus Luteum vs. Ovarian EP

- Extremely difficult to differentiate from ovarian EP unless YS or embryo is seen
- Corpus luteum wall less echogenic than trophoblast
- Very rare compared to ubiquitous corpus luteum

CLINICAL ISSUES

Presentation

- Most common signs/symptoms
  - o Pelvic/abdominal pain; vaginal bleeding, palpable mass
- Other signs/symptoms
  - o Hypotension and shock if presenting with rupture
  - o May be an incidental or subtle finding on early US
- Risk factors
  - o Sexually transmitted disease or pelvic inflammatory disease; prior tubal surgery, especially salpingectomy; prior ectopic pregnancy; assisted reproductive technology pregnancies; previous uterine, cervical surgery, or dilatation and curettage; endometriosis; indwelling intrauterine contraceptive devices; Asherman syndrome; fibroids

Demographics

- Age

- o Majority of EP are detected in women > 35 years
- Epidemiology
  - o EP outside the fallopian tube occurs in 3-5% of cases
  - o Interstitial 2-4%; scar < 1%; cervical < 1%; ovarian 0.15-3%; abdominal 1-3%

Natural History & Prognosis

- Overall, ↑ morbidity and mortality than for usual tubal EP
  - o Mortality rate 0.14% for usual tubal EP vs. 2-2.5% for interstitial EP and up to 20% for abdominal EP
  - o Improved blood supply from myometrium, cervix, or parasitized visceral arterial supply allow EP to grow larger and present later
  - o Increased risk of uterine rupture and hemorrhage
  - o Potential exsanguination
- Good outcome with preserved future fertility often possible with appropriate treatment
- Important to distinguish cornual EP from interstitial EP or angular pregnancy → different outcomes
  - o Cornual EP: High risk of recurrence
  - o Angular pregnancy: Can progress to live birth; ↑ risk for spontaneous abortion (38%) and uterine rupture (23%)

Treatment

- Tailored to individual patients based on clinical presentation, size of GS, presence of cardiac activity, and maternal hemodynamic stability
- Conservative treatments: Generally favored for interstitial EP due to ↑ complication risk with surgery
  - o Systemic methotrexate: Requires close follow-up and possibly additional doses
    - – Failed treatment goes to surgery
  - o Local sac injection: Methotrexate or potassium chloride; etoposide also used
    - – Via laparoscopy or ultrasound guidance
- Surgical intervention: Laparoscopy or laparotomy
  - o Recommended treatment for cornual EP because of suggested increased risk of recurrence
  - o Rupture may require hysterectomy
- Uterine artery embolization may be coupled with other treatments to control or reduce hemorrhage
- Expectant management
  - o Considered only if small sac and no living embryo

DIAGNOSTIC CHECKLIST

Consider

- 3D ultrasound for improved spatial orientation of sac to endometrial cavity

Image Interpretation Pearls

- Diagnosis of unusual ectopic pregnancy can be difficult
  - o Need high degree of suspicion, especially in a high-risk patient
  - o Short term follow-up for any eccentric or unusually located GS

SELECTED REFERENCES

1. Ghaneie A et al: Unusual Ectopic Pregnancies: Sonographic Findings and Implications for Management. J Ultrasound Med. 34(6):951-962, 2015
2. Parker RA 3rd et al: MR imaging findings of ectopic pregnancy: a pictorial review. Radiographics. 32(5):1445-60; discussion 1460-2, 2012

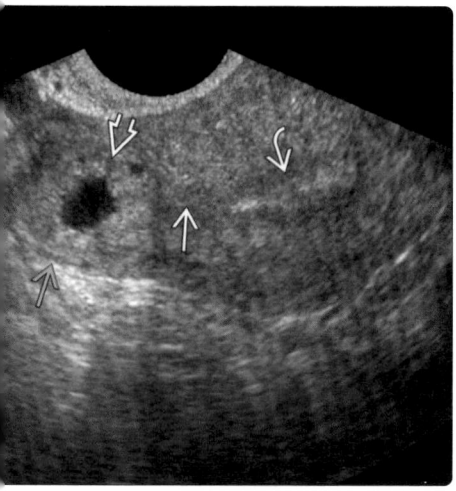

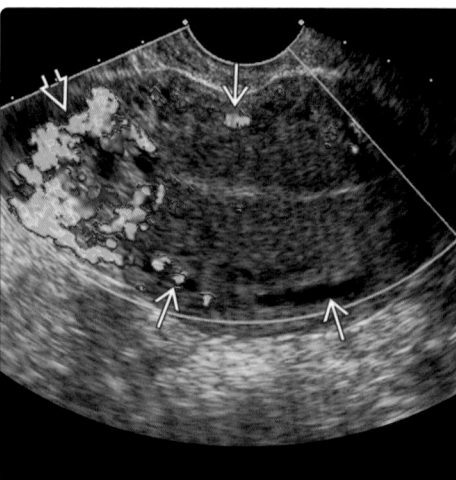

(Left) *Transverse transvaginal ultrasound shows the interstitial line sign ➡, a thin line extending from the eccentric gestational sac ➡ to the empty endometrial cavity ➡. Note thinning of the myometrium ➡ overlying the interstitial EP.* (Right) *Transverse transvaginal color Doppler ultrasound shows increased flow ➡ surrounding an interstitial EP. Note prominent arcuate vessels ➡ in the outer 1/3 of myometrium.*

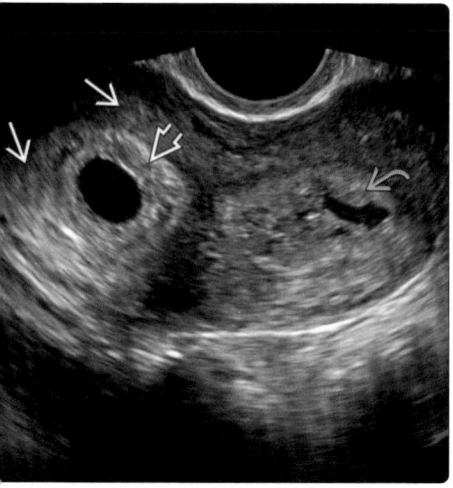

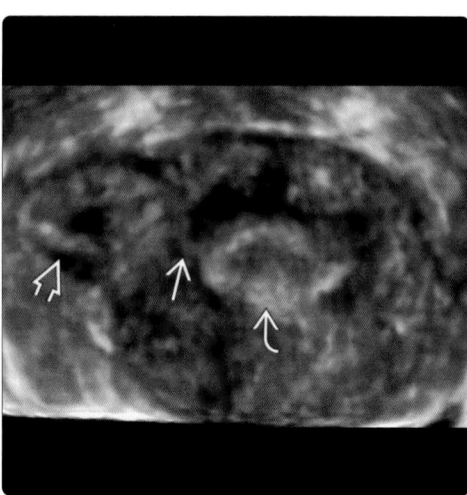

(Left) *Transverse transvaginal ultrasound shows an intrauterine pregnancy in one horn of a septate uterus ➡ with myometrium completely surrounding the sac ➡. The endometrium in the left horn is thickened with fluid ➡. This should not be mistaken for an interstitial pregnancy.* (Right) *Volume-rendered coronal 3D ultrasound clearly demonstrates an ectopically located interstitial gestational sac ➡ protruding from the uterus, separate from the empty endometrial cavity ➡. Note thin intervening interstitial line sign ➡.*

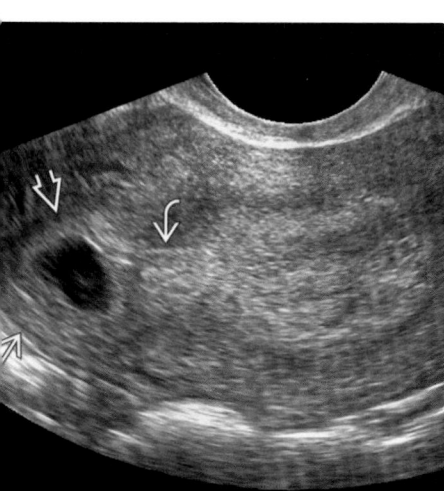

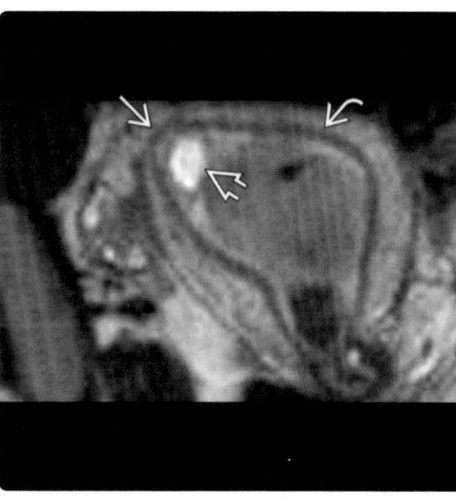

(Left) *Transverse transvaginal ultrasound shows an eccentrically located gestational sac ➡ abutting the echogenic endometrium medially ➡ with thinning of the overlying myometrium laterally ➡, suspected to be an interstitial pregnancy.* (Right) *Reconstructed coronal T2 HASTE MR shows an oval T2-hyperintense gestational sac ➡ in the right uterine angle with thinning of the overlying myometrium ➡ most compatible with an angular pregnancy. Note T2 hypointense junctional zone ➡.*

(Left) *Longitudinal transabdominal ultrasound shows an eccentrically located GS* ➔, *centered in the lower anterior uterine wall, with marked thinning of the myometrium between the bladder and the GS.* **(Right)** *Longitudinal transvaginal ultrasound in the same patient shows a triangular shaped defect* ➔ *compatible with a C-section scar, adjacent to the EP* ➔ *in the lower anterior uterine wall. Note separate empty uterine cavity* ➔.

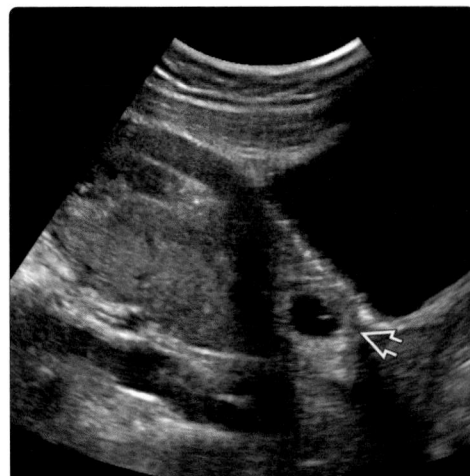
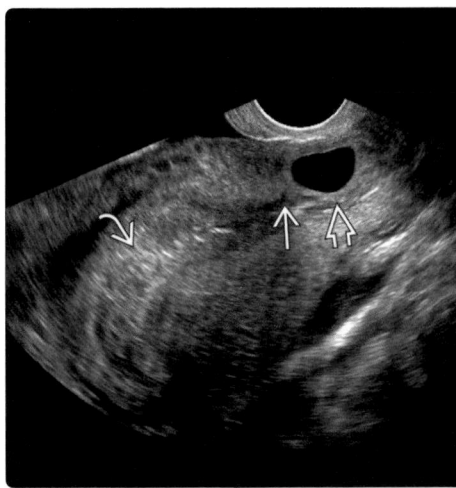

(Left) *Corresponding longitudinal oblique color Doppler US shows vascular flow within the wall of the EP* ➔ *and in the fetal pole* ➔. **(Right)** *Oblique transvaginal M-mode ultrasound in the same patient shows cardiac activity in the live scar ectopic pregnancy.*

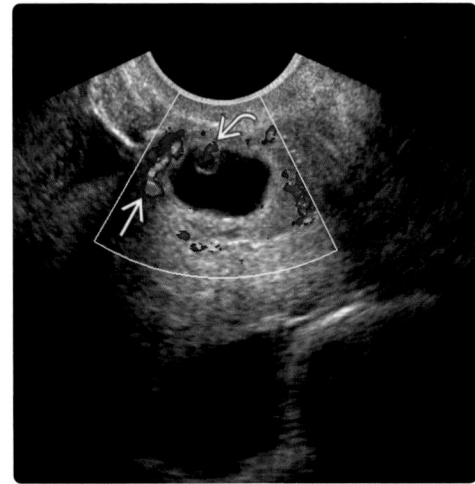
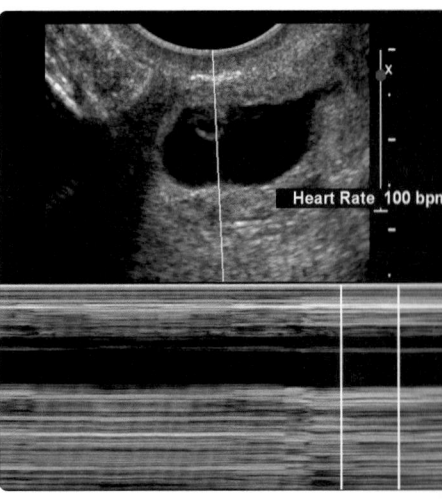

Heart Rate 100 bpm

(Left) *Sagittal T2 HASTE MR in the same patient shows a T2-bright structure* ➔ *with a thick T2-hyperintense wall, eccentrically located in the lower anterior uterine wall. Note the lack of intervening myometrium* ➔ *between the sac & the bladder and the normal cervical stroma* ➔. **(Right)** *Longitudinal transvaginal ultrasound obtained after targeted ultrasound-guided injection of potassium chloride shows new low-level internal echoes* ➔ *in sac. The yolk sac & fetal pole were no longer seen.*

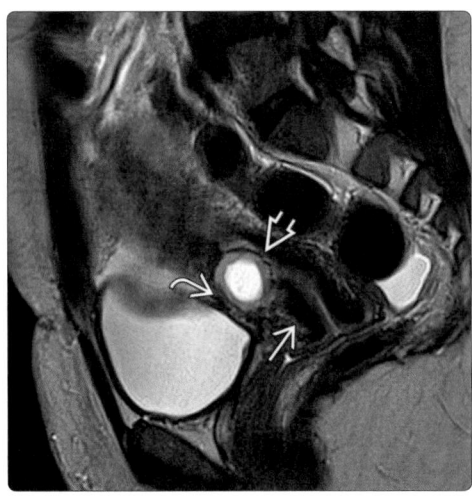
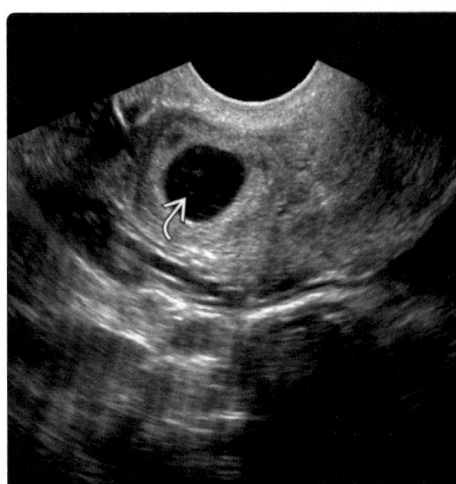

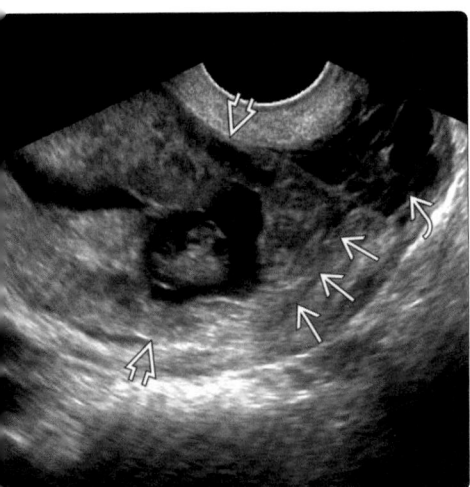

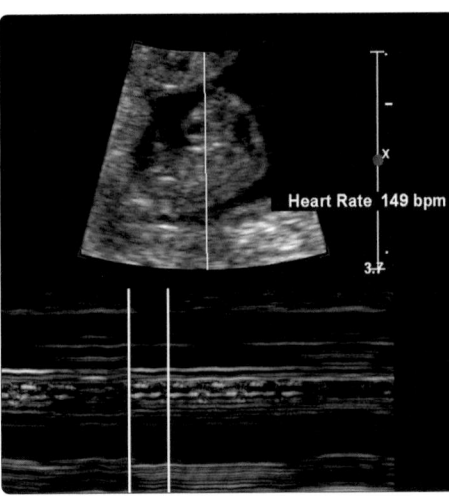

(Left) *Longitudinal transvaginal ultrasound shows a gestational sac with a fetal pole ➡ implanted in the anterior wall of the cervix. Note the large tortuous vessels around the implantation site ➡ and the endocervical canal posterior to the EP ➡.* (Right) *Corresponding longitudinal M-mode ultrasound shows cardiac activity in the live cervical ectopic pregnancy*

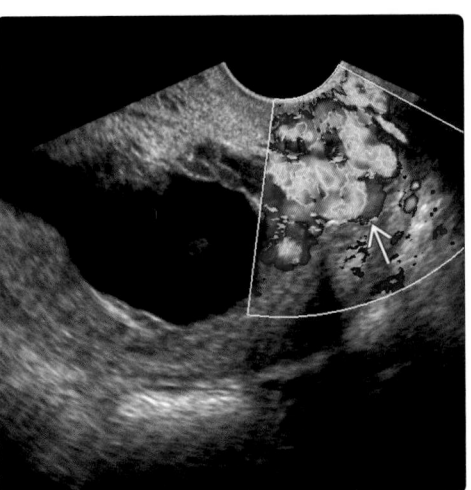

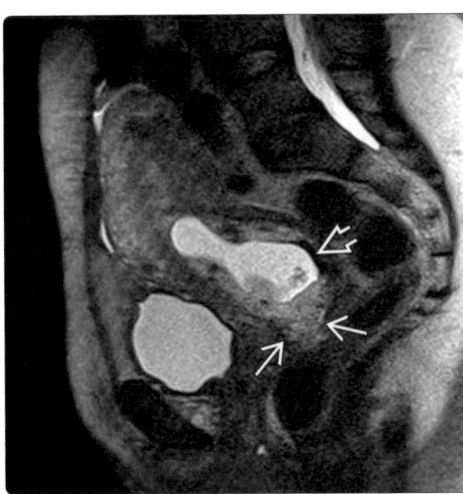

(Left) *Color Doppler ultrasound in the same patient shows marked vascularity around the implantation site ➡.* (Right) *Sagittal T2 HASTE MR shows an hourglass configuration of the uterus with a gestational sac ➡ containing a fetal pole centered in the cervix. T2-hyperintense trophoblastic tissue is seen extending into the cervical wall ➡.*

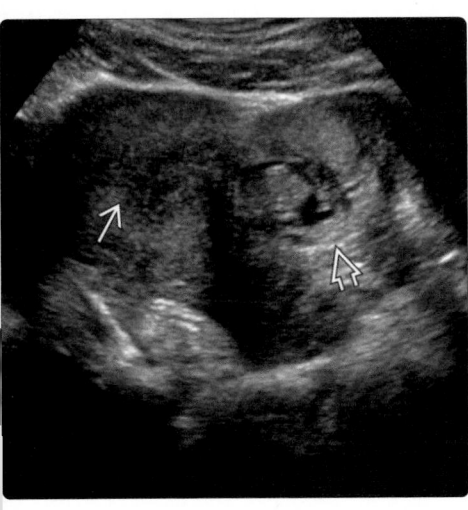

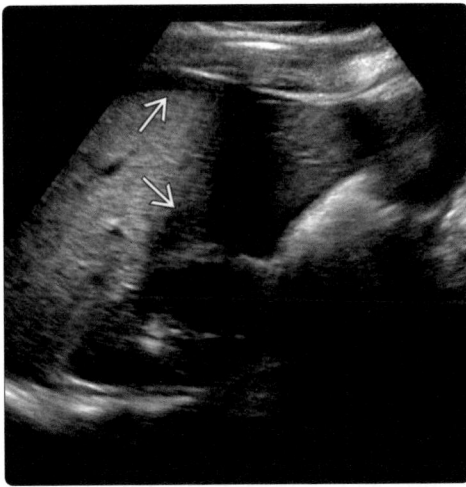

(Left) *Longitudinal transabdominal ultrasound shows an empty uterus ➡ and a large extrauterine gestational sac ➡ which contained a live fetus. Surgical exploration confirmed a secondary abdominal ectopic pregnancy which had ruptured from the tube and parasitized blood flow from the peritoneum.* (Right) *Longitudinal transabdominal ultrasound in the same patient shows echogenic free fluid around the liver ➡ indicating significant hemoperitoneum.*

Failed First Trimester Pregnancy

TERMINOLOGY

- Failed first trimester pregnancy: Collection of specific diagnoses of pregnancy failure

IMAGING

- Anembryonic pregnancy: Gestational sac (GS) with mean sac diameter ≥ 25 mm and no embryo
- Embryonic demise: Embryo with CRL ≥ 7 mm with no cardiac activity
- Spontaneous abortion: May be inevitable/impending, incomplete, or complete
  - Inevitable: GS herniating into or located centrally in cervical canal with open internal os
  - Incomplete: Heterogeneous endometrial thickening ± color Doppler flow, ± open cervical os
  - Complete: Thin, undistorted endometrial stripe; indistinguishable by US from ectopic or early nonvisualized IUP

- Must correlate with hCG trend, clinical presentation of bleeding, and possibly repeat US

TOP DIFFERENTIAL DIAGNOSES

- Normal early intrauterine pregnancy (IUP)
- Pseudosac of ectopic pregnancy (EP)
- Retained products of conception (RPOC)
- Gestational trophoblastic disease (GTD)
- Cervical ectopic pregnancy

CLINICAL ISSUES

- New guidelines for diagnosing failed pregnancy establish more stringent criteria to minimize potential of harming early IUP
- Single hCG measurement does not reliably distinguish between viable IUP, nonviable IUP, and ectopic pregnancy
- Follow-up hCG and ultrasound are often most prudent course when findings are not clear-cut

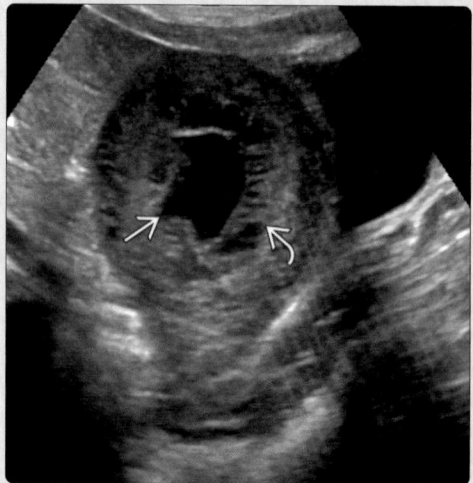
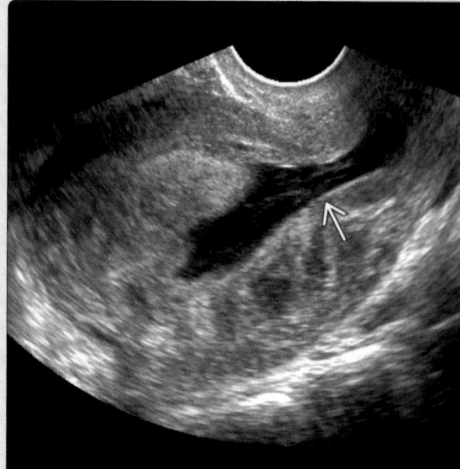

(Left) *Longitudinal transabdominal ultrasound shows an angular, enlarged gestational sac* ➡ *with a mean sac diameter (MSD) of 37 mm. There were no recognizable internal structures, which is compatible with an anembryonic pregnancy. Note the poorly echogenic cystic decidua* ➡. *(Right) Longitudinal transvaginal ultrasound shows an empty gestational sac herniating into the cervix through the open internal os* ➡. *Note internal echoes in the sac compatible with hemorrhage.*

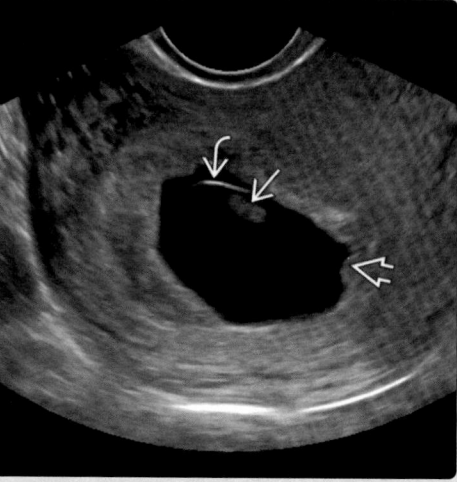
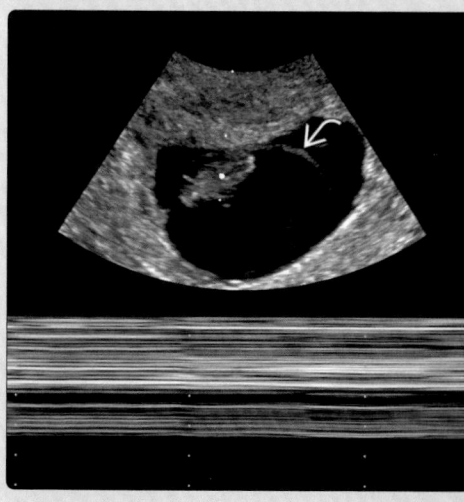

(Left) *Longitudinal transvaginal ultrasound shows a large intrauterine gestational sac (GS)* ➡ *with an embryo* ➡. *The sac is irregular in shape with poor decidual reaction. The amnion is seen surrounding the embryo* ➡. *(Right) M-mode ultrasound in the same patient shows the expanded amnion sign compatible with embryonic demise. The amnion* ➡ *is seen surrounding the embryo, which measures > 7mm and shows no cardiac activity.*

TERMINOLOGY

Definitions

Failed first trimester pregnancy refers to collection of specific diagnoses that are nonviable
- o Avoids confusion and simplifies terminology

Anembryonic pregnancy (AP): Failure of embryo to develop or early demise with resorption of embryonic pole (a.k.a. "blighted ovum," less favored term)

- Embryonic demise (ED): Embryo ≥ 7 mm in length with no heartbeat
- Spontaneous abortion: Involuntary pregnancy loss in 1st 20 weeks; may be inevitable, incomplete, or complete
- Missed abortion: General term for ED or AP; latter terms are more accurate and preferred

IMAGING

General Features

- Intrauterine pregnancy (IUP) with abnormal features that will not result in a live birth (nonviable)
  - o e.g., lack of embryonic development, lack of embryonic cardiac activity, or abnormal-appearing passing gestational sac (GS)

Ultrasonographic Findings

- Grayscale ultrasound
  - o Empty sac: Gestational sac with no embryo ± YS
    - – Empty amnion sign: GS with visible amnion, without visible embryo
    - – Specific sign of anembryonic gestation when mean sac diameter (MSD) ≥ 25 mm
      - □ Embryo usually seen at MSD of 18 mm (old criteria); however, not absolute
      - □ Lack of embryo with MSD 18-25 mm is worrisome and should prompt follow-up US in 2 weeks
      - □ Empty sac (i.e., no YS or embryo) on 2 scans performed 14 days apart is definitive for failed pregnancy
  - o Abnormal embryo
    - – Expanded amnion sign: Visible amnion surrounding embryo with no heartbeat
    - – Cardiac activity is usually visible when embryo is seen
    - – However, lack of cardiac activity at cutoff of 7 mm for crown rump length (CRL) is criterion for embryonic demise
    - – No cardiac activity at CRL < 7 mm is worrisome for failed IUP and should prompt follow-up US
  - o Spontaneous abortion
    - – Inevitable: GS herniating into or located centrally in cervical canal with open internal os
    - – Incomplete or in progress: Heterogeneous endometrial thickening ± color Doppler flow, ± open cervical os
    - – Complete: Thin, undistorted endometrial stripe
      - □ Indistinguishable by US from ectopic or early nonvisualized IUP
      - □ Conclusive if prior documentation of IUP
  - o Other findings that may indicate poor prognosis
    - – Abnormal yolk sac (YS) typically seen when MSD ≥ 10 mm (5 1/2 week gestation)
      - □ Normal YS is smooth, round, echogenic, < 6 mm

- □ Abnormal features: Pyknotic (collapsed), calcified, or large YS → poor prognosis
- □ Yolk stalk sign with YS distant from embryo
- – Irregular sac contour (e.g., angular or amoeboid shape)
- – Small sac size relative to embryo: < 5 mm difference between MSD and CRL
- – Poorly echogenic decidua ± cystic change
- – Abnormal GS location positioned low in uterus
- – Perigestational hemorrhage (a.k.a. subchorionic bleed)
  - □ Crescentic collection; echogenicity depends on age; usually anechoic or hypoechoic
  - □ Small (< 20% sac circumference): Common; often self-limited; > 90% pregnancy success when living embryo present
  - □ Large (> 50% sac circumference): ↑ risk pregnancy loss (20% with living embryo)
- Color Doppler
  - o Not necessarily useful: Variable findings and carries theoretical risks to developing embryo due to heating; use with caution to support abnormal diagnosis
  - o May see poor color Doppler signal around gestation sac

Imaging Recommendations

- Use magnified views to look carefully for yolk sac and embryo, and avoid missing multiple gestations
- Use M-mode US or video clips to document cardiac activity and M-mode to measure rate
- Correlate findings with clinical presentation and human chorionic gonadotropin (hCG) levels to guide interpretation and recommendations
  - o Use caution in interpreting single hCG measurement, does not reliably distinguish viable/nonviable IUP from ectopic pregnancy

DIFFERENTIAL DIAGNOSIS

Normal Early Intrauterine Pregnancy (IUP)

- GS appears at ~ 5 weeks: Smooth, round or oval, fundal, ± intradecidual sac sign (IDSS) or double sac sign (DSS)
  - o IDSS: Eccentric fluid collection in decidua, echogenic rim, curved edges
  - o DSS: Concentric echogenic bands around most of GS
  - o Signs absent in ≤ 35% of GS
  - o Helpful if seen; however, absence does not exclude IUP
  - o Normal IUP still possible if MSD 18-25 mm but no YS/embryo
- Prominent color flow around sac: Low resistance, high velocity on spectral analysis of chorion
  - o Variable and not necessarily useful, especially given theoretical risks to normal IUP with Doppler imaging

Pseudosac of Ectopic Pregnancy (EP)

- Tear drop-shaped fluid collection, centrally located, with no IDSS or DSS
- Nonspecific intrauterine fluid collection is more likely to be GS (normal or abnormal) than pseudogestational sac of ectopic pregnancy (seen in < 20% of EP)
- Search for specific findings (e.g., tubal ring in adnexa)
- Consider follow-up imaging in stable patient with indeterminate scan

Pregnancy of Unknown Location (PUL)

- Positive pregnancy test with no signs of intra- or extrauterine pregnancy on US
- Usually IUP when hCG > 2000 mIU/mL IRP
  - hCG <3000 mIU/mL, normal IUP still possible
  - hCG >3000 mIU/mL, viable IUP is unlikely, most likely diagnosis is nonviable IUP → follow-up hCG and US if increasing
    - hCG falls to zero with complete abortion

Retained Products of Conception (RPOC)

- Disorganized echogenic material in uterine cavity
- Color Doppler shows hypervascular pattern within endometrial contents
- Retained clot is usually hypoechoic, nonperfused
- No recognizable gestational sac

Gestational Trophoblastic Disease (GTD)

- Classic hydatidiform mole has "cluster of grapes" appearance
- May see abnormal-appearing gestational sac
  - Can mimic anembryonic sac
- Associated with ovarian theca lutein cysts

Cervical Ectopic Pregnancy

- Eccentric GS in wall of cervix; closed cervical os
- Cardiac activity more suggestive of cervical ectopic
- Passing abortion: Centrally located contents ± open internal os; may move during examination or on follow-up US

PATHOLOGY

General Features

- Etiology
  - 60% of spontaneous abortions < 12 weeks due to abnormal chromosomes
  - Less commonly: Uterine abnormalities, maternal infection, alcohol, smoking, immunologic and genetic defects

Microscopic Features

- Chorionic villi present in uterine curettings
  - Significant reduction in number of vessels per chorionic villus and abnormally located vessels suggests inadequate vasculogenesis
- Nuclear DNA abnormal in up to 40%
  - Suggests chromosomal aberrations → abnormal embryogenesis → anembryonic gestation

CLINICAL ISSUES

Presentation

- Most common signs/symptoms
  - Vaginal bleeding, pelvic pain, uterine contractions
    - May be heavy with incomplete or complete abortion
  - May be asymptomatic and diagnosed during routine US
  - Patient perception of diminished pregnancy symptoms
- Laboratory results
  - hCG > 3,000 mIU/mL IRP and no IUP
    - Failing IUP vs. early multiple gestation vs. EP
  - Lower hCG level and IUP not seen
    - Viable or nonviable IUP vs. EP

- Obtain follow-up hCG and US in indeterminate cases
  - hCG levels double every 2-3 days with normal IUP
  - Dropping levels suggest failing pregnancy
- Maternal serum progesterone levels
  - Helps predict normal IUP vs. EP/failing IUP
  - Cannot differentiate EP from failing IUP
  - < 5 ng/mL = nonviable pregnancy in 100%
  - > 25 ng/mL excludes ectopic with 97.5% sensitivity

Demographics

- Epidemiology
  - 30-60% documented hCG elevations end as failed pregnancy
  - Up to 20% of confirmed early pregnancies end in spontaneous abortion
    - 35% anembryonic, 54% early loss (cause not specified), 11% molar (partial or complete)
  - Groups with ↑ incidence of early pregnancy failure
    - Advanced maternal age; poor diabetic control; history of recurrent abortions

Natural History & Prognosis

- Threatened abortion → 1/2 abort
- Risk decreases to 5% if living embryo seen on US
- Random event with no specific recurrence risk if isolated
- Patients with recurrent abortion may be treated with aspirin, heparin, or progesterone supplementation (for luteal phase insufficiency)

Treatment

- "Wait and see" → most will pass without treatment
- Vaginal misoprostol
  - Many patients prefer definitive treatment to expectant management
  - Successful evacuation of uterus in majority of patients
  - Some will require curettage, but overall expect 50% reduction in need for surgical management
- Suction curettage
  - Small associated risk of excessive bleeding, uterine rupture, Asherman syndrome

DIAGNOSTIC CHECKLIST

Image Interpretation Pearls

- Empty amnion + MSD ≥ 25 mm → anembryonic gestation
- Lack of cardiac activity and CRL ≥ 7 mm → embryonic demise
- Be cautious when categorizing nonspecific intrauterine fluid collection as pseudosac
  - Nonspecific intrauterine fluid collection is more likely to be GS than pseudosac
  - Make diagnosis of ectopic pregnancy with definitive signs, not by lack of IUP, to minimize risk of harming IUP

SELECTED REFERENCES

1. Doubilet PM: Ultrasound evaluation of the first trimester. Radiol Clin North Am. 52(6):1191-9, 2014
2. Doubilet PM et al: Diagnostic criteria for nonviable pregnancy early in the first trimester. N Engl J Med. 369(15):1443-51, 2013
3. Lane BF et al: ACR appropriateness Criteria® first trimester bleeding. Ultrasound Q. 29(2):91-6, 2013

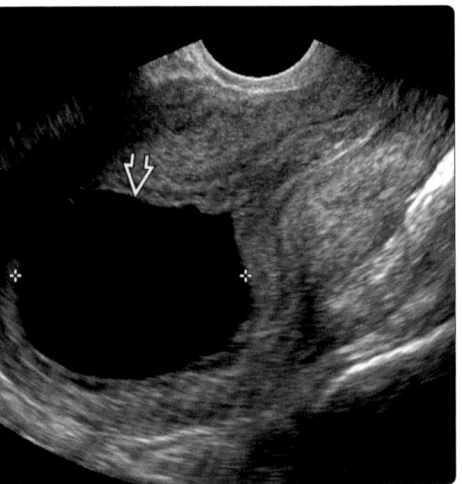

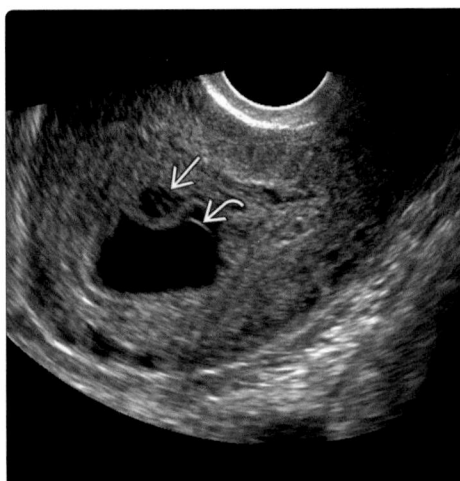

(Left) Longitudinal transvaginal ultrasound shows a large empty gestational sac ⮞ with a MSD of 40 mm and poor decidual reaction. A yolk sac and embryo were not seen, compatible with anembryonic pregnancy. (Right) Longitudinal transvaginal ultrasound shows another example of an anembryonic pregnancy with an enlarged angular empty gestational sac showing an empty amnion ⮞ and cystic decidual change ⮞.

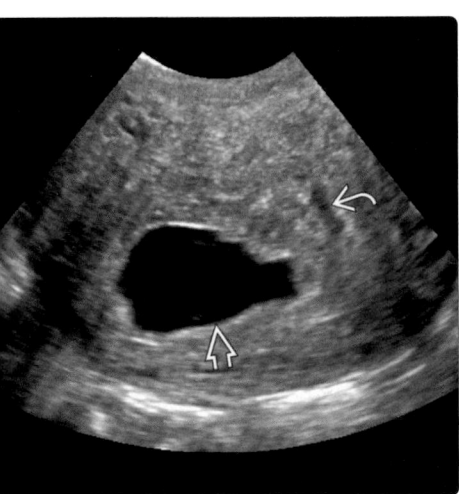

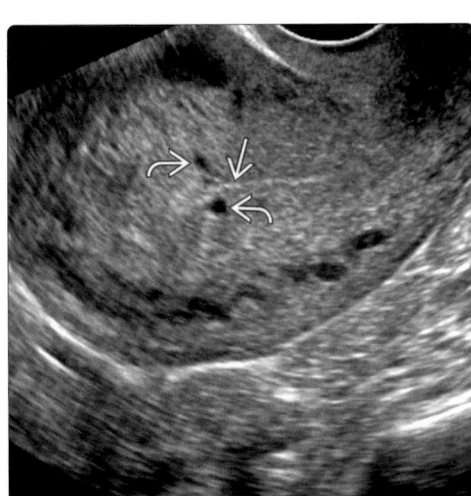

(Left) Transverse transvaginal ultrasound shows an irregular empty sac ⮞, poor decidual reaction, and cystic change ⮞. Findings were suspicious for failed pregnancy; however, MSD was < 25 mm and follow-up was obtained. (Right) Follow-up transvaginal ultrasound in the same patient shows findings compatible with interval complete abortion. There is a thin endometrial strip with no residual endometrial contents ⮞. Note small persistent decidual cysts ⮞.

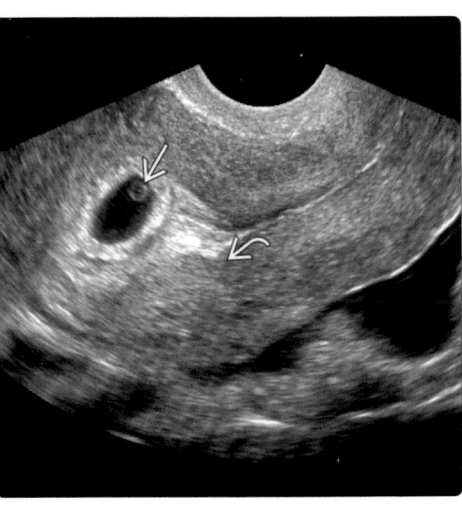

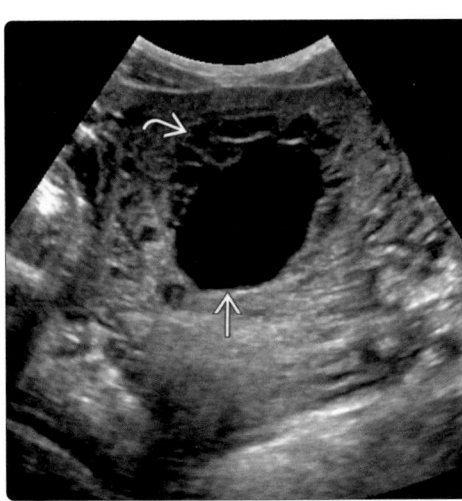

(Left) Transvaginal ultrasound of a retroflexed uterus (fundus better seen in a different plane) shows a GS with a YS ⮞ abnormally positioned in the lower uterus just above the internal os, which is beginning to dilate ⮞. Prognosis is guarded. (Right) Longitudinal transabdominal ultrasound performed for follow-up in the same patient shows interval pregnancy failure with enlargement of the GS ⮞ and development of marked cystic change ⮞ in the decidua. No recognizable internal contents were seen.

(Left) *Transverse transvaginal color Doppler ultrasound in a patient with embryonic demise shows lack of embryonic vascular flow, supporting this diagnosis.* (Right) *Transverse transvaginal ultrasound shows yolk sac abnormalities, which indicate a poor prognosis for this pregnancy. A small calcified YS* ➡ *is seen separated from the embryo by a thin stalk* ↗, *termed, the yolk stalk sign.*

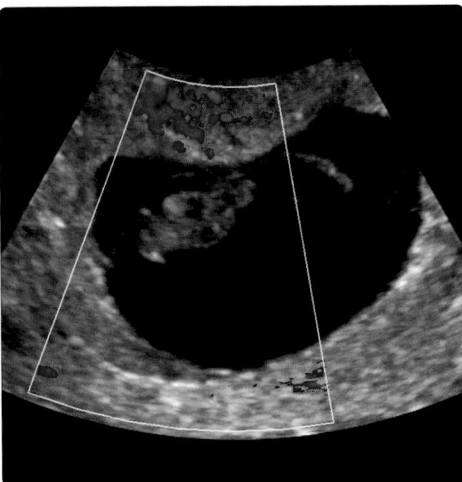
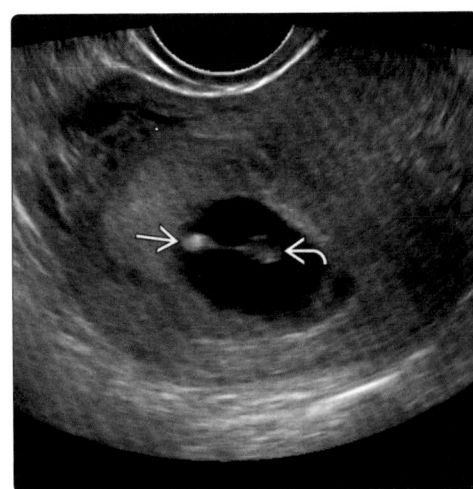

(Left) *Transverse transvaginal ultrasound shows an enlarged yolk sac (9 mm) with a thin wall* ➡, *findings suggesting a guarded prognosis. Note the tiny embryo* ➡ *growing on the yolk sac. Though cardiac activity was not seen, the embryo is below < 7 mm, and follow-up was recommended.* (Right) *Magnified view of a gestational sac shows an enlarged yolk sac with irregular wall thickening, which are poor prognostic features.*

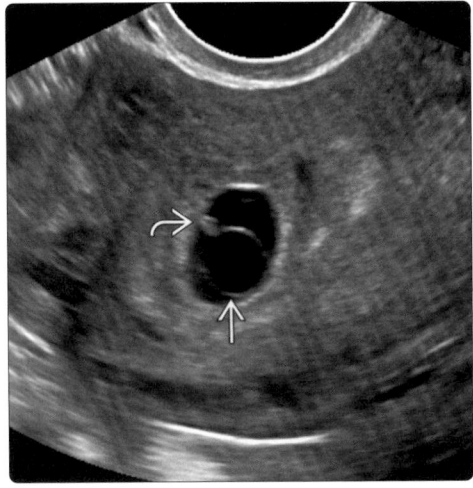
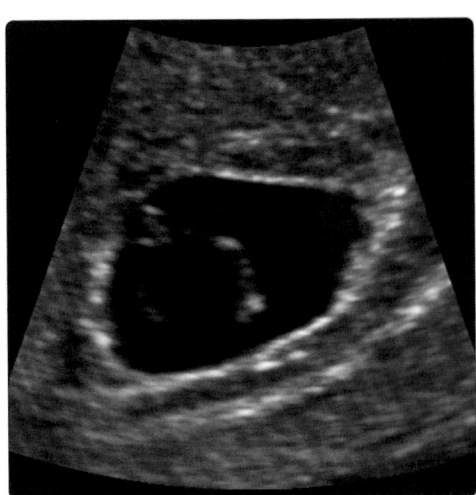

(Left) *Longitudinal transvaginal ultrasound of the uterus shows a small amount of nonspecific, centrally-located fluid* ➡ *in the endometrial cavity in the setting of a failed intrauterine pregnancy.* (Right) *Compared to the previous image, the intradecidual sac sign of early intrauterine pregnancy is a small, round collection* ➡ *with an echogenic rim, eccentrically located in the thickened decidua. Often absent, this sign is not required for diagnosis of an IUP.*

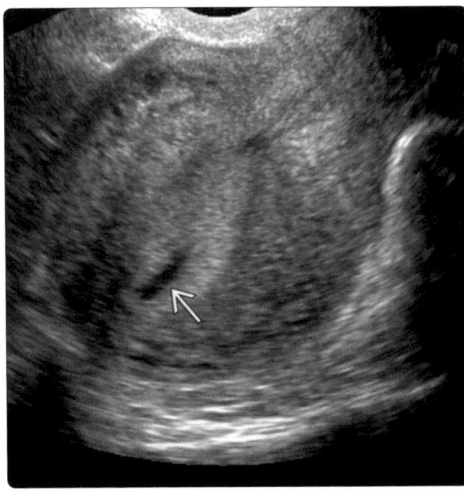
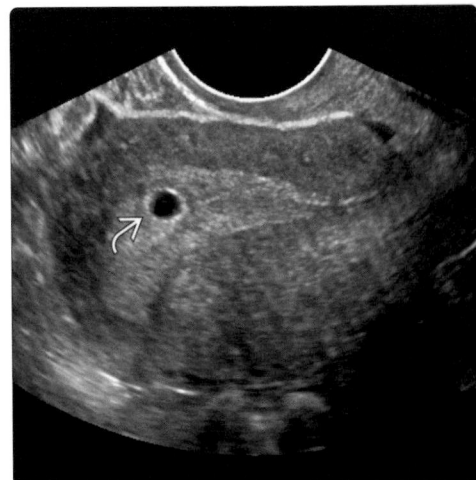

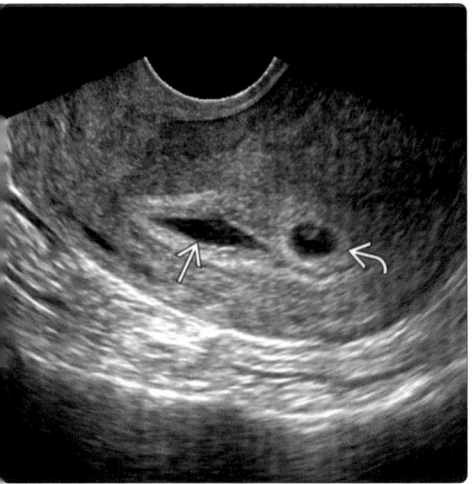

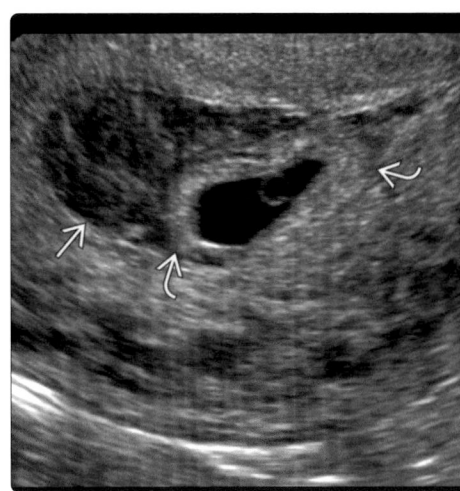

(Left) *Longitudinal transvaginal ultrasound shows an elongated anechoic perigestational fluid collection* ➡ *adjacent to a small gestational sac* ➡. **(Right)** *Longitudinal transvaginal ultrasound shows a large crescentic perigestational fluid collection* ➡ *with internal echoes surrounding at least 50% of the circumference of the gestational sac* ➡.

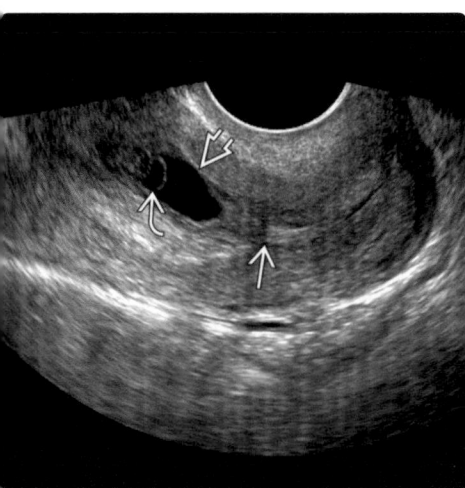

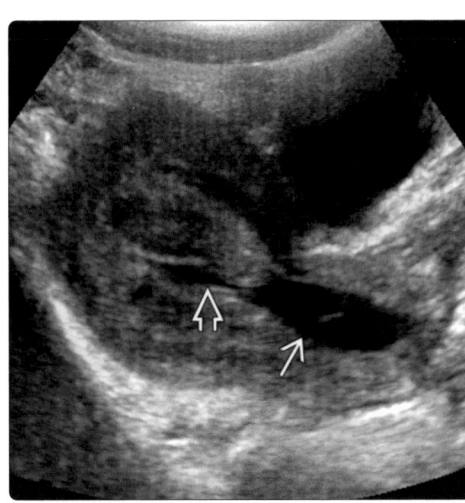

(Left) *Longitudinal transvaginal ultrasound shows an irregular elongated gestational sac* ➡ *positioned low in the endometrial cavity just above the internal os* ➡, *which is mildly dilated, compatible with an impending spontaneous abortion. The sac contains a flattened yolk sac* ➡ *with a thin wall.* **(Right)** *Longitudinal transabdominal ultrasound shows a heterogeneous elongated abnormal sac* ➡ *extending into the open cervix* ➡, *compatible with an abortion in progress*

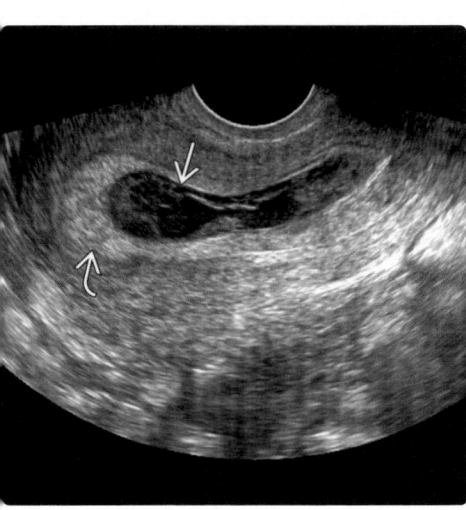

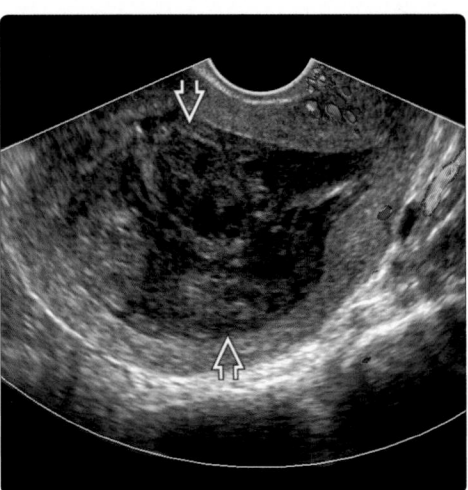

(Left) *Longitudinal transvaginal ultrasound shows a flattened GS* ➡ *and decidual tissue* ➡ *centrally located in a patient with spontaneous abortion. Amorphous echogenicity in the sac is compatible with hemorrhage and debris.* **(Right)** *Longitudinal transvaginal color Doppler ultrasound in a patient presenting with vaginal bleeding shows a heterogeneous, avascular collection* ➡ *in the uterus, compatible with blood clot and debris. A gestational sac was not seen.*

Retained Products of Conception

TERMINOLOGY

- Retained trophoblastic tissue
- Occurs after delivery or termination of pregnancy

IMAGING

- Grayscale ultrasound
  - Thickened endometrial echo complex or echogenic intrauterine mass
- Color Doppler ultrasound
  - Presence of vascularity in thickened endometrial echo complex or mass substantially increases likelihood of retained products of conception (RPOC)
  - Degree of vascularity may range from hypovascular to markedly hypervascular compared to normal uterine myometrium

TOP DIFFERENTIAL DIAGNOSES

- Normal postpartum uterus
- Uterine atony

- Intrauterine blood/clot
- Endometritis
- Invasive molar pregnancy
- Arteriovenous malformation (AVM)
- Subinvolution of placental implantation site
- Enhanced myometrial vascularity

PATHOLOGY

- Presence of chorionic villi indicates persistence of placental tissue

CLINICAL ISSUES

- More frequent following termination and 2nd trimester deliveries

(Left) Transverse color Doppler endovaginal US of the uterus shows a hypoechoic mass ⇨ with moderate ⇨ internal vascularity, consistent with retained products of conception (RPOC). (Right) Longitudinal color Doppler US of the uterus in a different patient shows a thickened endometrial echo complex ⇨ with marked vascularity ⇨ at the fundus, consistent with RPOC. Vascularity in the endometrium is a helpful clue to the presence of RPOC.

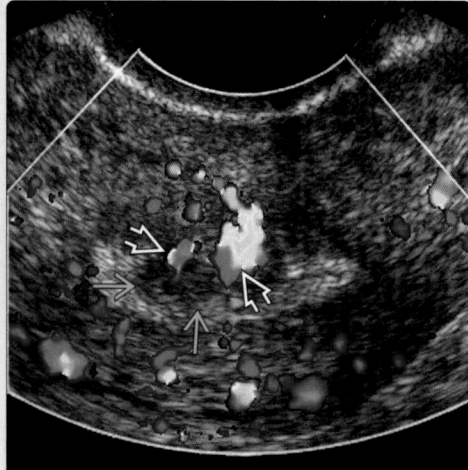
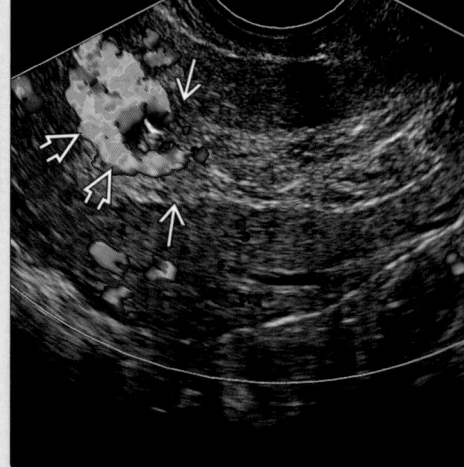

(Left) Transverse endovaginal US of the uterus shows a markedly thickened and heterogeneous endometrial echo complex ⇨, which was pathologically proven to represent RPOC. (Right) Transverse endovaginal color Doppler US in the same patient shows the thickened endometrial echo complex is markedly vascular ⇨, a common imaging appearance of RPOC, which should not be mistaken for arteriovenous malformation (AVM) particularly if there is a focal endometrial mass.

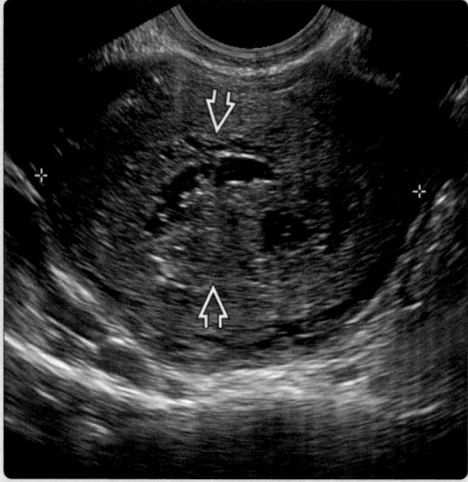
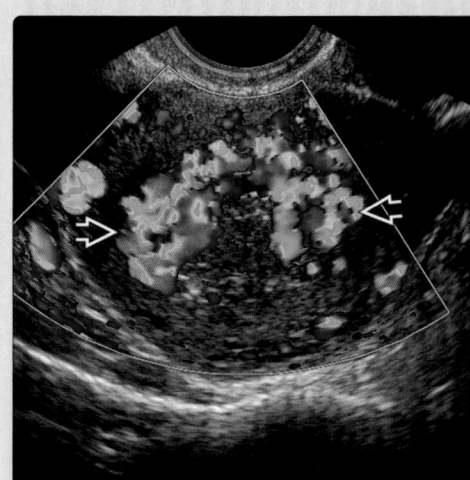

TERMINOLOGY

Abbreviations

Retained products of conception (RPOC)

Synonyms

- Retained trophoblastic tissue
- Retained placenta
- Placental polyp

Definitions

Retained placental tissue
- o Occurs after delivery or termination of pregnancy

IMAGING

General Features

Best diagnostic clue
- o Thickened endometrial echo complex or echogenic endometrial mass plus internal vascularity
  - – Vascularity + endometrial mass = high positive predictive value for RPOC
    - □ Less likely to be RPOC if endometrial echo complex < 10 mm in thickness and sonographically avascular
  - – Vascularity often low-resistance, high-velocity flow

Ultrasonographic Findings

- Grayscale ultrasound
  - o Thickened endometrial echo complex > 10 mm
  - o Solid, heterogeneous, or echogenic endometrial or intrauterine mass
    - – Sensitivity of this finding is variable: 29-79%
  - o Irregular interface between endometrium and myometrium
  - o Intrauterine fluid common
- Pulsed Doppler
  - o Pulsed Doppler may show high-velocity, low-resistance flow
    - – Peak systolic velocity varies but can be as high as 100 cm/sec
- Color Doppler
  - o Presence of vascularity in thickened endometrial echo complex or mass substantially increases likelihood of RPOC (PPV 96%)
  - o Degree of vascularity may range from hypovascular to markedly hypervascular compared to normal uterine myometrium
    - – Pitfalls
      - □ Markedly hypervascular RPOC may mimic arteriovenous malformation (AVM)
      - □ Avascular RPOC may mimic clot

CT Findings

- CECT
  - o Intrauterine endometrial mass with variable contrast enhancement

MR Findings

- T1WI C+
  - o Intrauterine soft tissue mass with variable contrast enhancement
    - – No extrauterine invasion

Imaging Recommendations

- Best imaging tool
  - o Grayscale and color Doppler ultrasound for evaluation of uterus and detection of internal vascularity
  - o MR for problem solving is occasionally necessary

DIFFERENTIAL DIAGNOSIS

Normal Postpartum Uterus

- Highly variable, from smooth to irregular endometrium
- Small echogenic foci and fluid common
- Foci of gas may be seen in up to 21% in 1st 3 weeks post partum
- Endometrial thickness < 2 cm initially and should decrease to < 8 mm with uterine involution

Uterine Atony

- Primary differential consideration for immediate postpartum hemorrhage (PPH)
- Should not see any sonographic evidence of retained products within endometrial cavity
  - o Blood/clot may potentially be confusing

Intrauterine Blood/Clot

- No flow with color Doppler
- Changes or resolves on follow-up scans

Endometritis

- Clinical diagnosis
- Postpartum fever and pelvic pain
- May see gas in endometrium but findings are typically nonspecific
- Patient may have both RPOC and coexisting endometritis

Invasive Molar Pregnancy

- Benign tumor arising from myometrial invasion of hydatidiform mole
- 10-17% of hydatidiform moles result in invasive moles
- Heterogeneous cystic and solid placental mass with hypervascular components in invasive mole
- Persistently elevated beta hCG levels
- May have extrauterine extension (metastasize to lungs or vagina)
- Chemosensitive

Arteriovenous Malformation (AVM)

- Marked vascularity isolated to myometrium
  - o Vascularity should not extend to endometrium in uterine AVM
  - o No tissue in endometrial cavity
  - o Hypervascular RPOC often misdiagnosed as uterine AVM
  - o Enhanced myometrial vascularity (a.k.a. uterine non-AVM) can have similar appearance
- Most develop secondary to uterine tissue injury, most commonly from prior D&C for termination of pregnancy
- Serum beta-hCG is usually negative or minimal
- Potential risk of life-threatening hemorrhage
- Definitive diagnosis made by identification of early draining vein on angiography
- True incidence of AVM unknown

Subinvolution of Placental Implantation Site

- Idiopathic cause of postpartum hemorrhage

- Delayed involution of superficial modified spiral arteries at placental attachment site
  - Leads to delayed postpartum hemorrhage
- Diagnosed during pathological analysis of D&C or hysterectomy specimens of placenta after excluding presence of chorionic villi, endometritis, and gestational trophoblastic disease
- Etiology remains poorly understood

Enhanced Myometrial Vascularity

- Presence of marked vascularity over full thickness of myometrium related to involution of placental bed after pregnancy and miscarriage
  - Myometrial hypervascularity represents involuting peri-trophoblastic flow
- Occur in 50% of normal postpartum patients at day 3
- Also known as uterine non-AVM
- Disappears spontaneously

Submucosal Leiomyoma

- Submucosal mass protruding into endometrium with increased vascularity
- May be contiguous with underlying myometrium

Endometrial Polyp

- Intraluminal pedunculated endometrial mass
- Typically ovoid and echogenic
- Single vascular pedicle

PATHOLOGY

General Features

- Presence of chorionic villi indicates persistence of placental tissue

Staging, Grading, & Classification

- Grading for degree of endometrial vascularity of RPOC with respect to myometrium
  - Type 0: Avascular
  - Type 1: Minimal vascularity
    - Vascularity < myometrium
  - Type 2: Moderate vascularity
    - Vascularity = myometrium
  - Type 3: Marked vascularity
    - Vascularity > myometrium

CLINICAL ISSUES

Presentation

- Most common signs/symptoms
  - Postpartum hemorrhage
    - RPOC may present as primary or secondary PPH
      - Primary PPH (within 1st 24 hours)
      - Secondary PPH (24 hours to 6 months post partum)
    - May rarely present weeks after delivery or termination with vaginal bleeding or infection
  - Pain
  - Fever

Demographics

- Epidemiology
  - ~ 1% of all pregnancies

- More frequent following termination and 2nd trimester deliveries
- ↑ incidence with
  - Placenta accreta
  - Instrumentation during delivery
  - Failure to progress during delivery

Treatment

- Options, risks, complications
  - May monitor 24-48 hours, especially if ultrasound findings are equivocal
    - May repeat ultrasound to reevaluate
    - Correlation with human chorionic gonadotropin (hCG) levels may be helpful to distinguish RPOC from invasive molar pregnancy
  - Expectant management
    - RPOC may pass spontaneously or with uterotonic medications
  - D&C
    - Performed in cases of persistent bleeding or obvious RPOC
    - Failure to evacuate may lead to prolonged hemorrhage and infection
  - Uterine artery embolization
    - Treatment of choice for excessive bleeding
    - May be diagnostic as well as therapeutic for both RPOC and AVM
  - Hysteroscopy
    - Directed visualization of intrauterine cavity may be necessary in cases of incomplete D&C

DIAGNOSTIC CHECKLIST

Image Interpretation Pearls

- Uterine atony vs. RPOC: Primary differential for immediate postpartum hemorrhage
  - Atony: Normal-appearing cavity
  - RPOC: Thickened endometrial echo complex or echogenic, intracavitary mass
- If endometrial thickness < 10 mm and without internal vascularity, RPOC unlikely

SELECTED REFERENCES

1. Goyal S et al: Acquired uterine arteriovenous malformation developing in retained products of conception: a diagnostic dilemma. J Obstet Gynaecol Res. 40(1):271-4, 2014
2. Zubor P et al: Recurrent secondary postpartum hemorrhages due to placental site vessel subinvolution and local uterine tissue coagulopathy. BMC Pregnancy Childbirth. 14:80, 2014
3. Sellmyer MA et al: Physiologic, histologic, and imaging features of retained products of conception. Radiographics. 33(3):781-96, 2013
4. Atri M et al: Best predictors of grayscale ultrasound combined with color Doppler in the diagnosis of retained products of conception. J Clin Ultrasound. 39(3):122-7, 2011
5. Kitahara T et al: Management of retained products of conception with marked vascularity. J Obstet Gynaecol Res. 37(5):458-64, 2011
6. Kamaya A et al: Retained products of conception: spectrum of color Doppler findings. J Ultrasound Med. 28(8):1031-41, 2009
7. Weydert JA et al: Subinvolution of the placental site as an anatomic cause of postpartum uterine bleeding: a review. Arch Pathol Lab Med. 130(10):1538-42, 2006
8. Durfee SM et al: The Sonographic and Color Doppler Features of Retained Products of Conception. J Ultrasound Med. 24(9):1181-1186, 2005
9. Sadan O et al: Role of sonography in the diagnosis of retained products of conception. J Ultrasound Med. 23(3):371-4, 2004

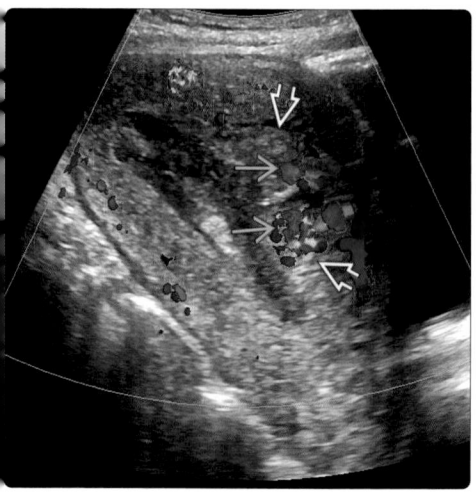

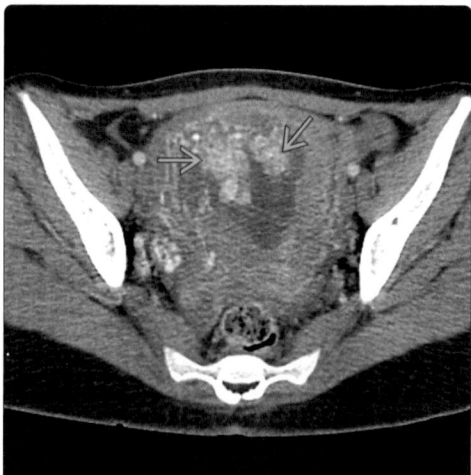

(Left) *Sagittal color Doppler US of the uterus in a patient with RPOC shows 2 rounded echogenic areas ➡ in the endometrial cavity with internal vascularity ➡, which are foci of retained placenta.* (Right) *Axial CECT in the same patient confirms that the endometrial masses ➡ are enhancing and compatible with retained products of conception. In this case, contrast-enhanced CT did not provide any additional information.*

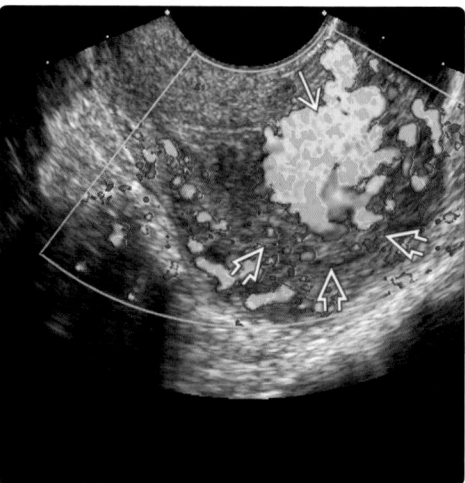

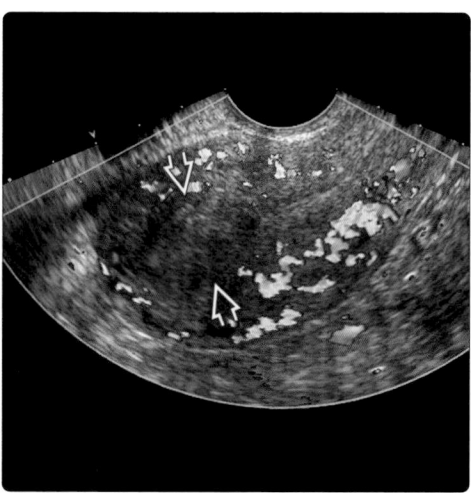

(Left) *Sagittal color Doppler US shows marked vascularity ➡ within a large RPOC, which distends the endometrial cavity ➡. Degree of vascularity is so pronounced that it can be confused for AVM. However, vascularity involves endometrium as well as myometrium, a helpful finding in correctly diagnosing RPOC.* (Right) *Longitudinal color Doppler US shows avascular RPOC with thickened endometrial echo complex ➡. Avascular RPOC may be difficult to distinguish from blood clot but both are likely to pass spontaneously.*

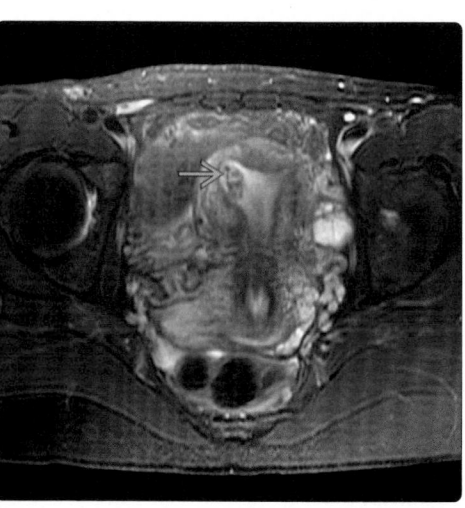

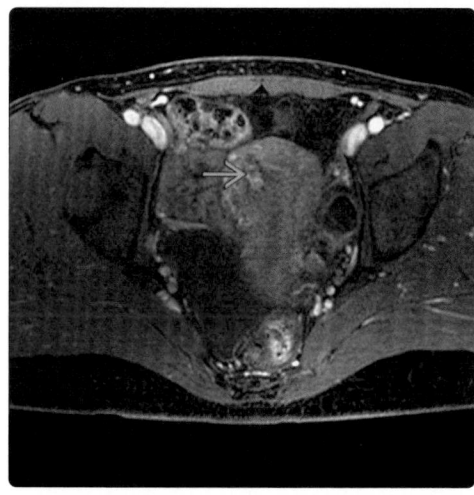

(Left) *Axial T2WI MR with fat saturation in a patient with RPOC shows a heterogeneous hypointense mass ➡ in the right uterine cavity.* (Right) *Axial post-contrast T1WI MR with fat saturation in the same patient confirms the rounded area is enhancing ➡, consistent with RPOC.*

Gestational Trophoblastic Disease

IMAGING

- **Hydatidiform moles**
  - **Partial hydatidiform mole**: Thickened placenta with cystic change and peripheral vascularity, may be associated with fetal parts
  - **Complete hydatidiform mole**: Enlarged placenta with multiple cysts
    - "Snowstorm" appearance or "bunch of grapes"
    - No embryo
- **Malignant Gestational Trophoblastic Disease**
  - **Invasive mole**: Heterogeneous intrauterine mass with extension into myometrium
  - **Choriocarcinoma**: Heterogeneous uterus with complex hypervascular mass invading myometrium and extrauterine extension
  - **Placental site trophoblastic tumor**: Intrauterine echogenic mass with myometrial involvement and extrauterine extension

TOP DIFFERENTIAL DIAGNOSES

- Placental hydropic degeneration
- Placental sonolucencies (pseudomole)
- Retained products of conception (RPOC)
- Androgenic biparental mosaicism with placental mesenchymal dysplasia (PMD)

PATHOLOGY

- Partial mole (triploidy)
  - Karyotypes: 69,XXY (most common); 69,XXX; 69,XXY
- Complete hydatidiform mole
  - 46, XX more common than 46, XY
  - No fetal tissue present

CLINICAL ISSUES

- ↑ risk at extremes of reproductive age

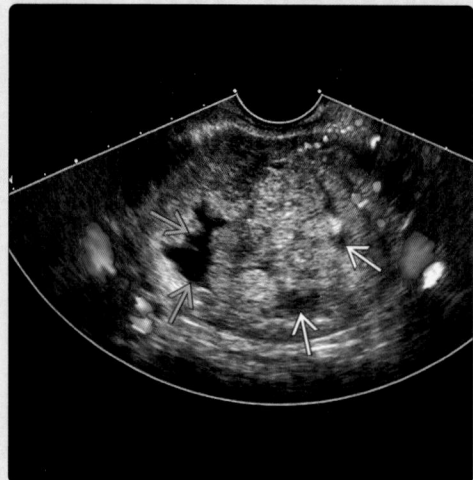

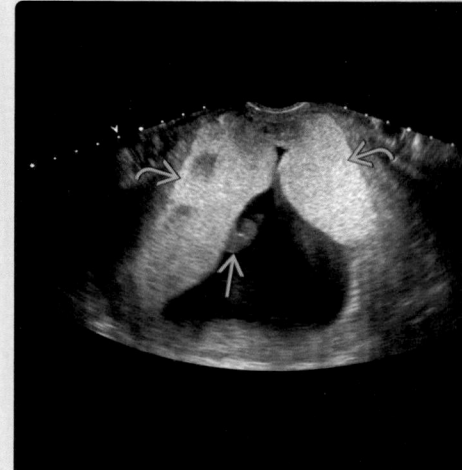

(Left) Coronal color Doppler US through the uterine body shows a partial molar pregnancy. Note the empty irregular gestational sac ➡ and associated enlarged placenta with cystic components ➡. (Right) Transverse grayscale US of a partial mole shows an intrauterine gestation with fetal pole ➡. No fetal cardiac activity was seen in real-time. The placenta ➡ is markedly thickened and echogenic in appearance, greater than expected for gestational age.

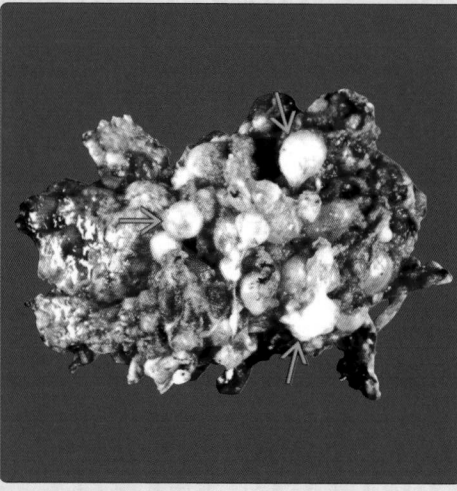

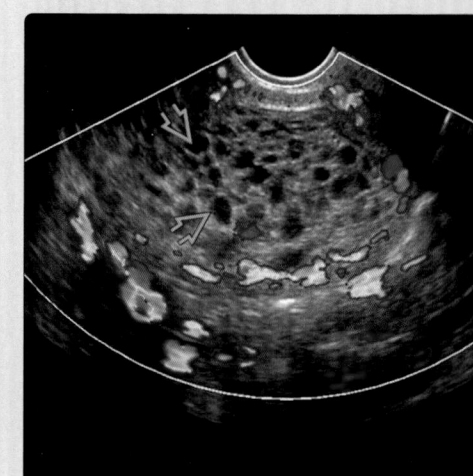

(Left) Gross pathology of a partial molar placenta shows typical trophoblastic hydropic villi and cluster of molar vesicles ➡, compatible with a "cluster of grapes" appearance. (Right) Longitudinal color Doppler US of a complete hydatidiform mole shows a heterogeneous multicystic mass ➡ resembling a "cluster of grapes." Note that the multicystic areas are relatively avascular, a helpful clue to differentiate from an invasive mole.

Gestational Trophoblastic Disease

TERMINOLOGY

Abbreviations
- Gestational trophoblastic disease (GTD)

Synonyms
- Gestational trophoblastic neoplasm
- Molar pregnancy

Definitions
- Abnormal proliferation of trophoblastic tissue
- GTD subtypes
  - Hydatidiform moles
    - Partial hydatidiform mole (triploidy)
    - Complete hydatidiform mole (CHM)
  - Malignant GTD
    - Invasive mole (chorioadenoma destruens)
    - Choriocarcinoma
    - Placental site trophoblastic tumor (PSTT)

IMAGING

General Features
- Best diagnostic clue
  - Markedly elevated beta human chorionic gonadotropin (hCG)
  - Enlarged placenta with cysts
  - ± ovarian theca lutein cysts
- Location
  - Complete and partial hydatidiform moles confined to endometrium
  - Invasive mole invades myometrium
  - Choriocarcinoma often metastatic

Ultrasonographic Findings
- **Partial hydatidiform mole**
  - Thickened placenta with cystic changes and peripheral vascularity
    - May be associated with fetal parts
    - Abnormal gestational sac
- **Complete hydatidiform mole**
  - Enlarged placenta with multiple cysts of varying shapes and sizes
    - Best imaging clue: "Snowstorm" appearance or "bunch of grapes"
  - Color Doppler shows increased vascularity
    - High-velocity, low-impedance flow
    - Mean resistive index (RI) of 0.55
  - No embryo or fetus
  - **Ovarian theca lutein cysts** present in 25-55 % of cases
    - 2° to ovarian hyperstimulation
    - ↑ hCG hormone
- **Malignant GTD**
  - Invasive mole
    - Enlarged, heterogeneous cystic intrauterine mass with increased vascularity extending into myometrium
    - Rarely metastasizes
  - Choriocarcinoma
    - Enlarged, heterogeneous uterus with complex solid and cystic mass with increased vascularity

  - □ May invade myometrium and have extrauterine extension
    - Lungs: Most common site of metastasis
  - PSTT
    - Focal echogenic intrauterine mass with myometrial involvement and extrauterine extension
    - Variable vascularity
    - Hypovascular PSTT: More difficult to diagnose on ultrasound

CT Findings
- NECT
  - Useful in detection of hemorrhagic brain metastasis in malignant GTD
- CECT
  - Enlarged, enhancing heterogeneous uterine mass
    - Malignant GTD may have extrauterine extension
  - Helpful for metastatic work-up and surveillance

MR Findings
- Heterogeneous, enhancing intrauterine mass with variable signal intensity
  - Malignant GTD may show disruption of junctional zone with abnormal uterine vasculature
- Helpful for determining extent of extrauterine invasion

Imaging Recommendations
- Best imaging tool
  - Pelvic ultrasound: Imaging modality of choice
  - MR with gadolinium for invasive mole
  - CT for metastatic choriocarcinoma work-up
- Protocol advice
  - Suspect GTD if hCG levels are atypical
    - Too high for gestational age
    - Persistently elevated
  - Look for heterogenous cystic intrauterine mass
  - Look for signs of invasion

DIFFERENTIAL DIAGNOSIS

Placental Hydropic Degeneration
- Hydropic change without proliferation
- Seen after pregnancy failure
  - Embryonic demise
  - Anembryonic gestation
- Less vascular than CHM
- Low hCG levels

Placental Sonolucencies (Pseudomole)
- Occasional sonolucencies are normal
  - Placental lakes
  - Intervillous thrombus
  - Often seen > 25 weeks
- "Swiss cheese" variant mimics CHM
  - Often with placentomegaly
  - ↑ maternal serum α-fetoprotein (MSAFP)
  - Associated with maternal/fetal morbidity
    - ↑ risk of placental insufficiency

Retained Products of Conception (RPOC)
- Retained placental or fetal tissue after normal delivery, abortion, or miscarriage

- Complex echogenic mass with increased vascularity
- Normal to slightly elevated hCG levels
  - Helps differentiate from invasive molar pregnancy

Androgenic Biparental Mosaicism With Placental Mesenchymal Dysplasia (PMD)

- Rare placental disorder
- Associated with Beckwith-Wiedemann syndrome (BWS)
  - Absence of trophoblastic hyperplasia distinguishes PMD from molar pregnancy

PATHOLOGY

General Features

- Etiology
  - Complete hydatidiform mole
    - Abnormal trophoblast proliferation
  - Theca lutein cysts
    - Ovarian hyperstimulation by ↑ hCG
    - Only present in 50%
    - Rare < 13 weeks
- Genetics
  - Partial mole (triploidy)
    - Karyotypes: 69,XXY (most common); 69,XXX; 69,XXY
      - Normal ovum + 2 normal (haploid) sperm
      - Normal ovum + 2 abnormal (diploid) sperm
  - Complete hydatidiform mole
    - Androgenetic pregnancy: 100% paternal genetic make-up
    - 46,XX more common than 46,XY
    - No fetal tissue present

Staging, Grading, & Classification

- Choriocarcinoma
  - Stage I: Confined to uterus
  - Stage II: Limited to pelvis
  - Stage III: Lung metastases
  - Stage IV: Other metastases

Gross Pathologic & Surgical Features

- Cystic villi resemble "cluster of grapes"

Microscopic Features

- Trophoblastic hyperplasia
- Hydropic villi

CLINICAL ISSUES

Presentation

- Most common signs/symptoms
  - Partial mole (triploidy)
    - Vaginal bleeding
    - Abnormal fetal tissue + thickened, cystic placenta
  - 1st trimester CHM
    - Variable appearance
      - hCG levels may be normal
    - Rapid uterine enlargement
    - Hyperemesis 2° to ↑ hCG levels
  - 2nd trimester CHM
    - ↑ hCG levels
    - Preeclampsia symptoms
  - Invasive mole

- Persistent ↑ hCG levels after CHM treatment
  - Choriocarcinoma
    - Symptoms of metastatic disease
    - ↑ hCG levels
  - PSTT
    - ↓ hCG levels and ↑ human placental lactogen (hPL) level
      - Minimal syncytiotrophoblastic tissue
- Other signs/symptoms
  - Adnexal pain or mass
    - Theca lutein cysts

Demographics

- Age
  - ↑ risk at extremes of reproductive age
- Ethnicity
  - ↑ risk for Asian women
- Epidemiology
  - Partial mole (triploidy)
    - 2-4% become invasive
  - Complete hydatidiform mole
    - Most common type of GTD
    - 0.5:1,000 in United States
    - 8:1,000 in Asia
    - 12-15% become invasive
    - Coexistent mole and fetus is variant of CHM
  - Choriocarcinoma
    - 50% originate from CHM
    - 25% occur after failed pregnancy
    - 25% after normal pregnancy

Natural History & Prognosis

- CHM has excellent prognosis
  - Evacuation often curative
- Invasive disease
  - Near 100% cure with chemotherapy
  - 75% remission even if extensive metastases

Treatment

- Complete hydatidiform mole
  - Dilation and curettage with serial hCG measurements
- Invasive disease
  - Low-risk malignant cases: Single agent chemotherapy with methotrexate or actinomycin D
  - High-risk malignant cases: Multiagent chemotherapy
  - Hysterectomy in nonresponsive cases or if fertility preservation is not desired

SELECTED REFERENCES

1. Lane BF et al: ACR Appropriateness Criteria® first trimester bleeding. Ultrasound Q. 29(2):91-6, 2013
2. Kohorn EI: Imaging practices in the diagnosis and management of gestational trophoblastic disease: an assessment. J Reprod Med. 57(5-6):207-10, 2012
3. Emoto M et al: Clinical usefulness of contrast-enhanced color Doppler ultrasonography in invasive and noninvasive gestational trophoblastic diseases: a preliminary study. J Reprod Med. 56(5-6):224-34, 2011
4. Lurain JR: Gestational trophoblastic disease I: epidemiology, pathology, clinical presentation and diagnosis of gestational trophoblastic disease, and management of hydatidiform mole. Am J Obstet Gynecol. 203(6):531-9, 2010
5. Betel C et al: Sonographic diagnosis of gestational trophoblastic disease and comparison with retained products of conception. J Ultrasound Med. 25(8):985-93, 2006

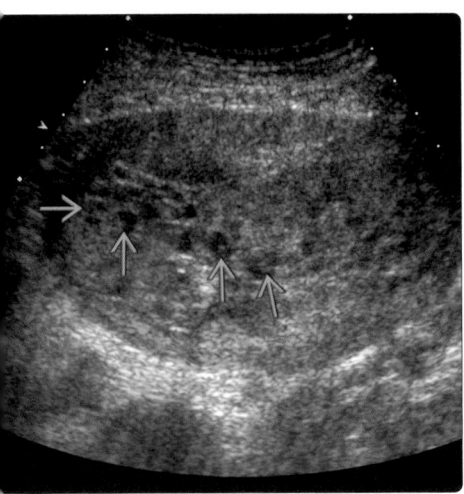

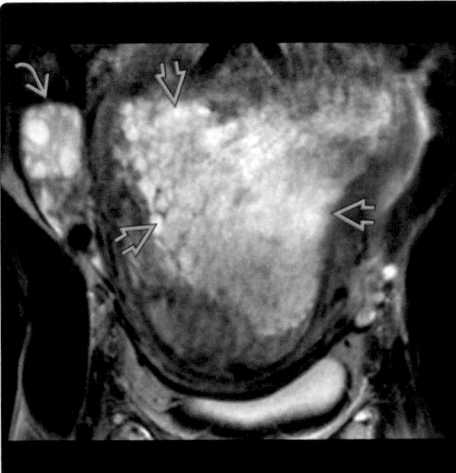

(Left) Transverse transabdominal grayscale US of the uterus in a 17-year-old female shows multiple cystic ➡ areas in the uterine cavity that are consistent with a complete hydatidiform mole. (Right) Coronal T2WI MR of a complete hydatidiform molar pregnancy shows an enlarged uterus markedly expanded by multiple cystic structures ➡, which creates a "cluster of grapes" appearance. The right ovary is enlarged with multiple theca lutein cysts ➡, often seen in the setting of a complete mole.

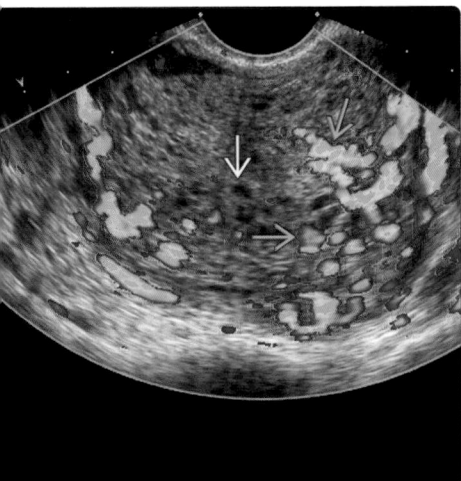

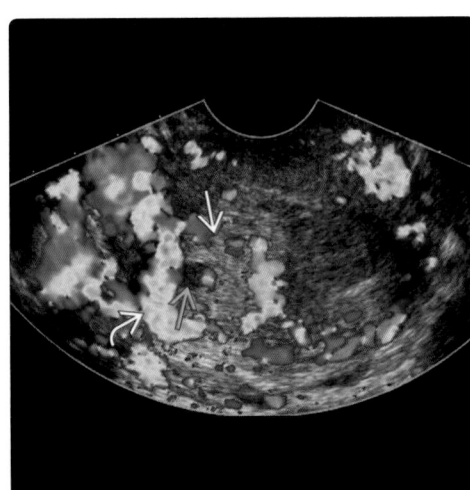

(Left) Transverse color Doppler ultrasound of the pelvis in a patient with an invasive molar pregnancy after complete mole evacuation shows multiple cystic areas ➡ as well as abnormal vascularity ➡. This patient was treated with chemotherapy with complete resolution. (Right) Coronal color Doppler US of the lower uterine segment of a choriocarcinoma shows a highly vascular heterogenous mass ➡ with cystic degeneration ➡ and invasion into the posterior uterine wall ➡.

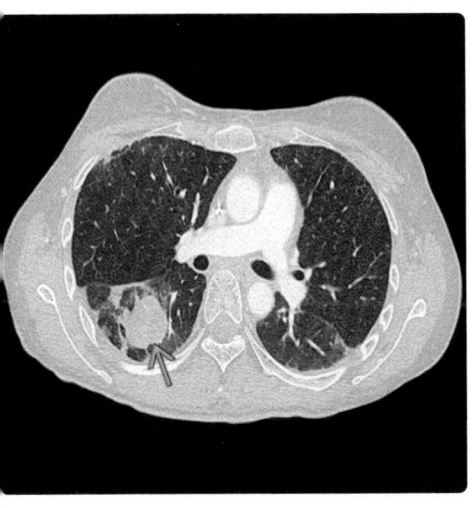

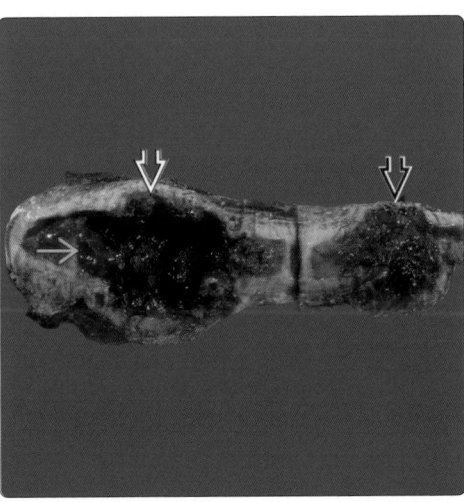

(Left) Axial CECT of chest in a patient with metastatic choriocarcinoma to the lungs shows a 3.1 x 2.7 cm mass ➡ in the right lower lobe. (Right) Gross pathologic specimen of a placental site trophoblastic tumor involving the endometrium ➡, myometrial wall ➡, and cervix ➡ is shown.

Functional Ovarian Cyst

TERMINOLOGY

- Follicular cyst (FC) forms from persistent follicle, ovulation does not occur
- Corpus luteum cyst (CLC) forms from graafian follicle following ovulation

IMAGING

- Follicular cyst
  - Intraovarian cystic lesion with thin walls
- Corpus luteum cyst
  - Occur after ovulation in latter part of menstrual cycle
  - Thick, hyperechoic wall
  - Central anechoic/hypoechoic cavity
  - Marked vascular flow within CLC wall: "Ring of fire" appearance
  - Commonly complicated by hemorrhage

TOP DIFFERENTIAL DIAGNOSES

- Ectopic pregnancy

- "Ring of fire" but separate from ovary, usually tubal
- Ovarian neoplasm

CLINICAL ISSUES

- Follicular and CL cysts occur during reproductive years
  - FL and CLC ≤ 5 cm: No follow-up necessary
  - FL and CLC > 5 and ≤ 7 cm: Annual follow-up ultrasound
- Further imaging or surgical evaluation recommended with simple cyst > 7 cm
- CLC may enlarge initially with fertilization and pregnancy
  - Most no longer seen by sonography by early 2nd trimester (16 weeks)
- Malignancy rate in unilocular simple cysts < 1%

DIAGNOSTIC CHECKLIST

- Majority of functional ovarian cysts will resolve spontaneously
- Even if CLC is persistent, may monitor through pregnancy if no malignant features

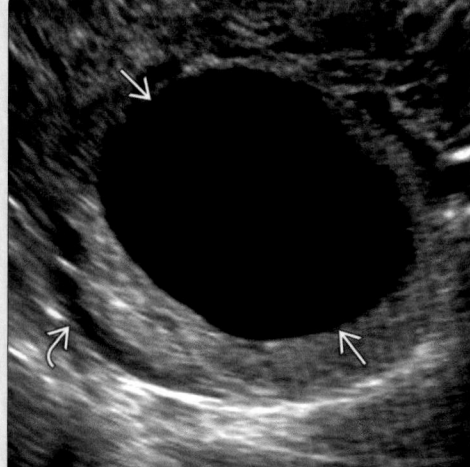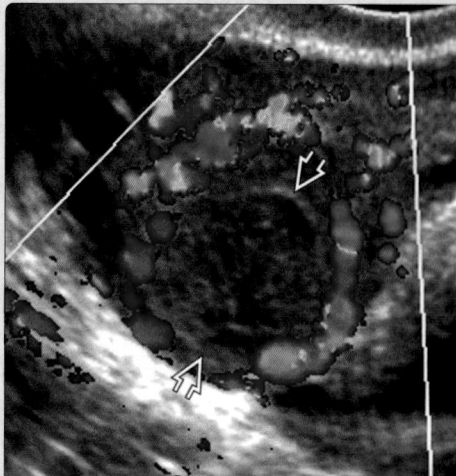

(Left) Typical appearance of a simple functional ovarian cyst ➡ is shown. The peripheral follicles within the surrounding parenchyma ➡ confirm this is an intraovarian cyst. (Right) The "ring of fire" appearance is associated with marked vascular flow within the corpus luteum cyst (CLC) wall on color Doppler. In this case, the CLC is centrally hypoechoic due to internal hemorrhage ➡.

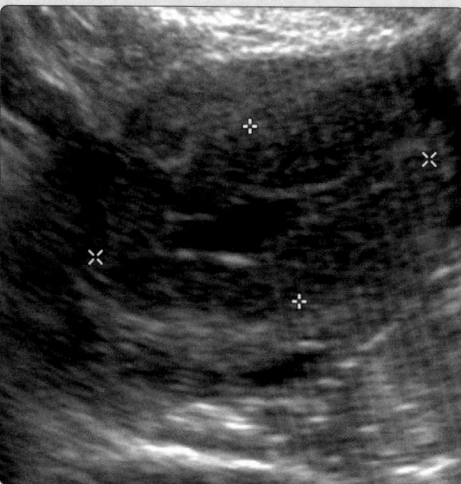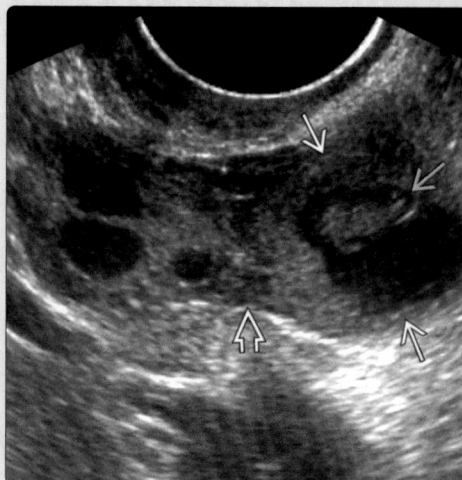

(Left) A thick-walled CLC can appear crenulated or decompressed after ovulation (calipers) is seen here on grayscale transvaginal US. (Right) CLC can be exophytic from the ovary ➡; look for the bridging ovarian parenchyma ➡. Commonly associated hemorrhage, retracted clot can also be present within a CLC ➡.

TERMINOLOGY

Abbreviations

- Follicular cyst (FC)
- Corpus luteum cyst (CLC)

Definitions

- 2 types of functional cysts
  - Follicular cyst forms from persistent follicle, ovulation does not occur
    - Associated with elevated serum estrogen
  - Corpus luteum cyst forms from graafian follicle following ovulation

IMAGING

General Features

- Best diagnostic clue
  - FC: Thin-walled cyst persisting after ovulation expected to occur
  - CLC: Thick-walled cyst seen after ovulation

Ultrasonographic Findings

- FC
  - Intraovarian cystic lesion with thin walls
  - No increased flow on Doppler evaluation
  - Tend to occur in 1st half of menstrual cycle or after missed ovulation
- CLC
  - Occur after ovulation in latter part of menstrual cycle
  - Intraovarian cystic lesion
    - Thick, hyperechoic wall
    - Central anechoic/hypoechoic cavity
  - May appear solid if significant hemorrhage or sac collapse
    - Retracting clot seen on follow-up scans
  - Commonly complicated by hemorrhage
    - Look for fluid-fluid level
    - Thin septations with lacy, reticular pattern
    - No internal flow on Doppler evaluation
  - Doppler findings
    - Marked vascular flow within CLC wall: "Ring of fire" appearance
    - Low-resistance waveform on pulsed Doppler

CT Findings

- In nonpregnant population presenting with acute pain, CT is often performed
- Low-attenuation adnexal mass unless hemorrhagic
  - If so, may see high-attenuation blood products or fluid-fluid level
- CT poor at evaluation of internal architecture of fluid attenuation structures
- CECT may show enhancing wall of CLC corresponding to "ring of fire"

MR Findings

- Appearances are highly variable depending on presence of associated hemorrhage

Imaging Recommendations

- Best imaging tool
  - Transvaginal ultrasound
- For thick-walled cysts, use Doppler to exclude solid component
  - Blood flow in solid tissues, not in clot
  - "Ring of fire" commonly seen around corpus luteum
  - Follow-up masses of concern in 6-12 weeks
    - Decreasing size and clot retraction confirm diagnosis of corpus luteum cyst
- Exophytic CLC may be difficult to differentiate from ectopic pregnancy
  - Use transvaginal ultrasound probe with gentle abdominal pressure to better evaluate adnexa
  - CL cyst moves with ovary
    - Tubal ectopic can be separated from ovary

DIFFERENTIAL DIAGNOSIS

Ectopic Pregnancy

- Extraovarian
- "Ring of fire" in adnexa, separate from ovary
  - Slide test: Ectopic mass can often be displaced away from ovary using gentle transvaginal probe pressure
  - Ring is typically more echogenic in ectopic than in CLC
- Adnexal mass (hematoma) with echogenic free fluid

Ovarian Neoplasm

- Benign cystic tumors
  - Serous cystadenoma
  - Mucinous cystadenoma
  - Cystic teratoma
- Solid tumors
  - Thecoma-fibroma
- Ovarian malignancy

Heterotopic Pregnancy

- Usually history of fertility treatments
- Intrauterine pregnancy documented
- Additional ectopic pregnancy, usually tubal

Normal Follicle

- Ovulation generally occurs when dominant follicle reaches about 22 mm diameter
- Correlate with menstrual history ± serum hormone levels if concern

PATHOLOGY

Gross Pathologic & Surgical Features

- Corpus luteum cyst
  - Rim of bright yellow luteal tissue
    - Corpus luteum means "yellow body"
  - If no embryo implants, CLC degenerates after about 14 days and becomes corpus albicans
  - Highly variable in size
    - Pathologists use > 3 cm diameter for definition of CLC

Microscopic Features

- Corpus luteum cyst
  - Contains luteinized granulosa cells
  - Central cystic cavity with fluid and fibrin
    - Often with hemorrhage
  - With conception, granulosa-lutein cells enlarge

- Placental human chorionic gonadotropin stimulates CL progesterone production by granulosa-lutein cells
- Maintains uterine endometrium to receive embryo for implantation
- CL progesterone production declines by end of 2nd month of gestation
  - □ Placenta takes over production of progesterone
- CL present throughout pregnancy, though significantly reduced in metabolic activity
  - □ Obliteration begins by 5th month of pregnancy and is complete by term

CLINICAL ISSUES

Presentation

- Most common signs/symptoms
  - Majority of functional cysts are asymptomatic
  - Clinical presentation with pelvic pain due to
    - Large size → capsular distension
    - Rupture: 25% of women experience mittelschmerz or ovulation pain
    - Hemorrhage: Occurs into FC or CLC, acute bleed may → rupture/hemoperitoneum
    - Torsion: Cyst enlarges ovary, may → torsion, infarction
- Other signs/symptoms
  - Palpable ovarian enlargement on clinical examination
  - FC may be discovered during infertility work-up
  - CLC incidentally noted on 1st trimester scan

Demographics

- Age
  - Follicular and CL cysts occur during reproductive years
  - Most fetal ovarian cysts are follicular
- Epidemiology
  - ~ 30% of menstruating women will have functional cyst at some point
  - 25-60% of ovarian lesions in children are functional ovarian cysts

Natural History & Prognosis

- Follicular cyst
  - May be associated with infertility: Oligo/anovulation
  - Estrogen levels are elevated: May interfere with ovulation induction for assisted reproduction
  - When seen in female fetus, may be present with intrauterine torsion
    - Look for fluid-fluid level
    - Most infants are asymptomatic at birth even if torsion occurred
    - Elective surgery may be indicated to fix contralateral ovary
- Corpus luteum cyst
  - May enlarge initially with fertilization and pregnancy
    - Peak size usually around 7 weeks
  - Should diminish in size with progression of pregnancy
  - Most no longer seen by sonography by early 2nd trimester (16 weeks)
  - If cystic mass persists after pregnancy, consider ovarian epithelial neoplasm
- Majority of functional ovarian cysts will resolve spontaneously

- Torsion more common on right side and with cysts > 4 cm in diameter
- Malignancy rate in unilocular simple cysts < 1%

Treatment

- Society of Radiologists in Ultrasound (SRU) consensus statement on ovarian cyst management
  - Simple cyst
    - Reproductive age women
      - □ No follow-up necessary ≤ 5 cm
      - □ > 5 and ≤ 7 cm: Annual follow-up ultrasound
    - Postmenopausal
      - □ > 1 and ≤ 7 cm: Annual ultrasound
    - Any age group with simple cyst > 7 cm
      - □ Refer for further imaging (MR) or surgical evaluation
- Symptomatic treatment if painful
  - Oral contraceptive pill helpful if recurrent cysts
- If persistent may require laparoscopic surgery
  - Fenestration vs. cystectomy
  - Goal is preservation of normal ovarian tissue

DIAGNOSTIC CHECKLIST

Consider

- Functional cysts are common in reproductive age women
- Most do not require follow-up ultrasound

Image Interpretation Pearls

- CLC may have "ring of fire" appearance; located within ovary
  - Beware of incorrectly diagnosing ectopic or heterotopic pregnancy, which should be outside ovary
  - If uncertain whether intraovarian or adjacent to ovary, use slide test
    - Ectopic mass can often be displaced away from ovary using gentle transvaginal probe pressure
- Even if CLC is persistent, may monitor through pregnancy if no malignant features
  - Most likely a persistent functional cyst

SELECTED REFERENCES

1. Rosenkrantz AB et al: US of incidental adnexal cysts: adherence of radiologists to the 2010 Society of Radiologists in Ultrasound guidelines. Radiology. 271(1):262-71, 2014
2. Ghosh E et al: Recommendations for adnexal cysts: have the Society of Radiologists in Ultrasound consensus conference guidelines affected utilization of ultrasound? Ultrasound Q. 29(1):21-4, 2013
3. Valentin L et al: Risk of malignancy in unilocular cysts: a study of 1148 adnexal masses classified as unilocular cysts at transvaginal ultrasound and review of the literature. Ultrasound Obstet Gynecol. 41(1):80-9, 2013
4. Faschingbauer F et al: Subjective assessment of ovarian masses using pattern recognition: the impact of experience on diagnostic performance and interobserver variability. Arch Gynecol Obstet. 285(6):1663-9, 2012
5. Levine D et al: Management of asymptomatic ovarian and other adnexal cysts imaged at US: Society of Radiologists in Ultrasound Consensus Conference Statement. Radiology. 256(3):943-54, 2010
6. Timmerman D et al: Simple ultrasound rules to distinguish between benign and malignant adnexal masses before surgery: prospective validation by IOTA group. BMJ. 341:c6839, 2010

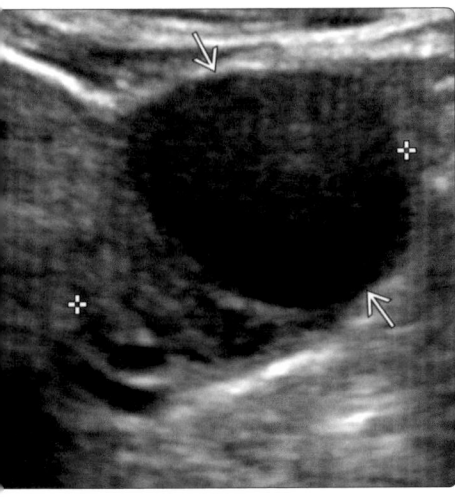
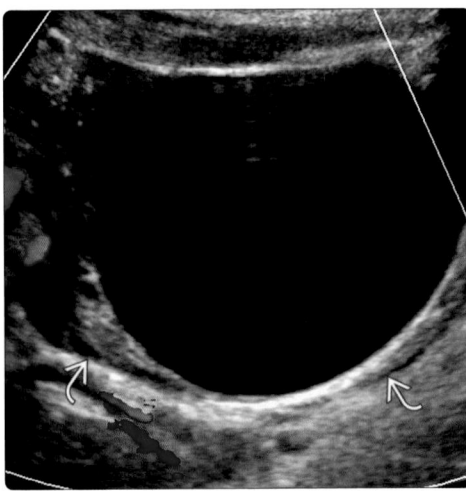

(Left) *Typical anechoic appearance of the functional cyst* ➡ *is shown on routine pelvic ultrasound, with surrounding ovarian parenchyma (calipers).* (Right) *Functional ovarian cysts can become large and the surrounding parenchyma compressed to a thin rim* ➡*. When presenting with pelvic pain, pulse Doppler should be used to confirm arterial and venous waveforms.*

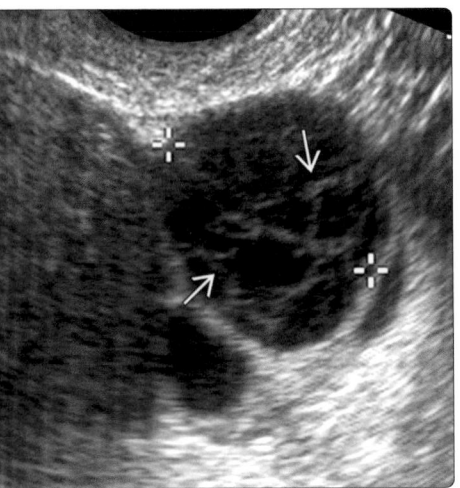
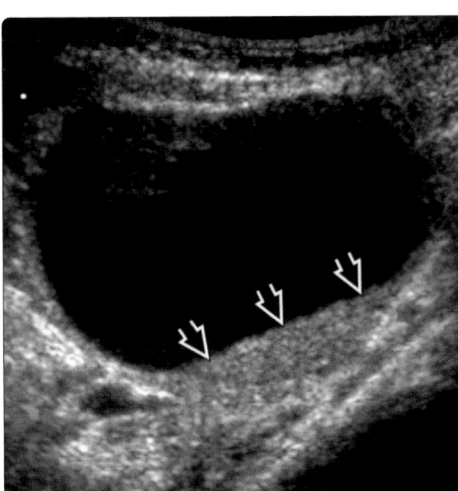

(Left) *CLC are often complicated by hemorrhage (calipers). Hemorrhagic CLC can have lace-like echoes and thin septations* ➡*, and typically spontaneously resolve, as demonstrated on this endovaginal grayscale ultrasound of the ovary.* (Right) *In this CLC, careful evaluation of the posterior cyst wall reveals a fluid/debris level* ➡*. The appearance is consistent with a resolving hemorrhagic cyst.*

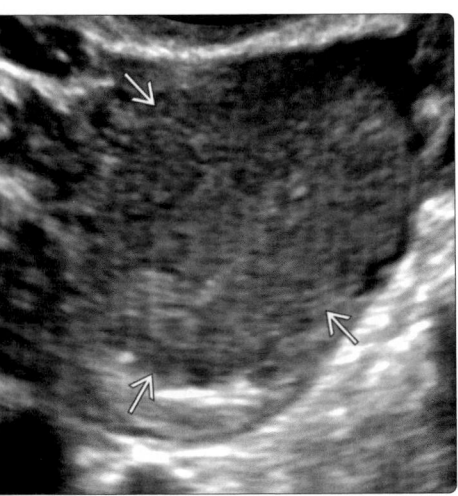
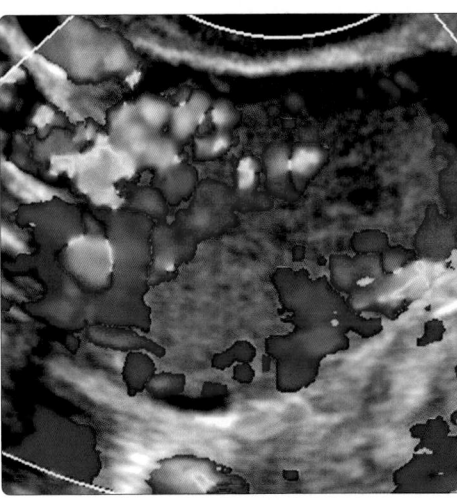

(Left) *CLC can also appear solid due to hemorrhage and collapse of the cyst after ovulation* ➡*.* (Right) *Color Doppler ultrasound shows the solid-appearing CLC has increased vascularity, similar in appearance to the "ring of fire."*

Hemorrhagic Cyst

KEY FACTS

TERMINOLOGY

- Hemorrhage into cystic space in ovarian parenchyma

IMAGING

- Avascular hypoechoic ovarian "mass" with fine lacy interstices
  - Lacy interstices due to fibrin strands → acute clot
- Majority resorb quickly and leave no sequela on 6-12 week follow-up scans
- May appear as mixed echogenicity mass
  - Color Doppler shows clot is avascular
- Hemorrhagic cyst (HC) may rupture
  - Adjacent echogenic free fluid

TOP DIFFERENTIAL DIAGNOSES

- Endometrioma
  - Uniform low-level internal echoes from blood breakdown products rather than lacy fibrin strands in clot

  - Will not change much on follow-up
- Solid ovarian mass
  - Papillary projections more likely than angular fragments
- Torsion

CLINICAL ISSUES

- May be asymptomatic and incidentally seen, or present with acute pelvic pain
- Majority resolve spontaneously
- Larger cysts more likely to cause acute pain/presentation with acute abdomen
- Surgical treatment for severe symptoms
  - Ovarian torsion
  - HC rupture with significant intraperitoneal hemorrhage

DIAGNOSTIC CHECKLIST

- 90% of hemorrhagic ovarian cysts will exhibit fibrin strands or retracting clot

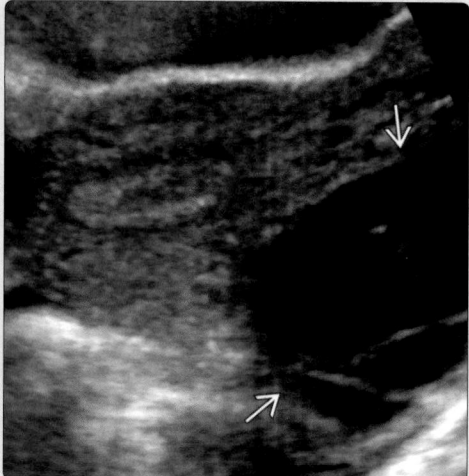
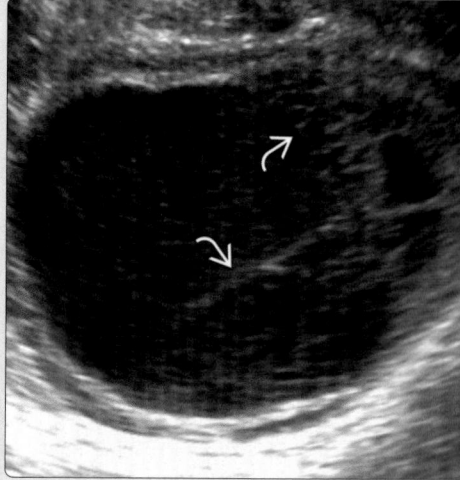

(Left) In this patient presenting with pelvic pain, there is a septated cystic mass in the left adnexa, which appears anechoic ➡ on transabdominal grayscale US. (Right) When further evaluated with transvaginal US, the typical hypoechoic and lace-like echoes are seen with retracted clot ➡, confirming a hemorrhagic cyst in a premenopausal patient. In general, a hemorrhagic cyst < 5 cm does not require additional follow-up US according to the Society of Radiologists in Ultrasound (SRU) recommendations.

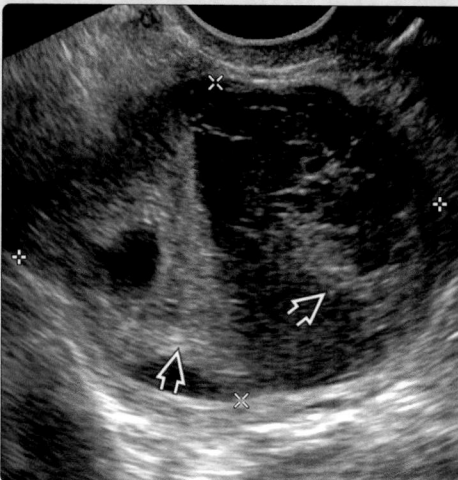
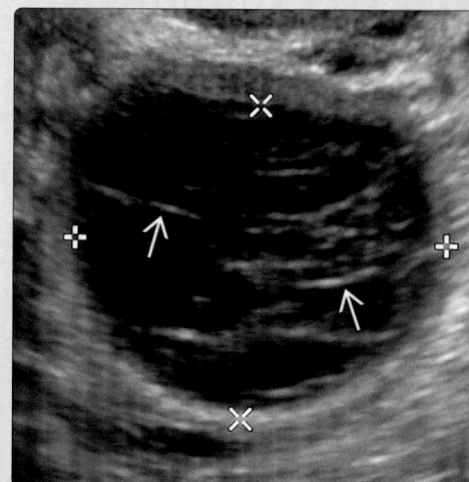

(Left) Endovaginal US shows a hemorrhagic cyst (HC), with areas of more echogenic clot ➡. These should not be confused with papillary projections in ovarian neoplasms, which generally have more convex margins and internal vascularity. (Right) Endovaginal grayscale US shows typical areas of reticular or lacy internal echoes are due to fibrin strands within the hemorrhagic cyst ➡.

TERMINOLOGY

Abbreviations

Hemorrhagic cyst (HC)

Definitions

Hemorrhage into cystic space in ovarian parenchyma
- o Most common at time of ovulation → hemorrhagic corpus luteum (HCL)
- o May occur into follicular cyst
- o Acute hemorrhage may occur into established endometrioma

IMAGING

General Features

Best diagnostic clue
- o Avascular hypoechoic ovarian "mass" with fine lacy interstices

Location
- o Intraovarian

Size
- o Variable, up to 8 cm diameter

Ultrasonographic Findings

Grayscale ultrasound
- o Lacy interstices due to fibrin strands are characteristic of acute clot
- o May appear as mixed or variable echogenicity mass
  - – Clot retraction → echogenic clot with surrounding cyst fluid
  - – Clot fragmentation → angular/concave margins of clot fragments
    - □ Fragments adhere to cyst wall
    - □ Float in fluid component
    - □ Jelly-like motion with transducer compression
- o ~ 90% of hemorrhagic cysts have fibrin strands or retracting clot
- o 92% show increased through transmission
  - – Indicates "cystic" nature even though initial assessment may suggest solid mass
- o As clot resorbs, HC appears more like simple cyst
- o Majority resorb quickly and leave no sequela on 6-12 week follow-up scans
- o HC may rupture
  - – Look for echogenic fluid in cul-de-sac
  - – With significant hemorrhage may see hemoperitoneum
    - □ Check for fluid in hepatorenal fossa/subphrenic spaces, which indicates large amount of hemoperitoneum
- o Cyst wall often appears thick

Color Doppler
- o Clot is avascular
- o May see increased flow at margins of corpus luteum: "Ring of fire" appearance
- o Look for flow in ovarian parenchyma stretched around hemorrhagic cyst

CT Findings

Cyst may appear simple on CT

- Fluid-fluid level or high-attenuation material may be seen in HC
- May show ring enhancement

MR Findings

- T1WI
  - o Typically intermediate to high signal blood products with no loss of signal on FS images
    - – In 1 study, however, 64% of 22 confirmed HC were hypointense on T1-weighted images
    - – 18% were also hyperintense on T2-weighted images
  - o Hematocrit effect: High signal layering blood akin to sonographic fluid-fluid level
- T2WI
  - o Typically intermediate to low signal

Imaging Recommendations

- Best imaging tool
  - o Transvaginal US

DIFFERENTIAL DIAGNOSIS

Endometrioma

- Uniform low-level internal echoes from blood breakdown products rather than lacy fibrin strands in clot
- Walls often contain punctate high echogenic foci
- More likely to have history of chronic pelvic pain
- Will not change much on follow-up
  - o HC would be expected to resolve or decrease significantly in size
- Occasionally acute bleed into endometrioma, may produce confusing picture
  - o Follow-up will show resolution of acute clot with persistent background endometrioma

Solid Ovarian Mass

- Papillary projections more likely than angular fragments
- Solid masses reflect sound equally with ovarian parenchyma
  - o No increased through transmission
- Internal vascularity with Doppler interrogation

Torsion

- Tender, enlarged ovary with peripheral follicles, parenchymal inhomogeneity, and abnormal position
- Variable vascularity: Low-pressure venous system affected earlier than arterial

Ectopic Pregnancy

- Positive pregnancy test
- Hemorrhagic **extraovarian** adnexal mass
- Use real-time observation during transducer pressure
  - o Ovary will "slide" separately from adnexal mass
  - o Intraovarian mass moves with ovary
- May see "ring of fire" sign of increased flow in trophoblastic tissue
  - o Make sure it is extraovarian and not around corpus luteum within ovary
  - o Not all ectopics demonstrate this sign

Pelvic Abscess

- Febrile patient

- May see echogenic fluid in cul-de-sac due to inflammatory exudate
- Pelvic inflammatory disease → edema → loss of tissue planes → difficulty identifying structures
  - May be associated with purulent discharge
  - Often extremely tender during sonography
- Appendix abscess may form in pelvis (remember nongynecologic causes)

PATHOLOGY

General Features

- Majority occur as result of bleeding into functional ovarian cyst; follicular/corpus luteum

CLINICAL ISSUES

Presentation

- Most common signs/symptoms
  - Acute pelvic pain
- Other signs/symptoms
  - May be asymptomatic
    - In 1 series of 112 patients, only 38% presented with acute pain
    - Remaining cases detected during sonography for other indications, most commonly palpable mass on pelvic examination
  - Mittelschmerz
    - Ovulation pain
  - May complicate ovulation induction in assisted reproduction
    - Rupture may lead to significant hemorrhage
    - Acute pain related to hemorrhagic cyst can be confused for torsion or hyperstimulated ovary
  - Neonatal presentation
    - Fetal ovarian cysts are well described
      - Usually appear in 3rd trimester
    - Development of fluid-fluid level in utero is very suspicious for hemorrhage/torsion

Demographics

- Epidemiology
  - 1 series of 112 patients
    - 71% in nulliparous patients
    - 29% multiparous
    - 77% in luteal phase of menstrual cycle
    - 12% in proliferative phase
    - 11% in early gestation

Natural History & Prognosis

- Majority resolve spontaneously
  - Severe pain resolves within hours in > 90%
  - Mass will disappear in > 90% within 8 weeks
- Larger cysts more likely to cause acute pain/presentation with acute abdomen
- If large may predispose to adnexal torsion
- May rupture
  - Supportive treatment adequate in most

Treatment

- Society of Radiologists in Ultrasound (SRU) consensus statement on ovarian cyst management
  - Hemorrhagic cyst
    - Reproductive age
      - ≤ 5 cm: No follow-up needed
      - > 5 cm: 6-12 week follow-up
    - Early postmenopausal
      - Follow-up US to ensure resolution
    - Late postmenopausal
      - Consider surgical evaluation
- Surgical treatment for severe symptoms
  - Ovarian torsion
  - HC rupture with significant intraperitoneal hemorrhage
- If recurrent consider ovulation suppression

DIAGNOSTIC CHECKLIST

Consider

- Look for rind of ovarian tissue containing follicles: "Claw" sign around hemorrhagic cyst
  - Confirms intraovarian process
- Increased through transmission suggests cystic entity rather than solid mass
- Hemorrhage can be cause or effect of ovarian torsion

Image Interpretation Pearls

- 90% of hemorrhagic ovarian cysts will exhibit fibrin strands or retracting clot
  - Lacy interstices due to fibrin strands are characteristic of acute clot
  - "Mass" with angular margins suggests fragmented clot rather than papillary projections from neoplasm
- Beware of ring-of-fire sign
  - If intraovarian, related to corpus luteum
  - If extraovarian, consider ectopic pregnancy
  - Majority of hemorrhagic cysts can be managed conservatively, unlike ruptured ectopic pregnancies
- Reported cause or false-positive F-18 FDG uptake in PET scans
  - Consider US for any unexpected ovarian mass on PET scans

SELECTED REFERENCES

1. Nakamura M et al: Postnatal Outcome in Cases of Prenatally Diagnosed Fetal Ovarian Cysts under Conservative Prenatal Management. Fetal Diagn Ther. ePub, 2014
2. Valentin L et al: Risk of malignancy in unilocular cysts: a study of 1148 adnexal masses classified as unilocular cysts at transvaginal ultrasound and review of the literature. Ultrasound Obstet Gynecol. 41(1):80-9, 2013
3. Patel MD: Pitfalls in the sonographic evaluation of adnexal masses. Ultrasound Q. 28(1):29-40, 2012
4. Alcázar JL et al: Diagnostic performance of transvaginal gray-scale ultrasound for specific diagnosis of benign ovarian cysts in relation to menopausal status. Maturitas. 68(2):182-8, 2011
5. Levine D et al: Management of asymptomatic ovarian and other adnexal cysts imaged at US: Society of Radiologists in Ultrasound Consensus Conference Statement. Radiology. 256(3):943-54, 2010
6. Patel MD et al: The likelihood ratio of sonographic findings for the diagnosis of hemorrhagic ovarian cysts. J Ultrasound Med. 24(5):607-14; quiz 615, 2005
7. Swire MN et al: Various sonographic appearances of the hemorrhagic corpus luteum cyst. Ultrasound Q. 20(2):45-58, 2004

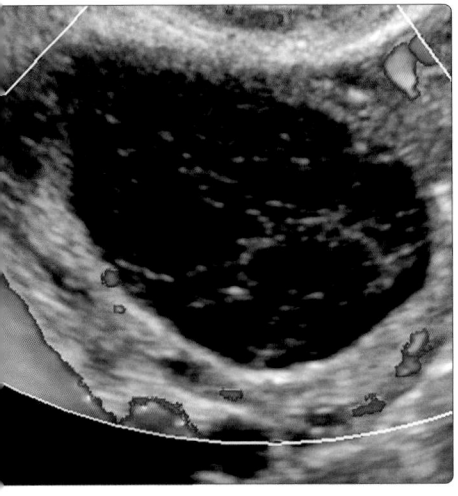

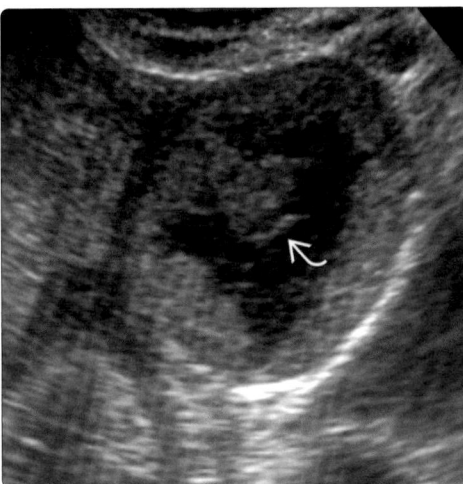

(Left) *Using color Doppler can help confirm the benign etiology of the ovarian hemorrhagic cyst. In this color Doppler US, the internal reticular echoes seen in this hemorrhagic cyst are not vascular.* (Right) *Hemorrhagic corpus lutea (HCL) may have a collapsed appearance, with central hemorrhage and a thickened, redundant wall ⮡, as seen on this endovaginal grayscale US. This should not be mistaken for an ovarian neoplasm, as real-time imaging will show the wall folding inward.*

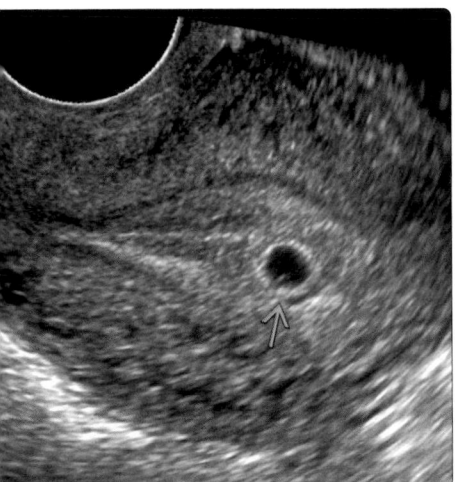

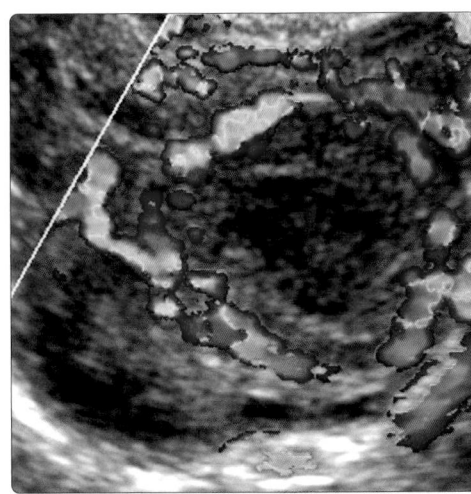

(Left) *US in early pregnancy shows a small intrauterine gestational sac embedded within the endometrium of a retroverted uterus, with a double decidual sac sign ➡.* (Right) *In the adnexa of the same patient, a hemorrhagic corpus luteum with thick wall and peripheral blood flow is seen on this color Doppler US. This should not be mistaken for the "ring of fire" associated with tubal ectopic pregnancies. With HCL, the cyst is clearly within the ovarian parenchyma.*

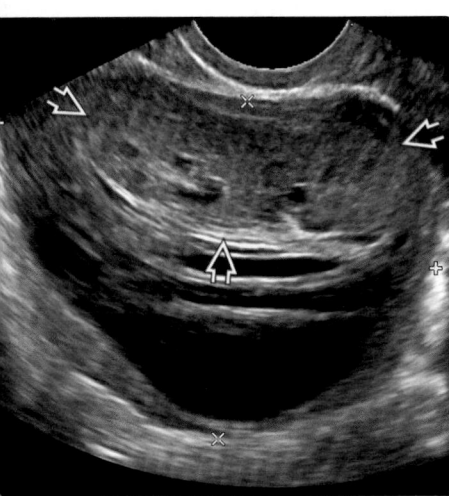

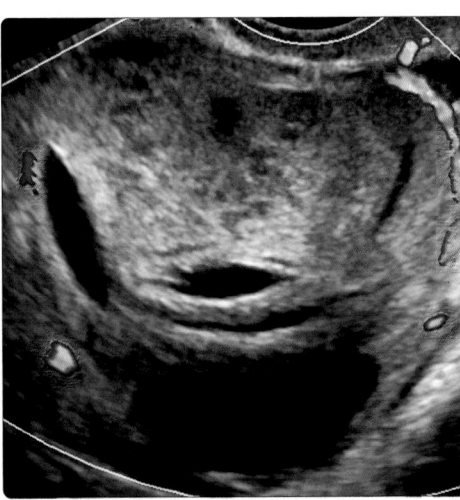

(Left) *Grayscale endovaginal US shows a hyperacute hemorrhagic cyst which can appear solid, with a dense hyperechoic component ➡.* (Right) *Color Doppler US is helpful to confirm there is no central vascularity, and interval follow-up US should be considered to demonstrate resolution especially if > 5 cm in diameter.*

Ovarian Hyperstimulation Syndrome

TERMINOLOGY

- Ovarian hyperstimulation syndrome (OHSS)
- Clinical syndrome generally associated with ovulation induction

IMAGING

- Bilaterally enlarged, cystic ovaries
  - Heterogeneous complex ovarian cysts with debris and septa if hemorrhagic component present
  - Typical "spoke-wheel" appearance
- Ascites
  - Occasionally will find hemorrhagic pelvic fluid
- Pleural effusion

TOP DIFFERENTIAL DIAGNOSES

- Theca lutein cysts
  - Not associated with ascites, pleural effusions, or oliguria
- Hyperreactio luteinalis
  - More mild, indolent course within spectrum of OHSS

PATHOLOGY

- Exaggerated response to ovulation induction
- Relative hemoconcentration due to fluid leaking into peritoneal/pleural spaces

CLINICAL ISSUES

- Typical clinical symptoms
  - Abdominal pain
  - Nausea/vomiting/diarrhea
  - Weight gain
  - Oliguria
- Should be self-limiting as long as supportive care started early in process

DIAGNOSTIC CHECKLIST

- Avoid aggressive transvaginal imaging as ovaries can be friable
- Correlate imaging appearance of ovaries with clinical history for diagnosis

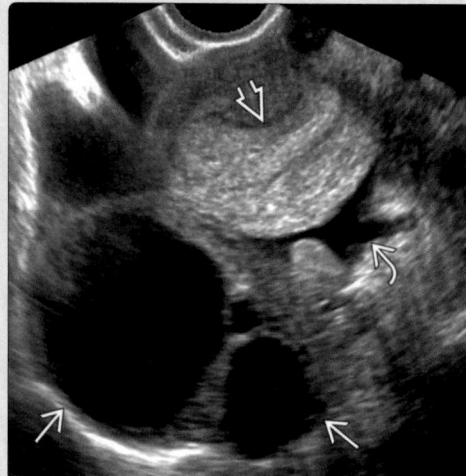
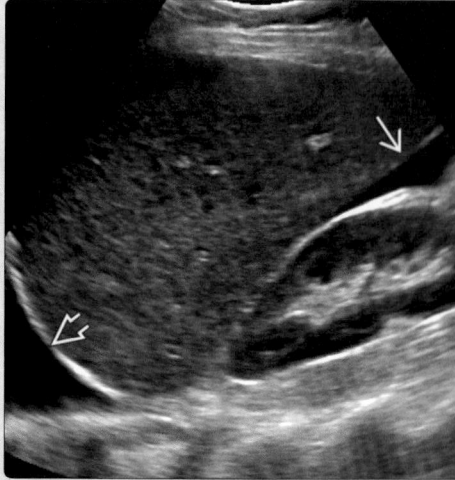

(Left) Endovaginal transverse sonographic view of the pelvis shows typical ovarian hyperstimulation syndrome (OHSS), in which decidual reaction is present in the uterus ➡, with anechoic free fluid ➡ and enlarged ovaries containing multiple cysts ➡ (right ovary). (Right) Transabdominal US of the right upper quadrant shows ascites ➡ and a pleural effusion ➡ in this patient with early OHSS.

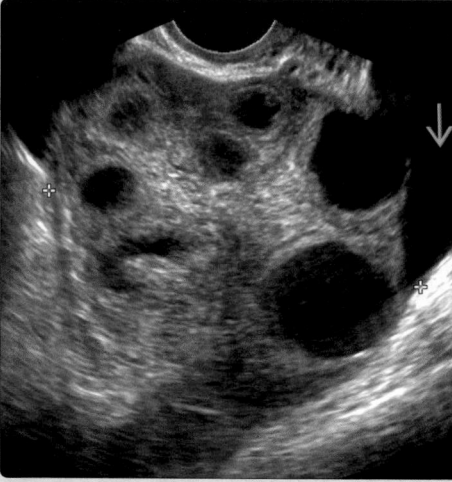
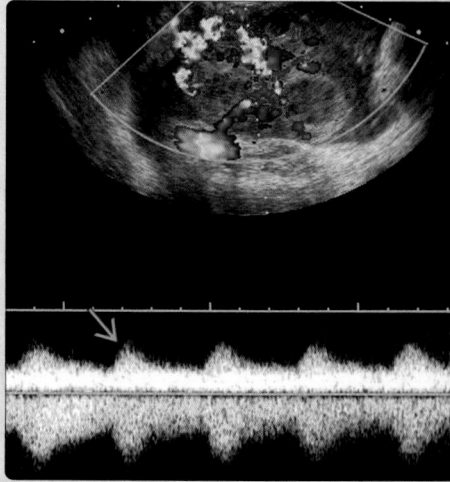

(Left) Transvaginal US shows a markedly enlarged ovary measuring up to 8 cm (calipers) in diameter with multiple follicles and ascites ➡ in a patient with OHSS. (Right) Spectral Doppler in the same patient shows normal low-resistance arterial flow in the ovary ➡. Color Doppler and spectral Doppler should be used to evaluate the ovarian parenchyma in patients with OHSS to document good blood flow in patients presenting with pain due to the risk of superimposed adnexal torsion.

Ovarian Hyperstimulation Syndrome

TERMINOLOGY

Abbreviations

- Ovarian hyperstimulation syndrome (OHSS)

Definitions

- Clinical syndrome generally associated with ovulation induction
  - Hyperstimulated, enlarged ovaries
  - Increased vascular permeability
    - Ascites
    - ± pleural effusion

IMAGING

Ultrasonographic Findings

- Bilaterally enlarged, cystic ovaries
  - > 5-10 cm diameter
  - Multiple cysts in ovary
  - Cysts may be simple or complex if hemorrhagic component present
- Ascites
  - May have internal echoes due to high protein content
- Pleural effusion

MR Findings

- Not usually required for diagnosis
  - Most often used to distinguish hyperstimulated ovaries from ovarian neoplasm
    - Cysts typically high signal on T2WI if simple
    - Cysts may be intermediate to low signal on T2WI if hemorrhagic components present
- Typical "spoke-wheel" appearance of ovaries
  - Enlarged follicles separated by thin septa
  - Centrally located stromal tissue
- Ascites
  - May be simple or hemorrhagic secondary to oocyte retrieval or rupture of follicle

DIFFERENTIAL DIAGNOSIS

Theca Lutein Cysts

- Multiple cysts within enlarged ovaries
- Not associated with ascites, pleural effusions, or oliguria
- Multiple etiologies
  - Multiple gestation
  - Exogenous hormonal stimulation
  - Gestational trophoblastic disease
  - Triploidy

Hyperreactio Luteinalis

- More mild, indolent course within spectrum of OHSS
- Bilateral ovarian enlargement with multiple theca lutein cysts
- Always associated with pregnancy
- High maternal human chorionic gonadotropin (hCG) serum levels
  - No exogenous hCG administered
  - May be response to chronic exposure to elevated hCG levels

Cystic Ovarian Neoplasm

- Usually unilateral
- Serous cystadenoma/cystadenocarcinoma
- Mucinous cystadenoma/cystadenocarcinoma
- Cystic germ cell tumors

Polycystic Ovarian Syndrome

- Bilateral enlarged ovaries with hyperechoic central stroma
- Multiple small peripheral follicles ("string of pearls")
- Chronic anovulation
- Associated with obesity and insulin resistance

Heterotopic Pregnancy

- Echogenic peritoneal fluid
- Adnexal mass
- Higher risk in women undergoing ovulation induction

PATHOLOGY

General Features

- Exaggerated response to ovulation induction
  - Almost exclusively associated with exogenous gonadotropin use
  - Numerous potential pathophysiologic mediators
    - Cytokines
    - Growth factors
- Most likely associated with vascular endothelial growth factor (VEGF)
  - Granulosa cells are 1 site of production
  - hCG and VEGF serum levels correlate with severity of OHSS
- Paradoxical arterial dilation and ↓ peripheral vascular resistance
  - Leads to compensatory release of vasoactive substances
    - Aldosterone
    - Antidiuretic hormone
    - Norepinephrine
    - Renin
  - Increased permeability of peritoneal and pleural surfaces
    - Protein-rich fluid leaks out of intravascular space
    - Leads to ascites and pleural effusions

Gross Pathologic & Surgical Features

- Ovaries appear similar to changes seen with theca lutein cysts
  - Bilaterally enlarged
  - Multiple follicular cysts with prominent luteinization of theca interna layer
- Corpus luteum present
  - May be more than 1

CLINICAL ISSUES

Presentation

- Most common signs/symptoms
  - Abdominal pain
  - Nausea/vomiting/diarrhea
  - Weight gain
  - Oliguria
- Other signs/symptoms
  - Abdominal distention from ascites

- o Shortness of breath from pleural effusion
- o Hypotension
- o Electrolyte imbalance
- o Hepatic dysfunction
- Relative hemoconcentration due to fluid leaking into peritoneal/pleural spaces
  - o Oliguria
  - o Hypercoagulability
- Rarely associated with venous occlusive disease or thromboembolic events
  - o Usually only with severe OHSS

Demographics

- Epidemiology
  - o Typically seen in women undergoing ovulation induction
    - More commonly with gonadotropin stimulation for in vitro fertilization (IVF)
    - Less commonly seen with clomiphene induction
      - □ Severe form rarely seen
  - o Mild OHSS: 20-33% of IVF cases
  - o Moderate OHSS: 3-6% of IVF cases
  - o Severe OHSS: 0.1-2.0% of IVF cases
- Risk factors
  - o Polycystic ovarian syndrome major risk factor
    - May be related to increased number of follicles/oocytes produced when stimulated
    - Oligomenorrhea itself also risk factor
  - o Greater number of follicles stimulated during IVF
    - High or rapidly increasing serum estradiol
  - o Younger age
  - o Previous OHSS history
  - o Low body mass index

Natural History & Prognosis

- Occurs after ovulation
  - o Early type occurs < 5 days after oocyte retrieval
    - Induced by exogenous hCG administration
  - o Late type occurs ≥ 5 days (range 5-15 days) after oocyte retrieval
    - Induced by endogenous hCG from implanted pregnancy
    - Late type always associated with pregnancy
- Should be self-limiting as long as supportive care started early in process
- Usually regresses over 10-14 days unless pregnancy implantation occurs
  - o Subsequently can have increase in endogenous hCG
  - o May prolong OHSS or initiate late form of OHSS
- More severe in patients who become pregnant
- Severe OHSS potentially life-threatening
  - o Mortality estimated at 1:45,000 cases of OHSS

Treatment

- No known therapy to immediately reverse OHSS
- Avoid pelvic trauma to ovaries
  - o No intercourse, pelvic exams, strenuous exercise
- Conservative therapy with observation warranted
  - o May be monitored as outpatient
    - Frequent vital sign and electrolyte checks
  - o Maintain intravascular volume and urine output
    - 24 urine volume measurements

- Daily weights
- o Consider US-guided paracentesis or thoracentesis for symptoms
  - Serial abdominal girth measurements
- o Prophylactic anticoagulation
  - Useful due to relative hemoconcentration
- Some advocate proactive management to shorten course of symptoms
  - o Most often considered if moderate to severe OHSS
  - o Actively administer fluids &/or albumin
    - Diuretics considered when adequate intravascular volume achieved
  - o Benefits of US-guided paracentesis
    - ↓ hospitalization
    - ↓ hemoconcentration
    - ↑ urine output
    - Ameliorates electrolyte abnormalities
- May require hospitalization for management of severe symptoms
  - o Intractable pain
  - o Intractable nausea/vomiting
  - o Respiratory difficulties
  - o Suspected infection/hemorrhage
- Surgical intervention only rarely required
  - o Ovarian torsion
  - o Cyst rupture with hemoperitoneum
- Partial oophorectomy for severe cases reported

DIAGNOSTIC CHECKLIST

Image Interpretation Pearls

- Avoid aggressive transvaginal imaging as ovaries can be friable
- Correlate imaging appearance of ovaries with clinical history for diagnosis

SELECTED REFERENCES

1. Mathur RS et al: British fertility society policy and practice committee: prevention of ovarian hyperstimulation syndrome. Hum Fertil (Camb). 17(4):257-68, 2014
2. Nastri CO et al: Ovarian hyperstimulation syndrome: physiopathology, staging, prediction and prevention. Ultrasound Obstet Gynecol. ePub, 2014
3. Thornton KG et al: Ovarian Hyperstimulation Syndrome and Arterial Stroke. Stroke. ePub, 2014
4. Baron KT et al: Emergent complications of assisted reproduction: expecting the unexpected. Radiographics. 33(1):229-44, 2013
5. Tan BK et al: Management of ovarian hyperstimulation syndrome guidelines. Produced on behalf of the BFS Policy and Practice Committee. Hum Fertil (Camb). 16(3):160-1, 2013
6. Kumar P et al: Ovarian hyperstimulation syndrome. J Hum Reprod Sci. 4(2):70-5, 2011
7. Nastri CO et al: Ovarian hyperstimulation syndrome: pathophysiology and prevention. J Assist Reprod Genet. 27(2-3):121-8, 2010
8. Zivi E et al: Ovarian hyperstimulation syndrome: definition, incidence, and classification. Semin Reprod Med. 28(6):441-7, 2010
9. Bartkova A et al: Acute ischaemic stroke in pregnancy: a severe complication of ovarian hyperstimulation syndrome. Neurol Sci. 29(6):463-6, 2008
10. Kim IY et al: Ovarian hyperstimulation syndrome. US and CT appearances. Clin Imaging. 21(4):284-6, 1997

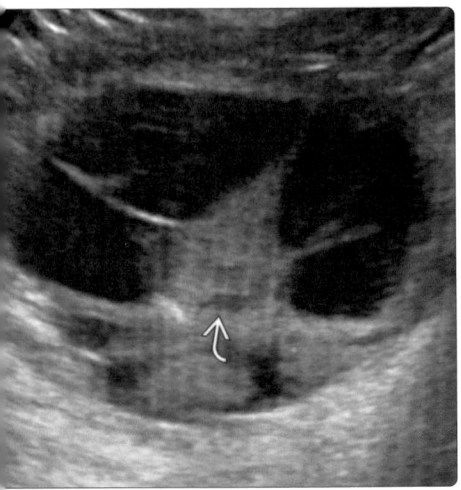

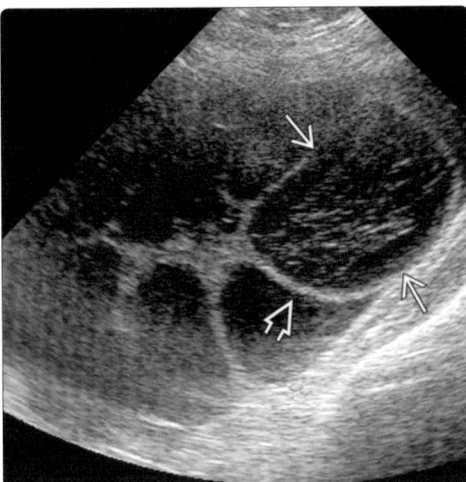

(Left) *Closer evaluation with grayscale US of a hyperstimulated ovary shows a "spoke-wheel" appearance due to the central area of stromal tissue* ➜ *with enlarged peripheral follicles.* **(Right)** *In some cases, the enlarged follicles can have reticular echogenicities on grayscale US, indicating internal hemorrhage* ➜. *Note the follicles are separated by thin septa* ➜, *as opposed to the thick papillary projections typically seen in ovarian neoplasm.*

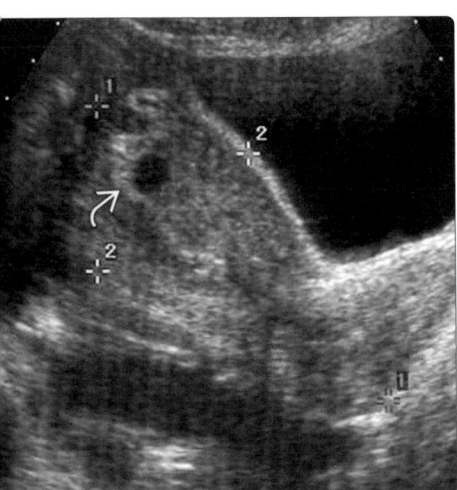

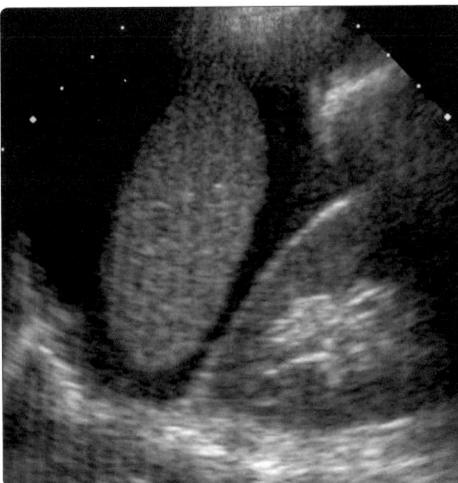

(Left) *In late OHSS, there is typically an implanted pregnancy* ➜ *(calipers mark the uterus) as seen in this patient on a transabdominal US longitudinal view of the pelvis.* **(Right)** *Anechoic fluid at the inferior margin of the liver on grayscale US reflects increased permeability of the peritoneal surfaces with leakage of fluid out of the intravascular space in this patient with OHSS.*

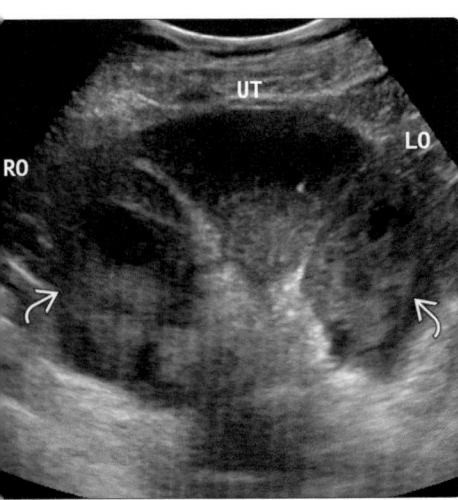

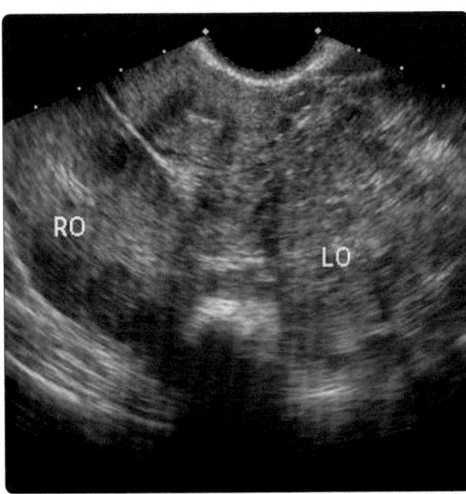

(Left) *In this case, transabdominal US shows the uterus surrounded by bilateral adnexal "masses"* ➜ *(labeled RO and LO), which are the enlarged hyperstimulated ovaries.* **(Right)** *At times the enlarged ovaries appear solid if there are multiple hemorrhagic follicles (ovaries labeled RO and LO). Often the ovaries can be found in close approximation at the midline pelvis as seen on grayscale US in this patient with hyperstimulated ovaries.*

TERMINOLOGY

- Serous epithelial neoplasm, which can be benign (serous cystadenoma), borderline (low malignant potential) or malignant (serous cystadenocarcinoma)

IMAGING

- Large, thin-walled, unilocular mass ± papillary projections
- Bilateral in 25% of benign tumors and 65% of malignant tumors
- Variable size but often large
- Typically unilocular or with few septations even in malignant tumors
- May see ascites and peritoneal implants in metastatic disease
- Ultrasound ideal method for lesion detection and characterization
- CT preferred for tumor staging
  - Evaluate along paracolic gutters and capsule of liver for peritoneal disease

TOP DIFFERENTIAL DIAGNOSES

- Mucinous cystadenoma/carcinoma

PATHOLOGY

- Metastatic spread
  - Intraperitoneal dissemination most common
  - Direct extension into surrounding organs
  - Lymphatic spread to paraaortic and pelvic nodes

CLINICAL ISSUES

- Pelvic discomfort/pain from large tumors
- 70% of patients with malignant tumors have peritoneal involvement at time of diagnosis
- Serous tumors most common epithelial neoplasm
- Malignant 25%, borderline 15%, benign 60%

DIAGNOSTIC CHECKLIST

- Serous cystadenoma is most likely diagnosis for large, anechoic, unilocular cyst in postmenopausal woman

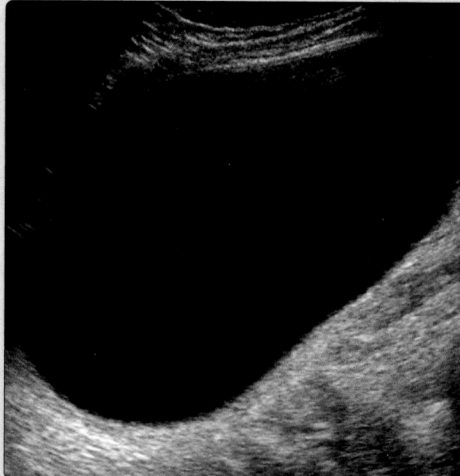
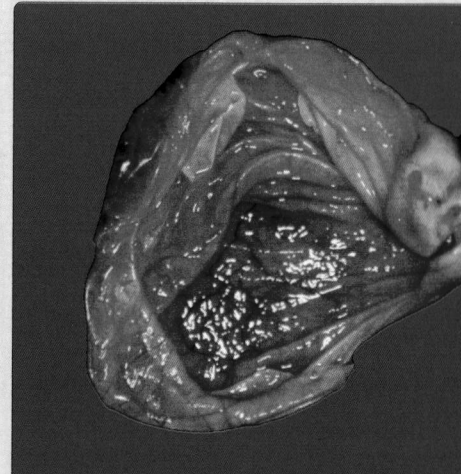

(Left) *Typical serous epithelial neoplasms are large with thin walls and unilocular. This ovarian serous cystadenoma measured up to 18 cm in diameter on this transabdominal grayscale ultrasound.* (Right) *Gross pathology after the fluid has been drained shows the thin wall typical of a serous cystadenoma. They are typically unilocular or have few septations.*

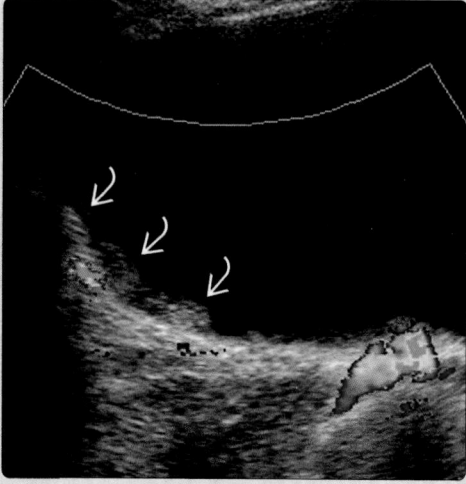
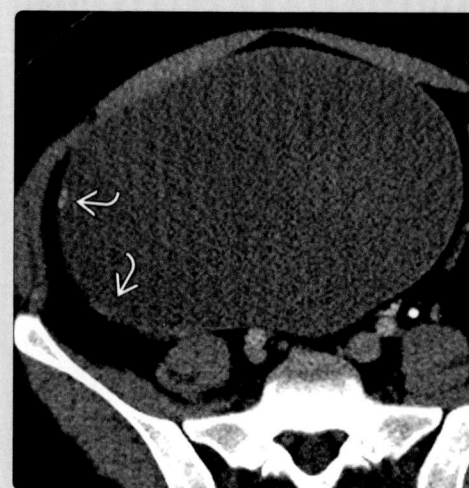

(Left) *Close evaluation of this serous cystadenoma reveals subtle nodularity along the right lateral margin of the wall ➡. (Right) Axial CECT of the same patient shows subtle enhancing nodules ➡ at the site of the sonographic finding, which correlated with areas of focal borderline neoplasm.*

Serous Ovarian Cystadenoma/Carcinoma

TERMINOLOGY

Abbreviations

- Benign or malignant serous tumor

Definitions

- Serous epithelial neoplasm, which can be benign (serous cystadenoma), borderline (low malignant potential), or malignant (serous cystadenocarcinoma)

IMAGING

General Features

- Best diagnostic clue
  - Large, thin-walled, unilocular mass ± papillary projections
- Location
  - Bilateral in 25% of benign tumors and 65% of malignant tumors
- Size
  - Variable but often large

Ultrasonographic Findings

- Grayscale ultrasound
  - Typically unilocular or few septations, even in malignant tumors
  - Cyst fluid is clear to mildly echogenic
    - Usually less echogenic than mucinous counterpart
  - Septa often thin but may be thick, especially in malignant tumors
  - Papillary projections common
    - Does not necessarily indicate malignancy
    - Likelihood of malignancy increases with increased amount of solid components
  - May see ascites and peritoneal implants in metastatic disease
    - Ascites very concerning for metastatic disease (positive predictive value of 72-80% as sign of peritoneal metastases)
  - ~ 1/3 have microcalcifications (psammoma bodies) in primary tumor and peritoneal metastases
    - Usually not discernible by ultrasound
- Doppler ultrasound
  - Flow seen in solid components
  - Central flow within mass is more suggestive of malignancy than peripheral flow
  - Malignant lesions often have increased flow but quantitative parameters, such as pulsatility index and resistive index, are not reliable in differentiating benign from malignant

CT Findings

- Calcifications may be present
- Soft tissue components enhance with contrast
- Study of choice for tumor staging

Imaging Recommendations

- Best imaging tool
  - Ultrasound ideal method for lesion detection and characterization
    - Always use Doppler to evaluate for flow
  - CT preferred for tumor staging
- Protocol advice

  - Evaluate along paracolic gutters and capsule of liver for possible peritoneal implants

DIFFERENTIAL DIAGNOSIS

Mucinous Cystadenoma/Carcinoma

- Multilocular masses with low-level echoes

Other Epithelial Tumors

- Significant overlap in imaging findings
- All less common than serous tumors

Ovarian Metastases

- Look for upper abdominal malignancy

PATHOLOGY

General Features

- Etiology
  - Not completely understood
  - One theory is "incessant ovulation": Repeated microtrauma with cellular repair to surface epithelium
    - Increased risk: Nulliparity, early menarche, late menopause (more ovulatory cycles)
    - Reduced risk: Multiparity, late menarche, early menopause, oral contraceptive use (fewer ovulatory cycles)
  - High-grade serous adenocarcinoma now thought to arise from epithelium of fimbriated end of fallopian tube rather than ovary itself
- Genetics
  - Hereditary causes in 5-10% of ovarian cancers
    - Low-grade serous adenocarcinoma
      - *KRAS, BRAF* mutations
    - High-grade serous adenocarcinoma
      - *P53* mutation
      - *BRCA1/BRCA2 (most common)*
    - Lynch syndrome
- Associated abnormalities
  - May occasionally be hormonally active producing estrogen
- **Ovarian neoplasms**
  - Epithelial tumors 60-70% of all tumors: 85-90% of malignancies
  - Germ cell tumors 15-20% of all tumors: 3-5% of malignancies
  - Sex cord-stromal tumors 5-10% of all tumors: 2-3% of malignancies
  - Metastases and lymphoma 5-10% of all tumors: 5-10% of malignancies
- **Methods of spread**
  - Intraperitoneal dissemination most common
    - Greater omentum, right subphrenic region, and pouch of Douglas most common sites found at surgery
  - Direct extension into surrounding organs
  - Lymphatic spread to paraaortic and pelvic nodes
  - Hematogenous spread least common
    - Liver and lung most common sites

Staging, Grading, & Classification

- FIGO staging system of ovarian carcinoma
  - Stage I: Tumor limited to ovaries

- IA: Unilateral, no malignant ascites
- IB: Bilateral, no malignant ascites
- IC: Tumor limited to 1 or both ovaries with any of the following
  - IC1: Surgical spill intraoperatively
  - IC2: Capsule rupture before surgery or tumor on ovarian/fallopian tube surface
  - IC3: Malignant cells in ascites or peritoneal washings
  - Stage II: Tumor involves 1 or both ovaries with pelvic extension
    - IIA: Extension to uterus or fallopian tubes, no malignant ascites
    - IIB: Extension to other pelvic tissues, no malignant ascites
  - Stage III: Peritoneal implants outside pelvis &/or retroperitoneal nodal metastases
    - IIIA1: Positive retroperitoneal lymph nodes only
    - IIIA2: Microscopic metastasis outside pelvis &/or positive retroperitoneal lymph nodes
    - IIIB: Macroscopic extrapelvic implants ≤ 2 cm ± positive nodes
    - IIIC: Macroscopic extrapelvic implants > 2 cm or ± positive nodes
  - Stage IV: Distant metastases (excluding peritoneal implants)
    - IVA: Pleural effusion with positive cytology
    - IVB: Hepatic &/or splenic parenchymal metastasis, or metastasis to extraabdominal organs (including inguinal nodes and nodes outside of abdomen)

CLINICAL ISSUES

Presentation

- Most common signs/symptoms
  - Often asymptomatic: Incidentally discovered on physical exam
  - Pelvic discomfort/pain from large tumors
  - Symptoms from metastatic disease
    - 70% of patients with malignant tumors have peritoneal involvement at time of diagnosis
- Abnormal CA-125: Strongest association with serous cystadenocarcinoma (compared to other histologic types)
  - False-positives occur (especially in premenopausal women) with benign neoplasms, endometriosis
  - False-negative in 50% of stage I tumors (inadequate as screening tool)
  - Most commonly used to follow known disease

Demographics

- Age
  - Serous cystadenoma in 30s and 40s
  - Serous cystadenocarcinoma in peri- and postmenopausal age group
- Epidemiology
  - Serous tumors most common epithelial neoplasm
  - Malignant 25%, borderline (low malignant potential) 15%, benign 60%
  - Bilateral in 25% of benign tumors, 30% of borderline tumors, and 65% of malignant tumors

Natural History & Prognosis

- 95% 5-year survival for low malignant potential tumors
  - If metastatic, prognosis is similar to those with frankly malignant histology
- 5-year survival rate for malignant epithelial tumors
  - Stage I: 90%
  - Stage II: 70%
  - Stage III: 39%
  - Stage IV: 17%

Treatment

- Primary treatment is surgery
  - Complete staging laparotomy and tumor debulking (cytoreduction)
    - Staging laparotomy includes hysterectomy with bilateral salpingo-oophorectomy, pelvic and paraaortic node biopsies, omentectomy, peritoneal biopsies and washings
- Chemotherapy after cytoreductive surgery
- Neoadjuvant chemotherapy before cytoreductive surgery in patients with unresectable disease
  - Includes bulky disease in difficult to reach areas (porta hepatis, lesser sac, root of mesentery), extensive surrounding organ or sidewall invasion, or stage IV disease

DIAGNOSTIC CHECKLIST

Consider

- Multiple parameters should be considered in determining benign from malignant ovarian masses
  - Morphologic appearance: Septations, papillary projections, solid components
  - Doppler: Presence of flow, location, and quantitative parameters
  - Age and hormonal status
  - Clinical history
  - Ancillary findings (e.g., ascites)

Image Interpretation Pearls

- Serous cystadenoma is most likely diagnosis for large, anechoic, unilocular cyst in postmenopausal woman

SELECTED REFERENCES

1. Trillsch F et al: Surgical staging and prognosis in serous borderline ovarian tumours (BOT): A subanalysis of the AGO ROBOT study. Br J Cancer. ePub, 2015
2. Prat J et al: Staging classification for cancer of the ovary, fallopian tube, and peritoneum. Int J Gynaecol Obstet. 124(1):1-5, 2014
3. Alcázar JL et al: Clinical and ultrasound features of type I and type II epithelial ovarian cancer. Int J Gynecol Cancer. 23(4):680-4, 2013
4. Xie M et al: Application of real-time ultrasound elastography for discrimination of low- and high-grade serous ovarian carcinoma. J Ultrasound Med. 32(2):257-62, 2013
5. Moyle P et al: Radiological staging of ovarian carcinoma. Semin Ultrasound CT MR. 31(5):388-98, 2010
6. Woodward PJ et al: From the archives of the AFIP: radiologic staging of ovarian carcinoma with pathologic correlation. Radiographics. 24(1):225-46, 2004
7. Wagner BJ et al: From the archives of the AFIP. Ovarian epithelial neoplasms: radiologic-pathologic correlation. Radiographics. 14(6):1351-74; quiz 1375-6, 1994

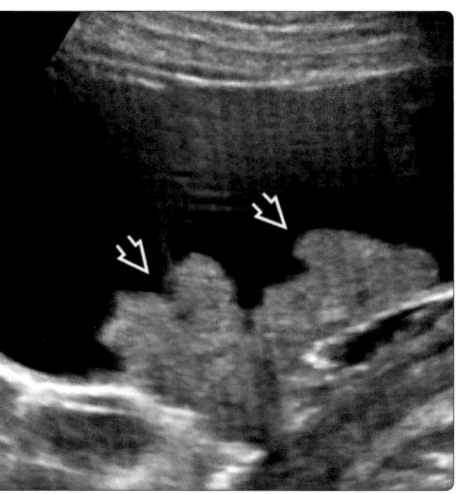

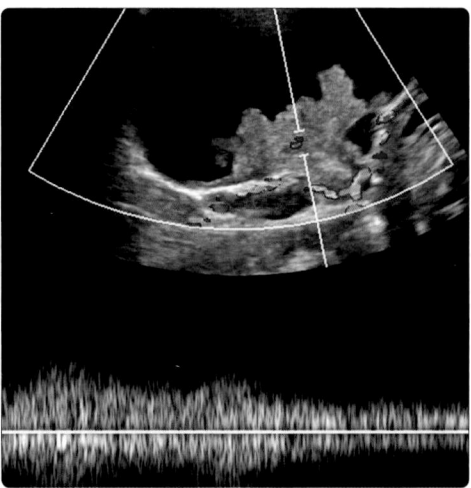

(Left) *Transabdominal grayscale ultrasound of a unilocular adnexal mass in a 28-year-old patient shows suspicious papillary projections* ➡ *along the wall of the otherwise cystic lesion.* (Right) *Color and pulsed Doppler ultrasound helps to prove vascularity in the solid component and exclude hematoma. In this case, pathology showed papillary serous borderline tumor.*

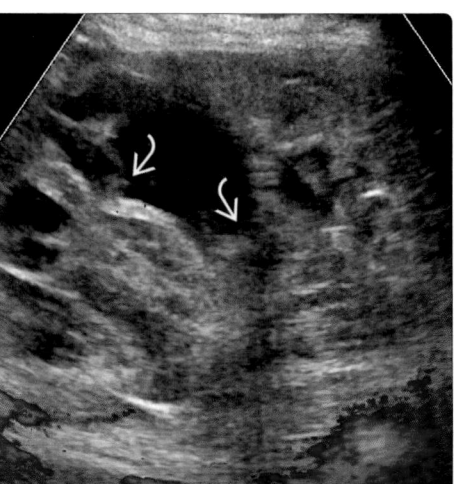

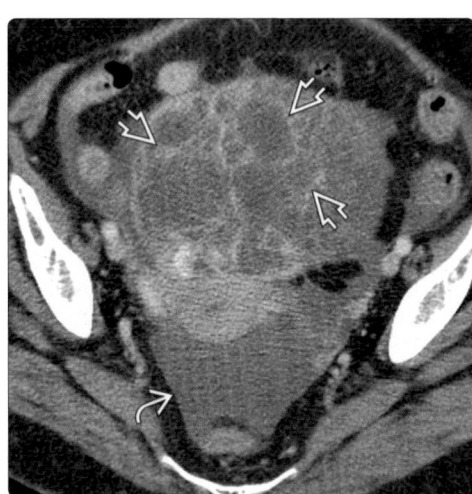

(Left) *Abundant solid-appearing material is present in this complex mixed solid and cystic ovarian mass* ➡; *however, there is no detectable internal vascularity on this power Doppler ultrasound.* (Right) *Axial CECT of the same mass shows multiple septations* ➡ *and pelvic free fluid* ➡. *Pathology showed serous cystadenoma with necrosis due to torsion.*

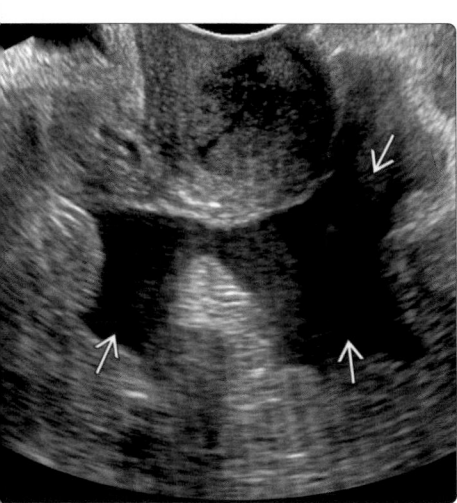

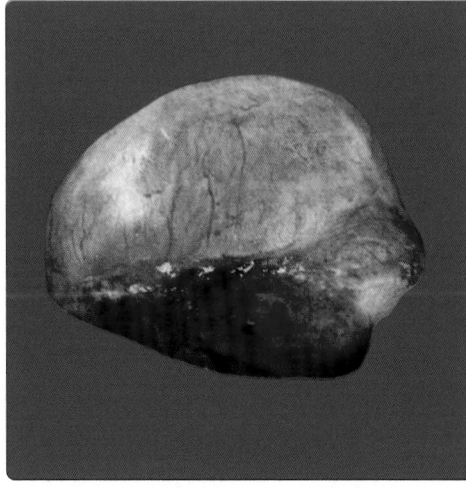

(Left) *The presence of ascites is very concerning for metastatic disease. When free fluid is identified* ➡, *close examination should be performed to assess for peritoneal implants. None were found in this case.* (Right) *In most cases ovarian masses are removed without rupture of the cyst to prevent contamination of the peritoneum. Typically, soft tissue and node biopsies are obtained at the time of surgery, as well as pelvic peritoneal washings for cytology.*

TERMINOLOGY

- Mucinous epithelial neoplasm, which can be benign (mucinous cystadenoma), borderline (low malignant potential), or malignant (mucinous cystadenocarcinoma)

IMAGING

- Multilocular cystic mass with low-level echoes
  - Papillary projections much less common than in serous tumors
  - Solid components increase suspicion for malignancy
- Variable in size, but often large; may fill entire pelvis and extend into upper abdomen
- Pseudomyxoma peritonei is potential form of peritoneal spread
  - Amorphous, mucoid material insinuating itself around mesentery, bowel, and solid organs

TOP DIFFERENTIAL DIAGNOSES

- Endometrioma

- Serous cystadenoma/carcinoma

PATHOLOGY

- Method of spread
  - Intraperitoneal dissemination most common (pseudomyxoma peritonei)
  - Direct extension to surrounding organs
  - Lymphatic spread to paraaortic and pelvic nodes

CLINICAL ISSUES

- Massive tumors can cause weight gain and distended abdomen
- Mucinous tumors 2nd most common epithelial neoplasm
- Gelatinous, insinuating nature of pseudomyxoma peritonei makes complete resection difficult

DIAGNOSTIC CHECKLIST

- Mucinous tumors are less commonly malignant than serous tumors

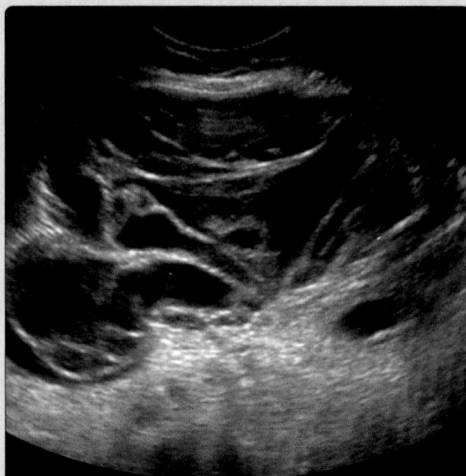
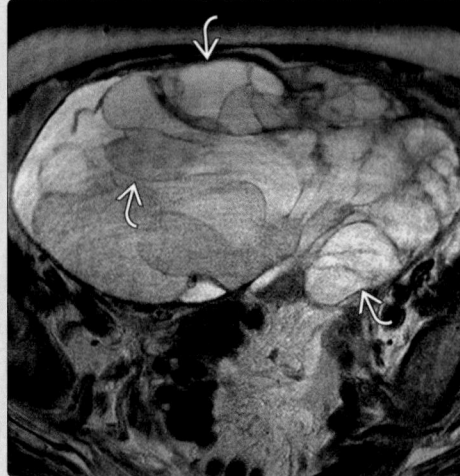

(Left) *Septations within a mucinous tumor are typically thin, creating multiple intervening locules, as seen in this transverse transabdominal ultrasound.* (Right) *Axial T2WI MR shows varying signal within the locules of the mass, due to differing concentrations of mucin ➨. Loculi with a high concentration of mucin will be higher signal on T1WI and lower signal on T2WI.*

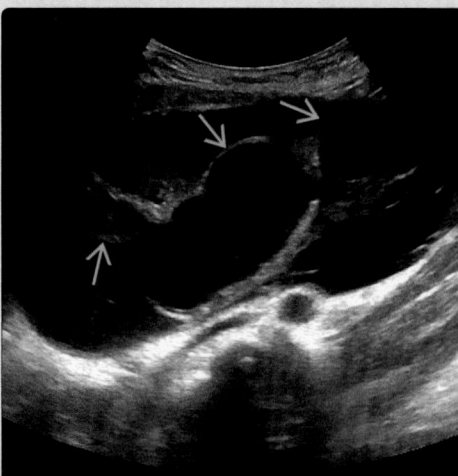
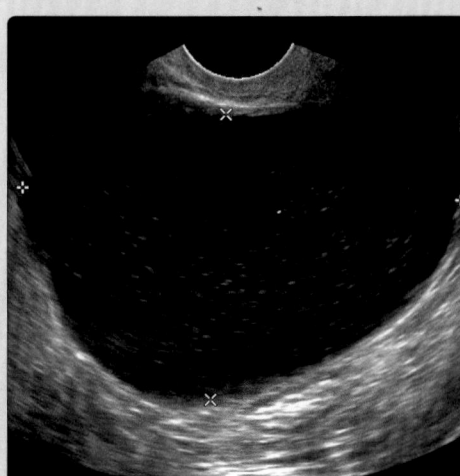

(Left) *Sagittal grayscale US of the right adnexa shows a large multiloculated mucinous cystadenoma. Multiple septations ➡ separate locules with varying degrees of internal low level echoes, creating a characteristic stained glass appearance.* (Right) *Closer inspection with transvaginal imaging in a different patient shows low-level echoes within the largest locule (calipers), consistent with mucin.*

Mucinous Ovarian Cystadenoma/Carcinoma

TERMINOLOGY

Abbreviations
- Benign or malignant mucinous tumor

Definitions
- Mucinous epithelial neoplasm, which can be benign (mucinous cystadenoma), borderline (low malignant potential), or malignant (mucinous cystadenocarcinoma)

IMAGING

General Features
- Best diagnostic clue
  - Multilocular cystic mass with low-level internal echoes
- Location
  - Bilateral in 5% of benign and 20% of malignant tumors
- Size
  - Variable in size, but often large, filling entire pelvis and extending into upper abdomen
  - Some of the largest tumors ever reported are mucinous cystadenomas
    - Massive size alone can suggest mucinous etiology

Ultrasonographic Findings
- Grayscale ultrasound
  - Typically multiloculated with thin septations
  - Papillary projections much less common than in serous tumors
  - Mucin creates low-level echoes within loculi
    - Typically have multiple loculi of varying echogenicity
    - Echogenicity variable depending on concentration of mucin
  - Solid components increase suspicion for malignancy
  - Pseudomyxoma peritonei: Potential form of peritoneal spread with amorphous, mucoid material insinuating itself around mesentery, bowel, and solid organs
    - More echogenic than simple ascites
    - Has mass effect with scalloping along solid organs (especially liver) and bowel matted posteriorly (rather than free floating)
    - May have subtle septations
- Color Doppler
  - Vascularity seen within solid components

CT Findings
- Variable attenuation of loculi, depending on concentration of mucin
- Peritoneal metastases often low attenuation
  - May be difficult to differentiate from fluid-filled bowel
- Enhancement of solid portions with contrast

MR Findings
- Signal intensity varies depending on concentration of mucin
- Loculi with high concentration of mucin will be higher signal on T1WI and lower signal on T2WI
  - Creates a stained glass appearance

DIFFERENTIAL DIAGNOSIS

Endometriomas
- Also contain low-level echoes
- MRI helpful: Blood high signal on T1WI with T2 shading

Serous Cystadenoma/Carcinoma
- More often unilocular
- Cyst contents not as echogenic
- Papillary projections common

Germ Cell Tumors
- Can have low-level echoes similar to mucin
- Typically more complicated with calcifications, fluid-fluid levels, etc.

Hemorrhagic Cyst
- Smaller and unilocular
- Resolves on follow-up scan

Mucocele
- Dilated appendix filled with mucinous material

PATHOLOGY

General Features
- Etiology
  - Not completely understood
  - 1 theory is "incessant ovulation": Repeated microtrauma with cellular repair to surface epithelium
    - Increased risk: Nulliparity, early menarche, late menopause (more ovulatory cycles)
    - Reduced risk: Multiparity, late menarche, early menopause, oral contraceptive use (fewer ovulatory cycles)
- Genetics
  - Hereditary causes in 5-10% of ovarian cancers (mutations in *BRCA1* and *BRCA2* tumor suppressor genes)
- Associated abnormalities
  - May occasionally be hormonally active, producing estrogen
- Ovarian neoplasms
  - Epithelial tumors: 60-70% of all tumors; 85-90% of malignancies
  - Germ cell tumors: 15-20% of all tumors; 3-5% of malignancies
  - Sex cord-stromal tumors: 5-10% of all tumors; 2-3% of malignancies
  - Metastases and lymphoma: 5-10% of all tumors; 5-10% of malignancies
- Benign epithelial tumors
  - Serous cystadenoma: 20-25%
  - Mucinous cystadenoma: 20-25%
- Malignant epithelial tumors
  - Serous cystadenocarcinoma: 40-50%
  - Endometrioid carcinoma: 20-25%
  - Mucinous cystadenocarcinoma: 5-10%
  - Clear cell carcinoma: 5-10%
  - Brenner tumor: 1-2%
  - Undifferentiated carcinoma: 4-5%
- Method of spread
  - Intraperitoneal dissemination most common
    - Greater omentum, right subphrenic region, and pouch of Douglas most common sites found at surgery
  - Direct extension to surrounding organs
  - Lymphatic spread to paraaortic and pelvic nodes
  - Hematogenous spread least common

– Liver and lung most common sites

Staging, Grading, & Classification

- FIGO staging system of ovarian carcinoma
  - Stage I: Tumor limited to ovaries
    - IA: Unilateral, no malignant ascites
    - IB: Bilateral, no malignant ascites
    - IC: Tumor limited to 1 or both ovaries with any of the following
      - ☐ IC1: Surgical spill intraoperatively
      - ☐ IC2: Capsule rupture before surgery, or tumor on ovarian/fallopian tube surface
      - ☐ IC3: Malignant cells present in ascites or peritoneal washings
  - Stage II: Tumor involves 1 or both ovaries with pelvic extension
    - IIA: Extension to uterus or fallopian tubes, no malignant ascites
    - IIB: Extension to other pelvic tissues, no malignant ascites
  - Stage III: Peritoneal implants outside pelvis &/or retroperitoneal nodal metastases
    - IIIA1: Positive retroperitoneal lymph nodes only
    - IIIA2: Microscopic metastasis outside pelvis &/or positive retroperitoneal lymph nodes
    - IIIB: Macroscopic extrapelvic implants ≤ 2 cm ± positive nodes
    - IIIC: Macroscopic extrapelvic implants > 2 cm or ± positive nodes
  - Stage IV: Distant metastases (excluding peritoneal implants)
    - IVA: Pleural effusion with positive cytology
    - IVB: Hepatic &/or splenic parenchymal metastasis, or metastasis to extra-abdominal organs (including inguinal nodes and nodes outside of abdomen)

Microscopic Features

- Ovarian origin of pseudomyxoma peritonei called into question
  - Most cases now thought to be appendiceal with metastases to ovary
  - Appendix should be thoroughly examined with special tissue staining in every case

CLINICAL ISSUES

Presentation

- Most common signs/symptoms
  - Incidental mass discovered on exam
  - Pelvic discomfort/pain from large tumors
    - Massive tumors can actually cause weight gain and distended abdomen
  - Symptoms from metastatic disease
- CA-125 not useful for mucinous tumors: False-negative in 30%

Demographics

- Age
  - Mucinous cystadenoma 3rd-5th decade
  - Mucinous cystadenocarcinoma in peri- and postmenopausal age group
- Epidemiology

- Mucinous tumors 2nd most common epithelial neoplasm (serous most common)
- Malignant: 10%; borderline: (Low malignant potential) 10%; benign 80%
- Bilateral in 5% of benign tumors, 10% of borderline tumors and 20% of malignant tumors

Natural History & Prognosis

- 95% 5-year survival for low malignant potential tumors
  - If metastatic, prognosis is similar to those with frankly malignant histology
- 5-year survival for malignant epithelial tumors
  - Stage I: 90%
  - Stage II: 70%
  - Stage III: 39%
  - Stage IV: 17%

Treatment

- Primary treatment is surgery
  - Complete staging laparotomy and tumor debulking (cytoreduction)
    - Staging laparotomy includes hysterectomy with bilateral salpingo-oophorectomy, pelvic and paraaortic node biopsies, omentectomy, peritoneal biopsies and washings
    - More conservative surgery may be done for women with stage I disease in reproductive age group
    - Care taken to avoid intraoperative rupture
      - ☐ May increase potential for recurrence
  - Gelatinous, insinuating nature of pseudomyxoma peritonei makes complete resection difficult
    - Recurrence common and multiple laparotomies required
  - Chemotherapy after cytoreductive surgery
  - Neoadjuvant chemotherapy before cytoreductive surgery in patients with unresectable disease
    - Includes bulky disease in difficult to reach areas (porta hepatis, lesser sac, root of mesentery), extensive surrounding organ or sidewall invasion, or stage IV disease

DIAGNOSTIC CHECKLIST

Image Interpretation Pearls

- Mucinous tumors are less commonly malignant than serous tumors

SELECTED REFERENCES

1. Sayasneh A et al: The characteristic ultrasound features of specific types of ovarian pathology (Review). Int J Oncol. 46(2):445-58, 2015
2. Ledermann JA et al: Gynecologic Cancer InterGroup (GCIG) consensus review for mucinous ovarian carcinoma. Int J Gynecol Cancer. 24(9 Suppl 3):S14-9, 2014
3. Alcázar JL et al: Clinical and ultrasound features of type I and type II epithelial ovarian cancer. Int J Gynecol Cancer. 23(4):680-4, 2013
4. Lalwani N et al: Histologic, molecular, and cytogenetic features of ovarian cancers: implications for diagnosis and treatment. Radiographics. 31(3):625-46, 2011

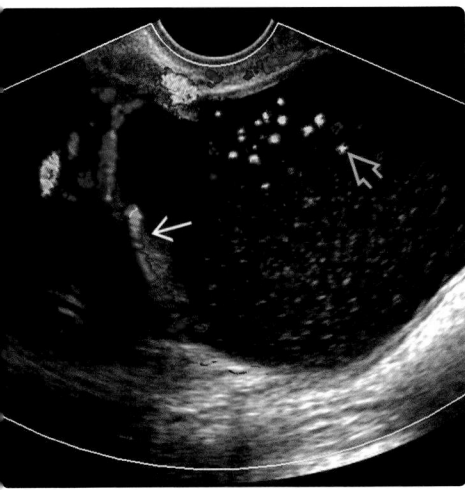

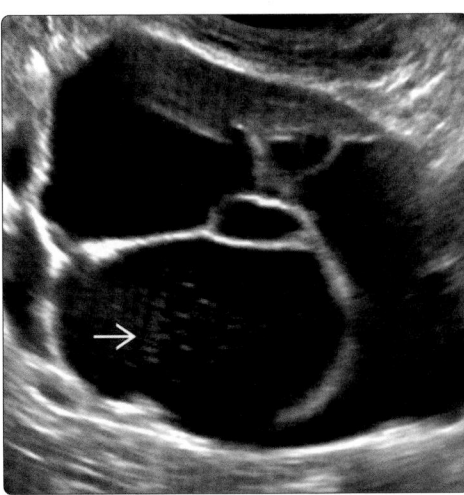

(Left) *Septations* ➡ *and diffuse low-level echoes are typical of mucinous cystadenomas. Transvaginal longitudinal Doppler ultrasound shows vascularity in the septations, and streaming artifact* ➡ *due to the mobile mucin.* (Right) *Within the locules of this mucinous cystadenoma, varying degrees of low-level echoes reflect differing concentrations of mucin* ➡ *on transabdominal ultrasound.*

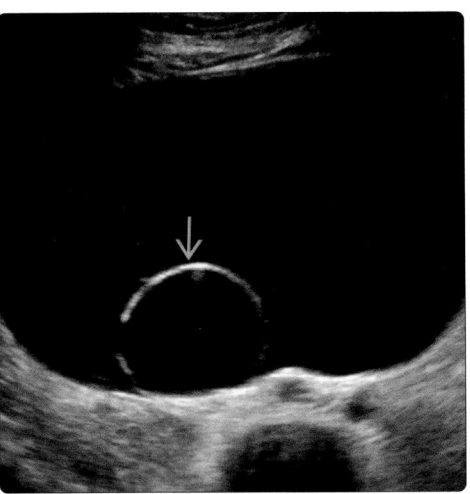

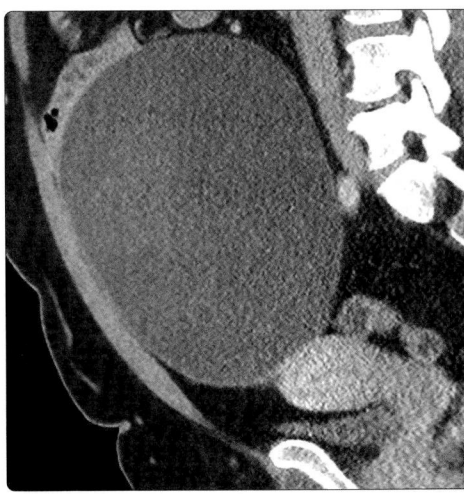

(Left) *A single thin-walled loculation* ➡ *is present in this cystic ovarian mass. Relatively few internal echoes are present in either compartment as seen on transvaginal ultrasound.* (Right) *CECT shows the full extent of the ovarian mass, which extends out of the pelvis and into the midabdomen. A large ovarian mass in a peri- or postmenopausal patient is the typical presentation for mucinous cystadenoma.*

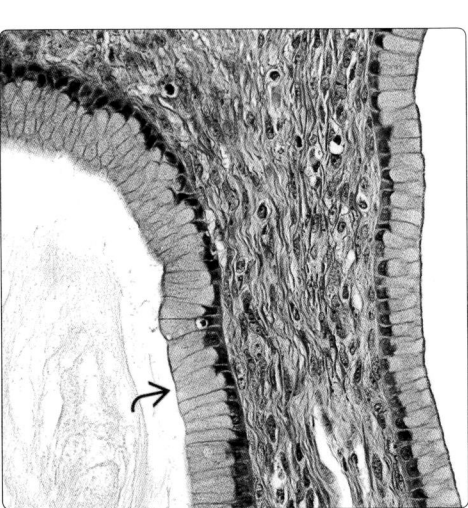

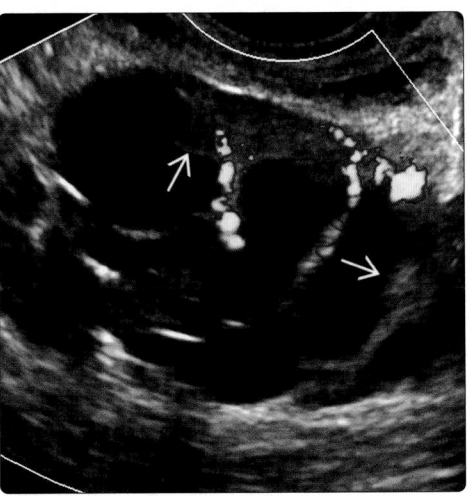

(Left) *Acellular mucin is present within a mucinous cystadenoma, and the lining cells have abundant mucinous cytoplasm* ➡. (Right) *Solid vascular components* ➡ *are suggestive of mucinous cystadenocarcinoma on transvaginal ultrasound.*

TERMINOLOGY

- Mature cystic teratoma (MCT) = dermoid cyst
- Immature teratoma (IT)
- Monodermal teratoma in which 1 cell line predominates

IMAGING

- **Mature cystic teratomas have a variety of appearances**
  - Heterogeneous cystic ovarian mass with echogenic shadowing mural nodule (Rokitansky nodule) on US
  - ± fat-fluid level
  - Highly echogenic focus/foci with distal acoustic shadowing represent teeth
  - Hair within mucin creates characteristic dot-dash-dot appearance
- Fat-containing adnexal mass is diagnostic on CT

TOP DIFFERENTIAL DIAGNOSES

- Hemorrhagic cyst
- Endometrioma

- Bowel

PATHOLOGY

- Mature tissues of endodermal, mesodermal, and ectodermal origin
- 88% unilocular, fat content liquid at body temperature, semisolid at room temperature

CLINICAL ISSUES

- Most common ovarian tumor
- 10-20% bilateral
- Rarely undergo malignant degeneration
- Rupture in < 1% of cases
- May act as lead point for adnexal torsion

DIAGNOSTIC CHECKLIST

- Rokitansky nodule (dermoid plug) is diagnostic

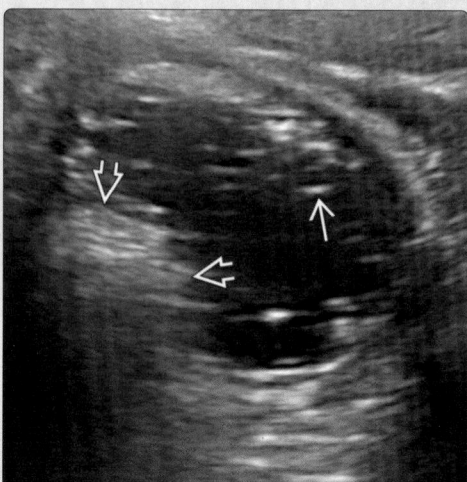
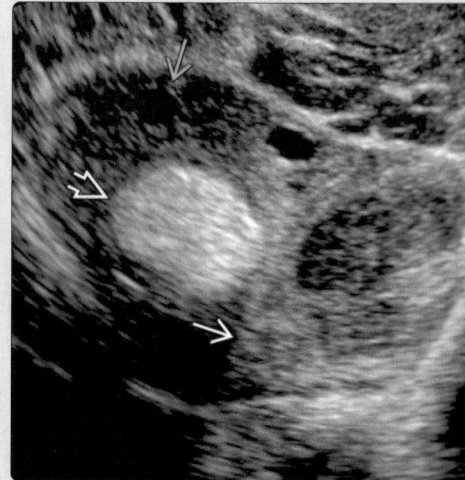

(Left) Dermoids may be mostly cystic, with linear floating echoes consistent with hair ➡. The echogenic shadowing Rokitansky nodule ➡ along the periphery is diagnostic for a dermoid. (Right) Ultrasound shows that this dermoid has a more heterogeneous appearance due to differing fat ➡ and echogenic fluid content ➡. The Rokitansky nodule ➡ is present as well.

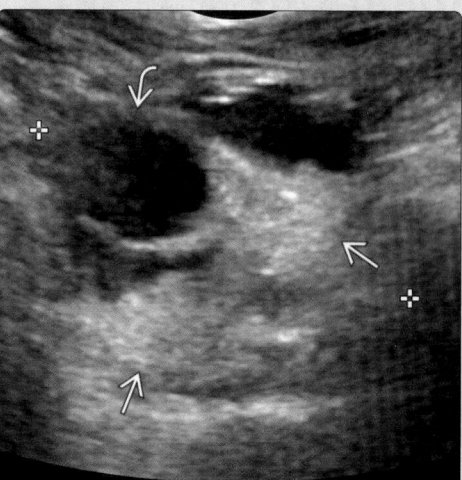
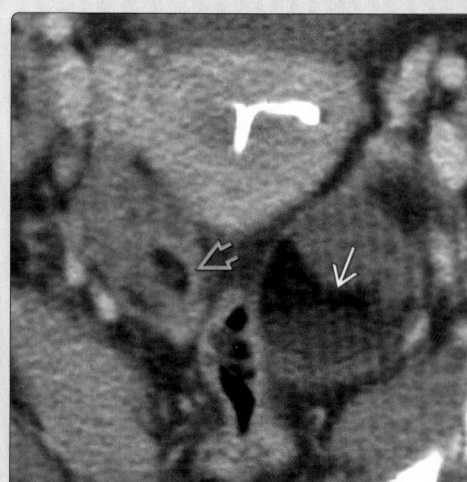

(Left) Within the same mass (calipers), there may be areas of highly echogenic semisolid fat ➡, with anechoic areas of more liquid fat ➡. (Right) Axial CECT in the same patient shows the layering areas of fat density in the left ovarian dermoid ➡. A smaller dermoid is also present in the right ovary ➡. 10-20% of dermoids are bilateral.

TERMINOLOGY

Synonyms

- Dermoid cyst

Definitions

- Ovarian teratoma includes
  - Mature cystic teratoma (MCT) = dermoid cyst
  - Immature teratoma (IT)
  - Monodermal teratoma in which 1 cell line predominates
    - Struma ovarii
    - Carcinoid tumor

IMAGING

General Features

- Best diagnostic clue
  - Ovarian mass with echogenic shadowing mural nodule (Rokitansky nodule) on US

Ultrasonographic Findings

- Grayscale ultrasound
  - **Mature cystic teratomas have a variety of appearances**
    - Heterogeneous cystic mass with echogenic component
    - Highly echogenic components due to fat content
    - ± fat-fluid level
    - Shadowing echogenic mural nodule (sebaceous material)
      - Rokitansky nodule (a.k.a. dermoid plug)
    - Hair
      - Punctate echoes in 1 plane
      - Elongate to become linear echoes in orthogonal plane
      - Hair will move through more fluid component with transducer pressure
      - Creates "dot-dash-dot" appearance
    - Teeth
      - Highly echogenic focus/foci with distal acoustic shadowing
    - "Tip of the iceberg" sign: Only leading edge of mass identified
      - Distal acoustic shadowing prevents assessment of deep edge
      - Size cannot be measured
      - Mass may be much larger than suggested by leading edge echoes
  - **Immature teratoma**: Heterogeneous, mainly solid, scattered calcification (i.e., nonspecific)
  - **Monodermal teratoma**: Nonspecific sonographic appearances
- Color Doppler
  - Look for flow in solid components
    - Typically avascular
  - Beware of "twinkling" artifact, as sound reverberates on calcified components
    - Always perform pulsed Doppler evaluation of apparent flow seen with color Doppler

Radiographic Findings

- May see associated calcification (e.g., "tooth" in pelvis)

CT Findings

- Fat-containing adnexal mass is diagnostic on CT
- 56% of MCT cases diagnosed on CT show teeth/calcification
- IT: Characteristic appearance is mass with large irregular solid component containing foci of fat and coarse calcifications
  - Hemorrhage often present
- If ruptured, characteristic low density fat-containing intraperitoneal fluid present
  - May lead to chemical peritonitis with mesenteric stranding, peritoneal surface thickening

MR Findings

- T1WI
  - High signal components = fat
- T1WI FS
  - With fat saturation, loss of high T1 signal differentiates fat from blood products
    - ↓ signal = fat within teratoma
- T2WI
  - Variable intensity of fatty component, can be confused with blood products
- IT: Characteristic appearance is mass with large irregular solid component containing foci of fat and coarse calcifications
  - Hemorrhage often present

Imaging Recommendations

- Best imaging tool
  - Ultrasound
    - No ionizing radiation

DIFFERENTIAL DIAGNOSIS

Hemorrhagic Cyst

- Fine network of fibrin strands rather than floating hair
- Distal acoustic enhancement
  - Fat content in MCT causes sound attenuation (i.e., acoustic shadowing)

Endometrioma

- Homogeneous low-level internal echoes
- Often history of chronic cyclical pelvic pain, endometriosis
- No Rokitansky nodule

Torsion

- Complex enlarged adnexal mass
- Characteristically avascular but may occasionally see arterial flow
- Any adnexal mass can act as lead point for torsion

Abscess

- Appendix abscess with appendicolith may mimic sonographic appearance of ovarian teratoma
- Clinical presentation with pain/fever should suggest diagnosis
- Infarcted dermoid may become infected

Bowel

- Use of TV sonography may help differentiate bowel from normal ovary

- Large bowel may contain echogenic feces mimicking teratoma
- Colon does not undergo peristalsis as much as small bowel
- May require repeat exam or alternate modalities, such as MR, to clarify

PATHOLOGY

Gross Pathologic & Surgical Features

- MCT
  - Mature tissues of endodermal, mesodermal, and ectodermal origin
  - 88% unilocular, fat content liquid at body temperature, semisolid at room temperature
  - Rokitansky nodule: Nodule protrudes into cyst cavity
    - Most hair arises from nodule; if teeth/bone present, will be in this protuberance
  - 31% of MCTs contain teeth
- IT: Often show capsular perforation
- Monodermal teratoma
  - Thyroid tissue in struma ovarii
    - Amber-colored thyroid tissue with hemorrhage, necrosis, fibrosis; no fat present
  - Neuroectodermal tissue in carcinoid tumor
    - Unlike MCT, these occur in postmenopausal women

Microscopic Features

- MCT
  - Scant mitotic activity, no cytologic atypia
  - Walls lined by squamous epithelium
  - Malignant degeneration may give rise to squamous cell cancer, malignant melanoma, sarcoma
- IT: Contain embryonic/immature tissues as well as mature line seen in MCT
  - Amount of yolk sac tumor correlates with stage, grade, and recurrence rate
  - Overgrowth of immature neural elements → primitive neuroectodermal tumor

CLINICAL ISSUES

Presentation

- Most common signs/symptoms
  - MCTs are often asymptomatic
    - Most common ovarian tumor
      - 50% of all ovarian tumors
    - Most common incidentally discovered ovarian mass during cesarean section delivery

Demographics

- Age
  - MCT: Mean age at presentation is 30 yrs.
    - Most common ovarian mass in children
  - IT: 0-20 years
- Epidemiology
  - Most commonly excised ovarian neoplasm
  - 95% ovarian germ cell tumors are MCT

Natural History & Prognosis

- MCT
  - 10-20% bilateral
  - Often asymptomatic

- May rupture: Reported in < 1% of cases
- May act as lead point for adnexal torsion
- Rarely undergo malignant degeneration
  - ~ 1-3%
  - Squamous cell carcinoma (most common), malignant melanoma, sarcoma
  - Older patients (6th-7th decades)
  - Tumor diameter > 10 cm
  - Rapid growth
- Rarely present with prolactinemia, hypercalcemia, autoimmune hemolytic anemia, erythrocytosis, or paraneoplastic syndrome (secondary to NMDA receptor antibodies)
- IT
  - Primitive neuroectodermal tumors have poor prognosis
  - IT treated with chemotherapy may "retroconvert" (i.e., take on MCT appearance)
    - May remain stable for long duration

Treatment

- Surgical resection for definitive diagnosis and to avoid potential complications
- Ovarian cystectomy
  - With laparoscopy or laparotomy
  - Care taken to prevent cyst rupture and copious irrigation performed to avoid peritonitis

DIAGNOSTIC CHECKLIST

Consider

- "Tip of the iceberg" sign prevents accurate estimation of size
  - Size may be important to operating surgeon

Image Interpretation Pearls

- Rokitansky nodule (dermoid plug) is diagnostic
- 10-20% MCTs are bilateral
  - Look for small contralateral tumor

SELECTED REFERENCES

1. Young RH: Ovarian tumors and tumor-like lesions in the first three decades. Semin Diagn Pathol. 31(5):382-426, 2014
2. Baser E et al: Adnexal masses encountered during cesarean delivery. Int J Gynaecol Obstet. 123(2):124-6, 2013
3. Hursitoglu BS et al: A clinico-pathological evaluation of 194 patients with ovarian teratoma: 7-year experience in a single center. Ginekol Pol. 84(2):108-11, 2013
4. Yun NR et al: Squamous cell carcinoma arising in an ovarian mature cystic teratoma complicating pregnancy. Obstet Gynecol Sci. 56(2):121-5, 2013
5. Fossey SJ et al: Sclerosing encapsulating peritonitis secondary to dermoid cyst rupture: a case report. Ann R Coll Surg Engl. 93(5):e39-40, 2011
6. Alotaibi MO et al: Imaging of ovarian teratomas in children: a 9-year review. Can Assoc Radiol J. 61(1):23-8, 2010
7. Choudhary S et al: Imaging of ovarian teratomas: appearances and complications. J Med Imaging Radiat Oncol. 53(5):480-8, 2009
8. Saba L et al: Mature and immature ovarian teratomas: CT, US and MR imaging characteristics. Eur J Radiol. 72(3):454-63, 2009
9. Park SB et al: Imaging findings of complications and unusual manifestations of ovarian teratomas. Radiographics. 28(4):969-83, 2008

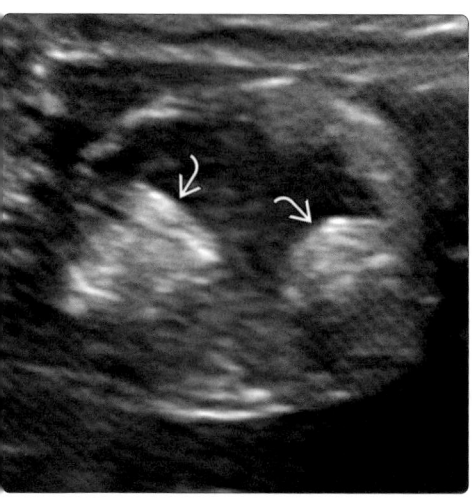

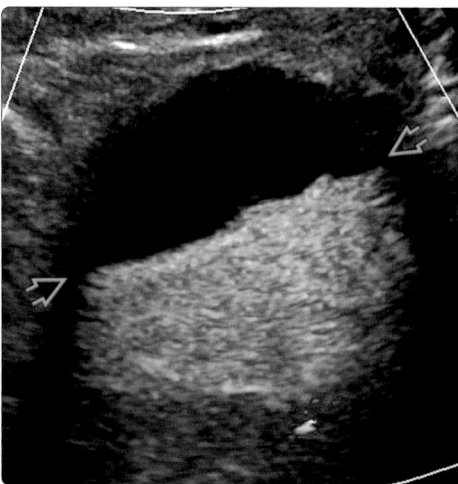

(Left) *Ultrasound shows that there are 2 Rokitansky nodules ➔ within the otherwise cystic-appearing fat of this dermoid.* (Right) *Color Doppler ultrasound shows that depending on the semisolid vs. liquid state of the fat within a dermoid, a fat-fluid level ➔ may be present.*

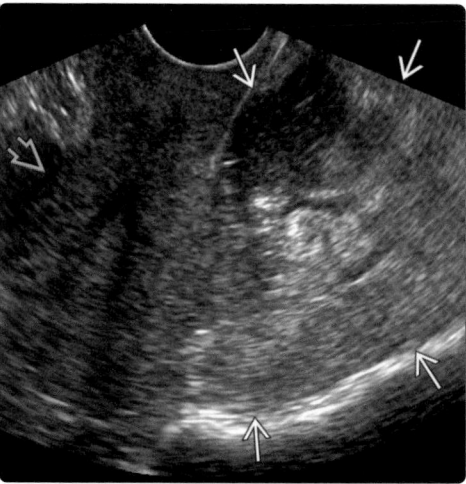

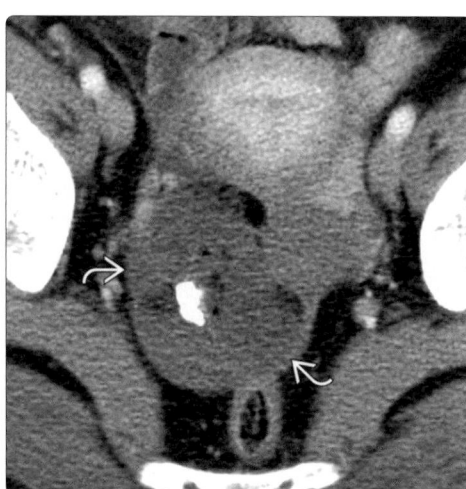

(Left) *Transvaginal ultrasound shows that dermoids can appear atypical on ultrasound when there is more soft tissue than fat within the mass. This dermoid is heterogeneously echogenic and fills the cul-de-sac ➔ posterior to the uterus ➔.* (Right) *Axial CECT of the same mass shows there is relatively little fat ➔, with a predominance of soft tissue creating the appearance on ultrasound.*

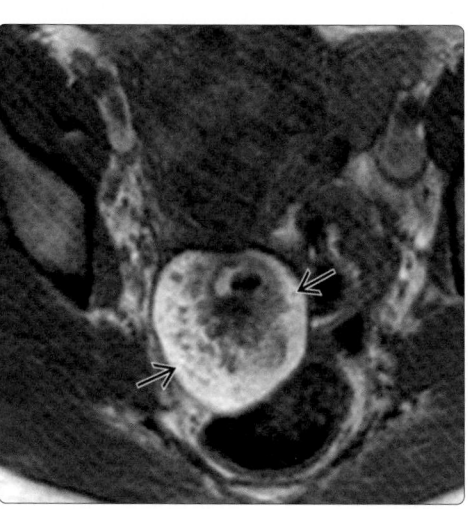

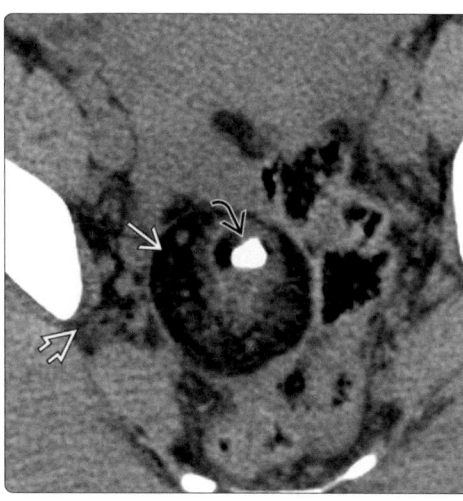

(Left) *On T1 MR, dermoids have internal high signal that is consistent with fat ➔.* (Right) *Axial CECT of the same dermoid shows the calcified tooth ➔, which is present in about 1/3 of cases. Notice the fat ➔ within the dermoid is markedly hypodense compared to normal extraperitoneal fat ➔.*

Polycystic Ovarian Syndrome

TERMINOLOGY

- Complex heterogenous syndrome of ovulatory dysfunction, menstrual irregularity, and androgen excess
- Rotterdam criteria for polycystic ovarian syndrome (PCOS) developed in 2003: 2 of 3 criteria must be present
  - Oligo- or anovulation
  - Hyperandrogenism (clinical or biochemical)
  - Polycystic ovaries (by ultrasound)

IMAGING

- Enlarged ovaries with volume > 10 mL **or** ≥ 12 follicles per ovary measuring 2-9 mm in diameter
- Calculate volume using formula for prolate ellipsoid (longitudinal x transverse x AP diameter x 0.5233)
- Ovarian stromal ↑ echogenicity
- If dominant follicle (> 10 mm diameter) or corpus luteum seen, repeat scan during next cycle to avoid false elevation of volume

TOP DIFFERENTIAL DIAGNOSES

- Normal
  - Ovarian morphology alone is insufficient for diagnosis of PCOS
  - PCOM seen in ~ 22% of women, PCOS prevalence is only 5-10%
- Suppressed ovary
- Other causes of hyperandrogenism

CLINICAL ISSUES

- Anovulation → oligo/amenorrhea
- Hyperandrogenism → hirsutism
- Obesity with associated hyperinsulinemia/insulin resistance

DIAGNOSTIC CHECKLIST

- Features seen in 1 ovary are sufficient to diagnose PCOS

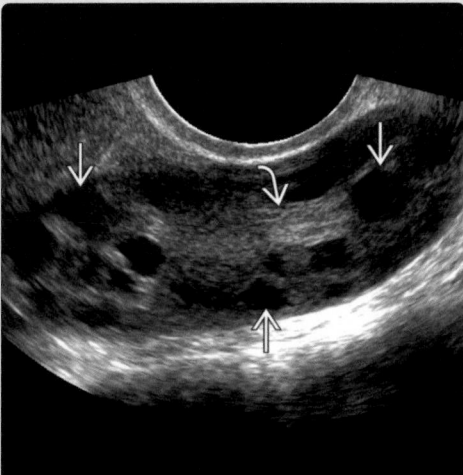
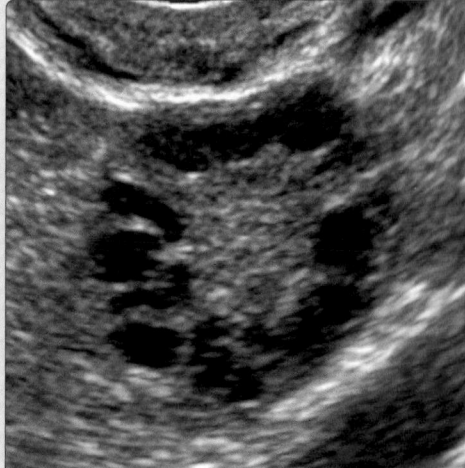

(Left) Transvaginal US demonstrates an enlarged right ovary with a volume of 19 mL and multiple follicles ➡ between 2-9 mm in size in a patient with polycystic ovarian syndrome (PCOS). Note the echogenic central stroma ➡. (Right) Transvaginal US demonstrates a normal size ovary with a volume < 10 mL. However, Rotterdam criteria are met because there are ≥ 12 follicles measuring between 2-9 mL.

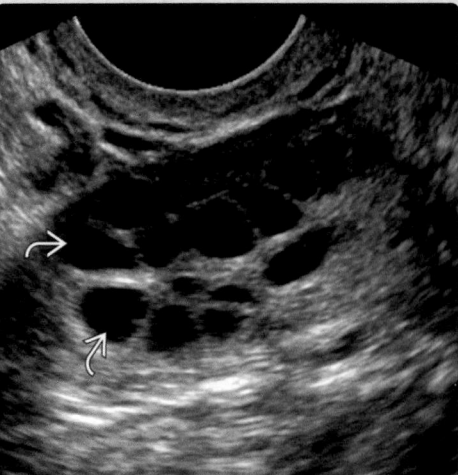
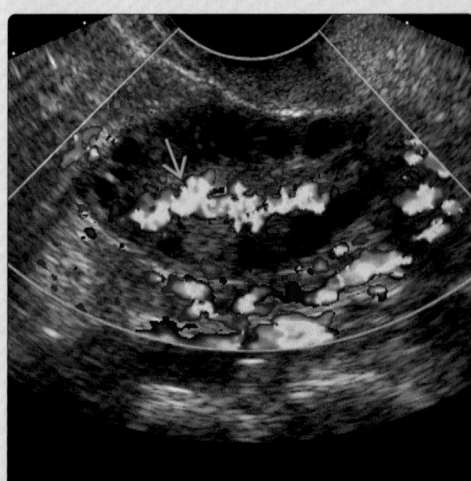

(Left) Transvaginal US demonstrates the typical appearance of polycystic ovarian morphology with an enlarged ovary containing multiple small follicles ➡. (Right) Color Doppler longitudinal transvaginal US shows the central stroma of the ovary is well vascularized ➡, which is not a diagnostic criterion but has been noted in polycystic ovarian morphology.

TERMINOLOGY

Abbreviations
- Polycystic ovarian syndrome (PCOS)

Synonyms
- Stein-Leventhal syndrome: Hyperandrogenemia → polycystic ovaries, hirsutism, menstrual abnormalities, obesity

Definitions
- Complex heterogenous syndrome of ovulatory dysfunction, menstrual irregularity, and androgen excess
- Rotterdam criteria for PCOS developed in 2003: 2 of 3 criteria must be present
  - Oligo- or anovulation
  - Hyperandrogenism (clinical or biochemical)
  - Polycystic ovaries (by ultrasound)
- Polycystic ovarian morphology (PCOM) is better term for ovaries meeting criteria on ultrasound because many women do not have PCOS

IMAGING

General Features
- Best diagnostic clue
  - Enlarged ovaries with volume > 10 mL or
  - ≥ 12 follicles per ovary measuring 2-9 mm in diameter

Ultrasonographic Findings
- Grayscale ultrasound
  - Uterus often enlarged due to estrogenization
  - Ovarian stromal ↑ echogenicity
  - ↑ ovarian stromal volume
    - ↑ stromal volume is main cause of ↑ ovarian volume (follicles do not contribute significantly)

Imaging Recommendations
- Best imaging tool
  - Transvaginal ultrasound because of ↑ resolution
- Protocol advice
  - Measure ovarian diameters in 3 planes
  - Calculate volume using formula for prolate ellipsoid (longitudinal x transverse x AP diameter x 0.5233)
    - Normal women 7.94 ± 2.34 cc
    - PCOS patients 10.04 ± 7.36 cc
  - Follicle numbers should be assessed in at least 2 planes to confirm size and position
  - Follicle diameter should be measured as mean of 3 planes
  - If dominant follicle (> 10 mm diameter) or corpus luteum seen, repeat scan during next cycle to avoid false elevation of volume
  - Regularly menstruating women should be scanned day 3-5, oligo/amenorrheic women can be scanned at random or 3-5 days after progestogen-induced bleed

DIFFERENTIAL DIAGNOSIS

Normal
- Ovarian morphology alone is insufficient for diagnosis of PCOS

- Polycystic ovarian morphology (PCOM) seen in ~ 22% of women, PCOS prevalence is only 5-10%

Suppressed Ovary
- Oral contraceptive pills suppress ovulation → multiple small follicles

Other Causes of Hyperandrogenism
- Hyperthecosis, congenital adrenal hyperplasia, 21-hydroxylase deficiency, Cushing syndrome, androgen producing neoplasm

PATHOLOGY

General Features
- Etiology
  - No single etiologic factor identified, no responsible gene as yet isolated
  - Likely complex interaction between genetics and environmental/metabolic factors
- Associated abnormalities
  - Obesity, hirsutism

CLINICAL ISSUES

Presentation
- Most common signs/symptoms
  - PCOS phenotype has 3 components
    - Anovulation → oligo/amenorrhea
    - Hyperandrogenism → hirsutism
    - Obesity with associated hyperinsulinemia/insulin resistance

Demographics
- Epidemiology
  - Most common cause of anovulatory infertility in USA
  - Affects 6-10% of females in reproductive age group

Natural History & Prognosis
- Associated with dysmetabolic syndrome
  - 3-7x ↑ risk maturity onset diabetes, some studies suggest ↑ cardio/cerebrovascular events

Treatment
- Traditional treatment centers on ovulation induction, treatment of acne/hirsutism, prevention of endometrial cancer, diabetes, and heart disease risk

DIAGNOSTIC CHECKLIST

Image Interpretation Pearls
- Features seen in 1 ovary are sufficient to diagnose PCOS
- Ovarian volume is suppressed in women taking oral contraceptives but appearance may still be polycystic

SELECTED REFERENCES

1. Dewailly D et al: Definition and significance of polycystic ovarian morphology: a task force report from the Androgen Excess and Polycystic Ovary Syndrome Society. Hum Reprod Update. 20(3):334-52, 2014
2. Lujan ME et al: Updated ultrasound criteria for polycystic ovary syndrome: reliable thresholds for elevated follicle population and ovarian volume. Hum Reprod. 28(5):1361-8, 2013

TERMINOLOGY

- Endometriosis: Ectopic endometrial glands outside of uterine cavity
- Endometrioma: Cystic collection of mixed blood products

IMAGING

- US
  - Diffuse low-level internal echoes in 95%
  - Increased through transmission
  - Homogeneous echotexture
  - Cyst wall with variable appearance
  - Endometrioma may look anechoic transabdominally
  - May see fluid-fluid level in cyst
- MR
  - T1WI: Homogeneous high signal
  - T2WI: Shading is distinguishing feature
- Cesarean section endometrioma
  - Abdominal wall mass
- Deep invasive endometriosis

- Scarring, aggressive implants
- Decidualization during pregnancy can lead to solid-appearing adnexal masses

TOP DIFFERENTIAL DIAGNOSES

- Hemorrhagic cyst
  - Acute hemorrhage can mimic endometrioma
  - Fibrin strands
  - Resolves in 4-6 weeks
- Dermoid cyst (teratoma)
  - Hyperechoic, dirty shadowing, "tip of the iceberg" sign
  - Fat-fluid level
- Cystic neoplasm
  - Typically postmenopausal

CLINICAL ISSUES

- Infertility
- Cyclical or chronic pain

(Left) Endovaginal US demonstrates small homogeneously isoechoic round endometrioma ⮕ adjacent to normal ovarian parenchyma ⮕ containing follicles ⮕. Doppler US (not shown) showed no internal flow. (Right) Transverse endovaginal US demonstrating coexistent hemorrhagic cyst ⮕ and endometrioma ⮕. Note the homogenous appearance of the echoes in the endometrioma in contradistinction to the fine fibrin strands ⮕ and mixed echogenicity of the hemorrhagic cyst.

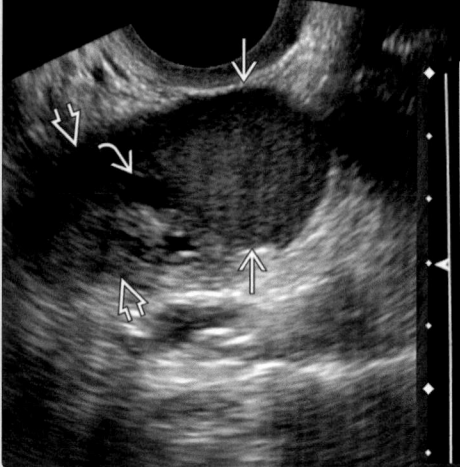
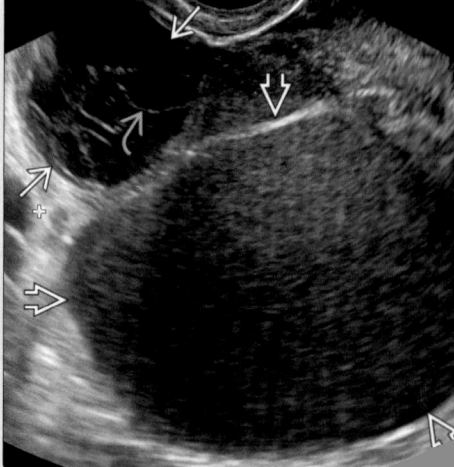

(Left) Transverse transabdominal US shows bilateral cystic adnexal masses ⮕ with homogeneous low level internal echoes. Endometriomas are bilateral in up to 50% of cases. (Right) Color Doppler endovaginal US demonstrates scattered minimal areas of flow in the mildly thickened wall of this endometrioma which is typical.

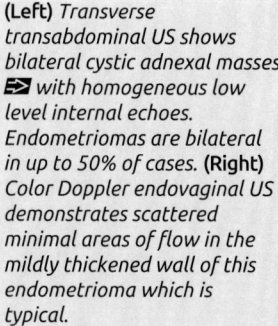
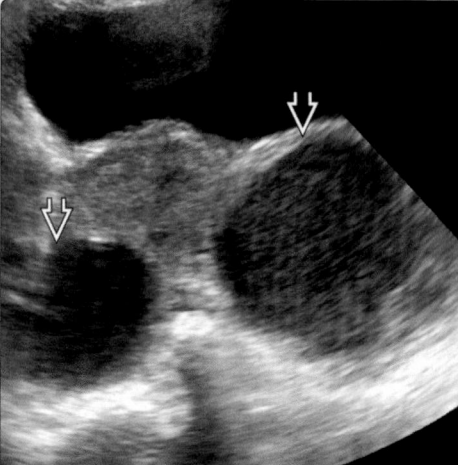
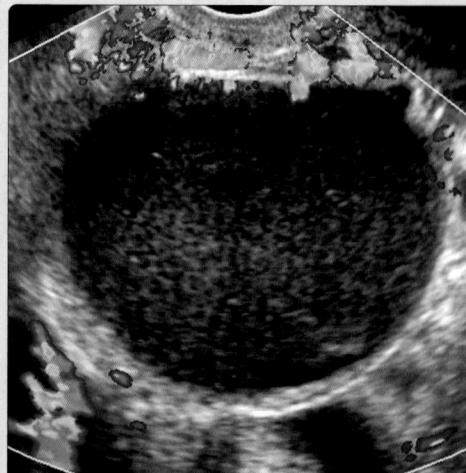

Endometrioma

TERMINOLOGY

Synonyms

- Endometriosis, endometriotic cysts, chocolate cyst

Definitions

- Functional endometrium outside of uterus
  - Cyclical hemorrhage
- Ectopic endometrial cells

IMAGING

General Features

- Location
  - Ovarian in 75%, bilateral 50%
  - Cul-de-sac involvement in 70%
  - Posterior broad ligament in 45%
  - Uterine serosa in 10%
  - Bowel, ureter, bladder in 8%
  - Multiple lesions often seen
- Size
  - Variable from implants to large cysts
  - Endometriomas up to 15 cm reported
  - Small endometriosis implants are < 1 cm
    - Rarely seen well by imaging
- Morphology
  - Varies from unilocular cyst to multilocular mass
  - Adhesions distort normal pelvic anatomy

Ultrasonographic Findings

- Diffuse low-level internal echoes in 95%
  - Homogeneous echotexture
  - Unilocular complex cyst
  - Increased through transmission
  - Most often within or arising from ovary
  - Often characterized as "ground glass"
- Cyst wall with variable appearance
  - Diffuse thickening common
  - Wall nodularity in 20%
    - May mimic neoplasm
  - Tiny bright foci in cyst wall is specific finding (35%)
    - Smaller and more echogenic than true nodule
    - Formed from cholesterol deposits in cyst wall
    - May have ring-down artifact
- May see fluid-fluid level in cyst
  - Blood of different ages will layer
    - Echogenic blood is dependent
    - Hypoechoic blood is supernatant
    - DDx: Dermoid, has opposite layering appearance
- Calcifications are rare
- Endometrioma may be multilocular
  - Thin or thick septations between loculi
  - Mimics neoplasia
- Nonovarian endometrioma/endometriosis
  - Not necessarily same appearance as ovarian
    - May be solid enhancing masses with infiltrative borders
  - Cesarean section endometrioma
    - Subcutaneous along scar
  - Deep invasive endometriosis

- Surface of uterus
- Peritoneal surface of cul-de-sac
- Bowel serosa
  - Bladder serosa
  - Ureter
    - Can cause hydronephrosis
- Decidualized endometrioma in pregnancy
  - Cystic adnexal mass with solid vascularized components
- Ruptured endometrioma
  - Collapsed cyst wall
  - Echogenic pelvic free fluid
- Malignant transformation
  - Cystic and solid mass with vascular solid component

MR Findings

- T1WI
  - Homogeneous high signal from repeated hemorrhage
    - Similar to or greater T1 signal than fat
- T1WI FS
  - Very hyperintense
- T2WI
  - T2 shading is distinguishing feature
    - Loss of signal within lesion on T2 compared to T1
    - Variable amounts of shading seen
  - T2 dark fibrosis with adhesions/deep infiltrating endometriosis

Imaging Recommendations

- Best imaging tool
  - Ultrasound is 1st imaging tool
    - Classic appearance is diagnostic
  - MR has greater specificity
- Protocol advice
  - Endometrioma may look anechoic transabdominally
    - Need transvaginal ultrasound and ↑ gain settings to see internal echoes
  - Look carefully at cyst wall for echogenic foci with "comet tail" artifact
    - Cholesterol in cyst wall
    - Do not confuse for nodules
  - True nodules and thick septations raise suspicion for malignancy

DIFFERENTIAL DIAGNOSIS

Hemorrhagic Cyst

- Functional ovarian cyst
  - Resolves in 6-12 weeks
- Acute hemorrhage can mimic endometrioma
  - Diffuse low or medium-level echoes
- Evolution of hemorrhage over time
  - Fibrin strands; thinner than septations
  - Clot retraction; surrounding seroma
- Complete resolution rules out endometrioma
- More likely to present with acute pain

Dermoid Cyst (Mature Cystic Teratoma)

- Common benign mass
  - Endoderm, ectoderm, mesoderm components
- Typical imaging
  - Rokitansky nodule

– Calcification (teeth)
– Focal echogenicity with shadowing along cyst wall
○ Liquefied fat
– Hyperechoic, dirty shadowing, "tip of the iceberg" sign
○ Fat-fluid level
– Echogenic fluid on top of hypoechoic fluid (floating fat)
○ Hair: Thin echogenic lines and dots
- 20-30% bilateral
- Symptomatic if rupture or torsion

Cystic Neoplasm
- Typically postmenopausal
- Multilocular mass
- Thick septations
- Wall nodularity
- Blood flow in septations and nodules
- Associated ascites
- More likely to be unilateral mass

PATHOLOGY

General Features
- Etiology
  ○ Retrograde menstruation (RM)
    – Metastatic implantation
    – 2° to hematogenous or lymphatic spread
  ○ Metaplasia of coelomic epithelium
    – Peritoneal cells become endometrial cells
  ○ Induction theory
    – Combination of previous 2 theories
    – RM induces metaplasia
  ○ Abnormal immunity
    – RM occurs in majority of women but implantation of functioning endometrium is rare
    – ↓ immunity results in implantation
- Associated abnormalities
  ○ Adhesions
  ○ Bowel, ureter, bladder involvement
  ○ Endometriosis can spread outside of pelvis

Gross Pathologic & Surgical Features
- Chocolate cyst
  ○ Dark brown viscous blood
- Endometriotic implant appearance variable
  ○ Immature foci are pale yellow or pink
  ○ Mature foci are dark brown or white scars

Microscopic Features
- Endometrial glands and stroma

CLINICAL ISSUES

Presentation
- Most common signs/symptoms
  ○ Infertility
  ○ Cyclical or chronic pain
  ○ Palpable mass
  ○ Incidentally noted mass on ultrasound
- Other signs/symptoms
  ○ Unusual symptoms for atypical locations

– Gastrointestinal bleeding
– Ureteral obstruction
– Pneumothorax
– Seizure

Demographics
- Age
  ○ Women of childbearing age
  ○ Mean age at diagnosis: 25-29 years
- Epidemiology
  ○ Overall prevalence 5-10%
    – 4% of all tubal ligation cases
    – 20% of infertility cases
    – 25% of chronic pelvic pain cases

Natural History & Prognosis
- Burns out with menopause
  ○ May remerge with estrogen replacement therapy

Treatment
- Medical treatment
  ○ Hormonal manipulation of menstrual cycle
  ○ Best evidence for using levonorgestrel-releasing IUD and GnRH analogues to decrease pain
- Conservative surgery
  ○ Laparoscopic: Ablation, excision of implants or endometrioma cyst wall
  ○ Reproductive function retained
  ○ 30-40% recurrence rates
- Definitive surgery
  ○ Hysterectomy and oophorectomy
  ○ May recur with exogenous estrogen
- Infertility from endometriosis
  ○ Conservative surgery increases spontaneous pregnancy and live birth rates
  ○ Improves assisted reproductive techniques
  ○ Monthly fecundity rates of 9-18%

DIAGNOSTIC CHECKLIST

Consider
- Endometrioma if unilocular adnexal cyst with diffuse low-level echoes

Image Interpretation Pearls
- Endometrioma can mimic dermoid and neoplasm
- Multiple lesions are common
- MR findings more specific than ultrasound

SELECTED REFERENCES
1. Brown J et al: Endometriosis: an overview of Cochrane Reviews. Cochrane Database Syst Rev. 3:CD009590, 2014
2. Groszmann Y et al: Decidualized endometrioma masquerading as ovarian cancer in pregnancy. J Ultrasound Med. 33(11):1909-15, 2014
3. McDermott S et al: MR imaging of malignancies arising in endometriomas and extraovarian endometriosis. Radiographics. 32(3):845-63, 2012
4. Siegelman ES et al: MR imaging of endometriosis: ten imaging pearls. Radiographics. 32(6):1675-91, 2012
5. Chamié LP et al: Findings of pelvic endometriosis at transvaginal US, MR imaging, and laparoscopy. Radiographics. 31(4):E77-100, 2011

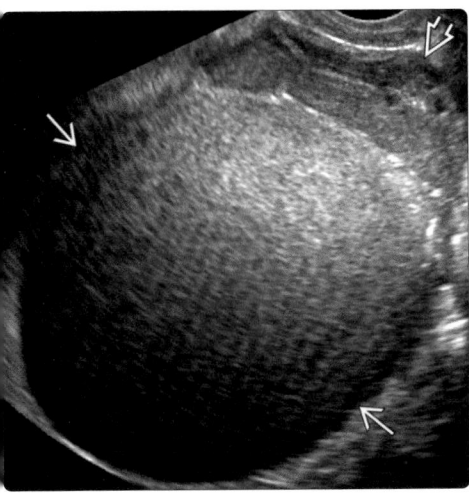

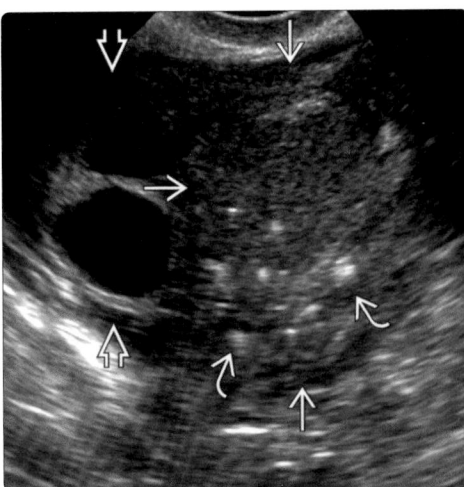

(Left) *Longitudinal endovaginal US shows a large right adnexal endometrioma as a complex cystic mass* ➡ *with a thin wall and diffuse homogenous low-level internal echoes. The large endometrioma displaces the uterus inferiorly* ➡. **(Right)** *Transabdominal US shows a large endometrioma* ➡ *with adjacent normal ovarian stroma* ➡ *containing follicles. Note echogenic foci with "comet-tail" artifact* ➡ *in the wall of the endometrioma from cholesterol deposits.*

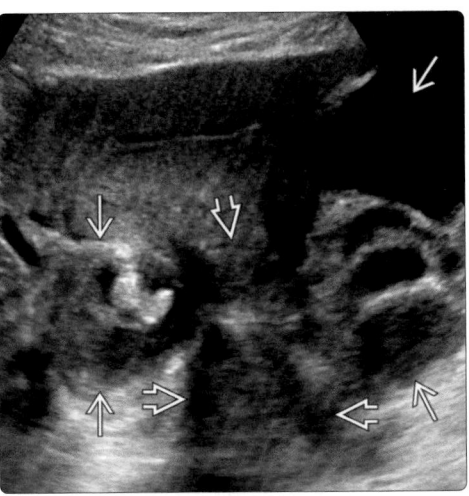

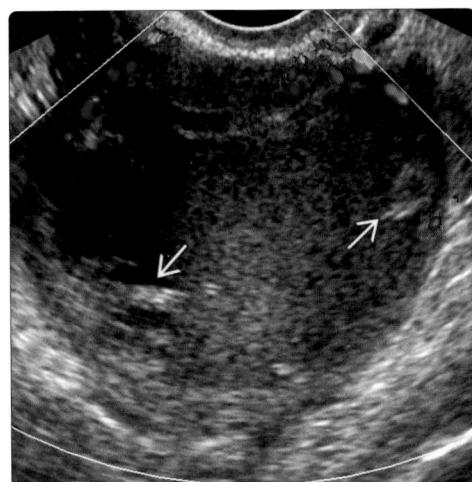

(Left) *Transverse transabdominal US shows bilateral endometriomas* ➡. *In the cul-de-sac, a spiculated mass* ➡ *representing deep invasive endometriosis pulls both ovaries together posterior to the uterus (so-called "kissing ovaries").* **(Right)** *Endovaginal US in a premenopausal woman demonstrates a thick-walled cystic mass with diffuse internal echoes. The irregular wall thickening is atypical* ➡ *and may be mistaken for malignancy; the lack of Doppler flow and clinical history are helpful features.*

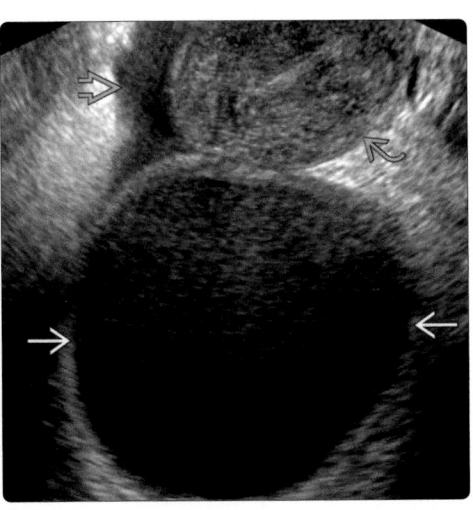

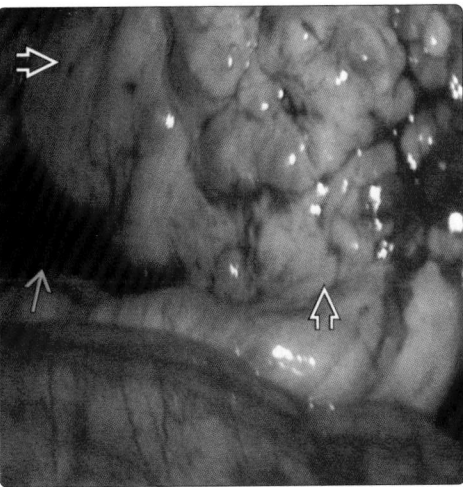

(Left) *Endovaginal US in a woman presenting with acute severe pelvic pain demonstrates a large adnexal complex cyst with homogeneous low-level internal echoes* ➡, *consistent with endometrioma. Complex free fluid* ➡ *is present adjacent to the uterus* ➡. **(Right)** *Caudal laparoscopic photo demonstrates the large adnexal mass* ➡ *seen on previous ultrasound. Note leaked old blood* ➡ *("chocolate fluid") into the peritoneal space. Pathologic findings confirmed ruptured endometrioma.*

Hydrosalpinx

TERMINOLOGY

- Fluid-filled dilatation of fallopian tubes resulting from tubal obstruction
- Must be distinguished from pyosalpinx or hematosalpinx based on tubal content and clinical picture

IMAGING

- Dilated tubular or oval structure separate from uterus and ovaries
- Cystic pelvic mass or complex fluid collection
- Convoluted or S-shaped, containing incomplete septa
- Waist sign: Indentation of opposing walls of dilated tubal structure resulting in appearance of a waist
- "Beads on a string" sign: Small hyperechoic mural nodules on transverse imaging
- "Cogwheel" sign: Thicker endosalpingeal folds in acute PID

TOP DIFFERENTIAL DIAGNOSES

- Pyosalpinx (acute PID)

- Tubo-ovarian complex
- Cystic ovarian neoplasm
- Paraovarian cyst
- Peritoneal inclusion cyst
- Dilated bowel

PATHOLOGY

- Tube obstruction from PID
- Also associated with endometriosis, appendicitis, or post pelvic surgery

CLINICAL ISSUES

- Usually asymptomatic
- Can present with pelvic or lower abdominal pain
- Can result in infertility

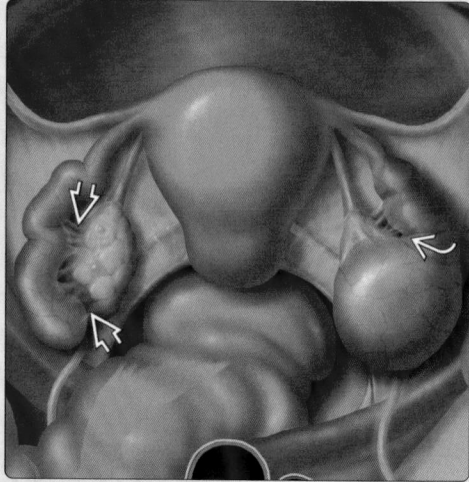
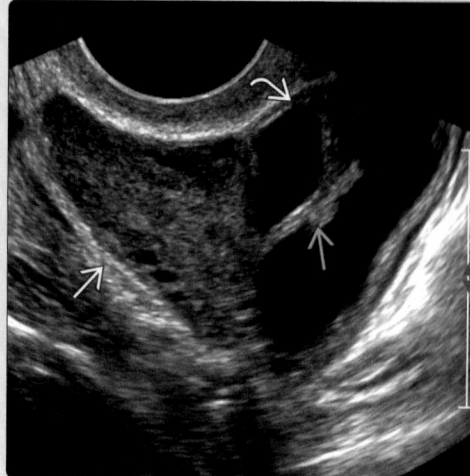

(Left) *Graphic shows bilateral hydrosalpinx. The left tube folds upon itself ⤼, which appears as an incomplete septum on ultrasound. Adhesions ⇒ and hydrosalpinx are sequelae of PID.* (Right) *Coronal transvaginal ultrasound shows a normal ovary ➡ with a dilated fallopian tube ⤼. The septa ⇨ are the walls of the folded tube.*

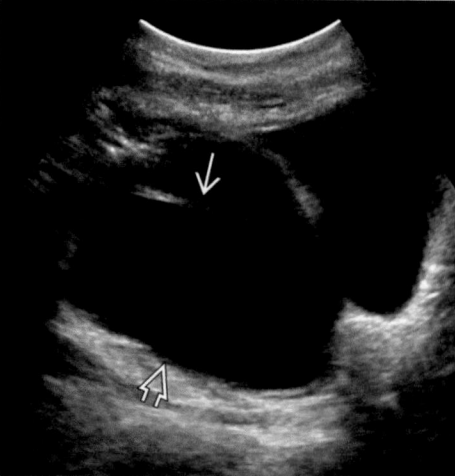
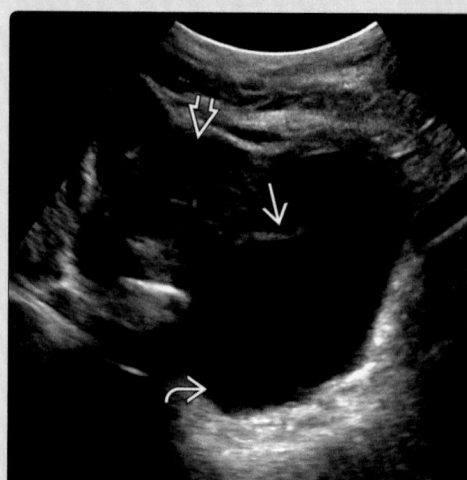

(Left) *Transabdominal longitudinal ultrasound shows a markedly dilated, thin-walled hydrosalpinx ⇨ with a thin incomplete septum ➡.* (Right) *Transverse transabdominal ultrasound of the same patient demonstrates the more dilated distal end of the tube ⤼. The uterus ⇨ was normal. The incomplete septum ➡ is better seen as a kink in the tube.*

TERMINOLOGY

Definitions

- Fluid-filled dilatation of fallopian tubes resulting from tubal obstruction
- Must be distinguished from pyosalpinx or hematosalpinx based on tubal content and clinical picture
- May /be isolated finding or bilateral or part of a complex adnexal pathologic process

IMAGING

General Features

- Best diagnostic clue
  - Dilated tubular structure in adnexa separate from uterus and ovaries containing incomplete septa, which are due to dilated tube folding upon itself
- Location
  - Adnexal but separate from ovary
- Morphology
  - Cystic pelvic mass or complex fluid collection
  - Oval
  - Pear shaped
  - Convoluted or S-shaped, dilated tubular structure
  - More dilated at fimbriated end
  - Content anechoic or may contain low-level echoes (debris)

Ultrasonographic Findings

- Thin-walled distended tube
  - Tube wall < 3 mm
  - Walls well defined and echogenic
  - Wall could be thicker in setting of chronic dilation (due to fibrotic changes)
- Waist sign: Indentation of opposing walls of dilated tubal structure, resulting in appearance of a waist
- Thin endosalpingeal folds
  - "Beads on a string" sign: Small hyperechoic mural nodules on transverse imaging
  - ~ 2-3 mm in size
  - Form due to flattened and fibrotic tubal folds as result of progressive (and chronic) dilation
  - Folds could also be flattened and effaced, resulting in smooth appearance of wall
    - Difficult to distinguish from other pelvic cystic masses
- Thicker endosalpingeal folds produce cogwheel sign in acute PID
  - Cogwheels represent thickened longitudinal folds of dilated tube
- Incomplete septa
  - Short linear echogenic projections into lumen from tubal kinking
- Fluid in tube and cul-de-sac is anechoic
  - Debris or echoes suggest PID
- Separate and distinguishable normal ovary and uterus
  - If extensive pelvic adhesions are present, dilated tube can be deformed and simulate other pelvic masses
- Doppler findings
  - High resistance flow in wall of hydrosalpinx
    - Resistive index (RI): ≥ 0.7
    - Higher resistance than acute PID

  - No flow in endosalpingeal folds
- Adnexal torsion is complication

Imaging Recommendations

- Best imaging tool
  - Transvaginal ultrasound
- Protocol advice
  - Look for intact separate ovary
  - Use high gain settings to look for echoes in fluid
  - Cine clips can be very helpful to confirm tortuous folded tube
  - 3D-rendered US can help see tortuous structure, which is difficult to follow with 2D imaging
- Inconclusive findings can be better assessed with MR
- Hysterosalpingogram (HSG) is mainstay of tubal patency evaluation

MR Findings

- If ultrasound findings are atypical, incompletely evaluated or another associated adnexal mass is seen, proceed to MR
  - T1WI
    - Tubular dilated structure separate from ovaries and uterus
    - Tube content has low SI if simple fluid
    - Proteinaceous or hemorrhagic fluid is intermediate to high signal intensity depending on content of tube
    - High SI is correlated to pelvic and tubal endometriosis
  - T2WI
    - Tube content is high SI
    - Incomplete septa are of low SI
    - T2* helpful in identifying hemorrhagic content
    - Heavily T2 FSE (long effective echo time of 250-350 msec) result in significantly hyperintense simple fluid, while layering debris or clot will appear low SI within fluid content
  - T1WI with contrast material
    - Mild enhancement of tubal wall and septa, which could also be thickened
    - Significant enhancement suggestive of active inflammatory process
- MR hysterosalpingography has been reported in literature
  - Diluted contrast agent instilled into uterine cavity via a cannula followed by multiplanar imaging

Fluoroscopic Findings

- HSG
- Dilated fallopian tube without spillage of contrast material into peritoneal cavity from fimbriated end
- Can be bilateral

DIFFERENTIAL DIAGNOSIS

Pyosalpinx (Acute PID)

- Tube distended with echogenic material
- Tube wall > 5 mm and thick endosalpingeal folds
  - Hypervascular on Doppler imaging
- Low resistive flow in walls and folds (RI ≤ 0.5)
- Patient is symptomatic with tenderness during transvaginal exam
- May be accompanied with adnexal inflammatory changes, ovarian enlargement, endometritis, and parovarian fluid collections

Tubo-Ovarian Complex

- More severe manifestation of PID
- Pyosalpinx adherent to ovary

Paraovarian Cyst

- Unilocular anechoic broad ligament cyst
- More round than hydrosalpinx and thin walled

Ectopic Tubal Pregnancy

- Echogenic ring in adnexa with ↑ flow
- Cul-de-sac fluid contains echoes if bleeding/rupture

Cystic Ovarian Neoplasm

- Usually not tubular; associated with ovary
  - Exception: High-grade serous ovarian carcinomas now believed to arise from distal tube
- May have papillary projections of variable sizes and locations
- May have multiple septations of various locations and thickness
- May have variable degree of internal debris and echogenic fluid and ovarian enlargement

Dilated Bowel

- Distinct bowel wall layers with peristalsis seen during imaging

Peritoneal Inclusion Cyst

- Pseudocyst formed by entrapped peritoneal fluid by peritoneal adhesions without true walls
- Ovary is entrapped by cystic structure, which may be surrounded by complete septations

Acute Appendicitis

- Thicker wall with gut signature
- Appendicolith, surrounding echogenic fat
- Traced to cecum

PATHOLOGY

General Features

- Etiology
  - Tube obstruction from PID
  - Usually at ampullary or infundibular segments due to adhesions
  - Most common pathogens: *Chlamydia trachomatis, Neisseria gonorrhoeae*
  - Also associated with endometriosis, appendicitis, or post pelvic surgery
- Associated abnormalities
  - Infertility
  - Ectopic pregnancy
  - Endometriosis and chronic pelvic pain

Microscopic Features

- Chronic salpingitis
- Fibrotic thickened endosalpingeal folds, small lumen

CLINICAL ISSUES

Presentation

- Most common signs/symptoms
  - Commonly asymptomatic

  - Can present with lower abdominal or pelvic pain
- Other signs/symptoms
  - Acute pain if adnexal torsion
    - Isolated tubal torsion is rare
  - Can be discovered during work-up for infertility

Demographics

- Age
  - Any age

Treatment

- None necessary if asymptomatic
- For those with infertility, recommended treatment by American Society for Reproductive Medicine is salpingectomy or proximal tubal occlusion

DIAGNOSTIC CHECKLIST

Image Interpretation Pearls

- Tubular fluid-filled structure with incomplete septa and mural nodules separate from uterus and ovaries
- Look for signs of acute PID

SELECTED REFERENCES

1. Kaproth-Joslin K et al: Imaging of female infertility: a pictorial guide to the hysterosalpingography, ultrasonography, and magnetic resonance imaging findings of the congenital and acquired causes of female infertility. Radiol Clin North Am. 51(6):967-81, 2013
2. Matorras R et al: Hysteroscopic hydrosalpinx occlusion with Essure device in IVF patients when salpingectomy or laparoscopy is contraindicated. Eur J Obstet Gynecol Reprod Biol. 169(1):54-9, 2013
3. Ma L et al: Fallopian tubal patency diagnosed by magnetic resonance hysterosalpingography. J Reprod Med. 57(9-10):435-40, 2012
4. Rezvani M et al: Fallopian tube disease in the nonpregnant patient. Radiographics. 31(2):527-48, 2011
5. Carrascosa PM et al: Virtual hysterosalpingography: a new multidetector CT technique for evaluating the female reproductive system. Radiographics. 30(3):643-61, 2010
6. Moyle PL et al: Nonovarian cystic lesions of the pelvis. Radiographics. 30(4):921-38, 2010
7. Timor-Tritsch IE et al: Three-dimensional ultrasound inversion rendering technique facilitates the diagnosis of hydrosalpinx. J Clin Ultrasound. 38(7):372-6, 2010
8. Kim MY et al: MR Imaging findings of hydrosalpinx: a comprehensive review. Radiographics. 29(2):495-507, 2009
9. Potter AW et al: US and CT evaluation of acute pelvic pain of gynecologic origin in nonpregnant premenopausal patients. Radiographics. 28(6):1645-59, 2008
10. Bontis JN et al: Laparoscopic management of hydrosalpinx. Ann N Y Acad Sci. 1092:199-210, 2006
11. Patel MD et al: Likelihood ratio of sonographic findings in discriminating hydrosalpinx from other adnexal masses. AJR. 186:1033-8, 2006
12. Simpson WL Jr et al: Hysterosalpingography: a reemerging study. Radiographics. 26(2):419-31, 2006
13. Benjaminov O et al: Sonography of the abnormal fallopian tube. AJR Am J Roentgenol. 183(3):737-42, 2004
14. Dohke M et al: Comprehensive MR imaging of acute gynecologic diseases. Radiographics. 20:1551-66, 2000

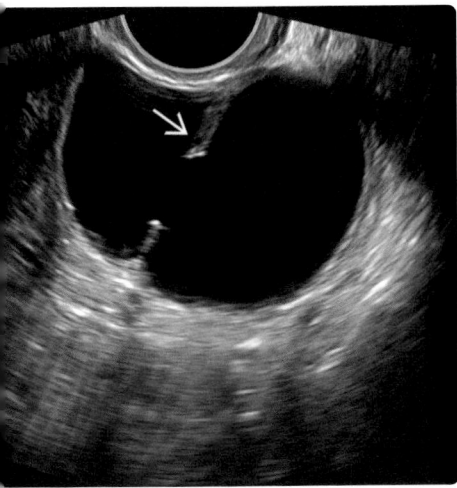
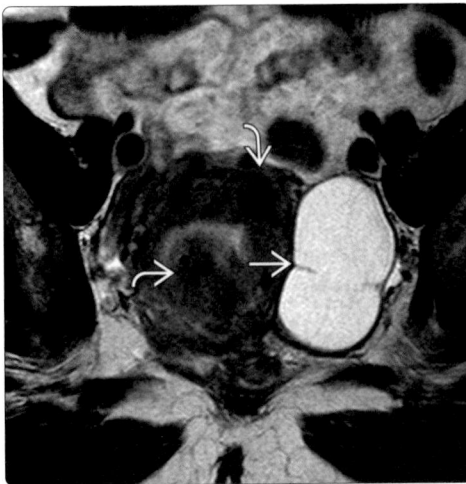

(Left) *Longitudinal transvaginal ultrasound shows an elongated, thin-walled, fluid-filled structure with an incomplete septum ➡. This was unchanged on follow-up examination and asymptomatic.* (Right) *Axial oblique T2 TSE MR confirms the tubular shape, internal fluid content, and incomplete septum ➡. Fibroids ➡ were also present.*

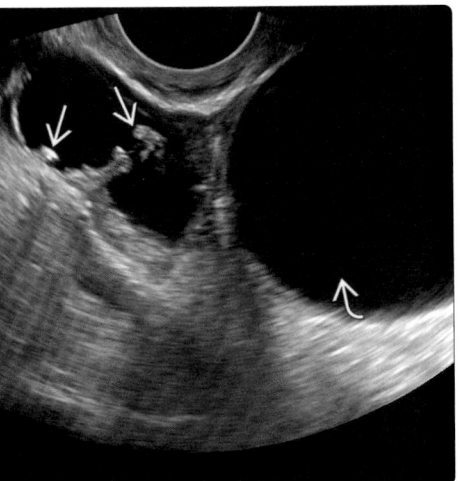
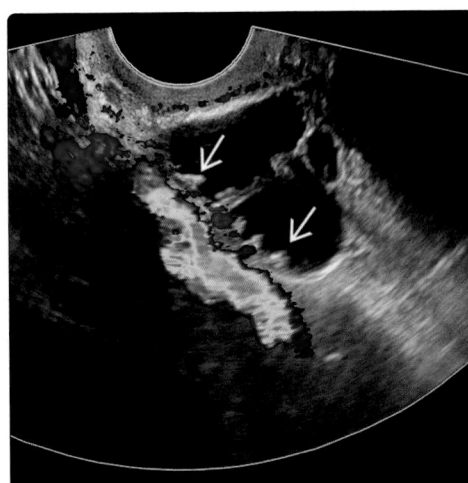

(Left) *Longitudinal transvaginal ultrasound shows a dilated, thin-walled fallopian tube with mural nodules (beads on a string) ➡. The distal end of the hydrosalpinx was much larger ➡.* (Right) *Coronal transvaginal color Doppler ultrasound shows no increased vascularity in the wall of the hydrosalpinx or in the nodules ➡ in this chronic hydrosalpinx.*

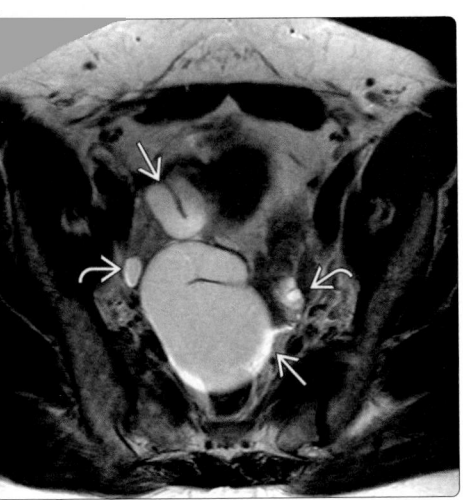
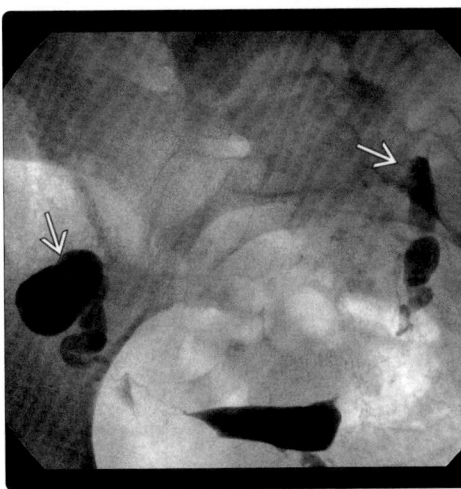

(Left) *Axial T2 TSE performed for staging cervical carcinoma shows bilateral asymptomatic hydrosalpinges ➡, the left greater than the right. The ovaries ➡ were seen separately.* (Right) *Hysterosalpingogram performed for infertility shows blunted fimbrial ends ➡ of the dilated fallopian tubes with no free spill, indicating bilateral tubal occlusion.*

Tubo-Ovarian Abscess

TERMINOLOGY

- Pelvic inflammatory disease (PID), tubo-ovarian abscess (TOA), tubo-ovarian complex (TOC)

IMAGING

- Transvaginal ultrasound is first-line modality
  - Early disease may be subtle
  - Distended serpiginous, ovoid or pear-shaped tube
  - Thickened tube walls, often > 5 mm
  - Thickened endosalpingeal folds: Cogwheel sign in cross section
  - Incomplete septa: Distended tube folding on itself
  - Tubo-ovarian abscess
  - Enlarged edematous ovary
  - Complex pelvic fluid collection
- CT useful for diffuse nonspecific symptoms, large abscesses, extensive infection
- MR helpful if other modalities are equivocal

TOP DIFFERENTIAL DIAGNOSES

- Endometrioma ± rupture
- Hemorrhagic cyst ± rupture
- Paraovarian cyst
- Appendicitis

PATHOLOGY

- Ascending infection damages endocervical canal and its mucus barrier, ascends into upper genital tract, involves tube and ovary
- Advanced disease results in abscess collections

CLINICAL ISSUES

- Associated with STD
  - Usually present with pain, fever, vaginal discharge
- Can result in tubal scarring
  - Infertility, ectopic pregnancy, chronic pelvic pain

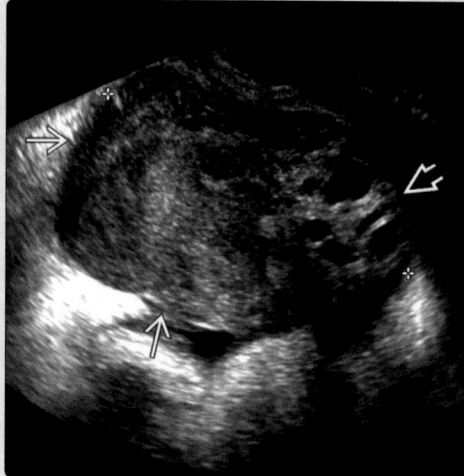
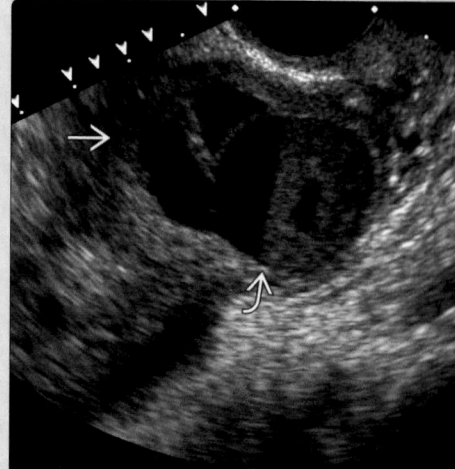

(Left) Longitudinal ultrasound of a left tubo-ovarian complex is shown. There is complex fluid in the abscess ➡, which is distinct from the ovary ➡. (Right) Coronal transvaginal ultrasound shows a tubo-ovarian abscess ➡ with a pus level ➡.

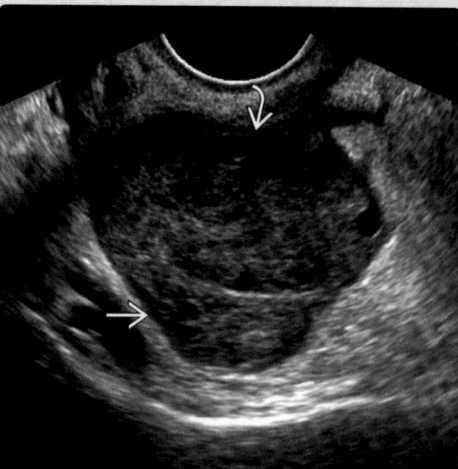
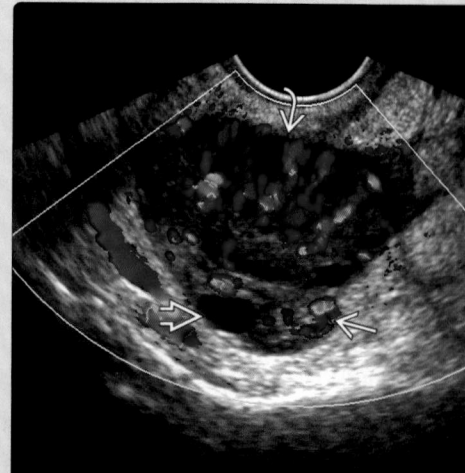

(Left) Coronal transvaginal ultrasound of the right ovary ➡ and thickened tender fallopian tube ➡ secondary to acute salpingitis is shown. (Right) Coronal transvaginal color Doppler ultrasound of the same patient shows increased color flow in the right salpingitis ➡. Fluid was seen in the tube ➡. The ovary ➡ was hyperemic.

TERMINOLOGY

Definitions

Pelvic inflammatory disease (PID)
- Spectrum of disease including endometritis, salpingitis, tubo-ovarian abscess, and oophoritis
- Usually sexually transmitted disease involving organism such as *Chlamydia trachomatis* or *Neisseria gonorrhoeae* but can also be polymicrobial
- Can occur from extension of inflammation from adjacent organs such as appendicitis, diverticulitis, and colitis

Pyosalpinx
- Tube distended with pus

Tubo-ovarian complex (TOC)
- Abscess adherent to tube
- Distinguishable separate ovary

Tubo-ovarian abscess (TOA)
- Abscess involving tube and ovary
- Separate ovary no longer distinguishable

IMAGING

General Features

Best diagnostic clue
- Pyosalpinx: Tubular fluid-filled structure with incomplete septa
- TOA: Painful complex cystic adnexal mass

Location
- TOA often bilateral, infection spreads from 1 side to other, often in posterior cul-de-sac
- Early PID is unilateral

Ultrasonographic Findings

- Thickened dilated fallopian tubes
  - Distal obstruction causes distention
    - Distended serpiginous, ovoid or pear-shaped tube
  - Complex fluid
    - Layering debris common ± gas
  - Thickened tube walls, often > 5 mm
  - Thickened endosalpingeal folds: Cogwheel sign in cross section
  - Incomplete septa: Distended tube folding on itself
- Inflammation of ovaries
  - Enlarged edematous ovary
    - Separate from tube but may be adherent to tube in later stage
    - ↑ number and size of follicles
  - Tubo-ovarian abscess
    - Complex adnexal mass, ovary not recognizable
    - May still see components of pyosalpinx
- Complex pelvic fluid collection
  - Can be seen early
  - Can form pelvic abscess
- Doppler ultrasound findings
  - Increased color Doppler flow of walls and folds of tube or ovary
  - Pulsed Doppler: Low-resistive flow
- Sonographic findings resolve quickly with treatment
  - Pyosalpinx → hydrosalpinx → ± resolution
  - Complex pelvic fluid resolution

CT Findings

- CT often ordered 1st with generalized or vague lower abdominal pain
  - Early findings subtle
    - Mild pelvic edema resulting in thickening of uterosacral ligament
    - Haziness of pelvic fat, obscured pelvic fascial planes
  - Inflammation/thickening of tube due to mild salpingitis
  - Enlarged abnormally enhancing ovaries due to oophoritis
  - Endometritis: Fluid in uterine cavity with abnormal uterine enhancement
- More advanced disease: Inflammatory changes seen better
  - Difficult to differentiate between pyosalpinx, TOC, and TOA
  - TOA and pelvic abscess
    - Thick-walled complex fluid collection
- Involvement of adjacent structures
  - Ureteral obstruction
  - Secondary inflammation of other organs
- Fitz-Hugh-Curtis syndrome
  - Peritoneal spread of infection to perihepatic surfaces and right lobe of liver
    - Pouch of Douglas → paracolic gutter → peritoneum
    - Right upper quadrant pain presentation
    - Hepatic capsular enhancement
    - Transient hepatic attenuation difference on anterior hepatic surface
    - Hepatic capsular retraction and adhesions
- Complicated ascites

Imaging Recommendations

- Best imaging tool
  - Transvaginal ultrasound
  - Transabdominal ultrasound of pelvis for large/extensive abscesses
- Protocol advice
  - Acute PID has subtle, nonspecific findings
  - Use probe pressure to diagnose tubo-ovarian complex
    - Do ovary and tube move together or apart?
    - Increase gain settings to see echoes of complex fluid collection in pelvis
  - Evaluate abdomen with US when pelvic findings are extensive
    - Consider CT to evaluate full extent of abnormalities or for complex disease
    - Complex fluid may ascend: Evaluate perihepatic region
    - Look for hydronephrosis

MR Findings

- T1WI
  - ± fat suppression useful for differentiation of blood/pus from simple fluid
    - Addition of contrast helps distinguish collections, inflammation, pyosalpinx
- T2WI
  - High signal fluid in dilated tubes and abscesses
  - Improved conspicuity of inflammation and free fluid
  - Pyosalpinx: Fluid-filled, dilated tortuous tubular structure
  - Abscess: Thick-walled complex cystic mass in the adnexa

- Wall and adjacent structures have increased enhancement
- May contain gas, best seen on T2*

DIFFERENTIAL DIAGNOSIS

Endometrioma ± Rupture

- Lack signs of infection, different clinical picture
- Multiple and bilateral lesions common
- Often ovarian
  - ± tube involvement, ± other pelvic organ involvement
- Round masses more often than tubular
  - Diffuse low-level echoes
  - Thick wall and nodularity common
  - May have fluid-fluid levels

Hemorrhagic Ovarian Cyst ± Rupture

- Usually single thin-walled cystic structure in ovary, separate from tube
  - Internal debris or classic reticular echoes, which may also be seen in pelvis if ruptured
  - Color Doppler: Halo of increased vascularity

Paraovarian Cyst

- Unilocular anechoic cyst, no endosalpingeal folds
- Thin wall, adjacent to but separate from ovary

Appendicitis

- Inflamed blind-ending tubular structure in right lower quadrant
  - If ruptured can see adjacent collections

PATHOLOGY

General Features

- Etiology
  - Infectious organism damages endocervical canal and its mucus barrier and ascends into upper genital tract
    - Coinfection with other organisms such as *Escherichia coli*, *Haemophilus influenza*, and *Streptococcus* are common
    - Extension of cervical columnar epithelium beyond cervix, and cervical mucosal changes in mid-cycle and during menstruation, increases risk of ascending infection
- Associated abnormalities
  - Salpingitis can progress to hydrosalpinx or pyosalpinx if left untreated; late sequela is tubo-ovarian abscess

CLINICAL ISSUES

Presentation

- Most common signs/symptoms
  - Pelvic pain and cervical motion tenderness
  - Fever, vaginal discharge
- Other signs/symptoms
  - Elevated WBC, ESR, or CRP
  - Right upper quadrant pain rare
    - Fitz-Hugh-Curtis syndrome
- Clinical profile
  - Risk factors are similar to those for STDs and include exposure to STD, multiple sexual partners, use of illicit drugs or smoking, and young age

Demographics

- Age
  - Women < 25 years at ↑ risk

Natural History & Prognosis

- Sequelae of fallopian tube scarring
  - Tubal infertility
  - Ectopic pregnancy
  - Salpingitis isthmica nodosa
    - Diverticula of fallopian tube, mostly at isthmus
- Chronic pelvic pain

Treatment

- Prompt antibiotic therapy
- Goal of treatment is to cure acute state of infection with short-term antibiotics as well as prevent long-term sequelae
- If adequate clinical response to outpatient antibiotic treatment is not achieved, patients may require parenteral antibiotics, additional diagnostic and laboratory testing, and possibly surgical intervention
- TOA may require drainage/surgery
- Presence of IUD does not alter treatment, and empirical removal is not indicated

DIAGNOSTIC CHECKLIST

Image Interpretation Pearls

- Acute PID may have subtle findings
  - Pain will be disproportionate to findings
  - Look for mild inflammatory change
  - Look in posterior cul-de-sac for pus
- TOA: Nonspecific complex cystic adnexal mass
  - Use color Doppler to show increased flow
- Abdominal ultrasound or CT important to assess extent of disease

SELECTED REFERENCES

1. Romosan G et al: The sensitivity and specificity of transvaginal ultrasound with regard to acute pelvic inflammatory disease: a review of the literature. Arch Gynecol Obstet. 289(4):705-14, 2014
2. Kaproth-Joslin K et al: Imaging of female infertility: a pictorial guide to the hysterosalpingography, ultrasonography, and magnetic resonance imaging findings of the congenital and acquired causes of female infertility. Radiol Clin North Am. 51(6):967-81, 2013
3. Romosan G et al: Ultrasound for diagnosing acute salpingitis: a prospective observational diagnostic study. Hum Reprod. 28(6):1569-79, 2013
4. Chappell CA et al: Pathogenesis, diagnosis, and management of severe pelvic inflammatory disease and tuboovarian abscess. Clin Obstet Gynecol. 55(4):893-903, 2012
5. Rezvani M et al: Fallopian tube disease in the nonpregnant patient. Radiographics. 31(2):527-48, 2011
6. Moyle PL et al: Nonovarian cystic lesions of the pelvis. Radiographics. 30(4):921-38, 2010
7. Kim JY et al: Perihepatitis with pelvic inflammatory disease (PID) on MDCT: characteristic findings and relevance to PID. Abdom Imaging. 34(6):737-42, 2009
8. Potter AW et al: US and CT evaluation of acute pelvic pain of gynecologic origin in nonpregnant premenopausal patients. Radiographics. 28(6):1645-59, 2008
9. Horrow MM: Ultrasound of pelvic inflammatory disease. Ultrasound Q. 20(4):171-9, 2004
10. Sexually Transmitted Diseases Treatment Guidelines, 2015

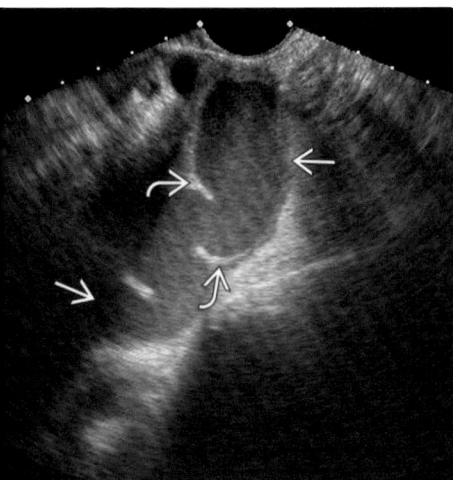

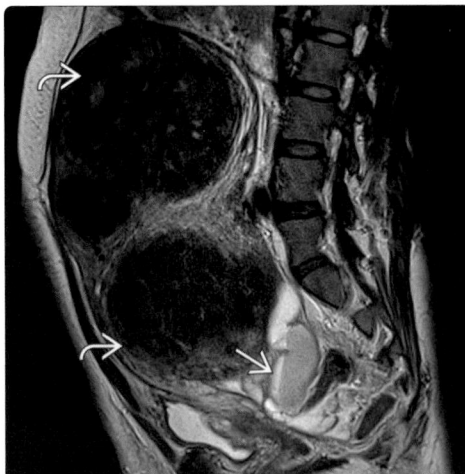

(Left) *Longitudinal transvaginal ultrasound shows a dilated tender fallopian tube* ➡ *containing low-level echoes and incomplete septa* ➡ *representing a pyosalpinx.* (Right) *Sagittal T2 TSE MR of the same patient shows a debris level in the pyosalpinx* ➡. *Numerous large fibroids* ➡ *were difficult to assess with ultrasound.*

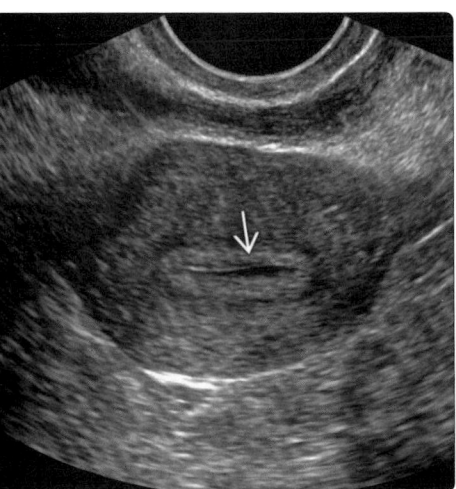

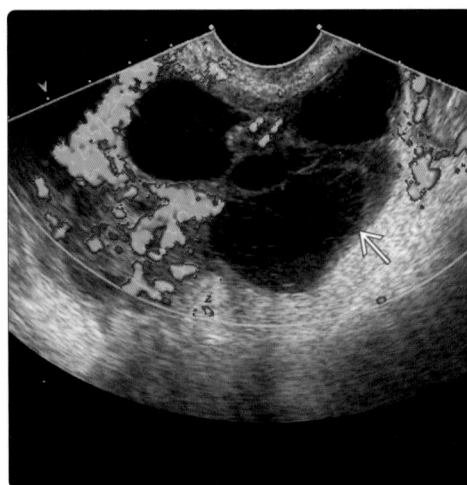

(Left) *Coronal transvaginal ultrasound of the uterus in a patient with pelvic inflammatory disease (PID) shows endometrial fluid* ➡ *indicating endometritis.* (Right) *Coronal transvaginal color Doppler ultrasound shows a multiloculated tubo-ovarian abscess with debris* ➡ *and surrounding hyperemia.*

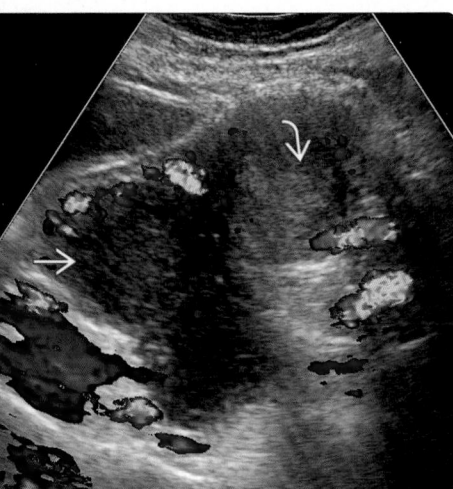

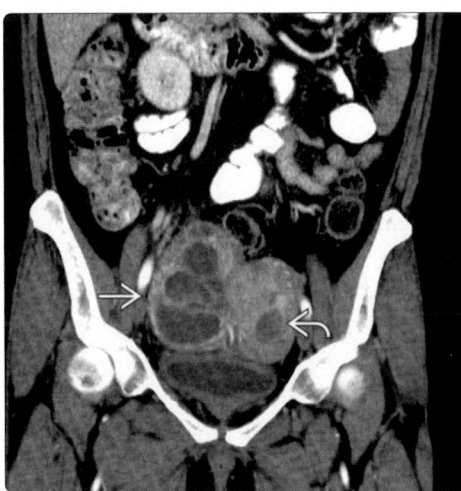

(Left) *Transverse transabdominal color Doppler ultrasound of the pelvis shows a right tubo-ovarian abscess (TOA) after dilatation and curettage. The abscess* ➡ *has no central color flow. The endometrium was thick* ➡. (Right) *Coronal CECT of the same patient shows the extent of the TOA* ➡. *Low density endometrium is noted* ➡.

Parovarian Cyst

TERMINOLOGY

- Cyst originating from wolffian duct in mesosalpinx or broad ligament

IMAGING

- Transvaginal ultrasound is study of choice
  - Round or oval cystic structure separate from ovary
  - Thin outer wall (< 3 mm)
  - Often unilateral
  - Lack of follicles distinguishes from ovary
  - Usually does not indent the ovary
  - Mean diameter: 40 mm (range: 15-120 mm)
  - Fluid is anechoic in 91%
  - May contain septa that are thin, smooth, complete
  - Rarely may be complicated by torsion or hemorrhage
- MR
  - Hypointense on T1WI and hyperintense on T2WI
  - If complicated by torsion or hemorrhage, hyperintense on T1WI with thick walls

- If soft tissue component, consider neoplasm

TOP DIFFERENTIAL DIAGNOSES

- Peritoneal inclusion cyst (PIC)
- Hydrosalpinx
- True ovarian cyst

PATHOLOGY

- Benign serous cyst in 98%
- Malignant features in 2%

CLINICAL ISSUES

- Asymptomatic in most women

DIAGNOSTIC CHECKLIST

- MR superior for identification of normal ovary when origin of large lesion cannot be determined with ultrasound

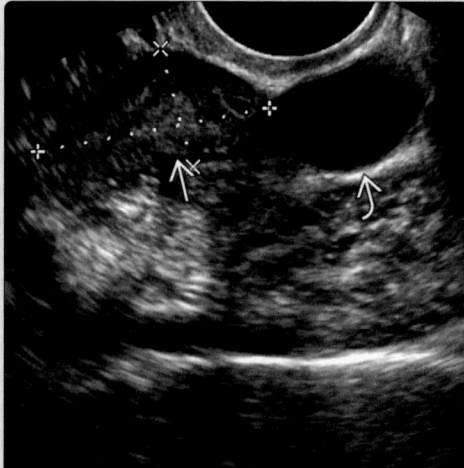
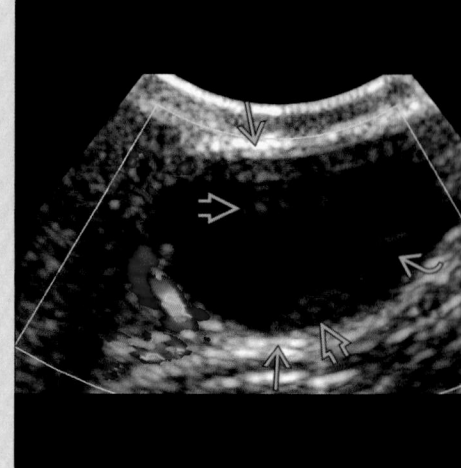

(Left) Longitudinal transvaginal ultrasound shows the right ovary ➡ with an adjacent paraovarian cyst ➡. On real-time scanning, they were separable with probe pressure. (Right) Longitudinal color Doppler ultrasound of the same paraovarian cyst ➡ now shows mural nodules ➡ and debris ➡ related to recent hemorrhage.

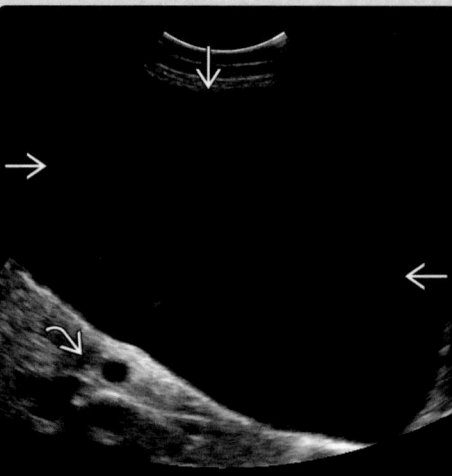
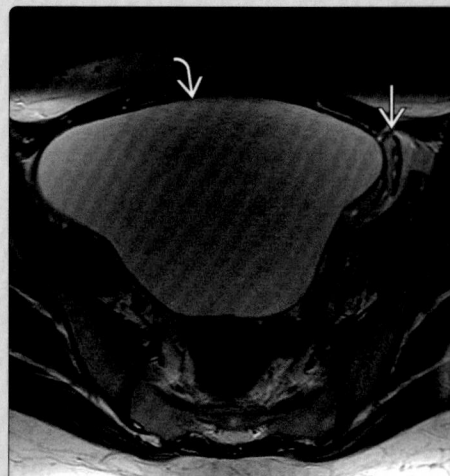

(Left) Transverse transabdominal ultrasound shows a large simple cyst ➡ arising out of the pelvis. The origin could not be determined. The normal aorta and vena cava ➡ are seen. (Right) Axial T2 TSE of the large cystic mass in the pelvis shows that the left ovary ➡ is normal and separate from the very large paraovarian cyst ➡. The right ovary was also seen to be separate and normal (not shown).

TERMINOLOGY

Abbreviations

Paratubal cyst

Definitions

Cyst originating from wolffian duct in mesosalpinx or broad ligament

IMAGING

General Features

Best diagnostic clue
- Unilocular cyst near but separate from ovary
  - Often unilateral

Size
- Mean diameter: 40 mm (range: 15-120 mm)

Morphology
- Well-defined, round or oval cystic mass
  - Rarely may be complicated by torsion or hemorrhage

Ultrasonographic Findings

Adnexal cyst medial to ovary
- Lack of follicles distinguishes from ovary
- Separate from ovary
- Usually does not indent ovary

Unilocular in 95%

Multilocular in 5%
- May contain septa that are thin, smooth, complete
- May represent multiple cysts on same side

Fluid is anechoic in 91%

Small, floating echoes (probably hemorrhage) in 9%

Thin outer wall (< 3 mm)
- Some with 2-5 mm papillae

Imaging Recommendations

Best imaging tool
- Transvaginal ultrasound

Protocol advice
- Study any adnexal mass from border to border
  - Decide ovarian vs. extraovarian
    - Evaluate cyst characteristics
- Study cyst mobility with vaginal probe
  - "Split" sign or "pelvic slide test" (cyst moves separate from ovary)

CT Findings

- Round or oval cystic structure, close but separate from ovary

MR Findings

- Round or oval cystic structure, close but separate from ovary
- Hypointense on T1WI and hyperintense on T2WI
  - If complicated by torsion or hemorrhage, may be hyperintense on T1WI and have thick walls
  - If soft tissue component, consider neoplasm

DIFFERENTIAL DIAGNOSIS

Peritoneal Inclusion Cyst (PIC)

Loculated, peritoneal fluid producing unilocular or multilocular cystic mass

- May be ovoid or irregular in contour
- May contain internal echoes or septa
- No perceptible walls
- Surrounds normal ovary

Hydrosalpinx

- Tubular morphology with separate ovary
- Hyperechoic mural nodules common

True Ovarian Cyst

- Unilocular or complex
- Look for ovarian tissue at cyst borders
  - Inseparable from ovary

PATHOLOGY

Gross Pathologic & Surgical Features

- 98% benign serous cyst
- 2% with malignant features
  - Cystadenoma or cystadenocarcinoma

CLINICAL ISSUES

Presentation

- Most common signs/symptoms
  - Asymptomatic
    - Found at time of imaging of pelvis for other reasons
  - Adnexal mass
- Other signs/symptoms
  - Torsion, growth, and malignancy are rare complications

Demographics

- Epidemiology
  - 10-20% of all adnexal masses
    - Most common in 3rd and 4th decade

Treatment

- Surgery avoided if cyst < 5 cm and no papillae

DIAGNOSTIC CHECKLIST

Consider

- Often misdiagnosed as true ovarian cyst

Image Interpretation Pearls

- Do not assume every cystic adnexal mass is ovarian
- Correct diagnosis important to avoid surgery
- MR superior for identification of normal ovary when origin of large lesion cannot be determined with ultrasound

SELECTED REFERENCES

1. Suzuki S et al: Two cases of paraovarian tumor of borderline malignancy. J Obstet Gynaecol Res. 39(1):437-41, 2013
2. Damle LF et al: Giant paraovarian cysts in young adolescents: a report of three cases. J Reprod Med. 57(1-2):65-7, 2012
3. Kiseli M et al: Clinical diagnosis and complications of paratubal cysts: review of the literature and report of uncommon presentations. Arch Gynecol Obstet. 285(6):1563-9, 2012
4. Laing FC et al: US of the ovary and adnexa: to worry or not to worry? Radiographics. 32(6):1621-39; discussion 1640-2, 2012
5. Patel MD: Pitfalls in the sonographic evaluation of adnexal masses. Ultrasound Q. 28(1):29-40, 2012
6. Moyle PL et al: Nonovarian cystic lesions of the pelvis. Radiographics. 30(4):921-38, 2010

Peritoneal Inclusion Cyst

TERMINOLOGY

- Synonyms: Peritoneal pseudocyst, benign cystic mesothelioma
- Not true cyst but peritoneal or ovarian fluid trapped by peritoneal adhesions

IMAGING

- Unilocular or multilocular pelvic cystic lesion
- Boundaries defined by pelvic structures
- Unilateral 65%, bilateral 35%, midline if large
- Normal ovary surrounded or displaced by fluid and septations
- Entrapped ovary: "Spider in web" appearance
- Fine septations most common
- Thick septations with nodules possible
- Blood flow can be seen in septations, especially if thick
- Transvaginal ultrasound first-line to localize ovary and exclude signs of malignancy

- MR most useful if peritoneal inclusion cyst (PIC) is large and normal ovaries cannot be found using ultrasound
- CT useful for large PIC and for excluding malignant peritoneal disease but less sensitive at locating ovaries

TOP DIFFERENTIAL DIAGNOSES

- Ovarian cystic neoplasm
- Hydrosalpinx
- Paraovarian cyst
- Endometriosis

PATHOLOGY

- PIC development requires functioning ovary and peritoneal adhesions

CLINICAL ISSUES

- Almost exclusively premenopausal women
- Pelvic pain, palpable mass, abdominal distension
- Tend to recur after drainage

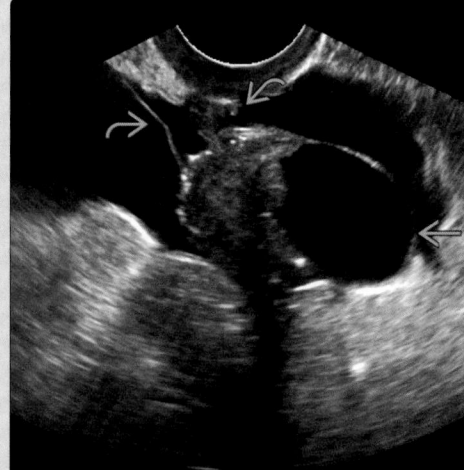
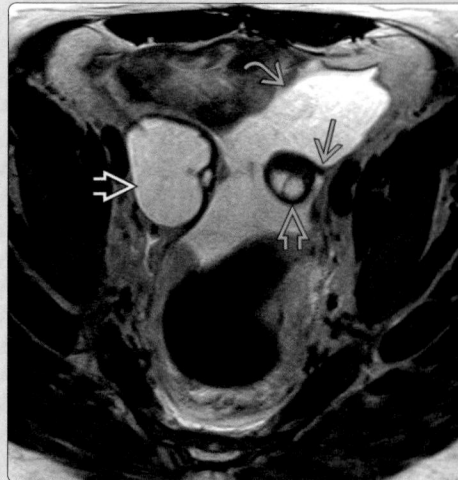

(Left) Coronal transvaginal ultrasound of the left ovary shows a dominant follicle ➡. The ovary is surrounded by simple fluid with thin septa ➡. (Right) Axial T2 TSE MR of the same patient at a later time shows the fluid conforming to the peritoneal cavity ➡. A thin adhesion is present ➡. The left ovarian follicle ➡ is smaller; the right ovary has developed a larger cyst ➡.

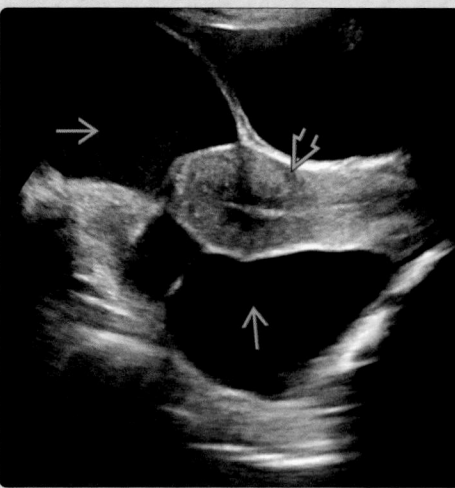
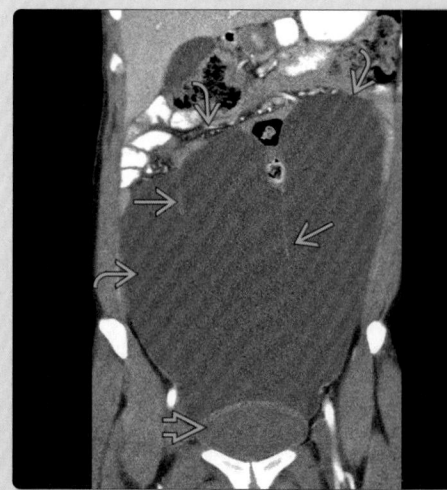

(Left) Sagittal transabdominal ultrasound shows a peritoneal inclusion cyst ➡ superior and posterior to the uterus ➡. Internal echoes were found to be from hemorrhage at surgery. (Right) Coronal CECT of the same patient shows the extent of the huge peritoneal inclusion cyst ➡, displacing bowel. Thin septa ➡ are present. The bladder was normal ➡.

Peritoneal Inclusion Cyst

TERMINOLOGY

Abbreviations
- Peritoneal inclusion cyst (PIC)

Synonyms
- Peritoneal pseudocyst
- Benign cystic mesothelioma
- Inflammatory cysts of pelvic peritoneum
- Benign encysted fluid
- Multilocular inclusion cyst

Definitions
- Not true ovarian cyst
- Peritoneal or ovarian fluid trapped by peritoneal adhesions

IMAGING

General Features
- Best diagnostic clue
  - Normal ovary surrounded or displaced by fluid containing septations
- Location
  - Adnexal
    - Unilateral 65%
    - Bilateral 35%
  - Midline if large
- Size
  - Variable
- Morphology
  - Lacks true wall
  - Boundaries defined by pelvic structures
  - Displaces structures without invasion

Ultrasonographic Findings
- Grayscale ultrasound
  - Irregular cystic lesion: Unilocular or multilocular
  - Soft and deformable
  - Lacks mass effect
    - Passive lesion conforming to shape of pelvis
      - Lateral border from pelvic sidewall
  - Anechoic content
    - Echoes with hemorrhage or proteinaceous debris
  - Variable number and thickness of septa (in 81%)
    - Fine septations most common
      - Mobile with transducer pressure
      - "Flapping sail" sign
    - Thick septations with nodules possible
  - Intact ovary present
    - Entrapped ovary
      - Ovary surrounded by fluid and septations
      - "Spider in web" appearance
    - Displaced ovary
      - External/adjacent to PIC
      - Along pelvic sidewall
      - Stuck to pelvic organ
    - Distorted ovary
      - May lose normal contour
      - Pulled by adhesions but intact
- Color Doppler
  - Blood flow can be seen in septations, especially if thick

CT Findings
- Multiseptated pelvic fluid collection
- Mass respects pelvic structure boundaries
  - Pelvic sidewall as lateral boundaries
  - Bladder, bowel, uterus, fallopian tubes serve as boundaries
- Thin septations not seen by CT
  - Mass appears unilocular
- Thicker septations resolved by CT
  - May enhance
- Associated ovary often not seen
- Useful for large PIC and for excluding malignant peritoneal disease

MR Findings
- Simple fluid characteristics
  - Low signal on T1
  - High signal on T2
- Blood products sometimes present
  - High signal on T1
- Enhancement helps define borders and septa
  - Walls of PIC formed by surrounding structures
    - Pelvic walls, pelvic organs, bowel loops
  - No true cyst wall
- MR may help find intact ovary if not seen by ultrasound

Nonvascular Interventions
- Therapeutic or diagnostic aspiration using transabdominal or transvaginal approach

Imaging Recommendations
- Best imaging tool
  - Transvaginal ultrasound first-line to localize ovary and exclude signs of malignancy
  - MR most useful if PIC is large and normal ovaries cannot be found using ultrasound
  - CT may be suggestive but less sensitive at locating ovaries
- Protocol advice
  - Suspect diagnosis in right clinical setting
    - Premenopausal patient with history of multiple pelvic surgeries
  - Look for otherwise normal ovary surrounded by septated fluid collection
    - May be displaced to periphery of mass
    - Consider MR to find ovary
  - Use transvaginal probe to displace pelvic structures
    - PIC is not invasive
  - Exclude solid components to differentiate from cancer

DIFFERENTIAL DIAGNOSIS

Ovarian Cystic Neoplasm
- Cystadenoma/cystadenocarcinoma
- Separate normal ovary not seen
- Unilocular or multilocular
- Papillary projections, solid nodules
- Thicker or irregular septa
- ± ascites, ± calcification
- Mass effect on adjacent structures

Hydrosalpinx

- Serpiginous morphology
  - May look multiloculated in short axis
- Look for mural nodules or cogwheel
- Adjacent normal ovary
- Bilateral common

Paraovarian Cyst

- Unilocular adnexal cyst
  - Anechoic with no septations
  - Well-defined cyst wall
- Rarely multiple
- Does not resolve with time
- Separate from ovary

Endometriosis

- Endometrioma has diffuse internal low-level echoes
- More complex multilocular appearance
- May have punctate mural echogenic foci
- Different history: Cyclical pain or infertility
- Can be seen in association with PIC

Pseudomyxoma Peritonei

- Mucinous fluid with low-level echoes
- Mass effect with scalloping of liver and spleen
- Thicker irregular septa

Peritoneal Carcinomatosis

- Ascites, peritoneal thickening and nodules, omental cake

Lymphangioma/Mesenteric Cyst

- Congenital infiltrative multilocular cystic peritoneal lesion
- Different age group and history

PATHOLOGY

General Features

- Etiology
  - PIC development requires functioning ovary and peritoneal adhesions
  - Ovaries normally produce peritoneal fluid
  - In patients with adhesions from prior pelvic surgery, inflammation, or endometriosis, there is impaired absorption resulting in loculated peritoneal fluid
  - Also seen with peritoneal dialysis, inflammatory bowel disease, pelvic inflammatory disease

Microscopic Features

- Septations
  - Single layer of flat to cuboidal mesothelial cells
    - Benign mesothelial proliferation
  - Occasional squamous metaplasia
- No true cyst wall

CLINICAL ISSUES

Presentation

- Most common signs/symptoms
  - Pelvic pain
  - Palpable mass
  - Abdominal distension
  - Incidentally noted on imaging
- Other signs/symptoms

- Pressure symptoms: Urinary frequency or hesitancy, constipation

Demographics

- Age
  - Almost exclusively premenopausal women
    - Functioning ovary required for PIC formation

Natural History & Prognosis

- Indolent course: May grow, remain stable, or regress
- Tend to recur after drainage

Treatment

- Hormonal therapy: Suppression of ovulation
- Ultrasound- or CT-guided drainage
  - ± sclerosant
- Surgery: Laparoscopic or open, avoid if possible
  - 30-50% recurrence risk with surgical resection

DIAGNOSTIC CHECKLIST

Consider

- PIC in appropriate clinical setting
  - Premenopausal patient with other pelvic pathology
    - Endometriosis
    - Surgery
    - Trauma
    - PID
- Differentiating from ovarian malignancy may be difficult
  - Must have high level of clinical suspicion for PIC
  - PIC: Absence of solid components and normal ovary

Image Interpretation Pearls

- Do not diagnose PIC in postmenopausal patient
  - Ovarian cancer much more likely
- Must see otherwise intact ovary
  - Ovary may be distorted
  - May be located at periphery of mass
- Ovarian neoplasm morphology
  - Thicker, more irregular septations
  - Mural nodules or papillary excrescences
  - More complex fluid

SELECTED REFERENCES

1. Bharwani N et al: Peritoneal pseudocysts: aetiology, imaging appearances, and natural history. Clin Radiol. 68(8):828-36, 2013
2. Veldhuis WB et al: Peritoneal inclusion cysts: clinical characteristics and imaging features. Eur Radiol. 23(4):1167-74, 2013
3. Laing FC et al: US of the ovary and adnexa: to worry or not to worry? Radiographics. 32(6):1621-39; discussion 1640-2, 2012
4. Moyle PL et al: Nonovarian cystic lesions of the pelvis. Radiographics. 30(4):921-38, 2010
5. Vallerie AM et al: Peritoneal inclusion cysts: a review. Obstet Gynecol Surv. 64(5):321-34, 2009
6. Tamai K et al: MR features of physiologic and benign conditions of the ovary. Eur Radiol. 16(12):2700-11, 2006
7. Guerriero S et al: Role of transvaginal sonography in the diagnosis of peritoneal inclusion cysts. J Ultrasound Med. 23(9):1193-200, 2004
8. Savelli L et al: Transvaginal sonographic appearance of peritoneal pseudocysts. Ultrasound Obstet Gynecol. 23(3):284-8, 2004
9. Hanbidge AE et al: US of the peritoneum. Radiographics. 23(3):663-84; discussion 684-5, 2003

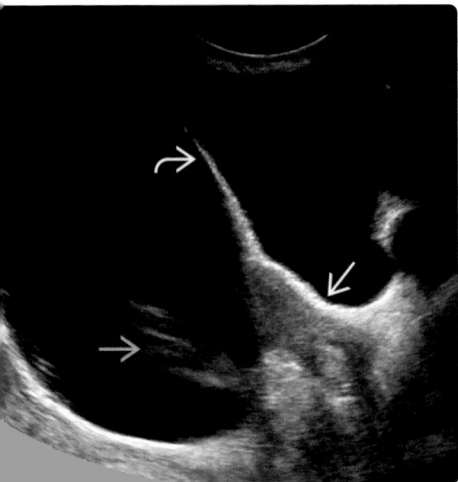

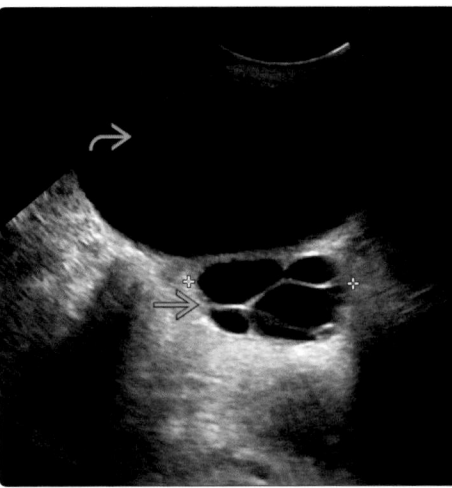

(Left) *Sagittal transabdominal ultrasound performed for abdominal distension in a patient with a history of peritonitis shows voluminous pelvic fluid with septa ⮞ anterior and posterior to the uterus ➡. Internal echoes ➡ were artifactual. The ovaries were displaced by the fluid.* (Right) *Parasagittal transabdominal ultrasound of the same patient shows an ovary ➡ displaced posteriorly by the large peritoneal inclusion cyst ⮞.*

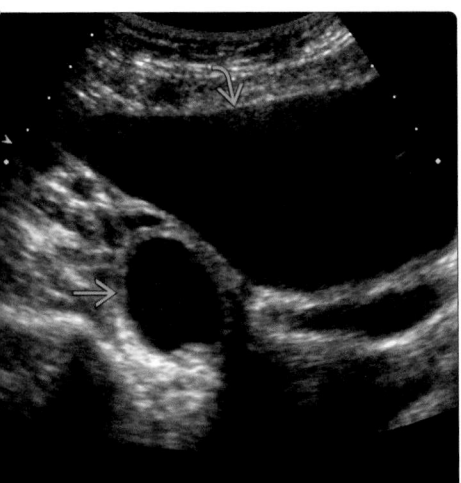

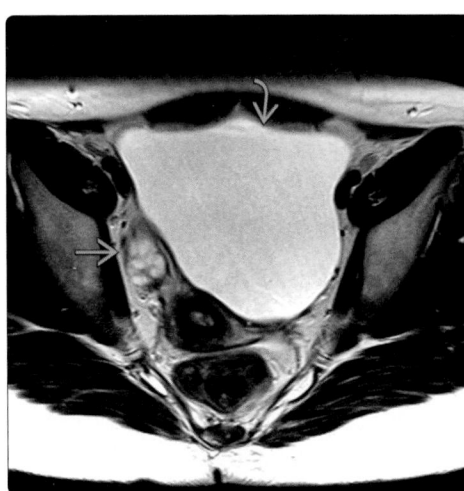

(Left) *Transverse transabdominal ultrasound of an adolescent post left oophorectomy for a mature teratoma shows a peritoneal inclusion cyst ➡ displacing the right ovary ➡, which contains a hemorrhagic functional cyst.* (Right) *Axial T2 TSE of the same patient shows the peritoneal inclusion cyst ➡ separate from the normal right ovary ➡. The cyst takes the shape of the peritoneal cavity.*

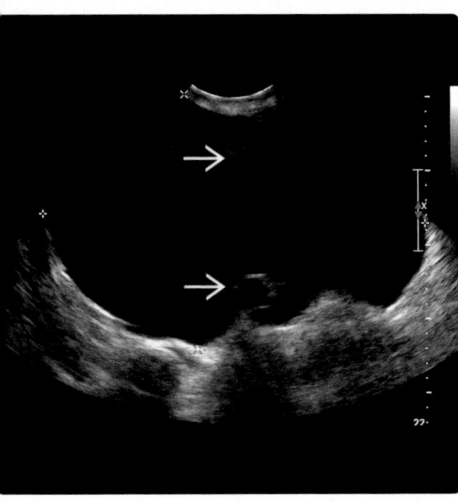

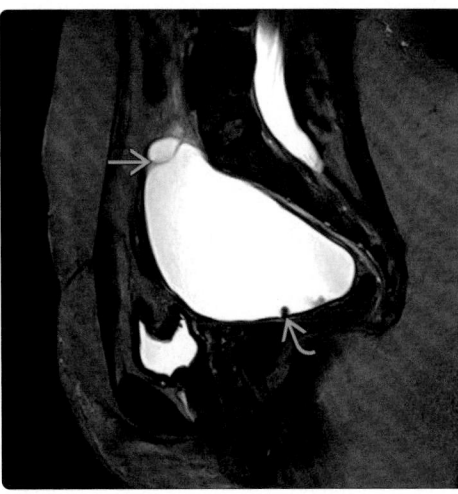

(Left) *Transverse transabdominal ultrasound shows a 26 cm peritoneal inclusion cyst with thin septa ➡. When cysts are this large, CT or MR is better for complete evaluation.* (Right) *Sagittal fat-suppressed T2 MR post hysterectomy shows loculated fluid in the pelvis. A thin adhesion is noted superiorly ➡ with thicker incomplete septa inferiorly ⮞.*

Bartholin Cyst

TERMINOLOGY

- Occlusion of Bartholin glands results in cyst formation

IMAGING

- Can be seen with all imaging modalities (CT, US, MR)
  - Usually found incidentally
- US: Cystic structure: Anechoic to mixed echogenicity if complicated by hemorrhage or infection
  - May contain septations
  - Thick walled if infected

TOP DIFFERENTIAL DIAGNOSES

- Sebaceous cyst
- Thrombophlebitis/other infections/varices
- Hematoma, endometrioma
- Gartner duct cyst
- Skene gland cyst
- Malignancy

PATHOLOGY

- Usually asymptomatic
  - Superimposed infection can develop
    - Increase in size; painful
- Malignancy very rare
  - Squamous and adenocarcinoma most common types

CLINICAL ISSUES

- Simple drainage can result in recurrence up to 38%
  - Incision/drainage ± silver nitrate cautery, marsupialization or excision, placement of Word catheter

DIAGNOSTIC CHECKLIST

- 1-4 cm cystic lesion located in vulvar vestibule, just lateral and inferior to vaginal introitus
- Usually asymptomatic

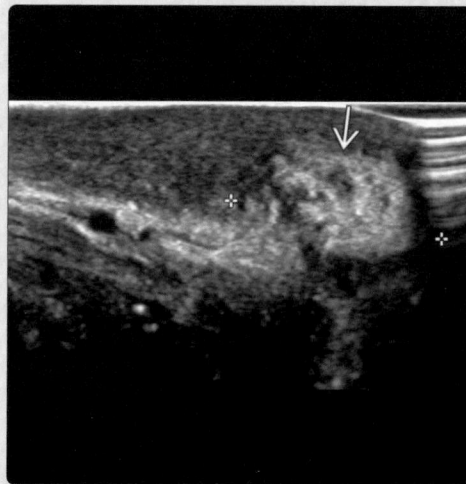
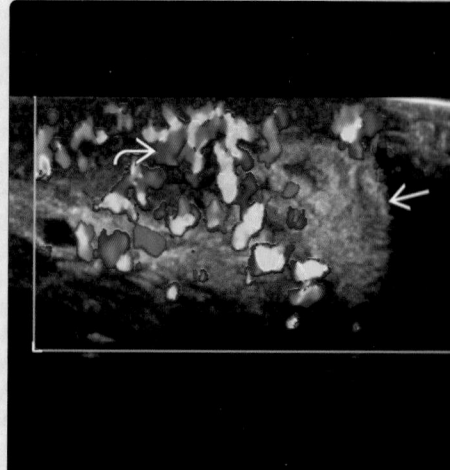

(Left) Longitudinal ultrasound shows an infected right Bartholin cyst ➡, which contains echogenic debris. (Right) Longitudinal color Doppler ultrasound of the infected right Bartholin cyst ➡ shows surrounding hyperemia ➡.

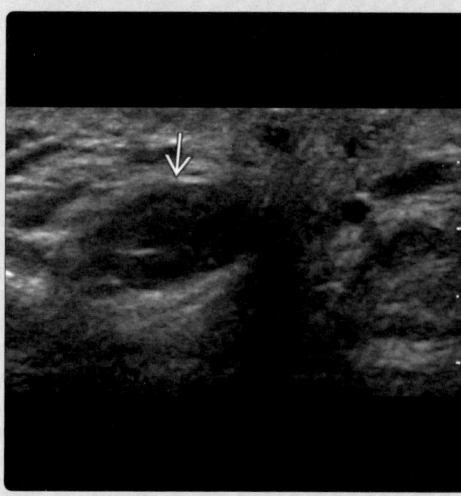
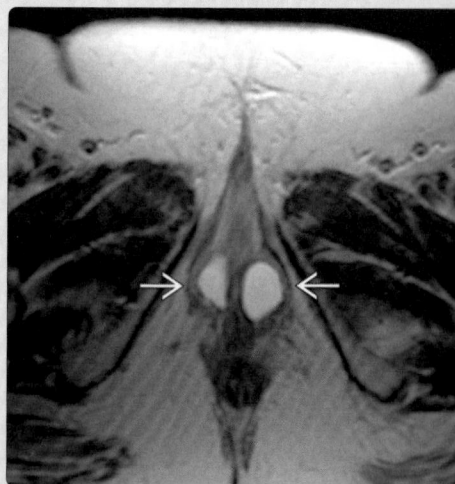

(Left) Transverse ultrasound shows a hemorrhagic right Bartholin cyst ➡ in a patient who presented with acute pain but no signs of infection. (Right) T2 MR shows the typical location of Bartholin cysts ➡, which are often an incidental finding. Note the high T2 signal from internal fluid.

Bartholin Cyst

TERMINOLOGY

Definitions

- Bartholin glands (or greater vestibular glands) are mucus-secreting glands located in vulvar vestibule, just lateral and inferior to vaginal introitus
- Drain via narrow duct 2.5 cm in length
- Cystic dilatation of Bartholin gland occurs secondary to duct obstruction

IMAGING

General Features

- Best diagnostic clue
  - Palpable, and sometimes visible mass lateral and inferior to vaginal introitus
  - Most common vulvar cystic mass
  - Size ranges 1-4 cm
- Location
  - Posterolateral distal vaginal wall, medial to labia minora, and at level of introitus

Ultrasonographic Findings

- Grayscale ultrasound
  - Cystic structure: Anechoic to mixed echogenicity if complicated by hemorrhage or infection; may contain septations
  - Thick walled if infected
- Power Doppler
  - No internal vascularity, may see reactive hyperemia around Bartholin abscess

MR Findings

- T1WI
  - Low signal fluid if uncomplicated, signal may ↑ with infection or hemorrhage
- T2WI
  - High signal fluid if uncomplicated, proteinaceous fluid may be lower signal than simple fluid

Imaging Recommendations

- Protocol advice
  - Clinical diagnosis: Imaging generally not required unless complications suspected

CT Findings

- Hypo- to hyperdense cystic lesion near vaginal introitus
  - Any solid component within should raise concern for malignancy

DIFFERENTIAL DIAGNOSIS

Other Labial Masses

- Sebaceous cyst: Epidermal inclusion cysts, may become infected, respond well to incision and drainage
- Thrombophlebitis or other infections
- Hematoma: Straddle injury, abuse
- Tumors: Rare, usually clinically obvious
- Endometriosis/endometrioma

Vulval Varices

- Associated with pelvic congestion syndrome
- Throughout vulva, not limited to vestibule

Gartner Duct Cyst

- Similar in appearance but in anterolateral wall of proximal vagina

Skene Gland Cyst

- Periurethral in origin and separate from vaginal wall

PATHOLOGY

General Features

- Etiology
  - Obstruction of normal Bartholin gland duct

Microscopic Features

- Body of gland contains mucinous acini, duct has mixed squamous, mucinous, and transitional epithelial cells, and duct orifice is mostly squamous cells

CLINICAL ISSUES

Presentation

- Most common signs/symptoms
  - Usually asymptomatic
  - 1-4 cm, but can increase in size with repeated sexual stimulation
  - Can result in dyspareunia
  - Can become painful due to infection

Demographics

- Epidemiology
  - Approximately 2% of women
  - Can typically become symptomatic in 2nd to 3rd decade of life, but seen in all ages

Natural History & Prognosis

- Most are uncomplicated
- If infected → Bartholin abscess
  - Perineal pain, tender labial mass
  - Multimicrobial or related to gonorrhea/chlamydia
  - Increased size of preexisting mass
- Carcinomas are rare (1% of all gynecologic malignancies and 0.1-0.5% of vulvar carcinomas)
  - 80% are either squamous or adenocarcinoma

Treatment

- Abscess
  - Incision/drainage ± silver nitrate cautery
  - Marsupialization or excision for recurrent cases
    - Broad-spectrum antibiotics after surgical drainage
  - Placement of Word catheter
    - Outpatient or ER treatment
    - Limited by tendency to dislodge

SELECTED REFERENCES

1. Hosseinzadeh K et al: Imaging of the female perineum in adults. Radiographics. 32(4):E129-68, 2012
2. Kushnir VA et al: Novel technique for management of Bartholin gland cysts and abscesses. J Emerg Med. 36(4):388-90, 2009
3. Ergeneli MH: Silver nitrate for Bartholin gland cysts. Eur J Obstet Gynecol Reprod Biol. 82(2):231-2, 1999
4. Hill DA et al: Office management of Bartholin gland cysts and abscesses. Am Fam Physician. 57(7):1611-6, 1619-20, 1998
5. Yuce K et al: Outpatient management of Bartholin gland abscesses and cysts with silver nitrate. Aust N Z J Obstet Gynaecol. 34(1):93-6, 1994

KEY FACTS

TERMINOLOGY

- Gartner duct cyst (GDC) is an embryonic remnant of wolffian (mesonephric) duct, lined with nonmucinous low columnar cells
  - Associated with renal/ureteral/müllerian anomalies
  - Located in anterolateral vaginal wall

IMAGING

- Ultrasound is 1st modality of choice
  - Cyst with thin walls, separate from cervix
    - May contain echogenic material and septations
- MR provides better resolution and spatial differentiation from other organs
  - Usually low T1 signal intensity and high T2 signal intensity
    - Hemorrhage or proteinaceous debris results in high T1 and T2 signal intensity

TOP DIFFERENTIAL DIAGNOSES

- Nabothian cysts
- Vaginal inclusion cysts
- Endometriosis
- Urethral diverticulum
- Ectopic ureterocele
- If solid appearing, consider vaginal tumors or cervical/vaginal polyp

DIAGNOSTIC CHECKLIST

- Cystic lesion in anterolateral vaginal wall, distinct from cervix and no internal flow on Doppler
- In females with ipsilateral renal dysgenesis, a ureterocele-like "cyst" without associated ureteric dilatation is highly suspicious for GDC

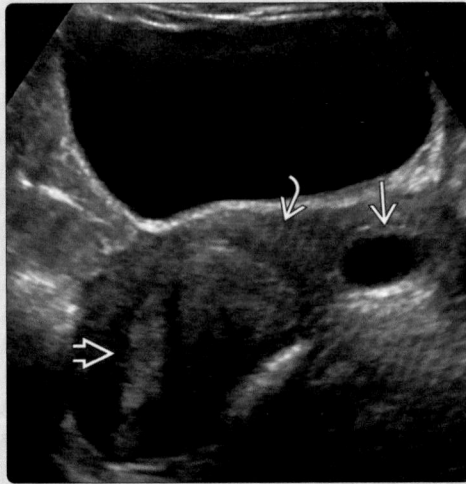
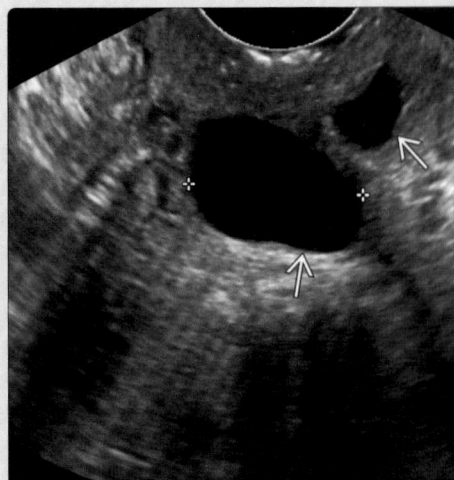

(Left) Longitudinal transabdominal ultrasound shows an ovoid cyst ➡ inferior to the cervix ➡. The endometrium ➡ is normal in this retroverted uterus. (Right) Coronal transvaginal ultrasound in the same patient shows 2 ovoid cysts ➡ in the upper vagina, consistent with Gartner duct cysts.

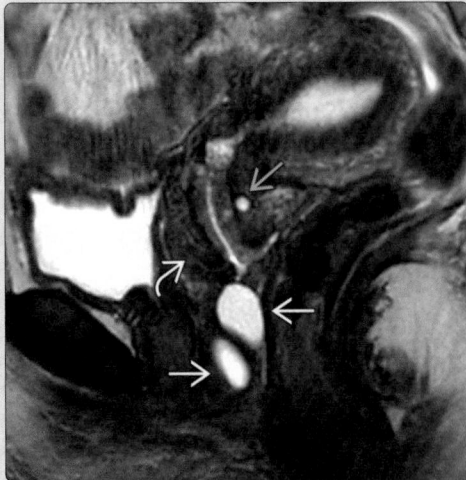
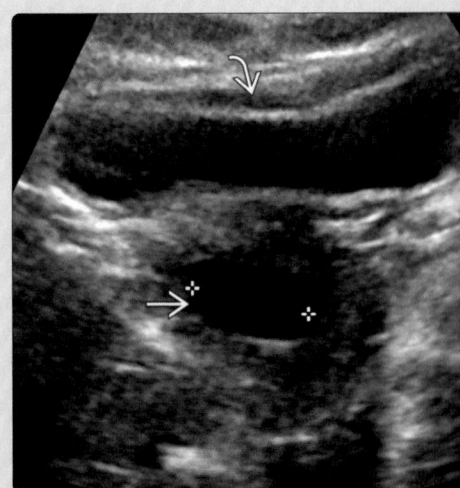

(Left) Sagittal T2 TSE MR, in the same patient, confirms the location of the Gartner duct cysts ➡, inferior to the cervix ➡, which contains a nabothian follicle ➡. (Right) Transverse transabdominal ultrasound shows a Gartner duct cyst ➡ inferior and posterior to the bladder ➡.

TERMINOLOGY

Abbreviations

- Gartner duct cyst (GDC)
- Gartner duct (GD)

Definitions

- Secretory retention cysts
  o Remnant of embryonic mesonephric (wolffian) ducts
  o Can occur anywhere along course of duct, most commonly anterolateral part of proximal 1/3 of vaginal wall

IMAGING

General Features

- Best diagnostic clue
  o Solitary fluid-filled structure in anterolateral vaginal wall
  o Does not communicate with urethra
- Size
  o Generally < 2 cm diameter
- Same appearance as müllerian cysts: Remnants of paramesonephric duct, cannot be distinguished from each other

Ultrasonographic Findings

- Grayscale ultrasound
  o Cyst characteristics
    – Anechoic to hypoechoic
    – Increased through transmission
    – Well-defined wall separate from cervix
  o Infection or hemorrhage → increased echogenicity of fluid component
  o May contain septa
  o In rare cases, can become quite large and can cause urethral obstruction
- Color/power Doppler
  o No internal flow on Doppler
  o Helps to confirm cystic nature rather than solid mass, such as vaginal tumor

Radiographic Findings

- GD may opacify on hysterosalpingography (HSG) if associated with fistula to vagina
  o Will opacify as focal dilated duct
- GD runs parallel to cervical canal

MR Findings

- T1WI
  o Low signal intensity if simple fluid content
  o Intermediate to high signal intensity if content is hemorrhagic or proteinaceous in nature
- T2WI
  o High signal fluid content
- In anterolateral vaginal wall
- When large or recurrent, may be multiloculated

Imaging Recommendations

- Best imaging tool
  o Transvaginal sonography is 1st modality of choice

  – Ultrasound may fail to differentiate GDC from urethral diverticulum if connection between diverticulum and urethra is not well seen
  – Light pressure with transducer will minimize compression of cyst
  – Partial withdrawal of transvaginal probe is helpful
  – Transperineal sonography is alternative
- Protocol advice
  o Pelvic MR helpful to show location within vaginal wall/relationship to surrounding tissues
    – Always include kidneys on coronal scout images
    – Introduction of water-soluble gel into vagina immediately prior to study improves delineation of vaginal fornices
  o Improved imaging with endoluminal coil is reported in literature

DIFFERENTIAL DIAGNOSIS

Cystic Appearance

- Nabothian cysts
  o Within cervix
  o Eccentric to cervical canal
  o GDC is adjacent to but separate from cervix
- Vaginal inclusion cysts
  o Occur as result of obstetric or gynecologic trauma
  o Usually posterior wall
    – GDC are anterolateral in location
  o Ask patient about prior deliveries/surgeries
- Endometriosis implant
  o More complex architecture
  o Thick wall, low-level internal echoes
  o Likely to have other manifestations of endometriosis
  o MR likely to show evidence of blood products
- Urethral diverticulum
  o In midurethra, arising in posterolateral wall facing vagina
    – Communicates with urethra
    – Associated with frequency, urgency, postvoid dribbling
    – When large enough, wraps around urethra in horseshoe configuration
- Ectopic ureterocele
  o Can occur any where between bladder neck and external urethral orifice
  o Associated with incontinence and urinary tract infection
  o Can present as cystic vaginal mass,
  o May produce filling defect on voiding cystourethrography (VCUG)

Solid Appearance

- Vaginal tumor
  o Extremely rare
  o Usually symptomatic
  o Solid mass; palpable, visible on speculum exam
    – Squamous cell carcinoma may undergo cystic degeneration
    – Vaginal sarcoma
- Uterine/cervical fibroid
  o Prolapsed submucosal fibroid
    – Solid, protrudes though cervix
    – Visible on speculum exam

- o Cervical fibroid
  - – Solid, arises from cervical stroma

PATHOLOGY

General Features

- Associated abnormalities
  - o Müllerian duct anomalies
    - – Unicornuate, bicornuate, didelphys, or septate uterus
    - – Carry ↑ risk for infertility, spontaneous abortion
    - – May present with hematocolpos/primary amenorrhea in setting of müllerian anomalies
  - o Renal anomalies
    - – Ipsilateral renal dysgenesis/agenesis
    - – Cross-fused ectopia/ectopic ureter
  - o Diverticulosis of fallopian tubes (salpingitis isthmica nodosa)
    - – Associated with increased incidence of infertility/increased risk for ectopic
- Embryology
  - o Mesonephric ducts normally resorb in females
  - o Remnants form interrupted channel along genital tract → GD
  - o Dilatation of lower portion of mesonephric duct remnants → GDC
    - – Commonest in vaginal wall
  - o Ureteral bud also develops from mesonephric duct
    - – Associated renal/ureteric anomalies are common

CLINICAL ISSUES

Presentation

- Most common signs/symptoms
  - o Usually asymptomatic
  - o Incidental finding on transvaginal ultrasound
  - o Incidental finding on pelvic examination
    - – Usually soft to palpation
- Other signs/symptoms
  - o May be symptomatic if large
    - – Pelvic pressure symptoms
    - – Dyspareunia
    - – Obstructed labor
    - – Mass at introitus described in neonate
  - o May present with urologic symptoms
    - – Cyst may be seen posterior to bladder or protrude into bladder, mimicking ureterocele
    - – May cause ureteric or urethral obstruction
    - – Reported cases of recurrent urinary retention in children requiring surgical resection of GDC
    - – Urinary incontinence
    - – Large GDC may mimic cystocele or urethral diverticulum

Demographics

- Epidemiology
  - o Remnants of GD can be detected in 25% of adult women
  - o GDC reported to occur in 1-2% of women

Natural History & Prognosis

- No specific treatment required if asymptomatic
- Infection/hemorrhage may cause acute pain

- Large cysts tend to be symptomatic
- GDC may recur postoperatively
  - o Recurrences tend to be multilocular
    - – May be mistaken for ovarian carcinoma, lymphocele, abscess
  - o Pelvic MR will show location inferior to levator plate
- Clear cell adenocarcinoma or malignant female adnexal tumor of wolffian origin (FATWO) from GDC are very rare; can present with vaginal bleeding and irritation

Treatment

- If symptomatic
  - o Aspiration
  - o Sclerotherapy
    - – Aspirate fluid
    - – Inject with 5% tetracycline solution in volume equal to aspirate
    - – Tetracycline solution reaspirated after 24 hours
  - o Marsupialization
  - o Surgical excision
- Check uterine/renal anatomy for possible associated malformations

DIAGNOSTIC CHECKLIST

Consider

- In young females with ipsilateral renal dysgenesis, a ureterocele-like "cyst" without associated ureteric dilatation is highly suspicious for GDC
  - o Strong association with other wolffian duct as well as müllerian duct anomalies
  - o Reported obstructing vaginal septum

Image Interpretation Pearls

- In infant with pelvic cyst, distension of vagina with saline allows confirmation that cyst arises in vaginal wall
- Associated with müllerian duct/renal/ureteral anomalies
  - o If cyst seen on pelvic imaging, check kidneys

SELECTED REFERENCES

1. Shobeiri SA et al: Evaluation of vaginal cysts and masses by 3-dimensional endovaginal and endoanal sonography. J Ultrasound Med. 32(8):1499-507, 2013
2. Surabhi VR et al: Magnetic resonance imaging of female urethral and periurethral disorders. Radiol Clin North Am. 51(6):941-53, 2013
3. Dwarkasing RS et al: MRI evaluation of urethral diverticula and differential diagnosis in symptomatic women. AJR Am J Roentgenol. 197(3):676-82, 2011
4. Chaudhari VV et al: MR imaging and US of female urethral and periurethral disease. Radiographics. 30(7):1857-74, 2010
5. Bats AS et al: Malignant transformation of Gartner cyst. Int J Gynecol Cancer 19(9):1655-7, 2009
6. Dwyer PL et al: Congenital urogenital anomalies that are associated with the persistence of Gartner's duct: a review. Am J Obstet Gynecol. 195(2):354-9, 2006
7. Macura KJ et al: MR imaging of the female urethra and supporting ligament in assessment of urinary incontinence: spectrum of abnormalities. Radiographics. 26(4):1135-49, 2006
8. Prasad SR et al: Cross-sectional imaging of the female urethra: technique and results. Radiographics. 25(3):749-61, 2005
9. Hahn WY et al: MRI of female urethral and periurethral disorders. AJR 182:677-82, 2004
10. Eilber KS et al: Benign cystic lesions of the vagina: a literature review. J Urol. 170(3):717-22, 2003
11. Sherer DM et al: Transvaginal ultrasonographic depiction of a Gartner duct cyst. J Ultrasound Med. 20(11):1253-5, 2001

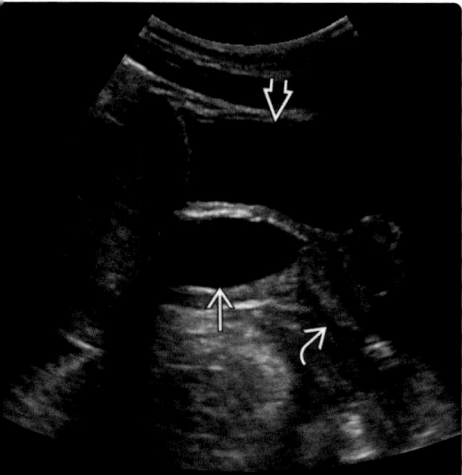

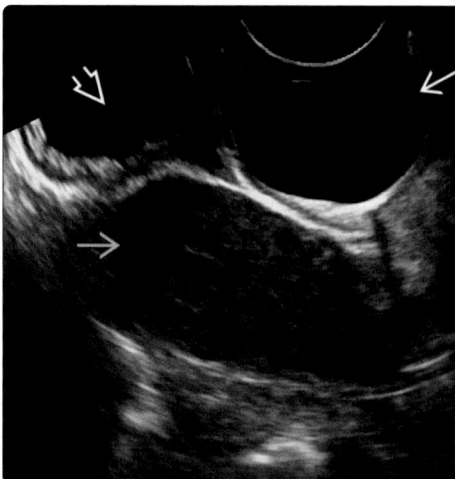

(Left) *Longitudinal sagittal transabdominal ultrasound of the pelvis shows an ovoid cyst ➡ in the upper vagina. The lower vagina ➡ and bladder ➡ are normal.* (Right) *Longitudinal transvaginal ultrasound (same patient) with minimal pressure shows the cyst to be more round ➡. The uterus ➡ and bladder ➡ are normal.*

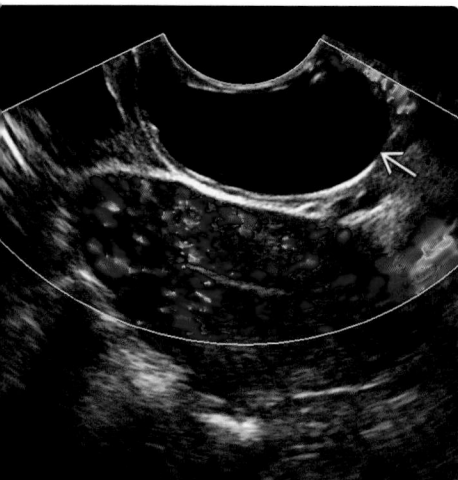

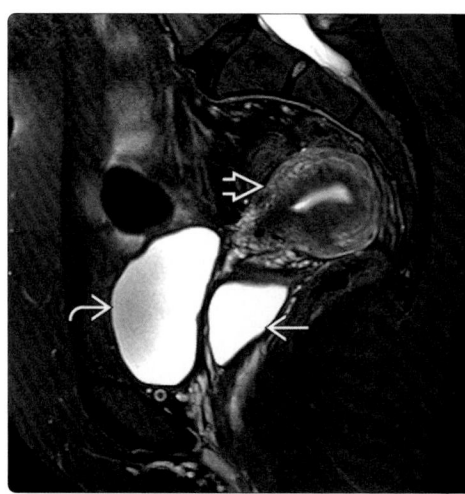

(Left) *Longitudinal transvaginal color Doppler ultrasound of the same patient shows no color flow in the Gartner duct cyst ➡.* (Right) *Parasagittal T2 FS MR shows a unilocular T2 bright Gartner duct cyst ➡ in the upper vagina. The bladder ➡ and uterus ➡ were normal.*

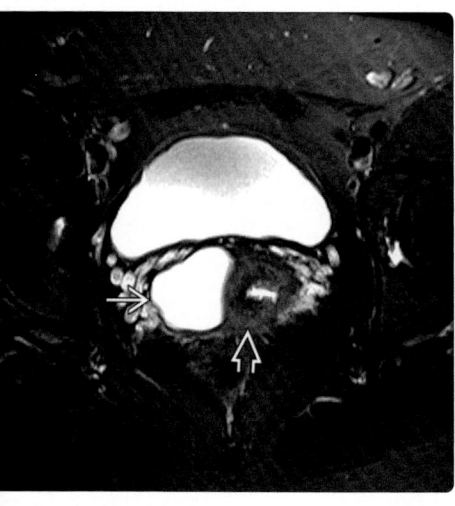

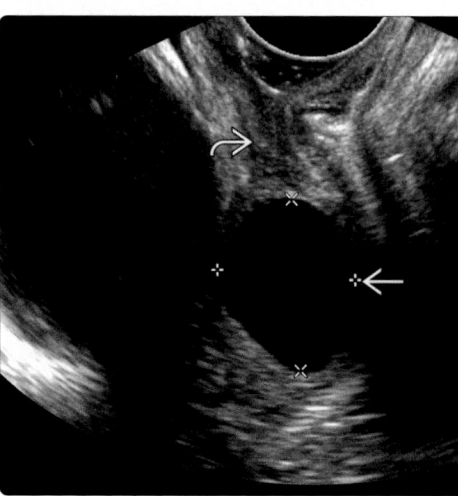

(Left) *Axial T2 FS MR shows a Gartner duct cyst ➡ lateral to the cervix ➡.* (Right) *Longitudinal transvaginal ultrasound shows a Gartner duct cyst ➡ in the upper vagina. The probe has been retracted to show the lower vagina ➡.*

Sex Cord-Stromal Tumor

TERMINOLOGY

- Group of ovarian tumors arising from either embryonic sex cords or mesenchyme
  - Fibroma, thecoma, fibrothecoma
  - Granulosa cell tumor
  - Sertoli-Leydig tumor (androblastoma)
  - Sclerosing stromal tumor, steroid cell tumors, gynandroblastoma, and sex cord tumor with annular tubules

IMAGING

- Ultrasound findings of sex cord-stromal tumors are diverse and nonspecific
- Range from small, solid tumors to large, multicystic masses
- Sex cord-stromal tumors are generally solid or have significant solid components
- Hormonally active tumors may be small and difficult to find
- **Granulosa cell tumors**
  - More often contain cysts with sponge-like appearance

- Cysts may be complex and contain hemorrhagic fluid
- **Fibrothecomas**
  - Hypoechoic with posterior acoustic attenuation
  - May have appearance similar to uterine leiomyoma

TOP DIFFERENTIAL DIAGNOSES

- Ovarian carcinoma
  - Sex cord-stromal tumors less likely to have papillary projections
- Germ cell tumors
  - Much more heterogeneous with calcifications, fluid-fluid levels, etc.

CLINICAL ISSUES

- Symptoms related to hormone production
- Some are estrogen producing tumors: Bleeding in postmenopausal patient
- May be associated with Meigs syndrome

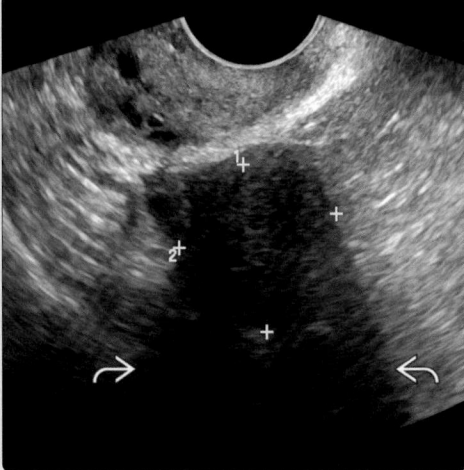
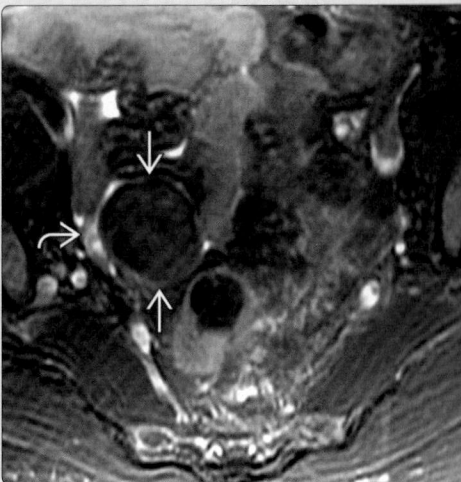

(Left) *Endovaginal US shows right adnexal hypoechoic solid mass (calipers) with dense posterior acoustic shadow* ⬈, *greater than expected given hypoechoic appearance of the mass. The ovary is not identified separately and the imaging appearance is most consistent with an ovarian fibroma. (Courtesy A. Kamaya, MD.)* **(Right)** *Axial T2 FS MR in the same patient shows the mass* ⮕ *is homogenously T2 dark and associated with a small claw of normal ovarian tissue* ⬈ *consistent with an ovarian fibroma.*

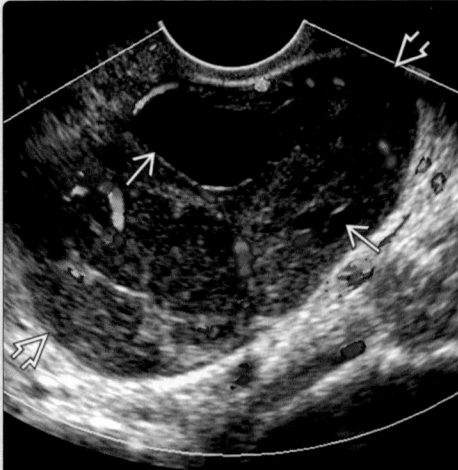
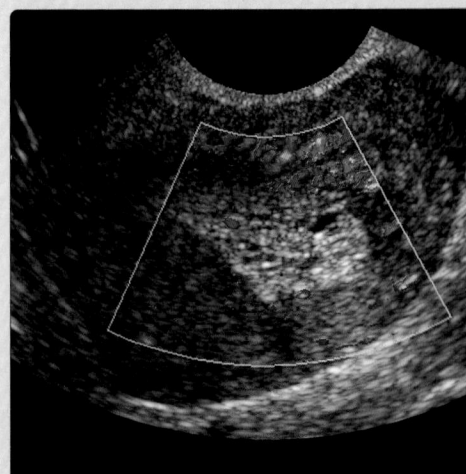

(Left) *Color Doppler endovaginal US in a perimenopausal woman with heavy vaginal bleeding shows a heterogeneous left adnexal mass* ⮕, *which is predominately solid and vascular but also contains small cystic foci* ⮕. *This was confirmed to be granulosa cell tumor at pathology.* **(Right)** *Color Doppler endovaginal ultrasound in the same patient shows a thickened endometrium with multiple cysts consistent with hyperplasia in the setting of a granulosa cell tumor.*

Sex Cord-Stromal Tumor

TERMINOLOGY

Definitions

- Group of ovarian tumors arising from either embryonic sex cords or mesenchyme
  - Fibroma, thecoma, fibrothecoma
  - Granulosa cell tumor: Occurs in both adult and juvenile forms
  - Sertoli-Leydig tumor (androblastoma)
  - Sclerosing stromal tumor, steroid cell tumors, gynandroblastoma, and sex cord tumor with annular tubules

IMAGING

General Features

- Sex cord-stromal tumors are generally solid or have significant solid components
- Hormonally active tumors may be small and difficult to find

Ultrasonographic Findings

- Ultrasound findings of sex cord-stromal tumors are diverse and nonspecific
  - Range from small, solid tumors to large, multicystic masses
- **Granulosa cell tumors**
  - More often contain cysts, with a sponge-like, Swiss cheese appearance
  - Cysts may be complex and contain hemorrhagic fluid
    - May rupture and cause hemoperitoneum
  - Adult and juvenile forms have similar appearance
  - Cysts will be thick-walled
  - Calcifications are rare
  - May be bilateral in 5%
- **Sertoli-Leydig tumors**
  - Significant overlap with granulosa cell tumors
  - Not as frequently cystic as granulosa cell tumors
    - 70% purely solid
    - 95% have solid component
  - Less likely to have hemorrhage
- **Fibrothecomas**
  - Hypoechoic with dense posterior acoustic attenuation
    - Similar to uterine leiomyoma
  - 1% associated with Meigs syndrome
- **Steroid cell tumors**
  - Typically small, without cysts

MR Findings

- T1WI
  - May see high signal from hemorrhage in granulosa cell tumor
  - High lipid content may cause steroid tumors to be high signal
- T2WI
  - Most intermediate signal with cystic area being high signal
    - Granulosa cell tumors may have network of smaller cysts creating sponge-like appearance
    - Fibrothecomas tend to be mild to markedly hypointense (compared to myometrium)
- T1WI C+

- Most enhance avidly except fibrothecomas

Imaging Recommendations

- Protocol advice
  - Evaluate uterus carefully
    - Hormonal stimulation may cause uterine enlargement and endometrial thickening (hyperplasia, polyps, or carcinoma) and can be tip-off to correct pathology

DIFFERENTIAL DIAGNOSIS

Ovarian Carcinoma

- Most epithelial tumors have dominant cystic component
- Confusion may occur if there is large, solid component

Germ Cell Tumors

- Much more heterogeneous with calcifications, fluid-fluid levels, dirty posterior shadow

Ovarian Torsion

- Edematous, enlarged ovary with peripheral cysts
- Patient is acutely symptomatic

Hormonally Functioning Ovarian Masses

- Patients may present with symptoms related to hormone production rather than mass
- May present with either hyperandrogenism or hyperestrogenism (some may do both)
- **Hyperandrogenism** (virilization with hirsutism, male pattern baldness, loss of female body contour, clitoromegaly)
  - Sertoli-Leydig tumor
  - Sclerosing stromal tumor
  - Gonadoblastoma
  - Brenner tumor
  - Polycystic ovarian disease
  - Stromal hyperplasia
  - Stromal hyperthecosis
  - Hyperreactio luteinalis
  - Nonovarian causes
    - Pituitary (Cushing disease)
    - Adrenal (Cushing syndrome)
- **Hyperestrogenism** (pseudoprecocious puberty, postmenopausal bleeding)
  - Granulosa cell tumor
  - Thecoma
  - Serous tumors
  - Mucinous tumors
  - Endometrioid tumors
  - Autonomously functioning follicular cyst most common in isosexual pseudoprecocious puberty

PATHOLOGY

General Features

- Etiology
  - Derive from 2 embryologically distinct groups of cells
    - Stromal cells: Fibroblasts, theca cells, and Leydig cells
    - Sex cords: Granulosa cells and Sertoli cells
  - Most tumors have more than 1 cell type
- Associated abnormalities
  - **Adult granulosa cell tumor**

- Endometrial hyperplasia, polyps, and carcinoma
  o **Juvenile granulosa cell tumor**
    - Pseudoprecocious puberty
    - Ollier disease (multiple enchondromas)
    - Maffucci syndrome (multiple enchondromas and hemangiomas)
  o **Sertoli-Leydig** most common virilizing tumor
    - Amenorrhea, hirsutism, deepening voice, male pattern baldness
  o **Sex cord tumor with annular tubules**
    - Peutz-Jeghers syndrome (autosomal dominant disorder with multiple gastrointestinal hamartomas and mucocutaneous pigmentation); ovarian tumors often bilateral
  o **Fibrothecoma**
    - Gorlin syndrome (odontogenic keratocysts of jaw, basal cell carcinoma, intracranial calcification, plantar and palmer pits, and craniofacial anomalies)

Microscopic Features

- Granulosa cell tumors are composed of granulosa cells growing in numerous patterns
  o Frequently accompanied by theca cells and fibroblasts
- Sertoli-Leydig cell tumors are composed of Sertoli cells, Leydig cells, and fibroblasts
  o May have tumors from single cell line
- Steroid cell tumors contain lutein cells, Leydig cells, and adrenocortical cells

CLINICAL ISSUES

Presentation

- Smaller masses may be incidental findings
- Pelvic pain/discomfort from larger masses
- Symptoms related to hormone production
- Fibromas may have elevated CA125
- May be associated with Meigs syndrome (pleural effusion, ascites, which resolve upon removal of benign mass)
- Granulosa cell tumors and thecomas are estrogen producing tumors
  o Clinical effects depend on patient age
  o Pseudoprecocious puberty in pediatric population
    - Not true precocious puberty because no ovulation or progesterone production
    - Present in 80% of juvenile granulosa cell tumors
    - Juvenile granulosa cell tumors account for 10% of precocious puberty cases
  o Uterine bleeding in postmenopausal patient
    - Endometrial stimulation with hyperplasia or carcinoma
    - 30-50% have hyperplasia
    - 3-25% have endometrial carcinoma
  o Women in reproductive age group may have irregular, heavy periods
- Sertoli-Leydig tumors are androgen-producing
  o Symptoms in 30% of patients

Demographics

- Epidemiology
  o Sex cord-stromal tumors represent 5-10% of ovarian neoplasms and 2% of ovarian malignancies
  o Distribution of sex cord-stromal tumors

- ~ 50% are fibrothecomas
- 10-20% granulosa cell tumors
- 5% Sertoli-Leydig tumors
- Remainder include sclerosing stromal tumor, steroid cell tumors, gynandroblastoma, and sex cord tumor with annular tubules
o Granulosa cell tumors occur in 2 distinct groups (juvenile and adult)
  - 5% are juvenile granulosa cell tumor and present < 30 years
  - Mean age for juvenile granulosa cell tumors is 13 years, with many presenting before puberty
  - 95% are adult granulosa cell tumors and present in perimenopausal and postmenopausal women (mean age: 52 years)
o Sertoli-Leydig tumor, mean age: 25 years

Natural History & Prognosis

- Many are low-grade malignancies and surgery is curative
- Juvenile granulosa cell tumors have excellent prognosis
  o Most are stage 1
- Adult granulosa cell tumors may act in more aggressive fashion with late recurrences (potentially decades) not uncommon
  o > 90%: Stage 1
  o 90-95%: 5-year survival for stage 1
  o 25-50%: 5-year survival for advanced disease
  o Mean survival after recurrence: 5 years
- 80-90% of Sertoli-Leydig cell tumors are stage 1 and are cured with resection
  o 10-20%: Behave in more malignant fashion
  o Most recurrences are in 1st 5 years
- Fibrothecomas are benign

DIAGNOSTIC CHECKLIST

Consider

- Key features differentiating sex cord-stromal tumors from more common epithelial neoplasms
  o More likely to present with symptoms from hormone production
  o Most are stage 1 with good prognosis
  o Affect all age groups, including pediatrics
  o More often solid
  o Cystic masses less likely to have papillary projections

Image Interpretation Pearls

- Multicystic lesion with hemorrhage in patient under 30 strongly suggests juvenile granulosa cell tumor
- Granulosa tumors are most common hormonally active tumor and produce estrogen
  o Thecomas: 2nd most common estrogen producing ovarian tumor
- Sertoli-Leydig cell tumor most common virilizing ovarian tumor

SELECTED REFERENCES

1. Heo SH et al: Review of ovarian tumors in children and adolescents: radiologic-pathologic correlation. Radiographics. 34(7):2039-55, 2014
2. Yen P et al: Ovarian fibromas and fibrothecomas: sonographic correlation with computed tomography and magnetic resonance imaging: a 5-year single-institution experience. J Ultrasound Med. 32(1):13-8, 2013

Sex Cord-Stromal Tumor

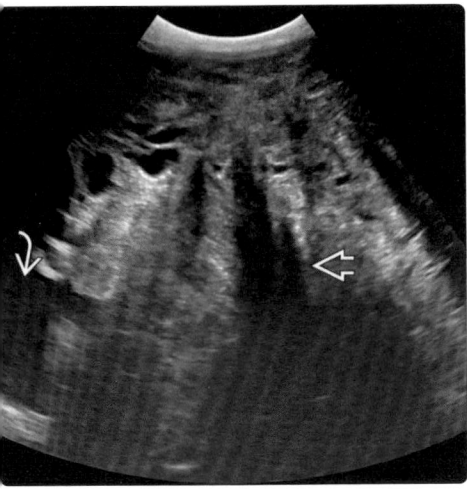
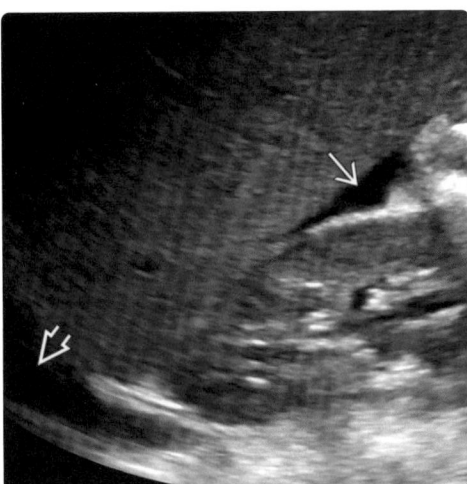

(Left) Transabdominal ultrasound shows a large midline pelvic mass that is mostly solid. A small amount of ascites is present ⟶. Note the linear shading areas ⟹ in the mass. Pathology revealed a large ovarian fibroma. (Right) Longitudinal ultrasound in the same patient shows ascites in the Morison pouch ⟶ and right pleural effusion ⟹. Fluid resolved with resection of the mass. Constellation of findings is consistent with Meigs syndrome, which is a triad of ovarian fibroma, pleural effusion, and ascites.

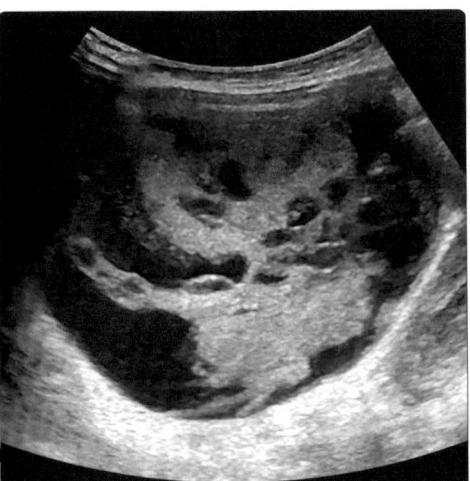
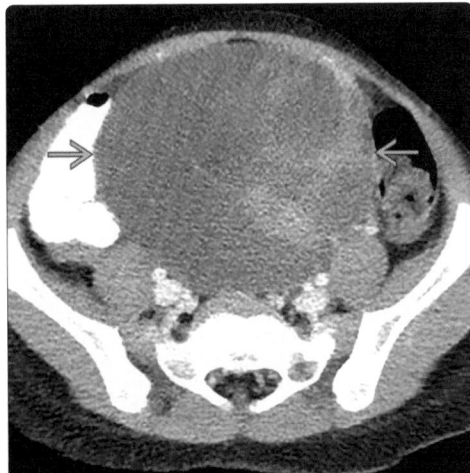

(Left) Transabdominal ultrasound in a 4-year-old girl shows a large mixed cystic and solid midline pelvic mass. The uterus and right ovary were identified separately and normal (not shown). (Right) Axial CECT in the same patient shows the midline large, heterogeneously enhancing, cystic and solid pelvic mass ⟶, which was confirmed to be a Sertoli-Leydig cell tumor at pathology.

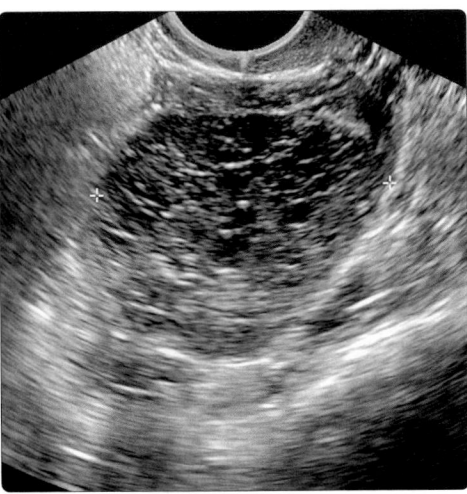
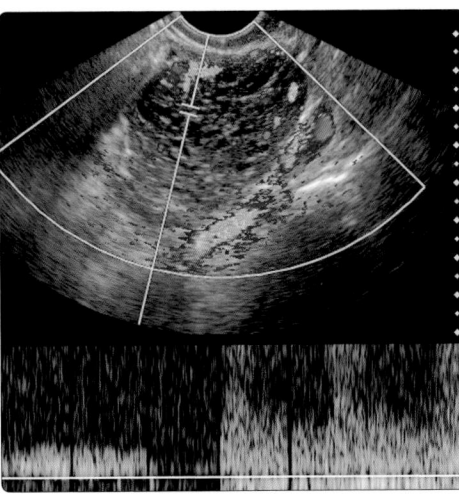

(Left) Endovaginal ultrasound in a patient with granulosa cell tumor shows a complex adnexal mass with multiple small cystic spaces and intervening septa giving the lesion a Swiss cheese appearance. (Right) Endovaginal color and pulse Doppler image in the same patient shows flow within the mass and helps distinguish this granulosa cell tumor from a hemorrhagic cyst.

(Left) *Transabdominal ultrasound shows a hypoechoic solid mass ➡ in the left adnexa with dense posterior acoustic shadowing. The ovary was not seen separately.* **(Right)** *Endovaginal ultrasound in the same patient shows the shadowing hypoechoic mass ➡ adjacent to a rim of normal ovarian tissue ➡. The imaging appearance is typical of fibroma/fibrothecoma.*

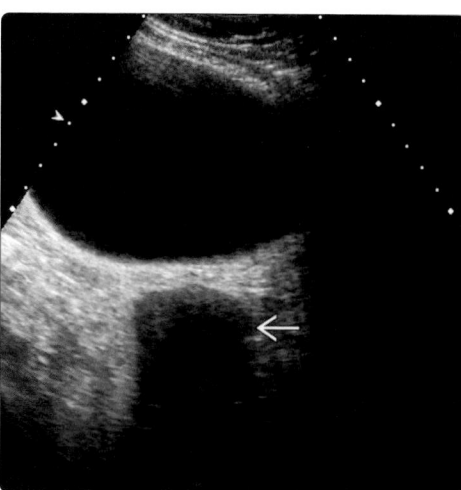
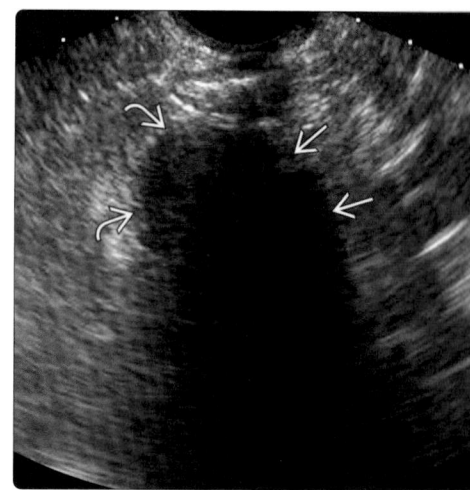

(Left) *Transabdominal ultrasound shows a large, homogenously hypoechoic pelvic mass with no color Doppler flow in this patient with a large fibrothecoma.* **(Right)** *Endovaginal ultrasound in the same patient shows a solid large mass with areas of linear refractive shadowing ➡, similar to that seen in a fibroid because of similar histology. A small cyst representing a normal follicle is seen at the periphery ➡.*

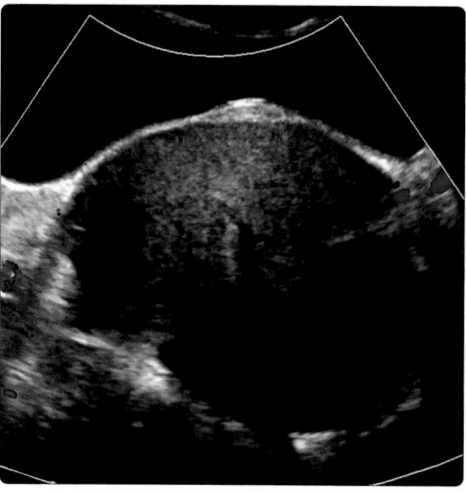
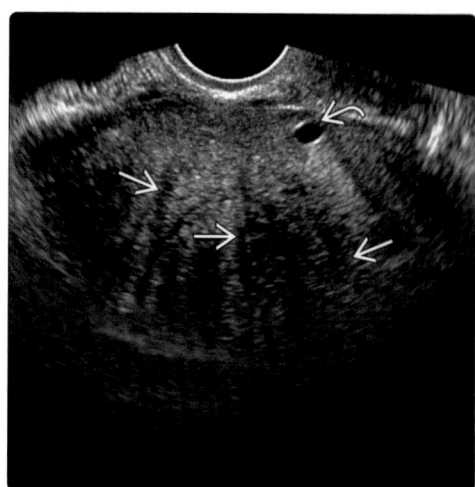

(Left) *Sagittal T2WI in the same patient from the above panel shows the large hypointense fibrothecoma ➡ posterior to the uterus with a claw of normal hyperintense ovarian parenchyma ➡.* **(Right)** *Coronal T1WI post gadolinium in the same patient shows hypoenhancement of the fibrothecoma ➡. A claw of normal ovary ➡ is again seen containing a follicle ➡, helping to distinguish this from a pedunculated fibroid. Chronic torsion was suspected given edematous ovarian parenchyma.*

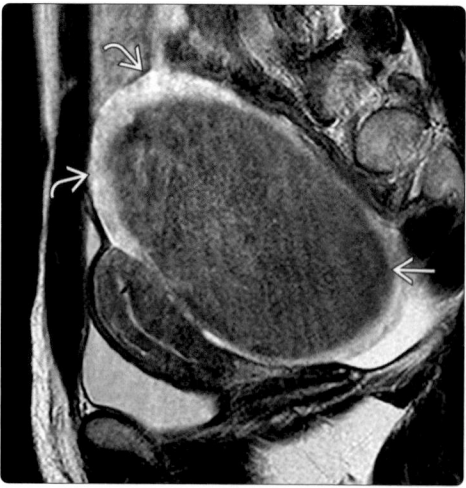
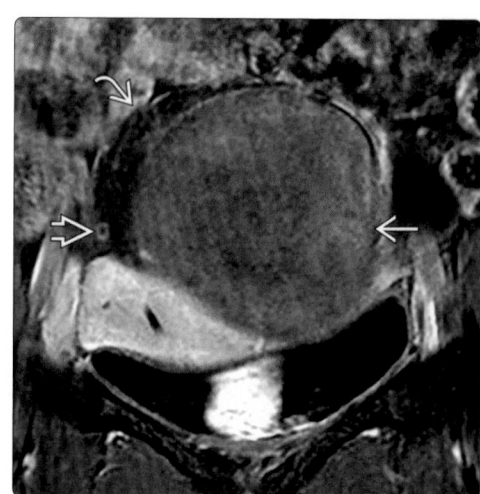

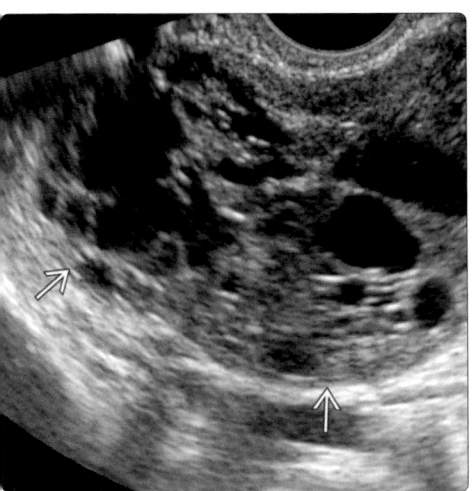

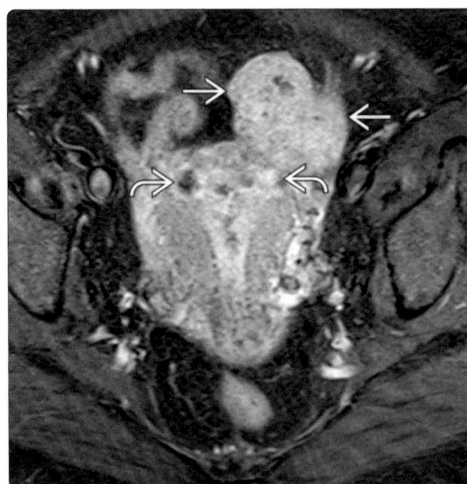

(Left) *Sagittal endovaginal ultrasound in a 33-year-old woman with a granulosa cell tumor shows a right ovarian mass ⇥ that is solid but with numerous small cystic spaces, exhibiting a Swiss cheese appearance.* (Right) *Axial T1WI C+ FS MR in a 55-year-old postmenopausal woman shows a left ovarian mass ⇥ displaying enhancement and containing small cystic spaces. Cystic changes are also seen within the thickened endometrium ⇥. Endometrial hyperplasia associated with a left ovarian granulosa cell tumor was found.*

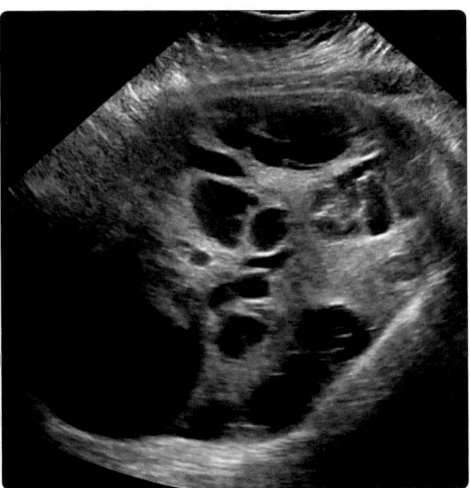

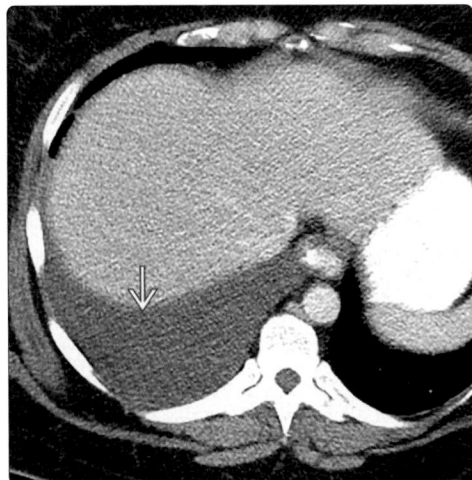

(Left) *Endovaginal US in a 38-year-old woman with a Sertoli-Leydig cell tumor shows a solid adnexal mass with multiple small and medium-sized cystic spaces. Note the lack of papillary projections and closely packed cystic spaces differentiating this from an epithelial tumor.* (Right) *CECT of the upper abdomen in the same patient shows a large right pleural effusion ⇥ in the setting of Meigs syndrome, which most commonly occurs in fibrothecomas but can also occur in other tumors, such as Sertoli-Leydig.*

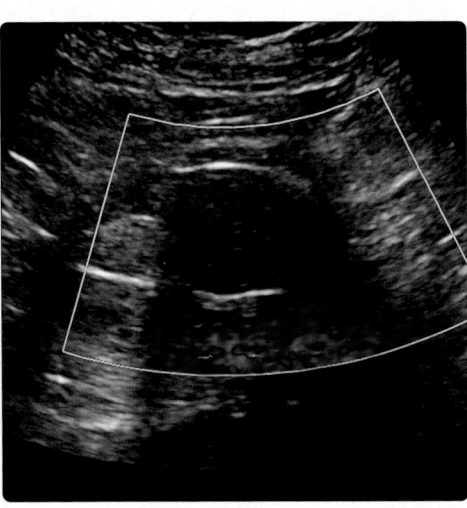

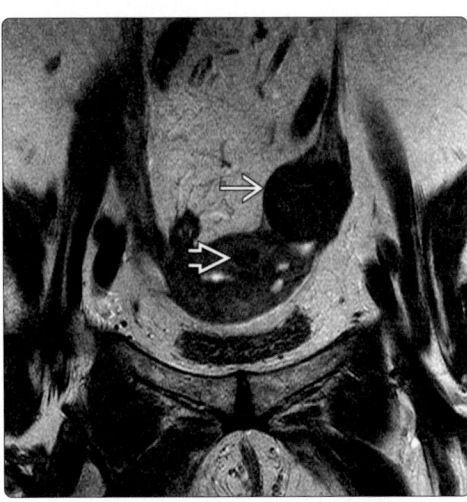

(Left) *Transabdominal US shows a hypoechoic adnexal mass with some internal echoes and no Doppler flow. It is unclear if this is a cystic mass, such as endometrioma, or a solid mass based on this single image. (Courtesy A. Kamaya, MD.)* (Right) *Coronal T2WI in the same patient shows the left adnexal mass ⇥ to be very hypointense, similar to the intramural fibroid ⇥. T1WI (not shown) shows similar hypointensity and after contrast the lesion is hypoenhancing. This is typical of a fibrothecoma. (Courtesy A. Kamaya, MD.)*

KEY FACTS

TERMINOLOGY

- Adnexal torsion is more accurate term than ovarian torsion, as torsion usually also includes fallopian tube

IMAGING

- Ovary > 4 cm long or > 20 cm³ in volume
- Ultrasound
  - Enlarged, heterogeneously echogenic ovarian stroma
  - Multiple small, peripheral, fluid-filled follicles displaced due to edematous stroma &/or mass
  - Whirlpool sign: Coiled, twisted pedicle
  - Flow pattern depends on degree of vascular obstruction and chronicity of torsion
  - Venous flow affected 1st
  - Due to dual arterial blood supply to ovary, arterial flow may be preserved
- CT
  - Twisted pedicle most specific sign but seen in < 1/3 of cases (use multiplanar reformations)

- Heterogeneous, minimal, or absent enhancement indicates evolution from ischemia to infarction

TOP DIFFERENTIAL DIAGNOSES

- Hemorrhagic corpus luteum
- Pelvic inflammatory disease
- Ectopic pregnancy

PATHOLOGY

- In adults, 50-90% have associated ovarian mass that serves as lead point
  - Large physiologic follicular cyst or corpus luteum cyst most common, followed by dermoid
- Presence of venous flow indicates viable ovary

DIAGNOSTIC CHECKLIST

- Presence of normal blood flow does **not** exclude torsion
- Always look for underlying mass

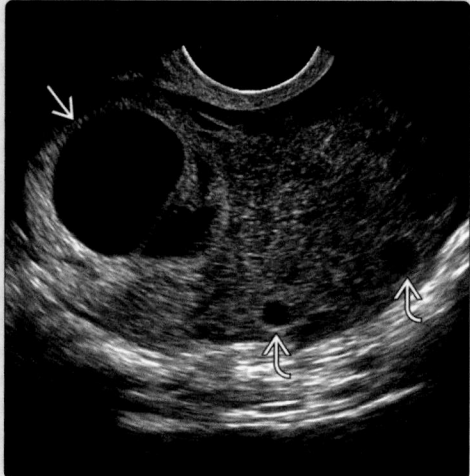
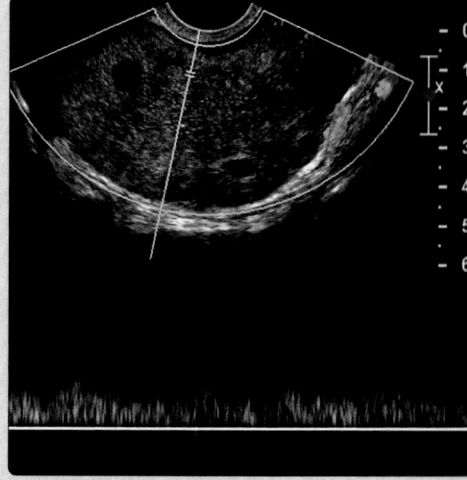

(Left) Longitudinal endovaginal ultrasound with adnexal torsion shows an enlarged, 6 cm ovary ➡ containing a hemorrhagic cyst with multiple peripheral follicles ➡. *(Right)* Endovaginal pulse wave Doppler ultrasound in the same patient with adnexal torsion shows low-resistance arterial flow in the ovary. It is important to remember that the presence of blood flow does not exclude ovarian torsion.

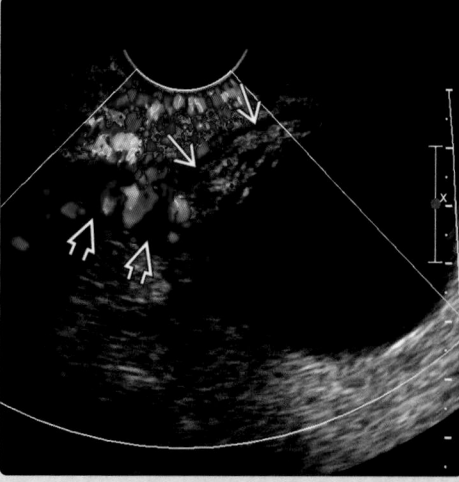
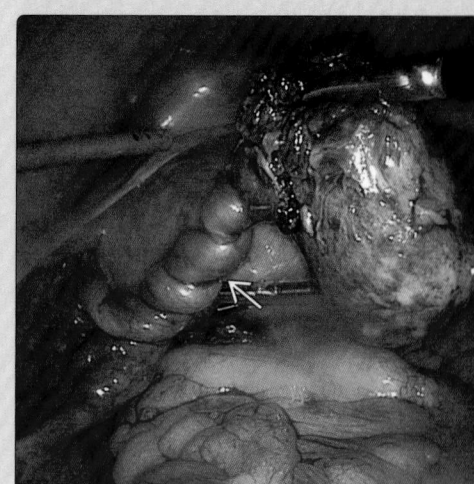

(Left) Endovaginal ultrasound in a woman with acute pelvic pain shows a large cyst in the ovary with adjacent edematous parenchyma ➡ with no color Doppler signal. Alternating red and blue color signal ➡ represents a twisted vascular pedicle, which is best seen during real time. *(Right)* Intraoperative photo in the same patient looking caudally confirms torsion and shows dusky infarcted right ovary (grasped) and twisted vascular pedicle ➡.

TERMINOLOGY

Synonyms

- Ovarian torsion
  - Adnexal torsion is more accurate term, as torsion usually also includes fallopian tube
    - Isolated fallopian tube torsion may also rarely occur

Definitions

- Rotation of ovary on its vascular pedicle resulting in venous congestion and ultimately infarction of ovary

IMAGING

General Features

- Best diagnostic clue
  - Enlarged ovary, often echogenic, with prominent peripheral follicles and absent venous flow on endovaginal color Doppler sonography
  - Twisted vascular pedicle
- Location
  - Torsed ovary/tube is often displaced from normal location
    - Midline, cephalad, anterior to uterine fundus, or in cul-de-sac
- Size
  - Enlarged ovary: > 4 cm in longest dimension or > 20 cm³ in volume
    - > 10 cm³ in postmenopausal women
  - Torsed ovary averages 28x normal volume
- Morphology
  - Swollen, rounded contour

Ultrasonographic Findings

- Grayscale ultrasound
  - Enlarged, heterogeneously echogenic ovarian stroma
  - Multiple small peripheral fluid-filled follicles displaced due to edematous stroma &/or mass
  - Follicle walls may become thickened and echogenic as torsion progresses
  - Ovarian cystic or solid mass
  - Ovary tends to be displaced midline, superior to uterus or down into cul-de-sac
  - Ovary is tender to touch by ultrasound probe
  - Pelvic free fluid; low-level echoes indicate hemoperitoneum
  - Twisted vascular pedicle (broad ligament, fallopian tube, ovarian vessels)
    - Sweep through pedicle with dynamic clip shows whirlpool sign
    - Target sign: Round hyperechoic structure, multiple hypoechoic concentric stripes
    - Beaked structure: Twisted fallopian tube
    - Heterogeneous tubular structure: Edematous fallopian tube
  - Isolated fallopian tube torsion: Often adnexal cyst separate from ovary, dilated tube with normal ovary
- Pulsed Doppler
  - Flow pattern depends on degree of vascular obstruction and chronicity of torsion
  - Normal arterial and venous waveforms may be present, especially in acute torsion
    - May also be seen with incomplete (< 360°) twist
  - Venous flow affected 1st
  - Due to dual arterial blood supply to ovary, arterial flow may be preserved
    - Resistive indices may be elevated
  - Absent venous and arterial flow in late torsion/ovarian infarction
- Color Doppler
  - Whirlpool sign: Coiled, twisted pedicle

CT Findings

- NECT
  - Ovarian hematoma/hematosalpinx best seen (> 50 HU)
- CECT
  - Enlarged displaced ovary
  - Use multiplanar reformations to better see twisted pedicle
    - Most specific sign, but only seen in < 1/3 of cases
  - Deviation of uterus toward side of torsion ± displaced ovary towards midline
  - Hypodense edematous stroma with peripherally placed cysts
  - Heterogeneous, minimal, or absent enhancement indicates evolution from ischemia to infarction

MR Findings

- T1WI
  - Hypointense ovarian edema
  - Hyperintensity indicates hemorrhagic infarction or hemorrhagic cyst
    - Look for hyperintense rim typical of subacute hematoma
  - Hyperintense fallopian tube/vascular pedicle (hemorrhage)
- T2WI
  - Hyperintense small peripheral cysts with background of increased ovarian signal intensity
- T1WI C+
  - Degree of enhancement variable depending on severity of ischemia and infarction
  - Best for twisted pedicle and evaluating for underlying mass

Imaging Recommendations

- Best imaging tool
  - Endovaginal US with both grayscale and color Doppler is best initial imaging examination
    - Reported accuracy of US varies among studies (23-75%)
  - CT/MR more likely to show twisted pedicle

DIFFERENTIAL DIAGNOSIS

Hemorrhagic Corpus Luteum

- Most common entity to be confused for torsion
- Variable appearance of cyst in otherwise normal-appearing ovary
  - "Fishnet" or lace-like fibrinous strands
  - Retracting clot
  - Fluid-fluid level
  - Diffuse low-level echoes similar to endometrioma
- Increased flow around cyst on color Doppler

Pelvic Inflammatory Disease

- Uniformly thickened and dilated fallopian tubes
- Pyosalpinx
  - Contains low-level echoes or fluid-fluid level
- ± enlarged ovaries secondary to oophoritis
  - Normal or increased flow pattern on color Doppler
- ± tubo-ovarian abscess
  - Complex cystic/solid masses
- "Indefinite uterus" sign
  - Obscuration of posterior margin of myometrium by inflammation

Ectopic Pregnancy

- Positive β-hCG
- No evidence of intrauterine pregnancy on endovaginal sonography
- Adnexal mass separate from ovary
  - Tubal ring with increased flow ("ring of fire")
- Visualization of embryo or yolk sac within tubal gestational sac
- Free fluid in pelvis and Morison pouch from hemoperitoneum

PATHOLOGY

General Features

- Etiology
  - In adults, 50-90% have associated ovarian mass, usually benign
    - Large physiologic follicular cyst or corpus luteum cyst is most common
    - Dermoid, paraovarian cyst, and epithelial and stromal tumors can also serve as lead points for torsion
  - Infants and children rarely have associated mass
    - Hypermobility due to long mesosalpinx
  - Isolated tubal torsion may occur due to hydrosalpinx, hematosalpinx, tubal neoplasms, tubal ligation, tubal hypermotility, and hydatid of Morgagni

Gross Pathologic & Surgical Features

- Torsion of both ovary and fallopian tube most commonly found at surgery
  - Isolated torsed fallopian tube possible
- Ovarian torsion occurs around suspensory ligament of ovary
  - Posterior fold of broad ligament that contains ovarian vessels
- Twist ranges 180-720°
- Sequential venous, lymphatic, and arterial obstruction
- Earliest pathologic changes include edema and microscopic hemorrhage within ovary
  - Begins centrally
- Prominent fluid-filled follicles displaced peripherally by central edema
- Late findings include hemorrhagic infarction
  - Cystic spaces filled with blood and associated hemoperitoneum
- Calcified mass in chronic cases

CLINICAL ISSUES

Presentation

- Most common signs/symptoms
  - Severe unremitting acute pelvic pain is most common symptom
    - Pain may be intermittent torsion/detorsion
  - Adnexal mass may or may not be palpable
  - Vomiting is common
  - Fever if ovary is infarcted

Demographics

- Epidemiology
  - 2-3% of all gynecologic emergencies
  - Most common in first 3 decades
  - More common during pregnancy
    - Usually before 20 weeks
    - As uterus enlarges, ovaries are pushed out of pelvis increasing risk of torsion
  - Increased risk in women undergoing ovarian stimulation
  - Increased risk in women with prior pelvic or abdominal surgery

Natural History & Prognosis

- Spontaneous detorsion can recur
  - Massive ovarian edema felt to result from episodes of intermittent torsion with detorsion
    - Usually long history of intermittent pain
- Presence of venous flow indicates viable ovary
- If no flow seen, ovary is infarcted

Treatment

- Surgical untwisting in noninfarcted adnexa either with laparoscopy or open surgery
  - Preservation of ovary is possible if normal blood flow is restored after detorsing ovary
- Careful examination and removal of any mass serving as lead point
- Salpingo-oophorectomy in infarcted ovary

DIAGNOSTIC CHECKLIST

Consider

- Ectopic pregnancy in pregnant patient

Image Interpretation Pearls

- Absent venous flow in enlarged echogenic ovary with prominent peripheral follicles is earliest reliable sign
- Presence of normal blood flow does **not** exclude torsion
- Always look for underlying mass

SELECTED REFERENCES

1. Lourenco AP et al: Ovarian and tubal torsion: imaging findings on US, CT, and MRI. Emerg Radiol. 21(2):179-87, 2014
2. Narayanan S et al: Fallopian tube torsion in the pediatric age group: radiologic evaluation. J Ultrasound Med. 33(9):1697-704, 2014
3. Sasaki KJ et al: Adnexal torsion: review of the literature. J Minim Invasive Gynecol. 21(2):196-202, 2014
4. Duigenan S et al: Ovarian torsion: diagnostic features on CT and MRI with pathologic correlation. AJR Am J Roentgenol. 198(2):W122-31, 2012
5. Sibal M: Follicular ring sign: a simple sonographic sign for early diagnosis of ovarian torsion. J Ultrasound Med. 31(11):1803-9, 2012
6. Wilkinson C et al: Adnexal torsion – a multimodality imaging review. Clin Radiol. 67(5):476-83, 2012

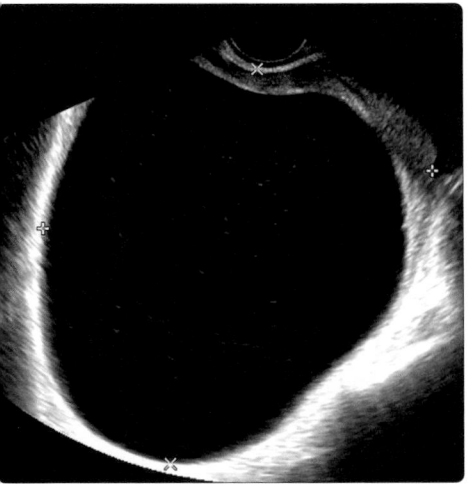

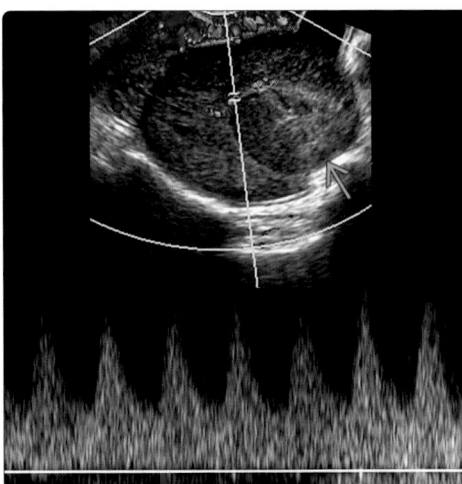

(Left) *Longitudinal endovaginal ultrasound shows a 11 cm unilocular adnexal cyst with scattered internal echoes. A torsed ovary from a mature cystic teratoma was found at surgery. Most cases of adult torsion have an underlying mass, which acts as a lead point.* (Right) *Transverse endovaginal ultrasound shows an enlarged heterogenous ovary ⊟ in a patient with adnexal torsion. Doppler ultrasound shows preserved arterial flow. It is important to remember that normal Doppler waveforms may be present in torsion.*

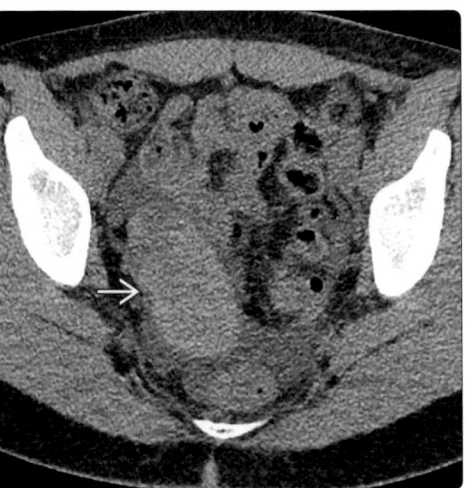

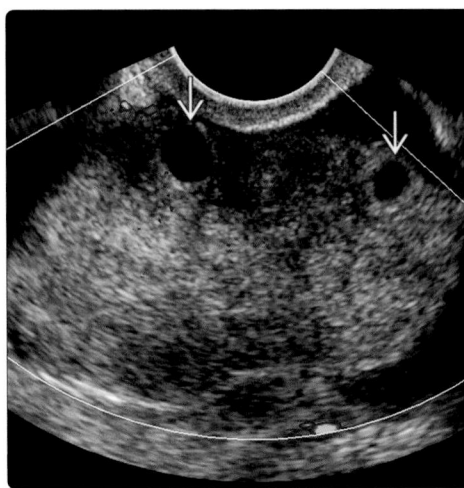

(Left) *Axial NECT obtained in a woman with acute pelvic pain initially thought to be a renal stone shows an oval 6 cm right adnexal hyperdense mass ⟹ a surrounded by small volume of free fluid.* (Right) *Subsequent endovaginal ultrasound in the same woman shows an enlarged ovary ⟹ with heterogenous stroma, peripheral follicles, and no color Doppler flow, which is consistent with adnexal torsion.*

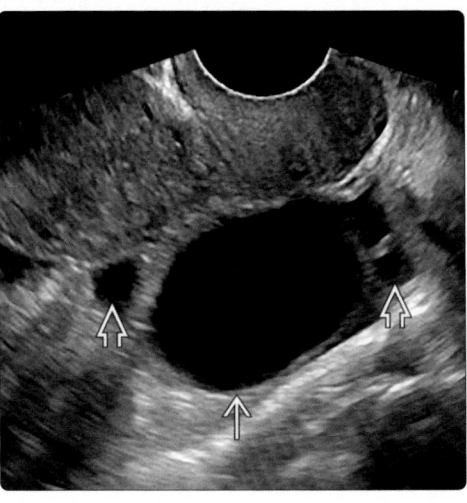

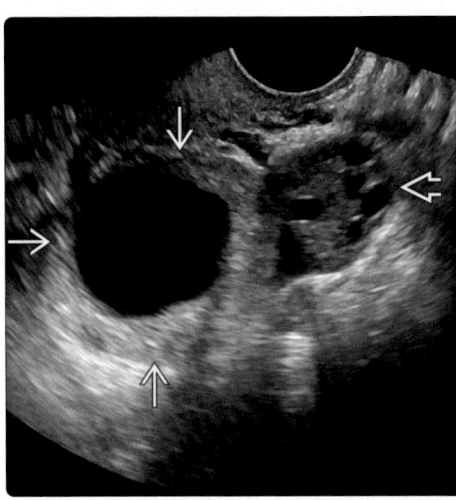

(Left) *Longitudinal endovaginal ultrasound in a 32-year-old woman with acute severe pain shows a large, thick-walled large cyst ⟹ in the cul-de-sac surrounded by a dilated fallopian tube seen in cross section ⟹.* (Right) *Transverse endovaginal US of the left adnexa in the same woman shows the large cyst with a thick wall ⟹ along the broad ligament, separate from a normal left ovary ⟹. Fallopian tube torsion was suspected preoperatively and confirmed at surgery. Fallopian tube torsion is rare, but can occur in isolation.*

Ovarian Metastases Including Krukenberg Tumor

TERMINOLOGY

- Secondary (metastatic) neoplasms to ovary
- Krukenberg tumor: Subtype of metastatic tumors that contain > 10% mucin-filled signet cells in cellular stroma
- High-stage mucinous tumors involving ovary frequently represent metastases from extraovarian primary sites and are often misdiagnosed as primary ovarian mucinous tumors

IMAGING

- Bilateral ovarian masses in patients with known primary carcinoma
- Metastases to ovary are usually solid masses
- Often large
- Lobulated masses with smooth external contour
- US
  - Solid or cystic and solid
  - Solid components demonstrate vascularity on Doppler evaluation

- Typically heterogeneous
  - May be complicated by hemorrhage
- CECT
  - Solid components often demonstrate heterogeneous enhancement
  - Cystic and necrotic areas do not enhance
- MR
  - T2WI: Solid components demonstrate heterogeneous signal intensity
  - T1WI C+: Solid components show marked heterogeneous enhancement
- PET/CT is modality of choice for tumor staging and shows increased metabolic uptake in ovarian metastases

TOP DIFFERENTIAL DIAGNOSES

- Primary ovarian cancer
- Ovarian lymphoma

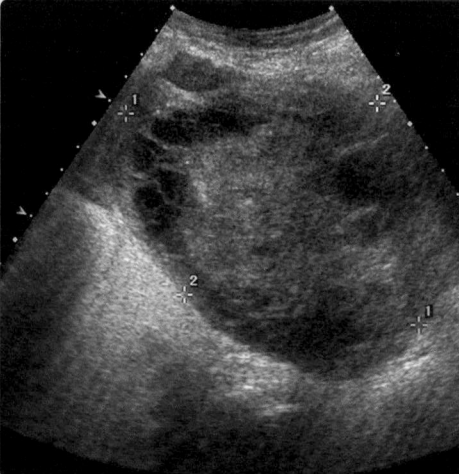
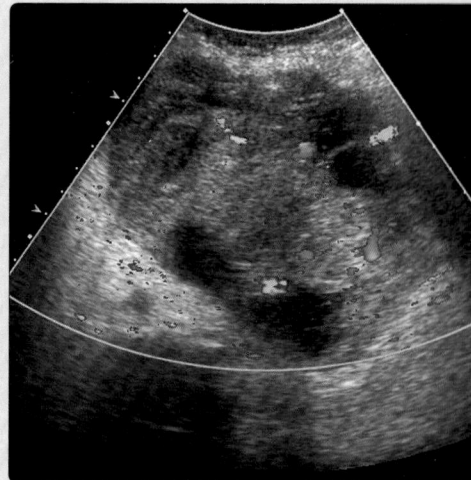

(Left) Transabdominal US in a woman with metastatic gastric adenocarcinoma shows large adnexal mass with a solid center and peripheral cystic areas. (Right) Longitudinal color Doppler US in the same patient shows flow in the solid component of the adnexal mass.

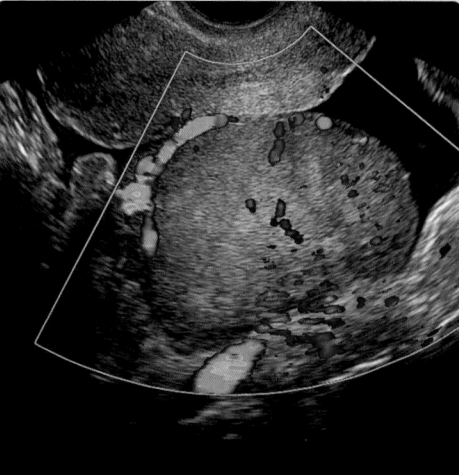
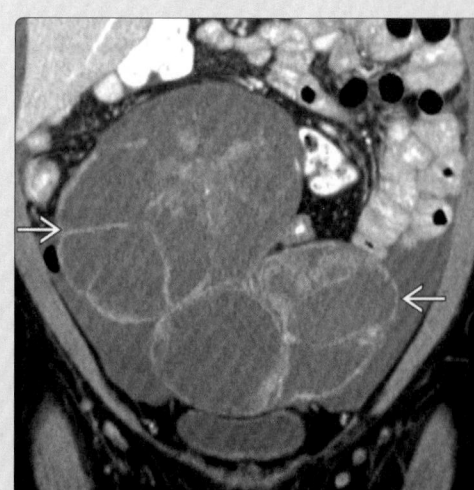

(Left) Longitudinal color Doppler US shows flow within a solid large right adnexal mass in a patient with metastatic melanoma to the ovary. Note the free fluid in the cul-de-sac. (Right) Coronal CECT in a 45-year-old woman shows large bilateral complex cystic and solid adnexal masses ➡. The patient had a recent history of colon cancer and these were confirmed metastases at oophorectomy.

TERMINOLOGY

Definitions

- Secondary (metastatic) neoplasms to ovary
- Krukenberg tumor
  - Subtype of metastatic tumors that contain > 10% mucin-filled signet cells in cellular stroma
  - Usually from gastrointestinal tract, with 76% arising from stomach
  - Krukenberg tumor is sometimes used inappropriately by some to include all metastatic ovarian carcinomas
- High-stage mucinous tumors involving ovary frequently represent metastases from extraovarian primary sites and are often misdiagnosed as primary ovarian mucinous tumors

IMAGING

General Features

- Best diagnostic clue
  - Bilateral ovarian masses in patients with known primary carcinoma
  - Metastases to ovary are usually solid masses
    - However, cystic and necrotic areas can be seen and tumors may resemble primary ovarian cancer
- Location
  - Usually bilateral
  - Majority of metastases from colon are bilateral (80%)
    - If unilateral, more common in right ovary
- Size
  - Often large masses
- Morphology
  - Lobulated masses with smooth external contour
    - 92% of ovarian metastases from colon cancer show smooth margin compared with 45% of primary ovarian cancers
  - Nonspecific imaging features in isolation

Ultrasonographic Findings

- Grayscale ultrasound
  - Ovarian mass
  - Solid or cystic and solid
    - Rarely unilocular cyst
    - May be complicated by hemorrhage
    - May mimic mucinous cystadenocarcinoma with multiple locules
- Color Doppler
  - Solid components demonstrate variable vascularity

CT Findings

- NECT
  - Metastatic ovarian tumors often have soft tissue density but may demonstrate low-attenuation cystic or necrotic areas
- CECT
  - Solid components often demonstrate heterogeneous enhancement
  - Cystic and necrotic areas do not enhance
  - Metastatic colorectal carcinoma may appear as multilocular cystic lesion with stained-glass appearance
    - Loculi with variable attenuation

- Mimics primary mucinous ovarian cancer

MR Findings

- T1WI
  - Solid components demonstrate intermediate signal intensity
- T2WI
  - Solid components demonstrate heterogeneous signal intensity
  - Cystic and necrotic components demonstrate high signal intensity
  - Loculi within multilocular tumors may show variable signal intensities
- T1WI C+
  - Solid components show marked heterogeneous enhancement

Nuclear Medicine Findings

- PET
  - PET/CT is modality of choice for tumor staging and shows variable increased metabolic uptake in ovarian metastases

Imaging Recommendations

- Best imaging tool
  - Ultrasound is usually 1st modality to demonstrate ovarian involvement in patient with known malignancy
  - CT and MR can be used to assess extent of disease

DIFFERENTIAL DIAGNOSIS

Primary Ovarian Cancer

- Most primary ovarian carcinomas are predominantly cystic masses
  - Multilocularity of cystic mass suggests primary ovarian tumor
- Most secondary malignancies of ovary are predominantly solid or mixture of solid and cystic areas

Ovarian Lymphoma

- Ovarian lymphomas are often homogeneous solid masses
- Extensive involvement of lymph node chains is seen in lymphoma

PATHOLOGY

General Features

- Etiology
  - Metastases to ovary occur by hematogenous, lymphatic, transperitoneal, or direct extension
  - Primary sites of nongynecologic tumors
    - Colon (30%)
      - Metastatic colon cancers to ovary usually arise from distal lesions, most commonly rectosigmoid, followed in decreasing order by transverse colon, ascending colon, cecum, and descending colon
    - Stomach (16%), appendix (13%), breast (13%), pancreas (12%), biliary tract (15%), and liver (4%)
  - Common gynecologic primary sites
    - Uterine body (23%), uterine cervix (4%)

Staging, Grading, & Classification

- Staging is based on staging system of primary malignancy

Gross Pathologic & Surgical Features

- Cut surfaces of ovaries may be solid, solid-cystic, or multicystic
- Have tendency to preserve contour of ovary
- Hemorrhage or necrosis may be present within mass

Microscopic Features

- Hyperplasia of ovarian stromal cells with significant number of signet ring cells
- Features favoring metastatic rather than primary ovarian neoplasm include
  - Bilaterality
  - Nodular pattern of ovarian involvement
  - Infiltrative pattern of stromal invasion
  - Microscopic surface deposits of tumor
  - Marked lymphovascular invasion (especially in hilum and outside ovary)
  - Signet ring cells
  - Cells floating in mucin
  - Variation in growth pattern from 1 nodule to another

CLINICAL ISSUES

Presentation

- Most common signs/symptoms
  - Abdominal pain
  - Palpable pelvic masses
- Other signs/symptoms
  - Occasionally associated hormonal activity can be seen due to reactive ovarian stromal hyperplasia
- Clinical profile
  - In many cases, there is known history of primary neoplasm
  - Usually symptoms of primary disease precede symptoms secondary to ovarian metastasis
  - On occasion, presentation is with symptoms related to ovarian mass in patient with no known history of malignancy

Demographics

- Age
  - More common in premenopausal women due to vascularity of ovaries
- Epidemiology
  - 5-15% of malignant ovarian tumors are metastatic tumors to ovary
  - 5-30% of cancer patients have ovarian metastases at autopsy
  - Only 30-40% of ovarian metastases are true Krukenberg tumors

Natural History & Prognosis

- Poor prognosis with mortality rate of ~ 90% 1 year after ovarian metastasis is discovered
- Krukenburg tumors: Mean survival 23 months
  - Premenopausal patients and metachronous lesions fair better

Treatment

- Radical tumor-reductive surgery
- Often have poor response to chemotherapy

- Due to high risk of ovarian metastasis, palliative bilateral oophorectomy may be performed during surgery for colon cancer

DIAGNOSTIC CHECKLIST

Consider

- Imaging findings of primary ovarian cancer and metastases to ovaries overlap in many cases, and confident imaging distinction between the 2 may be challenging
- In patients with metastases to ovaries, primary tumor is often clinically overt and associated with findings of widespread metastatic disease
- Investigation of gastrointestinal tract is recommended in patient without known primary cancer

Image Interpretation Pearls

- **Features that are more often seen in metastases to ovary include**
  - Bilateral ovarian masses
  - Predominantly solid appearance of mass

SELECTED REFERENCES

1. Jeung YJ et al: Krukenberg tumors of gastric origin versus colorectal origin. Obstet Gynecol Sci. 58(1):32-9, 2015
2. Nakamura Y et al: A Krukenberg Tumor from an Occult Intramucosal Gastric Carcinoma Identified during an Autopsy. Case Rep Oncol Med. 2014:797429, 2014
3. Alvarado-Cabrero I et al: Metastatic ovarian tumors: a clinicopathologic study of 150 cases. Anal Quant Cytol Histol. 35(5):241-8, 2013
4. La Fianza A et al: Intralesional hemorrhage in Krukenberg tumor: a case report and review of the literature. J Ultrasound. 16(2):89-91, 2013
5. Guerriero S et al: Preoperative diagnosis of metastatic ovarian cancer is related to origin of primary tumor. Ultrasound Obstet Gynecol. 39(5):581-6, 2012
6. Ho L et al: Bilateral ovarian metastases from gastric carcinoma on FDG PET/CT. Clin Nucl Med. 37(5):524-7, 2012
7. Willmott F et al: Radiological manifestations of metastasis to the ovary. J Clin Pathol. 65(7):585-90, 2012
8. Kitajima K et al: FDG PET/CT features of ovarian metastasis. Clin Radiol. 66(3):264-8, 2011
9. Maeda-Taniguchi M et al: Metastatic mucinous adenocarcinoma of the ovary is characterized by advanced patient age, small tumor size, and elevated serum CA125. Gynecol Obstet Invest. 72(3):196-202, 2011
10. de Waal YR et al: Secondary ovarian malignancies: frequency, origin, and characteristics. Int J Gynecol Cancer. 19(7):1160-5, 2009
11. Koyama T et al: Secondary ovarian tumors: spectrum of CT and MR features with pathologic correlation. Abdom Imaging. 32(6):784-95, 2007
12. Testa AC et al: Imaging in gynecological disease (1): ultrasound features of metastases in the ovaries differ depending on the origin of the primary tumor. Ultrasound Obstet Gynecol. 29(5):505-11, 2007
13. Chang WC et al: CT and MRI of adnexal masses in patients with primary nonovarian malignancy. AJR Am J Roentgenol. 186(4):1039-45, 2006
14. Khunamornpong S et al: Primary and metastatic mucinous adenocarcinomas of the ovary: Evaluation of the diagnostic approach using tumor size and laterality. Gynecol Oncol. 101(1):152-7, 2006
15. Kiyokawa T et al: Krukenberg tumors of the ovary: a clinicopathologic analysis of 120 cases with emphasis on their variable pathologic manifestations. Am J Surg Pathol. 30(3):277-99, 2006
16. Alcazar JL et al: Transvaginal gray scale and color Doppler sonography in primary ovarian cancer and metastatic tumors to the ovary. J Ultrasound Med. 22(3):243-7, 2003
17. Jung SE et al: CT and MR imaging of ovarian tumors with emphasis on differential diagnosis. Radiographics. 22(6):1305-25, 2002
18. Brown DL et al: Primary versus secondary ovarian malignancy: imaging findings of adnexal masses in the Radiology Diagnostic Oncology Group Study. Radiology. 219(1):213-8, 2001
19. Hann LE et al: Adnexal masses in women with breast cancer: US findings with clinical and histopathologic correlation. Radiology. 216(1):242-7, 2000

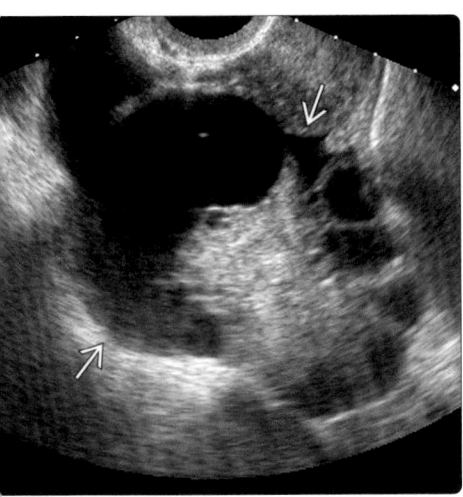

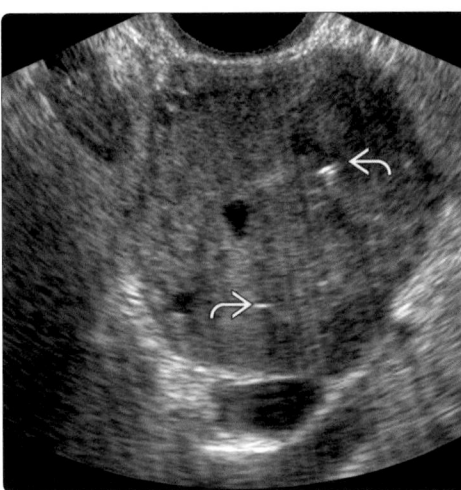

(Left) *Sagittal transvaginal US in a 63-year-old woman with history of rectal cancer shows an enlarged mixed solid and cystic right ovarian mass ➡.* (Right) *Longitudinal endovaginal US shows a large solid adnexal mass in a patient with gastric cancer. Note the small foci of calcification ➡, which can rarely be seen in mucinous gastric adenocarcinomas.*

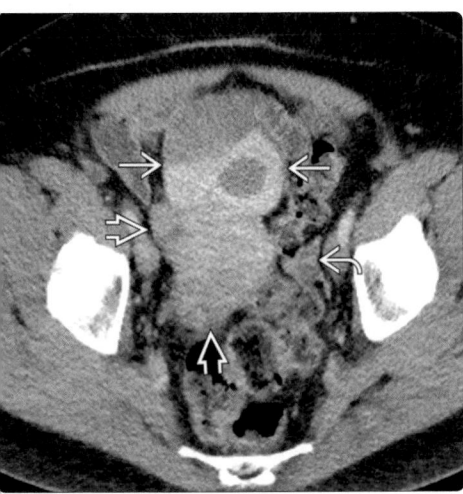

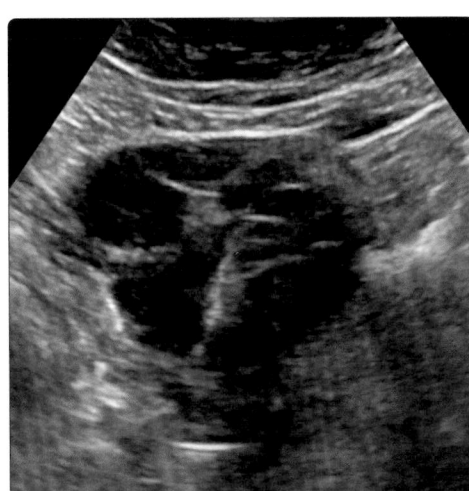

(Left) *Axial CECT in a 61-year-old woman undergoing restaging CT for colon cancer shows a heterogeneous adnexal mass ➡ anterior to the uterus ➡. The mass contains foci of high density suggesting blood products. Note the normal left ovary ➡.* (Right) *Transabdominal US in the same patient shows a multiseptated cyst without obvious large solid component. Although the imaging could represent a hemorrhagic cyst, this would be unusual in a postmenopausal woman.*

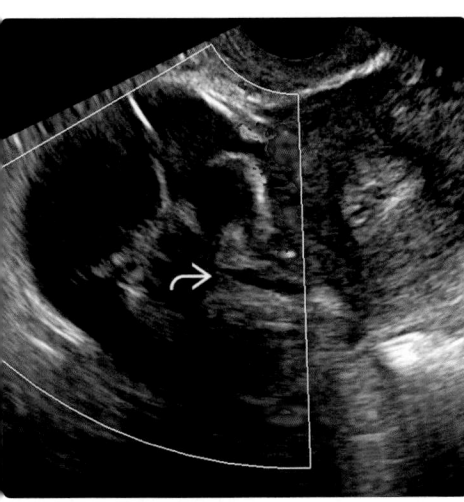

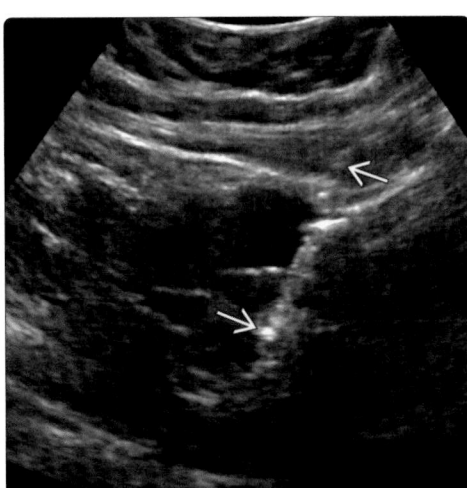

(Left) *Endovaginal color Doppler US in the same patient better shows solid irregular components ➡ of the complex cystic mass that have little color Doppler signal.* (Right) *Image from US-guided percutaneous fine needle aspiration shows needle ➡ in the most heterogenous solid component. Cytology showed malignant cells consistent with metastatic colon cancer. Percutaneous biopsy is not typically used to diagnose suspicious adnexal masses but is appropriate in cases of suspected metastatic disease.*

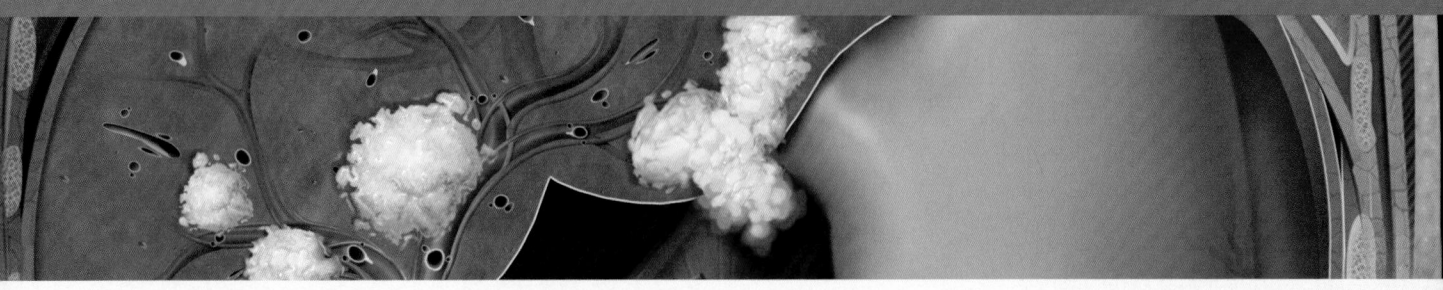

PART III
SECTION 1
Liver

DIFFERENTIAL DIAGNOSIS

Common

- Congested Liver
  - Congestive Heart Failure
  - Budd-Chiari Syndrome
- Acute Hepatitis
- Fatty Liver
- Steatohepatitis
- Fatty Cirrhosis
- Venoocclusive Disease
- Diffuse Neoplastic Infiltration
  - Infiltrative Hepatocellular Carcinoma
  - Lymphoma
  - Leukemia
  - Metastases

Less Common

- Sarcoidosis
- Glycogen Storage Disease

ESSENTIAL INFORMATION

Key Differential Diagnosis Issues

- Hepatomegaly
  - Commonly accepted to be > 15-16 cm long in mid clavicular line
    - Size varies depending on gender and body size
  - Volumetric measurements are time consuming and may not be suitable for everyday practice
- Ancillary signs used to identify hepatomegaly
  - Enlargement of caudate lobe
    - Differential diagnosis of cirrhosis
  - Extension of right lobe below right kidney
    - Differential diagnosis of Riedel lobe
  - Biconvex/rounded hepatic surface contour
  - Blunted, obtuse angle; rounded, inferior tip of right lobe
- Enlargement of left lobe (normally smaller than right)
  - Considered when left lobe is present between spleen and diaphragm

Helpful Clues for Common Diagnoses

- **Congested Liver**
  - **Congestive Heart Failure**
    - Dilated hepatic veins and inferior vena cava (IVC)
    - Venous "star" appearance at IVC-hepatic vein junction (instead of "rabbit ears")
    - Dilated hepatic veins may extend to periphery of liver
    - Hepatic venous flow: Turbulent appearance and pulsatile waveform on Doppler ultrasound
    - Marked pulsatility of portal vein
    - Hypoechoic parenchyma, increased posterior enhancement, soft consistency (dynamic indentation by cardiac motion)
    - Ancillary findings: Ascites, pleural effusion, thickened visceral walls (gallbladder, bowel, stomach), splenomegaly
    - Cardiomegaly
  - **Budd-Chiari Syndrome**
    - Acute phase

    - Hepatomegaly and parenchymal heterogeneous echogenicity due to congestion
    - Hepatic veins/IVC: Normal or distended caliber, partially/completely filled with hypoechoic material
    - Absent or restricted flow in hepatic veins/IVC
    - Aliasing or reversed flow in patent portions of IVC due to stenosis
    - Development of small intrahepatic venous collaterals
    - Chronic phase
      - Stenotic or occluded hepatic veins/IVC
      - Compensatory hypertrophy of caudate lobe, atrophy of involved segments
      - Large regenerative nodules
- **Acute Hepatitis**
  - Diffuse decrease in echogenicity
  - Echogenicity similar to renal cortex and spleen
  - "Starry sky" appearance
    - Increased echogenicity of portal triad walls against background hypoechoic liver
    - Variably seen
  - Periportal hypo-/anechoic areas due to edema
  - Marked circumferential gallbladder wall edema/thickening
    - Associated with hepatitis A virus
  - Elevated hepatic artery peak velocity on Doppler US
- **Fatty Liver**
  - Increase in size of liver and change in shape as volume of infiltration increases
    - Inferior margin of right lobe has rounded contours
    - Left lobe becomes biconvex
  - Increased echogenicity
    - Liver significantly more echogenic than kidney
    - Echogenicity may vary between segments (areas of focal fatty sparing)
  - Preservation of hepatic architecture
  - Blurred margins of hepatic veins due to increased refraction and scattering of sound
  - Vessels course through liver without distortion
    - May be spread apart secondary to expansion of liver parenchyma
  - Posterior segments of liver not clearly seen due to acoustic attenuation
  - Focal fatty sparing may simulate hypoechoic lesion
  - Soft consistency: Dynamic indentation by cardiac motion
- **Steatohepatitis**
  - Characterized by inflammation accompanying fat accumulation
    - Definitive diagnosis made by liver biopsy
  - May occur in alcoholic hepatitis and nonalcoholic steatohepatitis (NASH)
  - Etiology of NASH unknown but frequently seen in following conditions
    - Obesity
    - Diabetes
    - Hyperlipidemia
    - Drugs and toxins
  - Ultrasound findings
    - Signs of fatty liver

– Firm consistency (due to inflammation) on dynamic scanning during cardiac cycle
– Irregular borders of hepatic veins due to hepatic inflammation
– Intermittent loss of visualization of hepatic veins

Fatty Cirrhosis

o Enlarged left and caudate lobes and atrophic right lobe
o Hyperechoic but heterogeneous liver echo pattern
o Irregular hepatic veins
o Portal venous collaterals
o Stiff consistency
o Ancillary signs of portal hypertension
 – Ascites, varices, hepatofugal flow, splenomegaly

Venoocclusive Disease

o Hepatosplenomegaly and ascites
o Periportal and gallbladder wall edema
o Narrowing and monophasic waveform of hepatic veins due to hepatic edema
o Slow or reversed flow in portal vein
o Prominent hepatic arteries and elevated arterial peak systolic velocity
o Abnormal hepatic arterial resistive index
 – < 0.55 or > 0.75 (variably seen)

Diffuse Neoplastic Infiltration

o **Infiltrative Hepatocellular Carcinoma**
 – Ill-defined area of markedly heterogeneous echotexture
  □ Often indistinguishable from underlying cirrhosis
 – Color Doppler: Malignant portal vein thrombosis
  □ Absence of normal blood flow and presence of hypoechoic thrombus extending into portal vein
  □ Presence of arterialized flow in portal vein thrombus: High PPV but moderate sensitivity
o **Lymphoma**
 – Diffuse/infiltrative form presents as innumerable subcentimeter hypoechoic foci
 – Miliary pattern
 – Periportal location
 – Infiltrative pattern may be indistinguishable from normal liver

– Also look for lymphadenopathy, splenomegaly or splenic lesions, bowel wall thickening, ascites
o **Metastases**
 – Discrete nodules and masses or infiltrative pattern
 – Lung or breast cancer: Common primary showing infiltrative pattern hepatic metastases
 – Infiltrative pattern shows heterogeneous echotexture and simulates cirrhosis

Helpful Clues for Less Common Diagnoses

● **Sarcoidosis**
 o Hepatosplenic involvement
  – Most common finding: Nonspecific hepatosplenomegaly
  – Diffuse parenchymal heterogeneous echotexture
  – Numerous small nodular pattern
  – Advanced disease may cause or simulate cirrhosis
 o Can affect almost every organ
  – Most common site: Lung
 o Upper abdominal lymphadenopathy often present
● **Glycogen Storage Disease**
 o Hepatomegaly and multiple hepatic adenomas in chronically ill young patients
 o Liver may appear diffusely echogenic
  – Indistinguishable from fatty liver
 o Requires biopsy for diagnosis

SELECTED REFERENCES

1. Faraoun SA et al: Budd-Chiari syndrome: a prospective analysis of hepatic vein obstruction on ultrasonography, multidetector-row computed tomography and MR imaging. Abdom Imaging. ePub, 2015
2. Reynolds AR et al: Infiltrative hepatocellular carcinoma: what radiologists need to know. Radiographics. 35(2):371-86, 2015
3. Heller MT et al: The role of ultrasonography in the evaluation of diffuse liver disease. Radiol Clin North Am. 52(6):1163-75, 2014
4. Kratzer W et al: Factors affecting liver size: a sonographic survey of 2080 subjects. J Ultrasound Med. 22(11):1155-61, 2003

Congested Liver

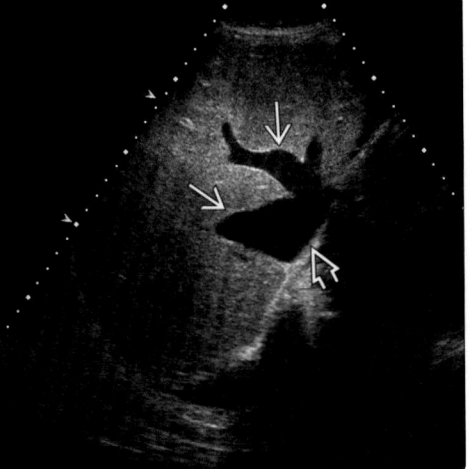

Budd-Chiari Syndrome

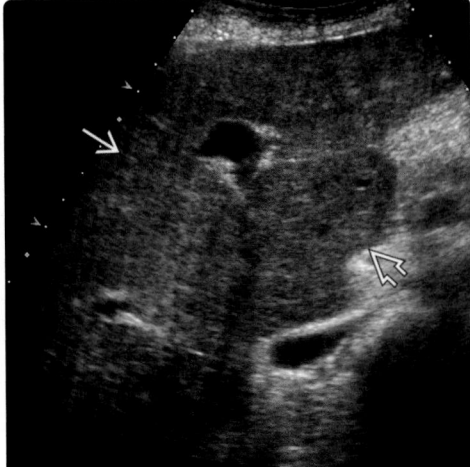

(Left) *Oblique ultrasound of the liver at the level of the hepatic venous confluence shows an enlarged liver with marked dilatation of hepatic veins ➡ and IVC ➡ indicating hepatic congestion in a patient with right heart failure.*
(Right) *Transverse abdominal ultrasound in a patient with Budd-Chiari syndrome shows heterogeneous hepatic parenchymal echogenicity ➡ and hypertrophied caudate lobe ➡. The caudate is often hypertrophied in the setting of Budd-Chiari due to its separate venous drainage into the IVC.*

(Left) *Longitudinal abdominal ultrasound in a patient with severe hepatic steatosis shows an enlarged liver measuring 21 cm in length, diffusely echogenic liver → compared to the right kidney ➜, and marked attenuation of the US beam which results in poor visualization of the diaphragm ➡. **(Right)** Longitudinal abdominal ultrasound in a patient who presented with acute liver failure from acute alcoholic hepatitis shows a markedly enlarged liver ➡ extending well below the inferior renal margin.*

Fatty Liver

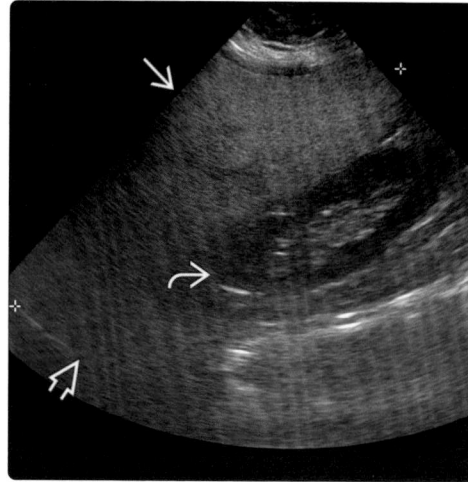

Steatohepatitis

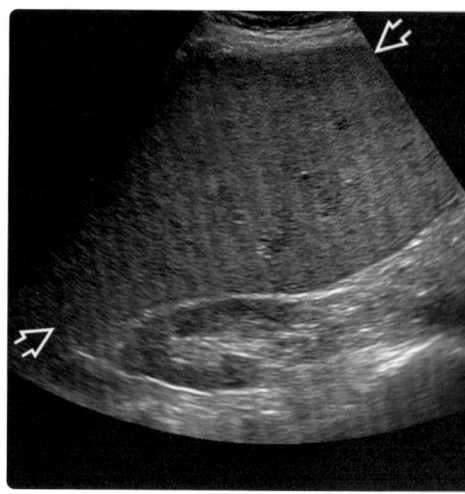

(Left) *Transverse abdominal ultrasound in a patient with venoocclusive disease shows a markedly enlarged and edematous liver resulting in narrowed hepatic veins ➜ and small-caliber inferior vena cava ➡. A small right pleural effusion is also evident ➡. **(Right)** Longitudinal abdominal ultrasound in a patient with venoocclusive disease shows marked hepatomegaly with craniocaudal length of the liver measuring 22.6 cm ➡. Liver extension well beyond the edge of the kidney is indicative of hepatomegaly.*

Venoocclusive Disease

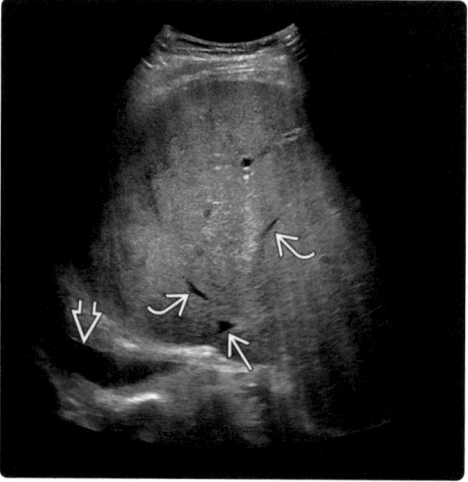

Venoocclusive Disease

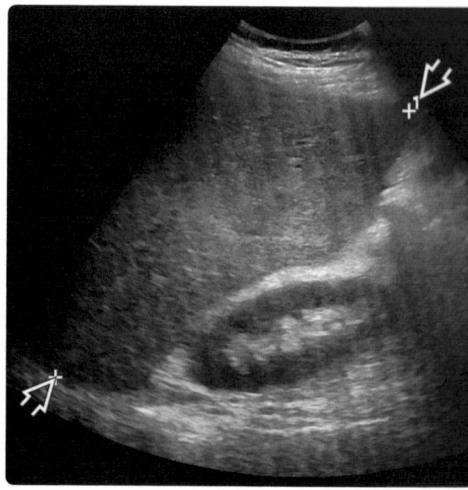

(Left) *Transverse grayscale ultrasound of the liver shows a markedly heterogeneous and enlarged liver with multiple refractive shadows ➡ caused by diffuse, infiltrative HCC. Focal echogenic lesion ➡ was shown to be a fat-containing focus of HCC. **(Right)** Transverse abdominal color Doppler ultrasound shows the right portal vein filled with echogenic material ➡, consistent with portal vein tumor thrombosis. Underlying liver is markedly heterogeneous because of diffuse HCC.*

Infiltrative Hepatocellular Carcinoma

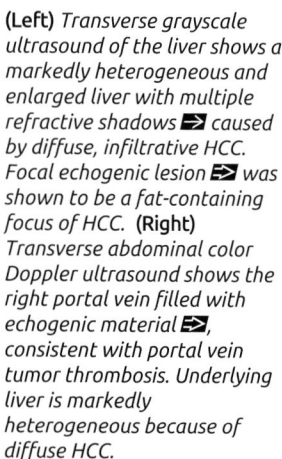
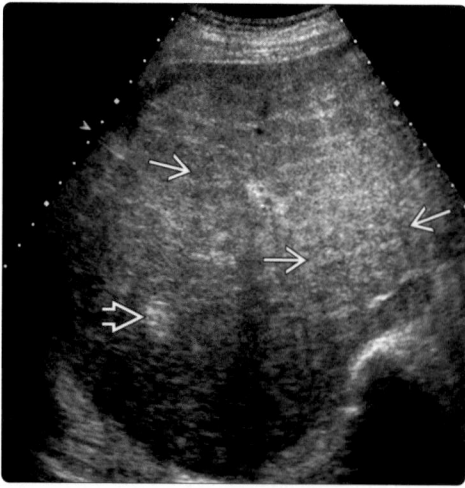

Infiltrative Hepatocellular Carcinoma

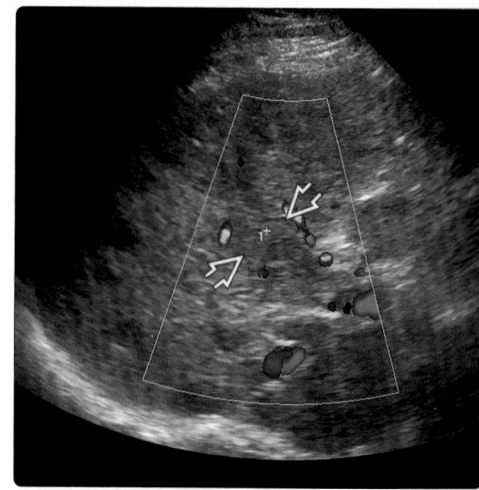

Lymphoma

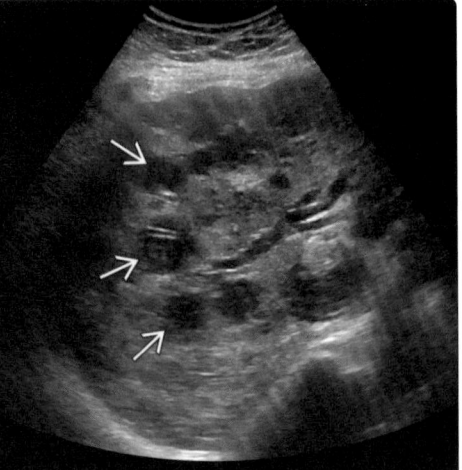

Lymphoma

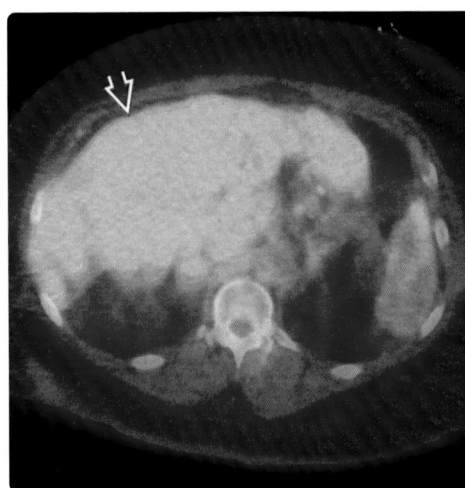

(Left) *Transverse abdominal ultrasound in a patient with lymphoma shows multiple markedly hypoechoic masses ➡ throughout the right lobe of the liver.* (Right) *FDG PET in the same patient with lymphoma shows the liver is enlarged and diffusely hypermetabolic throughout the entire liver parenchyma ➡.*

Metastases

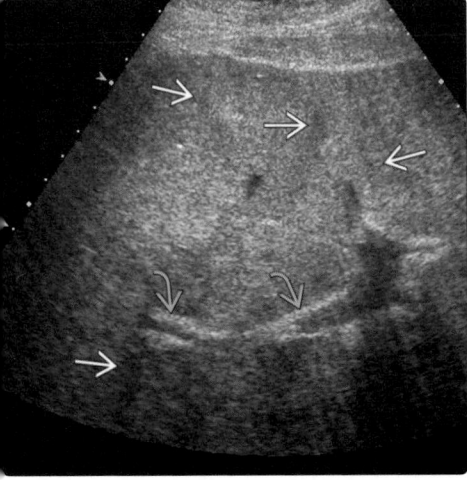

Metastases

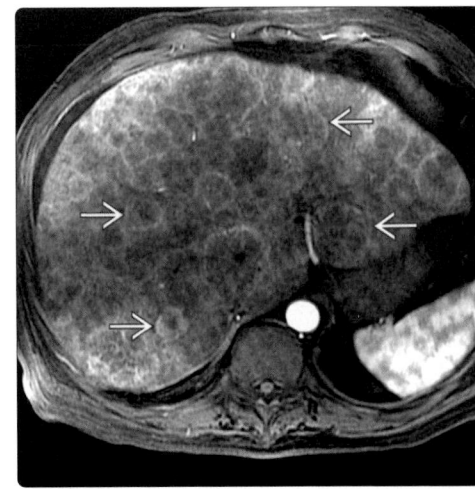

(Left) *Transverse abdominal ultrasound in a patient with hepatic metastasis from neuroendocrine tumor demonstrates enlarged and markedly heterogeneous appearance of the liver with numerous refractive shadows ➡ caused by underlying isoechoic metastasis. The portal veins are distorted ➡ by mass effect.* (Right) *T1WI C+ FS MR in the same patient demonstrates that the heterogeneous liver appearance on ultrasound is due to numerous masses ➡, which virtually replace the entire liver parenchyma.*

Metastases

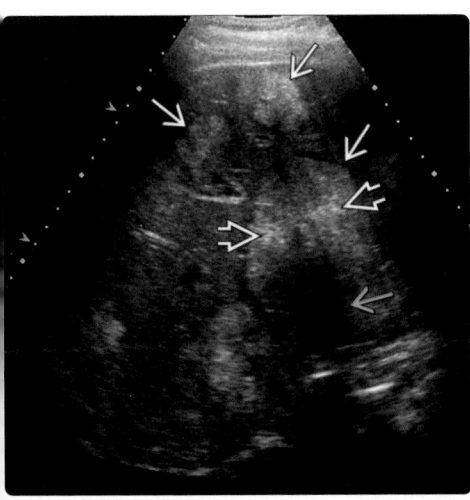

Sarcoidosis

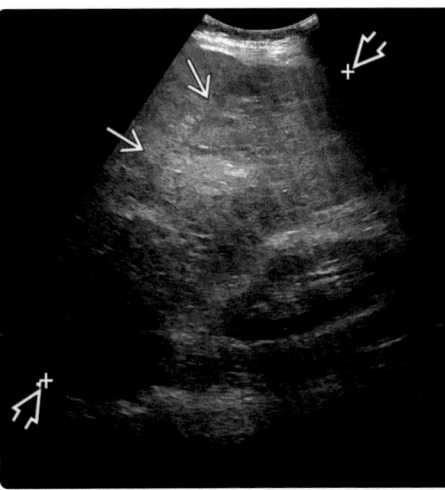

(Left) *Transverse abdominal ultrasound in a patient with colon cancer metastases in the liver shows multiple hyperechoic masses ➡, which enlarge the liver. Posterior acoustic shadowing ➡ associated with the largest mass is caused by calcifications ➡ in the liver metastasis.* (Right) *Transverse abdominal ultrasound in a patient with sarcoidosis shows hepatomegaly (26 cm in length) ➡ and heterogeneous hepatic parenchyma ➡ due to hepatic involvement by sarcoidosis.*

DIFFERENTIAL DIAGNOSIS

Common

- Steatosis (Fatty Liver)
- Cirrhosis
- Acute/Chronic Hepatitis
- Hepatocellular Carcinoma (Diffuse/Infiltrative)
- Infiltrative Metastasis
- Hepatic Lymphoma (Diffuse/Infiltrative)
- Biliary Hamartomas
- Technical Artifact (Mimic)

Less Common

- AIDS
- Hepatic Sarcoidosis
- Amyloidosis
- Schistosomiasis
- Glycogen Storage Disease
- Wilson Disease
- Venoocclusive Disease

ESSENTIAL INFORMATION

Key Differential Diagnosis Issues

- Diffusely increased echogenicity: Steatosis and cirrhosis account for most cases

Helpful Clues for Common Diagnoses

- **Steatosis (Fatty Liver)**
  - Diffuse increased echogenicity with acoustic attenuation
  - Liver often large with smooth contour
  - With increasing infiltration, vessels are pushed apart and hepatic veins take more curved course
- **Cirrhosis**
  - Heterogeneous parenchymal echogenicity
  - Liver surface nodularity, volume shrinkage
  - Altered flow dynamics in hepatic vasculature
- **Acute Hepatitis**
  - Decreased parenchymal echogenicity due to edema
    - Acute alcoholic hepatitis: Increased echogenicity

  - Hepatomegaly, periportal/gallbladder edema, ascites
- **Chronic Hepatitis**
  - Increased and heterogeneous parenchymal echogenicity
- **Hepatocellular Carcinoma (Diffuse/Infiltrative)**
  - Heterogeneous liver echotexture with refractive shadows
  - May accompany portal vein tumor thrombosis
- **Infiltrative Metastasis**
  - Lung or breast primary
  - May simulate cirrhosis
- **Hepatic Lymphoma (Diffuse/Infiltrative)**
  - Hepatomegaly
  - Numerous small hypoechoic foci, miliary in pattern and periportal in location
  - May be indistinguishable from normal liver
- **Biliary Hamartomas**
  - Tiny (< 1.5 cm) echogenic nodules with "comet-tail" artifacts
  - Numerous tiny lesions lead to inhomogeneous and coarse liver echotexture
- **Technical Artifact (Mimic)**
  - Improper transducer or gain setting

Helpful Clues for Less Common Diagnoses

- **AIDS**
  - Microabscesses from opportunistic infection (cytomegalovirus, mycobacterium, etc.)
- **Hepatic Sarcoidosis**
  - Diffuse heterogeneous echo pattern
  - Granulomas seen as hypoechoic nodules
- **Schistosomiasis**
  - Increased echogenicity caused by diffuse periportal septal thickening
- **Amyloidosis**
  - Hepatomegaly
  - Heterogeneous parenchymal echogenicity

SELECTED REFERENCES

1. Heller MT et al: The role of ultrasonography in the evaluation of diffuse liver disease. Radiol Clin North Am. 52(6):1163-75, 2014

Steatosis (Fatty Liver)

Cirrhosis

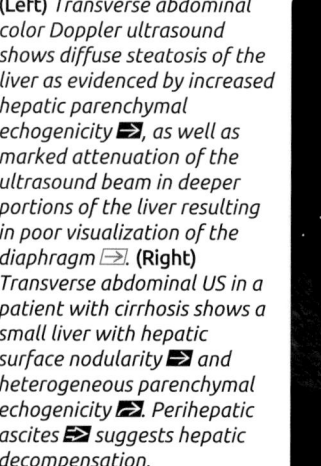

(Left) Transverse abdominal color Doppler ultrasound shows diffuse steatosis of the liver as evidenced by increased hepatic parenchymal echogenicity ➡, as well as marked attenuation of the ultrasound beam in deeper portions of the liver resulting in poor visualization of the diaphragm ➡. (Right) Transverse abdominal US in a patient with cirrhosis shows a small liver with hepatic surface nodularity ➡ and heterogeneous parenchymal echogenicity ➡. Perihepatic ascites ➡ suggests hepatic decompensation.

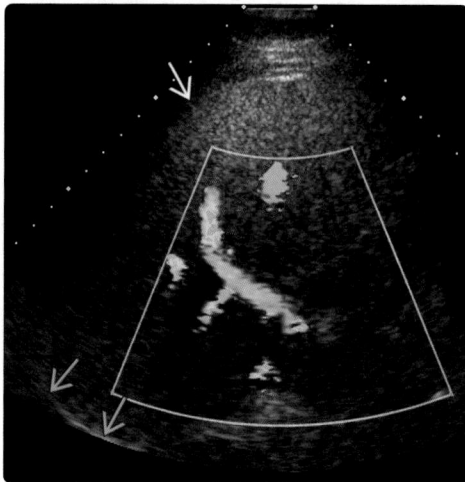

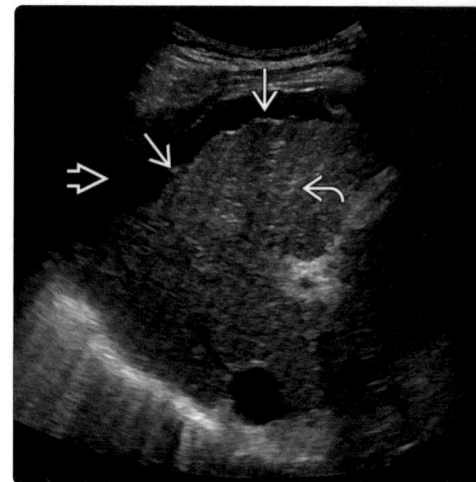

Acute/Chronic Hepatitis

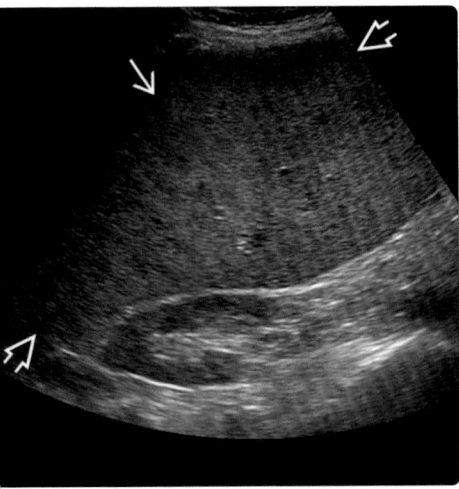

Hepatocellular Carcinoma (Diffuse/Infiltrative)

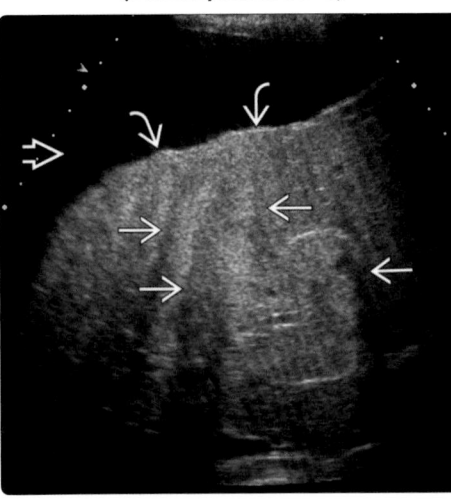

(Left) *Longitudinal abdominal ultrasound in a patient who presented with acute liver failure from acute alcoholic hepatitis shows marked hepatomegaly* ➡ *and slightly echogenic liver parenchyma* ➡. (Right) *Transverse abdominal ultrasound shows diffusely increased hepatic parenchymal echogenicity with multiple refractive shadows* ➡ *caused by diffuse, infiltrative hepatocellular carcinoma (HCC). Hepatic surface nodularity* ➡ *and ascites* ➡ *indicate underlying cirrhosis.*

Infiltrative Metastasis

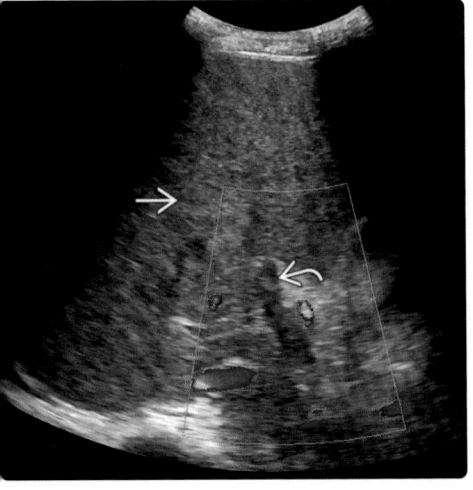

Biliary Hamartomas

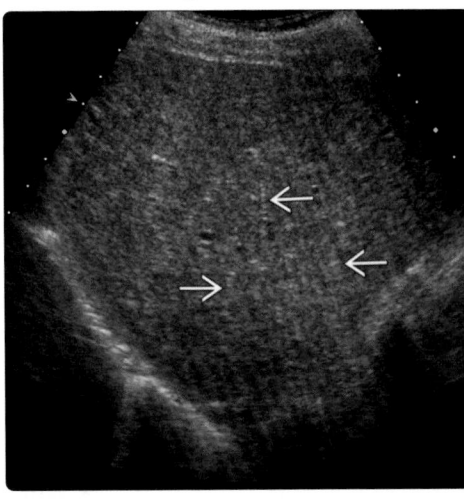

(Left) *Abdominal color Doppler ultrasound in a patient with renal cell carcinoma shows diffusely heterogeneous liver echogenicity caused by diffuse hepatic metastases* ➡. *Main portal vein is filled with hypoechoic material and shows no blood flow, suggesting thrombosis* ➡. (Right) *Oblique abdominal ultrasound shows diffuse and coarse liver parenchymal echotexture with multiple echogenic foci, some with associated "comet-tail artifacts"* ➡ *in a patient with numerous biliary hamartomas.*

Hepatic Sarcoidosis

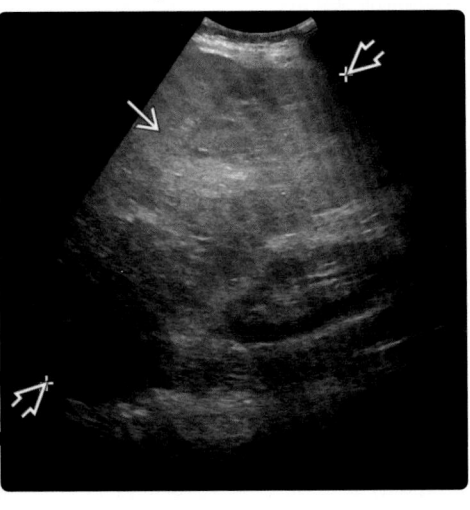

Amyloidosis

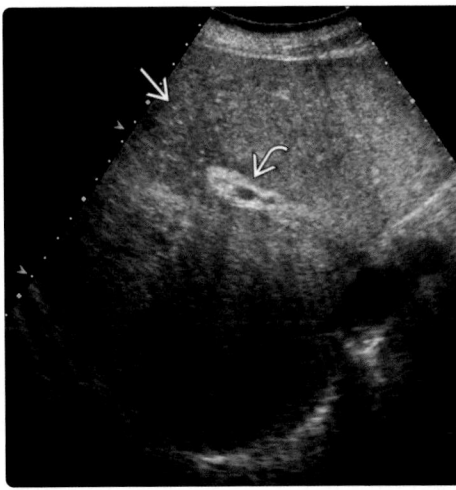

(Left) *Longitudinal abdominal ultrasound in a patient with sarcoidosis shows hepatomegaly (26 cm length)* ➡ *and heterogeneous liver parenchymal echogenicity* ➡ *due to hepatic involvement of sarcoidosis.* (Right) *Transverse abdominal ultrasound in a patient with amyloidosis shows heterogeneous and coarse liver echotexture* ➡ *and periportal edema* ➡ *due to hepatic involvement of amyloidosis.*

DIFFERENTIAL DIAGNOSIS

Common

- Hepatic Cyst
- Polycystic Liver Disease
- Pyogenic Hepatic Abscess
- Recent Hepatic Hemorrhage
- Biloma
- Vessels
- Biliary Cystadenoma/Cystadenocarcinoma
- Hepatic Echinococcal Cyst
- Peribiliary Cyst
- Biliary Hamartoma
- Amebic Abscess
- Dilated Bile Ducts

Less Common

- Hepatic Lymphoma
- Hepatic Metastases
- Ciliated Hepatic Foregut Cyst

Rare but Important

- Caroli Disease

ESSENTIAL INFORMATION

Key Differential Diagnosis Issues

- Lesions have few to no echoes within them
- Termed "simple"
  - When unilocular with no internal septa and not lobulated or irregular in contour
- Anechoic lesions tend to be round or oval-shaped with smooth contour on all surfaces
- Degree of posterior acoustic enhancement or shadowing and thickness of wall help limit differential diagnoses

Helpful Clues for Common Diagnoses

- **Hepatic Cyst**
  - Anechoic
  - Smooth borders but occasionally lobulated
  - Thin or imperceptible wall with no mural nodule
  - Well-defined back wall
  - Posterior acoustic enhancement
  - Often subcapsular and may bulge liver contour
  - Do not cross liver segments
  - Do not communicate with each other or bile ducts
  - No internal or mural vascularity but may distort adjacent vessels
  - May have internal echoes or septations after hemorrhage or infection
- **Polycystic Liver Disease**
  - May have concomitant autosomal dominant polycystic kidney disease
    - May make diagnosis of polycystic liver disease easier
    - Less likely to have pancreatic cysts as well
  - Individual cysts look identical to simple hepatic cysts
  - Number of cysts increases with age
  - When numerous and sizable, liver architecture is distorted, making diagnosis easier
  - Some cysts may be complicated by hemorrhage
    - Become hyperechoic or contain debris or septa

- **Pyogenic Hepatic Abscess**
  - Anechoic (50%), hyperechoic (25%), hypoechoic (25%)
  - Small or microabscesses closely simulate small cysts
    - May have internal echogenic debris when large
  - Variable in shape with thin or thick walls
  - Borders range from well defined to irregular
  - Tendency to cluster
    - Group of small pyogenic abscesses coalesce into single large cavity
  - May have adjacent hepatic parenchymal edema
    - Appears hypoechoic with coarse echo pattern ± vascularity
    - Vascularity may be seen in thick-walled portion
  - Diagnosis based on combination of clinical and sonographic features
- **Recent Hepatic Hemorrhage**
  - May be due to direct trauma, coagulopathy, surgery/biopsy
  - Initially traumatic hematoma is usually echogenic
    - Becomes anechoic after a few days
    - May have pseudowall of compressed liver parenchyma
  - Contour may be smooth or irregular
  - May be secondary hemorrhage into preexisting mass
    - Adenoma, hepatocellular carcinoma, metastasis, etc.
    - Usually not completely anechoic
- **Biloma**
  - Almost always secondary to trauma
    - Difficult to differentiate from traumatic hematoma
      - Hematomas show debris, septations over time
      - Bilomas remain anechoic
  - Round or oval in shape
  - Fluid content may be anechoic with posterior acoustic enhancement
    - Suggests fresh biloma
  - Thin capsule wall usually not discernible
  - Larger lesions may compress adjacent liver surface/architecture
  - Communicates with biliary tree
  - No vascularity within lesion
- **Vessels**
  - Portal veins: Venectasia, varicosities, collaterals from portal hypertension
  - Hepatic veins: Venectasia, Budd-Chiari, etc.
  - Hepatic arteries: Aneurysms, shunts, vascular malformation
  - Use of color Doppler
    - Confirm vascular nature and vessel type
- **Biliary Cystadenoma/Cystadenocarcinoma**
  - Well-defined, multiloculated, anechoic or hypoechoic mass
  - Highly echogenic septa
  - May see internal echoes with complex fluid, calcifications, mural/septal nodules, or papillary projections
    - More commonly associated with biliary cystadenocarcinoma
  - Color Doppler: Septal vascularity
  - Most commonly seen in middle-aged women
- **Hepatic Echinococcal Cyst**

- o May be solitary or multiple
- o Large, well-defined, cystic liver mass with numerous peripheral daughter cysts
- o Cyst-within-cyst appearance
- o Floating membrane within cyst
- o Layered cyst wall is diagnostic
  - – Thickness reduces posterior acoustic enhancement

Peribiliary Cyst
- o Well-defined cystic lesions of round/oval/tubular shape along portal triads
- o Usually multiple; discrete or confluent configuration
- o Smooth and thin walls without internal echoes
- o Variable size from 2 mm to 2 cm
- o No communication with biliary tree

Biliary Hamartoma
- o Numerous small hypoechoic/hyperechoic foci uniformly distributed throughout liver
  - – Leads to inhomogeneous and coarse appearance of liver echotexture
- o Multiple echogenic foci often associated with "comet tail" artifacts
- o Typically smaller lesions appear as echogenic foci while larger lesions appear cystic
  - – Extent of echogenic foci on US is greater than anticipated
  - – Small lesions are too small to resolve sonographically
- o Color Doppler US: Twinkling artifact may be associated with echogenic foci

Amebic Abscess
- o Sharply demarcated, round or ovoid mass
- o Hypoechoic with low-level internal echoes
- o May see internal septa or wall nodularity
- o May see posterior acoustic enhancement

Dilated Bile Ducts
- o Ducts may simulate anechoic nodules when viewed on cross section
- o Ducts follow periportal distribution
  - – Long axis orientation with hepatic artery/portal vein provide clues to its nature

Helpful Clues for Less Common Diagnoses
- **Hepatic Lymphoma**
  - o May be irregular or round/oval in shape
  - o ± posterior acoustic enhancement, "pseudocystic" appearance
  - o Extrahepatic signs such as lymphadenopathy, splenomegaly (± splenic infiltration)
- **Hepatic Metastases**
  - o Anechoic hepatic metastasis
    - – Suggests low degree of differentiation and high-grade malignancy
  - o Usually no posterior acoustic enhancement
  - o May have debris, mural nodularity, &/or thick septations
  - o May have irregular margins and contour
  - o Wall vascularity
- **Ciliated Hepatic Foregut Cyst**
  - o Unilocular subcapsular solitary cyst located in segment 4a

Helpful Clues for Rare Diagnoses
- **Caroli Disease**
  - o Central dot sign: Portal radicles within dilated intrahepatic bile ducts on color Doppler ultrasound

Technical Issues
- Important to make sure that gain settings are correct
- Gallbladder or inferior vena cava can be used as internal references for gain settings
  - o These anatomic structures should normally look anechoic

SELECTED REFERENCES
1. Corvino A et al: Contrast-Enhanced Ultrasound in the Characterization of Complex Cystic Focal Liver Lesions. Ultrasound Med Biol. ePub, 2015
2. Borhani AA et al: Cystic hepatic lesions: a review and an algorithmic approach. AJR Am J Roentgenol. 203(6):1192-204, 2014
3. Lantinga MA et al: Evaluation of hepatic cystic lesions. World J Gastroenterol. 19(23):3543-54, 2013
4. Vachha B et al: Cystic lesions of the liver. AJR Am J Roentgenol. 196(4):W355-66, 2011

Hepatic Cyst

Polycystic Liver Disease

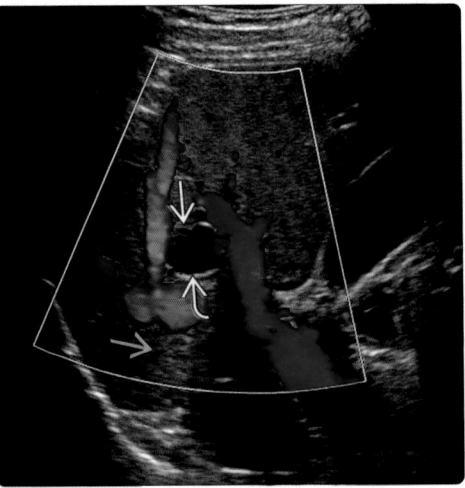
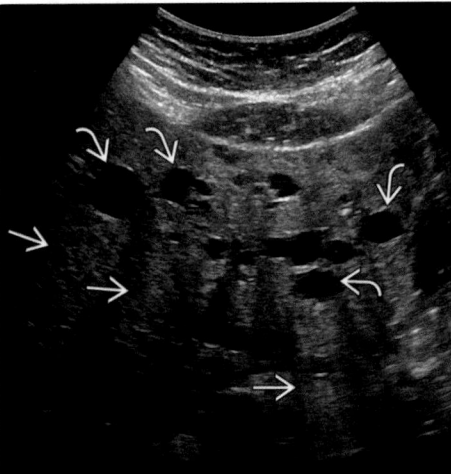

(Left) Transverse color Doppler US shows a well-defined round hepatic cyst with no internal vascularity ➡, well-defined back wall ➡, and posterior acoustic enhancement ➡, confirming the cystic nature of the lesion. (Right) Transverse grayscale US of the liver shows numerous cysts ➡ throughout the liver in a patient with polycystic liver disease. Posterior acoustic enhancement ➡ is associated with each of the cysts, confirming cystic nature of lesions.

Pyogenic Hepatic Abscess

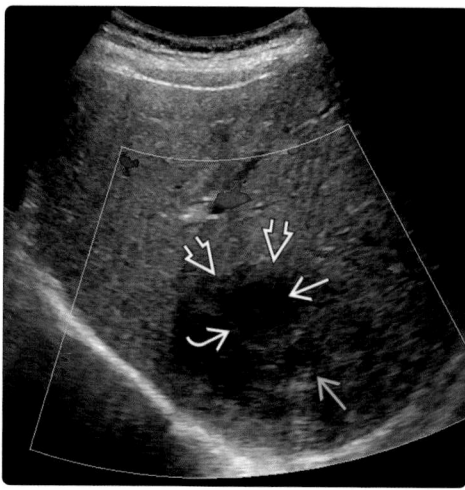

Biloma

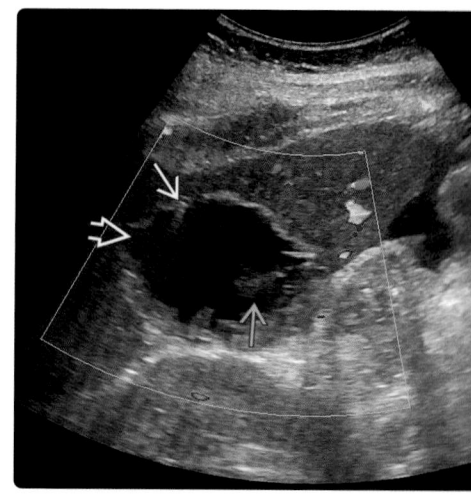

(Left) *Oblique transabdominal color Doppler ultrasound shows a centrally cystic hepatic abscess* ➡ *with surrounding hypoechoic hepatic parenchyma* ➡ *in the right lobe of liver. Central internal septations* ➡ *and echogenic debris* ➡ *are seen within the hepatic abscess.* (Right) *Transverse color Doppler US of the liver shows a biloma* ➡ *in a resection cavity with peripheral echogenic foci* ➡ *and ring-down artifact related to surgical clips. A small amount of internal debris is seen in the periphery of the biloma* ➡.

Vessels

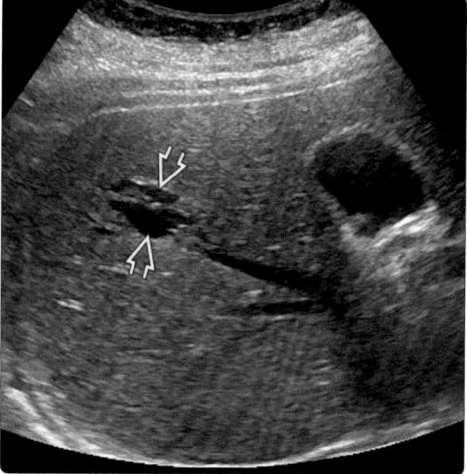

Vessels

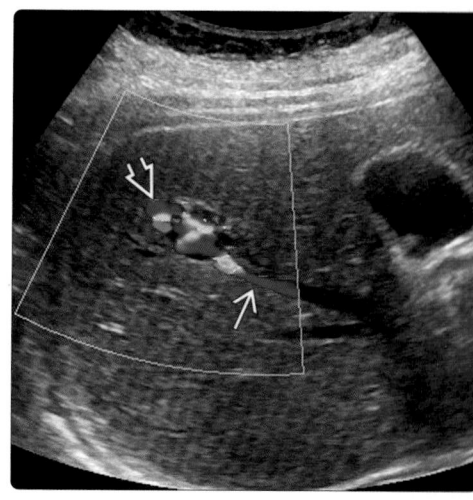

(Left) *Transverse grayscale US of the liver shows 2 adjacent well-defined tubular shaped anechoic lesions* ➡ *in the right lobe of the liver.* (Right) *On color Doppler US in the same patient the lesion is found to represent a vascular structure* ➡, *which drains into the middle hepatic vein* ➡. *Color Doppler US should always be used to evaluate anechoic appearing lesions as they may in fact be vascular, as in this case of a spontaneous intrahepatic portosystemic shunt.*

Biliary Cystadenoma/Cystadenocarcinoma

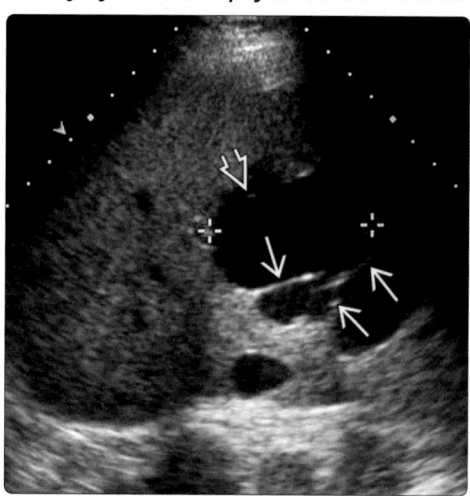

Hepatic Echinococcal Cyst

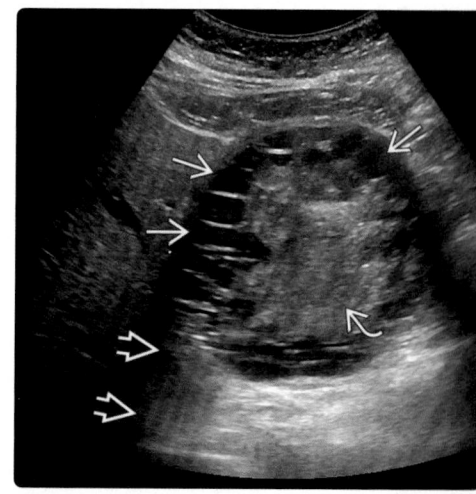

(Left) *Transverse grayscale US of the liver shows a biliary cystadenoma with sonographic imaging appearance of a complex cyst* ➡ *with multiple septations* ➡. *Most biliary cystadenomas are seen in middle-aged females.* (Right) *Transverse abdominal US shows an echinococcal cyst containing multiple peripheral daughter cysts* ➡ *and central heterogeneous content* ➡ *in the left lobe of the liver. Associated posterior acoustic enhancement* ➡ *is seen.*

Peribiliary Cyst

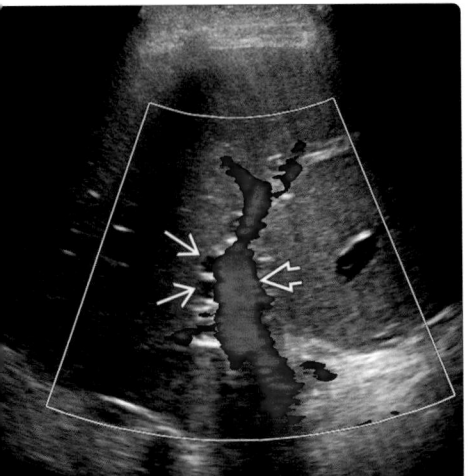

Biliary Hamartoma

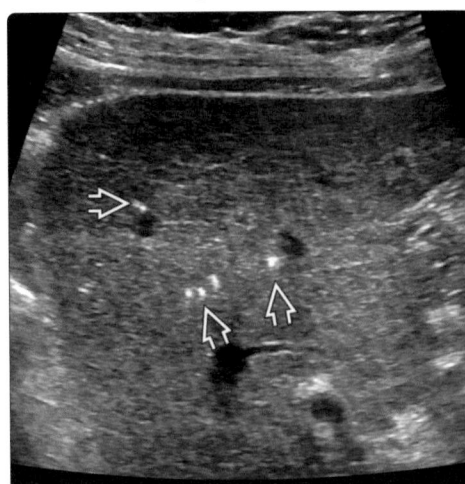

(Left) *Color Doppler US shows peribiliary cysts* ➡ *located adjacent to the portal vein* ➡. *Peribiliary cysts should not be confused with biliary ductal dilatation, which would have a more tubular and continuous appearance adjacent to the portal vein.* (Right) *Grayscale ultrasound of the liver shows multiple tiny, echogenic foci* ➡ *with "comet tail" artifacts generated from biliary hamartomas.*

Amebic Abscess

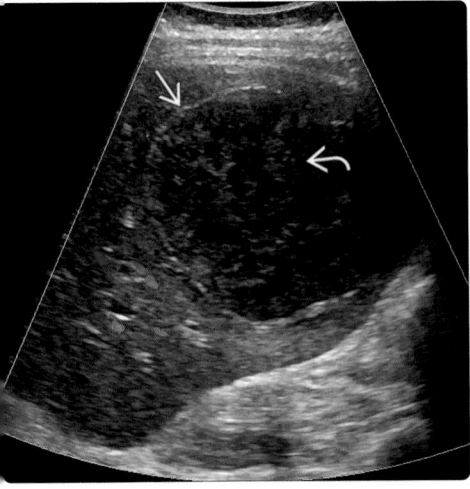

Hepatic Lymphoma

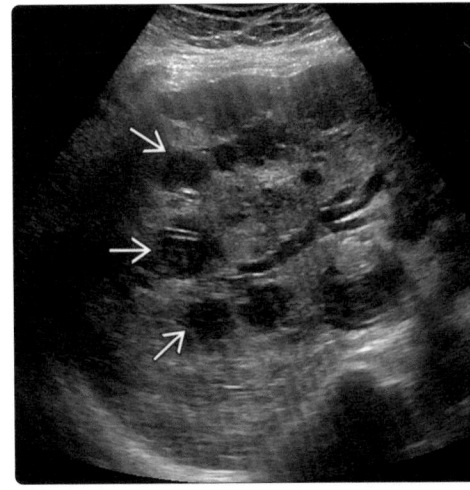

(Left) *Sagittal grayscale ultrasound of the liver shows a large, well-demarcated and encapsulated hypoechoic amebic abscess* ➡. *The contents are heterogeneous due to floating debris* ➡. *No vascularity is seen within the abscess.* (Right) *Transverse abdominal ultrasound in a patient with lymphoma shows multiple markedly hypoechoic nodules* ➡ *throughout the right lobe of the liver, which have a pseudocystic appearance.*

Hepatic Metastases

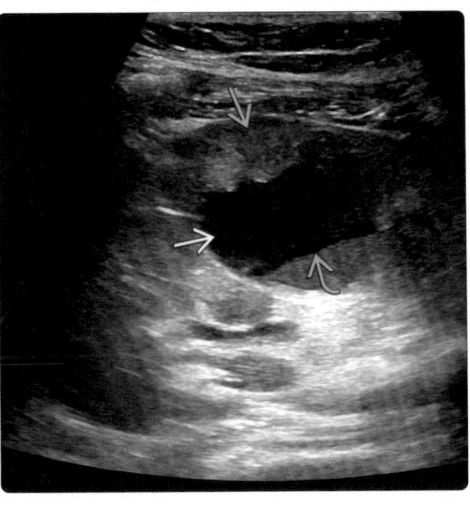

Ciliated Hepatic Foregut Cyst

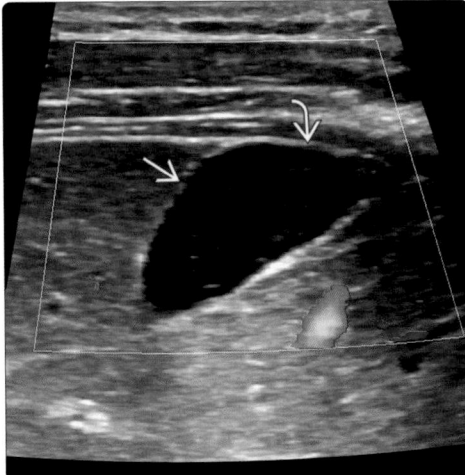

(Left) *Cystic liver metastasis in a patient with metastatic cervical cancer displays a central cystic area* ➡ *as well as an echogenic soft tissue rim* ➡ *and layering debris* ➡ *within the dependent portion of the mass.* (Right) *Oblique abdominal color Doppler US in a patient with a ciliated hepatic foregut cyst shows a well-defined, ovoid, subcapsular cystic mass* ➡ *in segment IV of the liver* ➡. *Internal content of the cystic lesion is relatively homogeneous, and no vascularity is seen.*

DIFFERENTIAL DIAGNOSIS

Common

- Complicated Benign Hepatic Cyst
- Hepatic Metastases
- Infection
  - Pyogenic Hepatic Abscess
  - Amebic Hepatic Abscess
  - Fungal Hepatic Abscess
- Focal Fatty Sparing
- Hepatocellular Carcinoma
- Infected Biloma

Less Common

- Hepatic Lymphoma
- Hepatic Adenoma
- Focal Nodular Hyperplasia
- Atypical Hemangioma
- Hepatic Hematoma
- Abnormal Bile Ducts
- Abnormal Vessels

ESSENTIAL INFORMATION

Key Differential Diagnosis Issues

- Lesions of lower echogenicity than liver parenchyma (compared to purely anechoic lesions)
  - With some low-level internal echogenicity
  - Solid lesion vs. complex cystic lesion

Helpful Clues for Common Diagnoses

- **Complicated Benign Hepatic Cyst**
  - Superimposed hemorrhage or infection in hepatic cyst
  - Septation/thickened wall ± mural calcification
  - Posterior acoustic enhancement
  - Solid appearance
    - If internal debris (clots or fibrin strands) dispersed within cyst
  - Fluid-debris level
    - If debris settles under influence of gravity
  - No mural nodule
  - Color Doppler
    - Absence of internal or mural vascularity
    - Adjacent vessels distorted by large cyst
- **Hepatic Metastases**
  - Hypoechoic metastases tend to be numerous and small
    - Larger lesions tend to have heterogeneous echogenicity
  - May have irregular or ill-defined borders
  - Hypoechogenicity
    - May reflect poor cellular differentiation and active growth
  - Suggest hypovascular and hypercellular tumor origin
    - Lung, breast, lymphoma
  - No posterior acoustic enhancement
  - Causes architectural distortion
    - If large or numerous
  - Color Doppler may show no vascularity
    - Most are hypovascular
  - Difficult to differentiate from lymphoma without history of known primary lesion

- **Pyogenic Hepatic Abscess**
  - Cystic mass with irregular border and debris
  - Posterior acoustic enhancement
  - Multiple thick or thin septations
  - Mural nodularity & vascularity
  - Adjacent parenchyma may be coarse & hypoechoic due to inflammation
  - "Cluster" sign: Coalescence of group of abscesses
  - May contain gas within abscess
    - Reverberation artifact or air-fluid level
  - Changes to anechoic when center becomes necrotic as center enlarges
  - Periportal distribution suggests dissemination along biliary tree
  - Random distribution suggests hematogenous spread
- **Amebic Hepatic Abscess**
  - Abuts liver capsule, under diaphragm
  - More likely to be round or oval-shaped than pyogenic abscess
  - Hypoechoic with fine internal echoes
    - More common in amebic than pyogenic abscess
  - Internal septa may be present
  - Posterior acoustic enhancement
  - No vascularity seen in wall or septa of abscess
  - Subdiaphragmatic rupture in presence of adjacent hepatic abscess
    - Suggests amebic nature of abscess
- **Focal Fatty Sparing**
  - Geographic hypoechoic area within echogenic liver
  - Due to direct drainage of hepatic flow into systemic circulation
  - Typical locations
    - Gallbladder fossa
      - Drained by cystic vein
    - Inferior aspect of segment 4b
      - Drained by aberrant gastric vein
    - Anterior to bifurcation of portal vein
      - Drained by aberrant gastric vein
    - Around hepatic veins
  - No architectural distortion
    - Vessels course through mass undistorted
    - No mass effect
  - Does not cross segments
- **Hepatocellular Carcinoma (HCC)**
  - Hypoechoic: Most common US appearance of HCC
    - Solid tumor
    - May be surrounded by thin, hypoechoic halo (capsule)
  - Background cirrhotic liver
  - Associated signs of portal hypertension
    - Ascites, splenomegaly, portosystemic collaterals
  - Color Doppler
    - Irregular hypervascularity
    - Portal vein thrombus with arterial neovascularity
- **Infected Biloma**
  - Fluid collection within liver, close to biliary tree, or in gallbladder fossa
  - Debris or septa suggest infected biloma
  - Color Doppler
    - No vascularity within lesion

– Adjacent hepatic parenchyma may demonstrate reactive hypervascularity

Helpful Clues for Less Common Diagnoses

- **Hepatic Lymphoma**
  o Hypoechoic mass with irregular margins
  o Marked hypoechogenicity
    – Probably due to high cellular density and lack of background stroma
  o Large/conglomerate masses may appear to contain septa and mimic abscesses
    – May have a "pseudocystic" appearance
  o Other sites of involvement commonly seen
    – Lymphadenopathy, splenomegaly ± focal splenic lesions provide clues to diagnosis
- **Hepatic Adenoma**
  o Only slightly hypoechoic compared to normal liver parenchyma
    – May be isoechoic
  o May have hypoechoic rim
  o Complications: Hemorrhage, central necrosis, and rupture may be present
  o Color Doppler shows distinct venous vascularity at borders
- **Focal Nodular Hyperplasia**
  o Usually homogeneous and isoechoic to liver
    – Occasionally hypoechoic or hyperechoic
  o Central hypoechoic stellate scar with radiating fibrous septa
  o Mass effect
    – Displacement of normal hepatic vessels and ducts
  o Color Doppler: Hypervascularity
    – "Spoke-wheel" pattern
      □ Large central feeding artery with multiple small vessels radiating peripherally
    – Large draining veins at tumor margin
    – Hemorrhage is rare
- **Atypical Hemangioma**
  o < 10% of hemangiomas are hypoechoic to liver parenchyma

– Usually with hyperechoic rim
    – "Typical atypical" appearance
  o May appear hypoechoic in fatty liver
    – Due to background hyperechoic liver
  o Hypoechoic areas within large lesions
    – May represent necrosis, hemorrhage, scar, or vessels
  o Smooth, well-defined borders
  o May see posterior acoustic enhancement
  o No visible color Doppler flow
    – Flow too slow to be detected
    – May be detected with power Doppler
- **Hepatic Hematoma**
  o Echogenicity evolves over time
    – Initially: Echogenic
    – After 4-5 days: Hypoechoic
    – After 1-4 weeks: Internal echoes and septations
- **Abnormal Bile Ducts**
  o Dilated duct with sludge or tumor
  o Interrogate in perpendicular plane to show its tubular nature
- **Abnormal Vessels**
  o Dilated portal or hepatic vein with hypoechoic thrombus
  o Interrogate in perpendicular plane to show its tubular nature

SELECTED REFERENCES

1. Corvino A et al: Contrast-Enhanced Ultrasound in the Characterization of Complex Cystic Focal Liver Lesions. Ultrasound Med Biol. ePub, 2015
2. Kunze G et al: Contrast-enhanced ultrasound in different stages of pyogenic liver abscess. Ultrasound Med Biol. 41(4):952-9, 2015
3. Klotz T et al: Hepatic haemangioma: common and uncommon imaging features. Diagn Interv Imaging. 94(9):849-59, 2013
4. Bhatnagar G et al: The varied sonographic appearances of focal fatty liver disease: review and diagnostic algorithm. Clin Radiol. 67(4):372-9, 2012
5. Bartolotta TV et al: Focal liver lesions: contrast-enhanced ultrasound. Abdom Imaging. 34(2):193-209, 2009
6. Wang ZL et al: Undetermined focal liver lesions on gray-scale ultrasound in patients with fatty liver: characterization with contrast-enhanced ultrasound. J Gastroenterol Hepatol. 23(10):1511-9, 2008
7. D'Onofrio M et al: Hypoechoic focal liver lesions: characterization with contrast enhanced ultrasonography. J Clin Ultrasound. 33(4):164-72, 2005

Complicated Benign Hepatic Cyst

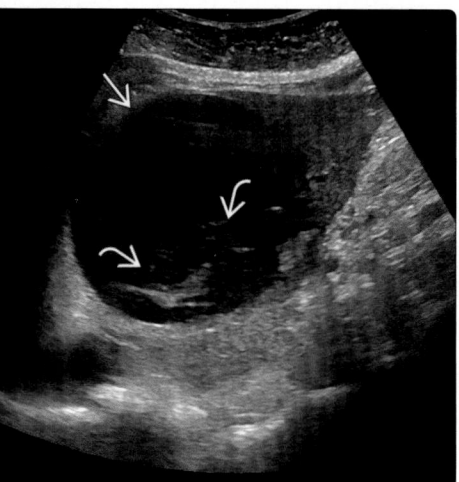

Hepatic Metastases

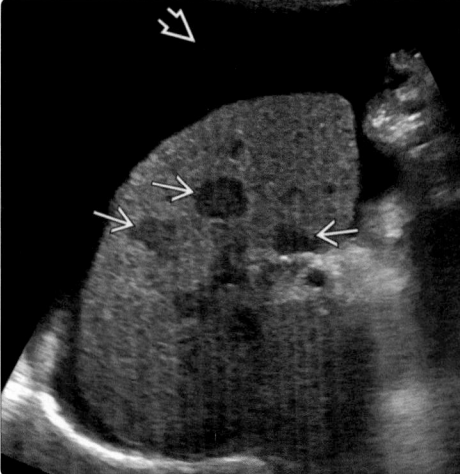

(Left) *Longitudinal oblique US of the liver shows a complicated liver cyst* ➡ *with internal layering debris* ➡ *from hemorrhage. Depending on age and amount internal hemorrhage, degree of echogenicity in a complicated cyst may vary.* **(Right)** *Grayscale abdominal US in a patient with breast cancer shows multiple well-defined hypoechoic metastatic lesions* ➡ *in the liver. Large amount of ascites is seen* ➡.

Hepatic Metastases

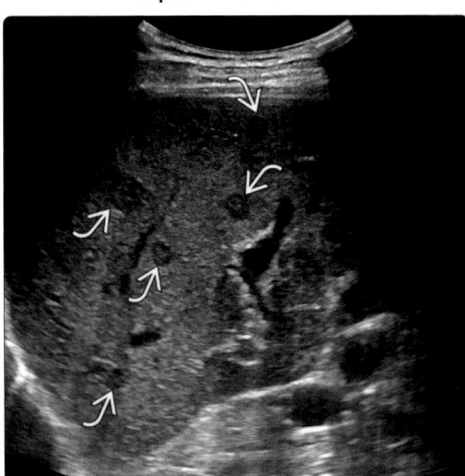

Pyogenic Hepatic Abscess

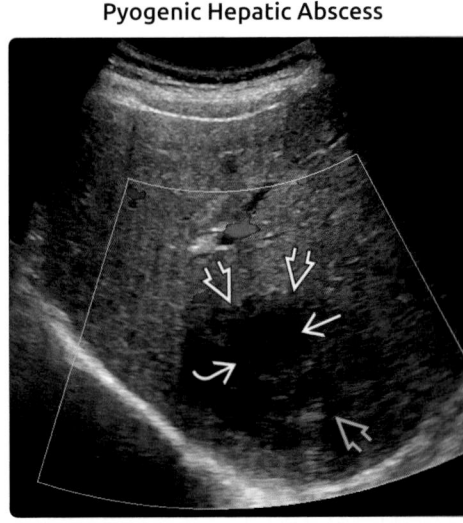

(Left) *Transverse abdominal US in a patient with colon cancer shows multiple small hypoechoic metastatic nodules in the right lobe of the liver* ➔. *(Right) Oblique abdominal color Doppler US shows a centrally cystic hepatic pyogenic abscess* ➔ *with surrounding hypoechoic hepatic parenchyma* ➔ *in the right lobe of the liver. Internal septations* ➔ *and echogenic debris* ➔ *are seen within the abscess.*

Amebic Hepatic Abscess

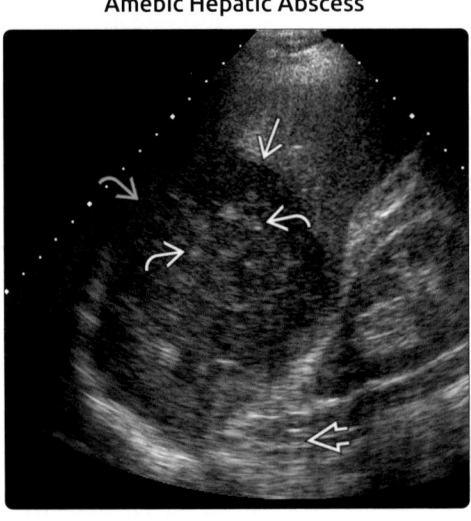

Fungal Hepatic Abscess

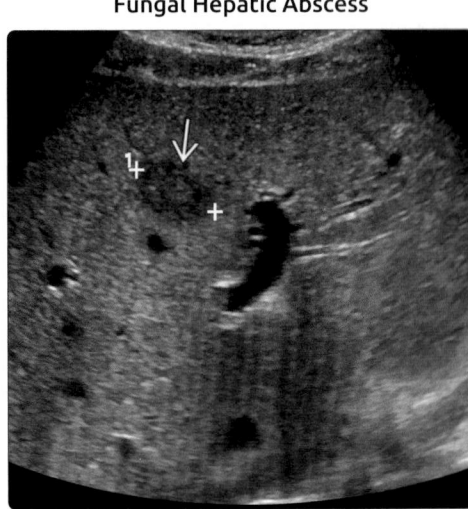

(Left) *Longitudinal abdominal US shows a large, round, hypoechoic amebic abscess in the right lobe of the liver* ➔ *abutting the liver capsule* ➔. *Internal contents are hypoechoic with heterogeneously echogenic scattered foci* ➔. *Mild posterior acoustic enhancement is seen* ➔. *(Right) Transverse abdominal US shows a hypoechoic fungal abscess in segment 4 of the liver* ➔.

Focal Fatty Sparing

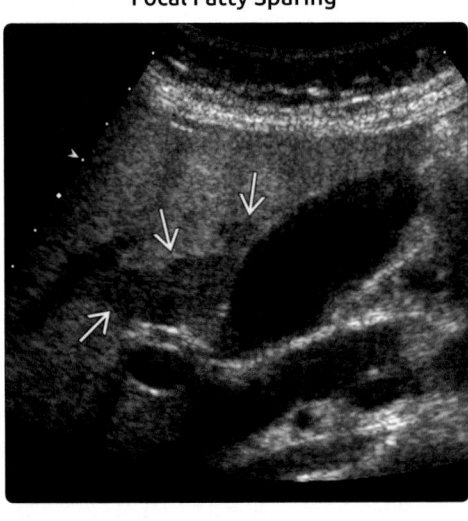

Hepatocellular Carcinoma

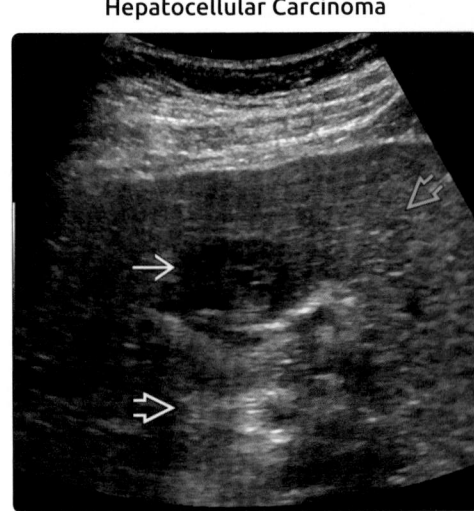

(Left) *Longitudinal abdominal US shows focal fatty sparing adjacent to the gallbladder fossa as a geographic area of decreased echogenicity* ➔ *in an otherwise echogenic liver due to diffuse steatosis. Liver adjacent to the gallbladder fossa is a typical location for fatty sparing.* **(Right)** *Transverse abdominal US shows a hypoechoic HCC* ➔. *Posterior acoustic enhancement is seen* ➔. *Underlying liver shows heterogeneous echotexture* ➔ *indicating background cirrhosis.*

Infected Biloma

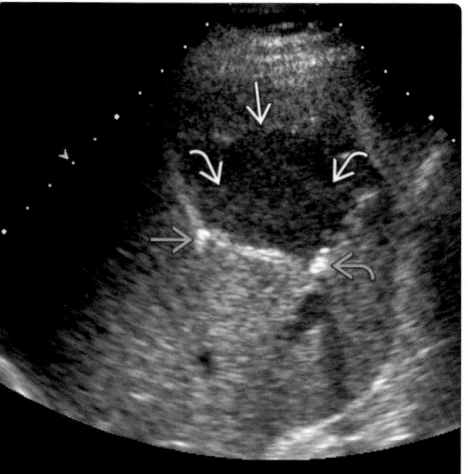

Hepatic Lymphoma

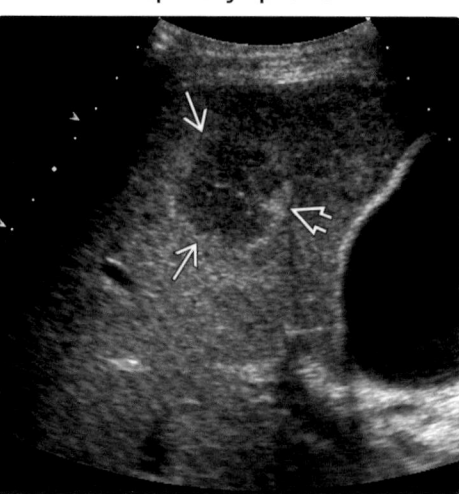

(Left) *Grayscale US shows a biloma ➡ after surgical removal of a liver mass. Low-level internal echoes ➡ suggest infected bile. Peripheral surgical suture with ring-down artifact ➡ and clip with posterior shadowing ➡ are seen along the cut liver edge.* **(Right)** *Transverse abdominal US in a patient with hepatic lymphoma shows a well-defined hypoechoic mass ➡ with thin hyperechoic rim ➡ in segment 5 of the liver.*

Hepatic Lymphoma

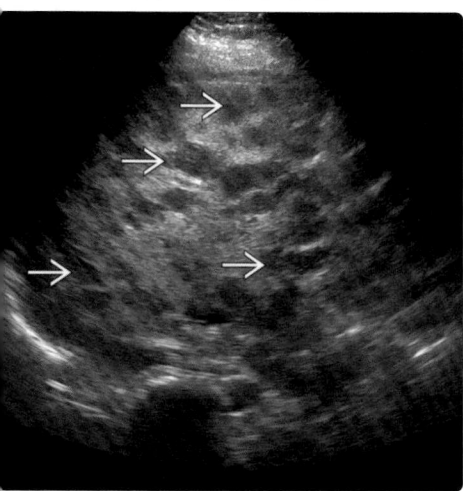

Hepatic Adenoma

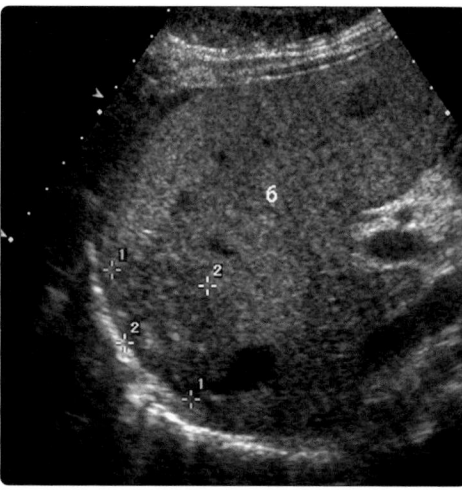

(Left) *Transverse abdominal US in a patient with hepatic lymphoma shows multiple hypoechoic nodules ➡ throughout the liver, consistent with diffuse hepatic involvement of lymphoma.* **(Right)** *Longitudinal abdominal US of the liver shows a heterogeneous slightly hypoechoic hepatic adenoma (demarcated by calipers) abutting the dome of the liver.*

Focal Nodular Hyperplasia

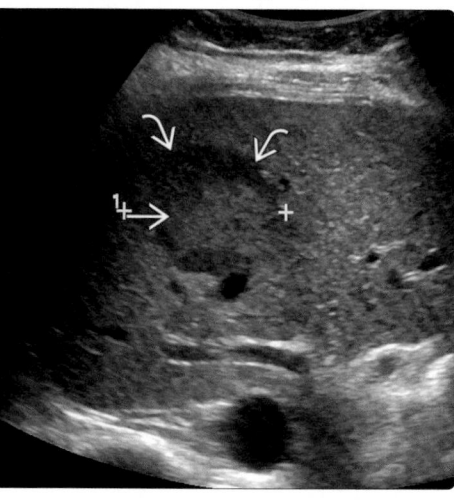

Atypical Hemangioma

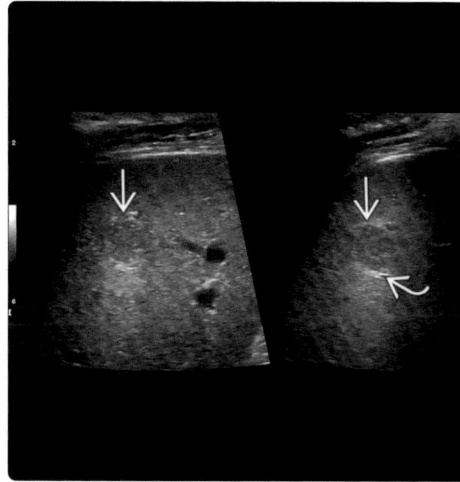

(Left) *Transverse abdominal US shows a predominantly hypoechoic focal nodular hyperplasia (FNH) ➡ with isoechoic center ➡ in the right lobe of the liver. In contrast to this case, most FNHs are isoechoic to background liver, making sonographic identification often challenging and earning the moniker "stealth lesion."* **(Right)** *Transverse abdominal US shows a hypoechoic hemangioma ➡ with thin hyperechoic rim ➡ in the right lobe of the liver, which is a "typical atypical" US finding of hepatic hemangioma.*

DIFFERENTIAL DIAGNOSIS

Common

- Focal Steatosis
- Hepatic Cavernous Hemangioma
- Hepatic Metastases
- Pyogenic Hepatic Abscess
- Normal Anatomic Pitfalls
  - Hepatic Ligaments and Fissures
  - Diaphragmatic Leaflets
  - Refractile Artifact
- Hepatocellular Carcinoma (HCC)

Less Common

- Cholangiocarcinoma (Intrahepatic)
- Hepatic Adenoma
- Fibrolamellar Carcinoma
- Amebic Hepatic Abscess
- Hepatic Angiomyolipoma (AML)
- Biliary Hamartoma
- Hepatic Hydatid/*Echinococcus* Cyst
- Hepatic Epithelioid Hemangioendothelioma (HEHE)
- Hepatic Lipoma

ESSENTIAL INFORMATION

Key Differential Diagnosis Issues

- Is echogenic lesion mass or echogenic focus?
  - Mass: Usually spherical
  - Echogenic focus: Often linear, such as surgical device, pneumobilia, portal vein gas, etc.
- Significant overlap in appearance of many echogenic masses
  - Contrast-enhanced triphasic CT or MR may be needed for further characterization

Helpful Clues for Common Diagnoses

- **Focal Steatosis**
  - No mass effect, with vessels running undisplaced through lesion
  - Varied appearances
    - Hyperechoic nodule/confluent hyperechoic lesions
      - May simulate metastases
    - Fan-shaped lobar/segmental distribution
  - CT or MR are good problem-solving tools
- **Hepatic Cavernous Hemangioma**
  - Typically homogeneously hyperechoic
    - Probably due to slow blood flow rather than multiple interfaces
    - Smooth or lobulated well-defined borders
    - May have acoustic enhancement
  - Echogenicity may vary
    - Echogenicity may change over time during imaging
    - Direction and angle of insonation may alter echogenic appearance
    - May appear hypoechoic in underlying fatty liver
    - Large lesions more heterogeneous
- **Hepatic Metastases**
  - Hyperechoic metastases: Most commonly from GI tract
  - Vascular metastases

- Neuroendocrine tumors, melanoma, choriocarcinoma, renal cell carcinoma
  - Target or bull's-eye appearance
    - Iso- or hyperechoic metastatic nodule with hypoechoic rim or halo
    - Usually from aggressive primary tumors
    - Bronchogenic carcinoma: Classic example
  - Calcified metastasis
    - Markedly echogenic interface with acoustic shadowing or diffuse small echogenic foci
    - Mucinous primary: Colon, ovary, breast
    - Calcific/ossific primary: Osteosarcoma, chondrosarcoma, neuroblastoma, malignant teratoma
    - Treated metastasis
- **Pyogenic Hepatic Abscess**
  - Echogenicity of abscess
    - Anechoic (50%), hyperechoic (25%), hypoechoic (25%)
    - Early lesions tend to be echogenic and poorly demarcated
    - May evolve into well-defined, nearly anechoic lesions
  - "Cluster" sign
    - Cluster of small pyogenic abscesses coalesce into single large cavity
  - Fluid level or debris, internal septa
  - Abscess wall: Hypoechoic or mildly echogenic
  - Gas within abscess: Bright echogenic foci with posterior reverberation artifact
- **Normal Anatomic Pitfalls**
  - **Hepatic Ligaments & Fissures, Diaphragmatic Leaflets**
    - Infolding of fat along these normal structures creates echogenic focus near surface of liver
    - In short axis section, "lesions" can appear spherical and resemble masses
    - Turn US beam perpendicular to show linear shape of "lesion"
  - **Refractile Artifact**
    - Lateral edge shadows at junction of vessels or gallbladder neck
- **Hepatocellular Carcinoma (HCC)**
  - Hyperechoic appearance indicates fatty metamorphosis/hypervascularity
    - Simulates hemangioma or focal steatosis
      - Look for background cirrhotic liver, portal vein thrombosis, risk factors (hep B, C, alcohol)
      - Generally irregular intratumoral vascularity
  - Small lesions more likely to be hyperechoic

Helpful Clues for Less Common Diagnoses

- **Cholangiocarcinoma (Intrahepatic)**
  - Heterogeneous mass with ill-defined margin and satellite nodules
    - Mostly hyperechoic (75%); iso-/hypoechoic (14%)
  - Isolated intrahepatic ductal dilatation upstream to mass without extrahepatic duct dilatation
- **Hepatic Adenoma**
  - Young woman with oral contraceptive use
  - Heterogeneous and hypervascular mass with hemorrhage
  - Complex hyper-/hypoechoic mass with anechoic areas
    - Due to fat, hemorrhage, necrosis or calcification
  - Well-defined border, round or lobulated

- **Fibrolamellar Carcinoma**
  - Large heterogeneous mass in adolescent or young adult
  - Well-defined and partially or completely encapsulated mass
  - Prominent central fibrous scar (hypo- or hyperechoic)
    - Calcification within scar common
  - Intratumoral necrosis/hemorrhage
  - Background cirrhosis or hepatitis in < 5% of patients
- **Amebic Hepatic Abscess**
  - Usually homogeneous and hypoechoic
    - Hyperechoic if complicated by bacterial superinfection or bowel fistula
  - Low-level internal echoes due to debris
  - Peripheral location: Abuts liver capsule, under diaphragm
- **Hepatic Angiomyolipoma (AML)**
  - Homogeneous/heterogeneous echogenic mass
    - Hyperechoic due to fat
  - May be hypoechoic if muscle, vascular elements, or hemorrhage predominate
- **Biliary Hamartoma**
  - Numerous small hypo/hyperechoic foci uniformly distributed throughout liver
    - When small, appear hyperechoic due to inability to resolve tiny cysts
    - Leads to inhomogeneous and coarse appearance of liver echotexture
  - Multiple echogenic foci
    - Often with associated "comet tail" artifacts
  - Typically smaller lesions appear as echogenic foci, whereas larger lesions appear cystic
    - Extent of echogenic foci on US is greater than anticipated, based on comparison CT or MR
- **Hepatic Hydatid/*Echinococcus* Cyst**
  - Membranes ± daughter cysts in complex heterogeneous mass
  - Anechoic cyst with internal debris, hydatid sand
  - *E. multilocularis*
    - Single or multiple echogenic lesions
    - Irregular necrotic areas and microcalcifications
    - Infiltrative solid masses

- – Invasion of IVC and diaphragm
- **Hepatic Epithelioid Hemangioendothelioma (HEHE)**
  - Variable echogenicity pattern
    - Predominantly hypoechoic
    - Hyper-/isoechoic lesions; may have peripheral hypoechoic rim
  - Often associated with adjacent retracted capsule
- **Hepatic Lipoma**
  - Extremely uncommon lesion
  - Contain mature adipose tissue

Alternative Differential Approaches

- Vascular masses
  - Cavernous hemangioma, HCC, hemangioendothelioma, angiosarcoma
- Fat-containing masses
  - Focal fatty infiltration, hepatic adenoma, HCC, lipid-containing metastases, angiomyolipoma, lipoma, liposarcoma, teratoma (primary or metastatic to liver)
- Gas-containing masses
  - Abscess, infarction, treated hepatic tumors with resulting sudden necrosis
- Solid masses
  - Primary liver tumors, metastases, cholangiocarcinoma
- Masses with calcified rim
  - Chronic cystic masses
- Masses with calcified scar
  - Fibrolamellar, HCC, cavernous hemangioma (large ones)

SELECTED REFERENCES

1. Bhatnagar G et al: The varied sonographic appearances of focal fatty liver disease: review and diagnostic algorithm. Clin Radiol. 67(4):372-9, 2012
2. Kamaya A et al: Hypervascular liver lesions. Semin Ultrasound CT MR. 30(5):387-407, 2009
3. Basaran C et al: Fat-containing lesions of the liver: cross-sectional imaging findings with emphasis on MRI. AJR Am J Roentgenol. 184(4):1103-10, 2005
4. Prasad SR et al: Fat-containing lesions of the liver: Radiologic-pathologic correlation. Radiographics 25:321-331; 2005

Focal Steatosis

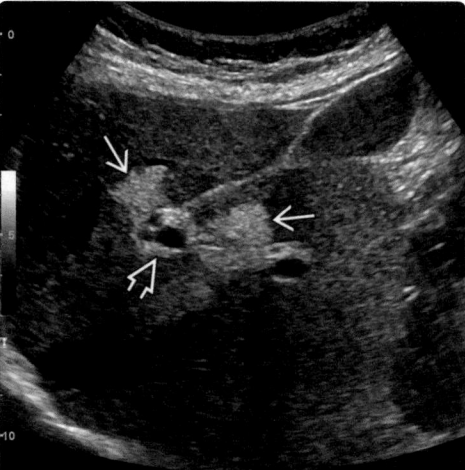

Hepatic Cavernous Hemangioma

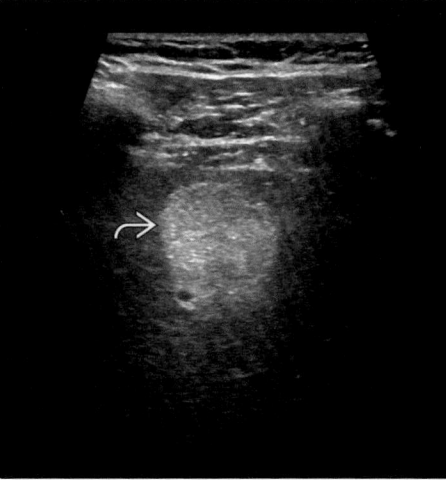

(Left) Abdominal grayscale ultrasound shows focal fat deposition as geographic areas of increased echogenicity ➡ around portal vein ➡. The lesion shows no mass effect and vessels run through the lesion, features that are helpful in the diagnosis of focal steatosis. (Right) Transverse high-frequency ultrasound of the liver shows a well-defined, homogeneously echogenic cavernous hemangioma ➡.

Hepatic Cavernous Hemangioma

Hepatic Metastases

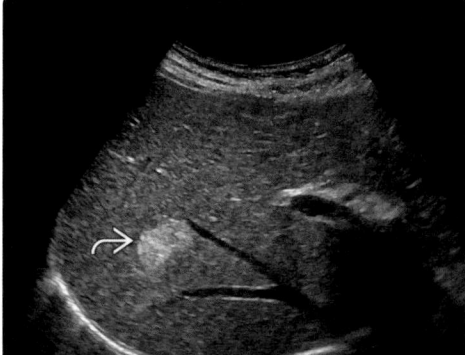

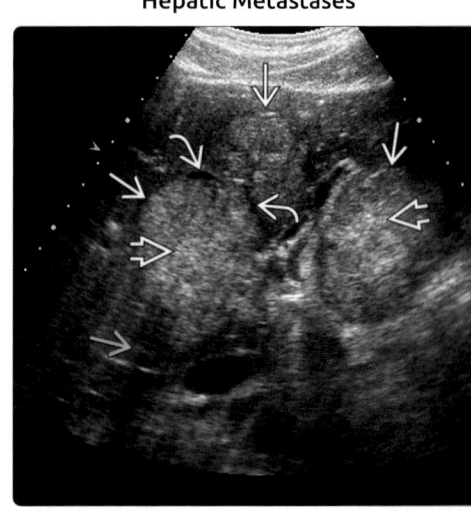

(Left) *Transverse ultrasound of the right lobe of the liver shows a typical hemangioma* ➽*, which is homogeneously echogenic with well-defined margins.* **(Right)** *Transverse ultrasound in a patient with mucinous colon cancer demonstrates multiple large, hyperechoic metastases* ➡ *in the liver, containing diffuse echogenic foci* ➾ *related to subtle calcifications that exhibit posterior acoustic shadowing* ➘*. Masses distort and compress the right portal vein* ➽*.*

Hepatic Metastases

Hepatic Metastases

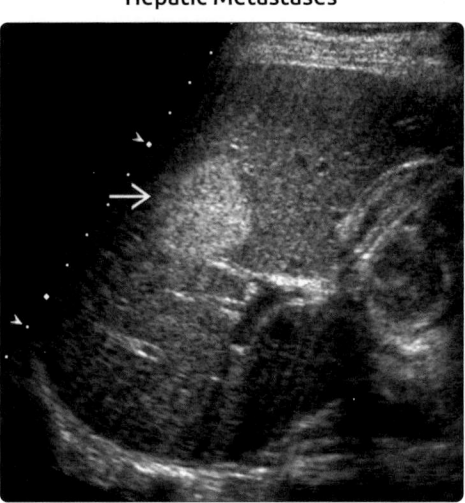

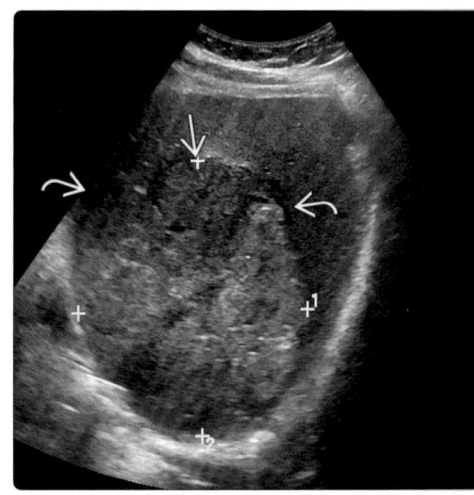

(Left) *Transverse abdominal grayscale ultrasound in a patient with carcinoid tumor shows a round, homogeneously hyperechoic metastasis in the right lobe of liver* ➡*.* **(Right)** *Oblique abdominal ultrasound in a patient with melanoma shows a large, heterogeneously hyperechoic metastasis* ➡ *in the liver abutting the hepatic capsule. Thin, hypoechoic peritumoral halo is present* ➽*, a finding often seen with hepatic metastases.*

Hepatic Metastases

Hepatic Metastases

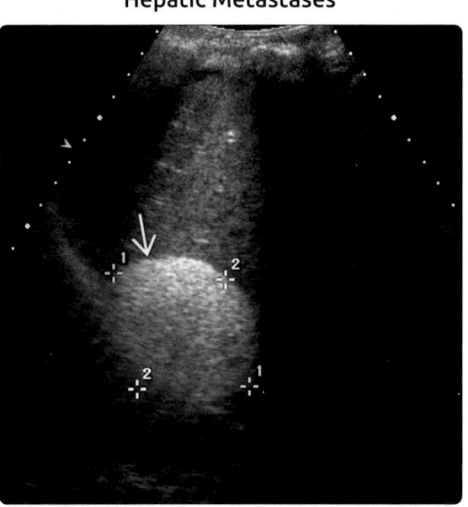

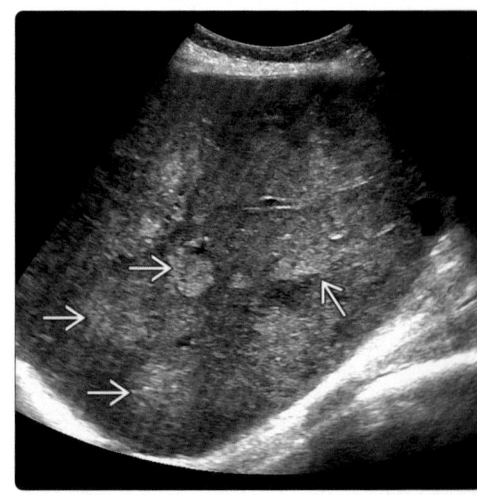

(Left) *Oblique abdominal grayscale ultrasound in a patient with liposarcoma shows a round, homogeneously hyperechoic metastasis along the margin of right lobe of liver* ➡*.* **(Right)** *Longitudinal abdominal ultrasound in a patient with bladder cancer shows multiple ill-defined, hyperechoic metastasis in the liver* ➡*.*

Hepatic Ligaments and Fissures

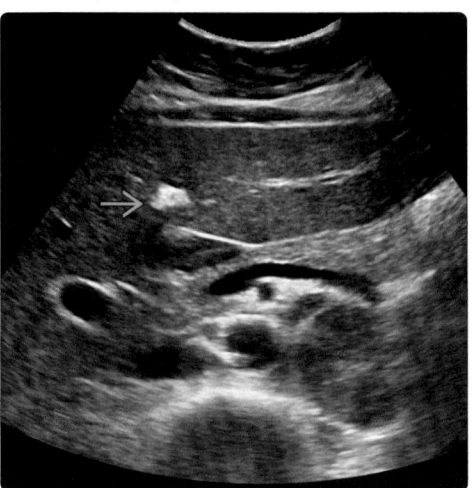

Hepatocellular Carcinoma (HCC)

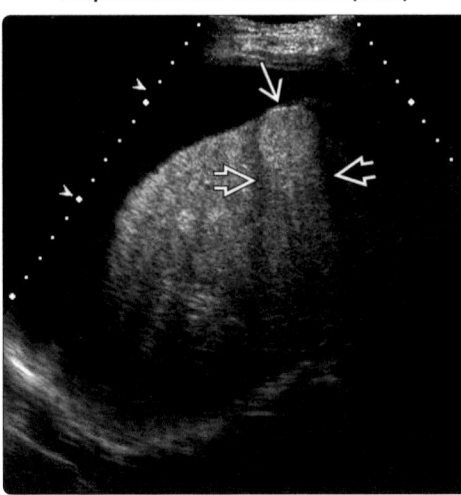

(Left) *Transverse grayscale ultrasound of the left lobe of the liver shows an echogenic falciform ligament ➡. The falciform ligament attaches the liver to the anterior body wall and often contains fat, which appears echogenic.* (Right) *Grayscale abdominal ultrasound shows a hyperechoic HCC in the subcapsular portion of the liver ➡. Lateral edge shadowing and posterior acoustic enhancement ➡ are seen associated with the HCC.*

Hepatic Adenoma

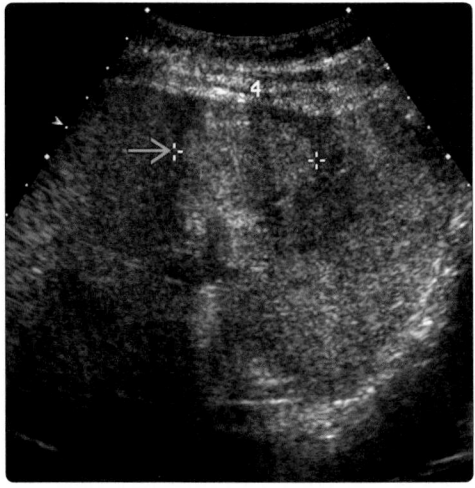

Hepatic Angiomyolipoma (AML)

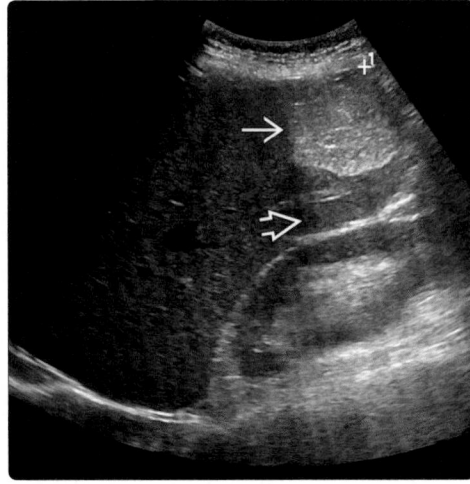

(Left) *Transverse grayscale ultrasound of the left lobe of the liver in a 22-year-old woman shows an echogenic solid mass ➡, which was proven to represent a hepatic adenoma.* (Right) *Longitudinal abdominal ultrasound shows a well-defined, homogeneously hyperechoic angiomyolipoma in the liver ➡. Slight posterior acoustic enhancement ➡ is seen associated with the AML.*

Hepatic Angiomyolipoma (AML)

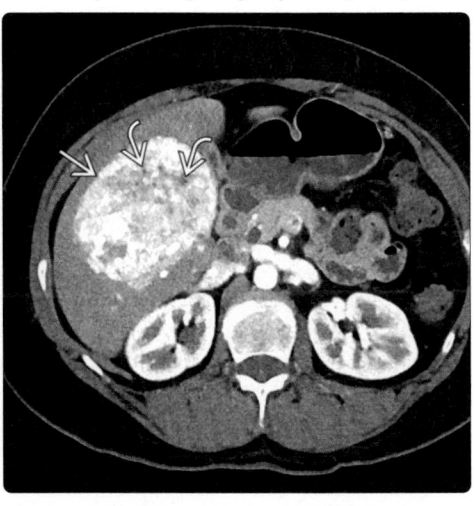

Hepatic Lipoma

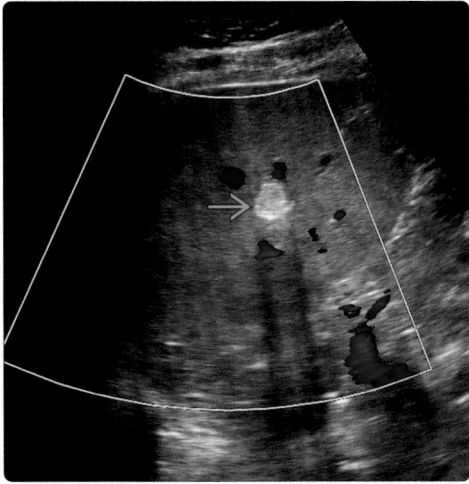

(Left) *Axial arterial phase of abdominal CECT in the same patient shows the large hypervascular angiomyolipoma in the right lobe of liver ➡. The mass contains tiny hypodense foci ➡ indicating fatty components.* (Right) *Color Doppler ultrasound shows a well-defined, uniformly echogenic avascular mass ➡ in the liver shown to represent an intrahepatic lipoma.*

DIFFERENTIAL DIAGNOSIS

Common

- Hepatic Metastases
- Hepatocellular Carcinoma (HCC)
- Hepatic Lymphoma
- Hepatic Adenoma
- Fungal Hepatic Abscess
- Amebic Hepatic Abscess
- Pyogenic Hepatic Abscess

Less Common

- Hepatic Atypical Hemangioma
- Hepatic Hematoma

Rare but Important

- Sarcoidosis
- Kaposi Sarcoma

ESSENTIAL INFORMATION

Key Differential Diagnosis Issues

- Target sign: Echogenic center surrounded by hypoechoic rim
  - a.k.a. "bull's-eye" lesions
  - Malignancy far outnumbers other causes
- "Reverse target": Hypoechoic core with hyperechoic rim

Helpful Clues for Common Diagnoses

- **Hepatic Metastases**
  - Solid central tumor with hypoechoic halo
    - Halo most likely related to compressed hepatic tissue along with zone of cancer cell proliferation
  - Alternating layers of hyper- and hypoechoic tissue
  - Usually from aggressive primary tumors
    - Classic example: Bronchogenic carcinoma
- **Hepatocellular Carcinoma (HCC)**
  - Background of cirrhosis, portal hypertension, ascites
  - Rare for cirrhotic livers to develop metastases from nonhepatic primary

- Any mass in cirrhotic liver is more likely HCC than metastasis
- **Hepatic Lymphoma**
  - Vast majority are uniformly hypoechoic
  - Splenomegaly or splenic lesions, lymphadenopathy, thickened bowel wall provide clues toward diagnosis
- **Hepatic Adenoma**
  - Usually isoechoic or slightly hypoechoic
  - Complications such as hemorrhage, central necrosis make center echogenic
  - Occasional hypoechoic rim forms target-like appearance
- **Fungal Hepatic Abscess**
  - Often multiple lesions
  - Typically in immunocompromised patient
- **Amebic Hepatic Abscess**
  - Iso- to mildly hyperechoic center with hypoechoic halo
  - Abuts liver capsule
- **Pyogenic Hepatic Abscess**
  - Central hyperechoic inflammatory nodule surrounded by hypoechoic halo of fibrosis
  - Cluster sign: Cluster of small pyogenic abscesses that coalesce into single large cavity
  - Lobulated or irregular contour

Helpful Clues for Less Common Diagnoses

- **Hepatic Atypical Hemangioma**
  - Hypoechoic center with thick or thin hyperechoic rim
    - "Typical atypical" appearance (up to 40%)
    - Hypoechogenicity seem to be related to predominant fibrous stroma
- **Hepatic Hematoma**
  - May have laceration tract leading to hepatic surface
  - Multiple organs involved if traumatic cause

SELECTED REFERENCES

1. Virmani J et al: Characterization of primary and secondary malignant liver lesions from B-mode ultrasound. J Digit Imaging. 26(6):1058-70, 2013
2. Kraus GJ et al: The reverse target sign in liver disease: a potential ultrasound feature in cirrhotic liver nodules characterization. Br J Radiol. 78(928):355-7, 2005

Hepatic Metastases

Hepatic Metastases

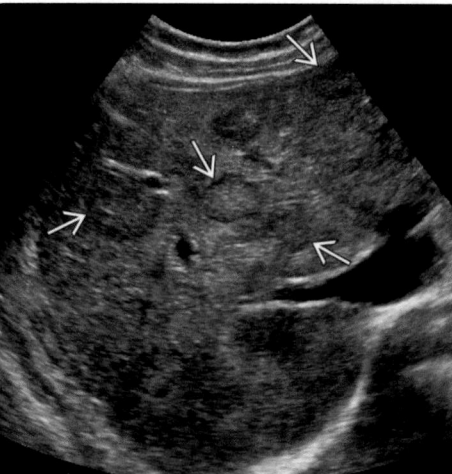
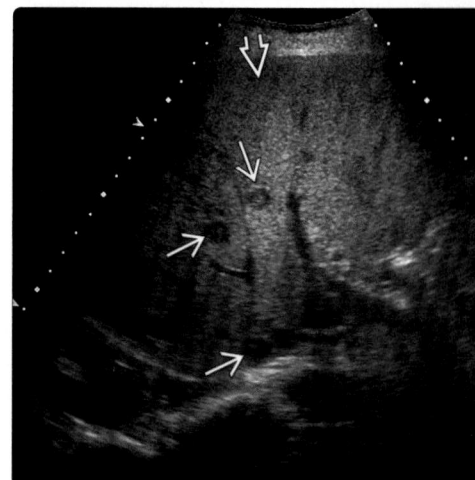

(Left) *Transverse abdominal US in a patient with breast cancer metastases to the liver shows that the metastases have a classic target appearance* ➡ *in which rounded echogenic lesions are surrounded by a hypoechoic rim.* **(Right)** *Transverse abdominal US in a patient with sarcoma metastases to the liver shows multiple small hepatic metastases have a target appearance* ➡ *in which echogenic rounded lesions are surrounded by a hypoechoic rim. Background liver shows diffuse steatosis* ➡.

Hepatic Metastases

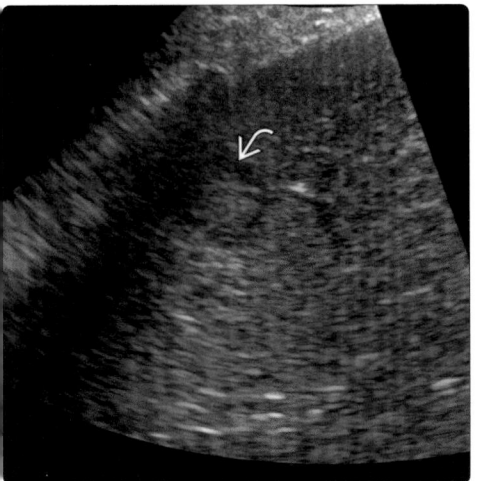

Hepatocellular Carcinoma (HCC)

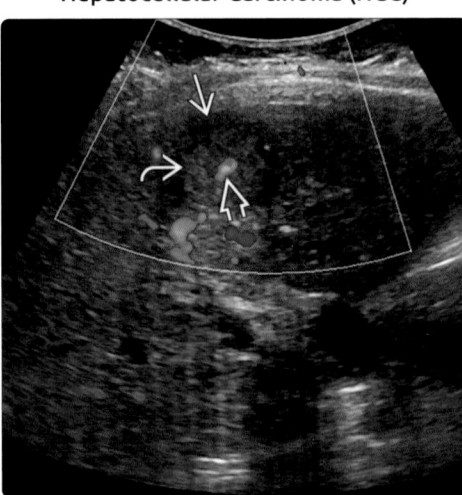

(Left) *Transverse abdominal US in a patient with lung cancer metastases to the liver shows a hepatic metastasis with a target appearance in which an isoechoic lesion is surrounded by a hypoechoic rim ➡. (Right) Transverse color Doppler US of the liver shows a hyperechoic HCC ➡ with a hypoechoic halo ➡, which creates a target appearance. Detectable internal vascularity ➡ within the tumor is seen.*

Hepatic Lymphoma

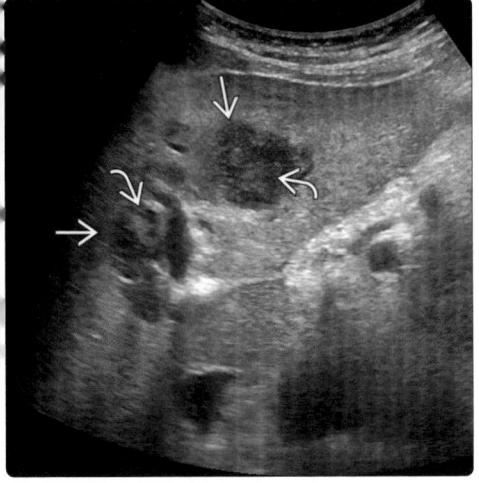

Fungal Hepatic Abscess

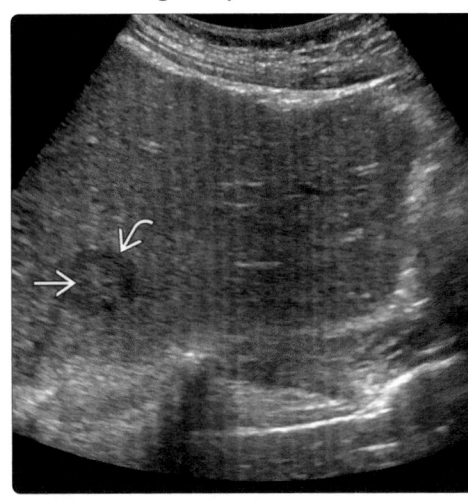

(Left) *Transverse abdominal grayscale ultrasound in a patient with lymphoma shows several hypoechoic masses with central echogenic cores ➡ surrounded by a hypoechoic rim ➡. (Right) Longitudinal grayscale US of the liver shows a fungal abscess that has an echogenic center ➡ surrounded by a hypoechoic rim ➡, which creates a target appearance.*

Pyogenic Hepatic Abscess

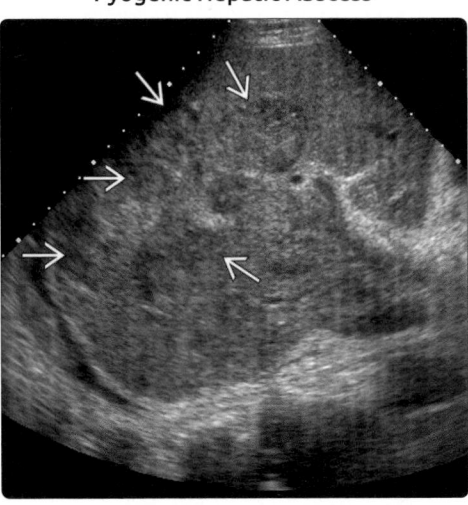

Hepatic Atypical Hemangioma

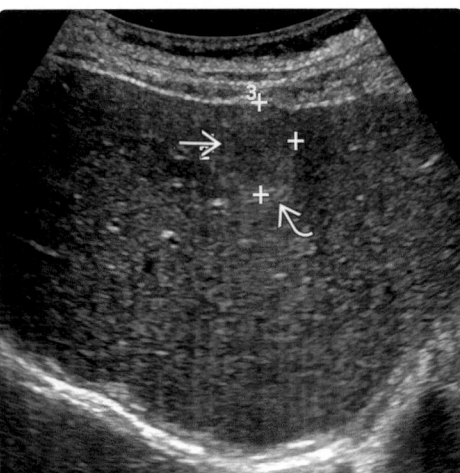

(Left) *Transverse abdominal US shows multiple hepatic abscesses ➡ that appear as isoechoic masses surrounded by thin hypoechoic rims. (Right) Longitudinal grayscale US of the liver shows an atypical hemangioma with "reverse target" appearance, which is a hypoechoic mass ➡ surrounded by hyperechoic rim ➡.*

DIFFERENTIAL DIAGNOSIS

Common

- Hepatic Cysts
- Hepatic Metastases
- Hepatic Steatosis (Multifocal)
- Hepatic Hemangioma
- Hepatic Lymphoma (Discrete Form)
- Cirrhosis With Regenerative/Dysplastic Nodules
- Hepatocellular Carcinoma
- Pyogenic Hepatic Abscess
- Hepatic Microabscesses
- Cholangitis
- Vessels

Less Common

- Hepatic *Echinococcus* Cyst
- Hepatic Hematoma
- Biliary Hamartoma

Rare but Important

- Caroli Disease

ESSENTIAL INFORMATION

Helpful Clues for Common Diagnoses

- **Hepatic Cysts**
  - Uncomplicated simple cyst
    - Anechoic rounded
    - Smooth or lobulated borders
    - Posterior acoustic enhancement
    - Thin or nondetectable wall
    - No septation/mural nodule/wall calcification
  - Hemorrhagic or infected cyst
    - Internal debris (clots or fibrin strands)
    - Septations/thickened wall, ± calcification
  - Autosomal dominant polycystic liver disease
    - Numerous cysts
    - Anechoic or with debris due to hemorrhage or infection
    - Calcification of some cyst walls
    - May have barely perceptible septations
    - No mural nodularity
    - Liver often distorted by innumerable cysts
    - Look for presence of renal cysts (adult polycystic kidney disease)
  - Do not demonstrate saccular configuration
    - vs. Caroli disease
  - Not associated with biliary duct dilatation
    - vs. hydatid cysts or Caroli disease
- **Hepatic Metastases**
  - Hypoechoic necrotic metastases
    - Usually from hypovascular tumors
    - Simulate cysts or abscesses
    - Abnormal intratumoral vascularity contains debris, mural nodules, or septa
  - Hyperechoic metastases
    - Simulate hemangioma or focal steatosis
    - Distort vessels and bile ducts
    - Vascular metastasis; from neuroendocrine tumors, choriocarcinoma, renal cell carcinoma, melanoma

- Target metastatic lesions
  - Solid echogenic mass with hypoechoic rim or halo
  - Usually from aggressive primary tumors
- Cystic metastasis
  - May demonstrate posterior acoustic enhancement
  - Mural nodules, thick walls, fluid-fluid levels, internal septa, or debris
- Calcified metastasis
  - Markedly echogenic interface with acoustic shadowing or diffuse small echogenic foci
  - Treated metastasis
- **Hepatic Steatosis (Multifocal)**
  - Focal fatty infiltration
    - Location: Right lobe, caudate lobe, perihilar
    - Hyperechoic area
  - Focal fatty sparing
    - Location: Gallbladder bed, segment 4 anterior to portal bifurcation
    - Hypoechoic areas within echogenic liver
  - Geographic or fan-shaped
  - In some cases may appear as multiple echogenic nodules throughout liver
  - No mass effect
  - Vessels run undisplaced through lesion
- **Hepatic Hemangioma**
  - Well-defined margins
  - Hyperechoic mass, typically homogeneous
  - Posterior acoustic enhancement
  - Atypical features
    - Hypoechoic ± hyperechoic rim
    - Heterogeneous, calcification, irregular borders
- **Hepatic Lymphoma (Discrete Form)**
  - Well-defined nodules or masses
  - Hypoechoic or anechoic
    - Low echogenicity due to high cellular density
  - Large/conglomerate masses may appear to contain septa
    - Mimic abscesses
  - Background vascular architecture ± distortion
  - More common in immunocompromised patients
    - e.g., AIDS patients and organ transplant recipients
- **Cirrhosis With Regenerative/Dysplastic Nodules**
  - Coarse echo pattern, increased parenchymal echogenicity, other signs of cirrhosis
  - Regenerating nodules (siderotic)
    - Iso-/hypoechoic nodules (regenerating nodules)
    - Hyperechoic rim (surrounding fibrosis)
  - Dysplastic nodules
    - Hypoechoic nodule > 1 cm diameter
    - Smooth or irregular borders
    - Difficult to differentiate from small hepatocellular carcinoma
      - Should be further investigated with CECT or MR
- **Hepatocellular Carcinoma**
  - Most commonly hypoechoic
    - Less commonly hyperechoic or isoechoic to liver
  - Irregular hypervascularity within mass
  - Cirrhotic background liver
  - May see portal vein invasion or tumor thrombosis
- **Pyogenic Hepatic Abscess**

- Cluster sign
  - Cluster of small abscesses coalesce into single septated cavity
- Complex cyst with septa and debris
- ± ill-defined borders
- Mural nodularity and vascularity
- May contain gas within abscess
  - Seen as echogenic foci of air or air-fluid level
- Adjacent parenchyma may be coarse and hypoechoic
- Color Doppler may show hypervascularity in inflamed surrounding liver parenchyma

- **Hepatic Microabscesses**
  - Multiple, small, hypo-/iso-/hyperechoic lesions
  - Central hypoechoic area of necrosis within hyperechoic lesion
  - Target sign
    - Central hyperechoic inflammation surrounded by hypoechoic "halo" of fibrosis
  - Similar lesions may be found in spleen
- **Cholangitis**
  - Circumferential bile duct wall thickening
  - Dilatation of intra- and extrahepatic ducts
  - Periportal hypo-/hyperechogenicity
    - Due to periductal edema/inflammation
  - Ascending cholangitis
    - Obstructing calculus in extrahepatic duct
  - Recurrent pyogenic cholangitis
    - Biliary calculi: Cast-like and often fill duct lumen
    - Atrophy of affected lobe/segment
- **Vessels**
  - Portal veins: Venectasia, varicosities, collaterals from portal hypertension
  - Hepatic veins: Venectasia, Budd-Chiari syndrome
  - Hepatic arteries: Aneurysms, shunts, vascular malformation
  - Use color Doppler to confirm vascular nature

Helpful Clues for Less Common Diagnoses

- **Hepatic *Echinococcus* Cyst**
  - Large, well-defined hypoechoic masses
  - Numerous peripheral daughter cysts
  - Intrahepatic duct dilatation may be seen
  - May show curvilinear or ring-like pericyst calcification
- **Hepatic Hematoma**
  - Lesions commonly in segments 6, 7, 8
  - Round, hyper-/hypoechoic foci
  - Echogenicity evolves over time
    - Echogenic initially
    - Hypoechoic after 4-5 days
    - Internal echoes and septations after 1-4 weeks
  - Ancillary signs: Subcapsular hematoma, hemoperitoneum, renal or splenic laceration
- **Biliary Hamartoma (von Meyenburg Complexes)**
  - Numerous small, hypo-/hyperechoic foci uniformly distributed throughout liver
    - Leads to inhomogeneous and coarse appearance of liver echotexture
  - Multiple echogenic foci
    - Often with associated "comet tail" artifacts
  - Typically smaller lesions appear as echogenic foci, whereas larger lesions appear cystic
    - Often extent of echogenic foci on US is greater than anticipated, based on comparison CT or MR

Helpful Clues for Rare Diagnoses

- **Caroli Disease**
  - Hypoechoic masses
  - Saccular or fusiform shape
  - Central dot sign
    - Small portal venous branches partially or completely surrounded by dilated ducts
  - May contain calculi, which do not form casts of ducts

SELECTED REFERENCES

1. Forner A et al: Lack of arterial hypervascularity at contrast-enhanced ultrasound should not define the priority for diagnostic work-up of nodules < 2 cm. J Hepatol. 62(1):150-5, 2015
2. Kim TK et al: Contrast-enhanced ultrasound in the diagnosis of nodules in liver cirrhosis. World J Gastroenterol. 20(13):3590-6, 2014
3. Friedrich-Rust M et al: Contrast-Enhanced Ultrasound for the differentiation of benign and malignant focal liver lesions: a meta-analysis. Liver Int. 33(5):739-55, 2013

Hepatic Cysts

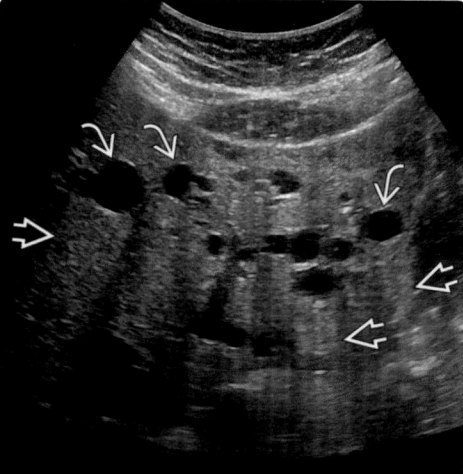

Hepatic Metastases

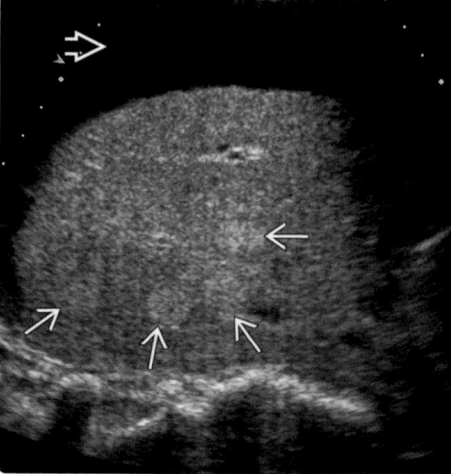

(Left) *Transverse grayscale US of the liver shows innumerable cysts ➔ throughout the liver in a patient with polycystic liver disease. Posterior acoustic enhancement ⇨ is seen associated with each cyst.* **(Right)** *Transverse abdominal US in a patient with carcinoid metastases to the liver shows multiple round and homogeneous hyperechoic metastatic nodules in the liver ➔. Large amount of perihepatic ascites ⇨ is seen.*

Hepatic Metastases

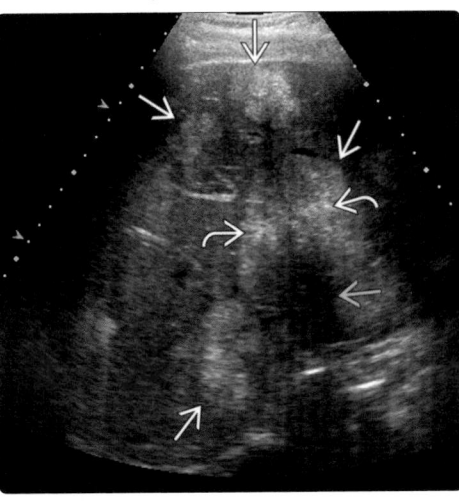

Hepatic Metastases

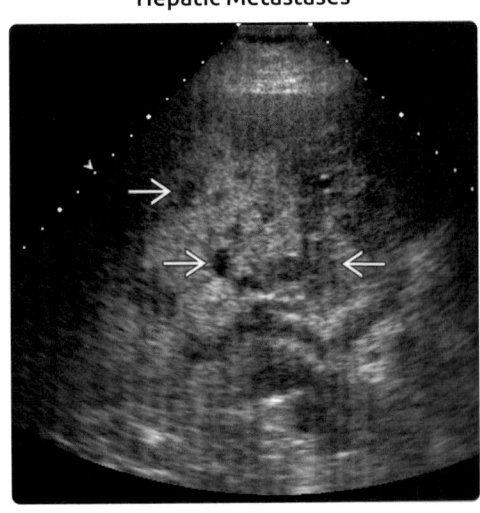

(Left) *Transverse US in a patient with mucinous colon cancer demonstrates multiple large, hyperechoic metastases ➡ containing diffuse echogenic foci ➡ related to subtle calcifications. Note posterior acoustic shadowing caused by the calcifications ➡. (Right) Transverse abdominal US in a patient with pancreatic cancer shows numerous small, hypoechoic metastases ➡ throughout the liver. The background liver is echogenic from hepatic steatosis, a common finding in the setting of chemotherapy.*

Hepatic Steatosis (Multifocal)

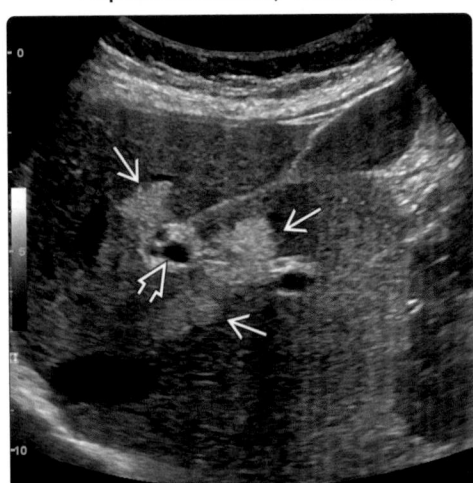

Hepatic Hemangioma

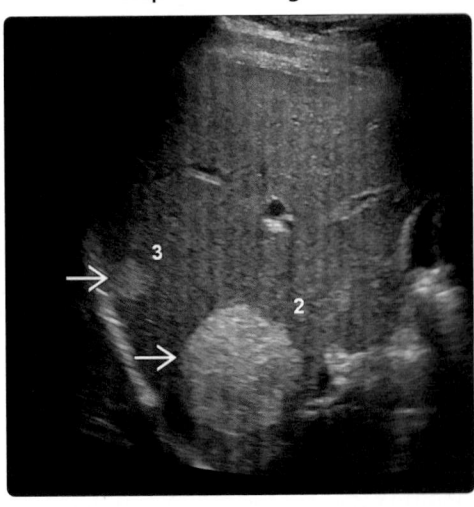

(Left) *Abdominal grayscale US shows multifocal fat deposition, which appears as geographic areas of increased echogenicity ➡ around the portal vein ➡. The lesion shows no mass effect, and vessels run through the lesion, characteristic features of fatty infiltration. (Right) Transverse abdominal US shows 2 well-defined, homogeneously hyperechoic hemangiomas in the right lobe of liver ➡.*

Hepatic Hemangioma

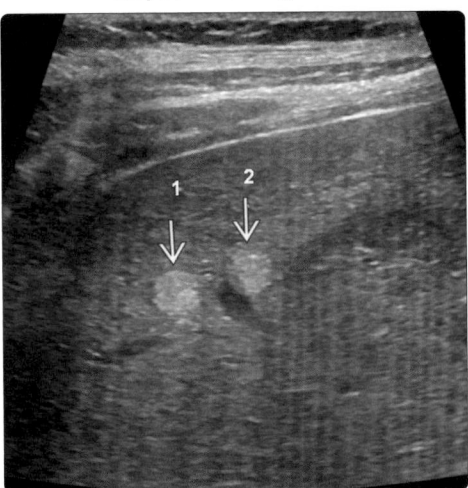

Hepatic Lymphoma (Discrete Form)

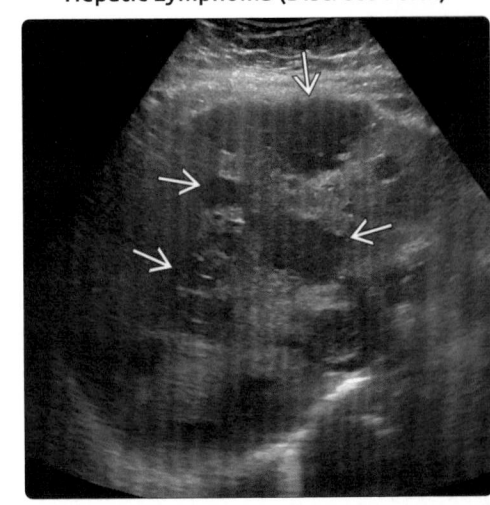

(Left) *Transverse abdominal US shows 2 well-defined and homogeneously hyperechoic hemangiomas in the liver ➡. Hemangiomas in the liver are often multiple. (Right) Transverse abdominal US in a patient with lymphoma shows multiple hypoechoic masses ➡ throughout the liver. Lesions are markedly hypoechoic, resulting in a pseudocystic appearance characteristic of lymphoma.*

Cirrhosis With Regenerative/Dysplastic Nodules

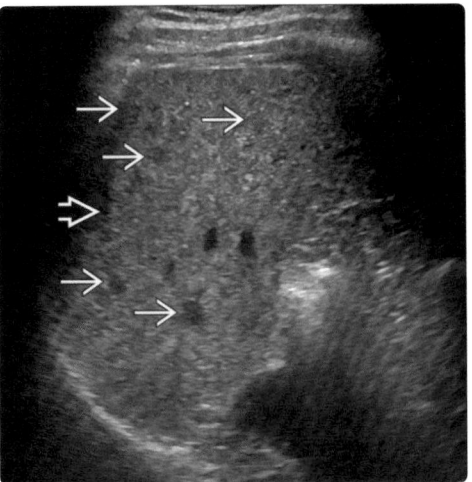

Hepatocellular Carcinoma

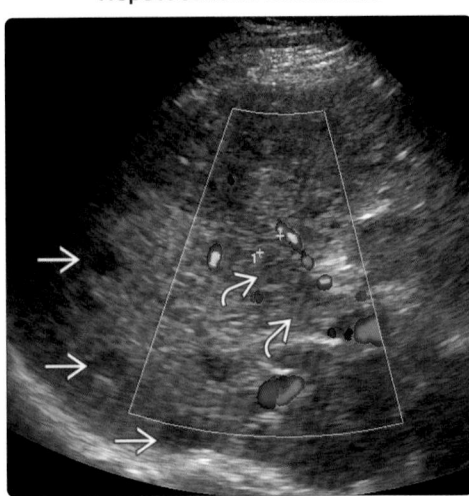

(Left) *Abdominal US in a patient with hepatitis B shows numerous small hypoechoic nodules in the liver ➡, indicating regenerative or dysplastic nodules. Coarse and heterogeneous echogenicity of liver parenchyma is consistent with underlying cirrhosis ➡.* **(Right)** *Abdominal US shows multifocal hypoechoic HCCs ➡ throughout the liver. The right portal vein is thrombosed and filled with echogenic material that was found to represent tumor thrombus ➡.*

Pyogenic Hepatic Abscess

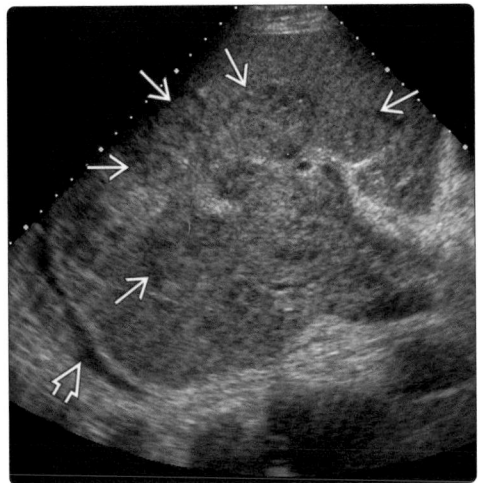

Hepatic Microabscesses

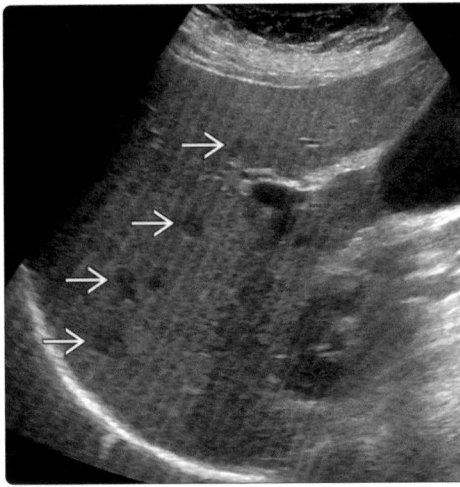

(Left) *Transverse abdominal grayscale US shows multiple hepatic abscesses ➡ in the liver, seen as ill-defined isoechoic masses surrounded by thin hypoechoic rims. A small amount of perihepatic ascites ➡ is present as well.* **(Right)** *Longitudinal abdominal grayscale US shows multiple small hypoechoic fungal microabscesses ➡ in the right lobe of liver.*

Hepatic Echinococcus Cyst

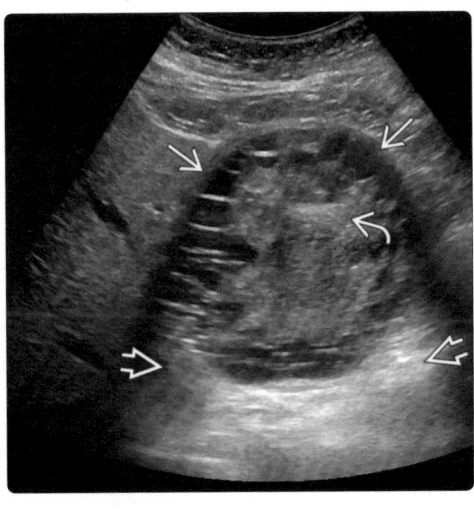

Caroli Disease

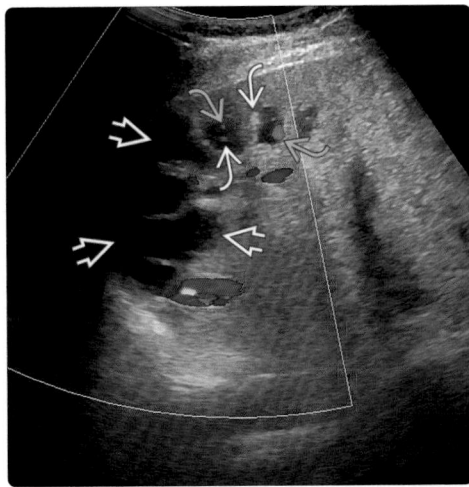

(Left) *Transverse abdominal ultrasound shows an echinococcal cyst containing multiple peripheral daughter cysts ➡ and heterogeneous material centrally ➡. Note the associated posterior acoustic enhancement ➡.* **(Right)** *Oblique abdominal ultrasound in a young patient with Caroli disease shows multiple dilated intrahepatic ducts ➡. Echogenic portal radicles ➡ are surrounded by dilated ducts. Some of the portal radicles within dilated ducts show color flow ➡, which creates the "central dot" sign appearance.*

DIFFERENTIAL DIAGNOSIS

Common

- Focal Nodular Hyperplasia
- Fibrolamellar Carcinoma
- Hepatocellular Carcinoma
- Hepatic Adenoma
- Hepatic Metastases

Less Common

- Atypical Hemangioma
- Hepatic *Echinococcus* Cyst

ESSENTIAL INFORMATION

Helpful Clues for Common Diagnoses

- **Focal Nodular Hyperplasia**
  - Mass: Typically homogeneous and isoechoic to liver
    - Occasionally hypoechoic or hyperechoic
  - Central scar: Typically hypoechoic (18% hyperechoic)
    - Contains central feeding artery
  - Color Doppler: "Spoke-wheel" pattern
    - Prominent central feeding artery with multiple small vessels radiating peripherally
    - Large draining veins at tumor margins
- **Fibrolamellar Carcinoma**
  - Presents in otherwise healthy young adults
    - Background cirrhosis or hepatitis in < 5% of patients
  - Well-defined, partially/completely encapsulated large mass
  - Prominent central fibrous scar
  - Calcification within scar common
  - Intralesional necrosis/hemorrhage
  - Vascular, biliary, and nodal invasion may be present
- **Hepatocellular Carcinoma**
  - Background cirrhosis ± signs of portal hypertension
  - Central tumor necrosis/fibrosis produces apparent central scar
  - Color Doppler may show irregular tumor hypervascularity or tumor thrombus in portal vein

- **Hepatic Adenoma**
  - Well-defined round or mildly lobulated contour
  - Hypo-/iso-/hyperechoic mass
  - Central fat, hemorrhage, necrosis, and calcification
    - May simulate central scar
  - Color Doppler shows hypervascular tumor supplied by hepatic artery
- **Hepatic Metastases**
  - Necrotic or treated metastases with necrotic center may simulate central scar
  - Necrotic center may be lined with irregular walls and contain debris
  - Color Doppler may not show vascularity as many metastases are hypovascular

Helpful Clues for Less Common Diagnoses

- **Atypical Hemangioma**
  - Hypoechoic center with hyperechoic rim may simulate central scar
    - "Typical atypical" hemangioma (up to 40%)
  - Posterior acoustic enhancement
  - No visible color Doppler flow in center of lesion
    - Flow too slow to be sonographically detected
- **Hepatic *Echinococcus* Cyst**
  - Honeycombed cyst
    - Multiple septations between daughter cysts in mother cyst
  - "Spoke-wheel" appearance of septa simulating central scar

SELECTED REFERENCES

1. Kong WT et al: Contrast-Enhanced Ultrasound in Combination with Color Doppler Ultrasound Can Improve the Diagnostic Performance of Focal Nodular Hyperplasia and Hepatocellular Adenoma. Ultrasound Med Biol. 41(4):944-51, 2015
2. Kim T et al: Liver masses with central or eccentric scar. Semin Ultrasound CT MR. 30(5):418-25, 2009

Focal Nodular Hyperplasia

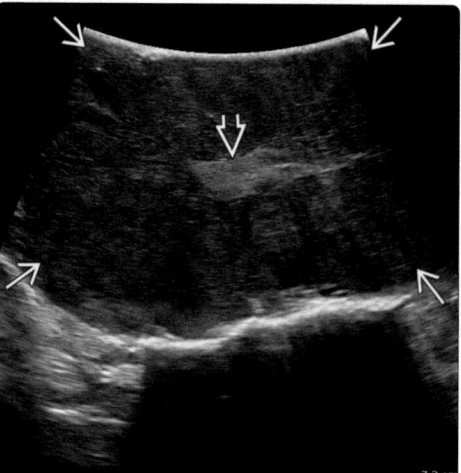

Focal Nodular Hyperplasia

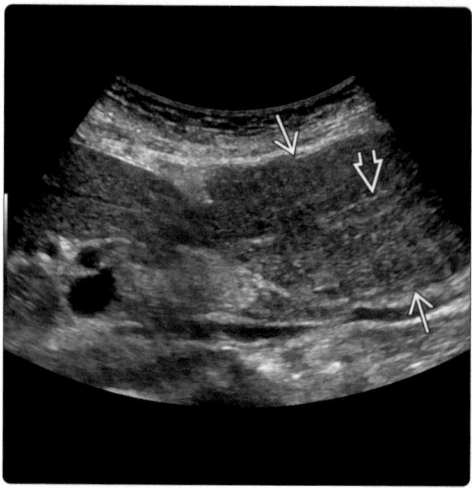

(Left) *Intraoperative abdominal US using a high-frequency transducer shows a hypoechoic focal nodular hyperplasia (FNH) in the liver ➡ with a hyperechoic central scar ➡.* **(Right)** *Transverse abdominal ultrasound shows a pedunculated FNH ➡ with a slightly hyperechoic central scar ➡ arising from the lateral segment of the left lobe of the liver.*

Focal Nodular Hyperplasia

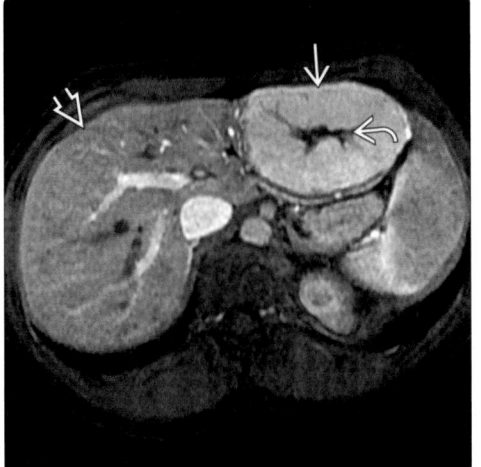

Focal Nodular Hyperplasia

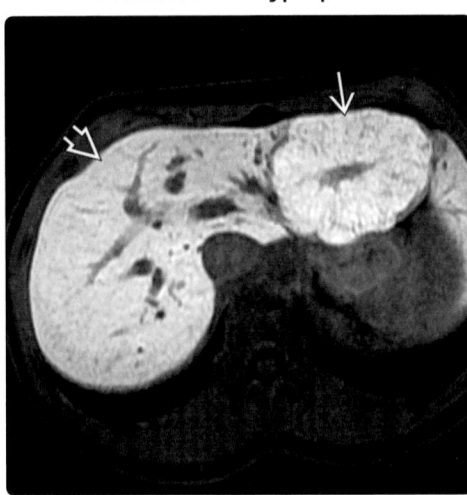

(Left) Axial arterial phase T1 contrast-enhanced MR shows a hyperenhancing FNH ➡, which is hyperintense compared to adjacent liver parenchyma ➡. Hypointense stellate central scar ➡ is characteristic of FNH. (Right) Axial hepatobiliary phase MR obtained 20 minutes after gadoxetate injection in the same patient shows the FNH retains contrast to slightly greater degree ➡ than the background liver ➡, confirming the presence of hepatocytes in the FNH.

Fibrolamellar Carcinoma

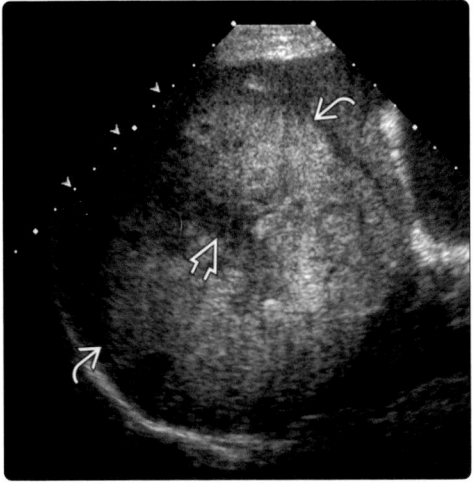

Hepatocellular Carcinoma

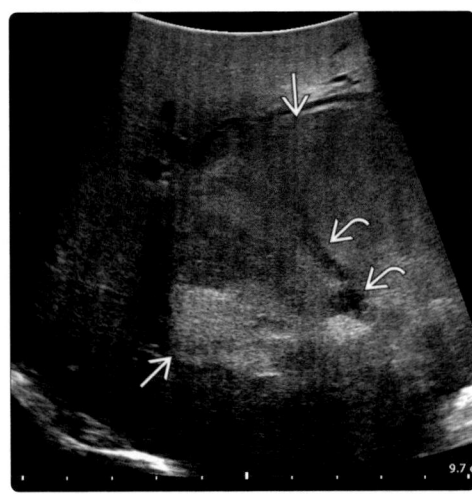

(Left) Transverse grayscale US of the liver shows a large, predominantly echogenic mass ➡ with a thick, hypoechoic central scar ➡. The mass was proven to be a fibrolamellar carcinoma. (Right) Intraoperative grayscale ultrasound of the liver shows a large, heterogeneous, isoechoic hepatocellular carcinoma ➡ with hypoechoic central scar ➡.

Hepatic Metastases

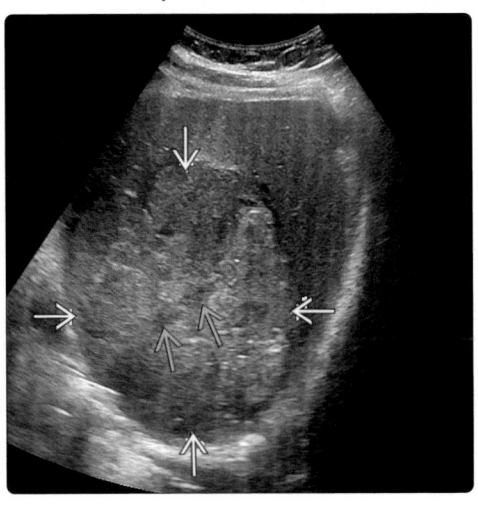

Atypical Hemangioma

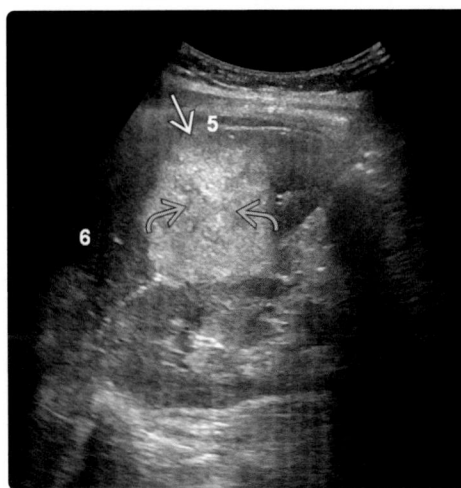

(Left) Oblique abdominal grayscale US in a patient with melanoma shows a large, heterogeneous, hyperechoic metastasis ➡ in the right lobe of the liver. Central hypoechoic areas simulate a central scar ➡. (Right) Longitudinal grayscale abdominal US shows a hyperechoic hemangioma in the liver ➡. The ill-defined hypoechoic area in the center ➡ simulates a central scar.

DIFFERENTIAL DIAGNOSIS

Common

- Ascending Cholangitis
- Cavernous Transformation of Portal Vein
- Portosystemic Collaterals
- Hepatic Trauma
- Acute Viral Hepatitis
- Fatty Sparing, Liver
- Diffuse/Infiltrative Hepatic Lymphoma
- Pneumobilia
- Choledocholithiasis
- Metastases

Less Common

- Peribiliary Cyst
- Hepatic Schistosomiasis
- Recurrent Pyogenic Cholangitis
- Iatrogenic Material
- Caroli Disease
- Hepatic Artery Calcification
- Cystic Duct Remnant

ESSENTIAL INFORMATION

Helpful Clues for Common Diagnoses

- **Ascending Cholangitis**
  - Periportal hypo- or hyperechogenicity adjacent to dilated intrahepatic ducts
    - Due to periductal edema/inflammation
  - Dilatation of intrahepatic bile ducts
  - Purulent bile/sludge as intraluminal echogenic material in dilated ducts
  - Circumferential thickening of bile duct wall
  - Obstructing stone in common bile duct
- **Cavernous Transformation of Portal Vein**
  - Collateralization due to portal vein occlusion
  - Usually in subacute or chronic portal vein obstruction
  - Serpiginous tubular channels along expected course of portal vein
  - Color Doppler shows hepatopetal flow
  - Signs of portal vein occlusion
    - Acute: Enlarged portal vein
    - Chronic: Small/imperceptible portal vein
    - Color Doppler: Lack of flow in portal vein
- **Portosystemic Collaterals**
  - Serpiginous hypoechoic channels in or around portal triad
  - Location
    - Intrahepatic: Portal to portal veins, portal to hepatic veins, portal to systemic veins
    - Paraumbilical vein (recanalization)
    - Gastroesophageal: Coronary and right gastric, left gastric and splenogastric
    - Lienorenal/mesenteric/retroperitoneal
  - Color Doppler
    - Shows hepatofugal flow in vessels (opposite to cavernous transformation)
    - Extent of collaterals
  - Background changes of cirrhosis/portal hypertension/portal vein thrombosis

- **Hepatic Trauma**
  - Lesions are commonly located in segments 6, 7, 8
  - Echogenicity evolves over time
    - Initially echogenic
    - Becomes hypoechoic after 4-5 days
    - Internal echoes with septa may develop after 1-4 weeks
  - Hematoma tracking along portal triad
    - Linear, focal, or diffuse periportal lesion
  - Ancillary signs of trauma
    - Subcapsular hematoma; hemoperitoneum, renal, or splenic laceration/hematoma
  - Better evaluated by MDCT
- **Acute Viral Hepatitis**
  - Increased echogenicity of fat in periportal tissues, ligamentum venosum, and falciform ligament
  - Hepatomegaly with diffuse decrease in echogenicity
  - "Starry sky" appearance
    - Increased echogenicity of portal triad walls against background of hypoechoic liver
  - Periportal hypo-/anechoic area
    - Due to hydropic swelling of hepatocytes
- **Fatty Sparing, Liver**
  - Focal hypoechoic area within otherwise echogenic liver
  - No mass effect: Vessels run undisplaced through lesion
  - Due to direct drainage of hepatic blood into systemic circulation
  - Typical location
    - Next to gallbladder: Drained by cystic vein
    - Segment 4/anterior to portal bifurcation: Drained by aberrant gastric vein
- **Diffuse/Infiltrative Hepatic Lymphoma**
  - Subcentimeter periportal hypoechoic foci, miliary in pattern
  - Other evidence of lymphoma
    - Lymphadenopathy, splenomegaly/splenic lesions, bowel wall thickening, ascites
- **Pneumobilia**
  - Highly echogenic linear foci in portal triad
  - Rises to nondependent portion of liver (left lobe if patient lying supine)
  - Change in position of gas with change in patient position
  - Posterior acoustic shadowing
  - Reverberation artifact deep to lesion
  - Causes
    - Recent passage of stone from or instrumentation of biliary tree
    - Choledochoenteric fistula
    - Biliary infection by gas-forming organism
- **Choledocholithiasis**
  - Multiple echogenic foci along portal triad
  - Posterior acoustic shadowing
    - Small (< 5 mm) or soft pigmented stones may not produce posterior shadowing
  - Large stones may cause biliary obstruction, resulting in focal bile duct dilatation
- **Metastases**
  - May be located anywhere in liver
  - Usually multiple

Helpful Clues for Less Common Diagnoses

- **Peribiliary Cyst**
  - Well-defined small cystic structures adjacent to portal triads
  - More common in cirrhotic patients
  - Usually multiple
  - No communication with biliary tree
- **Hepatic Schistosomiasis**
  - Periportal fibrosis
    - Most severe at porta hepatis
    - Widened portal tracts
    - "Clay-pipestem" fibrosis
      - □ Hyperechoic and thickened walls of portal venules
    - Bull's-eye lesion
      - □ Anechoic portal vein surrounded by echogenic mantle of fibrous tissue
  - Mosaic pattern
    - Network of echogenic septa outlining polygonal areas of normal-appearing liver
    - Represents complete septal fibrosis
      - □ Inflammation & fibrosis in reaction to embolized eggs
    - May be discontinuous and appear mottled, nodular, or sieve-like
      - □ Partial septal fibrosis or calcification
- **Recurrent Pyogenic Cholangitis**
  - Lateral segment of left lobe and posterior segment of right lobe more commonly involved
  - Early disease with active biliary sepsis
    - Periportal hypo- or hyperechogenicity due to periductal edema/inflammation
    - Biliary duct wall thickening due to edema
    - Floating echoes within dilated ducts due to inflammatory debris
  - Late-stage disease
    - Severe atrophy of affected segment/lobe, biliary cirrhosis
    - Crowded stone-filled ducts
      - □ May appear as single heterogeneous mass

- Stones may form casts of duct
- **Iatrogenic Material**
  - Shunt, stent, embolization material, drainage tube, staples, etc.
  - Echogenic material with strong reflective surface or smooth outline
- **Caroli Disease**
  - Anechoic masses: Saccular or fusiform shape
  - Central dot sign
    - Small portal venous branches partially/completely surrounded by dilated ducts
- **Hepatic Artery Calcification**
  - Branching linear echogenic structures along portal triads
  - Often marked calcifications of splenic artery and other smaller arteries
  - Risk factors
    - Longstanding diabetes
    - Chronic renal failure
    - Conditions that predispose to heavy vascular calcifications
- **Cystic Duct Remnant**
  - History of prior cholecystectomy
  - Remnant cystic duct may be dilated

SELECTED REFERENCES

1. Shin SW et al: Usefulness of B-mode and doppler sonography for the diagnosis of severe acute viral hepatitis A. J Clin Ultrasound. ePub, 2014
2. Spârchez Z et al: Role of contrast enhanced ultrasound in the assessment of biliary duct disease. Med Ultrason. 16(1):41-7, 2014
3. Trenker C et al: Contrast-enhanced ultrasound (CEUS) in hepatic lymphoma: retrospective evaluation in 38 cases. Ultraschall Med. 35(2):142-8, 2014
4. Wu S et al: Characteristics suggestive of focal fatty sparing from liver malignancy on ultrasound in liver screening. Ultrasound Q. 30(4):276-81, 2014
5. Kobayashi S et al: Intrahepatic periportal high intensity on hepatobiliary phase images of Gd-EOB-DTPA-enhanced MRI: imaging findings and prevalence in various hepatobiliary diseases. Jpn J Radiol. 31(1):9-15, 2013
6. Meacock LM et al: Evaluation of gallbladder and biliary duct disease using microbubble contrast-enhanced ultrasound. Br J Radiol. 83(991):615-27, 2010
7. Passos MC et al: Ultrasound and CT findings in hepatic and pancreatic parenchyma in acute schistosomiasis. Br J Radiol. 82(979):e145-7, 2009

Ascending Cholangitis

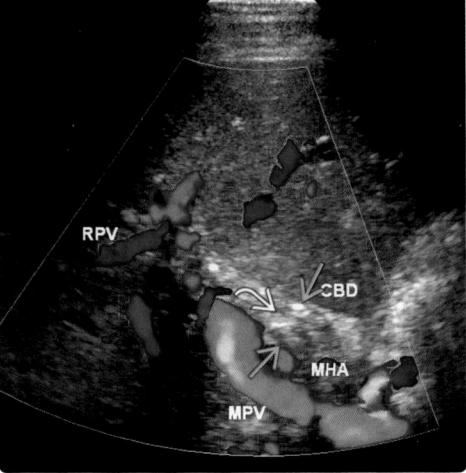

Cavernous Transformation of Portal Vein

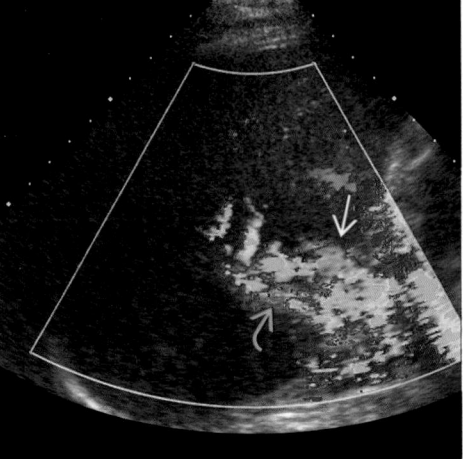

(Left) *Transverse color Doppler US in a patient with ascending cholangitis shows circumferential wall thickening of the common bile duct ➡ as well as echogenic debris ➤ within the lumen.* **(Right)** *Color Doppler US shows collateralized flow ➡ in the porta hepatis in a patient with chronic portal vein thrombosis ➡. Color Doppler signal is heterogeneous because portal vein collaterals are tortuous, resulting in vessels directed toward as well as away from the transducer.*

Differential Diagnoses: Liver

Portosystemic Collaterals

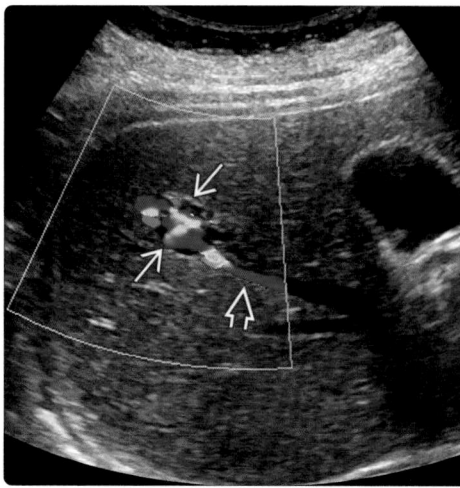

Portosystemic Collaterals

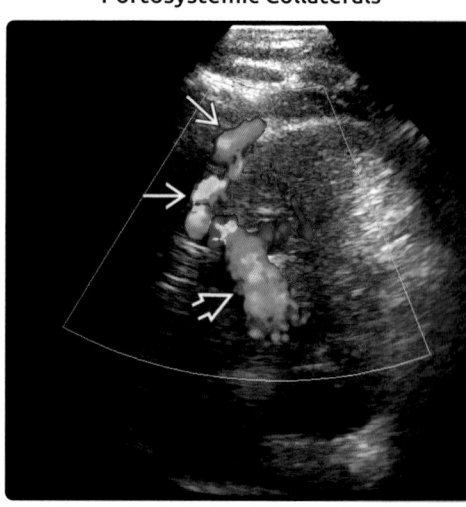

(Left) *Transverse abdominal US shows an intrahepatic portosystemic shunt between the right portal vein and right hepatic vein ➡, which appears as an entangled vascular structure that drains into the right hepatic vein ➡.* **(Right)** *Transverse abdominal color Doppler US in a patient with hepatic cirrhosis shows a recanalized paraumbilical vein ➡ arising from the left portal vein ➡ and traveling anteriorly along the falciform ligament toward the inferior epigastric vein.*

Diffuse/Infiltrative Hepatic Lymphoma

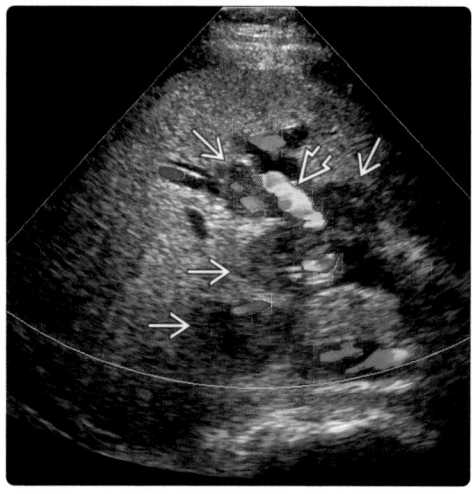

Pneumobilia

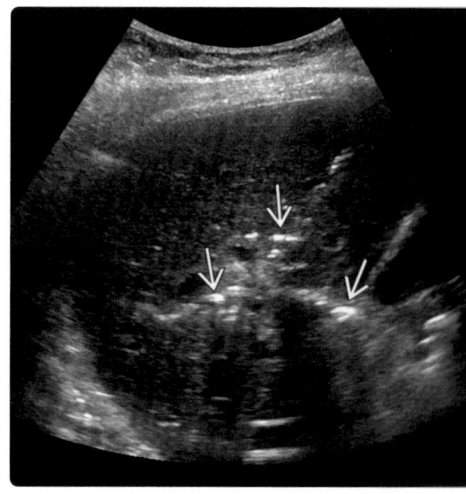

(Left) *Transverse color Doppler US in a patient with lymphoma involving the liver shows multiple markedly hypoechoic masses ➡ in a periportal distribution (right anterior portal vein ➡) in the liver. Lesions are predominantly hypovascular, a characteristic imaging appearance of lymphoma.* **(Right)** *Transverse abdominal ultrasound shows linear bright hyperechoic foci ➡ caused by pneumobilia along the expected course of the biliary tree.*

Choledocholithiasis

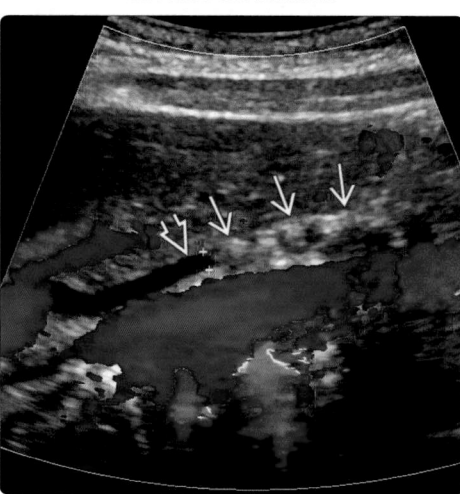

Metastases

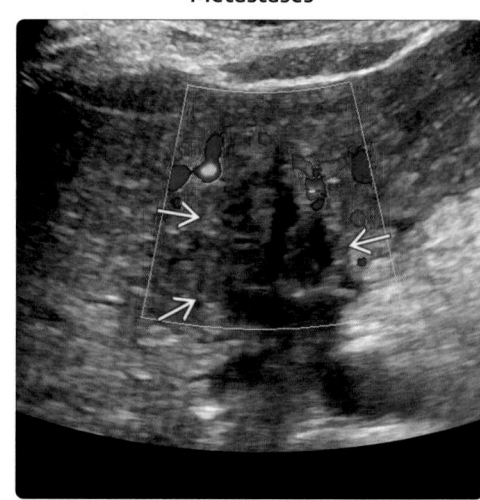

(Left) *Longitudinal color Doppler US shows multiple echogenic stones ➡ within the common bile duct, causing upstream biliary ductal dilation ➡. Color Doppler is helpful to distinguish avascular ducts from adjacent vasculature.* **(Right)** *Transverse abdominal color Doppler US in a patient with ovarian cancer shows an ill-defined, hypoechoic metastasis ➡ that infiltrates the left periportal region, occluding the left portal vein, which should normally be present in this region.*

Peribiliary Cyst

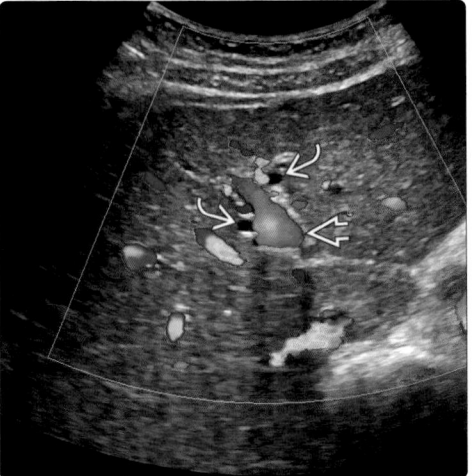

Hepatic Schistosomiasis

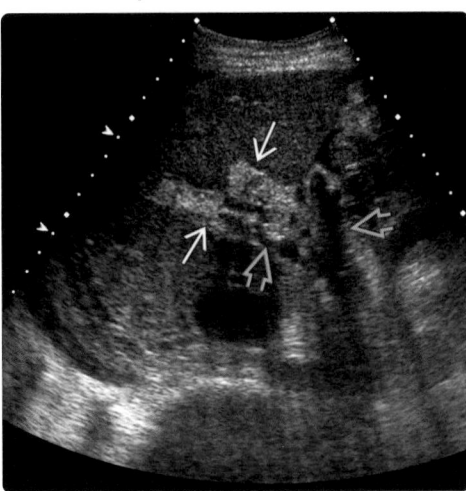

(Left) *Transverse abdominal color Doppler US shows several well-defined small peribiliary cysts* ➡ *along the left portal vein* ➡. **(Right)** *Transverse abdominal US in a patient with hepatic Schistosomiasis shows thick echogenic mantle of fibrotic tissue* ➡ *in the periportal area, encasing the portal veins* ➡. *(Courtesy W. Chong, MD.)*

Recurrent Pyogenic Cholangitis

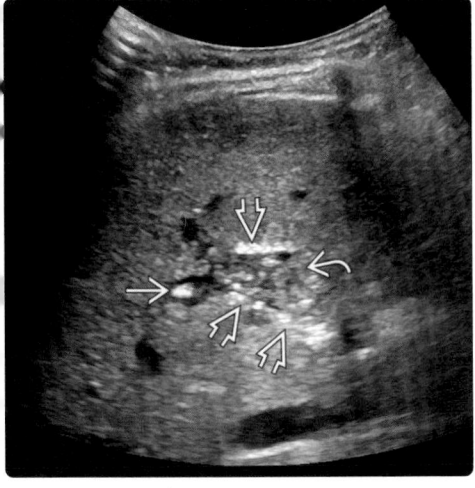

Recurrent Pyogenic Cholangitis

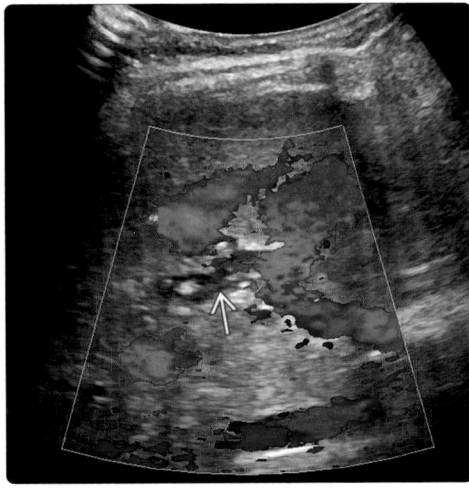

(Left) *Transverse abdominal US in a patient with recurrent pyogenic cholangitis shows echogenic intrahepatic stones* ➡ *and sludge* ➡ *within moderately dilated intrahepatic biliary ducts. Note the periductal hyperechogenicity* ➡, *related to periductal inflammation.* **(Right)** *Color Doppler US in the same patient demonstrates no flow within the dilated intrahepatic duct* ➡, *confirming the findings are indeed in the biliary tree rather than the portal or hepatic arterial system.*

Hepatic Artery Calcification

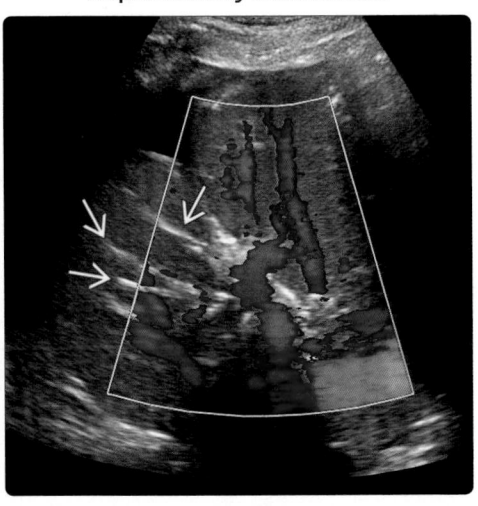

Cystic Duct Remnant

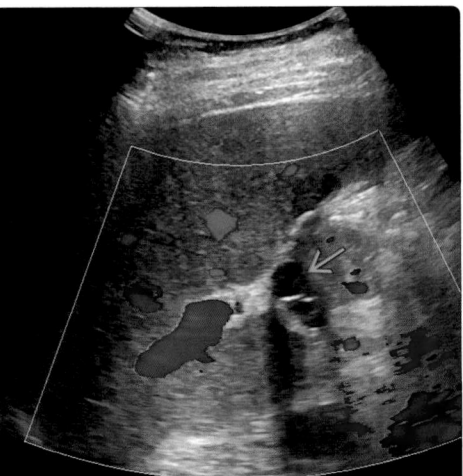

(Left) *Transverse abdominal color Doppler US shows multifocal linear branching echogenic structures* ➡ *that are hepatic artery calcifications related to end-stage renal disease.* **(Right)** *Longitudinal color Doppler US in a patient who underwent cholecystectomy shows a cystic duct remnant* ➡ *that appears as a round cystic lesion in the region of the porta hepatis.*

DIFFERENTIAL DIAGNOSIS

Common

- Cirrhosis
- Subcapsular Hepatic Neoplasm
- Hepatic Metastasis
- Infiltrative Hepatocellular Carcinoma
- Postsurgical Hepatic Resection

Less Common

- Hepatic Rupture
- Schistosomiasis

ESSENTIAL INFORMATION

Helpful Clues for Common Diagnoses

- **Cirrhosis**
  - Nodular surface contour
    - Micronodular (< 1 cm diameter): Due to alcoholism
    - Macronodular: Due to viral hepatitis
  - Hypertrophy of caudate lobe and lateral segment of left lobe
  - Atrophy of right lobe and medial segment of left lobe
  - Widening of fissures
  - Coarse/nodular/heterogeneous parenchymal echotexture
- **Subcapsular Hepatic Neoplasm**
  - Primary or secondary subcapsular neoplasm may distort surface contour when large or numerous
  - Lesions cause architectural distortion of liver parenchyma
- **Hepatic Metastasis**
  - Commonly due to gastric, ovarian, breast, or pancreatic primary
  - Treated metastases (e.g., from breast) may shrink and fibrose, simulating nodular contour of cirrhotic liver
- **Infiltrative Hepatocellular Carcinoma**
  - Margins of tumor often indistinct
  - May see refractive shadows emanating from hepatic parenchyma

- Portal triads may be effaced or invaded
- Often associated with tumor thrombus in the portal vein or hepatic vein (less common)
- **Postsurgical Hepatic Resection**
  - Combination of surgical defect and surrounding scarring causes irregularity of contour
  - Surgical material ± fat in surgical defect causes further heterogeneity of surgical site

Helpful Clues for Less Common Diagnoses

- **Hepatic Rupture**
  - Echogenic blood clot on surface of liver
  - May see breach of hepatic capsule or irregularity of capsular surface if underlying lesion is hepatocellular carcinoma
  - Hemoperitoneum may be present
    - More echogenic than ascites
  - Underlying cause
    - Large or exophytic hepatocellular carcinoma or other tumor
    - Spontaneous hepatic rupture associated with HELLP (hemolysis, elevated liver enzymes, and low platelets) syndrome
      - □ Thought to be secondary to endothelial dysfunction and thrombotic microangiopathy
- **Schistosomiasis**
  - Irregular/notched, liver surface
  - Echogenic periportal fibrotic bands (most severe at porta hepatis)
  - Mosaic pattern: Network of echogenic septa outlining polygonal areas of normal-appearing liver
    - Represents complete septal fibrosis (inflammation and fibrosis as reaction to embolized eggs)

SELECTED REFERENCES

1. Goel A et al: Pregnancy-related liver disorders. J Clin Exp Hepatol. 4(2):151-62, 2014
2. Irshad A et al: Current role of ultrasound in chronic liver disease: surveillance, diagnosis and management of hepatic neoplasms. Curr Probl Diagn Radiol. 41(2):43-51, 2012
3. Tchelepi H et al: Sonography of diffuse liver disease. J Ultrasound Med. 21(9):1023-32; quiz 1033-4, 2002

Cirrhosis

Cirrhosis

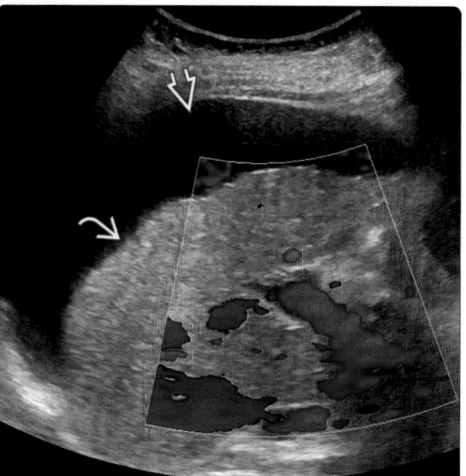
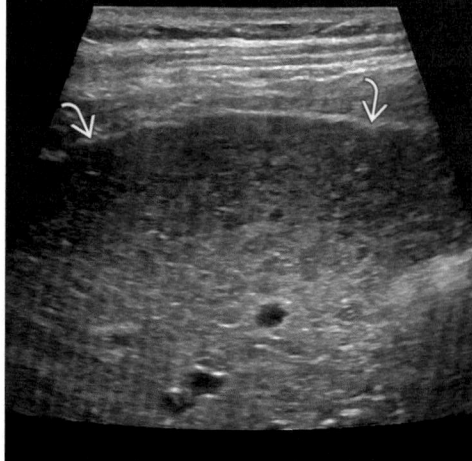

(Left) *Transverse color Doppler ultrasound in a patient with cirrhosis shows a nodular and irregular liver surface ⬈. A large amount of simple ascites ⬌ is consistent with portal hypertension related to underlying liver disease.* **(Right)** *Longitudinal high-resolution US in a patient with liver cirrhosis shows a nodular and irregular liver capsule ⬈ and heterogeneous echotexture of the underlying liver parenchyma. Imaging at higher frequencies focused at the level of liver capsule may help identify early or subtle cirrhosis.*

Subcapsular Hepatic Neoplasm

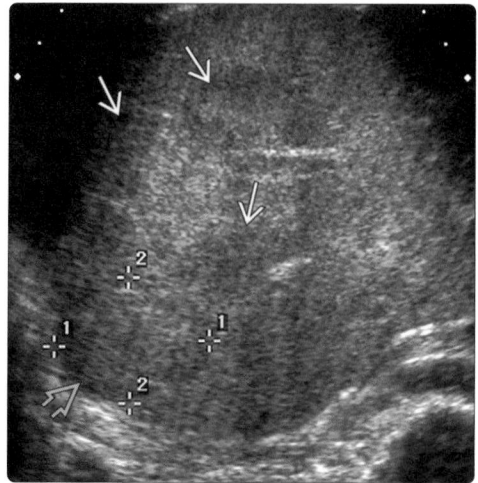

Subcapsular Hepatic Neoplasm

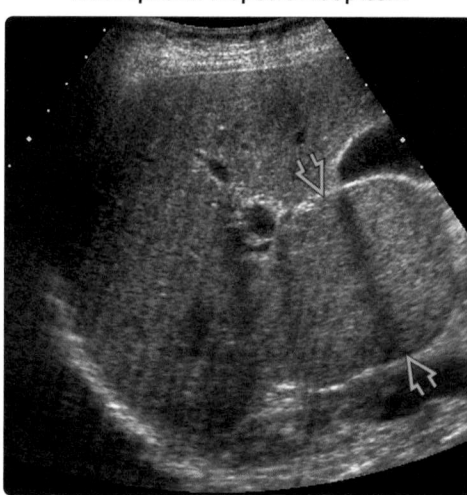

(Left) *Transverse grayscale ultrasound of the liver shows an isoechoic liver metastasis ⇨ from breast cancer that bulges and slightly distorts the liver surface. Multiple other subtle hypoechoic breast cancer metastases are seen throughout the rest of the liver ⇨.* (Right) *Transverse grayscale ultrasound of the liver shows a large isoechoic mass in the caudate lobe of the liver which creates a rounded bulge upon the hepatic surface in this area. This mass was a focal nodular hyperplasia (FNH) ⇨.*

Hepatic Metastasis

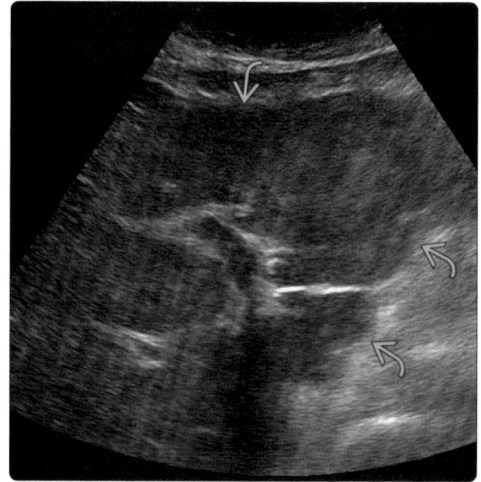

Infiltrative Hepatocellular Carcinoma

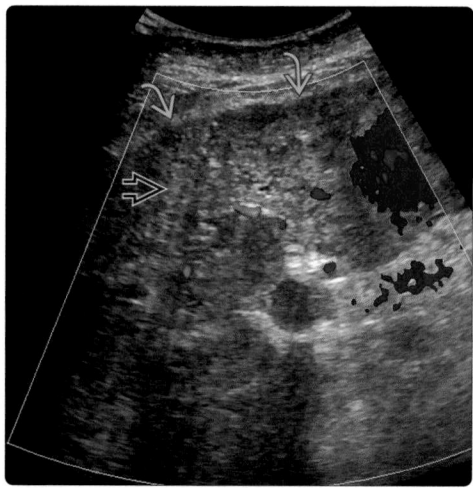

(Left) *Transverse grayscale ultrasound of the left lobe of the liver in a patient with breast cancer shows markedly irregular and nodular liver surface due to diffuse hepatic involvement with metastases ⇨.* (Right) *Transverse color Doppler ultrasound in a patient with infiltrative HCC throughout the liver shows the infiltrative tumor causes both markedly heterogeneous echotexture ⇨ as well as irregular hepatic surface ⇨.*

Hepatic Rupture

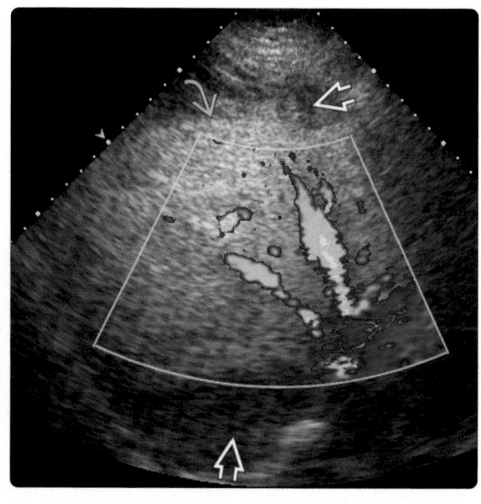

Schistosomiasis

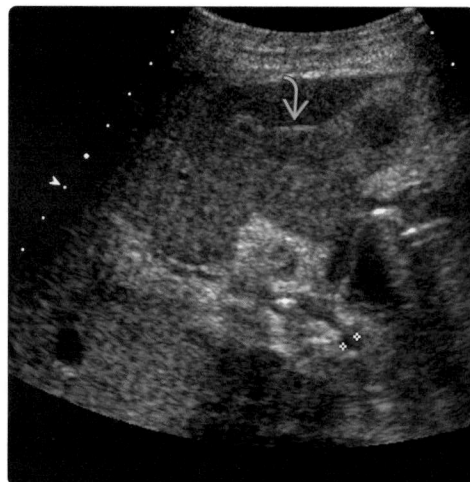

(Left) *Transverse color Doppler image in a patient with liver rupture from HELLP syndrome shows a large amount of perihepatic and subcapsular blood ⇨ which causes the liver margin ⇨ to appear irregular. Acute blood can be so echogenic that the liver margin can be obscured by the blood.* (Right) *Transverse grayscale ultrasound of a patient with schistosomiasis and periportal fibrosis as well as hepatic capsular irregularity ⇨ is shown. (Courtesy W. Chong, MD.)*

DIFFERENTIAL DIAGNOSIS

Common

- Portal Hypertension
- Portosystemic Collaterals
- Bland Portal Vein Thrombosis
- Portal Vein Tumor Thrombus
- Pulsatile Portal Vein

Less Common

- Portal Vein Gas

ESSENTIAL INFORMATION

Helpful Clues for Common Diagnoses

- **Portal Hypertension**
  - Decreased portal vein mean velocity (< 16 cm/s)
  - Portal venous pressure ≥ 10 mm Hg more than inferior vena cava pressure
  - Hepatofugal portal vein flow in severe portal hypertension
  - Absent (aphasic) portal venous flow due to stagnation
    - Lack of respiratory phasicity
    - Severe portal hypertension
  - Development of portosystemic shunts
  - Background cirrhosis, splenomegaly, ascites, thickened bowel wall
- **Portosystemic Collaterals**
  - Common locations
    - Inferior hepatic margin via gastroepiploic vein
    - Gastroesophageal junction via left gastric vein
    - Anterior abdominal wall via ligamentum teres (recanalized paraumbilical vein)
    - Lienorenal ligament via lienorenal collaterals
  - Color Doppler shows low velocity hepatofugal flow
- **Bland Portal Vein Thrombosis**
  - Echogenic material within portal vein (acute thrombosis)
  - Poor visualization of portal vein (chronic thrombosis)
  - Cavernous transformation of portal vein in chronic thrombosis

- Color Doppler: Interrupted/irregular flow in portal vein
- Signs of liver dysfunction or portal hypertension
  - Cirrhosis, ascites, splenomegaly, portosystemic collaterals
- **Portal Vein Tumor Thrombus**
  - Majority arise from hepatocellular carcinoma
  - Echogenic material within portal vein
  - Suspect tumor thrombus in case of adjacent hepatic malignancy
  - Color Doppler may show tumor neovascularity within thrombus
- **Pulsatile Portal Vein**
  - Normal portal vein waveform
    - Hepatopetal and mildly phasic (gentle undulation)
  - Increased pulsatility (pulsatile waveform)
    - When there is large difference between peak systolic velocity and end diastolic velocity
      - Tricuspid regurgitation
      - Right-sided congestive heart failure
      - Arterioportal shunting in cirrhosis
      - Arteriovenous fistula in hereditary hemorrhagic telangiectasia

Helpful Clues for Less Common Diagnoses

- **Portal Vein Gas**
  - Highly reflective foci (gas) travels within portal vein
  - Poorly defined, highly reflective parenchymal foci
  - Gas moves to periphery of liver (as opposed to biliary gas, which moves towards liver hilum)
  - High intensity transient signals (HITS) with spectral Doppler
    - Strong transient spikes superimposed on portal venous flow pattern

SELECTED REFERENCES

1. Manzano-Robleda Mdel C et al: Portal vein thrombosis: What is new? Ann Hepatol. 14(1):20-7, 2015
2. McNaughton DA et al: Doppler US of the liver made simple. Radiographics. 31(1):161-88, 2011
3. Abboud B et al: Hepatic portal venous gas: physiopathology, etiology, prognosis and treatment. World J Gastroenterol. 15(29):3585-90, 2009

Portal Hypertension

Portosystemic Collaterals

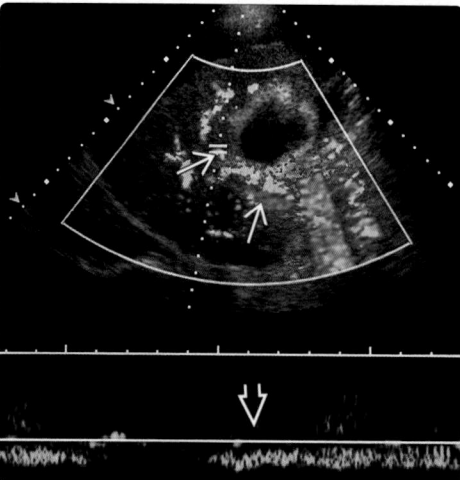
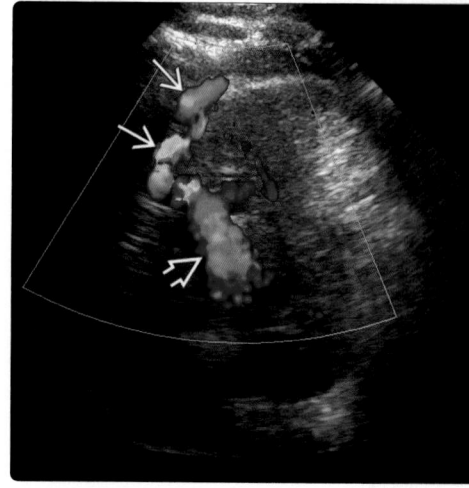

(Left) *Spectral Doppler ultrasound of the liver in a patient with portal hypertension shows retrograde (hepatofugal) flow in the portal vein ➡, a finding that appears blue on the color Doppler US and is displayed below the baseline on the spectral waveform ➡.* **(Right)** *Transverse abdominal color Doppler US in a patient with hepatic cirrhosis shows a recanalized paraumbilical vein ➡ arising from the left portal vein ➡ and traveling anteriorly along the falciform ligament towards the inferior epigastric vein.*

Bland Portal Vein Thrombosis

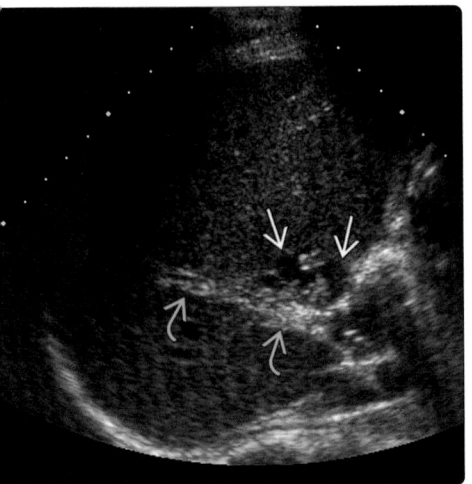

Bland Portal Vein Thrombosis

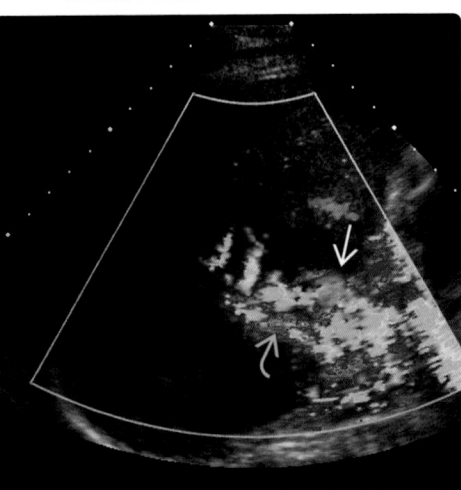

(Left) *Grayscale ultrasound shows an echogenic, chronically thrombosed main portal vein ⊿ and adjacent collateralized flow ➡ indicating cavernous transformation of the portal vein.* **(Right)** *Color Doppler ultrasound in the same patient shows collateralized flow ➡ in the porta hepatis in this patient with chronic portal vein thrombosis ⊿. Color Doppler signal is heterogeneous because portal vein collaterals are tortuous, resulting in vessels directed towards as well as away from the transducer.*

Portal Vein Tumor Thrombus

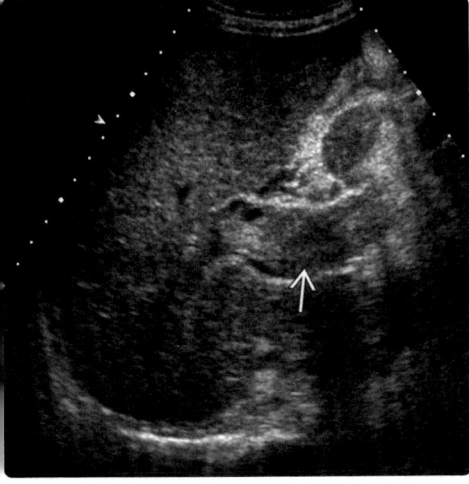

Portal Vein Tumor Thrombus

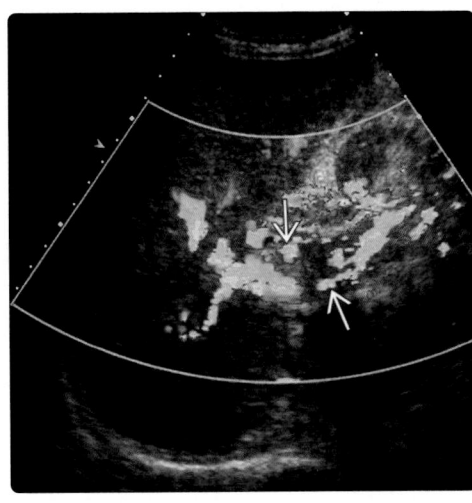

(Left) *Transverse grayscale ultrasound of the liver in a patient with hepatocellular carcinoma shows an expansile echogenic tumor thrombus in the main portal vein ➡.* **(Right)** *Color Doppler US in the same patient shows multiple small feeding vessels ➡ in the tumor thrombus with a dot-dash pattern. Tumor thrombus in the setting of hepatocellular carcinoma is almost always associated with infiltrative tumor and carries a poor prognosis.*

Pulsatile Portal Vein

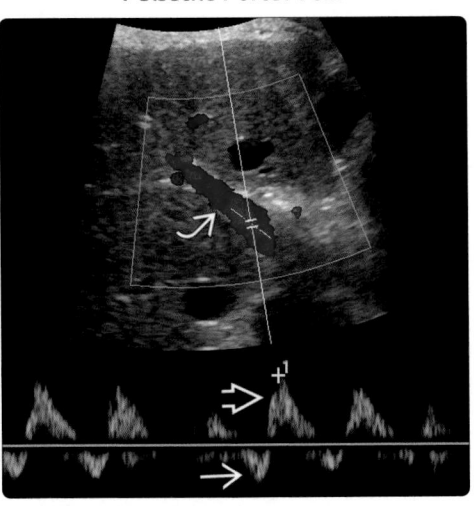

Portal Vein Gas

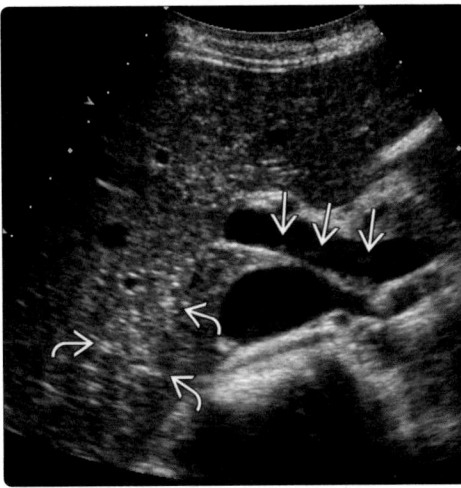

(Left) *Spectral Doppler US in a patient with right heart failure shows a pulsatile waveform with flow above ➡ and below ➡ baseline in the main portal vein ⊿. The waveform is characterized as predominantly antegrade, pulsatile, and biphasic-bidirectional.* **(Right)** *Oblique ultrasound of the liver shows several echogenic foci in the main portal vein ➡ representing gas bubbles. Bright echogenic patches ➡ in the liver parenchyma more peripherally represent intraparenchymal portal venous gas.*

**PART III
SECTION 2**

Biliary System

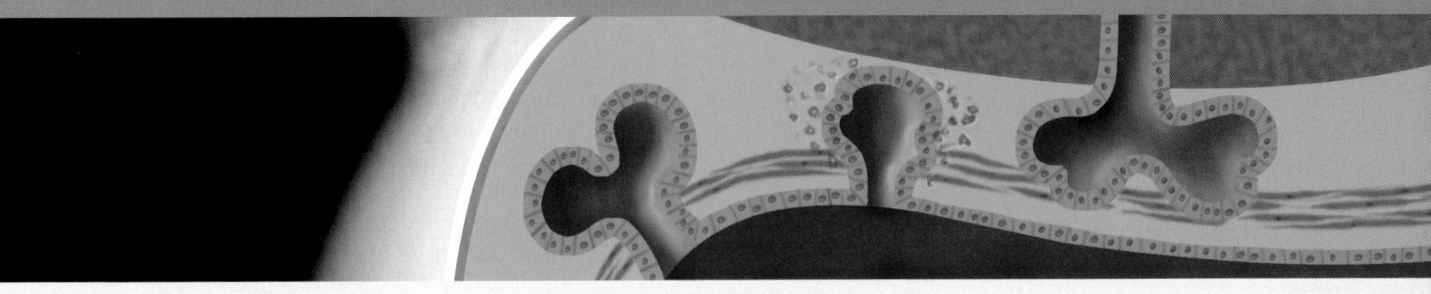

DIFFERENTIAL DIAGNOSIS

Common

- Acute Calculous Cholecystitis
- Chronic Cholecystitis
- Hyperplastic Cholecystosis (Adenomyomatosis)
- Wall Thickening due to Systemic Diseases
  - Congestive Heart Failure
  - Renal Failure
  - Hepatic Cirrhosis
  - Hypoalbuminemia

Less Common

- Acute Acalculous Cholecystitis
- Acute Pancreatitis
- Acute Hepatitis
- Perforated Peptic Ulcer
- Gallbladder Carcinoma
- Lymphoma
- AIDS-Related Cholangiopathy
- Gallbladder Varices

Rare

- Xanthogranulomatous Cholecystitis
- Dengue Fever

ESSENTIAL INFORMATION

Key Differential Diagnosis Issues

- Clinical information is essential to derive differential diagnosis
- Presence of sepsis and right upper quadrant (RUQ) pain favor acute cholecystitis
- Presence of known systemic diseases: Congestive heart failure, renal failure, hypoalbuminemia are important considerations
- Presence of regional disease: Acute hepatitis or pancreatitis, cirrhosis affect gallbladder wall
- Known malignancy

Other Info

- Fever, leucocytosis, liver function tests

Helpful Clues for Common Diagnoses

- **Acute Calculous Cholecystitis**
  - Clinical: RUQ pain, fever, positive Murphy sign
  - Acute gallbladder (GB) inflammation secondary to calculus obstructing cystic duct
  - Gallstones ± impaction in GB neck
  - Diffuse GB wall thickening (> 3 mm)
    - Striated appearance: Alternating bright and dark bands within thick GB wall
    - GB wall lucency "halo" sign: Sonolucent middle layer due to edema
  - Distended gallbladder (GB hydrops)
  - Positive sonographic Murphy sign
  - Presence of pericholecystic fluid
  - Complicated cholecystitis
    - Gangrenous cholecystitis
      - Asymmetric wall thickening
      - Marked wall irregularities
      - Intraluminal membranes

- GB perforation
  - Defect in GB wall
  - Pericholecystic abscess or extraluminal stones
- Emphysematous cholecystitis
  - Gas in GB wall/lumen
- Empyema of GB
  - Intraluminal echoes, purulent exudate/debris

- **Chronic Cholecystitis**
  - Mostly asymptomatic
  - Diffuse GB wall thickening
    - Mean thickness ~ 5 mm
    - Smooth/irregular contour
  - Contracted GB
    - GB lumen may be obliterated in severe cases
  - Presence of gallstones in nearly all cases

- **Hyperplastic Cholecystosis (Adenomyomatosis)**
  - Adenomyomatosis of GB
  - Clinically asymptomatic, usually incidental US finding
  - Focal or diffuse GB wall thickening
  - Tiny echogenic foci in GB wall producing "comet-tail" artifacts
  - Presence of cystic spaces within GB wall
  - Fundal adenomyomatosis: Smooth thickening or focal mass in fundal region ± ring down artifact
  - Hourglass GB: Narrowing of mid portion of GB

- **Wall Thickening due to Systemic Diseases**
  - Clinical correlation is key to explain presence of GB wall thickening
  - Appearance of wall thickening is nonspecific
  - Other ancillary US findings
    - **Congestive heart failure**: Engorged hepatic veins and IVC, diffuse hypoechoic liver echo pattern
    - **Renal failure**: Small kidneys with increased parenchymal echogenicity
    - **Hepatic cirrhosis**: Coarse liver echo pattern, irregular/nodular liver contour, signs of portal hypertension (e.g., ascites, splenomegaly, varices)
    - **Hypoalbuminemia**: Presence of ascites, diffuse bowel wall thickening

Helpful Clues for Less Common Diagnoses

- **Acute Acalculous Cholecystitis**
  - More commonly seen in critically ill patients (e.g., post major surgery, severe trauma, sepsis, etc.)
  - US features are similar to acute calculous cholecystitis except for absence of impacted gallstone
    - GB wall thickening: Hypoechoic, layered/striated appearance
    - GB distension: Often filled with sludge
    - Positive sonographic Murphy sign
    - Pericholecystic fluid

- **Acute Pancreatitis**
  - Spread of inflammation to GB fossa
  - Nonspecific GB wall thickening
  - Diffuse/focal, swollen, hypoechoic pancreas

- **Acute Hepatitis**
  - Clinical history: General malaise, vomiting, deranged liver function test with hepatitic pattern
  - Hepatomegaly with diffuse decrease in echogenicity

- o "Starry sky" appearance: Increased echogenicity of portal triad walls against hypoechoic liver parenchyma
- o Periportal hypo-/anechoic area
- o Gallbladder lumen less dilated than in acute cholecystitis

- **Perforated Peptic Ulcer**
  - o Penetrating ulcer in duodenal wall causes sympathetic GB wall thickening
  - o Presence of extraluminal fluid/gas

- **Gallbladder Carcinoma**
  - o Asymmetric or irregular GB wall thickening
  - o Mass replacing GB with locally advanced tumor
  - o Presence of gallstones
  - o Invasion of adjacent structures (e.g., liver, duodenum)
  - o Regional nodal and liver metastases

- **Lymphoma**
  - o Rare involvement of GB by secondary lymphoma
  - o Nonspecific diffuse GB wall thickening
  - o Presence of intraabdominal lymphomatous lymph nodes

- **AIDS-Related Cholangiopathy**
  - o Biliary inflammatory lesions caused by AIDS-related opportunistic infections leading to biliary stricture/obstruction or cholecystitis
  - o Diffuse GB wall thickening
  - o Bile duct wall thickening/inflammation
    - Periductal hyper-/hypoechoic areas
  - o Focal biliary stricture and dilatation

- **Gallbladder Varices**
  - o Usually seen in portal hypertension or cavernous transformation of main portal vein
  - o Tubular structures in GB wall readily confirmed with color/power Doppler and pulsed Doppler

- **Xanthogranulomatous Cholecystitis**
  - o Rare form of chronic cholecystitis
  - o Diffuse irregular wall thickening, may appear infiltrative; mimics GB carcinoma

- **Dengue Fever**
  - o Rash, fever, headache and joint pains after travel to endemic area
  - o GB thickening from acute viral hepatic infection leading to hepatic failure

Alternative Differential Approaches

- Etiology of GB wall thickening
  - o Inflammatory conditions
    - Acute calculous cholecystitis
    - Acute acalculous cholecystitis
    - Chronic cholecystitis
    - AIDS-related cholangiopathy
    - Secondary causes: Acute hepatitis, perforated peptic ulcer, pancreatitis
  - o Systemic diseases
    - Congestive heart failure
    - Renal failure
    - Liver cirrhosis
    - Hypoalbuminemia
  - o Neoplastic infiltration
    - GB carcinoma
    - Leukemic/lymphomatous infiltration

SELECTED REFERENCES

1. Garg PK et al: Xanthogranulomatous Inflammation of Gallbladder and Bile Duct Causing Obstructive Jaundice Masquerades Gallbladder Cancer: a Formidable Diagnostic Challenge Continues. J Gastrointest Cancer. ePub, 2014
2. Runner GJ et al: Gallbladder wall thickening. AJR Am J Roentgenol. 202(1):W1-W12, 2014
3. Zemour J et al: Gallbladder tumor and pseudotumor: Diagnosis and management. J Visc Surg. 151(4):289-300, 2014
4. Teefey SA et al: Acute cholecystitis: do sonographic findings and WBC count predict gangrenous changes? AJR Am J Roentgenol. 200(2):363-9, 2013
5. Charalel RA et al: Complicated cholecystitis: the complementary roles of sonography and computed tomography. Ultrasound Q. 27(3):161-70, 2011
6. O'Connor OJ et al: Imaging of cholecystitis. AJR Am J Roentgenol. 196(4):W367-74, 2011
7. Ito K et al: Imaging findings of unusual intra- and extrahepatic portosystemic collaterals. Clin Radiol. 64(2):200-7, 2009
8. Furlan A et al: Gallbladder carcinoma update: multimodality imaging evaluation, staging, and treatment options. AJR Am J Roentgenol. 191(5):1440-7, 2008
9. van Breda Vriesman AC et al: Diffuse gallbladder wall thickening: differential diagnosis. AJR Am J Roentgenol. 188(2):495-501, 2007
10. Levy AD et al: Gallbladder carcinoma: radiologic-pathologic correlation. Radiographics. 21(2):295-314; questionnaire, 549-55, 2001

Acute Calculous Cholecystitis

Congestive Heart Failure

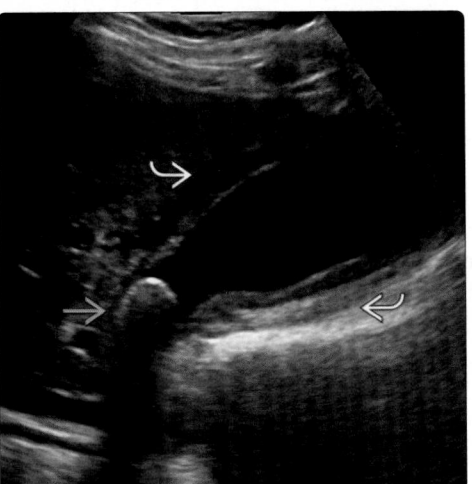
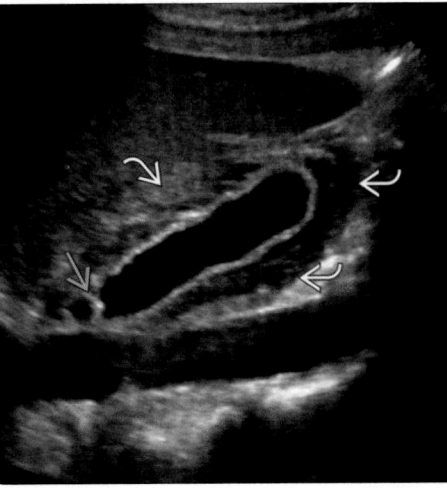

(Left) *Longitudinal oblique ultrasound of acute calculous cholecystitis shows an impacted stone ⟶ in the gallbladder neck. There is diffuse edema and thickening of the gallbladder wall ⟶.* **(Right)** *Longitudinal oblique ultrasound shows diffuse gallbladder wall edema secondary to heart failure. There is striated wall thickening ⟶ and a fold in the gallbladder neck ⟶.*

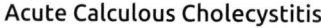

Acute Calculous Cholecystitis

Acute Hepatitis

(Left) *Longitudinal oblique ultrasound in gangrenous acute calculous cholecystitis shows a markedly abnormal gallbladder with shadowing stones ➡. There is asymmetric wall thickening with intramural fluid collections ➡ and focal thinning of the wall at the fundus ➡.* (Right) *Transverse ultrasound in a patient with acute hepatitis and fulminant liver failure shows that the gallbladder wall is circumferentially thickened ➡ with striations. Ascites ➡ is noted.*

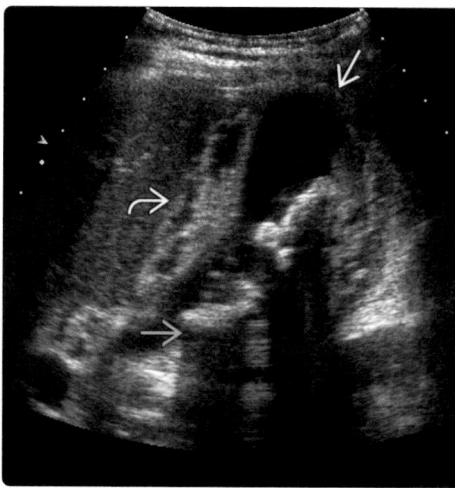

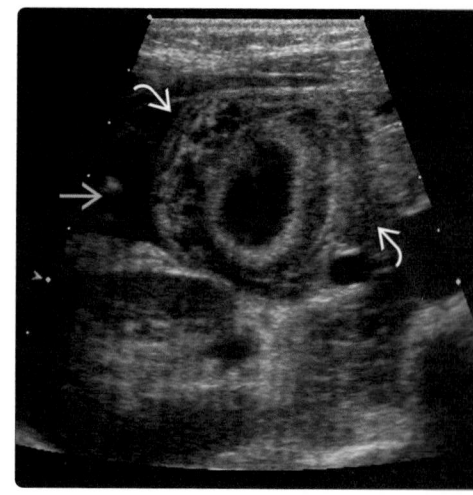

Acute Calculous Cholecystitis

Acute Calculous Cholecystitis

(Left) *Longitudinal ultrasound shows the gallbladder in a patient with perforated acute calculous cholecystitis. The gallbladder wall is asymmetrically thickened ➡ and there is intraluminal debris with linear membranes ➡.* (Right) *Axial CECT of the same patient shows multiple calcified gallstones ➡ in an abscess cavity ➡ outside the perforated gallbladder ➡.*

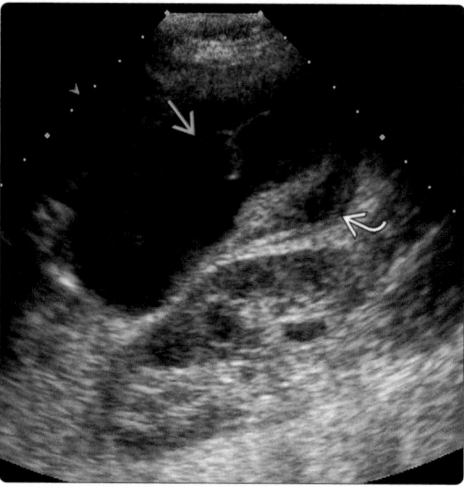

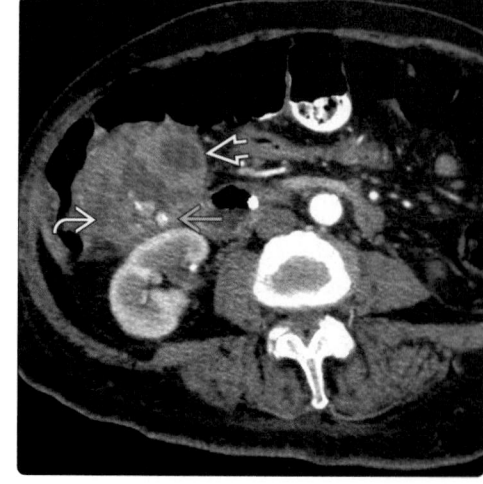

Hyperplastic Cholecystosis (Adenomyomatosis)

Hyperplastic Cholecystosis (Adenomyomatosis)

(Left) *Longitudinal ultrasound in a patient with adenomyomatosis shows diffuse thickening of the gallbladder wall ➡ with several tiny focal polypoid lesions ➡.* (Right) *Longitudinal ultrasound in a patient with segmental adenomyomatosis shows diffuse thickening of the gallbladder wall in the fundus ➡ with multiple small, echogenic foci. There is a transition zone ➡ (waisting) in the body with normal wall thickness in the neck ➡.*

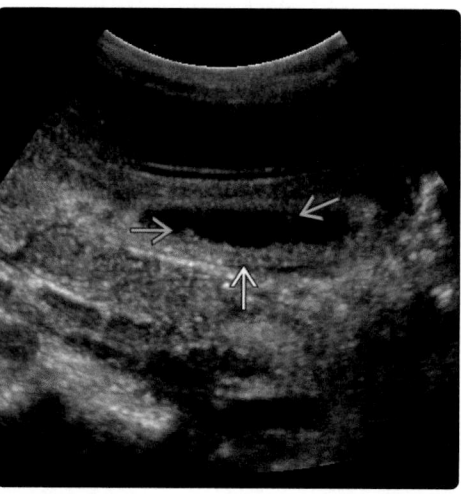

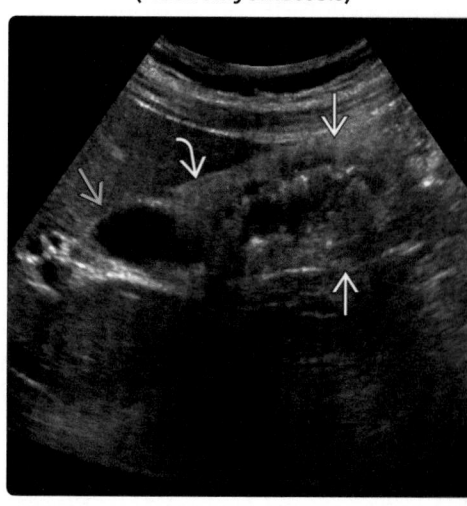

Hepatic Cirrhosis

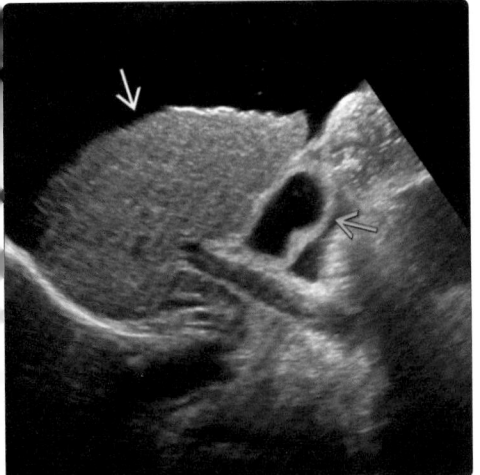

AIDS-Related Cholangiopathy

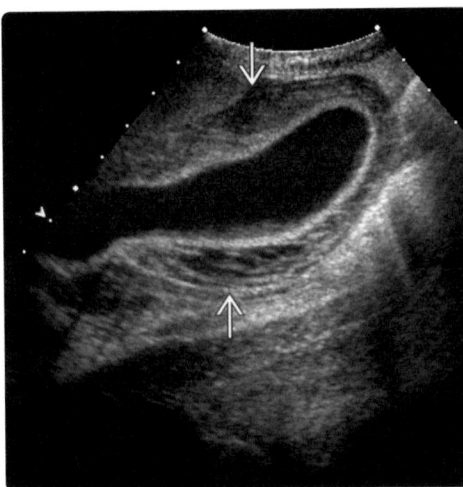

(Left) *Longitudinal oblique ultrasound through the liver and gallbladder shows a nodular cirrhotic liver* ➡ *surrounded by ascites. The gallbladder wall* ➡ *is mildly uniformly thickened. There were no stones.* (Right) *Longitudinal oblique ultrasound in a patient with HIV/AIDS shows a thick-walled gallbladder with no gallstones. There are linear strands in the edematous wall* ➡ *compatible with striated edema.*

Gallbladder Carcinoma

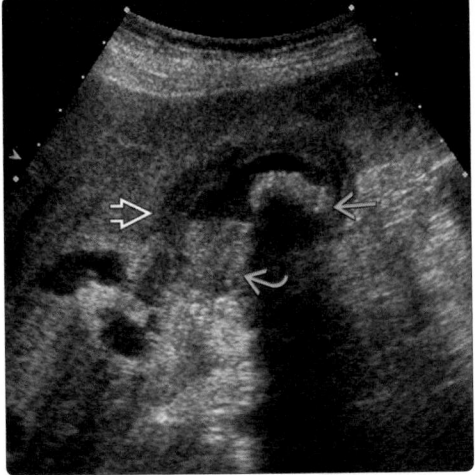

Gallbladder Carcinoma

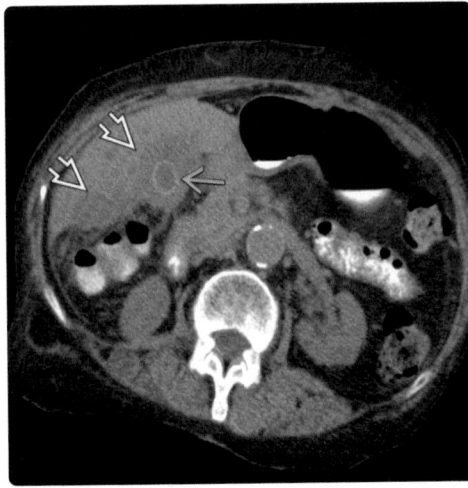

(Left) *Transverse ultrasound of gallbladder carcinoma shows a shadowing stone* ➡ *with sludge* ➡. *The gallbladder wall was thick and indistinct with loss of echogenicity* ➡ *at its interface with the liver.* (Right) *Axial NECT of the same patient shows a gallstone* ➡. *The gallbladder wall is thick and hypodense, with infiltration of the adjacent liver* ➡.

Gallbladder Varices

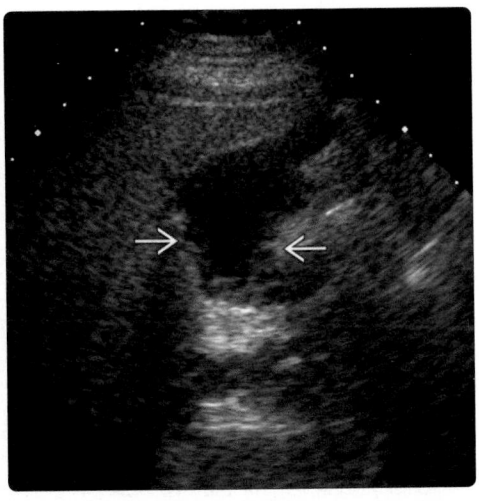

Gallbladder Varices

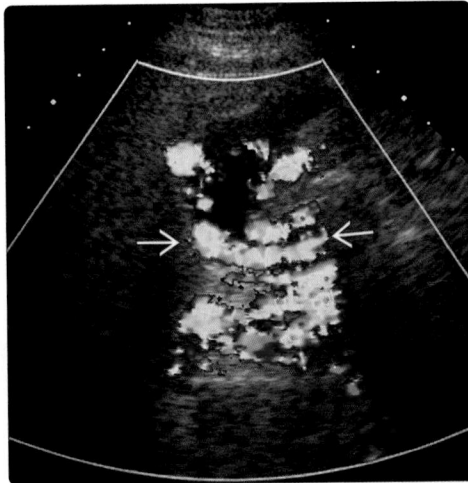

(Left) *Transverse ultrasound in a patient with cavernous transformation of the main portal vein secondary to pancreatitis shows small cystic spaces in the wall at the gallbladder neck and body* ➡. *(Right) Transverse color Doppler ultrasound in the same patient shows multiple collateral veins* ➡ *in the gallbladder wall and around the porta hepatis.*

DIFFERENTIAL DIAGNOSIS

Common

- Large Gallstone
- Porcelain Gallbladder
- Contracted Gallbladder With Gallstones
- Gas-Filled Duodenal Bulb

Less Common

- Hyperplastic Cholecystosis
- Adherent Gallstones
- Emphysematous Cholecystitis
- Fistula to Gallbladder
- Iatrogenic: Post Endoscopic Retrograde Cholangiopancreatography (ERCP)

ESSENTIAL INFORMATION

Key Differential Diagnosis Issues

- Differentiate gas-filled duodenum from abnormal gallbladder by location and repositioning patient
- Duodenum may be mistaken for gallbladder post cholecystectomy
  - Relevant surgical history is key
  - Look for cholecystectomy scars if no history is available
  - Correlate with other imaging
- Gas in gallbladder may be a surgical emergency
  - If unclear, confirm with CT

Helpful Clues for Common Diagnoses

- **Large Gallstone**
  - Strong acoustic impedance at wall-stone interface with posterior shadowing
  - Wall-echo-shadow appearance (optimize technique)
  - Mobile on changing patient's position unless stone is very large and gallbladder is contracted around it
- **Contracted Gallbladder With Gallstones**
  - Multiple, closely packed echogenic stones without bile mimic echogenic gallbladder wall
  - Thickened gallbladder wall

- Gallstones may not move on changing patient's position if gallbladder is severely contracted
- **Gas-Filled Duodenal Bulb**
  - Observe peristalsis
  - Move patient to move gas or have patient drink water to confirm
- **Porcelain Gallbladder**
  - Diffuse gallbladder wall calcification
    - Echogenic curvilinear line in gallbladder fossa
    - Dense posterior acoustic shadowing
  - Segmental form: Interrupted echogenic line on anterior wall
    - Or multiple separate coarse echogenic foci/clumps in wall with posterior acoustic shadowing

Helpful Clues for Less Common Diagnoses

- **Hyperplastic Cholecystosis**
  - Focal, diffuse or segmental gallbladder wall thickening
  - Tiny echogenic foci in gallbladder wall with characteristic "comet tail" artifacts
  - Segmental form: Transition from normal to thick wall in mid gallbladder producing "hourglass" gallbladder
- **Adherent Gallstones**
  - Not curvilinear in configuration or mobile
- **Emphysematous Cholecystitis**
  - Complicated form of acute cholecystitis
  - Clinical evidence of fulminant biliary sepsis is usually present
  - Gas in gallbladder wall/lumen
    - Echogenic crescent in gallbladder with reverberation artifacts ("dirty" shadowing)
  - More common in diabetes and immunosuppressed patients
- **Gallbladder Fistula**
  - Spontaneous fistula from erosion of gallstone into duodenum: Gallstone ileus
  - Fistula to gallbladder from adjacent bowel malignancy
- **Post ERCP or Biliary Stent**
  - Known history of intervention
  - Gas in gallbladder without signs of cholecystitis

(Left) *Transverse oblique ultrasound shows a large, curved, echogenic structure ➡ within the gallbladder casting a dense posterior acoustic shadow. The gallbladder wall ➡ is seen separately. This is the wall-echo-shadow sign, which differentiates a large gallstone from a porcelain gallbladder.* **(Right)** *Oblique transabdominal ultrasound shows numerous small shadowing echogenic gallstones ➡ filling a contracted gallbladder ➡. The gallbladder wall is thick suggesting chronic cholecystitis.*

Large Gallstone

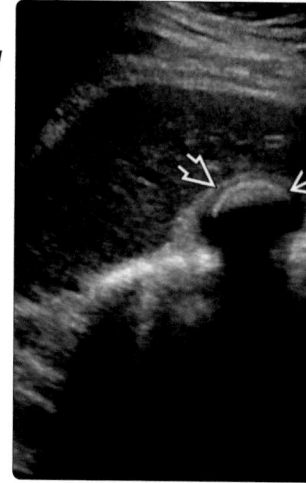

Contracted Gallbladder With Gallstones

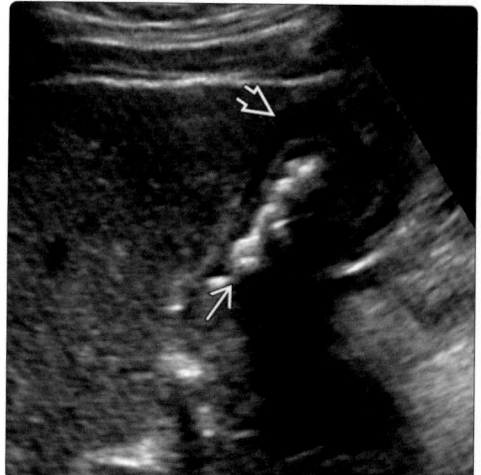

Porcelain Gallbladder

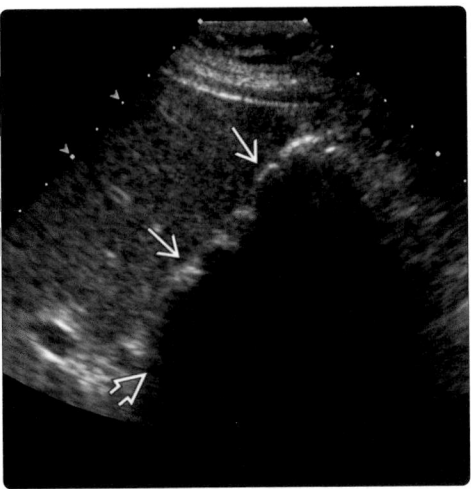

Porcelain Gallbladder

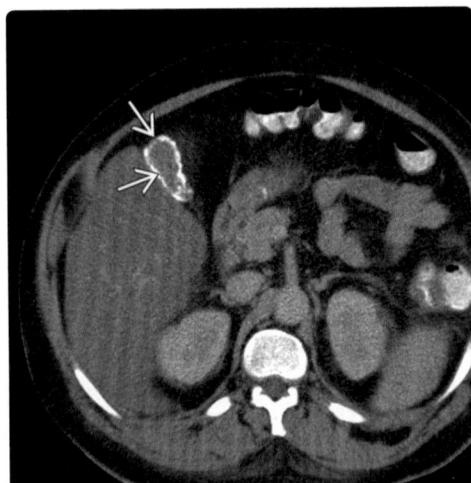

(Left) *Oblique transabdominal ultrasound shows curvilinear echogenicity ➡ in the gallbladder wall casting dense posterior acoustic shadowing ⇉. Absence of wall-echo-shadow sign suggests porcelain gallbladder.* (Right) *Axial CECT of the same patient confirms the thin diffuse gallbladder wall calcification ➡ in a contracted gallbladder.*

Gas-Filled Duodenal Bulb

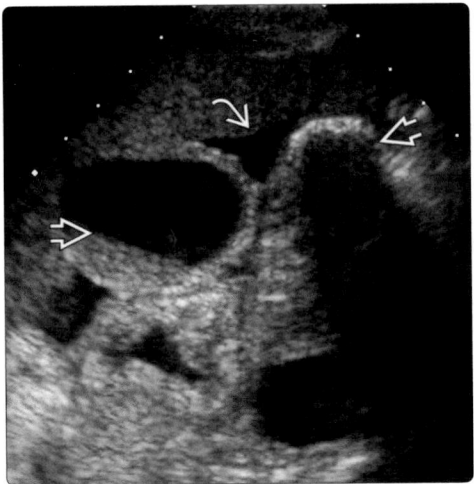

Hyperplastic Cholecystosis

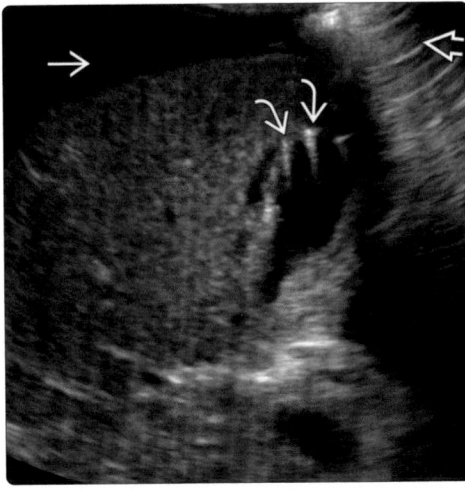

(Left) *Transverse ultrasound shows the duodenal bulb containing gas ⇉. The gallbladder contains sludge in this patient with ascites ➡ and cirrhosis. The duodenum may be mistaken for a gallbladder.* (Right) *Transverse oblique ultrasound shows multiple areas of "comet tail" artifact ➡ emanating from the thick wall of the gallbladder. Reverberation artifact is noted from bowel ⇉ and there is ascites ➡ in this patient with chronic liver disease.*

Emphysematous Cholecystitis

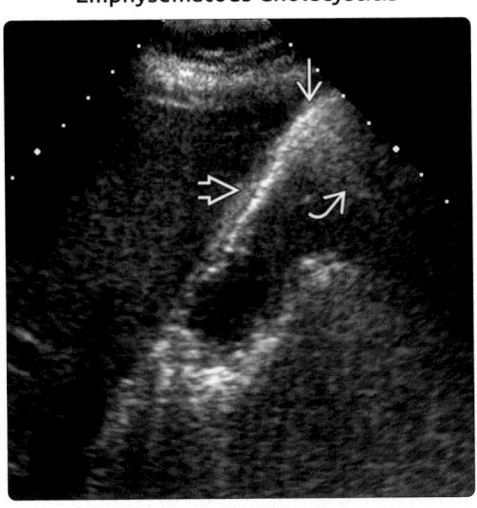

Iatrogenic: Post Endoscopic Retrograde Cholangiopancreatography (ERCP)

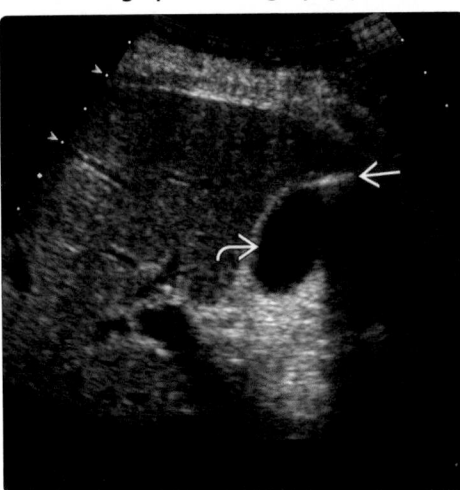

(Left) *Longitudinal ultrasound shows the gallbladder fundus in a diabetic patient with fever and right upper quadrant pain. A linear bright echo ➡ within a thick wall ⇉ produces dirty shadowing ➡ that is highly suggestive of gas. This was confirmed with CT. Surgery was performed for emphysematous cholecystitis.* (Right) *Transverse oblique ultrasound shows a bright linear echo with dirty shadowing ➡ representing gas in the gallbladder fundus post ERCP. The gallbladder ➡ was normal.*

DIFFERENTIAL DIAGNOSIS

Common

- Gallbladder Cholesterol Polyp
- Hyperplastic Cholecystosis (Adenomyomatosis)
- Adenomatous Polyp
- Adherent Gallstone

Less Common

- Gallbladder Adenocarcinoma
- Adjacent Liver or Colonic Tumor
- Metastases to Gallbladder
- Other Primary Gallbladder Neoplasms
- Gastric or Pancreatic Heterotopia/Foregut Cysts

Rare but Important

- Xanthogranulomatous Cholecystitis

ESSENTIAL INFORMATION

Key Differential Diagnosis Issues

- Most lesions are benign; key is to detect gallbladder (GB) carcinoma early
- Carcinoma: Large irregular soft tissue mass
  - Circumferential or eccentric wall thickening ± internal color flow
  - Ill-defined margin, infiltration of gallbladder wall and adjacent liver parenchyma
  - Presence of regional nodal/liver metastases

Helpful Clues for Common Diagnoses

- **Gallbladder Cholesterol Polyp**
  - Multiple, small, nonshadowing lesions with soft tissue echogenicity
  - Smooth in contour, sometimes multilobulated in outline
  - Round or ovoid shape; broad base is attached to gallbladder wall
  - Nonmobile on decubitus positioning
  - Overlying GB wall is intact and normal
  - Cholesterolosis: Diffuse nodular wall thickening from cholesterol deposits

- **Hyperplastic Cholecystosis (Adenomyomatosis)**
  - Tiny echogenic foci within thick GB wall with "comet tail" artifacts
  - Fundal adenomyomatosis: Smooth sessile mass/thickening in fundus
    - Look for comet tail artifacts/color Doppler twinkling artifact
  - Diffuse adenomyomatosis: Diffuse wall thickening with tiny intramural diverticula
  - Segmental form: Wall thickening of midportion to fundus with hourglass appearance
- **Adenomatous Polyp**
  - Larger size (> 10 mm), solitary lesion
  - Usually pedunculated in appearance

Helpful Clues for Less Common Diagnoses

- **Gallbladder Adenocarcinoma**
  - Asymmetric GB wall thickening
  - Intramural polypoid mass protruding into gallbladder lumen
  - Ill-defined infiltrative mass in gallbladder fossa
  - Invasion of adjacent liver parenchyma: Indistinct separation between GB mass and liver capsule
  - Presence of regional nodal/liver metastases ± intratumoral vascularity
- **Metastases to Gallbladder**
  - Most common: melanoma, renal and breast cancer
  - Usually have other metastases
  - Multiple, sessile, hypoechoic, internal color flow
- **Other Primary Gallbladder Neoplasms**
  - Epithelial and nonepithelial benign and malignant tumors such as leiomyoma, leiomyosarcoma

Helpful Clues for Rare Diagnoses

- **Xanthogranulomatous Cholecystitis**
  - Irregular gallbladder wall thickening, infiltration into liver
  - Hypoechoic bands or nodules in thick gallbladder wall on ultrasound
  - Coexisting gall stones
  - May be indistinguishable from GB carcinoma

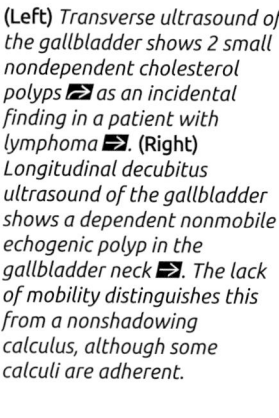

(Left) Transverse ultrasound of the gallbladder shows 2 small nondependent cholesterol polyps ⇗ as an incidental finding in a patient with lymphoma ⇗. (Right) Longitudinal decubitus ultrasound of the gallbladder shows a dependent nonmobile echogenic polyp in the gallbladder neck ⇗. The lack of mobility distinguishes this from a nonshadowing calculus, although some calculi are adherent.

Gallbladder Cholesterol Polyp

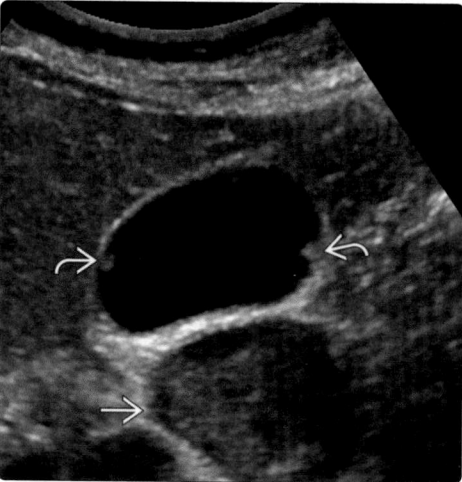

Gallbladder Cholesterol Polyp

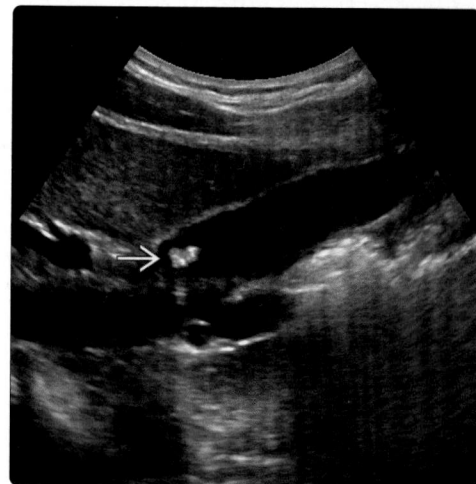

Adenomatous Polyp

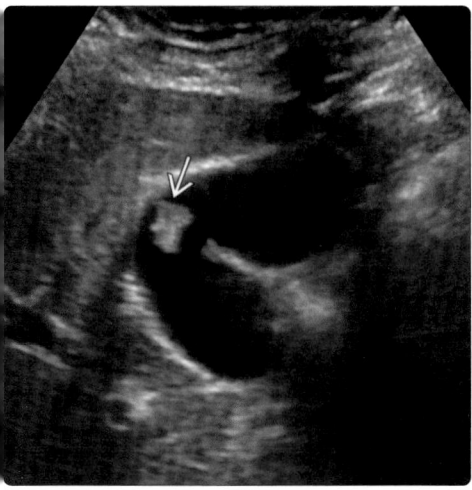

Hyperplastic Cholecystosis (Adenomyomatosis)

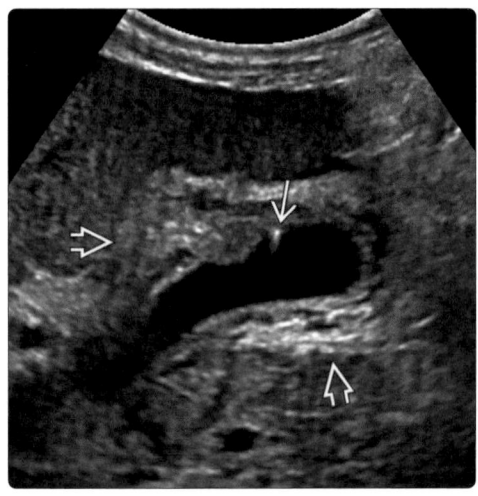

(Left) *Longitudinal oblique ultrasound shows a well-circumscribed homogeneous polypoid mass ➡ with a lobulated margin arising from the gallbladder wall. When larger than 10 mm, surgery should be considered.* **(Right)** *Longitudinal ultrasound of the gallbladder in a patient with cirrhosis shows diffuse wall-striated thickening ➡ and a "comet tail" artifact ➡ consistent with adenomyomatosis and secondary wall thickening. There was no tenderness.*

Hyperplastic Cholecystosis (Adenomyomatosis)

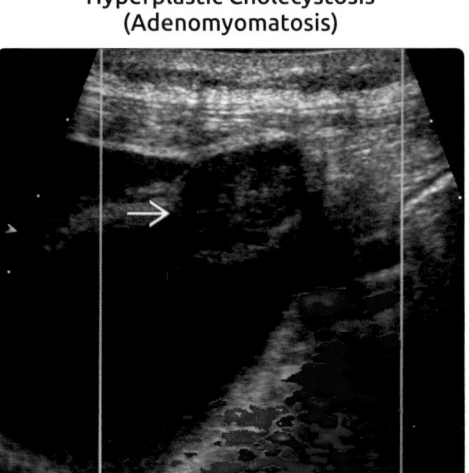

Hyperplastic Cholecystosis (Adenomyomatosis)

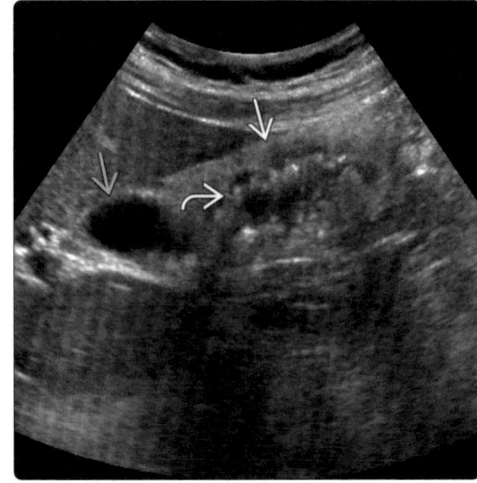

(Left) *Longitudinal oblique color Doppler ultrasound of the gallbladder fundus shows a round, hypovascular mass with internal cystic spaces ➡ consistent with fundal adenomyomatosis.* **(Right)** *Longitudinal ultrasound shows segmental fundal gallbladder adenomyomatosis. The distal gallbladder wall is thick ➡ with numerous echogenic foci ➡. The neck was normal ➡.*

Gallbladder Adenocarcinoma

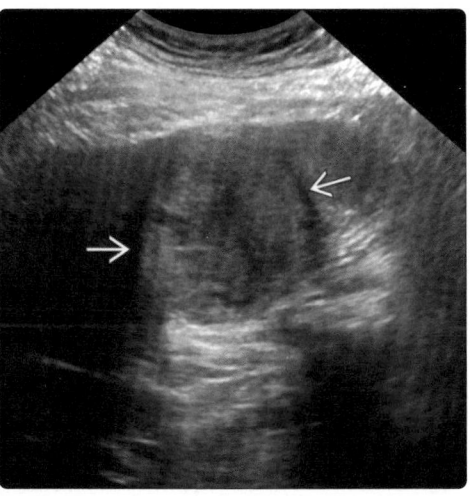

Xanthogranulomatous Cholecystitis

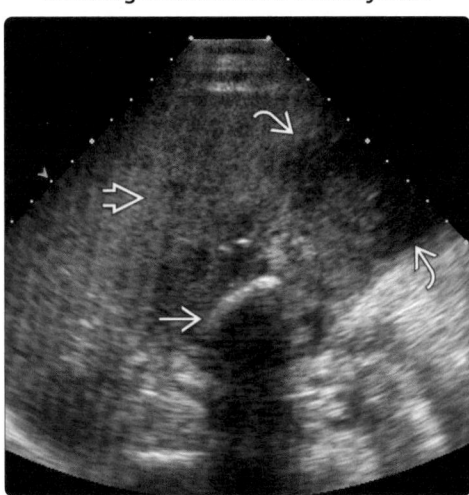

(Left) *Transverse ultrasound shows a soft tissue mass in the gallbladder ➡ obliterating the lumen representing gallbladder carcinoma.* **(Right)** *Longitudinal oblique ultrasound of the gallbladder fossa shows an indistinct soft tissue mass with hypoechoic components ➡ infiltrating into liver ➡. This was proven to be xanthogranulomatous cholecystitis. Gallstones were present ➡.*

DIFFERENTIAL DIAGNOSIS

Common

- Cholelithiasis
- Sludge/Sludge Ball/Echogenic Bile

Less Common

- Blood Clot
- Complicated Cholecystitis
- Gas Within Gallbladder Lumen
- Drainage Catheter
- Tumor: Primary or Secondary
- Parasitic Infestation

ESSENTIAL INFORMATION

Helpful Clues for Common Diagnoses

- **Cholelithiasis**
  - Highly reflective intraluminal structure within gallbladder lumen
  - Posterior acoustic shadowing
  - Gravity-dependent and mobile
  - Variants
    - Bright echoes with acoustic shadowing in gallbladder fossa representing gallbladder packed with stones
    - Nonshadowing gallstones, usually small (< 5 mm)
    - Double-arc shadow sign or wall-echo-shadow (WES) sign
    - Immobile adherent/impacted gallstones
  - Complication: Acute calculous cholecystitis: Gallbladder distension and wall thickening, sonographic Murphy sign, pericholecystic fluid
- **Sludge/Sludge Ball/Echogenic Bile**
  - Amorphous, mid-/high-level echoes within gallbladder, lack of shadowing
  - Sediment in dependent portion
  - Mobile on changing patient's position without posterior acoustic shadowing
  - Sludge ball: Aggregate with well-defined, round contour, moves slowly

- Can be isoechoic to liver resulting in "hepatization" of gallbladder

Helpful Clues for Less Common Diagnoses

- **Blood Clot**
  - Echogenic/mixed echoes or blood fluid level within gallbladder
  - Occasionally retractile, conforming to gallbladder shape
  - Post trauma, post surgery, or after hepatobiliary intervention; associated with gastrointestinal bleed
- **Complicated Cholecystitis**
  - Gangrenous cholecystitis: Intraluminal echogenic debris and membranes
    - Asymmetric wall thickening, marked wall irregularities
  - Emphysematous cholecystitis: Gas in gallbladder wall and lumen
  - Gallbladder empyema
    - Distended pus filled gallbladder, echogenic contents, no shadowing
- **Gas in Lumen**
  - Iatrogenic from interventional procedure or endoscopy
  - Secondary to fistula with bowel as in gallstone ileus
    - Small bowel obstruction and pneumobilia, CT more definitive
- **Catheter**
  - History of percutaneous or endoscopic drainage
  - Tubular, parallel echogenic lines, ± "pig tail" loop, man-made configuration
- **Tumor**
  - Primary cancers involve wall ± endoluminal mass, stones, and extension to liver
  - Hematogenous metastases most commonly from melanoma
    - Multiple > single broad-based, hypoechoic, polypoid lesions, ± wall thickening
  - Look for color Doppler flow in mass, confirm with spectral Doppler

Helpful Clues for Rare Diagnoses

- **Parasitic Infestation**
  - Tubular, parallel echogenic lines

(Left) *Longitudinal decubitus ultrasound of the gallbladder shows a fundal curvilinear echo ➡ with a strong acoustic shadow ⤴. Note the normal wall with no cholecystitis.* **(Right)** *Transverse decubitus ultrasound of the gallbladder shows a thick wall ➡, shadowing stones ➡, and sludge ➡ in a patient with acute cholecystitis.*

Cholelithiasis

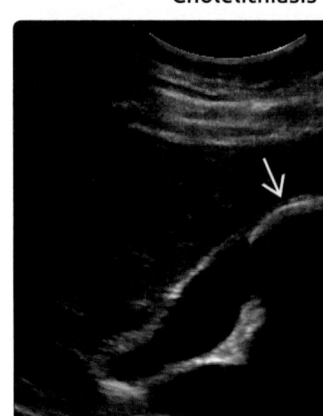

Cholelithiasis

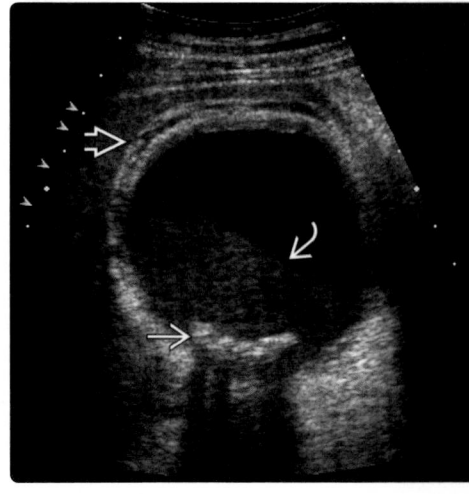

Sludge/Sludge Ball/Echogenic Bile

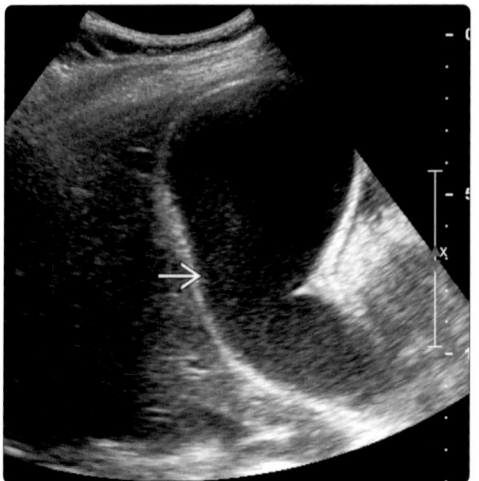

Sludge/Sludge Ball/Echogenic Bile

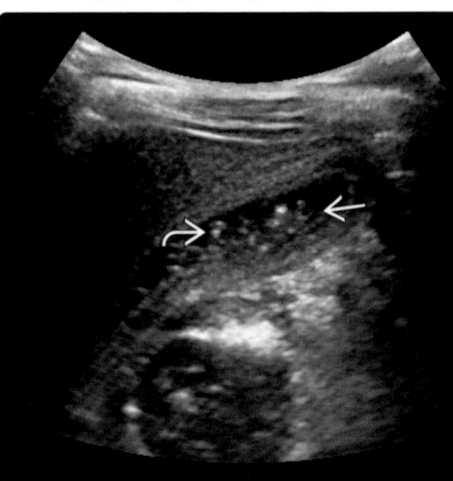

(Left) Transverse ultrasound of the right upper quadrant shows a markedly distended sludge-filled gallbladder ➡ in acalculous cholecystitis. Although the wall was not thick, the patient was treated with percutaneous drainage. (Right) Longitudinal decubitus ultrasound of a nondistended gallbladder shows intraluminal echoes from small nonshadowing sludge balls ➡. Some display the "comet tail" artifact ➡.

Complicated Cholecystitis

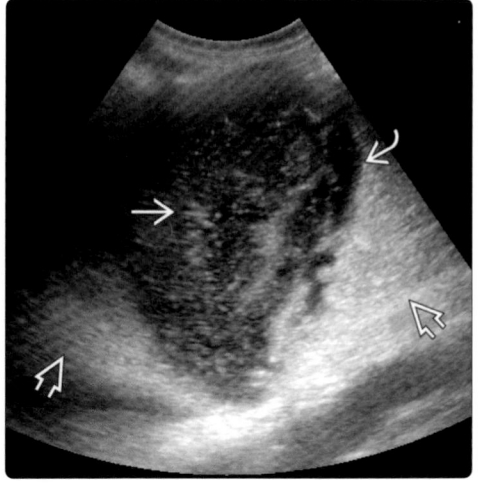

Complicated Cholecystitis

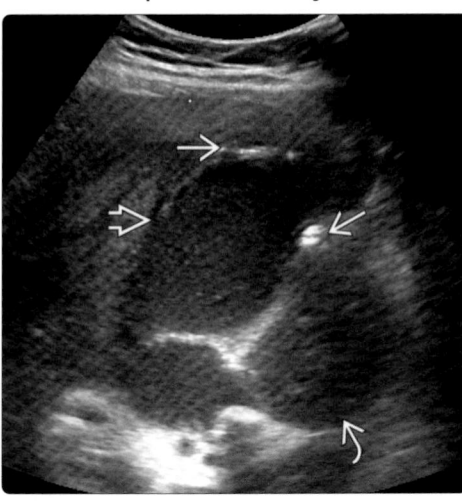

(Left) Transverse ultrasound of the gallbladder fossa shows the gallbladder lumen to be filled with membranes ➡ with no wall. There is pericholecystic fluid ➡ and echogenic fat ➡ in this diabetic patient with gangrenous cholecystitis. (Right) Transverse ultrasound shows a distended gallbladder with intraluminal sludge, discontinuous wall ➡, pericholecystic abscess ➡, and gas in the wall ➡ from emphysematous cholecystitis.

Drainage Catheter

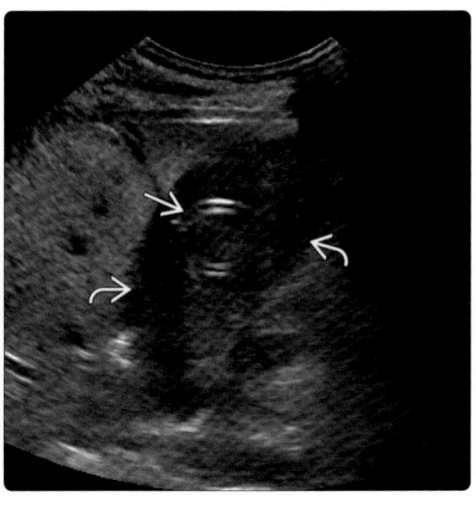

Tumor: Primary or Secondary

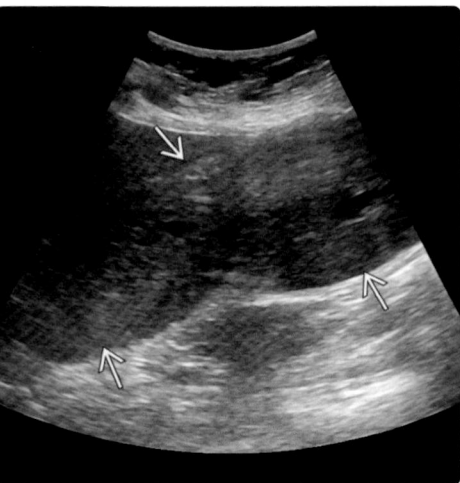

(Left) Transverse ultrasound following percutaneous drainage for acalculous cholecystitis in a sick patient. The pig tail catheter ➡ is looped in the gallbladder lumen, which contains sludge ➡. The wall is indistinct. (Right) Longitudinal ultrasound shows a markedly distended gallbladder (15 cm) with low level intraluminal echoes ➡. The lumen was filled with necrotic adenocarcinoma with muscle invasion in the neck only.

DIFFERENTIAL DIAGNOSIS

Common
- Physiologic
- Acute Calculous Cholecystitis
- Acute Acalculous Cholecystitis

Less Common
- Mucocele/Hydrops
- Drugs
- Post Vagotomy
- Choledochal Cyst
- Gallbladder Carcinoma
- Gallbladder Hemorrhage
- Acute Hemorrhagic Cholecystitis
- Other Causes of Cholecystitis
  - Obstruction post biliary stenting
  - Ischemia post transarterial hepatic chemoembolization or in the setting of severe hypotension or sepsis
  - Infections

Rare but Important
- Mucin Producing Gallbladder Carcinoma
- Torsion/Volvulus
- Systemic Lupus Erythematosus

ESSENTIAL INFORMATION

Key Differential Diagnosis Issues
- Determine if the gallbladder is obstructed or not
  - Look for an intrinsic lesion such as stone, polyp, or mass
  - Look for an extrinsic mass, collection, or inflammation
- Differentiate acute surgical from nonsurgical gallbladder distension
- Look for secondary signs of inflammation
  - Wall thickness, pericholecystic fluid, or inflamed fat
- Correlate with patient history, signs, and laboratory results

Physiologic Dilatation
- Distended > 5 x 5 x 10 cm
- Otherwise normal appearing gallbladder
- Secondary to
  - Prolonged fasting
  - Postoperative state
  - Total parenteral nutrition
  - Post vagotomy

Acute Calculous Cholecystitis
- Distension with
  - Gallstones
  - Wall thickening
  - Pericholecystic fluid
- Presence of sonographic Murphy sign is key for diagnosis of acute cholecystitis

Acute Acalculous Cholecystitis
- Distension without gallstones
- Sludge, wall thickening and gallbladder
- Ill patient with sepsis, postoperative or post trauma
- Increased risk of wall necrosis and gangrene
- Difficult diagnosis as sonographic Murphy sign may not be elicited in obtunded or sedated patients

- Confirm with HIDA
- Or diagnostic/therapeutic percutaneous cholecystotomy

Drugs
- Various drugs may decrease gallbladder contraction
  - Including atropine, somatostatin, arginine, nifedipine, progesterone, trimebutine, loperamide, and ondansetron

Unusual Causes of Acute Cholecystitis
- Ischemic cholecystitis
  - Following transarterial hepatic chemoembolization for liver malignancy
  - Following prolonged hypotension post trauma, hemorrhage, sepsis
- Following metal bile duct stent placed for malignant biliary stricture
  - Cholecystitis from cystic duct obstruction

Gallbladder Hemorrhage
- Mobile internal echoes
- Increasing echogenic luminal content over time if active bleeding
- Retracting clot
- Post hepatobiliary intervention or biopsy
- Post trauma or surgery
- Secondary to neoplasms, anticoagulation or bleeding disorder
- Post aneurysm rupture
- Present with
  - Pain
  - Jaundice
  - Hemobilia
  - Hematemesis
  - Hematochezia

Acute Hemorrhagic Cholecystitis
- Intraluminal hemorrhage with signs of acute cholecystitis
- Underlying
  - Atherosclerosis
  - Diabetes
  - Bleeding diathesis
  - Anticoagulation therapy

Gallbladder Carcinoma
- Typically thick irregular wall or solid tumor in lumen
- Extension into liver
- Gallstones typically present
- Mucin producing variant may produce distended mucin filled gallbladder
  - Smaller mural/polypoid mass

Mucocele/Hydrops
- Distended gallbladder filled with watery mucoid material
- Thin gallbladder wall
- Secondary to Gallbladder outlet obstruction
  - Obstructing polyp or stone
  - Obstructing masses such as pancreaticobiliary and ampullary carcinoma
  - Acute or chronic pancreatitis
- Courvoisier sign

- Distended nontender palpable gallbladder in the setting of jaundice is rarely due to obstructing gallstones
  - Stones are associated with chronic inflammation and lack of gallbladder distensibility
  - Or they produce acute obstruction with less gallbladder distension
- Neoplasms such as pancreatic carcinoma are more likely as they produce chronic lower grade obstruction

Choledochal Cyst

- Large cyst may compress or obstruct the gallbladder or mimic a distended gallbladder
- Associated with biliary dilatation
- Can be confirmed with MRCP or ERCP

Infections Causing Acalculous Cholecystitis

- Ultrasound findings similar to acute acalculous cholecystitis
- Bacteria
  - Salmonella typhi: Acute and chronic infection
  - Escherichia coli, Klebsiella, Staphylococcus species
  - Leptospirosis
- Viral
  - Hepatitis A, B viruses, CMV, dengue virus
- Diagnoses made by clinical picture and laboratory tests
- Hydatid
  - In endemic regions
  - Intraluminal gallbladder membranes or cysts
  - Curvilinear calcifications
  - Typically associated with liver cysts
- Ascariasis
  - Intraluminal living or dead worms
  - Obstruct cystic duct causing cholecystitis
- Malaria
  - Can cause acalculous cholecystitis

Henoch-Schönlein Purpura

- Associated with gallbladder hydrops or acalculous cholecystitis
- Characteristic skin rash

Gallbladder Torsion/Volvulus

- Elderly thin women with wandering gallbladder
- Features of cholecystitis but difficult preoperative diagnosis
- Markedly dilated gallbladder
- May be displaced from normal location
- Twisting of the cystic duct and artery
  - Whirl sign on color Doppler

Systemic Lupus Erythematosus

- Acalculous cholecystitis due to vasculitis of gallbladder wall and bile ducts
- Treated nonsurgically with corticosteroids

SELECTED REFERENCES

1. Eachempati SR et al: Acute cholecystitis in the sick patient. Curr Probl Surg. 51(11):441-66, 2014
2. Revzin MV et al: The gallbladder: uncommon gallbladder conditions and unusual presentations of the common gallbladder pathological processes. Abdom Imaging. Epub ahead of print, 2014
3. Sebastian S et al: Managing incidental findings on abdominal and pelvic CT and MRI, Part 4: white paper of the ACR Incidental Findings Committee II on gallbladder and biliary findings. J Am Coll Radiol. 10(12):953-6, 2013
4. Boonstra EA et al: Torsion of the gallbladder. J Gastrointest Surg. 16(4):882-4, 2012
5. Charalel RA et al: Complicated cholecystitis: the complementary roles of sonography and computed tomography. Ultrasound Q. 27(3):161-70, 2011
6. Gore RM et al: Gallbladder imaging. Gastroenterol Clin North Am. 39(2):265-87, ix, 2010

Physiologic

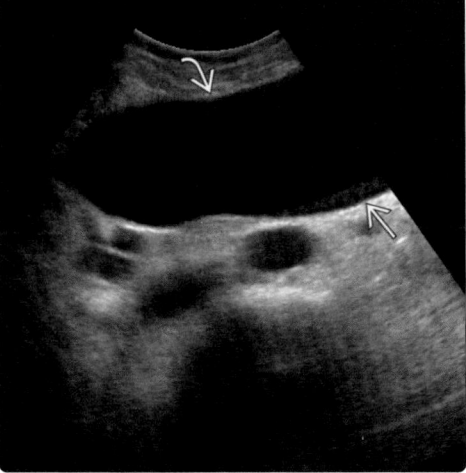

Physiologic

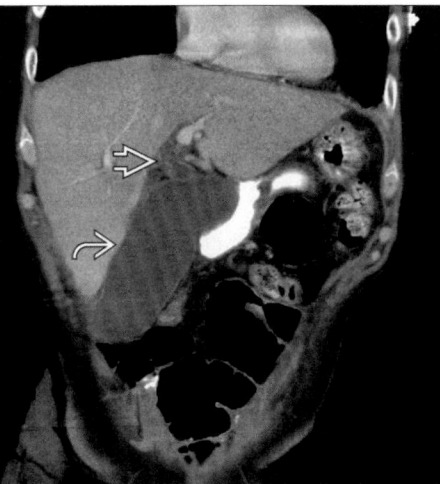

(Left) Transverse oblique ultrasound of the gallbladder in a ventilated patient on total parenteral nutrition. The gallbladder is distended ➡ with minimal sludge ➡. There is no wall thickening. (Right) CECT of the same patient shows the distended gallbladder ➡ and cystic duct ➡ without signs of inflammation or obstructing lesion.

Acute Calculous Cholecystitis

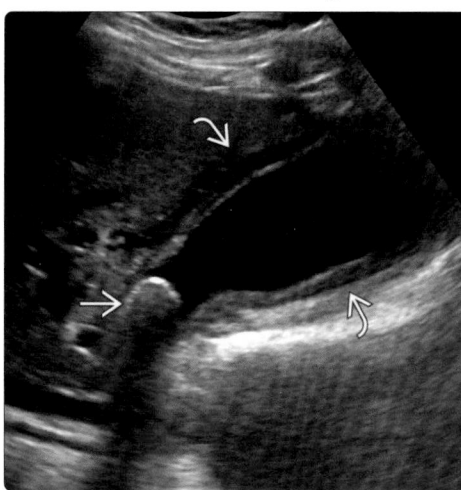

Acute Calculous Cholecystitis

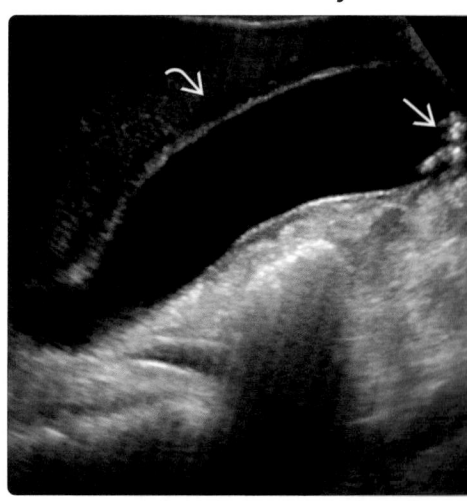

(Left) *Longitudinal oblique ultrasound of the gallbladder shows an obstructing stone in the neck ➡. The gallbladder is distended with diffuse hypoechoic wall thickening ➡ in this patient with acute calculous cholecystitis.* (Right) *Longitudinal oblique ultrasound shows a distended gallbladder with fundal stones ➡ and wall thickening ➡. The patient had a positive Murphy sign consistent with acute calculous cholecystitis.*

Acute Calculous Cholecystitis

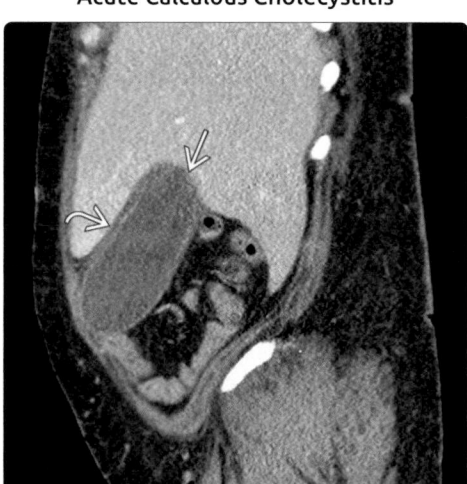

Acute Acalculous Cholecystitis

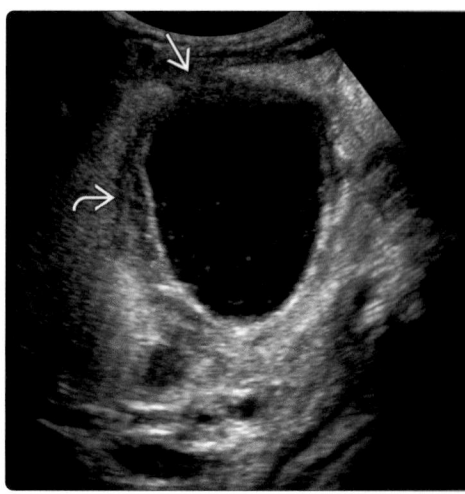

(Left) *Sagittal CECT of the same patient shows a distended gallbladder ➡ with diffuse wall thickening ➡. The stones were not visible on CT.* (Right) *Transverse ultrasound shows a gangrenous gallbladder with no stones. The wall is edematous ➡ with a focal defect anteriorly ➡. A pericholecystic abscess had developed (not shown).*

Gallbladder Carcinoma

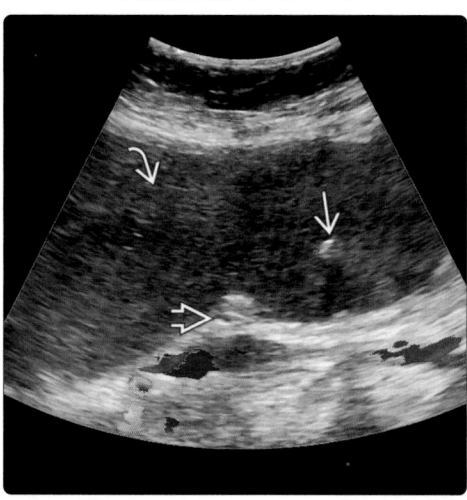

Gallbladder Carcinoma

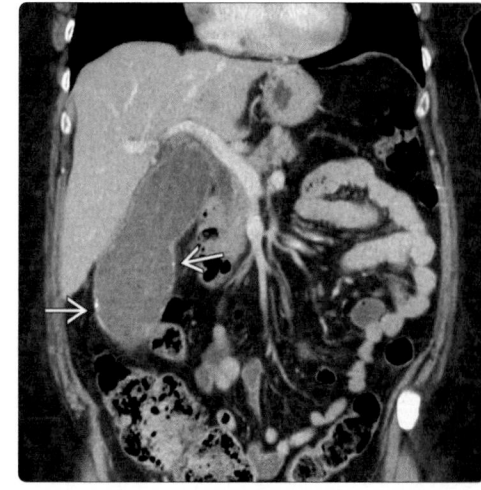

(Left) *Oblique color Doppler ultrasound of a distended gallbladder filled with avascular low level echoes ➡ with one small stone ➡. The posterior wall is irregular ➡. The lumen was filled with necrotic adenocarcinoma.* (Right) *CECT shows a dilated gallbladder with low density contents. There is subtle wall calcification ➡ and internal heterogeneity. This was largely necrotic adenocarcinoma with a small invasive tumor in the gallbladder neck.*

Mucocele/Hydrops

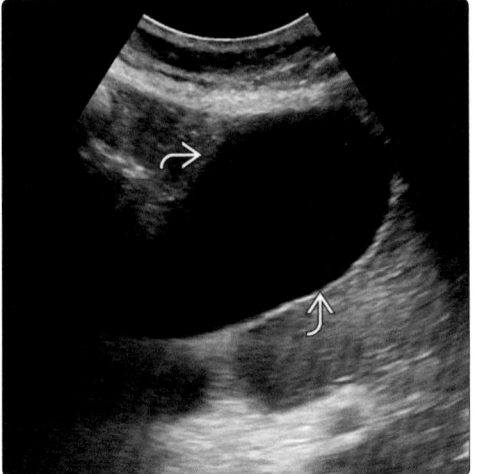

Mucocele/Hydrops

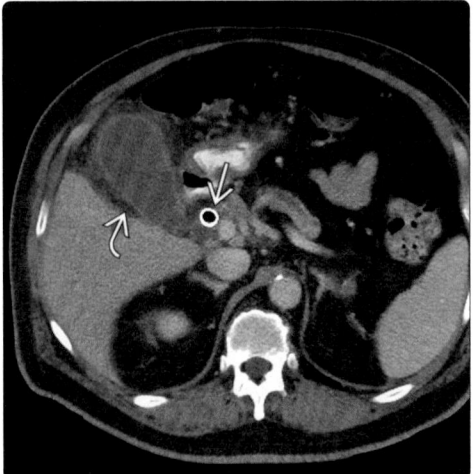

(Left) *Longitudinal oblique ultrasound of the gallbladder in a patient with obstructive jaundice from a pancreatic head carcinoma shows a distended but otherwise normal gallbladder ➘, the Courvoisier sign.* (Right) *Axial CECT of the same patient after placement of a metal bile duct stent ➡ to relieve biliary obstruction. There is now edema of the gallbladder wall and pericholecystic stranding ➩ from acute cholecystitis which later perforated.*

Mucocele/Hydrops

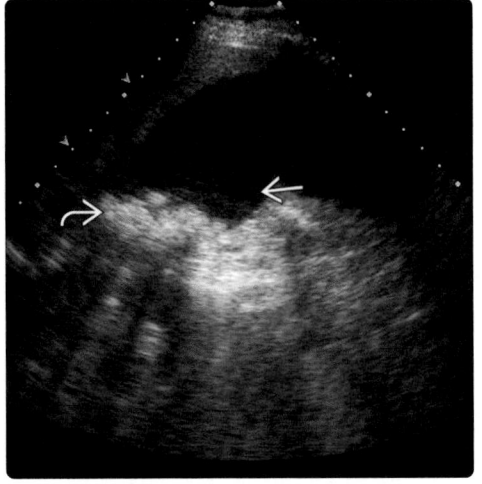

Mucocele/Hydrops

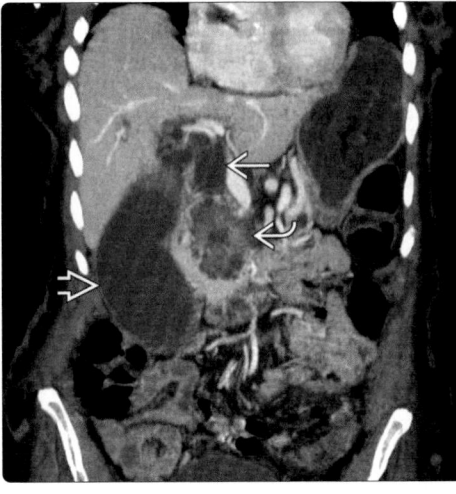

(Left) *Longitudinal oblique ultrasound of the gallbladder in an elderly patient with jaundice shows a dilated gallbladder with stones ➘ and sludge ➡. The wall was normal. The common bile duct was dilated secondary to a pancreatic lesion.* (Right) *CECT of the same patient better demonstrates the obstructing multicystic serous cystadenoma in the head of pancreas ➩ obstructing the bile duct ➡ and causing gallbladder distension ➘.*

Acute Hemorrhagic Cholecystitis

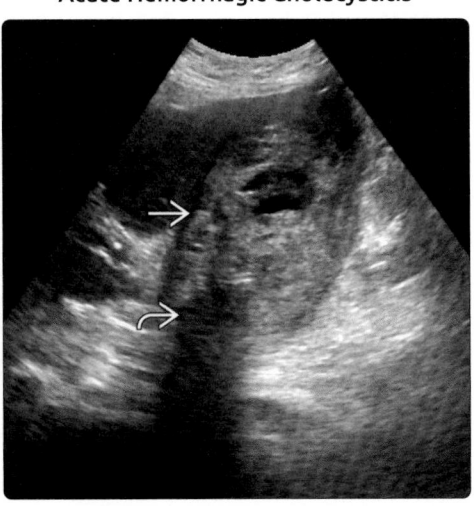

Acute Hemorrhagic Cholecystitis

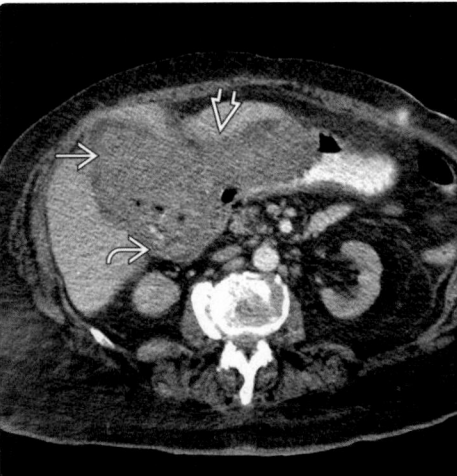

(Left) *Longitudinal oblique ultrasound shows a markedly abnormal gallbladder filled with bright echoes ➡ in a patient with a dropping hematocrit and signs of infection. Shadowing is noted ➘ but the stone is indistinct.* (Right) *Axial CECT of the same patient shows a perforated gallbladder with gallstones ➘ and luminal hemorrhage ➡. There is an adjacent hematoma ➩. Active bleeding was treated by embolization.*

DIFFERENTIAL DIAGNOSIS

Common

- Choledocholithiasis
- Ascending Cholangitis
- Recurrent Pyogenic Cholangitis
- Pancreatic Ductal Carcinoma
- Cholangiocarcinoma
- Choledochal Cyst

Less Common

- Sludge
- Periampullary Tumor
- Sclerosing Cholangitis
- Parasitic Infestation
- AIDS-Related Cholangiopathy
- Biliary Intraductal Papillary Mucinous Neoplasm

ESSENTIAL INFORMATION

Helpful Clues for Common Diagnoses

- **Choledocholithiasis**
  - Most common location is in common bile duct (CBD)
  - Round echogenic focus with marked posterior acoustic shadowing
- **Ascending Cholangitis**
  - Imaging may reveal biliary duct wall thickening, intraluminal debris, or obstructing biliary stone
  - Periportal inflammatory hypo-/hyperechogenicity may be seen
- **Recurrent Pyogenic Cholangitis**
  - Bacterial colonization of brown pigment stones in both intrahepatic and extrahepatic bile ducts
  - Densely packed intrahepatic stones
  - Atrophy of involved lobe/segment of liver in later stages
- **Pancreatic Ductal Carcinoma**
  - Ill-defined, solid mass in pancreatic head
  - Pancreatic duct dilatation that abruptly tapers at point of pancreatic carcinoma
  - Vascular encasement ± regional nodal/liver metastases

- **Cholangiocarcinoma**
  - Extrahepatic cholangiocarcinoma involves biliary ducts in hepatoduodenal ligament
    - Intra- and extrahepatic biliary dilatation
    - May see: Irregular soft tissue thickening of extrahepatic bile duct or polypoidal mass within CBD
  - Intrahepatic cholangiocarcinoma: Ill-defined, infiltrative, iso-/hyperechoic mass often with capsular retraction
- **Choledochal Cyst**
  - Congenital biliary malformation characterized by fusiform duct dilatation
  - Most commonly involves CBD
  - Cystic extrahepatic mass separated from gallbladder and communicating with CHD or intrahepatic ducts
  - Fusiform dilatation of extra- ± intrahepatic bile ducts
  - Abrupt change in caliber at junction of dilated segment to normal ducts

Helpful Clues for Less Common Diagnoses

- **Sclerosing Cholangitis**
  - Autoimmune disease that causes multiple intra- and extrahepatic biliary strictures with dilatation
- **Biliary Intraductal Papillary Mucinous Neoplasm**
  - Ductal intraluminal mass with frond-like papillary projections
  - Hypersecretion of mucin as well as anatomic obstruction leads to markedly dilated intra- and extrahepatic biliary ducts

SELECTED REFERENCES

1. Plentz RR et al: Clinical presentation, risk factors and staging systems of cholangiocarcinoma. Best Pract Res Clin Gastroenterol. 29(2):245-252, 2015
2. Raman SP et al: Abnormalities of the Distal Common Bile Duct and Ampulla: Diagnostic Approach and Differential Diagnosis Using Multiplanar Reformations and 3D Imaging. AJR Am J Roentgenol. 203(1):17-28, 2014
3. Attasaranya S et al: Choledocholithiasis, ascending cholangitis, and gallstone pancreatitis. Med Clin North Am. 92(4):925-60, x, 2008
4. Lim JH et al: Biliary intraductal papillary-mucinous neoplasm manifesting only as dilatation of the hepatic lobar or segmental bile ducts: imaging features in six patients. AJR Am J Roentgenol. 191(3):778-82, 2008

Choledocholithiasis

Ascending Cholangitis

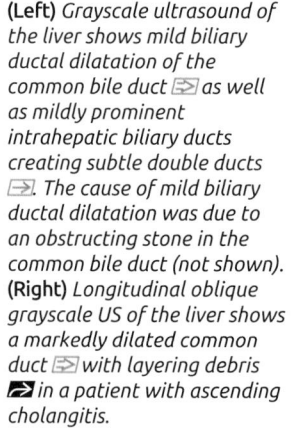

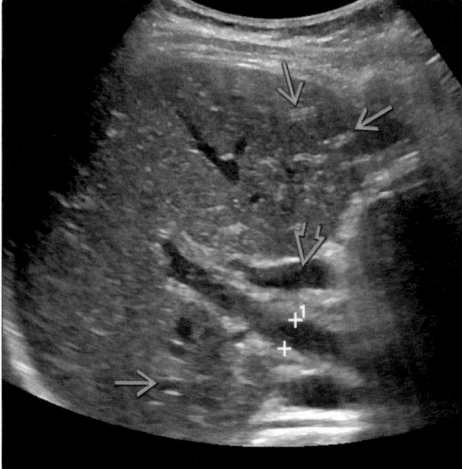

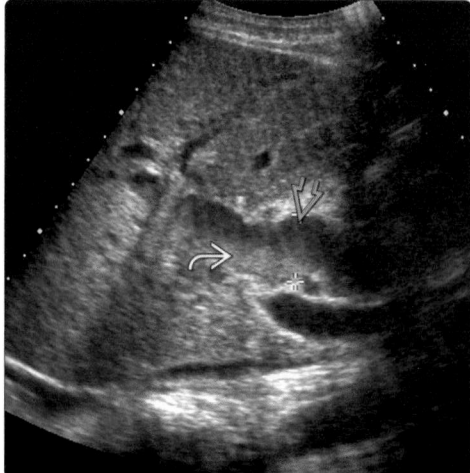

(Left) *Grayscale ultrasound of the liver shows mild biliary ductal dilatation of the common bile duct ⊟ as well as mildly prominent intrahepatic biliary ducts creating subtle double ducts ⊟. The cause of mild biliary ductal dilatation was due to an obstructing stone in the common bile duct (not shown).* **(Right)** *Longitudinal oblique grayscale US of the liver shows a markedly dilated common duct ⊟ with layering debris ➡ in a patient with ascending cholangitis.*

Recurrent Pyogenic Cholangitis

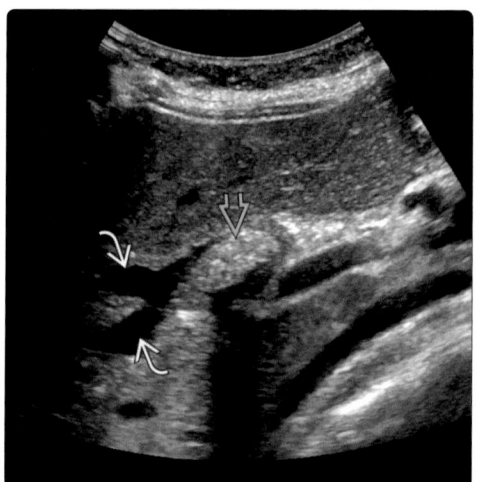

Cholangiocarcinoma

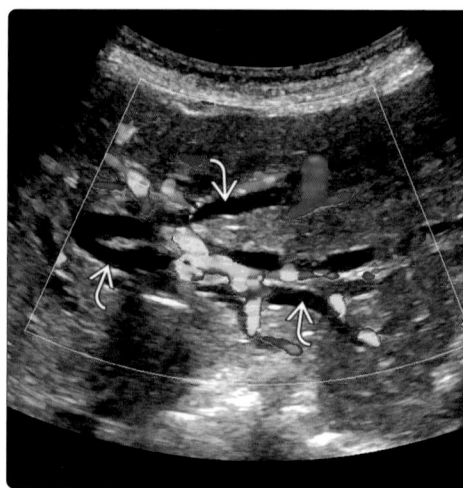

(Left) *Grayscale US of the liver shows a large intrahepatic stone ⇨ causing upstream biliary ductal dilatation ⇨ in a patient with recurrent pyogenic cholangitis.* (Right) *Transverse color Doppler US of the left lobe of the liver shows moderate biliary ductal dilatation ⇨ caused by an obstructing central cholangiocarcinoma.*

Cholangiocarcinoma

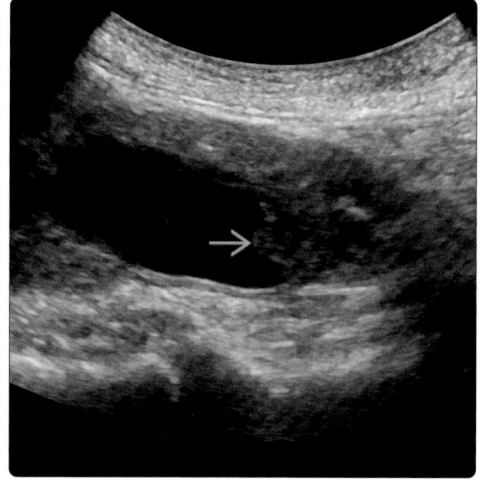

Choledochal Cyst

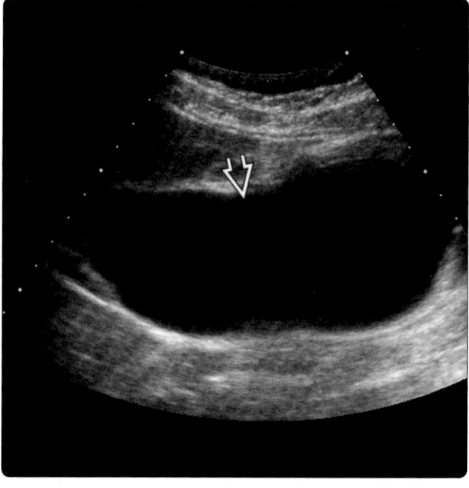

(Left) *Longitudinal oblique US of the common bile duct demonstrates an obstructing soft tissue mass ⇨, which was proven to represent an intraluminal cholangiocarcinoma.* (Right) *Longitudinal oblique US of the right upper quadrant in a 14-year-old girl shows a markedly dilated tubular structure ⇨, which was found to be a large type I choledochal cyst.*

Biliary Intraductal Papillary Mucinous Neoplasm

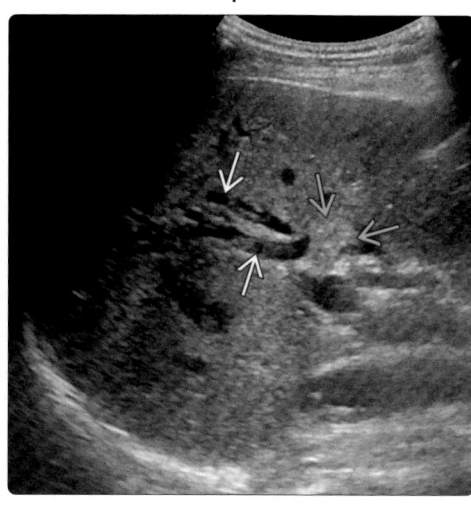

Biliary Intraductal Papillary Mucinous Neoplasm

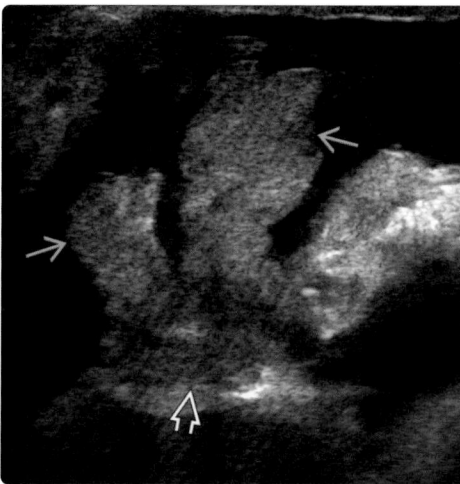

(Left) *Transverse US of the liver shows moderate intrahepatic ductal dilatation ⇨, which was caused by a biliary intraductal papillary mucinous neoplasm. ⇨ Biliary ductal dilatation was seen both proximal as well as distal to the lesion due to copious mucin production.* (Right) *Intraoperative grayscale ultrasound in the same patient shows the biliary intraductal papillary neoplasm has frond-like projections ⇨ into the biliary tree. The point where the biliary IPMN arises from the biliary duct wall ⇨ is evident on this image.*

PART III
SECTION 3
Pancreas

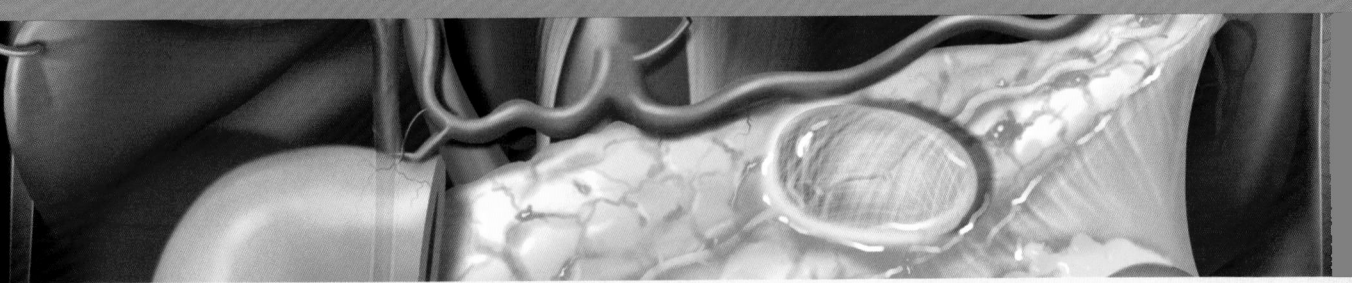

DIFFERENTIAL DIAGNOSIS

Common

- Pancreatic Pseudocyst
- Serous Cystadenoma of Pancreas
- Mucinous Cystic Neoplasm (MCN)
- Intraductal Papillary Mucinous Neoplasm (IPMN)

Less Common

- Necrotic Pancreatic Ductal Carcinoma
- Solid Pseudopapillary Neoplasm
- Cystic Pancreatic Neuroendocrine Tumor
- Congenital Cyst
- Lymphoepithelial Cyst
- Cystic Metastases

ESSENTIAL INFORMATION

Key Differential Diagnosis Issues

- US can characterize simple or macrocystic pancreatic lesions
  - Most represent pancreatic pseudocysts
- Remaining benign and malignant cystic pancreatic lesions may appear echogenic due to numerous microcystic interfaces, soft tissue components, or complex content
- CECT or CEMR is necessary to adequately characterize internal features that are not well assessed with transabdominal ultrasound
- Endoscopic ultrasound (EUS) also provides high-resolution imaging but is invasive and requires conscious sedation
  - Can be used for biopsy or fluid aspiration in indeterminate cases
- Key features which guide differential diagnosis
  - Location and size
  - Wall thickness
  - Loculation and number of locules
  - Internal septations and septal thickness
  - Presence of solid components and vascularity
  - Central scar
  - Calcification and location
  - Communication with pancreatic duct
  - Fluid characterization/presence of hemorrhage
  - Pancreatic and biliary diameter
  - Upstream pancreatic atrophy
  - Evidence of acute or chronic pancreatitis
  - Locoregional adenopathy and hepatic metastases
- Consider clinical context
  - Patient demographics, pancreatitis, obstructive symptomatology, familial syndromes

Helpful Clues for Common Diagnoses

- **Pancreatic Pseudocyst**
  - Common late complication of pancreatitis
    - Develops 4-6 weeks after onset of acute pancreatitis
    - Evolves over time, whereas neoplastic lesions persist without change
  - Generally well circumscribed, smooth-walled, unilocular, anechoic with posterior acoustic enhancement
  - May be complicated
    - Multilocular
    - Internal echoes with fluid-debris level or septations
    - Wall calcification

  - But shows no vascularized soft tissue elements
  - Associated with other findings of acute or chronic pancreatitis
    - Parenchymal atrophy or calcification, fat stranding on CT, ductal strictures on MR
    - Generally not seen with MCN, the primary mimic of pseudocyst
- **Serous Cystadenoma of Pancreas**
  - Benign pancreatic tumor
  - Commonly in pancreatic body and tail; 30% occur in pancreatic head
  - Typically composed of small cystic areas separated by internal septations
  - Septa coalesce to form central echogenic scar with "sunburst" calcification
  - Can mimic nonspecific solid and cystic tumor
    - Heterogeneous echogenic appearance due to numerous interfaces
    - Intralesional color Doppler flow in fibrovascular septa
  - Characteristic honeycomb appearance on CT, MR, and endoscopic ultrasound
  - Less commonly, may see oligocystic variant that may be indistinguishable from MCN by imaging
    - EUS-guided cyst aspiration may be helpful in making diagnosis
  - Usually seen in older women (mean age: 61 years)
- **Mucinous Cystic Neoplasm (MCN)**
  - Tumors range in grade from benign with malignant potential to invasive carcinoma
  - More common location: Pancreatic body and tail
  - Anechoic or hypoechoic, thick-walled, cystic mass ± mildly thickened septa
  - Can demonstrate peripheral calcification
  - May be indistinguishable from pseudocyst
  - Lacks additional findings/history of pancreatitis
  - EUS-guided biopsy may be helpful in making diagnosis
  - Solid components or marked septal thickening suggests carcinoma
  - Seen almost exclusively in middle-aged women (mean age: 50 years)
- **Intraductal Papillary Mucinous Neoplasm (IPMN)**
  - Tumor with varying malignant potential: Branch type generally benign with low malignant potential; main duct IPMN thought to be precursor to invasive pancreatic ductal adenocarcinoma
  - Typically in head of pancreas/uncinate process
  - Main duct type: Marked pancreatic ductal dilatation
    - When diffuse, may simulate chronic pancreatitis
      - However, calcification and parenchymal atrophy are not typically seen
    - If segmental, can mimic fluid collection or mucinous cystic tumor
  - Side branch type: Collections of dilated side branches
    - Anechoic or hypoechoic cyst or collection of small anechoic cysts
    - Look for communication with pancreatic duct, which is a distinguishing feature compared to other cystic neoplasms
    - May be multifocal, whereas serous cystadenoma and MCN are typically solitary
  - Occur most frequently in older men (mean age: 65 years)

Helpful Clues for Less Common Diagnoses

- **Necrotic Pancreatic Ductal Carcinoma**
  - Most common pancreatic neoplasm
  - Malignant lesion
  - Commonly in head of pancreas
  - Typically appears as an ill-defined, solid, hypoechoic mass with ductal obstruction
  - May show complex cystic areas due to tumor necrosis, side branch obstruction or adjacent pseudocyst
    - Uncommon form of common neoplasm
  - Infiltrative appearance ± vascular invasion distinguishes this entity from other solid malignancies that may show cystic change
  - Obstructive symptomatology
- **Solid Pseudopapillary Neoplasm**
  - Tumor with low-grade malignant potential
  - Commonly in the pancreatic tail
  - Well-defined, large heterogeneous echogenic solid and cystic mass
  - Cystic areas are secondary to tumor degeneration and vary in size and morphology
  - Prominent vascular soft tissue components
  - Often shows intratumoral hemorrhage
  - Typically seen in young women (< 35 years)
- **Cystic Pancreatic Neuroendocrine Tumor**
  - All tumors > 5 mm considered malignant
  - Typically round, solid, hypoechoic mass with internal color Doppler flow
  - Central cyst formation may occur due to tumor degeneration
    - Uncommon form of uncommon neoplasm
  - Identification of hypervascular rim can be challenging
  - Familial syndromes: Multiple endocrine neoplasia type I; von Hippel-Lindau; neurofibromatosis type I; tuberous sclerosis
    - May have multiple lesions
    - Occurs in younger patients (< 40 years)
- **Congenital Cyst**
  - True epithelial lining with serous fluid
  - Consider in patients with autosomal dominant polycystic kidney disease, von Hippel-Lindau and cystic fibrosis
    - Usually multiple; can replace entire pancreas (e.g., in cystic fibrosis)
- **Lymphoepithelial Cyst**
  - Rare, benign, lesion usually in tail of pancreas
  - Nonneoplastic, no malignant behavior
  - Macrocystic morphology, multilocular or unilocular cysts
  - May see characteristic T1 hyperintensity and low T2 signal due to keratin content
  - Almost exclusively in middle-aged to elderly men
- **Cystic Metastases**
  - Pancreatic metastases are uncommon
  - Can occur with renal cell carcinoma, melanoma, breast cancer, lung cancer, gastric cancer, colorectal carcinoma

SELECTED REFERENCES

1. Kim YS et al: Rare nonneoplastic cysts of pancreas. Clin Endosc. 48(1):31-8, 2015
2. Goh BK et al: Are the Sendai and Fukuoka consensus guidelines for cystic mucinous neoplasms of the pancreas useful in the initial triage of all suspected pancreatic cystic neoplasms? A single-institution experience with 317 surgically-treated patients. Ann Surg Oncol. 21(6):1919-26, 2014
3. Sahani DV et al: Diagnosis and management of cystic pancreatic lesions. AJR Am J Roentgenol. 200(2):343-54, 2013
4. Megibow AJ et al: The incidental pancreatic cyst. Radiol Clin North Am. 49(2):349-59, 2011
5. Hutchins G et al: Diagnostic evaluation of pancreatic cystic malignancies. Surg Clin North Am. 90(2):399-410, 2010
6. Kalb B et al: MR imaging of cystic lesions of the pancreas. Radiographics. 29(6):1749-65, 2009

Pancreatic Pseudocyst

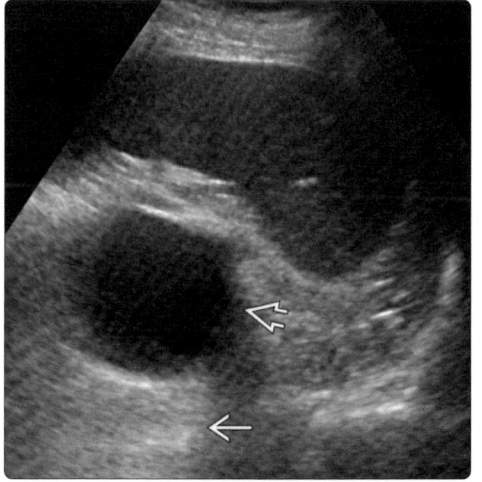

Pancreatic Pseudocyst

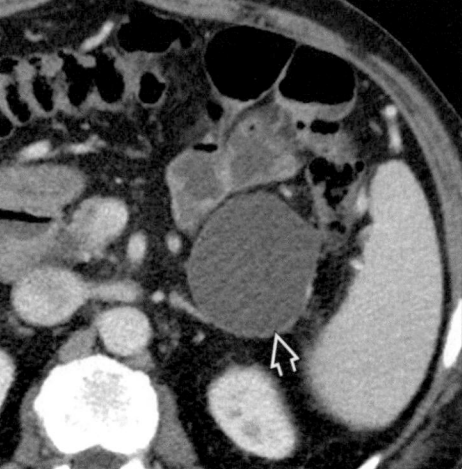

(Left) *Transverse transabdominal ultrasound shows a well-demarcated, anechoic lesion* ➡ *with through transmission* ➡ *in the tail of the pancreas, compatible with a pseudocyst.* (Right) *Axial CECT in the same patient demonstrates a well-demarcated, low-density cystic lesion* ➡ *with a thin wall in the tail of the pancreas. Note the lack of enhancing components and marked pancreatic atrophy.*

Pancreatic Pseudocyst

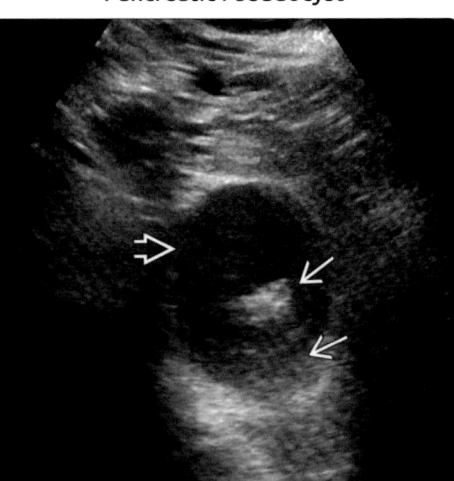

Pancreatic Pseudocyst

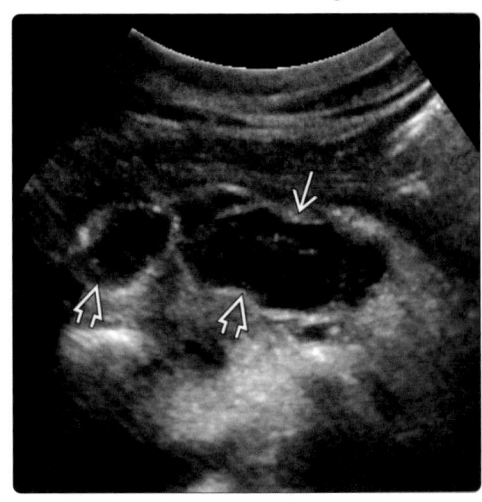

(Left) *Transverse transabdominal ultrasound in the region of the pancreas shows a well-circumscribed, unilocular cystic lesion* ➡ *with through transmission. Note the echogenic internal contents and layering debris* ➡ *compatible with a complex pseudocyst.* (Right) *Transverse transabdominal ultrasound shows pancreatic ductal dilation* ➡ *and 2 well-circumscribed, elongated fluid collections* ➡ *with internal echoes in the neck and body of the pancreas, compatible with complex pseudocysts from severe pancreatitis.*

Serous Cystadenoma of Pancreas

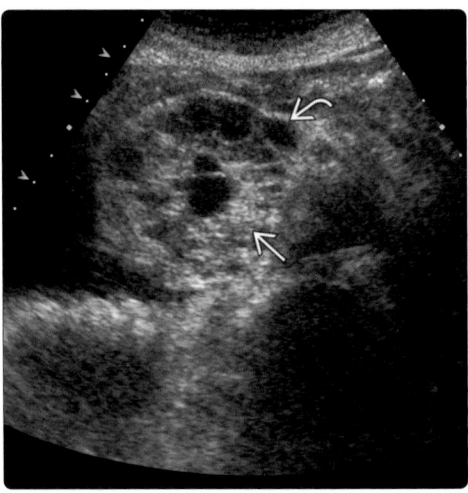

Serous Cystadenoma of Pancreas

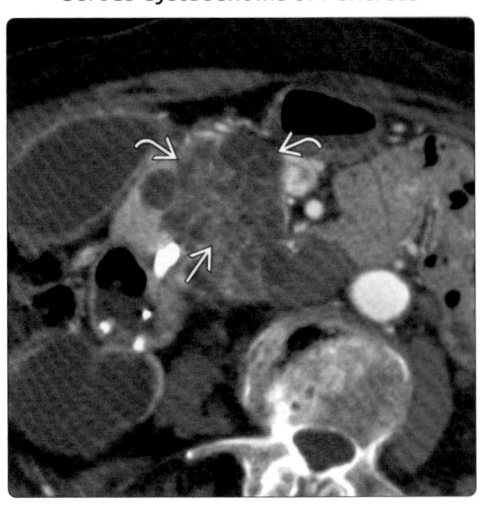

(Left) *Transverse transabdominal ultrasound shows a hyperechoic, solid-appearing mass in the head of the pancreas with small cystic components* ➡ *and more echogenic center* ➡. (Right) *Corresponding axial CECT better characterizes numerous small cysts* ➡ *within the lesion, separated by thin septa, which appear more coalescent centrally* ➡.

Serous Cystadenoma of Pancreas

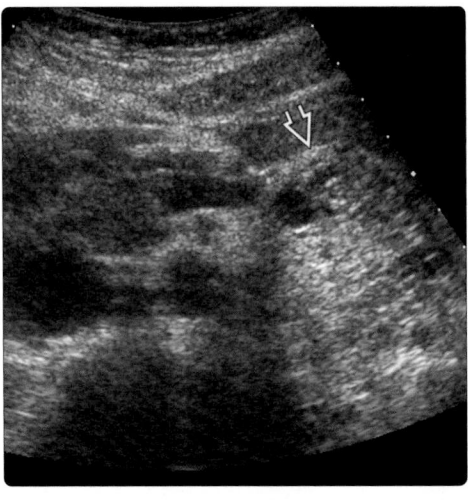

Serous Cystadenoma of Pancreas

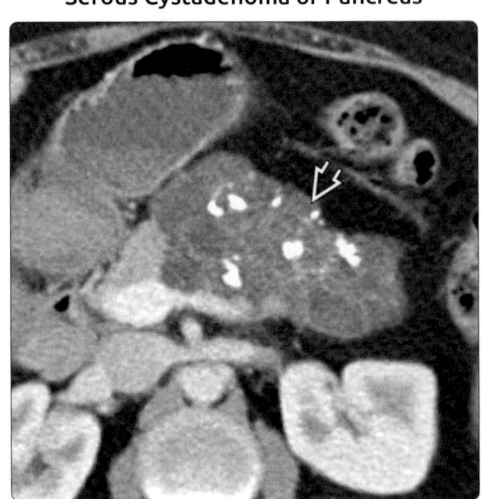

(Left) *Transverse transabdominal ultrasound shows a heterogeneous lesion* ➡ *in the tail of the pancreas composed of innumerable tiny cysts separated by linear septations, which result in a hyperechoic appearance due to the highly reflective interfaces* (Right) *Axial CECT shows the classic honeycomb appearance of a serous cystadenoma* ➡: *A microcystic lesion with thin enhancing septa delineating small cysts. Note the scattered central calcifications and lack of wall thickening, which are also typical features.*

Mucinous Cystic Neoplasm (MCN)

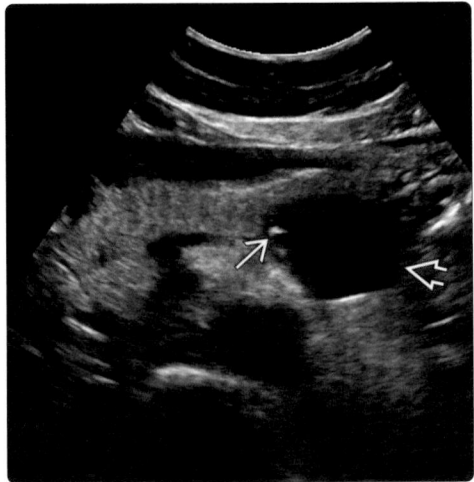

Mucinous Cystic Neoplasm (MCN)

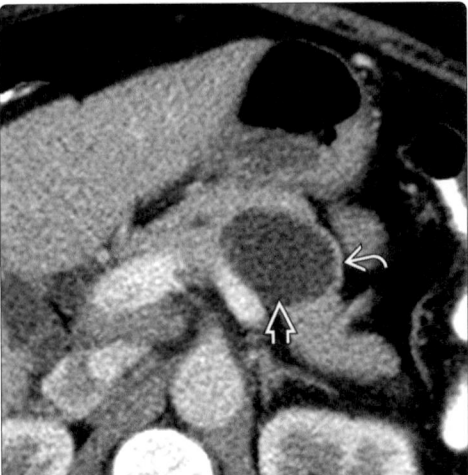

(Left) *Transverse transabdominal ultrasound shows a well-defined, anechoic cystic lesion* ➡ *in the body of the pancreas with a few hyperechoic peripheral foci* ➡. (Right) *Corresponding axial CECT shows an encapsulated oval, hypodense mass* ➡ *in the body of the pancreas with a thickened enhancing cyst wall* ➡. *The lesion contained internal septations, not seen on CT.*

Intraductal Papillary Mucinous Neoplasm (IPMN)

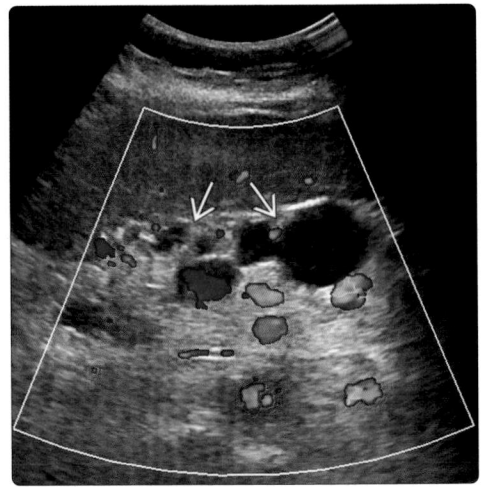

Intraductal Papillary Mucinous Neoplasm (IPMN)

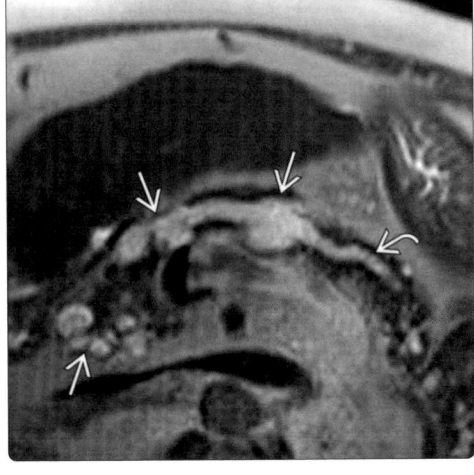

(Left) *Transverse transabdominal color Doppler ultrasound shows a collection of multiple small, round and oval cysts* ➡ *within the body of the pancreas.* (Right) *Axial T2 HASTE MR in the same patient better demonstrates multifocal involvement of the pancreas. Numerous T2-bright cysts* ➡ *are seen throughout the pancreas, several of which appear contiguous with a dilated pancreatic duct* ➡, *compatible with a mixed, branch, and main duct IPMN.*

Cystic Pancreatic Neuroendocrine Tumor

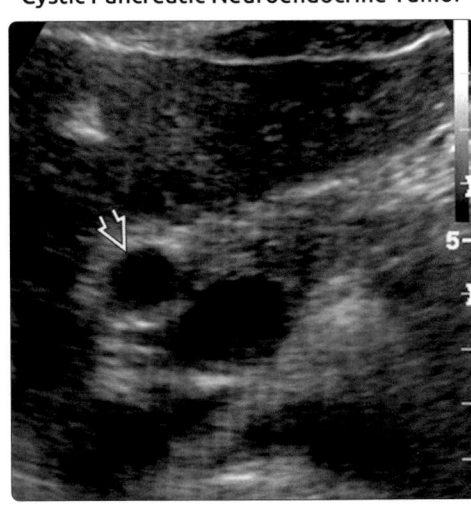

Cystic Pancreatic Neuroendocrine Tumor

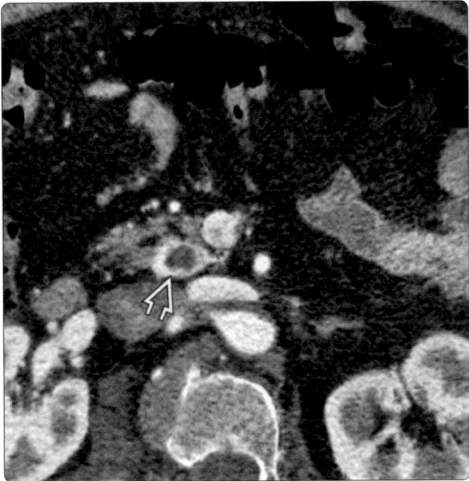

(Left) *Transverse transabdominal ultrasound of the pancreas shows a round, well-circumscribed, cystic lesion* ➡ *extending exophytically from the neck of the pancreas. This was amenable to EUS-guided biopsy, which showed a cystic neuroendocrine tumor.* (Right) *Axial CECT in a different patient, shows a round cystic lesion* ➡ *in the uncinate process with a peripheral rim of hypervascular enhancement, a typical appearance for a small cystic neuroendocrine tumor.*

DIFFERENTIAL DIAGNOSIS

Common

- Pancreatic Ductal Carcinoma
- Focal Acute Pancreatitis
- Chronic Pancreatitis
- Pancreatic Neuroendocrine Tumor
- Serous Cystadenoma of Pancreas
- Mucinous Cystic Neoplasm of Pancreas

Less Common

- Metastasis
- Lymphoma
- Solid Pseudopapillary Neoplasm
- Intrapancreatic Splenule

ESSENTIAL INFORMATION

Key Differential Diagnosis Issues

- Correlate with clinical information (e.g., history of pancreatitis, obstructive symptomatology)
- Pancreatic duct dilatation favors diagnosis of pancreatic ductal carcinoma
  - Biliary dilatation present as well in pancreatic head ductal carcinoma
- Other ancillary findings to look for include
  - Cystic component
  - Internal septation
  - Presence of intralesional calcification
  - Vascular encasement
  - Regional lymph node and liver metastases
- Clues to detection of small tumor
  - Focal contour irregularity
  - Subtle pancreatic duct/bile duct dilatation
- CECT or CEMR improves ability to detect and characterize solid pancreatic lesions
  - Can evaluate for vascular encasement
- Endoscopic ultrasound is invasive; however, increases sensitivity for lesion detection and can be used to guide biopsy for diagnosis

Helpful Clues for Common Diagnoses

- **Pancreatic Ductal Carcinoma**
  - Arises from ductal epithelium of exocrine pancreas
  - Location: Head of pancreas (60-70%), body (20%), diffuse (15%), tail (5%)
  - Average size ~ 2-3 cm
  - Pathology: Scirrhous infiltrative adenocarcinoma with dense cellularity and sparse vascularity
  - Typical US findings
    - Poorly defined, homogeneous or heterogeneous, hypoechoic mass
    - Pancreatic duct dilatation upstream from tumor with abrupt tapering at site of obstruction
    - Bile duct dilatation seen in pancreatic head tumor
    - Necrosis/cystic component is rarely seen
    - Displacement/encasement of adjacent vascular structures (e.g., superior mesenteric vessels, splenic artery, hepatic artery, gastroduodenal artery)
    - Presence of liver and regional nodal metastases
    - Ascites due to peritoneal metastases

- **Focal Acute Pancreatitis**
  - Clinical information very important for correct imaging interpretation
    - Acute onset of epigastric pain, fever, and vomiting
    - Raised serum amylase and lipase
    - Presence of underlying predisposing factors: Biliary stone, alcoholism, drugs (e.g., steroid), trauma, etc.
  - Focal, ill-defined, hypoechoic enlargement of pancreatic parenchyma
    - Heterogeneous appearance in cases with intrapancreatic necrosis/hemorrhage
  - Blurred pancreatic outline/margin
  - Presence of peripancreatic fluid collection
  - Lack of pancreatic duct dilatation
  - No parenchymal calcification

- **Chronic Pancreatitis**
  - Longstanding clinical symptoms, recurrent attacks of epigastric pain, typically radiates to back
  - Most common US features
    - Diffuse atrophy
    - Main pancreatic duct beading and side branch dilatation
    - Parenchymal and ductal calcifications
  - Can have focal involvement with mass-like appearance
  - Look for smoothly stenotic or normal main duct penetrating abnormal region on MRCP

- **Pancreatic Neuroendocrine Tumor**
  - Functioning and nonfunctioning subtypes have distinct appearances
    - Functioning tumor usually small, solid, well-circumscribed, hypo-/isoechoic mass
    - Nonfunctioning tumors tend to be larger with more heterogeneous echo pattern due to necrosis, calcification, and cystic change
    - Solid components are typically hypervascular on power Doppler US and hyperenhancing on CT and MR
  - Detection may be difficult with small functioning tumors
  - Endoscopic US detects tumors in pancreatic head and body
  - Intraoperative US is useful for tumor localization
  - Liver and regional lymph node metastases seen in 60-90% at clinical presentation
    - Hyperechoic liver metastases more suggestive of neuroendocrine tumors than ductal carcinoma

- **Serous Cystadenoma of Pancreas**
  - Commonly in pancreatic body and tail; 30% occur in pancreatic head
  - Composed of tiny cysts separated by internal septations
  - Septa coalesce to form central echogenic scar with "sunburst" calcification
  - US appearance depends on size of individual cysts
    - Slightly echogenic, solid-appearing mass (small cysts provide numerous acoustic interfaces)
    - Partly solid-appearing mass with anechoic cystic areas; cysts usually at periphery due to central scar
    - Multicystic mass with internal septations and solid component
  - Typically no pancreatic duct dilatation
    - However, large lesions in head of pancreas can behave more aggressively
  - Intralesional color Doppler flow in fibrovascular septa

- o Usually seen in older women (6th decade)
- **Mucinous Cystic Neoplasm of Pancreas**
  - o More common in pancreatic body and tail
  - o Well-demarcated, anechoic or hypoechoic, thick-walled, cystic mass
    - − Uni-/multilocular cysts separated by thick echogenic septations
  - o Solid papillary tissue protruding into tumor suggests malignancy
  - o Liver metastases appear as thick-walled cystic hepatic lesions
  - o Seen almost exclusively in middle-aged women

Helpful Clues for Less Common Diagnoses

- **Metastasis**
  - o Nonspecific imaging findings
  - o Focal or diffuse involvement
  - o Renal cell carcinoma: Most common primary; often solitary
  - o Other sources: Lung, GI, breast, melanoma, ovary, liver; typically disseminated disease
- **Lymphoma**
  - o Secondary lymphoma more common than primary lymphoma
    - − Known clinical history of systemic lymphomatous involvement
  - o Large, homogeneous, solid mass
  - o Presence of peripancreatic nodal masses
  - o Peripancreatic vessels displaced or stretched
- **Solid Pseudopapillary Neoplasm**
  - o Most common in pancreatic tail
  - o Well-demarcated, large, heterogeneous echogenic solid and cystic mass
  - o Small cystic areas often present due to tumor degeneration
    - − Often with intratumoral hemorrhage
  - o Dystrophic calcification occasionally seen
  - o No pancreatic duct dilatation or calcification
  - o Prominent vascular soft tissue components
    - − → hypervascular pattern with color Doppler

- o Liver metastases seen in ~ 4% of patients
- o Typically seen in young women (< 35 years)
- **Intrapancreatic Splenule**
  - o Congenital anomaly arising from aberrant splenic embryologic fusion
  - o Second most common location for accessory spleens is in the pancreatic tail
  - o Appears as small, well-circumscribed solid mass, usually at tip and not > 3 cm from tail
  - o Can easily be mistaken for primary pancreatic mass, particularly neuroendocrine tumor
  - o Follows attentuation of spleen on all phases of CT imaging and intensity of spleen on all MR sequences
  - o Confirm with Tc-99m labeled heat damaged red blood cells

SELECTED REFERENCES

1. Al-Hawary MM et al: Mimics of pancreatic ductal adenocarcinoma. Cancer Imaging. 13(3):342-9, 2013
2. Bhosale PR et al: Vascular pancreatic lesions: spectrum of imaging findings of malignant masses and mimics with pathologic correlation. Abdom Imaging. 38(4):802-17, 2013
3. Dimcevski G et al: Ultrasonography in diagnosing chronic pancreatitis: new aspects. World J Gastroenterol. 19(42):7247-57, 2013
4. Coakley FV et al: Pancreatic imaging mimics: part 1, imaging mimics of pancreatic adenocarcinoma. AJR Am J Roentgenol. 199(2):301-8, 2012
5. Raman SP et al: Pancreatic imaging mimics: part 2, pancreatic neuroendocrine tumors and their mimics. AJR Am J Roentgenol. 199(2):309-18, 2012

Pancreatic Ductal Carcinoma

Pancreatic Ductal Carcinoma

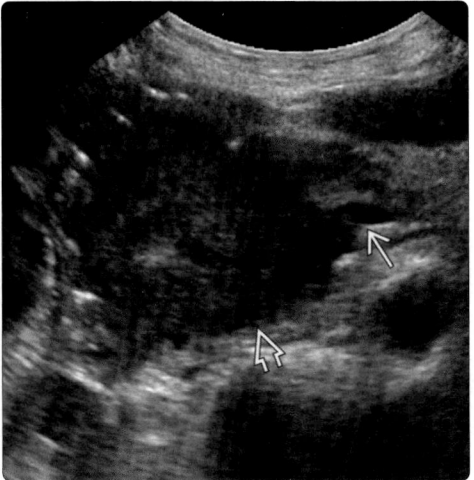

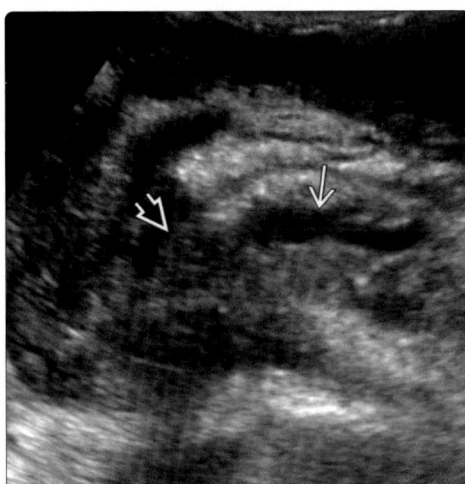

(**Left**) *Transverse transabdominal ultrasound shows a large infiltrative, solid, hypoechoic mass in the head of the pancreas ➡ abutting the superior mesenteric vein ➡, raising concern for vascular encasement.* (**Right**) *Transverse transabdominal ultrasound shows a poorly defined infiltrative hypoechoic mass ➡ in the head of the pancreas, obstructing the pancreatic duct, which is dilated upstream ➡.*

Pancreatic Ductal Carcinoma

Pancreatic Ductal Carcinoma

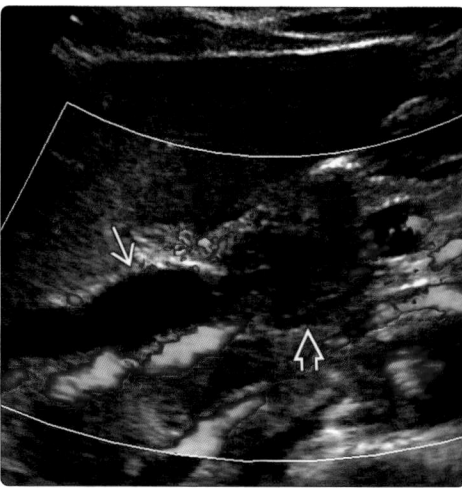

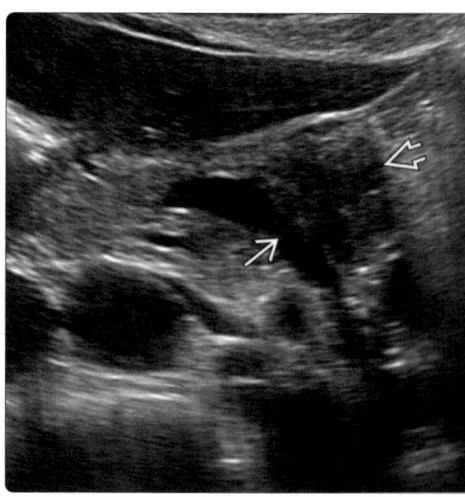

(Left) *Longitudinal oblique power Doppler ultrasound shows an ill-defined, solid hypoechoic mass ➡ in the pancreatic head resulting in obstruction of the terminal portion of the common bile duct ➡. (Right) Transverse transabdominal ultrasound shows a poorly marginated, solid, hypoechoic mass ➡ in the body of the pancreas, narrowing the splenic vein ➡.*

Focal Acute Pancreatitis

Chronic Pancreatitis

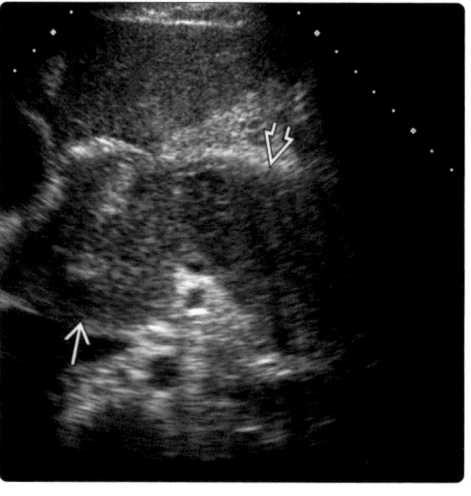

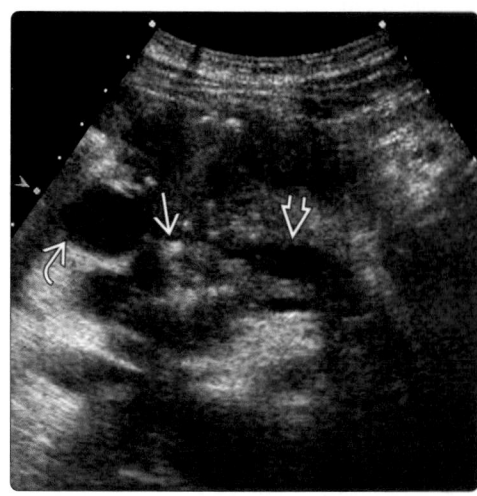

(Left) *Transverse transabdominal ultrasound shows focal enlargement ➡ of the distal pancreas with a homogeneous hypoechoic appearance relative to the normal pancreas ➡. Note the absence of ductal dilatation. (Right) Transverse ultrasound shows parenchymal calcifications ➡ in the enlarged pancreatic head. Note dilated pancreatic ➡ and common bile ➡ ducts and the pancreatic margins are indistinct.*

Pancreatic Neuroendocrine Tumor

Serous Cystadenoma of Pancreas

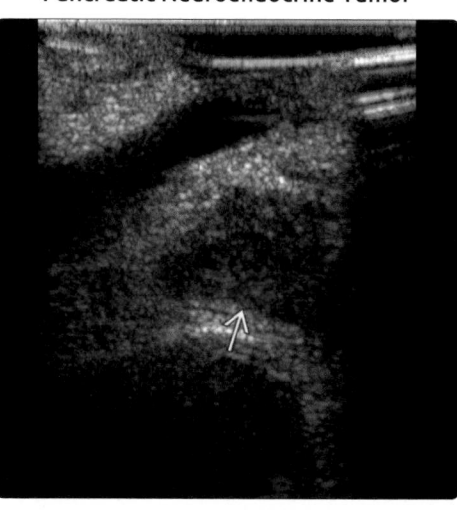

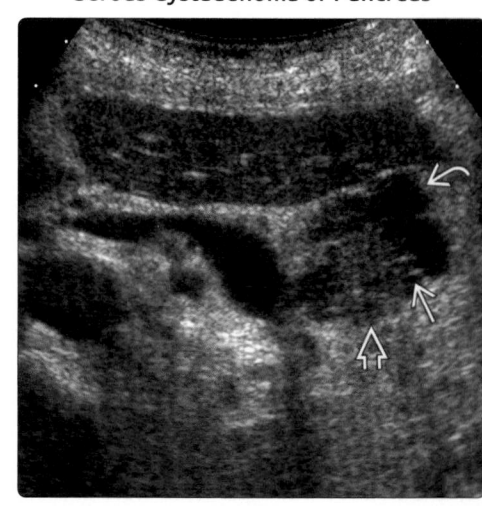

(Left) *Transverse intraoperative ultrasound shows a well-defined, hypoechoic, solid mass ➡ in the body of the pancreas, which was a biopsy-proven pancreatic neuroendocrine tumor. (Right) Transverse transabdominal ultrasound shows a well-circumscribed solid and cystic mass ➡ with peripheral loculations ➡. There are also tiny cystic spaces with thin linear septations ➡.*

Solid Pancreatic Lesion

Serous Cystadenoma of Pancreas

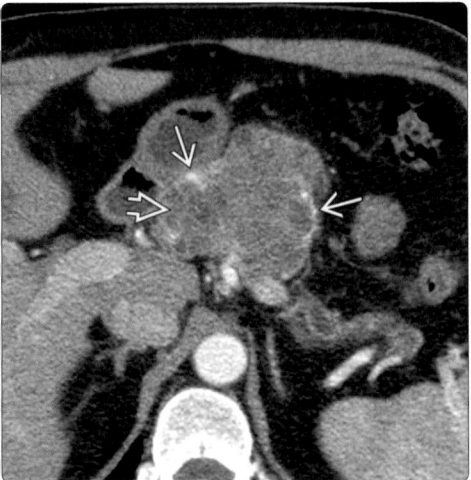

Mucinous Cystic Neoplasm of Pancreas

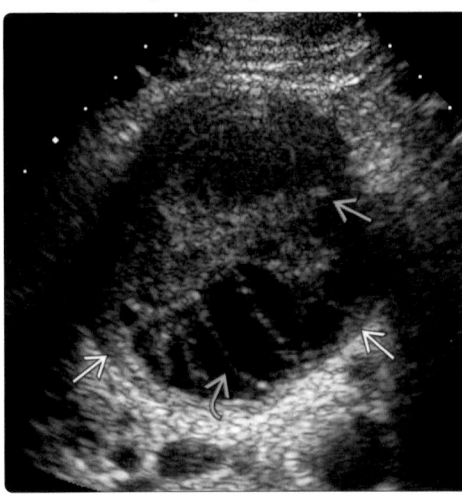

(Left) *Axial CECT demonstrates clusters of tiny cysts ⮕ separated by thin enhancing septations, in a honeycomb pattern characteristic of serous cystadenoma. Note the thin calcifications ⮕.* (Right) *Transverse transabdominal ultrasound shows a well-circumscribed, heterogeneous, multilocular cystic mass in the pancreas with thick ⮕ and thin ⮕ internal septations and a thick wall ⮕.*

Metastasis

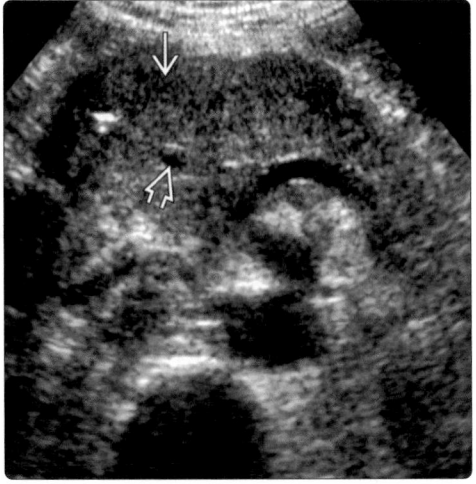

Lymphoma

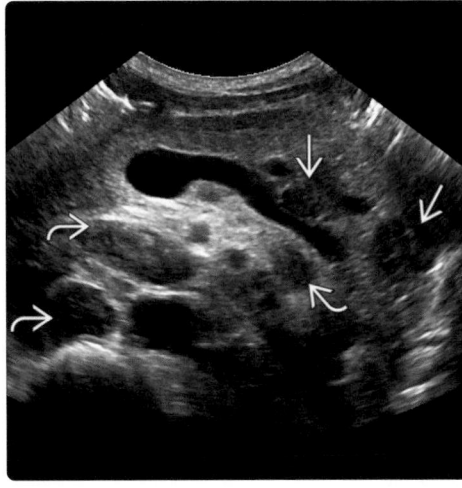

(Left) *Transverse transabdominal ultrasound shows an ill-defined, solid, hypoechoic mass ⮕ involving the head and body of the pancreas. The common hepatic artery is encased ⮕. Note the absence of pancreatic duct dilatation.* (Right) *Transverse ultrasound of the pancreas shows multiple round masses in the pancreatic tail ⮕, compatible with lymphomatous involvement. Other abnormal nodes were present in the retroperitoneum ⮕ from disseminated non-Hodgkin lymphoma.*

Solid Pseudopapillary Neoplasm

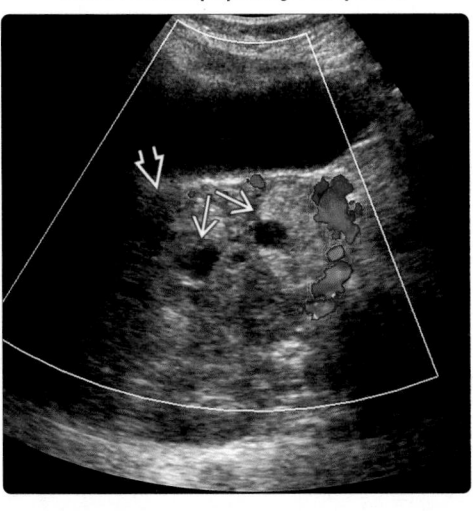

Intrapancreatic Splenule

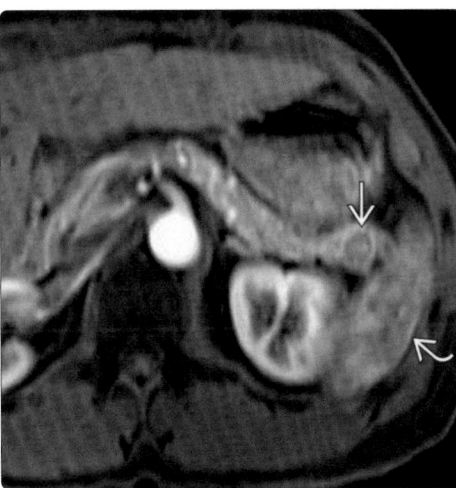

(Left) *Longitudinal ultrasound demonstrates a well-circumscribed, large, heterogeneous, echogenic solid mass ⮕ in a 17-year-old female. Note color Doppler flow in the periphery of the lesion and heterogeneous cystic areas of degeneration ⮕.* (Right) *Axial post-contrast T1 FS MR in the arterial phase shows a small, round, well-circumscribed lesion in the tip of the tail of the pancreas ⮕. The lesion demonstrates heterogeneous arterial phase enhancement, which matches that of the spleen ⮕.*

DIFFERENTIAL DIAGNOSIS

Common

- Chronic Pancreatitis
- Pancreatic Ductal Carcinoma
- Periampullary Tumor

Less Common

- Obstructing Distal Common Bile Duct Stone
- Intraductal Papillary Mucinous Neoplasm (IPMN)

ESSENTIAL INFORMATION

Key Differential Diagnosis Issues

- Pancreatic ductal dilatation: > 3 mm possibly with tortuous configuration
  - May see abrupt tapering at site of obstruction
  - Should prompt thorough search for obstructing lesion at the papilla or in pancreatic head
    - US may not provide adequate visualization due to overlying bowel gas or body habitus
    - CT, MR &/or endoscopic US should be considered
- Isolated pancreatic duct dilatation
  - Most commonly due to chronic pancreatitis
  - High possibility of pancreatic cancer if no evidence of chronic pancreatitis
  - Mild, idiopathic dilatation without tortuosity, frequently seen in elderly patients
- When associated with biliary duct dilatation, termed "double duct" sign
  - Etiology more likely malignant disease; most commonly pancreatic ductal adenocarcinoma
  - Obstructing common bile duct stone or benign stenosis are also possibilities if patient does not have jaundice or mass

Helpful Clues for Common Diagnoses

- **Chronic Pancreatitis**
  - Clinical history of longstanding recurrent attacks of epigastric pain; typically radiates to back
  - Atrophic pancreas with irregular outline and heterogeneous, hypo-/hyperechoic echo pattern
  - Pancreatic calcification: Intraductal and parenchymal
  - May see dilated side branches when severe
  - MR may show duct dilatation with strictures → more suggestive of chronic pancreatitis than IPMN
- **Pancreatic Ductal Carcinoma**
  - Causes pancreatic duct obstruction as tumor arises from ductal epithelium of exocrine pancreas
  - Irregular, ill-defined, solid, hypoechoic mass
  - Pancreatic duct dilatation upstream from tumor
  - Bile duct dilatation with tumor in pancreatic head
  - Lack of pancreatic calcification or ductal calculus
  - May see liver and regional lymph node metastases

Helpful Clues for Less Common Diagnoses

- **Obstructing Distal Common Bile Duct Stone**
  - Obstructive jaundice and epigastric pain
  - Presence of bile duct dilatation
- **Intraductal Papillary Mucinous Neoplasm (IPMN)**
  - Main duct type shows marked diffuse pancreatic ductal dilatation ± pancreatic atrophy
    - Calcification not typically seen and is more suggestive of chronic pancreatitis
    - Mural/intraluminal nodularity or associated soft tissue mass is suggestive of malignancy
  - Side branch duct type may show mild ductal dilatation communicating with cystic pancreatic lesion
    - Grape-like cluster of cysts with IPMN vs. unilocular cyst with chronic pancreatitis

SELECTED REFERENCES

1. Cohen J et al: Double-duct sign in the era of endoscopic ultrasound: the prevalence of occult pancreaticobiliary malignancy. Dig Dis Sci. 59(9):2280-5, 2014
2. Kim JH et al: Intraductal papillary mucinous neoplasm of the pancreas: differentiate from chronic pancreatits by MR imaging. Eur J Radiol. 81(4):671-6, 2012
3. Tanaka S et al: Slight dilatation of the main pancreatic duct and presence of pancreatic cysts as predictive signs of pancreatic cancer: a prospective study. Radiology. 254(3):965-72, 2010

(Left) *Transverse transabdominal ultrasound shows pancreatic ductal dilatation* ➡ *in the atrophic body of the pancreas with parenchymal* ⤴ *and intraluminal calcifications* ➘. (Right) *Axial transabdominal color Doppler ultrasound shows the double duct sign of biliary (calipers) and pancreatic duct* ➡ *dilatation due to an ill-defined mass in the head of the pancreas* ➘ *better seen on a more inferior plane.*

Chronic Pancreatitis

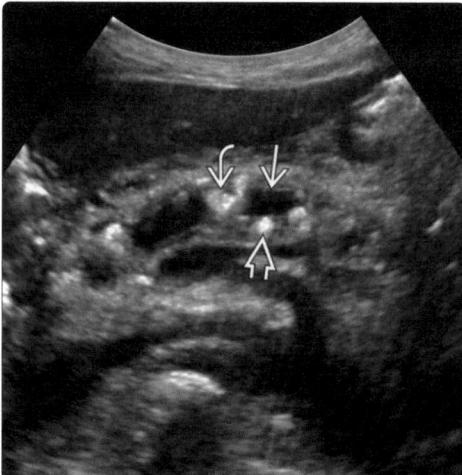

Pancreatic Ductal Carcinoma

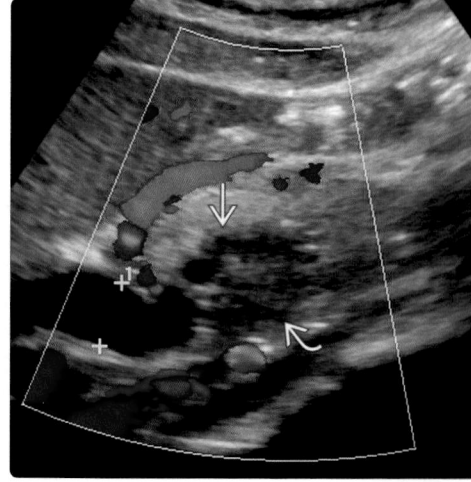

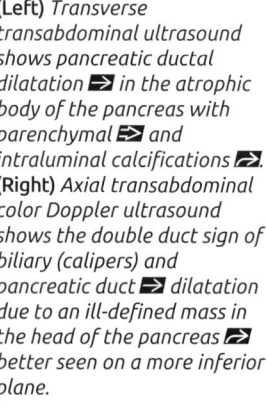

Chronic Pancreatitis

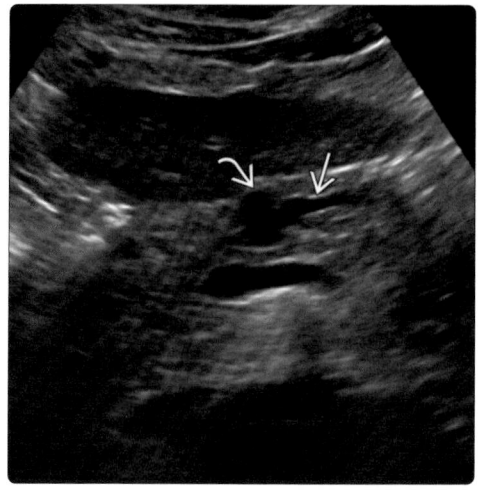

Chronic Pancreatitis

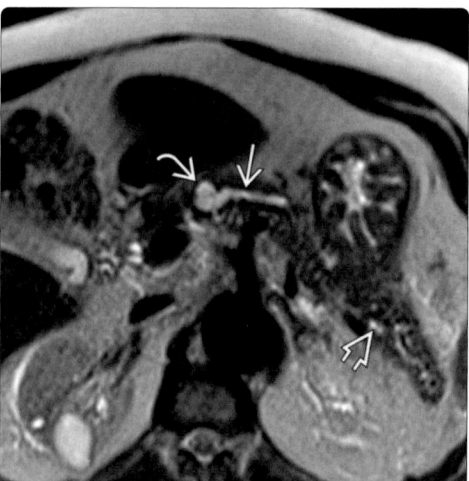

(Left) *Transverse transabdominal ultrasound shows a dilated pancreatic duct* ➡ *communicating with a small pseudocyst* ➡ *in the body of the pancreas.* (Right) *Axial T2 HASTE MR better demonstrates mild pancreatic ductal dilatation* ➡ *communicating with the small pseudocyst* ➡. *Note tiny dilated side branches* ➡ *in the tail of the pancreas. Pancreatic duct strictures were also seen (not shown) in this patient with a history of pancreatitis.*

Pancreatic Ductal Carcinoma

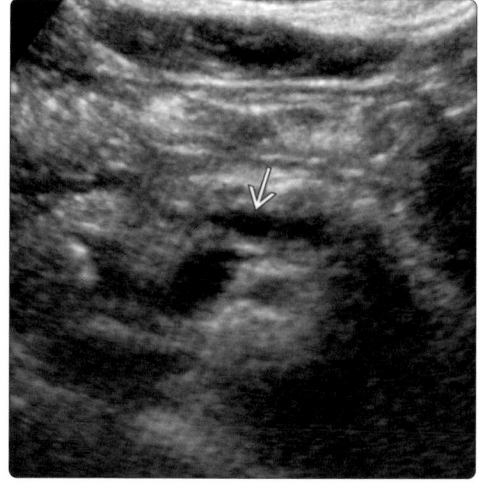

Pancreatic Ductal Carcinoma

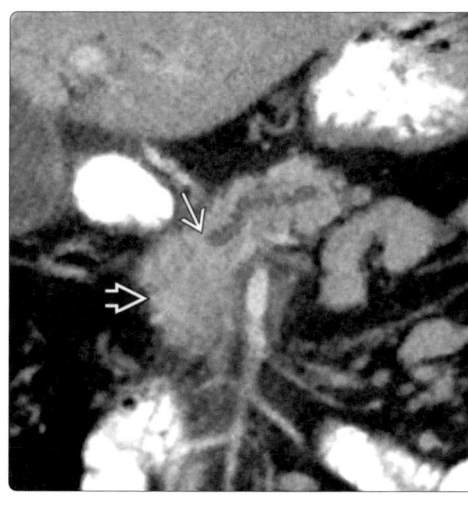

(Left) *Transverse oblique transabdominal ultrasound shows pancreatic ductal dilation in the body of the pancreas* ➡. (Right) *Coronal CECT was performed in the same patient to further characterize the cause of the pancreatic ductal dilatation. The dilated duct terminates abruptly* ➡ *at the site of a large, ill-defined mass in the pancreatic head* ➡.

Intraductal Papillary Mucinous Neoplasm (IPMN)

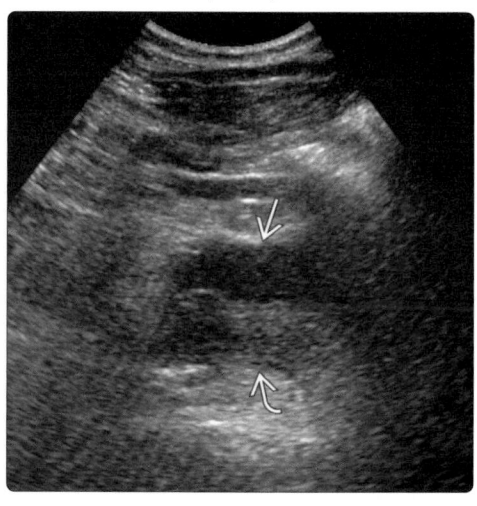

Intraductal Papillary Mucinous Neoplasm (IPMN)

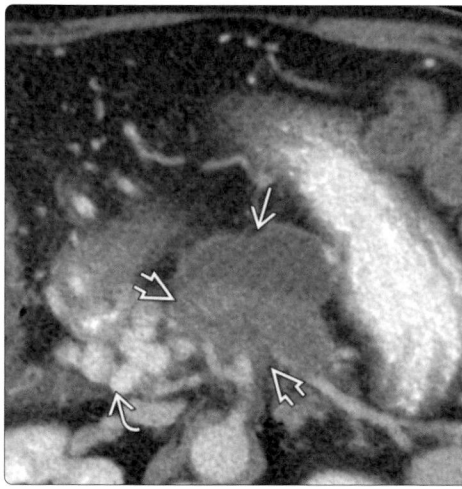

(Left) *Transverse transabdominal ultrasound shows marked pancreatic ductal dilatation* ➡ *with low-level internal echoes and an ill-defined hypoechoic mass posteriorly* ➡. (Right) *Axial CECT demonstrates marked pancreatic ductal dilatation* ➡ *with an infiltrative soft tissue mass posteriorly* ➡, *encasing the celiac axis. Note cavernous transformation of the portal vein* ➡ *due to venous occlusion from the mass which was proven by biopsy to be malignant transformation of a main duct type IPMN.*

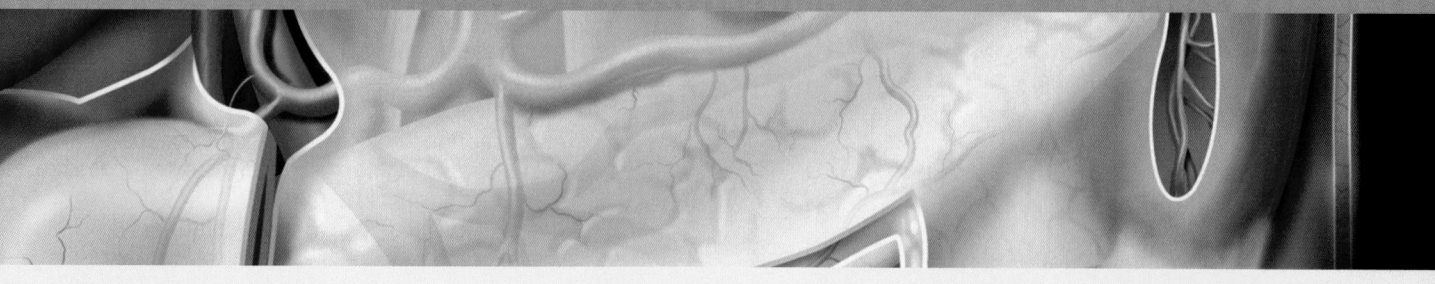

DIFFERENTIAL DIAGNOSIS

Common

- Acquired Splenic Cyst

Less Common

- Congenital (Epidermoid) Cyst
- Infected Cyst/Abscess
  - Pyogenic Abscess
  - Fungal Abscess
  - Parasitic Abscess (Hydatid Cyst)
  - Granulomatous Abscess
- Hemangioma
- Malignant Neoplasm
  - Lymphoma
  - Metastasis
- Splenic Infarct
- Splenic Hematoma/Laceration

Rare but Important

- Hamartoma
- Lymphangioma
- Primary Vascular Neoplasm
  - Littoral Cell Angioma
  - Angiosarcoma
- Sarcoidosis
- Peliosis
- Intrasplenic Pseudocyst

ESSENTIAL INFORMATION

Key Differential Diagnosis Issues

- Differentiate cystic from solid or vascular lesion
  - Clear fluid content is anechoic
  - Thick fluid content (proteinaceous fluid, hemorrhage, abscess) shows low-level internal echoes, mimics solid lesion
    - Grayscale movement of internal echoes and fluid level suggest fluid nature
    - Bright band sign of infarct could mimic internal echoes; assess shape
  - Use color or power Doppler
    - Presence of internal vascularity suggests solid nature rather than thick fluid content
    - Absence of color or power Doppler signal suggests cystic lesion or infarct; however, absent flow does not always exclude solid nature; may need further evaluation with contrast enhanced CT or MR
    - If anechoic component completely fills with color → high flow vascular space, e.g., intrasplenic aneurysm or pseudoaneurysm
  - Some lesions can have mixed cystic and solid appearance, for example
    - Early abscess formation in inflammatory phlegmon
    - Hemangioma, lymphangioma
    - Malignant tumor (irregular internal necrosis)
- If cystic, distinguish between unilocular and multilocular
  - Unilocular: Acquired or congenital cysts, abscess, cystic neoplasm
  - Multilocular: Septated or infected cysts, hydatid cysts, organizing hematoma, hemangioma, lymphangioma

- Determine if abnormality is solitary or multifocal
  - Solitary: Consider acquired or congenital cyst, pyogenic abscess, hydatid cyst, infarct or hematoma, benign or malignant tumors
  - Multiple: Consider pyogenic, fungal or granulomatous abscesses, benign or malignant tumors (particularly metastases, lymphoma), peliosis, sarcoidosis
- Note: There is considerable overlap in imaging appearance of focal splenic pathologies
  - Also, specific pathologies may have broad spectrum of appearances (ranging from hypo- to iso- to hyperechoic or from cystic to solid to mixed)
  - Often, CT or MR may be needed for further characterization

Helpful Clues for Common Diagnoses

- **Acquired Splenic Cyst**
  - Secondary cyst, due to liquefactive necrosis with cystic degeneration within lesions; 80% of cysts
    - Prior trauma (hematoma), infarction, infection, pancreatitis
    - Remote history of left upper quadrant injury can often be obtained (majority are post-traumatic)
  - Compared to primary (congenital) cysts, acquired cyst usually smaller, well defined; often anechoic with thicker fibrous wall; ± calcification, ± debris

Helpful Clues for Less Common Diagnoses

- **Congenital (Epidermoid) Cyst**
  - True cyst, lined by epithelium; 20% of cysts
  - Compared to secondary (acquired) cyst, epidermoid typically larger, well defined, anechoic, unilocular thin wall; ± calcification (uncommon); ± debris
- **Infected Cyst/Abscess**
  - **Pyogenic Abscess**
    - Solitary or multiple
    - Mobile low-level internal echoes to anechoic with posterior acoustic enhancement
    - Irregular wall, no capsule or pseudocapsule, ± internal gas
    - Rim enhancement on CT is less frequently seen than in hepatic abscesses
  - **Fungal Abscess**
    - Most common in immunocompromised patients, e.g., Candida
    - Multiple, small (few mm to 2 cm), hypoechoic foci representing microabscesses
    - Typically target appearance: Hypoechoic center = central necrotic hyphae, hyperechoic ring = concentric band of viable fungal element, outermost hypoechoic rim = inflammation
  - **Parasitic Abscess (Hydatid Cyst)**
    - Hydatid cysts rarely involve spleen (less than 2% of patients with echinococcosis)
    - Usually due to systemic dissemination and intraperitoneal spread from ruptured liver cyst
    - Appearances similar to hepatic hydatid cysts; majority are anechoic with thin wall ± septa, ± calc
  - **Granulomatous Abscess**
    - Due to TB, atypical mycobacterium (MAC); histoplasmosis; cat scratch disease

– Typically multiple well-defined, small, hypoechoic lesions (early); multifocal small calcifications (chronic/healed)

- **Hemangioma**
  - Most common benign tumor of spleen
  - Typically well-defined, hyperechoic solid lesion; echogenicity can be variable (range from solid to cystic to mixed); ± calc when complex
  - May be solitary or multiple (splenic hemangiomatosis, Klippel-Trenaunay-Weber syndrome, etc.)
- **Malignant Neoplasm**
  - **Lymphoma**
    - Most common malignant tumor of spleen; primary vs. secondary/systemic
    - Focal, multifocal, or diffuse; hypoechoic or cystic/pseudocystic
      - May contain internal irregular cystic area representing necrosis
      - Occasionally, markedly hypoechoic lymphoma infiltrate has pseudocystic appearance
      - Hyperechoic lesions less common
    - Indistinct boundary echo pattern
    - Evidence of disease elsewhere in liver, adenopathy
  - **Metastasis**
    - Multifocal lesions with variable size & appearance; iso-/hypo-/hyperechoic; solid, cystic, or mixed
      - Common primary sites = breast, lung, ovary, stomach, melanoma
      - Cystic metastases from melanoma, adenocarcinoma of breast, pancreas, ovaries, and endometrium
      - May be hyperechoic due to coagulative necrosis (hemorrhage), seen in melanoma, or calcification, as in mucinous adenocarcinomas
    - Target lesions with hypoechoic halo
    - Other evidence of disseminated disease
- **Splenic Infarct**
  - Classically peripheral, wedge-shaped, hypoechoic & hypo- or avascular; bright band sign
- **Splenic Hematoma/Laceration**

- History of trauma is crucial
- Peripheral (extending from capsular margin), band-like or wedge-shaped, hypo- or hyperechoic depending on stage of hematoma, avascular

Helpful Clues for Rare Diagnoses

- **Hamartoma**
  - Typically well-defined, homogeneous, hyperechoic
  - Variable echogenicity, vascularity; ± cystic change or calc
- **Lymphangioma**
  - Most occur in childhood; typically subcapsular location
  - Well-defined anechoic or hypoechoic complex cystic mass ± internal septations & intralocular debris; ± wall calc
  - Avascular on color Doppler, unless along cyst walls
- **Littoral Cell Angioma**
  - Commonly benign, though malignant has been reported
  - Variable echogenicity & vascularity; solitary or multiple; almost always with splenomegaly, hypersplenism
- **Angiosarcoma**
  - Heterogenous solid mass; majority (> 70%) have associated metastasis in liver
- **Sarcoidosis**
  - Hepatic involvement more common than splenic
  - Splenomegaly; multiple hypoechoic nodules (or iso/hyper); calcified in chronic phase
- **Peliosis**
  - Rare, idiopathic; associated with malignant hematologic disease, disseminated metastases, TB, etc.
  - Widespread blood-filled cystic spaces of varying size ± endothelial lining
  - Thrombosis within blood-filled spaces may occur
- **Intrasplenic Pseudocyst**
  - Pancreatic pseudocyst (1-5% of patients with pancreatitis)
  - Well-defined, rounded, cystic splenic lesion; associated inflammatory changes of pancreas

Acquired Splenic Cyst

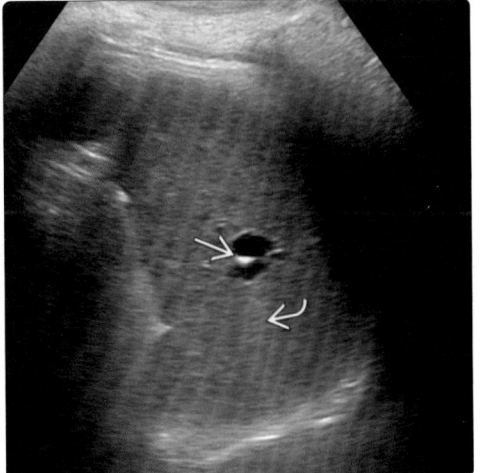

Acquired Splenic Cyst

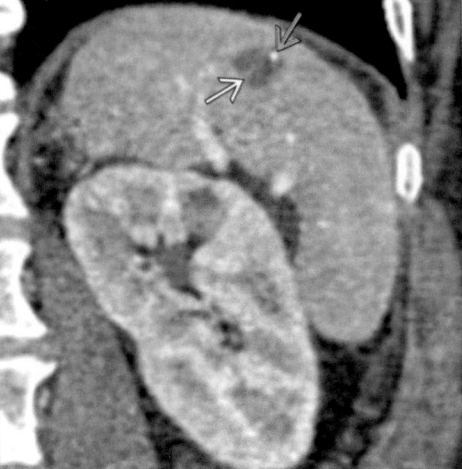

(Left) Transverse US of a splenic pseudocyst demonstrates posterior through transmission ⊿ and internal septation ⊒. Note that this appearance is nonspecific; a congenital epidermoid cyst may have a similar appearance. A history of trauma may aid in diagnosis of acquired pseudocyst. (Right) Corresponding coronal CECT shows the cyst with internal septation ⊒ and calcification ⊡ (not seen on the US). Both acquired and congenital cysts may have calcification, though more common in acquired cysts.

(Left) *Longitudinal US shows dense curvilinear calcification of a longstanding splenic cyst ➡ in a patient with a remote history of left upper quadrant injury. CT (not shown) revealed clear cystic content. The features are suggestive of a calcified pseudocyst.* **(Right)** *Longitudinal US of the spleen shows a thin-walled, anechoic cyst ➡ with thin internal septa ➡ and posterior enhancement ➡. This appearance is nonspecific. At histology, an epidermoid cyst has an epithelial lining, distinguishing it from other splenic cysts.*

Acquired Splenic Cyst

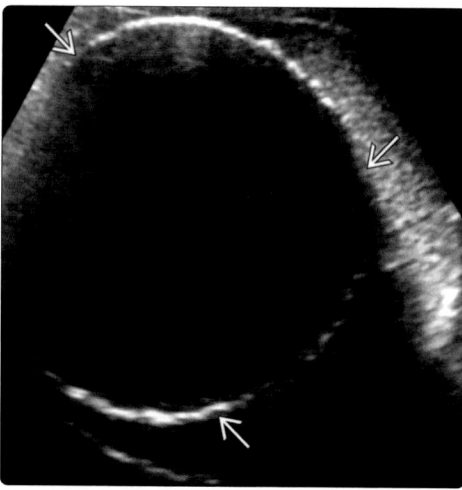

Congenital (Epidermoid) Cyst

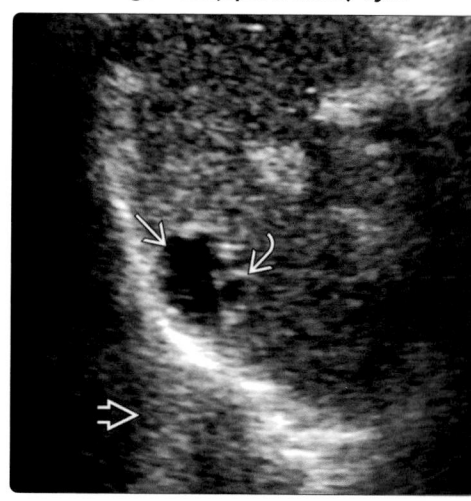

(Left) *Longitudinal transabdominal US shows an early splenic abscess ➡ with nonspecific, rounded, well-defined, hypoechoic appearance.* **(Right)** *Longitudinal splenic US shows a large, splenic cyst ➡ with internal debris ➡, forming a fluid level. Drainage revealed purulent material.*

Infected Cyst/Abscess

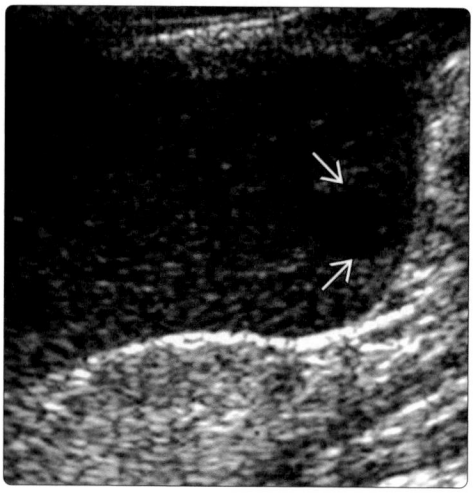

Pyogenic Abscess

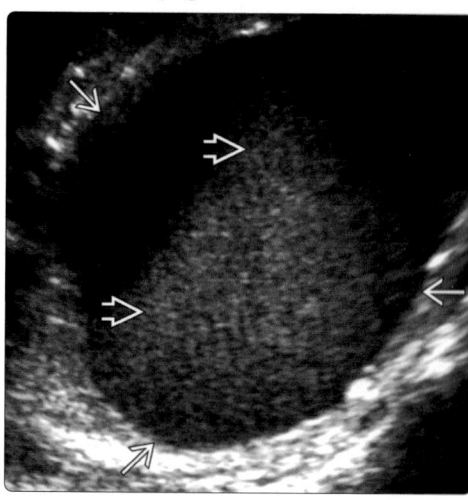

(Left) *Longitudinal transabdominal US of the spleen shows a rounded splenic abscess with partial liquefaction ➡. A thick irregular rim of inflammatory tissue ➡ remains in the periphery.* **(Right)** *Color Doppler US of the spleen shows a large, irregular-shaped, avascular, and largely anechoic collection in the mid spleen, with internal debris ➡. This was confirmed to represent pyogenic abscess.*

Pyogenic Abscess

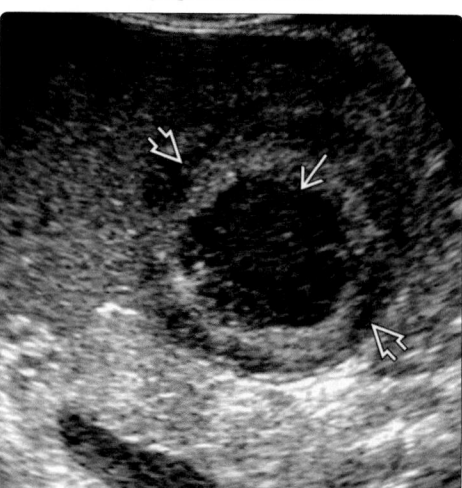

Pyogenic Abscess

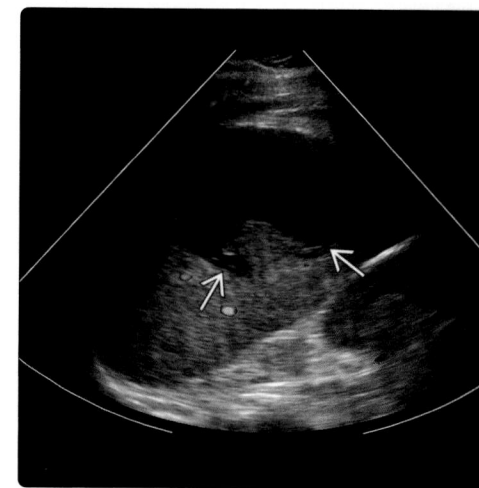

Pyogenic Abscess

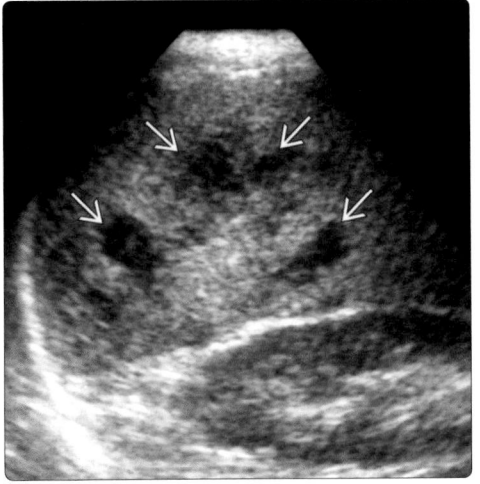

Parasitic Abscess (Hydatid Cyst)

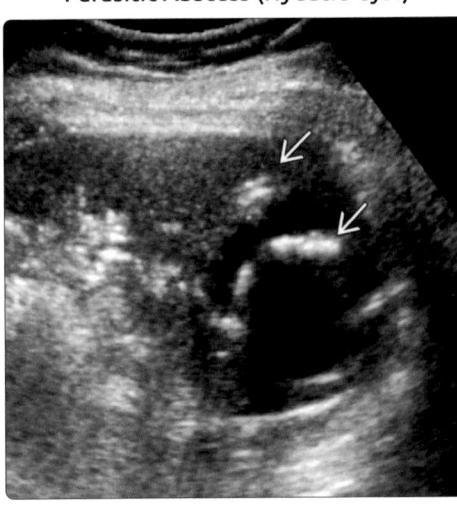

(Left) *Longitudinal transabdominal US of the spleen shows multifocal splenic abscesses* ➡. *They are irregular, some with surrounding hypoechoic areas (inflammatory edema). Multifocal fungal or granulomatous abscesses are typically smaller than pyogenic types.* (Right) *Transverse US of the spleen shows a multiloculated, thin-walled, anechoic cyst with a "cyst-within-cyst" appearance. Curvilinear calcification* ➡ *is seen in the cyst wall. This represents a chronic, healed hydatid cyst.*

Granulomatous Abscess

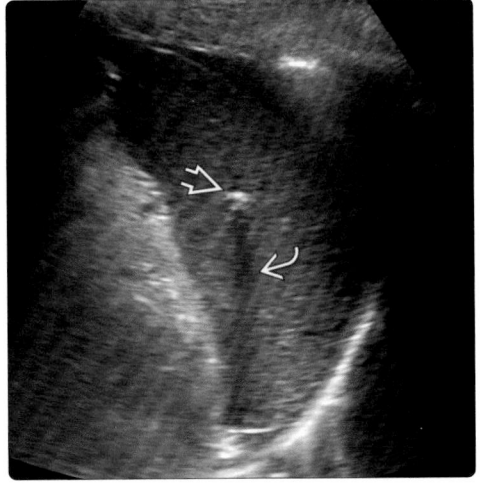

Hemangioma

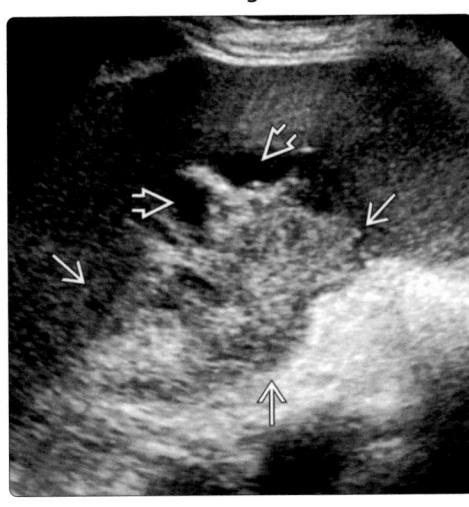

(Left) *Transverse splenic US shows a small echogenic focus* ➡ *with posterior acoustic shadowing* ➡, *consistent with a healed calcified granuloma (typically due to prior TB, MAC, histoplasmosis, or sarcoidosis). Mimics may include vascular calcifications or Gamna-Gandy bodies of portal hypertension.* (Right) *Longitudinal US shows a large hemangioma* ➡ *with hyperechoic solid and anechoic cystic components* ➡. *On occasion, cystic areas may be as large as entire lesion, giving the lesion a predominantly cystic appearance.*

Hemangioma

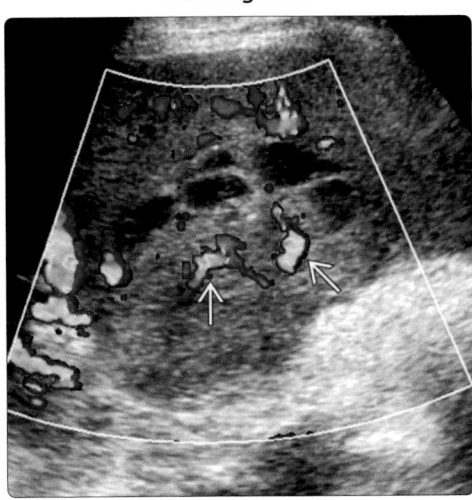

Lymphoma

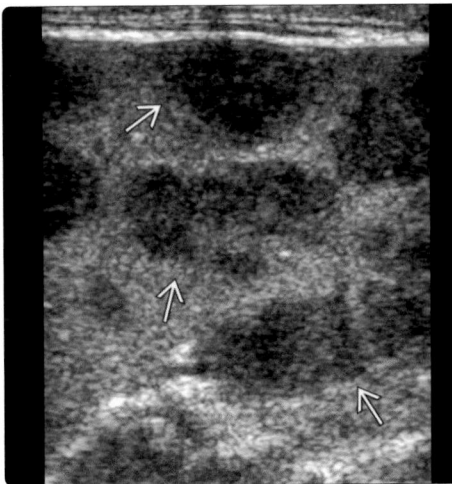

(Left) *Color Doppler US in the same patient shows prominent internal vascularity* ➡ *in the solid portion of the splenic hemangioma.* (Right) *Longitudinal US shows multiple hypoechoic lesions* ➡ *in a patient with multifocal lymphomatous involvement of the spleen. The differential would also include metastasis and granulomatous diseases.*

(Left) *A single lesion* ➡ *in the mid spleen is shown, predominately hypoechoic with some internal peripheral vascularity. This was confirmed to be lymphomatous involvement of the spleen.* (Right) *Longitudinal US shows an exophytic gastric MALT lymphoma with direct invasion* ➡ *into the spleen. Portions of the mass are cystic* ➡ *(due to internal necrosis). Solid components range from hyperechoic* ➡ *to hypoechoic* ➡.

Lymphoma

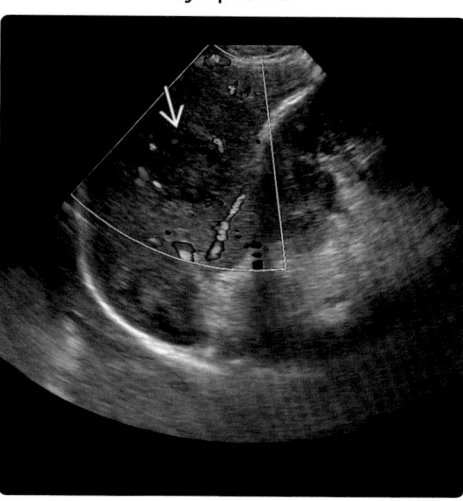

Lymphoma

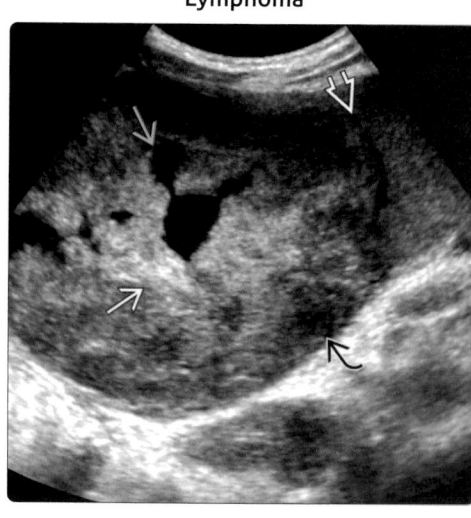

(Left) *Power Doppler US show a heterogeneously hyperechoic mass representing secondary lymphoma involvement. Note that the absence of internal Doppler signal does not always exclude solid nature.* (Right) *Transverse US shows lymphomatous deposits* ➡ *in the spleen. The markedly hypoechoic appearance may be confused with cystic lesions (in the left kidney* ➡*).*

Lymphoma

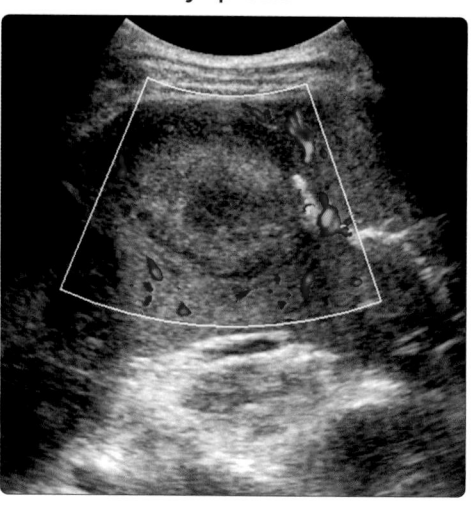

Lymphoma

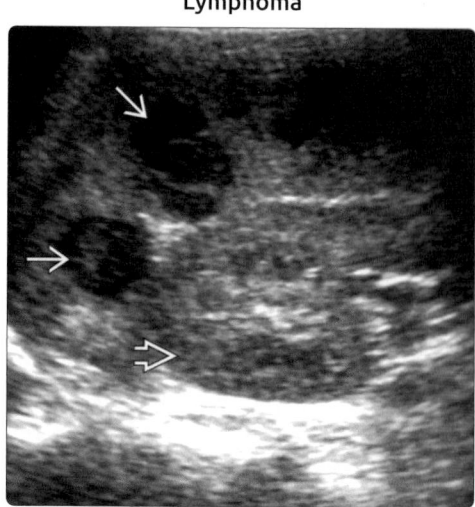

(Left) *Color Doppler US shows a similar heterogeneously hyperechoic mass with hypoechoic rim, here representing a metastasis from conjunctival melanoma. Hyperechoic mets may be from melanoma (hemorrhage) or mucinous adenocarcinomas (calcification).* (Right) *Longitudinal US shows irregular, echogenic nodules* ➡ *of varying sizes (mets from hepatocellular carcinoma), hypodense on CECT. Echogenic appearance may represent coagulative necrosis. Mimics include granulomas, hemangiomatosis.*

Metastasis

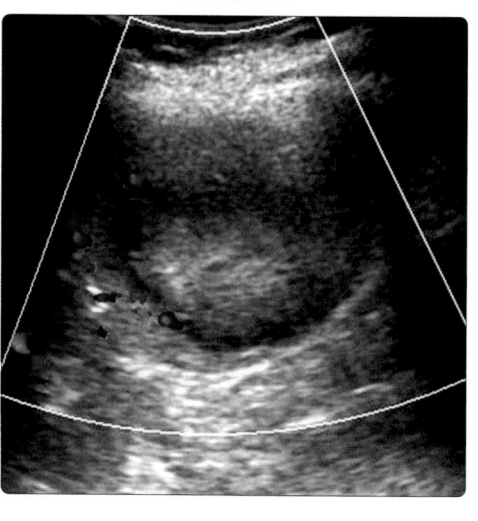

Metastasis

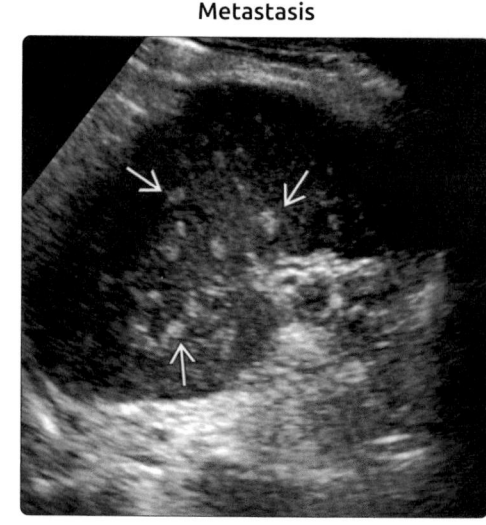

Splenic Infarct

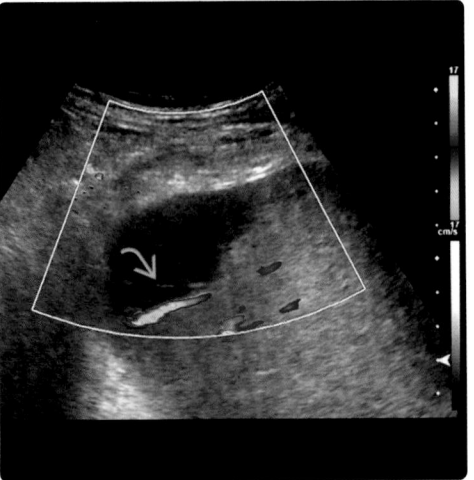

Splenic Infarct

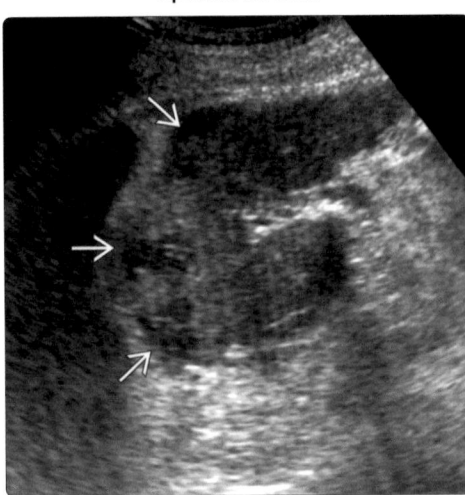

(Left) *Color Doppler US shows a splenic infarct, predominately anechoic. This can mimic a cyst or hematoma; take note of the shape (peripheral, wedge-like) with a few parallel echogenic bands (bright band sign)* ➔ *more characteristic of infarct.* **(Right)** *US shows a small spleen an with irregular contour. Multiple cystic areas* ➔ *with echogenic bands are present in the subcapsular region, consistent with liquefactive necrosis from previous splenic infarcts. Multifocal infarcts may be due to embolic processes.*

Splenic Hematoma/Laceration

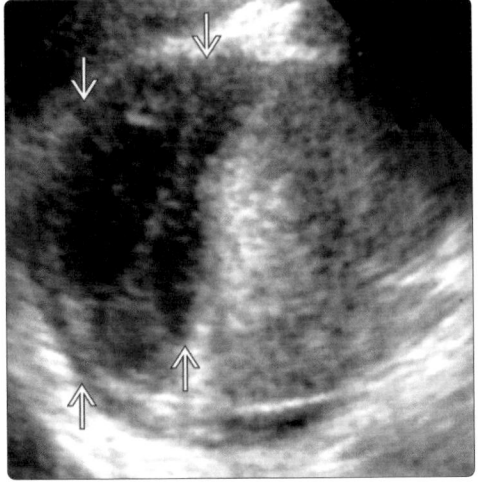

Splenic Hematoma/Laceration

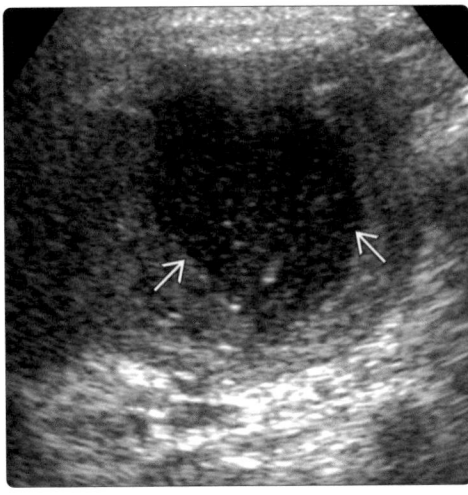

(Left) *Longitudinal US shows cystic change* ➔ *in a splenic hematoma. Note that part of the hematoma remains echogenic, representing acute component.* **(Right)** *Longitudinal US shows liquefactive necrosis with cystic change* ➔ *in the subacute stage of a splenic laceration. The history of trauma is important to make the diagnosis of laceration.*

Hamartoma

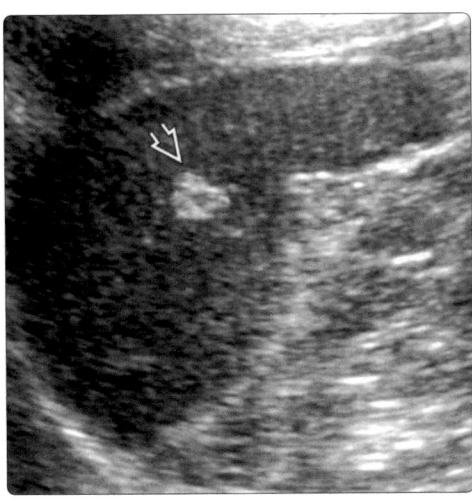

Lymphangioma

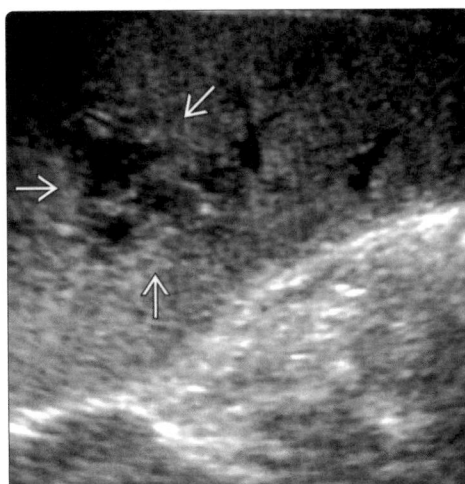

(Left) *Longitudinal US shows a calcified splenic hamartoma* ➔; *it is well defined and echogenic. The echogenicity is higher than that seen in a solid tumor, e.g., hemangioma, and is suggestive of a calcified lesion.* **(Right)** *Longitudinal US of the spleen shows a splenic lymphangioma* ➔. *Note its multiloculated, thin-walled, cystic appearance and the normal surrounding parenchyma.*

PART III
SECTION 5
Urinary Tract

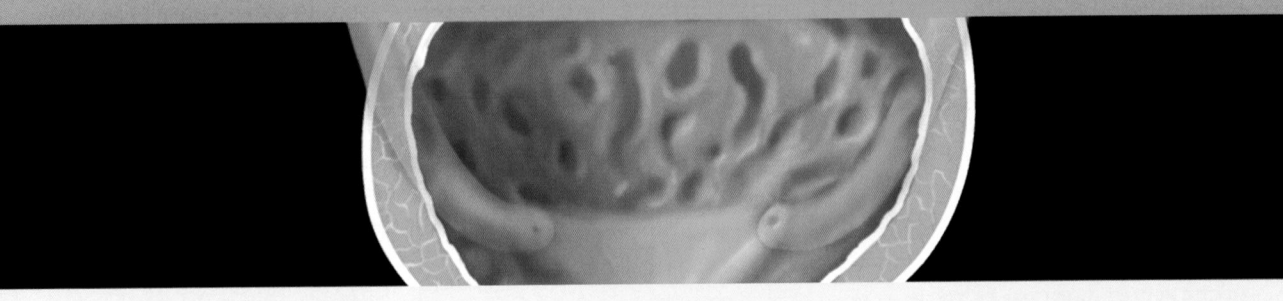

DIFFERENTIAL DIAGNOSIS

Common

- Bladder Calculi and Sludge
- Blood Clot
- Foley Catheter
- Bladder Carcinoma
- Benign Prostatic Hyperplasia
- Ureterocele

Less Common

- Foreign Body
- Fungal Ball

ESSENTIAL INFORMATION

Key Differential Diagnosis Issues

- Confirm mobile vs. immobile intraluminal masses by scanning in different position (e.g., decubitus)
- Assess for posterior acoustic shadowing seen with stone and calcified masses
- Assess intralesional vascularity to differentiate tumor from non-tumor masses
- Enlarged prostate seen as indentation on bladder base

Helpful Clues for Common Diagnoses

- **Bladder Calculi and Sludge**
  - Bladder calculi seen as mobile, avascular, echogenic mass with posterior acoustic shadowing
  - Bladder calculi may be present in bladder diverticulum assessment with optimally distended bladder useful
  - Bladder sludge is sand-like, echogenic, mobile debris with no posterior shadowing; can be seen associated with cystitis
  - Sludge balls are mobile, avascular, echogenic mass with less acoustic shadowing than calculi
- **Blood Clot**
  - Clinical history of frank hematuria favors diagnosis
    - Causes: Spontaneous, post instrumentation, renal biopsy, or tumor

  - Seen as heterogenous or echogenic, avascular mobile mass lacking posterior acoustic shadowing
  - May be associated with layering debris (blood-urine level)
- **Foley Catheter**
  - Round anechoic structure with echogenic rim, often centrally located
  - Bladder often underdistended/decompressed
- **Bladder Carcinoma**
  - Often pedunculated polypoidal, rarely broad-based, frond-like immobile mass with mixed echogenicity
  - Color Doppler shows intralesional vascularity
- **Benign Prostatic Hyperplasia**
  - Can cause mass-like nodular protrusion of median lobe at bladder base
  - Difficult to entirely exclude bladder carcinoma on imaging
- **Ureterocele**
  - Thin-walled, anechoic/cystic, intravesical mass near vesicoureteric junction
  - Changes in size based on ureteric peristalsis and distension

Helpful Clues for Less Common Diagnoses

- **Foreign Body**
  - Broken Foley catheter, or other foreign bodies; echogenicity depends on material and may range from isoechoic to hyperechoic masses ± posterior shadowing
- **Fungal Ball**
  - Seen in immunosuppressed or diabetic patient
  - Seen as mixed echogenicity, well-defined, mobile, avascular mass lacking posterior acoustic shadowing

SELECTED REFERENCES

1. Byler TK et al: Incidental computed tomographic bladder wall abnormalities: harbinger or herring? Urology. 85(2):288-91, 2015
2. Shinagare AB et al: Urinary bladder: normal appearance and mimics of malignancy at CT urography. Cancer Imaging. 11:100-8, 2011
3. Lieber MM et al: Intravesical prostatic protrusion in men in Olmsted County, Minnesota. J Urol. 182(6):2819-24, 2009

Bladder Calculi and Sludge

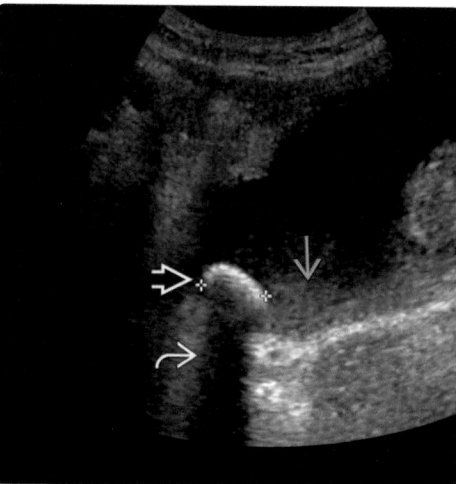

Foley Catheter

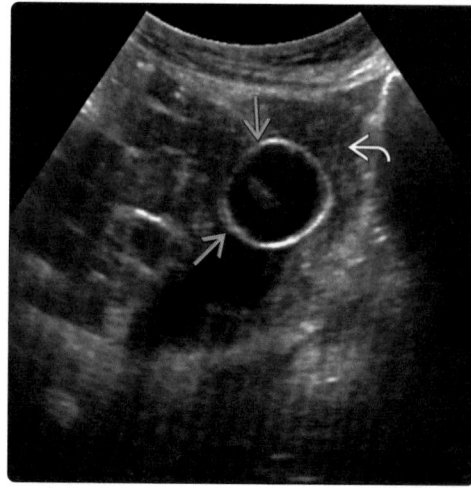

(Left) Transverse transabdominal ultrasound shows a large, echogenic stone ➡ with posterior acoustic shadowing ➡ within the urinary bladder. Also note dependent debris ➡. (Right) Longitudinal transabdominal ultrasound through the bladder shows a Foley catheter ➡ with underdistended bladder. The underdistention is often associated with pseudothickening of the bladder wall ➡.

Bladder Carcinoma

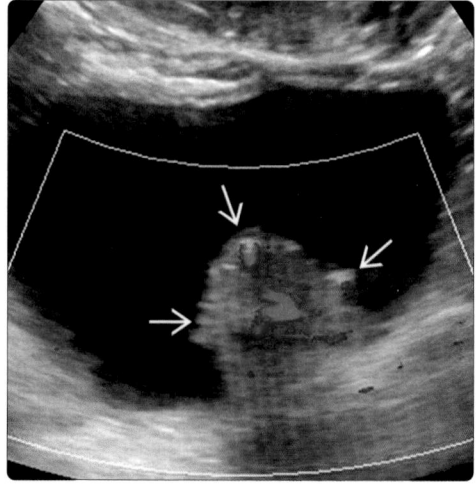

Bladder Carcinoma

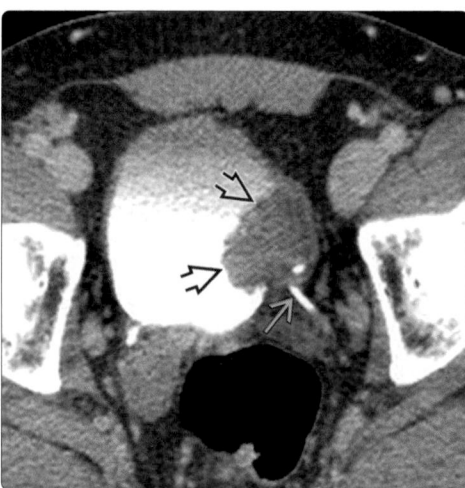

(Left) Transverse transabdominal color Doppler ultrasound of the urinary bladder shows an intraluminal bladder mass with intralesional vascularity ⮕ arising from the left posterolateral bladder wall. (Right) Axial CT urography image through the bladder in the same patient confirms the intraluminal polypoidal mass arising from the left posterolateral bladder wall ⮕, abutting the left ureterovesical junction (UVJ) ⮕ and confirmed as urothelial carcinoma.

Fungal Ball

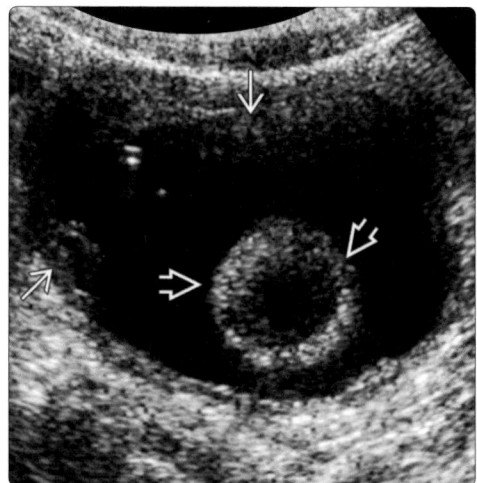

Benign Prostatic Hyperplasia

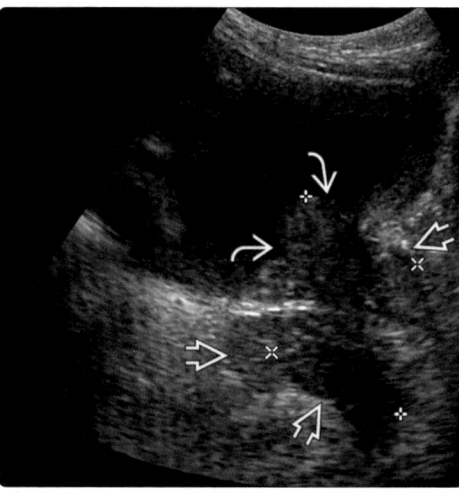

(Left) Transverse transabdominal ultrasound shows diffuse bladder wall thickening ⮕ and a fungal ball ⮕ in the bladder of a patient with fungal cystitis. (Right) Longitudinal transabdominal ultrasound through the urinary bladder shows an enlarged prostate gland ⮕ with median lobe hypertrophy indenting the bladder base seen as a lobulated, intraluminal mass ⮕.

Blood Clot

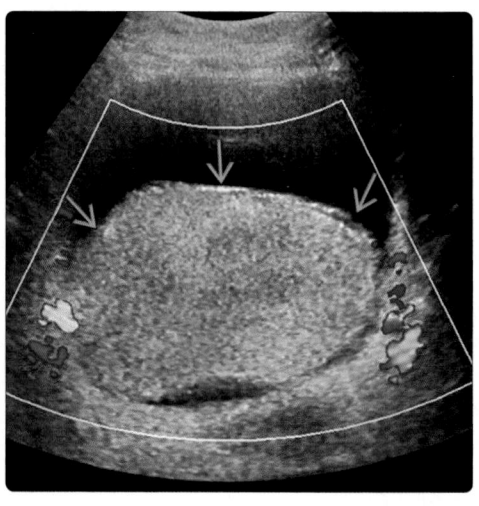

Ureterocele

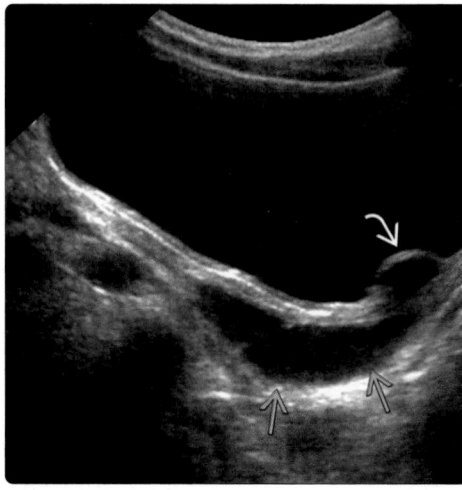

(Left) Transverse transabdominal Doppler ultrasound of the urinary bladder in this patient with recent renal biopsy and gross hematuria shows a large, avascular, mixed-echogenicity blood clot ⮕ in the bladder with no posterior shadowing. (Right) Longitudinal oblique transabdominal grayscale ultrasound at the suprapubic region shows a dilated ureter ⮕ terminating in the ureterocele ⮕. The patient had a complete duplicated collecting system.

DIFFERENTIAL DIAGNOSIS

Common

- Underfilled/Underdistended Bladder
- Normal Trigone
- Bacterial Cystitis
- Chronic Cystitis
- Neurogenic Bladder
- Chronic Bladder Outlet Obstruction
- Bladder Carcinoma
- Invasion by Pelvic Neoplasm

Less Common

- Fungal Cystitis
- Tuberculous Cystitis
- Bladder Schistosomiasis
- Emphysematous Cystitis
- Invasion by Pelvic Inflammatory Disease

ESSENTIAL INFORMATION

Key Differential Diagnosis Issues

- Bladder wall thickness should be commented on optimally distended bladder
- Be aware of sites of normal thickening near trigone
- Classify bladder wall thickening as focal or diffuse pattern
  - Focal suspicious for neoplastic process
- Color Doppler (including power Doppler) helps to identify intralesional vascularity in malignant conditions
- Check kidneys and ureters for hydronephrosis, other clues of infectious causes, such as TB and schistosomiasis
- Bladder echoes and debris often seen with cystitis

Helpful Clues for Common Diagnoses

- **Underfilled/Underdistended Bladder**
  - Common cause for pseudothickening of the bladder wall
    - Rescan with optimal distension
- **Normal Trigone**
  - Normal mild thickening between ureteral orifices (interureteric ridge)
  - May pose diagnostic challenge in patients with prostatomegaly
- **Bacterial Cystitis**
  - Most common etiology: *Escherichia coli* (E. coli)
    - Transurethral invasion of bladder by perineal flora in women
    - Bladder outlet obstruction and urinary stasis in men
  - Usually smooth diffuse bladder wall thickening
  - Recurrent bacterial infection: Malakoplakia
    - Granulomatous inflammatory process
    - Associated with E. coli
- **Chronic Cystitis**
  - Associated with vesicoureteric reflux
  - Associated with decreased bladder capacity
  - Other complications associated with chronic cystitis
    - Hyperplastic uroepithelial cell clusters (Brunn nests) form in bladder submucosa
    - Cystitis cystica
      - Fluid accumulation → pseudocysts
      - Malignant potential
    - Cystitis glandularis

- Transformation into glands
  - Radiation cystitis: Sequelae of radiation therapy for pelvic malignant neoplasm (uterine, cervical, prostate, and rectal carcinoma)
    - Small volume bladder with diffuse irregular wall thickening
    - May be associated with obstructive hydronephrosis
    - May have fistulous communication with adjacent viscera secondary to necrosis (from obliterative endarteritis)
  - Chemotherapeutic agents induced cystitis, often causing hemorrhagic cystitis
    - Common agents: Cyclophosphamide (cytoxan), ifosfamide, bacillus Calmette-Guérin (BCG) instillation for Ca bladder
- **Neurogenic Bladder**
  - Dysfunctional bladder secondary to neural injury regulating the bladder
  - Diffuse bladder thickening ± trabeculations
    - Muscular hypertrophy leading to irregular outline of inner bladder wall
  - Typical Christmas tree-shaped bladder
  - Detrusor hyperreflexia
    - Gross trabeculation and abnormal shape
- **Chronic Bladder Outlet Obstruction**
  - Usually in males secondary to benign prostatic hypertrophy
  - Diffuse bladder wall thickening with trabeculations
  - ± focal pseudopolyps, which are indistinguishable from tumor
- **Bladder Carcinoma**
  - Commonly appears as focal bladder wall thickening
    - Polypoidal or broad-based most common
    - May see frond-like projections
  - Best diagnostic clue
    - Focal immobile mass with mixed echogenicity arising from bladder wall
      - Scan patient in decubitus position to differentiate from mobile blood clot or debris
    - Absent posterior acoustic shadowing
  - Color Doppler shows increased vascularity in most large tumors
  - Reported sensitivity for bladder tumor detection by US range from 50-95%
  - US may be useful in detecting tumor in bladder diverticulum, often inaccessible by cystoscopy
  - Tumor near bladder base in male may be confused with prostatic enlargement
    - Transrectal US differentiates bladder tumors from prostatic lesions
    - Bladder tumors and prostatic enlargement often coexist
    - Bladder tumors may invade prostate
- **Invasion by Pelvic Neoplasm**
  - Common tumors
    - Male
      - Rectal carcinoma
      - Prostate carcinoma
    - Female
      - Cervical carcinoma

- □ Uterine carcinoma
- □ Vaginal carcinoma
- □ Ovarian carcinoma
- ○ Loss of fat plane between the bladder wall and the adjacent pelvic neoplasm
- ○ May have direct intramural and intralesional extension
  - − May be associated with fistulous communication
- ○ Color Doppler
  - − Vascularity of tumor outside bladder cavity may be demonstrated

Helpful Clues for Less Common Diagnoses

- **Fungal Cystitis**
  - ○ *Candida albicans* is most common organism
  - ○ May be associated with fungal ball within bladder
- **Tuberculous Cystitis**
  - ○ Hematogenous spread of primary tubercular infection, usually lungs (caused by *Mycobacterium tuberculosis*)
  - ○ Secondary to renal ± ureteric involvement
  - ○ Earliest form of bladder tuberculous cystitis starts around ureteral orifice
  - ○ Typically low-volume bladder with diffuse wall thickening ("thimble bladder") ± wall calcification
  - ○ Fibrotic changes near ureteric orifice result in vesicoureteric reflux
  - ○ Associated with localized or generalized pyonephrosis
- **Bladder Schistosomiasis (Bilharziasis of Bladder)**
  - ○ Infection of urinary system by parasite *Schistosoma hematobium*
  - ○ Thick-walled fibrotic bladder
  - ○ Echogenic calcification within bladder wall
  - ○ Small capacity bladder with inability to completely empty
  - ○ ± hydronephrosis and hydroureter due to distal ureteric stricture
  - ○ Late complication
    - − Squamous cell carcinoma of bladder
  - ○ Often difficult to differentiate from tuberculosis based on imaging
- **Emphysematous Cystitis**

- ○ Infection of the bladder wall by gas-forming bacterial or fungal organism
  - − *E. coli, Enterobacter aerogenes, Klebsiella pneumonia, Proteus mirabilis*
- ○ Echogenic foci within area of bladder wall thickening with ring-down artifact
- ○ Plain radiograph or CT for confirmation
- **Invasion by Pelvic Inflammatory Disease**
  - ○ Crohn disease: Inflamed bowel or fistula formation
  - ○ Sigmoid colonic diverticulitis
  - ○ Endometriotic pelvic implants
    - − Diffuse of focal bladder wall thickening, surrounding inflammatory changes
    - − Increased vascularity in the inflammatory tissue

SELECTED REFERENCES

1. Lee G et al: Cystitis: from urothelial cell biology to clinical applications. Biomed Res Int. 2014:473536, 2014
2. Manack A et al: Epidemiology and healthcare utilization of neurogenic bladder patients in a US claims database. Neurourol Urodyn. 30(3):395-401, 2011
3. Manikandan R et al: Hemorrhagic cystitis: A challenge to the urologist. Indian J Urol. 26(2):159-66, 2010
4. Vikram R et al: Imaging and staging of transitional cell carcinoma: part 1, lower urinary tract. AJR Am J Roentgenol. 192(6):1481-7, 2009
5. Figueiredo AA et al: Urogenital tuberculosis: update and review of 8961 cases from the world literature. Rev Urol. 10(3):207-17, 2008
6. Thomas AA et al: Emphysematous cystitis: a review of 135 cases. BJU Int. 100(1):17-20, 2007
7. Wein AJ et al: Overactive bladder: a better understanding of pathophysiology, diagnosis and management. J Urol. 175(3 Pt 2):S5-10, 2006
8. Wong-You-Cheong JJ et al: From the archives of the AFIP: Inflammatory and nonneoplastic bladder masses: radiologic-pathologic correlation. Radiographics. 26(6):1847-68, 2006
9. Abrams P: Bladder outlet obstruction index, bladder contractility index and bladder voiding efficiency: three simple indices to define bladder voiding function. BJU Int. 84(1):14-5, 1999

Underfilled/Underdistended Bladder

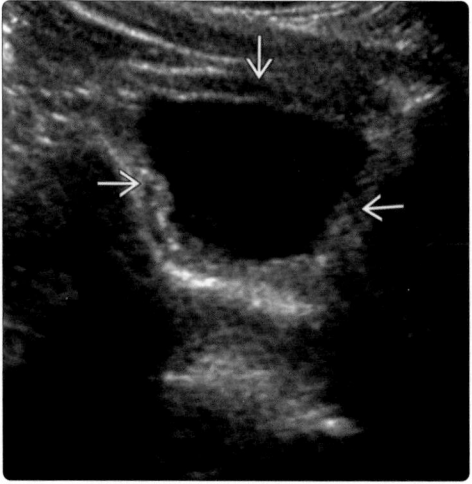

Normal Trigone

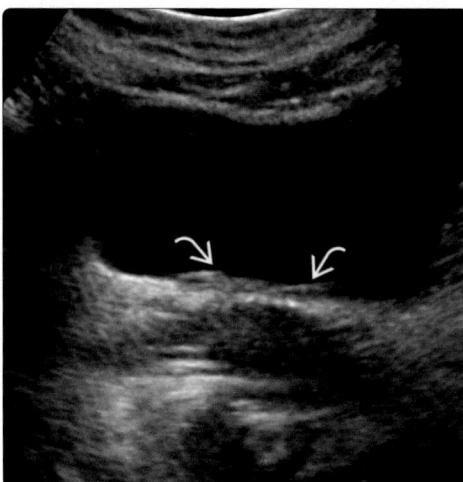

(Left) *Transverse transabdominal ultrasound shows an apparent uniformly thickened wall of an underdistended bladder →. The bladder wall was normal after optimal distension.* **(Right)** *Transverse transabdominal ultrasound shows a focal thickening → at the interureteric ridge (trigone), a normal finding.*

Bacterial Cystitis

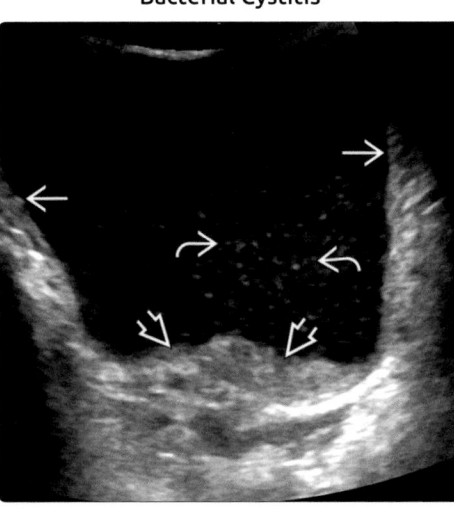

Chronic Cystitis

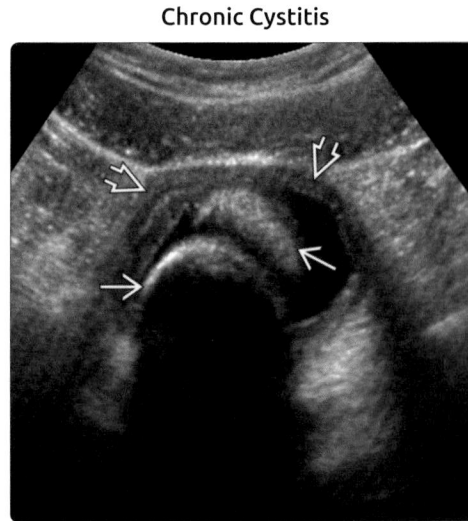

(Left) *Transverse transabdominal ultrasound shows diffuse bladder wall thickening* ➡ *with internal debris* ➡ *and echoes* ➡ *in a patient with a urinary tract infection, with positive bacterial growth on urine culture.* (Right) *Transverse transabdominal ultrasound of the urinary bladder shows multiple large stones* ➡ *with diffuse wall thickening* ➡*, suggesting chronic cystitis.*

Neurogenic Bladder

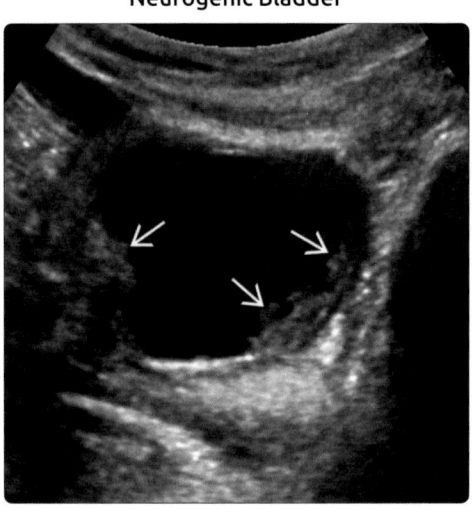

Chronic Bladder Outlet Obstruction

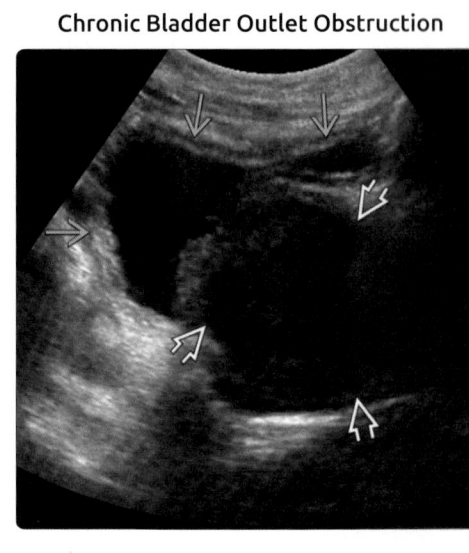

(Left) *Transverse transabdominal ultrasound shows a small capacity bladder with wall thickening and an irregular inner bladder surface (trabeculations)* ➡ *in a neurogenic bladder.* (Right) *Longitudinal transabdominal ultrasound shows diffuse bladder wall thickening* ➡ *secondary to benign prostatic hyperplasia* ➡ *with a lobulated contour, indenting the bladder base. A common cause of chronic bladder outlet obstruction in elderly male patients.*

Bladder Carcinoma

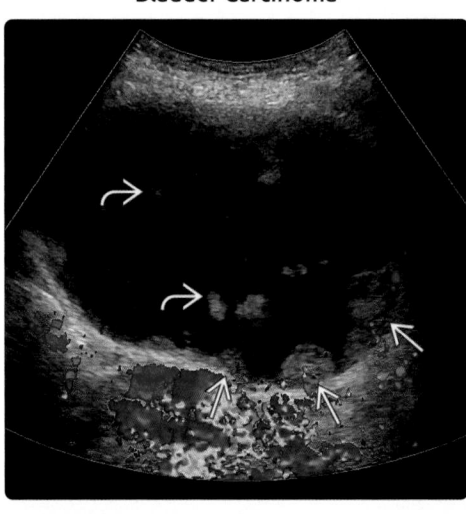

Bladder Carcinoma

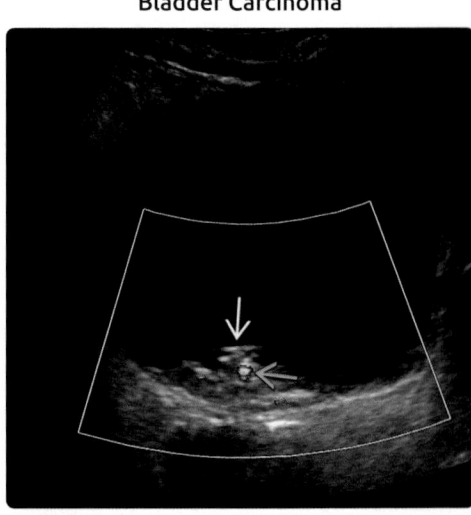

(Left) *Longitudinal color Doppler US of the bladder shows multiple solid masses* ➡ *arising from the posterior wall of the bladder with internal vascularity consistent with transitional cell carcinoma of the bladder. Note the echogenic debris* ➡ *within the bladder caused by associated hematuria.* (Right) *Transverse color Doppler image of the bladder shows an irregular echogenic mass* ➡ *arising from the posterior wall of the bladder with internal vascularity* ➡ *consistent with bladder carcinoma.*

Invasion by Pelvic Neoplasm

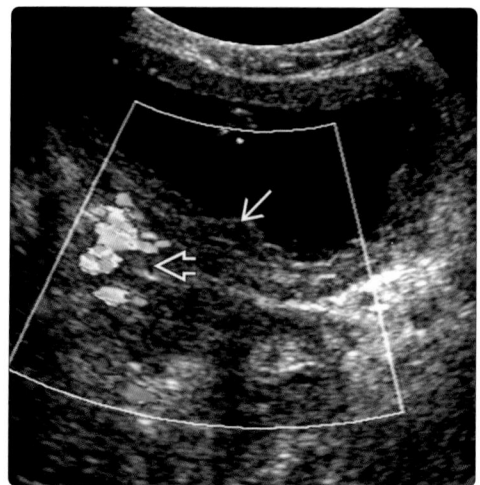

Tuberculous Cystitis

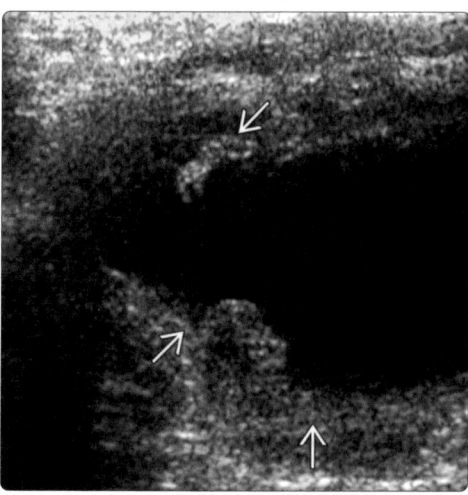

(Left) *Longitudinal color Doppler ultrasound shows bladder wall thickening ➡ due to local invasion by uterine cancer. Increased vascularity is present in the tumor tissue ➡. (Right) Transverse transabdominal ultrasound shows a bladder infected by TB with an irregularly thickened bladder wall ➡. Tuberculous cystitis may be indistinguishable from other forms of bacterial cystitis.*

Emphysematous Cystitis

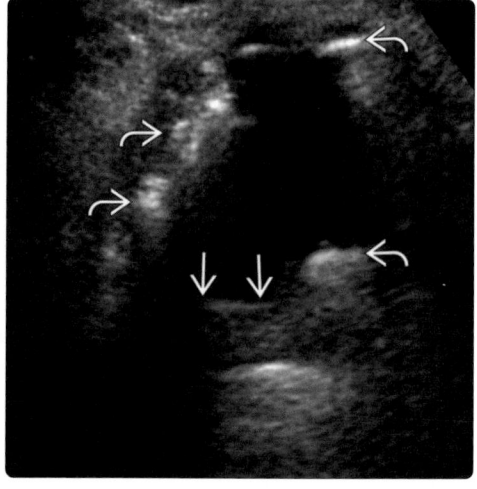

Emphysematous Cystitis

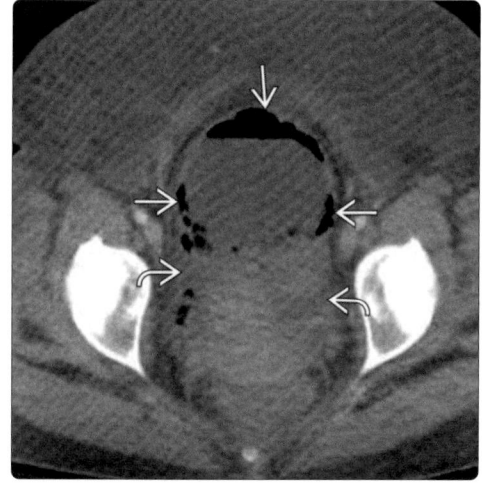

(Left) *Transverse transabdominal ultrasound of the bladder shows diffuse wall thickening with several echogenic foci in the bladder wall (dependent and nondependent) ➡ with debris ➡ suggesting emphysematous cystitis. (Right) Axial contrast enhanced CT through the pelvis shows gas within the bladder wall with ➡ perivesical/pelvic stranding ➡ (emphysematous cystitis).*

Invasion by Pelvic Inflammatory Disease

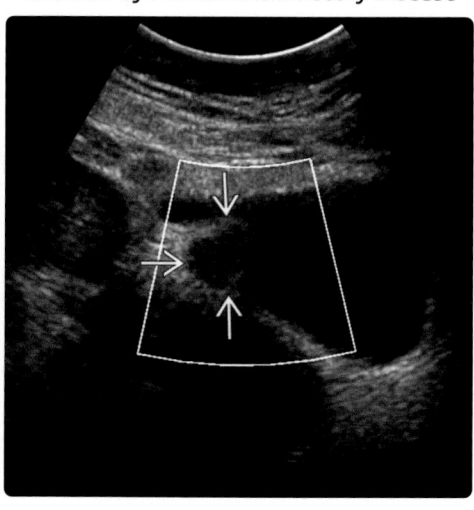

Invasion by Pelvic Inflammatory Disease

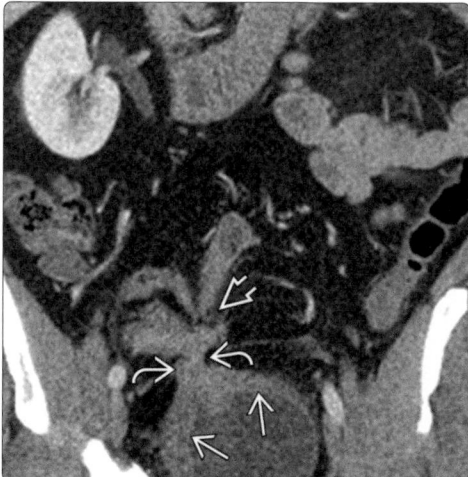

(Left) *Transverse oblique transabdominal ultrasound shows focal hypoechoic mass in the right bladder wall ➡ confirmed as endometriotic implant. (Right) Coronal reformat CECT in this patient with known Crohn disease, shows asymmetric right bladder wall thickening ➡ secondary to fistulous communication ➡ with small bowel loops ➡ (enterovesical fistula).*

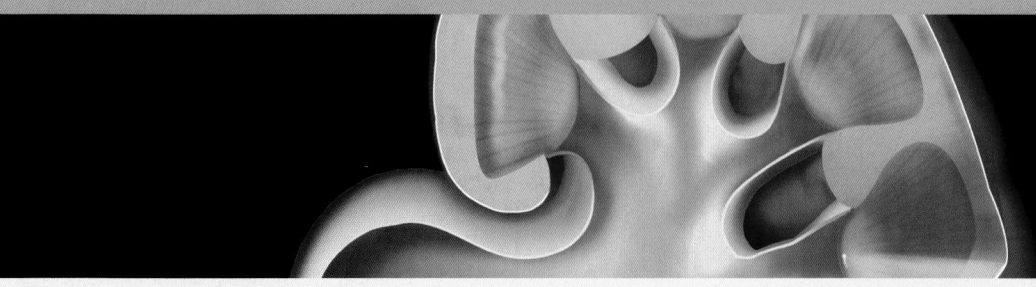

DIFFERENTIAL DIAGNOSIS

Common

- Hydronephrosis
- Acute Pyelonephritis
- Primary Renal Tumors: Benign and Malignant
- Compensatory Renal Hypertrophy
- Duplex Kidney
- Renal Parenchymal Diseases
  - Acute Glomerulonephritis, Lupus Nephritis, Diabetic Nephropathy, Acute Tubular Necrosis
- Renal Vascular Diseases
  - Acute renal vein thrombosis, acute renal infarction, acute cortical necrosis
- Renal Abscess
- Pyonephrosis
- Perinephric Fluid Collections
- Renal Trauma

Less Common

- HIV Nephropathy
- Autosomal Dominant Polycystic Kidney Disease (ADPKD)
- Multicystic Dysplastic Kidney (MDK)
- Horseshoe Kidney
- Crossed Fused Renal Ectopia

Rare but Important

- Autosomal Recessive Polycystic Kidney Disease (ARPKD)
- Renal Lymphoma
- Renal Leukemia
- Xanthogranulomatous Pyelonephritis
- Renal Amyloidosis
- Renal Tuberculosis
- Exercise-Induced Nonmyoglobinuric Acute Renal Failure

ESSENTIAL INFORMATION

Key Differential Diagnosis Issues

- Establish if renal enlargement is unilateral or bilateral and if enlargement is focal or diffuse
- Acute causes: Obstruction, infection, inflammation
- Chronic causes: Cellular hypertrophy, abnormal protein deposition, malignancies, infection, glomerular or microvascular proliferation

Helpful Clues for Common Diagnoses

- **Hydronephrosis**
  - Splitting of central renal echocomplex by branching fluid filled pelvis
  - Dilated calyces may be variable in size
  - Cortical thinning in chronic hydronephrosis
  - Look for dilated ureter and determine if simply dilated or truly obstructed (VCUG/MAG 3 renogram)
  - Gross hydronephrosis may mimic multicystic dysplastic kidney, ovarian or mesenteric cyst (in infants), or large collection
  - Causes include stones, tumors, congenital malformations, clot, infection, extrinsic compression, bladder outlet obstruction, and vesico ureteral reflux
- **Acute Pyelonephritis**
  - Normal renal size or diffuse enlargement
  - Echogenicity variable: Decreased or increased

- Focal pyelonephritis
  - Focal alteration of cortical echogenicity
  - Wedge shaped, triangular, or round
  - May produce a focal external cortical bulge
  - Wedge-shaped perfusion defect extending from papilla on color and power Doppler or contrast-enhanced ultrasound
    - Cortical vascularity decreased secondary to cortical vasoconstriction and edema
- **Primary Renal Tumors: Benign and Malignant**
  - **Renal Cell Carcinoma**
    - Varied size and appearance
    - Exophytic echogenic renal mass when large
    - Hypoechoic rim, cystic change from necrosis, calcification
    - Diffuse infiltration is less common
  - **Upper Tract Urothelial Carcinoma**
    - Hydronephrosis and dilated calyces secondary to pelvic or ureteral tumor
    - Infiltrating soft tissue mass in renal pelvis or pelvic wall thickening
  - **Renal Angiomyolipoma (AML)**
    - Echogenic mass with posterior shadowing, single or multiple
    - Variable size and lipid content
      - Lipid poor are less echogenic
      - Usually require confirmation with CT or MR
    - Large AML may be indistinguishable from other renal solid tumors
  - **Multilocular Cystic Nephroma**
    - Multilocular encapsulated cystic lesion, which may herniate into renal pelvis
  - **Mesoblastic Nephroma**
    - Typically solid unilateral mass in neonate or fetus
- **Compensatory Renal Hypertrophy**
  - Enlarged, otherwise unremarkable kidney
  - Occurs with contralateral renal disease, aplasia/dysplasia, or nephrectomy
- **Duplex Kidney**
  - Splitting of central echogenic renal sinus into upper and lower pole moieties
  - 2 distinct draining ureters may be seen if they are dilated
- **Renal Parenchymal Diseases**
  - **Acute Glomerulonephritis**
    - Bilateral enlarged kidneys with hyperechoic cortex and prominent pyramids
  - **Lupus Nephritis**
    - Acute: Normal or increased size bilaterally; cortical echogenicity increased or normal
    - May also have multiple focal infarcts
  - **Diabetic Nephropathy**
    - Bilateral enlarged bright kidneys in early stage
  - **Acute Tubular Necrosis**
    - Normal or diffuse bilateral renal swelling
    - Prominent pyramids due to edema
- **Renal Vascular Diseases**
  - **Acute Renal Vein Thrombosis**
    - Common in membranous glomerulonephritis

Enlarged Kidney

- Nonneoplastic causes: Dehydration and fever in children; hypercoagulability and nephrotic syndrome in adults
- Renal enlargement with ↓ echogenicity, renal vein thrombus ± collaterals
- Unilateral > bilateral
- ○ **Acute Renal Infarction**
  - Embolic or traumatic arterial occlusion
  - Unilateral flank pain
  - Normal or enlarged kidneys with wedge-shaped defect on color Doppler
- ○ **Acute Cortical Necrosis**
  - Caused by abruptio placentae, postpartum hemorrhage, shock, sepsis, and toxins
  - Results from microvascular thrombosis with cortical ischemia
  - Bilateral enlarged echogenic kidneys with hypoechoic subcapsular rim
- **Renal Abscess**
  - ○ Solitary or multiple thick-walled intrarenal cystic lesions in the setting of infection
  - ○ More common in patients with diabetes mellitus, drug abuse, vesicoureteral reflux, renal calculi
- **Pyonephrosis**
  - ○ Swollen obstructed kidney with debris or dependent echoes in collecting system
- **Perinephric Fluid Collections**
  - ○ May represent abscess, blood, urine, and lymph
  - ○ May mimic large renal mass or compress the kidney causing "page kidney"
- **Renal Trauma**
  - ○ Perirenal and renal hematomas, renal fracture, contusion

Helpful Clues for Less Common Diagnoses

- **HIV Nephropathy**
  - ○ Normal or enlarged kidneys
  - ○ Typically increased echogenicity with decreased corticomedullary differentiation
  - ○ Later small
- **Autosomal Dominant Polycystic Kidney Disease (ADPKD)**

- ○ Usually presents in adulthood
- ○ Bilateral large kidneys with innumerable cysts of varying sizes that distort normal renal architecture
- **Multicystic Dysplastic Kidney (MDK)**
  - ○ Multiple noncommunicating renal cysts of varying size with echogenic intervening parenchyma
  - ○ Initially enlarged kidney, later atrophy
  - ○ Association with contralateral renal disease common
- **Horseshoe Kidney**
  - ○ Lower poles joined by isthmus of functioning renal tissue or fibrous band
  - ○ Lower in position with medially deviated lower poles
- **Crossed Fused Renal Ectopia**
  - ○ Enlarged kidney with malrotation
  - ○ Absence of contralateral kidney

Helpful Clues for Rare Diagnoses

- **Autosomal Recessive Polycystic Kidney Disease (ARPKD)**
  - ○ Detected in utero or in infancy
  - ○ Bilaterally enlarged kidneys with increased echogenicity and multiple tiny cysts
- **Renal Lymphoma**
  - ○ Focal or diffuse renal enlargement: Unilateral or bilateral
  - ○ Infiltrative: Diffuse renal enlargement with disruption of internal architecture
  - ○ Perirenal soft tissue rind
- **Renal Leukemia**
  - ○ Gross renal involvement uncommon
  - ○ Symmetrically enlarged kidneys with distorted central sinus and ↓ corticomedullary differentiation
- **Xanthogranulomatous Pyelonephritis**
  - ○ Pelvicalyceal obstruction by stone, (usually staghorn)
  - ○ Diffuse unilateral renal enlargement with echogenic debris in dilated calyces and cortical thinning
  - ○ Diabetes, recurrent urinary tract infections, immunocompromise
- **Renal Amyloidosis**
  - ○ Abnormal protein deposition in kidneys
- **Renal Tuberculosis**
  - ○ Dilated calyces and granulomatous abscesses

Hydronephrosis

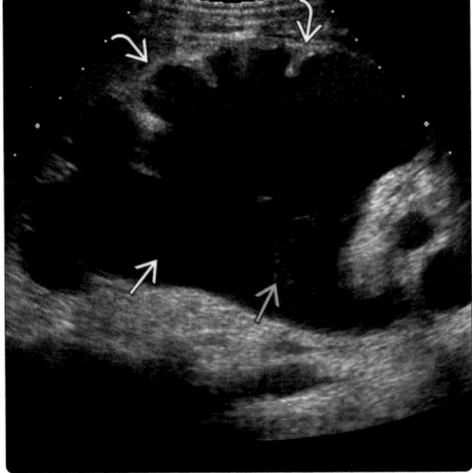

Acute Pyelonephritis

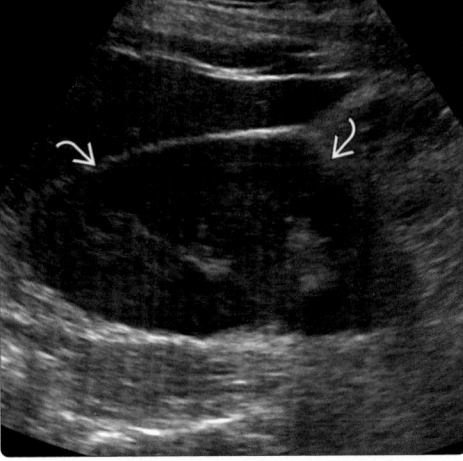

(Left) Longitudinal ultrasound of a markedly enlarged right kidney with severe hydronephrosis ➡, hydroureter and cortical thinning ➡ in a patient with a history of posterior urethral valves and severe reflux. Renal pelvis echoes ➡ could represent infection, blood, or cellular debris. (Right) Longitudinal ultrasound in a patient with acute pyelonephritis and diabetes shows an enlarged hypoechoic right kidney ➡ with loss of corticomedullary differentiation.

Acute Pyelonephritis

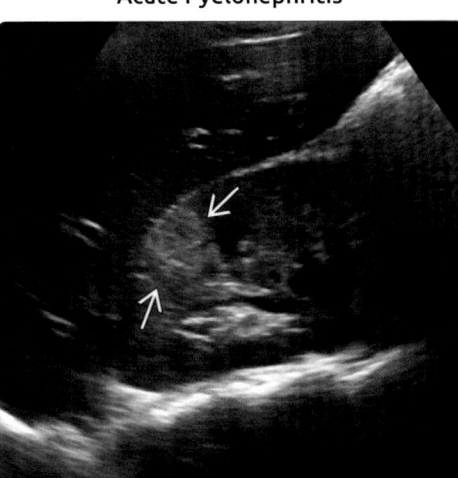

Primary Renal Tumors: Benign and Malignant

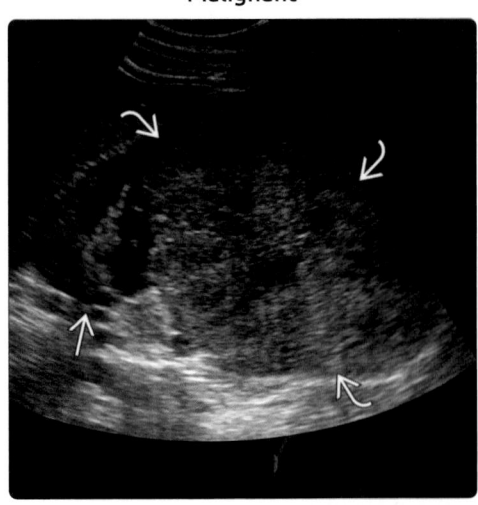

(Left) *Longitudinal transabdominal ultrasound shows focal acute pyelonephritis in a pregnant woman. There is a wedge-shaped area of increased echogenicity ➜ in the upper pole.* **(Right)** *Longitudinal ultrasound shows an enlarged kidney ➜ with a large solid mass in the lower pole ➜. Given the size of this mass, renal cell carcinoma was suspected but it was an oncocytoma at surgery.*

Compensatory Renal Hypertrophy

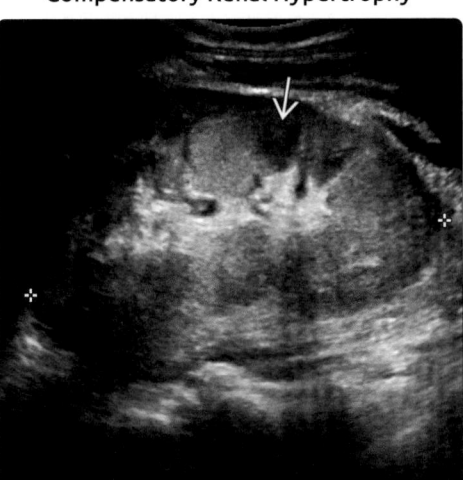

Duplex Kidney

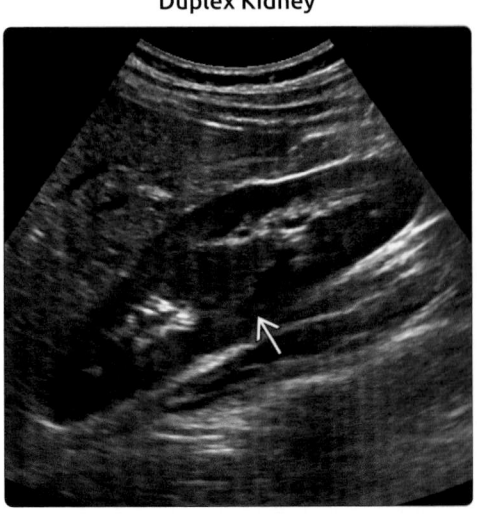

(Left) *Longitudinal ultrasound shows an enlarged kidney measuring 14 cm. The kidney is increased in echogenicity with increased prominence of the pyramids ➜ in this patient with a contralateral, severely hydronephrotic, poorly functioning kidney.* **(Right)** *Longitudinal ultrasound shows a nonobstructed duplex kidney with splitting of central sinus echoes by a hypoechoic band of tissue ➜. Duplex kidneys are normal variants, which are longer than normal kidneys.*

Renal Abscess

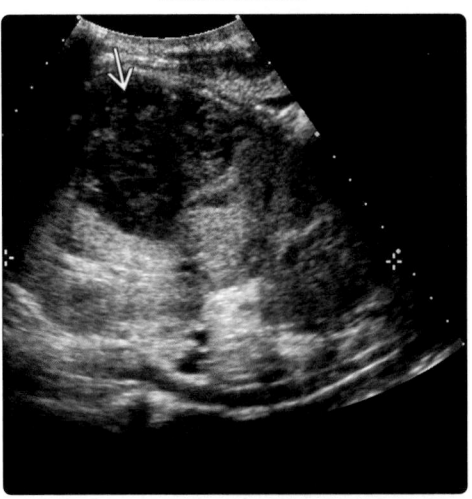

Pyonephrosis

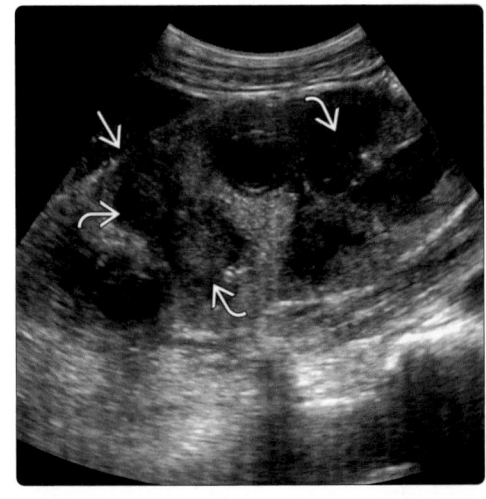

(Left) *Longitudinal ultrasound shows an enlarged (14 cm), hyperechoic kidney in a diabetic patient with fever, flank pain, and positive blood cultures. There is a large renal abscess ➜ with acoustic enhancement.* **(Right)** *Longitudinal ultrasound shows the right kidney in a patient with lupus nephritis, fever, and bacteriuria. There is severe hydronephrosis and cortical thinning ➜. The calyces are filled with low-level echoes representing pus ➜.*

Perinephric Fluid Collections

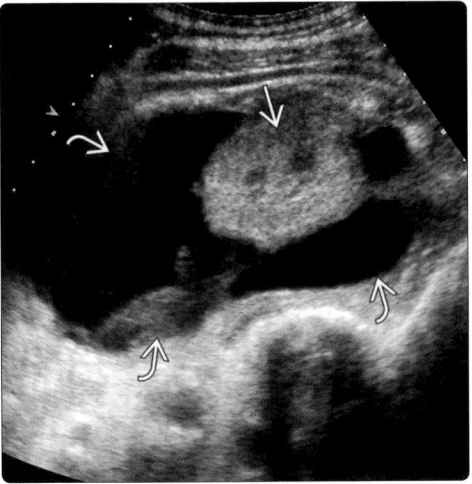

HIV Nephropathy

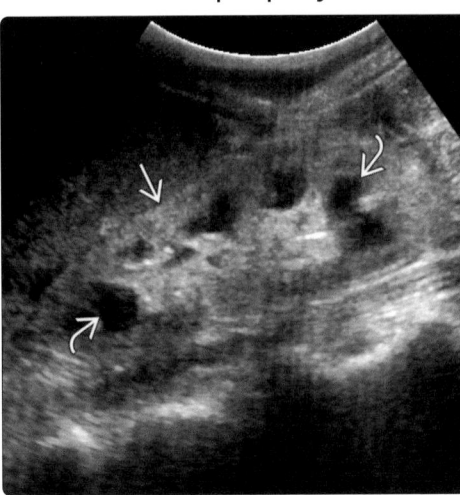

(Left) *Transverse ultrasound shows the right renal lower pole* ➔*, which is surrounded by a perinephric collection* ➔ *containing debris. Differential diagnosis includes hematoma, seroma, urinoma, or lymphocele.* (Right) *Longitudinal ultrasound shows a large right kidney with echogenic cortex* ➔ *and prominent pyramids* ➔ *in a patient with HIV nephropathy. Many pathologic processes cause increased cortical echogenicity.*

Autosomal Dominant Polycystic Kidney Disease (ADPKD)

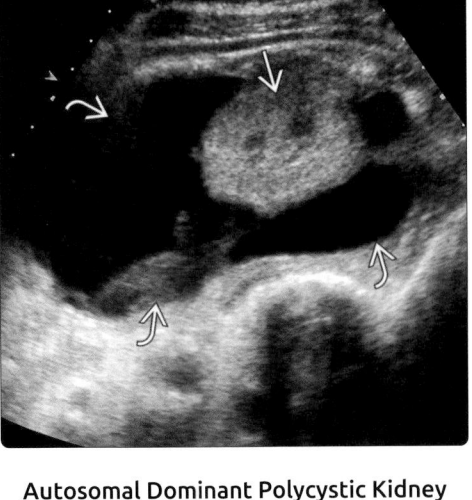

Multicystic Dysplastic Kidney (MDK)

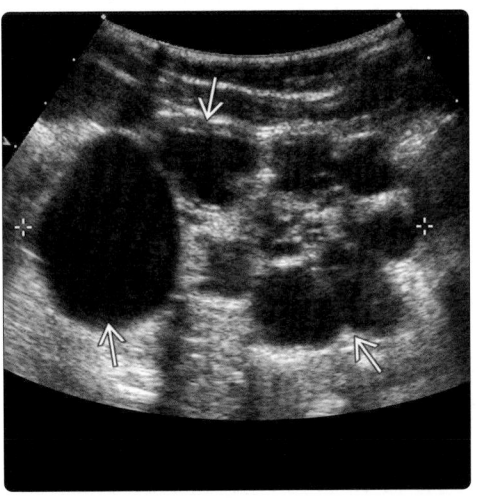

(Left) *Longitudinal ultrasound shows an enlarged left kidney (16 cm) with multiple cysts* ➔ *of varying sizes. There is no normal intervening parenchyma. The right kidney was similar. Liver cysts were also present.* (Right) *Longitudinal ultrasound of an infant with multicystic dysplastic kidney shows an enlarged left kidney with multiple noncommunicating cysts of varying sizes* ➔ *with no normal cortex. This was a nonfunctioning kidney.*

Crossed Fused Renal Ectopia

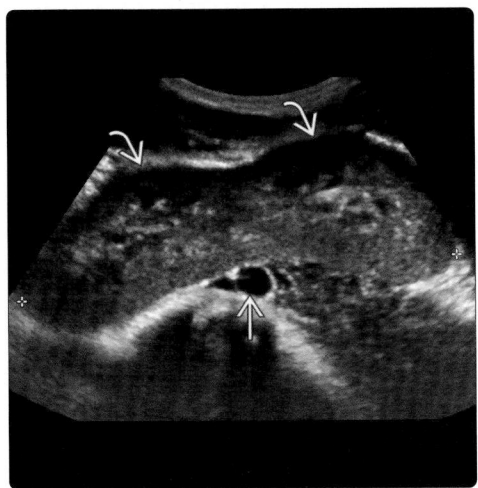

Autosomal Recessive Polycystic Kidney Disease (ARPKD)

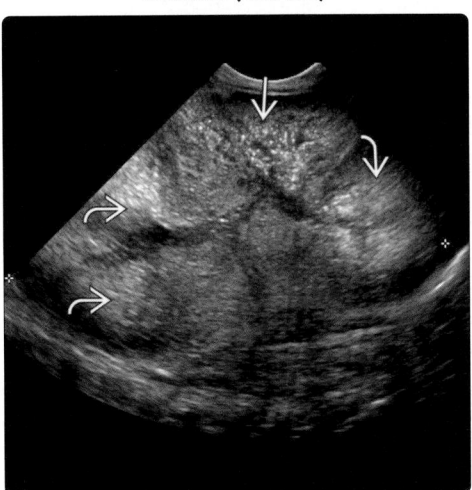

(Left) *Transverse oblique ultrasound shows a crossed fused ectopia with the 2 renal moieties* ➔ *fused in the upper pelvis anterior to the aorta* ➔*.* (Right) *Longitudinal ultrasound of the right kidney in a neonate with abnormal kidneys detected in utero. The kidney is large (10.1 cm) and echogenic with innumerable tiny cysts* ➔*. These produce areas of increased reflectivity* ➔ *when too small to be resolved.*

DIFFERENTIAL DIAGNOSIS

Common

- Chronic Diabetic Nephropathy
- Chronic Glomerulonephritis
- Chronic Hypertensive Nephropathy
- Chronic Lupus Nephritis
- Chronic Reflux Nephropathy
- Postobstructive Atrophy
- Partial Nephrectomy/Post Ablative Therapy/Post Surgery
- Chronic Renal Allograft Rejection/Chronic Allograft Nephropathy

Less Common

- Chronic HIV Nephropathy
- Multicystic Dysplastic Kidney
- Recurrent Infection
- Chronic Renal Artery Stenosis
- Chronic Renal Infarction
- Chronic Vascular Injury
- Post-Traumatic Renal Atrophy
- Following Acute Cortical Necrosis or Acute Tubular Necrosis
- Post Chemotherapy

Rare but Important

- Chronic Radiation Nephropathy
- Chronic Nephritis (Alport Syndrome)
- Renal Cystic Dysplasia
- Medullary cystic disease complex
- Tuberculous Autonephrectomy
- Renal Hypoplasia
- Supernumerary Kidney
- Chronic Lead Poisoning

ESSENTIAL INFORMATION

Key Differential Diagnosis Issues

- Renal atrophy is end result of many pathologic processes
- Causes of loss of renal parenchyma include
  - Acquired: Infection, inflammation, obstruction, reflux, trauma, necrosis/ischemia, fibrosis, surgical intervention
  - Congenital: Hypoplasia, dysplasia
- Ultrasound findings are not specific for cause
- Renal size and cortical thickness are useful in differentiating acute from chronic kidney disease
- Determine if abnormality is unilateral or bilateral, global or focal/multifocal
- Hydronephrosis suggests ureteral obstruction or vesicoureteral reflux
- Renal echogenicity is variable but commonly increased in medical renal renal disease
- Usually not possible to determine cause of small echogenic scarred kidney
- Clinical history is essential for diagnosis
- Biopsy usually not indicated if kidneys are small

Helpful Clues for Common Diagnoses

- **Chronic Diabetic Nephropathy**
  - Small kidneys + ↑ cortical echogenicity
  - Corticomedullary differentiation (CMD) usually preserved, unless patient is in overt renal failure

- **Chronic Glomerulonephritis**
  - Small kidneys + smooth renal outline
  - Parenchyma remains echogenic
- **Chronic Hypertensive Nephropathy**
  - Due to progressive nephrosclerosis
  - Small kidneys + irregular cortical thinning
  - ↓ cortical vascularity due to arteriolar fibrosis and hyaline degeneration
- **Chronic Lupus Nephritis**
  - Small kidneys
  - Variable renal echogenicity and CMD
- **Chronic Reflux Nephropathy**
  - Unilateral or bilateral vesicoureteral reflux in childhood
  - May cause focal/diffuse renal scarring and atrophy
  - Cortical scars are common in upper and lower pole
  - Dilated calyces next to scar suggest diagnosis
  - Calyces and pelvis may be dilated initially but shrink as kidney atrophies
  - Focal areas of compensatory hypertrophy seen adjacent to cortical scars
  - Small kidneys + irregular renal outline
- **Postobstructive Atrophy**
  - Caused by longstanding ureteropelvic junction (UPJ), ureteric, or bladder outlet obstruction
  - Results in progressive decrease in renal blood flow and glomerular filtration
  - Small kidney with cortical thinning and variable hydronephrosis
- **Partial Nephrectomy/Post Ablative Therapy/Post Surgery**
  - Small residual kidney with preserved CMD
  - Compensatory hypertrophy of contralateral kidney may be evident
  - History is essential
- **Chronic Renal Allograft Rejection/Chronic Allograft Nephropathy**
  - Irreversible cause of renal allograft dysfunction
  - Small transplant kidney with cortical thinning and increased cortical echogenicity
  - Decreased color Doppler flow
  - Decreased arterial diastolic flow

Helpful Clues for Less Common Diagnoses

- **Chronic HIV Nephropathy**
  - Normal or enlarged kidneys becoming small with progressive renal failure
  - Increased cortical echogenicity, loss of CMD and sinus fat
  - Thickened urothelium
- **Multicystic Dysplastic Kidney**
  - Initially unilateral enlarged kidney replaced by noncommunicating cysts of varying sizes
  - Undergoes partial or complete involution in infancy
  - Later appears small and echogenic kidney ± cysts
  - Contralateral diseases common such as vesicoureteric reflux, UPJ obstruction, and ureteric stenosis
- **Recurrent Infection**
  - Risk factors: Calculi, urinary tract obstruction, neurogenic bladder, and urinary diversion
  - Small kidney, parenchymal scarring
  - Focal cortical thinning causing irregular outline

- o Pseudotumors from adjacent hypertrophy
- **Chronic Renal Artery Stenosis**
  - o Mostly atherosclerosis affects main, interlobar, or interlobular renal arteries or arterioles
  - o Progressive generalized reduction in kidney size caused by ischemia
  - o Produces renal atrophy or collateralization
  - o Smooth contour
- **Chronic Renal Infarction**
  - o Renal atrophy after acute renal infarction caused by embolism or thrombosis
  - o Atrophy may be focal (segmental) or global
  - o Parenchymal loss depends on distribution of occluded artery
  - o Infarcted area may be contracted, producing renal scar
  - o More common in transplanted than native kidneys
- **Chronic Vascular Injury**
  - o Sequela of vasculitides such as polyarteritis nodosa or ischemia from fibromuscular dysplasia
  - o End result of nonspecific small echogenic kidneys
- **Post-Traumatic Renal Atrophy**
  - o Caused by segmental renal infarction due to renal artery thrombosis after blunt renal trauma or after embolization for bleeding
  - o Contracted kidney + irregular outline
  - o Collateralization may be demonstrated
- **Following Acute Cortical Necrosis or Acute Tubular Necrosis**
  - o May be associated with cortical or medullary calcification
- **Post Chemotherapy**
  - o Scarring after therapy for renal lymphoma, leukemia, or metastases

Helpful Clues for Rare Diagnoses

- **Chronic Radiation Nephropathy**
  - o Occurs after renal irradiation for bone marrow transplantation
  - o Begins months to years after irradiation
  - o Areas of diminished perfusion may be seen
  - o Small kidneys with increased renal echogenicity

- **Chronic Nephritis (Alport Syndrome)**
  - o Chronic hereditary nephritis
  - o Small kidneys + smooth renal outline
  - o ↑ cortical echogenicity due to cortical nephrocalcinosis
- **Renal Cystic Dysplasia**
  - o May be bilateral
  - o Associated with posterior urethral valve, renal duplication, crossed-fused ectopia, horseshoe and pelvic kidneys
  - o Unilateral small kidney with increased echogenicity and small cortical cysts
- **Medullary Cystic Disease Complex**
  - o Inherited cystic renal disease
  - o Progressive tubular atrophy with glomerulosclerosis
  - o Echogenic kidneys with progressive decrease in size
  - o Multiple small medullary cysts
- **Tuberculous Autonephrectomy**
  - o Calcified caseous pyonephrosis with UPJ fibrosis
  - o Shrunken kidney + extensive calcification
  - o Dilated calyces
- **Renal Hypoplasia**
  - o At least 50% smaller than normal
  - o Has fewer calyces and papillae
  - o Renal function normal for its size
  - o Usually unilateral
  - o Differentiation from obstruction, chronic pyelonephritis, and ischemia difficult
- **Supernumerary Kidney**
  - o Extremely rare, hypoplastic 3rd kidney
  - o Connected to dominant kidney either completely or by loose areolar connective tissue
  - o Most are caudal to orthotopic kidney
- **Chronic Lead Poisoning**
  - o Bilateral small kidneys
  - o Indistinguishable sonographically from other causes of renal atrophy
  - o Blood level of lead useful for diagnosis

Chronic Diabetic Nephropathy

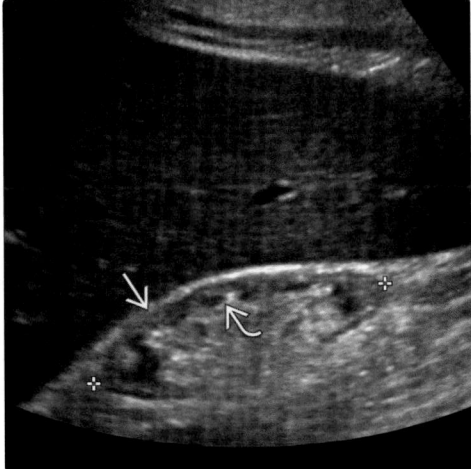

Chronic Glomerulonephritis

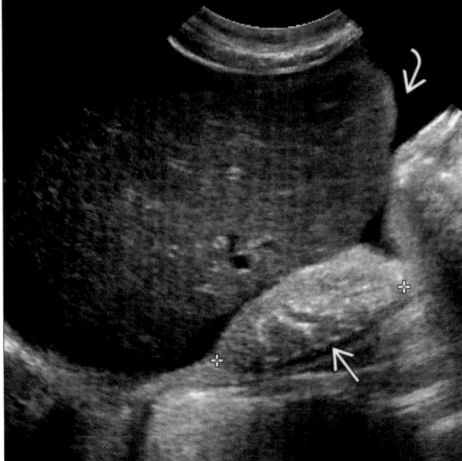

(Left) Longitudinal ultrasound of the right kidney in end-stage renal disease and diabetes. There is diffuse cortical thinning ➜ with increased echogenicity and preserved corticomedullary differentiation ➡. (Right) Longitudinal ultrasound of the right kidney in end-stage renal disease and cirrhosis. The kidney ➜ is small (8 cm) with increased echogenicity and loss of corticomedullary differentiation. Ascites and nodular liver contour ➡ is present.

Chronic Hypertensive Nephropathy

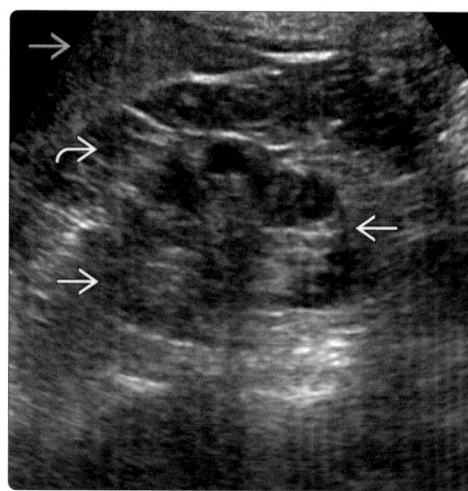

Chronic Reflux Nephropathy

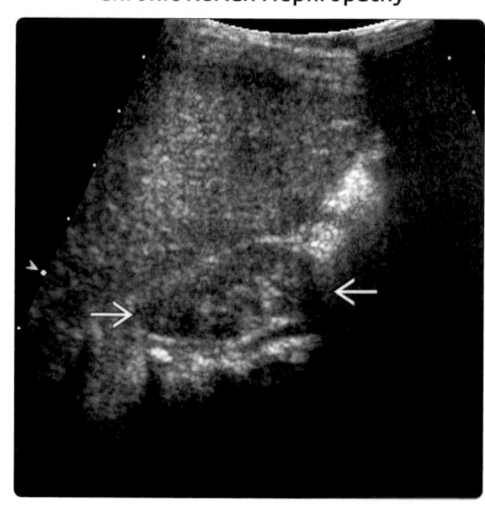

(Left) *Longitudinal ultrasound of the right kidney in end-stage renal disease. The kidney ➡ is small and lobulated, a nonspecific appearance, which can be the end result of many disorders. Note the prominent perinephric fat ➡ between the liver ➡ and kidney.* (Right) *Longitudinal ultrasound of the right kidney in a 1 year old with a history of grade III-IV reflux on the right shows an atrophic kidney ➡ with no hydronephrosis. No focal scars were detected.*

Chronic Reflux Nephropathy

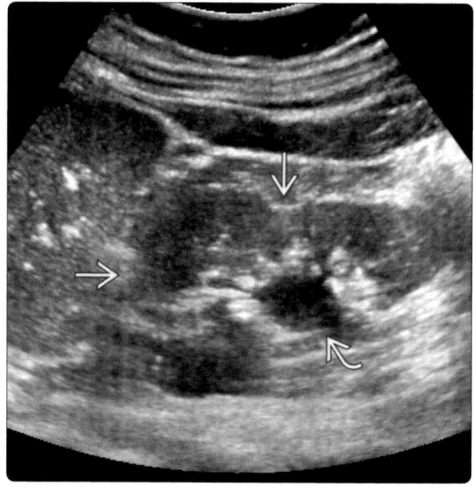

Chronic Reflux Nephropathy

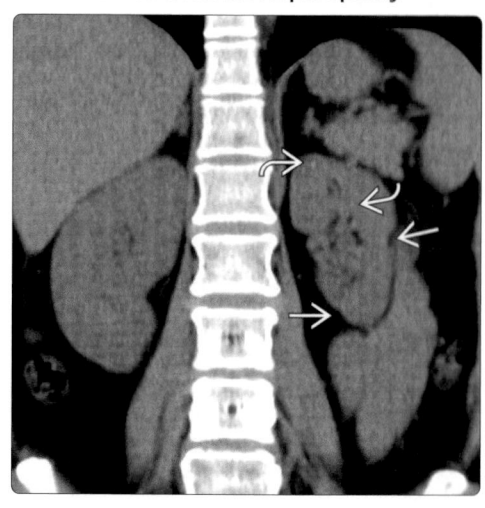

(Left) *Longitudinal ultrasound of the left kidney shows a lobulated contour with cortical loss ➡ in the upper and mid to lower poles. There is mild pelvic dilatation ➡.* (Right) *NECT of the same patient confirms the atrophy of the left kidney with cortical loss ➡. A few tiny calcifications ➡ were noted, not seen on the ultrasound.*

Chronic Reflux Nephropathy

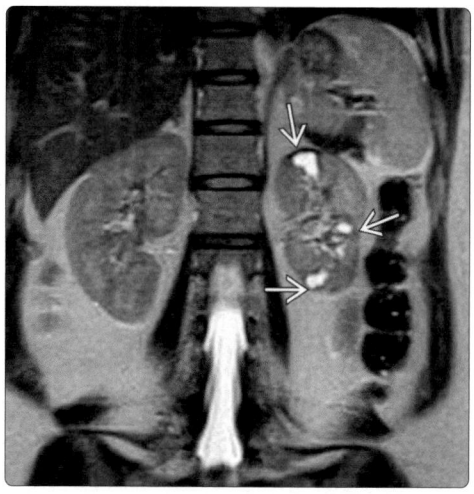

Chronic HIV Nephropathy

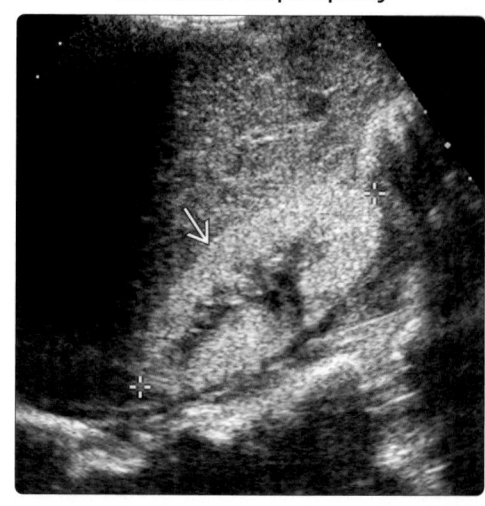

(Left) *T2 HASTE MR of the same patient performed for gallbladder disease shows calyceal dilatation under areas of cortical loss ➡. MR has superior contrast resolution to CT and is less affected by body habitus than ultrasound.* (Right) *Longitudinal ultrasound of the right kidney in a patient with established HIV nephropathy. The renal cortex is markedly echogenic ➡ and small with loss of sinus fat.*

Postobstructive Atrophy

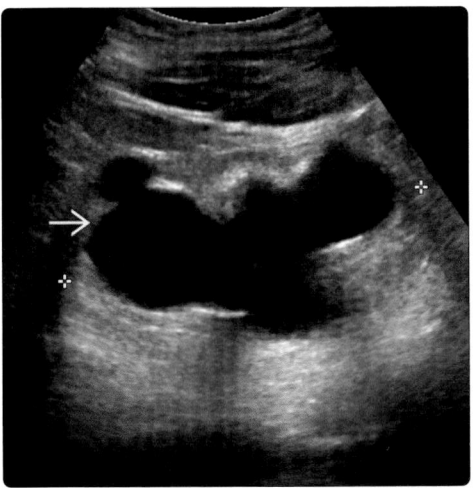

Postobstructive Atrophy

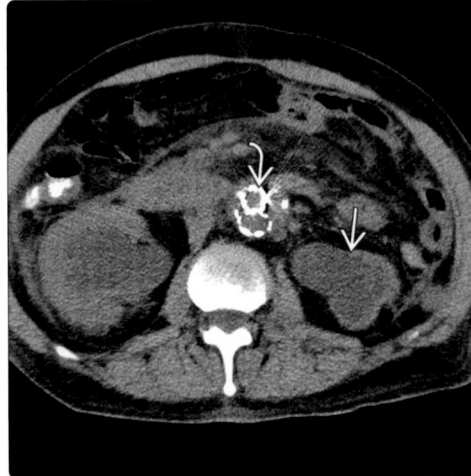

(Left) *Longitudinal ultrasound of the left kidney shows severe hydronephrosis* ➡ *and cortical thinning, which was secondary to chronic ureteral obstruction. However, severe reflux can also produce this appearance.* (Right) *Axial NECT of the same patient shows bilateral hydronephrosis with more atrophy on the left* ➡ *and an aortic stent graft* ➡. *Renal failure precluded the use of intravenous contrast.*

Partial Nephrectomy/Post Ablative Therapy/Post Surgery

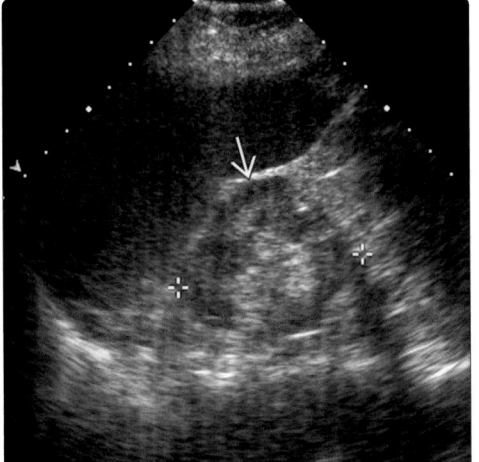

Partial Nephrectomy/Post Ablative Therapy/Post Surgery

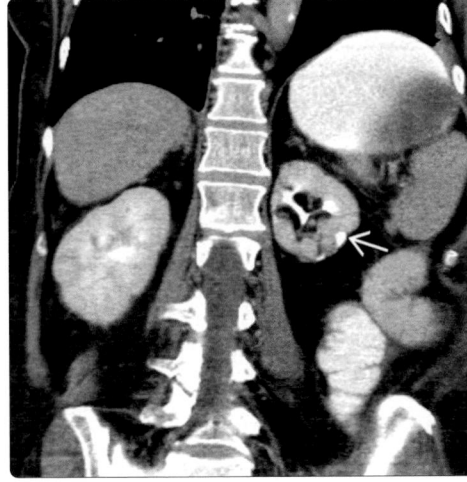

(Left) *Longitudinal ultrasound of a left kidney* ➡ *post partial nephrectomy 20 years prior. The kidney is small (6 cm) with preserved corticomedullary differentiation.* (Right) *CECT of the same patient shows loss of cortex overlying mid pole calyces* ➡ *status post lower pole resection.*

Partial Nephrectomy/Post Ablative Therapy/Post Surgery

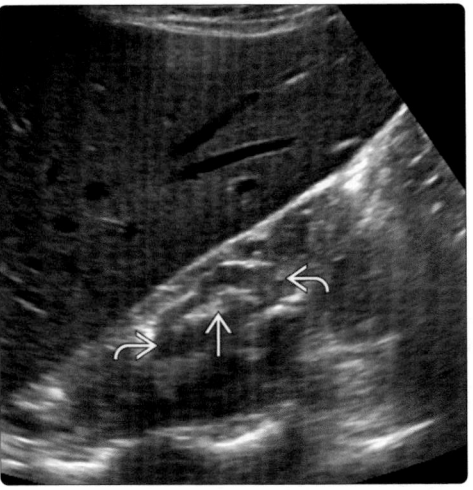

Chronic Renal Infarction

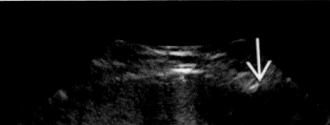
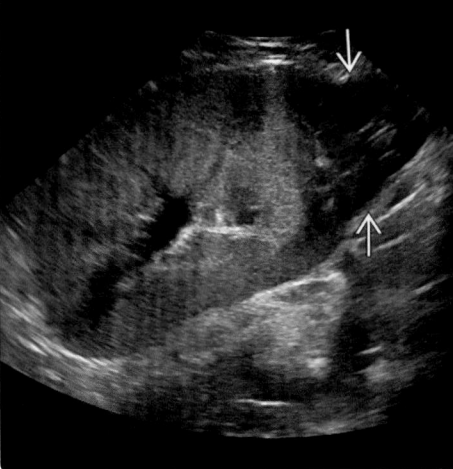

(Left) *Longitudinal ultrasound of the liver and atrophic right kidney in a patient with testicular cancer post retroperitoneal lymph node dissection. The right kidney* ➡ *is very small with global cortical thinning. Renal sinus fat* ➡ *is preserved* (Right) *Longitudinal ultrasound of a renal transplant with scarring of the lower pole* ➡, *a sequela of thrombosis of a lower pole accessory artery.*

DIFFERENTIAL DIAGNOSIS

Common

- Acute Pyelonephritis
- Severe Fatty Liver (Mimic)
- Renal Parenchymal Disease

Less Common

- Perinephric Hematoma or Other Fluid Collection
- Acute Renal Transplant Rejection
- Acute Renal Vein Thrombosis
- Acute Renal Artery Thrombosis
- Renal Cell Carcinoma
- Upper Tract Urothelial Carcinoma
- Multiple Myeloma
- Renal Leukemia
- Renal Lymphoma
- Hypoechoic Renal Fat With Atrophic Kidneys

Rare but Important

- Acute Amyloidosis
- Acute Cortical Necrosis
- Xanthogranulomatous Pyelonephritis

ESSENTIAL INFORMATION

Key Differential Diagnosis Issues

- Determine if there is diffuse hypoechogenicity or focal hypoechoic lesion
  - And if there is distortion of normal architecture by infiltration
- Use color Doppler to look for vascular flow or distortion of normal vessels
- Most commonly related to nonneoplastic conditions
  - Infection
  - Inflammation
  - Vascular thrombosis or arteritis
  - Deposition of abnormal proteins
- Neoplasms
  - Typically of infiltrative type
    - Renal lymphoma, leukemia and multiple myeloma
  - Less commonly renal cell or urothelial carcinoma
    - May be large and infiltrative
    - Tend to be more heterogeneous

Helpful Clues for Common Diagnoses

- **Acute Pyelonephritis**
  - Ascending bacterial infection
  - Manifestations include
    - Diffuse hypoechoic renal parenchyma
    - Focal hypoechoic or hyperechoic round or wedge-shaped lesions
    - May progress to thick-walled abscesses
    - Urothelial thickening
    - Decreased color Doppler flow secondary to vasoconstriction
- **Severe Fatty Liver (Mimic)**
  - Highly attenuating fatty liver may cause spurious decreased echogenicity of kidney
  - Attempt ultrasound imaging directly and posteriorly
- **Renal Parenchymal Disease**
  - Acute forms of glomerulonephritis and lupus nephritis
  - May cause enlarged hypoechoic kidney but typically hyperechoic
  - Diseases affecting tubules and interstitium tend to increase cortical echogenicity

Helpful Clues for Less Common Diagnoses

- **Perinephric Hematoma or Other Fluid Collection**
  - May occur spontaneously in patients with coagulopathy
    - Or after spontaneous forniceal rupture in acute ureteral obstruction
  - Also after trauma, surgery, interventional procedure
  - May compress kidney and cause renal dysfunction
  - Perirenal or subcapsular collection of blood, urine, lymphatic or serous fluid
  - Hematomas have variable echogenicity
  - Other collections are hypoechoic to anechoic
  - Color/power Doppler helpful to identify kidney
- **Acute Renal Transplant Rejection**
  - Swollen and hypoechoic kidney
  - Urothelial thickening
  - Resistive index may be elevated
  - Color perfusion may be decreased
  - Diagnosis requires biopsy
- **Acute Renal Vein Thrombosis**
  - Enlarged and relatively hypoechoic native or transplant kidney
  - Usually segmental or subsegmental venous thrombus
  - Abnormally high resistive index with reversal of arterial flow in diastole
  - Absence of venous flow, complete or partial
  - Secondary to hypercoagulability
    - Direct tumor invasion from renal or adrenal carcinoma
    - Nephrotic syndrome
    - Dehydration and sepsis in children particularly
  - After renal transplantation
    - May be iatrogenic from surgical injury or technical difficulties
    - May be due to fluid collections or compartment syndrome
- **Acute Renal Artery Thrombosis**
  - May affect main or segmental artery of native or transplant renal artery
  - Main renal artery embolism results in swollen kidney with decreased renal echogenicity
  - Absence of color flow may be segmental or total
  - Secondary to dissection, trauma, embolism, hypotension
  - After renal transplantation
    - Etiologic factors as above
    - Additionally associated with severe acute or chronic rejection
- **Renal Cell Carcinoma**
  - Variable size and echogenicity
  - Large tumors tend to be hypoechoic and can be necrotic
  - Smaller tumors are more echogenic
- **Upper Tract Urothelial Carcinoma**
  - Typically soft tissue mass in renal pelvis
  - Causes obstruction, resulting in hydronephrosis
  - Aggressive tumors can diffusely infiltrate kidney with preservation of renal contour

- **Multiple Myeloma**
  - Bilateral nephromegaly
  - Decreased echogenicity
  - Nephrocalcinosis or urate calculi may be present
- **Renal Leukemia**
  - Leukemia may cause diffuse hypoechoic enlargement or focal masses
- **Renal Lymphoma**
  - Hypoechoic enlarged kidneys represent one phenotype of renal lymphoma
  - Associated with lymphadenopathy and perirenal rind
  - Rarely confined to kidneys
- **Hypoechoic Renal Fat With Atrophic Kidneys**
  - Prominent hypoechoic perirenal fat may be mistaken for kidneys when kidneys are atrophic and indistinct

Helpful Clues for Rare Diagnoses

- **Acute Amyloidosis**
  - Uncommon disease
  - Amyloid deposition is common in kidneys, particularly glomeruli
  - Amyloid nephropathy associated with proteinuria and renal insufficiency
  - Enlarged hypoechoic kidney due to deposition of amyloid fibrils
  - Later, kidneys may be echogenic and small
- **Acute Cortical Necrosis**
  - Hypoechoic cortex
  - Loss of corticomedullary differentiation
  - May subsequently become calcified
- **Xanthogranulomatous Pyelonephritis**
  - Enlarged kidney with dilated calyces
  - Staghorn calculus, perinephric collection
  - Hypoechoic/anechoic round collections
  - Chronic obstruction secondary to calculus with infection and development of cystic spaces

SELECTED REFERENCES

1. Hammond NA et al: Imaging of adrenal and renal hemorrhage. Abdom Imaging. ePub, 2015
2. Rodgers SK et al: Ultrasonographic evaluation of the renal transplant. Radiol Clin North Am. 52(6):1307-24, 2014
3. Dedekam E et al: Primary renal lymphoma mimicking a subcapsular hematoma: a case report. J Radiol Case Rep. 7(8):18-26, 2013
4. Bach AG et al: Prevalence and patterns of renal involvement in imaging of malignant lymphoproliferative diseases. Acta Radiol. 53(3):343-8, 2012
5. Herts BR: Renal lymphoma presenting as an incidental renal mass. J Urol. 188(1):271-3, 2012
6. Le O et al: Common and uncommon adult unilateral renal masses other than renal cell carcinoma. Cancer Imaging. 12:194-204, 2012
7. Piscaglia F et al: The EFSUMB Guidelines and Recommendations on the Clinical Practice of Contrast Enhanced Ultrasound (CEUS): update 2011 on non-hepatic applications. Ultraschall Med. 33(1):33-59, 2012
8. Raman SP et al: Beyond renal cell carcinoma: rare and unusual renal masses. Abdom Imaging. 37(5):873-84, 2012
9. Roy A et al: Common and uncommon bilateral adult renal masses. Cancer Imaging. 12:205-11, 2012
10. Smith AD et al: Bosniak category IIF and III cystic renal lesions: outcomes and associations. Radiology. 262(1):152-60, 2012
11. Taneja R et al: Common and less-common renal masses and masslike conditions. Radiol Clin North Am. 50(2):245-57, v-vi, 2012
12. Elsayes KM et al: Imaging of renal transplant: utility and spectrum of diagnostic findings. Curr Probl Diagn Radiol. 40(3):127-39, 2011
13. Israel GM et al: The incidental renal mass. Radiol Clin North Am. 49(2):369-83, 2011
14. Kitazono MT et al: CT of unusual renal masses invading the pelvicaliceal system: potential mimics of upper tract transitional cell carcinoma. Clin Imaging. 35(1):77-80, 2011

Acute Pyelonephritis

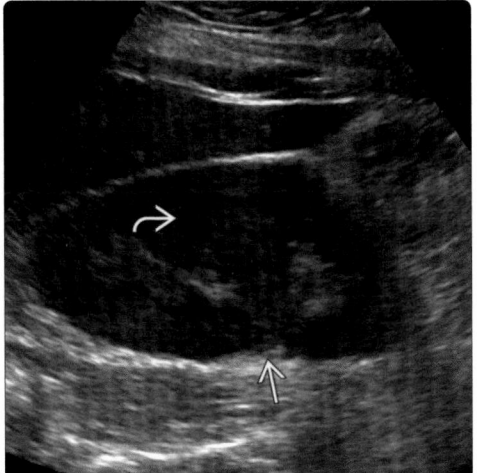

Severe Fatty Liver (Mimic)

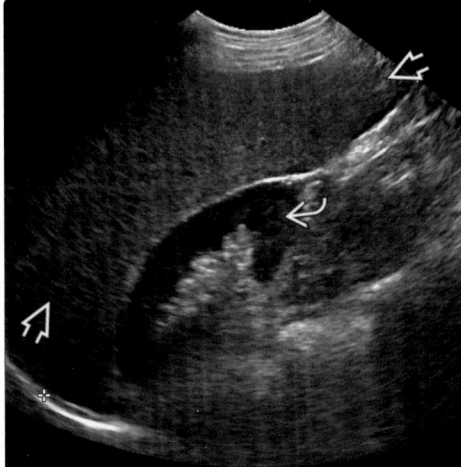

(Left) Longitudinal ultrasound of the right kidney in acute uncomplicated pyelonephritis shows an enlarged hypoechoic kidney ➡ with loss of corticomedullary differentiation ➡. (Right) Longitudinal ultrasound shows a large fatty liver ➡ causing the normal right kidney to appear hypoechoic ➡.

(Left) *Longitudinal ultrasound of the right kidney in a patient with sepsis, liver disease, and acute kidney injury shows loss of corticomedullary differentiation and a perirenal rind of fluid* ➡ *in addition to ascites* ➡. **(Right)** *Longitudinal ultrasound of a renal transplant with delayed graft function from acute tubular necrosis shows loss of corticomedullary differentiation* ➡.

Renal Parenchymal Disease

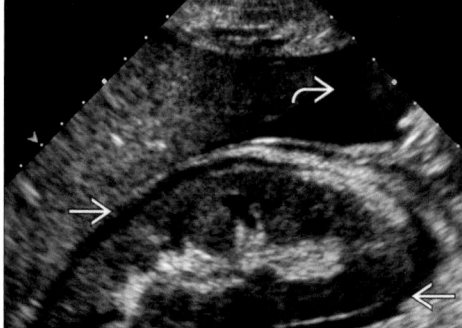

Renal Parenchymal Disease

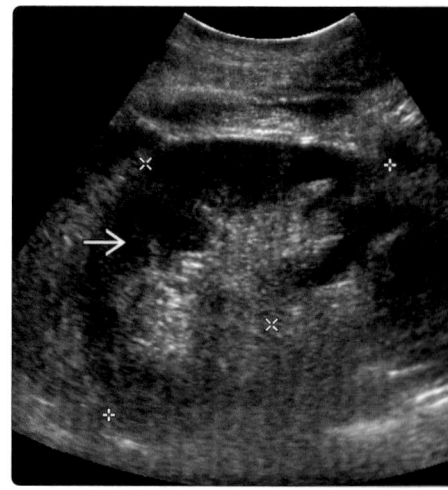

(Left) *Longitudinal ultrasound of the right renal fossa shows a hypoechoic reniform structure* ➡ *with some posterior acoustic enhancement* ➡. *Normal kidney could not be seen.* **(Right)** *Axial T2 HASTE MR in the same patient shows a large subcapsular collection* ➡ *compressing the kidney* ➡. *Drainage of the collection revealed abscess.*

Perinephric Hematoma or Other Fluid Collection

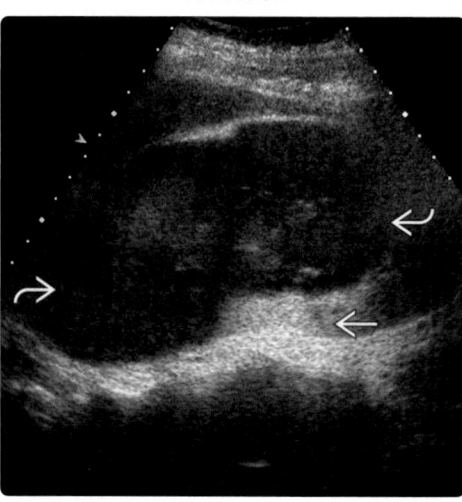

Perinephric Hematoma or Other Fluid Collection

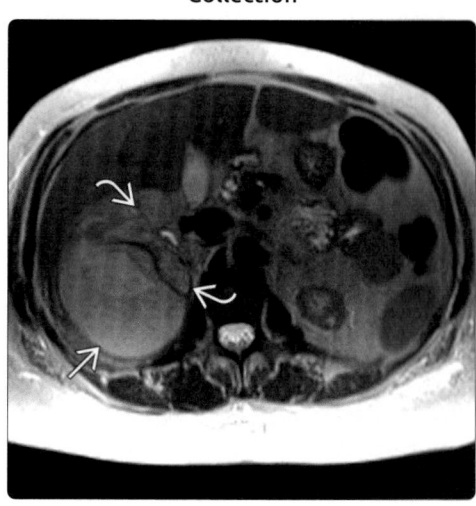

(Left) *Longitudinal ultrasound of a renal transplant with acute renal vein thrombosis shows renal edema* ➡ *and urothelial thickening* ➡. *Percutaneous ultrasound-guided biopsy showed cell-mediated rejection.* **(Right)** *Longitudinal power Doppler ultrasound of a renal transplant shows almost complete absence of intrarenal flow with a patent segmental artery* ➡. *The kidney is swollen and hypoechoic.*

Acute Renal Transplant Rejection

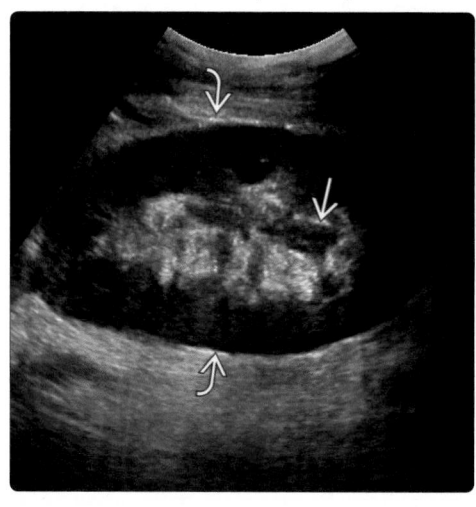

Acute Renal Vein Thrombosis

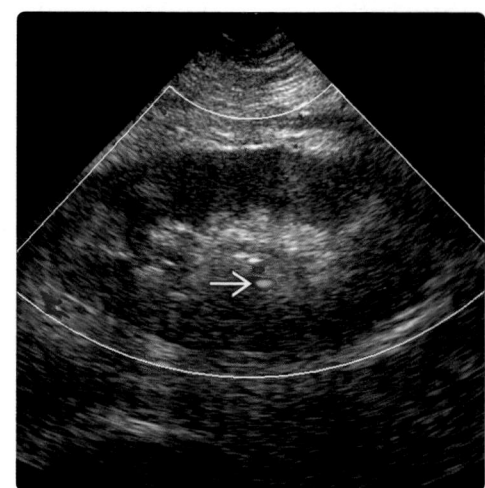

Acute Renal Artery Thrombosis

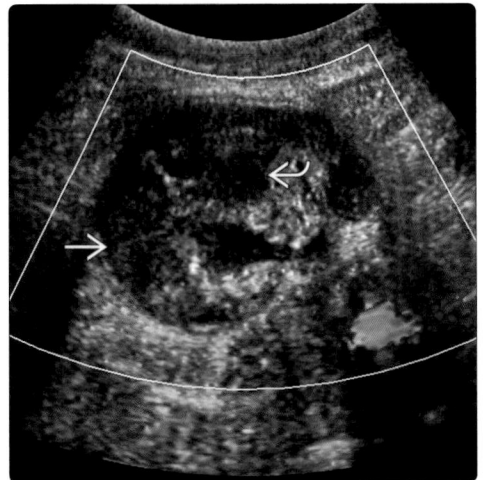

Renal Cell Carcinoma

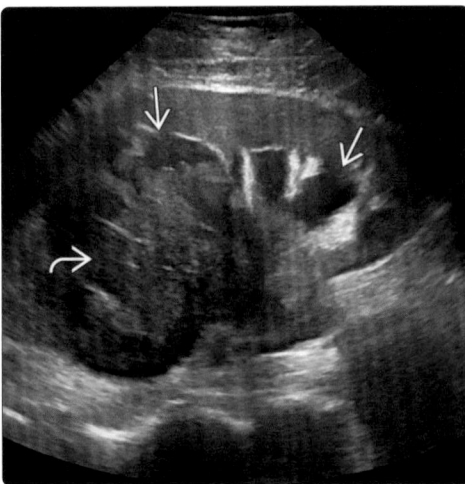

(Left) Transverse color Doppler ultrasound of a renal transplant shows complete absence of intrarenal color flow secondary to renal artery thrombosis. The cortex ➡ and pyramids ➡ are hypoechoic. (Right) Longitudinal ultrasound of the right kidney shows an isoechoic solid mass in the upper to mid pole ➡ extending into the sinus and causing hydronephrosis ➡. Top differential diagnoses are renal cell and urothelial carcinoma. Biopsy showed renal cell carcinoma.

Upper Tract Urothelial Carcinoma

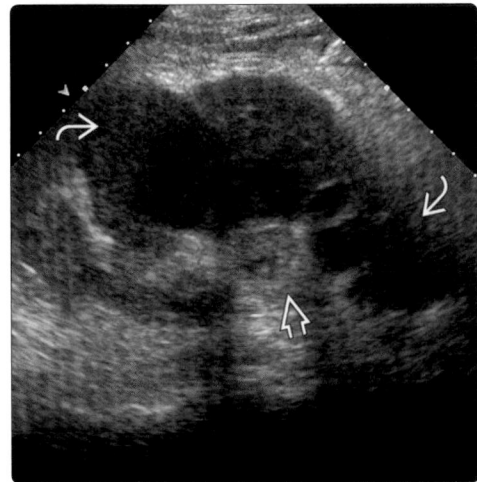

Renal Leukemia

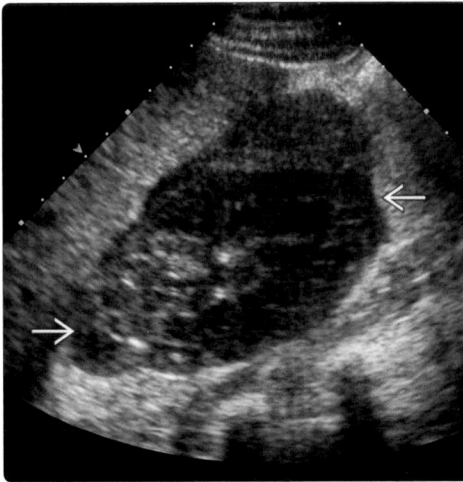

(Left) Longitudinal ultrasound of the left kidney shows hydronephrosis and cortical thinning ➡. The obstruction was caused by a solid mass in the renal pelvis ➡ representing urothelial cancer. (Right) Longitudinal oblique ultrasound shows an enlarged hypoechoic kidney ➡ with loss of corticomedullary differentiation and sinus echogenicity. Biopsy showed acute myeloid leukemia.

Renal Lymphoma

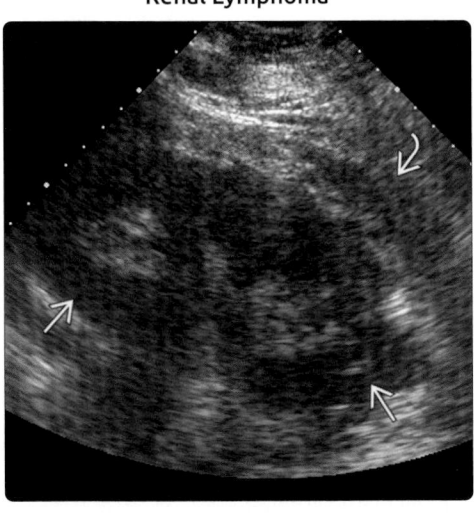

Xanthogranulomatous Pyelonephritis

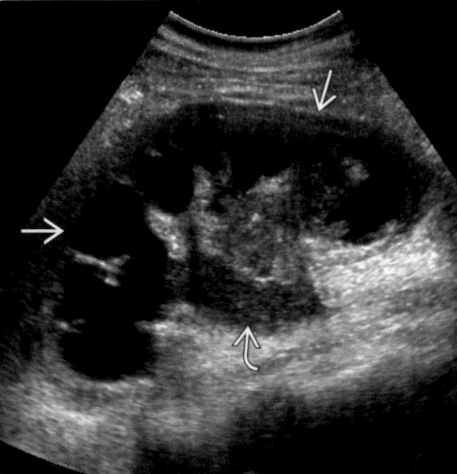

(Left) Longitudinal ultrasound of the left kidney ➡ shows an enlarged (14 cm) hypoechoic kidney secondary to infiltrating lymphoma. Note the perirenal soft tissue rind ➡. (Right) Longitudinal ultrasound of the kidney shows hydronephrosis and cortical atrophy ➡ with avascular soft tissue ➡ in the renal pelvis. There were stones as well. These findings are indistinguishable from pelvic urothelial carcinoma and further evaluation is needed.

DIFFERENTIAL DIAGNOSIS

Common

- Diabetic Nephropathy
- Chronic Glomerular Diseases
- Hypertensive Nephrosclerosis
- Acute Interstitial Nephritis
- Acute Tubular Necrosis
- Medullary Nephrocalcinosis
- Cortical Nephrocalcinosis
- Acute Pyelonephritis
- Reflux Nephropathy

Less Common

- Vasculitis
- Ischemia
- Lupus Nephritis
- Chronic Renal Transplant Rejection/Chronic Allograft Nephropathy
- Sarcoidosis
- Multicystic Dysplastic Kidney
- HIV Nephropathy
- Acute Cortical Necrosis

Rare but Important

- Emphysematous Pyelonephritis
- Autosomal Recessive Polycystic Kidney Disease
- Oxalosis
- Alport Syndrome
- Renal Amyloidosis
- Renal Tuberculosis
- Lithium Nephropathy
- Renal Cystic Dysplasia

ESSENTIAL INFORMATION

Key Differential Diagnosis Issues

- Increased renal echogenicity is most commonly diffuse and secondary to medical renal disease
- Cortical echogenicity greater than liver is abnormal
- Progresses through loss of corticomedullary differentiation (CMD)
- Pyramids may be dark, later bright
- Cortical echogenicity equal to sinus fat is markedly abnormal
- Secondary to multiple diseases
  - Tubular, glomerular or interstitial intrinsic renal disease
  - End result of obstruction, ischemia
  - Calcification: Cortical, medullary, interstitial, vascular
- Increased renal echogenicity indicates abnormal kidneys but not any particular cause
- Echogenicity correlates well with interstitial disease but not with glomerular disease
- Degree of echogenicity correlates poorly with severity of renal impairment
- Renal biopsy indispensable in diagnosis of renal parenchymal disease
- Role of ultrasound
  - Determine renal size and cortical thickness
    - Differentiating acute from chronic renal insufficiency
  - Exclude ureteral obstruction

- Large hyperechoic kidneys: Diabetes, HIV, acute inflammation
- Small hyperechoic kidneys nonspecific
- Differentiate from focal areas of increased echogenicity e.g., medullary, cortical, or lesional

Helpful Clues for Common Diagnoses

- **Diabetic Nephropathy**
  - Single most important cause of renal failure in adults
  - Diabetes involves glomerulus, interstitium and vessels
  - Early: Normal or enlarged kidneys with preserved cortical thickness
  - Chronic: Small echogenic kidney with thin cortex and variable CMD
  - ↑ resistive index (RI) on Doppler studies with ↑ cortical echogenicity
- **Chronic Glomerular Diseases**
  - Multiple pathologic entities and multiple diseases
    - Immunoglobulin A (IgA) disease most common type of idiopathic glomerulonephritis (GN)
    - Focal segmental glomerulosclerosis may be idiopathic or secondary to hypertension or reflux nephropathy
    - Membranous nephropathy most common cause of idiopathic nephrotic syndrome in Caucasians
  - Acute: Normal/enlarged kidney with normal or ↑ renal echogenicity
  - CMD disappears with chronic disease: Small echogenic kidney
- **Hypertensive Nephrosclerosis**
  - 25% of end-stage renal disease
  - Renal echogenicity depends on chronicity
  - ↑ RI with ↑ cortical echogenicity
- **Acute Interstitial Nephritis**
  - Hypersensitivity reaction to drug or infective antigen
  - Mimics acute tubular necrosis clinically
  - Kidney size may be normal or enlarged
  - Cortical echogenicity may be increased depending on severity of reaction
- **Acute Tubular Necrosis**
  - May be normal or increased in echogenicity
- **Medullary Nephrocalcinosis**
  - Cause: Hyperparathyroidism, renal tubular acidosis, medullary sponge kidney, vitamin D excess, gout, sarcoidosis, bone metastases
  - ↑ echogenicity of renal medullae compared to hypoechoic cortex, reversal of normal
  - Acoustic shadowing
- **Cortical Nephrocalcinosis**
  - Focal: Caused by trauma, infarction, or infection
  - Diffuse: Due to renal cortical necrosis, kidney transplant rejection, chronic GN, Alport syndrome
  - Characterized by peripheral parenchymal calcifications and ↑ cortical echogenicity
- **Acute Pyelonephritis**
  - Normal/swollen kidney with typically decreased echogenicity and loss of normal CMD
  - Focal areas of increased echogenicity may be seen but more commonly hypoechoic
  - Thickened urothelium and mild hydronephrosis
- **Reflux Nephropathy**
  - Secondary to interstitial nephritis caused by reflux

o Echogenic cortex, dilated calyces with overlying cortical scarring

Helpful Clues for Less Common Diagnoses

- **Vasculitis**
  o Polyarteritis nodosa, Wegener granulomatosis
  o Small kidneys with ↑ cortical echogenicity
  o May have focal scarring and fibrosis
- **Ischemia**
  o Renal artery stenosis or fibromuscular dysplasia
    - Low intrarenal RI, tardus parvus waveform
  o Renal vein thrombosis
    - Absent venous flow, reversal of arterial diastolic flow
  o Renal artery thrombosis
    - Global or segmental loss of arterial flow
  o Asymmetrical, initially enlarged and hypoechoic
  o Later, small and hyperechoic with global decreased perfusion
  o May have segmental wedge-shaped areas of scarring and decreased perfusion
- **Lupus Nephritis**
  o Acute: Renal echogenicity and size are nonspecific
  o Chronic: Small and echogenic kidney
- **Chronic Renal Transplant Rejection/Chronic Allograft Nephropathy**
  o End result of rejection and other insults
  o Occurs months to years after transplantation
  o Results in interstitial fibrosis
  o Echogenic kidney with decrease in size and perfusion ± calcifications
- **Multicystic Dysplastic Kidney**
  o Initially unilateral multicystic lesion with hyperechoic dysplastic renal parenchyma
  o Later cysts shrink and parenchyma remains echogenic
- **HIV Nephropathy**
  o Occurs almost exclusively in African American descent
  o Present with nephrotic syndrome and may progress rapidly to end-stage renal disease
  o Typically **large** echogenic kidneys with preserved CMD
  o Later sinus blends with cortex and kidneys become small

- **Acute Cortical Necrosis**
  o Subcapsular area spared, hypoechoic rim initially
  o Rapid cortical calcification may ensue: Curvilinear/shadowing
  o Diffuse ↑ parenchymal echogenicity

Helpful Clues for Rare Diagnoses

- **Emphysematous Pyelonephritis**
  o Diabetes, immunocompromise, clinical picture of sepsis
  o Gas-forming necrotizing renal infection
  o Diffuse or segmental
  o Bright echoes with posterior dirty shadowing
- **Autosomal Recessive Polycystic Kidney Disease**
  o Detected prenatally by ultrasound
  o Symmetrically enlarged echogenic kidneys
  o Innumerable small cysts
  o Echogenicity increased due to multiple reflections from small cyst walls
- **Oxalosis**
  o Characterized by combined cortical and medullary nephrocalcinosis
  o Hyperechoic kidneys; absent CMD
- **Alport Syndrome**
  o Inherited disease with hematuria, proteinuria, hypertension, and deafness
  o Initially normal kidneys, later small and echogenic
- **Renal Amyloidosis**
  o Enlarged kidneys in acute phase, ↓ cortical echogenicity
  o Chronic: ↓ renal size & ↑ echogenicity
- **Renal Tuberculosis**
  o Chronic parenchymal atrophy, hydronephrosis, calcifications
  o Calcified small kidney "autonephrectomy"
- **Lithium Nephropathy**
  o Innumerable tiny cysts in cortex and medulla of **normal-sized** kidneys
  o Cysts produce bright punctate echoes

Diabetic Nephropathy

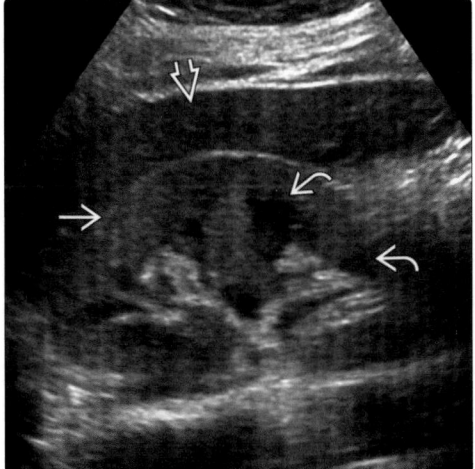

Chronic Glomerular Diseases

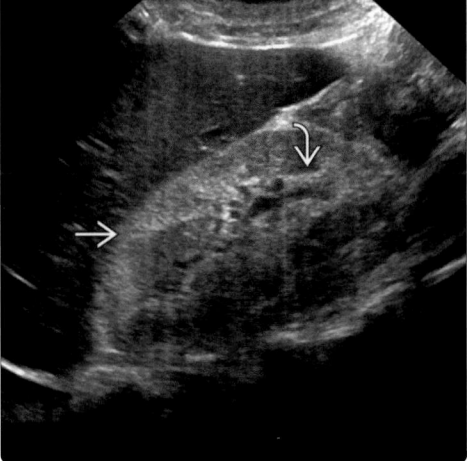

(Left) *Longitudinal ultrasound of a normal-sized right kidney in early chronic kidney disease is shown. The renal cortex ➡ is isoechoic to slightly hyperechoic to the liver ➡. Pyramids ➡ are prominent. These findings are common in medical renal disease and not specific as to cause.* **(Right)** *Longitudinal ultrasound of a normal-sized right kidney with diffuse increase in cortical echogenicity ➡ is shown. Pyramids are not conspicuous. The renal sinus ➡ is barely seen.*

Chronic Glomerular Diseases

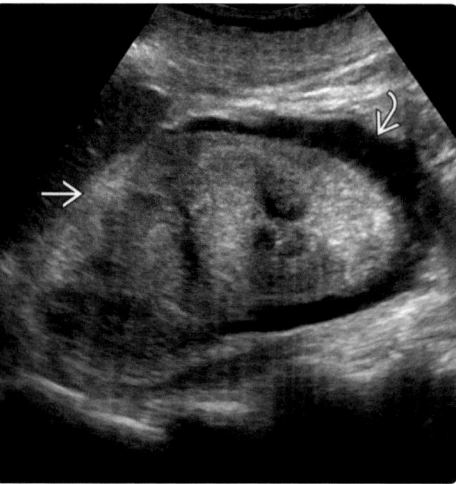

Hypertensive Nephrosclerosis

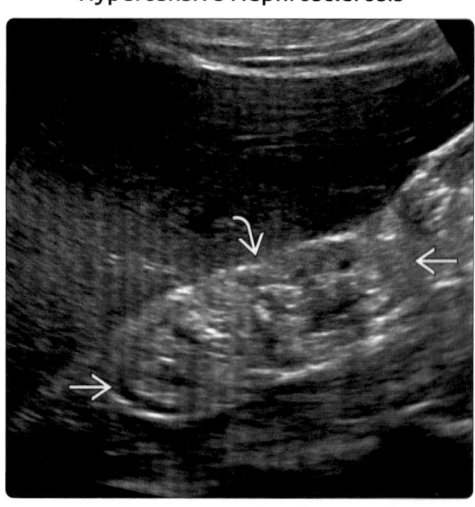

(Left) *Longitudinal ultrasound shows increased cortical and medullary echogenicity* ➡, *equal to sinus fat in an enlarged kidney. There is perinephric fluid* ➡ *in a patient with nephrotic syndrome and HIV. Biopsy showed focal glomerulosclerosis.* (Right) *Longitudinal ultrasound of a small right kidney* ➡ *with diffuse increase in cortical echogenicity is shown. The cortex is thin and slightly lobulated* ➡. *This is compatible with established renal failure.*

Medullary Nephrocalcinosis

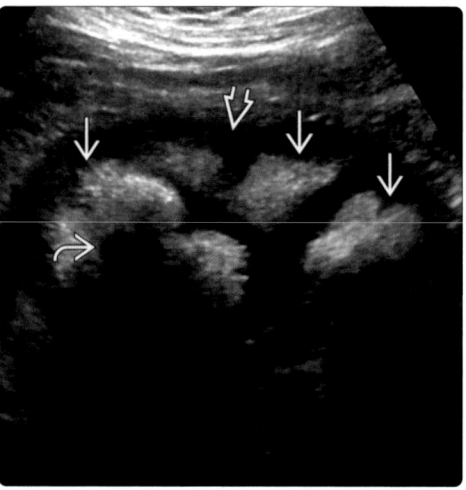

Cortical Nephrocalcinosis

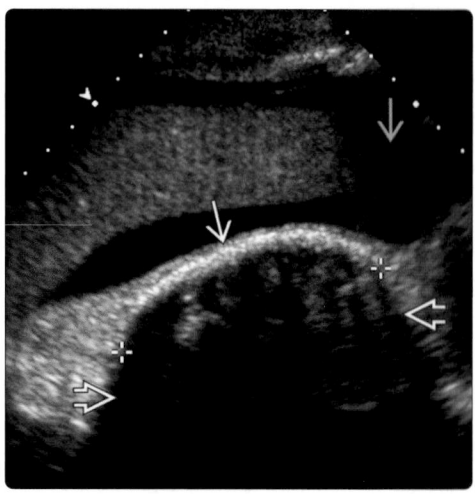

(Left) *Longitudinal ultrasound shows hyperechoic pyramids* ➡ *with some shadowing* ➡. *The cortex* ➡ *is less echogenic than the pyramids in medullary sponge kidney.* (Right) *Longitudinal ultrasound of the right kidney in a patient with end-stage renal failure and ascites* ➡ *is shown. There is calcification of the renal cortex* ➡ *causing significant shadowing* ➡.

Chronic Renal Transplant Rejection/Chronic Allograft Nephropathy

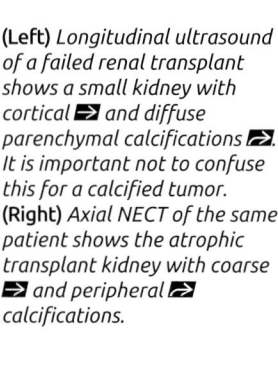

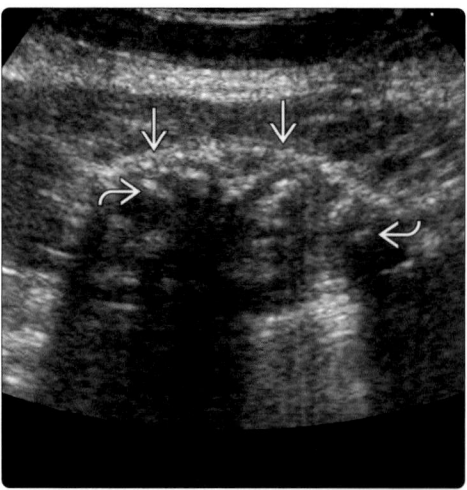

Chronic Renal Transplant Rejection/Chronic Allograft Nephropathy

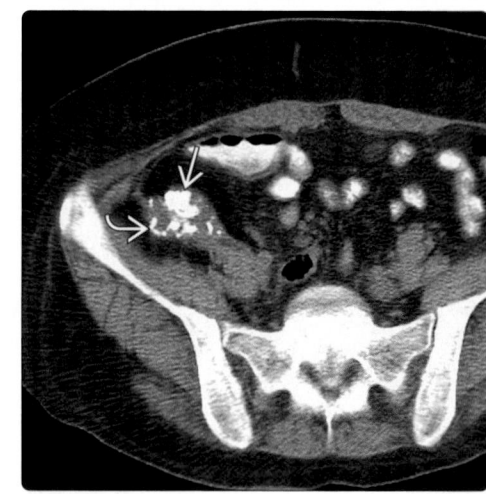

(Left) *Longitudinal ultrasound of a failed renal transplant shows a small kidney with cortical* ➡ *and diffuse parenchymal calcifications* ➡. *It is important not to confuse this for a calcified tumor.* (Right) *Axial NECT of the same patient shows the atrophic transplant kidney with coarse* ➡ *and peripheral* ➡ *calcifications.*

Chronic Glomerular Diseases

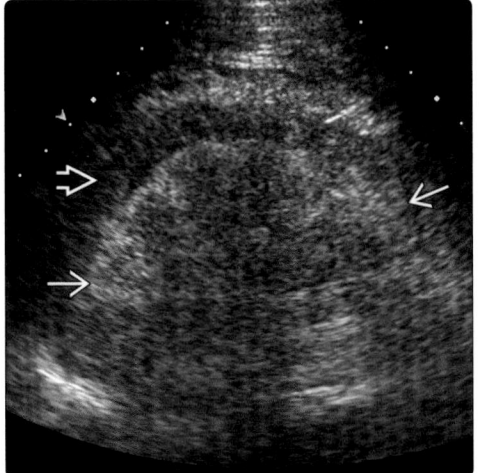

HIV Nephropathy

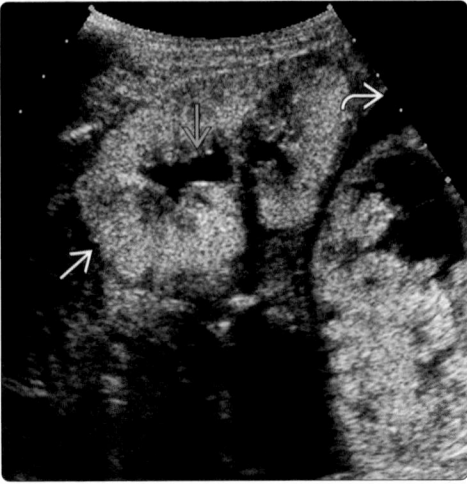

(Left) *Longitudinal ultrasound after biopsy of the kidney is shown. There is a very echogenic kidney* ➡️ *with a hypoechoic perinephric hematoma* ➡️ *which was managed conservatively. Biopsy revealed focal glomerulosclerosis. The noisy image results from diffuse edema/nephrotic syndrome.* (Right) *Longitudinal US of the left kidney in a patient with AIDS & renal failure is shown. The left kidney* ➡️ *is small and markedly increased in echogenicity with pelviectasis* ➡️. *There is a small amount of ascites* ➡️.

Emphysematous Pyelonephritis

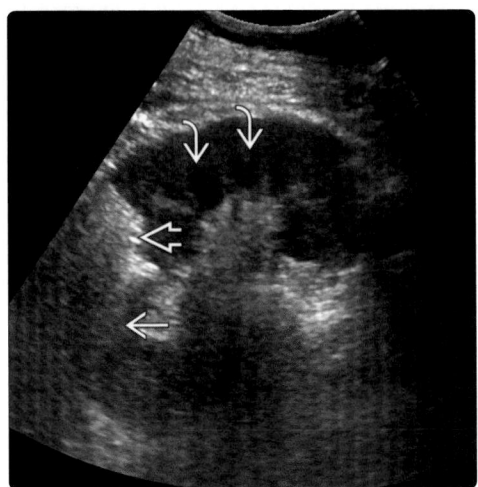

Autosomal Recessive Polycystic Kidney Disease

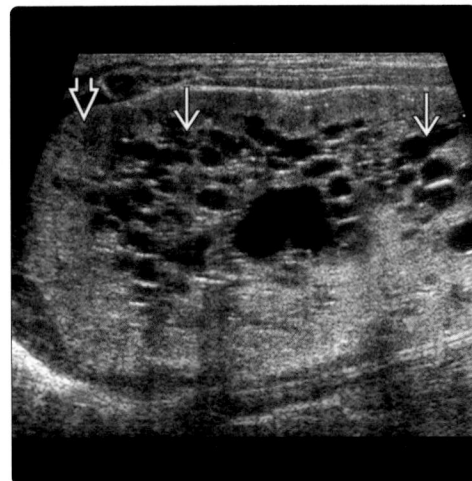

(Left) *Longitudinal ultrasound of a renal transplant shows normal pyramids* ➡️ *in the lower pole. In the upper pole, there is an area of increased echogenicity* ➡️ *with shadowing* ➡️ *representing gas from segmental emphysematous pyelonephritis.* (Right) *Longitudinal ultrasound of the kidney in a neonate shows an enlarged hyperechoic kidney* ➡️ *with innumerable tiny cysts* ➡️. *The other kidney was the same.*

Lithium Nephropathy

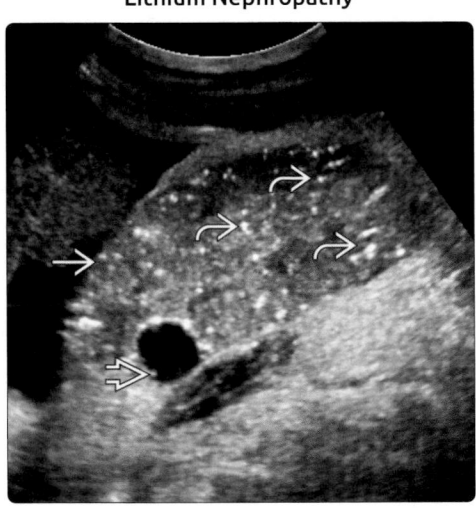

Ischemia

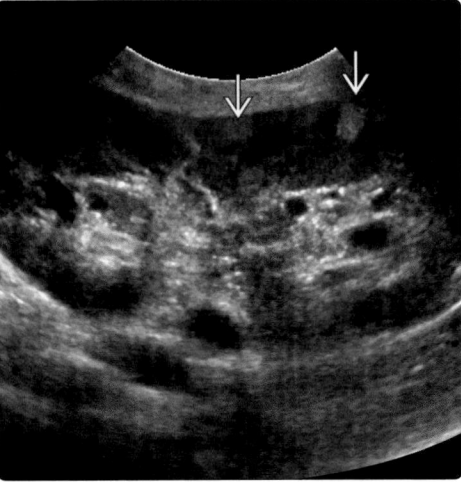

(Left) *Longitudinal ultrasound shows a hyperechoic right kidney* ➡️ *with innumerable tiny echogenic nonshadowing foci* ➡️ *representing microcysts. A larger cyst* ➡️ *was also present.* (Right) *Longitudinal ultrasound of a renal transplant shows hyperechoic wedge-shaped cortical lesions* ➡️. *Multiple cortical infarcts were found on biopsy.*

DIFFERENTIAL DIAGNOSIS

Common

- Simple Renal Cyst
- Complex Cysts: Hemorrhagic, Infected, or Proteinaceous
- Renal Sinus Cysts
- Hydronephrosis
- Cystic Disease of Dialysis
- Autosomal Dominant Polycystic Kidney Disease
- Multicystic Dysplastic Kidney
- Cystic Renal Cell Carcinoma
- Localized Cystic Renal Disease
- Renal Abscess
- Renal Hematoma

Less Common

- Multilocular Cystic Nephroma
- Mixed Epithelial and Stromal Tumor
- Primary Renal Synovial Sarcoma
- Lymphangioma
- Perinephric Collection
- Tuberous Sclerosis
- von Hippel-Lindau Disease
- Arteriovenous Fistula/Malformation; Intrarenal Aneurysm
- Congenital Megacalyces
- Renal Lymphoma or Metastases
- Hydatid Cyst

ESSENTIAL INFORMATION

Key Differential Diagnosis Issues

- Cystic renal masses run the gamut from simple cyst to cystic renal carcinoma
- Simple cysts are benign and require no follow-up
- Ensure that the lesion is truly a simple cyst
- Beware of technical artifacts producing internal echoes within cysts such as
  - Reverberation from skin-transducer interfaces superficial to cyst
  - High gain settings
  - Side lobe artifacts from adjacent tissue
- Posterior acoustic enhancement typically occurs with larger lesions
  - May not be seen if cyst is very small
- Multiple tiny cysts may not be resolved
  - Instead may appear as an echogenic lesion due to multiple reflective surfaces
- Complex cysts may represent complicated benign cysts or cystic neoplasms including renal cell carcinoma
- Therefore, it is imperative to detect features that indicate further imaging or follow-up
  - Look for solid components or mural nodules
  - Evaluate the entire wall of large cysts
  - Evaluate septa
  - CECT: CEMR or CEUS for further evaluation
  - Bosniak classification helps in guiding management
- May difficult to confirm origin of exophytic or large renal cysts
- Cysts in upper pole of kidney may be difficult to differentiate from suprarenal, hepatic (right), or splenic (left) cysts
  - Try to delineate relationship during real-time imaging
- Determine if single cystic lesion or multiple lesions
- Consider syndromes with cysts if multiple bilateral renal cysts in young patients

Helpful Clues for Common Diagnoses

- **Simple Renal Cyst**
  - Extremely common; increases with age
  - Well-defined, round or oval, smooth, and thin walled
  - Entirely echo free with posterior acoustic enhancement
  - No septum or solid component; no color Doppler flow
  - May exert mass effect on calyces if large
  - Location: Renal cortex, deep or superficial
- **Complex Cysts: Hemorrhagic, Infected, or Proteinaceous**
  - Thin, smooth internal septa
  - Internal echoes from hemorrhage, infection, or proteinaceous debris
  - Calcified wall or septa
- **Renal Sinus Cysts**
  - Include peripelvic cysts and lymphangiectasia
  - Located in renal hilum
  - Surround and may compress renal pelvis but do not communicate with collecting system
  - Can mimic hydronephrosis
  - Most are asymptomatic; rarely associated with hematuria or hypertension
- **Hydronephrosis**
  - Dilated calyces connecting to dilated pelvis
  - Use color Doppler to distinguish from prominent vessels
- **Cystic Disease of Dialysis**
  - 3 or more cysts per kidney in patient with chronic kidney disease and no history of hereditary cystic disease
  - May precede dialysis, almost inevitable after long-term dialysis
  - Atrophic echogenic kidneys with loss of corticomedullary differentiation
  - Cysts in both renal cortex and medulla, especially at site of renal scars
  - Renal size may be enlarged due to multiple large cysts
    - May resemble polycystic kidney disease, clinical correlation needed
  - Increased risk of renal cell carcinoma (RCC): 3-7%
- **Autosomal Dominant Polycystic Kidney Disease**
  - Autosomal dominant inheritance, spontaneous mutation in 10%
  - Massively enlarged, echogenic kidneys with lack of corticomedullary differentiation
  - Multiple bilateral cysts of varying size
  - Intracystic hemorrhage/infection/milk of calcium
  - Mural calcification
  - Associated with cysts of other organs: Liver (75%), pancreas (10%), spleen (5%)
- **Multicystic Dysplastic Kidney**
  - Congenital lesion discovered on prenatal ultrasound or incidental finding
  - Multiple noncommunicating cysts of varying size
  - No communication to ureter
  - Usually unilateral, may be complete or segmental

- Associated with contralateral renal abnormalities such as ureteropelvic junction obstruction and vesicoureteric reflux
- **Cystic Renal Cell Carcinoma**
  - 15% of RCC are cystic
  - Unilocular or multilocular unencapsulated cystic lesion
  - Thin and thick septa and solid components
  - ± tumor nodules, ± tumor necrosis
- **Localized Cystic Renal Disease**
  - Cluster of simple cysts, not encapsulated, normal intervening parenchyma
- **Renal Abscess**
  - Thick walled with internal debris and septation
  - Perinephric extension
  - Clinical picture of infection
- **Renal Hematoma**
  - History of trauma, intervention, surgery, bleeding diathesis
  - Spontaneous bleeding from renal mass such as RCC or angiomyolipoma
  - Avascular complex cystic lesion of variable echogenicity in kidney and perinephric space

Helpful Clues for Less Common Diagnoses

- **Multilocular Cystic Nephroma (MLCN)**
  - Encapsulated multilocular cystic lesion
  - Thin and thick septa, lacking solid nodules
  - Classically herniating into renal pelvis or renal vein
  - Unilateral, middle-aged women
- **Mixed Epithelial and Stromal Tumor**
  - Benign tumor of perimenopausal women
  - Similar appearance to MLCN
- **Primary Renal Synovial Sarcoma**
  - Typically solid but may have large cystic components
  - Rare tumor with poor prognosis
- **Lymphangioma**
  - Benign
  - Asymptomatic
  - Unilateral or bilateral renal sinus or perinephric fluid-filled lesions

- Unilocular or multilocular
- **Perinephric Collection**
  - Results from ruptured hydronephrosis or pyonephrosis or ruptured cyst
  - Occasionally direct extension of peritoneal or retroperitoneal infection
  - Fluid collection outside renal parenchyma
    - May cause indentation or distortion of renal contour
- **Tuberous Sclerosis**
  - Autosomal dominant inherited disease with developmental delay, seizures and multiple hamartomas
  - Renal lesions include multiple cysts and angiomyolipomas
  - Risk of renal cell carcinoma not increased but develops at a younger age
- **von Hippel-Lindau Disease**
  - Autosomal dominant disease with multiorgan manifestations
  - Renal lesions include multiple renal cysts and multifocal renal carcinoma (clear cell most common)
- **Arteriovenous Fistula/Malformation; Intrarenal Aneurysm**
  - Tubular, serpiginous fluid filled lesions ± aneurysms ± collateral vessels
  - Use color and spectral Doppler to prove vascular nature
  - Acquired more common than congenital
  - Present with hematuria and flank pain or may be asymptomatic
- **Congenital Megacalyces**
  - Rare nonobstructive enlargement of calyces
  - May be associated with megaureter
  - Usually unilateral
- **Renal Lymphoma or Metastases**
  - Lymphoma may be hypoechoic
  - Metastases may be cystic
  - Diagnosis based on presence of other lesions or biopsy

Simple Renal Cyst

Complex Cysts: Hemorrhagic, Infected, or Proteinaceous

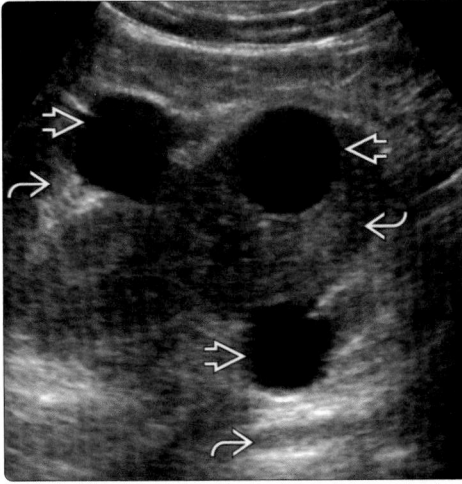 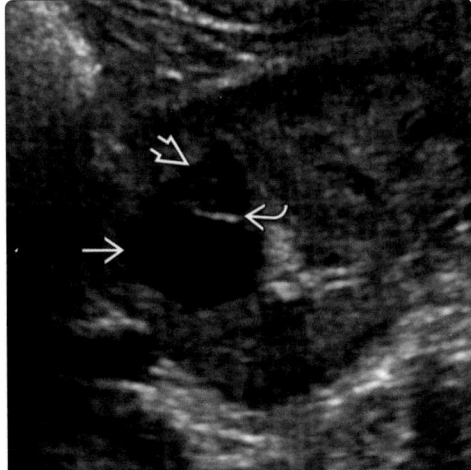

(Left) Transverse oblique ultrasound shows multiple simple renal cortical cysts ➡. Two are exophytic. All cysts are round, thin walled, anechoic with posterior acoustic enhancement ➡. (Right) Longitudinal ultrasound of a renal transplant is shown. The cyst ➡ in the upper pole is complex because there is a thin septum ➡ with low-level echoes ➡ in the anterior component. This requires further evaluation with color Doppler and contrast-enhanced CT, MR, or ultrasound.

Complex Cysts: Hemorrhagic, Infected, or Proteinaceous

Complex Cysts: Hemorrhagic, Infected, or Proteinaceous

(Left) *Longitudinal color Doppler ultrasound of the kidney demonstrates an exophytic cortical lesion* ➡, *apparently solid but with no internal color flow. Further evaluation with MR showed that this was a hemorrhagic cyst.* **(Right)** *Longitudinal ultrasound of the right kidney shows a cyst* ➡ *with dependent highly echogenic milk of calcium* ➡. *The layer moved on repositioning the patient.*

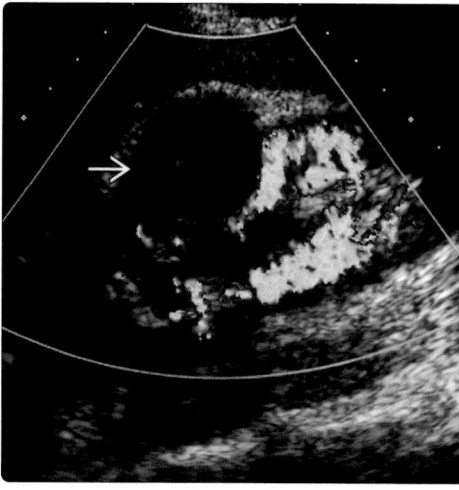

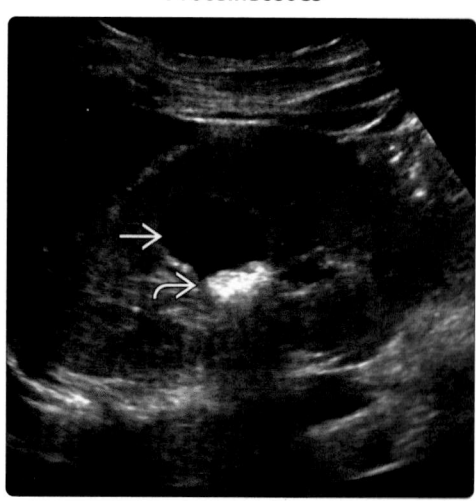

Renal Sinus Cysts

Hydronephrosis

(Left) *Transverse ultrasound shows a multiseptated, fluid-filled lesion* ➡ *in the renal sinus. It may be difficult to distinguish from hydronephrosis if the calyces appear dilated; however, enhanced CT or MR can be definitive.* **(Right)** *Longitudinal ultrasound of the kidney shows an exophytic lower pole cyst* ➡, *which did not communicate with the moderate hydronephrosis* ➡.

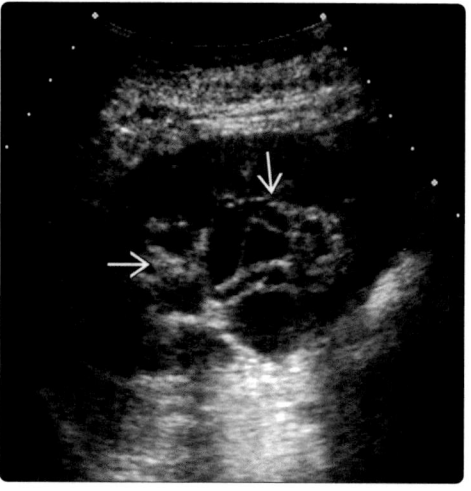

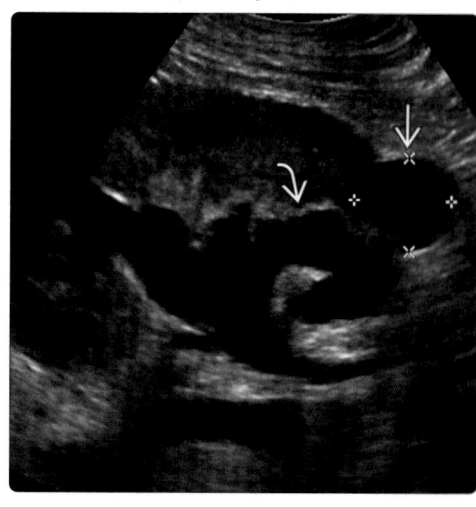

Cystic Disease of Dialysis

Autosomal Dominant Polycystic Kidney Disease

(Left) *Longitudinal ultrasound of the right kidney shows a small right kidney with multiple cysts of various sizes* ➡ *in a patient on dialysis. Ascites is present* ➡. **(Right)** *Longitudinal ultrasound of the right abdomen shows a large kidney with multiple cysts* ➡ *abutting the upper pole of a renal transplant* ➡. *Cysts* ➡ *were also present in the enlarged liver.*

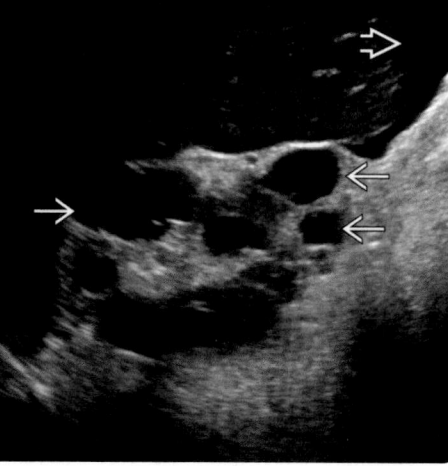

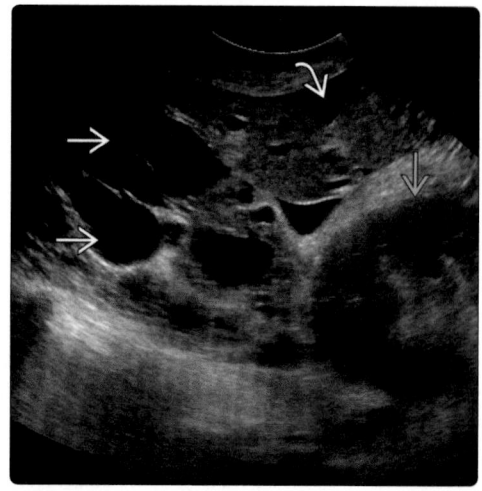

Multicystic Dysplastic Kidney

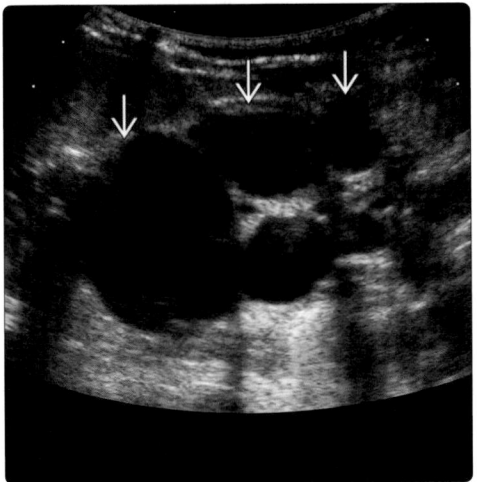

Cystic Renal Cell Carcinoma

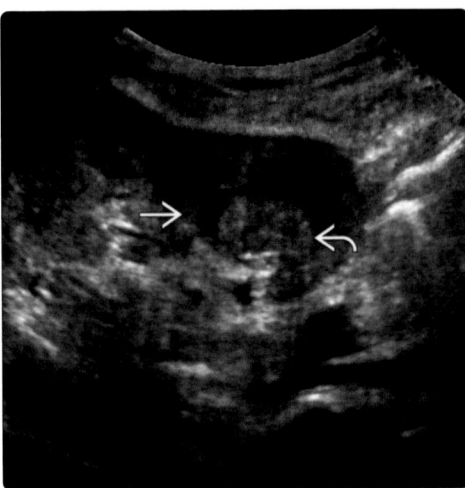

(Left) *Longitudinal ultrasound of the kidney in an infant shows multiple noncommunicating cysts* ➡ *with no normal intervening parenchyma.* **(Right)** *Longitudinal ultrasound of a failing renal transplant is shown. A thick-walled cystic lesion* ➡ *in the lower pole contains a solid nodule* ➡ *with internal color Doppler flow (not shown). Enhanced CT confirmed that this was enhancing and nephrectomy was performed.*

Renal Abscess

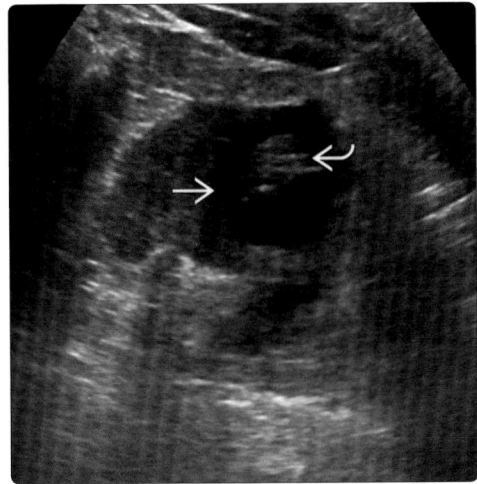

von Hippel-Lindau Disease

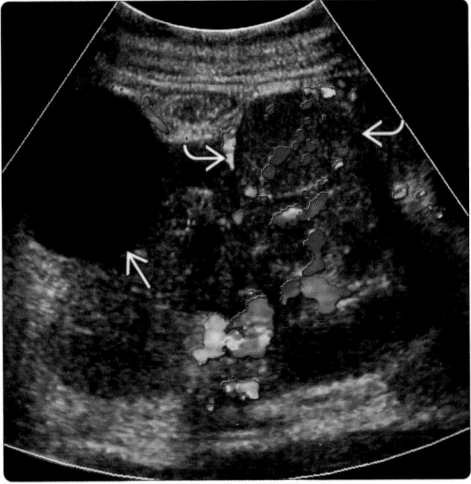

(Left) *Transverse ultrasound of the left kidney in a patient with fever, chills and bacteruria is shown. A cystic lesion* ➡ *with internal debris* ➡ *represents an abscess. Knowledge of the clinical picture is essential for diagnosis.* **(Right)** *Longitudinal ultrasound shows an exophytic upper pole simple cyst* ➡ *and a mid pole exophytic renal carcinoma* ➡ *with internal color Doppler flow.*

Arteriovenous Fistula/Malformation; Intrarenal Aneurysm

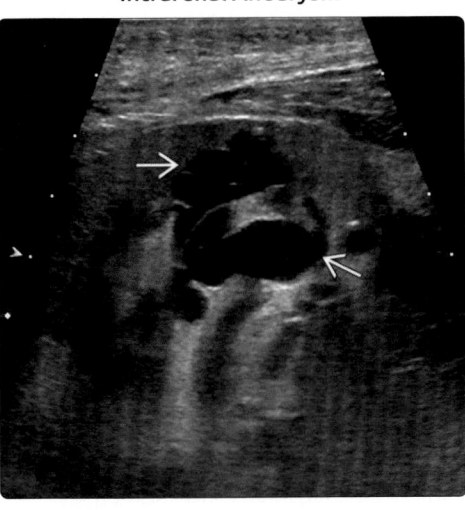

Arteriovenous Fistula/Malformation; Intrarenal Aneurysm

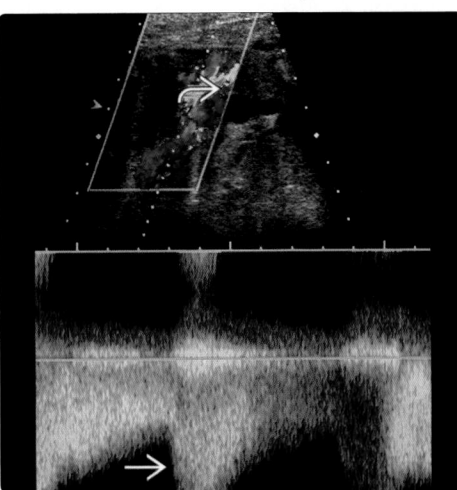

(Left) *Transverse ultrasound of a renal transplant shows a tubular, serpiginous, fluid-filled structure* ➡ *extending from sinus to cortex representing a large, post-biopsy arteriovenous fistula. Color Doppler should be used to evaluate all cystic lesions.* **(Right)** *Transverse Doppler ultrasound of the same patient shows high-velocity turbulent flow* ➡ *in the arteriovenous fistula* ➡.

DIFFERENTIAL DIAGNOSIS

Common

- Renal Cell Carcinoma
- Renal Angiomyolipoma
- Upper Tract Urothelial Cancer
- Renal Pseudotumor
  - Column of Bertin
  - Dromedary Hump
  - Focal Hypertrophy
- Focal Pyelonephritis
- Horseshoe Kidney
- Crossed Fused Ectopia
- Renal Lymphoma
- Renal Leukemia and Myeloma
- Renal Metastases
- Other Renal Tumors
  - e.g., Oncocytoma
- Wilms Tumor

Less Common

- Xanthogranulomatous Pyelonephritis (XGP)
- Renal Sinus/Replacement Lipomatosis
- Renal Tuberculosis
- Renal Papillary Necrosis

ESSENTIAL INFORMATION

Key Differential Diagnosis Issues

- Major role of grayscale US is to characterize simple cysts
- For noncystic lesions, evaluate margin and echogenicity
- Highly echogenic shadowing lesions suggestive of fat
  - Also consider calcification or gas
- Solid lesions should be carefully evaluated for intrinsic blood flow
- Use color or power Doppler for internal vascular flow
  - Color flow in solid areas, septa, nodules, or debris
  - Presence of internal flow highly suspicious for malignancy
- CECT or CEMR usually next line for solid renal mass characterization and staging
- Contrast-enhanced ultrasound increases sensitivity for tumor perfusion
  - Complementary to enhanced CT or MR
  - Substitute for CT and MR when patient cannot receive iodinated or gadolinium-based contrast
- Look for other lesions ipsilateral and contralateral
- Beware of pseudotumors
  - Pseudotumors are isoechoic to normal parenchyma and have normal kidney architecture
  - Pseudotumors are identical to normal kidney on CT and MR before and after contrast
- Look for signs of malignancy
  - Renal vein invasion, inferior vena cava (IVC) tumor thrombosis, regional lymphadenopathy, and liver metastasis
- Interpret findings with clinical information, e.g., fever, trauma, known malignancy
- Consider risk factors, e.g., dialysis, von Hippel-Lindau disease

Helpful Clues for Common Diagnoses

- **Renal Cell Carcinoma**
  - Most common primary renal malignancy
  - Variable grayscale US appearances: Solid, heterogeneous cystic and solid or predominantly cystic
  - Hyperechoic (48%), isoechoic (42%), hypoechoic (10%)
  - Large tumors tend to be hypoechoic, exophytic with anechoic necrotic areas
  - Hypoechoic pseudocapsule
  - Smaller tumors tend to be hyperechoic, overlapping with angiomyolipoma (which shadow)
  - May contain dystrophic coarse calcification
  - Color Doppler: Peripheral, intratumoral vascularity
  - Associated with renal vein thrombosis (23%) and IVC tumor extension (7%)
- **Renal Angiomyolipoma**
  - Benign tumor containing fat, smooth muscle and dysmorphic vascular tissue
  - Sporadic when single
  - Multiple in tuberous sclerosis complex
  - Echogenic lesion but can be variable depending upon relative amounts of fat and soft tissue
  - Small lesions (< 3 cm) are well marginated and hyperechoic
  - Acoustic shadowing in 21-33%; distinguishing feature from RCC
  - Internal vascularity and aneurysms
  - May be complicated by hemorrhage, which confounds imaging diagnosis on US, CT, and MR
  - Confirm fat with CT or MR
- **Upper Tract Urothelial Cancer**
  - Hypovascular soft tissue lesion centered in renal pelvis
  - Associated with hydronephrosis
  - Infiltrative, preserving renal contour when large
  - Synchronous and metachronous bladder and upper tract tumors
- **Renal Pseudotumor**
  - **Column of Bertin**
    - Hypertrophied band of cortical tissue that separates pyramids of renal medulla
    - Isoechoic mass like lesion continuous with renal cortex
    - Normal external renal outline but indent renal sinus fat
    - Normal vascularity on Doppler
  - **Dromedary Hump**
    - Focal bulge in lateral border of left kidney mid-pole
    - Similar to rest of kidney
    - Calyces extend into hump with normal vascular supply
  - **Focal Hypertrophy**
    - Hypertrophied kidney next to scar
    - Similar appearance to rest of normal kidney
- **Focal Pyelonephritis**
  - Loss of corticomedullary differentiation, enlarged kidney
  - Hypoechoic round or wedge-shaped lesions
  - May have increased echogenicity due to hemorrhage
  - Other features of inflammation: Renal enlargement, urothelial thickening of renal pelvis
  - Later liquefaction and abscess formation
  - Decreased color Doppler flow
  - Clinical picture of infection

Solid Renal Mass

- **Horseshoe Kidney**
  - Congenital renal anomaly where lower poles of kidneys are fused by isthmus
  - Elongated kidneys with medially located lower poles
  - Lower poles curve away from transducer
  - Isthmus can consist of normal parenchyma or fibrous band
    - Usually anterior to aorta and IVC at L3/5 level
- **Crossed Fused Ectopia**
  - Mass with renal type morphology arising from lower renal pole
  - Absence of kidney in contralateral renal fossa
- **Renal Lymphoma**
  - Variable manifestations
    - Solitary or multiple hypoechoic hypovascular masses
    - Direct invasion from retroperitoneal lymphoma
    - Diffuse infiltration with renal enlargement
    - Perinephric soft tissue rind
    - Renal sinus dominant
  - Lesions are often hypoechoic or near anechoic (pseudocystic)
  - Less vascular than renal cell carcinoma
  - Infrequently associated with renal vein and IVC tumor thrombosis
- **Renal Leukemia and Myeloma**
  - Multifocal or infiltrative hypoechoic masses
  - Associated with tumor elsewhere and lymphadenopathy
- **Renal Metastases**
  - Most commonly secondary to lung cancer followed by breast, gastrointestinal tract cancers, and melanoma
  - Typically small and round; occasionally wedge-shaped
  - Usually cortical, rarely disrupting renal contour or capsule
  - Variable echogenicity and may be isoechoic
  - Mostly avascular or hypovascular on color Doppler
  - Look for other evidence of disseminated disease, e.g., liver, lymph node, lung involvement
- **Other Renal Tumors**
  - No specific imaging findings
  - Oncocytomas may have central scar

- **Wilms Tumor**
  - Most common primary renal tumor in children > 1 year old, most presenting < 5 years of age
  - Similar to renal cell carcinoma

Helpful Clues for Less Common Diagnoses

- **Xanthogranulomatous Pyelonephritis (XGP)**
  - Chronic renal inflammation associated with longstanding urinary calculus and obstruction
  - Destruction and replacement of renal parenchyma by lipid-laden macrophages
  - Anechoic/hypoechoic masses replacing normal parenchyma ± abscesses
  - Associated with highly reflective central echocomplex containing calculus
  - Hydronephrosis and cortical thinning
  - Clinical context essential
- **Renal Sinus/Replacement Lipomatosis**
  - Severe renal atrophy with proliferation of fat in renal hilum and perirenal space
  - Hypoechoic poorly defined masses in renal sinus
  - Associated with calculus disease, chronic inflammation, and hydronephrosis
  - Confirm with CT or MR
  - Distinct from XGP as renal parenchyma does not contain lipid-laden foamy cells
- **Renal Tuberculosis**
  - Hematogenous spread of *Mycobacterium tuberculosis* from primary focus, usually lungs
  - Hydronephrosis, infundibular strictures, caseating cavities, calcification
- **Renal Papillary Necrosis**
  - Edematous papilla surrounded by fluid
  - Hydronephrosis from sloughed papilla
  - Later fluid-filled cavity communicating with renal pelvis

Renal Cell Carcinoma

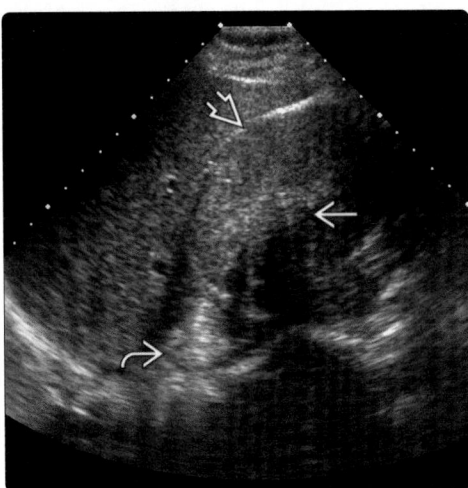

Renal Cell Carcinoma

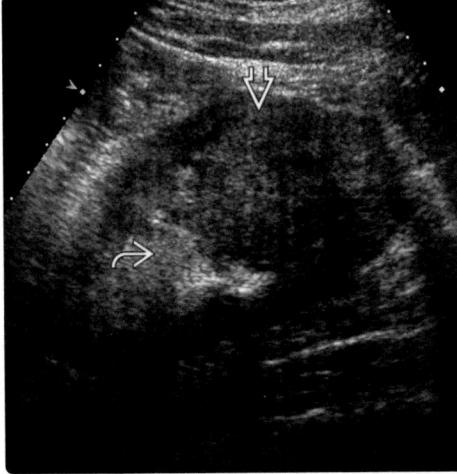

(Left) *Longitudinal ultrasound shows a large, solid renal mass* ➡, *which contains central shadowing calcifications* ➡. *The upper pole of the kidney* ➡ *is atrophic and increased in echogenicity secondary to chronic kidney disease.* (Right) *Longitudinal ultrasound shows a solid, hypoechoic renal mass* ➡, *which exerts mass effect on the renal sinus fat* ➡. *The patient presented with diffuse metastatic disease, and tissue diagnosis was made by percutaneous renal mass biopsy.*

Renal Angiomyolipoma

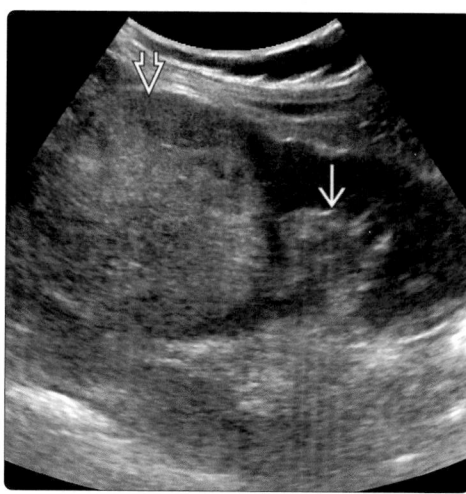

Renal Angiomyolipoma

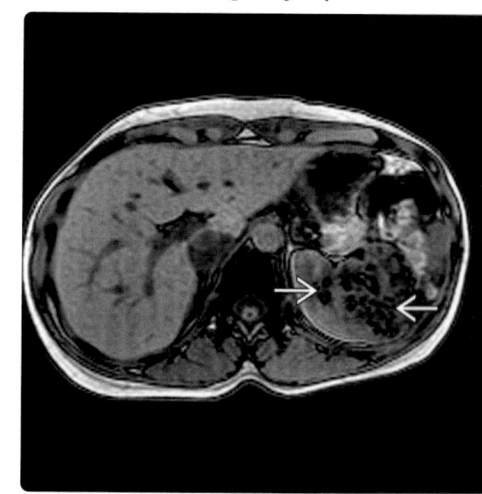

(Left) *Longitudinal ultrasound shows a large, homogeneous, hyperechoic renal mass ⇒ similar in echogenicity to the renal sinus fat ⇒. While suggestive of angiomyolipoma, confirmation with CT or MR is necessary.* **(Right)** *Axial T1 opposed-phase MR of the same patient shows multiple regions of low signal ⇒ within the mass indicating fat next to soft tissue. This confirms angiomyolipoma.*

Upper Tract Urothelial Cancer

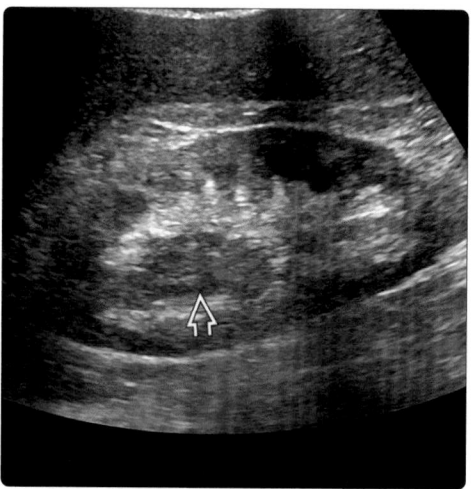

Column of Bertin

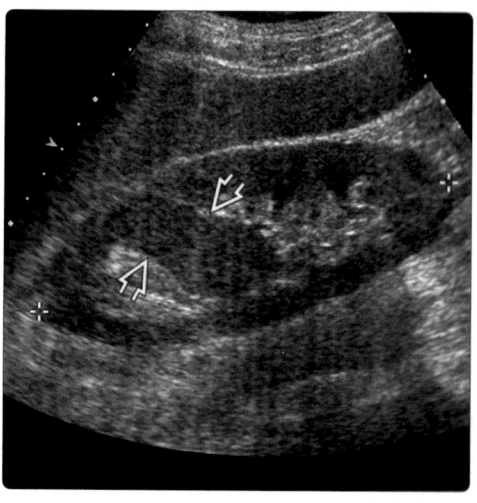

(Left) *Longitudinal ultrasound performed for hematuria shows a hypoechoic solid mass in the upper renal sinus ⇒, which did not have detectable color flow. Absence of color flow does not exclude tumor, presence of color flow is suggestive of tumor. Unlike the column of Bertin, this mass did not arise from the cortex.* **(Right)** *Longitudinal ultrasound shows a solid renal pseudolesion ⇒ extending from cortex to renal sinus. The echogenicity is identical to cortex.*

Focal Pyelonephritis

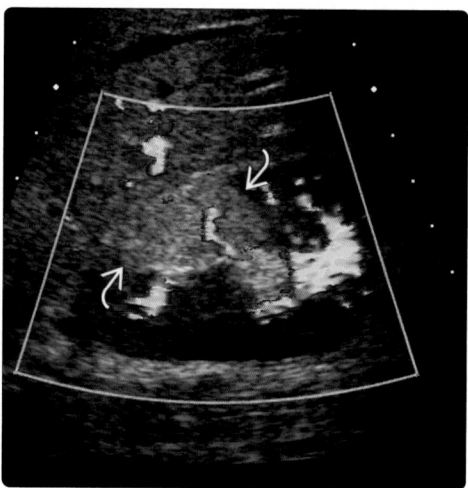

Crossed Fused Ectopia

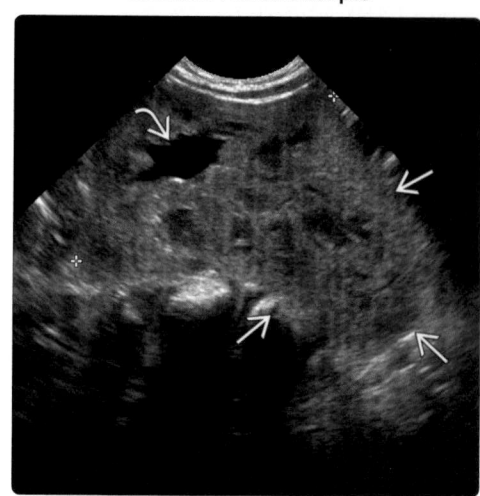

(Left) *Longitudinal color Doppler ultrasound shows a hyperechoic, wedge-shaped cortical lesion ⇒ with decreased internal color flow.* **(Right)** *Longitudinal ultrasound shows the left kidney (between calipers) with mild pelvic diltation ⇒. A solid "mass" ⇒ projects from the lower pole. The "mass" resembles normal kidney. No kidney was seen in the right renal fossa.*

Renal Lymphoma

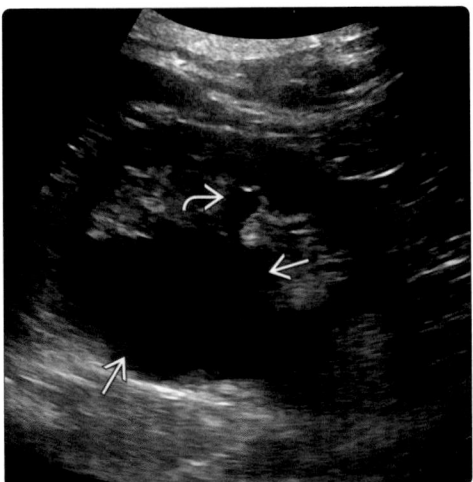

Renal Leukemia and Myeloma

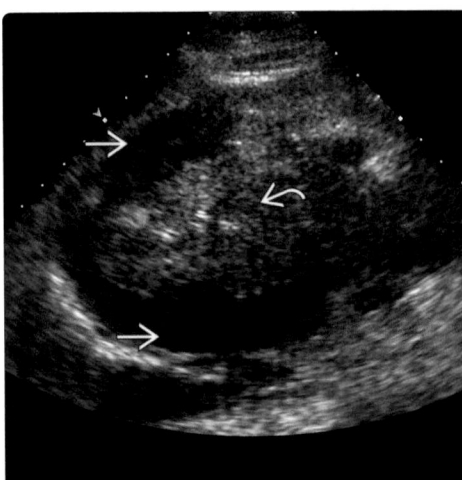

(Left) *Longitudinal ultrasound of the kidney demonstrates a very hypoechoic central lesion* ➡ *with focal calyceal dilatation* ➡. *Lymphoma may have a pseudocystic appearance as in this case.* (Right) *Longitudinal ultrasound shows hypoechoic enlargement of the upper pole of the kidney* ➡ *from myeloma. The renal sinus fat is still discrete* ➡ *but likely involved.*

Other Renal Tumors

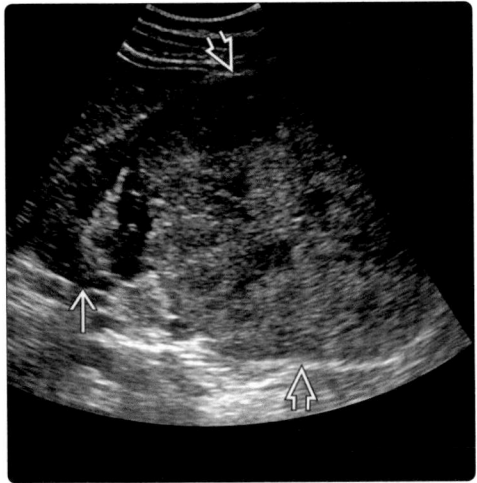

Other Renal Tumors

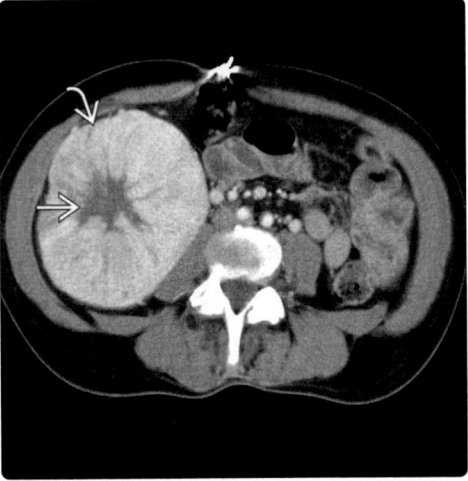

(Left) *Longitudinal ultrasound shows a large, solid lower pole renal mass* ➡, *which is hyperechoic to normal kidney* ➡. *Given its size, nephrectomy was performed.* (Right) *Axial CECT of the same patient shows a large, enhancing, solid renal mass* ➡ *with a central scar* ➡ *classic for oncocytoma.*

Renal Sinus/Replacement Lipomatosis

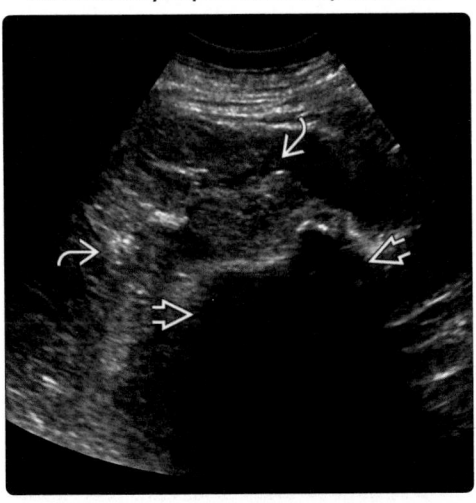

Renal Sinus/Replacement Lipomatosis

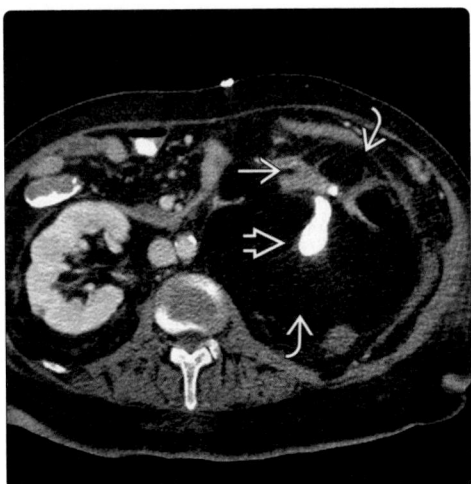

(Left) *Longitudinal ultrasound of the renal fossa reveals no normal kidney. There is a large shadowing stone* ➡ *surrounded by soft tissue of intermediate echogenicity* ➡. (Right) *Axial CECT of the same patient confirms a staghorn calculus* ➡ *surrounded by fat* ➡. *There is barely any residual renal parenchyma* ➡.

DIFFERENTIAL DIAGNOSIS

Common

- Column of Bertin
- Renal Junction Line, Junctional Parenchymal Defect
- Fetal Lobulation
- Dromedary Hump
- Hypertrophy Next to Scar
- Focal Pyelonephritis/Abscess

Less Common

- Crossed Fused Ectopia
- Hematoma
- Arteriovenous Malformation
- Focal Xanthogranulomatous Pyelonephritis
- Extramedullary Hematopoiesis
- Splenorenal Fusion

ESSENTIAL INFORMATION

Key Differential Diagnosis Issues

- Differentiate pseudotumors composed of normal variants from nonneoplastic lesions mimicking renal masses
- Note typical locations of normal variant pseudotumors
- Rare to have mass effect or distortion of normal architecture/vessels

Helpful Clues for Common Diagnoses

- **Column of Bertin**
  - Isoechoic, continuous with renal cortex, normal renal outline
  - No abnormal vascularity on color Doppler
  - Junction of upper and middle 1/3 of kidney
  - Changing sonographic window may clarify nature
- **Renal Junction Line, Junctional Parenchymal Defect**
  - Echogenic line at anterosuperior aspect of kidney without disruption of renal contour or cortical loss
  - Junction of upper and middle 1/3 of kidney and right side most common location
  - Junctional parenchymal defect: Triangular echogenic defect in renal cortex, upper to mid 1/3

- Cine clips are helpful for confirmation
- **Fetal Lobulation**
  - Multiple indentations in renal outline, between renal pyramids or calyces; preserved cortical thickness
  - Distinguished from scars of pyelonephritis, which are directly over calyces with thinned cortex
- **Dromedary Hump**
  - Only occurs in left kidney: "Splenic hump"
  - Focal bulge in lateral border of midpole of left kidney with similar echogenicity as rest of kidney
  - Calyces extend laterally into hump, which contains normal vessels, unlike tumor
- **Hypertrophy Next to Scar**
  - Hypertrophied normal renal tissue adjacent to an area of cortical loss
  - Similar echogenicity to normal parenchyma without vascular distortion
- **Focal Pyelonephritis/Abscess**
  - Pyelonephritis: Cortical hypo-/hyperechoic lesion with decreased color Doppler flow, lacking external bulge
  - Abscess: Thick-walled cystic lesion, clinical correlation essential, may need aspiration

Helpful Clues for Less Common Diagnoses

- **Crossed Fused Ectopia**
  - Kidney-like morphology, absence of contralateral kidney
- **Hematoma**
  - Echogenicity varies with age, avascular
- **Arteriovenous Malformation**
  - Tubular, internal color flow
- **Focal Xanthogranulomatous Pyelonephritis**
  - Hypoechoic lesion with calculi
- **Extramedullary Hematopoiesis**
  - Single or multiple lesions in patients with hematolologic disease, may require biopsy for diagnosis

Alternative Differential Approaches

- Consider CECT, CEUS or CEMR if ultrasound is nondiagnostic
- Clinical correlation is essential

Column of Bertin

Column of Bertin

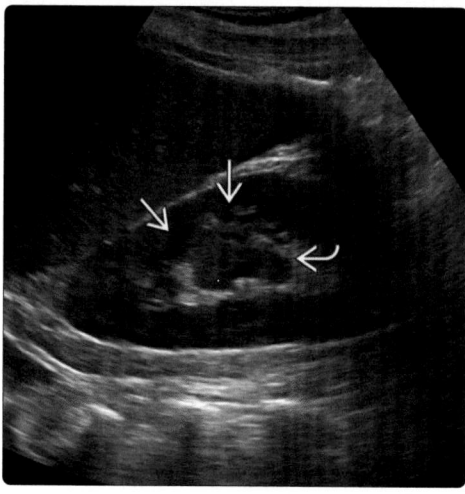
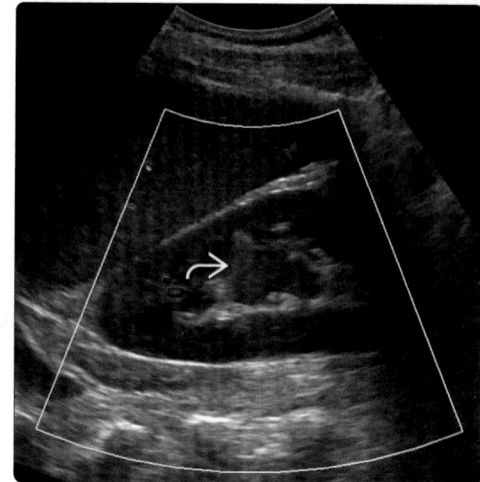

(Left) *Longitudinal ultrasound of the right kidney shows a lobulated lesion in the mid kidney ⇗ between pyramids ➥. The lesion is continuous with renal cortex and slightly hyperechoic to renal cortex secondary to anisotropy.* **(Right)** *Longitudinal color Doppler ultrasound of the same lesion ➥ shows no increase in color flow as might be seen in a solid renal tumor.*

Column of Bertin

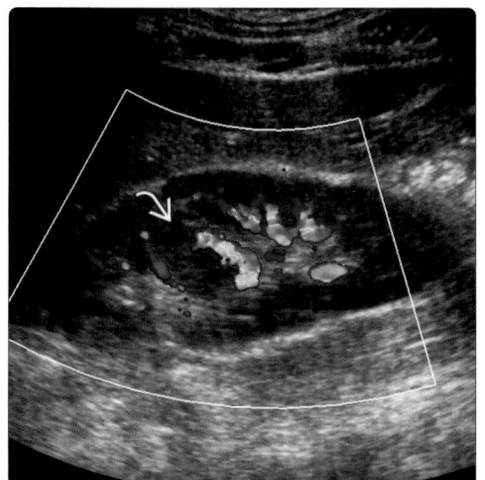

Column of Bertin

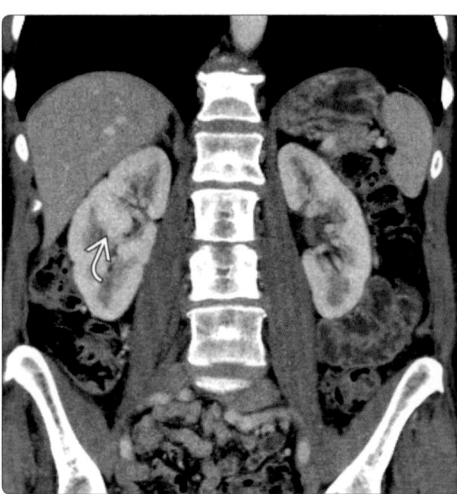

(Left) *Longitudinal color Doppler ultrasound of the right kidney shows a lesion ➦ that is isoechoic to cortex with no internal color flow.* (Right) *Coronal CECT of the same patient confirms that the lesion ➦ represents cortical tissue as it was isodense to cortex on all phases of the multiphasic CECT.*

Fetal Lobulation

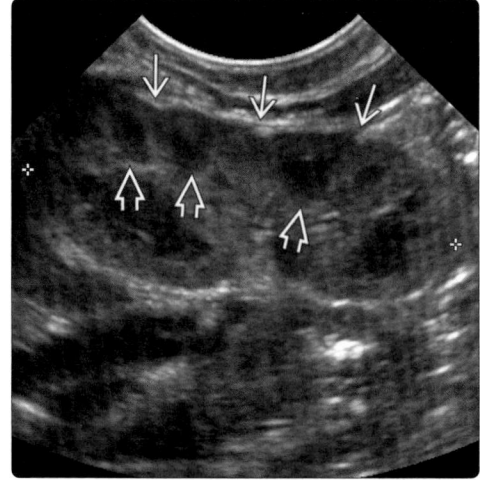

Focal Pyelonephritis/Abscess

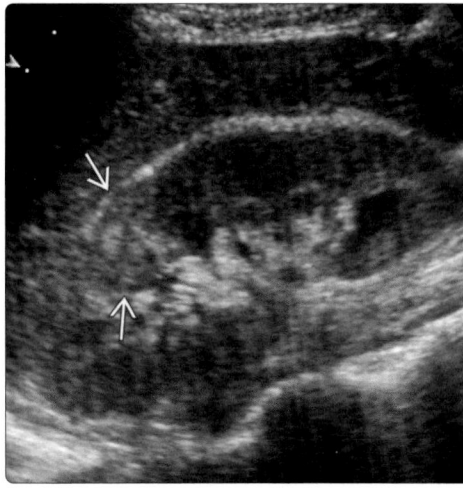

(Left) *Longitudinal ultrasound of the left kidney in a neonate shows fetal lobulation. The cortical indentations ➦ are located between pyramids ➦.* (Right) *Longitudinal ultrasound of right kidney shows a focal wedge-shaped area of increased cortical echogenicity ➦ in a patient with fever and pain from acute pyelonephritis.*

Dromedary Hump

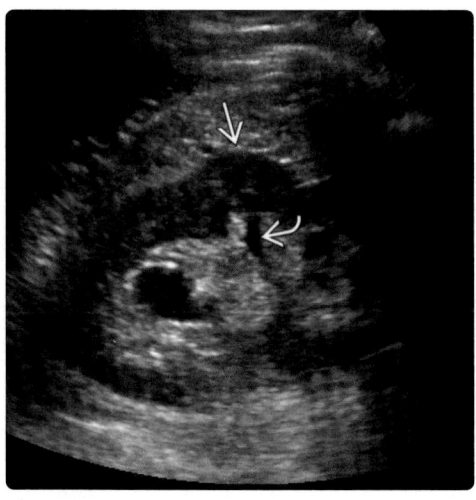

Dromedary Hump

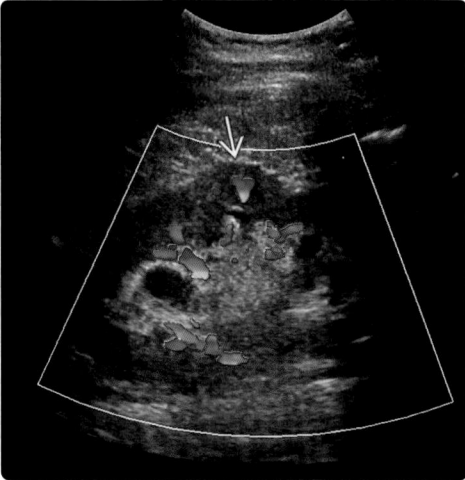

(Left) *Longitudinal ultrasound of the left kidney shows an exophytic hump on the anterior mid pole ➦. There is mild hydronephrosis with a calyx ➦ extending into the hump.* (Right) *Longitudinal color Doppler ultrasound of the same kidney shows no distortion of vascular supply in the dromedary hump ➦.*

DIFFERENTIAL DIAGNOSIS

Common

- Obstructed Renal Pelvis
- Reflux Into Dilated Renal Pelvis
- Extrarenal Pelvis
- Physiologic Distention of Renal Pelvis
- Parapelvic Cyst
- Prominent Renal Vessel
- Urothelial Carcinoma

Less Common

- Pyonephrosis
- Hemonephrosis
- Renal Sinus Hemorrhage
- Pararenal Fluid Collections
- Peripelvic Cyst
- Intrarenal Abscess
- Calyceal Diverticulum
- Acute Renal Vein Thrombosis

Rare but Important

- Pyelogenic Cyst
- Multilocular Cystic Nephroma
- Lucent Sinus Lipomatosis
- Renal Lymphoma
- Retroperitoneal Lymphoma
- Renal Artery Aneurysm
- Arteriovenous Malformation (AVM)
- Intrarenal Varices
- Renal Lymphangiomatosis

ESSENTIAL INFORMATION

Key Differential Diagnosis Issues

- Important to differentiate between obstruction and nonobstruction
  - Follow ureter to level of obstruction to determine cause
- Ultrasound is first-line modality for detection but other modalities such as CT, MR, VCUG, and retrograde pyelography may be required for definitive diagnosis
- Nuclear scintigraphy differentiates obstruction from nonobstructive dilatation

Helpful Clues for Common Diagnoses

- **Obstructed Renal Pelvis**
  - Isolated dilatation of renal pelvis is uncommon
  - Dilatation elsewhere in GU tract determined by level of obstruction
    - For example, ureteropelvic junction obstruction manifests with pelvic dilatation and (to lesser degree) calyceal dilatation
    - Ureterovesical junction obstruction presents with hydroureter as well as pelvicalyceal dilatation
  - Determine if unilateral or bilateral
  - Level of obstruction helps narrow differential diagnosis
  - Most common cause of unilateral obstruction is stone disease
  - Other causes include bladder, ureteral or other pelvic mass, retroperitoneal mass or hemorrhage, aortic aneurysm, retroperitoneal fibrosis, iatrogenic injury
- **Reflux Into Dilated Renal Pelvis**
  - Hydroureter may be present in addition to renal pelvic dilatation
  - VCUG essential in determining reflux
    - In future, contrast-enhanced voiding urosonography may be used in place of VCUG to evaluate for reflux without use of ionizing radiation
- **Extrarenal Pelvis**
  - Common finding in neonates and often incidentally noted in other age groups
    - Renal pelvis projects medial to renal sinus
  - Appearance may simulate early obstruction but calyces are not dilated
- **Physiologic Distension of Renal Pelvis**
  - Commonly noted when bladder is distended
    - Frequent in pregnant patients, most commonly in 3rd trimester; R > L
    - Fetal pyelectasis can result in mild pelvic dilatation in neonates, which subsequently resolves
- **Parapelvic Cyst**
  - 1-3% of renal parenchymal cysts; usually solitary
  - May be mixed picture, as parapelvic cysts can compress collecting system resulting in true dilatation
- **Prominent Renal Vessel**
  - May mimic pelvic dilatation but color Doppler denotes flow
    - Protocol advice: Always remember to use color Doppler when concerned about pelvic dilatation or cystic lesion to distinguish from vessel
- **Urothelial Carcinoma**
  - Hypoechoic mass in dilated pelvis, though usually slightly hyperechoic to renal parenchyma
  - Can mimic hemorrhage or pus
  - On color Doppler, note internal vascularity within urothelial carcinoma

Helpful Clues for Less Common Diagnoses

- **Pyonephrosis**
  - Debris (pus) in dilated pelvicalyceal system
  - Look for presence of urothelial thickening and cause such as stone
- **Hemonephrosis**
  - Blood within dilated pelvicalyceal system ± blood in bladder
  - Echogenicity variable depending upon age of blood products
- **Renal Sinus Hemorrhage**
  - In absence of trauma, most often secondary to anticoagulation, but can be secondary to occult neoplasm, vasculitis, or blood dyscrasia
  - Cystic lesion of variable echogenicity disrupting normal central echocomplex, with mass effect upon renal pelvis and tension upon infundibula
  - Should spontaneously resolve in 3-4 weeks
- **Pararenal Fluid Collections**
  - May occur in setting of infection, obstruction, or transplantation; include urinoma, hematoma, abscess, and lymphocele near renal hilum
- **Peripelvic Cyst**
  - Lymphatic collection in renal sinus, distinct from parapelvic cyst, which is intraparenchymal
  - Often multiple and bilateral (unlike parapelvic cyst)

- **Intrarenal Abscess**
  - Hypoechoic parenchymal lesion, which may mimic collecting system dilatation
  - May also be associated with hydronephrosis and urothelial thickening
  - Most often secondary to acute pyelonephritis, but relatively rare
- **Calyceal Diverticulum**
  - Typically upper pole, connects with calyx
    - Lined with transitional cell epithelium
  - May appear like simple cyst or dilated calyx
  - Prone to calculus formation and infection: Containing milk of calcium and debris
  - On excretory phase CT/ MR, VCUG, or retrograde pyelography, diagnostic filling of diverticulum with contrast
- **Acute Renal Vein Thrombosis**
  - Dilated vein with hypoechoic thrombus
    - Chronic thrombosis often demonstrates greater internal echogenicity and organized clot along walls
  - Absent venous color Doppler flow

Helpful Clues for Rare Diagnoses

- **Pyelogenic Cyst**
  - Similar to calyceal diverticulum but communicates with pelvis rather than calyx
- **Multilocular Cystic Nephroma**
  - Encapsulated multilocular cystic renal lesion with internal septa
    - On MR/CT, note enhancement of septa
  - May herniate into renal pelvis, mimicking pelviectasis, or may cause hydronephrosis
- **Lucent Sinus Lipomatosis**
  - Very rarely, renal sinus fat may appear less echogenic than normal and mimic hydronephrosis or hypoechoic mass
    - Secondary to chronic steroid use, obesity, diabetes, renal atrophy, and inflammation
  - More evident when there is chronic kidney disease and hyperechoic kidneys

- **Renal Lymphoma**
  - Multiple forms, including hypoechoic infiltration of renal sinus
    - May mimic dilated renal pelvis or cause hydronephrosis
- **Retroperitoneal Lymphoma**
  - Retroperitoneal adenopathy may demonstrate contiguous extension into renal pelvis, mimicking dilatation of collecting system
  - Distinct from renal lymphoma
- **Renal Artery Aneurysm**
  - Pulsatile fluid-filled structure with diagnostic color/power Doppler
  - Typically small < 2 cm and saccular
  - Located at bifurcation of main renal artery
- **Arteriovenous Malformation (AVM)**
  - Congenital malformation which appears hypoechoic on grayscale ultrasound
  - Color Doppler flow reveals hypervascular mass with aliasing
- **Intrarenal Varices**
  - May present as cystic renal mass
  - May mimic hydronephrosis
  - Associated with AVM
- **Renal Lymphangiomatosis**
  - Multiple cystic lesions in both parapelvic and perirenal areas
  - Related to lymphatic obstruction

SELECTED REFERENCES

1. Ma TL et al: Parapelvic cyst misdiagnosed as hydronephrosis. Clin Kidney J. 6(2):238-9, 2013
2. Darge K et al: Pediatric uroradiology: state of the art. Pediatr Radiol. 41(1):82-91, 2011
3. Sheth S et al: Imaging of renal lymphoma: patterns of disease with pathologic correlation. Radiographics. 26(4):1151-68, 2006
4. Browne RF et al: Transitional cell carcinoma of the upper urinary tract: spectrum of imaging findings. Radiographics. 25(6):1609-27, 2005
5. Rha SE et al: The renal sinus: pathologic spectrum and multimodality imaging approach. Radiographics. 24 Suppl 1:S117-31. Review, 2004
6. Nahm AM et al: The renal sinus cyst-the great imitator. Nephrol Dial Transplant. 15(6):913-4, 2000

Obstructed Renal Pelvis

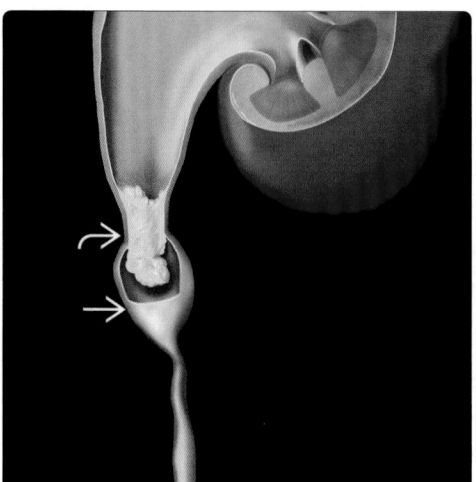

Obstructed Renal Pelvis

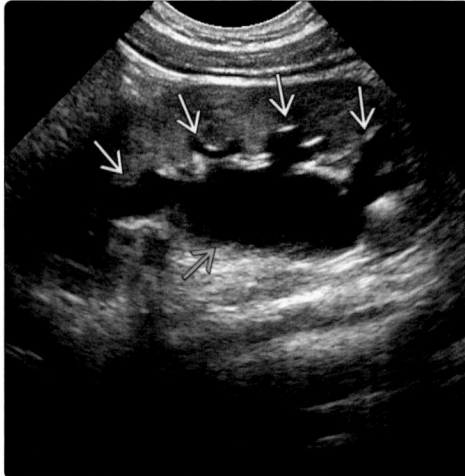

(Left) *Graphic shows an obstructing polypoid tumor* ➡ *at the ureteropelvic junction. The proximal ureter is dilated around the tumor, producing the goblet sign* ➡. **(Right)** *Longitudinal ultrasound demonstrates hydronephrosis, with pelvic dilatation* ➡ *to a greater degree than calyceal dilatation* ➡, *consistent with UPJ obstruction.*

Reflux Into Dilated Renal Pelvis

(Left) *Longitudinal ultrasound of the left kidney demonstrates pelvic ⇥ and calyceal ⇥ dilatation.* (Right) *VCUG evaluation in the same patient reveals left grade 4 reflux.*

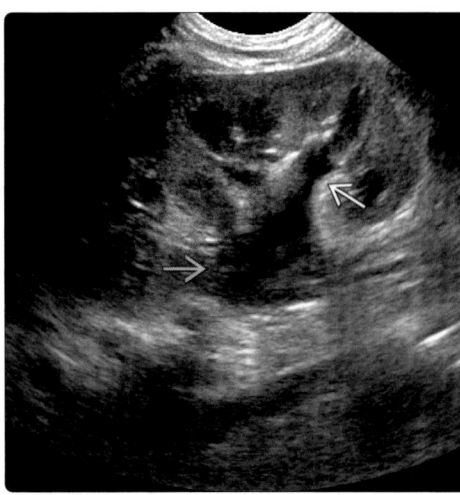

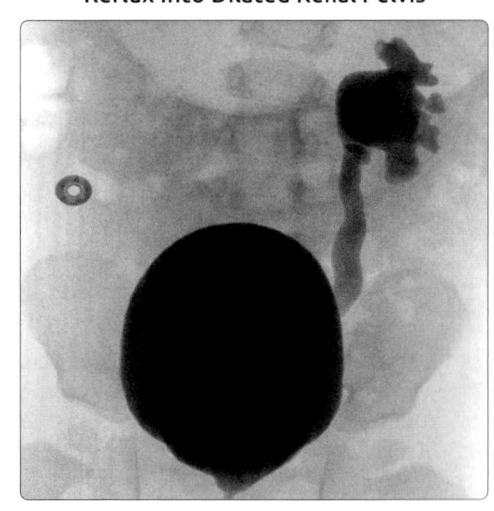

Extrarenal Pelvis

(Left) *Longitudinal color Doppler ultrasound demonstrates an anechoic central structure in the left kidney without flow ⇥ distinct from the central sinus fat ⇗, representing extrarenal pelvis.* (Right) *Axial contrast-enhanced CT obtained in the same patient demonstrates left extrarenal pelvis ⇥.*

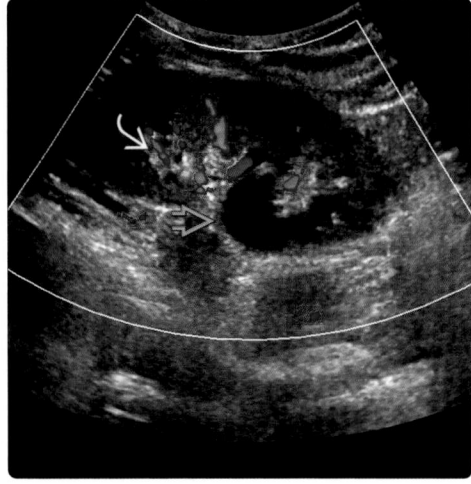

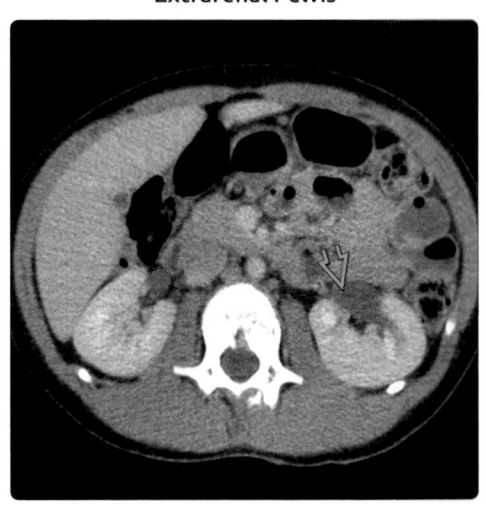

Parapelvic Cyst

(Left) *On longitudinal ultrasound, note large anechoic structure in the upper pole and interpolar region ⇥.* (Right) *Coronal contrast-enhanced CT in the same patient reveals a discrete cyst in the upper pole of the left kidney ⇥ approaching the pelvis representing parapelvic cyst.*

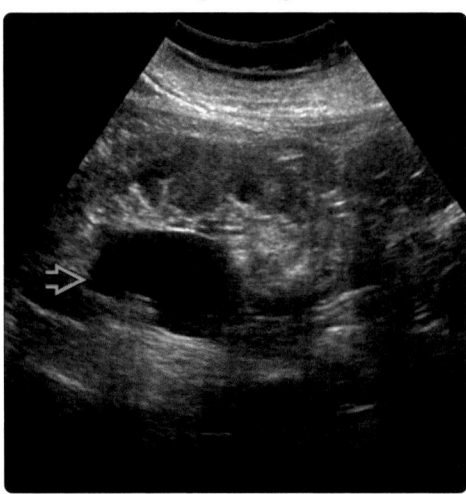

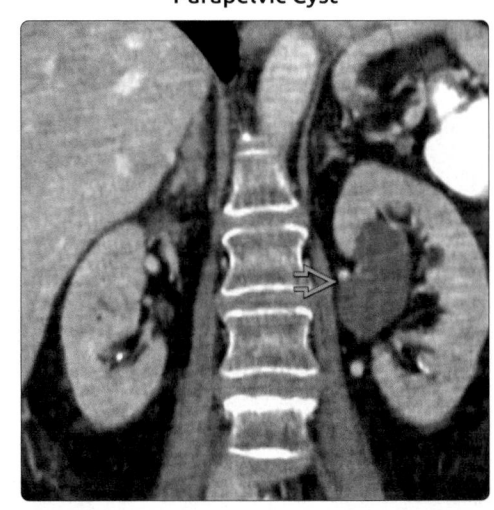

Pyonephrosis

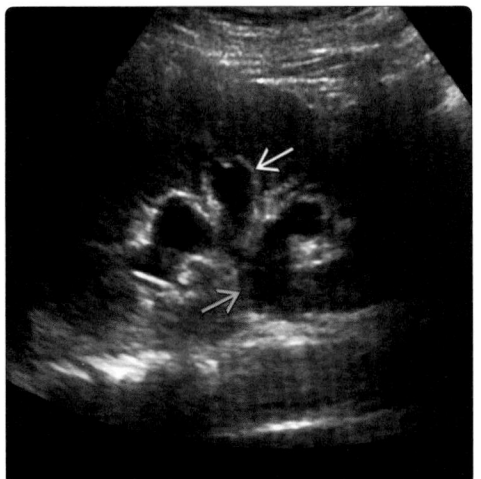

Pyonephrosis

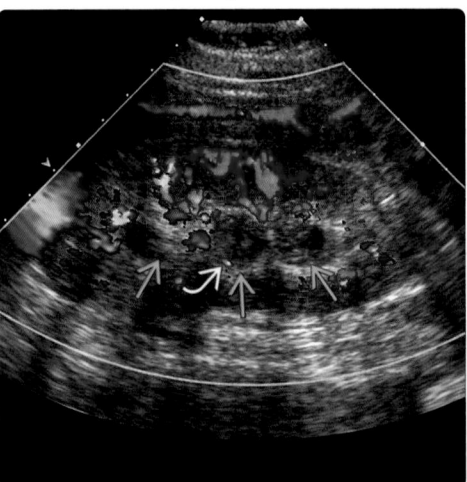

(Left) *Longitudinal ultrasound of the right kidney demonstrates low-level echoes in the dilated renal pelvis* ➡ *representing pyonephrosis. Note urothelial thickening* ➡, *an ancillary finding of urinary tract infection.* (Right) *Longitudinal color Doppler ultrasound shows hypoechoic tissue filling the dilated renal collecting system* ➡ *with internal color flow* ➡ *distinguishing this material as neoplasm rather than avascular pus or clot.*

Calyceal Diverticulum

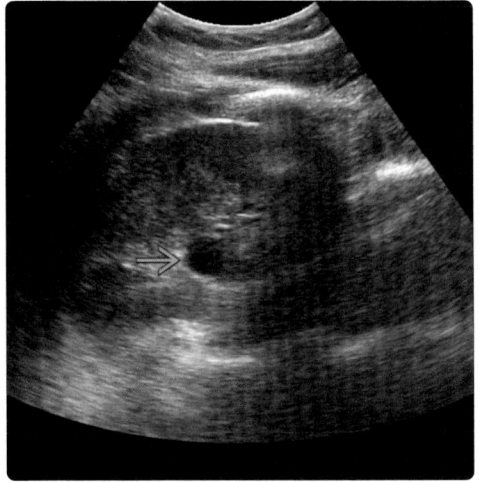

Calyceal Diverticulum

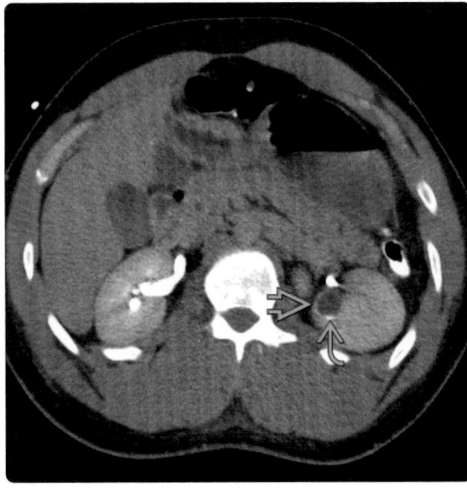

(Left) *Longitudinal ultrasound demonstrates an anechoic structure in the interpolar region of the left kidney* ➡. *Given this image alone, one might suspect pelviectasis or a simple cyst.* (Right) *In this CT obtained in the same patient, however, one can appreciate a small amount of layering contrast* ➡ *within the lesion* ➡ *on excretory phase imaging, confirming calyceal diverticulum.*

Multilocular Cystic Nephroma

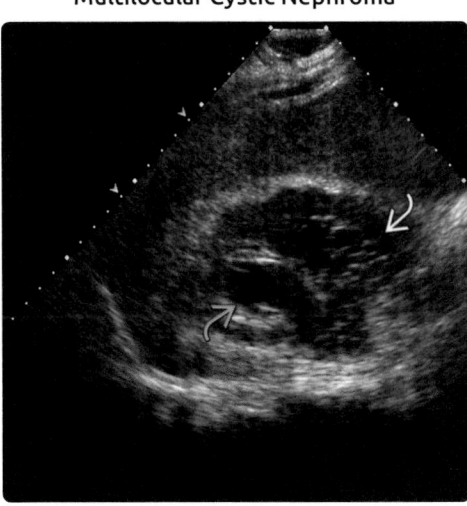

Multilocular Cystic Nephroma

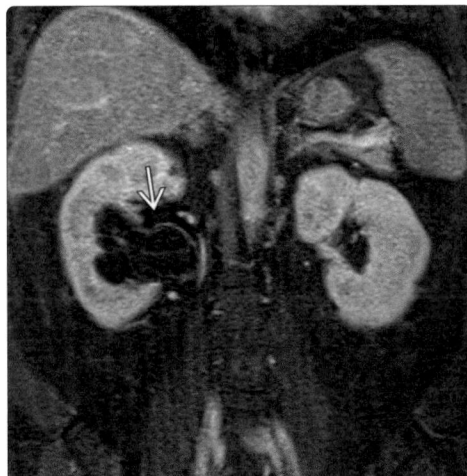

(Left) *Longitudinal ultrasound demonstrates dilatation of the renal pelvis* ➡, *which contains a cystic mass with thin internal septa* ➡. (Right) *Coronal contrast-enhanced T1-weighted MR in the same patient shows a mass demonstrating septal enhancement* ➡ *entering the renal pelvis. Histopathology revealed multilocular cystic nephroma.*

Abdominal Wall/Peritoneal Cavity

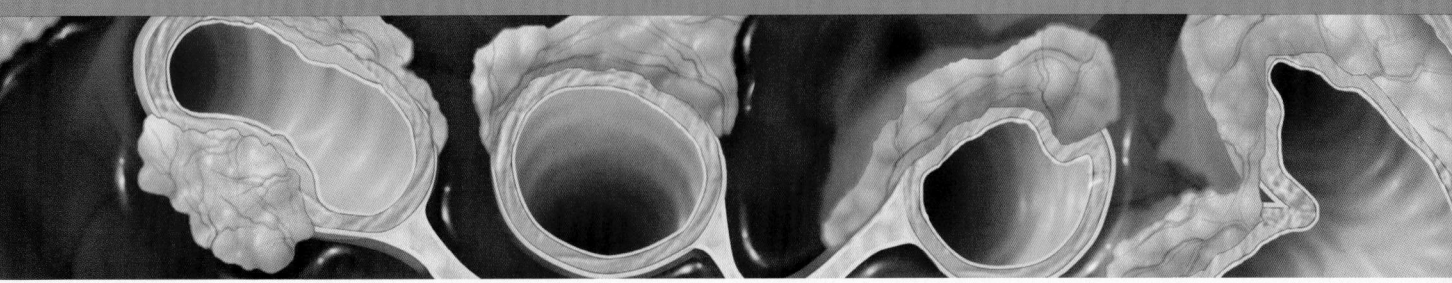

DIFFERENTIAL DIAGNOSIS

Common

- Transudate
  - Portal Hypertension
    - Cirrhosis
    - Portal Vein Thrombosis
    - Budd-Chiari Syndrome
  - Heart Failure
  - Renal Failure: Acute or Chronic
  - Fluid Overload

Less Common

- Exudate
  - Peritoneal Inflammation
    - Pancreatitis, Polyserositis
  - Peritonitis
    - Pyogenic Peritonitis
    - Tuberculosis Peritonitis
  - Carcinomatosis
- Hemoperitoneum
  - Post-Traumatic or Ruptured Aneurysm
  - Ruptured Ovarian Cyst or Ectopic Pregnancy
  - Ruptured Intraabdominal Tumor
    - Hepatic, Splenic, and Ovarian are Most Common

Rare but Important

- Chylous Ascites
- Urine, Bile, CSF

ESSENTIAL INFORMATION

Key Differential Diagnosis Issues

- Simple ascites = anechoic fluid = transudate
  - Other causes: Dialysate fluid, CSF from ventriculo-peritoneal shunt
- Complicated ascites = exudate or complicated transudate
  - Infection, malignancy, hemorrhage, or chylous ascites
    - Echogenic fluid and debris
    - Septa suggest subacute to chronic nature

Helpful Clues for Common Diagnoses

- Transudate
  - Look for cause: Cirrhotic liver, engorged hepatic veins from heart failure, chronic renal parenchymal disease

Helpful Clues for Less Common Diagnoses

- Hemoperitoneum
  - History of trauma ± solid organ laceration/fracture, aortic injury
  - Irregular or collapsed ovarian cyst in a female of reproductive age
  - Ruptured tumors (hepatic, ovarian, splenic) are usually large and present with acute severe abdominal pain
- Pyogenic Peritonitis
  - Marked echogenic peritoneal fluid
  - Dilated, fluid-filled bowel with ↓ peristalsis
  - Clinical pictures of infection
- Carcinomatosis
  - Peritoneal deposits, omental cake, other evidence of metastases or primary
- Tuberculosis Peritonitis
  - Diffuse omental thickening, nodules or mass, debris, septation; may closely mimic carcinomatosis

Helpful Clues for Rare Diagnoses

- Chylous Ascites
  - Disruption of abdominal lymphatics can be traumatic or atraumatic
    - Congenital lymphatic anomalies most frequent in childhood
    - Malignancy 2nd most common cause (lymphoma most common)
    - Trauma, surgical injury, radiation
    - Cirrhosis: Increased abdominal pressure resulting in leakage of lymph
    - Inflammatory: Pancreatitis, mycobacterial infection

Cirrhosis   **Peritoneal Inflammation**

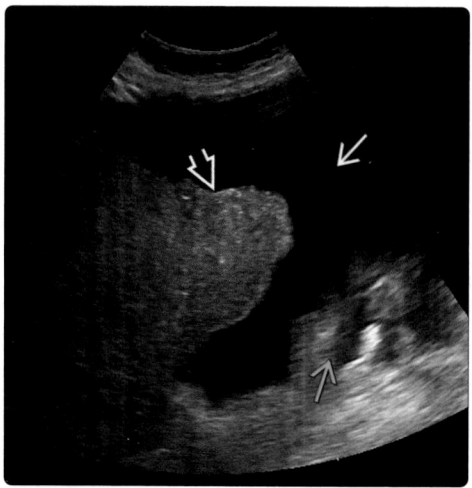
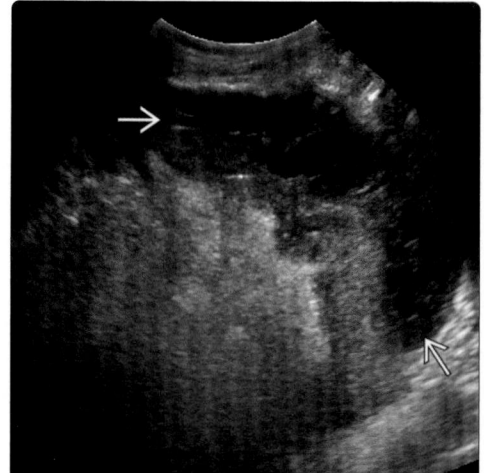

(Left) *Longitudinal ultrasound of the right upper quadrant shows anechoic ascites* ➡ *in a patient with a nodular cirrhotic liver* ➡. *Bowel loops are noted* ➡. **(Right)** *Transverse ultrasound of the left lower quadrant shows complex septated ascites* ➡. *Aspiration is required for diagnosis.*

Hemoperitoneum

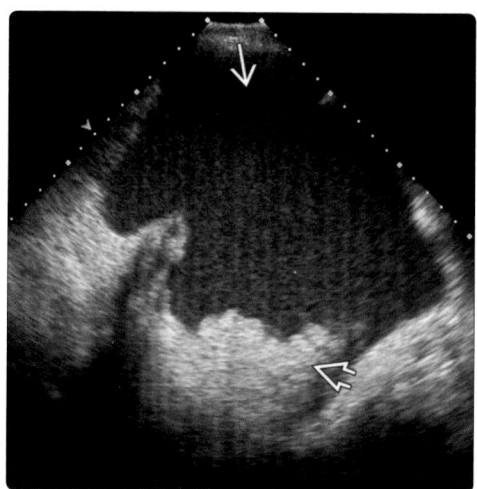

Hemoperitoneum

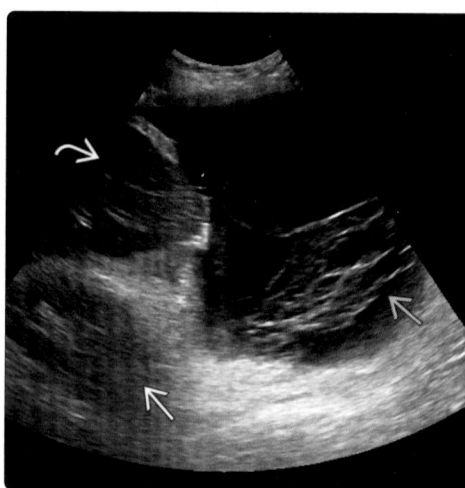

(Left) *Transverse ultrasound of the left lower quadrant in a liver transplant recipient is shown. Low-level echoes* ➡ *in the nonseptated ascites were shown to be secondary to hemorrhage at paracentesis. Bowel* ➡ *was not floating, secondary to mass effect.* (Right) *Longitudinal ultrasound of the left upper quadrant after liver transplantation is shown. There are multiple avascular fibrinous septa* ➡ *within chronic hemorrhagic ascites inferior to the spleen* ➡ *and left kidney* ➡.

Pyogenic Peritonitis

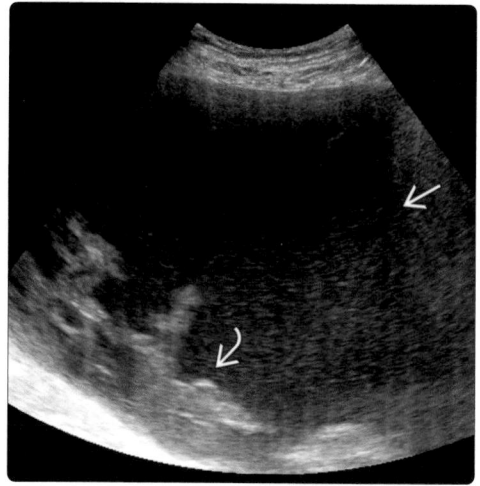

Carcinomatosis

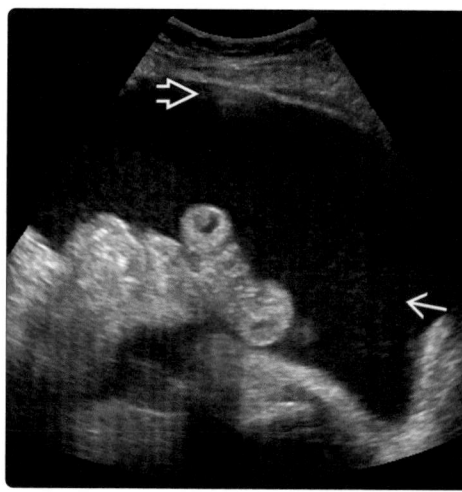

(Left) *Transverse ultrasound of the mid abdomen in a patient with heart failure and fever is shown. Fluid with layering low-level echoes* ➡ *is noted with dependent, more solid debris* ➡. *Aspiration showed pus.* (Right) *Transverse ultrasound of the pelvis shows complex ascites with low-level echoes* ➡ *in a patient with liver and renal transplants. Aspiration showed malignant cells from ovarian carcinoma. Subtle peritoneal nodularity* ➡ *was present.*

Carcinomatosis

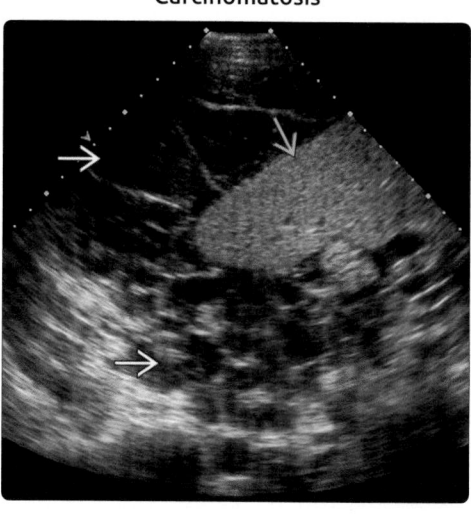

Ruptured Ovarian Cyst or Ectopic Pregnancy

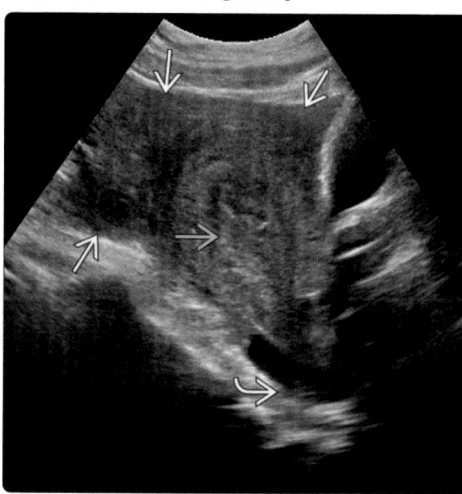

(Left) *Transverse ultrasound of the right upper quadrant in a patient with appendiceal pseudomyxoma peritonei is shown. There are numerous septa in the gelatinous fluid* ➡ *surrounding the liver* ➡. (Right) *Longitudinal transabdominal pelvic ultrasound shows echogenic hemorrhagic fluid* ➡ *superior to the uterus, and less echogenic fluid in the cul-de-sac* ➡ *from a ruptured ectopic pregnancy. Note the endometrial thickening* ➡. *Ruptured ovarian cysts may present similarly. Knowledge of pregnancy status is key.*

DIFFERENTIAL DIAGNOSIS

Common

- Peritoneal Carcinomatosis
- Lymphadenopathy
- Secondary Inflammatory Changes
- Mesenteric Hematoma
- Mimics
  - Pedunculated Mass From Abdominal Solid Organs or Bowel

Less Common

- Peritoneal Lymphomatosis
- Peritoneal Sarcomatosis
- Peritoneal Tuberculosis
- Malignant Peritoneal Mesothelioma
- Malignant Fibrous Histiocytoma

Rare but Important

- Primary Malignant Peritoneal Tumors
  - Papillary Serous Carcinoma
  - Desmoplastic Small Round Cell Tumor
- Carcinoid
- Benign Mesenchymal Tumor
  - Disseminated Intraperitoneal Leiomyomatosis
- Tumor-Like Conditions
  - Desmoid Tumor
  - Castleman Disease
  - Inflammatory Pseudotumor
  - Endometriosis
- Systemic Diseases
  - Extramedullary Hematopoiesis
  - Systemic Amyloidosis

ESSENTIAL INFORMATION

Key Differential Diagnosis Issues

- Peritoneal tumors generally lack specific features for definitive diagnosis
- Secondary peritoneal tumor much more common than primary peritoneal or mesenchymal tumor
  - However, primary peritoneal tumors are generally more aggressive
- Image-guided biopsy for histological type

Helpful Clues for Common Diagnoses

- **Peritoneal Carcinomatosis**
  - Metastatic tumoral seeding of peritoneal surface, peritoneal ligaments, omentum, and mesentery
  - Known malignancy, common sites of origin: Ovary, stomach, colon, and pancreas
  - Morphological forms
    - Nodular peritoneal masses: Multiple hypoechoic nodules or plaques on peritoneal surface; commonly involve pouch of Douglas, Morrison pouch, right subphrenic space
    - Plaque-like involvement of omentum (omental cake), diffuse or nodular
    - Mesenteric and peritoneal infiltration
    - Ascites
- **Lymphadenopathy**

- Solid nodules along lymphatic distribution
- Metastasis, lymphoma, leukemia > sarcoidosis, tuberculosis, mastocytosis, Crohn disease, Whipple disease, and nontropical sprue

- **Secondary Inflammatory Changes**
  - Local peritoneal inflammation secondary to adjacent inflammatory process, e.g., pancreatitis or appendicitis
  - Ill-defined echogenic/hypoechoic mass due to inflamed mesentery with adhesion or omental infiltration
  - Identification of underlying cause important
- **Mesenteric Hematoma**
  - Traumatic or spontaneous hemorrhage in patients with clotting abnormality
  - Echogenicity depends on age of hematoma, from echogenic to heterogeneously hypoechoic over time
  - Ill-defined border ± hemoperitoneum or ascites

Helpful Clues for Less Common Diagnoses

- **Peritoneal Lymphomatosis**
  - Rare presentation of aggressive non-Hodgkin lymphoma (diffuse large B-cell or Burkitt)
  - Unusual to have peritoneum as only site of involvement at presentation
  - Significant mesenteric and retroperitoneal adenopathy, splenic and bowel involvement favor lymphoma
    - Important to distinguish from peritoneal carcinomatosis as treatment is nonsurgical
- **Peritoneal Sarcomatosis**
  - Intraabdominal or extremity primary sarcomas
  - Most common: Gastrointestinal stromal tumor and leiomyosarcoma
  - Variable imaging findings
  - Larger, well-defined heterogeneous vascular masses ± necrosis and adjacent invasion
    - Less ascites, omental caking, peritoneal thickening and lymphadenopathy than carcinomatosis
- **Malignant Peritoneal Mesothelioma**
  - Asbestos exposure is risk factor, but < 1/2 patients have significant asbestos exposure
  - Adult predominance, middle-aged men
  - Rapid fatal course, median survival 6-12 months
  - Appearance similar to peritoneal carcinomatosis but calcification and lymphadenopathy is less common
  - Biopsy with immunohistochemical markers useful for diagnosis
- **Malignant Fibrous Histiocytoma**
  - Most common primary adult sarcoma, 5-10% are intraperitoneal
  - Large, solid hypoechoic, hypervascular ± central necrosis, which may appear cystic with thick septations
  - May present with intraperitoneal hemorrhage
- **Peritoneal Tuberculosis**
  - 2% of extrapulmonary tuberculosis
  - Consider *Mycobacterium avium-intracellulare* in AIDS patients
  - Wet, fibrotic, or dry types
  - Distinguishing features from peritoneal carcinomatosis
    - Thickening of ileocecal segment and matted hypoperistaltic small bowel
    - Necrotic mesenteric lymphadenopathy ± calcification
    - Splenomegaly and splenic calcifications

- Higher density ascites
- Smooth peritoneal thickening
- No omental cake

Helpful Clues for Rare Diagnoses

- **Primary Malignant Peritoneal Tumors**
  - **Papillary Serous Carcinoma**
    - Postmenopausal women with elevated CA125
    - Imaging appearance and histology closely mimic metastatic papillary serous ovarian carcinoma, but with much worse prognosis
    - Ovaries are normal with at most surface involvement by tumor
    - Extensive calcification in up to 30%
  - **Desmoplastic Small Round Cell Tumor**
    - Highly aggressive malignancy of adolescents and young adults
    - Multiple hypoechoic, round bulky peritoneal masses ± internal necrosis ± ascites
- **Carcinoid**
  - Arises within bowel wall; strong fibrotic reaction of mesentery causing radiating appearance of mesenteric vessels on color Doppler study
- **Benign Mesenchymal Tumors**
  - Leiomyomatosis peritonealis disseminata primarily affects reproductive-age females
    - Absence of ascites and omental cake
  - Mesenteric plexiform neurofibroma in NF1 is most common manifestation
  - Solitary fibrous tumor
    - Rare, usually benign spindle cell neoplasm
    - Well-defined, hypervascular soft tissue mass
- **Tumor-Like Conditions**
  - **Desmoid Tumor**: Benign, locally aggressive proliferative process with tendency to recur locally; irregular solid hypoechoic mass
    - 30% have mesenteric infiltration; 13% of these patients have Gardner syndrome

- **Castleman Disease**: Hypertrophic lymphadenopathy ± hypervascular soft tissue masses; foci of coarse calcification (5-10%); hepatosplenomegaly
- Inflammatory pseudotumor: Idiopathic chronic inflammatory disorder, children and young adults
  - Omental and mesenteric masses or infiltration, increased vascularity, ± tiny calcifications
- Splenosis: History of splenic rupture or splenectomy
  - Multiple small solid nodules, similar to spleen, no ascites, peritoneal thickening or omental cake
- Sclerosing mesenteritis
  - Idiopathic condition; variants: Mesenteric panniculitis and retractile mesenteritis
  - Soft tissue masses with varying amounts of echogenic fat with shadowing ± calcification
- Omental infarction/epiploic appendagitis
  - Vascular compromise to omentum or epiploic appendage respectively
  - Hyperechoic tender fat containing "mass"
- Endometriosis
  - Women of childbearing age
  - Fibrotic implants on bowel serosa, adhesions, endometriomas
- Gliomatosis peritonei
  - Implantation of glial tissue on peritoneum from rupture of teratoma, ventriculoperitoneal shunt, or metaplasia
  - Masses, peritoneal thickening, omental cake, ascites
- **Systemic Diseases**
  - **Extramedullary Hematopoiesis**
    - Infiltrative form (spleen, liver, mesentery) > mass-like form (paraspinal)
    - Hypoechoic, hypovascular masses
  - **Systemic Amyloidosis**: Rarely multifocal or diffuse mesenteric infiltration, dystrophic Ca++ important clue but not always present

Peritoneal Carcinomatosis

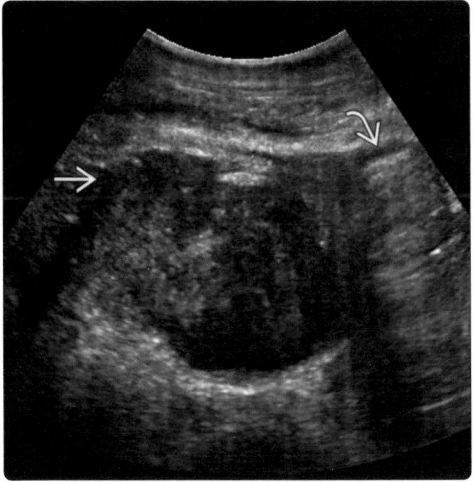

Peritoneal Carcinomatosis

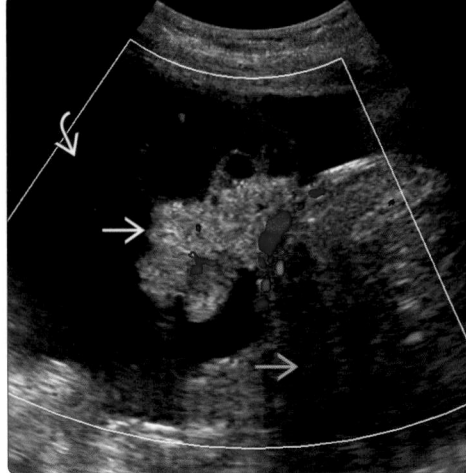

(Left) Transverse ultrasound of the right lower quadrant in a patient with a history of perforated colon carcinoma shows a heterogeneous peritoneal metastasis ➡ lateral to ileum ➡. (Right) Longitudinal color Doppler of the pelvis in a patient with endometrial cancer shows an ovarian metastasis ➡ and surrounding ascites ➡. A fibroid is also noted ➡.

Peritoneal Carcinomatosis

Peritoneal Carcinomatosis

(Left) *Transverse high-resolution ultrasound of the right upper quadrant shows ascites* ➡ *and nodular peritoneal metastases* ➡ *from pancreatic mucinous carcinoma. The liver* ➡ *was not involved.* (Right) *Longitudinal ultrasound of the left pelvis shows a round, solid mass* ➡ *and ascites* ➡ *from recurrent metastatic endometrial carcinoma post hysterectomy and salpingo-oophorectomy.*

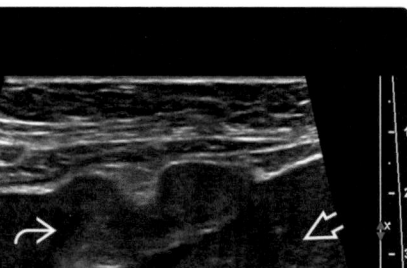
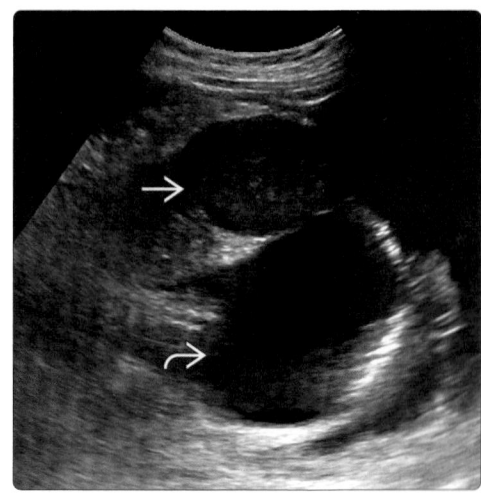

Lymphadenopathy

Mesenteric Hematoma

(Left) *Transverse color Doppler ultrasound of the mid abdomen shows adenopathy* ➡ *sandwiching mesenteric vessels* ➡ *in a patient with lymphoma.* (Right) *Color Doppler ultrasound of the lower abdomen shows a mixed echogenicity subacute hematoma* ➡*. No internal color flow was found. Note the patent common iliac vessels* ➡*.*

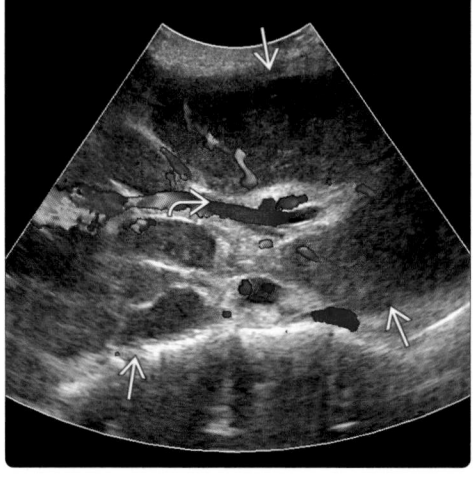
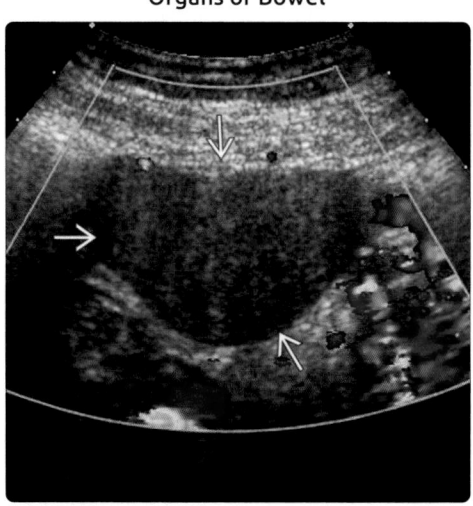

Pedunculated Mass From Abdominal Solid Organs or Bowel

Pedunculated Mass From Abdominal Solid Organs or Bowel

(Left) *Longitudinal color Doppler ultrasound of the right lower quadrant shows a solid mobile hypovascular mass* ➡ *with no demonstrable attachment to any organ. This proved to be a leiomyoma on biopsy.* (Right) *Longitudinal ultrasound of the mid abdomen shows a large, solid mass with internal heterogeneity and acoustic shadowing* ➡*. This was an infarcted gastrointestinal stromal tumor.*

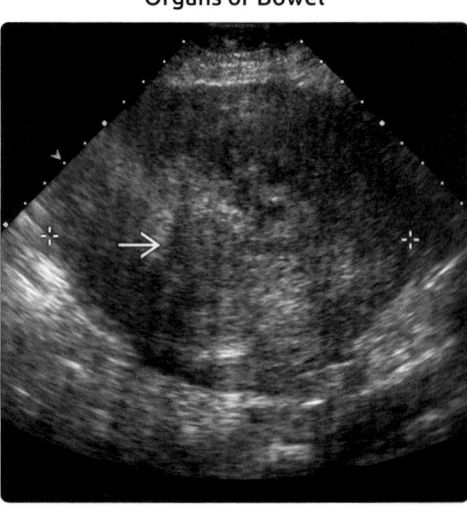

Mimics

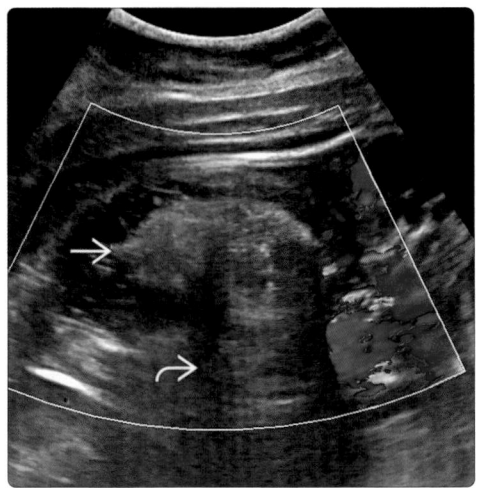

Benign Mesenchymal Tumor

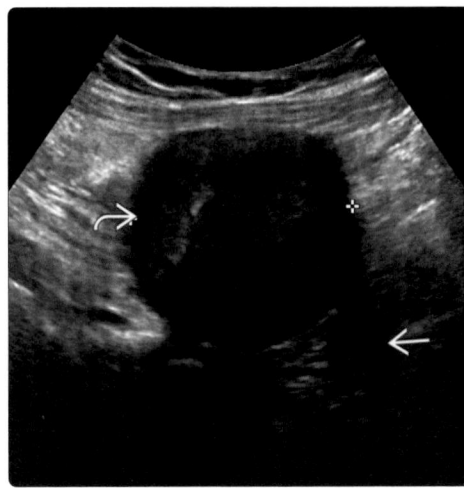

(Left) *Transverse color Doppler ultrasound of the pelvis shows an ovoid, hypoechoic lesion with central echogenic fat ➜ representing a mature teratoma. No color flow is seen in the fatty component, which exhibits shadowing ➡. (Right) Transverse ultrasound of the right lower quadrant in a patient status post-hysterectomy shows a hypoechoic solid mass ➡ with posterior acoustic shadowing ➡ and no color flow. This was a leiomyoma at surgical excision. Biopsy was not possible due to firmness.*

Peritoneal Sarcomatosis

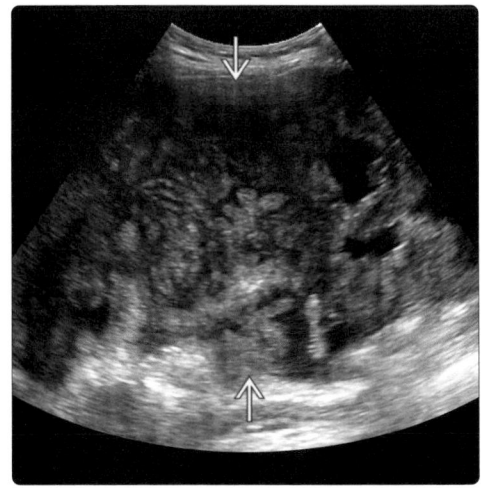

Peritoneal Lymphomatosis

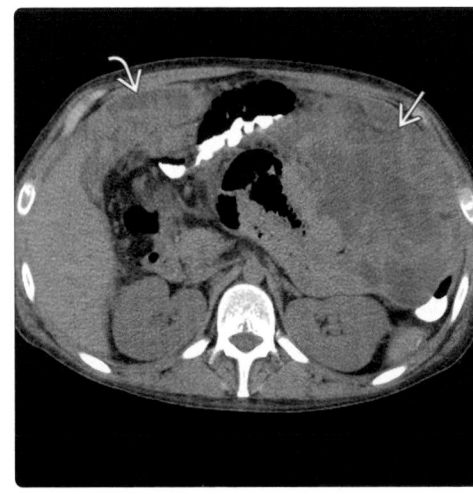

(Left) *Transverse ultrasound of the left upper abdomen in a patient with Burkitt lymphoma shows a large, heterogeneous, predominantly solid mass ➡. There was ascites inferiorly. (Right) Axial NECT of the same patient shows the mixed density lymphomatous mass ➡ as well as lymphomatous deposits in the right abdomen ➡. There was ascites on other images.*

Peritoneal Tuberculosis

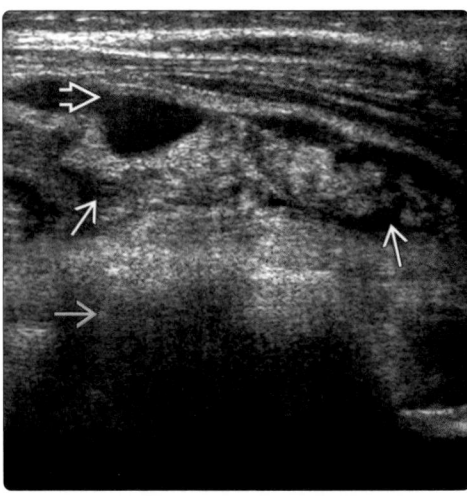

Papillary Serous Carcinoma

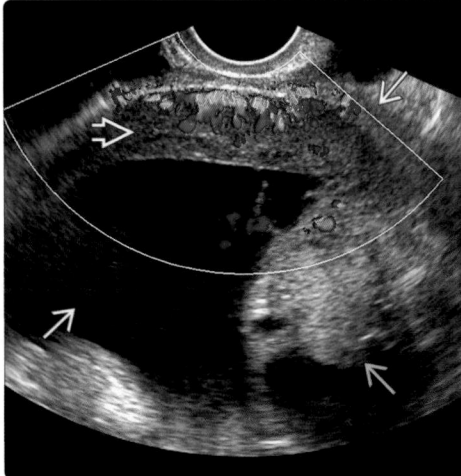

(Left) *Transverse transabdominal ultrasound in a patient with peritoneal tuberculosis shows omental thickening ➡ superficial to matted bowel ➡. There is a small amount of ascites ➡. (Right) Coronal transvaginal color Doppler ultrasound of the left adnexa shows ascites ➡, thick malignant peritoneum with color flow ➡, and a solid peritoneal mass ➡. This was primary peritoneal serous carcinoma.*

DIFFERENTIAL DIAGNOSIS

Common

- Abscess
- Organizing Hematoma
- Complicated Ascites
- Pancreatic Pseudocyst
- Cystic Ovarian Masses

Less Common

- Paraovarian/Paratubal Cyst
- Localized Collections
  - Biloma, Urinoma, CSF Pseudocyst
- Pedunculated Cyst/Diverticula
- Peritoneal Inclusion Cyst
- Cystic Non Ovarian Malignant Neoplasm
  - Cystic Metastasis
  - Pseudomyxoma Peritonei
  - Pedunculated Cystic Tumor
    - Gastrointestinal Stromal Tumor (GIST)
    - Cystic Leiomyosarcoma
    - Pancreatic Mucinous Cystadenoma/Cystadenocarcinoma
  - Cystic Mesenchymal Tumor
    - Malignant Fibrous Histiocytoma
    - Synovial Sarcoma
- Cystic Benign Neoplasm
  - Mesenteric Teratoma
  - Multicystic Mesothelioma
- Cystic Lymph Nodes

Rare but Important

- Mesenteric/Omental Cyst
  - Lymphangioma
  - Nonpancreatic Pseudocyst
  - Enteric Duplication Cyst
  - Enteric Cyst
  - Mesothelial Cyst
- Urachal Cyst/Abscess
- Infarcted Accessory Spleen

ESSENTIAL INFORMATION

Key Differential Diagnosis Issues

- Lesions with relevant history
  - Abscess, organizing hematoma
- Lesions with characteristic appearances
  - Peritoneal inclusion cyst, pseudomyxoma peritonei, mature teratoma (dermoid), enteric duplication cyst
- Lesions with thin-walled cystic appearance unless complicated
  - Mesenteric/omental cysts
  - Pedunculated cyst from adjacent organs
- Lesions with complicated appearance
  - Any cystic neoplasm mentioned above or cystic lesion with complication (infection/hemorrhage)
  - Bowel wall origin suggests GIST
  - Other lesions nonspecific, need clinical information to make specific diagnosis and biopsy/aspiration to confirm

Helpful Clues for Common Diagnoses

- **Abscess**
  - Pyogenic
    - Unilocular/multiloculated; thin-/thick-walled plus debris-fluid level
    - Echogenic foci with "ring-down" artifacts/"dirty" shadow = gas
      - Consider infection with gas forming organism or bowel leak
    - Occasionally, surgical hemostatic agents (cellulose) will mimic gas-containing collection, surgical history is key
  - Tuberculous
    - With features of TB peritonitis or GI/renal/mesenteric lymph node involvement
  - Parasitic
    - Hydatid disease: 12% affects peritoneum
    - Variable appearance ranging from heterogeneous solid-looking mass to complex cystic mass
- **Organizing Hematoma**
  - History of trauma, coagulopathy, or anticoagulant therapy
  - Organization with liquefaction in subacute to chronic stage
  - Localized collection with multiple thick septa horizontally aligned ± layering debris
  - May be difficult to determine origin with ultrasound
- **Complicated Ascites**
  - Infection, hemorrhage, inflammation
  - Septations and loculation develop over time
    - Multiple, thick, irregular septa in chronic cases
- **Cystic Ovarian Masses**
  - Benign and malignant cystic neoplasms
  - Mucinous and serous cystadenoma and cystadenocarcinoma
  - Mature cystic teratoma
  - Variable appearances depending on pathology

Helpful Clues for Less Common Diagnoses

- **Paraovarian/Paratubal Cyst**
  - Typically small and simple, separate from ovary
- **Localized Collections**
  - Urinomas, lymphoceles, bilomas
  - CSF pseudocyst associated with ventriculoperitoneal shunt, due to inflammation or infection
    - Cysts are close to shunt tip and contain tubing
- **Pedunculated Cyst/Diverticula**
  - Hepatic, splenic, renal cyst, or GI diverticula
  - Origin may be difficult to trace
  - May cause abdominal pain and palpable mass if hemorrhagic or infected
- **Peritoneal Inclusion Cyst**
  - Fluid conforming to peritoneal cavity with internal septa producing multilocular lesion
  - Low-resistance flow sometimes present in septa from vessels in mesothelial lining
  - May appear complicated if containing debris/hemorrhage
  - Loculated fluid may surround normal ipsilateral ovary and produce characteristic "spider in web" appearance

○ Women of reproductive age with history of surgery, pelvic inflammation, or pelvic adhesions

- **Cystic Non Ovarian Malignant Neoplasm**
  - ○ **Cystic Metastasis**
    - – Most common: ovarian or endometrial carcinoma, GIST
    - – Thick irregular wall to thin-walled (especially after imatinib treatment for GIST)
  - ○ **Pseudomyxoma Peritonei**
    - – Characteristic appearance of voluminous, septated pseudoascites containing punctate poorly mobile echoes
    - – Irregular soft tissue mass with cystic spaces
    - – Typically from cystadenocarcinoma of ovary or appendix; also associated with several other tumors
  - ○ **Pedunculated Cystic Tumor**
    - – GIST: Exophytic from bowel or arising in omentum and mesentery
      - □ Often solid with varying necrosis
    - – Cystic pancreatic neoplasm
  - ○ **Cystic Mesenchymal Tumor**
    - – Rare, but malignant fibrous histiocytoma is most common histologic type
    - – Varies from thick irregular wall (with central necrosis) to completely cystic ± mural nodule plus debris/hemorrhage
  - ○ **Malignant Cystic Mesothelioma**
    - – Dry or wet types
    - – Confluent peritoneal tumor with ascites, peritoneal masses, and omental cake
- **Cystic Benign Neoplasm**
  - ○ **Mesenteric Teratoma**
    - – Purely cystic (10-15%), complex cystic (66%), predominantly solid (10-13%)
    - – Fat-fluid level is characteristic (chylous pseudocyst is mimic)
    - – Tooth (calcification) and hair are specific
- **Cystic Lymph Nodes**
  - ○ Tuberculosis, metastatic (cervix, ovary), inflammatory (celiac disease)

Helpful Clues for Rare Diagnoses
- **Mesenteric/Omental Cyst**
  - ○ **Lymphangioma**
    - – Pediatric patients; mesenteric more common than bowel lymphangioma
    - – insinuate between bowel loops and mesentery exerting mass effect
    - – Multilocular, thin walled, thin septa; anechoic > hypoechoic or fluid fluid debris levels
  - ○ **Nonpancreatic Pseudocyst**
    - – Rare septated cysts with thick fibrous capsule and internal debris (hemorrhage, pus, serous, or chylous fluid
    - – Sequelae of infection, trauma, surgery
  - ○ **Enteric Duplication Cyst**
    - – Uncommon congenital abnormality
    - – Anywhere in alimentary tract along mesenteric side; ileum is most common site
    - – Unilocular thick-walled cyst with mucosa and muscle layer producing double layer in wall ± peristalsis
  - ○ **Enteric Cyst**
    - – Thin-walled unilocular cyst within mesentery or mesocolon
    - – Single mucosal layer without muscle layer
  - ○ **Mesothelial Cyst**
    - – Anechoic, thin-walled, nonseptated cysts on small bowel, mesentery, or mesocolon
- **Urachal Cyst/Abscess**
  - ○ In midline, anywhere between dome of urinary bladder and umbilicus
  - ○ Complicated appearance of abscess may mimic urachal carcinoma
- **Hydatid Infection**
  - ○ Peritoneal seeding from hepatic, splenic, mesenteric cysts
  - ○ Uni or multilocular cysts with internal daughter cysts, membranes or matrix

Abscess

Abscess

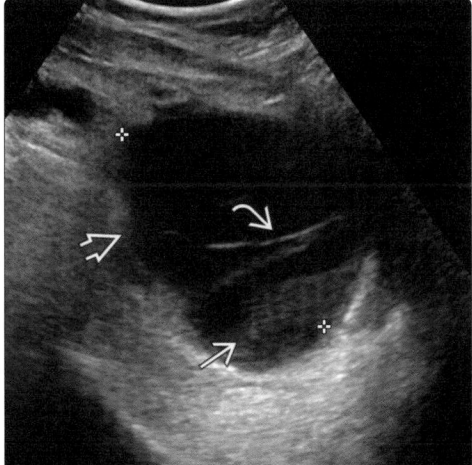

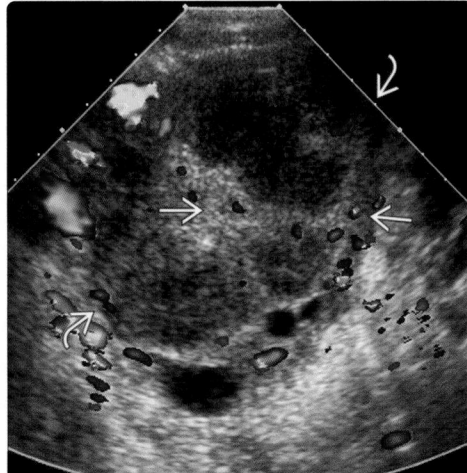

(Left) *Longitudinal transabdominal ultrasound of the pelvis shows a loculated abscess ➡ with layering dependent debris ➡ and septa ➡. **(Right)** Transverse ultrasound of a tubo-ovarian abscess in a teenager shows a multiloculated collection ➡ with internal debris. Color flow is noted in the thick wall and thick septa ➡.*

Organizing Hematoma

Complicated Ascites

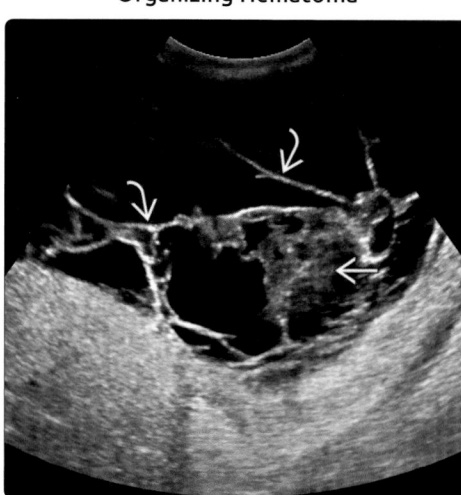
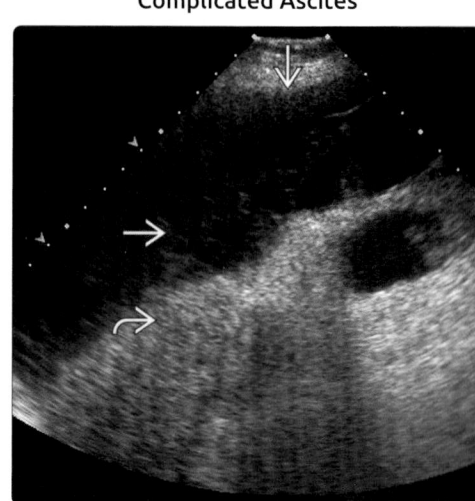

(Left) *Transverse ultrasound of the pelvis post renal transplant shows a complex fluid collection with multiple internal septa of varying thickness ➡. Avascular clot is also noted ➡ in this organizing hematoma.* **(Right)** *Longitudinal ultrasound of peritonitis secondary to a perforated gastric ulcer in patient with cirrhosis. The omental fat ➡ is echogenic and inflamed. There are septa in the ascites ➡.*

Pancreatic Pseudocyst

Cystic Ovarian Masses

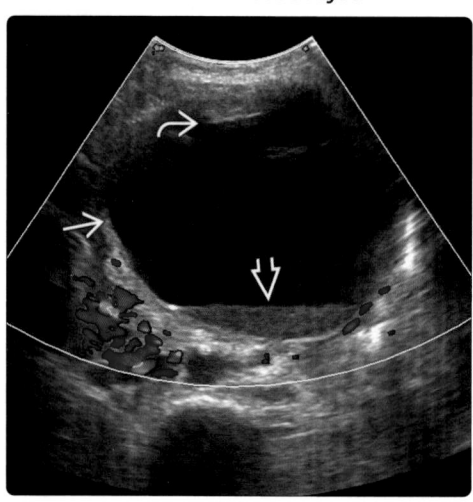
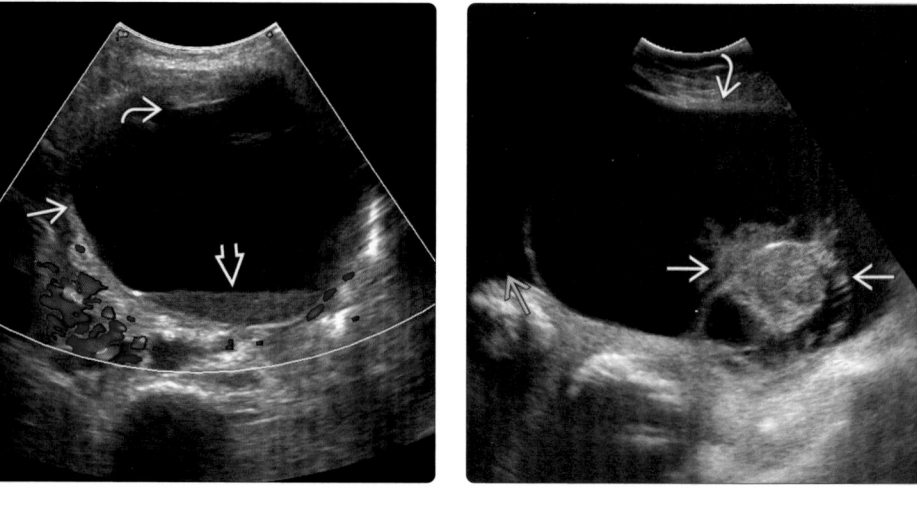

(Left) *Transverse color Doppler ultrasound of the upper abdomen shows a unilocular pancreatic pseudocyst ➡ with avascular dependent debris ➡. There is reverberation artifact ➡ in the near field.* **(Right)** *Transverse pelvic ultrasound in patient with diffuse metastatic disease and elevated CA125 shows a cystic mass ➡ with lobulated solid components ➡ and ascites ➡. Biopsy of an inguinal node showed poorly differentiated adenocarcinoma.*

Paraovarian/Paratubal Cyst

Peritoneal Inclusion Cyst

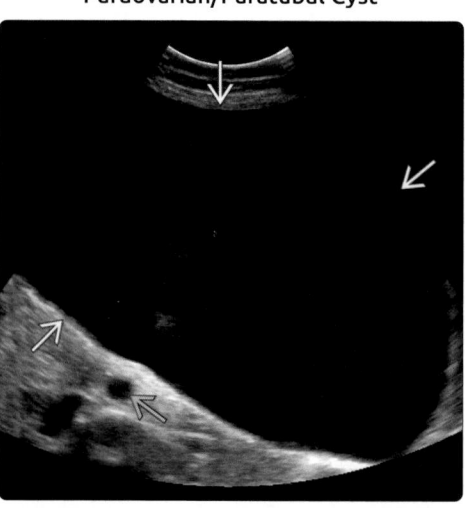
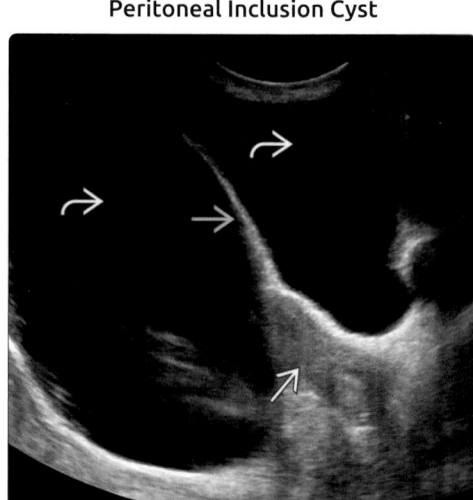

(Left) *Transverse ultrasound shows a very large, unilocular, thin-walled paraovarian cyst ➡ in the central abdomen. Due to its size, the origin could not be determined but the ovaries were normal. Note the aorta ➡.* **(Right)** *Longitudinal ultrasound of pelvic peritoneal inclusion cysts shows large fluid collections ➡ with intervening septa ➡ conforming to the peritoneal cavity and surrounding the uterus ➡. The ovaries were normal. The fluid was drained successfully.*

Pseudomyxoma Peritonei

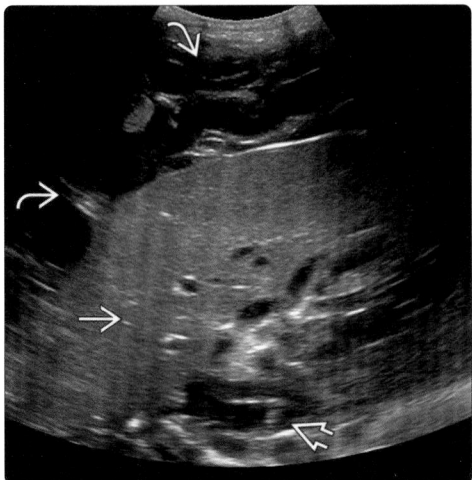

Gastrointestinal Stromal Tumor (GIST)

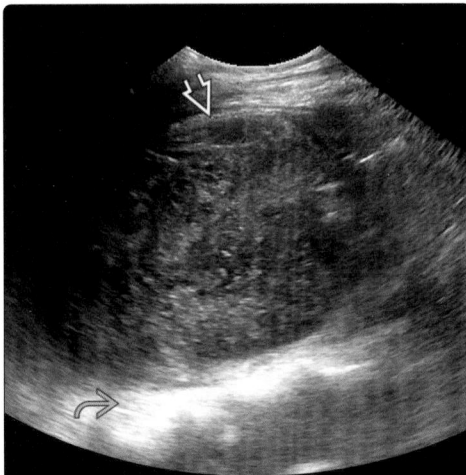

(Left) *Transverse ultrasound demonstrates multiple septa and low-level echoes in pseudomyxoma peritonei anterior ➔ and posterior ➔ to the liver ➔.* (Right) *Longitudinal ultrasound of the left upper quadrant shows a recurrent gastric leiomyosarcoma ➔ post surgery and protein kinase inhibitor. Posterior acoustic enhancement ➔ and lack of internal color flow indicate necrosis and response to treatment.*

Mesenteric Teratoma

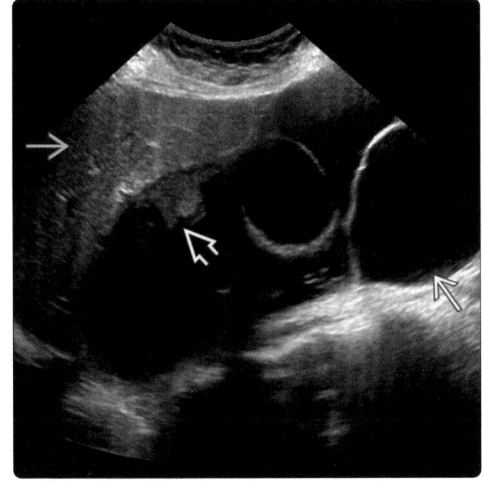

Mesenteric/Omental Cyst

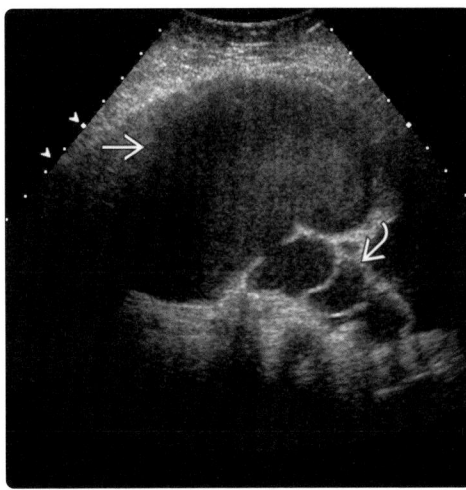

(Left) *Longitudinal ultrasound shows a large cystic ➔ lesion inferior to the liver ➔. Mural nodules ➔ were present and there was fat in this teratoma. It can be difficult to differentiate intraperitoneal from retroperitoneal masses when they are very large.* (Right) *Transverse ultrasound of the mid abdomen region shows a mesenteric cyst ➔ containing low-level echoes with more tubular lymphangiectasia ➔. The wall of the cyst is thin and has a single layer.*

Enteric Duplication Cyst

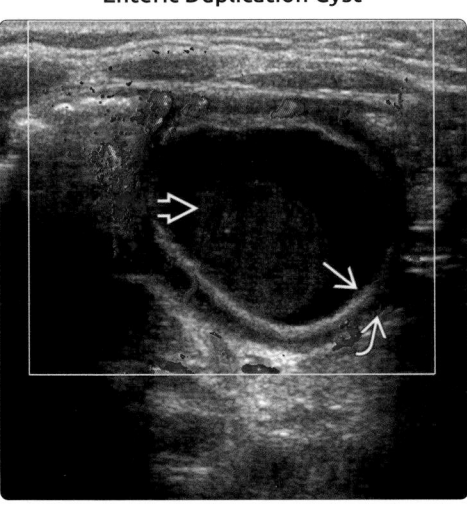

Urachal Cyst/Abscess

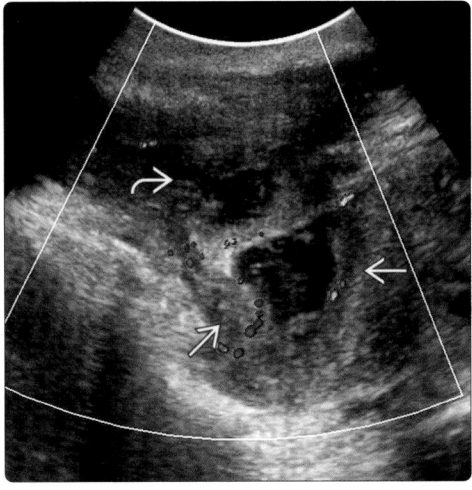

(Left) *Transverse ultrasound shows an ileal duplication cyst with internal debris ➔, The echogenic mucosal ➔ and hypoechoic muscularis ➔ layers confirm that this is of bowel origin.* (Right) *Longitudinal ultrasound of the midline pelvis shows a thick walled urachal abscess ➔ extending to the thickened rectus muscle ➔. Urachal cancer may appear similar, tissue diagnosis is required.*

PART III
SECTION 8
Prostate

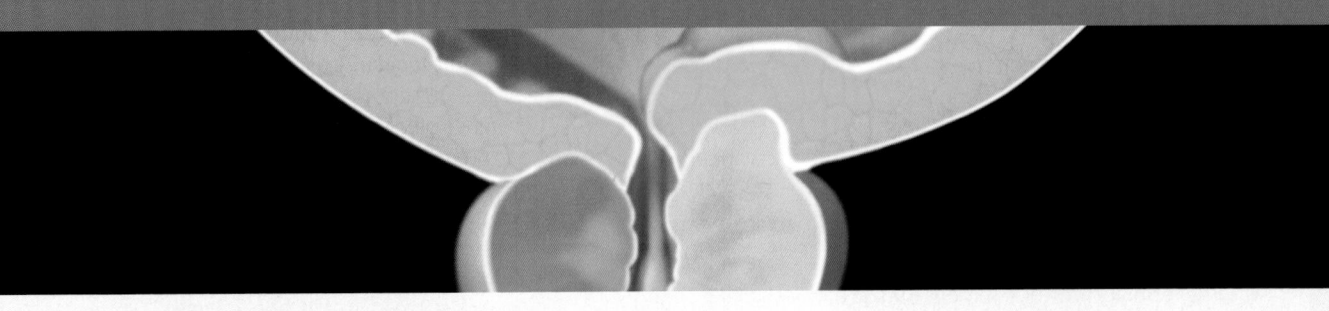

DIFFERENTIAL DIAGNOSIS

Common

- Benign Prostatic Hyperplasia

Less Common

- Prostatic Adenocarcinoma
- Prostatitis ± Abscess
- Prostatic Cyst
- Secondary Involvement of Periprostatic Tumors: Bladder Cancer, Colorectal Adenocarcinoma, or Gastrointestinal Stromal Tumour

Rare but Important

- Other Primary Prostatic Tumors: Benign and Malignant

ESSENTIAL INFORMATION

Helpful Clues for Common Diagnoses

- **Benign Prostatic Hyperplasia**
  - By far, most common cause of prostatomegaly
  - Epithelial and stromal hyperplasia in transition zone (TZ) and periurethral glands
  - Heterogeneously enlarged TZ compressing peripheral and central zones

Helpful Clues for Less Common Diagnoses

- **Prostate Adenocarcinoma**
  - Most cases of prostate cancer do not cause global enlargement
- **Prostatitis ± Abscess**
  - Prostatitis: Diffusely enlarged prostate (but may be normal in size), global vs. focal hypoechogenicity, ↑ glandular or perilesional vascularity
    - Often coexists with urinary tract infection
  - Prostatic abscess: Uni- or multilocular cyst with thick walls/septa and peripheral hyperemia
    - More common in elderly, diabetic, or immunocompromised patients
- **Prostatic Cyst**
  - Large müllerian duct cysts often extend above base

- **Secondary Involvement of Periprostatic Tumors**
  - Urothelial carcinoma of bladder is most common tumor to secondarily infiltrate prostate

Helpful Clues for Rare Diagnoses

- **Other Primary Prostatic Tumors**
  - **(Giant) Multilocular Prostatic Cystadenoma**
    - Large multiseptated cystic pelvic mass
    - Evidence of local invasion excludes this diagnosis
    - Can regenerate and cause recurrent symptoms if incomplete resection
  - **Prostatic Phyllodes Tumor**
    - Large, well-circumscribed mass with variable amounts of cystic and solid components
    - Despite aggressive resection, up to 65% locally recur
    - Up to 39% undergo sarcomatous transformation and may spread to contiguous organs (bladder, colon)
  - **Small Cell and Squamous Cell Carcinomas**
    - Both are very aggressive and do not change serum prostate specific antigen; usually already advanced at time of diagnosis
  - **Prostate Sarcomas**
    - Most common type in children: Rhabdomyosarcoma
    - Most common type in adults: Leiomyosarcoma
    - Predominantly solid, heterogeneous, vascular mass; high-grade tumors show tumor necrosis; occurs more often in younger men (between ages of 35-60)
  - **Prostate Lymphoma**
    - Usually secondary prostate involvement
      - Most reported is chronic lymphocytic leukemia (CLL) or small lymphocytic lymphoma (SLL)
    - Primary prostate lymphomas even more rare

SELECTED REFERENCES

1. Chu LC et al: Prostatic stromal neoplasms: differential diagnosis of cystic and solid prostatic and periprostatic masses. AJR Am J Roentgenol. 200(6):W571-80, 2013
2. Rusch D et al: Giant multilocular cystadenoma of the prostate. AJR Am J Roentgenol. 179(6):1477-9, 2002
3. Warrick JI et al: Diffuse large B-cell lymphoma of the prostate. Arch Pathol Lab Med. 138(10):1286-9, 2014

Benign Prostatic Hyperplasia

Benign Prostatic Hyperplasia

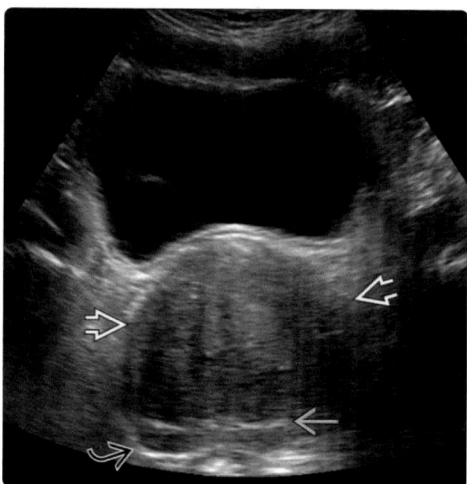
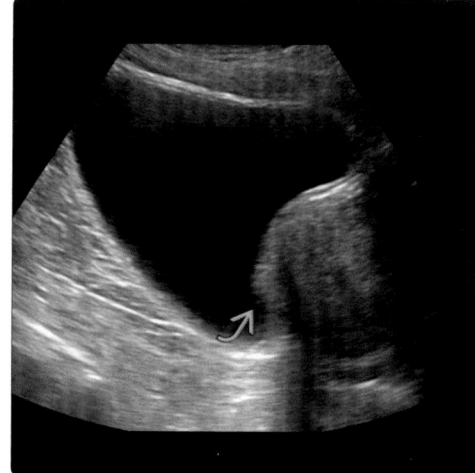

(Left) *Transverse transabdominal sonogram shows marked enlargement of the transition zone (TZ) ➡ causing compression of the peripheral zone (PZ) ➡. Echogenic line represents the pseudocapsule ➡ separating the TZ from PZ.* **(Right)** *Sagittal ultrasound from the same patient shows elevation of the bladder base ➡ by the enlarged TZ.*

Benign Prostatic Hyperplasia

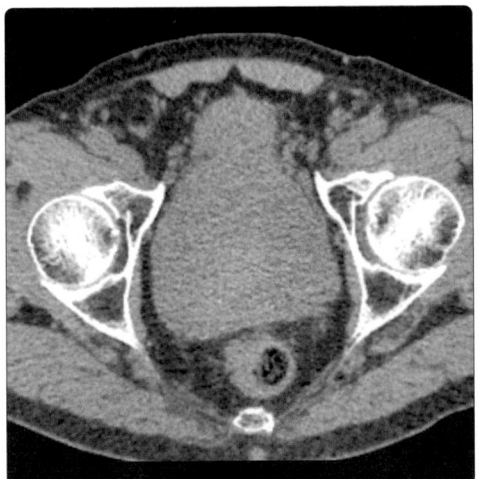

Benign Prostatic Hyperplasia

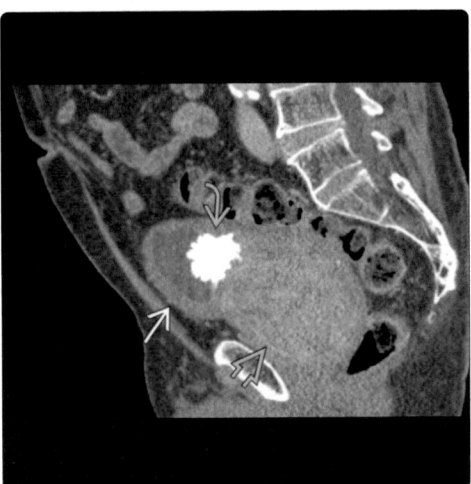

(Left) *Axial NECT shows a markedly enlarged prostate, which is homogeneous with well-defined margins.* (Right) *Sagittal CT in the same patient shows mildly heterogeneous enhancement of the markedly enlarged TZ ⊟. Associated severe bladder wall trabeculation ➡ is consistent with bladder outlet obstruction. Presence of a large jackstone ⊟ within the bladder indicates bladder decompensation.*

Benign Prostatic Hyperplasia

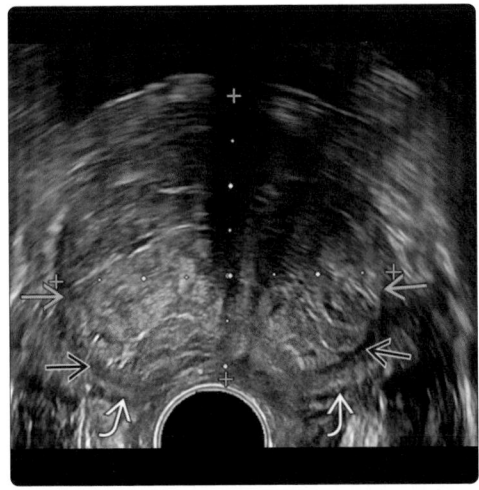

Prostatic Adenocarcinoma

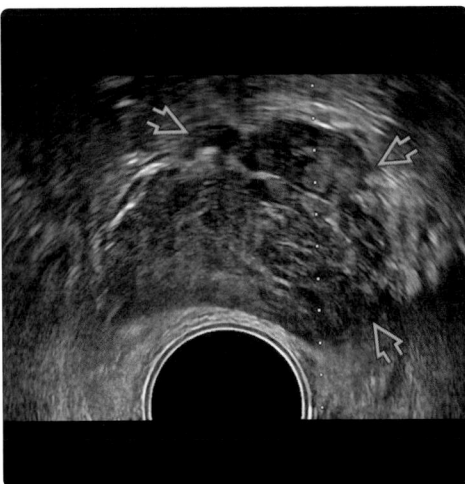

(Left) *Transverse transrectal ultrasound (TRUS) shows heterogeneous enlargement of both lobes of the TZ ⊟. The peripheral zone is severely compressed ➡. Hypoechoic line represents the pseudocapsule ⊟.* (Right) *Transverse TRUS at the level of the apex shows a slightly hypoechoic mass causing asymmetric, nodular enlargement of the left 1/2 of the prostate ⊟. Targeted MR-US fusion biopsy of this mass revealed Gleason 4+5 prostate adenocarcinoma.*

Prostatic Adenocarcinoma

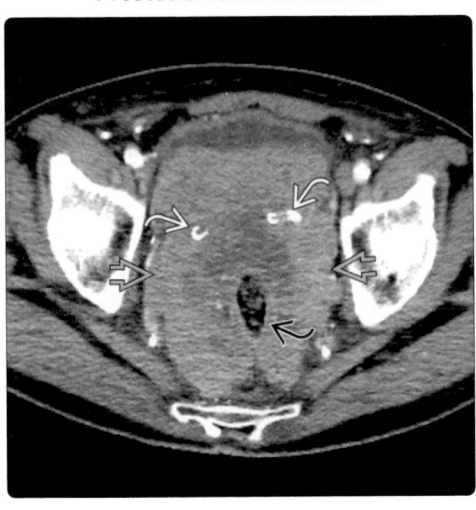

Other Primary Prostatic Tumors: Benign and Malignant

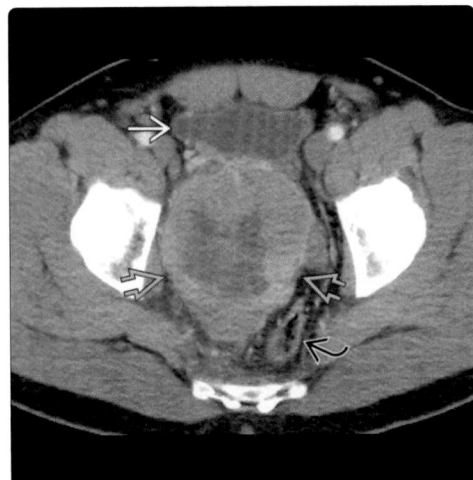

(Left) *Large, centrally necrotic pelvic mass ⊟ encases the rectum ⊿ and calcified vas deferens ⊅. Pathology from TRUS-guided biopsy showed Gleason 5+5 adenocarcinoma.* (Right) *Centrally necrotic, enhancing pelvic mass ⊟ arising from the prostate anteriorly displaces the bladder ⊿. The rectum ⊿ is separate. Surgical pathology from surgical resection revealed prostate sarcoma, not otherwise specified.*

DIFFERENTIAL DIAGNOSIS

Common

- Benign Prostatic Hyperplasia (BPH) Nodules
- Prostatic Calcification
- Prostate Carcinoma (PCa)
- Atypical Small Acinar Proliferation
- Prostatic Intraepithelial Neoplasia (PIN)
- Prostatitis
- Retention Cyst
- Focal Atrophy/Fibrosis

Less Common

- Prostatic Abscess
- Müllerian Duct Cyst
- Utricle Cyst
- Seminal Vesicle Cyst

Rare but Important

- Ejaculatory Duct Cyst
- Vas Deferens Cyst
- Other Primary Prostate Neoplasms
  - Multilocular prostatic cystadenoma, sarcoma, small and squamous cell carcinomas, stromal tumors of uncertain malignant potential
- Secondary Tumors of Prostate

ESSENTIAL INFORMATION

Key Differential Diagnosis Issues

- Focal lesion may be discovered by digital rectal exam (DRE) as incidental finding or part of screening
  - Or in patient with symptoms, signs, or abnormal lab/microbiology studies
    - Fever, pain, dysuria, hematospermia, painful ejaculation, obstructive urinary symptoms
    - ↑ PSA, abnormal urinalysis, UTI
- Location of cystic lesion may help in diagnosis

Helpful Clues for Common Diagnoses

- **BPH Nodules**
  - Enlarged gland with hyper- and hypoechoic nodules; echogenicity dependent on composition
  - Arise in transition zone (TZ) and periurethral glands
  - ± cystic degeneration, which is common, accounts for most cystic prostatic lesions; irregular shapes, various sizes, may contain hemorrhage or calcification
- **Prostatic Calcification**
  - Often incidental finding in asymptomatic men; seen in benign (prostatitis) and malignant (PCa) diseases; significance is poorly understood, possibly dependent on zonal distribution
  - Laminated bodies of secretions and desquamated cells are called corpora amylacea → deposition of calcium crystals → calculi
- **Prostatic Carcinoma (PCa)**
  - ~ 70% originate from peripheral zone (PZ)
  - Often indistinguishable from BPH nodules in TZ
  - Historically, PCa on TRUS described as hypoechoic PZ lesion, but other nonmalignant entities (prostatitis, atrophy, PIN) are also hypoechoic; hypoechoic lesion has 17-57% change of being cancer

- > 30% of PCa are isoechoic
  - Due to earlier cancer detection with PSA, study showed only 9% of hypoechoic nodules contained PCa compared with 10% of isoechoic areas
- **Atypical Small Acinar Proliferation**
  - When needle biopsy shows foci that are probably PCa but either lack definitive diagnostic features or are too small to be certain, they do not represent edge of benign lesion
  - If other cores are negative, rebiopsy is performed
  - ~ 40% of men diagnosed with atypia will have PCa diagnosed on rebiopsy
- **PIN**
  - Prostatic glandular epithelial dysplasia
  - Management of high-grade PIN is controversial; PCa diagnosis on rebiopsy is similar to that in men whose initial biopsies showed normal tissue
- **Prostatitis**
  - Acute: Bacterial infection, *E. coli* is most common causative organism; enlarged gland, but may be normal size; global or focal hypoechogenicity; ↑ global or perilesional vascularity
  - Chronic: Normal-sized gland; heterogeneous ± Ca++
    - Chronic bacterial: Insidious onset; relapsing, recurrent UTI due to persistent infection despite antibiotics
    - Cavitary prostatitis: Fibrosis causes ductal stenoses and acinar dilation → multiple cysts of varying sizes throughout gland → Swiss cheese appearance
    - Granulomatous prostatitis: Rare nodular form of chronic prostatitis; mimics PCa on DRE and imaging; may be seen after BCG therapy for bladder cancer; diagnosis by biopsy
- **Retention Cyst**
  - Common; often asymptomatic; due to obstructed acini
  - Round, unilocular cyst with smooth walls; size ~ 1-2 cm; lateral location
  - May be indistinguishable from cystic BPH nodule

Helpful Clues for Less Common Diagnoses

- **Prostatic Abscess**
  - Most commonly due to acute bacterial prostatitis
  - Complex fluid collection with thick walls/septa and peripheral hyperemia ± internal debris ± gas
  - TRUS is preferred method of evaluation; can perform aspiration for diagnosis and therapy
- **Müllerian Duct Cyst**
  - Failure of regression of müllerian duct remnants
  - Typically diagnosed in patients between 20-40 years; reported prevalence of 5%
  - Midline but may be slightly paramidline; classically teardrop-shaped cyst; no communication with urethra
  - Usually large, can extend above prostatic base ± calculi; malignancy reported
  - Differentiation from utricle cyst is difficult; not associated with GU anomalies
- **Utricle Cyst**
  - Dilation of müllerian duct remnant
  - Typically diagnosed in patients < 20 years; reported prevalence 1-5%
  - Midline arising from verumontanum

- o Variable size but usually smaller (< 10 mm) than müllerian duct cysts; does not extend above prostate base
- o Associated with GU anomalies: Hypospadias, undescended testes, and unilateral renal agenesis; malignancy reported
- o Complications: Infection, hemorrhage, may cause postvoid dribbling (communicates with urethra)
- **Seminal Vesicle Cyst**
  - o Lateral cyst; variable size; congenital or acquired
  - o Unilateral → associated with ipsilateral renal agenesis/dysgenesis, ectopic ureteral insertion, vas deferens agenesis
  - o Bilateral → associated with autosomal dominant polycystic kidney disease

Helpful Clues for Rare Diagnoses

- **Ejaculatory Duct Cyst**
  - o Congenital or acquired obstruction of ejaculatory duct
  - o Paramedian cyst at base, may appear midline at or just above level of verumontanum ± intracystic calculi
  - o Spermatozoa in cyst fluid
- **Vas Deferens Cyst**
  - o Extraprostatic, superior to gland; congenital or acquired
- **Other Primary Prostate Neoplasms**
  - o **Multilocular prostatic cystadenoma**
    - – Rare benign tumor; large multiseptated cystic pelvic mass
  - o **Prostate sarcoma**
    - – Occurs more often in younger men (35-60 years)
    - – Predominantly solid, heterogeneous, vascular mass; high-grade tumors show necrosis
  - o **Cystic prostatic adenocarcinoma**
    - – Very rare, 0.6% prostatic carcinomas
    - – Thick-walled cystic mass with mural nodularity
- **Secondary Tumors of Prostate**
  - o Extension of periprostatic malignancy, lymphoma, metastases
  - o Bladder cancer is most common tumor to secondarily infiltrate prostate

- o Prostate lymphoma and metastases to prostate are both very rare
- o Prostate lymphoma is usually secondary; primary prostatic lymphoma is exceedingly rare
- o Metastases to prostate described in melanoma, lung cancer, and testicular cancer

Other Essential Information

- **Mimics of prostatic and periprostatic cysts**
  - o TURP defect
  - o Bladder diverticula
  - o Ectopic ureteral insertion, ureterocele
  - o Malpositioned Foley catheter balloon

Alternative Differential Approaches

- **Cystic lesion**
  - o Intraprostatic
    - – Median: Müllerian and utricle duct cysts
    - – Paramedian: Ejaculatory duct cyst
    - – Lateral: Retention cysts, cystic degeneration of BPH
    - – Variable: Cystic neoplasms, abscess
  - o Extraprostatic
    - – Seminal vesicle and vas deferens cysts
- **Solid lesion**
  - o Central: BPH nodules, PCa
  - o Peripheral: PCa, atypia, PIN, prostatitis, fibrosis/atrophy

SELECTED REFERENCES

1. Dorin RP et al: Prostate atypia: Does repeat biopsy detect clinically significant prostate cancer? Prostate. 75(7):673-8, 2015
2. Smolski M et al: Prevalence of prostatic calcification subtypes and association with prostate cancer. Urology. 85(1):178-81, 2015
3. Chu LC et al: Prostatic stromal neoplasms: differential diagnosis of cystic and solid prostatic and periprostatic masses. AJR Am J Roentgenol. 200(6):W571-80, 2013
4. Shebel HM et al: Cysts of the lower male genitourinary tract: embryologic and anatomic considerations and differential diagnosis. Radiographics. 33(4):1125-43, 2013
5. Schull A et al: Imaging in lower urinary tract infections. Diagn Interv Imaging. 93(6):500-8, 2012
6. Galosi AB et al: Cystic lesions of the prostate gland: an ultrasound classification with pathological correlation. J Urol. 181(2):647-57, 2009
7. Curran S et al: Endorectal MRI of prostatic and periprostatic cystic lesions and their mimics. AJR Am J Roentgenol. 188(5):1373-9, 2007

Benign Prostatic Hyperplasia (BPH) Nodules

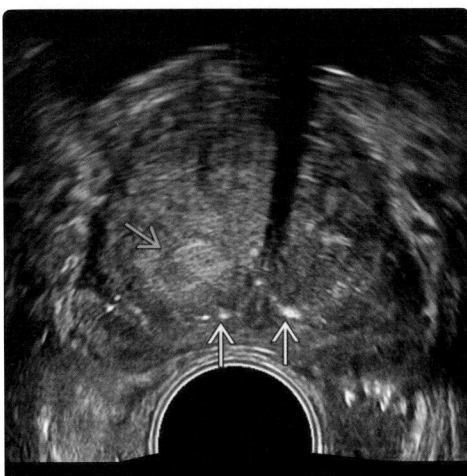

Benign Prostatic Hyperplasia (BPH) Nodules

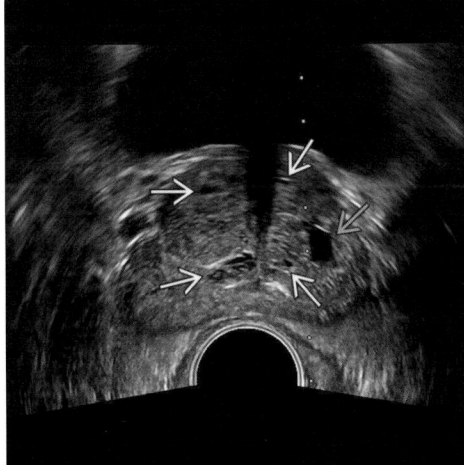

(Left) Transverse TRUS image shows a well-defined relatively homogeneous hyperechoic nodule in the right transition zone (TZ) ➡ consistent with a benign prostatic hypertrophy nodule. Calcifications ➡ are seen in the periurethral region and along the surgical capsule. (Right) Transverse transrectal ultrasound (TRUS) shows multiple small cystic lesions within the enlarged TZ, most consistent with retention cysts ➡. A larger anechoic, simple cyst in the left TZ likely represents cystic degeneration of a BPH nodule ➡.

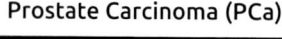

Prostate Carcinoma (PCa)

Prostate Carcinoma (PCa)

(Left) *TRUS image shows a hypoechoic left peripheral zone (PZ) lesion* ⇨ *with bulging of the left lateral prostate contour* ⇨ *& thickening of the left neurovascular bundle (NVB)* ⇨*. A smaller hypoechoic lesion is in the right PZ* ⇨*.* (Right) *Color Doppler shows focal hypervascularity of the left PZ lesion & mild hypervascularity of the right PZ lesion. Prostatectomy pathology showed multifocal cancer, including left PZ Gleason 5+5 adenocarcinoma with left extraprostatic extension and NVB invasion.*

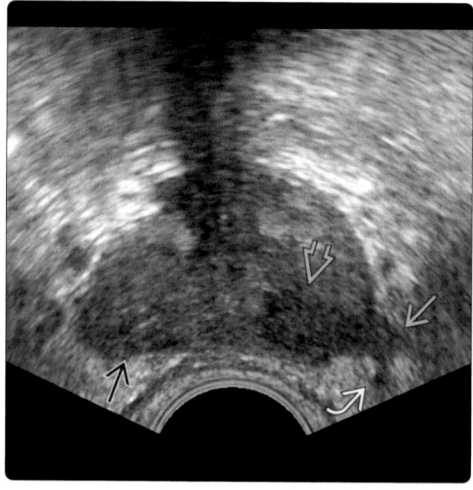

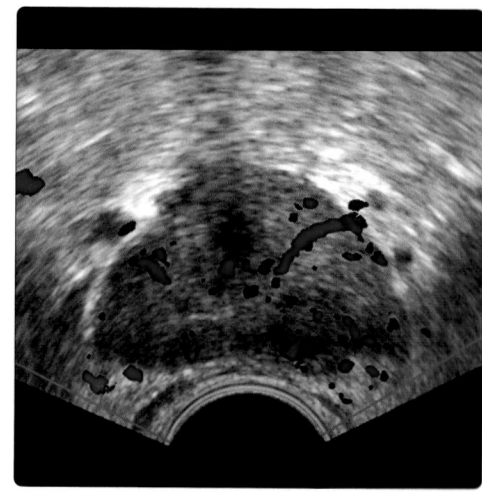

Prostate Carcinoma (PCa)

Prostate Carcinoma (PCa)

(Left) *TRUS image performed during MR-US fusion biopsy shows a hypoechoic target (outlined in red) within the left transition zone. Ruler shows the planned biopsy tract. Pathology showed Gleason 4+5 adenocarcinoma.* (Right) *Transverse transabdominal image demonstrates multiple, small, shadowing, bright reflectors* ⇨ *scattered throughout the prostate corresponding to brachytherapy seeds.*

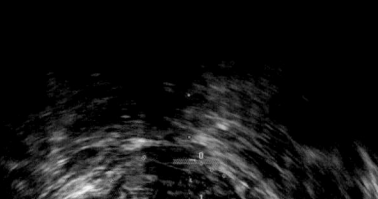

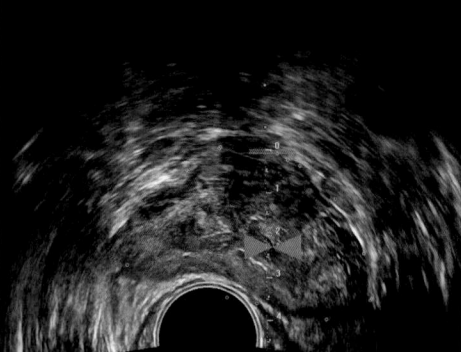

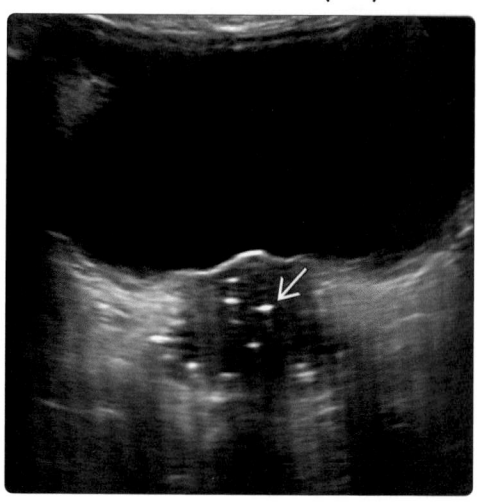

Prostatitis

Prostatitis

(Left) *TRUS image shows focal hypoechogenicity in the left peripheral zone* ⇨ *with mild bulging of the contour* ⇨*. Periurethral and transition zone calcifications* ⇨ *are present.* (Right) *Color Doppler image shows focal hypervascularity in this region* ⇨*. Pathology from targeted biopsies of this region showed focal prostatitis.*

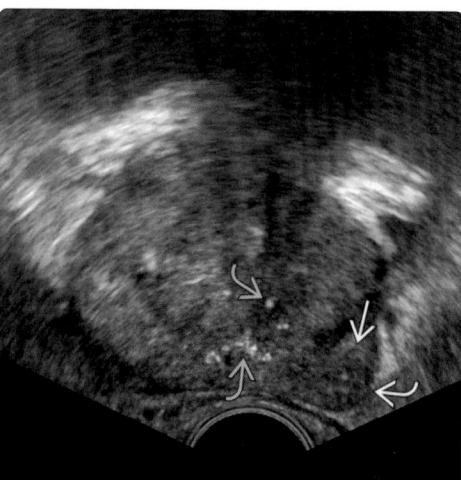

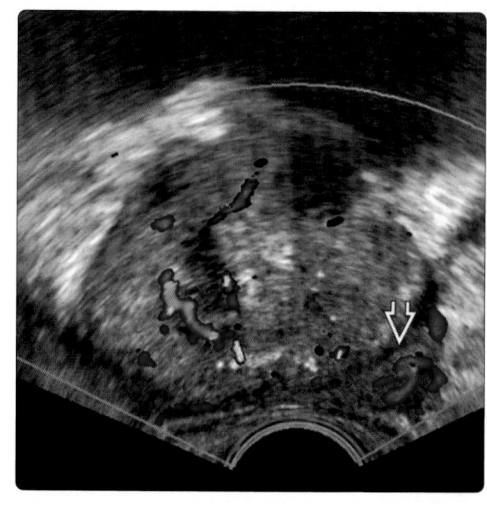

Müllerian Duct Cyst

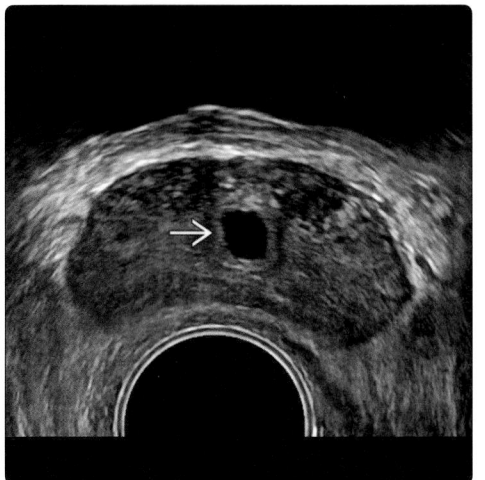

Müllerian Duct Cyst

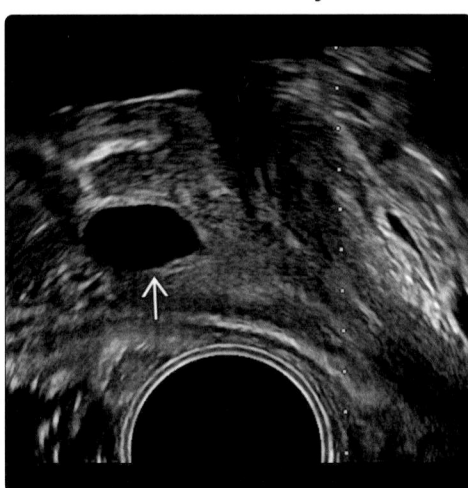

(Left) *TRUS at the level of the prostate base shows a midline unilocular cystic structure* ➡. (Right) *Sagittal image in the same patient shows the teardrop shape of the cyst* ➡ *with extension just beyond the prostate base. Findings are most consistent with a müllerian duct cyst.*

Müllerian Duct Cyst

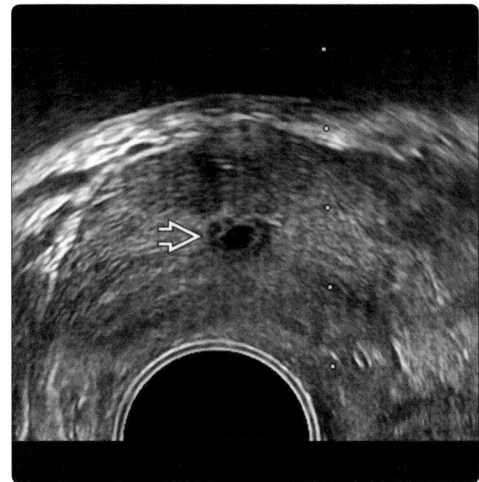

Müllerian Duct Cyst

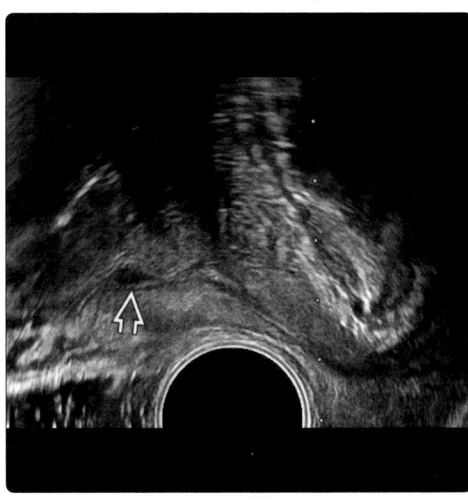

(Left) *TRUS image in a 65-year-old man at the level of the prostate base shows a small midline cyst with hypoechoic halo* ➡. (Right) *On sagittal image, this cyst has a teardrop shape* ➡ *but does not extend beyond the prostate base and possibly communicates with the urethra. Patient's age and absence of other GU abnormalities favor a müllerian duct cyst rather than utricle cyst, but these are often indistinguishable. Mild wall thickening may be due to inflammation or superimposed infection.*

Retention Cyst

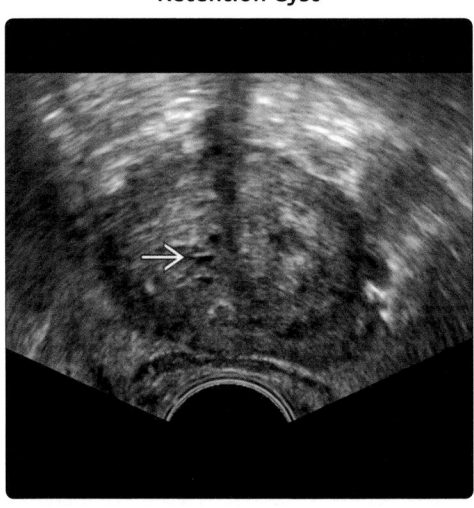

Prostatic Abscess

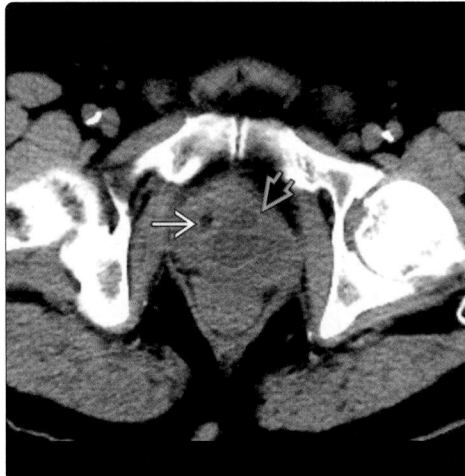

(Left) *TRUS shows several tiny cysts within the enlarged transition zone* ➡, *likely reflecting retention cysts.* (Right) *Axial noncontrast CT shows a lobulated, cystic mass within the left prostate gland* ➡, *causing rightward deviation of a urethral catheter* ➡. *In this patient with fever and UTI, findings are consistent with a prostatic abscess. The patient subsequently underwent TRUS-guided drainage.*

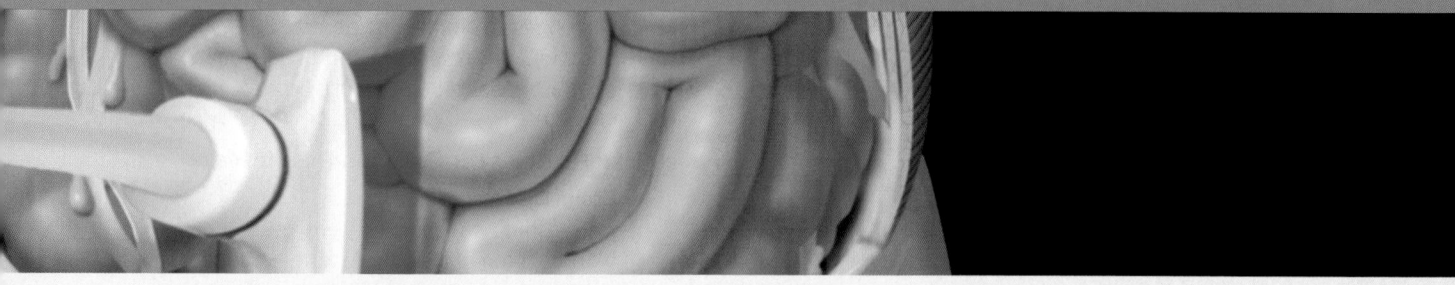

Bowel Wall Thickening   1000

DIFFERENTIAL DIAGNOSIS

Common

- Inflammatory Bowel Disease (IBD)
  - Crohn Disease
  - Ulcerative Colitis
- Bowel Neoplasms
  - Adenocarcinoma
  - Lymphoma
  - Carcinoid
  - Gastrointestinal Stromal Tumors
- Diverticulosis/Diverticulitis
- Intussusception
- Intestinal Ischemia
  - Primary
    - Acute Arterial Ischemia
    - Acute Venous Ischemia
  - Secondary
    - Secondary to Closed Loop Obstruction
  - Ischemic Colitis
- Acute Infective Enteritis/Colitis
- Reactive Thickening Adjacent to Inflammatory Process
  - Appendicitis, Cholecystitis
- Chronic Edema
  - Portal Hypertension
  - Hypoproteinemia
- Acute Edema
  - Prestenotic in Acute Bowel Obstruction

Less Common

- Tuberculosis
- Clostridium Difficile Colitis
- Mural Hemorrhage
- Deep Infiltrative Endometriosis
- Post-Radiation Enteritis
- Excess Fat Deposition in Bowel Wall
- Cystic Fibrosis

Rare but Important

- Vasculitis
  - Systemic Lupus Erythematosus
- Graft-vs.-Host Reaction
- Intestinal Amyloidosis
- Systemic Mastocytosis
  - Inflammatory Bowel Disease (Mimic)
- Behçet Disease
  - Crohn Colitis (Mimic)
- Intestinal Lymphangiectasia

ESSENTIAL INFORMATION

Key Differential Diagnosis Issues

- Clinical presentation is important
  - Overlapping findings from different causes
- Identify site of involvement
  - Stomach, small bowel, or large bowel
- When there is thickening, map bowel upstream and downstream
- Comment on
  - Diffuse or focal thickening

- When diffuse, length involved, and degree of thickening
- Mural flow and surrounding vascularity with color flow and power Doppler
- Assess for preservation/absence of mural stratification
- Assess and comment on the perienteric/pericolonic fat
- Observe and comment on peristalsis
- Comment on presence of peritoneal free fluid
- Contrast-enhanced US useful is assessing activity of IBD, inflammatory thickening, and bowel wall ischemia

Helpful Clues for Common Diagnoses

- **Crohn Disease**
  - Transmural inflammatory process
  - Most commonly occurs in terminal ileum
  - Usually noncompressible, rigid, and fixed
  - Wall thickening is symmetrical and circumferential
    - May be continuous or skipped
  - Hypertrophy of the mesenteric fat
  - Echogenic tissue "creeping fat" extending to antimesenteric surface of bowel
  - Mural stratification gut signature is usually preserved
    - Prominent widened echogenic submucosal layer is seen due to fibrofatty proliferation
    - In some, there is loss of gut signature, which is more common in active disease
  - Associated luminal narrowing
    - Inflammatory or fibrotic
  - Power Doppler useful in showing mural increased vascularity and engorged vasa recta: Comb sign
  - Bowel fistulation and abscess formation from deep penetrating ulcers can be detected
  - Involved segment shows aperistalsis or moderately reduced peristalsis
- **Ulcerative Colitis**
  - Mucosal inflammatory process
    - Thickening is mild with loss of haustra coli
    - Mural stratification is preserved
  - Continuous involvement of colon
  - Suspect toxic megacolon when
    - Wall thickness reduced, gaseous distension, ascites
- **Adenocarcinoma**
  - Segmental annular lesion
    - Affects short segment
    - May be associated with bowel obstruction
  - Focal mass ± ulceration
  - Loss of mural stratification
  - Extra mural tumor infiltration may be visible
- **Lymphoma**
  - Most commonly occurs in stomach, small intestine, colon, and esophagus in decreasing order of frequency
  - Loss of gut signature
  - Morphology
    - Segmental circumferential, focal mass, or multifocal bowel wall involvement
    - Extramural spread into mesentery
  - Dilatation of bowel lumen may be seen
    - Rarely results in bowel obstruction
  - ± hepatosplenomegaly, lymph node enlargement
- **Carcinoid**
  - Most common small bowel tumor

- – Distal ileum is most frequent site
- o Initially seen as hypoechoic mass confined to submucosal layer
  - – In late stages, extramural tumor extension with infiltration into mesentery and desmoplastic reaction giving characteristic "sunburst" pattern
  - – Mesenteric masses similar echogenicity to primary
    - ▫ Can demonstrate calcification
- **Gastrointestinal Stromal Tumors**
  - o Most commonly located in stomach, followed by small bowel
  - o May be seen intraluminal or as exophytic mass
    - – May show central necrosis with cavitation, which may be in communication with bowel lumen
    - – Variable echogenicity on ultrasound
  - o Lymph node metastases rare
- **Diverticulosis/Diverticulitis**
  - o Thickened muscularis propria
  - o Presence of diverticula
    - – Thin-walled outpouching containing gas or feces
  - o Diverticulitis
    - – Thick-walled diverticulum
    - – Surrounding inflamed echogenic fat
    - – Increased mural and peri colonic vascularity
- **Intussusception**
  - o Telescoping of proximal segment of bowel into adjacent distal segment of bowel
  - o Bowel within bowel appearance
    - – Target sign in cross section
  - o Proximal bowel dilatation may be seen
    - – Complete obstruction rare
- **Intestinal Ischemia**
  - o Clinical findings important
  - o Long segment involved
  - o Mural stratification preserved (unless becoming hemorrhagic)
  - o Assess adjacent structures, mesenteric vasculature, obstruction, predisposing conditions
- **Acute Infective Enteritis/Colitis**

- o Clinical presentation important with microbiologic confirmation
- o Edematous bowel wall; mural stratification preserved
- o Usually long segment involved
- o Findings overlap with radiation enteritis, reactive thickening, & prestenotic edema

Helpful Clues for Less Common Diagnoses

- **Tuberculosis**
  - o Preferential thickening of cecum and ileocecal valve
  - o Necrotic lymph nodes
  - o Inflammatory mass or stricturing
  - o Loss of mural stratification
- **Clostridium Difficile Colitis**
  - o Usually pancolitis
  - o Marked mural edema with widened submucosal layer
  - o Pronounced haustral pattern; accordion sign
- **Mural Hemorrhage**
  - o Long segment involved
  - o Homogeneous hypoechoic symmetric thickening
  - o Associated with luminal effacement
  - o Mural stratification may or may not be preserved
  - o Vascularity variable from normal to absent on Doppler assessment
  - o Causes
    - – Anticoagulant treatment, vasculitis, ischemic bowel, coagulation disorders
- **Deep Infiltrative Endometriosis**
  - o Rectosigmoid, appendix, caecum, and distal ileum
  - o Focal eccentric thickening & widening of muscular layer

SELECTED REFERENCES

1. Muradali D et al: US of gastrointestinal tract disease. Radiographics. 35(1):50-68, 2015
2. Razzaq R et al: Ultrasound diagnosis of clinically undetected Clostridium difficile toxin colitis. Clin Radiol. 61(5):446-52, 2006
3. Di Mizio R et al: Small bowel Crohn disease: sonographic features. Abdom Imaging. 29(1):23-35, 2004
4. O'Malley ME et al: US of gastrointestinal tract abnormalities with CT correlation. Radiographics. 23(1):59-72, 2003

Crohn Disease

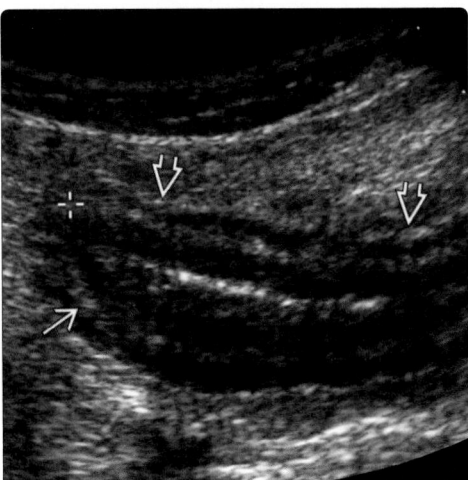

Crohn Disease

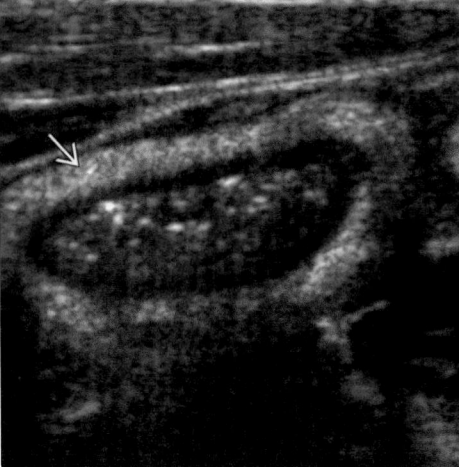

(Left) Oblique axial US through the right iliac fossa shows an inflamed thickened segment ➡ of the distal ileum from Crohn disease. Note symmetrical thickening with preservation of the gut signature. Prominent echogenic submucosal layer ➡ is seen. (Right) Short axis US of an inflamed segment of bowel with Crohn disease shows a target-like appearance due to the preserved mural stratification (gut signature). The echogenic layer ➡ represents thickened submucosal layer from fibrofatty proliferation.

(Left) *Oblique axial US through the right iliac fossa (RIF) shows symmetrical thickening of the terminal ileum* ➡ *with preservation of gut signature.* **(Right)** *Power Doppler US in the same patient shows increased flow. Note the surrounding echogenic fat* ➡ *and deep penetrating ulcer* ➡, *appearances representing active Crohn disease.*

Crohn Disease
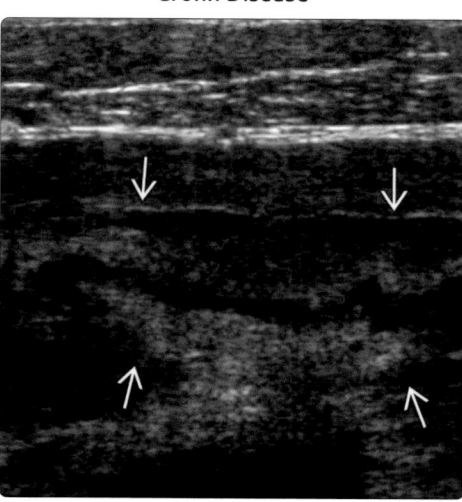

Crohn Disease
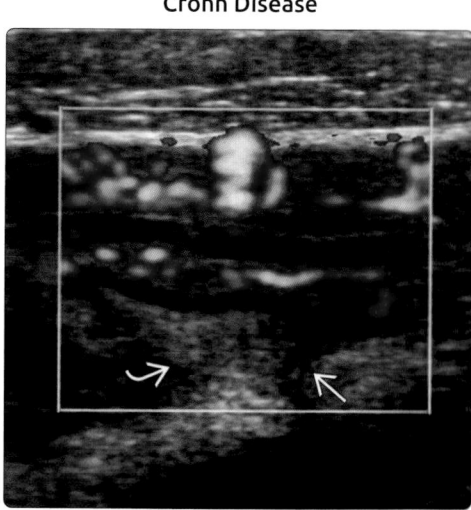

(Left) *Long axis US of terminal ileum shows marked mural thickening with loss of normal mural stratification, appearances representing active Crohn disease with acute inflammatory infiltration. Note the central luminal narrowing* ➡ *from gross inflammatory thickening* ➡. **(Right)** *Short axis US of the same segment shows loss of mural stratification. Note central luminal narrowing* ➡ *and surrounding echogenic inflamed fat* ➡.

Crohn Disease
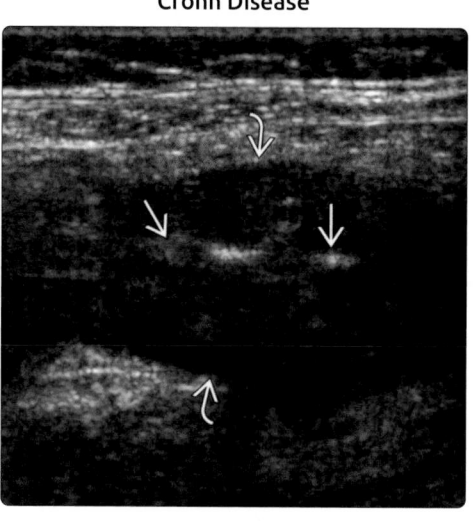

Crohn Disease
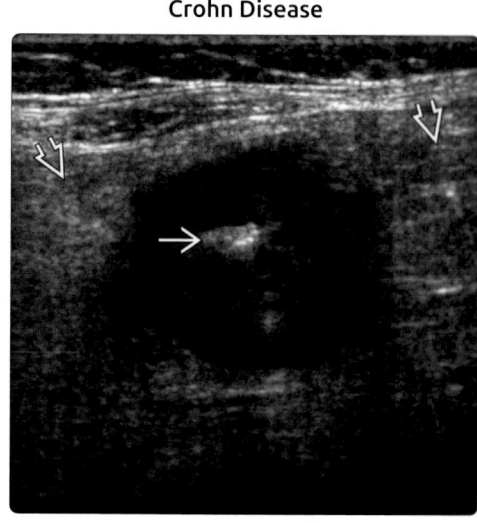

(Left) *Power Doppler US of the same segment shows increased mural flow* ➡, *supporting active disease.* **(Right)** *Power Doppler US in the same patient shows engorged vasa recta, representing ultrasound equivalent of comb sign* ➡.

Crohn Disease
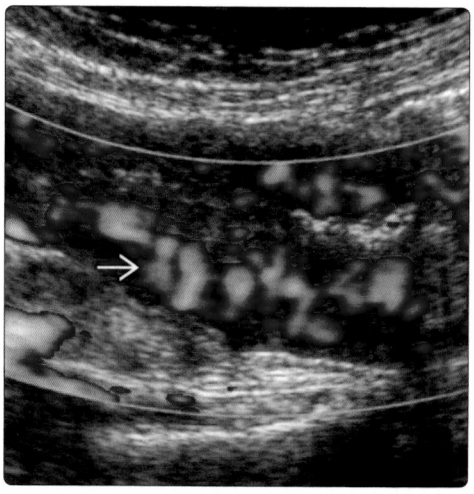

Crohn Disease
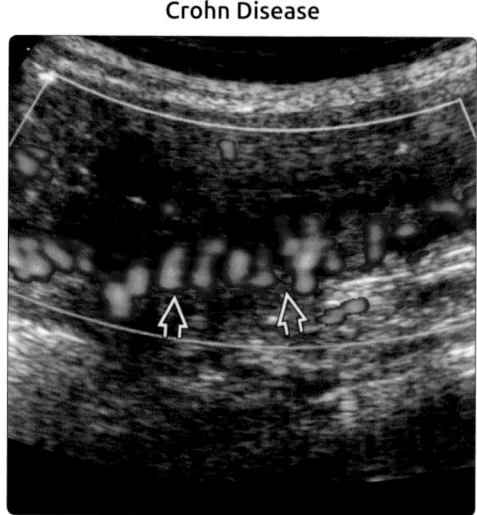

Crohn Disease

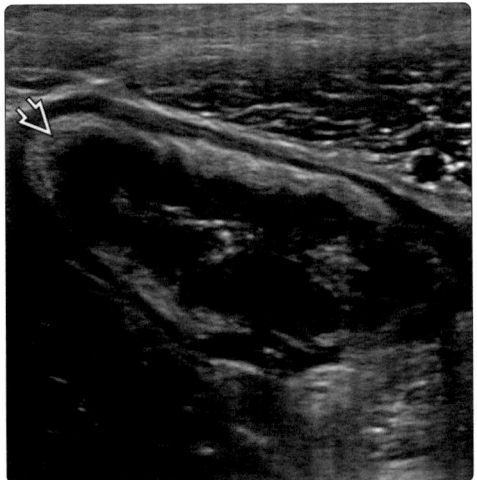

Crohn Disease

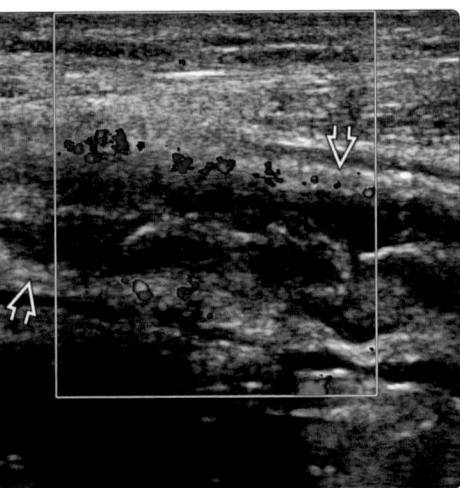

(Left) *Axial transabdominal US of the descending colon shows circumferential thickening with preservation of the gut signature. Note the echogenic prominent submucosal layer ➡. This was histologically proven to be Crohn colitis.*
(Right) *Long axis US shows the same thickened segment of descending colon with preservation of the gut signature and prominent echogenic submucosal layer ➡, representing fibrofatty proliferation in chronic Crohn disease. Note some increased flow on color flow mapping.*

Adenocarcinoma

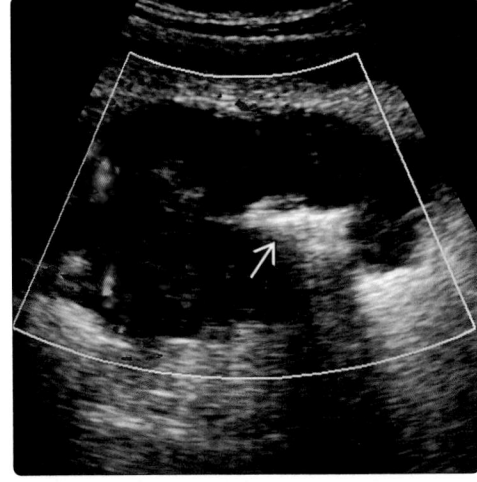

Adenocarcinoma

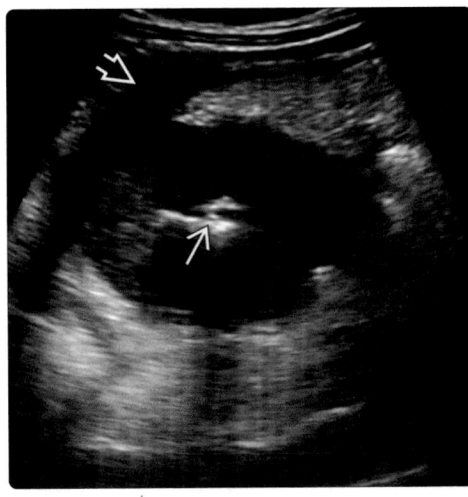

(Left) *Asymmetrical lobular thickening of a short segment of proximal transverse colon is shown, representing colonic carcinoma. Note the loss of the gut signature. The central lumen has an irregular outline ➡, representing ulceration.*
(Right) *Short axis US of hepatic flexure shows infiltrative carcinoma with loss of mural stratification and central luminal narrowing ➡. Note extramural tumor infiltration of the anterior abdominal wall ➡.*

Lymphoma

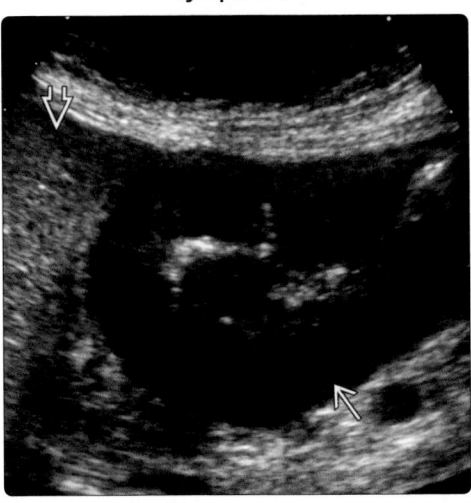

Lymphoma

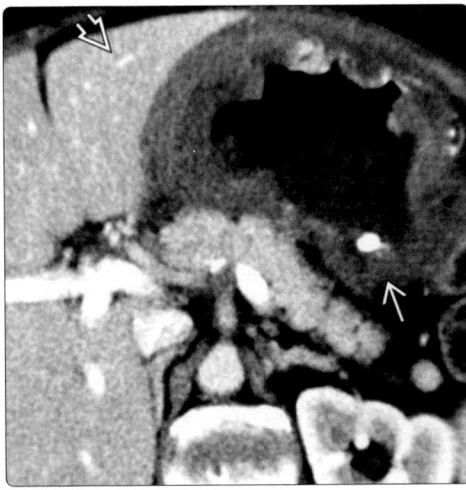

(Left) *Circumferential hypoechoic wall thickening ➡ of the gastric wall with loss of the gut signature is shown. This was histologically proven to be lymphoma, abutting the left lobe of the liver ➡.*
(Right) *Axial CECT in the same patient shows circumferential thickening ➡. There is no luminal narrowing. The left lobe of the liver ➡ is noted.*

Carcinoid

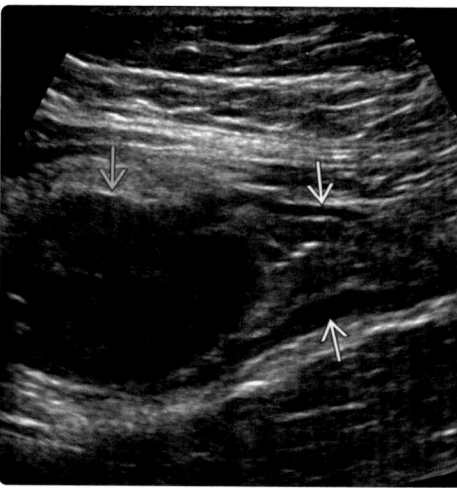

Carcinoid

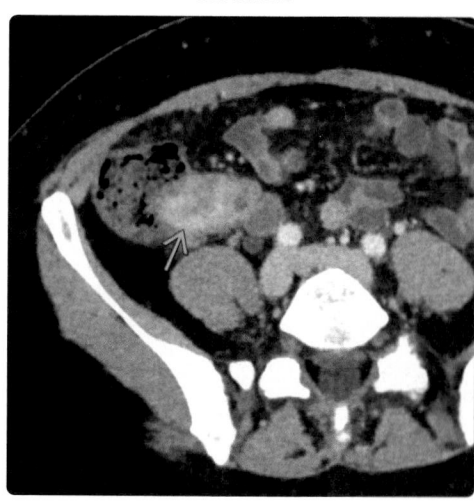

(Left) *Oblique axial US through the right iliac fossa shows an oval hypoechoic focal mural mass ➡ in the terminal ileum, histologically proven to be a carcinoid. Note the gut signature in the remainder of the bowel. The hypoechoic outer layer represents the muscularis propria layer ➡. (Right) Axial CT in the same patient shows the enhancing tumor in the terminal ileum ➡.*

Diverticulosis/Diverticulitis

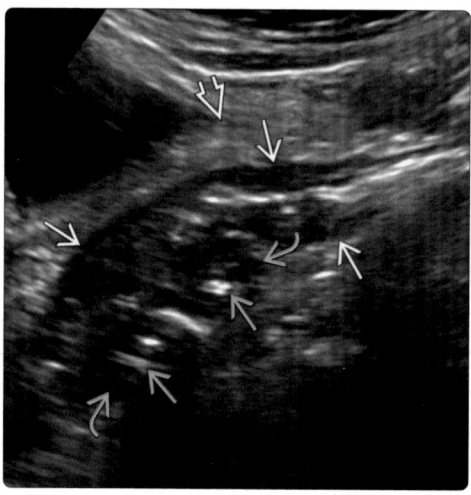

Intussusception

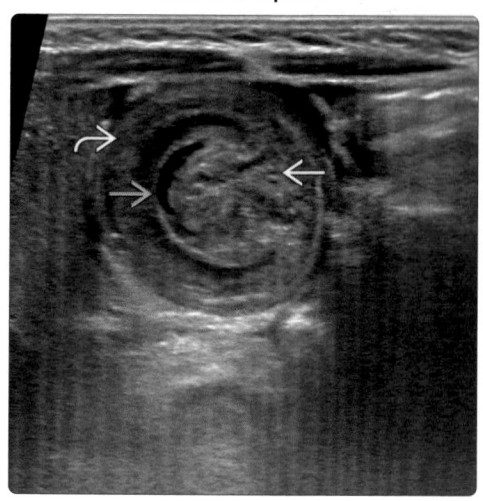

(Left) *Oblique US of the left iliac fossa through the long axis of sigmoid colon shows thickening of the outer hypoechoic muscular layer ➡ and thick-walled inflamed diverticula ➡ with echogenic material ➡ (air/fecal material). Note the surrounding inflamed echogenic fat ➡. (Right) Short axis US shows the "bowel within bowel" appearance from intussusception. Note the outer edematous intussuscipiens ➡, the central intussusceptum ➡, and intervening fluid ➡.*

Acute Venous Ischemia

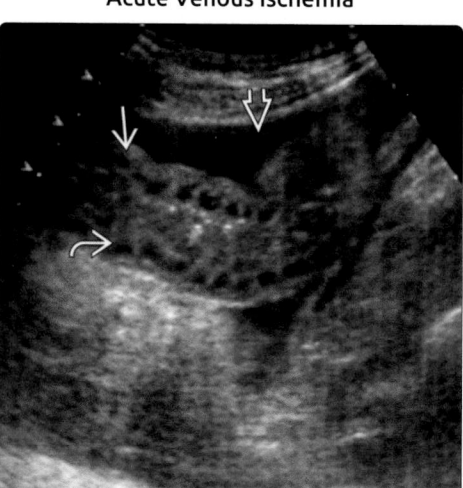

Acute Venous Ischemia

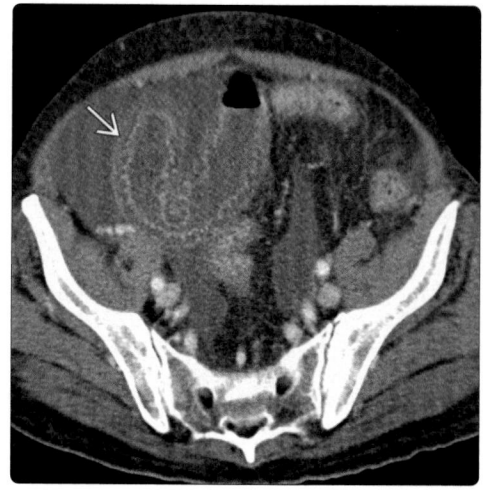

(Left) *Longitudinal US shows a long segment of small bowel with acute mural edema ➡ (note edematous hypoechoic submucous layer ➡), resulting in thickening secondary to acute superior mesenteric venous thrombosis. There is ascites ➡. (Right) Axial CECT in the same patient shows the same segment with acute mural edema ➡. Note the presence of ascites in this patient with known cirrhosis of the liver.*

Clostridium Difficile Colitis

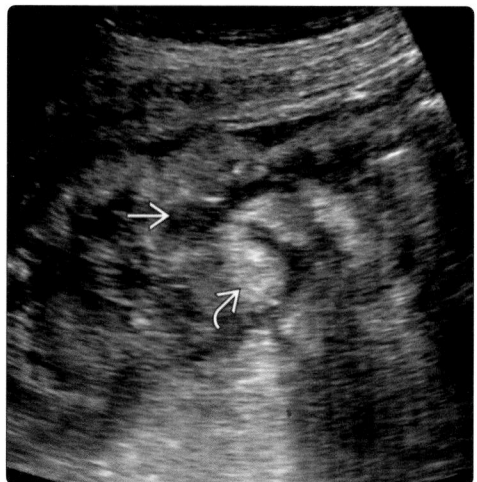

Clostridium Difficile Colitis

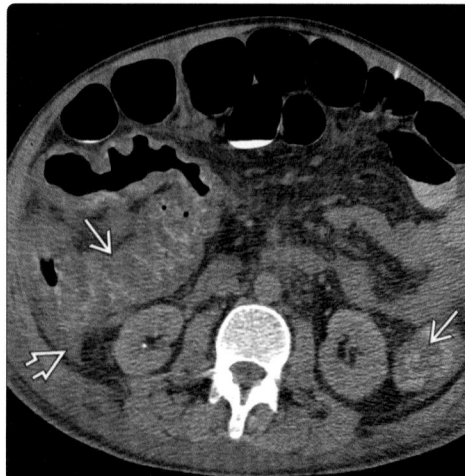

(Left) *Oblique sagittal US in right flank demonstrates markedly thickened ascending colon due to clostridium difficile colitis. Note the marked submucosal layer edema ➡ and pronounced haustral pattern ➤, giving rise to the accordion sign.* (Right) *Corresponding CECT reflects the described ultrasound findings. The colonic wall is markedly thickened ➡; this is typically a pancolitis. Ascites ➡ is usually present.*

Mural Hemorrhage

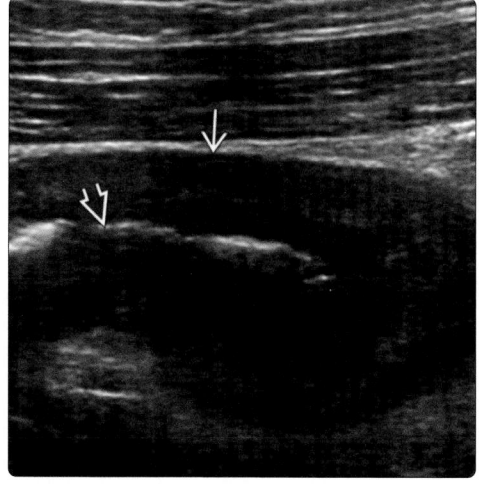

Mural Hemorrhage

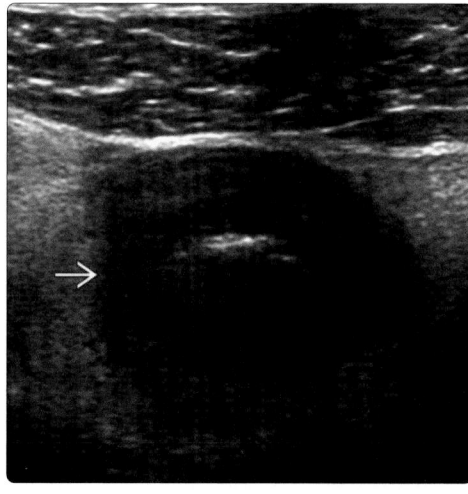

(Left) *Longitudinal US of the small bowel shows homogeneous hypoechoic symmetric thickening ➡ and luminal narrowing ➡. The mural stratification is almost lost in this case, appearances representing intramural hemorrhage in a patient with Henoch-Schönlein purpura.* (Right) *Axial US of the same segment shows the symmetrical circumferential thickening ➡ with loss of the mural stratification.*

Deep Infiltrative Endometriosis

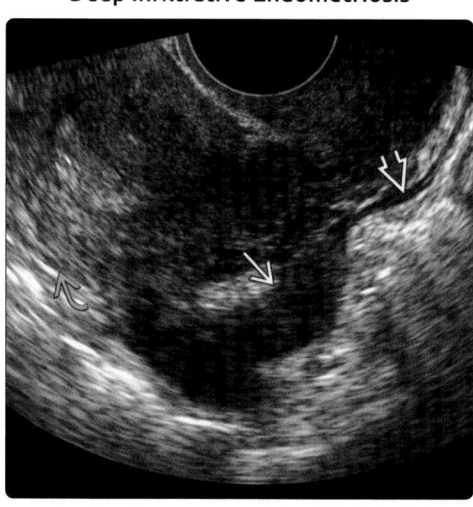

Deep Infiltrative Endometriosis

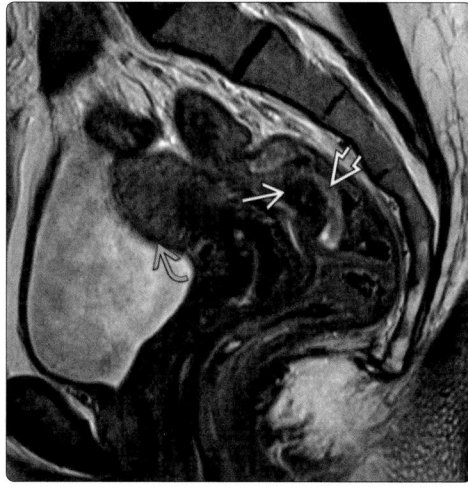

(Left) *Sagittal transvaginal US shows deep infiltrative endometriosis ➡ in the posterior compartment of the pelvic cul-de-sac. Note the focal eccentric thickening of anterior rectosigmoid wall from endometriosis infiltration and widening of the muscularis propria layer ➡. The uterus ➔ is noted.* (Right) *Corresponding MR shows the focal anterior rectosigmoid wall thickening ➡ from infiltration and the edematous overlying mucosa giving the mushroom cap sign ➡. The uterus ➔ is noted.*

PART III
SECTION 10
Scrotum

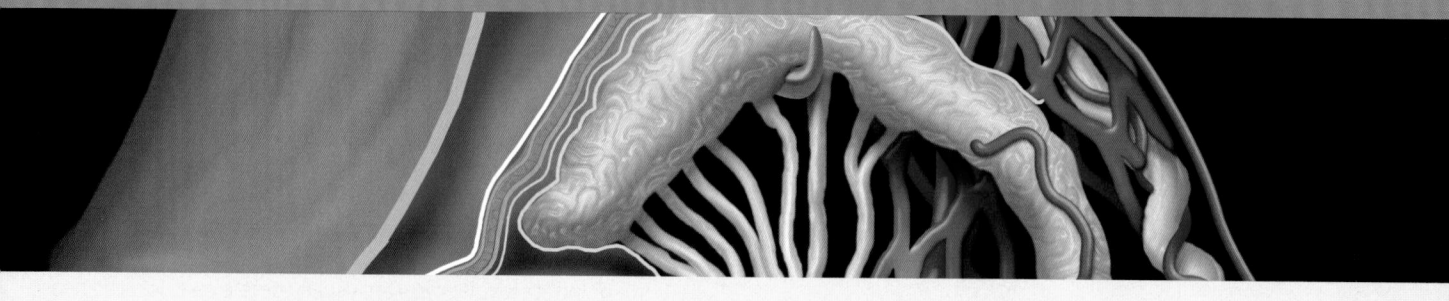

DIFFERENTIAL DIAGNOSIS

Common

- Orchitis
- Testicular Torsion/Infarction
- Testicular Carcinoma
- Scrotal Trauma

Less Common

- Testicular Lymphoma
- Testicular Metastases
- Testicular Cyst

ESSENTIAL INFORMATION

Key Differential Diagnosis Issues

- Diagnosis depends not on sonographic appearances alone, but on combination of clinical and ultrasound features

Helpful Clues for Common Diagnoses

- **Orchitis**
  - Characterized by edema of testes contained within rigid tunica albuginea
  - Heterogeneous parenchymal echogenicity and septal accentuation, seen as hypoechoic bands
  - Diffuse increase in testicular parenchymal vascularity on color Doppler ultrasound
- **Testicular Torsion/Infarction**
  - Acute infarction: Diffusely enlarged hypoechoic testis
  - Chronic infarction: Small, shrunken, heterogeneous testis
  - "Whirlpool" or "torsion knot" at level of spermatic cord; dampened or absent vascularity in testis
- **Testicular Carcinoma**
  - Discrete hypoechoic or mixed echogenic testicular mass ± vascularity
  - Although seminomas are usually discrete hypoechoic lesions, they may cause diffuse enlargement of involved testis
- **Scrotal Trauma**
  - History of scrotal trauma

- Focal hypoechoic area, discrete linear/irregular fracture plane within testis, tunica albuginea rupture, hematocele
- Abnormal testicular parenchymal echogenicity, avascular mass; echogenicity of hematoma depends on its age

Helpful Clues for Less Common Diagnoses

- **Testicular Lymphoma and Metastases**
  - Multiple >> solitary lesion(s); 50% of cases bilateral
  - Metastases are rare; most common sites include prostate, lung, and GI tract
  - Often large in size at time of diagnosis; associated with disseminated disease
    - Ill-defined, mostly hypoechoic lesions
- **Testicular Cyst**
  - Intratesticular cysts are usually simple cysts located near mediastinum testis
  - Need to differentiate them from cystic neoplasms
    - Search carefully for solid components and internal vascularity

SELECTED REFERENCES

1. Coursey Moreno C et al: Testicular tumors: what radiologists need to know–differential diagnosis, staging, and management. Radiographics. 35(2):400-15, 2015
2. Nicola R et al: Imaging of traumatic injuries to the scrotum and penis. AJR Am J Roentgenol. 202(6):W512-20, 2014
3. Bhatt S et al: Imaging of non-neoplastic intratesticular masses. Diagn Interv Radiol. 2011 Mar;17(1):52-63. Epub 2010 Jun 30. Review. Erratum in: Diagn Interv Radiol. 17(4):388, 2011
4. Loberant N et al: Striated appearance of the testes. Ultrasound Q. 26(1):37-44, 2010
5. Bhatt S et al: Role of US in testicular and scrotal trauma. Radiographics. 28(6):1617-29, 2008
6. Dogra VS et al: Torsion and beyond: new twists in spectral Doppler evaluation of the scrotum. J Ultrasound Med. 23(8):1077-85, 2004
7. Dogra V et al: Acute painful scrotum. Radiol Clin North Am. 42 (2): 349-63, 2004
8. Dogra VS et al: Sonography of the scrotum. Radiology. 227(1):18-36, 2003
9. Dogra VS et al: Benign intratesticular cystic lesions: US features. Radiographics. 21 Spec No:S273-81, 2001
10. Subramanyam BR et al: Diffuse testicular disease: sonographic features and significance. AJR Am J Roentgenol. 145(6):1221-4, 1985

Orchitis

Orchitis

(Left) Sagittal grayscale US of the left testis demonstrates an enlarged heterogeneous testis ⊟➙ with surrounding pyocele ⬈ and overlying skin thickening ⬊, suggestive of acute orchitis. (Right) Transverse color Doppler US of the left testis demonstrates an enlarged, heterogeneous testis with a striated ⊟➙ pattern and increased vascularity suggestive of acute orchitis.

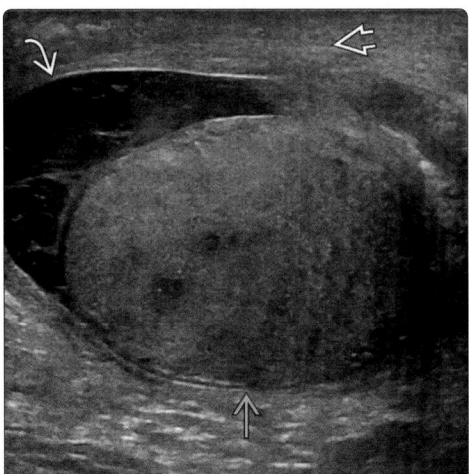

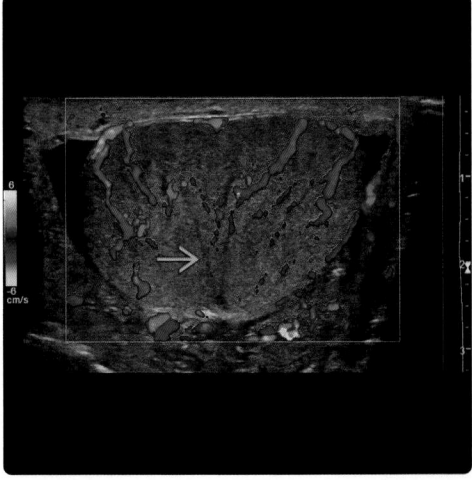

Diffuse Testicular Enlargement

Testicular Torsion/Infarction

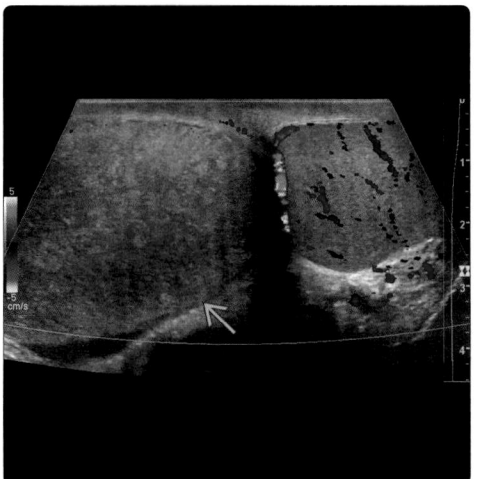

Testicular Carcinoma

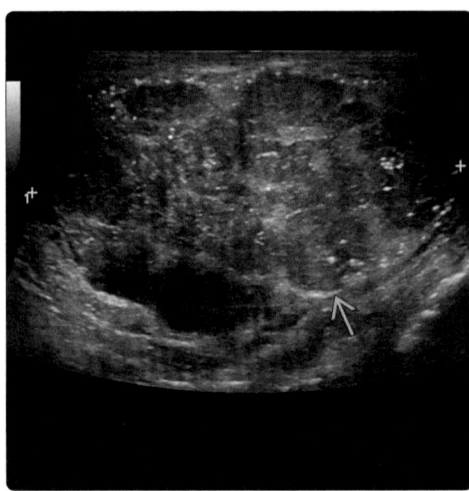

(Left) Transverse color Doppler US of bilateral testes demonstrates an enlarged heterogeneous right testis ⇨ with complete absence of blood flow suggestive of acute testicular torsion with infarction. (Right) Sagittal grayscale US of the right testis demonstrates an enlarged heterogeneous testis ⇨ with multiple hypoechoic masses in the background of testicular microlithiasis pathologically confirmed to be testicular seminoma.

Scrotal Trauma

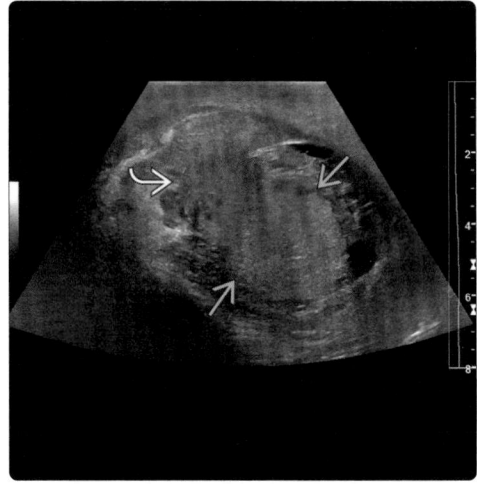

Testicular Lymphoma

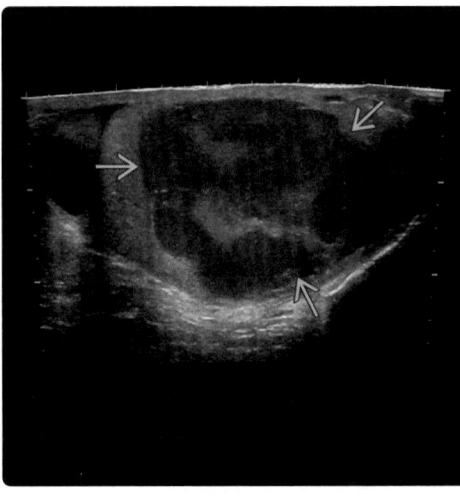

(Left) Sagittal grayscale US of the left testis in a young male recently involved in a motor vehicle accident demonstrates an enlarged heterogeneous irregular testis ⇨ with contour abnormality ⇨ suggestive of testicular rupture. (Right) Sagittal grayscale US of the left testis demonstrates an enlarged heterogeneous testis with a large hypoechoic mass ⇨ that was pathologically confirmed to be testicular lymphoma.

Testicular Metastases

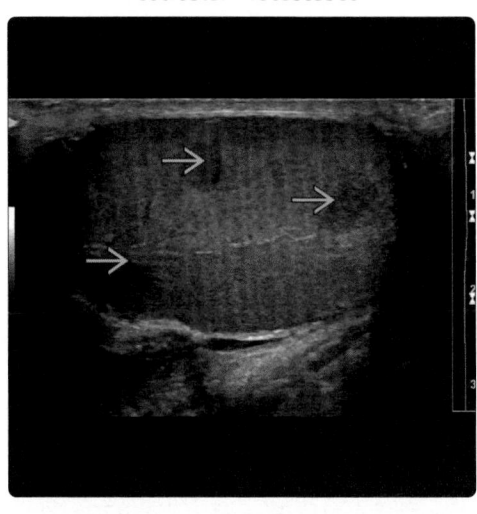

Testicular Cyst

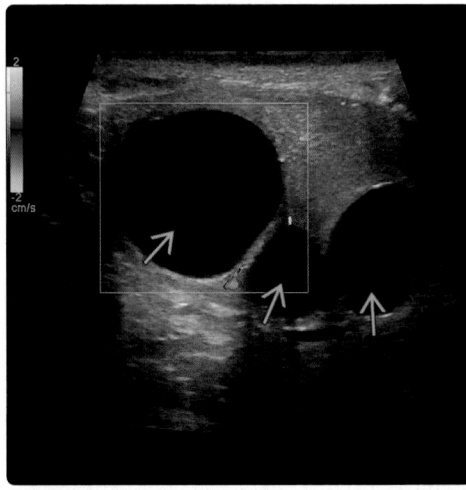

(Left) Transverse grayscale US of the right testis in a young male with history of rhabdomyosarcoma demonstrates an enlarged testis with multiple hypoechoic masses ⇨ that were pathologically confirmed to be metastases from rhabdomyosarcoma. (Right) Transverse color Doppler US demonstrates an enlarged left testis with multiple anechoic structures ⇨ without internal blood flow or solid components, compatible with testicular cysts.

DIFFERENTIAL DIAGNOSIS

Common

- Testicular Infarction
- Scrotal Trauma
- Chronic Mass Effect
- Undescended Testis

Rare but Important

- Hypogonadism
- Polyorchidism

ESSENTIAL INFORMATION

Key Differential Diagnosis Issues

- Consider testicular atrophy if combined axis measurements of testes differ by ≥ 10 mm, or if testicular size < 4 x 2 cm
- Reduction in size considered significant if volume of affected testis reduced to 50% of unaffected testis
- Critical to identify viability of testis to determine whether orchiopexy or orchiectomy is needed

Helpful Clues for Common Diagnoses

- **Testicular Infarction**
  - Ischemic orchitis is known complication of inguinal hernia surgery
  - Epididymoorchitis may result from severe inflammation/induration of cord
    - Venous infarction is a rare complication of orchitis
  - Missed torsion: In utero cord torsion (45%), or may present later in life
  - Uniformly hypoechoic or focal mixed echogenicity of testis, (or striated appearance) with absence of flow are features of diffuse or focal infarction, respectively
    - Reduced echogenicity is sensitive marker of poor outcome compared to clinical parameters
- **Scrotal Trauma**
  - Acute testicular hematoma may lead to ischemia/infarction of viable parenchyma due to raised intratesticular pressure

- Resorption of nonviable testicular tissue leads to atrophy or scarring
- **Chronic Mass Effect**
  - Longstanding extratesticular mass or hydrocele may compromise testicular blood flow and result in atrophy
- **Undescended Testis**
  - Exhibits different degrees of atrophy with altered parenchymal echogenicity
    - Less echogenic and smaller than normally descended testis
  - Testes < 1 cm often not detected by US

Helpful Clues for Rare Diagnoses

- **Hypogonadism**
  - Pituitary neoplasm, Kallmann syndrome, hypogonadotrophic hypogonadism
  - Diffuse heterogeneous echogenicity
- **Polyorchidism**
  - Supernumerary or duplicated testis
    - Tunica albuginea surrounds and separates bifid testis
    - Epididymis may also duplicate
    - Homogeneously echogenic oval structure with echogenicity identical to that of normal testis, but smaller in size

SELECTED REFERENCES

1. Loberant N et al: Striated appearance of the testes. Ultrasound Q. 26(1):37-44, 2010
2. Patel SR et al: Prevalence of testicular size discrepancy in infertile men with and without varicoceles. Urology. 75(3):566-8, 2010
3. Chu L et al: Testicular infarction as a sequela of inguinal hernia repair. Can J Urol. 16(6):4953-4, 2009
4. Bhatt S et al: Role of US in testicular and scrotal trauma. Radiographics. 28(6):1617-29, 2008
5. Pinto KJ et al: Varicocele related testicular atrophy and its predictive effect upon fertility. J Urol. 152(2 Pt 2):788-90, 1994
6. Desai KM et al: Fate of the testis following epididymitis: a clinical and ultrasound study. J R Soc Med. 79(9):515-9, 1986

Testicular Infarction

Undescended Testis

(Left) Transverse color and spectral Doppler view of bilateral testes shows the right testicle ⟶ is atrophic and hypoechoic compared to the left testicle in a 35-year-old male with prior history of right epididymoorchitis. (Right) Sagittal color Doppler ultrasound in a 8-year-old boy with tenderness in his right suprapubic region demonstrates an avascular hypoechoic small undescended testis ⟶. Patients who have an undescended testis have an increased risk of development of seminoma.

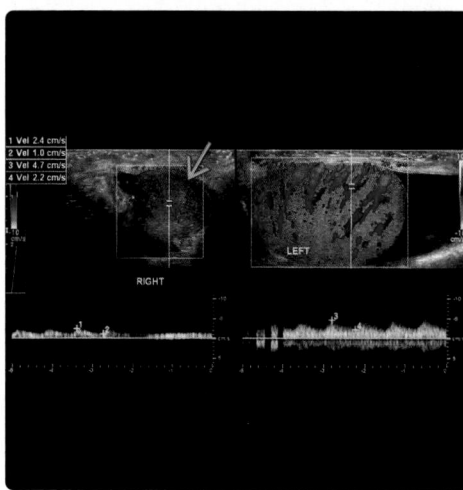

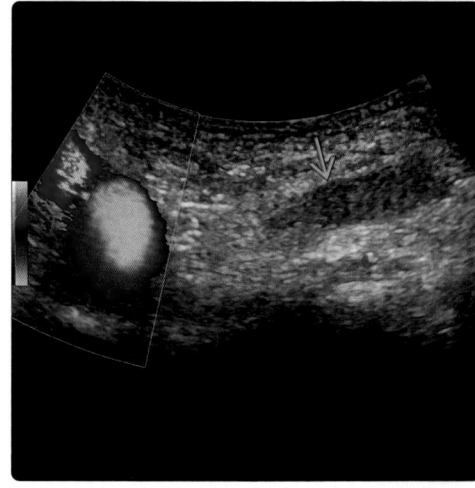

Testicular Infarction

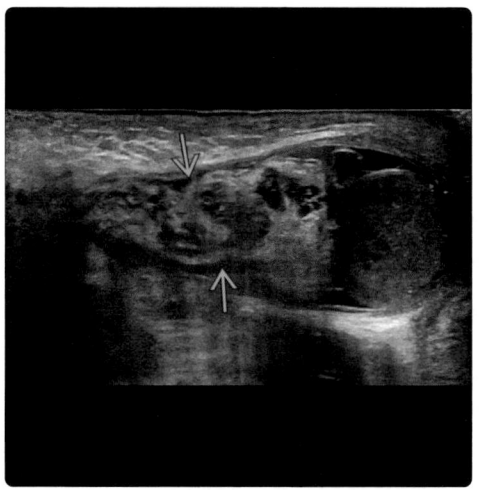

Testicular Infarction

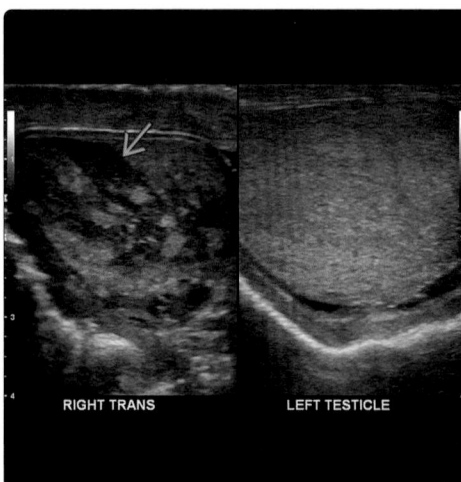

(Left) *Sagittal grayscale US of the right scrotum in a 42-year-old man with recent history of right inguinal hernia surgery who presented with worsening right scrotal pain is shown. Color Doppler US demonstrates complete absence of flow in the testis and an edematous cord ➡.* (Right) *Transverse grayscale ultrasound image of bilateral testes shows an atrophic right testis with a striated pattern ➡. Patient had a remote history of right-sided epididymoorchitis.*

Chronic Mass Effect

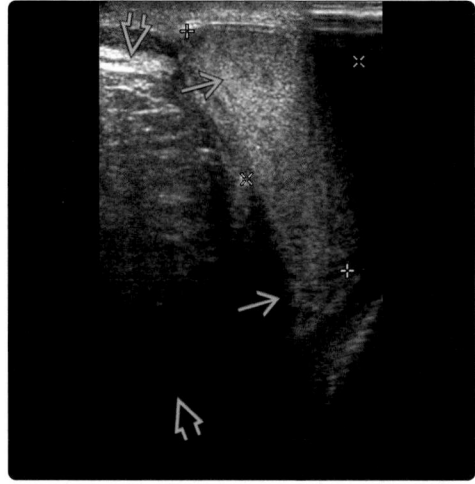

Chronic Mass Effect

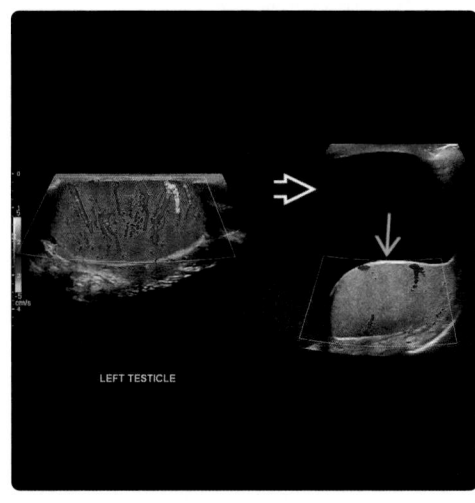

(Left) *Sagittal grayscale ultrasound of the left scrotum shows a small left testis ➡ pushed to 1 side by the large echogenic "mass" confirmed to be an omental inguinal hernia ➡.* (Right) *Sagittal color Doppler ultrasound images of bilateral testis shows an atrophic right testis ➡, secondary to a large hydrocele ➡.*

Testicular Infarction

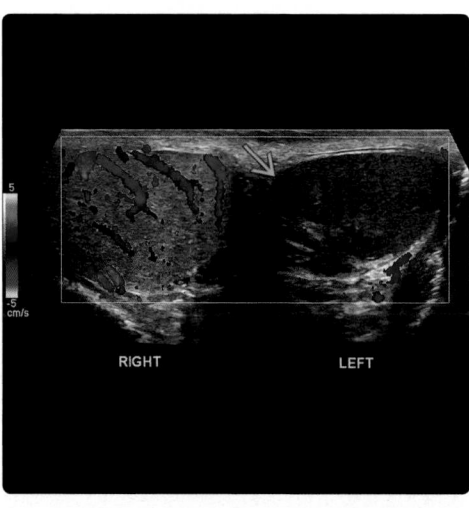

Testicular Infarction

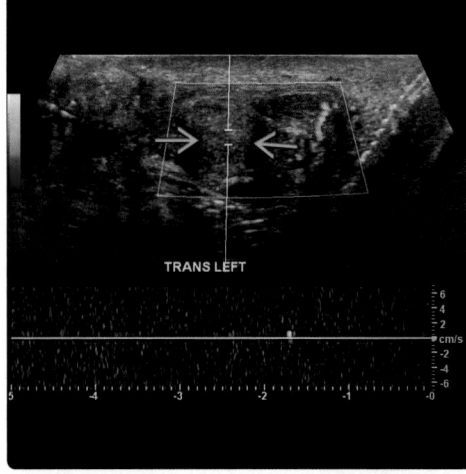

(Left) *Transverse color Doppler view of bilateral testicles shows that the left testis is atrophic ➡ with reduced vascularity. The patient had a prior history of mumps orchitis.* (Right) *Follow-up power Doppler image of a 50-year-old patient with prior history of orchitis demonstrates a severely atrophic and avascular left testis ➡, consistent with infarction, a rare complication of orchitis.*

DIFFERENTIAL DIAGNOSIS

Common

- Testicular Microlithiasis
- Nonseminomatous Germ Cell Tumor
- Sertoli Cell Tumor

Less Common

- Scrotal Trauma
- Scrotal Pearl
- Epidermoid Cyst
- Scrotal Abscess or Epididymoorchitis
- Tunica Albuginea Cyst

ESSENTIAL INFORMATION

Key Differential Diagnosis Issues

- Correlation between clinical and sonographic features essential
  - Incidental finding: Testicular microlithiasis, scrotal pearl
  - History of pain: Abscess, chronic infections, tumors
  - Mass with intrinsic calcification: Testicular tumors, epidermoid cyst
  - Associated with trauma: Testicular hematoma, hematocele

Helpful Clues for Common Diagnoses

- **Testicular Microlithiasis**
  - Multiple small (2-3 mm), discrete, nonshadowing, echogenic intratesticular foci
  - Unilateral or bilateral involvement
  - Concurrent germ cell tumor in up to 40%
- **Nonseminomatous Germ Cell Tumor**
  - Complex solid-cystic testicular mass
  - Heterogeneous echogenic foci due to calcification ± fibrosis, along with retroperitoneal lymphadenopathy can be seen with burnt out testicular tumor
  - Calcifications more common in tumors that contain teratomatous components
- **Sertoli Cell Tumor**
  - Small, hypoechoic, solid-cystic mass

- Punctate calcification may be present
- Occasionally, tumoral calcification may form large calcified mass, known as large calcifying Sertoli cell tumor

Helpful Clues for Less Common Diagnoses

- **Scrotal Trauma**
  - Chronic hematocele
    - Complex echogenic fluid
    - If chronic, appears as heterogeneous echogenic mass, ± calcification
    - No intrinsic vascularity on Doppler
- **Scrotal Pearl**
  - Calcification of detached testicular epididymal appendages due to previous inflammation or torsion of appendages
  - Solitary, discrete, echogenic focus in tunica vaginalis
- **Epidermoid Cyst**
  - Lamellated appearance on ultrasound
  - May have peripheral calcified rim
- **Scrotal Abscess or Epididymoorchitis**
  - Tuberculous infections may produce intrascrotal calcifications, scrotal sinuses
  - Granulomas appear as small echogenic foci, ± calcification
- **Calcified Tunica Albuginea Cyst**
  - Typically located at anterosuperior aspect of testis
  - Within tunica albuginea; may cause mass effect on testicular parenchyma if large
  - Avascular

SELECTED REFERENCES

1. Richenberg J et al: Testicular microlithiasis imaging and follow-up: guidelines of the ESUR scrotal imaging subcommittee. Eur Radiol. 25(2):323-30, 2015
2. Alvarez DM et al: Sonographic spectrum of tunica albuginea cyst. J Clin Imaging Sci. 1:5, 2011
3. Woodward PJ et al: From the archives of the AFIP: tumours and tumorlike lesions of the testis:radiologic-pathologic correlation. Radiographics. 22(1):189-216, 2002
4. Taghizadeh AK et al: Calcified epidermoid cyst in the testis: an unusual finding on ultrasound. Eur J Ultrasound. 11(3):199-200, 2000

Testicular Microlithiasis   **Nonseminomatous Germ Cell Tumor**

(Left) Sagittal grayscale ultrasound of the right testis demonstrates multiple tiny calcific foci consistent with testicular microlithiasis. (Right) Transverse grayscale ultrasound of the right testis demonstrates a partially calcified heterogeneous mass ⮞. Pathology confirmed a mixed germ cell tumor with 75% embryonal cell, 15% teratoma, and 10% yolk cell components.

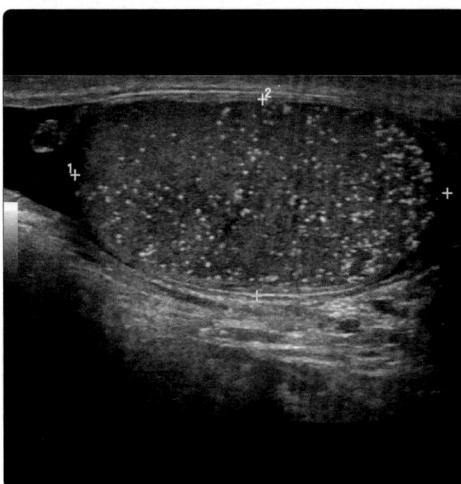
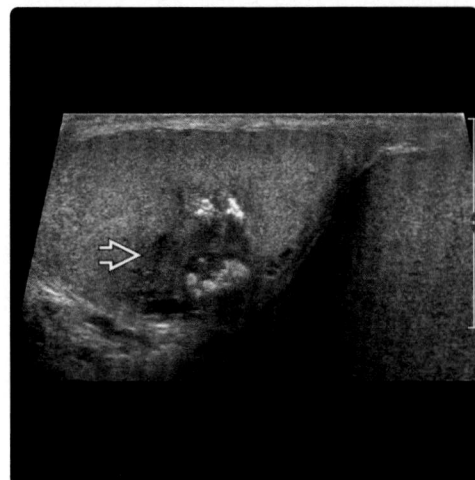

Sertoli Cell Tumor

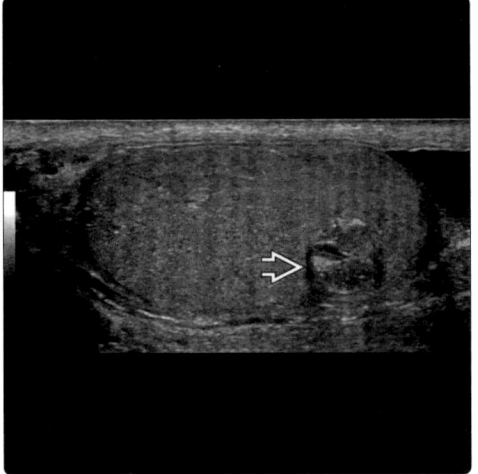

Scrotal Trauma

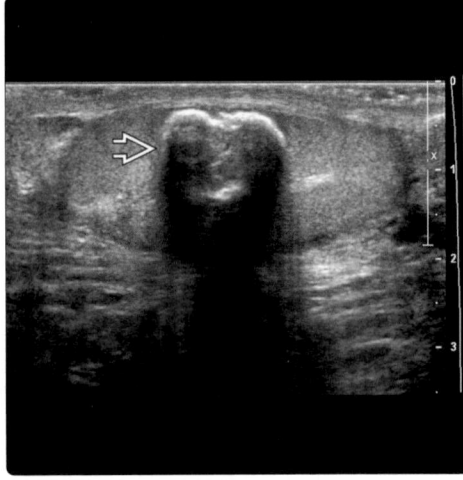

(Left) *Sagittal grayscale ultrasound of the right testis demonstrates a partially calcified mass ⮞. Pathology confirmed Sertoli cell tumor.* (Right) *Sagittal grayscale ultrasound of the right testis demonstrates a densely calcified mass ⮞. Pathology confirmed fibrosis with heterotopic ossification likely secondary to prior traumatic injury.*

Scrotal Pearl

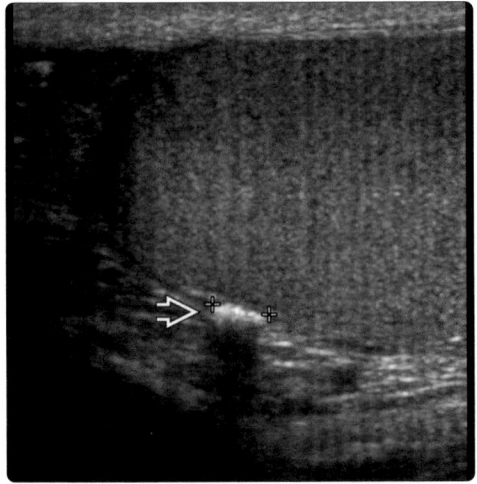

Epidermoid Cyst

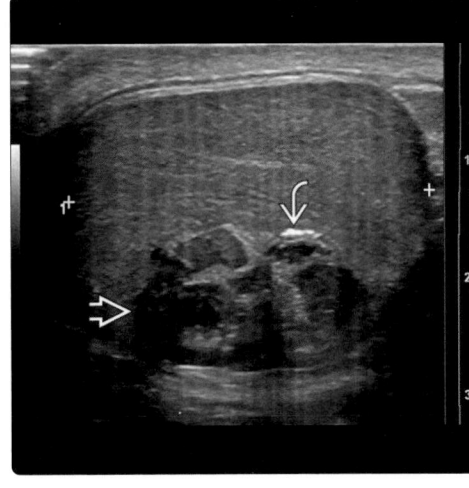

(Left) *Sagittal grayscale ultrasound of the superior pole of the right testis demonstrates a small extratesticular calcific focus ⮞. This is suggestive of a scrotal pearl or scrotolith.* (Right) *Transverse grayscale ultrasound of the left testis demonstrates a heterogeneous complex cystic mass ⮞ with areas of calcification ⮡. Pathology confirmed epidermoid cyst.*

Scrotal Abscess or Epididymoorchitis

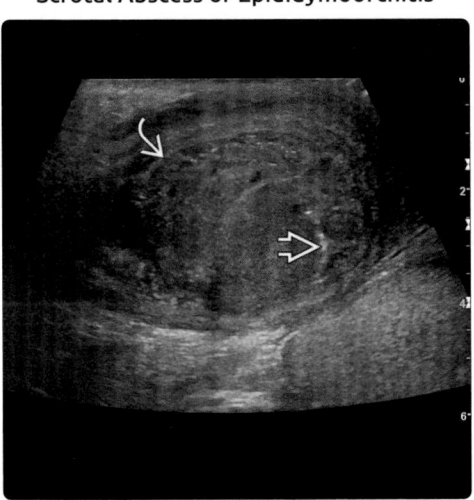

Tunica Albuginea Cyst

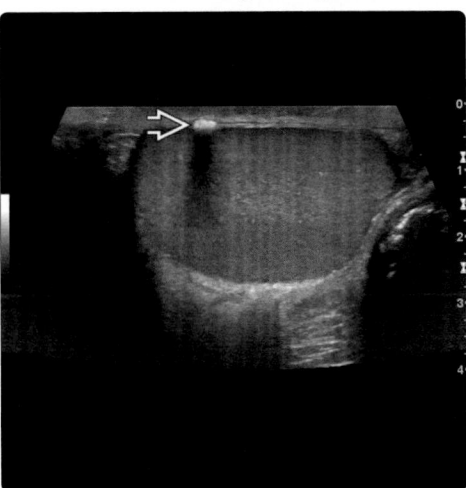

(Left) *Sagittal grayscale ultrasound of the right testis demonstrates a heterogeneous left testis ⮞ with calcification ⮞. Findings represent sequela of prior epididymoorchitis.* (Right) *Sagittal grayscale ultrasound of the right testis demonstrates a calcified lesion in the tunica albuginea ⮞. Findings represent a calcified tunica albuginea cyst.*

DIFFERENTIAL DIAGNOSIS

Common

- Testicular Carcinoma
- Orchitis (Epididymoorchitis)
- Testicular Torsion/Infarction
- Testicular Hematoma

Less Common

- Testicular Abscess
- Testicular Lymphoma, Leukemia, and Metastases
- Gonadal Stromal Tumor
- Testicular Epidermoid Cyst
- Testicular Adrenal Rests
- Testicular Sarcoid

ESSENTIAL INFORMATION

Key Differential Diagnosis Issues

- Correlate ultrasound with age and clinical features
- Sonographic findings are key but overlap among various tumors
- Histopathological correlation needed

Helpful Clues for Common Diagnoses

- **Testicular Carcinoma**
  - Best diagnostic clue: Discrete hypoechoic or mixed echogenicity testicular mass, ± vascularity
    - Tumor ≤ 1.5 cm is commonly hypovascular
    - Tumor > 1.5 cm is more often hypervascular
    - Discrete mass on grayscale ultrasound with abnormal intrinsic vascularity on color Doppler should raise suspicion of testicular carcinoma
  - Seminoma
    - Most common neoplasm in males 15-39 years old
    - Well-defined, lobulated, hypoechoic, solid lesion without calcification
    - May undergo necrosis and appear partly cystic (rare)
  - Teratoma/teratocarcinoma
    - Heterogeneous, complex, solid-cystic mass
    - Calcification (cartilage, immature bone) ± fibrosis characterizes teratoma/teratocarcinoma
  - Embryonal cell carcinoma
    - Heterogeneous, predominantly solid, mixed echogenicity mass
    - Poorly marginated; 1/3 have cystic necrosis
    - May invade tunica albuginea and distort testicular contour
  - Choriocarcinoma
    - Mixed echogenicity, heterogeneous mass
    - Cystic areas and calcification common
    - Hemorrhage with focal necrosis is typical feature of choriocarcinoma
    - May invade tunica albuginea
    - Early hematogenous spread, especially to brain
- **Orchitis (Epididymoorchitis)**
  - Primarily involves epididymis
    - Orchitis is usually secondary, occurring in 20-40% of cases with epididymitis due to contiguous spread of infection
    - Primary orchitis is typically viral (mumps) and bilateral

- Orchitis is characterized by inflammation, edema, and hyperemia of testis
  - Diffuse orchitis: Testis is diffusely enlarged with heterogeneous echo pattern
  - Focal orchitis: Hypoechoic focal area, usually adjacent to inflamed epididymis
    □ Can be differentiated from neoplasm by demonstrating resolution on interval follow-up
  - Associated with other findings of epididymoorchitis including skin thickening, hydrocele, or pyocele
  - Increase in vascularity on color Doppler without displacement of vessels
- **Testicular Torsion/Infarction**
  - Findings of torsion vary with duration and degree of cord rotations
    - Grayscale appearance in early torsion may be normal
    - Decreased abnormal flow or absent flow on color Doppler (always compare to contralateral normal side)
    - Diffusely hypoechoic small testis/focal mass in infarcted testis
    - Hyperechoic regions (hemorrhage, fibrosis)
  - Segmental infarction may be sequela of inflammatory process (orchitis) or surgical complication (hernia repair)
    - Focal infarctions may be round or wedge shaped or may have linear striated appearance
  - Infarction may occur in patients with hypercoagulable states or advanced atherosclerosis, such as diabetes, or as a sequela of epididymoorchitis or funiculitis
- **Testicular Hematoma**
  - History of scrotal trauma is present in majority of cases
  - Abnormal testicular parenchymal echogenicity
    - Echogenicity depends on age of hematoma
  - Discrete linear or irregular fracture plane within testis
  - May or may not be associated with ruptured tunica albuginea
  - Color Doppler
    - Hematoma forms avascular mass within testis
    - Distorted intratesticular vascularity with interruption of vessels in area of hematoma or injury
  - Spontaneous testicular hemorrhage is rare entity where intratesticular hemorrhage has no identifiable risk factors
    - Mixed echogenicity solid or cystic mass with lack of significant internal color Doppler flow signals
    - Changes in appearance, as clot resolution occurs over time

Helpful Clues for Less Common Diagnoses

- **Testicular Abscess**
  - Epididymal abscess (6%)
  - Testicular abscess (6%)
  - Microabscess formation is usually seen in low-grade infections (e.g., tuberculosis)
    - Also seen in immunocompromised hosts
  - Well-defined, discrete, round, hypoechoic lesion(s) in testicular parenchyma
  - Necrotic center shows no vascularity on color Doppler studies
- **Testicular Lymphoma, Leukemia, and Metastases**
  - Lymphoma

- Most common testicular tumor in men older than 60 years; multiple lesions; 50% of cases bilateral
- Often large at time of diagnosis
- Commonly occurs in association with disseminated disease
- Ill-defined, predominantly hypoechoic lesions
- Increased vascularity on color Doppler
- Involvement of epididymis and spermatic cord is common
- Hemorrhage or necrosis is rare
○ Leukemia
- Most often seen in children
- Testis is often the 1st site of extramedullary relapse
- Diffuse testicular infiltration appears diffusely hypoechoic with increased vascularity; may be indistinguishable from orchitis on ultrasound
  □ Clinical correlation with signs of inflammation may help identify orchitis
○ Metastases are rare
- Most common primaries include prostate, lung, and GI tract
○ Testis is frequent site of recurrence in male patients with lymphoma and acute leukemia
- **Gonadal Stromal Tumor**
○ Bilateral in 3%
- < 3 cm usually benign
- > 5 cm usually malignant
○ Leydig cell tumor
- Small solid hypoechoic testicular mass
- In larger tumor, hemorrhage or necrosis leads to heterogeneous echo pattern
○ Sertoli cell tumor
- Small hypoechoic mass
- Solid and cystic components
- Punctate calcification may be present; large calcified mass in calcifying Sertoli cell tumor
- Hemorrhage may lead to heterogeneity
○ Indistinguishable from other testicular tumors by ultrasound findings
- **Testicular Epidermoid Cyst**

○ Cystic cavity lined by stratified squamous epithelium
○ Onion skin appearance on ultrasound due to alternating layers of keratin and desquamated squamous cells
○ May have peripheral calcified rim
- **Testicular Adrenal Rests**
○ Described in patients with congenital adrenal hyperplasia
○ May be associated with impaired spermatogenesis
○ Usually bilateral hypoechoic lesions; typically located at the mediastinum testis
○ If left untreated may lead to fibrosis and testicular destruction
- **Testicular Sarcoid**
○ Usually bilateral involvement of epididymii and testes
○ Hypoechoic nodule(s)
○ Associated chest findings on radiograph or CT may be helpful clue

SELECTED REFERENCES

1. Coursey Moreno C et al: Testicular tumors: what radiologists need to know–differential diagnosis, staging, and management. Radiographics. 35(2):400-15, 2015
2. Piton N et al: Focal non granulomatous orchitis in a patient with Crohn's disease. Diagn Pathol. 10(1):39, 2015
3. Rajkanna J et al: Large testicular adrenal rest tumours in a patient with congenital adrenal hyperplasia. Endocrinol Diabetes Metab Case Rep. 2015:140080, 2015
4. Thompson JP et al: Identify Before Orchiectomy: Segmental Testicular Infarct. Ultrasound Q. ePub, 2015
5. Bhatt S et al: Imaging of non-neoplastic intratesticular masses. Diagn Interv Radiol. 2011 Mar;17(1):52-63. Epub 2010 Jun 30. Review. Erratum in: Diagn Interv Radiol. 17(4):388, 2011
6. Gaur S et al: Spontaneous intratesticular hemorrhage: two case descriptions and brief review of the literature. J Ultrasound Med. 30(1):101-4, 2011
7. Loberant N et al: Striated appearance of the testes. Ultrasound Q. 26(1):37-44, 2010
8. Bhatt S et al: Role of US in testicular and scrotal trauma. Radiographics. 28(6):1617-29, 2008
9. Bhatt S et al: Sonography of benign intrascrotal lesions. Ultrasound Q. 22(2):121-36, 2006
10. Dogra V et al: Acute painful scrotum. Radiol Clin North Am. 42 (2): 349-63, 2004
11. Mazzu D et al: Lymphoma and leukemia involving the testicles: findings on gray-scale and color Doppler sonography. AJR Am J Roentgenol. 164(3):645-7, 1995

Testicular Carcinoma
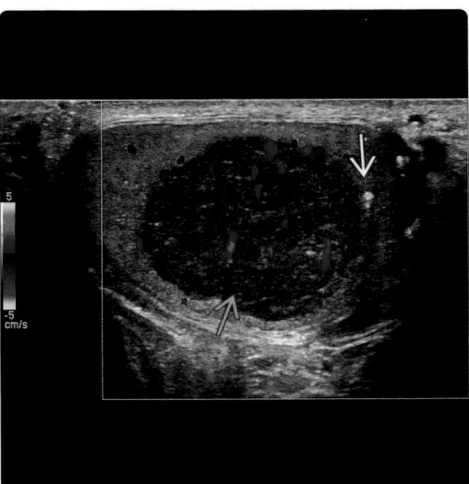

Orchitis (Epididymoorchitis)
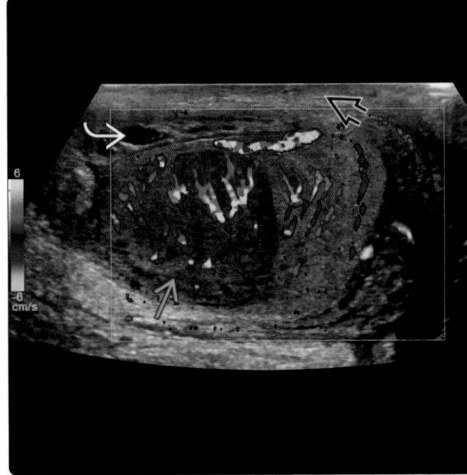

(Left) Sagittal color Doppler ultrasound of the right testis in a 30-year-old man shows a focal well-defined hypoechoic mass ➡ with increased vascularity. Associated testicular microliths ➡ are noted. Pathologically, this was confirmed to be a seminoma. (Right) Sagittal color Doppler ultrasound of right testis in a 22-year-old man with acute right scrotum shows a focal hypervascular hypoechoic mass ➡. Associated overlying skin ➡ thickening and complex hydrocele ➡ are seen. Patient was found to have focal orchitis.

Testicular Torsion/Infarction

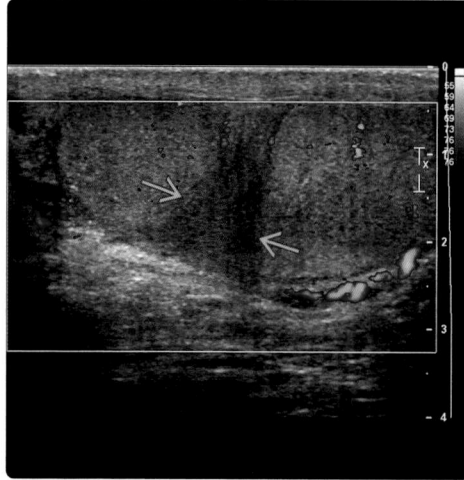

Testicular Hematoma

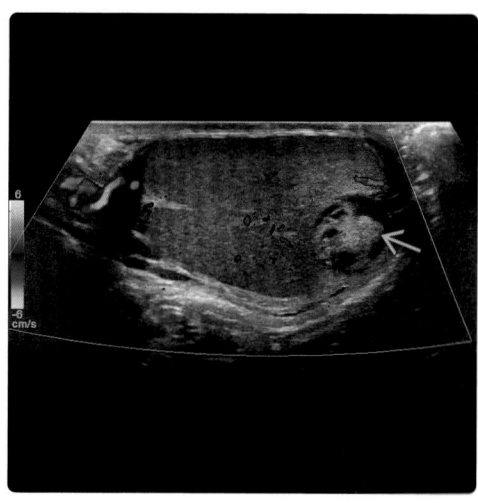

(Left) *Sagittal power Doppler ultrasound of the right testis in an 18-year-old man shows a focal wedge-shaped hypoechoic region* ⇨ *with absent vascularity consistent with segmental infarct in the presence of prior history of torsion.* (Right) *Sagittal color Doppler ultrasound of the right testis in a young man after trauma shows a focal avascular heterogeneous mass* ⇨. *Follow-up images demonstrated resolution consistent with a focal hematoma.*

Testicular Hematoma

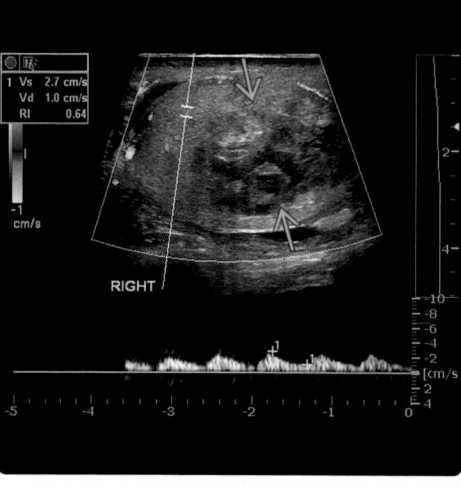

Testicular Abscess

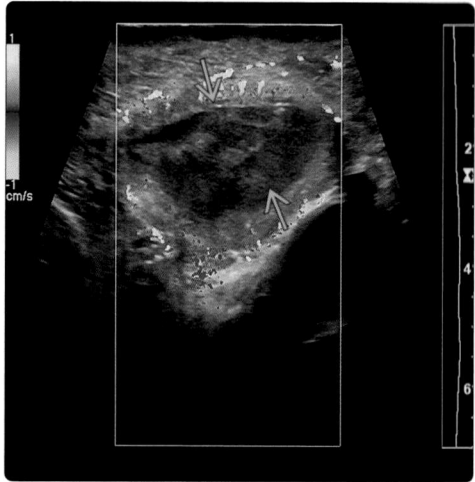

(Left) *Transverse color Doppler ultrasound of the right testis in a young man with acute onset pain without preceding history of trauma shows a heterogeneous avascular mass* ⇨, *which was confirmed to be a spontaneous testicular hemorrhage.* (Right) *Transverse color Doppler ultrasound in a 23-year-old man with fever and scrotal pain, shows a hypoechoic avascular area* ⇨ *in the testis, confirmed to be a testicular abscess.*

Testicular Lymphoma, Leukemia, and Metastases

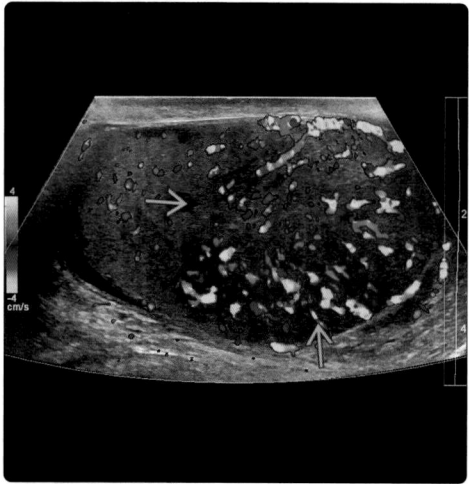

Testicular Lymphoma, Leukemia, and Metastases

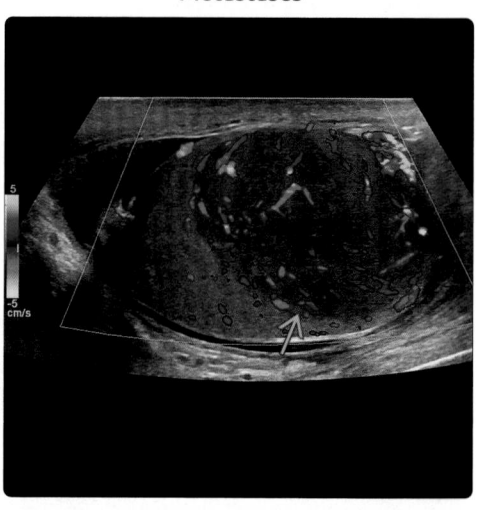

(Left) *Sagittal color Doppler ultrasound of the right testis in a 65-year-old man with scrotal mass shows a focal hypoechoic mass* ⇨ *with increased vascularity, which was confirmed to be lymphoma.* (Right) *Sagittal color Doppler ultrasound of the right testis in a 45-year-old man with acute lymphoblastic leukemia shows a hypervascular focal hypoechoic mass* ⇨ *confirmed to be leukemic infiltration.*

Testicular Lymphoma, Leukemia, and Metastases

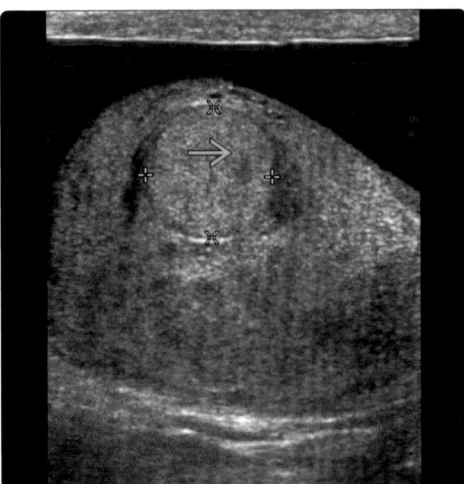

Gonadal Stromal Tumor

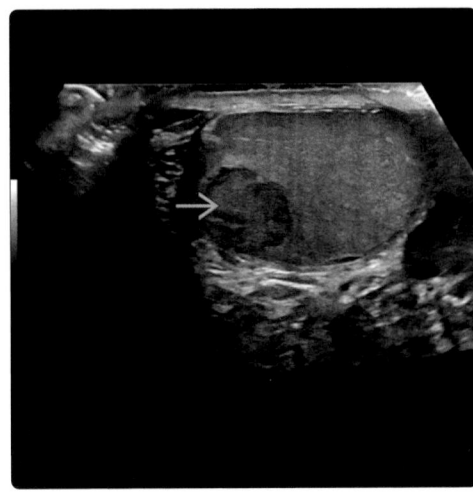

(Left) *Sagittal grayscale ultrasound of the testis in a patient with multiple myeloma shows a focal well-defined echogenic mass ➡, surgically confirmed to be a metastatic lesion.* (Right) *Transverse grayscale ultrasound of the testis in a 25-year-old man shows a focal well-defined hypoechoic mass ➡, surgically confirmed to be a Leydig cell tumor.*

Gonadal Stromal Tumor

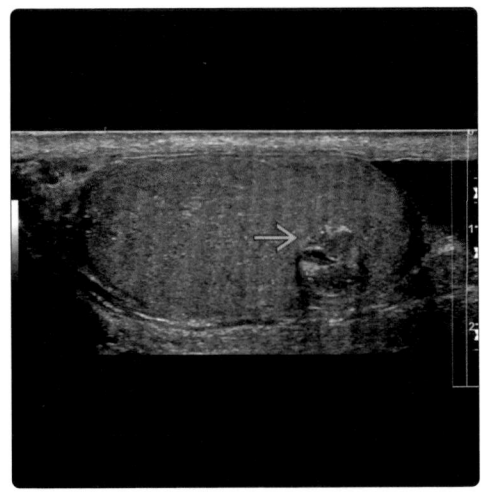

Testicular Epidermoid Cyst

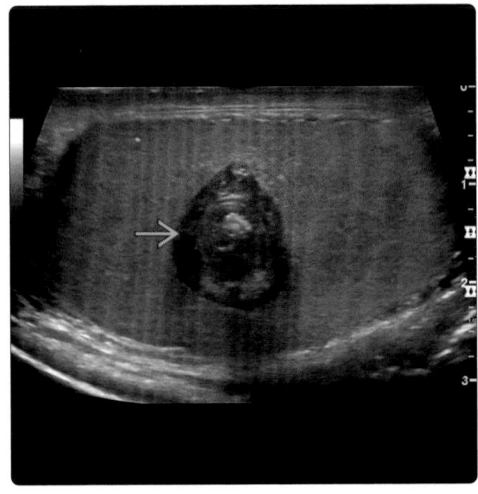

(Left) *Sagittal grayscale ultrasound of the testis in a 30-year-old man shows a focal well-defined heterogeneous mass ➡, with calcifications and cystic areas, surgically confirmed to be a Sertoli cell tumor.* (Right) *Sagittal grayscale ultrasound of the testis in a 15-year-old male shows a focal well-defined hypoechoic mass ➡, with concentric onion skin pattern, surgically confirmed to be epidermoid cyst.*

Testicular Adrenal Rests

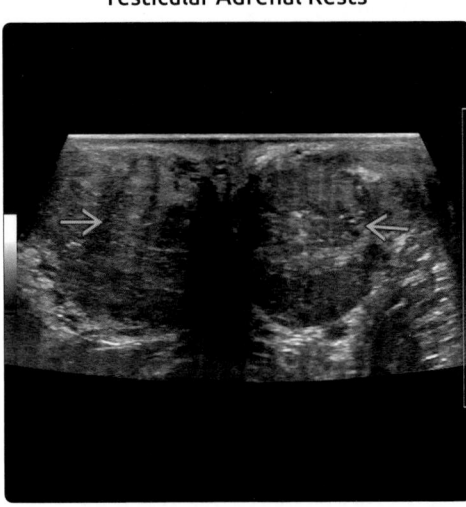

Testicular Sarcoid

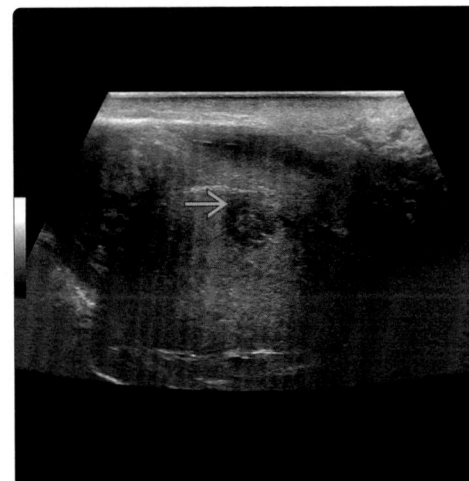

(Left) *Transverse grayscale ultrasound of both testes in a 16-year-old male with congenital adrenal hyperplasia shows bilateral hypoechoic masses ➡, consistent with intratesticular hyperplastic adrenal rests.* (Right) *Sagittal grayscale ultrasound of the testis in a patient with known sarcoidosis shows a focal well-defined hypoechoic mass ➡, surgically confirmed to be testicular sarcoid.*

DIFFERENTIAL DIAGNOSIS

Common

- Epididymitis
- Spermatocele
- Epididymal Cyst
- Varicocele
- Spermatic Cord Torsion

Less Common

- Hematoma
- Adenomatoid Tumor
- Inguinal Hernia
- Fatty Deposition
- Encysted Hydrocele of Cord
- Papillary Cystadenoma
- Lipoma
- Epididymal/Scrotal Wall Abscess
- Fibrous Pseudotumor
- Leiomyoma

Rare but Important

- Sarcoidosis
- Rare Tumors
  - Liposarcoma of Spermatic Cord
  - Sclerosing Lipogranuloma
  - Leiomyosarcoma
  - Malignant Schwannoma
  - Epididymal Rhabdomyosarcoma
- Metastases
- Tuberculous Epididymitis
- Funiculitis
- Vasitis

ESSENTIAL INFORMATION

Key Differential Diagnosis Issues

- Diagnosis based on combination of clinical and sonographic features
- Acute pain
  - Epididymitis
  - Hematoma
  - Torsion
  - Strangulated inguinoscrotal hernia
- Chronic pain
  - Varicocele
  - Tumors
- Incidental finding
  - Epididymal cyst
  - Spermatocele

Helpful Clues for Common Diagnoses

- **Epididymitis**
  - Most common cause of acutely painful scrotum
  - Hyperemic epididymis &/or testis on color Doppler ultrasound
    - Compare with contralateral side
    - Epididymis appears hypervascular compared to adjacent testicle
  - Acute epididymitis

- Enlarged, heterogeneous, predominantly hypoechoic epididymis
- Reactive thickening of scrotal wall ± hydrocele
- Urinary tract pathogens typical in older men
- STDs in younger men
  - Chronic epididymitis
    - Granulomatous infection caused by tuberculosis, brucellosis, syphilis, and fungal infection
    - Usually bilateral involvement
    - Enlarged epididymis with heterogeneous appearance, ranging from hypoechoic to hyperechoic, ± calcification
- **Spermatocele**
  - Size: 1-2 cm, may be very large
  - Retention cyst of tubules connecting rete testis to head of epididymis
    - Obstruction and dilatation of efferent ductal system
    - Usually seen in individuals with previous vasectomy
  - Appearance
    - Cystic with low-level mobile internal echoes
    - Contain nonviable sperm
    - Rarely spermatoceles may be hyperechoic
    - Large spermatoceles may have internal septations
    - Acoustic streaming of low level internal echoes: Falling snow sign on color Doppler sonography
- **Epididymal Cyst**
  - Usually ≤ 1 cm
  - Well-defined anechoic lesion with posterior acoustic enhancement
  - Large cysts (true cysts or spermatocele) may have septation and may be confused with hydroceles
    - Cysts displace testis, while hydrocele envelop it
- **Varicocele**
  - Dilatation of veins of pampiniform plexus > 3 mm in diameter due to reflux in internal spermatic vein
  - Best imaging tool: Color Doppler US
    - Dilated serpiginous veins behind superior pole of testis
    - Veins enlarge with Valsalva maneuver
- **Spermatic Cord Torsion**
  - Twisting of testicle and spermatic cord within scrotum leads to testicular ischemia and infarction
  - Twisted spermatic cord cranial to testis and epididymis often becomes edematous and mass-like, which can appear as extratesticular torsion knot with whirlpool appearance
    - Surgical emergency requiring emergent reduction to preserve viable testis

Helpful Clues for Less Common Diagnoses

- **Hematoma**
  - Associated with trauma, torsion
  - Complex echogenic fluid with layering debris ± internal septation; varies with chronicity
  - Must confirm intact testicular vascularity as enlarging hematoma may compress testicular vessels
  - Carefully evaluate tunical albungina of testicle for associated testicular rupture (surgical emergency)
- **Adenomatoid Tumor**
  - Most common tumor of epididymis
    - 1/3 of all paratesticular neoplasms

- 3-50 mm
- Most common in men over 20 years old
- Usually unilateral, more common on left side
  - Variable US appearance
    - Typically seen as well-circumscribed, round to oval, homogeneous mass, variable echogenicity
- **Inguinal Hernia**
  - Herniation of abdominal contents into scrotum
  - Accentuated by Valsalva maneuver, real-time evaluation essential
  - Solid, irreducible mass if obstruction/strangulation
  - Ill-defined echogenic structure representing mesentery ± bowel in herniated sac
    - Obstruction at neck of hernia sac leads to strangulation of herniated contents
- **Encysted Hydrocele of Cord**
  - Patent processus vaginalis seen in infants; associated ascites may also be seen
  - Elongated fluid collection within layers of spermatic cord located above level of testis and epididymis
- **Papillary Cystadenoma**
  - On US, variable appearance
    - Large, solid tumors, echogenic, ± cystic spaces
  - Typically 1-4 cm
  - Identified in men with von Hippel-Lindau disease (50-70%)
- **Lipoma**
  - Among most common extratesticular neoplasms
  - Usually involves spermatic cord
  - Homogeneous, well-circumscribed, variable-sized, hyperechoic, solid mass
- **Epididymal/Scrotal Wall Abscess**
  - Abscess involving epididymis or scrotal wall as complication of severe epididymoorchitis
- **Fibrous Pseudotumor**
  - Reactive fibrous proliferation in epididymis
    - Tunica albuginea may be another site for such fibrous proliferation
    - Lesions may be as large as 8 cm
  - Generally hypoechoic ± posterior acoustic shadowing

- **Leiomyoma**
  - 2nd most common epididymal neoplasm
  - Slow growing, hence delayed presentation (generally 5th decade)
  - Solid or cystic, variable US appearance, ± calcifications

Helpful Clues for Rare Diagnoses

- **Liposarcoma of Spermatic Cord**
  - Aggressive fat-containing malignancy derived from mesenchymal tissue
  - Present as painless inguinal mass which may be mistaken for inguinal hernia
- **Sclerosing Lipogranuloma**
  - Rare, hypoechoic paratesticular mass, histopathological correlation
- **Metastases**
  - 25% of solid tumors of epididymis are malignant; majority of these are metastases
  - On ultrasound, most metastatic lesions are hypoechoic, but no other specific feature differentiates them from other epididymal neoplasms
- **Funiculitis**
  - Inflammation of the entire spermatic cord
  - Presents with pain and swelling
  - Hypoechoic soft tissue around vas deferens extending into inguinal canal
- **Vasitis**
  - Inflammation of only vas deferens

SELECTED REFERENCES

1. Annam A et al: Extratesticular masses in children: taking ultrasound beyond paratesticular rhabdomyosarcoma. Pediatr Radiol. ePub, 2015
2. Inokuchi R et al: Noninfectious Funiculitis. J Emerg Med. ePub, 2015
3. Mirochnik B et al: Ultrasound evaluation of scrotal pathology. Radiol Clin North Am. 50(2):317-32, vi, 2012
4. Philips S et al: Benign non-cystic scrotal tumors and pseudotumors. Acta Radiol. 53(1):102-11, 2012
5. Wasnik AP et al: Scrotal pearls and pitfalls: ultrasound findings of benign scrotal lesions. Ultrasound Q. 28(4):281-91, 2012
6. Cassidy FH et al: MR imaging of scrotal tumors and pseudotumors. Radiographics. 30(3):665-83, 2010

Epididymitis

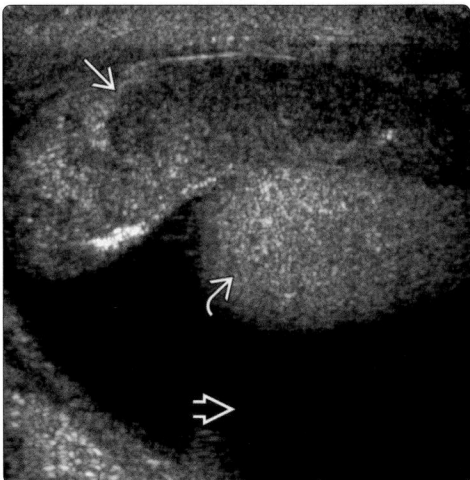

Epididymitis

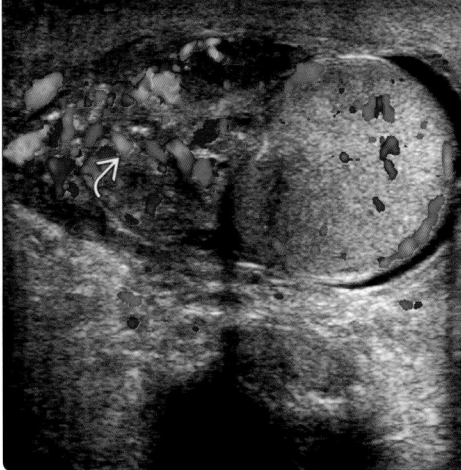

(Left) Longitudinal ultrasound shows a markedly enlarged, predominantly hypoechoic head of the epididymis ➡️, features suggestive of acute epididymitis. Note the preserved size, echo pattern of testis ➡️, and moderate reactive hydrocele ➡️. *(Right)* Transverse color Doppler ultrasound in another patient shows marked increase in intrinsic vascularity ➡️ of an inflamed epididymis. Note the undistorted pattern of the vessels, which helps to differentiate diffuse inflammation from a neoplasm.

Spermatocele

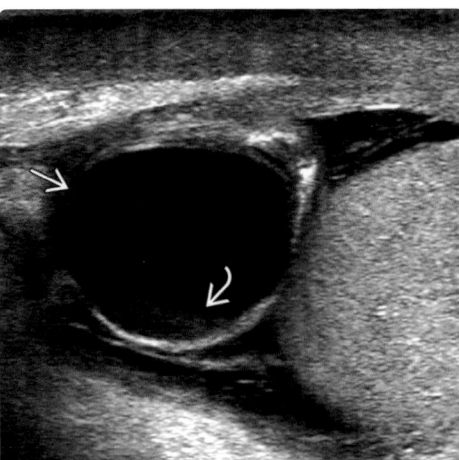

Epididymal Cyst

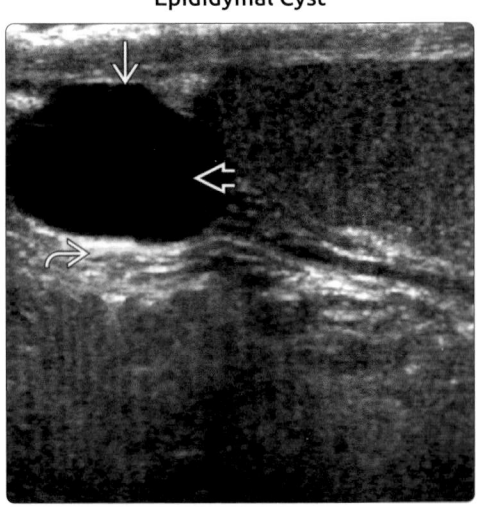

(Left) *Longitudinal ultrasound shows a well-circumscribed cystic lesion ➡ in the head of the epididymis. Note layering of internal echoes ➡ due to spermatozoa within the spermatocele.* (Right) *Oblique ultrasound shows a well-circumscribed anechoic lesion ➡ in the head of the epididymis, features suggestive of a simple epididymal cyst. Note the anechoic internal contents ➡ and posterior acoustic enhancement ➡.*

Varicocele

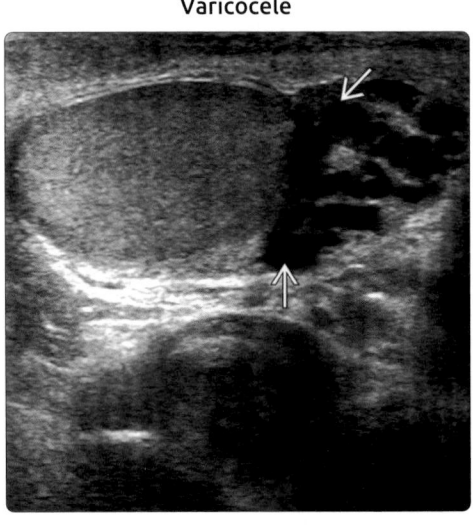

Spermatic Cord Torsion

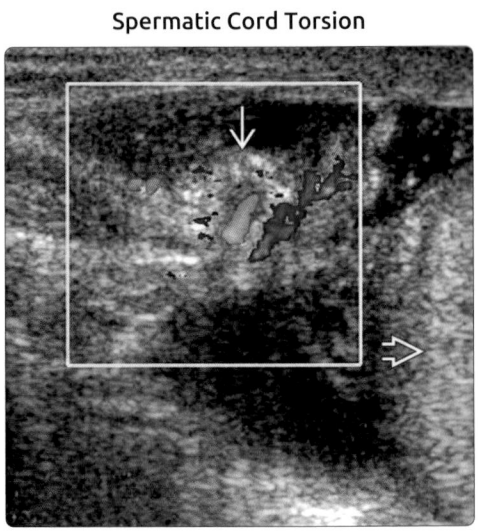

(Left) *Oblique ultrasound shows dilated, tortuous varicose veins of the pampiniform plexus ➡ in the spermatic cord, along the posterosuperior aspect of the testis, features of a varicocele.* (Right) *Oblique color Doppler ultrasound shows a "torsion knot" ➡ or "whirlpool" pattern of spermatic cord just immediately cranial to the testis ➡, features suggesting an acute torsion of spermatic cord. The testis is prone to infarct due to compromised vascularity.*

Hematoma

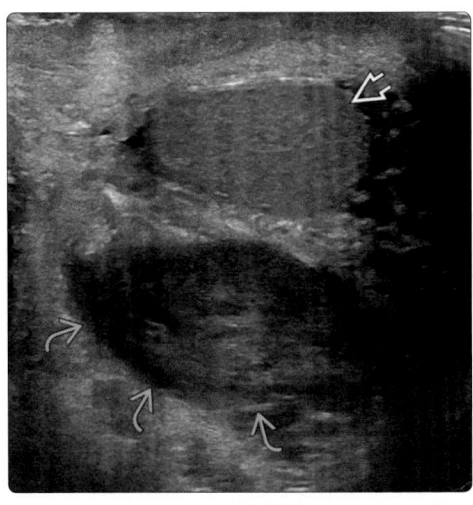

Adenomatoid Tumor

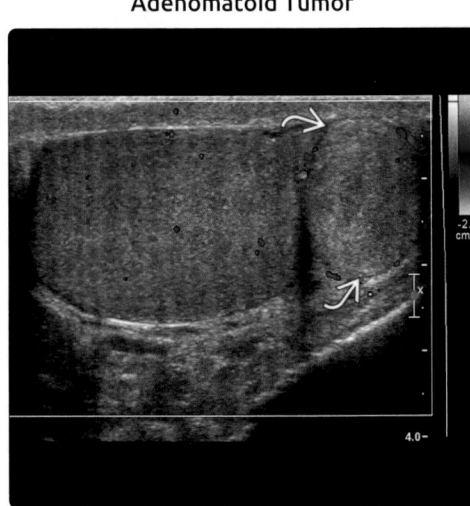

(Left) *Hypoechoic extratesticular hematoma ➡ in a patient with straddle injury to groin is shown. No injury to ipsilateral testicle ➡ was seen in this patient.* (Right) *This solid, well-circumscribed slightly hyperechoic adenomatoid tumor in the epididymal tail ➡ has little internal vascularity.*

Inguinal Hernia

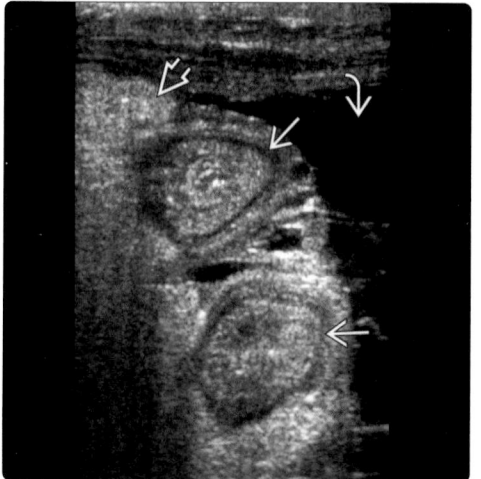

Inguinal Hernia

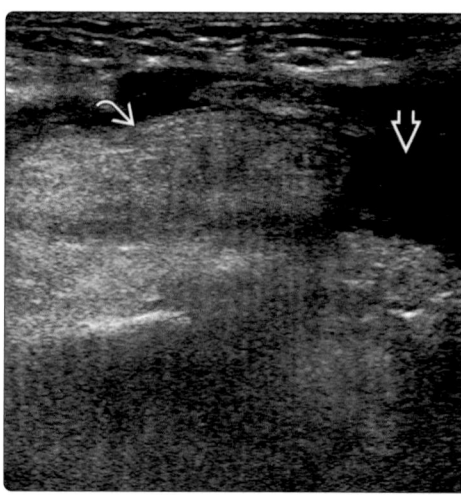

(Left) *Oblique ultrasound shows an inguinoscrotal hernia, containing small bowel loops ➡, and mesentery ⇉. Note the bowel wall (gut signature), which distinguishes this from a cord or epididymal mass. Note the fluid in the hernia sac ⬈.* **(Right)** *Longitudinal ultrasound shows an ill-defined, lobulated, echogenic ➡ structure herniating into the scrotum ⇉, features suggestive of an omentocele.*

Fatty Deposition

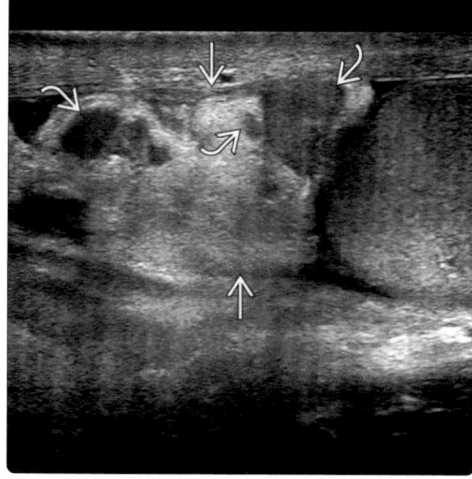

Fatty Deposition

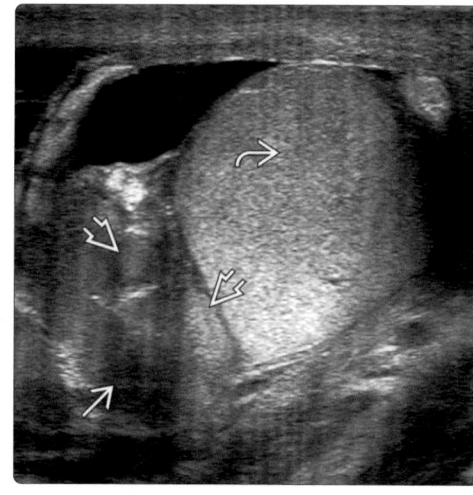

(Left) *Longitudinal ultrasound shows an ill-defined hyperechoic structure ➡ surrounding the epididymis ⬈. This "pseudomass" is due to the deposition of fat.* **(Right)** *Transverse ultrasound shows an ill-defined, hyperechoic structure ➡ in the region of the body and head of the epididymis. No obvious discrete mass is identifiable. This "pseudomass" is likely due to the deposition of fat. Parts of epididymis can be seen as small hypoechoic areas ⇉ within the "pseudomass." Note the normal testis ⬈.*

Encysted Hydrocele of Cord

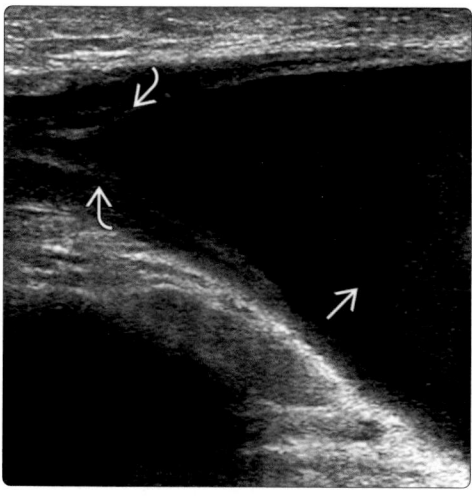

Encysted Hydrocele of Cord

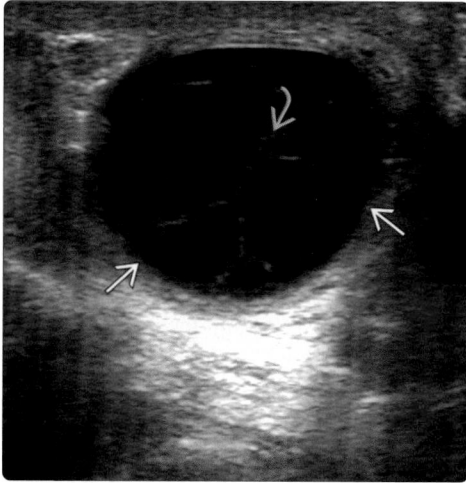

(Left) *Longitudinal ultrasound shows an elongated anechoic fluid collection ➡ within layers of the distal spermatic cord in the inguinoscrotal region. Note the splayed layers ⬈ of the proximal spermatic cord, features suggestive of an encysted hydrocele of the spermatic cord.* **(Right)** *Transverse ultrasound shows a chronic, fluid collection ➡ with multiple fine septations ⬿ in the inguinoscrotal region representing an encysted hydrocele of the spermatic cord.*

Papillary Cystadenoma

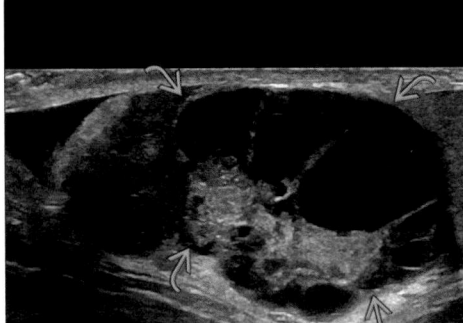

Papillary Cystadenoma

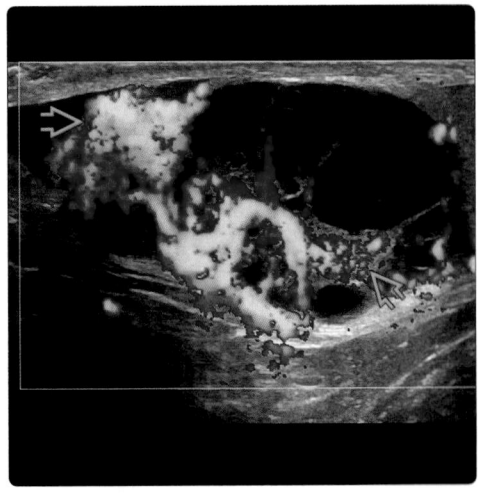

(Left) *Solid and cystic extratesticular mass in a patient with with VHL ➔ is compatible with a papillary cystadenoma.* (Right) *Power Doppler shows brisk flow within the solid components ➔ of a papillary cystadenoma.*

Lipoma

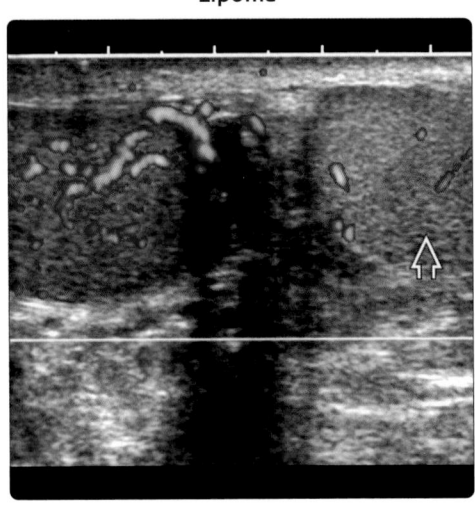

Epididymal/Scrotal Wall Abscess

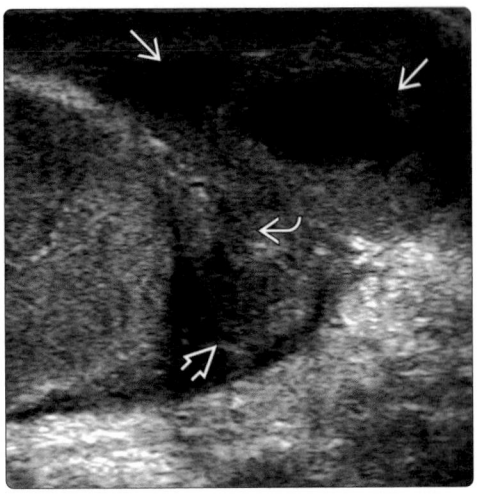

(Left) *Power Doppler ultrasound shows relative hypovascularity within a hyperechoic, well-circumscribed epididymal lipoma ➔.* (Right) *Oblique ultrasound shows a poorly defined, hypoechoic abscess ➔ within the layers of the scrotum, due to the spread of infection from the adjacent inflamed epididymis ➔. Note the track ➔ along which the infection has reached the scrotal wall.*

Epididymal/Scrotal Wall Abscess

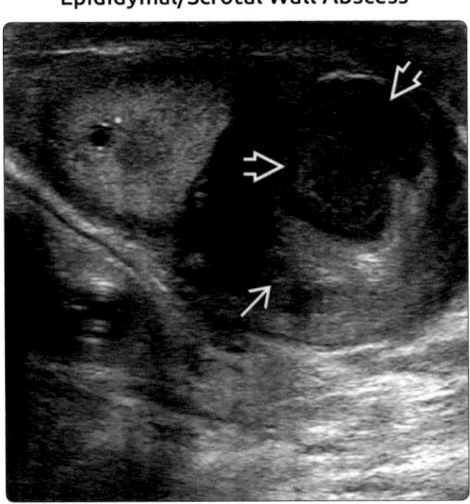

Epididymal/Scrotal Wall Abscess

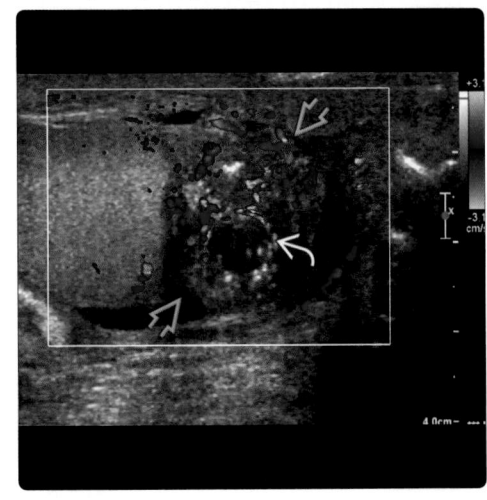

(Left) *A markedly enlarged epididymis ➔ with central liquefactive necrosis ➔ indicating abscess formation in a patient with subacute epididymitis not responding to antibiotic therapy.* (Right) *Round hypoechoic collection ➔ representing abscess within an enlarged and hyperemic epididymis ➔ in a patient with chronic urinary tract infections and bilateral epididymitis. Note the Doppler flow surrounding, but not within, the collection.*

Liposarcoma of Spermatic Cord

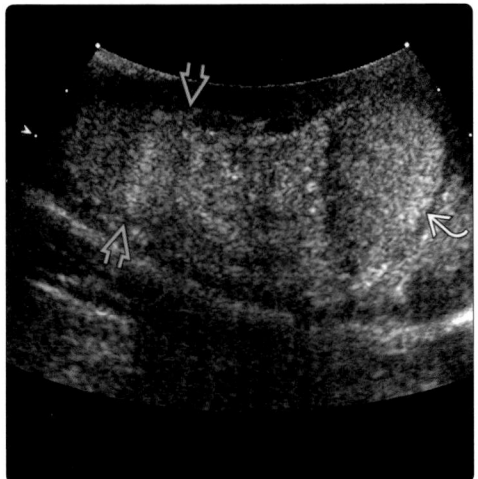

Liposarcoma of Spermatic Cord

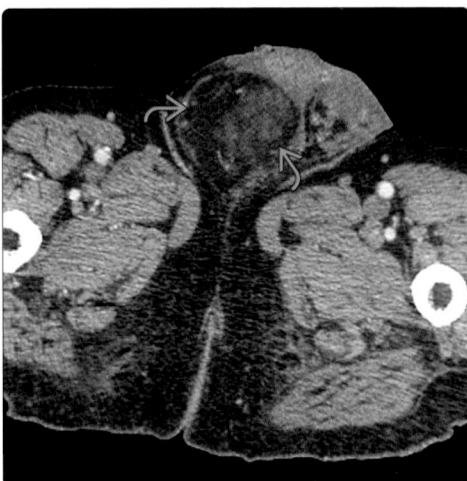

(Left) *Proliferative fat within the inguinal canal ⮥ inferiorly displaces the right testis ➘ in a patient with right inguinal liposarcoma.* (Right) *CECT in the same patient shows bulky adipose tissue with soft tissue elements ⮥ in the upper scrotum in this spermatic cord liposarcoma.*

Epididymal Rhabdomyosarcoma

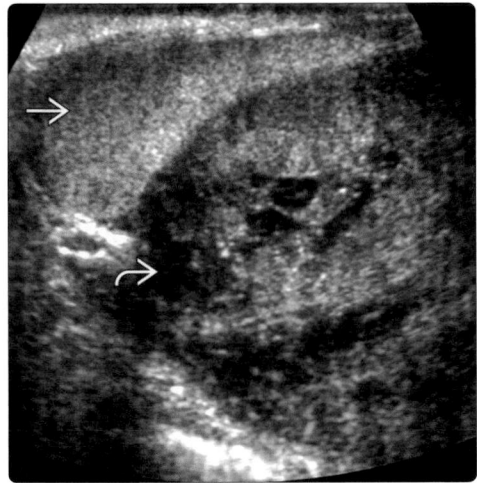

Metastases

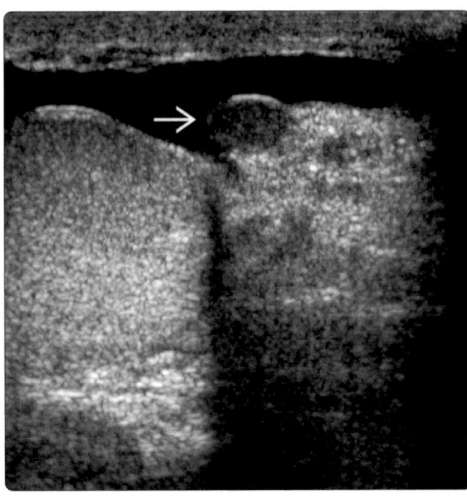

(Left) *Longitudinal ultrasound shows a large, heterogeneous, paratesticular mass ➘ compressing the testis ➘. The epididymis could not be seen separately in this patient with epididymal rhabdomyosarcoma.* (Right) *Oblique ultrasound shows a small, well-defined, hypoechoic lesion ➘ within the head of the epididymis in this patient with known disseminated malignancy. The final diagnosis was epididymal metastases.*

Tuberculous Epididymitis

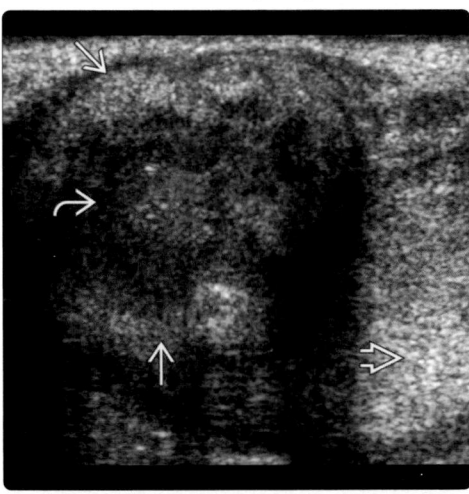

Tuberculous Epididymitis

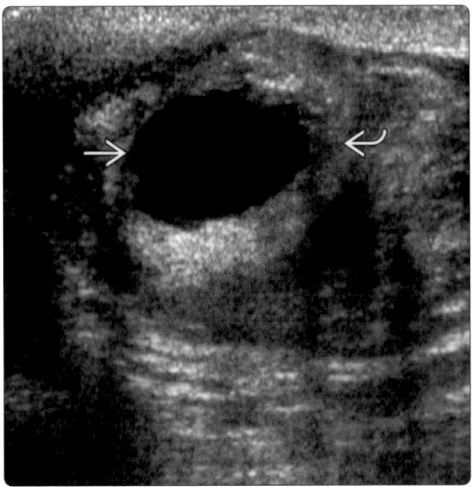

(Left) *Transverse ultrasound shows an enlarged, lobulated, epididymal head ➘. Note the heterogeneous intrinsic echo pattern ➘, features suggestive of a chronic granulomatous inflammatory mass in this patient with tuberculous epididymitis. Note the normal testis ➘.* (Right) *Oblique ultrasound follow-up performed 2 years later in the same patient shows a well-developed area of necrosis ➘ within the chronically inflamed epididymal head ➘.*

DIFFERENTIAL DIAGNOSIS

Common

- Hydrocele
- Varicocele
- Spermatocele
- Epididymal Cyst

Less Common

- Tunica Albuginea Cyst
- Acute Hematocele
- Pyocele
- Epididymal or Scrotal Wall Abscess
- Inguinal Hernia Containing Bowel

Rare but Important

- Papillary Cystadenoma of Epididymis

ESSENTIAL INFORMATION

Helpful Clues for Common Diagnoses

- **Hydrocele**
  - Congenital or acquired
  - Fluid collection in tunica vaginalis
    - May be simple or complex
  - Envelops testis except for "bare area" where tunica vaginalis is deficient
- **Varicocele**
  - Dilation of veins of pampiniform plexus > 3 mm, due to retrograde flow in internal spermatic vein
  - Enlargement and "color flash" with Valsalva maneuver
  - Left (78%), right (6%), bilateral (16%)
- **Spermatocele**
  - Retention cyst of tubules connecting rete testis to head of epididymis
  - Located in head of epididymis; contains spermatozoa
  - Often associated with tubular ectasia of rete testis
- **Epididymal Cyst**
  - Simple cyst in epididymal head, body, tail
  - Anechoic, does not contain spermatozoa

Helpful Clues for Less Common Diagnoses

- **Tunica Albuginea Cyst**
  - Invested between layers of tunica albuginea
    - May appear as intra-/extratesticular cyst
  - Usually solitary but can be multiple
    - 2-3 mm diameter
  - Asymptomatic
- **Acute Hematocele**
  - Associated with trauma, torsion, and infarction
  - Varies in appearance with evolution of blood products
  - Look for associated testicular injury
- **Pyocele**
  - Sequela of scrotal infections
  - Septate fluid with low-level internal echoes
  - Chronicity may lead to thickening of tunica and scrotal wall
- **Epididymal or Scrotal Wall Abscess**
  - Associated with chronic epididymitis or orchitis
  - No central vascularity but surrounding hyperemia
  - Internal contents complex, rarely simple
- **Inguinal Hernia Containing Bowel**
  - Varies with Valsalva
  - Multilaminar gut signature present
  - May show peristalsis

Helpful Clues for Rare Diagnoses

- **Papillary Cystadenoma of Epididymis**
  - Rare benign lesion associated with von Hippel-Lindau syndrome
  - Cystic and solid epididymal mass

SELECTED REFERENCES

1. Mirochnik B et al: Ultrasound evaluation of scrotal pathology. Radiol Clin North Am. 50(2):317-32, vi, 2012
2. Wasnik AP et al: Scrotal pearls and pitfalls: ultrasound findings of benign scrotal lesions. Ultrasound Q. 28(4):281-91, 2012
3. Valentino M et al: Cystic lesions and scrotal fluid collections in adults: Ultrasound findings. J Ultrasound. 14(4):208-15, 2011

Hydrocele

Spermatocele

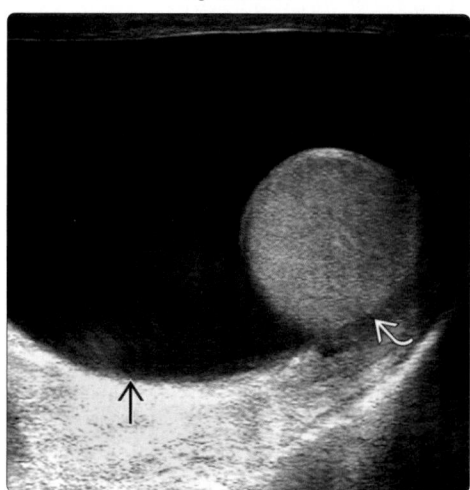
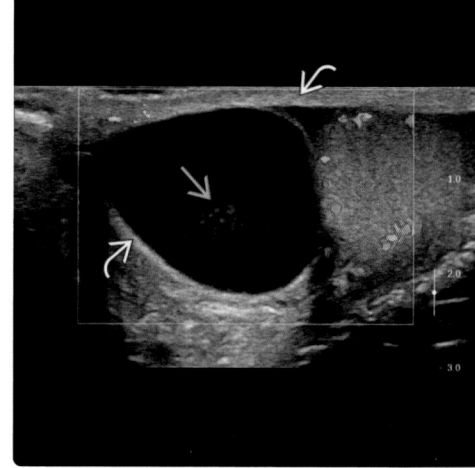

(Left) *Longitudinal ultrasound of scrotum shows anechoic fluid ➡ within the tunica vaginalis, indicative of a simple hydrocele. Fluid in the tunica vaginalis envelops the testis except posteriorly ➡ at the "bare area."* (Right) *Well-circumscribed cystic collection ➡ superior to the right testis contains punctate echogenic spermatozoa and debris, which is mobile and generates Doppler artifact ➡ in real time.*

Extratesticular Cystic Mass

Varicocele

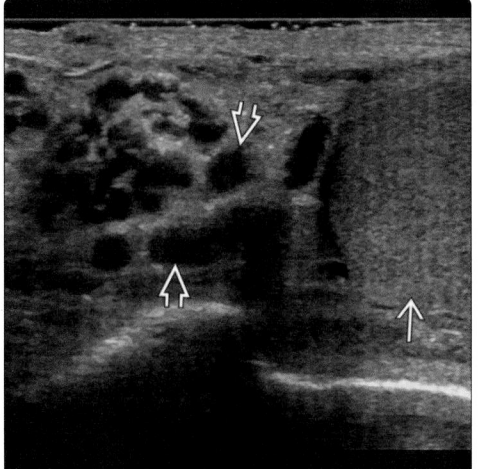

Varicocele

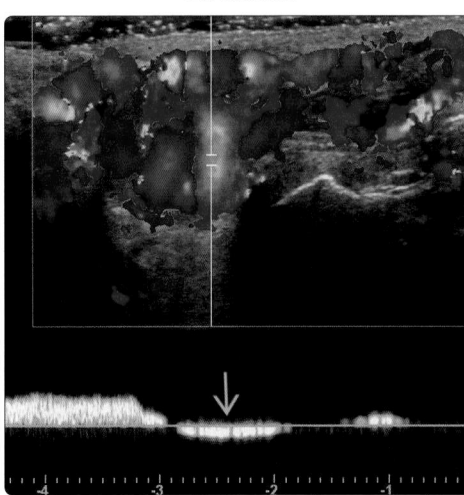

(Left) *Longitudinal ultrasound shows multiple serpiginous, dilated vessels ➡, just cephalad to the testis ➡.* (Right) *Color Doppler ultrasound in the same patient shows flow within these vessels. The scan was performed during a Valsalva maneuver, which caused retrograde filling ➡ due to incompetent valves.*

Epididymal Cyst

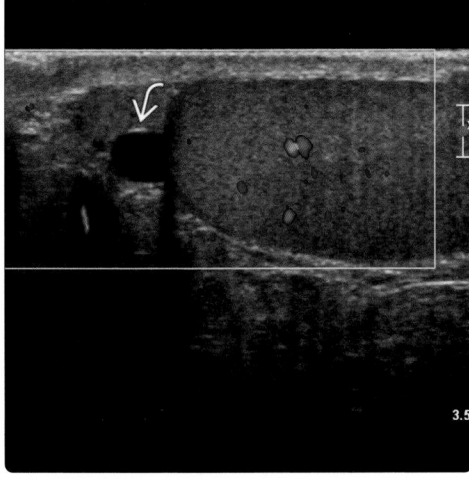

Acute Hematocele

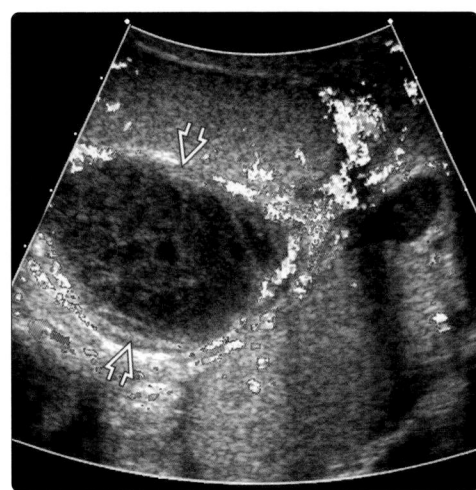

(Left) *Subcentimeter epididymal head cysts ➡ are often incidentally detected or may be palpable as a painless mass.* (Right) *Color Doppler ultrasound of the scrotum shows an avascular, complex, extratesticular fluid collection ➡ in a man who recently had a vasectomy. The hematoma resolved on follow-up studies.*

Tunica Albuginea Cyst

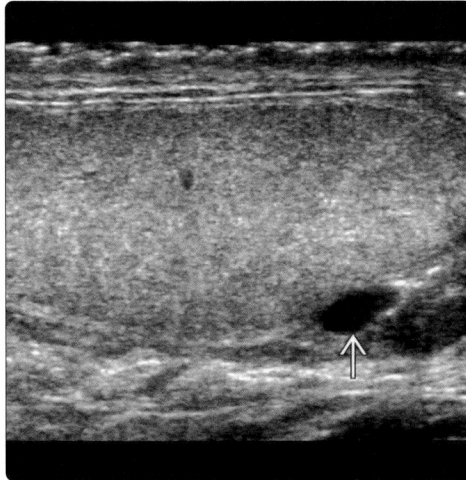

Epididymal or Scrotal Wall Abscess

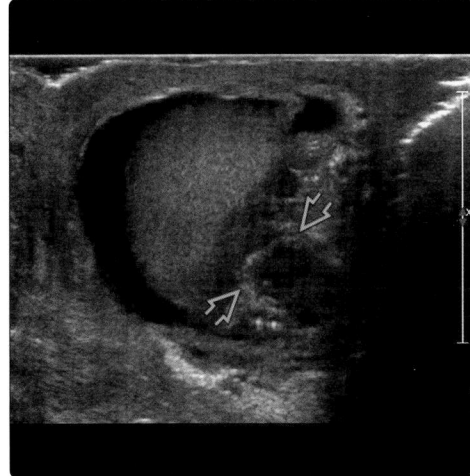

(Left) *Longitudinal ultrasound shows a small, well-defined, anechoic cyst ➡ along the periphery of the testis, classic appearance of a tunica albuginea cyst.* (Right) *Complex cystic collection within the epididymis ➡ is compatible with abscess in this patient with a history of several months of epididymitis poorly responsive to antibiotics.*

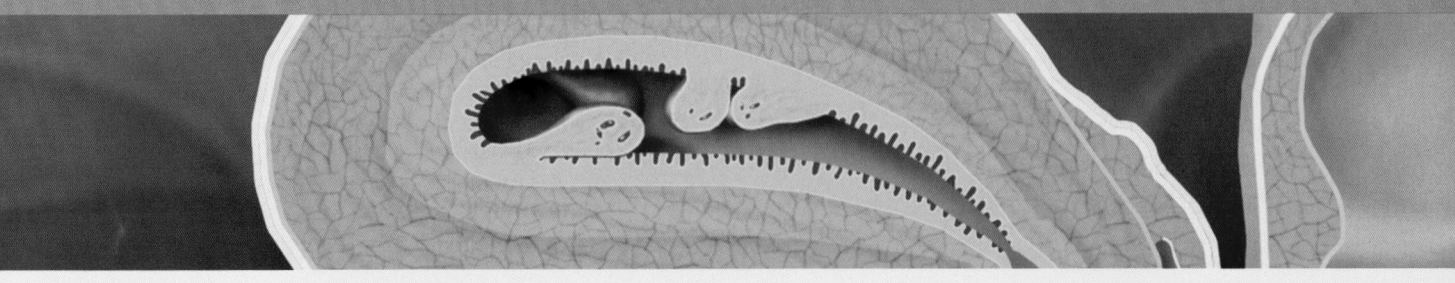

PART III
SECTION 11
Female Pelvis

DIFFERENTIAL DIAGNOSIS

Common

- Physiologic Cysts
  - Follicular Cyst
  - Corpus Luteal Cyst
- Paraovarian/Paratubal Cyst
- Postmenopausal Adnexal Cyst
- Inclusion Cyst, Ovary

Less Common

- Serous Cystadenoma
- Hydrosalpinx
- Theca Lutein Cysts
- Peritoneal Inclusion Cysts
- Dermoid (Mature Cystic Teratoma)

Rare but Important

- Serous Cystadenocarcinoma
- Anechoic Adnexal Cyst (Mimic)
  - Loop of Bowel
  - Bladder Diverticulum
  - Tarlov Cyst
  - GI Duplication Cyst
  - Complex Cyst (Mimic)
  - Solid Lesion (Mimic)
  - Nabothian Cyst
- Adnexal Torsion

ESSENTIAL INFORMATION

Key Differential Diagnosis Issues

- Thin-walled, anechoic cysts are benign
  - Solid elements increase risk of malignancy
- Rule of 1-2-3
  - 1 cm cyst in 1st week of menstrual cycle is follicle
  - 2 cm cyst in 2nd week of menstrual cycle is dominant follicle
  - 3 cm cyst in 3rd week of menstrual cycle is corpus luteum
- Size is important
  - Cyst < 3 cm in premenopausal woman is likely physiologic
  - Cyst > 7 cm is potentially neoplastic
- Follow-up sonogram in 6 weeks often shows resolution of physiologic cysts but is almost always unnecessary
- Pain can be due to size of cyst or torsion of cyst
- Is cyst separate from ovary?
  - Paraovarian cyst
  - Hydrosalpinx
  - Loop of bowel

Helpful Clues for Common Diagnoses

- **Physiologic Cysts**
  - Premenopausal women
    - Resolve over time
  - Birth control pills can decrease formation of new cysts while current cyst resolves
- **Paraovarian/Paratubal Cyst**
  - Separate from ovary
  - Thin walled
  - Anechoic

- Tend to not change in size over time
- **Postmenopausal Adnexal Cyst**
  - Cysts may be present in postmenopausal women
  - If thin walled and anechoic (simple), highly likely benign (99%) up to 10 cm (many are serous cystadenomas)
  - May change in size over time
  - Use of tamoxifen associated with adnexal cysts
- **Inclusion Cyst, Ovary**
  - Invagination of ovarian cortical surface epithelium with lost connection to surface
  - Typically small caliber (1-13 mm) but may be up to 10 cm
  - Thin, smooth wall
  - Typically within 1-2 mm of outer surface of ovary

Helpful Clues for Less Common Diagnoses

- **Serous Cystadenoma**
  - Thin-walled cyst
  - Usually unilocular
  - May have thin septation
- **Hydrosalpinx**
  - Elongated "cyst" with tubular or coiled shape
  - "Cysts" connect
  - Prior pelvic inflammatory disease or endometriosis
  - Longitudinal folds show classic cogwheel appearance when tube imaged in cross section
- **Peritoneal Inclusion Cyst**
  - History of prior surgery, endometriosis, pelvic inflammatory disease
  - Ovary at edge or surrounded by cyst
  - Irregularly shaped with poorly defined walls (formed by adjacent organs)
- **Dermoid (Mature Cystic Teratoma)**
  - Rare for dermoid to present as purely anechoic cyst but can occur if predominately sebum component
  - Calcifications in wall or echogenic nodule (dermoid plug) raise suspicion of dermoid
  - May see
    - "Dot-dash-dot" appearance of hair in sebum
    - "Tip of the iceberg" sign in which "dirty" shadowing from dermoid obscures visualization of deep margins of mass

Helpful Clues for Rare Diagnoses

- **Serous Cystadenocarcinoma**
  - Extremely rare for serous cystadenocarcinoma to present as anechoic cyst
  - If cyst is large, small solid element could be missed at imaging
- **Anechoic Adnexal Cyst (Mimic)**
  - Use transvaginal scanning to assess for internal echotexture to exclude solid elements or septations
  - At real-time scanning assess for peristalsis
  - Ensure that gain is set appropriately to detect solid elements
  - Assess for flow within presumed cyst to ensure it is not homogeneous, hypoechoic, solid lesion
  - Ensure that lesion is in adnexa and not related to bowel or spine
  - **Complex Cyst (Mimic)**
    - May appear anechoic due to transabdominal technique or gain set too low

    □ Hemorrhagic cyst or endometrioma may be mistaken for simple cyst
- Solid Lesion (Mimic)
  - May appear as anechoic cyst if gain set too low and color Doppler not used
- Nabothian Cyst
  - Can be confused for adnexal cyst if location in cervix is not noted
- **Adnexal Torsion**
  - Rare for adnexal torsion to present as anechoic cyst
  - Cyst 5-10 cm in size can act as lead point for torsion
  - Ipsilateral pain out of proportion to size of cyst suggests torsion
  - Blood flow analysis typically not helpful, because anechoic cysts do not demonstrate flow

Alternative Differential Approaches

- Multiple cysts
  - Multiple physiologic cysts
  - Hydrosalpinx folded on itself
  - Peritoneal inclusion cyst
  - Ovarian inclusion cysts
  - Theca lutein cysts
  - Hyperstimulated ovaries
- Bilateral cysts
  - Peritoneal inclusion cyst
  - Theca lutein cysts
  - Hyperstimulated ovaries
  - Hydrosalpinx
  - Cystadenoma
- Pregnant patient
  - Corpus luteum
  - Serous cystadenoma
  - Theca lutein cysts
  - Hyperstimulated ovaries

Society of Radiologists in Ultrasound Consensus Criteria for Reporting of Simple Cyst

- Premenopausal

    ○ ≤ 3 cm: Best to refer to these as dominant follicles and not necessary to report

    ○ > 3 and ≤ 5 cm: Mention in the report; state almost certainly benign; no follow-up needed

    ○ > 5 and ≤ 7 cm: 1-year follow-up

    ○ > 7cm: Surgical evaluation

        – Some seemingly simple cysts may have complex features missed by US when over 7.5 cm

- Peri- or postmenopausal
  - ≤1 cm: Benign; no follow-up; discretion of radiologist wether to mention in report
  - >1 and ≤7 cm: Almost certainly benign; 1-year follow-up
  - >7 cm: Surgical evaluation

American College of Radiology Incidental Cystic Adnexal Findings Detected at CT/MR

- Benign appearing cyst (defined as oval/round, unilocular, uniform fluid attenuation/signal, thin wall, no solid area or mural nodule, < 10 cm maximum diameter)
  - Premenopausal
    - ≤ 5 cm: No follow-up
    - > 5 cm: US follow-up in 6-12 weeks
  - Early postmenopausal
    - ≤ 3 cm: No follow-up
    - > 3 and ≤ 5 cm: US follow-up in 6-12 weeks
    - > 5 cm: US
  - Late postmenopausal
    - ≤ 3 cm: Benign, no follow-up
    - > 3 cm: US
    - Note: Higher threshold of 3 cm was adopted which decreases sensitivity; some groups may want to adopt 1 cm similar to SRU guidelines

SELECTED REFERENCES

1. Patel MD et al: Managing incidental findings on abdominal and pelvic CT and MRI, part 1: white paper of the ACR Incidental Findings Committee II on adnexal findings. J Am Coll Radiol. 10(9):675-81, 2013
2. Levine D et al: Management of asymptomatic ovarian and other adnexal cysts imaged at US: Society of Radiologists in Ultrasound Consensus Conference Statement. Radiology. 256(3):943-54, 2010

Follicular Cyst

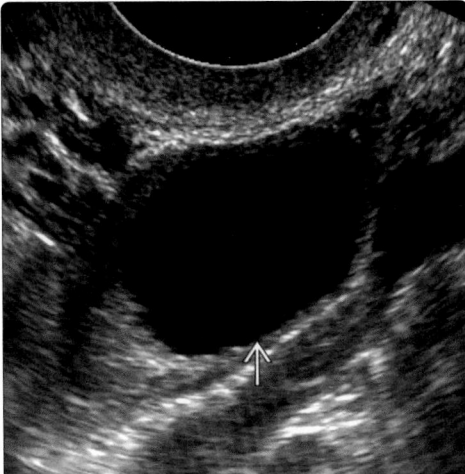

Follicular Cyst

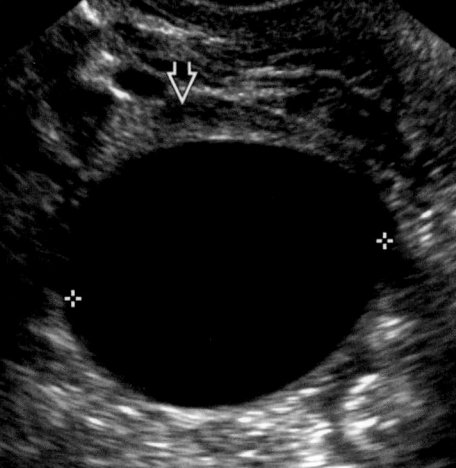

(Left) *Longitudinal endovaginal US in a 27-year-old woman shows a 2.5 cm anechoic cyst* ➡ *in the left ovary consistent with a follicular cyst, a normal finding. These do not have to be mentioned in the radiology report as it may elicit inappropriate follow-up and patient anxiety.* (Right) *Endovaginal US in a premenopausal asymptomatic woman shows thin-walled anechoic ovarian cyst, measuring 3.5 cm compressing adjacent ovarian parenchyma* ➡. *This is typical of a follicular cyst.*

Corpus Luteal Cyst

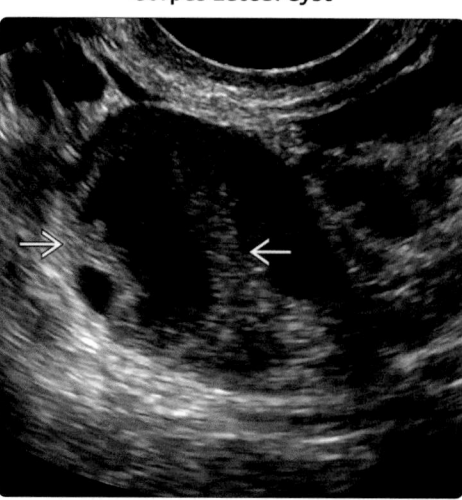

Paraovarian/Paratubal Cyst

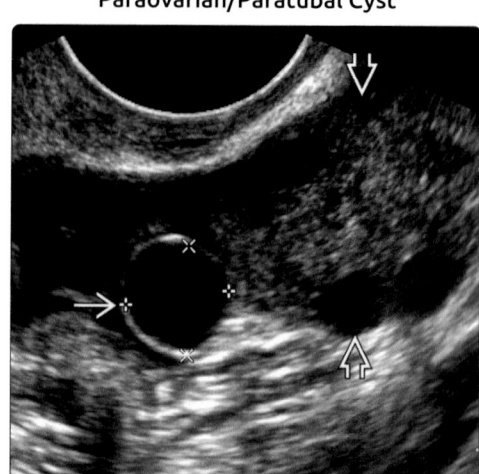

(Left) *Longitudinal endovaginal US shows a typical corpus luteum as an anechoic cyst ➡ with a thick and crenulated wall. Corpus lutea may show variable degrees of simple or complex internal fluid hemorrhagic cyst.* (Right) *Transverse endovaginal US of the left adnexa shows a thin-walled, anechoic cyst ➡, surrounded by free fluid, separate from the normal follicle containing ovary ➡. Applying transducer pressure in real-time can often help in distinguishing a lesion arising from ovary versus broad ligament.*

Serous Cystadenoma

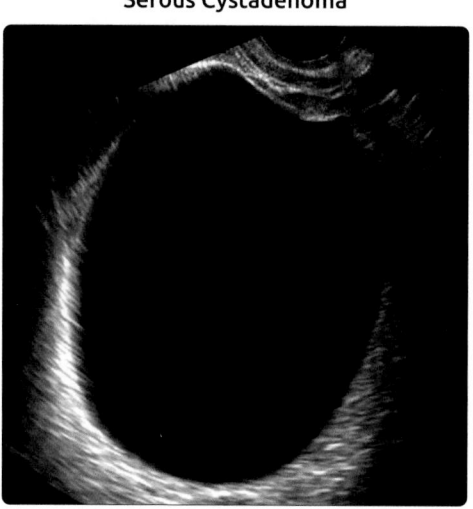

Hydrosalpinx

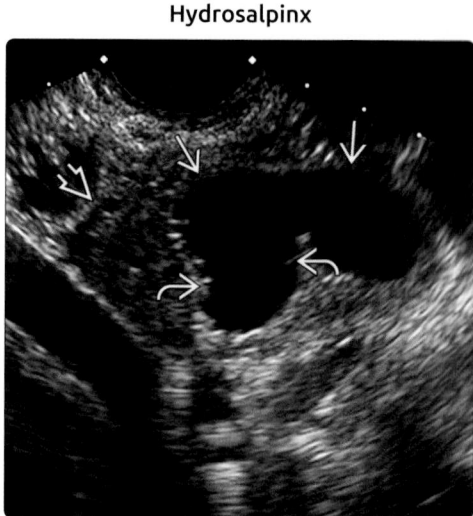

(Left) *Endovaginal US shows large simple cyst measuring 10 cm, typical of a serous cystadenoma. A cystadenocarcinoma would contain mural nodules/solid components, which would typically be large.* (Right) *Longitudinal endovaginal US shows a cyst ➡ adjacent to the left ovary ➡. Note the tubular shape and longitudinal folds ➡ in cross section giving the cogwheel appearance typical of hydrosalpinx*

Theca Lutein Cysts

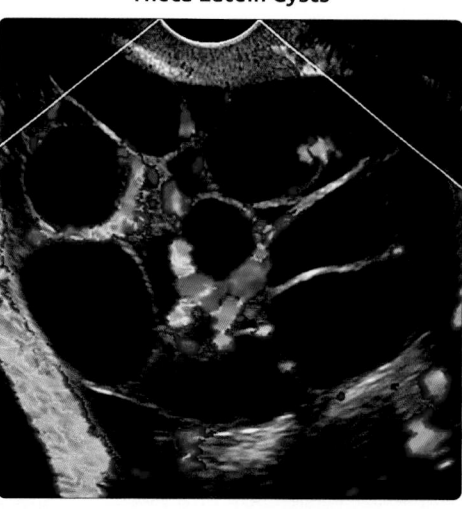

Peritoneal Inclusion Cysts

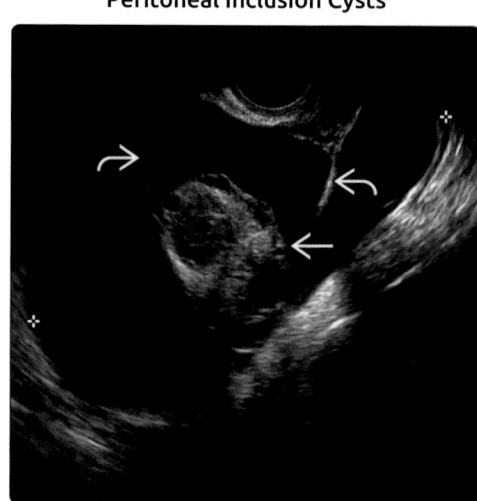

(Left) *Endovaginal US in a 26-year-old woman with a molar pregnancy shows numerous large cysts within an enlarged, 8 cm right ovary. The left ovary was the same. Note the difference between this and ovarian torsion where the cysts are small and peripheral with central ovarian edema.* (Right) *Longitudinal endovaginal US in a woman with prior pelvic surgery shows large a cyst surrounding the left ovary ➡ with thin septations ➡. This is typical of a peritoneal inclusion cyst.*

Dermoid (Mature Cystic Teratoma)

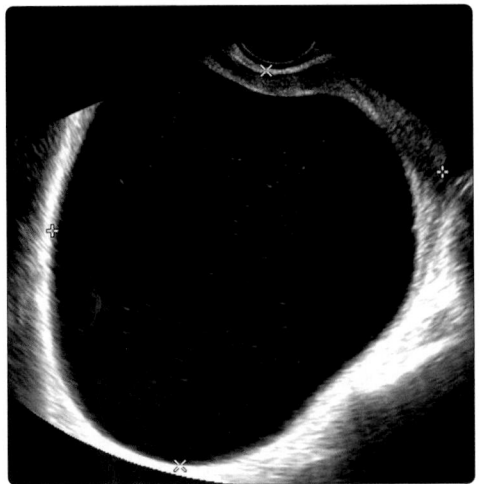

Complex Cyst (Mimic)

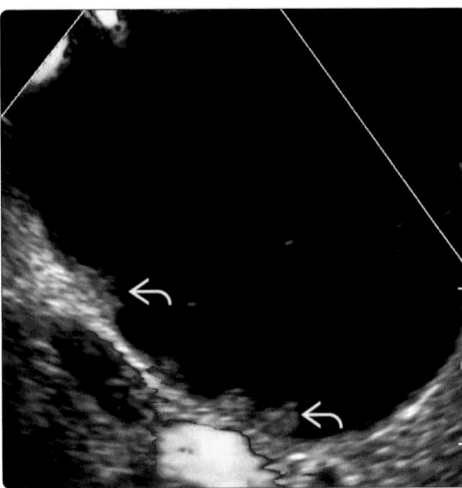

(Left) *Endovaginal US in a premenopausal woman shows a large thin-walled, adnexal cyst, which is predominately anechoic but contains a few specular reflectors. Dermoids can rarely mimic an anechoic cyst if they are predominately filled with sebum.* (Right) *Transverse endovaginal power Doppler US in a premenopausal woman shows a large, anechoic cyst with several small avascular mural nodules ➘. Pathology revealed a serous borderline tumor. Careful search for mural nodules should be performed.*

Complex Cyst (Mimic)

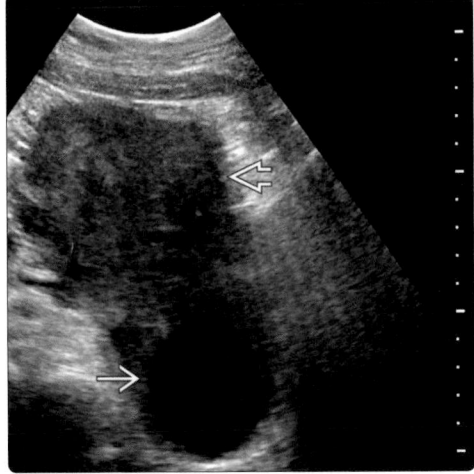

Complex Cyst (Mimic)

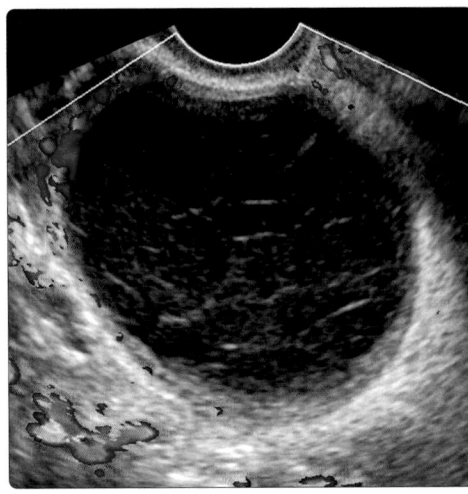

(Left) *Longitudinal transabdominal US in a premenopausal woman shows an anechoic left ovarian cyst ➡ at 10 cm depth posterior to a fibroid uterus ➡. (Right) Transverse endovaginal US in the same patient shows classic findings of a hemorrhagic cyst with lacy interstices/cobweb appearance. Note that transabdominal ultrasound may not show the detailed architecture of a cyst and transvaginal ultrasound should always be performed when feasible.*

Complex Cyst (Mimic)

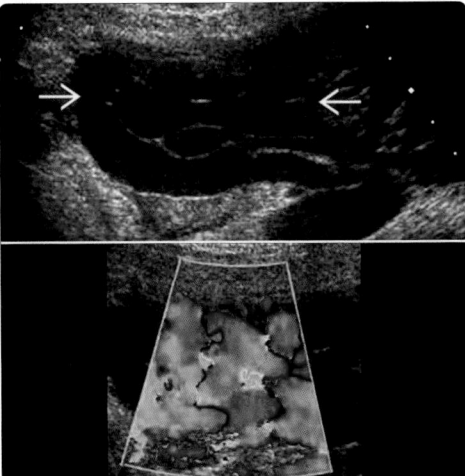

Adnexal Torsion

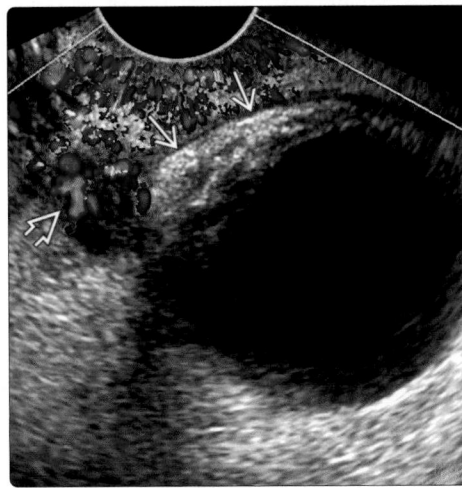

(Left) *Transverse transabdominal US of the right adnexa in the 3rd trimester shows dilated adnexal veins ➡, which should not be mistaken for a complex cystic adnexal mass.* (Right) *Endovaginal color Doppler US in a woman with acute pelvic pain shows a simple cyst with surrounding claw of edematous ovarian parenchyma ➡ with no Doppler flow. A twisted pedicle ➡ could be seen in real time. Cysts may act as a lead point for ovarian torsion.*

DIFFERENTIAL DIAGNOSIS

Common

- Leiomyoma
- Ectopic Pregnancy
- Mature Teratoma (Dermoid)

Less Common

- Adnexal Torsion
- Metastases, Ovary
- Ovarian Fibroma
- Solid Adnexal Mass (Mimics)
  - Hemorrhagic Ovarian Cyst
  - Endometrioma
  - Obstructed Uterine Duplication
  - Pelvic Kidney
  - Rectosigmoid Carcinoma
- Primary Ovarian Malignancy
  - Mucinous Cystadenocarcinoma
  - Serous Cystadenocarcinoma
  - Endometrioid Carcinoma

Rare but Important

- Ovarian Lymphoma
- Tubo-Ovarian Abscess
- Tubal Carcinoma
- Luteoma of Pregnancy
- Adenofibroma
- Granulosa Cell Tumor
- Brenner Tumor
- Atypical Germ Cell Tumors
  - Immature Teratoma
  - Dysgerminoma
  - Choriocarcinoma
- Massive Ovarian Edema and Fibromatosis

ESSENTIAL INFORMATION

Key Differential Diagnosis Issues

- Understanding typical appearance of benign lesions and mimics of malignant solid masses is important to avoid unnecessary work-up or surgery
- Ovaries visualized separate from mass suggests nonovarian etiology
- If mass appears fibrotic with shadowing, tends to be benign fibrous lesions
  - Pedunculated or broad ligament leiomyoma
  - Ovarian fibroma
  - Adenofibroma
- Bilateral lesions
  - Primary ovarian malignancy
  - Metastases
  - Endometrioid carcinoma
  - Lymphoma
- Hormonally active lesion
  - Thecoma
  - Granulosa cell tumor

Helpful Clues for Common Diagnoses

- **Leiomyoma**
  - May be subserosal, exophytic, pedunculated

- Ovaries are seen separate from mass
  - Using transducer pressure to push away ovary can confirm this
- Fibrous appearance with edge shadowing
- Blood flow is seen connecting mass to uterus
- MR helpful in establishing etiology if uncertain (leiomyoma vs. fibrous ovarian tumor)
- Can grow/degenerate during pregnancy due to hormonal stimulation
  - Causes pain
  - Appears as growing, solid adnexal mass
- **Ectopic Pregnancy**
  - Always should be suspected in premenopausal woman with pelvic pain and adnexal mass
  - Typically, small round adnexal mass (tubal ring) separate from ovary
    - With absent intrauterine pregnancy
    - Hypervascular rim on color Doppler
      - Do not confuse with increased flow around corpus luteum
  - May see yolk sac or fetal pole but typically do not
  - When ruptured, if adherent, adnexal clot can be confused for large solid adnexal mass
    - Ovary and tubal pregnancy may not be seen separately from clot
- **Mature Teratoma (Dermoid)**
  - Cystic mass with variety of imaging appearances that can mimic solid lesion
    - Typical: Heterogeneous cystic ovarian mass with echogenic shadowing mural nodule (Rokitansky nodule)
    - Posterior "dirty" shadowing, tip of iceberg sign
    - ± fat-fluid level
    - Dot-dash sign from hair
    - Rarely entirely echogenic and solid appearing but should lack central Doppler flow
      - Beware of twinkling artifact mimicking true flow; use pulsed Doppler if unsure

Helpful Clues for Less Common Diagnoses

- **Adnexal Torsion**
  - Unilateral lesion in patient with severe ipsilateral pain
  - Enlarged ovary
  - Multiple, small, peripheral follicles or mass acting as lead point
  - Blood flow may be absent on affected side, but not all cases of torsion have abnormal blood flow
- **Metastases, Ovary**
  - Patient with known primary carcinoma, most commonly from colon, gastric, breast, lung, or contralateral ovary
  - Krukenberg tumors are metastatic ovarian tumors that contain mucin-secreting signet-ring cells, usually of GI origin
- **Ovarian Fibroma**
  - Typically seen in women age 40-60
  - May be associated with hirsutism and amenorrhea if it secretes androgen
  - May be associated with endometrial thickening if it secretes estrogen
- **Solid Adnexal Mass (Mimics)**
  - **Hemorrhagic Ovarian Cyst**

- May masquerade as solid lesion when acute
- Clues to diagnosis are increased through transmission and lack of blood flow within lesion
- Short-term follow-up often required and will show rapid change in appearance of blood products

○ **Endometrioma**
- May be echogenic and mimic solid mass, especially if gain high
- Should have no color Doppler flow except for wall

○ **Obstructed Uterine Duplication**
- Look for deviation of uterus/endometrial stripe away from side of obstructed horn
- Look for duplication of cervix

○ **Pelvic Kidney**
- Look for reniform shape, corticomedial differentiation, collecting system, and ipsilateral empty renal fossa

- **Primary Ovarian Malignancy**
○ May have other signs of malignancy such as ascites, omental thickening, serosal metastases on liver &/or spleen

○ **Endometrioid carcinoma**
- 30% are bilateral
- Typical mixed cystic and solid adnexal mass but may appear solid
- Associated with endometriosis in 15-20%

Helpful Clues for Rare Diagnoses

- **Ovarian Lymphoma**
○ Most cases of ovarian involvement are in patients with systemic disease
○ Primary ovarian lymphoma is rare
○ Homogeneous, bilateral, solid masses with lack of ascites

- **Tubo-Ovarian Abscess**
○ Patient with pelvic pain, vaginal discharge, elevated white blood cell count

- **Tubal Carcinoma**
○ May be associated with hydrosalpinx
○ Seen between uterus and ovary

○ Tube may be dilated containing tubular-shaped, solid mass
○ Often advanced and indistinguishable from primary ovarian carcinoma

- **Luteoma of Pregnancy**
○ Solid, ovarian, nonneoplastic mass that occurs during pregnancy
○ Elevated androgen levels
○ Regresses postpartum

- **Adenofibroma**
○ Fibrous lesion with shadowing

- **Granulosa Cell Tumor**
○ Due to estrogen secretion, associated with postmenopausal bleeding and precocious puberty, depending on patient age

- **Brenner Tumor**
○ Almost always benign
○ May have calcifications

- **Massive Ovarian Edema and Fibromatosis**
○ MOE: Tumor-like ovarian enlargement secondary to edema
○ OF: Tumor-like ovarian enlargement due to fibromatous growth of ovarian stroma

Alternative Differential Approaches

- Patient age/menstrual status aids in differential diagnosis
○ Prepubertal girls
- Granulosa cell tumor
- Germ cell tumor
- Immature teratoma, ovary
○ Reproductive age
- Leiomyoma, subserosal
- Dermoid (mature teratoma)
- Primary ovarian malignancy
- Ovarian fibroma
○ Postmenopausal
- Ovarian fibroma
- Primary ovarian malignancy
- Metastases, ovary
- Leiomyoma

Leiomyoma

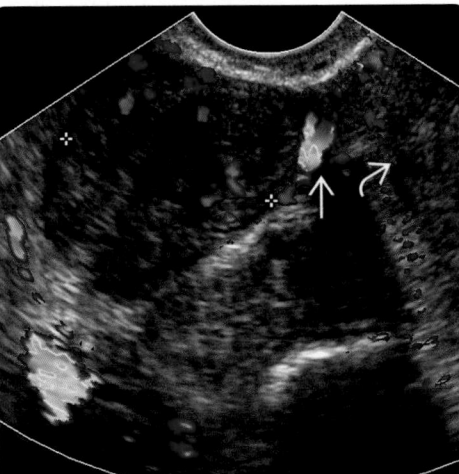

Leiomyoma

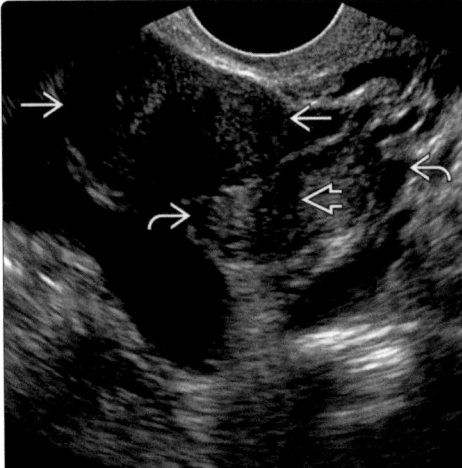

(Left) Transverse color Doppler US shows heterogeneous right adnexal hypoechoic mass (calipers). Note the vascular supply ➡ running within the stalk arising from the anterior uterine fundus ➡, typical of a pedunculated fibroid. (Right) Longitudinal endovaginal US in a 41-year-old woman with known fibroids shows a hypoechoic adnexal mass ➡ adjacent to, but separate from the right ovary ➡. Edge shadowing from the mass is seen through the ovary in the far field ➡.

Leiomyoma

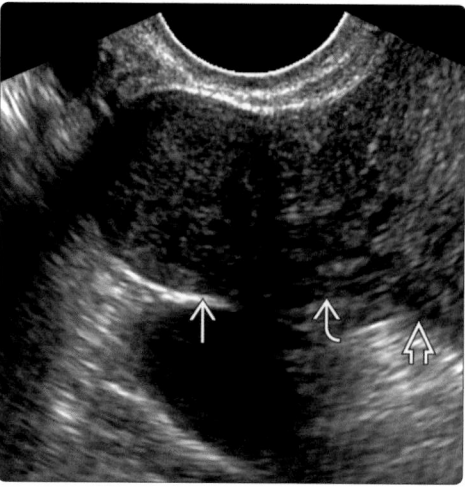

Ectopic Pregnancy

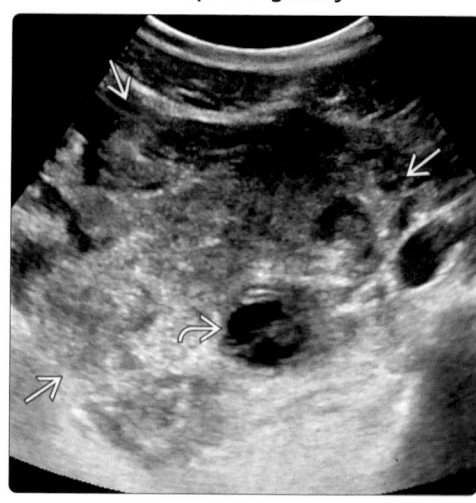

(Left) *Transverse endovaginal US in the same patient shows the pedunculated fibroid* ➡ *projecting into the right adnexa with a broad based stalk* ➡ *connecting it to the uterine body* ➡. **(Right)** *Transverse transabdominal US shows a large, heterogenous, echogenic mass* ➡ *in the left adnexa surrounding a small cystic component* ➡. *The patient was 7 weeks pregnant by LMP and no IUP was seen. A large clot surrounding a ruptured tubal ectopic was confirmed at surgery.*

Mature Teratoma (Dermoid)

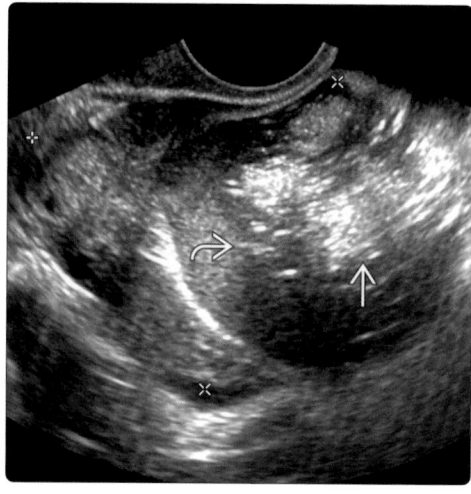

Adnexal Torsion

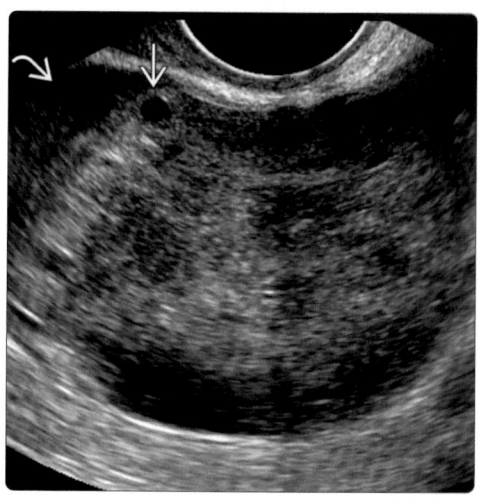

(Left) *Endovaginal US in a 19-year-old woman with a pelvic mass on exam shows a large, complex, heterogeneous mass (calipers) with echogenic Rokitansky nodule* ➡, *dot-dash sign* ➡ *from hair, and echogenic fluid. This is the most common ovarian tumor and should not be mistaken for carcinoma.* **(Right)** *Longitudinal endovaginal US in a 34-year-old woman with acute pain shows an enlarged, 6 cm, heterogeneous ovary with peripheral follicles* ➡. *Echogenic free fluid is present* ➡, *not uncommonly seen.*

Metastases, Ovary

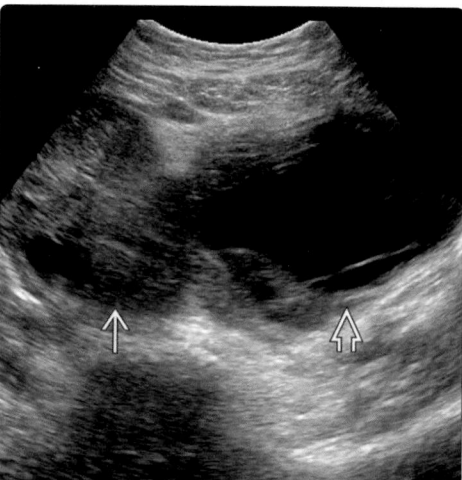

Metastases, Ovary

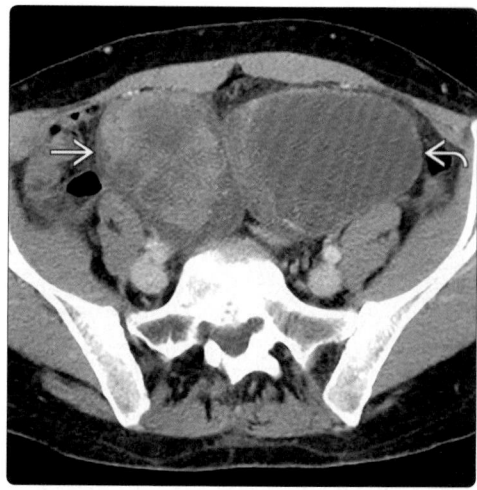

(Left) *Transverse transabdominal US in a 45-year-old woman with colon cancer shows bilateral adnexal masses, solid on the right* ➡ *and predominately cystic on the left* ➡. **(Right)** *Axial CECT in the same patient shows an enhancing solid right adnexal mass* ➡ *and a mixed cystic and solid left adnexal mass* ➡, *pathologically confirmed to be metastatic colon cancer. Ovarian metastases are often bilateral, large, and heterogeneous.*

Fibrothecoma

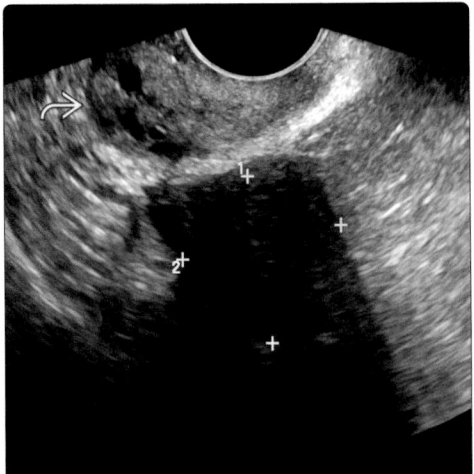

Hemorrhagic Ovarian Cyst

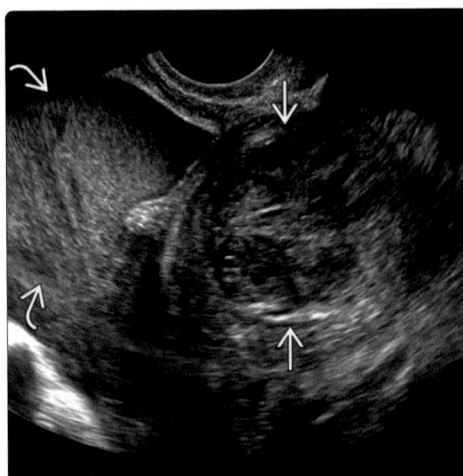

(Left) *Longitudinal endovaginal US shows a homogeneous hypoechoic mass (calipers) with posterior acoustic shadowing. While it resembles a leiomyoma, there is no stalk connecting the mass to the uterus/cervix ➡.* (Right) *Longitudinal endovaginal US in a 22-year-old woman with acute pelvic pain shows a large, heterogenous adnexal mass ➡. Large-volume echogenic pelvic free fluid ➡ indicates a ruptured hemorrhagic cyst. Lack of Doppler flow centrally is useful in distinguishing this from a solid mass.*

Endometrioma

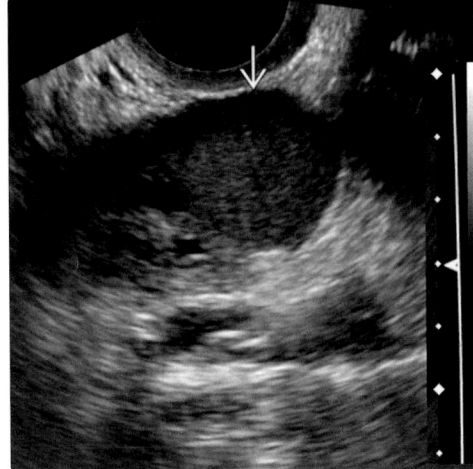

Endometrioma

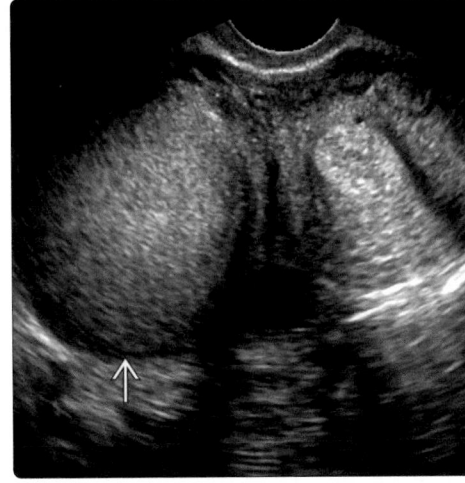

(Left) *Longitudinal endovaginal US in this asymptomatic woman shows a homogeneous small ovarian mass ➡. Lack of Doppler flow (not shown) and homogeneous echoes are typical of an endometrioma.* (Right) *Transverse endovaginal US shows a large, hyperechoic adnexal mass ➡. While Doppler flow will be seen in the wall, there should be no flow centrally, helping to distinguish this from a solid mass. Occasionally, endometriomas appear hyperechoic, which may in part be technical (↑ gain).*

Endometrioid Carcinoma

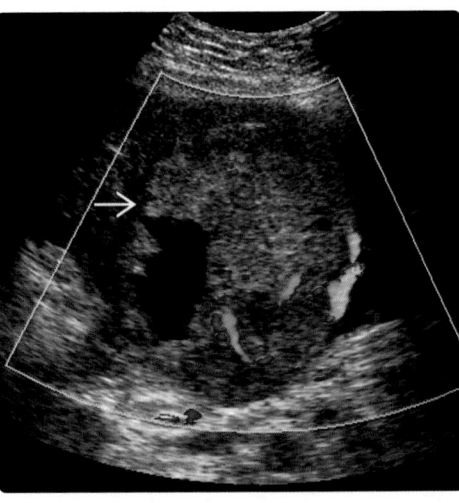

Tubo-Ovarian Abscess

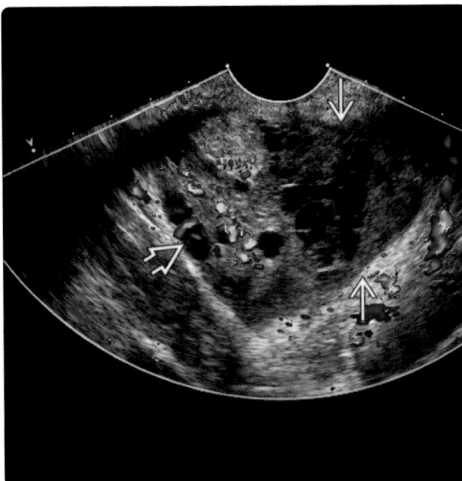

(Left) *Transabdominal US shows a cystic and solid adnexal mass ➡ with Doppler flow. The presence of a solid mass, aside from findings of carcinomatosis, is the most specific finding of ovarian carcinoma.* (Right) *Coronal endovaginal color Doppler US of the right adnexa shows the right ovary ➡ with adjacent avascular hypoechoic mass with mixed solid and cystic areas ➡ representing small pockets of pus and fibrin strands.*

DIFFERENTIAL DIAGNOSIS

Common

- Subserosal Leiomyoma/Broad Ligament Fibroid
- Hydrosalpinx/Hematosalpinx/Pyosalpinx
- Peritoneal Inclusion Cyst
- Paraovarian/Peritubal Cyst
- Endometrioma
- Ectopic Pregnancy

Less Common

- Gastrointestinal
  - Bowel Loop
  - Appendicitis
  - Appendicular Mucocele
  - Gastrointestinal Stromal Tumor (GIST)
- Lymphatics
  - Lymphocele
  - Lymph Nodes
- Vascular
  - Hematoma
  - Aneurysm
  - Pelvic Varices
- Urinary Tract
  - Bladder Diverticulum
  - Pelvic Kidney
- Neurogenic
  - Perineural/Arachnoid Cyst
  - Neurofibroma

Rare but Important

- Tubal Torsion
- Müllerian Duct Anomaly
- Malignant
  - Malignant Transformation of Endometrioma
  - Tubal Carcinoma
- Risk of Malignancy
  - Tail Gut Cyst
- Mimics of Malignancy
  - Endosalpingiosis
  - Actinomycosis

ESSENTIAL INFORMATION

Key Differential Diagnosis Issues

- Is the mass ovarian or extraovarian?
  - Ovarian origin can be confirmed by relationship to gonadal vessels and round ligament
  - Identifying separate ipsilateral ovary confirms extraovarian origin
  - In larger ovarian lesions, splayed ovarian stroma and ovarian blood supply confirm ovarian origin
- Is the mass intra- or extraperitoneal?
  - Relationship to iliac vessels will help to establish extraperitoneal location
  - Extraperitoneal lesions have flattened interfaces with pelvic wall
- Is the mass gynecological or non-gynecological?
  - Establishing uterine or tubal origin narrows differential diagnosis
- Is there a typical clinical history?

- Pregnancy status and features of sepsis are crucial diagnostic clues
- Transvaginal ultrasound is superior to transabdominal for demonstrating these features
  - See separate movement of mass from ovary with "slide test"
- MR is excellent where ultrasound is inconclusive

Helpful Clues for Common Diagnoses

- **Subserosal Leiomyoma/Broad Ligament Fibroid**
  - Oval or round extraovarian mass
  - Multiple refractory and acoustic shadows due to fibrous and calcific components
  - Demonstrable attachment to uterus with serpiginous feeding vessels
  - Acute pain and inflammation suggests torsion
  - Broad ligament fibroids have similar characteristics but no uterine feeding vessels
- **Hydrosalpinx/Pyosalpinx**
  - Coexist with pelvic inflammatory disease (PID), endometriosis, adhesions
  - C- or S-shaped interconnecting tubular cystic structures
  - Incomplete internal septations represent folds
  - Internal echoes suggests hematosalpinx or pyosalpinx
  - Real-time ultrasound essential to demonstrates tubular morphology
  - Wall thickening and complexity suggest pyosalpinx
    - Often bilateral and may contain gas
    - Clinical features of sepsis and cervical motion tenderness
- **Peritoneal Inclusion Cyst**
  - Develop in presence of functioning ovary
  - History of pelvic inflammation, endometriosis or surgery
  - Fluid-filled cavity engulfing ovary
  - Ovary may be suspended by adhesions (spider web sign) or eccentrically placed within fluid
  - Conform to pelvic contours
- **Paraovarian/Peritubal Cysts**
  - Thin-walled, unilocular anechoic cyst
  - Ipsilateral ovary demonstrated separately
  - Usually < 2 cm in diameter
  - If multiple, consider endosalpingiosis
- **Endometrioma**
  - Homogeneous low-level internal echoes represent hemorrhagic debris
  - Demonstrate acoustic enhancement
  - Multilocularity and hyperechoic wall deposits can be present
  - Often located in pelvic cul-de-sac
  - Associated with adenomyosis and solid fibrotic endometriosis
  - May coexist with tubal distension or inclusion cysts
- **Ectopic Pregnancy**
  - Tubal ring sign; extrauterine hypoechoic cystic structure with concentric hyperechoic wall
  - Extrauterine live pregnancy pathognomonic but seen in minority
  - Uterine pseudogestational sac or decidual cyst may be present

Helpful Clues for Less Common Diagnoses

- **Bowel Loop**
  - Gut signature and peristalsis
- **Appendicitis**
  - Clinical features of infection, local pain, peritonism
  - Noncompressible blind ending tubular structure > 7 mm diameter
  - Appendicolith may be visible
- **Appendicular Mucocele**
  - Pear-shaped or tubular mass arising from cecum
  - Wall calcification common
- **Gastrointestinal Stromal Tumor (GIST)**
  - Feeding vessels from mesentery or attached to bowel
- **Lymphocele**
  - History of nodal dissection
  - Extraperitoneal cysts flattened against pelvic sidewall
  - Surgical clips may be visible as echogenic foci
- **Lymph Nodes**
  - Malignant nodes can be anechoic and mistaken for cysts
  - Necrotic nodes can appear cystic (squamous cell carcinoma or tuberculosis)
- **Hematoma**
  - Poorly defined hypoechoic mass with internal echoes and complex septations
  - Consider in presence of corpus luteal cyst or ectopic
- **Aneurysm**
  - Tubular extraperitoneal structure in continuity with vessels
  - May have crescentic echogenic mural thrombus
  - Doppler assessment confirms arterial flow
- **Pelvic Varices**
  - Multiple dilated veins in adnexa
  - Reversal of flow and increased caliber on Valsalva
  - May coexist with vulval or thigh varices
- **Bladder Diverticulum**
  - Demonstrable connection with bladder lumen
  - May be thick walled and contain debris
- **Pelvic Kidney**
  - Reniform morphology

- Absent ipsilateral kidney elsewhere
- **Perineural/Arachnoid Cyst**
  - Simple cystic lesions related to sacral nerve roots
  - Communication with sacral foramina may be visible

Helpful Clues for Rare Diagnoses

- **Isolated Tubal Torsion**
  - Acute pain with previous tubal ligation, PID, hydrosalpinx
  - Dilated thick walled tubular mass medial to normal ovary
  - Sonographic whirlpool sign
- **Müllerian Duct Anomaly**
  - Accumulated blood products in non-communicating rudimentary horn simulates adnexal mass
  - Stratified appearance of myometrium/endometrium
- **Malignant Transformation of Endometrioma**
  - As for endometrioma but with solid nodular components
- **Tubal Carcinoma**
  - Solid mass between uterus and ovary
  - Latzko triad of intermittent colicky pain and palpable mass relieved by profuse vaginal discharge
- **Tail Gut Cyst**
  - Thin walled uni- or multilocular para-/retro-rectal cyst
  - Mucoid fluid with internal echoes
  - May be adherent to sacrum
- **Endosalpingiosis**
  - Multiple small cysts in relation to peritoneal surfaces of pelvic viscera
- **Actinomycosis**
  - Prolonged placement of intrauterine device
  - Fibrotic thickening of pelvic peritoneum forms hypoechoic mass-like lesions
  - May be associated with tubo-ovarian abscesses

SELECTED REFERENCES

1. Laing FC et al: US of the ovary and adnexa: to worry or not to worry? Radiographics. 32(6):1621-39; discussion 1640-2, 2012
2. Moyle PL et al: Nonovarian cystic lesions of the pelvis. Radiographics. 30(4):921-38, 2010
3. Saksouk FA et al: Recognition of the ovaries and ovarian origin of pelvic masses with CT. Radiographics. 24 Suppl 1:S133-46, 2004

Subserosal Leiomyoma/Broad Ligament Fibroid

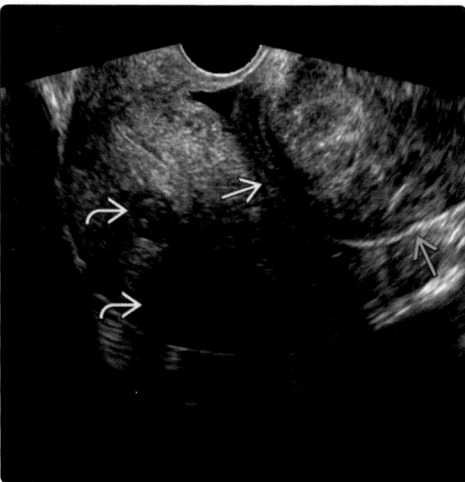

Subserosal Leiomyoma/Broad Ligament Fibroid

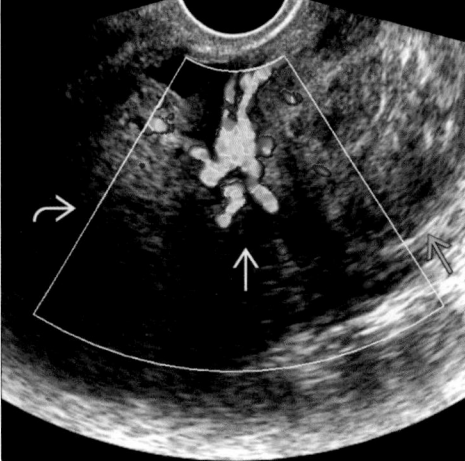

(Left) Transvaginal ultrasound demonstrates an ovoid mass ➡ with a narrow base of contact with the posterior aspect of the retroverted uterus ➡. The mass representing an exophytic fibroid has a heterogenous texture. Other fibroids ➡ are seen with refractory shadows. (Right) Transvaginal color Doppler US demonstrates multiple serpiginous feeding vessels ➡ coursing between the mass (fibroid) ➡ and the uterus ➡, confirming the uterine origin of the mass.

Subserosal Leiomyoma/Broad Ligament Fibroid

(Left) *Sagittal MR in the same patient demonstrates a well-demarcated, ovoid, retro-uterine mass ⇨ with heterogeneous internal signal. Note feeding vessels ➡.*
(Right) *MR clearly depicts the pedicle ⇨ between the retro-uterine mass and the myometrium, with multiple internal low signal serpiginous feeding vessels that were visible sonographically. The ovaries are seen separately ➡.*

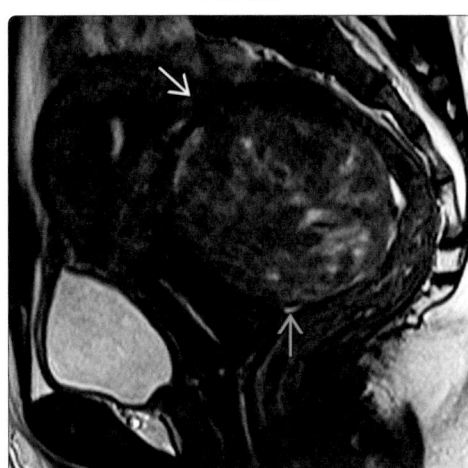

Subserosal Leiomyoma/Broad Ligament Fibroid

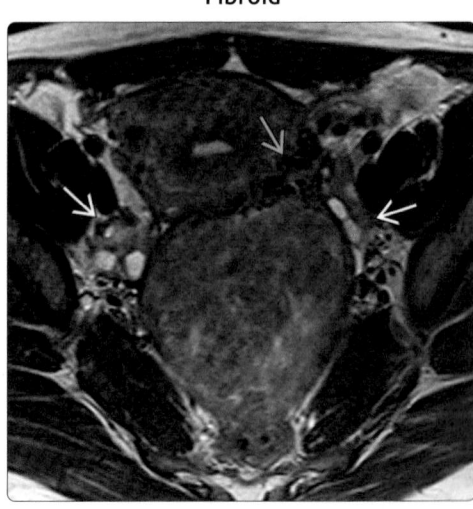

Subserosal Leiomyoma/Broad Ligament Fibroid

Hydrosalpinx/Hematosalpinx/Pyosalpinx

(Left) *The interconnecting nature of the C- or S-shaped tubular cystic structures seen here ⇨ is readily demonstrated by real-time ultrasound. The anechoic nature of the internal fluid is consistent with hydrosalpinx.*
(Right) *T2-weighted MR shows incomplete internal septations representing the folds in the walls of fallopian tube ➡. Note internal T2 shading ⇨ in the dependent/widest part of the dilated tube. Appearances are compatible with hematosalpinx. Adjacent Infiltrative endometriosis ➡ is seen.*

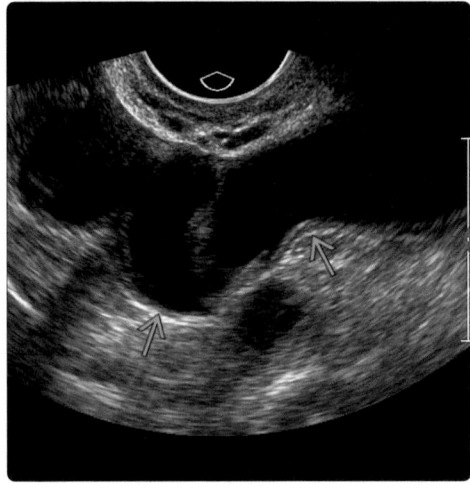

Hydrosalpinx/Hematosalpinx/Pyosalpinx

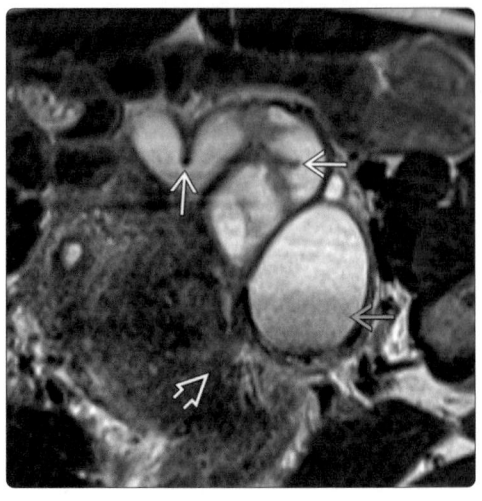

Peritoneal Inclusion Cyst

(Left) *The normal ovary ⇨ is suspended in the center of a fluid-filled cavity by band-like adhesions ⇨. Appearances represent a peritoneal inclusion cyst.* **(Right)** *Axial T2WI MR in the same patient demonstrates the conformal nature of the fluid to the pelvic peritoneal contours, confirming the diagnosis. The left ovary is again seen suspended within the fluid by bands of septations ⇨ (spider web sign).*

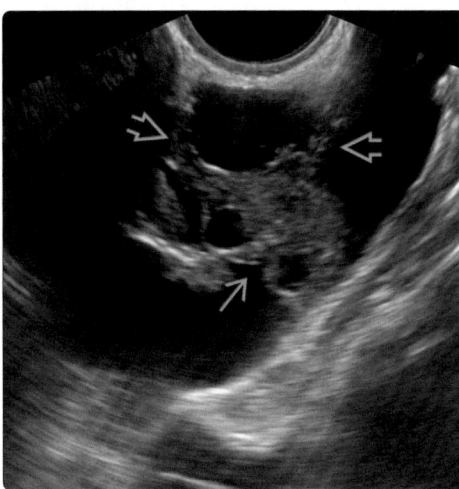

Peritoneal Inclusion Cyst

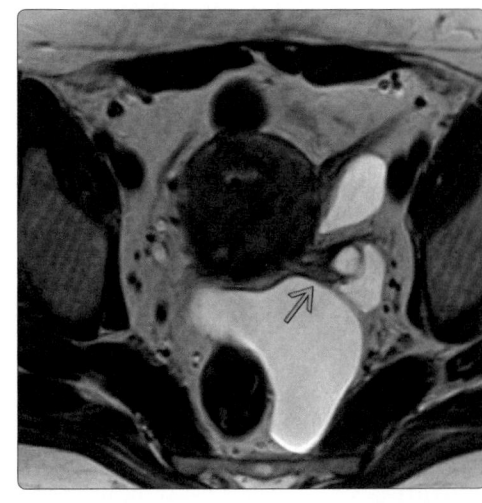

Paraovarian/Peritubal Cyst

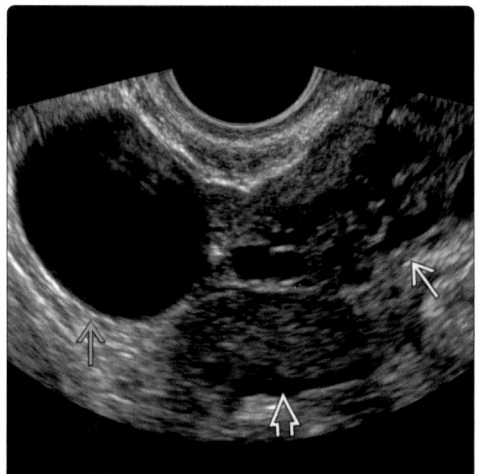

Pelvic Varices

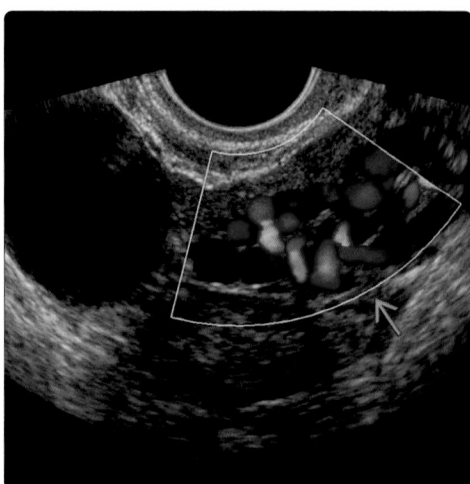

(Left) *Grayscale ultrasound depicts a thin-walled anechoic cyst ⇨ separate from the ipsilateral ovary ⇥ and uterus, consistent with a paraovarian cyst. Appearances also raise the possibility of an adjacent complex adnexal mass ⇥.* (Right) *US with color flow mapping in the same patient shows that the mass-like lesion ⇨ is composed of multiple dilated veins representing pelvic varices.*

Endometrioma

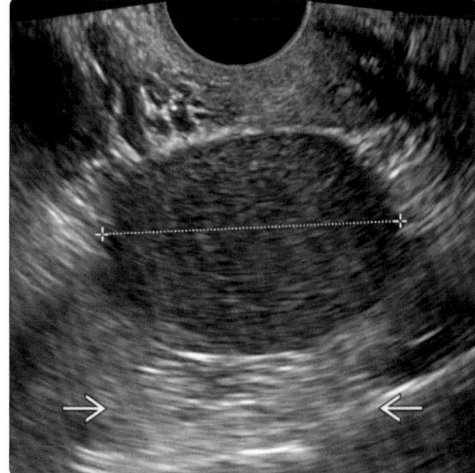

Endometrioma

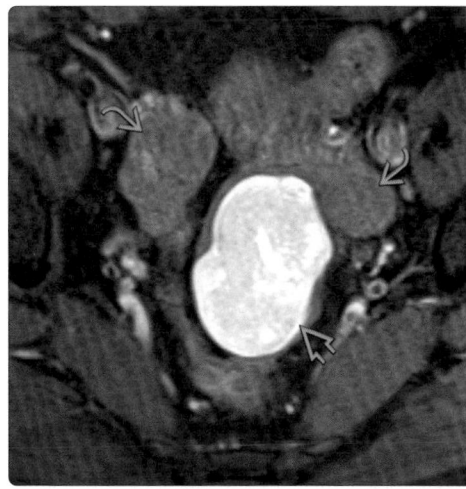

(Left) *TV US demonstrates a mass with homogeneous low-level internal echoes and posterior acoustic enhancement ⇥. The ipsilateral ovary was identified separately (not shown).* (Right) *Internal high signal on T1-weighted fat saturation MR confirms the hemorrhagic nature of the lesion's contents, in keeping with the diagnosis of endometrioma ⇨. Ovaries ⇥ are noted.*

Ectopic Pregnancy

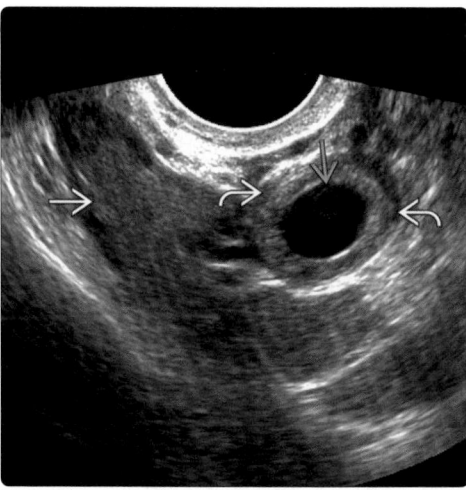

Ectopic Pregnancy

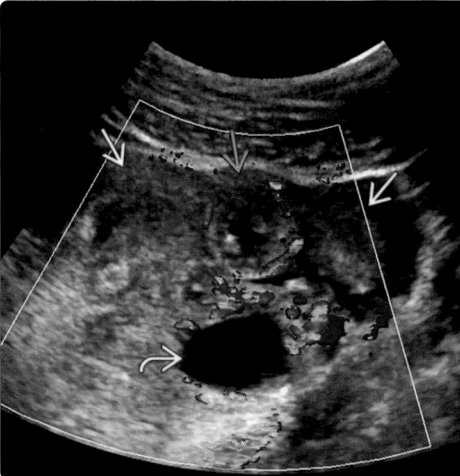

(Left) *Coronal ultrasound of the right adnexa shows a right tubal ectopic separate from the normal right ovary ⇥. There is an echogenic tubal ring ⇥ with central fluid and a yolk sac ⇨.* (Right) *Transverse transabdominal color Doppler ultrasound shows an echogenic vascular ring ⇨ surrounded by hemorrhage ⇥, consistent with a bleeding ectopic pregnancy. The left ovary contains a luteal cyst ⇥.*

Appendicitis

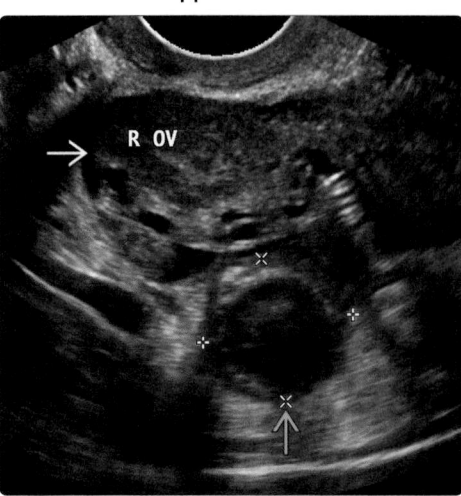

Appendicitis

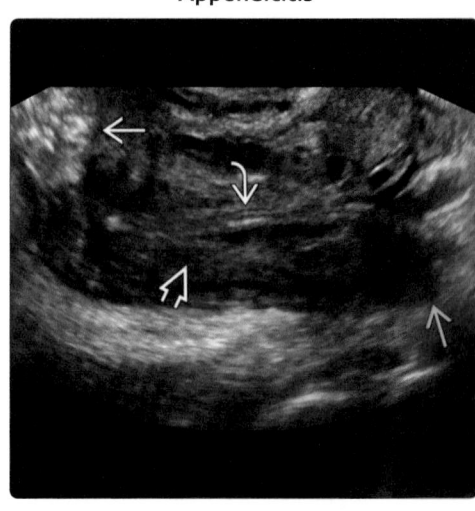

(Left) *Coronal ultrasound shows a tender, incompressible, thick-walled tubular mass ⇥ adjacent to the normal right ovary ➔. Low-level echoes are seen in the lumen.* (Right) *Longitudinal ultrasound of the same patient confirms the tubular structure to be blind ending ⇥ and traceable to the cecum ➔, consistent with an inflamed appendix. Mural stratification ⇲ and intraluminal debris ⇨ are noted.*

Appendicular Mucocele

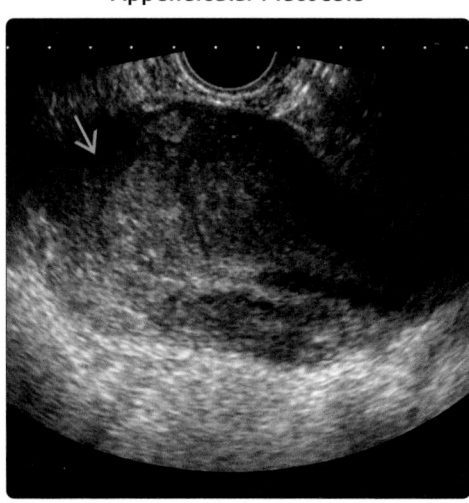

Appendicular Mucocele

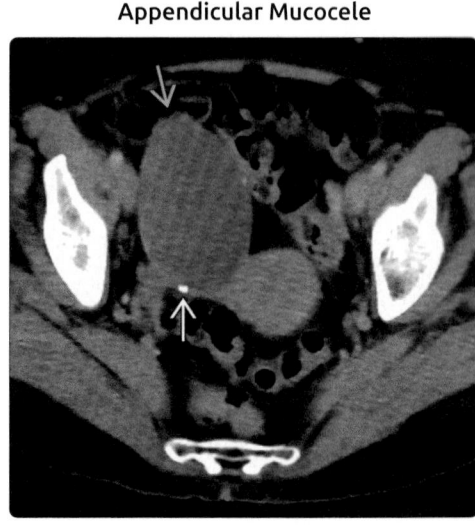

(Left) *This well-marginated, pear-shaped mass has echogenic contents with a typical onion skin appearance ⇥ centrally, representing a pelvic appendicular mucocele.* (Right) *CT in the same patient shows the mass to be inseparable from the base of the appendix/cecum ⇥, representing an appendicular mucocele. Also note the typical wall calcification ➔.*

Gastrointestinal Stromal Tumor (GIST)

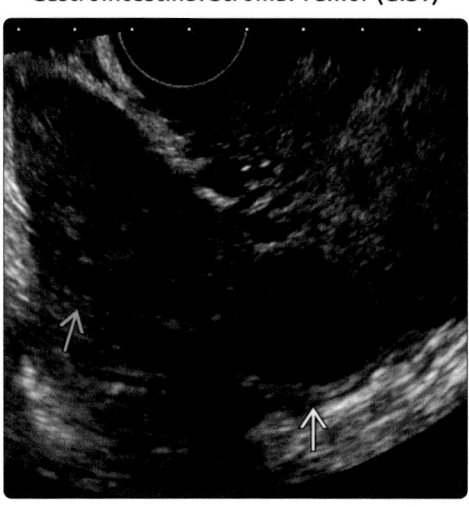

Gastrointestinal Stromal Tumor (GIST)

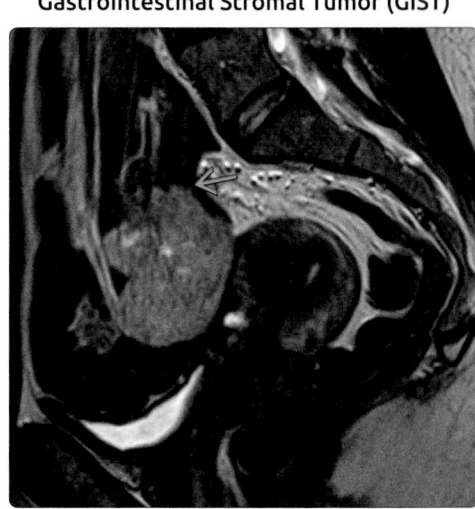

(Left) *US demonstrates a solid adnexal mass ⇥ abutting the ovary (physiological ovarian cyst ➔). Note the absence of typical refractory and acoustic shadows of a fibroid/fibroma.* (Right) *MR in the same patient demonstrates an intimate relationship between the mass, adjacent small bowel loops, and mesenteric vessels, supporting the diagnosis of gastrointestinal stromal tumor. Note the loss of fat plane with the small bowel loops ⇥. The diagnosis was confirmed after resection.*

Lymph Nodes

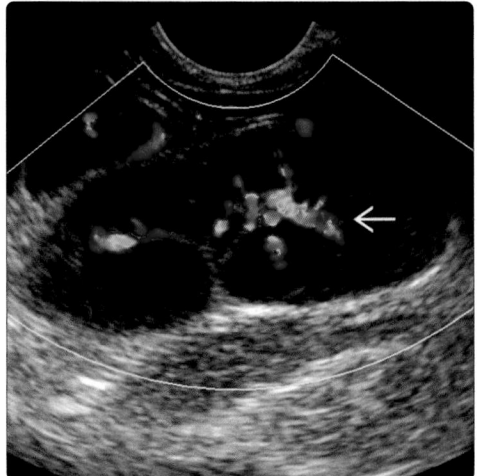

Lymph Nodes

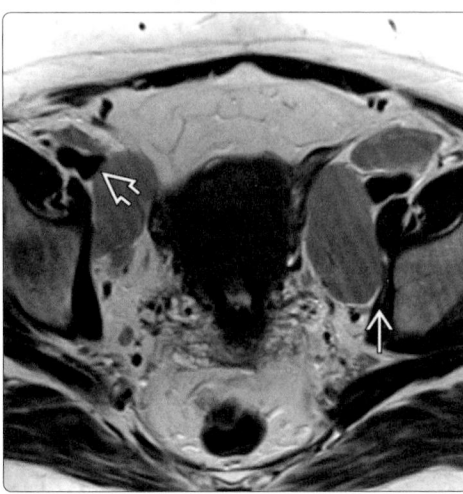

(Left) *Hypoechoic enlarged nodes can be mistaken for cystic lesions on grayscale ultrasound. The absence of posterior acoustic enhancement and presence of internal blood flow ➡ on color Doppler confirm their solidity.* (Right) *MR in the same patient confirms the extraperitoneal location. Features localizing lesions to this space include flattening against the pelvic sidewall ➡ and loss of the fat plane with the external iliac vessels ➡.*

Hematoma

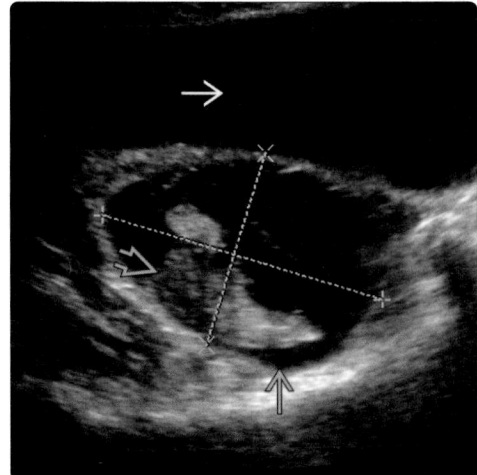

Hematoma

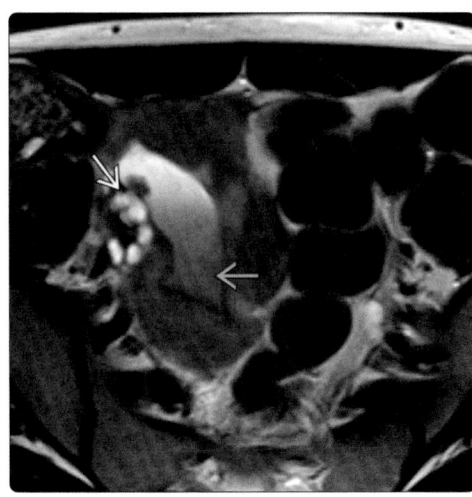

(Left) *US demonstrates a heterogeneous, septated adnexal mass ➡ adjacent to the urinary bladder ➡. The central echogenic region ➡ represents a retracting clot.* (Right) *MR in the same patient demonstrates characteristic dependent T2 shading ➡, confirming the diagnosis of pelvic hematoma. Hemorrhagic corpus luteal cyst is the likely source of bleeding. At the periphery of the collection is the ipsilateral ovary ➡.*

Tail Gut Cyst

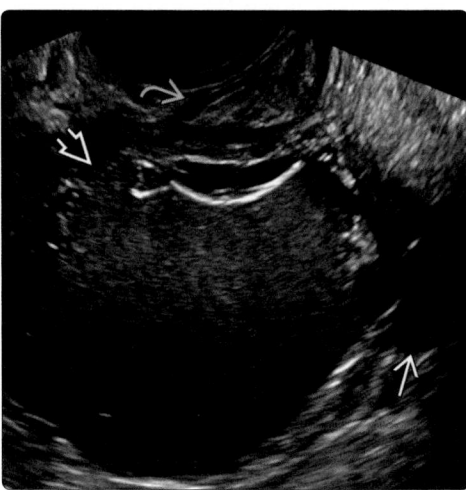

Tail Gut Cyst

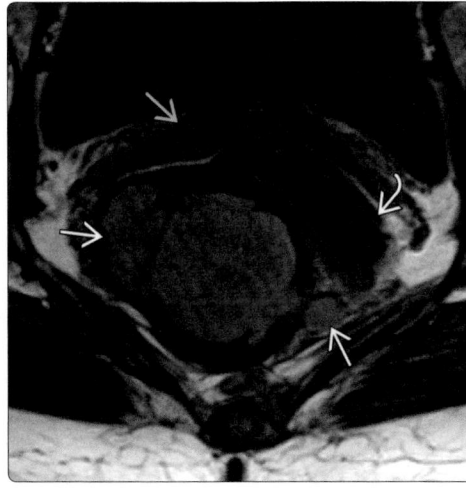

(Left) *Oblique axial endovaginal US shows a retro-rectal cyst ➡ containing uniform intermediate-level echoes representing mucinous content. Axial section of rectum ➡ is noted. The outer hypoechoic rim represents the muscularis propria layer of the rectal wall. Note adjacent smaller locules ➡.* (Right) *Axial T1 MR in the same patient shows a multilocular extraperitoneal retro-rectal cyst ➡. Contents are of T1-intermediate signal intensity, representing mucinous material. Rectum ➡ & vagina ➡ are noted.*

DIFFERENTIAL DIAGNOSIS

Common

- Polycystic Ovarian Syndrome (PCOS)
- Functional Ovarian Cyst
- Hemorrhagic Cyst
- Corpus Luteum/Luteal Cyst

Less Common

- Adnexal Torsion
- Benign Masses
  - Teratoma
  - Serous Cystadenoma
  - Mucinous Cystadenoma
  - Fibroma/Fibrothecoma
  - Endometrioma
- Ovarian Hyperstimulation
- Theca Lutein Cysts
- Tubo-ovarian Abscess

Rare but Important

- Malignant Masses
- Massive Ovarian Edema (MOE) and Ovarian Fibromatosis (OF)

ESSENTIAL INFORMATION

Key Differential Diagnosis Issues

- Size
  - Normal ovary is typically 3 x 2 x 2 cm or ~ 10 ± 6 mL, max 22 mL
  - Postmenopausal ovary ~ 2-6 mL
- Generally differential categories
  - Endocrine
  - Neoplasm
  - Vascular
  - Iatrogenic
  - Infectious
- 1 approach is to think about differential as 2 major groups
  - Enlarged ovary with maintained architecture
  - Enlarged ovary because of lesion

Helpful Clues for Common Diagnoses

- **Polycystic Ovarian Syndrome (PCOS)**
  - Normal architecture with multiple small follicles of uniform size
  - Echogenic stroma
  - Diagnostic criteria for polycystic ovarian morphology
    - Volume ≥ 10 mL **or**
    - ≥ 12 follicles measuring 2-9 mm
  - Polycystic ovarian morphology is seen in 22% of women and is not diagnostic of PCOS alone
    - Hyperandrogenism **or** oligo- or anovulation also needed to fulfil Rotterdam criteria
  - Several other causes of polycystic ovarian morphology
- **Functional Ovarian Cyst**
  - Reproductive-aged women (premenopausal)
    - Every month, 1 or more follicles are stimulated and enlarge typically to 2.0-2.5 cm prior to ovulation
  - Thin wall, anechoic, no thick septa
  - Early postmenopausal women may have functional cyst

- Late postmenopausal women should not have functional cyst though may have inclusion or epithelial cyst
- **Hemorrhagic Cyst**
  - Typically, corpus luteum that has bled centrally
  - Avascular hypoechoic ovarian mass with fine, lacy interstices
  - May have hyperechoic retracted clot at periphery
  - Avascular strands/septa
  - Majority resolve in 6-12 weeks
  - Follow-up ultrasound
    - Premenopausal women follow-up at > 5 cm
    - Postmenopausal women follow-up at any size
- **Corpus Luteum/Luteal Cyst**
  - Very commonly encountered ovarian lesion
  - Occur after ovulation in latter part of menstrual cycle
  - Thick, crenulated wall
  - Centrally may have anechoic fluid, hemorrhagic fluid, or little fluid and may be mostly solid-appearing
  - Hypervascular rim/wall

Helpful Clues for Less Common Diagnoses

- **Adnexal Torsion**
  - Enlarged ovary: > 4 cm in longest dimension or > 20 cm³ in volume
  - Peripheral follicles, heterogenous stroma
  - Presence of normal blood flow does **not** exclude torsion
- **Benign Masses**
  - Teratoma
    - Most common ovarian tumor
    - 10-20% bilateral
    - Heterogeneous cystic mass
    - Echogenic shadowing mural nodule (Rokitansky nodule)
    - "Dirty" posterior acoustic shadow
    - Dot-dash sign from hair suspended in sebum
    - Shadowing calcification from teeth
  - Serous Cystadenoma
    - Large unilocular cystic mass
    - Typically > 7-10 cm
    - Minimal to no septa
  - Mucinous Cystadenoma
    - Often very large, filling entire pelvis, extending into upper abdomen
    - Multilocular unilateral cystic mass
    - Thin avascular to thick vascular septa
    - Echogenic fluid to variable degrees in each locule
  - Fibroma/Fibrothecoma
    - Most common sex cord-stromal tumor
    - Hypoechoic solid mass
    - Dense posterior acoustic shadowing
    - Meigs syndrome: Ascites and pleural effusion associated with benign adnexal mass
  - Endometrioma
    - Cystic adnexal mass with homogenous low-level echoes
    - Thick walled, may see echogenic foci in wall of cyst
    - Generally unilocular but may have septations/folds that are often incomplete
    - Range in size from small (1-2 cm) to very large (> 10 cm)

- – Often bilateral (50%)
  - ○ Cystadenofibroma
    - – Benign cystic adnexal mass
    - – Uni- or multilocular
    - – Unilocular with 1 or more small, shadowing, avascular, hyperechoic mural nodules in majority
- **Ovarian Hyperstimulation**
  - ○ Occurs in setting of ovulation induction
  - ○ Range of clinical severity from mild to severe requiring ICU support
  - ○ Bilateral enlarged ovaries with multiple cysts
    - – > 5-10 cm ovarian diameter
    - – Spoke wheel configuration
    - – Cysts may be simple or complex if hemorrhagic component present
  - ○ Ascites, pleural effusions, hemoconcentration, oliguria
- **Theca Lutein Cysts**
  - ○ Enlarged ovaries with multiple cysts
  - ○ Typically bilateral
  - ○ Thin septa between simple cysts
    - – May be complex cysts from hemorrhage
  - ○ Typically occurs in few clinical scenarios with common etiology of ↑ human chorionic gonadotropin
    - – Multiples
    - – Gestational trophoblastic disease
    - – Triploidy (partial mole)
    - – Fetal hydrops (immune type)
  - ○ PCOS may predispose
- **Tubo-Ovarian Abscess**
  - ○ Thickened Fallopian tubes containing fluid, often echogenic (pus)
  - ○ Complex fluid collection with thick hypervascular wall, septa, echogenic debris
  - ○ Tube often coiled around abscess
    - – Best appreciated with cine sweep imaging
  - ○ Pain, fever, and leukocytosis

Helpful Clues for Rare Diagnoses

- **Malignant Masses**
  - ○ Ascites often present

- ○ Ovarian cancer usually presents with advanced disease, stage III or IV
- ○ Ovarian cystadenocarcinoma: Complex cystic and solid mass, large, often bilateral
  - – Borderline tumors may present as unilocular cyst with papillary projections/mural nodules
- ○ Ovarian metastases: Bilateral cystic &/or solid masses most often occurring in setting of known malignancy
  - – Most often gastric, colon, pancreas, breast carcinomas
- **Massive Ovarian Edema (MOE) and Ovarian Fibromatosis (OF)**
  - ○ MOE: Tumor-like ovarian enlargement secondary to edema
  - ○ OF: Tumor-like ovarian enlargement due to fibromatous growth of ovarian stroma
  - ○ Both conditions are usually unilateral
  - ○ Diffuse ovarian enlargement with maintained ovarian configuration
    - – MOE: Enlarged ovary with edematous appearance and peripheral follicles
    - – OF: Enlarged ovary with segmental or peripheral areas of T1 and T2 low signal intensity

Alternative Differential Approaches

- Preserved ovarian architecture
  - ○ PCOS
  - ○ Functional Ovarian cyst
  - ○ Hemorrhagic cyst
  - ○ Corpus luteum/corpus luteal cyst
  - ○ Adnexal torsion
  - ○ Ovarian hyperstimulation
  - ○ Theca lutein cysts
  - ○ MOE and OF
- Enlarged ovary with altered architecture
  - ○ Benign masses
  - ○ Tubo-ovarian abscess
  - ○ Malignant masses

Polycystic Ovarian Syndrome (PCOS)

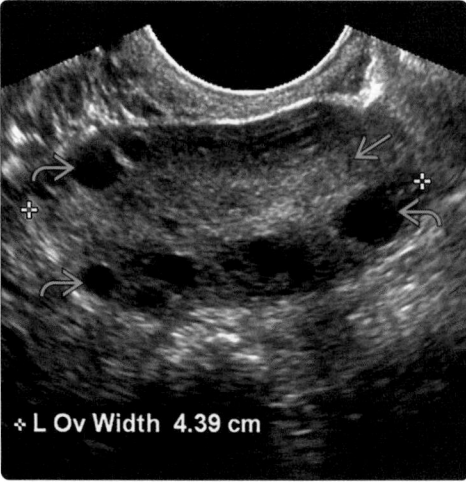

Hemorrhagic Cyst

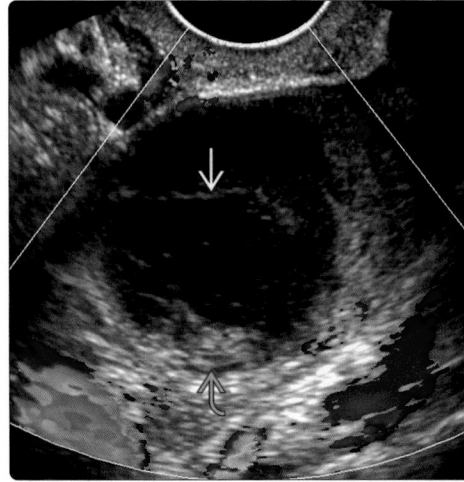

(Left) *Longitudinal endovaginal US shows an enlarged ovary with a length of 4.4 cm and a volume of 19 mL. Note the echogenic stroma ➡ and multiple small (< 1 cm) peripheral follicles ➡.* **(Right)** *Transverse endovaginal color Doppler US of an enlarged right ovary shows a hemorrhagic cyst with thin, lacy, nonvascular strands ➡ and a retracted clot along the periphery ➡.*

Corpus Luteum/Luteal Cyst

Adnexal Torsion

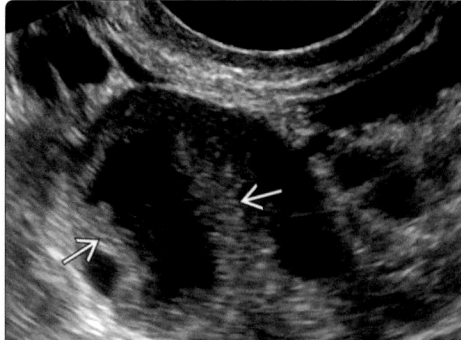
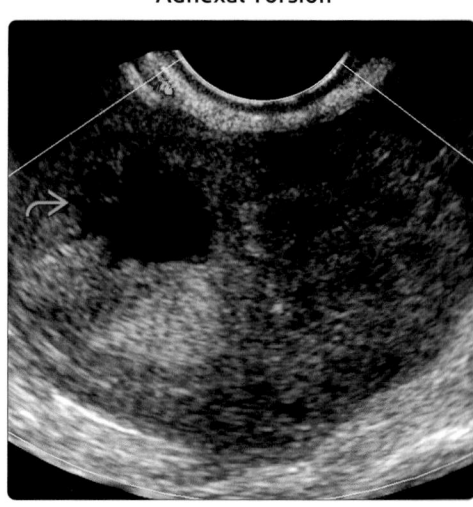

(Left) *Longitudinal endovaginal US shows a typical corpus luteum as an anechoic cyst with a thick and crenulated wall ➡. It is important to remember that corpus lutea may show variable degrees of simple or complex internal fluid.* (Right) *Endovaginal US in a 34-year-old woman with adnexal torsion presenting with acute pelvic pain shows an enlarged, 6-cm ovary with heterogeneous echogenicity and a corpus luteum ➡. Note the lack of power Doppler flow.*

Serous Cystadenoma

Endometrioma

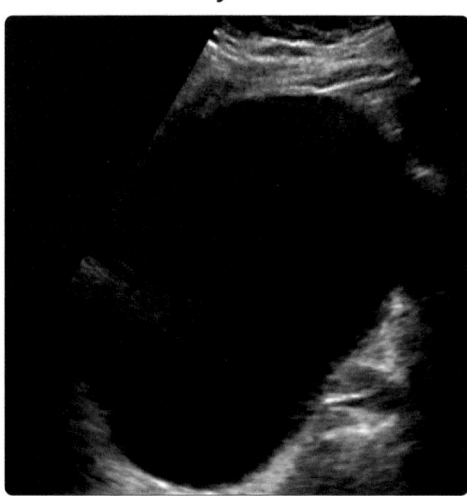
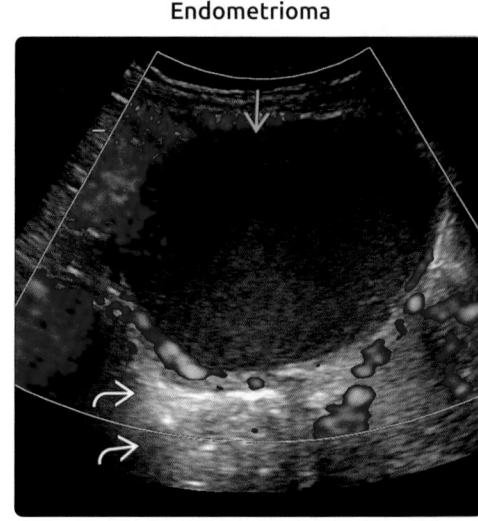

(Left) *Transabdominal US shows a large unilocular cystic mass in the right adnexa without septations or mural nodules.* (Right) *Power Doppler US of the left adnexa shows a large homogeneously hypoechoic endometrioma ➡ with no internal vascularity. Diffuse homogeneous low-level echoes within the mass as well as posterior acoustic enhancement ➡ are characteristic of an endometrioma.*

Ovarian Hyperstimulation

Ovarian Hyperstimulation

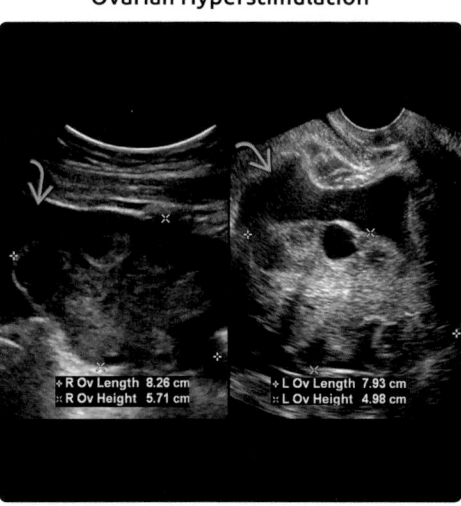
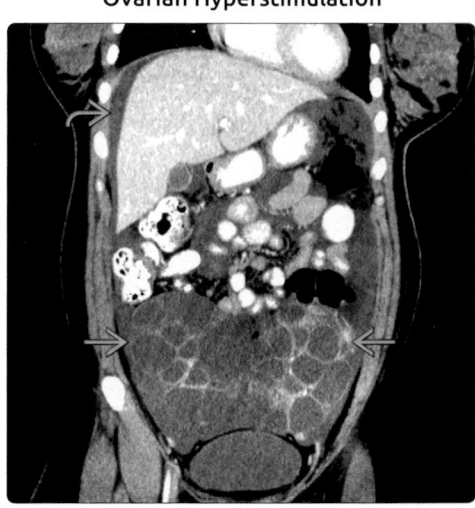

(Left) *US in a 31-year-old woman undergoing ovulation induction presenting with abdominal pain and distention shows bilateral enlarged heterogenous ovaries (calipers), both measuring 8 cm in length with multiple follicles. Note the echogenic ascites ➡ due to 3rd spacing or hemorrhage.* (Right) *Coronal CECT shows massive bilateral ovarian enlargement and replacement by multiple fluid-density cysts ➡ and moderate ascites ➡, consistent with ovarian hyperstimulation syndrome.*

Theca Lutein Cysts

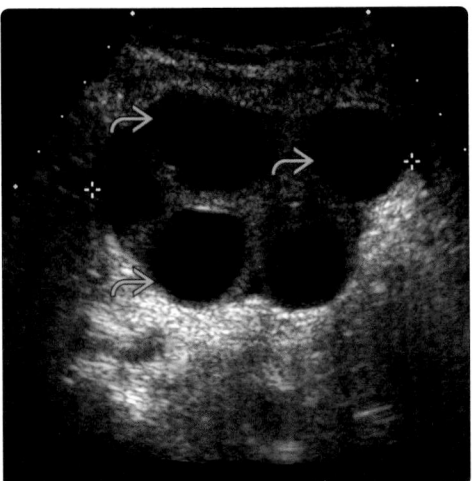

Theca Lutein Cysts

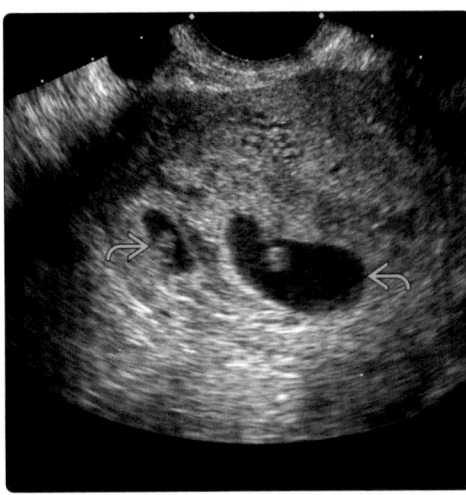

(Left) *Transverse transabdominal US in a woman in the 1st trimester shows multiple enlarged follicles ➔. The ovary measures 7 cm in diameter in this patient with multiple theca lutein cysts in the ovary.* (Right) *Endovaginal US in the same patient shows twin gestations with 2 intrauterine gestational sacs ➔ and fetal poles. Multiple gestations may elevate the β-human chorionic gonadotropin and cause theca lutein cysts in the ovary.*

Tubo-ovarian Abscess

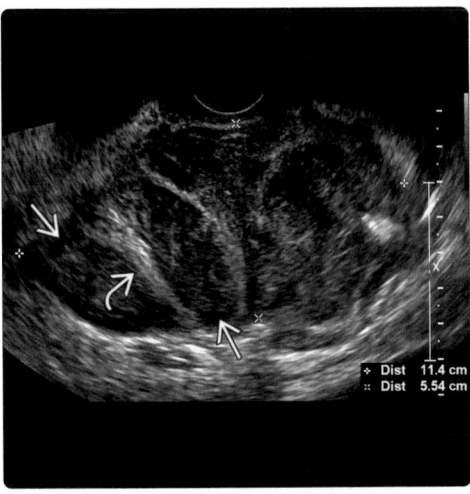

Malignant Masses

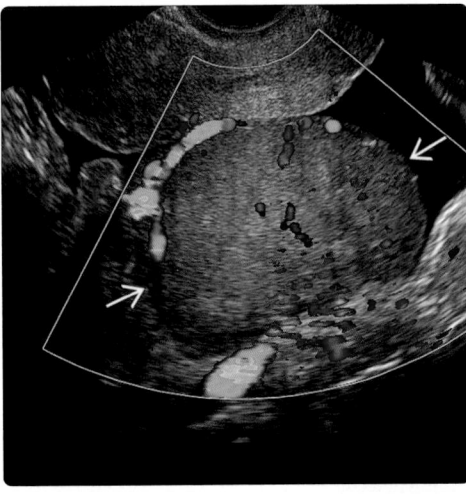

(Left) *Longitudinal endovaginal US shows an 11 cm complex adnexal mass (calipers) with thick septations ➔ and multiple loculations in a patient with a tubo-ovarian abscess. The locules contain echogenic fluid ➔. One month earlier, a CT was normal.* (Right) *Longitudinal endovaginal color Doppler US in a patient with metastatic melanoma shows an enlarged right ovary ➔ secondary to a solid vascular mass.*

Massive Ovarian Edema (MOE) and Ovarian Fibromatosis (OF)

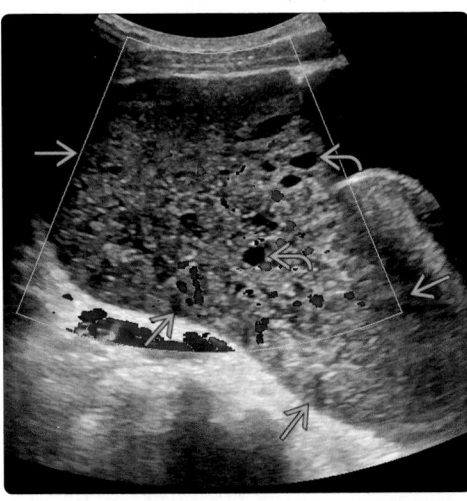

Massive Ovarian Edema (MOE) and Ovarian Fibromatosis (OF)

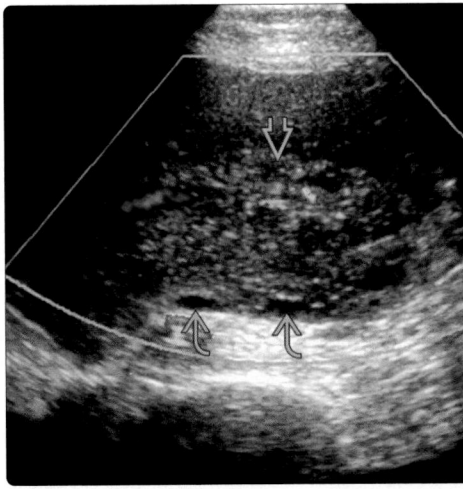

(Left) *Longitudinal transabdominal color Doppler US shows a marked ovarian enlargement ➔ with multiple small, peripheral cysts ➔. Both arterial and venous flow are seen within the enlarged ovary.* (Right) *Transverse color Doppler US shows massive ovarian enlargement with an edematous heterogenous ovarian stroma and small peripheral follicles ➔. Note the preserved blood flow centrally ➔.*

DIFFERENTIAL DIAGNOSIS

Common

- Pregnancy/Normal Postpartum
- Complications of Pregnancy/Abnormal Postpartum
- Multiparous Patient
- Leiomyoma
- Adenomyosis
- Focal Myometrial Contraction

Less Common

- Endometrial Cancer
- Cervical Stenosis
- Cervical Mass
- Hematometrocolpos

Rare but Important

- Uterine Leiomyosarcoma
- Uterine Lymphoma

ESSENTIAL INFORMATION

Key Differential Diagnosis Issues

- Is the patient pregnant or recently pregnant?
- Are there signs of infection?
- Enlarged uterus without focal mass
  - Diffuse adenomyosis
  - Multiparous patient
- Multiple masses
  - Round, well-defined masses: Intramural leiomyomas
  - Ovoid, ill-defined masses: Focal adenomyosis
- Fluid in endometrial cavity causing uterine enlargement
  - Obstructed outflow secondary to cervical stenosis or mass (carcinoma, leiomyoma)
  - Or secondary to congenital anomaly: Imperforate hymen, vaginal septum, cloacal abnormality
- Ill-defined mass in uterine cavity: Endometrial cancer

Helpful Clues for Common Diagnoses

- **Pregnancy/Normal Postpartum**
  - Presence of gestational sac or fetus

- **Complications of Pregnancy**
  - Retained products of conception, clot, failed pregnancy, molar pregnancy, endometritis
- **Leiomyoma**
  - Focal, well-defined hypoechoic masses
  - May have pseudocapsule
  - Lobulated contour of uterus
- **Adenomyosis**
  - Asymmetric myometrial thickening
  - Cystic spaces in endometrium and subendometrium
  - Alternating bands of increased through transmission and shadowing
- **Focal Myometrial Contraction**
  - Focal bulge of myometrium during pregnancy, resolves over time
  - Affects internal myometrial appearance more than external contour
  - Disruption of hypoechoic subendometrial halo
  - Isoechoic to surrounding myometrium

Helpful Clues for Less Common Diagnoses

- **Endometrial Cancer**
  - Patient typically presents with bleeding
  - Diffuse uterine enlargement
  - Ill-defined endometrium
- **Cervical Stenosis**
  - Patient with history of curettage or childbearing
  - Fluid in endometrial cavity, thin surrounding endometrium with no focal lesion
- **Cervical Mass**
  - Hypoechoic, ill-defined mass with necrosis suggests malignancy
  - Well-defined homogeneous mass suggests leiomyoma
- **Hematometrocolpos**
  - Hemorrhagic fluid in uterus &/or vagina
  - Acquired or congenital

Helpful Clues for Rare Diagnoses

- **Uterine Leiomyosarcoma**
  - Large heterogenous rapidly growing masses

Complications of Pregnancy/Abnormal Postpartum

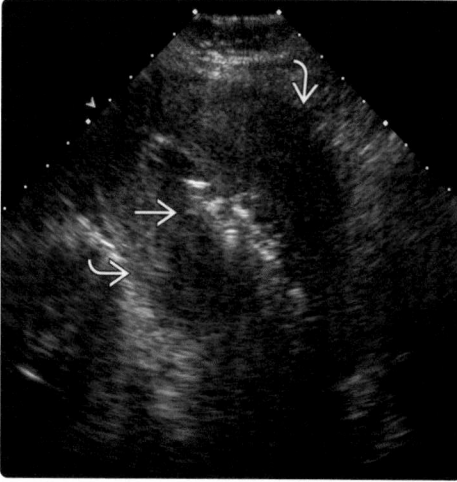

Leiomyoma

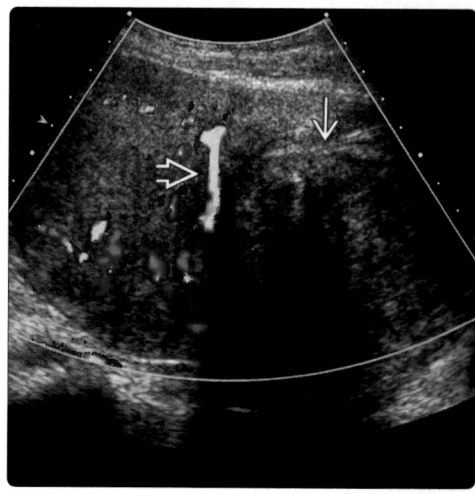

(Left) Longitudinal transabdominal ultrasound of a patient with postpartum endometritis shows an enlarged uterus ➡ with gas and debris ➡ in the endometrial cavity. (Right) Transverse color Doppler ultrasound shows a large, shadowing, painful subserosal fibroid ➡. Despite patent adjacent myometrial vessels ➡, there was no internal color flow.

Leiomyoma

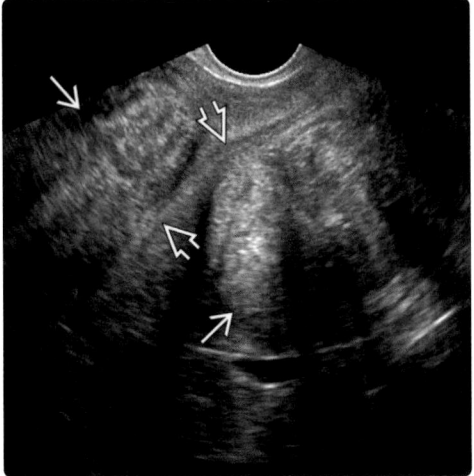

Adenomyosis

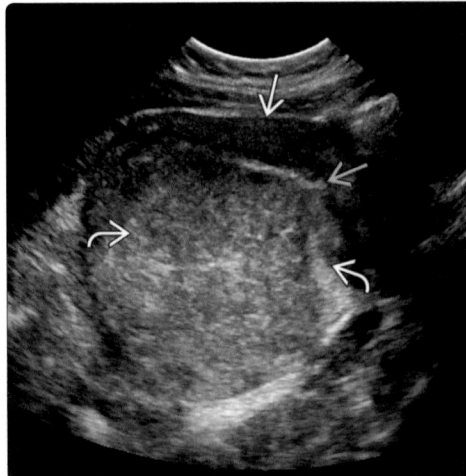

(Left) *Longitudinal US shows an enlarged uterus secondary to multiple leiomyomas. Two are visible* ➡ *on this image, with typical imaging findings including well-defined borders and internal heterogeneity and shadowing. The thin endometrium is visible centrally* ➡. **(Right)** *Transabdominal sagittal ultrasound shows a uterus with adenomyosis. The posterior myometrium* ➡ *is much thicker than the anterior myometrium* ➡. *The endometrium is normal* ➡.

Adenomyosis

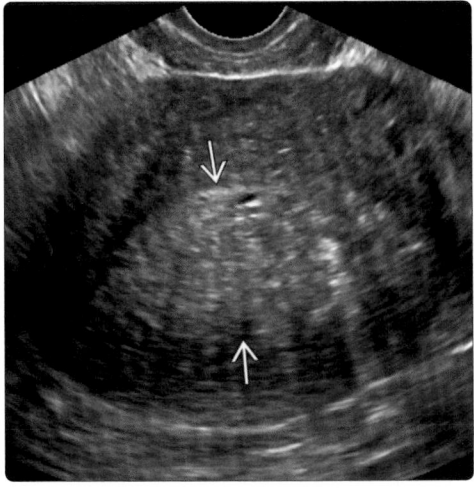

Cervical Stenosis

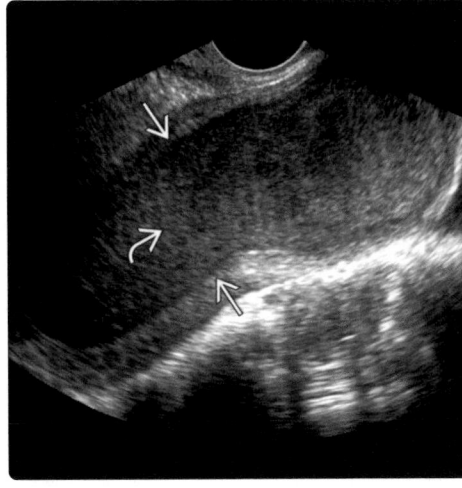

(Left) *Transverse US shows pseudothickening of the endometrium* ➡ *and uterine enlargement. Alternating bands of shadowing and increased through transmission are typical of adenomyosis.* **(Right)** *Longitudinal US of the lower uterine segment shows expansion of the endometrial cavity* ➡ *with echogenic material* ➡, *consistent with hematocolpos in this patient with cervical stenosis.*

Endometrial Cancer

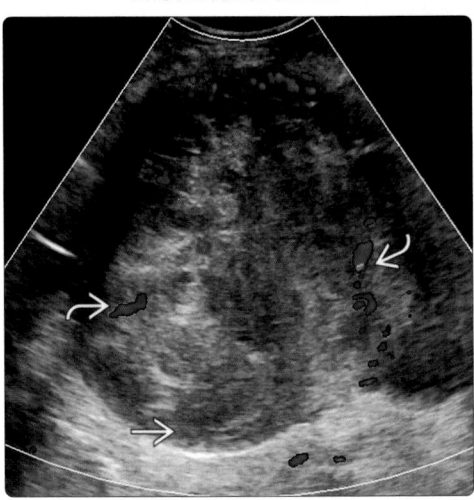

Cervical Mass

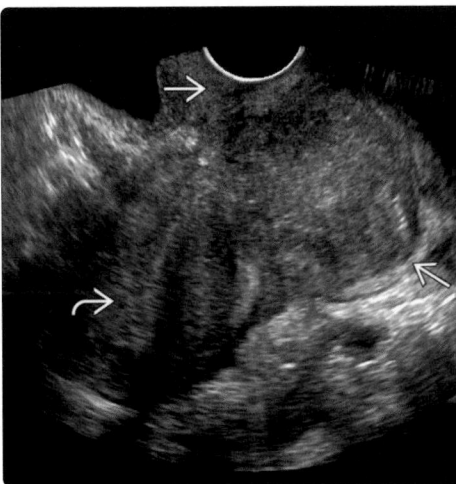

(Left) *Transverse US in the same patient shows a necrotic mass with peripheral color flow* ➡. *There is myometrial thinning* ➡, *suggesting deep muscle invasion.* **(Right)** *Longitudinal transvaginal ultrasound shows a large, lobulated, solid cervical mass* ➡ *representing cervical carcinoma. There was no endometrial cavity fluid* ➡.

DIFFERENTIAL DIAGNOSIS

Common

- Secretory Phase Endometrium
- Pregnancy and Complications
- Retained Products of Conception
- Mimic of Endometrial Thickening
  o Submucosal Leiomyoma
  o Intramural Leiomyoma
  o Adenomyosis
  o Hematometra
- Endometrial Polyps

Less Common

- Endometrial Hyperplasia
- Endometrial Cancer
- Tamoxifen-Induced Changes

Rare but Important

- Endometritis
- Unopposed Estrogen Use
- Polycystic Ovary Syndrome
- Endometrial Stromal Sarcoma

ESSENTIAL INFORMATION

Key Differential Diagnosis Issues

- Is patient postpartum?
  o Endometritis
  o Retained products of conception
- Is thickening focal?
  o Endometrial polyps
  o Leiomyoma, submucosal
  o Endometrial cancer
  o Endometrial hyperplasia
  o Retained products of conception
- Does patient have abnormal bleeding?
  o Endometrial polyps
  o Leiomyoma, submucosal
  o Leiomyoma, intramural
  o Endometrial hyperplasia
  o Endometrial cancer
  o Retained products of conception
- Is endometrial-myometrial interface indistinct?
  o Endometrial cancer
  o Leiomyoma, submucosal
  o Adenomyosis

Helpful Clues for Common Diagnoses

- **Secretory Phase Endometrium**
  o After ovulation in second 1/2 of menstrual cycle, endometrium can be thick, heterogeneous, and echogenic
  o Follow-up early in subsequent menstrual cycle will show thin endometrium
- **Pregnancy and Complications**
  o Positive urine/serum human chorionic gonadotropin
    - Normal early pregnancy
    - Miscarriage
    - Ectopic pregnancy
    - Hydatidiform mole, complete mole

- Hydatidiform mole, partial mole
- **Retained Products of Conception**
  o Focal endometrial echogenic lesion
  o Fluid ± clot
  o May have calcifications
  o May have low-resistance arterial flow, but lack of flow does not exclude diagnosis
- **Submucosal Leiomyoma**
  o Submucosal lesions > 50% within endometrium
  o Iso- or hypoechoic well-marginated lesion
  o Less echogenic than endometrium
  o Posterior shadowing
  o Multiple feeding vessels
- **Intramural Leiomyoma**
  o Not true endometrial lesion but can cause appearance of endometrial thickening
  o Iso- or hypoechoic lesion distorting or obscuring endometrium
  o Shadowing behind leiomyoma
- **Adenomyosis**
  o Poor definition of endometrial myometrial interface makes it difficult to evaluate and measure endometrium
  o Look for streaky linear hypoechoic myometrial bands and subendometrial cysts
  o Asymmetric uterine enlargement
  o Tender uterus
- **Hematometra**
  o Look for underlying cause of obstruction
    - Uterine duplication anomaly
    - Leiomyoma
    - Endometrial cancer
    - Cervical cancer
    - If thin surrounding endometrium and no obstructing lesion, cervical stenosis is diagnosis of exclusion
- **Endometrial Polyps**
  o Focal endometrial lesion
  o Typically more echogenic than surrounding endometrium
  o May have internal cysts
  o Stalk with single feeding vessel
  o May have broad base
  o Frequently multiple
  o Smooth margins

Helpful Clues for Less Common Diagnoses

- **Endometrial Hyperplasia**
  o Peri- or postmenopausal woman
  o Association with polycystic ovarian syndrome
  o ± cystic spaces
  o Typically diffuse but may be focal
- **Endometrial Cancer**
  o Early stage
    - Appears as focal endometrial lesion
  o Later stage
    - Invades myometrium, leads to indistinct endometrial-myometrial interface
  o Irregular thickened heterogeneous endometrium
- **Tamoxifen-Induced Changes**
  o Paradoxical estrogenic effect on endometrium increases with ↑ dose and time of treatment

- o Multiple effects include
  - – Polyps
  - – Endometrial hyperplasia
  - – Reactivation of foci of adenomyosis
  - – Cystic endometrial atrophy with subendometrial cysts
  - – Endometrial carcinoma
    - □ Endometrial cancer in patients taking tamoxifen is frequently in endometrial polyps

Helpful Clues for Rare Diagnoses

- **Endometritis**
  - o In postpartum patient, painful enlarged uterus
  - o In nonpregnant patient, associated with pelvic inflammatory disease
  - o Elevated white blood cell count
  - o Thick, heterogeneous endometrial contents ± gas in septic endometritis
- **Unopposed Estrogen Use**
  - o Estrogen use without progesterone → endometrial polyps, hyperplasia, and carcinoma
- **Polycystic Ovary Syndrome**
  - o Enlarged ovaries with multiple, small, peripheral follicles
  - o Central stroma may be echogenic but not a necessary component for diagnosis
  - o No dominant follicle
  - o Diffuse endometrial thickening due to prolonged proliferative phase or endometrial hyperplasia

Other Essential Information

- Transvaginal scanning is best for evaluation of endometrium
  - o Saline infused hysterosonography helpful to differentiate focal lesions from diffuse thickening
  - o Diffuse thickening can be sampled with blind biopsy
  - o Focal mass best assessed with hysteroscopic biopsy
- In some patients, orientation of endometrial cavity is such that transabdominal scan allows for better insonation and evaluation of endometrium
- Additionally fibroids or very large uteri may preclude assessment using transvaginal probes

- In uterine duplication anomalies, each endometrium must be separately evaluated

Alternative Differential Approaches

- Solid or complex ovarian lesion in association with endometrial lesion
  - o Estrogenic effect from granulosa cell tumor may produce endometrial hyperplasia or carcinoma
  - o Estrogen secretion from thecoma → endometrial lesions
  - o Synchronous ovarian and endometrial carcinoma
  - o Endometrioid ovarian carcinoma resembles endometrial carcinoma, associated with endometrial hyperplasia or carcinoma
  - o Metastatic disease to ovaries from endometrial carcinoma

SELECTED REFERENCES

1. Van den Bosch T et al: Intra-cavitary uterine pathology in women with abnormal uterine bleeding: a prospective study of 1220 women. Facts Views Vis Obgyn. 7(1):17-24, 2015
2. Langer JE et al: Imaging of the female pelvis through the life cycle. Radiographics. 32(6):1575-97, 2012
3. Sakhel K et al: Sonography of adenomyosis. J Ultrasound Med. 31(5):805-8, 2012
4. Sofoudis C et al: Endometrial stromal sarcoma in a 29-year-old patient. Case report and review of the literature. Eur J Gynaecol Oncol. 33(3):328-30, 2012
5. Allison SJ et al: saline-infused sonohysterography: tips for achieving greater success. Radiographics. 31(7):1991-2004, 2011
6. Bennett GL et al: ACR appropriateness criteria(®) on abnormal vaginal bleeding. J Am Coll Radiol. 8(7):460-8, 2011
7. Salim S et al: Diagnosis and management of endometrial polyps: a critical review of the literature. J Minim Invasive Gynecol. 18(5):569-81, 2011

Secretory Phase Endometrium

Secretory Phase Endometrium

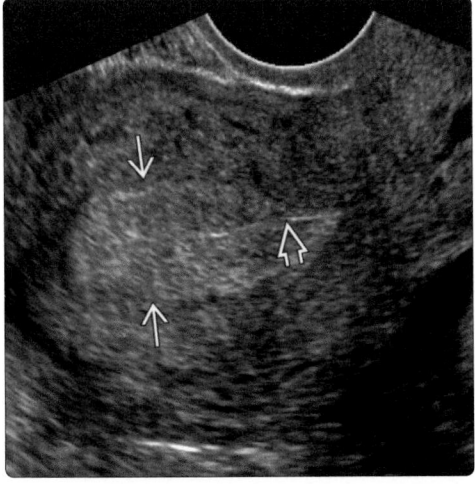
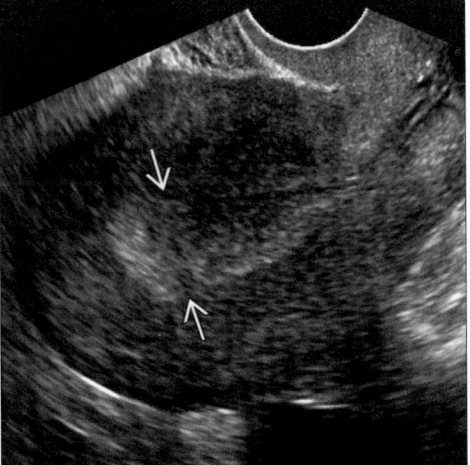

(Left) Longitudinal US in a patient on day 24 of her menstrual cycle shows secretory phase endometrium ➡. The coapted walls of the cavity remain partially visible as a thin echogenic line ➡. (Right) Longitudinal US in a patient late in her menstrual phase shows a thickened, slightly hyperechoic endometrium ➡ consistent with the secretory phase.

Secretory Phase Endometrium

Secretory Phase Endometrium

(Left) *The CT appearance of the endometrium is nonspecific. Low density was thought to represent fluid within an expanded endometrial cavity ➔; subsequent ultrasound confirmed normal secretory phase endometrium.* **(Right)** *US in the same patient shows a thickened echogenic endometrial complex ➔ consistent with secretory phase endometrium, which corresponds to the hypodensity on the CT scan. There is no fluid present.*

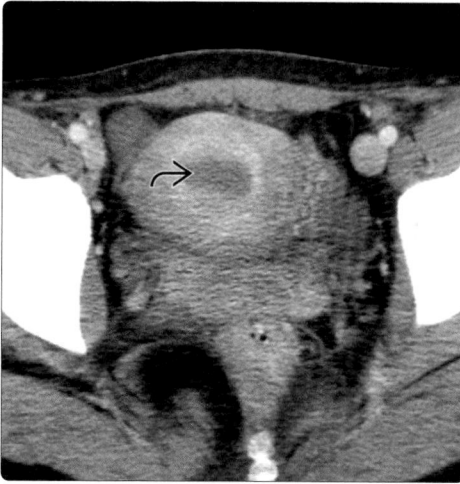

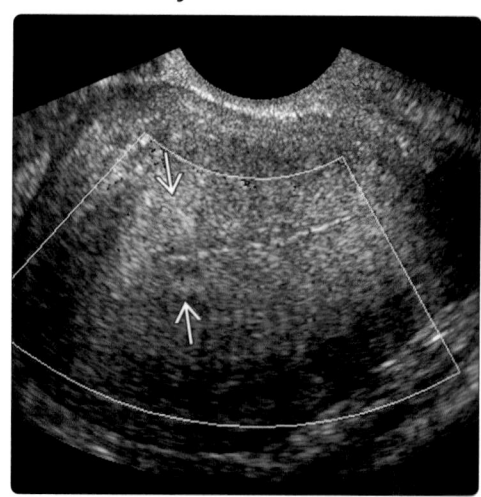

Secretory Phase Endometrium

Secretory Phase Endometrium

(Left) *Longitudinal US shows nonspecific endometrial thickening ➔ in a patient with irregular vaginal bleeding.* **(Right)** *US obtained during saline infusion sonohysterography in the same patient shows distention of the endometrial cavity without focal lesions. Slight lobularity of the endometrial lining is a normal finding ("endometrial wrinkles").*

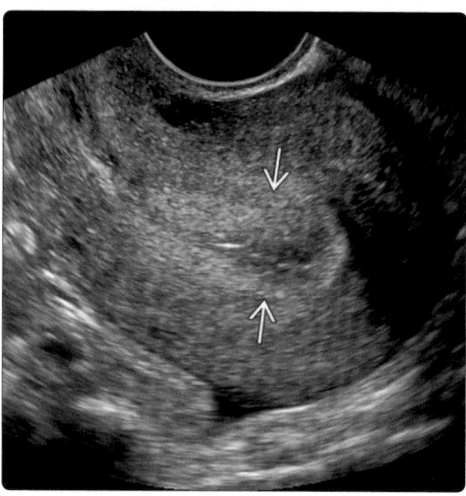

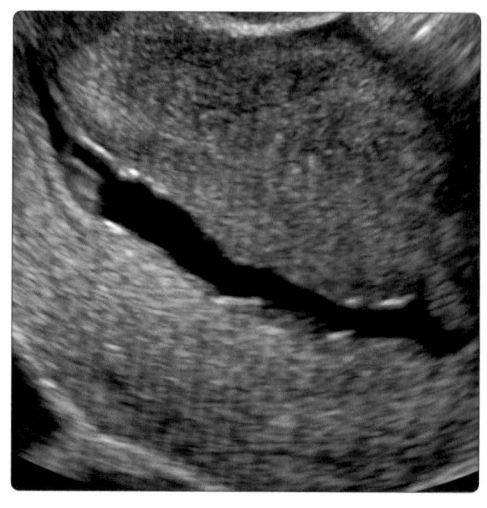

Retained Products of Conception

Retained Products of Conception

(Left) *Transverse color Doppler US in a patient status post recent medical abortion demonstrates a thickened endometrium ➔ with vascular flow ➔, consistent with retained products of conception.* **(Right)** *Pulsed Doppler US in the same patient shows low-resistance flow, typical of but not specific for retained products of conception.*

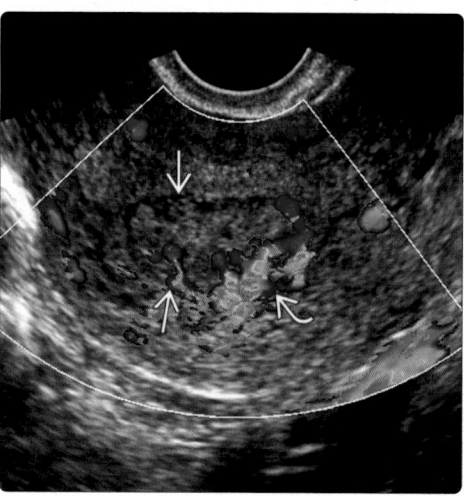

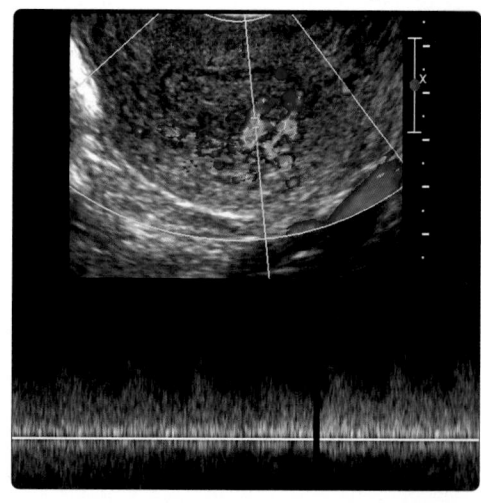

Pregnancy and Complications

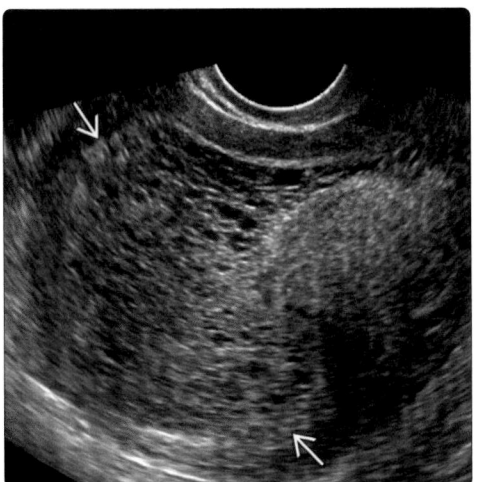

Pregnancy and Complications

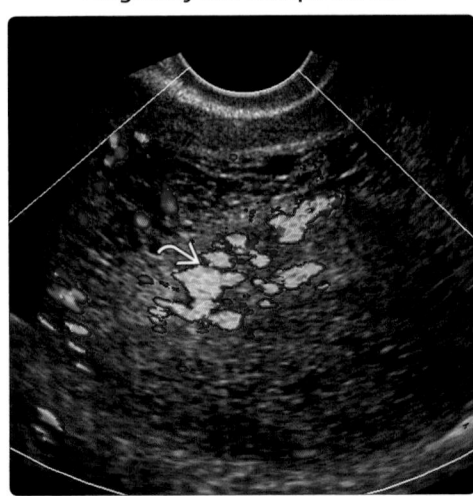

(Left) *Sagittal US in a patient in the 1st trimester with a serum HCG > 260,000 mIU/mL shows marked expansion of the endometrial cavity with echogenic tissue and numerous tiny cysts* ➡. *Pathology was consistent with a partial mole.* **(Right)** *Transverse color Doppler US in the same patient shows increased blood flow within the trophoblastic tissue* ➡.

Submucosal Leiomyoma

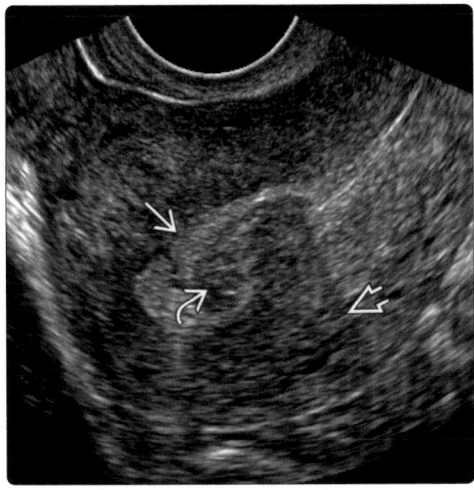

Adenomyosis

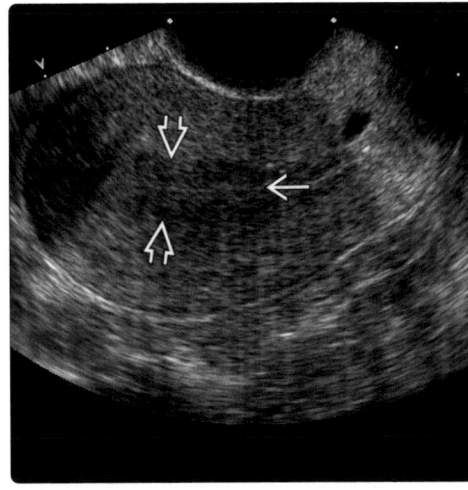

(Left) *Longitudinal US shows a hypoechoic intracavitary submucosal leiomyoma* ➡, *well delineated by the echogenic endometrium* ➡. *Also note partial shadowing* ➡. **(Right)** *Longitudinal US shows what appears to be a widened trilaminar endometrium; however, the echogenic line* ➡ *represents the thin endometrium, with the poorly delineated hypoechoic regions* ➡ *secondary to adenomyosis.*

Endometrial Polyps

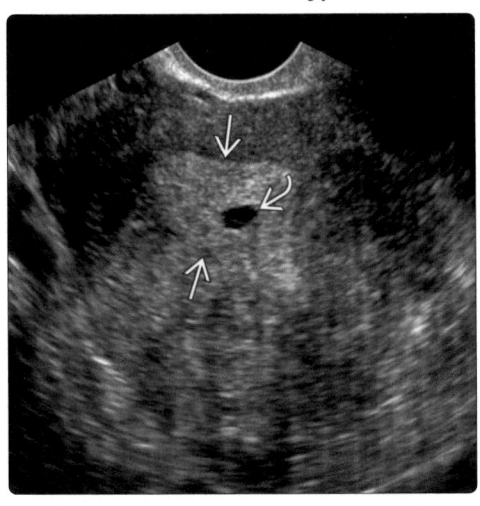

Endometrial Polyps

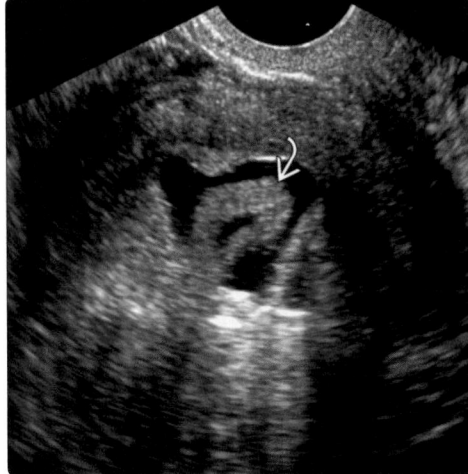

(Left) *Transverse US shows nonspecific endometrial thickening* ➡ *with an internal cyst* ➡. **(Right)** *Saline infusion sonohysterography in the same patient reveals a pedunculated endometrial polyp* ➡ *as the etiology of thickening.*

(Left) *Longitudinal US shows nonspecific thickening of the endometrium ➡ with heterogeneous echogenicity. Pathology revealed an endometrial polyp.* **(Right)** *Transverse US in a postmenopausal patient with bleeding shows a thickened endometrium ➡ with small heterogeneous areas of increased blood flow ➡. Pathology revealed polyps as well as inactive endometrium.*

Endometrial Polyps

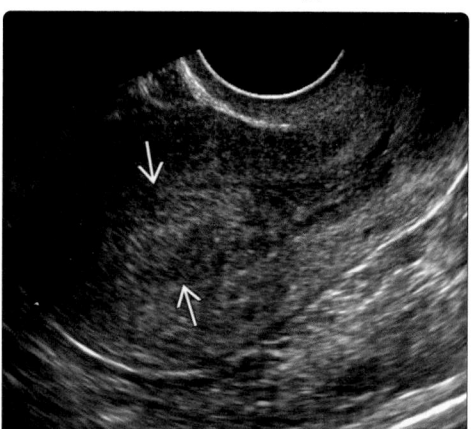

Endometrial Polyps

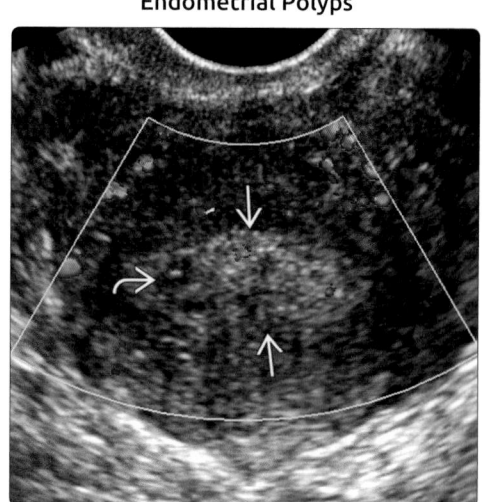

(Left) *Transverse color Doppler US shows a thickened endometrium ➡ with a single feeding vessel ➡, highly suggestive of an endometrial polyp.* **(Right)** *Additional imaging in the same patient shows fluid ➡ within the endometrial cavity surrounding the polyp ➡.*

Endometrial Polyps

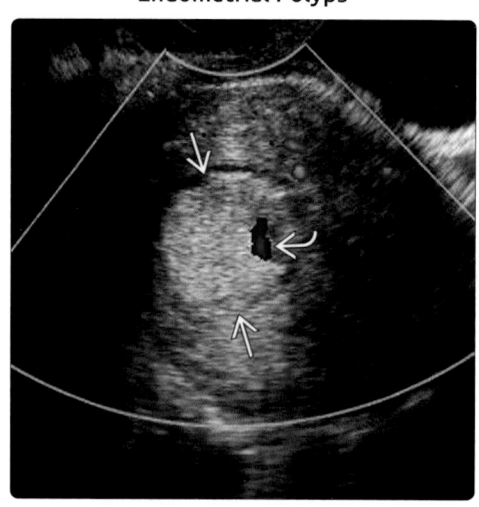

Endometrial Polyps

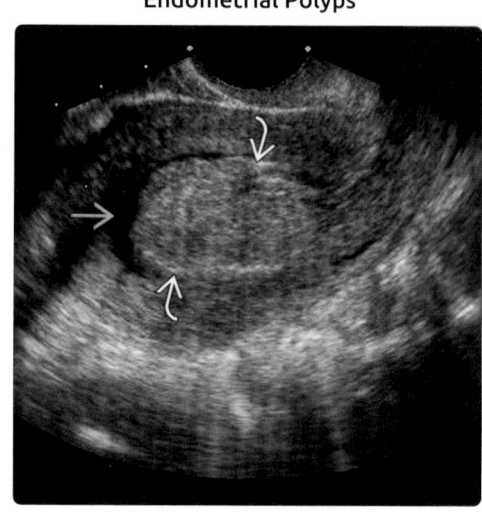

(Left) *Longitudinal US shows a thickened, slightly irregular endometrium ➡ with internal cystic components ➡. Pathology was consistent with hyperplasia.* **(Right)** *Nonspecific thickening of the endometrium ➡ is shown. Although the presence of a small cyst ➡ is suggestive of a benign etiology, the importance of biopsy is emphasized as this was shown on pathology to represent endometrioid carcinoma.*

Endometrial Hyperplasia

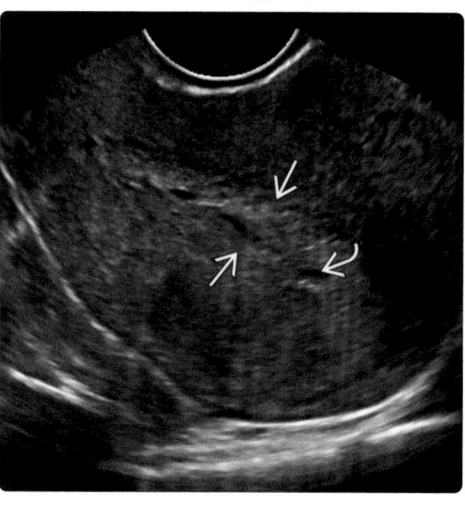

Endometrial Cancer

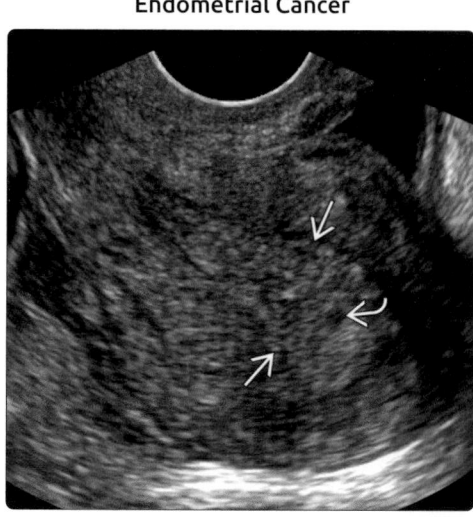

Tamoxifen-Induced Changes

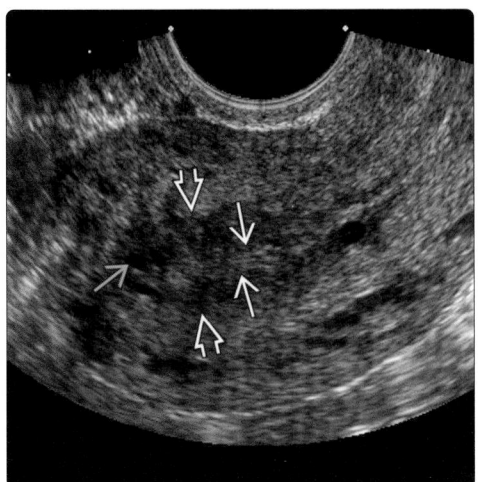

Tamoxifen-Induced Changes

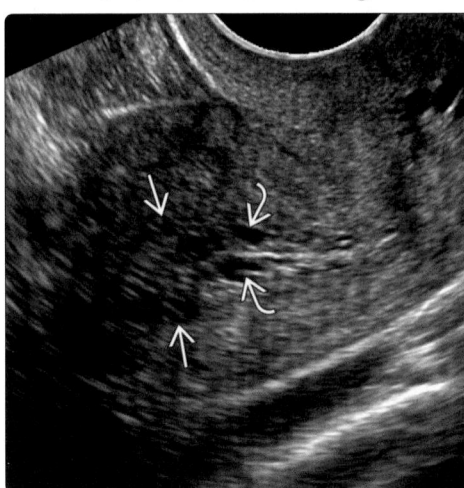

(Left) *Longitudinal US shows normal-thickness endometrium ➡ surrounded by ill-defined hypoechoic myometrium ⮕ secondary to tamoxifen therapy, which mimics a thickened endometrium. Subendometrial cysts ⤇ are visible.* (Right) *Longitudinal US shows a thickened, heterogeneous endometrium ➡ with internal cysts ⮕ in a patient on Tamoxifen therapy for breast cancer.*

Endometritis

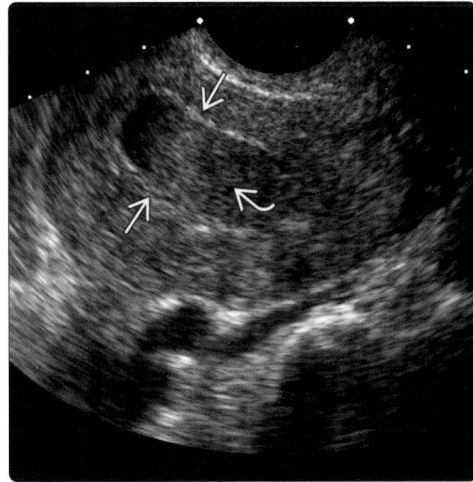

Polycystic Ovary Syndrome

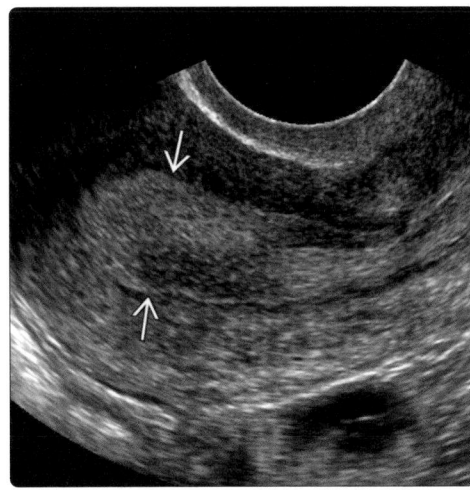

(Left) *Longitudinal US shows an expanded endometrium ➡ containing mixed-echogenicity material ⮕ in a patient with pelvic inflammatory disease and vaginal discharge, consistent with pyometra.* (Right) *Longitudinal US shows a thickened, predominantly echogenic secretory phase endometrium ➡ in a patient with polycystic ovarian syndrome.*

Endometrial Stromal Sarcoma

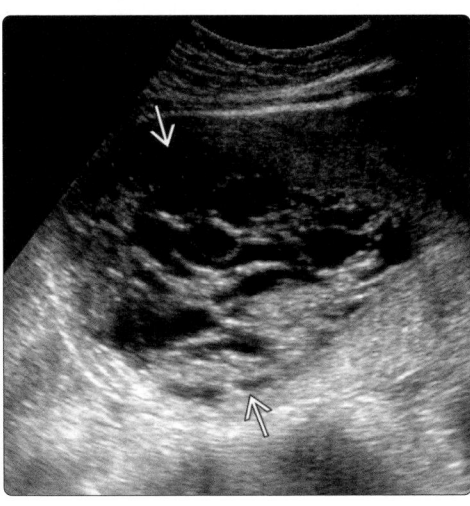

Endometrial Stromal Sarcoma

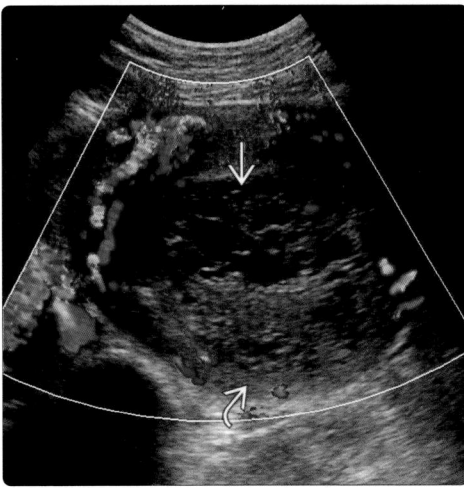

(Left) *Transabdominal US in the sagittal plane shows a markedly thickened endometrium with mixed solid and cystic components ➡. Pathology showed endometrial sarcoma.* (Right) *Transabdominal transverse color Doppler US in the same patient shows a markedly thickened endometrium with mixed solid and cystic components ➡. Although this appears hypovascular, pathology was consistent with endometrial sarcoma. Note the thinning of the posterior myometrium ⮕ from invasion.*

INDEX

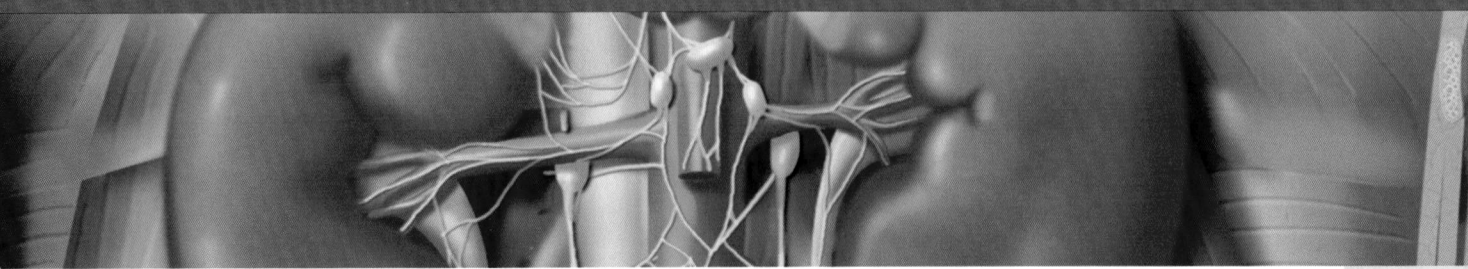

INDEX

INDEX

INDEX

INDEX

H

J

INDEX

INDEX

INDEX

INDEX

X